Dietary Reference Intakes (DRIs): Recommended Intakes for Individuals, Elements
Food and Nutrition Board, Institute of Medicine, National Academies

Life Stage Group	Calcium (mg/d)	Chromium (µg/d)	Copper (µg/d)	Fluoride (mg/d)	Iodine (µg/d)	Iron (mg/d)	Magnesium (mg/d)	Manganese (mg/d)	Molybdenum (µg/d)	Phosphorus (mg/d)	Selenium (µg/d)	Zinc (mg/d)
Infants												
0–6 mo	210*	0.2*	200*	0.01*	110*	0.27*	30*	0.003*	2*	100*	15*	2*
7–12 mo	270*	5.5*	220*	0.5*	130*	11	75*	0.6*	3*	275*	20*	3
Children												
1–3 y	500*	11*	340	0.7*	90	7	80	1.2*	17	460	20	3
4–8 y	800*	15*	440	1*	90	10	130	1.5*	22	500	30	5
Males												
9–13 y	1,300*	25*	700	2*	120	8	240	1.9*	34	1,250	40	8
14–18 y	1,300*	35*	890	3*	150	11	410	2.2*	43	1,250	55	11
19–30 y	1,000*	35*	900	4*	150	8	400	2.3*	45	700	55	11
31–50 y	1,000*	35*	900	4*	150	8	420	2.3*	45	700	55	11
51–70 y	1,200*	30*	900	4*	150	8	420	2.3*	45	700	55	11
>70 y	1,200*	30*	900	4*	150	8	420	2.3*	45	700	55	11
Females												
9–13 y	1,300*	21*	700	2*	120	8	240	1.6*	34	1,250	40	8
14–18 y	1,300*	24*	890	3*	150	15	360	1.6*	43	1,250	55	9
19–30 y	1,000*	25*	900	3*	150	18	310	1.8*	45	700	55	8
31–50 y	1,000*	25*	900	3*	150	18	320	1.8*	45	700	55	8
51–70 y	1,200*	20*	900	3*	150	8	320	1.8*	45	700	55	8
>70 y	1,200*	20*	900	3*	150	8	320	1.8*	45	700	55	8
Pregnancy												
≤18 y	1,300*	29*	1,000	3*	220	27	400	2.0*	50	1,250	60	13
19–30 y	1,000*	30*	1,000	3*	220	27	350	2.0*	50	700	60	11
31–50 y	1,000*	30*	1,000	3*	220	27	360	2.0*	50	700	60	11
Lactation												
≤18 y	1,300*	44*	1,300	3*	290	10	360	2.6*	50	1,250	70	14
19–30 y	1,000*	45*	1,300	3*	290	9	310	2.6*	50	700	70	12
31–50 y	1,000*	45*	1,300	3*	290	9	320	2.6*	50	700	70	12

NOTE: This table presents Recommended Dietary Allowances (RDAs) in bold type and Adequate Intakes (AIs) in ordinary type followed by an asterisk (*). RDAs and AIs may both be used as goals for individual intake. RDAs are set to meet the needs of almost all (97 to 98 percent) individuals in a group. For healthy breastfed infants, the AI is the mean intake. The AI for other life stage and gender groups is believed to cover needs of all individuals in the group, but lack of data or uncertainty in the data prevent being able to specify with confidence the percentage of individuals covered by this intake.

SOURCES: Dietary Reference Intakes for Calcium, Phosphorous, Magnesium, Vitamin D, and Fluoride (1997); Dietary Reference Intakes for Thiamin, Riboflavin, Niacin, Vitamin B_6, Folate, Vitamin B_{12}, Pantothenic Acid, Biotin, and Choline (1998); Dietary Reference Intakes for Vitamin C, Vitamin E, Selenium, and Carotenoids (2000); and Dietary Reference Intakes for Vitamin A, Vitamin K, Arsenic, Boron, Chromium, Copper, Iodine, Iron, Manganese, Molybdenum, Nickel, Silicon, Vanadium, and Zinc (2001). These reports may be accessed via www.nap.edu.

$\mathcal{P}$ERSPECTIVES IN
NUTRITION

ABOUT THE AUTHORS

Gordon M. Wardlaw, Ph.D., R.D., L.D., C.N.S.D. teaches nutrition to students in the Division of Medical Dietetics, School of Allied Medical Professions, The Ohio State University. Dr. Wardlaw is the author of many articles that have appeared in prominent nutrition, biology, physiology, and biochemistry journals and was the 1985 recipient of the American Dietetic Association's Mary P. Huddleson Award. Dr. Wardlaw is a full member of the presitgious American Society for Nutritional Sciences and is certified as a Specialist in Human Nutrition by the American Board of Nutrition and as a Nutrition Support Dietitian by the American Society of Parenteral and Enteral Nutrition.

Margaret Kessel, Ph.D., R.D., L.D., worked for many years as a dietitian in hospitals, a nursing home, and a large state institution. Since 1983, Dr. Kessel has taught in the Department of Human Nutrition at The Ohio State University. She has long been interested in the use of computers in nutrition. In recent years, her teaching has been concentrated in the introductory courses. A United States Department of Agriculture grant gave her the opportunity to combine these interests by designing and teaching an interactive nutrition course entirely on the web.

FIFTH EDITION

$\mathscr{P}$ERSPECTIVES IN
NUTRITION

GORDON M. WARDLAW
PH.D., R.D., L.D., C.N.S.D.

MARGARET W. KESSEL
PH.D., R.D., L.D.
THE OHIO STATE UNIVERSITY

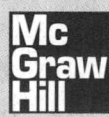

Boston   Burr Ridge, IL   Dubuque, IA   Madison, WI   New York   San Francisco   St. Louis
Bangkok   Bogotá   Caracas   Kuala Lumpur   Lisbon   London   Madrid   Mexico City
Milan   Montreal   New Delhi   Santiago   Seoul   Singapore   Sydney   Taipei   Toronto

McGraw-Hill Higher Education

A Division of The McGraw-Hill Companies

PERSPECTIVES IN NUTRITION, FIFTH EDITION

Published by McGraw-Hill, a business unit of The McGraw-Hill Companies, Inc., 1221 Avenue of the Americas, New York, NY 10020. Copyright © 2002, 1999, 1996, 1993, 1990 by The McGraw-Hill Companies, Inc. All rights reserved. No part of this publication may be reproduced or distributed in any form or by any means, or stored in a database or retrieval system, without the prior written consent of The McGraw-Hill Companies, Inc., including, but not limited to, in any network or other electronic storage or transmission, or broadcast for distance learning.

Some ancillaries, including electronic and print components, may not be available to customers outside the United States.

This book is printed on recycled, acid-free paper containing 10% postconsumer waste.

International   2 3 4 5 6 7 8 9 0 VNH/VNH 0 9 8 7 6 5 4 3 2
Domestic   3 4 5 6 7 8 9 0 VNH/VNH 0 9 8 7 6 5 4 3 2

ISBN 0–07–228784–5
ISBN 0–07–112286–9 (ISE)

Publisher: *Colin H. Wheatley*
Senior developmental editor: *Lynne M. Meyers*
Marketing manager: *Michelle Watnick*
Senior project manager: *Marilyn Rothenberger*
Production supervisor: *Enboge Chong*
Coordinator of freelance design: *Michelle M. Meerdink*
Cover/interior designer: *Diane Beasley*
Cover image: *PhotoDisc*
Photo research coordinator: *John C. Leland*
Photo research: *Mary Reeg*
Senior supplement producer: *David A. Welsh*
Media technology senior producer: *Barbara R. Block*
Compositor: *GAC—Indianapolis*
Typeface: *10/12 Galliard*
Printer: *Von Hoffmann Press, Inc.*

The credits section for this book begins on page C-1 and is considered an extension of the copyright page.

Library of Congress Cataloging-in-Publication Data

Wardlaw, Gordon M.
    Perspectives in nutrition / Gordon M. Wardlaw, Margaret W. Kessel. — 5th ed.
        p.   cm.
    Includes index.
    ISBN 0–07–228784–5
    1. Nutrition.   I. Kessel, Margaret Wagner.   II. Title.

    QP141 .W38   2002
    613.2—dc21   2001024012
                                                       CIP

INTERNATIONAL EDITION ISBN 0–07–112286–9
Copyright © 2002. Exclusive rights by The McGraw-Hill Companies, Inc., for manufacture and export. This book cannot be re-exported from the country to which it is sold by McGraw-Hill. The International Edition is not available in North America.

www.mhhe.com

Brief Contents

v

Contents

■ PART ONE NUTRITION BASICS 2

■ PART TWO THE ENERGY-YIELDING NUTRIENTS 160

■ PART THREE   THE VITAMINS AND MINERALS 322

■ PART FOUR   ENERGY PRODUCTION AND ENERGY BALANCE   506

13 ENERGY BALANCE AND WEIGHT CONTROL 506

■ PART FIVE   NUTRITION APPLICATIONS IN THE LIFE CYCLE   630

■ PART SIX PUTTING NUTRITION KNOWLEDGE INTO PRACTICE 748

A Visual Guide to
Perspectives in Nutrition, fifth edition

HUMAN PHYSIOLOGIC PROCESSES

chapter 3

■ **CHAPTER OUTLINE**

*A*ll fundamental activities referred to as nutrition occur within a variety of cells. Although each cell is comprised of the same components, there is enough variety within each cell to provide about 200 distinctive cell types. Each cell performs a specialized task. Groups of cells are organized to form tissues. Tissues unite to form organs. Organs are grouped together to carry out functions in the body and are known as systems.[12]

The integumentary system provides protection from the environment. The skeletal system is the body's structural framework. Movement depends on the muscle system. The circulatory system, composed of the heart and blood vessels, transports blood to all tissues throughout the body in order to deliver essential nutrients and pick up cellular waste. The lymph ... t also provides immunity, the ... aders. The respiratory system ... es with the external ... coordinates activities within ... he internal and external ... consciousness, learning, and ... oordinates activities to ... ve system chemically changes

Overview

Each chapter opens with an Overview that conveys the significance of the nutrition concepts to be covered in that chapter.

Outline

An opening Outline provides a detailed preview of the material to be covered next.

■ **KEY CHAPTER CONCEPTS**

- The cell is the structural and functional unit of all living organisms. Each cell contains a plasma or cell membrane and organelles, which carry out unique tasks related to the function of the cell.
- Cells join together to make up tissues, tissues unite to form organs, and organs work together as a system.
- The body has 11 organ systems, each controlling one aspect of human nutrition. (There are 12 if the immune and lymphatic systems are counted separately.)
- The integumentary system is the largest system in the body. It provides material (tissues) to cover body surfaces and is a source of vitamin D.
- The muscle and skeletal systems consist of muscles and bones, which permit movement and protection from injury. The skeletal system itself is a storehouse for important nutrients. The muscle system is a significant source of heat.
- The circulatory system delivers oxygen, nutrients, and fluid to all tissues in the body; maintains fluid balance; and removes waste materials, such as carbon dioxide, from the body. Another circulatory system, the lymph, also distributes nutrients and fluids throughout the body and acts as a defense system to protect the body from invading pathogens.
- The immune system coordinates the attack against invading pathogens. There are two types of immunity, specific and nonspecific. The body is exposed to dangerous bacteria, viruses, fungi, and parasites coming in through the skin, mouth (gastrointestinal tract), and respiratory tract. The immune system identifies the microorganisms and destroys them.
- The respiratory system picks up oxygen in the lungs from inhaled air and delivers it to the blood. The lungs recover carbon dioxide from the blood and disposes of it as we exhale.
- The nervous system is composed of cells called neurons, which act as communication links. In order to maintain homeostasis, receptors present throughout the body transmit information about the internal and external environment to the central nervous system (CNS). The CNS, in turn, responds by issuing commands to all the systems that will eventually maintain this homeostasis.
- Located in the body are endocrine glands, which produce chemicals called hormones. Hormones are transported to all parts of the body to help regulate cellular function.
- The gastrointestinal tract digests food and beverages and converts them into absorbable nutrients. This system acts as a barrier against invading pathogens.
- The kidneys filter the blood and remove waste, excess fluid, and substances not needed by the body. The filtrate is urine. Thus, the urinary system constantly maintains the composition of the blood.
- The reproductive system generates new humans. This replaces ones who are dying. Hormones produced by this system control many aspects of nutrition.

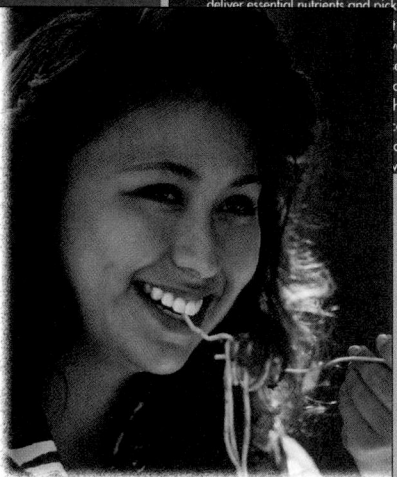

■ **CASE SCENARIO**

A fellow student complains to you about a gastrointestinal problem that "just won't go away." She is 20 years old, is very short, and complains of abdominal pain, diarrhea, and joint pain. Her family doctor says it's nothing, just the stress of being a high-achieving university student. She confides in you that she is worried about her health, as she has experienced a sudden weight loss of 5 pounds in the past week. You suggest she visit the Student Health Service immediately.

A barium enema X ray, colonoscopy, and CT scan reveal that the student is suffering from Crohn's disease. What is Crohn's disease? What happens to the intestinal tract when someone has this disease? Are there any treatments to alleviate the symptoms? What, if any, foods should she eat or avoid? Overall, how does she cope with this health problem?

■ **REFRESH YOUR MEMORY**

As you begin your study of anatomy and physiology in Chapter 3, you may want to review
- The classes of macronutrients in Chapter 1
- Cell structure and the function of various organelles, found from previous coursework in your university-level biology text

Key Chapter Concepts

A list of Key Chapter Concepts alerts students to major points they are expected to learn in the chapter.

Case Scenario

Each chapter begins with a Case Scenario that engages students by asking them to consider the nutritional implications of a real-life situation.

Refresh Your Memory

Refresh Your Memory directs students to topics in earlier chapter they may wish to revisit to reinforce their understanding of related material in the upcoming chapter.

Expert Opinion

WHY IS WEIGHT MANAGEMENT SO DIFFICULT?

Sachiko T. St. Jeor, Ph.D., R.D.

Currently we are expecting a worldwide epidemic of obesity; 97 million or approximately 60% of adults in the United States are overweight (body mass index, or BMI, ≥ 85th percentile of 25.0 to 29.9 kg/m²) or obese (BMI in the ≥ 95th percentile or > 30.0 kg/m²). This is a sad commentary on the history of weight gain over the years. Although Americans are weight conscious, it appears that they are not successful in weight management overall.

Why is weight management so difficult? The first reason is that small weight gains over time go unnoticed. According to the statistics of two nationally representative surveys, the National Health and Nutrition Examination Survey II, or NHANES II (1976–1980), and NHANES III (1988–1994), it appears that the average weight gain over 10 years is approximately 8 lbs (3.6 kg), or approximately 1 lb/year. We would rarely notice a 1-lb weight gain over a year but hopefully would notice a 10 to-20-lb weight gain over a 10- to 20-year period. In addition, many of us would rather not notice a small weight gain over time and certainly would

like to think that these small weight gains are temporary and will even out over time. Thus, new weight monitoring techniques may be of importance.

Second, little emphasis has been placed on weight maintenance or on the prevention of weight gain. This epidemic of obesity could have been partially halted if we did not gain so much weight and instead accept weight stability as our first goal. Since the conditions of overweight and obesity are associated with increased morbidity and mortality from at least five major diseases (hypertension, diabetes, dyslipidemia, cardiovascular disease, and stroke) as well as some types of cancers (endometrium, breast, prostate, and colon), the problem is of major significance. Our research group has defined weight maintenance as ± 5 lb between any two points in time. The reflects about a 3% change in body weight. However, there has been no standard definition broadly accepted for weight maintenance, and individual fluctuations vary widely.

Using this practical definition, only 20% of a group of both normal and overweight males and females of all ages

studied in my laboratory were weight maintainers over 4 years. Furthermore, more normal-weight individuals were weight maintainers (75%) than those who were overweight (25%). Older males, adults who experienced lower weight variability, and adults undergoing less dieting were also more successful at maintaining their weight. The weight maintainers tended to have better health profiles, were characterized by being more physically active, used more problem-solving and self-monitoring strategies, and had more "normalized" eating patterns, social support, and self-efficacy. These results point to the difficulty of implementing well-accepted strategies for weight management over the long term.

Third, we are a population with very unrealistic expectations. Weight maintenance is not a popular concept; instead, weight loss is always the goal. A fad diet is usually on the bestseller list, and losing large amounts of weight in short periods of time (10 lbs/10 days) is always attractive. Few individuals are really committed to putting in the long-term effort needed to lose weight gradually (1–3 lb/week) in a

The many new and updated Expert Opinion boxes are written by leaders in the field and acquaint students with topics of emerging interest and the latest research.

adolescent years also deserve attention. Adults should gene___ greater than about 10 to 16 pounds more than their weight ___ People who gain weight rapidly should closely monitor foo___ terns to discover the causes and then moderate the increase___ appropriate ways.[4]

Critical Thinking

As students study the text, Critical Thinking Questions are posed to challenge them to apply their newly acquired knowledge to real-life situations.

Concept Check

At key points in each chapter, brief Concept Checks allow students to mentally summarize what they have learned before proceeding to the next topic.

CRITICAL THINKING

David (age 34) would like to be a Goliath-like athlete, but he is only 5'7" and weighs 140 pounds. Recently, he has been surfing the Web, looking for a remedy for his small build. He has found a company that will sell him an extract of human liver and genital factors "guaranteed" to be a source of testosterone and a special growth hormone. He is assured that the product will change the chemistry of his bones, so that they will start growing, just as they did when he was an adolescent. He expects to be about 6 feet tall in just a year. What is your advice to him?

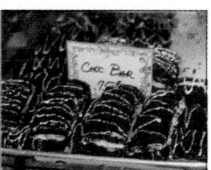

Most of the foods we eat consist of carbohydrates, protein, and fat. Our bodies break down each of these nutrients in a different way.

Neural and Endocrine Regulation

Whether a chemical is acting as a hormone or a neurotransmitter, the target cell must have a receptor protein to combine with it. This causes a change in the target cell. This also means that there must be a mechanism to turn off the action. Hormones are subject to control by an off switch. For example, when the blood sugar (glucose) concentration has been returned to normal by the action of the hormone insulin, insulin production is turned off. If it were not, the person would experience decreasing glucose concentrations until such time as the concentration drops so low the person goes into shock and dies.

How Hormones Act

Hormones are available to all cells in the body, but only those with the correct receptor protein on the cell membrane can bind the hormone. These binding sites are highly specific. For hormones that pass through the cell membrane, thyroxine and steroid hormones, the receptor protein is within the cytosol of the cell. This receptor guides the hormone into the nucleus of the cell, where the hormone binds to DNA and turns on the production mRNA to produce a specific enzyme.

Hormones that don't penetrate the cell membrane act by another mechanism. The hormone (the messenger) attaches to a receptor protein on the cell surface. This binding site activates a second messenger within the cell to carry out the assigned task, like the activation or inhibition of a specific enzyme. Many hormones activate a form of ATP as the second messenger. Another second messenger is calcium.

In summary, hormones in the blood can act directly with a target cell, can pass its instructions to the cell indirectly with the aid of a second messenger, can be inactivated by a metabolic process, or can be ignored and excreted from the body as they are.

CONCEPT CHECK

The nervous system consists of the central nervous system and the peripheral nervous system. The functional unit of the nervous system is the neuron, or nerve cell.

Hormones are regulatory substances that are produced by glands in response to a change in the internal environment of the body. The gland secretes the hormone into the blood, and the blood delivers it to target cells. The hormone either enters the cell and turns on the production of an enzyme within the cell or attaches to the exterior of the cell and, through the action of a second messenger, causes enzymatic changes within the cell.

■ Digestive System

The processes of digestion and absorption take place in a long tube, open at both ends, extending from the mouth to the anus. It is essentially part of our exterior environment. With the exception of water, almost all the food and beverages we ingest require some preparation before the nutrients are released and prepared for absorption (Fig. 3-11).[17]

How the Body Reacts to Food

You eat. You are aware of the contents in your mouth because of taste buds located on your tongue.[4] If a food or beverage tastes good, you begin to chew and swallow the food.

There are four types of taste: sweet, sour, salty, and bitter. The salty taste is due to Na^+ enhanced by Cl^-. The sour taste is due to the presence of hydrogen ions (H^+). Bitter and sweet tastes are generated by specific components in the food that interact with membrane receptors on the tongue. Some evidence exists for a fifth sense

A sixth taste sensation, called umami, has been proposed. This taste sensation is elicited by monosodium glutamate, a substance often added to Chinese and Japanese foods to enhance flavor. Brothy, meaty, and savory are ex-

Illustrations

Beautifully rendered Illustrations enhance students' understanding of complex concepts and processes. New diagrams and photographs are featured throughout this edition.

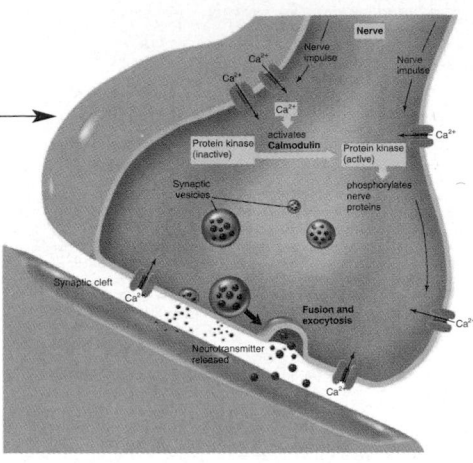

■ FIGURE 11-9 The release of a neurotransmitter. Nerve impulses, by opening Ca²⁺ channels, stimulate the fusion of synaptic vesicles with the cell membrane of the nerve terminals. This leads to exocytosis and the release of a neurotransmitter. The activation of protein kinase (an enzyme that adds a phosphate group to a molecule) by Ca²⁺ may also contribute to this process.

Definitions

Definitions of important terms and concepts are generally found in the margins as they are first introduced in the text. All appear in the glossary.

Cell Metabolism. Calcium ions help regulate metabolism in the cell by participating in the **calmodulin** system. When calcium enters a cell (often because of hormone action) and binds to the protein calmodulin, the resulting protein-calcium complex can regulate the activity for various enzymes, including one that breaks down glycogen to many units of glucose 1-phosphate (Fig. 11-10).

Other Attributes of a Diet Rich in Calcium. As discussed in the Nutrition Perspective at the end of this chapter, calcium may contribute to lower blood pressure values in some people. Calcium may also reduce the risk of colon cancer by binding bile acids and free fatty acids in the lumen of the colon; these stimulate colon cells, likely leading to colon cancer. There is also speculation that calcium may reduce the symptoms associated with premenstrual syndrome. A few studies have shown that [...] blood cholesterol by binding saturated fatty acids in the [...] bsorption. Finally, in some people, calcium may reduce the [...] a person should be under medical care if he or she has a [...] wants to experiment with higher calcium intakes. Overall, [...] o meet calcium needs on a regular basis.²²

calmodulin A cell protein that binds calcium ions. The resulting calmodulin-Ca²⁺ complex influences the activity of some enzymes in the cell.

[...]m-related disease is osteoporosis. Failure to maintain ade-[...]ody eventually leads to a state of **osteopenia**. Osteopenia [...]min D deficiency disease osteomalacia, the use of certain [...] If these or similar causes are not present, the diagnosis is [...] when the bone loss is quite marked. People who develop [...]thood can sustain greater age-related bone loss with less [...]th who have less bone. Thus, osteoporosis is considered to [...]th geriatric consequences.

osteopenia Decreased bone mass caused by cancer, hyperthyroidism, or other reasons.

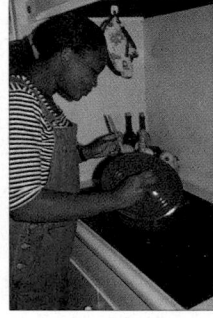

Attention to one's diet is especially important in pregnancy.

On the WIC program, participants' diets have improved markedly, as has the likelihood that women will have healthy babies. This program is credited with decreasing the cases of iron deficiency anemia and LBW infants within the population it serves. Studies have estimated that every dollar spent on the prenatal component of WIC saves about $3 in public health expenditures for the care of LBW babies.

The WIC program is available in all areas of the United States and has a staff trained to help women have healthy babies. More than 7 million women, infants, and young children are currently enrolled in the program. Many eligible pregnant women are not taking advantage of this program.

■ CASE SCENARIO
Follow-Up

From a dietary standpoint, Tracey is smart to take a close look at her protein intake because needs will increase slightly during pregnancy. More fruits and vegetables will provide some fiber to help prevent constipation, which is common in the later stages of pregnancy. These foods also supply folate, and her use of an over-the-counter vitamin and mineral supplement provides an ample amount of synthetic folate, the preferred form. Still, she should discuss this supplement use with her physician and would probably eventually benefit more from a prenatal supplement prescribed by her physician, as this will have more folate and iron than over-the-counter multivitamin and mineral supplements. Her diet may not have enough calcium, so she should pay as much attention to consuming some extra calcium as she does for protein. Avoiding alcohol is a smart move.

Many experts would say that she is consuming too much caffeine and would be wise to cut down to one to two cups of coffee per day, or possibly even eliminate coffee altogether. Her exercise routine is probably too vigorous if she hasn't already been practicing regular running. Tracey should not begin a new exercise routine upon becoming pregnant unless it is at a moderate pace, such as brisk walking or stationary biking.

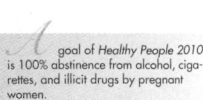

A goal of *Healthy People 2010* is 100% abstinence from alcohol, cigarettes, and illicit drugs by pregnant women.

■ CONCEPT CHECK

Infants born after 37 weeks of gestation and weighing more than 5.5 lb (2.5 kg) have the fewest medical problems at birth. Individual mothers and whole societies can attempt to reduce infant and maternal death and medical problems by limiting the factors that increase the risk of having a preterm or small-for-gestational-age infant. Such contributing factors, besides an inadequate diet in general, include low socioeconomic status; closely spaced births; obesity; inadequate or absent prenatal care; cigarette smoking; alcohol consumption; illegal drug use; teenage pregnancy; inadequate prenatal weight gain; heavy caffeine use; Listeria exposure; and prenatal ketosis. Adequate nutrition can reduce the risk of many medical problems in pregnancy.

■ PHYSIOLOGICAL CHANGES THAT CAN CAUSE DISCOMFORT IN PREGNANCY

During pregnancy, the fetus's needs for oxygen, nutrients, and excretion increase the burden on the mother's lungs, heart, and kidneys. Although a mother's digestive and metabolic systems work very efficiently, some discomfort accompanies the changes her body undergoes to accommodate the fetus.³²

Case Scenario Follow-Up

As students progress through the chapter, the Case Scenario Follow-Up revisits the real-life situation introduced at the beginning of the chapter to help students apply what they have just learned.

Margin Notes

Margin Notes highlight important facts and clarify essential concepts.

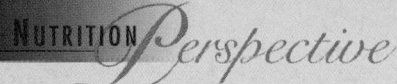

NUTRITION *Perspective*

VEGETARIAN DIETS

Vegetarianism has evolved over the centuries from a necessity into an option. Historically, vegetarianism was linked with specific philosophies and religions or with science. In the sixth century B.C., Pythagoras advocated a meatless diet for its physical health, ecological, religious, and philosophical benefits.

Today, there are about 12 million vegetarians in the United States, about double the number in 1985. Over the past two decades, vegetarian diets have gone from dull to delicious, with the inclusion of such new products as soy-based sloppy joes, chili, tacos, burgers, and more. In addition, cookbooks that feature the use of a variety of fruits, vegetables, and seasonings are enhancing food selection for vegetarians of all degrees.

Vegetarianism is popular among college students. Fifteen percent of college students in one survey said they select vegetarian options at lunch or dinner on any given day. In response, dining services offer vegetarian options at every meal, the most common being pastas with meatless sauce and pizza. Many teenagers are also turning to vegetarianism out of respect for animals. And a survey by the National Restaurant Association found that 20% of their customers want a vegetarian option when they eat out. Many customers cite health and taste as reasons for choosing vegetarian fare.

As nutrition science has grown, new information has enabled the design of adequate vegetarian diets. It is important for vegetarians to take advantage of this information because a diet of only plants can lead to various nutrient deficiencies and a substantial growth retardation in infants and children. People who choose a vegetarian diet can meet their nutritional needs by following a few basic rules and knowledgeably planning their diets[11] (Fig. 7-13).

Studies show that death rates from some chronic diseases, such as certain forms of heart disease, cancer, and type 2 diabetes, and obesity, are lower for vegetarians than for nonvegetarians.[1] Healthful lifestyles (not smoking, abstaining from alcohol and drugs, and increasing physical activity) and social class bias probably partially account for these findings.

These symbols show fats, oils, and added sugars in foods:
● Fat (naturally occuring and added)
▼ Sugars (added)

Fats, oils, and sweets
USE SPARINGLY

Milk, yogurt, and cheese
2-3 SERVINGS

Eggs*, legumes, nuts, and seeds
2-4 SERVINGS

Vegetables
3-5 SERVINGS

Fruit
2-4 SERVINGS

Bread, c

▓ FIGURE 7-13 Food Guide Pyramid for lactoovovegetarian. Base serving size on Food Guide Pyramid in Chapter 2.
*Lactovegetarians would omit eggs as a choice.

290

Nutrition Perspective

Nutrition Perspectives offer in-depth examination of a key topic of interest and facilitate further student exploration.

TAKE ACTION

II. A CLOSER LOOK AT SUPPLEMENT USE

With the current popularity of vitamin and mineral supplements, it is more important than ever to understand how to evaluate a supplement. Study the accompanying label and then answer the following questions. Then, by way of comparison, go to a store and examine a general multivitamin/mineral supplement. When you have done that, answer the set of questions again. How do the answers change? Which of the two do you think would be safer to take on a regular basis?

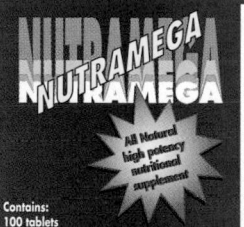

Our protective formula has been extensively researched to bring you the best answer to problems associated with changing seasons.

Suggested use: For best results, begin taking **Nutramega** tablets at the very first signs of imbalances in your well-being. During imbalances, take 2 to 3 tablets every three hours. For daily maintenance, take 1 or 2 tablets a day. Or, take as recommended by your health care professional.

WARNING: Not for use by pregnant or nursing women.
KEEP OUT OF THE REACH OF CHILDREN.

Contains:
100 tablets

Three tablets provide: Vitamins & Minerals		% Daily Value
Vit A activity (4,000 IU		
Beta Carotene, 1,000 IU)	5,000 IU	100%
Vit C (Ascorbic Acid, and Zinc, Calcium, & Magnesium Ascorbates)	1275 mg	2125%
Calcium (Ascorbate)	7.5 mg	1%
Copper (Sebocate)	300 mcg	15%
Magnesium (Ascorbate)	3.8 mg	1%
Selenium (Sodium Selenite)	25 mcg	30%
Zinc (Ascorbate)	23 mg	153%
Other ingredients		
Propolis	300 mg	
Garlic	360 mg	
Boneset	238 mg	
Polygonum Odoratum	200 mg	
Echinacea Extract	164 mg	
Isatis (Root & Leaf)	159 mg	
Horehound	150 mg	
Bioflavonoids	120 mg	
Angelica Archangelica Root	87 mg	
Mullein	80 mg	
Centenseed	75 mg	
Siberian Ginseng	66 mg	
Hawthorn Berry	58 mg	
Oregon Grape Root	55 mg	
Pau D'Arco Extract	36 mg	
Cayenne	30 mg	

NUTRAMEGA
All Natural high potency nutritional supplement

1. What is the recommended dosage of this supplement? _____

2. Based on the recommended dosage, are there any individual vitamins for which the intake would be greater than 100% of the Daily Value? List these vitamins. _____

3. Are any suggested intakes above the Upper Level for the nutrient? _____

4. Are there any superfluous ingredients, such as herbs or flavors, in the supplement? You can often tell this because these ingredients do not have a percent of Daily Value. _____

5. Does at least 50% of the vitamin A in the product come from beta-carotene or other provitamin A carotenoids (to reduce risk of preformed vitamin A toxicity)? _____

6. Are there any warnings on the label as to populations who should not consume this product? _____

7. Are there any other signs that tip you off that this may not be a safe product? _____

Take Action

Each chapter concludes with two Take Action activities that involve students with assessing their own nutritional status. These activities are perfect for in-class discussions or at-home assignments.

Preface

TO THE INSTRUCTOR

Since you teach nutrition, you undoubtedly find it a fascinating and challenging topic. However, nutrition can also be quite frustrating to teach. Claims and counterclaims abound regarding the need for certain dietary constituents. Sodium is a good example. One group of researchers promotes a reduction in salt intake for the general population as an effective preventive measure for hypertension. Other groups believe that normal blood pressure values can be maintained despite the excess intakes of salt common among Americans.

Your authors are aware of conflicting opinions in our field and thus draw on as many sources as possible in the continual updating of this textbook, now in its fifth edition. We have incorporated much new material, especially from recently published articles in major nutrition and medical journals; supplements to the *American Journal of Clinical Nutrition;* and the latest edition of *Modern Nutrition in Health and Disease,* edited by Shils, Olson, and Shike. In addition, available information as of January, 2001 on the ongoing DRI revision by the Food and Nutrition Board is incorporated where appropriate.

In all, the book strives to present many perspectives in current nutrition research so that you and your students can better understand and participate in debates about current nutrition issues.

■ PERSONALIZING NUTRITION

One prominent theme in nutrition research today is *individuality*. Not all of us, for example, find that saturated fat in our diets raises our blood cholesterol values above recommended standards. Each person responds individually, often idiosyncratically, to nutrients, and that is something we continually point out in this textbook.

Moreover, even at this basic level the book discussions do not assume that all nutrition students are alike. We ask students to learn more about themselves and their health status and to use this new knowledge to improve their health. After reading this textbook, students will understand much more clearly how the nutrition information given on the evening news, on cereal box labels, in popular magazines, and by government agencies applies to them. They will become sophisticated consumers of both food and nutrition information. They will understand that their knowledge of nutrition allows them to personalize information, rather than follow every guideline issued for an entire population. After all, a population by definition consists of

individuals with varying genetic and cultural backgrounds, and these individuals have varying responses to diet.

In addition, the book covers important questions that students often raise concerning ethnic diets, eating disorders, nutrient supplements, phytochemicals, vegetarianism, diets for athletes, food safety, fad diets, and alternative medical practices, with an overall emphasis on the importance of understanding one's food choices and changing one's diet as needed.

■ AUDIENCE

This book has been designed for a nutrition majors audience. The chemistry has been presented at an appropriate level. Health majors, home economics majors, nursing students, physical education students, and students in other health-related areas will also find this text appropriate. Because of the flexible chapter organization and content, this book can be adopted for students of diverse educational backgrounds. Although it is not absolutely necessary, most students will find that having taken a course in college-level biology or having an understanding of basic biological concepts provides a helpful background when using this book.

■ ORGANIZATION

The book is most suitable for a semester-length course; it can also be used in a quarter-length course by omitting chapters or by skipping various sections. A useful feature of this text is that it is presented in six segments:

Part One: Nutrition Basics
Part Two: The Energy-Yielding Nutrients
Part Three: The Vitamins and Minerals
Part Four: Energy Production and Energy Balance
Part Five: Nutrition Applications in the Life Cycle
Part Six: Putting Nutrition Knowledge into Practice

This organization makes it easy to tailor the text to specific course needs.

■ NEW TO THIS EDITION

The fifth edition of *Perspectives in Nutrition* incorporates several new features designed to enhance student learning and understanding. Many of these features are a direct result of feedback received from instructors using previous editions.

Refresh Your Memory

Each chapter after Chapter 1 begins with a box reminding students of previous chapter content that will be helpful to know for understanding the current chapter, such as reminding students to review the concept of glycemic index in Chapter 5 before beginning the Sports Nutrition material in Chapter 14.

Case Scenario

Each chapter contains a case scenario that allows students to apply knowledge gained from the chapter in a real-life setting. Answers to the case scenario are provided in the chapter at the point in which the specific content needed to answer the case scenario is covered.

New or Updated Expert Opinions

All of the expert opinions are either updated or are new. Among those that are new to this edition are the following: trans fatty acids (Dr. Bruce Holub), a prescription for exercise (Dr. Sheri Melton), and the safety of genetically modified foods (Dr. John Allred).

New Take Action Activities

Each chapter now contains two Take Action activities. Previous editions contained one. These activities are great assignments for students to complete in order to enhance nutrition knowledge and provide real world application of nutrition.

New Chapter on Alcohol

Chapter 8 expands content on both the benefits and risks associated with alcohol use and the treatment of alcoholism, compared with previous editions. The Nutrition Perspective covers the risks of binge drinking, a prevalent problem on college campuses.

Expanded Coverage on Human Physiology

Chapter 3 covers not only the gastrointestinal tract, as was done in previous editions, but also now reviews the other body systems that support nutrition-related functions and overall health.

Nutrition Perspective on Alternative Medical Practices

Chapter 18 contains a Nutrition Perspective on alternative medical practices. The implications of the 1994 Dietary Supplement and Health Education Act (DSHEA) are reviewed, as well as possible benefits and risks of the use of popular herbal remedies.

Latest Dietary Reference Intakes (DRIs)

All of the current DRIs for vitamins and minerals are included in this revision, including those for vitamin A, vitamin K, and many trace minerals published in January 2001.

Updated Illustration Program

Numerous new photos and illustrations, including colorful variations of the USDA Food Guide Pyramid, keep the text current and fresh, as well as help convey important concepts.

■ ADDITIONAL FEATURES

Overall Content, Especially Controversial Topics Current and Well-referenced

Much of the material is supported and referenced from sources published after the previous edition of this text was published late in 1998. Providing up-to-date research not only gives students the most accurate picture of nutrition today but also directs them to current materials for further study.

Separate Chapter on Eating Disorders

This chapter provides current and in-depth coverage of this popular topic.

Emphasis on Nutrient Density

Discussions of nutrients concentrate on the most nutrient-dense sources of foods. Leading food sources in the U.S. diet are identified for each nutrient when that data are available.

Application of the Exchange System

The latest version of the Exchange System is presented in Chapter 2 and summarized in Appendix D.

Summary Tables

Some chapters contain large summary tables detailing the major points. These tables are convenient capsules for reference.

URLs for Nutrition-Related Web Sites

URLs for a variety of credible nutrition-related web sites are included in the chapters. When available, toll-free telephone numbers and other resources are also listed.

Glossary

A comprehensive glossary of key terms, located at the end of the text, is included for students' reference. The glossary contains pronunciation keys for many unfamiliar words.

■ SUPPLEMENTARY MATERIALS

The latest supplementary materials are provided to both you and students to make better use of the text and the concepts presented in the course.

Instructor's Manual

This manual includes all the features of a useful instructor's manual, including learning objectives, suggested lecture outlines, suggested activities, media resources, and web links. Available to adopters of the book, it also includes suggestions for teaching difficult material; activities; suggested readings; activities to use with FoodWorks College Edition software; source lists of supplementary materials; and a "survival" section, addressed to the novice instructor, which discusses class organization, scheduling, and problem areas, such as cheating.

Test Bank

This printed manual includes the test bank and features approximately 2,000 test items (multiple choice, short answer, and matching questions), coded for level of difficulty and type of knowledge being tested.

Computerized Test Bank

Instructors who adopt the text may receive MicroTest, a computerized test bank package compatible with Windows and Macintosh computers. This test-generation software combines a number of user-friendly aids, enabling you to select, edit, delete, or add questions and construct and print tests and answer keys.

FoodWorks College Edition

Based on the widely tested professional version of Food-Works, this dietary analysis software has been developed for use in college courses. It offers a variety of functions based on the latest release of the USDA database. FoodWorks College Edition features a novice-friendly interface and contains approximately 7,500 foods. It generates a wide range of standard, easy-to-grade reports and allows you the opportunity to add additional foods to the database.

PowerWeb Nutrition

Add the Internet to your course with PowerWeb. *Power-Web: Nutrition* provides students with current articles from *Annual Editions,* curriculum-based materials, weekly updates with assessment, informative and timely world news, refereed web links, research tools, student study tools, and interactive exercises. Preview the site at www.dushkin.com/powerweb.

Visual Resource Library for Nutrition 2002

Available to qualified adopters, this CD-ROM, compatible with either Windows or Macintosh, contains key illustrations from the text. The VRL also includes a book-specific PowerPoint lecture presentation. Illustrations and the PowerPoint can also be printed full-size for use as acetates and may be exported for use with other programs and applications, such as the computerized test bank.

Transparency Acetates for Nutrition 2002

Text adopters may receive over 200 full-color transparency acetates. They feature key illustrations from *Perspectives in Nutrition,* as well as other McGraw-Hill nutrition texts, with large, easy-to-read labels.

Online Learning Center

This site contains a variety of text and web resources correlated specifically to *Perspectives in Nutrition.* As students are assigned text chapters, they also can access additional study support, such as online quizzes, learning objectives, and web links, directly related to the material you are covering in that week's class. Instructor resources will correlate *all* instructor supplements to the appropriate chapter and are password-protected. In addition, there will be an online version of the Visual Resource Library. McGraw-Hill content can be delivered through most of the popular course management systems, such as WebCT and Blackboard. www.mhhe.com/wardlaw

PageOut Course Website Development Center

PageOut is McGraw-Hill's exclusive tool for creating your own website for your Nutrition course. It requires no knowledge of coding. Simply type your course information into the templates provided. PageOut is hosted by McGraw-Hill.

McGraw-Hill Nutrition Web Site (www.mhhe.com/nutrition)

This website has been designed as an on-line nutrition resource for students and instructors using McGraw-Hill textbooks. It contains a wide variety of study materials, content enhancements, instructional supplements, and links to key nutrition information sites, as well as information on McGraw-Hill products.

Innovations: Nutrition Applications and Updates

Innovations is a newsletter devoted to nutrition education; is jointly sponsored by Novartis Nutrition and McGraw-Hill and will be published twice yearly. It provides current information on topics that will appeal to anyone interested in nutrition and health. It is available free of charge to adopters of McGraw-Hill textbooks.

Issues in Nutrition: Obesity and Weight Control Videotape

This video explores obesity and weight control, including the concept of energy balance and the importance of physical activity in the energy balance equation, body mass index, and safe vs. unsafe diets.

Issues in Nutrition: Eating Disorders Videotape

This video looks at three types of eating disorders: anorexia nervosa, bulimia, and compulsive overeating. Professionals define and discuss each of these eating disorders, and three people who have been in treatment for an eating disorder discuss their experiences. Running time: 11 min. 29 sec.

Annual Edition Nutrition

This publication contains an assortment of previously published, contemporary articles on many topics, such as nutrition through the life span, food safety, fat and weight control, health claims, and hunger and global issues.

Diet and Fitness Log

This logbook helps students track their diet and exercise programs. Students don't always have access to a computer, and this booklet provides the diary that helps them log their behaviors.

▪ SPECIAL ACKNOWLEDGMENTS

We would like to thank Julie Giarrana, Monica Stubler, Jana Meyer, and Marcella Sander for their help with this revision. Our editor, Lynne Meyers, supported and assisted us through every step of the revision, and facilitated the difficult decisions that frequently arose. Marilyn Rothenberger and Debra DeBord did excellent and careful production work and copyediting. All these individuals contributed key expertise to the project.

Contributors

A special thanks to all those who contributed to this book—especially the authors of the Expert Opinion commentaries. Their names are listed in the Table of Contents.

Reviewers

As with the earlier editions, the goal is to provide the most accurate, up-to-date, and useful introductory nutrition text available. We, along with our publishers, would like to recognize and thank those people whose direction and insight guided the latest edition.

Fifth Edition Reviewers

Alan B. Avakian, Reedley College
Beverly A. Benes, University of Nebraska–Lincoln
Michael Braun, Madison Area Technical College
K. Shane Broughton, University of Wyoming
Jo Carol Chezem, Ball State University
Jean Freeland-Graves, University of Texas–Austin
Nancy Harris, East Carolina University
Carolyn J. Hoffman, Central Michigan University
K-L. Catherine Jen, Wayne State University
Zaheer Ali Kirmani, Sam Houston State University
Allen Knehans, University of Oklahoma Health Sciences Center
Karen A. Kramer, San Juan College
Mary Beth Kuehn, St. Olaf College
Shiu-Ming Kuo, University of Buffalo, State University of New York
Glen F. McNeil, Fort Hays State University
Barbara Mikuszewski, Cuyahoga Community College
Diana-Marie Spillman, Miami Univeristy
H. Garrison Wilkes, University of Massachusetts Boston
Elizabeth Wilson, Harding Univeristy

Content Survey Contributors

Richard C. Baybutt, Kansas State University
Jacqueline R. Berning, University of Colorado-Colorado Springs
Jo M. Cornforth, Mesa State College
Sharon Gow, Central Florida Community College
Jackie Hedgpeth, Everett Community College
Catherine Hagen Howard, Texarkana College
Allen Knehans, University of Oklahoma Health Sciences Center
Frank Konishi, University of Colorado-Boulder
Lola McGourty, Bossier Parish Community College
Earle J. Meyers, Bucks County Community College
Judy Myhand, Louisiana State University
Diana-Marie Spillman, Miami University
Dana Wu Wassmer, Cosumnes River College
Suzy Weems, Stephen F. Austin State University
Harry Womack, Salisbury State University

■ A Request to Professors Who Use This Book

As you might imagine, it is difficult to range across the vast areas of nutrition science, following all of the various controversies and new developments. We try our best but realize that sometimes we miss a side of an argument that deserves attention. If you find content that you question or believe warrants a more detailed or broader look, feel free to contact us by mail, fax, or e-mail.

Gordon M. Wardlaw, Ph.D., R.D., L.D., C.N.S.D.
The Ohio State University
516H School of Allied Medical Professions
1583 Perry Street
Columbus, OH 43210
Fax: 614-292-0210
E-mail: wardlaw.1@osu.edu

Margaret W. Kessel, Ph.D., R.D., L.D.
The Ohio State University
Department of Human Nutrition and Food Management
1783 Neil Ave.
Columbus, OH 43210
Fax: 614-292-8880
E-mail: kessel.2@osu.edu

Preface

TO THE STUDENT

Cholesterol, sports drinks, food labeling, bulimia nervosa, alternative sweeteners, vegetarianism, *Salmonella* food-borne illness and genetically-engineered foods—we suspect you have heard about these topics. Which topics are important enough to be a consideration in your life or in the life of someone you know?

Americans pride themselves on their individuality. Nutritional advice should be given accordingly. For example, not all of us have high blood cholesterol and other significant risk factors for developing premature cardiovascular disease. The need to tailor dietary advice to each person's individual nature is the basic approach of this book. First, you are given a brief introduction to the study of nutrition; then, how to be a knowledgeable consumer is discussed. With so much information available—both accurate and inaccurate—you should know how to make informed decisions about your nutritional well-being. Second, you are encouraged to learn the basic principles of nutrition and to discover how to apply the concepts in this book that pertain specifically to you.

The text discusses some of the most interesting and important elements of nutrition and food consumption to help you understand both how your body works and how your food choices affect your health.

■ FEATURES

Planning a New Way of Eating

Early in the text, many of the basic guidelines for planning a healthy diet are presented, including a description of the USDA Food Guide Pyramid, in Chapter 2. Later, in Chapter 13, the steps involved in setting nutritional goals and designing a diet plan to attain those goals are reviewed.

Understanding the World Around Us

In a college environment, it is often difficult to envision how real the problem of world hunger is. Chapter 20 examines the tragedy of undernutrition and the conditions that create it. The chapter allows you to explore possible solutions that offer hope for the future of our world.

Chemistry Review

Appendix B discusses in detail the critical chemistry concepts you need to know for an introductory study of nutrition. This information will give you a better understanding of how nutrients function and how nutrition information applies to you.

Organization

The fifth edition of *Perspectives in Nutrition* incorporates some important tools to help you learn the nutrition concepts in this text. Following is a guide to those tools:

1. Each chapter after Chapter 1 begins with a Refresh Your Memory box reminding you of previous chapter content that will be helpful to know for understanding the current chapter. Following this is a case scenario, which allows you to apply knowledge gained from the chapter in a real-life setting. An answer to each case scenario is provided in the chapter at the point at which the specific content needed to answer the case scenario is covered.
2. **Key Chapter Concepts** then help you focus your attention on key ideas in the chapter.
3. Throughout each chapter are **boldfaced key terms,** many of which are defined in the margin. All boldfaced terms appear with their definitions and pronunciations in the glossary at the end of the text.
4. Also throughout each chapter are **margin notes,** which further explain ideas, provide references to other chapters. Some URLs to nutrition-related web sites are in these margin notes, as well as in the text itself.
5. The numerous **tables** throughout the text present major points.
6. The **Concept Checks,** which follow the major sections within each chapter, summarize key points. If you are having trouble understanding the material in the Concept Check, you should reread the preceding section.
7. Each chapter ends with a **summary,** which conveys the main ideas in the chapter, and **study questions**—both provide a review of chapter material.
8. **References** with annotations are provided to back up material presented in the chapter. Much of this material cited has been published since the previous edition of the text in late 1998. If you are preparing a research paper for your class, or would just like more information on specific topics, consult these sources.
9. Also at the end of each chapter are **Take Action** boxes, which make major concepts presented in the chapter relevant to daily life. For example, you may be asked to look more carefully at your own diet, examine your family history, or apply information you've learned to friends or family.

10. In the **Expert Opinion** boxes, experts in the field of nutrition and health discuss information you need to understand regarding nutrition issues of our day. Think of these boxed discussions as "visiting speakers" who come into your classroom to talk about their latest research findings.

11. **Critical Thinking questions** ask you to apply information as you learn it. This fosters understanding of the material.

12. **Nutrition Perspective essays** at the end of each chapter develop current topics in nutrition, often covered earlier in the chapter, in greater detail.

13. A variety of supplements to this text, including a *Food-Works* dietary analysis software, are available to you. These instructional aids are designed to help you learn the major concepts developed in the text and prepare for class examinations.

14. The web site http://www.mhhe.com/wardlaw contains an **online learning center,** with quizzes, flash cards, other activities, and web links designed to further help you learn about nutrition. This is organized according to each chapter in the book.

FoodWorks—Dietary Analysis Software

This user-friendly dietary analysis program provides a variety of useful features, which allow you to track daily food intake, energy expenditure, and establish weight or body mass index (BMI) goals. Several different reports and pie charts allow you to see how calories from a specific food, meal, day, or daily average break out. For example, you can click on the fat pie chart to see what percentage of calories from saturated, monounsaturated, or polyunsaturated fat were in this morning's breakfast.

Features

- *FoodWorks* has a database of nearly 7,500 foods; the database allows you to accurately record your intake, and to analyze a specific food, meal, day, or average.

- *FoodWorks* calculates recommended daily calories and body mass index (BMI) based on height, weight, and other personal information entered into the program.

- You can track your daily activities—from sleeping to jogging—and *FoodWorks* will calculate daily energy expenditure.

- You can view a "personalized" food label in standard food label format for a given food.

- This colorful program is intuitively designed, making it easy to maneuver from one screen to another.

- Additional features include an easily accessible "Help" function, the ability to add your own foods to the database, and a link to the Nutrition Analysis web site.

■ A REQUEST TO STUDENTS WHO USE THIS BOOK

We try our best but realize that sometimes we miss a side of an argument that deserves attention or do not make something perfectly clear. If as you read this book you find content that you question or needs a clearer explanation, feel free to contact us by mail, fax, or e-mail.

Gordon M. Wardlaw, Ph.D., R.D., L.D., C.N.S.D.
The Ohio State University
516H School of Allied Medical Professions
1583 Perry Street
Columbus, OH 43210
Fax: 614-292-0210
E-mail: wardlaw.1@osu.edu

Margaret W. Kessel, Ph.D., R.D., L.D.
The Ohio State University
Department of Human Nutrition and Food Management
1783 Neil Ave.
Columbus, OH 43210
Fax: 614-292-8880
E-mail: kessel.2@osu.edu

The Online Learning Center
Your Password to Success

www.mhhe.com/wardlaw

This text-specific website allows students and instructors from all over the world to communicate. Instructors can create a more interactive course with the integration of this site, and students will find tools that help them improve their grades and learn that nutrition can be fun.

Student Resources

Study questions
Quizzing with immediate feedback
Links to chapter-related websites
Nutrition newsletters
Critical thinking exercises
Crossword puzzles
Concentration vocabulary game

Instructor Resources

Instructor's Manual
Online image and animation library
Links to related websites to expand on
  popular topics
Classroom activities
PowerPoint Lecture outlines

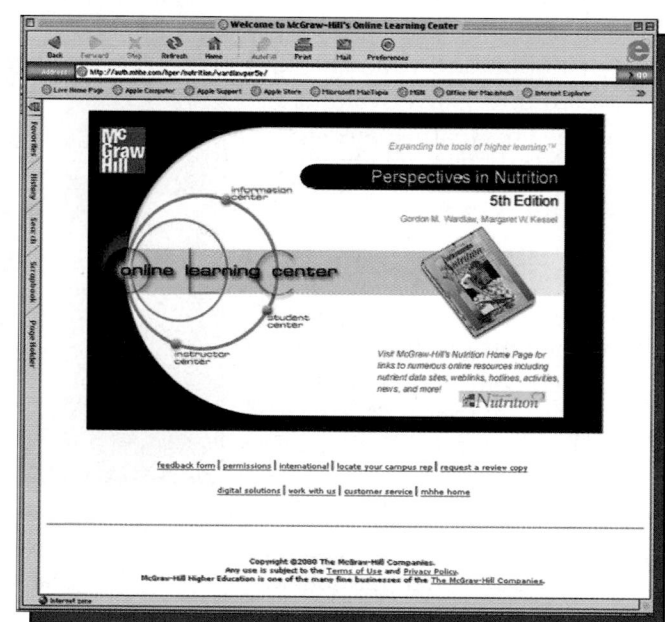

Imagine the advantages of having so many learning and teaching tools all in one place—all at your fingertips—FREE.

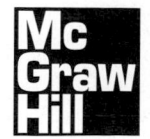

Contact your McGraw-Hill sales representative for more information or visit *www.mhhe.com*.

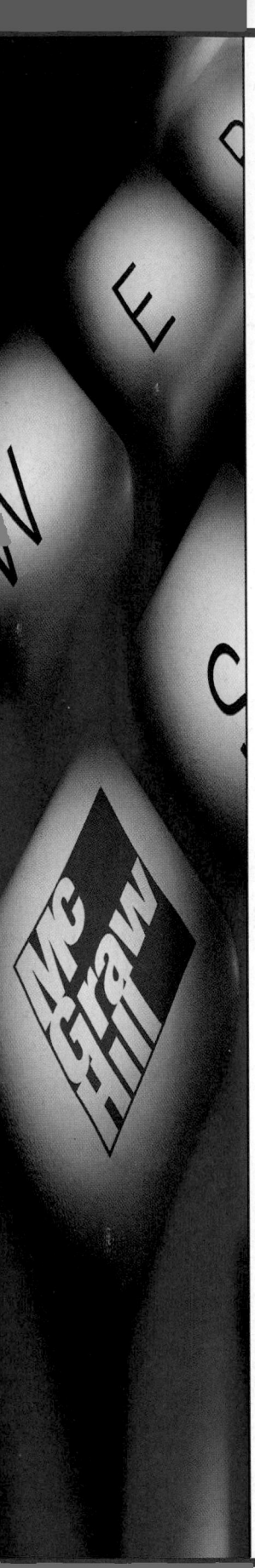

PageOut
Proven. Reliable. Class-tested.

Tens of thousands of professors have chosen **PageOut** to create course websites. And for good reason: **PageOut** offers powerful features, yet is incredibly easy to use.

Now you can be the first to use an even better version of **PageOut**. Through class-testing and customer feedback, we have made key improvements to the grade book, as well as the quizzing and discussion areas. Best of all, **PageOut** is still free with every McGraw-Hill textbook. And students needn't bother with any special tokens or fees to access your **PageOut** website.

Customize the site to coincide with your lectures.

Complete the **PageOut** templates with your course information and you will have an interactive syllabus online. This feature lets you post content to coincide with your lectures. When students visit your **PageOut** website, your syllabus will direct them to components of McGraw-Hill web content germane to your text, or specific material of your own.

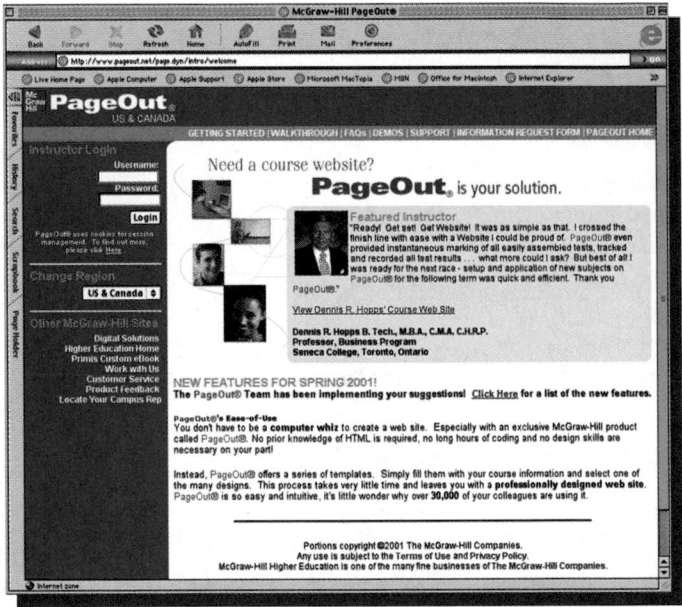

New Features based on customer feedback:

- Specific question selection for quizzes

- Ability to copy your course and share it with colleagues or use as a foundation for a new semester

- Enhanced grade book with reporting features

- Ability to use the **PageOut** discussion area, or add your own third party discussion tool

- Password protected courses

Short on time? Let us do the work.

Send your course materials to our McGraw-Hill service team. They will call you for a 30 minute consultation. A team member will then create your **PageOut** website and provide training to get you up and running. Contact your McGraw-Hill Representative for details.

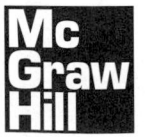

Contact your McGraw-Hill sales representative for more information or visit *www.mhhe.com*.

Visual Resource Library CD-ROMs

These CD-ROMs are electronic libraries of educational presentation resources that instructors can use to enhance their lectures. View, sort, search, and print catalog images, play chapter-specific slideshows using PowerPoint, or create customized presentations when you:

- Find and sort thumbnail image records by name, type, location, and user-defined keywords
- Search using keywords or terms
- View images at the same time with the Small Gallery View
- Select and view images at full size
- Display all the important file information for easy file identification
- Drag and place or copy and paste into virtually any graphics, desktop publishing, presentation, or multimedia application

Perspectives in Nutrition Visual Resource Library CD-ROM

This helpful CD-ROM contains hundreds of photographs and illustrations from the text as well as from several other McGraw-Hill nutrition texts. You'll be able to create interesting multimedia presentations with the use of these images, and students will have the ability to easily access the same images in their texts to later review the content covered in class. Additional resources include animations and sample Power-Point lecture outlines.

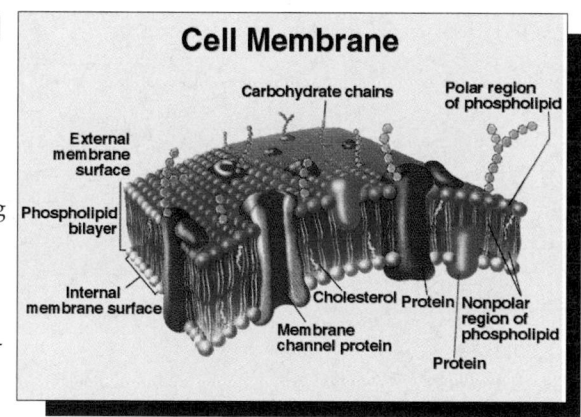

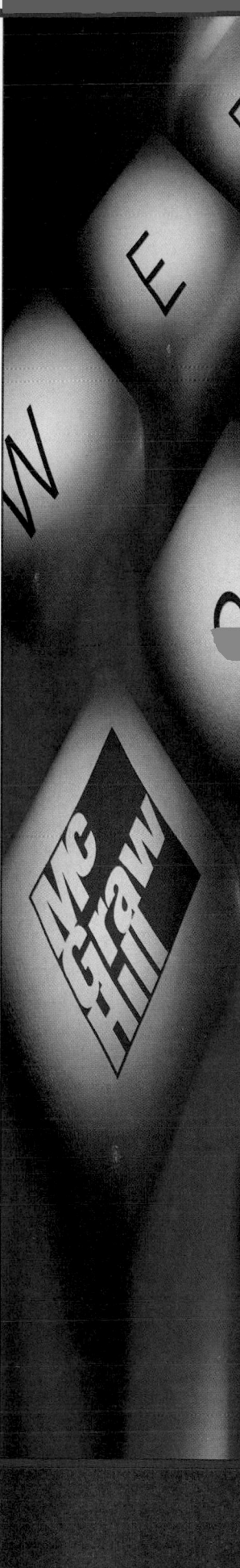

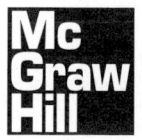

Contact your McGraw-Hill sales representative for more information or visit *www.mhhe.com*.

PERSPECTIVES IN NUTRITION

WHAT NOURISHES YOU?

chapter 1

*D*o you need to take vitamin and mineral supplements? Are you eating too much fat and cholesterol? Is much of what you eat unsafe? Are some foods actually *junk foods?* Should you become a vegetarian? If you're confused about what you should eat, you are not alone. This chapter will help you sort out some of these issues as you are introduced to the science of nutrition.

And, as you begin this study of nutrition, keep in mind what nutrition expert Dr. Irwin Rosenberg has written as his "bottom line" for a healthy lifestyle: "Research has shown no better way to slow or even reverse the progress of aging itself and of all the age-related degenerative conditions than through the combination of aerobic and strength-building exercise and a balanced, nutritious diet." Overall, it is clear that the nutritional lifestyles of some (but not all) Americans are out of balance with their physiology.[17] And, since we live longer than our ancestors, preventing the age-related diseases that develop later in life is a more important focus today than in the past.

By optimizing dietary choices, we can strive to bring the goal of a long, healthy life within reach.[26] This is the primary theme not just in this chapter but throughout this entire book.

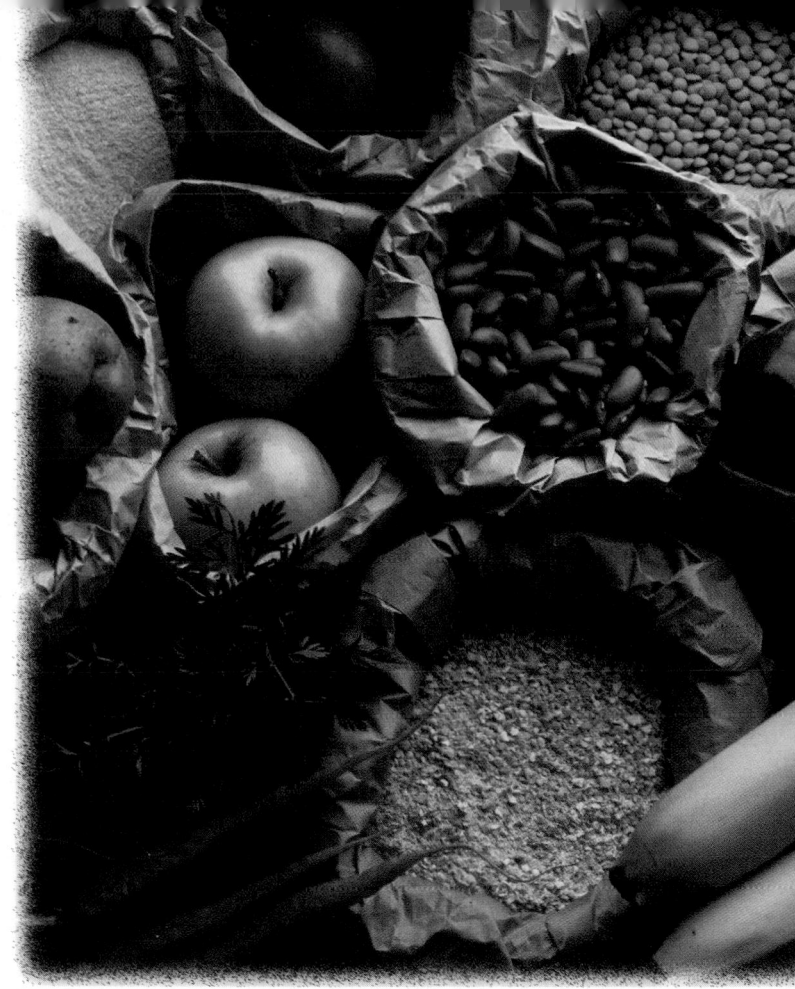

KEY CHAPTER CONCEPTS

- A varied diet coupled with regular physical activity contributes to good health.
- Unfortunately, poor nutrition contributes to much of the age-related disease Americans experience.
- Nutrients are classed into six major groups: carbohydrates, lipids (fats and oils), proteins, vitamins, minerals, and water. The lipids are especially rich in energy.
- Foods, rather than nutrient supplements, deserve the major focus in diet planning. Nutrition experts advocate eating more whole-grain breads and cereals, fruits, and vegetables.
- The scientific method is the procedure for testing the validity of possible explanations, called hypotheses. Only after we have much experimental information that supports a specific hypothesis should we embrace a concept and consider adopting the suggested dietary practice.
- There are no "junk" or "bad" foods per se. Focusing on one's total diet is the best approach for obtaining essential nutrients.
- Because genetic background influences health, family history for disease is important to consider. It is advisable to recognize this relationship and to take appropriate preventive action when possible.

CASE SCENARIO

Brendon listens to talk radio as he commutes to school each morning. He hears numerous advertisements for food supplements. Commentators also warn about the dangers of certain lifestyle practices. News briefs discuss the latest breakthroughs, touting new findings regarding both positive and negative health practices. Typical terms he hears are *heart disease, diabetes, cancer, obesity, vitamin E, omega-3 fatty acids, cholesterol,* and *creatine*. These are all topics generally covered in an introductory nutrition class. One advantage of taking such a class is to be able to decipher the health news that one reads in newspapers, hears on the radio, and is exposed to via television.

Start your exploration of nutrition by looking up these terms in the glossary at the back of this book. You will likely find this an interesting task, one that will heighten your awareness of nutrition and, so, help you in your study of nutrition. Also consider adding a few other words you are curious about and look those up as well in the glossary, or use the index if the glossary does not contain the word.

■ NUTRITION AND YOUR HEALTH

In your lifetime, you will eat about 70,000 meals and 60 tons of food. This opening chapter will take a close look at the general classes of nutrients supplied by this food intake, the role research plays in sorting out which food components are essential for the maintenance of health, and the powerful effect of genetic background in determining both nutrition-related and overall health.

■ What Actually Is Nutrition?

The Council on Food and Nutrition of the American Medical Association defines *nutrition* as "The science of food, the nutrients and the substances therein, their action, interaction, and balance in relation to health and disease, and the process by which the organism ingests, digests, absorbs, transports, utilizes, and excretes food substances."

■ Nutrients Come from Food

What is the difference among food, nutrients, and nutrition? Food provides both the energy and the materials needed to build and maintain all body cells. Nutrients are the nourishing substances we must obtain from food. These essential substances are vital for growth and maintenance of a healthy body throughout life. For a nutrient to be considered essential, two characteristics are needed. First, its omission from the diet must lead to a decline in certain aspects of human health, such as function of the nervous system. Second, if the omitted nutrient is restored to the diet before permanent damage occurs, those aspects of human health hampered by its absence should regain normal function.[12]

Some nutrients that perform life-sustaining functions can be produced by the body if they are missing from the diet. The essential nature of such nutrients sometimes is not clear-cut. For example, the body requires vitamin D, but the skin is capable of synthesizing its own vitamin D upon receiving sunlight. This reduces the need from dietary sources among people who experience regular sun exposure (see Chapter 9).

■ Why Study Nutrition?

Nutrition is one key to developing and maintaining a state of health that is optimal for you. In addition, a poor diet coupled with a sedentary lifestyle are known to be **risk factors** for life-threatening **chronic** diseases and deaths: **heart disease, stroke, hypertension, diabetes,** and some forms of **cancer** (Table 1-1). Together, these disorders account for two-thirds of all deaths in the United States (Table 1-2). Not consuming enough essential **nutrients** in younger years also makes us more likely to suffer consequences of poor nutrition habits in later years, such as bone fractures from the disease **osteoporosis.** Iron-deficiency **anemia** is another possibility. At the same time, taking too much of a nutrient supplement—such as vitamin A, vitamin D, vitamin B-6, calcium, or copper—can be harmful. Another dietary problem, drinking too much alcohol, is associated with **cirrhosis** of the liver, some forms of cancer, accidents, and suicides.

All of these consequences of modern living are partly an "affliction of affluence." Note, however, that these diseases are often preventable.[14] Age fast or age slowly: It is partly your choice. Government scientists have calculated that a poor diet combined with a lack of sufficient physical activity account for 300,000 fatal cases of heart disease, cancer, and diabetes each year. Thus, the combination of poor diet and lack of physical activity is indirectly the second leading cause of death. In addition, **obesity** is considered the second leading cause of preventable death (smoking is the first).

As you gain understanding about your nutritional habits and increase your knowledge about nutrition, you have the opportunity to dramatically reduce your risk for many common health problems.[5] To help U.S. citizens, the federal government provides two web sites that can link you to many sites providing health and nutrition information (http://www.healthfinder.gov and http://www.nutrition.gov).

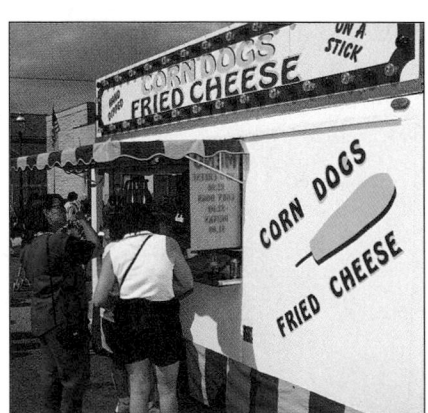

The major health problems in the United States are largely caused by excessive energy intake and not enough physical activity.

TABLE 1-1   Glossary Terms to Aid Your Introduction to Nutrition*

anemia Generally refers to a decreased oxygen-carrying capacity of the blood. This can be caused by many factors, such as iron deficiency or blood loss.

body mass index Weight (in kilograms) divided by height squared (in meters). A value of 25 or greater indicates a higher risk for body weight–related health disorders if one is overfat.

cancer A condition characterized by uncontrolled growth of abnormal cells.

cholesterol A waxy lipid found in all body cells; it has a structure containing multiple chemical rings (steroid structure). Cholesterol is found only in foods that contain animal products.

chronic Long-standing, developing over time. When referring to disease, this term indicates that the disease process, once developed, is slow and tends to remain; a good example is heart disease.

cirrhosis A loss of functioning liver cells, which are replaced by nonfunctioning connective tissue. Any substance that poisons liver cells can lead to cirrhosis. The most common cause is a chronic, excessive alcohol intake.

diabetes A disease characterized by high blood glucose (hyperglycemia), resulting from either insufficient or no insulin release by the pancreas or general inability of insulin to act on certain body cells, such as muscle cells.

heart disease A disease characterized by the deposition of fatty material in the blood vessels that serve the heart, often called hardening of the arteries. These deposits restrict blood flow through the heart, which in turn can lead to heart damage and death. Also termed *coronary heart disease* (CHD), as the vessels of the heart are the primary site of disease. The term **cardiovascular disease (CVD)** is also used, since in addition to the heart, the arteries that serve the rest of the body can experience the same deterioration.

hypertension A condition in which blood pressure remains persistently elevated. Obesity, inactivity, alcohol intake, and salt intake all can contribute to the problem.

kilocalorie (kcal) The heat energy needed to raise the temperature of 1000 g (1 liter) of water 1 degree Celsius. Also written as Calories, with a capital C.

nutrients Chemical substances in food, many of which are essential parts of a diet. Nutrients nourish us by providing energy, materials for building body parts, and factors to regulate necessary chemical processes in the body. The body either can't make these nutrients or can't make them in sufficient amounts for its needs.

obesity A condition characterized by excess body fat, typically defined in clinical settings as a body mass index (BMI) ≥ 30.

osteoporosis Decreased bone mass where no obvious causes can be found. This bone loss is related to the effects of aging, genetic background, poor diet, and hormonal effects of postmenopausal status in women.

risk factor A term used frequently when discussing diseases and factors contributing to their development. A risk factor is an aspect of our lives—such as heredity, lifestyle choices (i.e., smoking), or nutritional habits—that may make us more likely to develop a disease.

stroke The loss of body function that results from a blood clot or other change in arteries in the brain that affects blood flow. This in turn causes the death of brain tissue. Also called a *cerebrovascular accident*.

*All bold terms in the book are defined in a glossary, which follows Chapter 20. Many of these key terms are also defined in the chapter margin.

TABLE 1-2   Ten Leading Causes of Death in the United States

Rank	Cause of Death	Percent of Total Deaths
	All causes	100
1	Heart disease (primarily heart attack)*†	31
2	Cancer*†	23
3	Cerebrovascular diseases (stroke)*†	7
4	Chronic obstructive pulmonary diseases and allied conditions (lung diseases)†	5
5	Pneumonia and influenza	4
6	Accidents and adverse effects†	4
	Motor vehicle accidents	(2)
	All other accidents and adverse effects	(2)
7	Diabetes*	3
8	Suicide†	1
9	Kidney disease*†	1
10	Liver disease†	1

From Centers for Disease Control and Prevention, *National Vital Statistics Report,* accessed January 18, 2001.

*Causes of death in which diet plays a part

†Causes of death in which excessive alcohol consumption plays a part

†Causes of death in which tobacco use plays a part

Carbohydrate

Glycogen
Storage form of carbohydrate in the body

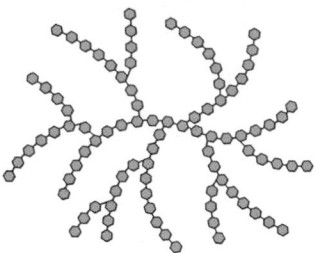

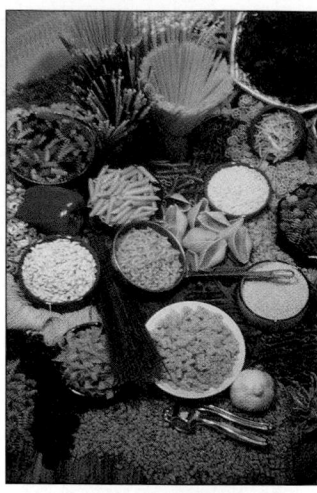

Each green circle represents one glucose molecule.

Lipid

Triglyceride

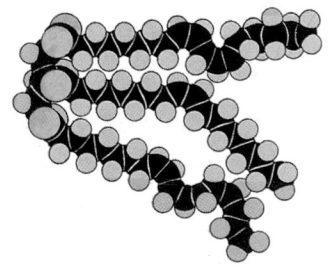

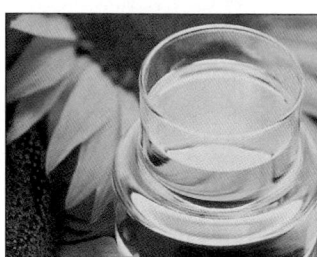

The black, blue, and yellow circles represent carbon, hydrogen, and oxygen atoms, respectively, in the triglyceride molecule.

Protein

Hemoglobin

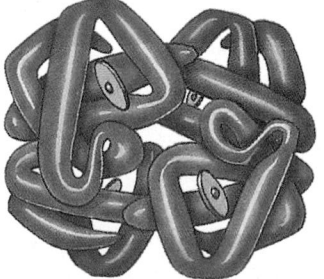

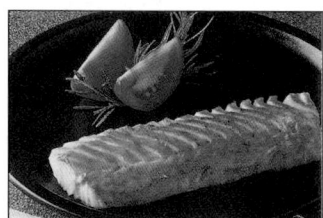

This protein, found in a red blood cell, is a structure formed of linked amino acids.

■ FIGURE 1-1 Two views of carbohydrates, lipids, and proteins—chemical and dietary perspectives.
Illustrations by William Ober.

carbohydrate A compound containing carbon, hydrogen, and oxygen atoms; most are known as *sugars*, *starches*, and *dietary fibers*.

protein Food and body components made of amino acids; proteins contain carbon, hydrogen, oxygen, nitrogen, and sometimes other atoms, in a specific configuration. Proteins contain the form of nitrogen most easily used by the human body.

lipid A compound containing much carbon and hydrogen, little oxygen, and sometimes other atoms. Lipids dissolve in ether or benzene, but not in water, and include fats, oils, and cholesterol.

vitamins Compounds needed in very small amounts in the diet to help regulate and support chemical reactions in the body.

minerals Elements used in the body to promote chemical reactions and to form body structures.

water The universal solvent; chemically, H_2O. The body is composed of about 60% water. Water (fluid) needs are about 8 cups per day; needs are greater if one exercises heavily (see Chapter 14).

■ CLASSES AND SOURCES OF NUTRIENTS

To begin the study of nutrition, let's start with an overview of the various classes of nutrients. You are probably already familiar with the terms **carbohydrates, lipids** (fats and oils), **proteins, vitamins,** and **minerals** (Figure 1-1). These, plus **water,** make up the six classes of nutrients found in food.

Nutrients can then be assigned to three functional categories: (1) those that primarily provide us with energy (typically expressed in **kilocalories [kcal]**); (2) those that are important for growth, development, and maintenance; and (3) those that act to keep body functions running smoothly. Some overlap exists among these groupings. The energy-yielding nutrients make up a major portion of most foods.

Provide Energy	Promote Growth and Development	Regulate Body Processes
Carbohydrates	Proteins	Proteins
Proteins	Lipids	Lipids
Lipids (fats and oils)	Vitamins	Vitamins
	Minerals	Minerals
	Water	Water

Let's now look more closely at these six classes of nutrients.

■ Carbohydrates

Carbohydrates are composed mainly of the elements carbon, hydrogen, and oxygen. Carbohydrates provide a major source of fuel for the body, on average 4 kcal per gram (kcal/g). Small carbohydrate structures are called sugars or simple sugars. Table sugar (sucrose) is an example. Some simple sugars, such as **glucose,** can link chemically to form large storage carbohydrates, called polysaccharides or complex carbohydrates (see Fig. 1-1). An example of this type of carbohydrate is the **starch** in potatoes.

Aside from enjoying their taste, we need sugars and other carbohydrates in our diets primarily to satisfy the energy needs of body cells. Glucose, which the body can produce from most carbohydrates, is a primary source of energy in most cells. When not enough carbohydrate is eaten to supply sufficient glucose, the body is forced to make glucose from proteins. However, a typical North American diet contains more than enough carbohydrate to prevent this from happening.[28]

Digestion of some dietary starch begins in the mouth. The digestive process continues in the small intestine until starches break down into single sugar molecules (such as glucose), which are absorbed into the bloodstream (see Chapter 3 for more on digestion). However, the links between the sugar molecules in certain complex carbohydrates cannot be broken down by human digestive processes. These carbohydrates are part of what is called **dietary fiber.** Such dietary fiber passes through the small intestine undigested to provide bulk for the stool (feces), which is formed in the large intestine (colon). Chapter 5 focuses on carbohydrates.

■ Lipids

Lipids (mostly fats and oils) are composed of the elements carbon and hydrogen; they contain fewer oxygen atoms than carbohydrates. Because of this difference in composition, lipids yield more energy per gram than carbohydrates—on average, 9 kcal/g. (See Chapter 4 for more details concerning the reason for the high-energy yield of lipids.) Lipids are insoluble in water but dissolve in certain organic solvents (e.g., ether and benzene).

The basic structure of most lipids is the three-carbon glycerol molecule with a fatty acid attached to each of the three carbons (see Fig. 1-1). This form of lipid is generally called a **triglyceride.** Triglycerides are a key energy source for the body and the major form of fat in foods. They are also the major form for energy storage in the body.

In this book, the more familiar term, *fats* or *fats and oils,* will generally be used, rather than *lipids* or *triglycerides.* Roughly speaking, fats are lipids that are solid at room temperature, and oils are lipids that are liquid at room temperature.

Most lipids can be separated into two basic types—saturated and unsaturated—based on the chemical structure of their dominant fatty acids. This property determines whether such a lipid is solid or liquid at room temperature. Plant oils tend to contain many unsaturated fatty acids, which makes them liquid. Animal fats are often rich in saturated fatty acids, which makes them solid. Almost all foods contain a variety of saturated and unsaturated fatty acids.

glucose A six-carbon carbohydrate found in blood and in table sugar bound to fructose; also known as *dextrose,* it is one of the simple sugars.

Many basic chemistry concepts are reviewed in Appendix B. If you are unfamiliar with chemistry terms, you will find the review quite helpful.

dietary fiber Substances in plant foods that are not digested by the processes that take place in the stomach or small intestine. These add bulk to feces.

triglyceride The major form of lipid in the body and in food. It is composed of three fatty acids bonded to glycerol, an alcohol. May also be called a triacylglycerol, since the form of fatty acid attached exists as an acyl group (see Appendix B).

Much attention has been given to saturated fat in the past few years. This is because saturated fat bears a great deal of the responsibility for raising blood cholesterol. High blood cholesterol leads to clogged arteries and, so, can eventually lead to heart disease. For this reason, it is recommended that people limit the amount of saturated fat in their diet.

Certain unsaturated fatty acids are essential nutrients. These key fatty acids that the body can't produce, called essential fatty acids, perform several important functions in the body: they help regulate blood pressure and play a role in the synthesis and repair of vital cell parts. However, we need only about 1 tablespoon of a common vegetable oil (such as the canola or soybean oil found in supermarkets) each day to supply the essential fatty acids. The average American diet supplies about three times the amount of essential fatty acids needed daily.[28] Adding fish in a diet twice a week adds to this benefit derived from the inclusion of vegetable oil. The unique fatty acids in fish complement the healthy aspects of vegetable oil. This will be explained in greater detail in Chapter 6, which focuses on lipids.

■ Proteins

Like carbohydrates and fats, proteins are composed of the elements carbon, oxygen, and hydrogen. But, unlike the other energy-yielding nutrients, all proteins also contain much nitrogen. Proteins are the main structural material in the body (see Fig. 1-1). For example, proteins constitute a major part of bone and muscle; they are also important components in blood, cell membranes, and immune factors. Furthermore, proteins can also provide energy for the body—on average, 4 kcal/g. Typically, the body uses little protein for that purpose of meeting daily energy needs. Proteins are formed by the linking of **amino acids.** Twenty common amino acids are found in food; nine of these are essential nutrients for adults, and one additional one for infants.

Most of us eat about one and a half to two times more protein than the body needs to maintain health.[28] In a healthy person (i.e., no evidence of heart disease, osteoporosis, kidney disease, or diabetes or family history of colon cancer), this amount of extra protein in the diet is generally not harmful—it simply reflects the standard of living and the dietary habits of most North Americans. The excess is used for fuel or converted into fat or carbohydrate. Chapter 7 focuses on proteins.

Three other classes of nutrients are vitamins, minerals, and water. Although vitamins and minerals are vital to good health, they are needed only in small amounts in the diet and provide no direct source of energy for the body.

■ Vitamins

Vitamins exhibit a wide variety of chemical structures and can contain the elements carbon, hydrogen, nitrogen, oxygen, phosphorus, sulfur, and others. The main function of vitamins is to enable many chemical reactions to occur in the body. Some of these reactions help release the energy trapped in carbohydrates, lipids, and proteins. Remember, however, that vitamins themselves provide no usable energy for the body.

The 13 vitamins are divided into two groups: four that are fat soluble (vitamins A, D, E, and K) and nine that are water soluble (vitamin C and the B vitamins). The two groups of vitamins often act quite differently. For example, cooking destroys water-soluble vitamins much more readily than it does fat-soluble vitamins. Water-soluble vitamins are also excreted from the body much more readily than are fat-soluble vitamins. Thus, the fat-soluble vitamins, especially vitamins A and D, are much more likely to accumulate in excessive amounts in the body, which then can cause toxicity. The vitamins are the focus of Chapters 9 and 10.

■ Minerals

The nutrients discussed so far are all **organic** compounds, whereas minerals are structurally very simple, **inorganic** substances, which exist as groups of one or more of the same atoms. These terms, *organic* and *inorganic,* have nothing to do with gardening but are based on simple chemistry concepts (see Chapter 2 for use of the term on food labels).

Minerals typically function as such in the body (Na^+, K^+), or as parts of simple mineral combinations, such as bone mineral [$Ca_{10}(PO_4)_6 OH_2$]. Because of their simple structure, minerals are not destroyed during cooking, but they can still be lost

---

*M*any health-food stores market protein powders and shakes for bodybuilders and other athletes. As noted in this section, the American diet contains nearly two times the required amount of protein. Thus, these products are unnecessary; diet can suffice.

amino acid The building block for proteins containing a central carbon atom with a nitrogen atom and other atoms attached.

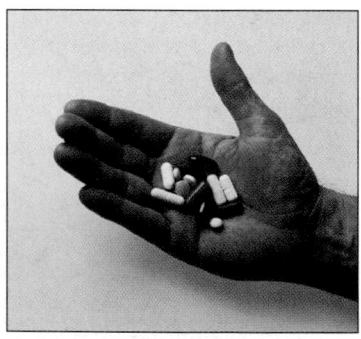

Taking a daily multivitamin and mineral supplement is generally a safe practice. However, uninformed nutrient supplement use can lead to health problems. Chapter 9 will explore the appropriate and safe use of supplements in detail.

organic Any substance that contains carbon atoms bonded to hydrogen atoms in the chemical structure.

inorganic Any substance lacking carbon atoms bonded to hydrogen atoms in the chemical structure.

if they leak into the water used for cooking and then are discarded if that water is not consumed. Although minerals themselves yield no energy as such for the body, they are critical players in nervous system functioning, other cellular processes, water balance, and structural (e.g., skeletal) systems.

The amounts of the 16 or more essential minerals that are required in the diet for good health vary enormously. Thus, they are divided into two groups: major minerals and trace minerals, based on dietary needs. If daily needs are less than 100 mg, the mineral is put in the trace mineral class. The actual dietary requirement for some trace minerals has yet to be determined. Minerals are the focus of Chapters 11 and 12.

▪ Water

Water is the sixth class of nutrients. Although sometimes overlooked as a nutrient, water (chemically, H_2O) has numerous vital functions in the body. It acts as a **solvent** and lubricant, as a medium for transporting nutrients and waste, and as a medium for temperature regulation and chemical processes. For these reasons, and because the human body is approximately 60% water, we require about 2 liters (L)—equivalent to 2000 g or 8 cups—of water and fluids containing water every day.

Water is not only available from the obvious sources, but it is also the major component in some foods, such as many fruits and vegetables (e.g., lettuce, grapes, and melons). The body even makes some water as a by-product of **metabolism.** Water is examined in detail in Chapter 11.

▪ NUTRIENT COMPOSITION OF DIETS AND THE HUMAN BODY

The quantities of the various nutrients that people consume vary widely, and the nutrient amounts present in different foods also vary a great deal. The total daily intake of protein, fat, and carbohydrate amounts to about 500 g. In contrast, the typical daily mineral intake totals about 20 g, and the daily vitamin intake totals less than 300 mg. Although each day we require nearly a gram of some minerals, such as calcium and phosphorus, we need only a few milligrams or less of other minerals. For example, we need about 10 mg of zinc per day, which is just a few specks of the mineral.

Figure 1-2 contrasts the relative concentrations of all the major classes of nutrients in a lean man and a lean woman with the composition of both a cooked steak and a cooked stalk of broccoli. Note how the nutrient composition of the body differs from the nutritional profiles of the foods we eat. This is because growth, development, and later maintenance of the human body are directed by the genetic material inside the cell nucleus.[23] This genetic blueprint determines how each cell uses the essential nutrients to perform body functions. These nutrients can come from a variety of sources. Cells are not concerned whether available amino acids come from animal or plant sources. The carbohydrate glucose can come from sugars or starches. Thus, you really aren't what you eat. Rather, what you eat provides cells with basic materials to function according to the directions supplied by the genetic material **(genes)** housed in the cell (see the Nutrition Perspective at the end of this chapter).

▪ ENERGY SOURCES AND USES

We obtain the energy we need to perform body functions and do work from carbohydrates, fats, and proteins. Foods generally provide more than one energy source. Vegetable oil is an exception; it is 100% fat. **Alcohol** is also a source of energy for some of us, supplying about 7 kcal/g. It is not considered a nutrient, however,

solvent A substance that other substances dissolve in.

metabolism Chemical processes in the body by which energy is provided in useful forms and vital activities are sustained.

genes The hereditary material on chromosomes that makes up DNA. Genes provide the blueprints for the production of cell proteins.

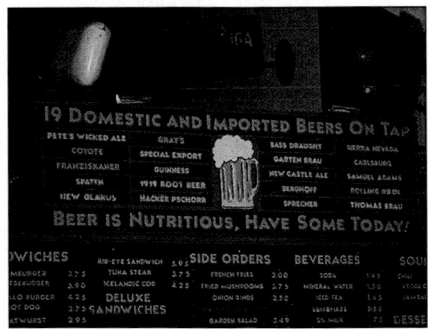

Alcoholic beverages are calorie rich, but alcohol is not a nutrient per se.

alcohol Ethyl alcohol (CH_3CH_2OH).

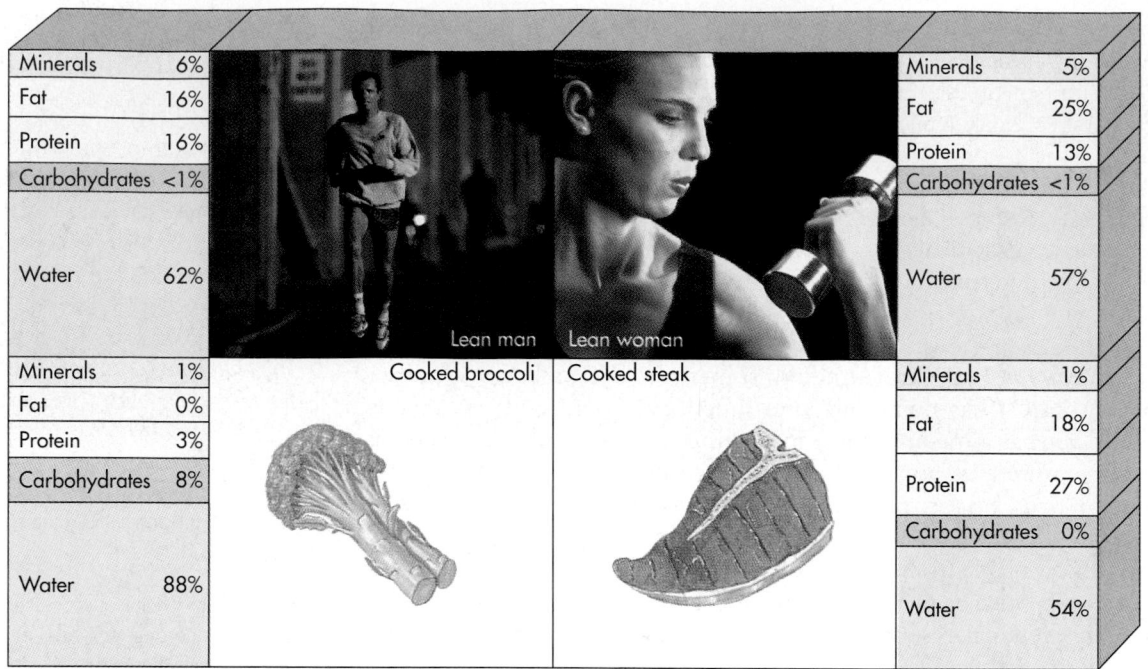

Minerals	6%
Fat	16%
Protein	16%
Carbohydrates	<1%
Water	62%

Lean man

Minerals	5%
Fat	25%
Protein	13%
Carbohydrates	<1%
Water	57%

Lean woman

Cooked broccoli

Minerals	1%
Fat	0%
Protein	3%
Carbohydrates	8%
Water	88%

Cooked steak

Minerals	1%
Fat	18%
Protein	27%
Carbohydrates	0%
Water	54%

FIGURE 1-2 You aren't what you eat. The proportions of nutrients in the human body do not match those found in typical foods—animal or vegetable.

ion An atom with an unequal number of electrons and protons. Negative ions have more electrons than protons; positive ions have more protons than electrons.

In many scientific journals, the kilojoule (kJ), rather than the kilocalorie, is used to express the energy content of food. A mass of 1 gram moving at a velocity of 1 meter/sec possesses the energy of 1 joule (J); 1000J = 1 kJ. Since heat and work are just two forms of energy, measurements expressed in terms of kilocalories (a heat measure) are interchangeable with measurements expressed in terms of kilojoules (a work measure): 1 kcal = 4.18 kJ.

digestibility Corresponds to the proportion of food substances eaten that can be broken down into individual nutrients in the intestinal tract for absorption into the body.

because it has no required function. Still, alcoholic beverages—generally also rich in carbohydrate—are typically a contributor of energy to the diet of adults.[28]

The body transforms the energy trapped in carbohydrate, protein, and fat (and alcohol) into other forms of energy in order to

- Build new compounds
- Perform muscular movements
- Promote nerve transmissions
- Maintain **ion** balance within cells

Chapter 4 describes how that energy is released from chemical bonds and then used by body cells to support the processes just described.

You have likely noticed on food labels that the energy in food is often expressed in terms of calories. Technically, a calorie is the amount of heat energy it takes to raise the temperature of 1 g of water 1 degree Celsius (1°C, centigrade scale). Because a calorie is such a tiny measure of heat, food energy is more accurately expressed in terms of the kilocalorie (kcal), which equals 1000 calories. A kcal is the amount of heat energy it takes to raise the temperature of 1000 g (1 L) of water 1°C. The term *kilocalorie* and its abbreviation *kcal* are used throughout this book. In everyday life, the word *calorie* is often used loosely to mean *kilocalorie*. The values given on food labels in calories are actually in kilocalories (Fig. 1-3). A suggested intake of 2000 calories per day on a food label is really 2000 kcal.

Carbohydrates, proteins, lipids, and alcohol provide the body with differing amounts of energy. Use the 4-9-4 estimates for carbohydrate, fat, and protein introduced over the last few pages to determine energy content of a food. Consider a typical deluxe hamburger sandwich:

Carbohydrate	39 grams × 4 = 156 kcal
Fat	32 grams × 9 = 288 kcal
Protein	30 grams × 4 = 120 kcal
Total	564 kcal

Note also that the 4-9-4 estimates have been adjusted for (1) **digestibility** and (2) substances not available for energy use. Such substances include waxes and some fibrous parts of plants. The energy estimates are then rounded to whole numbers.

Nutrition Facts

Serving Size 1 slice (36g)
Servings Per Container 19

Amount Per Serving

Calories 80   Calories from Fat 10

	% Daily Value*		% Daily Value*
Total Fat 1g	**2%**	**Total Carbohydrate** 15g	**5%**
Saturated Fat 0g	**0%**	Dietary Fiber 2g	**8%**
Cholesterol 0mg	**0%**	Sugars less than 1g	
Sodium 200mg	**8%**	**Protein** 3g	

Vitamin A 0%   Vitamin C 0%   Calcium 0%   Iron 4%

HONEY WHEAT BREAD

*Percent Daily Values (DV) are based on a 2,000 calorie diet. Your daily values may be higher or lower depending on your calorie needs:

		Calories:	2,000	2,500
Total Fat	Less than		65g	80g
Sat Fat	Less than		20g	25g
Cholesterol	Less than		300mg	300mg
Sodium	Less than		2,400mg	2,400mg
Total Carbohydrate			300g	375g
Dietary Fiber			25g	30g

INGREDIENTS: WHOLE WHEAT, WATER, ENRICHED WHEAT FLOUR [FLOUR, MALTED BARLEY, NIACIN, REDUCED IRON, THIAMINE MONONITRATE (VITAMIN B1) AND RIBOFLAVIN (VITAMIN B2)], CORN SYRUP, PARTIALLY HYDROGENATED COTTONSEED, OIL, SALT, YEAST.

FIGURE 1-3 Use the nutrient values on the Nutrition Facts label to calculate energy content of a food. A serving of this food contains 81 kcal ([15 × 4] + [3 × 4] + [1 × 9] = 81). The label lists 80, suggesting that the energy value was rounded down.

You can also use the 4-9-4 estimates to determine what portion of total energy intake is contributed by the various energy-yielding nutrients. Assume that one day you consume 290 g of carbohydrates, 60 g of fat, and 70 g of protein. This consumption yields a total of 1980 kcal ([290 × 4] + [60 × 9] + [70 × 4] = 1980). The percentage of your total energy intake derived from each nutrient can then be determined:

% of kcal as carbohydrate = (290 × 4) ÷ 1980 = 0.586 or 59%

% of kcal as fat = (60 × 9) ÷ 1980 = 0.273 or 27%

% of kcal as protein = (70 × 4) ÷ 1980 = 0.141 or 14%

Check your calculations by adding the percentages together. Do they total 100?

CONCEPT CHECK

Food contains vital nutrients that are essential for good health: carbohydrates, lipids (fats and oils), proteins, vitamins, minerals, and water. Nutrients have three general functions in the body: (1) to provide materials for building and maintaining the body; (2) to act as regulators for key metabolic reactions; and (3) to participate in metabolic reactions that provide the energy necessary to sustain life. A common unit of measurement for this energy is the kilocalorie (kcal).

INTEREST IN THE FIELD OF NUTRITION HAS A LONG HISTORY

The science of nutrition evolved primarily from the disciplines of physiology, chemistry, and medicine.[12] Our interest in the relationship between food and the maintenance of health has a long history, beginning some 2400 years ago in Greece, during the time of Hippocrates. The Bible even contains references to the importance of certain foods, such as beans, for maintaining health.

The science of nutrition began in the 1600s in Europe. A British physician, Sydenham, in 1674 showed that iron filings in wine can be used to treat anemia. In the 1740s, a British naval surgeon, Lind, found that the consumption of citrus fruits—lemons and limes—cures the disease scurvy in sailors. Between 1770 and 1794, Lavoisier and Laplace in France discovered that certain carbon-containing

In the fifth century BC, Hippocrates said "Let food be your medicine and medicine be your food."

compounds are the source of energy for body functions. Adding to this observation, in 1816 German scientist Magendie showed that dogs fed only carbohydrate and fat lost much body protein and died within a few weeks.

By 1830, it was known that foods contain three major constituents: proteins, carbohydrates, and fats. By 1850, at least six mineral elements—calcium, phosphorous, sodium, potassium, chloride, and iron—had been established as essential for the diets of higher animals. Nutrition as a scientific discipline was born. Scientists now realized that components in foods, some of which are present in very small amounts, contribute to health.

During the 1880s, a Japanese physician, Takaki, showed that a common disease of sailors, called beriberi, can be treated with evaporated milk and meat. Later research in the Dutch East Indies by both Eijkman and Grijns showed that the same disease is associated with the use of refined rice, whereas use of the whole rice grain prevented the problem. By 1901, it was assumed that refined rice lacks an essential nutrient (later called water-soluble B and then eventually found to be the vitamin thiamin), which was present in the whole-grain product.

In the 1890s, Rubner in Germany and Atwater in the United States established the energy (kcal) content of protein, carbohydrate, and fat. This research also quantified human energy output, showing that, on average, we expend about 2000 to 3000 kcal/day, with some variation at both ends of the range.

In 1906, the amino acid tryptophan was shown to be essential for mice by Willcock and Hopkins in Britain. By 1913, Osborne and Mendel in the United States had shown that food proteins are quite different in terms of their amino acid content.

The year 1912 was a banner year—the term *vitamine* was coined by Polish scientist Funk at this time to describe certain compounds present in very small amounts in foods that promote health. *Vita* came from the Latin for "life," and *amine* came from the term for nitrogen bonded to carbon (technically, called an amine). (The *e* was dropped from *vitamine* to form *vitamin* in the 1920s, when it was shown that some vitamins do not contain nitrogen.) Later, in 1913, American researchers McCollum and Davis showed that butterfat contains a protective dietary factor; this was called fat-soluble A.

By 1915, nutrition experts knew that six minerals, four amino acids, and three vitamins—A, B (later shown to be a group of vitamins), and the anti-scurvy factor (later shown to be ascorbic acid, which we also call vitamin C)—are essential nutrients. By 1918, the importance of consuming a wide variety of foods in order to consume an adequate quantity of nutrients had become a focus in dietary advice given throughout the United States and Europe.

From the 1920s to today, nutrition research has been a key part of the intense scientific inquiry that characterized the twentieth century. **Recommended Dietary Allowances (RDAs)** for nutrients were first published in the United States in 1943 in response to growing recognition of the poor nutritional health of many Americans. All vitamins we know of today had been characterized by 1949. The research on vitamins such as thiamin, vitamin K, vitamin C, and vitamin B-12 even led to Nobel prizes such as for Eijkman, Dam, and Szent-Gyorgyi. By 1950, some 35 nutrients had been shown to be necessary to maintain human health. Today we know that the minimum diet for humans must contain about 45 essential nutrients in order to maintain health (Table 1-3).

In the 1950s, British researchers Watson and Crick described the structure of genetic material in cells, DNA. Today the Human Genome Project is extending that work by deciphering the human DNA code. This should help us understand the genetic effects on individual health status, as well as the possible genetic differences that lead to differences in human nutritional needs (see the Nutrition Perspective at the end of this chapter).

In 1968, Dudrick in the United States was able to support the nutrient needs of dogs using only intravenous feedings of purified nutrients. Soon after, it was shown that this is also possible for humans. Thus, we had evidence that meeting the needs for nutrients known to be essential at that time sufficed to maintain health.

Recommended Dietary Allowances (RDAs) Recommended intakes of nutrients that are sufficient to meet the needs of almost all individuals (97%) of similar age and gender. These are established by the Food and Nutrition Board of the National Academy of Sciences.

TABLE 1-3 Essential Nutrients in the Human Diet and Their Classes*

Energy-Yielding Nutrients

Carbohydrate	Fat (Lipids)†	Protein (Amino Acids)	Water
Glucose† (or a carbo-hydrate that yields glucose) —	Linoleic acid (omega-6) α-Linolenic acid (omega-3)	Histidine Isoleucine Leucine Lysine Methionine Phenylalanine Threonine Tryptophan Valine	Water

Vitamins

Water-Soluble	Fat-Soluble
Thiamin	A
Riboflavin	D§
Niacin	E
Pantothenic acid	K
Biotin	
B-6	
B-12	
Folate	
C	

Minerals

Major	Trace	Some Questionable Varieties
Calcium	Chromium	Arsenic
Chloride	Copper	Boron
Magnesium	Fluoride‖	Nickel
Phosphorus	Iodide	Silicon
Potassium	Iron	Vanadium
Sodium	Manganese	
Sulfur	Molybdenum	
	Selenium	
	Zinc	

*This table includes nutrients that the current *Dietary Reference Intakes* and related publications list for humans. Some disagreement exists over the questionable varieties, and certain other minerals not listed. Dietary fiber could be added to the list of essential substances, but it is not a nutrient (see Chapter 5). Alcohol is a source of calories but is not a nutrient per se.
†The lipids listed are needed only in small amounts, about 2% of total energy needs (see Chapter 6).
‡To prevent ketosis and thus the muscle loss that would occur if protein were used to synthesize carbohydrate (see Chapter 5)
§Sunshine on the skin also allows the body to make vitamin D for itself (see Chapter 9).
‖Primarily for dental health (see Chapter 12)

The vitamin-like compound choline plays essential roles in the body but is not listed under the vitamin category at this time. Rough estimates of human needs for this water-soluble compound recently have been set (see the inside cover of the text). Note, however, that body synthesis suffices during many stages of life (see Chapter 10 for details).

Over the past 30 years, interest in nutrition has grown. Health-conscious consumers are especially interested in the topic. Government policymakers stepped up their interest after the 1970 White House conference on food, nutrition, and health, and support of federal feeding programs (see Chapter 20). Following this, more and more research, much of which was funded by the federal government, supported the role of nutrition in the maintenance of health, as well as showed a link between poor nutrition (both inadequate and excessive nutrient intakes) and various health problems. To date, we have made much progress in the field of nutrition, but work needs to be done, and nutrition problems still plague peoples around the world.[9] In fact, the Worldwatch Institute estimates that the number of overweight people now equals the number of undernourished people in the world; each group contains roughly 1.2 billion people.

■ CURRENT STATE OF THE AMERICAN DIET

Humans derive energy mostly from carbohydrates, fats, and proteins. If we ignore alcohol, American adults consume about 16% of their kcal as proteins, 50% as

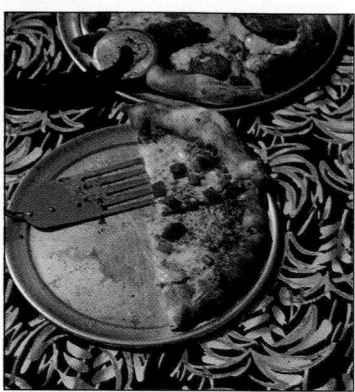

A market research firm surveyed the eating habits of people in 2000 American households. The top meal choice was pizza, followed by ham sandwich, hot dog, peanut butter and jelly sandwich, steak, macaroni and cheese, turkey sandwich, cheese sandwich, hamburger on a bun, and spaghetti.

salt Generally refers to a compound of sodium and chloride in a 40:60 ratio.

carbohydrates, and 33% as fats. These percentages are estimates and vary slightly from year to year and from person to person. As a rough estimate, changing to a 10 to 15%, 55 to 60%, and 25 to 30% distribution of calories from protein, carbohydrate, and fat, respectively, is widely advocated. This advice contributes to a lower fat intake, a change that can lead to many health benefits, as has been shown in women (see Chapters 6 and 13).[2] Note that recommendations for different distributions of calories among protein, carbohydrate, and fat come and go in the popular press. The pros and cons of these patterns—such as the 45%, 15%, 40% pattern of carbohydrate, protein, and fat calories in the popular book *Syndrome X*, authored by Dr. Gerald Reaven and colleagues—will be reviewed in future chapters.

Animal sources supply about two-thirds of protein intake for most Americans; plant sources supply only about one-third. In many other parts of the world, it is just the opposite: plant proteins—from rice, beans, corn, and other vegetables—dominate protein intake. About half the carbohydrate in American diets comes from simple sugars; the other half comes from starches (such as in pastas, breads, and potatoes). About 60% of our dietary fat comes from animal sources and 40% from plant sources.[17]

■ Assessing the Current American Diet

Information about the American diet comes from large surveys designed to find out what and when people eat.[30] The primary methods the federal government uses to collect data about food and nutrient consumption, and the relationship between diet and health are two survey programs: the Continuing Survey of Food Intakes by Individuals (CSFII) conducted by USDA and the National Health and Nutrition Examination Survey (NHANES) administered by the U.S. Department of Health and Human Services. CSFII, as the name implies, is a ongoing program that collects data on America's eating habits. The NHANES is an examination of the health status of Americans as related to their nutrient intake. Results from these surveys and other studies, show that we eat a wide variety of foods. Many people are meeting their nutrient needs; some are not. Chapter 2 will look at this situation in more detail. For now, note that studies show that some of us should choose more foods that are rich in iron, calcium, vitamin A, various B vitamins, vitamin C, zinc, and dietary fiber.[28] Almost all experts also recommend that we pay more attention to balancing energy intake with need. An excess intake of energy is usually tied to an overindulgence in sugar, fat, and alcoholic beverages. African-Americans may need to pay special attention to the amount of sodium (**salt** is a mixture of sodium and chloride) and alcohol in their diets. This is because they have a greater chance of developing hypertension than do other ethnic groups in America, and these substances are two of the many factors linked to that health problem. Actually, a careful look at sodium and alcohol intake—along with saturated and total fat and total energy intake—is a useful task for all adults.[15]

Many Americans would benefit from a more helpful balance of foods in their diets—greater moderation in the intake of some foods is needed, such as sugared soft drinks and fried foods, while increasing the variety of other foods, such as fruits and vegetables. Few adults currently meet the "five-a-day" minimum recommendation for total servings of vegetables and fruits, even though, when interviewed, 70% of the people said these are an important part of a diet.[9]

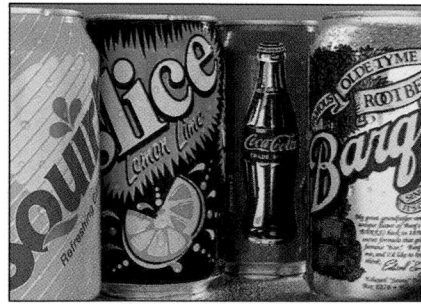

Today soft drinks are more popular than milk, although not as beneficial to the diet. Soft drinks account for on average 10% of the energy intake of teenagers and, in turn, contribute to generally poor calcium intakes in this age group.

■ Improving Our Diets

Our cultural diversity, varied cuisines, and generally high nutritional status should be points of pride for Americans. Today we can choose from a tremendous variety of food products, the result of continual innovation by food manufacturers.

During the past hundred years, the United States has led the world in creating new food products (Table 1-4). From toaster pastries to microwave popcorn, the variety of food products in a typical supermarket is nearly limitless. Even astronauts

TABLE 1-4 Years When Common American Foods Were Introduced

1875—Chocolate milk	1950—Sugar Corn Pops
1876—Heinz ketchup	1951—Duncan Hines cake mix
1891—Fig Newtons	1952—Kellogg's Sugar Frosted Flakes
1896—Tootsie Rolls	1953—Sugar Smacks, frozen pizza
1897—Jell-O	1956—Jif peanut butter
1897—Grape-Nuts	1957—Sweet 'n Low
1898—Graham crackers	1958—Tang
1907—Hershey's Kisses	1960—Instant potatoes
1912—Life Savers, Oreos	1963—Tab
1913—Fruit cocktail	1965—Shake 'n Bake
1916—All-Bran	1966—Cool Whip
1921—Mounds, Wonder bread	1968—Pringles, Care Free sugarless gum
1923—Milky Way, Sanka decaffeinated coffee	1976—Country Time lemonade
1927—Kool-Aid	1981—TCBY frozen yogurt
1928—Rice Krispies, Velveeta	1984—Diet Coke (with aspartame)
1930—Birds Eye frozen foods	1986—Pop Secret microwave popcorn
1930—Snickers, chocolate chip cookies	1987—Minute Maid calcium-fortified orange juice
1932—3 Musketeers, Fritos corn chips	1995—Hellman's (Best Foods) low-fat mayonnaise
1934—Ritz crackers, Bisquick	1996—Fat-free Pringle's potato chips (with Olestra)
1937—Spam, Kraft macaroni and cheese	1996—Vitamin-fortified fruit juice
1941—Cheerios, M&M's	1998—Vitamin-fortified vegetable juice
1944—Hawaiian Punch	1999—Margarine with Benechol (to lower blood cholesterol), chocolate candies fortified with vitamins and calcium
1946—Minute Rice, frozen orange juice, instant coffee	

Modified from Staten V: *Can you trust a tomato in January?* New York, 1993, Simon & Schuster, and from other sources.

in space have their unique food product: a plastic bag containing the nutritional equivalent of an entree, two side dishes, and a beverage, which is kneaded for several minutes and then squeezed into the mouth.

Today we are eating more breakfast cereals, pizza, pasta entrees, stir-fried meat and vegetables served on rice, salads, tacos, burritos, and fajitas than ever before.[24] Sales of whole milk are down, whereas in the same time period sales of nonfat and 1% low-fat milk have increased. Consumption of frozen vegetables, rather than canned vegetables, is also on the rise. Still, soft drinks are more popular than milk, although not as beneficial to the diet. Overall, many of these recent diet changes are advantageous; some are not.[17]

North Americans currently are living longer, and many enjoy better general health. Many also have more money, more diverse food and lifestyle choices to consider, and more time to relax and enjoy life. The nutritional consequences of these trends are not fully known. Deaths from heart disease and strokes, for example, have dropped dramatically since the late 1960s, partly because of better medical care and diets. Still, if affluence leads to sedentary lifestyles and high intakes of fat, sodium, and alcohol, it can lead to problems.[4] Obesity is also a growing problem in our population.[19] Because of better technology and greater choices, we can have a much better diet today than ever before—if we know what choices to make.

The goal of this book is to help you find the best path to good nutrition. There are no "junk" or bad foods, but some foods provide relatively few nutrients in comparison with energy content and, thus, contribute to less nutritious food habits. One's overall diet is the proper focus in a nutritional evaluation. Chapter 2 will emphasize this point and show you how to balance your diet. As you reexamine your nutritional goals, remember that your health is partly your responsibility (Table 1-5).[5]

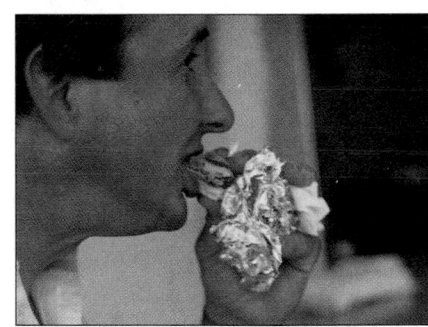

The fast-paced life for some of us requires eating on the run. What we choose should be as important as how fast it is served.

According to Dr. Andrew Weil, the primary danger from food is overindulgence.

TABLE 1-5   Recommendations for Health Promotion and Disease Prevention: What We Can Expect from Adequate Nutrition and Good Health Habits[1, 4, 6, 16, 18]

Diet

Eating enough essential nutrients and meeting energy needs help prevent
  Birth defects and low birth weight in infants
  Stunted growth and poor resistance to disease in infancy and childhood
  Poor resistance to disease in adulthood
  Deficiency diseases, such as cretinism (lack of iodine), scurvy (lack of vitamin C), and anemia
    (lack of iron, folate, or other nutrients)
Eating enough calcium helps
  Build bone mass in childhood and adolescence
  Prevent some adult bone loss, especially among older individuals
Obtaining adequate intake of fluoride and moderating sugar intake helps prevent
  Dental caries
Eating enough dietary fiber helps prevent
  Digestive problems, such as constipation and some intestinal problems
Eating enough vitamin A and related plant carotenoids may help reduce
  Susceptibility to some cancers
  Degeneration of the retina (intake of carotenoids in green and orange vegetables, specifically)
Moderating energy intake helps prevent
  Obesity and related diseases, such as type 2 diabetes, hypertension, cancer, and heart disease
Limiting intake of sodium helps prevent
  Hypertension and related diseases of the heart and kidney in susceptible people
Moderating intake of total fat, saturated fat, and cholesterol, while meeting folate needs, helps
prevent
  Heart disease
Moderating intake of essential nutrients when taking vitamin and mineral supplements, if practiced,
prevents
  Most chances for nutrient toxicities

Physical Activity

Adequate, regular physical activity (a minimum of 30 minutes per day) helps prevent
  Obesity
  Type 2 diabetes
  Heart disease
  Some adult bone loss and loss of muscle tone
  Premature aging

Lifestyle

Minimizing alcohol intake (no more than one to two drinks per day) helps prevent
  Liver disease
  Fetal alcohol syndrome
  Accidents
Not smoking cigarettes or cigars helps prevent
  Lung cancer, other lung disease, and kidney and heart disease

In addition, minimum use of medication, no illicit drug use, adequate sleep (7–8 hours), adequate
  fluid intake (about 8 cups per day) and a reduction in stress provide a more complete approach
  to good nutrition and health. Finally, consultation with health-care professionals on a regular basis is important. This is because early diagnosis is especially useful for controlling the damaging
  effects of many diseases. Overall, prevention of disease is an important investment of your time.

TABLE 1-6   A Sample of Nutrition-Related Objectives from *Healthy People 2010*

	Target	Current Estimate
Increase the proportion of adults who are at a healthy weight (defined as a body mass index between 18.5 and 25).	60%	39%
Reduce the proportion of adults who are obese (body mass index of 30 or more).	15%	23%
Reduce the proportion of children and adolescents who are overweight or obese.	5%	10%
Increase the proportion of persons age 2 years and older who consume at least two daily servings of fruit.	75%	28%
Increase the proportion of persons age 2 years and older who consume at least three daily servings of vegetables, with at least one-third being dark green or deep yellow vegetables.	50%	3%
Increase the proportion of persons age 2 years and older who consume at least six daily servings of grain products, with at least three being whole grains (e.g., whole wheat bread and oatmeal).	50%	7%
Increase the proportion of persons age 2 years and older who consume less than 10% of calories from saturated fat.	75%	36%
Increase the proportion of persons 2 years and older who consume no more than 30% of calories from fat.	75%	33%
Increase the proportion of persons age 2 years and older who consume 2400 mg or less of sodium daily.	65%	21%
Increase the proportion of persons age 2 years and older who meet dietary recommendations for calcium (see inside cover of this book).	75%	46%
Reduce iron deficiency among young children and females of childbearing age.	6%	10%

Note: Related objectives include those addressing osteoporosis, various forms of cancer, diabetes prevention and treatment, food allergies, heart disease and stroke, low birth weight, nutrition during pregnancy, breastfeeding, eating disorders, physical activity, and alcohol use (see later chapters).

■ Health Objectives for the United States for the Year 2010, Including Numerous Nutrition Objectives

Health promotion and disease prevention have been public health strategies in the United States since the late 1970s. One part of this strategy is *Healthy People 2010*, a report issued in 2000 by the U.S. Department of Health and Human Services' Public Health Service. This report consists of national health promotion and disease prevention objectives for the nation for the year 2010 and assigns each of the objectives to appropriate federal agencies to address. Many nutrition-related objectives are part of the overall plan (Table 1-6).[13]

The main objectives of *Healthy People 2010* are to promote healthful lifestyles and to reduce preventable death and disability in all Americans. Minority groups, in particular, are the focus of *Healthy People 2010* programs, as overall health status currently lags in these population groups, especially with respect to hypertension, diabetes, and obesity.[20]

The following Internet sites have resources for both patients and professionals on the *Healthy People* program:

Healthy People initiative:
http://www.health.gov/healthypeople
http://www.health.gov/partnerships
Healthy People data:
http://www.cdc.gov/nchs/hphome.htm

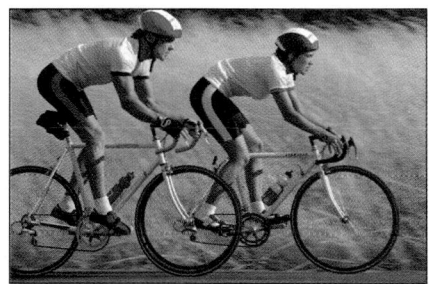

Regular physical activity complements a healthy diet; practice both each day.

CONCEPT CHECK

Surveys in the United States show that we generally have a variety of food available to us. However, some of us could improve our diets by focusing on rich food sources of iron, calcium, vitamin A, various B vitamins, vitamin C, zinc, and dietary fiber. In addition, many of us should reduce our consumption of energy, sugar, protein, fat, sodium, and alcoholic beverages. These recommendations are consistent with an overall goal to attain and maintain good health.

■ USING SCIENTIFIC RESEARCH TO DETERMINE NUTRIENT NEEDS

hypotheses "Educated guesses" by a scientist to explain a phenomenon.

People certainly are interested in nutrition (see the Expert Opinion by Dr. Finn). How do we know what we know about nutrition? How has this knowledge been gained? In a word, research. Like other sciences, the research that underpins nutrition has developed through the use of the *scientific method,* a procedure for testing designed to detect and eliminate error. The first step is the observation of a natural phenomenon. Scientists then suggest possible explanations, called **hypotheses,** about its cause. Distinguishing a true cause-and-effect relationship from mere coincidence can be difficult.[25] For instance, earlier in the past century, many patients in mental hospitals suffered from the disease *pellagra,* which suggested a possible relationship between mental illness and this disease. In time, it became clear that this supposed connection was simply coincidental; the real culprit was the poor diet common in mental institutions at that time.

experiments Tests made to examine the validity of a hypothesis.

theory An explanation for a phenomenon that has numerous lines of evidence to support it.

To test hypotheses and eliminate coincidental explanations, scientists perform controlled scientific **experiments.** The data gathered from these experiments may either support or refute each hypothesis (Fig. 1-4). If the results of many experiments support a hypothesis, the hypothesis becomes generally accepted by scientists and can be called a **theory** (such as the theory of gravity). Very often, the results from one experiment suggest a new set of questions to be answered.

The scientific method requires a skeptical attitude. Scientists must not accept proposed hypotheses and theories until they are supported by considerable evidence, and they must reject those that fail to pass critical analyses. Likewise, students should adopt a healthy skepticism and be critical of many current ideas about nutrition.[3, 32]

ulcer Erosion of the tissue lining, usually in the stomach (gastric ulcer) or the upper small intestine (duodenal ulcer). These are generally referred to as peptic ulcers.

A recent example of this need for skepticism involves stomach **ulcers.** Not so many years ago, "everyone knew" that stomach ulcers were caused by a stressful lifestyle and a poor diet. Then, in 1983, an Australian physician, Marshall, reported in a respected medical journal that ulcers are usually caused by a common microorganism called *Helicobacter pylori.* Furthermore, he stated that a cure is possible using antibiotics. At first, other physicians were skeptical about this finding and continued to prescribe medications that reduce stomach acid. But, as more studies were published, and patients were cured of ulcers using antibiotics, the medical profession eventually accepted the findings, and today, ulcers are managed for the most part by medications that destroy the pathogen. Overall, we can expect that scientific discoveries will always be subject to challenge and change.

■ Generating Hypotheses

Historical events have provided clues to important relationships in nutrition science. In the fifteenth and sixteenth centuries, for example, many European sailors on the long voyages to the Americas developed the disease scurvy. The sailors ate few fruits and vegetables, and eventually a British naval surgeon, Lind, as noted earlier,

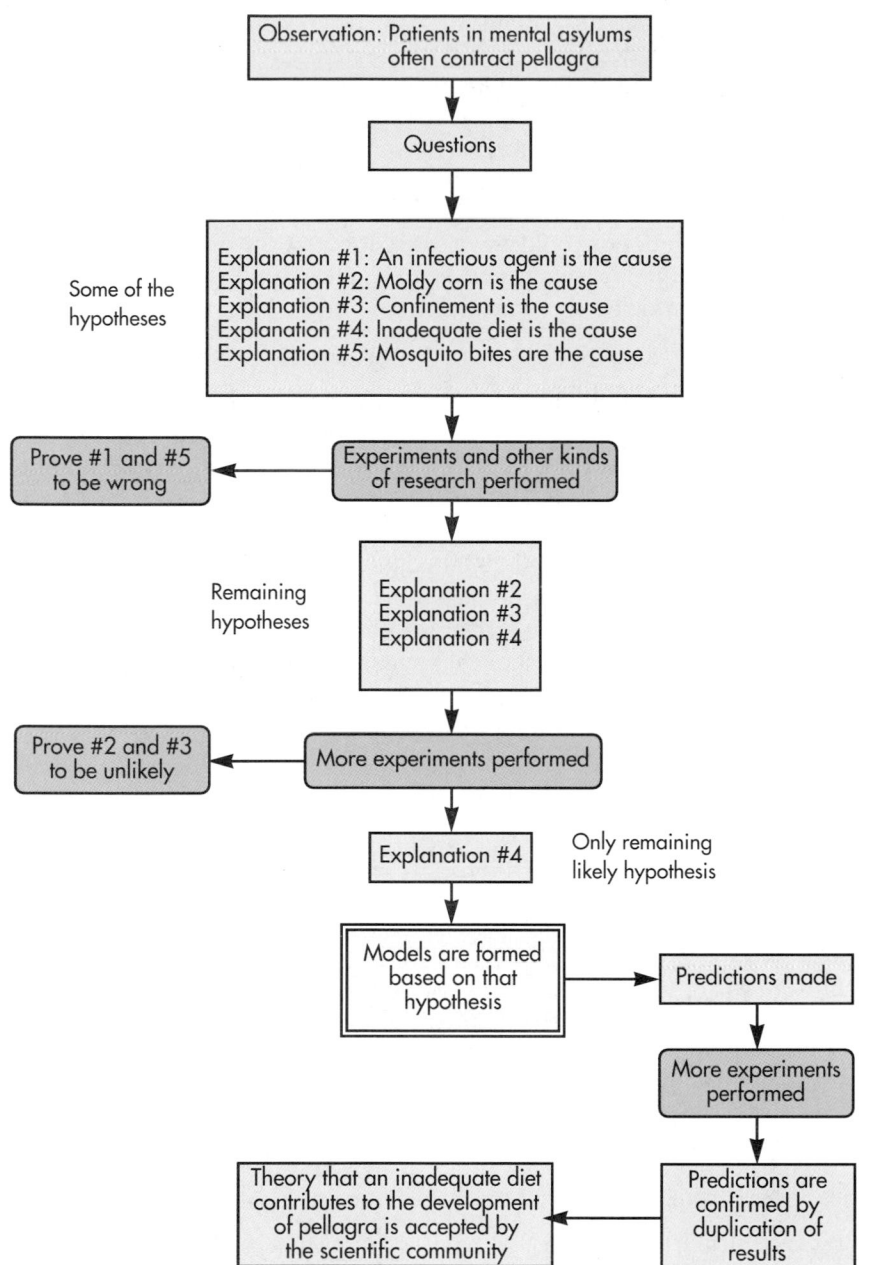

FIGURE 1-4 From question to theory—the process of science applied to nutrition. Only after careful and thorough analysis and repeated experimentation should a research finding influence our food choices, such as the need to consume the vitamin niacin to prevent the development of pellagra.

discovered that lime juice prevents or cures the scurvy. After this, sailors were given a ration of lime juice, earning them the nickname "limeys." This simple practice ensured a healthy workforce for the British navy and helped it dominate the seas worldwide. About 200 years later, scientists identified vitamin C, the nutrient present in fruits and vegetables that prevents scurvy.[12]

In a related approach to using historical observation, scientists establish nutritional hypotheses by studying the dietary and disease patterns among various populations in today's world. If one group tends to develop a certain disease but another group does not, scientists can speculate about the role diet plays in this difference. The study of diseases in populations is called **epidemiology.**

An example of this approach occurred in the 1920s, in the United States, when Goldberger noticed that prisoners in jail—but not their jailers—suffered from pellagra. He reasoned that, if pellagra were an **infectious disease,** both populations

epidemiology The study of how disease rates vary among different population groups. For example, the rate of stomach cancer in Japan could be compared with that in Germany.

infectious disease Any disease caused by invasion of the body by microorganisms, such as bacteria, fungi, or viruses.

CRITICAL THINKING

For thousands of years, early humans consumed a diet rich in vegetable products and low in animal products. These diets were generally lower in fat and higher in dietary fiber than modern diets. Do the differences in human diets throughout history necessarily tell us which diet is better—that of early humans or of modern humans? If not, what is a more reliable way to pursue this question of potential diet superiority?

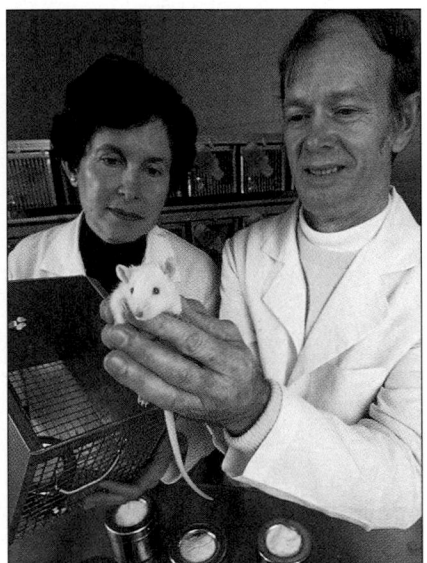

Research using laboratory animals contributes to our nutrition knowledge.

animal model Study of disease in animals that duplicates human disease. This can be used to understand more about human disease.

double-blind study An experimental design in which neither the participants nor the researchers are aware of each participant's assignment (test or placebo) or the outcome of the study until it is completed. An independent third party holds the code and the data until the study has been completed.

control group Participants in an experiment who are not given the treatment being tested.

would suffer from it. Since this was not the case, he concluded that pellagra is probably caused by a dietary deficiency.

Historical and epidemiological findings can suggest hypotheses about the role of diet in various health problems. To prove the role of particular dietary components, however, requires controlled experiments. For instance, once the high incidence of pellagra in mental institutions during the 1920s was linked to poor diet, various foods were given to patients who had the disease. These experiments showed that yeast and high-protein foods could cure these patients if the disease was not in its final stage, indicating that pellagra results from a deficiency of some nutrient present in these foods. Eventually, this nutrient was found to be the B vitamin called niacin.[12]

■ Laboratory Animal Experiments

When scientists cannot test their hypotheses by experiments with humans, they often use animals. Much of what we know about human nutritional needs and functions has been generated from animal experiments. Still, human experiments are the most convincing to scientists. In the 1930s, scientists showed that a pellagra-like disease seen in dogs, called *blacktongue,* is cured by nicotinic acid. Only when nicotinic acid actually cured the disease in humans were scientists convinced that nicotinic acid, later identified as the vitamin niacin, was the critical dietary factor.

Today, we know that low doses of the mineral fluoride can stimulate growth in rats. However, we still do not know whether this is true for humans, because it is not practical to control the fluoride intake of humans accurately enough to answer the question. Thus, fluoride might stimulate growth in humans, but real proof is lacking.

In addition, the use of humans in certain types of experiments is considered unethical. Although some people argue that animal experiments are also unethical, most people believe that the careful, humane use of animals is an acceptable alternative to using human subjects. For example, most people would think it is reasonable to feed rats a low-copper diet to study the importance of this mineral in the formation of blood vessels. Almost universally, however, people would object to a similar study in infants.

The use of animal experiments to study the role of nutrition in certain human diseases depends on the availability of an **animal model**—a disease in laboratory animals that closely mimics a particular human disease. If no animal model is available and human experiments are ruled out, scientific knowledge often cannot advance beyond what can be learned from epidemiological studies.

■ Human Experiments

Various experimental approaches are used to test research hypotheses in humans, including case-control and double-blind studies.[32]

Case-Control Study

In a case-control study, individuals who have the condition in question, such as lung cancer, are compared with individuals who do not have the condition. Comparisons are made only between groups that are matched for other major characteristics (e.g., age, race, and gender) not under study. This type of study may identify factors other than the disease in question, such as fruit and vegetable intake, that differ between the two groups, thus providing researchers with clues about the cause, progression, and prevention of the disease, but no specific evidence of cause and effect.

Double-Blind Study

An important approach for more definitive testing of hypotheses is the **double-blind study,** in which a group of participants—the experimental group—follows a specific protocol (e.g., consuming a certain food or nutrient), and participants in a corresponding **control group** conform to their normal habits. People are randomly assigned to each group, such as by the flip of a coin. Scientists then observe the experimental group over time to see if there is any effect that is not found in the control group. Sometimes individuals are used as their own control: First they are observed for a period of time, and then they are treated and their responses noted.

Two features of a double-blind study help reduce the introduction of bias (prejudice), which can easily affect the outcome of an experiment. First, neither the participants nor the researchers know which individuals are in the experimental group and which are in the control group. Second, the expected effects of the experimental protocol are not disclosed to the participants or researchers until after the entire study is completed. This approach reduces the possibility that researchers may see the change they want to see in the participants to prove a certain "pet" hypothesis, even though such a change did not actually occur. This approach also reduces the chance that the persons participating begin to feel better simply because they are involved in a research study or are receiving a new treatment, a phenomenon called the *placebo effect.*

Derived from the Latin word *placebo,* meaning "I shall please," the placebo effect cannot be explained by pharmacological or other direct physical action. It may instead be linked to a simple reduction in stress and anxiety. At least one-third of all patients show improvement after receiving a placebo (generally in the form of a fake medicine). Thus, it is critical to make allowances for the placebo effect in research studies.

In a double-blind experiment, the control group often receives a sugar pill or other placebo to camouflage who is in which group and thereby eliminate the bias introduced by the placebo effect. During the course of the experiment, neither the researchers nor the participants know who is getting the real treatment and who is getting a placebo. Sometimes only a single-blind protocol is possible, in which either the participants or the researchers are kept in the dark. Either way, now it is up to the experimental treatment—not just the practice of both groups taking a pill—to show an effect, if one is possible.

Drug studies lend themselves to double-blind protocols because it is often easy to substitute a placebo for the drug. However, food studies often cannot be placebo controlled. For example, disguising a diet high in fruits and vegetables from one low in them is difficult. In such a study, the experimenters should try to ensure that the results from blood assays or other measurements are not revealed until the end of the study. In addition, the results should be kept from the participants until the end of the study. These precautions can eliminate much potential bias. The more bias that is controlled in an experiment, the more confidence we can have in the results.

A recent example illustrates the need to test hypotheses based on epidemiological observations in double-blind studies. Epidemiologists using primarily case-control studies found that smokers who regularly consumed fruits and vegetables had a lower risk for lung cancer than smokers who ate few fruits and vegetables. Some scientists proposed that beta-carotene, a pigment present in many fruits and vegetables, could reduce the damage that tobacco smoke creates in the lungs. This hypothesis helped fuel sales of supplements of beta-carotene.

However, in double-blind studies involving heavy smokers, the risk of lung cancer was found to be higher for those who took beta-carotene than for those who did not. Some investigators criticized this research, arguing that the beta-carotene was given too late in the smokers' lives to be of much use, but even these critics did not suspect that the substance would increase cancer risk. Soon after these results were reported, the federal agency supporting two other large ongoing studies that employed beta-carotene supplements called a halt to the research, stating that these supplements are ineffective in preventing both lung cancer and heart disease.

Overall, health and nutrition advice provided by grandparents, parents, friends, and other well-meaning individuals can't be verified unless it is put to the ultimate scientific test—blinded studies. Until that is done, we can't be sure that the substance or procedure in question is truly effective.[32] One reason for this is the power of the placebo effect. In addition, many common symptoms, such as sneezing, lower back

---

Before researchers conduct any research process using humans (or laboratory animals), they must first obtain approval from the Human Use (or Animal Use) Committee at their university or company. The committee determines if the experimental protocol is valid and assesses the risks and benefits of the potential therapy to the subject and, when appropriate, society at large. In human studies, the committee insists that a document depicting the risks and benefits of the study be developed, which the participants must receive and sign. The process is called *informed consent,* meaning the participant knows what he or she is expected to do in the research study and the associated risks.

placebo Generally a fake medicine used to disguise the roles of participants in an experiment; if fake surgery is performed, it is called a *sham operation.*

Recently major nutrition organizations put together ten red flags that they consider signals for poor nutrition advice:

1. Recommendations that promise a quick fix
2. Dire warnings of dangers from a single product or regimen
3. Claims that sound too good to be true
4. Simplistic conclusions drawn from a complex study
5. Recommendations based on a single study
6. Dramatic statements that are refuted by reputable scientific organizations
7. Lists of "good" and "bad" foods
8. Recommendations made to help sell a product
9. Recommendations based on studies published without peer review
10. Recommendations from studies that ignore differences among individuals or groups

Expert Opinion

HOW TO FIND RELIABLE NUTRITION INFORMATION

Susan Calvert Finn, Ph.D., R.D., FADA

Life in the Information Age is never boring! Everywhere we turn, there is more to know and new ways to learn. With 150,000 books published in the United States every year, hundreds of thousands of Web sites and more than 10,000 periodicals—plus radio, television, CDs, fax and e-mail—we are bombarded with facts and figures. No wonder so many of us suffer from information anxiety!

But just because we have easy access to an abundance of information doesn't mean that all the "facts" we encounter are correct. Ironically, the easier and more fun information retrieval becomes, the more difficult our role as responsible consumers becomes. Nowhere is this irony more prevalent than in the nutrition and health arena.

According to The American Dietetic Association's Nutrition and You: Trends 2000, almost 50% of Americans look to television as their major source of nutrition information. And, not surprisingly, Health-Focus research reveals that approximately seven in 10 shoppers believe it is hard to follow the experts' advice because they keep changing their minds! Indeed, almost daily consumers are asked to judge the reliability of nutrition reports and studies that often seem contradictory. We are told that our diets should contain low fat, no fat, some fat. We've been advised to drink wine and to avoid wine. The virtues of fiber, phytochemicals and functional foods are extolled and refuted (see Chapter 2 for details). We've witnessed a resurgence in alternative health therapies, often promoted with little science to back them up. "Experts" advise gimmicks and gadgets, pills and potions. As the traveling medicine men of the nineteenth century liked to say, whatever is being sold is good for what ails you.

Our fascination with youth and our desire to stay vital, alert, and mobile as we age have propelled the field of nutritional health into a multibillion dollar business. In the Food Marketing Institute's (FMI) 1999 Trends in the United States, 95% of respondents said that nutrition is very or somewhat important when they shop for food. FMI's 1999 Shopping for Health survey revealed that half of all grocery shoppers actively seek information about health and nutrition. And as the Health-Focus 1999 Trend Report reveals, 80% of shoppers want to eat healthy foods more often. Despite this active interest in nutrition, however, close to 40% of Health-Focus survey respondents admit to being confused about what they should eat to stay healthy.

FINDING ACCURATE NUTRITION INFORMATION

With a number of potential pitfalls in your path, where and how do you find legitimate nutrition experts—trained professionals who offer valid diagnoses and prescribe safe and effective nutritional therapies? A number of avenues are available. If you have access to an accredited university, you may be able to obtain current and authoritative information from faculty members, particularly those who teach nutrition, dietetics, health, or medicine. Similarly, many hospital dietetics departments can be valuable references.

Most public, private and school libraries offer Web access to and stock nutrition books by experts on topics you may be researching. But be aware that appearing on the World Wide Web or in print does not necessarily make information credible. With all sources, it is essential to authenticate the background and training of the practitioner before accepting the material. A string of initials after a name does not automatically mean that the person is qualified. Even a legitimate

pain, and headache, go away within a month or so without any treatment, reflecting the natural course of the underlying diseases. When people say, "I get fewer colds now that I take vitamin C," they overlook the fact that many cold symptoms disappear quickly with no treatment; the apparent curative effect of vitamin C or any other remedy is often coincidental rather than causal to the natural healing process.

All consumers need to become more sophisticated about science, its accepted standards of evidence, and its current limitations. Failure to do so leads many to a frantic pursuit of fraudulent remedies. To ignore science is to follow an inferior path—the road of hard knocks. Those who follow this road learn about the dangers of various health practices primarily from the experiences of those harmed by them.

degree may be misleading. A Ph.D. in mathematics, for example, is irrelevant to nutrition.

It also is important to look out for danger signals, which include an overemphasis on "magic" pills or "unique" apparatuses; heavy reliance on testimonials from people you don't know, or who may not even exist; departure from established and legitimate medical practices; and performance of strange procedures, such as hair analysis or eye color tests.

As more and more consumers assume greater responsibility for their health and well-being, self-care communities and health-related web sites are becoming standard fare on the internet. In the year 2000, there were more than 25,000 (and counting) health-related web sites. Many of these online sources are credible; many are not. To protect yourself from erroneous information, stick with web sites sponsored by well-known health entities such as the American Heart Association, the American Dietetic Association or the National Institutes of Health. In addition, Tufts University School of Nutrition Science and Policy rates nutrition-related sites for accuracy and usability. Tufts has evaluated many of the most commonly visited sites. Check it out at: http://navigator.tufts.edu.

THE REGISTERED DIETITIAN

The most dependable source for up-to-date, accurate nutrition data is a registered dietitian (R.D.). There are more than 70,000 registered dietitians in the United States; they can be identified by the credential R.D. after their names. Registered dietitians are health-care professionals who are rigorously trained in a single specialty—nutrition science. Their goal is to promote health and fight illnesses by fostering the practice of proper nutrition. R.D.s are the most reliable disseminators of information and educational materials on food and nutrition. An R.D. analyzes each patient's situation, taking into account such factors as medical history, lifestyle, and eating habits, and tailors specific regimens to meet those unique needs. Because R.D.s do not make medical diagnoses, the patient is encouraged to consult a physician regularly.

What is it about registered dietitians that make them so qualified? An R.D. has both theoretical and practical experience, including a bachelor's degree in food and nutrition from an accredited university plus a thorough and extensive professional internship under expert supervision. R.D.s also must pass a comprehensive examination. Tough continuing education and recertification standards ensure that R.D.s keep up-to-date with the profession's science base.

Many states have enacted some form of statutory regulation of registered dietitians (certification or licensing). Unfortunately, in those states without regulation, anyone with little or no training, experience, a license, or specific qualifications can call himself or herself a dietitian or nutritionist.

As you seek nutrition information, you would do well to remember these two guidelines. Availability doesn't mean accuracy. Abundance doesn't mean reliability. A good measure of common sense, sound research and thorough verification of references and credentials will ensure that you have chosen an accurate and reliable source of information. The benefits you will receive are well worth the extra effort required to secure their advice.

Susan Calvert Finn is the director of nutrition and health services for Ross Products Division, Abbott Laboratories, a leading research facility and manufacturer of scientifically formulated nutritional products. She is a past president of the American Dietetic Association, author of The American Dietetic Association Guide to Women's Nutrition for Healthy Living *(Perigee 1997), and co-author of* The Real Life Nutrition Book *(Penguin Books 1992).*

Medical science does not ignore novel approaches to disease prevention and cure. Anecdotes and personal experiences are important clues to fruitful experimentation, but they are not credible evidence.[3]

■ Peer Review of Experimental Results

Once an experiment is complete, scientists summarize the findings and publish the results in scientific journals. At the end of each chapter in this book, many reports are listed, describing important experiments that have been published in scientific journals. Generally, before articles are published in scientific journals, they are critically reviewed by other scientists familiar with the subject. The objective of this peer review is to ensure that only high-quality research findings are published. This is an important step because most scientific research in this country is funded by the federal government, nonprofit foundations, drug companies, and other private industries. All these funding sources can have strong expectations about the research outcomes. In theory, the scientists conducting these research studies will be fair in evaluating their results and will not be influenced by the funding agency. Peer review helps ensure that the researchers are as objective as possible. This then helps ensure that results published in peer-reviewed journals, such as the *American Journal of Clinical Nutrition*, the *New England Journal of Medicine*, and the *Journal of the American Dietetic Association*, are much more reliable than those found in popular magazines or promoted on television talk shows. Unfortunately, reputable journals are not the main sources for the information presented in the popular media, and claims are seldom scrutinized by competent researchers for accuracy and scientific validity.[3]

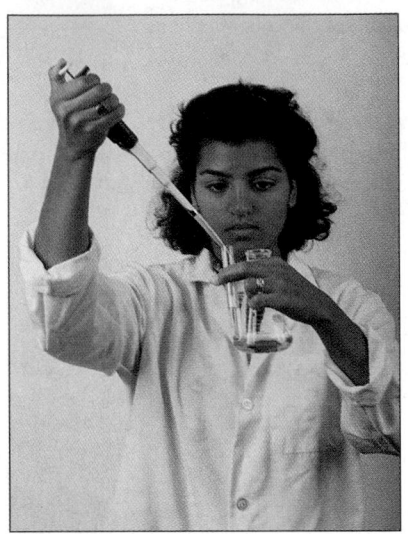

Careful research contributes to nutrition knowledge, more so than personal experience.

■ Follow-Up Studies

Even if an acceptable protocol has been followed and the results of a study have been accepted by the scientific community, one experiment is never enough to prove a particular hypothesis or provide a basis for nutritional recommendations. Rather, the results obtained in one laboratory must be confirmed by experiments conducted in other laboratories. Only then can we really trust and use the results. The more lines of evidence available to support an idea, the more likely it is to be true (Figure 1-5). It is important to avoid rushing to accept new ideas as fact or incorporating them into your health habits until they are proved by several lines of evidence.

Two other common types of studies are migrant and cohort. Migrant studies look at changes in health in people who move from one country to another. Cohort studies start with a healthy population and follow them, looking for the development of disease.

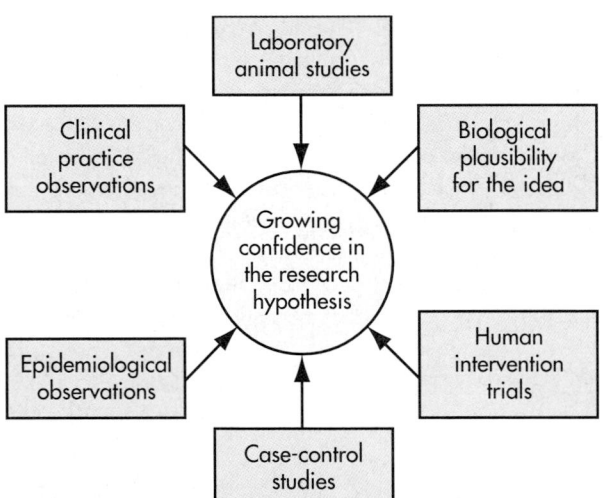

■ **FIGURE 1-5** Data from a variety of sources can come together to support a research hypothesis. For example, **epidemiological studies** show that type 2 diabetes is characteristically found in obese populations, compared with leaner populations. Physicians notice in **clinical practice** that type 2 diabetes is much more likely in their obese patients, compared with their leaner patients. **Laboratory animal studies** show that overfeeding that eventually leads to obesity often leads to the development of type 2 diabetes. **Case-control studies** show that obese patients are much more likely to have type 2 diabetes than the leaner comparison group that is matched for other characteristics. Finally, **human intervention trials** show that weight loss can correct type 2 diabetes in many people. Laboratory researchers also show that the enlarged fat cells associated with obesity are much less responsive to the hormonal signals involved in blood glucose regulation (see Chapter 5). All these lines of data come together with **biological plausibility** from various laboratory studies to support the research hypothesis that obesity can lead to type 2 diabetes.

CONCEPT CHECK

The scientific method is the procedure for testing the validity of possible explanations of a phenomenon, called hypotheses. Experiments are conducted to either support or refute a specific hypothesis. Once we have much experimental information that supports a specific hypothesis, it then can be called a theory. Ideally, experiments are conducted in a blinded fashion, where the subjects and researchers (preferably both) do not find out the results of an experiment until after the experiment is completed. This reduces bias in the results and minimizes the placebo effect. All of us need to be skeptical of new ideas in the nutrition field. We should wait until many lines of experimental evidence support a concept for adopting any suggested dietary practice.

SUMMARY

1. Nutrition is the study of the food substances vital for health and the study of how the body uses these substances to promote and support growth, maintenance, and reproduction of cells. Research in the field has been especially vigorous from the past century to present times.

2. Nutrients in foods fall into six classes: (1) carbohydrates, (2) lipids (mostly fats and oils), (3) proteins, (4) vitamins, (5) minerals, and (6) water. The first three, along with alcohol, provide energy for the body to use.

3. The body transforms the energy contained in carbohydrate, protein, and fat into other forms of energy, which allow the body to function. Fat provides, on average, 9 kcal/g, whereas protein and carbohydrate each provides, on average, 4 kcal/g. Vitamins, minerals, and water do not supply energy to the body but are essential for proper body function.

4. A basic plan for health promotion and disease prevention includes eating a varied diet, performing regular physical activity, not smoking, not abusing nutrient supplements (if used), getting adequate fluid and sleep, limiting alcohol intake (if consumed), and limiting or coping with stress.

5. The focus of nutrition planning should be on food, not primarily on dietary supplements. The focus on foods to supply nutrient needs avoids the possibility of severe nutrient imbalances.

6. Results from large nutrition surveys in the United States such as CSFII and NHANES suggest that some of us need to concentrate on consuming foods that supply more vitamin A, certain B vitamins, calcium, iron, zinc, and dietary fiber.

7. There are no true "junk" or "bad" foods. The focus should be on balancing a total diet by choosing many nutritious foods.

8. The scientific method is the procedure for testing the validity of possible explanations of a phenomenon, called hypotheses. Experiments are conducted to either support or refute a specific hypothesis. Once we have much experimental information that supports a specific hypothesis, it then can be called a theory. All of us need to be skeptical of new ideas in the nutrition field, waiting until many lines of experimental evidence support a concept before adopting any suggested dietary practice.

STUDY QUESTIONS

1. Name one chronic disease associated with poor nutrition habits. Now list a few corresponding risk factors.

2. Explain the concept of energy as it relates to foods. What are the fuel (energy) values used for a gram of carbohydrate, fat, protein, and alcohol?

3. Identify three ways that water is used in the body.

4. Wendy's Big Bacon Classic contains 44 g carbohydrate, 36 g fat, and 37 g protein. Calculate the percentage of energy derived from fat.

5. Describe two types of fat and explain why the differences are important in terms of overall health.

6. According to national nutrition surveys, which nutrients tend to be underconsumed by many adult Americans? Why is this the case?

7. List four health objectives for the United States for the Year 2010. How would you rate yourself in each area? Why?

8. List one food habit you should work on to improve your health. Indicate why and list three actions to take.

9. What nutrition-related disease is common in your family? What step(s) could you take at this point to minimize your risk?

10. List one nutrition claim you have heard recently that sounds too good to be true. What do you suspect is the motive of the person providing the advice?

■ ANNOTATED REFERENCES

1. Achievements in Public Health, 1900–1999: Changes in the public health system. *Journal of the American Medical Association* 283:735, 2000.

   Improvements cited as major advances in health promotion over the past century are safer and healthier foods, healthier mothers and babies, fluoridation of drinking water, and recognition of tobacco use as a health hazard.

2. ADA Reports: Position of the American Dietetic Association and dietitians of Canada: Women's health and nutrition. *Journal of the American Dietetic Association* 99:738, 1999.

   Chronic diseases that particularly affect women are reviewed, providing advice on prevention and treatment, such as daily physical activity and regular screening for chronic disease.

3. Blumenthal SJ: A top woman doctor tells how to get past the hype to the truth. *American Health*, p. 36, January/February 1998.

   The assistant U.S. surgeon general provides advice on how to interpret research findings that appear in the media, such as who paid for the study and whether the findings are supported by previous studies.

4. Breslow L: From disease prevention to health promotion. *Journal of the American Medical Association* 281:1030, 1999.

   Current concepts of health promotion are discussed, including goals such as increasing moderate daily physical activity and reducing excessive alcohol use as important health preventive measures.

5. Checkup for the new millennium. *Consumer Reports on Health*, p. 1, December 1999.

   A checklist of both healthy habits and not-so-healthy habits is given, along with suggested changes in habits to maximize wellness. The focus is on a balanced diet, maintaining a healthy weight, and performing regular physical activity.

6. Chidley E: Smoking: Butt in to help your clients kick the habit. *Today's Dietitian*, p. 35, January 2000.

   Risks of smoking are discussed, along with current therapies that can help smokers break the habit. Physicians now more than ever can prescribe effective medical approaches that aid success.

7. Collins FS: Shattuck lecture—Medical and societal consequences of the human genome project. *The New England Journal of Medicine* 341:28, 1999.

   The current human genome project and the many anticipated applications are discussed. This will lead to a better understanding of the personal health risks each individual faces.

8. Eisen A, Weber BL: Prophylactic mastectomy—the price of fear, *The New England Journal of Medicine* 340:137, 1999.

   Issues surrounding this radical procedure for reducing breast cancer in women at very high risk are reviewed. The procedure is effective, but the psychological effects also need to be considered.

9. Frazao E: High costs of poor eating patterns in United States. *CNI Nutrition Week*, p. 4, June 18, 1999.

   The many chronic diseases associated with the poor dietary and lifestyle habits seen in some Americans are discussed. Although genetics plays an important role in an individual's risk for chronic disease, environmental factors are also significant.

10. Garber J: A 40-year-old woman with a strong family history of breast cancer. *Journal of the American Medical Association* 280:1953, 1999.

    After a detailed discussion concerning one specific woman at high risk for breast cancer, physicians discuss the role of genetic testing and management of her disease. Overall, family history is a major risk factor for breast cancer.

11. Gene therapy setback. *Scientific American*, p. 36, February 2000.

    The death of an 18-year-old man who underwent gene therapy for a rare form of liver disease is discussed, including the possible reasons for his death. Intravenous delivery of the viral particle containing the gene into an artery leading directly to the liver is thought to be one reason.

12. Harper A: Defining the essentiality of nutrients. In Shills ME and others (eds), *Modern nutrition in health and disease*, 9th ed., Baltimore, MD: Williams & Wilkins, 1999.

    A short history of nutrition is provided in the context of the definition of an essential nutrient. Much of the progress in nutrition science has been made in the past 100 years.

13. *Healthy People 2010* targets healthy diet and healthy weight as critical goals. *Journal of the American Dietetic Association* 100:300, 2000.

    Many of the nutrition goals included in Healthy People 2010 *are enumerated. Two key goals are to reduce obesity and inactivity in the American population.*

14. Kant AK and others: A prospective study of diet quality and mortality in women. *Journal of the American Medical Association* 283:2109, 2000.

    Women whose diets included plenty of fruits, vegetables, whole grains, and low-fat meats and dairy products showed a 30% reduction in death, compared with those who ate the most unhealthy diets.

15. JAMA patient page: Maintaining good health. *Journal of the American Medical Association* 282:2092, 1999.

    Habits that are widely regarded as important for health maintenance are not using tobacco in any form, maintaining a healthy weight, exercising regularly, eating a healthy diet, and drinking alcohol only in moderation.

16. Jee SH and others: Smoking and atherosclerotic cardiovascular disease in men with low levels of serum cholesterol: The Korean Medical Insurance Corporation study. *Journal of the American Medical Association* 282:2149, 1999.

    Despite otherwise favorable cardiovascular disease risk factors, smoking still raises risk of cardiovascular disease over three times that seen in nonsmokers.

17. Liebman B: The changing American diet, *Nutrition Action Healthletter*, p. 8, April 1999.

    Both positive and negative trends in the American diet in the past 30 years are shown in graphic form, demonstrating that improvements have been made, such as a switch from whole milk to fat-reduced and nonfat milk, but much more work needs to be done.

18. Lifestyle and aging. *Mayo Clinic Health Letter*, p. 4, July 1999.

    Mayo Clinic physicians provide their advice for a healthy lifestyle, such as getting regular exercise, opting for many whole-grain choices, and drinking alcohol in moderation, if at all.

19. Moldad AH and others: The spread of the obesity epidemic in the United States, 1991–1998. *Journal of the American Medical Association* 282:1519, 1999.

    Statistics depicting the problem of obesity in the American population are provided. The United States has shown a rapid increase in the number of obese people in the past decade; this will likely contribute to much ill health in future years.

20. Nemeck S: Unequal health. *Scientific American*, p. 40, January 1999.

    Concerns surrounding the health of minority populations are discussed, along with the current government programs that are addressing these issues. Currently overall life expectancy has reached an all-time high of 76.1 years, but for black Americans it stands at just 70.2 years.

21. Patterson RE and others: Genetic revolution: Change and challenge for the dietetics profession. *Journal of the American Dietetic Association* 99:1412, 1999.

 Methods used in genetic therapy are reviewed. A detailed glossary of genetics-related terms is provided, along with a discussion of genetic counseling. Health professionals need to understand the basis behind this procedure in order to participate in today's health care.

22. Prepare for the future: Know your ancestors. *Consumer Reports on Health* p. 1, September 1999.

 Interpreting your family history as it potentially affects your health is discussed. Use of a family tree for health risks is described.

23. Simopoulos AP: Genetic variation and nutrition. *Nutrition Reviews* 57(5):S10, 1999.

 Many nutrition-related diseases that show genetic susceptibility, such as heart disease, hypertension, and osteoporosis, are reviewed, providing much evidence that genetic background must be considered in providing health advice to individuals.

24. Sloann AE: Top 10 trends to watch and work on for the new millennium. *Food Technology* 53(8):40, 1999.

 Current trends in the food supply that are described include more packaged, precooked meals; more foods undergoing less processing; more home-delivered foods; a greater variety of snack foods; and a growing number of foods fortified with vitamins, minerals, and other substances that may contribute to better health.

25. Solving the diet-and-disease puzzle. *Nutrition Action Health Letter*, p. 3, May 1999.

 Current nutrition research trials in the United States are described, along with the specific doses of vitamins and minerals used and the other health practices included. These trials are trying to determine if risks of diseases such as colon cancer, breast cancer, heart disease, cataracts, and strokes can be reduced through diet and lifestyle manipulation.

26. Stamler J and others: Low risk-factor profile and long-term cardiovascular and noncardiovascular mortality and life expectancy. *Journal of the American Medical Association* 282:2012, 1999.

 Individuals with favorable blood cholesterol and blood pressure values who did not smoke and did not have diabetes or evidence of existing cardiovascular disease showed much lower mortality and greater longevity (up to 9 years) than the comparison group.

27. Stephenson J: Gene therapy trials show clinical efficacy. *Journal of the American Medical Association* 283:589, 2000.

 Successful application of gene therapy in children with a rare immune deficiency disease is described, as well as potential uses of gene therapy for people with hemophilia.

28. Subar AF and others: Dietary sources of nutrients in the U.S. diet, 1989 to 1991. *Journal of the American Dietetic Association* 98:537, 1998.

 Leading contributors of the variety of nutrients consumed on a daily basis are described, such as the chief sources of fat, carbohydrate, and protein in the American diet. Currently cheese, beef, and milk are the major sources of saturated fat in our diets.

29. Thompson L: Human gene therapy: Harsh lessons, high hopes. *FDA Consumer*, p. 19, September–October 2000.

 FDA is hopeful that one day gene therapy will work in a wider number of diseases. Currently a person has to have the right disease, such that the appropriate gene can be inserted into the specific cell lacking the correct gene. The results also need to be positive.

30. Tippet KS and others: Food consumption surveys in the U.S. Dept. of Agriculture. *Nutrition Today* 34:33, 1999.

 The variety of food consumption surveys conducted over the past 80 years by the U.S. Department of Agriculture are described, including studies currently underway. These indicate few adults consume the recommended amounts of fruits and vegetables each day.

31. White MT and others: Genetic testing for disease susceptibility: Social, ethical, and legal issues for family physicians. *American Family Physician* 60:748, 1999.

 Guidelines for patient counseling concerning genetic testing are discussed, as well as the benefits and risks of genetic testing. It is best that people undergo genetic counselling before genetic tests are performed.

32. Yet another study—Should you pay attention? *Tufts University Nutrition Letter*, p. 4, September 1998.

 Types of studies used to investigate diet and health relationships are described, as well as how to interpret findings from various study designs. Overall a single study hardly ever tells the whole story.

TAKE ACTION

I. EXAMINE YOUR EATING HABITS MORE CLOSELY.

Choose one day of the week that is typical of your eating pattern. Using the first table found in Appendix E, list all foods and drinks you consumed for 24 hours. In addition, write down the approximate amounts of food you ate in units, such as cups, ounces, teaspoons, and tablespoons. Check the food composition table in Appendix A for examples of appropriate serving units for different types of foods, such as meat and vegetables. After completing this activity, you will use this list of foods for future assignments.

After you record the amount of each food and drink consumed, indicate in the table why you chose to consume the item. Use the following symbols to indicate your reasons. Place the corresponding abbreviation in the space provided to indicate why you picked that food or drink.

FLVR	Flavor/texture	ADV	Advertisement	PEER	Peers
CONV	Convenience	WTCL	Weight control	NUTR	Nutritive value
EMO	Emotions	HUNG	Hunger	$	Cost
AVA	Availability	FAM	Family/cultural	HLTH	Health

There can be more than one reason for choosing a particular food or drink.

Application

Now ask yourself what your most frequent reason is for eating or drinking. To what degree is health a reason for your food choices? Should you make it a higher priority?

II. CREATE YOUR FAMILY TREE FOR HEALTH-RELATED CONCERNS.

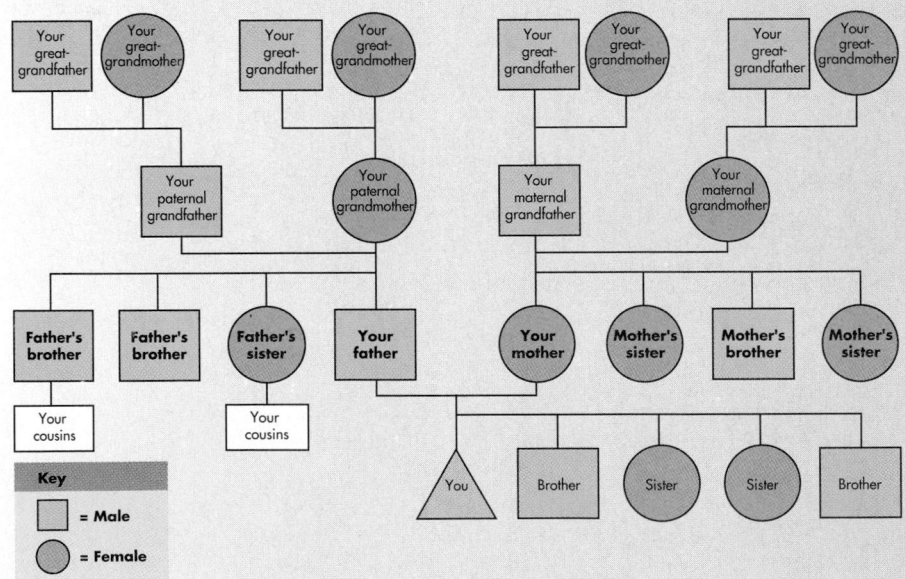

Under each heading, list year born, year died (if applicable), major diseases that developed during the person's lifetime, and cause of death (if applicable). Figure 1-6 in the Nutrition Perspective provides one such example.

Note that you are likely to be at risk for any diseases listed. Creating a plan for preventing such diseases when possible, especially those that developed in your family members before age 50–60 years, is advised. Speak with your physician about any concerns arising from this exercise.

GENETICS AND NUTRITION

The growth, development, and maintenance of cells, and ultimately of the entire organism, are directed by genes present in the cells. The genes contain the codes that control the expression of individual traits, such as height, eye color, and susceptibility to many diseases. An individual's genetic risk for a given disease is an important factor, although often not the only factor, in determining whether he or she develops that disease.[23]

Interest in the human genetic code and its relationship to specific diseases has exploded in recent years. Currently, the federal government is sponsoring a program to sequence the more than 30,000 genes present on human chromosomes.[7] This Human Genome Project is not actually sequencing the genes of just one person but is compiling a composite genome based on the DNA contributed by about 50 individuals. Each gene essentially represents a recipe, noting the ingredients (specifically, amino acids) and how those ingredients should be put together. The human genome then would be the cookbook.

It is likely that soon it will be relatively easy to screen a person's DNA for genes that increase the risk for disease. Currently, a woman can pay about $2600 to be tested for the BRCA1 and BRCA2 genes; these greatly increase the risk for breast cancer (see a later section in this feature).[10] To date, scientists have developed about 600 genetic tests. Many are for very rare diseases and fortunately often are much less expensive than for the BRCA genes. These genetic tests are especially valuable for families plagued by certain illnesses, but more routine testing of now-healthy people to predict future risks of cancer or other diseases is poised to grow rapidly. This is a brand new field and is about to mushroom into the significant part of medical practice, as almost every medical condition has a genetic component. Most, however, are not single gene disorders but, instead, arise from alterations in a number of genes.[21]

Each year new links between specific genes and diseases are reported. It is thought that the decoding of the human genome will ultimately transform the practice of medicine, allowing for the prediction years in advance of what illnesses will likely eventually develop in a person. The hope is then to replace genes that encourage diseases, such as cancer and Alzheimer's, with those that do not.[29]

An exciting application of the Human Genome Project are gene chips. About 100,000 pieces of DNA can be loaded onto a chip the size of a fingernail. Blood can be processed and then placed on the chip and rapidly tested for altered genes. Genetic material binding to certain areas on the chip can signal a healthy form of a specific gene or alternately a form that is associated with disease. Currently, about 75 laboratories in the United States are using gene chips to investigate disease risk. Information from gene chips provides opportunities for physicians in the future to diagnose disease more carefully and to prescribe individual medical therapies, instead of treating all patients with the same disease with essentially the same therapy. It is likely that many medications may be more appropriate in certain people given their genetic traits.[31]

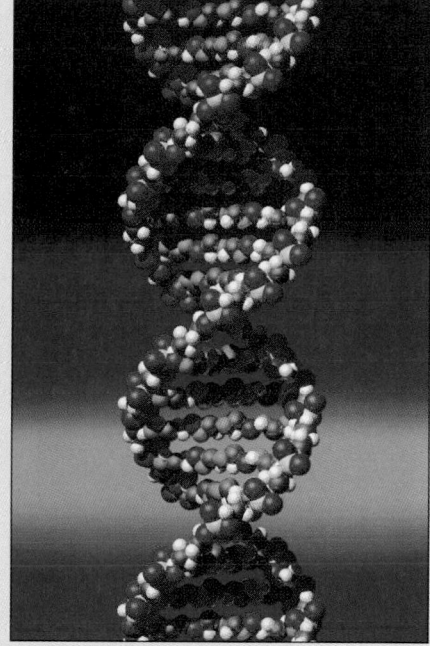

Genes are present on DNA—a double helix. The cell nucleus contains most of the DNA in the body.

NUTRITIONAL DISEASES WITH A GENETIC LINK

Most chronic diseases in which nutrition plays a role are also influenced by genetics.[23] The risks of developing heart disease, hypertension, obesity, diabetes, cancer, and osteoporosis are influenced by interactions between genetic and nutritional factors. Studies of families, including those with twins and adoptees, provide strong support for the effect of genetics in these disorders. In fact, family history is considered to be one of the important risk factors in the development of many nutrition-related diseases.

■ Heart Disease

About one of every 500 people in the American population has a defective gene that greatly delays cholesterol removal from the bloodstream. As you will learn in Chapter 6, this and other genetic effects lead to an increased risk of developing heart disease at a young age. Diet changes can help these people, but medications and possibly surgery may be needed to address these problems.

■ Hypertension

An estimated 10 to 15% of the American population is very sensitive to salt intake. When these salt-sensitive individuals consume too much salt, their blood pressure climbs above the desirable range. The fact that more of these people are African-American than White suggests a genetic component. At present, the only way to determine whether individuals with hypertension are salt sensitive is to place them on a salt-restricted diet and see if their blood pressure falls. Note also that many cases of hypertension are unrelated to salt sensitivity and are caused by other factors (see Chapter 11).

■ Obesity

Most obese Americans have at least one parent who is also obese. Findings from many human studies suggest that a variety of genes (likely 50 or more) are involved in the regulation of body weight (see Chapter 13 for more details). Little is known, however, about the specific nature of these genes in humans or how the actual changes in body metabolism (such as lower energy use in general or fat use in particular) are produced.

Still, although some individuals may be genetically predisposed to store body fat, whether they actually do so depends on how much excess energy—above energy needs—they ultimately consume. A common concept in nutrition is that *nurture*—how people live and the environmental factors that influence them—allows *nature*—each person's genetic potential—to be expressed. Although not everyone with a genetic tendency toward obesity develops this condition, he or she does have a higher lifetime risk than individuals without a genetic predisposition to obesity.

■ Diabetes

Both of the two common types of diabetes have genetic links, as revealed by family and twin studies. Only sensitive and expensive testing can determine who is at risk. The form of diabetes involved in about 90% of all cases, called type 2 diabetes, also has a strong link to obesity. A genetic tendency for type 2 diabetes is expressed once a person becomes obese but often not before, again illustrating that nurture affects nature (see Chapter 5 for more details).

■ Cancer

A few types of cancer (e.g., some forms of colon and breast cancer) have a strong genetic link, and genetics may play a role in others. Because obesity increases the risk of several forms of cancer, a diet with excess energy and fat is also a risk factor. And one-third of all cancers result from smoking. Again, genetics is often not enough—environment also contributes to the risk profile (see Chapter 10 for more details).

■ Osteoporosis

Bone mineral content, and in turn bone strength, is similar in twins, as well as in mothers and their daughters. The exact relative importance of genetic versus dietary factors is unknown, but a number of genes have been shown to contribute to a person's overall risk of low bone mineral content. In any case, children and adolescents need to consume sufficient calcium to build strong, dense bones, thus reducing the risk of osteoporosis in later life. Adults should then continue that practice. The porous bones that are a result of osteoporosis greatly increase the risk of fractures, especially in the wrist, spine, and hip. As discussed in Chapter 11, the risk of osteoporosis in women can be greatly reduced by a combination of medical and nutritional means if therapy is started at least by midlife.

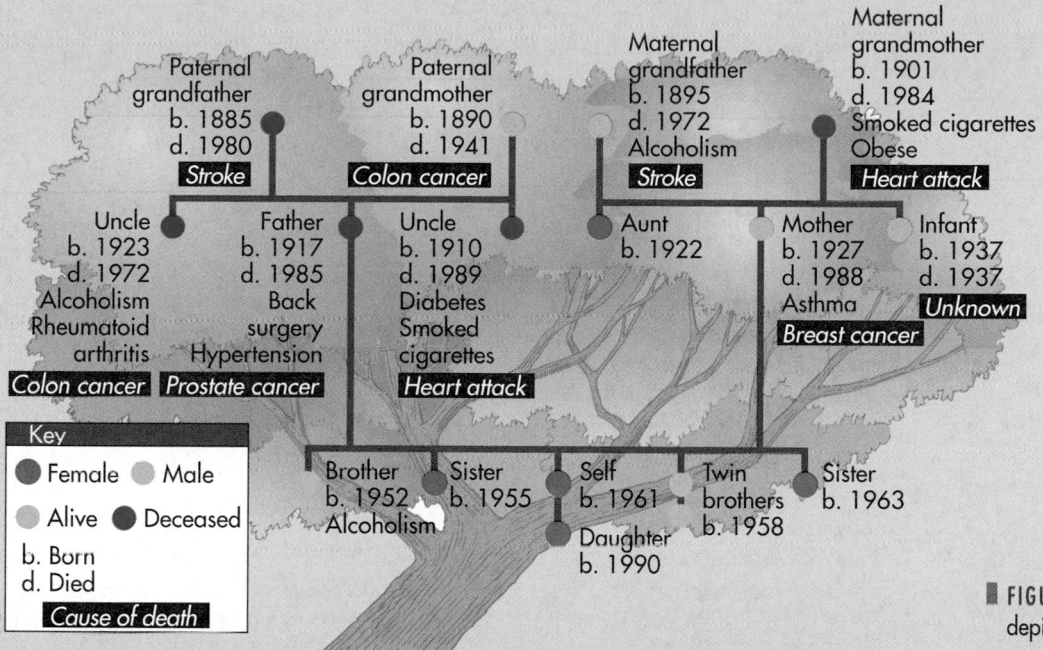

FIGURE 1-6 Example of a family tree depicting disease presentation in family members.

YOUR GENETIC PROFILE

From this discussion, you can see that a family history of certain diseases raises your risk of developing those diseases. By recognizing your potential for developing a particular disease, you can avoid behavior that contributes to it.[22] For example, women with a family history of breast cancer should avoid becoming obese, should minimize alcohol use, and should obtain mammograms regularly. In general, the more of your relatives who had a genetically transmitted disease and the closer they are related to you, the greater your risk. One way to assess your risk is to put together a family tree of illnesses and deaths by compiling a few key facts on your primary relatives: siblings, parents, aunts and uncles, and grandparents, as suggested in the Take Action section.

Figure 1-6 shows an example of a family tree (also called a genogram). High-risk conditions include two or more first-degree relatives in a family with a specific disease (first-degree relatives include one's parents, siblings, and offspring). Another sign of risk of inherited disease is development of the disease in a first-degree relative before age 50 to 60 years. In the family in Figure 1-6, prostate cancer killed the man's father. This means that the son should be tested regularly for prostate cancer. His sisters should consider frequent mammograms and other preventive practices because the mother died of breast cancer. Because heart attack and stroke are also common in the family, all the children should adopt a lifestyle that minimizes the risk of developing these conditions, such as a moderate fat and sodium intake. Colon cancer is also evident in the family, so careful screening throughout life is important.

GENE THERAPY

Scientists are currently developing therapies to correct some genetic disorders.[29] Typically, the gene of interest is inserted into a virus, and then this virus is injected into the target tissue. For example, a gene that stimulates blood vessel growth has been inserted into a **virus,** and this combination has been injected into the hearts of people with poor heart circulation. This gene therapy has led to improvement in health. In addition, in 1990 two girls were treated for a severe immune deficiency disease with genetic therapy. Both girls are alive and well today. Scientists hope that one day gene therapy applications such as these can be used to treat many

virus The smallest known type of infectious agent, many of which cause disease in humans. They do not metabolize, grow, or move by themselves. They reproduce by the aid of a living cellular host. Viruses are essentially a piece of genetic material surrounded by a coat of protein.

phenylketonuria (PKU) A disease caused by a defect in the ability of the liver to metabolize the amino acid phenylalanine into the amino acid tyrosine. Toxic by-products of phenylalanine can then build up in the body and lead to mental retardation.

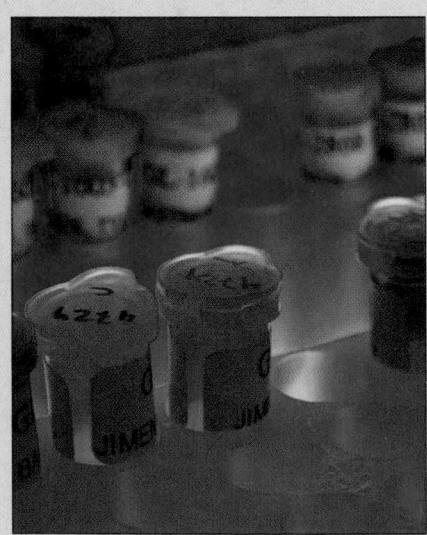

Genetic testing for disease susceptibility will be more common in the future as the genes that increase risk for various diseases are isolated and deciphered.

diseases, especially inherited diseases.[27] Still, much more research is needed for that to happen. For example, a young man in Pennsylvania died while involved in a gene therapy protocol that injected gene-laden viral particles into the main artery leading to the liver. This attempt to correct a defective enzyme in his liver shows that we need much more experience with this technology before it becomes widespread.[11]

GENETIC TESTING

In recent years, scientists have developed ways of testing a person's genes for the likelihood of developing certain diseases. For cases such as Huntington's disease, a degenerative brain disorder, a positive gene test guarantees the eventual development of the disease. However, with diseases such as cancer and Alzheimer's disease, a positive gene test simply indicates a greater risk for developing the disease. In addition to the diseases mentioned, risk factors for birth defects, cystic fibrosis, certain forms of muscular dystrophy, and a host of other diseases can be detected through genetic testing.

Today in the United States, newborns are routinely tested for **phenylketonuria,** an inherited metabolic disease that leads to mental retardation and other problems if appropriate treatment is not given. Infants found to have this disorder are put on a special diet, which reduces development of the disease (see Chapter 7 for details). In contrast to infants with phenylketonuria, individuals with genetic predispositions to many other diseases do not always develop disease.

Because genetic background does influence disease risk, certain dietary guidelines are more beneficial for some people than for others. For example, people prone to osteoporosis, as mentioned earlier, need to be more aware of calcium intake. Overall, the benefits of genetic testing include the potential for more individualized nutrition and health advice, more informed decisions by couples attempting to have children (i.e., alternatives such as adoption or therapeutic abortion), increased surveillance for the disease, and the ability to plan appropriately for the future. However, it is not possible, given the resources presently allocated to medical care in North America, to identify all people at genetic risk for the major chronic diseases and other health problems. In addition, in many cases genetic susceptibility does not equate to a guarantee of development of the disease. And, in almost all cases, there is no way to cure a specific gene alteration—only the health problems that result can be treated. Thus, the wisdom of genetic testing is an open question.[31] Perhaps preventive measures and careful scrutiny for the specific genetically linked diseases in one's family would suffice.

Researchers also are concerned that people who are found to have genetic alterations that increase disease risk may face job and insurance discrimination. Testing positive could also lead to unnecessary radical treatment. As well, a seemingly hopeless diagnosis could result in depression or withdrawal from life when a cure is out of reach.

Consider the following situations with regard to genetic testing.

- Using the family tree such as in the Take Action section, you realize that colon cancer runs in your family. Knowing that the mortality rate for colon cancer is quite high, would you be tested for specific colon cancer genes (note: these genes do not guarantee colon cancer but do indicate greater risk)? What factors would affect your decision?
- You as a female (or a female you care about, if you are a male) carry the breast cancer gene BRCA1 or BRCA2, or you have a family history of breast cancer. Would you consider mastectomies to try to make sure the disease does not develop? This has been shown to be effective therapy, reducing risk of breast cancer and death by 90%.[8] However, even some high-risk women never actually develop the disease.
- You and your (future) spouse would like to have children. You know that phenylketonuria has occurred in your family and would like to be tested as a carrier. It turns out that both you and your spouse carry the gene for phenylketonuria. Any offspring have a 1 in 4 chance of having the fatal disease. How would this affect your decision to have a child?

Some experts recommend that anyone considering genetic testing should first undergo genetic counseling.[31] Genetic counselors are trained to analyze family history and evaluate risk of developing or passing along an inherited disease. They can also help determine whether testing is worth the time and trouble, since genetic tests are primarily for people whose family history puts them at especially high risk of having a genetic defect. Genetic counselors can be found by contacting a local hospital or nearby university-affiliated hospital or medical school.

In the final analysis, would you rather know if you were at risk for a specific disease that a genetic test could point out? If so, ask your physician about the possibility and wisdom of testing you for the genetically linked diseases in your family tree. Also, be aware that, throughout this book, discussions will point out how you can personalize nutrition advice based on your genetic background. In this way, you can identify and avoid the "controllable" risk factors that would contribute to the development of genetically linked diseases present in your family.

The following web links will help you gather more information about genetic conditions and testing:

http://www.geneticalliance.org   Alliance of Genetic Support Groups.

http://www.kumc.edu/gec/support   Information on genetic conditions and rare conditions.

http://cancernet.nci.nih.gov/p_genetics.html   Genetics information from the National Cancer Institute.

http://www.nhgri.nih.gov   National Human Genome Research Institute (at the NIH) home page. Describes latest research findings, and ethics issues, and provides a talking glossary.

http://www.faseb.org/genetics   Compilation of major genetics societies throughout the world. Information on genetics meetings, society policy statements, etc.

http://vector.cshl.org   Cold Spring Harbor Labs DNA Learning Center home page; includes animation of genetic techniques.

http://www.ncgr.org   National Center for Genomic Resources home page.

THE BASIS OF A HEALTHY DIET

chapter 2

*H*ow many times have you heard wild claims about how healthful certain foods are for you? As consumers focus more and more on diet and disease, food manufacturers are asserting that their products have all sorts of health benefits. Supermarket shelves have begun to look like an 1800s medicine show.[20] "Take garlic capsules to avoid a heart attack." "Eat more olive oil and oat bran to lower blood cholesterol." Hearing these claims, you would think that food manufacturers have solutions to all of our health problems.

Advertising aside, nutrient intakes out of balance with nutrient needs—such as excess energy, saturated fat, sodium, and alcohol and sugar intake—are linked to many leading causes of death in the United States, including obesity, hypertension, heart disease, cancer, liver disease, and type 2 diabetes.[2, 26] In this chapter, you will explore the components of a healthy diet—a diet that will minimize your risks of developing nutrition-related diseases. The goal is to provide you with a firm understanding of basic diet-planning concepts before you study the nutrients in detail.

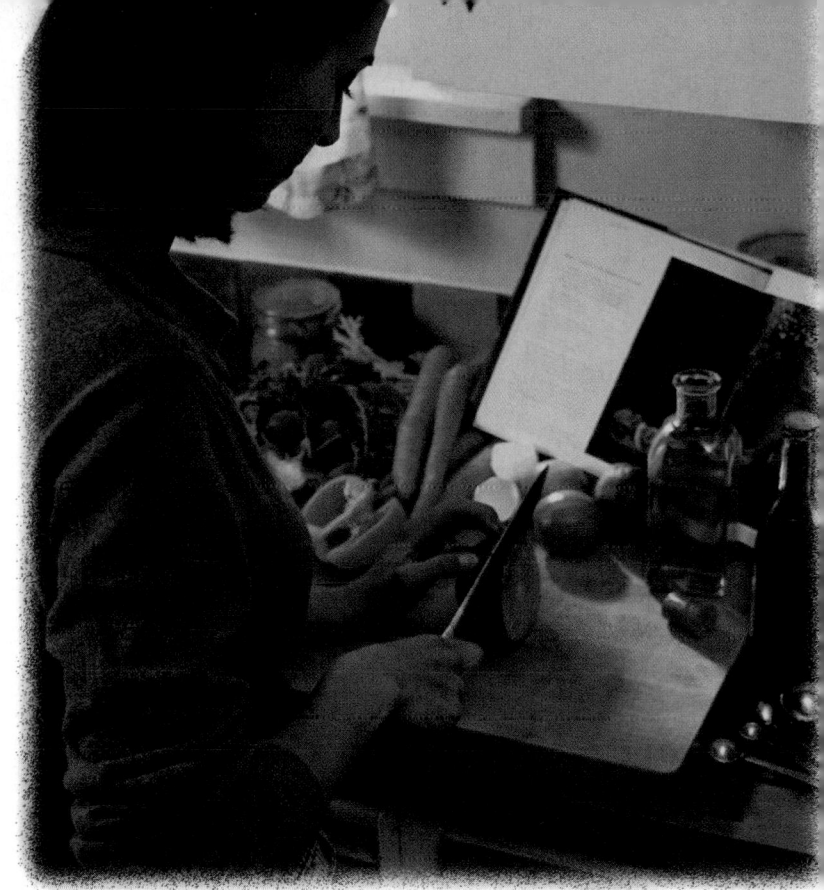

KEY CHAPTER CONCEPTS

- Three watchwords of nutrition are *variety, balance,* and *moderation* when it comes to designing a diet. To those we can also add *calorie control* and *regular exercise* to complement the diet.
- Nutrient density compares nutrient content of a food with nutrient needs. A nutrient-dense food is high in one or more nutrients, compared with energy content; for example, milk is a nutrient-dense source of calcium.
- Energy density of a food is determined by comparing energy content with the weight of food. A food rich in calories but weighs relatively very little is considered energy dense. Examples include nuts, cookies, fried foods in general, and fat-free snacks. Foods with low energy density include fruits, vegetables, and any food that incorporates lots of water during cooking, such as oatmeal. Having low-energy-density foods in a meal contributes to satiety without contributing many calories and, so, may aid in weight loss.
- Dietary Reference Intakes and associated nutrient standards provide a benchmark for estimating the nutrient needs of healthy individuals. These standards should be met primarily (or entirely) by consuming a variety of nutrient-rich foods—not by relying mostly on nutrient supplements.
- Daily Values are adapted from accepted nutrient standards. Daily Values are used to express the nutrient content of foods on the Nutrition Facts panel. Food labels are a valuable tool for tracking nutrient intakes.
- The Food Guide Pyramid provides one blueprint for a healthful diet and is an appropriate place to begin when evaluating daily food intake.
- Dietary Guidelines issued by the federal government encourage a varied diet; daily physical activity; plenty of fruits, vegetables, and grains; and moderation in fat, cholesterol, sugar, and sodium intake. Moderation in alcohol intake, if not complete abstinence, is also advised, along with safe cooking and food-storage practices.
- The Exchange System is a tool for estimating the carbohydrate, fat, protein, and energy content of a food or meal, and for planning a diet to correspond to specific goals for carbohydrate, fat, protein, and energy consumption.
- Dietary patterns in the United States have been influenced by the many ethnic diets seen around the world. Most ethnic diets show a basic dietary pattern as recommended by the Food Guide Pyramid—particularly, a diet rich in unrefined grains, fruits, and vegetables and low in sources of simple sugars. However, many ethnic diets include less milk and meat than the Food Guide Pyramid, focusing more on nuts, beans, and cheese.

REFRESH YOUR MEMORY

As you begin your study of diet planning in Chapter 2, you may want to review the terms in the margin in Chapter 1 and Table 1-1. This will help, as much of the same terminology appears in this chapter.

CASE SCENARIO

Andy is like many other college students. He grew up on a quick bowl of cereal and milk for breakfast and a hamburger, French fries, and cola for lunch, either in the school cafeteria or at a local fast-food restaurant. At dinner, he generally avoided eating any of his salad or vegetables, and by 9 o'clock he was deep into bags of chips and cookies. Andy has taken most of these habits to college. He prefers coffee for breakfast and possibly a chocolate bar. Lunch is still mainly a hamburger, French fries, and cola, but pizza and tacos now alternate more frequently than when he was in high school. One thing Andy really likes about the restaurants surrounding campus is that, for just about half a dollar more, he can *supersize* his meal. This helps him stretch his food dollar; searching out value meals for lunch and dinner now has become part of a typical day.

Provide some dietary advice for Andy. Start with his positive habits and then provide some constructive criticism. Use the concepts of variety, balance, and moderation, developed in the chapter, as well as the term *phytochemicals,* to frame your advice.

Variety—choose different types of foods within each food group.

Balance—choose foods from all five food groups.

Moderation—control portion size so that balance and variety are possible in your diet.

*S*ome people might like to live on pizza alone. What are pizza's nutrient strengths and inadequacies? Check the food composition table in Appendix A for the vitamin C content of cheese pizza. How many slices would you need to eat to yield the vitamin C RDA of 75–95 milligrams? (Answer: 30–40 slices)

phytochemical A chemical found in plants. Some phytochemicals may contribute to a reduced risk of cancer or heart disease in people who consume them regularly.

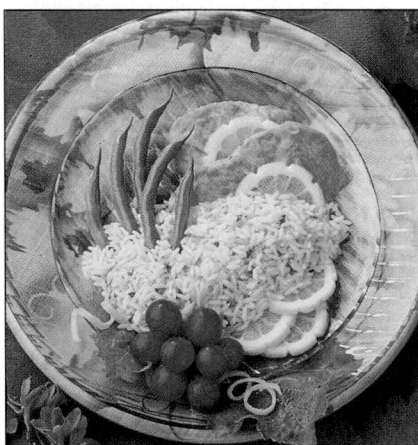

Focus on nutrient-rich foods as you strive to meet your nutrient needs.

■ A FOOD PHILOSOPHY THAT WORKS

You may be surprised to learn that what you should eat to minimize the risk of developing the common nutrition-related diseases seen in the United States is exactly what you've heard many times before: *Consume a variety of foods balanced by a moderate intake of each food.*[10] A variety of foods is best because no one food meets all your nutrient needs. Human milk comes close to meeting all of an infant's needs, except that it provides only limited amounts of iron, vitamin D, and fluoride. Cow's milk contains very little iron; neither form of milk provides dietary fiber. Meat provides protein but little calcium. Eggs have no vitamin C and provide little calcium because the calcium is mostly in the shell. Thus, you need variety in your diet because the required nutrients are scattered among many different foods.

Health professionals have recommended the same basic diet and health plan for the past 30 years: Watch how much you eat, focus on the major food groups, and stay physically active. Whole grains, fruits, and vegetables have always been among the foods emphasized for our diet for the past 30 years.[2]

It is disappointing, however, that, according to a survey conducted by the American Dietetic Association, two of five people in the United States believe that following a healthful diet means giving up foods they enjoy. To the contrary, a healthful diet requires only some simple planning and doesn't have to mean deprivation and misery. Besides, eliminating favorite foods typically doesn't work for "dieters" in the long run. The best plan consists of learning the basics of a healthful diet—a variety and balance of foods from all food groups and moderate consumption of all foods.[9] Let's now fine-tune this advice.

■ Variety Contributes to Diet Adequacy

Variety in your diet means choosing a number of different foods within any given food group, rather than eating the "same old thing" day after day. Variety makes meals more interesting and helps ensure that a diet contains sufficient nutrients. For example, carrots may be your favorite vegetable; however, if you choose carrots every day as your only vegetable source, you may miss out on the vitamin folate. Other vegetables, such as broccoli and asparagus, are rich sources of this nutrient. This concept is true of all classes of foods: fruits, vegetables, grains, and so on. Different foods within each class vary somewhat in the nutrients they contain, but they generally provide similar types of nutrients.

An added bonus of variety in the diet is the inclusion of a rich supply of what scientists call **phytochemicals.** These substances are not absolutely required elements of the diet. Still, many of these substances probably provide significant health benefits. Considerable research attention is focused on various phytochemicals in reducing the risk for certain diseases.[7] Because current vitamin and mineral supplements contain few or none of these potentially beneficial substances, they generally are available only from food.

Numerous population studies show reduced cancer among people who regularly consume fruits and vegetables. This is true for cancer of the gastrointestinal (GI) tract, breast, lung, and bladder. Researchers surmise that some phytochemicals present in the fruits and vegetables block the cancer process.[14, 18, 21, 23] The cancer process is described in the Nutrition Perspective in Chapter 10. For now, realize that cancer develops over many years via a multistep process. If an agent such as a phytochemical can block any one of the steps in this process, the chances that cancer will ultimately appear in the body are reduced. Other phytochemicals have been linked to a reduced risk of cardiovascular disease.[3, 4] Could it be that, because humans evolved on a wide variety of plant-based foods, the body developed with a need for these phytochemicals to maintain optimal health?

It will likely take many years for scientists to unravel the important effects of the myriad of phytochemicals in foods, and it is unlikely that all will ever be available in supplement form. For this reason, leading heart disease and cancer researchers suggest that a diet rich in fruits and vegetables is the most reliable way to obtain the potential benefits of phytochemicals.[27] Table 2-1 lists a variety of phytochemicals under study, with their common food sources. Table 2-2 provides a number of suggestions for including more phytochemicals—essentially, more fruits and vegetables, as well as more whole grains and legumes (beans)—in a diet.

■ Balance Means Not Overconsuming Any One Food

One way to balance your diet as you consume a variety of foods is to select foods from the five major food groups every day:

- Milk, yogurt, and cheese
- Meat, poultry, fish, dry beans, eggs, and nuts
- Vegetables
- Fruit
- Bread, cereal, rice, and pasta

A lunch consisting of a bean burrito with tomatoes accompanied by a glass of milk and an apple covers all groups. Fats, oils, and sweets can also be added to your diet in moderation to increase its flavor and to help deliver certain nutrients, such as vitamin E and essential fatty acids.

■ Moderation Refers Mostly to Portion Size

Eating moderately requires planning your entire day's diet, so that you don't overconsume nutrient sources. For example, if you eat something relatively high in fat, sugar, or energy, such as a bacon cheeseburger with a regular soft drink at a fast-food (quick-service) restaurant, you should eat other foods that are less concentrated sources of the same nutrients, such as fruits and salad greens, the same day. If you prefer whole milk to low-fat or nonfat milk, reduce the fat elsewhere in your meals. Try low-fat salad dressings, or use jam rather than butter or margarine on toast. Overall, strive to simply moderate—rather than eliminate—intake of some foods.

Some research suggests that increasing variety in a diet can lead to overeating. Thus as one incorporates a wide variety of foods in a diet, attention to total calorie intake is also important to consider.

A term has been coined to refer to foods rich in phytochemicals—*functional foods.*[15] This term indicates that the food provides health benefits beyond those supplied by the traditional nutrients it contains. Since a tomato contains the phytochemical lycopene, it can be called a functional food. The food industry especially has begun to use this term.

TABLE 2-1	Phytochemical Compounds Under Study.[1, 4, 16, 17, 18, 21]
Phytochemical	**Food Sources**
Allyl sulfides/organosulfurs	Garlic, onions, leeks
Saponins	Garlic, onions, licorice, legumes
Phenolic acids	All plants
Protease inhibitors	Soybeans and all other plants
Carotenoids	Orange, red, yellow fruits and vegetables (egg yolks are a source as well)
Monoterpenes	Oranges, lemons, grapefruit
Capsaicin	Chili peppers
Lignans	Flaxseed, berries, whole grains
Triterpenoids (glycyrrhizin)	Citrus fruit, mushrooms
Indoles	Cruciferous vegetables (broccoli, cabbage, kale)
Isothiocyanates	Cruciferous vegetables, especially broccoli
Phytosterols	Soybeans, other legumes, cucumbers, other fruits and vegetables
Flavonoids	Citrus fruit, onions, apples, grapes, wine, tea, chocolate
Isoflavones	Soybeans, other legumes
Catechins	Tea
Ellagic acid	Strawberries, raspberries, grapes, apples, bananas
Anthocyanosides	Red, blue, and purple plants (eggplant, blueberries)
Curcumin	Turmeric
Dithiolthiones	Carrots
Fructooligosaccharides	Onions, bananas, oranges

Some related compounds under study are found in animal products, such as sphingolipids (meat and dairy products) and conjugated linoleic acid (meat and cheese). These are not phytochemicals per se because they are not from plant sources, but they have been shown to have health benefits.[14, 25]

CRITICAL THINKING

Andy, described in the Case Scenario would benefit from more variety in his diet. What are some practical tips he can use to increase fruit and vegetable intake?

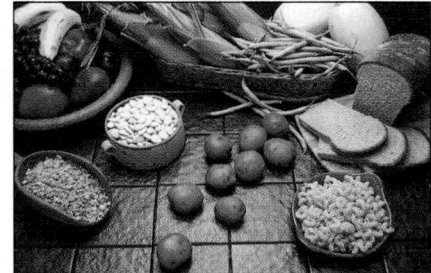

Fruits, vegetables, beans, and whole grains are typically rich in phytochemicals.

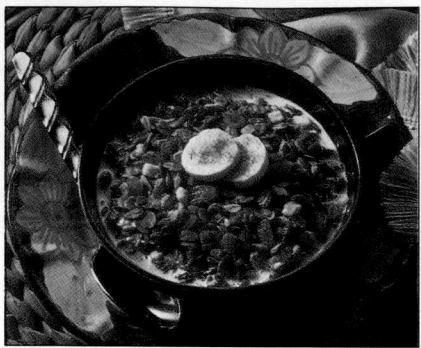

Choosing whole-grain cereals is an excellent way to increase nutrient value of a diet. Ideally, the cereal should have ≥3 g of dietary fiber per serving.

TABLE 2-2   Tips for Including Foods Rich in Phytochemicals in a Diet

- Include vegetables in main and side dishes. Add these to rice, omelets, potato salad, tuna salad, and pastas. Try broccoli or cauliflower florets, mushrooms, peas, carrots, corn, or peppers.
- Look for quick-fixing grain side dishes in the supermarket. Pilafs, couscous, rice mixes, and tabbouleh are just a few that you'll find.
- Choose fruit-filled cookies, such as fig bars. Use fresh or canned fruit as a topping for puddings, hot or cold cereal, pancakes, and frozen desserts.
- Put raisins, grapes, apple chunks, pineapples, grated carrots, zucchini, or cucumber into coleslaw, chicken salad, or tuna salad.
- Be creative at the salad bar: try fresh spinach, leaf lettuce, red cabbage, zucchini, yellow squash, cauliflower, peas, mushrooms, or red or yellow peppers.
- Pack fresh or dried fruit for snacks away from home instead of grabbing a candy bar or going hungry.
- Add slices of cucumber, zucchini, spinach, or carrot slivers to the lettuce and tomato on your sandwiches.
- Try one or two vegetarian meals per week, such as beans and rice or pasta; Chinese vegetable stir fry; or spaghetti, squash, and tomato sauce.
- When daily protein intake more than meets recommended amounts, reduce the meat, fish, or poultry in casseroles, stews, and soups by one-third to one-half and add more vegetables and legumes.
- In the refrigerator, keep a bowl of fresh vegetables handy for snacks.
- Choose 100% fruit or vegetable juices instead of soft drinks.
- Substitute tea for coffee or soft drinks on a regular basis.
- Have a bowl of fruit on hand.
- Switch from crisphead lettuce to leaf lettuce, such as romaine.
- Use salsa as a dip for chips.
- Choose whole-grain breakfast cereals, breads, and crackers.
- Flavor food with plenty of herbs and spices, including ginger, rosemary, basil, thyme, garlic, parsley, and chives.
- Experiment with soy products, such as tofu, soy milk, soy protein isolate, and roasted soybeans (see Chapter 7).

Although there are no "good" or "bad" foods as such, many Americans have diets overloaded with high-fat foods (e.g., whole milk, doughnuts, French fries, hot dogs), white bread and related refined-wheat products, and sugared soft drinks. Such diets lack the foundations of a healthy food plan—variety, balance, and moderation—and pose substantial risks for nutrition-related diseases.[11]

■ Nutrient Density Can Also Help Guide Food Choice

nutrient density The ratio derived by dividing a food's contribution to nutrient needs by its contribution to energy needs. When its contribution to nutrient needs exceeds its energy contribution, the food is considered to have a favorable nutrient density.

Nutrient density has gained acceptance in recent years for assessing the nutritional quality of an individual food. To determine the nutrient density of a food, simply compare its vitamin or mineral content with the amount of energy it provides. A food is said to be nutrient dense if it provides a large amount of a nutrient for a relatively small amount of kcal (compared with other food sources). The higher a food's nutrient density, the better it is as a nutrient source. Comparing the nutrient density of different foods is an easy way to estimate their relative nutritional quality. Generally, nutrient density is assessed with respect to individual nutrients. For example, many fruits and vegetables have a high content of vitamin C, compared with their modest energy content: That is, they are nutrient-dense foods for vitamin C. Moreover, as Figure 2-1 shows, nonfat milk is much more nutrient dense than sugared soft drinks for many nutrients.

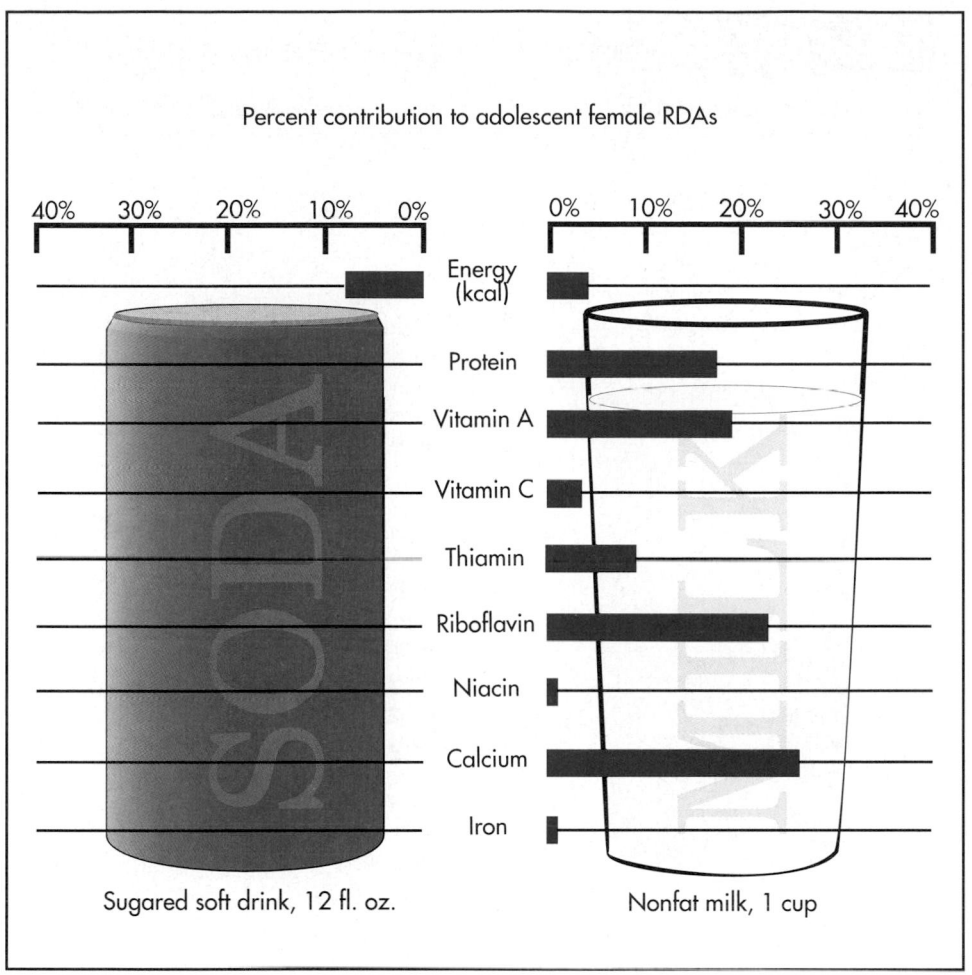

Percent contribution to adolescent female RDAs

Sugared soft drink, 12 fl. oz.

Nonfat milk, 1 cup

■ FIGURE 2-1 Comparison of the nutrient density of a sugared soft drink with that of nonfat milk. Both contribute fluid to the diet. However, choosing a glass of nonfat milk makes a significantly greater contribution to nutrient intake in comparison with a sugared soft drink. An easy way to determine nutrient density is to see how many of the nutrient bars in the graph are longer than the kcal bar. The soft drink has no longer nutrient bars. Nonfat milk has longer nutrient bars for protein, vitamin A, thiamin, riboflavin, and calcium. Including many nutrient-dense foods in your diet aids in meeting nutrient needs.

As we have noted before, menu planning focuses mainly on the total diet—not on the selection of one critical food as key to an adequate diet. Nonetheless, nutrient-dense foods—such as nonfat and low-fat milk, lean meats, beans, oranges, carrots, broccoli, whole-wheat bread, and whole-grain breakfast cereals—do help balance less nutrient-dense foods—such as cookies and potato chips—which many people like to eat. The latter are often called empty-calorie foods because they tend to supply much energy as sugar and/or fat but few other nutrients.

Searching for nutrient-dense foods is especially important in some cases. For example, this strategy can aid diet planning for people who tend to consume little food energy, including some older people and those following weight-loss diets.

■ Energy Density Especially Influences Energy Intake

Energy density is a concept that has captured the attention of nutrition scientists in recent years.[19] Energy density of a food is determined by comparing energy (kcal) content with the weight of food. A food that is rich in calories but that weighs relatively very little is considered energy dense. Examples include nuts, cookies, fried foods in general, and fat-free snacks, such as fat-free pretzels. Foods with low energy density include fruits, vegetables, and any food that incorporates lots of water during cooking, such as oatmeal (Table 2-3).

Researchers have shown that having low-energy-density foods in a meal contributes to satiety without contributing many calories. This is because we probably consume a constant weight of food at a meal, rather than a constant number of calories. How this constant weight of food is regulated is not known, but careful labo-

energy density A comparison of the energy (kcal) content of a food with the weight of the food. An energy-dense food is high in calories but weighs very little (e.g., many fried foods), whereas a food low in energy density has few calories but weighs a lot, such as an orange.

TABLE 2-3 Energy Density of Common Foods (Listed in Relative Order)

Very Low Energy Density (< 0.6 kcal/g)	Low Energy Density (0.6 to 1.5 kcal/g)
Lettuce	Whole milk
Tomatoes	Oatmeal
Strawberries	Cottage cheese
Broccoli	Beans
Salsa	Bananas
Grapefruit	Broiled fish
Nonfat milk	Fat-free yogurt
Carrots	Breakfast cereals with 1% low-fat milk
Vegetable soup	Plain baked potato
	Cooked rice
	Spaghetti noodles

Medium Energy Density (1.5 to 4 kcal/g)	High Energy Density (> 4 kcal/g)
Eggs	Graham crackers
Ham	Fat-free sandwich cookies
Pumpkin pie	Chocolate
Whole-wheat bread	Chocolate chip cookies
Bagels	Tortilla chips
White bread	Bacon
Raisins	Potato chips
Cream cheese	Peanuts
Cake with frosting	Peanut butter
Pretzels	Mayonnaise
Rice cakes	Butter or margarine
	Vegetable oils

Data adapted from Rolls B, Barnett RA: *Volumetrics.* New York: HarperCollins, 2000.

A useful diet/lifestyle acronym is *ABCDE:*

A adequacy of diet
B balance in diet
C calorie control
D diversity in food choice
E exercise on a regular basis

ratory studies show that people consume fewer calories in a meal if the food choices tend to be low in energy density, compared with foods high in energy density. A popular book now promotes following a diet low in energy density in order to lose weight.

Overall, foods with lots of water and dietary fiber provide a low-energy-density contribution to a meal and help one feel full, whereas foods with high energy density—especially those high in fat—must be eaten in greater amounts in order to contribute to fullness. This is one more reason to support a diet rich in fruits, vegetables, and whole grains, a pattern that also is typical of many ethnic diets throughout the world (see the Nutrition Perspective at the end of this chapter). Still, favorite foods, even if they are high in energy density, have a place in your dietary pattern, but you will have to plan for them. For example, chocolate is a very energy-dense food, but a small portion at the end of a meal can supply a satisfying finale. In addition, foods with high energy density can help people with poor appetites, such as older people, to maintain or gain weight.

CONCEPT CHECK

Basic diet-planning concepts include consuming a variety of foods, balancing a diet by consuming foods from each of the five food groups, and moderating portion size with each food choice, so that the diet is not excessive in energy. Choosing nutrient-dense foods, such as nonfat milk, fruits, vegetables, and whole grains, helps supply a diet with many nutrients but not excessive calories. Many of these foods are also rich sources of phytochemicals, supplying an even greater health benefit to the diet. Consuming foods of low energy density, such as fruits and vegetables, may also help in weight control, in that these provide satiety for a meal because of their large volume but few calories. As you will also see throughout this book, regular physical activity complements any diet plan.

■ SETTING NUTRIENT NEEDS— DIETARY REFERENCE INTAKES (DRIs)

Before designing a diet plan, such as the Food Guide Pyramid, it must be determined what frequency and amount of each nutrient are needed. People have puzzled over this question for centuries. During World War II, when many men were rejected from military service because of the effects of poor nutrition on their health, the need for official dietary recommendations was recognized. In 1941, a group of 25 scientists formed the first Food and Nutrition Board. These established dietary standards for evaluating the nutritional intakes of large populations and for planning agricultural production, first published in 1943.

The current Food and Nutrition Board was formed in 1993. It recognized the need for an overhaul of previously published nutrient standards for several reasons. New research has made it clear that some of the previous standards did not maximize human benefit from food components. The new recommendations that board members are now developing will include an additional amount of each nutrient when appropriate to help prevent chronic diseases, such as heart disease, osteoporosis, and cancer. Previous standards only accounted for the amount of each nutrient needed to reduce the risk of deficiency diseases, such as rickets and scurvy.[29]

The framework of these new recommendations are named **Dietary Reference Intakes (DRIs)** and have been released in stages through the last few years. So far, DRIs have been set for all vitamins and most minerals. There are other categories of nutrients for which recommendations are being developed. These include macronutrients (carbohydrates, proteins, and fats), electrolytes (sodium, potassium, and chloride), water, and other food components (for example, dietary fiber). Until these updates are available, older nutrient standards for such dietary components developed in 1989 will remain in place.

Under the umbrella of the DRIs, four sets of standards have been established: **Estimated Average Requirements (EARs), Recommended Dietary Allowances (RDAs), Adequate Intakes (AIs), and Tolerable Upper Intake Levels (Upper Levels or ULs)** (see the inside cover of this textbook). Following is a more detailed discussion of each of these standards.

■ Estimated Average Requirements (EARs)

Estimated Average Requirements are the nutrient intake that is estimated to meet the needs of 50% of the individuals in a certain age and gender group (Fig. 2-2). To set an Estimated Average Requirement, the Food and Nutrition Board must be able to agree on a specific measurable functional marker to use for establishing nutrient adequacy. Such markers are typically the activity of an **enzyme** in the body or the ability of a cell to maintain physiological health. (The specific markers used for various nutrients will be discussed in Chapters 9 through 12.) If no measurable functional marker is available, no Estimated Average Requirement can be set. This is the case for the mineral calcium. The Estimated Average Requirement also includes an adjustment for the amount of each nutrient that passes through the digestive tract unabsorbed. At this intake, though, the needs of the other 50% of the population would not be met. Thus, the Estimated Average Requirement can only be used to evaluate the adequacy of diets of a group of people.

*C*urrent revisions of U.S. dietary standards will apply to Canadians as well, as this revision is a joint venture of scientists from both countries (see Appendix C for details on Canadian standards).

Dietary Reference Intakes (DRIs) The term used to encompass the latest nutrient recommendations made by the Food and Nutrition Board of the National Academy of Sciences. These include RDAs and AIs.

enzyme A compound that speeds the rate of a chemical process but is not altered by the chemical process. Almost all enzymes are proteins.

Adequate intake (AI): a recommended intake value based on observed or experimentally determined approximations or estimates of nutrient intake by a group (or groups) of healthy people that is assumed to be adequate – used when an RDA cannot be determined. When set for a nutrient, aim for this intake.

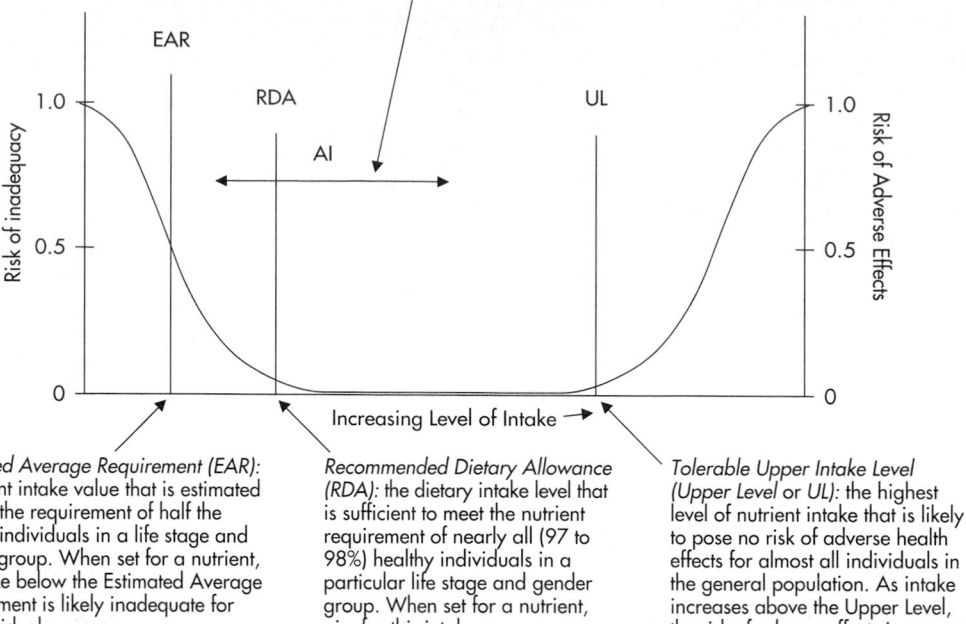

Estimated Average Requirement (EAR): a nutrient intake value that is estimated to meet the requirement of half the healthy individuals in a life stage and gender group. When set for a nutrient, an intake below the Estimated Average Requirement is likely inadequate for an individual.

Recommended Dietary Allowance (RDA): the dietary intake level that is sufficient to meet the nutrient requirement of nearly all (97 to 98%) healthy individuals in a particular life stage and gender group. When set for a nutrient, aim for this intake.

Tolerable Upper Intake Level (Upper Level or UL): the highest level of nutrient intake that is likely to pose no risk of adverse health effects for almost all individuals in the general population. As intake increases above the Upper Level, the risk of adverse effects increases.

FIGURE 2-2 Dietary Reference Intakes. This figure shows that 50% of North Americans would have an inadequate intake by consuming the *Estimated Average Requirement (EAR),* whereas 50% would have their needs met. Only about 2 to 3% of such people would have an inadequate intake if each were to meet the *Recommended Dietary Allowance (RDA),* whereas 97 to 98% would have their needs met. At intakes between the RDA and the *Tolerable Upper Intake Level (Upper Level or UL),* the risk of either an inadequate diet or adverse effects from the nutrient in question is close to 0. The Upper Level is then the highest level of nutrient intake that is likely to pose no risks of adverse health effects to almost all individuals in the general population. At intakes above the Upper Level, the risk of adverse effects increases. The *Adequate Intake (AI),* set for some nutrients instead of an RDA, lies somewhere between the Estimated Average Requirement and the Upper Level. In determining the Adequate Intake for a nutrient, it is expected that the amount exceeds the RDA for that nutrient, if an RDA were known. Thus, the Adequate Intake should cover the needs of more than 97 to 98% of individuals. The actual degree to which the Adequate Intake exceeds the RDA is likely to differ among the various nutrients and population groups. The Food and Nutrition Board states that there is no established benefit for healthy individuals if they consume nutrient intakes above the RDA or Adequate Intake.

▪ Recommended Dietary Allowances (RDAs)

The RDA is the nutrient intake that is sufficient to meet the needs of nearly all individuals (about 97%) in an age and gender group. RDAs are based on a multiple of the Estimated Average Requirements (generally the RDA = EAR × 1.2). Because of this relationship, RDAs can be set for nutrients only if the Food and Nutrition Board has enough information to determine an Estimated Average Requirement. Additional consideration in setting an RDA also can be given to a nutrient's ability to prevent chronic disease, rather than just prevent deficiency. A good example is vitamin C (see the next section titled Setting One RDA: Vitamin C).

Setting One RDA: Vitamin C

The amount of vitamin C needed each day to prevent scurvy is about 10 mg. However, as you will learn in Chapter 10, vitamin C has other functions as well, some of which are involved in the workings of the immune system. Based on this relationship, the concentration of vitamin C in one component of the immune system—notably, white blood cells (specifically neutrophils)—can be used as a marker for vitamin C adequacy in an individual. The Food and Nutrition Board feels that near-maximal saturation of neutrophils with vitamin C is, in fact, the best marker for optimal vitamin C status. Research published to date suggests that, for adults 19 to 30 years of age, it takes on average a daily intake of 75 mg for men and 60 mg for women for near-saturation of neutrophils. These average amounts then become the Estimated Average Requirement for young adult men and women.

The Estimated Average Requirement for vitamin C is multiplied by 1.2 to yield the RDA; in this case, the RDA becomes 90 mg for men and 75 mg for women. Other age groups have slightly different recommendations; smokers should add 35 mg to the RDA for their age and gender (see Chapter 10 for details).

Putting the RDA for Vitamin C to Use

If you total the amount of vitamin C you eat in 1 week and divide by 7, you will have your average daily vitamin C consumption. If that value is close to the RDA, you are most likely consuming enough vitamin C. Even if you eat less than the RDA, you will not likely suffer ill effects because your needs are most likely less than the RDA, as it is set to include almost all individuals, some of whom probably need more vitamin C than you do. As a general rule, however, the further you stray below the RDA—particularly as you approach the Estimated Average Requirement—the greater your risk of a nutritional deficiency. Symptoms of a vitamin C deficiency may be subtle and develop slowly. It takes a long time to detect problems such as a weakened immune system and even poor wound healing. If you suspect that your diet is not nutritious enough, don't wait for warning signs to develop. Start eating a diet that meets the RDAs set for vitamin C (and all the other nutrients listed for your age and gender), rather than risk the development of health problems from poor nutrition.

Setting RDAs for Energy Needs

RDAs for nutrients are set high enough to meet the needs of almost all healthy individuals. In contrast, the RDAs for energy, set last in 1989, refer to the average needs for various age groups (see the inside cover of this textbook). Unlike most vitamins and minerals, excess energy consumed (above energy needs) is not excreted. Thus, to promote weight maintenance, a more conservative standard was used for energy needs than for nutrient needs. Overall, an energy RDA is only a rough estimate, because energy needs depend on energy use. For most adults, the ability to obtain and maintain a healthy weight is the best yardstick of energy balance—energy intake matching energy output.

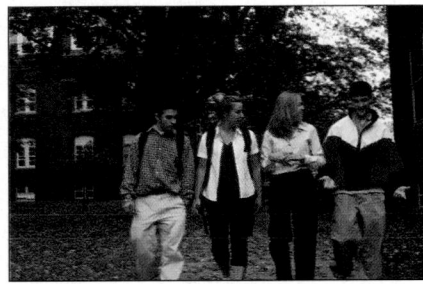

Energy needs in adulthood are based on the number of calories required to maintain weight.

■ Adequate Intakes (AIs)

Nutrients for which there is not enough information to establish an Estimated Average Requirement are assigned an Adequate Intake. Adequate Intakes are based on observed or experimentally determined estimates of the average nutrient intake that appears to maintain a defined nutritional state (for example, normal circulating nutrient values or bone health) in a certain population. Adequate Intakes have been set for two B-vitamins, the vitamin-like choline, vitamin D, and some minerals such as calcium and fluoride. In addition, Adequate Intakes are being set for all nutrients for infants under 1 year of age.

■ Tolerable Upper Intake Levels (Upper Levels or ULs)

The Upper Level is the maximum level of daily intake of a nutrient that is unlikely to cause adverse health effects in almost all people (97 to 98%) in a population. This number applies to chronic daily use and is set to protect even very susceptible people in the healthy general population. The Upper Level is not a goal for nutrient intake but, rather, is a ceiling below which nutrient intake should remain. Not enough information is available to set a Upper Level for all nutrients, but this does not mean that toxicity from these nutrients is impossible. Furthermore, there is no clear-cut evidence that intakes above the RDA or Adequate Intake confer any additional health benefits for most of us.

The Upper Level for most nutrients is based on the combined intake of food, water, supplements, and fortified foods. Two exceptions are magnesium and zinc, for which the Upper Level for each refers only to nonfood sources, such as medicines and supplements. This is because toxicity due to dietary intake of magnesium or zinc is unlikely.

*M*inimum requirements have been set for sodium, potassium, and chloride (see the inside cover of this textbook). These values represent minimum nutrient needs. Note that these amounts are much less than typical intakes of sodium or chloride but are about equal to Americans' typical intake of potassium. It is likely that these nutrients will be given AIs when re-evaluated by the Food and Nutrition Board in 2001.

■ Appropriate Uses of the DRIs

The DRIs are intended mainly for diet planning. Specifically, a diet plan should aim to meet any RDAs set. If no RDA has been determined, it is reasonable to use the Adequate Intake as a guide for nutrient intake. Finally, the Upper Level for a nutrient should not be exceeded.[29] Keep in mind also that none of these dietary standards are necessarily appropriate amounts for individuals who are already undernourished or for those with diseases that require higher intakes. This concept will be covered in Chapters 9 through 12.

CONCEPT CHECK

Dietary Reference Intakes are set for specific nutrients in order to guide food intake. These standards include Recommended Dietary Allowances (RDAs), Adequate Intakes (AIs), and Tolerable Upper Intake Levels (Upper Levels or ULs). Recommended Dietary Allowances represent the nutrient needs for healthy individuals. RDAs are established for specific age and gender categories. No one knows his or her own nutritional requirements; the best general rule is that, the further you stray from nutrient standards set for your age and gender, especially below the Estimated Average Requirement (EAR), the greater your chance of having a nutritional deficiency or toxicity. Adequate Intakes are set when there is not enough information to set a more precise RDA. Intakes above Upper Levels should not be consumed on a regular basis, as toxic effects are possible.

■ DAILY VALUES (DVs): THE STANDARDS USED FOR FOOD LABELING

The DRIs and accompanying nutrient standards are not used in food labeling because they are age and gender specific. We can't have different packages for men and women or for teens and adults. The Food and Drug Administration (FDA) has developed a set of generic standards, called **Daily Values,** which are used to express the nutrient content of foods for the Nutrition Facts panel on food labels. The content of a particular nutrient is listed on labels as a percentage of the Daily Value. These percentages serve as a benchmark for evaluating the nutrient content of foods. They do not, however, represent a set of tailor-made recommendations for an adult. You will see why once the method for setting Daily Values is described.

The Daily Values are based on two sets of dietary standards. The first, **Reference Daily Intakes (RDIs),** are for vitamins and minerals. The second, **Daily Reference Values (DRVs),** are standards for protein and various dietary components that have no RDA or other established nutrient standard (e.g., total fat, cholesterol, and dietary fiber). These two terms—*Reference Daily Intakes* and *Daily Reference Values*—do not appear on labels. To make reading labels less confusing for consumers, the term *Daily Value* is used to represent the combination of these two sets of dietary standards, since the differences between Reference Daily Intakes and Daily Reference Values for typical consumers are inconsequential. For health professionals and nutrition experts, though, it is important to understand how nutrition label information (Reference Daily Intakes vs. Daily Reference Values) is actually derived:

For food labels, standards are set for nutrients that have RDAs or other established nutrient standards, called RDIs.

For food labels, standards are set for many nutrients that do not have RDAs or other established nutrient standards, called DRVs.

Daily Values, used on food labels, are a combination of RDI and DRV standards.

Daily Values Standard nutrient-intake values developed by FDA and used as a reference for expressing nutrient content on nutrition labels. The Daily Values include two types of standards—RDIs and DRVs.

Reference Daily Intakes (RDIs) Nutrient-intake standards set by FDA based on the 1968 RDAs for various vitamins and minerals. RDIs have been set for four categories of people: infants, toddlers, people over 4 years of age, and pregnant or lactating women. Generally the highest RDA value in each category is used as the RDI. The RDIs constitute part of the Daily Values used in food labeling.

Daily Reference Values (DRVs) Nutrient-intake standards established for protein and some other dietary components lacking an RDA or a related nutrient standard, including fat, saturated fat, cholesterol, carbohydrate, dietary fiber, sodium, and potassium. The DRVs for cholesterol, sodium, and potassium are constant; those for the other nutrients increase as energy intake increases. The DRVs constitute part of the Daily Values used in food labeling.

■ Reference Daily Intakes (RDIs)

Reference Daily Intakes (RDIs) make up the majority of the Daily Values (DVs). The Reference Daily Intakes have been set by FDA using a compilation of the nutrient standards published in 1968. Essentially, Reference Daily Intakes use the highest RDA values of any age category set in 1968. For example, consider iron: In 1968, the RDA for adult men was 10 mg/day and that for adult women and adolescents was 18 mg/day. The iron Reference Daily Intake for adults is the higher value: 18 mg/day. Table 2-4 lists the Reference Daily Intakes used for various age groups.

The Reference Daily Intake values currently in use, which are based on the 1968 RDAs, are generally slightly higher than current RDAs and related nutrient

TABLE 2-4 Comparison of Daily Values with the Latest DRIs and Other Nutrient Standards*

Dietary Constituent	Unit of Measure	Current Daily Values for People Over 4 Years of Age	DRI or other current dietary standard	
			Males 19 Years Old	Females 19 Years Old
Fat[†]	g	<65	—	—
Saturated fatty acids[†]	"	<20	—	—
Protein[†]	"	50	58	46
Cholesterol[§]	mg	<300	—	—
Carbohydrate[†]	g	300	—	—
Fiber	"	25	—	—
Vitamin A	µg Retinol Activity Equivalents	1000	900	700
Vitamin D	International Units	400	200	200
Vitamin E	"	30	22–33	22–33
Vitamin K	µg	80	120	90
Vitamin C	mg	60	90	75
Folate	µg	400	400	400
Thiamin	mg	1.5	1.20	1.10
Riboflavin	"	1.7	1.30	1.10
Niacin	"	20	16	14
Vitamin B-6	"	2	1.30	1.30
Vitamin B-12	µg	6	2.40	2.40
Biotin	mg	0.3	0.03	0.03
Pantothenic acid	"	10	5	5
Calcium	"	1000	1000	1000
Phosphorus	"	1000	700	700
Iodide	µg	150	150	150
Iron	mg	18	8	18
Magnesium	"	400	400	310
Copper	"	2	0.9	0.9
Zinc	"	15	11	8
Sodium[†]	"	<2400	500	500
Potassium[†]	"	3500	2000	2000
Chloride[†]	"	3400	750	750
Manganese	"	2	2.3	1.8
Selenium	µg	70	55	55
Chromium	"	120	35	25
Molybdenum	"	75	45	45

Abbreviations: g = gram, mg = milligram, µg = microgram

*Daily Values are generally set at the highest nutrient recommendation in a specific age and gender category. Many Daily Values exceed current nutrient standards. This is in part because aspects of the Daily Values were originally developed in the early 1970s using estimates of nutrient needs published in 1968. The Daily Values have yet to be updated to reflect the current state of knowledge.

[†]Sodium, potassium, and chloride values are based on the minimum requirement for health. The considerably higher Daily Values for sodium and chloride are there to allow for more diet flexibility, but the extra amounts are not needed to maintain health.

[‡]No RDA has been set for these nutrients, except protein (see Chapter 7). These values are based, instead, on a 2000 kcal diet, with a caloric distribution of 30% from fat (and one-third of this total from saturated fat), 60% from carbohydrate, and 10% from protein.

[§]Based on recommendations of federal agencies

*N*utrition educators often instruct patients to look only at the total amount of a nutrient (shown on the left side of the Nutrition Facts panel) rather than the % Daily Value when watching a specific nutrient. This is because the % Daily Value is not correct unless that person consumes 2000 kcal/day. For example, if a person is to limit his or her saturated fat intake to 20 g per day, the % Daily Value does not provide adequate information to assess grams of saturated fat consumed in a day.

standards. FDA will likely revise the Reference Daily Intakes to reflect the latest nutrient standards once the current Food and Nutrition Board has completed its work on the DRIs.

■ Daily Reference Values (DRVs)

The Daily Values for some food constituents are based on Daily Reference Values (DRVs) rather than RDIs. Except for the protein Daily Reference Value, which is based on RDA values, the other Daily Reference Values cover certain dietary components that have no RDA or related nutrient standard at this time: total fat, saturated fatty acids, cholesterol, carbohydrate, fiber, sodium, and potassium. The Daily Reference Values are intended to help consumers evaluate their food choices by comparing their actual intakes of these food constituents with desirable (or maximum) intakes. Table 2-5 lists the Daily Reference Values. The amounts for energy-yielding nutrients are based on 30% of total kcal from fat, 60% from carbohydrate, and 10% from protein, which corresponds to the Dietary Guidelines and recommendations from various other major health-related associations (see the section entitled Dietary Guidelines—Another Planning Tool).

Note that many of the Daily Reference Values, such as those for saturated fat, total fat, and dietary fiber, are related to total energy intake. By accounting for this, you can evaluate your diet even if your energy intake is more or less than the standard energy intake, 2000 kcal, used on the label. For example, if you consume only 1600 kcal per day, the total percentage of Daily Value for each of these nutrients should add up to no more than 80% because 1600 ÷ 2000 = 0.8, or 80%. If you eat 2800 kcal, your total percentage of Daily Value for each nutrient in all the foods you eat in one day can add up to 140%, because 2800 ÷ 2000 = 1.4, or 140%. However, the % Daily Values for some dietary constituents, such as cholesterol and sodium, are not adjusted for differences in energy intake.

In the same way, you can calculate the amount of a certain nutrient you have left in a day by using the % Daily Value. For example, if you consume 2000 kcal per day, your total fat intake for the day should be 65 g or less. If you consume 10 g of fat at breakfast, you have 55 g, or 85%, of your Daily Value left for the rest of the day.

■ Daily Values in Perspective

The Nutrition Facts panel on the label of a food product lists various components of the food as a percentage of their Daily Values. Use this information to learn more about your food choices. Unfortunately most adults do not do this. To practice using this information, suppose that one serving of a macaroni and cheese product contains 15% of the Daily Value for iron. Since the Daily Value for iron is 18 mg, this product contains about 3 mg of iron per serving (18 × 0.15 = 2.7 mg).

TABLE 2-5   Daily Reference Values (DRVs)*

Food Component	Unit of Measure	DRV (2000 kcal Intake)	DRV (2500 kcal Intake)	DRV (3200 kcal Intake)
Fat	g	<65	<80	<107
Saturated fatty acids	g	<20	<25	<36
Protein	g	50	65	80
Cholesterol	mg	<300	<300	<300
Carbohydrate	g	300	375	480
Fiber	g	25	30	37
Sodium	mg	<2400	<2400	<2400
Potassium	mg	3500	3500	3500

*Daily Reference Values based on an energy intake of 2000 kcal constitute the Daily Values used as reference standards for food labeling. Note that the Daily Reference Values for some nutrients (e.g., total fat) increase as energy intake increases.

aily Values are currently used as a benchmark for representing the nutrient content of foods on nutrition labels. Nutrient content is expressed as percentages of the Daily Values, which in turn are based on Reference Daily Intakes (RDIs) or Daily Reference Values (DRVs). The Reference Daily Intakes for vitamins and minerals constitute the majority of Daily Values and are based on the 1968 RDA standards. The Daily Reference Values have been set for protein and some nutrients that don't have an RDA or Adequate Intake, such as fat, cholesterol, and dietary fiber. To decrease confusion, the Daily Value is the only term that appears on food labels.

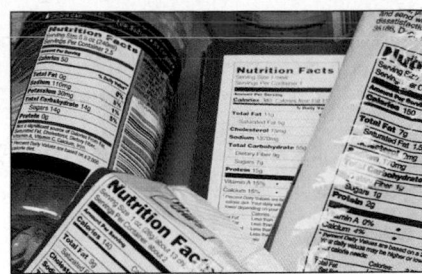

Use the Nutrition Facts label to learn more about the nutrient content of the foods you eat. Nutrient content is expressed as a % of Daily Value.

■ FROM NUTRIENT RECOMMENDATIONS TO FOOD CHOICES

The following sections of the chapter will describe various guidelines for planning healthy diets.

■ The Food Guide Pyramid—a Menu-Planning Tool

Since the early twentieth century, researchers have worked to clarify the science of nutrition into practical terms, so that people with no special training could estimate whether their nutritional needs were being met. A seven-food-group plan, based on foods traditionally eaten by Americans, was one of the first formats. Daily food choices had to include items from each group. This plan had been simplified by the mid-1950s to a four-food-group plan: a milk group, a meat group, a fruit and vegetable group, and a breads and cereals group. The entire plan was designed to provide a minimum foundation for a diet, and it represented about 1200 to 1400 kcal/day. Other food choices were to be added to meet daily energy needs.

Today, the Food Guide Pyramid, which is designed to represent a total diet providing sufficient protein, vitamins, and minerals, is widely advocated for diet planning (Fig. 2-3).[9] This pyramid goes beyond earlier guides to suggest a pattern of food choices for the entire day, rather than simply a foundation diet. The major changes from earlier food guides include an increase in total fruit and vegetable servings from 4 per day to 5 to 9 per day and an increase in bread and cereal servings from 4 per day to 6 to 11 per day. One goal of these changes is to provide the bulk of dietary energy intake from unrefined carbohydrates while moderating fat intake.

Components of the Food Guide Pyramid

The number of servings to consume from each food group in the current Food Guide Pyramid depends on a person's age and energy needs. Serving size is also adjusted downward for young children (see Chapter 17). Table 2-6 lists serving sizes and amounts for adults of various ages. The table also lists the major nutrients each food group supplies. Note the similarities and differences among the groups.

The plan for an adult over 18 essentially consists of the following:
- 2 servings from the milk, yogurt, and cheese group
- 2 to 3 servings from the meat, poultry, fish, dry beans, eggs, and nuts group (5 to 7 ounces total)
- 3 to 5 servings from the vegetable group
- 2 to 4 servings from the fruit group
- 6 to 11 servings from the bread, cereals, rice, and pasta group

For some population groups—children, teenagers, and pregnant or breastfeeding women—three servings of the milk, yogurt, and cheese group are recommended due to higher calcium needs.

The American Institute for Cancer Research is promoting a "plate" instead of a "pyramid" for menu planning. The plate should be covered ⅔ or more by vegetables, fruits, whole grains, and beans, and ⅓ or less by meat, fish, poultry, and low fat dairy products.

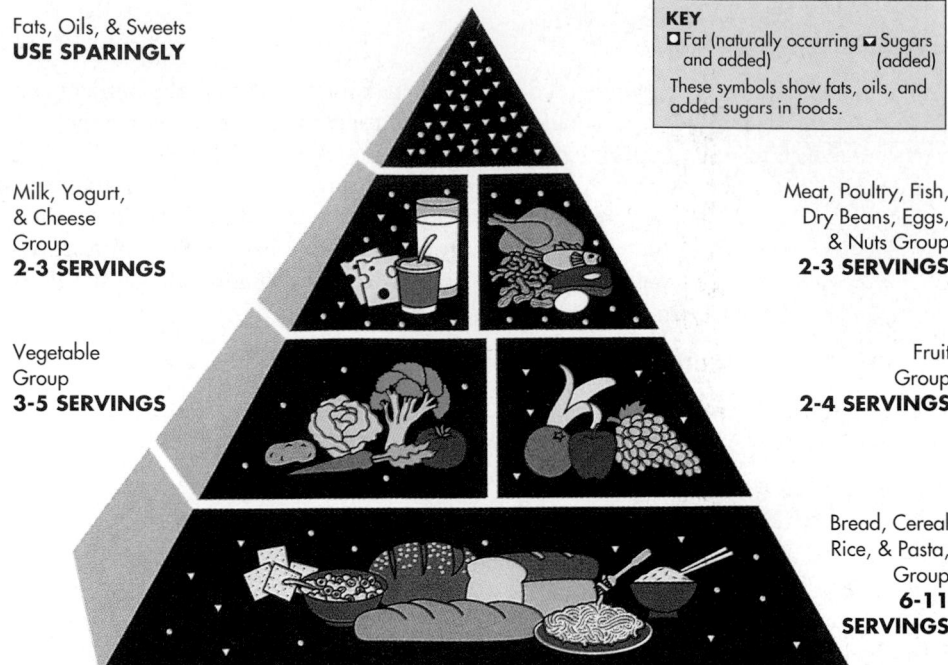

KEY
☐ Fat (naturally occurring ☑ Sugars and added) (added)
These symbols show fats, oils, and added sugars in foods.

Fats, Oils, & Sweets
USE SPARINGLY

Milk, Yogurt, & Cheese Group
2-3 SERVINGS

Meat, Poultry, Fish, Dry Beans, Eggs, & Nuts Group
2-3 SERVINGS

Vegetable Group
3-5 SERVINGS

Fruit Group
2-4 SERVINGS

Bread, Cereal Rice, & Pasta, Group
6-11 SERVINGS

FIGURE 2-3 USDA's Food Guide Pyramid. The Food Guide Pyramid lists the food groups and the amount to consume from each group. Note that, for children and teenagers, three servings should be chosen from the milk, yogurt, and cheese group. Once you have estimated your energy needs, recommended servings from the other groups with wider ranges are as follows:

Energy Intake	1600 kcal	2200 kcal	2800 kcal
Bread, etc. group	6	9	11
Vegetable group	3	4	5
Fruit group	2	3	4
Milk, etc. group	2–3	2–3	2–3
Meat, etc. group (ounces)	5	6	7
Total fat (grams)	53	73	93
Total added sugars (teaspoons)	6	12	18

Foods in a final category, which is not a group per se, include fats, oils, and sweets. These can be eaten to help meet individual energy needs but should not replace foods from other groups.

Menu Planning with the Food Guide Pyramid

Table 2-7 illustrates a 1-day menu based on the Food Guide Pyramid. Remember the following points when using the Food Guide Pyramid to plan daily menus:
1. The guide does not apply to infants or children under 2 years of age.
2. No one food is absolutely essential to good nutrition. Each food is deficient in at least one essential nutrient.
3. No one food group provides all essential nutrients in adequate amounts. Each food group makes an important, distinctive contribution to nutritional intake.
4. Variety is the key to the success of the guide and is first guaranteed by choosing foods from all the groups. Furthermore, one should consume a variety of foods within each group, except possibly in the milk, yogurt, and cheese group.
5. The foods within a group may vary widely with respect to nutrient and energy content. For example, the energy content of 3 ounces of baked potato is 98 kcal, whereas that of 3 ounces of potato chips is 470 kcal. Compare an orange and an apple with respect to vitamin C, using the food composition table in Appendix A.

TABLE 2-6   The Food Guide Pyramid—a Summary

Food Category	Major Contributions	Foods and Individual Serving Sizes†
Milk, yogurt, and cheese	Calcium Phosphorus Carbohydrate Protein Riboflavin Vitamin D Magnesium Zinc	1 cup milk (includes low-lactose products) 1½ oz cheese 2 oz processed cheese 1 cup yogurt 2 cups cottage cheese 1 cup soy-based beverage with added calcium
Meat, poultry, fish, dry beans, eggs, and nuts	Protein Thiamin Riboflavin Niacin Vitamin B-6 Folate§ Vitamin B-12‖ Phosphorus Magnesium§ Iron Zinc	2–3 oz cooked meat, poultry, or fish 1–1½ cups cooked dry beans 4 tbsp peanut butter 2 eggs 2/3–1 cup nuts 5 oz soyburger
Fruit	Carbohydrate Vitamin A (few varieties) Vitamin C Folate Magnesium Potassium Dietary fiber	¼ cup dried fruit ½ cup cooked or canned fruit ¾ cup juice 1 whole piece of fruit 1 melon wedge (about ¼) ½ cup berries
Vegetable	Carbohydrate Vitamin A Vitamin C Folate Magnesium Potassium Dietary fiber	½ cup raw or cooked vegetables 1 cup raw leafy vegetables ¾ cup vegetable juice
Bread, cereal, rice, and pasta	Carbohydrate Thiamin Riboflavin¶ Niacin Folate# Magnesium‡ Iron¶# Zinc# Dietary fiber#	1 slice of bread 1 oz (about 3/4 cup) ready-to-eat cereal ½ cup cooked cereal, rice, or pasta ½ hamburger roll, bagel, or English muffin 3–4 plain crackers 1 small roll, biscuit, or muffin 1 6" tortilla
Fats, oils, and sweets	Food from this category should not replace any from the other groups. Amounts consumed should be determined by individual energy needs.	

†May be reduced for child servings
§Primarily in plant protein sources
‖Only in animal foods
¶If enriched
#Whole grains and some enriched/fortified products
‡Whole grains

To quickly estimate serving sizes, use the following equivalents:
Thumb = 1 oz of cheese
4 stacked dice = 1 oz cheese
Thumb tip = 1 tsp
Matchbox = 1 oz meat
Bar of soap or pack of cards = 3 oz meat

Palm of a hand = 3 oz
1 ice cream scoop = 1/2 cup
Fist = 1 cup
Handful = 1 or 2 oz of a snack food
Tennis ball = 1 medium fruit serving

Computer mouse = 1 medium potato
Ping-pong ball = 2 tbsp peanut butter
Yo-yo = 1 bagel serving

Experts recommend that we pay close attention to the stated serving size for each choice when following the Food Guide Pyramid. This aids in controlling total energy intake.

TABLE 2-7   Putting the Food Guide Pyramid into Practice

Meal	Servings/Food Group*
Breakfast	
1 small peeled orange	1 fruit
¾ cup Healthy Choice Low-fat Granola	1 bread
with ½ cup nonfat milk	½ milk
½ small toasted raisin bagel	1 bread
with 1 tsp soft margarine	1 fat/sweet
Optional: coffee or tea	
Lunch	
Ham sandwich	
2 slices whole-wheat bread	2 bread
2 oz ham	1 meat
2 tsp mustard	
1 small apple	1 fruit
2 oatmeal-raisin cookies (small)	2 fat/sweet
Optional: diet soft drink	
3 P.M. Study break	
6 whole wheat crackers	2 bread
1 tbsp peanut butter	¼ meat
½ cup nonfat milk	½ milk
Dinner	
Lettuce salad	
1 cup romaine lettuce	1 vegetable
½ cup sliced tomatoes	1 vegetable
1½ tbsp Thousand Island dressing	1½ fat/sweet
½ cup grated carrot	1 vegetable
3 oz broiled salmon	1 meat
½ cup rice	1 bread
½ cup green beans	1 vegetable
with 1 tsp soft margarine	1 fat/sweet
Optional: coffee or tea	
Late-Night Snack	
1 cup "light" fruit yogurt	1 milk
Nutrient Breakdown	
1800 kcal	
Carbohydrate 56% of kcal	
Protein 18% of kcal	
Fat 26% of kcal	

This menu meets nutrient needs for all vitamins and minerals for an average adult. For adolescents and teenagers, add one additional serving from the milk, yogurt, and cheese group.

*Names of food groups are abbreviated as follows: milk = milk, yogurt, and cheese group; meat = meat, poultry, fish, dry beans, eggs, and nuts group; bread = bread, cereal, rice, and pasta group; fat/sweet = fats, oils, and sweets category.

Overall, the Food Guide Pyramid incorporates the foundations of a healthy diet: variety, balance, and moderation. The nutritional adequacy of diets planned using this tool, however, depends on the selection of a variety of foods. In addition, to ensure enough vitamin E, vitamin B-6, magnesium, and zinc—nutrients sometimes low in diets based on this plan—consider the following advice:

1. Choose primarily low-fat and nonfat items from the milk, yogurt, and cheese group. By reducing energy intake in this way, you can select more items from other food groups.
2. Include plant foods that are good sources of proteins, such as beans, at least several times a week because these are rich in minerals and dietary fiber.
3. For vegetables and fruits, try to include a dark green vegetable for vitamin A and a vitamin C–rich fruit, such as an orange, every day. Surveys show that only 25% of adults eat a green vegetable on any given day. Increased consumption of these foods is important because they contribute vitamins, minerals, dietary fiber, and phytochemicals.
4. Choose whole-grain varieties of breads, cereals, rice, and pasta often because they contribute dietary fiber. A plate about two-thirds covered by grains, fruits, and vegetables and one-third or less covered by protein-rich foods promotes this diet advice. As well, a daily serving of a whole-grain ready-to-eat breakfast cereal is an excellent choice because the vitamins and minerals typically added to it, along with dietary fiber, help fill in the potential gaps listed earlier.

Following the Food Guide Pyramid makes it possible to create daily diets containing as few as 1600 to 1800 kcal (review Table 2-7), sufficient for a sedentary adult or an older person. Not following this advice can leave a diet of 1600 to 1800 kcal short on the nutrients just mentioned. Recall that excessive consumption of any one food—even ones considered "healthy"—is also undesirable and possibly risky.

If 1600 to 1800 kcal represents too much food energy for you, you should first consider becoming more physically active rather than eating less. Obtaining enough nutrients from a diet that supplies fewer than 1600 kcal/day is very difficult. If you can't increase your energy output, you can make a special attempt to choose regularly some nutrient-fortified foods (e.g., breakfast cereals) or take a balanced nutrient supplement (see Chapter 9). In addition, for those whose diets do not include meat or other animal products, the Nutrition Perspective on vegetarianism in Chapter 7 provides advice on adapting the Food Guide Pyramid to that dietary practice.

Evaluation of the Current American Diet Using the Food Guide Pyramid

The average American diet, based on surveys, fails to meet the serving recommendations in the Food Guide Pyramid for many food groups. For example, the average diet includes only one to two fruit servings (rather than the recommended two to four servings) and only two to three vegetable servings (rather than three to five servings), and much of that comes from potatoes, not a particularly nutrient-dense vegetable choice. Overall, fruits and vegetables are the most underrepresented groups. In contrast, the fats, oils, and sweets are well represented.[11]

Criticisms of the Food Guide Pyramid

The Food Guide Pyramid has recently come under criticism on three accounts (excluding the call for the elimination of all animal products issued by some groups). First, some people have difficulty digesting large amounts of the sugar lactose; this is present in appreciable amounts in many dairy products. Singling out dairy products in the pyramid has been criticized as inappropriate for these people. Ways to address this concern are to consume moderate amounts of dairy products at any one time or to consume yogurt (most of the lactose is broken down in the small intestine by the bacteria in the yogurt; see Chapter 5 for other options). A second criticism is that refined grains and whole grains are lumped together; it would be healthier to emphasize primarily whole-grain choices because of their fiber content.[28] This is relatively easy to implement (see Chapter 5). Third, fat need not necessarily be placed at the top of the pyramid, indicating caution should be used with intake. Fat could be a more central part of the diet if the fat is primarily from plant oils. The Mediterranean diet discussed in the Nutrition Perspective at the end of this chapter is an example of one of such plan. And, as you will see in the next section, the latest Dietary Guidelines issued by the federal government recommend

Other food pyramids have been proposed by various nutrition organizations. The Nutrition Perspective at the end of this chapter discusses the Latin American, Asian, Mediterranean, and Soul Food pyramids.

Another criticism of the Food Guide Pyramid is the advice is not specific enough. For example, most vegetable servings could be potatoes, or none of the bread, cereal, rice, and pasta servings could be whole-grain. In either case, diet quality is compromised.

moderation in fat consumption (limitation is primarily directed to saturated fat in-take). This allows for more plant oil use than is suggested by the placement of fat at the top of the pyramid. Whole grains are also emphasized in the latest Dietary Guidelines.

In the final analysis, however, the Food Guide Pyramid provides enough latitude that one can make appropriate choices based on personal health concerns and still consume the recommended servings of the five food groups. Some additional fat from plant oils is fine, as long as overall calorie balance is maintained. Following a diet that avoids all animal products, which will be covered in Chapter 7, is another matter altogether.

How Does Your Current Diet Rate?

Regularly comparing your daily food intake with the Food Guide Pyramid recommendations is a relatively simple way to evaluate your overall diet. Strive to meet the recommendations. If that is not possible, identify the nutrients that are low in your diet based on the nutrients found in each food group (review Table 2-6). For example, if you do not consume enough servings from the milk, yogurt, and cheese group, your calcium intake is most likely too low. After completing the Take Action activities at the end of this chapter, you will be able to determine more accurately which nutrients are too low in your current diet and by how much. Armed with this knowledge, find foods that you enjoy that supply those nutrients, such as calcium-fortified orange juice. Customizing the Food Guide Pyramid to accommodate your own food habits may seem a daunting task now, but it is not difficult once you gain some additional nutrition knowledge. To learn more, see the web page sponsored by USDA (http://www.usda.gov/cnpp). At this site, you can view the entire booklet describing the pyramid.

CONCEPT CHECK

The Food Guide Pyramid translates the general needs for carbohydrate, protein, fat, vitamins, and minerals into the recommended number of daily servings from each of five major food groups. It is a convenient and valuable tool for planning daily menus.

■ Dietary Guidelines—Another Tool for Menu Planning

The Food Guide Pyramid was designed to help meet nutritional needs for carbohydrate, protein, fat, vitamins, and minerals. However, most of the major chronic "killer" diseases in America, such as cardiovascular disease, cancer, and alcoholism, are not primarily associated with deficiencies of these nutrients. Nor are deficiency diseases such as scurvy (vitamin C deficiency) and pellagra (niacin deficiency), still common. For many Americans, the primary dietary culprit is an overconsumption of one or more of the following: energy, saturated fat, cholesterol, alcohol, and sodium (salt). Underconsumption of calcium, iron, folate and other B-vitamins, zinc, or dietary fiber is also a problem for some people, but easy to remedy as the major dietary problems are addressed.[22]

In response to concerns regarding these killer disease patterns in the United States, since 1980 the USDA and Department of Health and Human Services (DHHS) have published **Dietary Guidelines** to aid diet planning. The latest Dietary Guidelines begin with three overarching messages and then list 10 specific guidelines:

Aim for Fitness

1. *Aim for a healthy weight* (body mass index of 18.5 to 24.9; see Chapter 13).
2. *Be physically active each day* (about 30 minutes per day as a minimum; see Chapter 14).

Dietary Guidelines General goals for nutrient intakes and diet composition set by the USDA and the Department of Health and Human Services (DHHS).

Build a Healthy Base

3. *Let the pyramid guide your food choices* (see the previous section on the Food Guide Pyramid).
4. *Choose a variety of grains daily, especially whole grains* (see the Food Guide Pyramid and Chapter 5).
5. *Choose a variety of fruits and vegetables daily* (see the Food Guide Pyramid).
6. *Keep foods safe to eat* (especially proper cooking and refrigeration of perishable foods; see Chapter 19).

Choose Sensibly

7. *Choose a diet that is low in saturated fat and cholesterol and moderate in total fat* (animal fats are the chief culprits; see Chapter 6).
8. *Choose beverages and foods to moderate your intake of sugars* (soft drinks, cookies, and candy are the chief culprits; see Chapter 5).
9. *Choose and prepare foods with less salt* (it is easy to adjust to a lower salt intake; see Chapter 11).
10. *If you drink alcoholic beverages, do so in moderation* (no more than one to two drinks per day; see Chapter 8).

These guidelines are intended for healthy children (2 years and older) and adults of any age. You can view the entire Dietary Guidelines booklet at http://www.usda.gov/cnpp.

Practical Use of the Dietary Guidelines

The Dietary Guidelines are designed to promote adequate vitamin and mineral intake. The guidelines also emphasize changes that will reduce the risk of obesity, hypertension, cardiovascular disease, type 2 diabetes, alcoholism, and food-borne illness.

The Dietary Guidelines are not difficult to implement (Table 2-8). In addition, this overall diet approach is not especially expensive, as some people suspect. Fruits, vegetables, and low-fat and nonfat milk are no more expensive than the chips, cookies, and sugared soft drinks they should in part replace.

Note also that diet recommendations for adults have been issued by other scientific groups, such as the American Heart Association, U.S. Surgeon General, National Academy of Sciences, American Cancer Society, Canadian Ministries of Health (see Appendix C), and World Health Organization. All are consistent with the spirit of the Dietary Guidelines. These groups encourage people to modify their eating behavior in ways that are both healthful and pleasurable.[2, 24]

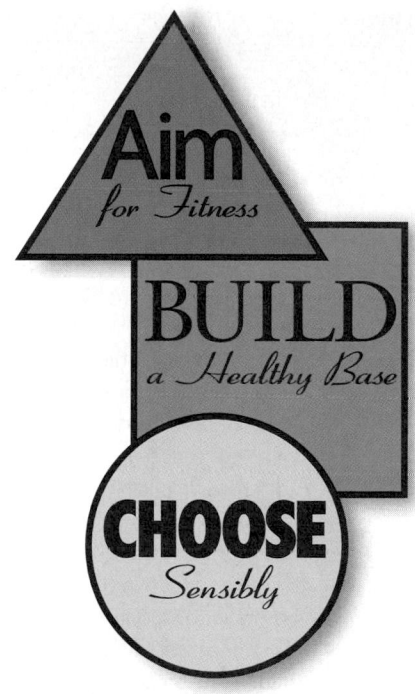

Logo for the current Dietary Guidelines.

*A*dvice from the American Dietetic Association suggests five basic principles with regard to diet and health. Be realistic, making small changes over time. Be adventurous, trying new foods regularly. Be flexible, balancing some sweet and fatty foods with physical activity. Be sensible, including favorite foods in smaller portions. Finally, be active, including physical activity in daily life.

TABLE 2-8   Advice for Applying the Dietary Guidelines to Practical Situations

You Usually Eat This	Reconsider and Eat This
White bread	Whole-wheat bread (fewer nutrients lost in refinement/processing and more fiber)
Sugared breakfast cereal	Low-sugar (and high-fiber) cereal (use the kcal you save for a side dish of fruit)
Cheeseburger and French fries	Hamburger (hold the mayonnaise) and baked beans (for less fat and cholesterol and the benefits of plant proteins)
Potato salad at the salad bar	Three-bean salad
Doughnut, chips, salty snack foods	Bran muffin or bagel (little or no cream cheese)
Soft drinks	Diet soft drinks (save the kcal for more nutritious foods)
Boiled vegetables	Steamed vegetables (for more nutrient retention)
Canned vegetables	Frozen vegetables (fewer nutrients lost in processing)
Fried meats	Broiled meats (watch the fat drain away)
Fatty meats, such as ribs	Lean meats, such as ground round (also, eat chicken and fish often)
Whole milk and ice cream	Low-fat or nonfat milk and sherbet or frozen yogurt (to reduce saturated fat intake)
Mayonnaise or sour cream salad dressing	Oil and vinegar dressings or diet varieties (to save kcal)
Cookies for a snack	Popcorn (air popped with minimal margarine or butter)
Heavily salted foods	Foods flavored primarily with herbs, spices, lemon juice

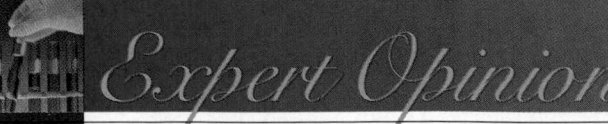

Expert Opinion

WHAT SHOULD I EAT TO LIVE LONGER?

David M. Klurfeld, Ph.D.

The fountain of youth emanates, according to popular culture, from a proper diet. This rosy view stems, in part, from the dietary recommendations made to reduce the risk of several chronic diseases. Implicit in the recommendations is the promise of longer life—but how long and for whom?

Cardiovascular disease and cancer account for almost three-fourths of all deaths in affluent societies. One reason for this is that many causes of premature death—infections, poor sanitation, and accidents—have been dramatically allayed. This change translates into a life expectancy at birth in the United States of 76.5 years. At the same time, more people are overweight, and health-care costs are a greater percentage of the economy than in any other country, so we have lots of room for improvement. In spite of our highly publicized "killer diet," deaths from cardiovascular disease, stroke, and cancer unrelated to tobacco have all declined markedly over the past 30 years.

We don't know for sure why this drop has occurred, but it has been attributed, in part, to less use of tobacco and reductions in hypertension and blood cholesterol, along with better medical care. These changes in risk factors point to the multifaceted causes of both cardiovascular disease and cancer. In addition, since many environmental factors interact with genetic predisposition to a disease, we simply don't know enough to attribute a specific portion of risk for chronic diseases to diet. Many of the estimates of dietary contribution to the risk of cancer are made by default; that is, cancers that are not traceable to other risk factors are often lumped as being caused by diet. Although many health recommendations emphasize a Mediterranean diet, there are markedly different diets in this region of the world that fall under the category (see the Nutrition Perspective at the end of this chapter for one example). In addition, there is no evidence that populations living around the Mediterranean Sea have a longer life expectancy than people in the United States, Japan, or Scandinavia, where diets differ substantially.

Actually, the only dietary change effective in reducing many types of cancer and increasing life span in animals is caloric restriction. When energy intake is reduced to about 70% of what would normally be eaten—but all nutrient requirements are met—the result is physiologically younger animals. Long-term studies of monkeys eating such low-calorie diets have found reduced body fat and lower blood glucose, insulin, and lipids when compared with animals given free access to food. These studies have been in progress long enough for some of the monkeys to have died from natural causes; far fewer in the low-calorie groups have died. Circumstantial evidence for a calorie effect in people includes the fact that the highest concentration of centenarians is found in Okinawa. The people over 100 years old have been found to consume less energy and to eat more fruits, vegetables, and meat than in the rest of Japan. In addition, most of the very elderly in *every* society tend to be slimmer and shorter than average.

Can we reduce cardiovascular disease by dietary means with some degree of certainty? Probably, according to epidemiological and animal data. But epidemiology offers only leads—it cannot prove cause and effect. Today, there's little controversy over increased risk of cardiovascular disease with elevated blood cholesterol. What is debated is at what point dietary or drug treatments should begin. And, although the consensus recommendation is to reduce blood cholesterol below 200 mg/dl (dl stands for 100 ml), some argue that this is too modest a target, whereas others contend that it's an unnecessary one. Still, the slope of cardiovascular disease versus blood cholesterol is quite steep at the upper concentrations (over 250 mg/dl) but shallow near 210 mg/dl, the average adult concentration. Thus, much less benefit is derived from lowering average cholesterol values.

Several prospective epidemiological studies have reported that a healthy dietary pattern, rather than an intake of individual nutrients predicts longer life expectancy. One study found a strong dose-response relationship evidenced by decreased mortality in subjects who consumed more fruits, vegetables, whole grains, low-fat dairy, and lean meats and poultry. Another large study implicated high consumption of cereal fiber, some fish, the vitamin folate, along with a high polyunsaturated-saturated fat ratio, and low consumption of trans fatty acids (present primarily in stick margarine, shortening, and deep-fat-fried foods; see Chapter 6), simple sugars, and refined carbohydrates as a dietary pattern linked to a reduced risk of cardiovascular disease. However, this dietary pattern strongly correlated with lower weight-for-height status, more exercise, nonsmoking, moderate alcohol intake, and daily use of vitamin/mineral supplements. Although scientists often attempt to sort out these factors to find the most important, it is becoming apparent that a combination of healthy habits achieves the desired benefits.

There's a strong statistical correlation of gross national product, telephones, flush toilets, and other signs of wealth with the incidence of cancer and cardiovascular disease because life expectancy is longer in more affluent countries. The chronic diseases are much more common among older individuals. Populations that can afford to eat a lot of fat, sugar, and salt do so because these three dietary components are what people think make food taste good.

Everyone in the country has been told to follow a low-sodium diet when only a minority of young and middle-aged adults are hypertensive, and only some of those are salt sensitive. There is also substantial evidence implicating low protein and high calcium, potassium, and magnesium intakes in controlling blood pressure.

A potential explanation for the lack of uniformity in response to dietary factors is that perhaps only some of the population shows elevated blood cholesterol from eating saturated fat, and only some people are genetically predisposed to colon cancer, whereas a fortunate few are destined to live long, healthy lives no matter what rules they violate. This observation does not discount the importance of nutrition in longevity but suggests that recommendations for dietary modification should not be blanket public health policies. Instead, these need to be made on individualized bases—that is, dietary guidelines for those who are at increased risk for specific diseases via family history or the presence of other risk factors may differ. This conclusion should not be taken to mean that a good diet is unimportant. High consumption of fruits, vegetables, and whole grains is associated with a lower incidence of obesity, type 2 diabetes, intestinal disorders, cardiovascular disease, and cancer.

Observational studies have implicated a high intake of vitamin E as a protective factor against cardiovascular disease.

However, increased survival has not been found in bottles of antioxidant supplements. Four of five intervention studies have failed to find a significant benefit of vitamin E on cardiovascular disease rates or mortality. However, diets low in this vitamin and other antioxidants are associated with excess mortality from both cancer and cardiovascular disease.

The explanation that diet modification wouldn't hurt may satisfy some, but it's certainly not scientific. The burden of proof falls on those who suggest specific dietary changes, rather than on those who question the efficacy of those changes. Although what is written today will surely be outdated in the future, there are two nutritional rules that will make sense over time: (1) Eat a variety of foods and (2) consume all foods in moderation. Combining these recommendations with adequate physical activity and the avoidance of tobacco and excess alcohol is a lifestyle that promotes good health and extra years, whereas dietary changes made in isolation may be doomed to failure—boring, perhaps, but advice one can take to heart.

Dr. Klurfeld is professor and chairman of the Department of Nutrition and Food Science at Wayne State University. His research interests include the reduction of cancer and cardiovascular disease through diet, lipid metabolism, and dietary fiber.

The Dietary Guidelines and You

When using the Dietary Guidelines, you should consider your own state of health. Dr. David Klurfeld discusses the importance of this concept in his Expert Opinion. Make specific changes and see whether they are effective. Note that results are sometimes disappointing, even when you are following a diet change very closely. Some people can eat a lot of saturated fat and still keep blood cholesterol under control. Other people, unfortunately, have high blood cholesterol even if they eat a diet low in saturated fat. Differences in genetic background are a key cause, as emphasized in Chapter 1. Thus, we have individual nutritional needs and risks of developing certain diseases. One's diet should be planned with this in mind, responding to one's current health status and family history for specific diseases. However, tailoring a unique nutrition program for every North American citizen is unrealistic. The Food Guide Pyramid and the Dietary Guidelines provide adults with simple advice, which can be actively practiced by anyone willing to take a step toward good health.

There is no "optimal" diet. Instead, there are numerous healthful diets. The web page http://www.ificinfo.health.org is a great source to lead you in that direction.

CONCEPT CHECK

Dietary Guidelines have been set by a variety of private and government organizations. These guidelines are designed to reduce the risk of developing obesity, hypertension, type 2 diabetes, cardiovascular disease, and alcoholism. To do so, they recommend eating a variety of foods, which is fostered by following the Food Guide Pyramid. They also recommend performing regular physical activity, aiming for a healthy weight, and moderating total fat, saturated fat, salt, sugar, and alcohol intake, while focusing more on fruits, vegetables, and grain products in daily menu planning. Safe food preparation and storage are also highlighted.

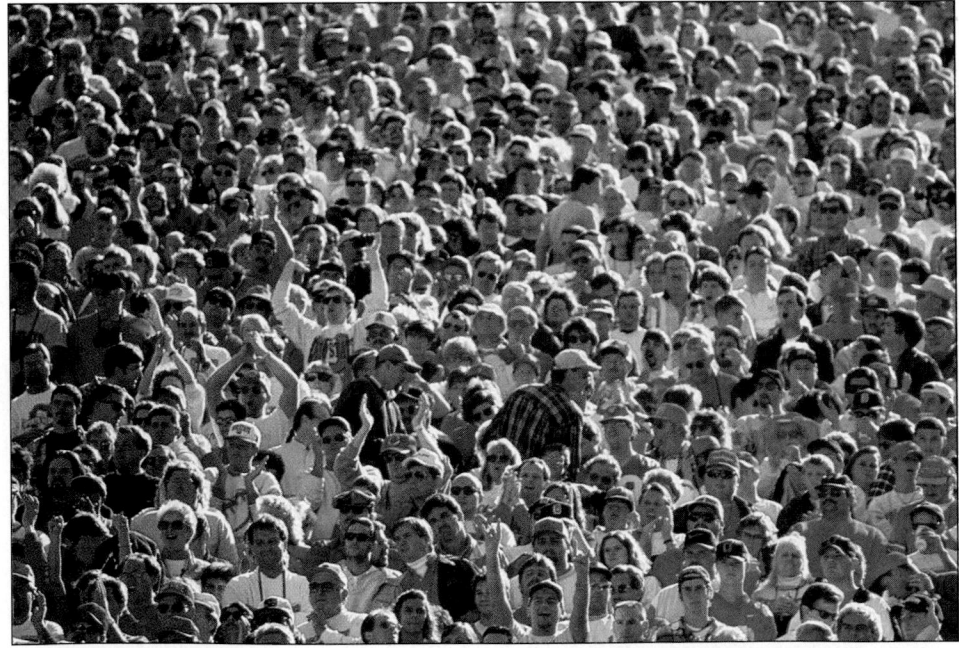

Nutrition recommendations are often made on a population-wide basis. However, in some cases, it would be more appropriate if we were evaluated on an individual basis.

The most positive aspect of Andy's diet is that it contains adequate protein, zinc, and iron because it is rich in animal protein. On the downside, his diet is low in calcium, some B-vitamins (such as folate), and vitamin C. This is because it is low in dairy products, fruits, and vegetables. It is also low in many of the phytochemical (plant-based) substances discussed at the beginning of this chapter. In addition, dietary fiber intake is low because fast-food restaurants primarily use refined grain products, rather than whole-grain products. And, since most super-sized options apply to foods rich in fat (French fries) and sugar (soft drinks), his diet is likely excessive in those two components.

He could alternate between tacos and bean burritos to gain the benefits of plant proteins in a diet. He could choose a low-fat granola bar instead of the candy bar for breakfast, or he could take the time to eat a bowl of whole-grain breakfast cereal with low-fat or nonfat milk to increase fiber intake (and calcium intake in the latter case). He could also order milk at least half the time at his restaurant visits and substitute diet soft drinks for the regular variety. This would help *moderate* his sugar intake. Overall, his diet is most lacking in a variety of fruit and vegetable choices and dairy products because it lacks *variety* in food choice and *balance* among the five food groups.

■ WHAT DO FOOD LABELS HAVE TO OFFER IN DIET PLANNING?

Today, nearly all foods sold in the grocery store must be labeled with the product name, name and address of the manufacturer, amount of product in the package, and ingredients listed in descending order by weight. This food and beverage labeling is monitored by government agencies such as Food and Drug Administration (FDA). The listing of certain food constituents also is required—specifically, on a Nutrition Facts panel (Fig. 2-4). Use this information to learn more about what you eat. The following components must be listed: total kcal, kcal from fat, total fat, saturated fat, cholesterol, sodium, total carbohydrate, dietary fiber, sugars, protein, vitamin A, vitamin C, calcium, and iron. In addition to these required components, manufacturers can choose to list polyunsaturated and monounsaturated fat, potassium, dietary fiber, and others. Listing these components is *required,* however, if a claim is made about the health benefits of the specific nutrient (see the section in this chapter entitled "Health Claims on Food Labels") or if the food is fortified with that nutrient.

The percentage of the Daily Value (% Daily Value) is usually given for each nutrient per serving. It is important to understand that these percentages are based on a 2000 kcal diet. In other words, they are not as applicable to people who require considerably more or less than 2000 kcal per day with respect to fat and carbohydrate intake.

Serving sizes on the Nutrition Facts panel must be consistent between similar foods. This means that all brands of ice cream, for example, must use the same serving size on their labels. In addition, food claims made on packages must follow legal definitions (Table 2-9). For example, if a product claims to be "low sodium," it must have 140 mg of sodium or less per serving.

Many manufacturers list the Daily Values set for dietary components such as fat, cholesterol, and carbohydrate on the Nutrition Facts panel. This can be useful as a reference point. As noted before they are based on 2000 kcal; if the label is large enough, amounts based on 2500 kcal are listed as well. Recall also from Chapter 1 that the term *calories* is used to express energy content on the labels; however, scientifically speaking this is an incorrect use of the term.

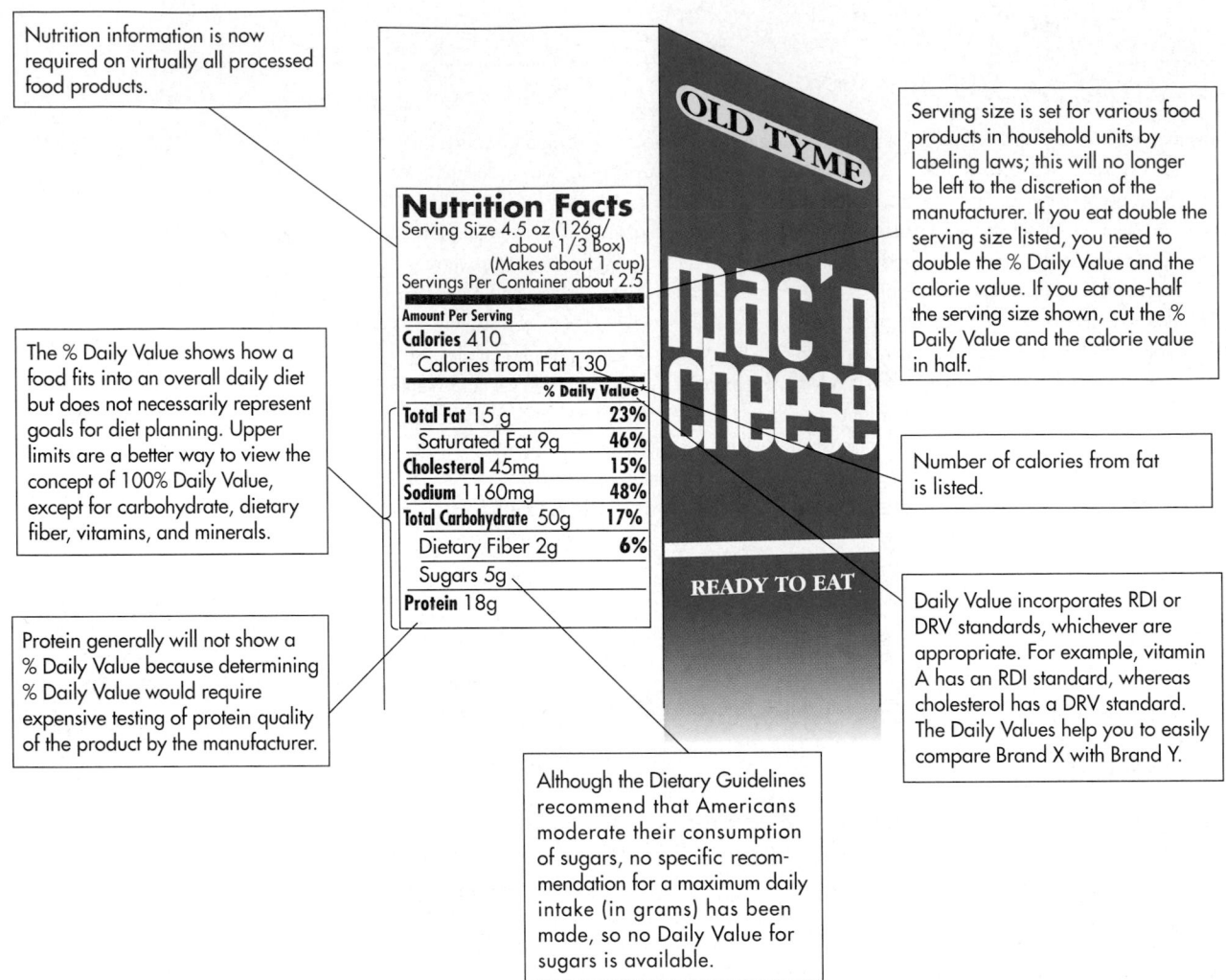

Nutrition information is now required on virtually all processed food products.

The % Daily Value shows how a food fits into an overall daily diet but does not necessarily represent goals for diet planning. Upper limits are a better way to view the concept of 100% Daily Value, except for carbohydrate, dietary fiber, vitamins, and minerals.

Protein generally will not show a % Daily Value because determining % Daily Value would require expensive testing of protein quality of the product by the manufacturer.

Serving size is set for various food products in household units by labeling laws; this will no longer be left to the discretion of the manufacturer. If you eat double the serving size listed, you need to double the % Daily Value and the calorie value. If you eat one-half the serving size shown, cut the % Daily Value and the calorie value in half.

Number of calories from fat is listed.

Daily Value incorporates RDI or DRV standards, whichever are appropriate. For example, vitamin A has an RDI standard, whereas cholesterol has a DRV standard. The Daily Values help you to easily compare Brand X with Brand Y.

Although the Dietary Guidelines recommend that Americans moderate their consumption of sugars, no specific recommendation for a maximum daily intake (in grams) has been made, so no Daily Value for sugars is available.

Nutrition Facts
Serving Size 4.5 oz (126g/ about 1/3 Box) (Makes about 1 cup)
Servings Per Container about 2.5

Amount Per Serving

Calories 410

Calories from Fat 130

% Daily Value*

Total Fat 15 g	**23%**
Saturated Fat 9g	**46%**
Cholesterol 45mg	**15%**
Sodium 1160mg	**48%**
Total Carbohydrate 50g	**17%**
Dietary Fiber 2g	**6%**
Sugars 5g	
Protein 18g	

OLD TYME
mac'n cheese
READY TO EAT

■ FIGURE **2-4a** The Nutrition Facts panel on a current food label. The box is broken into two parts: (*a*) the top and (*b*) the bottom. The % Daily Value listed on the label is the percentage of the generally accepted amount of a nutrient needed daily that is present in one serving of the product. You can use the % Daily Values to compare your diet with current nutrition recommendations for certain diet components. Let's consider dietary fiber. Assume that you consume 2000 kcal per day, which is the energy intake corresponding to the % Daily Values listed on labels. If the total % Daily Value for dietary fiber in all the foods you eat in one day adds up to 100%, your diet meets the recommendations for dietary fiber.
Illustration by William Ober.

■ Exceptions to Food Labeling

Foods such as fresh fruits and vegetables, fish, meats, and poultry currently are not required to have Nutrition Facts labels. However, many grocers and some meat packers have voluntarily chosen to provide their customers with information on these products. Nutrition Facts labels on meat products will also likely be required in the coming years. The next time you are at the grocery store, ask where you might find information on the fresh products that do not have a Nutrition Facts panel. You will likely find a poster or pamphlet near the product; often, these pamphlets contain recipes in which to use your favorite fruit, vegetable, or cut of meat. They may even assist you in your endeavor to improve your diet.

Because protein deficiency is not a public health concern in the United States, declaration of the % Daily Value for protein is not mandatory on foods for people over 4 years of age. If the % Daily Value is given on a label, FDA requires that the product be analyzed for protein quality. Because this procedure is expensive and time-

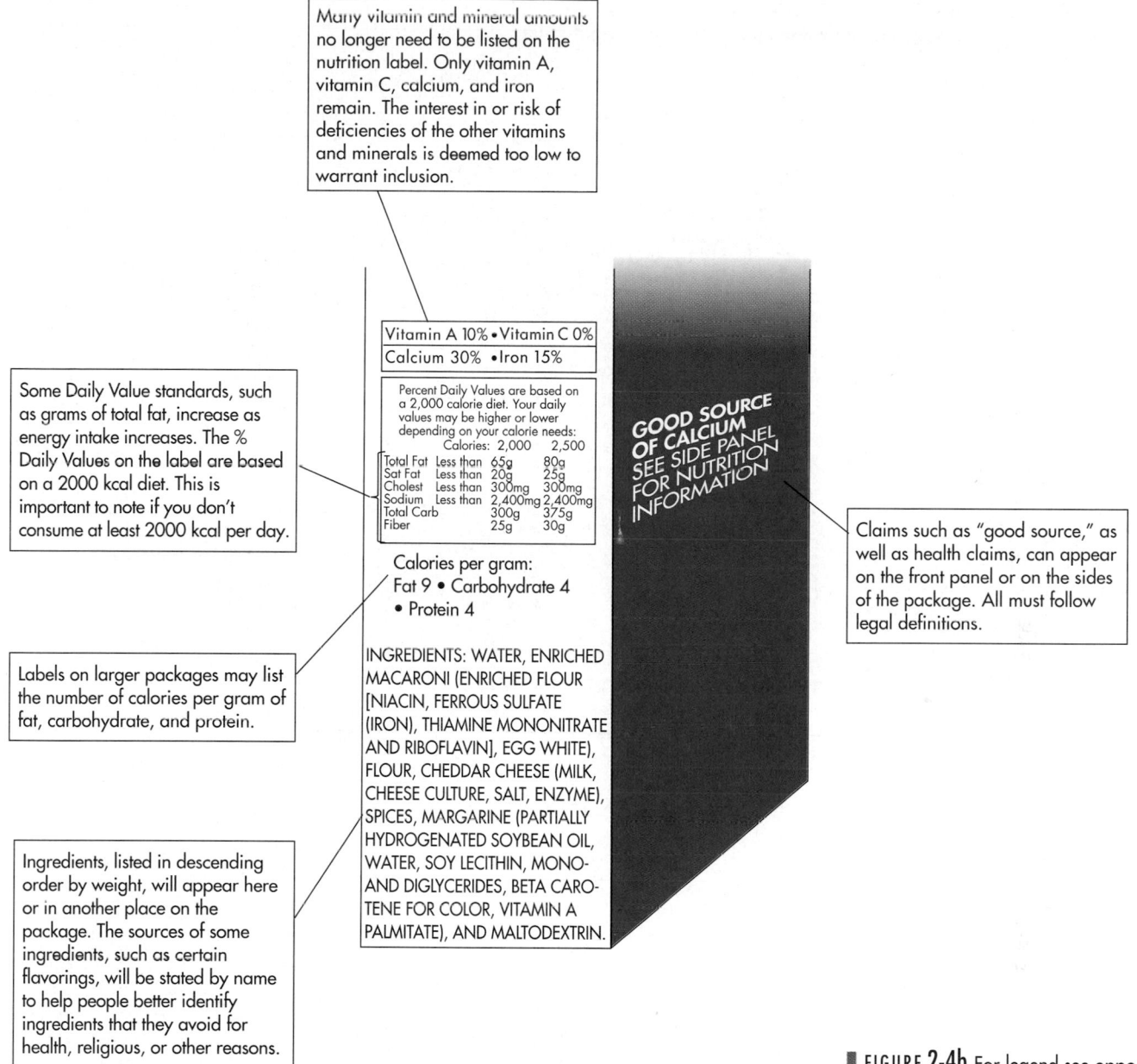

Many vitamin and mineral amounts no longer need to be listed on the nutrition label. Only vitamin A, vitamin C, calcium, and iron remain. The interest in or risk of deficiencies of the other vitamins and minerals is deemed too low to warrant inclusion.

Vitamin A 10% • Vitamin C 0%
Calcium 30% • Iron 15%

Some Daily Value standards, such as grams of total fat, increase as energy intake increases. The % Daily Values on the label are based on a 2000 kcal diet. This is important to note if you don't consume at least 2000 kcal per day.

Percent Daily Values are based on a 2,000 calorie diet. Your daily values may be higher or lower depending on your calorie needs:

		Calories:	2,000	2,500
Total Fat	Less than		65g	80g
Sat Fat	Less than		20g	25g
Cholest	Less than		300mg	300mg
Sodium	Less than		2,400mg	2,400mg
Total Carb			300g	375g
Fiber			25g	30g

Calories per gram:
Fat 9 • Carbohydrate 4
• Protein 4

Labels on larger packages may list the number of calories per gram of fat, carbohydrate, and protein.

INGREDIENTS: WATER, ENRICHED MACARONI (ENRICHED FLOUR [NIACIN, FERROUS SULFATE (IRON), THIAMINE MONONITRATE AND RIBOFLAVIN], EGG WHITE), FLOUR, CHEDDAR CHEESE (MILK, CHEESE CULTURE, SALT, ENZYME), SPICES, MARGARINE (PARTIALLY HYDROGENATED SOYBEAN OIL, WATER, SOY LECITHIN, MONO- AND DIGLYCERIDES, BETA CARO- TENE FOR COLOR, VITAMIN A PALMITATE), AND MALTODEXTRIN.

GOOD SOURCE OF CALCIUM SEE SIDE PANEL FOR NUTRITION INFORMATION

Claims such as "good source," as well as health claims, can appear on the front panel or on the sides of the package. All must follow legal definitions.

Ingredients, listed in descending order by weight, will appear here or in another place on the package. The sources of some ingredients, such as certain flavorings, will be stated by name to help people better identify ingredients that they avoid for health, religious, or other reasons.

■ FIGURE 2-4b For legend see opposite page.

consuming, many companies opt not to list a % Daily Value for protein rather than undergo the expense. However, labels on food for infants and children under 4 years of age must include the % Daily Value for protein, as must the labels on any food carrying a claim about protein content (see Chapter 17).

■ Health Claims on Food Labels

As a marketing tool directed toward the health-conscious consumer, food manufacturers are asserting that their products have all sorts of health benefits. This campaign began in earnest in 1984, when the Kellogg Company, in conjunction with The National Cancer Institute, printed a health claim on its "high-fiber" cereals, stating that fiber may help prevent certain forms of cancer. This type of label message was not allowed at the time and caused a heated debate among nutrition scientists. After reviewing hundreds of comments on the proposed rule allowing health claims, the Food and Drug Administration (FDA), which has legal oversight over

TABLE 2-9   Definitions for Comparative and Absolute Nutrient Claims on Food Labels

Sugar

- *Sugar free:* less than 0.5 grams (g) per serving
- *No added sugar; without added sugar; no sugar added:*
  - No sugars were added during processing or packing, including ingredients that contain sugars (for example, fruit juices, applesauce, or jam).
  - Processing does not increase the sugar content above the amount naturally present in the ingredients. (A functionally insignificant increase in sugars is acceptable for processes used for purposes other than increasing sugar content.)
  - The food that it resembles and for which it substitutes normally contains added sugars.
  - If the food doesn't meet the requirements for a low- or reduced-calorie food, the product bears a statement that the food is not low calorie or calorie reduced and directs consumers' attention to the nutrition panel for further information on sugars and calorie content.
- *Reduced sugar:* at least 25% less sugar per serving than reference food

Calories

- *Calorie free:* fewer than 5 kcal per serving
- *Low calorie:* 40 kcal or less per serving and, if the serving is 30 g or less or 2 tablespoons or less, per 50 g of the food
- *Reduced or fewer calories:* at least 25% fewer kcal per serving than reference food

Fiber

- *High fiber:* 5 g or more per serving (foods making high-fiber claims must meet the definition for low fat, or the level of total fat must appear next to the high-fiber claim)
- *Food source of fiber:* 2.5 to 4.9 g per serving
- *More or added fiber:* at least 2.5 g more per serving than reference food

Fat

- *Fat free:* less than 0.5 g of fat per serving
- *Saturated fat free:* less than 0.5 g per serving, and the level of trans fatty acids does not exceed 0.5 g per serving

- *Low fat:* 3 g or less per serving and, if the serving is 30 g or less or 2 tablespoons or less, per 50 g of the food. 2% milk can no longer be labeled low-fat, as it exceeds 3 g per serving. *Reduced fat* will be the term used instead.
- *Low saturated fat:* 1 g or less per serving and not more than 15% of kcal from saturated fatty acids
- *Reduced or less fat:* at least 25% less per serving than reference food
- *Reduced or less saturated fat:* at least 25% less per serving than reference food

Cholesterol

- *Cholesterol free:* less than 2 mg of cholesterol and 2 g or less of saturated fat per serving
- *Low cholesterol:* 20 mg or less cholesterol and 2 g or less of saturated fat per serving and, if the serving is 30 g or less or 2 tablespoons or less, per 50 g of the food
- *Reduced or less cholesterol:* at least 25% less cholesterol and 2 g or less of saturated fat per serving than reference food

Sodium

- *Sodium free:* less than 5 mg per serving
- *Very low sodium:* 35 mg or less per serving and, if the serving is 30 g or less or 2 tablespoons or less, per 50 g of the food
- *Low sodium:* 140 mg or less per serving and, if the serving is 30 g or less or 2 tablespoons or less, per 50 g of the food
- *Light in sodium:* at least 50% less per serving than reference food
- *Reduced or less sodium:* at least 25% less per serving than reference food

Other Terms

- *Fortified/enriched:* Vitamins and/or minerals have been added to the product in amounts in excess of at least 10% of that normally present in the usual product.
- *Healthy:* An individual food that is low fat and low saturated fat and has no more than 360 to 480 mg of sodium or 60 mg of cholesterol per serving can be labeled "healthy" if it provides at least 10% of vitamin A, vitamin C, protein, calcium, iron, or dietary fiber.
- *Light or lite:* The descriptor *light* or *lite* can mean two things: first, that a nutritionally

altered product contains one-third fewer kcal or half the fat of reference food (if the food derives 50% or more of its kcal from fat, the reduction must be 50% of the fat) and, second, that the sodium content of a low-calorie, low-fat food has been reduced by 50%. 2% milk can no longer be labeled low fat because it has more than 3 g of fat per serving. In addition, "light in sodium" may be used for foods in which the sodium content has been reduced by at least 50%. The term *light* may still be used to describe such properties as texture and color, as long as the label explains the intent—for example, "light brown sugar" and "light and fluffy."

- *Diet:* A food may be labeled with terms such as *diet, dietetic, artificially sweetened,* or *sweetened with nonnutritive sweetener* only if the claim is not false or misleading. The food can also be labeled *low calorie* or *reduced calorie.*
- *Good source: Good source* means that a food contains 10 to 19% of the Daily Value for a particular nutrient.
- *High: High* means that a food contains 20% or more of the Daily Value for a particular nutrient.
- *Organic:* Federal standards for organic foods allow claims when much of the ingredients do not use chemical fertilizers or pesticides, genetic engineering, sewage sludge, antibiotics, or irradiation in their production. At least 95% of ingredients must meet these guidelines to be labeled "organic" on the front of the package. For livestock, the animals need to be allowed to graze outdoors and as well be fed organic feed. They also cannot be exposed to antibiotics or growth hormones.
- *Natural:* The food must be free of food colors, synthetic flavors, or any other synthetic substance.

The following terms apply only to meat and poultry products regulated by USDA.

- *Extra lean:* less than 5 g of fat, 2 g of saturated fat, and 95 mg of cholesterol per serving (or 100 g of an individual food)
- *Lean:* less than 10 g of fat, 4.5 g of saturated fat, and 95 mg of cholesterol per serving (or 100 g of an individual food)

Many definitions are from FDA's *Dictionary of Terms,* as established in conjunction with the 1990 NLEA.

most food products, decided to permit this and other health claims with certain restrictions.

Currently, FDA limits the use of health messages to specific diseases in which there is significant scientific agreement concerning the relationship between a nutrient, food, or food constituent and the disease.[12] The claims allowed at this time may show a link between the following:

- A diet with enough calcium and a reduced risk of osteoporosis
- A diet low in total fat and a reduced risk of some cancers
- A diet low in saturated fat and cholesterol and a reduced risk of cardiovascular (heart) disease
- A diet rich in dietary fiber–containing grain products, fruits, and vegetables and a reduced risk of some cancers
- A diet low in sodium and high in potassium and a reduced risk of hypertension and stroke
- A diet rich in fruits and vegetables and a reduced risk of some cancers
- A diet adequate in the vitamin folate and a reduced risk of neural tube defects (a type of birth defect)
- Use of sugarless gum and a reduced risk of tooth decay, especially when compared with foods high in sugars and starches
- A diet rich in fruits, vegetables, and grain products that contain fiber and a reduced risk of cardiovascular disease. Oats (oatmeal, oat bran, and oat flour) and psyllium are two fiber-rich ingredients that can be singled out in reducing the risk of cardiovascular disease, as long as the statement also says the diet should also be low in saturated fat and cholesterol.
- A diet rich in whole-grain foods and other plant foods, as well as low in total fat, saturated fat, and cholesterol, and a reduced risk of cardiovascular disease and certain cancers
- A diet low in saturated fat and cholesterol that also includes 25 g of soy protein and a reduced risk of cardiovascular disease. The statement "one serving of the (name food) provides _____ g of soy protein" must also appear as part of the health claim.
- A diet rich in potassium and a reduced risk of stroke.
- Margarines containing plant stanol and sterol esters and a reduced risk of cardiovascular disease (see Chapter 6 for more details on plant stanol and sterol esters).

A "may" or "might" qualifier must be used in any statement.

In addition, before a health claim can be made for a food product, it must meet two general requirements. First, the food must be a "good source" (before fortification) of dietary fiber, protein, vitamin A, vitamin C, calcium, or iron. The legal definition of "good source" appeared in Table 2-9. Second, a single serving of the food product cannot contain more than 13 g of fat, 4 g of saturated fat, 60 mg of cholesterol, or 480 mg of sodium. If a food exceeds any one of these amounts, no health claim can be made for it, despite its other nutritional qualities. For example, even though whole milk is high in calcium, its label can't make the health claim about calcium and osteoporosis because whole milk contains 5 g of saturated fat per serving.

In addition, the product must meet criteria specific to the health claim being made. For example, a health claim regarding fat and cancer can be made only if the product contains 3 g or less of fat per serving, which is the standard for low-fat food.

The bottom line for health claims is honesty. FDA is vigilant in controlling the claims made about foods on supermarket shelves.[12]

Some products make so called "structure/function" claims, such as "improves blood circulation." These do not fall under FDA jurisdiction because of laws passed by Congress in 1994 (see Chapter 18). View any of these non-FDA-approved claims skeptically.

The Nutrition Facts panel on a food label provides key information for helping track one's food intake. Nutrient quantities are compared with the Daily Values and expressed on a percentage basis (% Daily Value). This information can be used to either increase or reduce intake of specific nutrients. Health claims on food labels are closely regulated by FDA. Fruits, vegetables, whole grains, soy, and rich sources of calcium are prominent among the foods that can make specific health claims.

■ EXCHANGE SYSTEM: A FINAL MENU-PLANNING TOOL

exchange system A system for classifying foods into numerous lists based on the foods' macronutrient composition and establishing serving sizes, so that one serving of each food on a list contains the same amount of carbohydrate, protein, fat, and energy content.

The **Exchange System** is a valuable tool for roughly estimating the energy, protein, carbohydrate, and fat content of a food or meal. This tool organizes many details of the nutrient composition of foods into a manageable framework. By using the Exchange System, you can plan daily menus to fall roughly within specific percentages of macronutrients without having to look up or memorize the nutrient values of numerous foods, so the time you spend now becoming familiar with the Exchange System will pay dividends in the future.

In the Exchange System, individual foods are placed into three broad groups: carbohydrate, meat and meat substitutes, and fat. Within these groups are lists that contain foods of similar macronutrient composition: various types of milk; fruit; vegetables; starch; other carbohydrates; meat and meat substitutes; and fat. These lists are designed so that, when the proper serving size is observed, each food on a list provides about the same amount of carbohydrate, protein, fat, and energy. This equality allows the exchange of foods on each list, hence the term *Exchange System*.

exchange The serving size of a food on a specific exchange list.

The Exchange System was originally developed for planning diabetic diets. Diabetes is easier to control if the person's diet has about the same composition day after day. If a certain number of **exchanges** from each of the various lists is eaten each day, that regularity is easier to achieve. However, because the Exchange System provides a quick way to estimate the energy, carbohydrate, protein, and fat content in any food or meal, it is a valuable menu-planning tool.

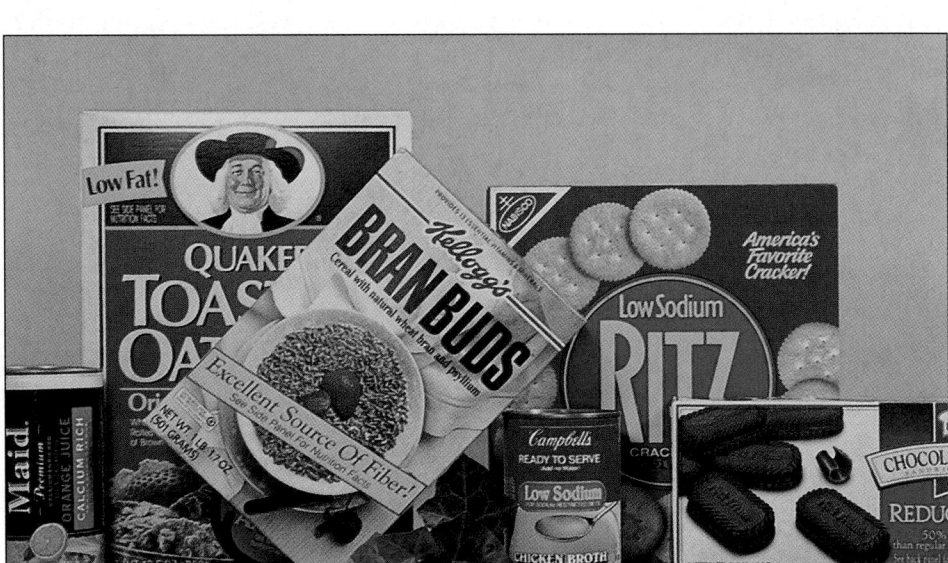

Many food products prominently feature health claims.

■ Becoming Familiar with the Exchange System

To use the Exchange System, you must know which foods are on each list and the serving sizes for each food.

Table 2-10 gives the serving sizes for foods on each exchange list, as well as the carbohydrate, protein, fat, and energy content per exchange. Note that the meat and milk lists are divided into subclasses, which vary in fat content and hence in the amount of energy they provide. Foods on the meat and fat lists contain essentially no carbohydrate; those on the fruit and fat lists lack appreciable amounts of protein; and those on the vegetables, fruit, and other carbohydrates lists contain essentially no fat. You need to study Table 2-10 to become familiar with the sizes of the exchanges (that is, serving sizes) on each list and the amounts of carbohydrate, protein, fat, and energy per exchange.

Before you can turn a group of exchanges into a daily meal plan, you must be aware of which foods are on each exchange list (Fig. 2-5). The entire U.S. Exchange System is presented in Appendix D, which you should consult frequently while exploring the system to discover its various peculiarities. For example, the starch list includes not only bread, dry cereal, cooked cereal, rice, and pasta but also baked beans, corn on the cob, and potatoes. These foods are not identical to those composing the bread, cereal, rice, and pasta group in the Food Guide Pyramid. The Exchange System is not concerned with the origin of a food, whether animal or vegetable. It is primarily concerned with the macronutrients carbohydrate, protein, and fat in each food on a specific list. For example, the carbohydrate composition of potatoes resembles that of bread more than that of broccoli, although potatoes are vegetables. In addition, several foods on the meat and meat substitutes list are not

TABLE 2-10   Nutrient Composition of Exchange System Lists (1995 Edition)

Groups/Lists	Household Measures*	Carbohydrate (g)	Protein (g)	Fat (g)	Energy (kcal)
Carbohydrate Group					
Starch	1 slice, ¾ cup raw, or ½ cup cooked	15	3	1 or less†	80
Fruit	1 small/medium piece	15	—	—	60
Milk	1 cup				
Nonfat/very-low-fat		12	8	0–3†	90
Low-fat		12	8	5	120
Whole		12	8	8	150
Other carbohydrates	Varies	15	Varies	Varies	Varies
Vegetables	1 cup raw or ½ cup cooked	5	2	—	25
Meat and Meat Substitutes Group	1 oz				
Very lean		—	7	0–1	35
Lean		—	7	3	55
Medium-fat		—	7	5	75
High-fat		—	7	8	100
Fat Group	1 tsp	—	—	5	45

*Just an estimate; see exchange lists for actual amounts

†Calculated as 1 g for purposes of energy contribution

■ FIGURE 2-5 Foods arranged according to the Exchange System lists.

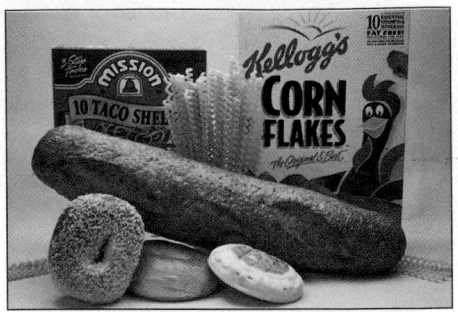

Starch exchange choices

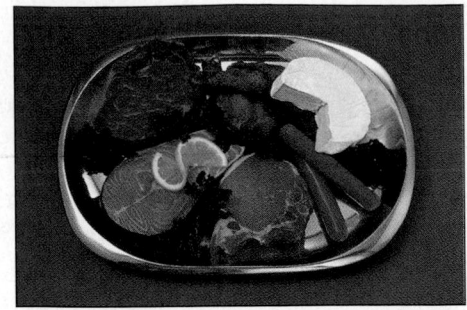

Meat and meat substitutes exchange choices

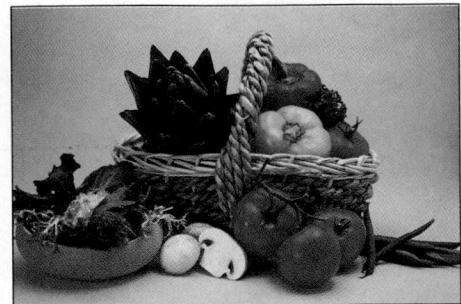

Vegetables exchange choices

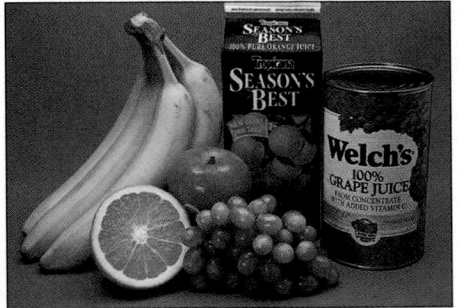

Fruit exchange choices

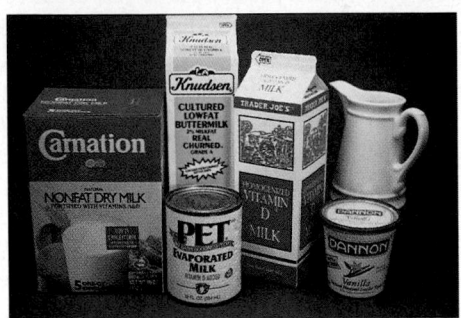

Milk exchange choices

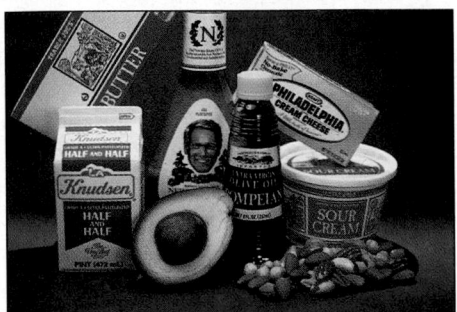

Fat exchange choices

meats. The list of other carbohydrates includes jam, angel food cake, fat-free frozen yogurt, and foods, such as frosted cake, that count as both other carbohydrate exchanges and fat exchanges. Bacon appears in the fat list, rather than the high-fat meat category.

Free foods (essentially calorie-free) include bouillon, diet soda, coffee, tea, dill pickles, and vinegar, as well as herbs and spices. Most vegetables, such as cabbage, celery, mushrooms, lettuce, and zucchini, also can be considered free foods; their minimal energy contribution need not count in the calculations when they are eaten in moderation (one to two servings per meal or snack).

■ Using the Exchange System to Develop Daily Menus

Now let's use the Exchange System to plan a 1-day menu. Let's target an energy content of 2000 kcal, with 55% derived from carbohydrates (1100 kcal), 15% from protein (300 kcal), and 30% from fat (600 kcal). This can be translated into 2 low-fat milk exchanges, 3 vegetable exchanges, 5 fruit exchanges, 11 starch exchanges, 4 lean meat exchanges, and 6 fat exchanges (Table 2-11). Note that this is only one of many possible combinations; the Exchange System offers great flexibility.

Table 2-12 arbitrarily separates these exchanges into breakfast, lunch, dinner, and a snack. Breakfast includes 1 low-fat milk exchange, 2 fruit exchanges, 2 starch exchanges, and 1 fat exchange. This total corresponds to 3/4 cup of cold cereal, 1 cup of reduced fat milk, 1 slice of bread with 1 teaspoon margarine, and 1 cup of orange juice.

Lunch consists of 2 fat exchanges, 4 starch exchanges, 1 vegetable exchange, 1 low-fat milk exchange, and 2 fruit exchanges. This translates into one slice of bacon with 1 teaspoon mayonnaise on two slices of bread, with tomato—in other words, a bacon and tomato sandwich. You can also add lettuce to the sandwich. This can be considered a free vegetable choice. Add to this meal a 9-inch banana (1 exchange = 1 small banana), 1 cup of reduced fat milk, and 6 graham crackers (2½″ by 2½″). Later add a snack ¾ oz of pretzels for another starch exchange.

TABLE 2-11	Possible Exchange Patterns That Yield 55% of Energy as Carbohydrate, 30% as Fat, and 15% as Protein for Energy Intakes ≥ 2000 kcal

kcal/Day

Exchange List	1200*	1600*	2000	2400	2800	3200	3600
Milk (low fat)	2	2	2	2	2	2	2
Vegetable	3	3	3	4	4	4	4
Fruit	3	4	5	6	8	9	9
Starch	5	8	11	13	15	18	21
Meat (lean)	4	4	4	5	6	7	8
Fat	2	4	6	8	10	11	13

This is just one set of options. More meat could be included if less milk were used, for example.

*Energy intakes of 1200 and 1600 kcal contain 20% of energy as protein and 50% energy as carbohydrate to allow for greater flexibility in diet planning.

TABLE 2-12	Sample 1-Day 2000 kcal Menu Based on the Exchange System Plan*

Breakfast

1 low-fat milk exchange	1 cup reduced-fat milk (some on cereal)
2 fruit exchanges	1 cup orange juice
2 starch exchanges	¾ cup cold cereal, 1 piece whole-wheat toast
1 fat exchange	1 tsp soft margarine on toast

Lunch

4 starch exchanges	2 slices whole-wheat bread, 6 graham crackers (2½" by 2½")
2 fat exchanges	1 slice bacon, 1 tsp mayonnaise
1 vegetable exchange	1 sliced tomato
2 fruit exchanges	1 banana (9 inches)
1 low-fat milk exchange	1 cup reduced-fat milk

Snack

1 starch exchange	¾ oz pretzels

Dinner

4 lean meat exchanges	4 oz lean steak (well trimmed)
2 starch exchanges	1 medium baked potato
1 fat exchange	1 tsp soft margarine
2 vegetable exchanges	1 cup cooked broccoli
1 fruit exchange	1 kiwifruit
	Coffee (if desired)

Snack

2 starch exchanges	1 bagel
2 fat exchanges	2 tbsp regular cream cheese

*The target plan was a 2000 kcal energy intake, with 55% from carbohydrate, 15% from protein, and 30% from fat. Computer analysis indicates that this menu yielded 2040 kcal, with 53% from carbohydrate, 16% from protein, and 31% from fat—in close agreement with the targeted goals.

CRITICAL THINKING

Leah is trying to lose a few extra pounds and is going to use the Exchange System to limit her energy intake to 1600 kcal/day. Her dietitian recommends that she begin with about 50% of her kcal from carbohydrate, 20% from protein, and 30% from fat. Design a 1-day sample menu for Leah. Hint: Use Table 2–11 as a starting place.

*C*heck out the *Perspectives in Nutrition* online learning center http://www.mhhe.com/wardlaw for quizzes, flash cards, other activities, and web links designed to further help you learn about various tools for diet planning.

Dinner consists of 4 lean meat exchanges, 1 fruit exchange, 2 vegetable exchanges, 1 fat exchange, and 2 starch exchanges. This total corresponds to a 4-ounce broiled steak (meat only, no bone), 1 medium baked potato (1 exchange = 1 small baked potato) with 1 teaspoon of margarine, 1 cup of broccoli, and 1 kiwifruit. Coffee (if desired) is not counted, since it contains no appreciable energy.

Finally, we have a snack containing 2 starch exchanges and 2 fat exchanges. This translates into 1 bagel with 2 tablespoons of regular cream cheese.

This 1-day menu is only one of many that are possible with the exchange lists. Apple juice could replace the orange juice; two apples could be exchanged for the banana. The choices are endless. Notice that an exchange diet is much easier to plan if you use individual foods, as was done here; however, the Exchange System tables list some combination foods to help you (see Appendix D). Using combination foods, such as pizza or lasagna, however, makes it more difficult to calculate the number of exchanges in a serving. For instance, lasagna typically has meat exchanges, vegetable exchanges, and starch exchanges. With experience, you will be able to tackle such complex foods. For now, using individual foods makes learning the Exchange System much easier.

CONCEPT CHECK

*T*he Exchange System makes it possible to design and follow a precise diet that yields desired ratios of carbohydrate, fat, and protein, while accounting for total energy intake. When the set serving sizes are observed, all the foods within each of the various Exchange System lists yield similar contributions of carbohydrate, fat, protein, and energy. Because of their similar nutrient profiles, the foods in each group can be exchanged for one another.

▌ EPILOGUE

The tools discussed in this chapter greatly aid in menu planning. Menu planning can start with the Food Guide Pyramid. The totality of choices made within the groups can then be evaluated using the Dietary Guidelines. Individual foods that make up a diet can be examined more closely using the comparison with the Daily Values listed on the Nutrition Facts panel of the product. For the most part, these Daily Values are in line with the Dietary Reference Intakes and related nutrient standards. The Nutrition Facts panel is especially useful in identifying nutrient-dense foods—foods that are high in a specific nutrient, such as the vitamin folate, but low in comparison with the relative amount of energy provided, as well as foods that fill you up without providing a lot of calories. The latter are described as foods with low energy density. Once mastered, the Exchange System is helpful for formulating a menu plan that meets specific carbohydrate, fat, and protein goals. Generally speaking, the more you learn about and use these tools, the more they will benefit your diet.

SUMMARY

1. *Variety*, *balance*, and *moderation* are three watchwords of diet planning.
2. Nutrient density is a useful concept. It reflects the nutrient content of a food in relation to its energy (kcal) content. Nutrient-dense foods are relatively rich in nutrients, in comparison with energy content.
3. Energy density of a food is determined by comparing energy content with the weight of food. A food that is rich in calories but that weighs relatively very little, such as nuts, cookies, fried foods in general, and fat-free snacks, is considered energy dense. Foods with low energy density include fruits, vegetables, and any food that incorporates much water during cooking, such as oatmeal.
4. Recommended Dietary Allowances (RDAs) are set for many nutrients. These amounts yield enough of each nutrient to meet the needs of healthy individuals within specific gender and age categories. Adequate Intake (AI) is the standard used when not enough information is available to set a revised RDA. Tolerable Upper Intake Levels (Upper Levels or ULs) for nutrient intake have been set for some vitamins and minerals. All of the many dietary standards fall under the term *Dietary Reference Intakes (DRIs)*.
5. Daily Values are used as a basis for expressing the nutrient content of foods on the Nutrition Facts panel. Reference Daily Intakes (RDIs), which are derived from the 1968 nutrient standards, constitute the majority of the Daily Values. Daily Reference Values (DRVs) have been set for some nutrients with no such RDA, as is true for fat and dietary fiber; Daily Reference Values compose the rest of the Daily Values.
6. The Food Guide Pyramid is designed to translate nutrient recommendations into a food plan that exhibits variety, balance, and moderation. The best results are obtained by using low-fat or nonfat dairy products; including some vegetable proteins in addition to animal-protein foods; including citrus fruits and dark green vegetables; and emphasizing whole-grain breads and cereals.
7. Dietary Guidelines have been issued to help reduce chronic diseases in our population. The guidelines emphasize eating a variety of foods; performing regular physical activity; maintaining or improving weight; moderating consumption of fats, cholesterol, sugar, salt, and alcohol; eating plenty of grain products, fruits, and vegetables; and safely preparing and storing foods, especially perishable foods.
8. The Exchange System is valuable for estimating the carbohydrate, fat, protein, and energy content of a food or meal and for planning a diet to correspond to specific goals for carbohydrate, fat, protein, and energy intake.

STUDY QUESTIONS

1. Describe the philosophy underlying the creation of the Food Guide Pyramid. What dietary changes would you need to make to meet the pyramid guidelines on a regular basis?
2. Describe the intent of the Dietary Guidelines. Point out one criticism for its general application to all American adults.
3. Based on the discussion of the Dietary Guidelines, suggest two key dietary changes the typical American adult should consider making.
4. What three key points should you make when explaining the significance of the DRIs to a friend?
5. How do RDAs and Adequate Intakes differ from Daily Values in intention and application?
6. How would you explain the concepts of nutrient density and energy density to a fourth-grade class?
7. Describe how the Exchange System can be used to help design a diet, based on what the system can predict and monitor.
8. Nutritionists encourage all people to read labels on food packages to learn more about what they eat. What four nutrients could easily be tracked in your diet if you were to read the Nutrition Facts panels regularly on food products?
9. Explain why consumers can have confidence in FDA-approved health claims on food packages.
10. Relate the importance of variety in a diet to the discovery of various phytochemicals in foods.

▪ ANNOTATED REFERENCES

1. ADA Reports: Position of the American Dietetic Association: Functional foods. *Journal of the American Dietetic Association*, 99:1278, 1999.

   The philosophy that food can be health promoting beyond its traditional nutritional value (i.e., phytochemical content) is gaining acceptance among scientists and health professionals. Never before have the health benefits of food had so much support.

2. American Heart Association Conference Proceedings: Unified dietary recommendations. *Circulation* 100:450, 1999.

   A variety of health-related organizations, such as the American Heart Association and American Cancer Society, provide support for the dietary pattern recommended by the Dietary Guidelines.

3. Beecher GR: Phytonutrients' role in metabolism: Effects on resistance to degenerative processes. *Nutrition Reviews* 57(9):S3, 1999.

   The roles of a variety of phytochemical substances is discussed—particularly, specific biochemical roles each may play in reducing chronic disease risk.

4. Bruce B and others: A diet high in whole and unrefined foods favorably alters lipids, antioxidant defenses and colon function. *Journal of the American College of Nutrition* 19:61, 2000.

   A diet abundant in phytochemical-rich foods beneficially affected blood lipids, the antioxidant defense mechanism in the body, and colon function.

5. Campbell TC, Chen J: Diet and health in rural China: Lessons learned and unlearned. *Nutrition Today* 34:116, 1999.

   Studies of rural Asian subjects show that their traditional, primarily plant-based diet contributes to their low risk for chronic degenerative diseases. These findings are consistent with the observations of Asian migrants; they experience more of these diseases when they switch to a more westernized approach.

6. Chidley E: Let food be your medicine. *Today's Dietitian*, p. 28, December 1999.

   No single functional food is a "magic bullet"; people should follow a diet rich in plant foods to gain the benefits of the many phytochemicals under study. The increasing interest in functional foods is being driven by consumers who are taking an active interest in issues of health and wellness.

7. Clairmont MA: Nutraceuticals, phytochemicals and functional foods: A field of dreams for dietitians. *Today's Dietitian*, p. 36, April 2000.

   Growing evidence supports the role of phytochemicals in disease prevention. Phytochemi- cal-rich foods discussed include broccoli, cabbage, tomatoes, tea, soy, whole grains, oranges, grapes, and onions.

8. de Lorgeril and others: Mediterranean diet, traditional risk factors, and the rate of cardiovascular complications after myocardial infarction: Final report of the Lyon Diet Heart Study. *Circulation* 99:779, 1999.

   People following a Mediterranean diet plan—in this case, based on canola oil products rather than the traditional source of fat, olive oil—showed a substantial reduction in heart attack risk. This study provides further evidence of the benefits of the Mediterranean diet.

9. JAMA Patient Page: A healthy diet. *Journal of the American Medical Association* 283:2198, 2000.

   The American Medical Association supports the Food Guide Pyramid as a way for reducing risk for certain forms of both cancer and heart disease. The study by A. K. Kant and others discussed in Chapter 1, showing greater longevity among people following such a diet, is highlighted.

10. JAMA Patient Page: Why you should eat more fruits and vegetables. *Journal of the American Medical Association* 282:1304, 1999.

    The benefits of consuming at least five servings of fruits and vegetables each day are considerable. For example, this reduces the risk of stroke, compared with people who consume few fruits and vegetables.

11. Kantor LS: A dietary assessment of the US food supply. *CNI Nutrition Week*, p. 4, January 22, 1999.

    The U.S. diet still falls short in fruit and vegetable intake, and the primary vegetable consumed is potatoes. Thus, many of us are not benefiting from the various health effects provided by fruits and vegetables. Sugar intake is also more than two times more than what it should be.

12. Kurtzweil P: Staking a claim to good health. *FDA Consumer*, p. 16, November–December 1998.

    Health claims on food labels are closely regulated by FDA. Substantial research information must be available to back up any health claim made.

13. Laudan R: Birth of the modern diet. *Scientific American*, p. 76, August 2000.

    Advances in knowledge concerning diet and nutrition have had a great effect on our diets over the last 300 years. Recognizing the importance of fruits and vegetables scores high marks for our current diet, while the central role of fat in our diets because of the importance given to meat and fat-based sauces is blamed for the high amounts of obesity in most developed nations.

14. McBean LD: Functional foods: An overview. *Dairy Council Digest* 70:31, 1999.

    Dairy products provide a number of components that can benefit health. The benefits from the bacteria in yogurt are getting much attention. As discussed in Chapter 3, these bacteria are termed probiotics, and they contribute to the health of the large intestine (colon).

15. Milner JA: Functional foods: The US perspective. *American Journal of Clinical Nutrition* 71(Suppl):1654S, 2000.

    Increased interest in functional foods is likely occurring for three reasons: increased healthcare costs, recent legislation allowing for structure/function claims, and scientific discoveries, primarily with phytochemicals. We need a greater understanding of how phytochemicals affect specific biological processes in the cells; this research is underway in many laboratories throughout the world.

16. Mukhtar H, Ahmad N: Tea polyphenols: Prevention of cancer and optimizing health. *American Journal of Clinical Nutrition* 71(Suppl):1698S, 2000.

    Results from laboratory animal studies show that tea consumption prevents many forms of intestinal cancer induced by cancer-causing substances. Other studies show the benefits of tea consumption against cardiovascular disease and hypertension. Much evidence supports the benefits of tea and the polyphenols present with regard to health.

17. Raloff J: Chocolate hearts: Yummy and good medicine? *Science News* 157:188, 2000.

    As long as people do not overindulge, chocolate provides health benefits, as it is a good source of some phytochemicals—notably, polyphenols.

18. Rao AV, Agarwal S: Role of the antioxidant lycopene in cancer in heart disease. *Journal of the American College of Nutrition* 19:563, 2000.

    Tomatoes and tomato products are a rich source of lycopene. It is a major carotenoid found in the bloodstream and in various body tissues. Regular intake of lycopene has been reported to reduce the risk of developing both cancer and heart disease.

19. Rolls BJ: The role of energy density in the overconsumption of fat. *Journal of Nutrition* 130:268S, 2000.

    Eating foods that have a low energy density is one way to feel full without consuming a lot of calories. If the food is high in fat, even small portions may have a high energy con-

tent; energy-dense foods are generally consumed in larger quantities in order to feel full at the end of a meal.

20. Sloan EA: The top ten functional food trends. *Food Technology* 54(4):33, 2000.

    Current trends in functional foods include more organic foods, more foods fortified with vitamins and minerals, including snack foods and energy bars, and the addition of compounds to foods to support growth of beneficial bacteria in the colon (see Chapter 3 for details). Overall, selling "healthy foods" to otherwise healthy people has spawned some of the most lucrative markets the food industry has ever seen.

21. Tea and health. *Harvard Health Letter*, p. 2, October 2000.

    Tea contains flavanoids that are excellent antioxidants. Tea however can impede the absorption of iron, but that problem can be avoided by consuming tea between meals.

22. Ten tips for putting healthy eating into practice. *Tufts University Health & Nutrition Letter*, p. 4, April 2000.

    Tips to improve eating practices include paying more attention to what is eaten, putting a greater emphasis on fruits and vegetables, making gradual changes, paying careful attention especially to food intake when eating out at restaurants, eating breakfast, trying new foods, and specifically monitoring one's progress toward nutrition goals.

23. The new foods: Functional or dysfunctional? *Consumer Reports on Health*, p. 1, June 1999.

    Some food manufacturers are adding herbal medicinal substances, such as Kava Kava, to foods (see Chapter 18 for details on this dubious practice). Other trends are fortifying juices with calcium and putting various forms of fiber into foods. Today, many so-called functional foods mainly boost manufacturers' profit, not consumer health. Consumers need to be careful about understanding the risks and benefits of the functional foods they purchase, especially foods to which herbs have been added.

24. Truswell AS: Dietary goals and guidelines: National and international perspectives. In Shils ME and others (eds.): *Modern nutrition in health and disease.* 9th ed. Baltimore MD: Williams & Wilkins, 1999.

    The basic recommendations of the U.S. Dietary Guidelines show overall good agreement, compared with those issued by other countries, particularly regarding moderating foods high in total fat and saturated fat, adjusting energy intake and physical activity to maintain a healthy weight, eating more fruits and vegetables, watching salt intake, and using alcohol in moderation, if at all.

25. Vesper H and others: Sphingolipids in food and the emerging importance of sphingolipids to nutrition. *Journal of Nutrition* 129:1239, 1999.

    Sphingolipids present in dairy foods, eggs, and soybeans have been shown to benefit the health of many types of cells, including those of the colon. These compounds are just another of what can be considered part of the functional food designation applied to certain foods.

26. Weisburger JH: Approaches for chronic disease prevention based on current understanding of underlying mechanisms. *American Journal of Clinical Nutrition* 71(Suppl):1710S, 2000.

    Consuming adequate fruits and vegetables, having a high fiber intake, and having an ample fluid intake reduce the risk for many chronic diseases. We should put these recommendations into practice.

27. Whole fruits and vegetables. *Harvard Heath Letter*, p. 6, October 2000.

    Despite the obvious pluses from a diet rich in fruits and vegetables, the fact remains that the average American consumes only about three servings—about half the half of the recommended 5 servings per day. As people cut down on fatty meats, high fat dairy products, and high calorie, refined carbohydrates they should look to fruits and vegetables along with whole grains to make up the bulk of their diet.

28. Willett WC: The dietary pyramid: Does the foundation need repair? *American Journal of Clinical Nutrition* 68:218, 1998.

    The choices from the bottom of the Food Guide Pyramid should emphasize whole grains. These forms of grains are rich sources of dietary fiber and have been shown to reduce the risk of heart disease. Less emphasis should be placed on refined grains.

29. Yates AA: Process and development of dietary reference intakes: Bases, need, and application of recommended dietary allowances. *Nutrition Reviews* 56(4):S5, 1998.

    The Food and Nutrition Board has revamped U.S. dietary standards, as this article discusses. For an update on the board's recent actions, see the web site: http://www4.nationalacademies.org/IOM/ IOMHome.nsf/Pages/Food+and+Nutrition +Board.

TAKEACTION

I. DOES YOUR DIET MEET NUTRIENT NEEDS, FOOD GUIDE PYRAMID RECOMMENDATIONS, AND THE DIETARY GUIDELINES?

Complete either Part I or Part II. Then complete Parts III, IV, and V. (For help in following the instructions for this activity, see the sample assessment in Appendix E.)

Part I

Manual RDA Analysis

A. Take the information from the 1-day food-intake record you completed in Chapter 1 and record it on the blank form provided in Appendix E or by your instructor. Be sure to record the food or drink ingested and the amount (e.g., weight) consumed. Note: Your instructor may require you to keep the food record for more than 1 day.

B. Review the various nutrient standards on the inside cover of this book and choose the appropriate recommendations for your gender and age. Write the appropriate value for each nutrient on the line on the form labeled "Nutrient Need." The values for sodium and potassium from the table on the inside cover of the book are labeled "Estimated Sodium, Chloride, and Potassium Requirements of Healthy Persons."

C. Look up the foods and drinks that you listed on the form in the food composition table, Appendix A. Record on the form the amounts of each nutrient and the kcal present in them, based on the serving size and the number of servings you ate. For example, if you drank 2 cups of milk and the serving size listed in Appendix A is 1 cup, double all nutrient values as you record them. If the food is not listed, choose a substitute, such as cola for root beer.

D. For each food and drink, add the amounts in each column and record the results on the line labeled "Totals."

E. Compare the totals with your nutrient needs. Divide the total for each nutrient by the specific amount and multiply that by 100. Record the result on the line labeled "% of Nutrient Needs."

F. Keep this assessment for use in subsequent activities in other chapters.

Part II

Computer Diet Analysis

A. Load the computer software shrink-wrapped with this book into the computer.

B. Choose RDAs and related nutrient standards based on your age and gender.

C. Enter the information from the 1-day food intake record you kept in Chapter 1. Be sure to enter each food and drink and the specific amount you ate.

D. This software program will give you the following results:

1. The appropriate DRI (or related standard) for each nutrient

2. The total amount of each nutrient and the kcal consumed for the day

3. The percentage of intake compared with needs for each nutrient you consumed

E. Keep this assessment for use in subsequent activities in other chapters.

Part III

Evaluation of Nutrient Intakes as a Percentage of Nutrient Needs

Remember that you don't necessarily need to consume your estimated nutrient needs every day. A general standard is meeting needs averaged over 5 to 8 days. It is best not to exceed the Upper Level (if set) to avoid potential toxic effects for some nutrients.

A. For which nutrients did your intakes fall below estimated nutrient needs?

B. Did you exceed the minimum requirements for sodium? to what degree?

C. For which nutrients did you exceed the Upper Level (if set)?

D. What dietary changes could you make to correct or improve your dietary profile? If you're not sure, Chapters 5 through 12 will help guide your decisions.

TAKE ACTION

Part IV

Food Guide Pyramid

Using the same food-intake record used in Part I or II, place each food item in the appropriate group of the Food Guide Pyramid in Appendix E. That is, for each food item, indicate how many servings it contributes to each group based on the amount you ate (see Table 2–6 for serving sizes). Note that many of your food choices may contribute to more than one group. For example, toast with margarine contributes to two categories: (1) the breads, cereals, rice, and pasta group and (2) fats, oils, and sweets. After entering all the values, add the number of servings consumed in each group. Finally, compare your total in each food group with the recommended number of servings shown in Figure 2-3. Enter a minus sign (–) if your total falls below the recommendation or a plus sign (+) if it equals or exceeds the recommendation.

Part V

Further Diet Evaluation

Do the weaknesses, if any, suggested in your nutrient analysis (see Part III) correspond to missing servings in the Food Guide Pyramid chart? If so, consider changing your food choices based on the Food Guide Pyramid to help improve your nutrient profile. Finally, indicate whether your day's diet did or did not conform to the following items in the Dietary Guidelines:

	Yes	No
Aim for Fitness		
• Aim for a healthy weight.	___	___
• Be physically active each day.	___	___
Build a Healthy Base		
• Let the pyramid guide your food choices.	___	___
• Choose a variety of grains daily, especially whole grains.	___	___
• Choose a variety of fruits and vegetables daily.	___	___
• Keep foods safe to eat.	___	___
Choose Sensibly		
• Choose a diet that is a low in saturated fat and cholesterol and moderate in total fat.	___	___
• Choose beverages and foods to moderate your intake of sugars.	___	___
• Choose and prepare foods with less salt.	___	___
• If you drink alcoholic beverages, do so in moderation.	___	___

If your diet comes up short on any of these evaluations, take appropriate action to improve your eating patterns.

II. APPLYING THE NUTRITION FACTS LABEL TO YOUR DAILY FOOD CHOICES

Imagine that you are at the grocery store, looking for a quick meal before a busy evening. In the frozen food section, you find two brands of frozen cheese manicotti (see labels a and b). Which of the two brands would you choose? What information on the Nutrition Facts label in the figure contributed to this decision?

_____

_____

_____

Nutrition Facts (a)
Serving Size 1 Package (260g)
Servings Per Container 1

Amount Per Serving
Calories 390 Calories from Fat 160

% Daily Value*
Total Fat 18g — 27%
Saturated Fat 9g — 45%
Cholesterol 45mg — 14%
Sodium 880mg — 36%
Total Carbohydrate 38g — 13%
Dietary Fiber 4g — 15%
Sugars 12g
Protein 17g

Vitamin A 10% • Vitamin C 4%
Calcium 40% • Iron 8%

*Percent Daily Values are based on a 2,000 calorie diet. Your daily values may be higher or lower depending on your calorie needs:

	Calories:	2,000	2,500
Total Fat	Less than	65g	80g
Sat Fat	Less than	20g	25g
Cholesterol	Less than	300mg	300mg
Sodium	Less than	2,400mg	2,400mg
Total Carbohydrate		300g	375g
Dietary Fiber		25g	30g

Nutrition Facts (b)
Serving Size 1 Package (260g)
Servings Per Container 1

Amount Per Serving
Calories 230 Calories from Fat 35

% Daily Value*
Total Fat 4g — 6%
Saturated Fat 2g — 10%
Cholesterol 15mg — 4%
Sodium 590mg — 24%
Total Carbohydrate 28g — 9%
Dietary Fiber 3g — 12%
Sugars 10g
Protein 19g

Vitamin A 10% • Vitamin C 10%
Calcium 35% • Iron 4%

*Percent Daily Values are based on a 2,000 calorie diet. Your daily values may be higher or lower depending on your calorie needs:

	Calories:	2,000	2,500
Total Fat	Less than	65g	80g
Sat Fat	Less than	20g	25g
Cholesterol	Less than	300mg	300mg
Sodium	Less than	2,400mg	2,400mg
Potassium		3,500mg	3,500mg
Total Carbohydrate		300g	375g
Dietary Fiber		25g	30g

ETHNIC INFLUENCES ON THE AMERICAN DIET

Human societies have developed under widely varying conditions. These conditions affected which foods were available (e.g., rice vs. wheat) and how long each food could be stored (e.g., tropical vs. temperate climates). This, in turn, influenced the dietary patterns of these various cultures. Then as these various cultures migrated to new locations, the migrants kept some traditional dietary habits, or *foodways;* changed some habits; and abandoned others. As people migrate and mingle with those of other cultures, their cuisines tend to mingle as well. Note that about 25% of all restaurants in the United States have an ethnic theme. Recent changes in affluence and technology also affect dietary habits, some for better and some for worse.

In this Nutrition Perspective, we will examine how the cuisines of various cultures throughout the world have affected the American diet. Examining the nutritional attributes of a number of ethnic diets will help you understand that no single cuisine is either completely healthful or unhealthful. The trick to finding healthful food is to evaluate individual dishes carefully. Let's look at six cuisines that contribute to food "American style." Note that almost all Americans sample at least one of these on a regular basis.

NATIVE AMERICANS

The size and varied geography of the American continent meant that different foods were available to people living in different locations. Some of these people were hunter-gatherers, depending on wild vegetation and wild game for subsistence. Others learned to grow vegetable crops. Depending on where they lived, Native American groups cultivated early forms of such plant foods as tomatoes, sweet potatoes, squash, vanilla, and cocoa. Their diets tended to be low in sodium and fat and high in dietary fiber. In the far north, populations subsisted on fish, sea mammals, other game, and a few plants, such as seaweed, willow leaves, and berries.

Studies have shown that the diseases that affected these societies differed significantly from the diseases common in American society today. For example, Alaskan natives who still eat the traditional diet have heart disease rates lower than those in the general United States population. Younger generations of Alaskan natives, however, who usually do not eat the traditional diet, have developed heart disease at rates similar to those in the U.S. population in general. These and other studies indicate that, as societies become more uniform, so, too, do disease patterns.

HISPANIC-AMERICANS

When Spanish colonists arrived in what is now called Latin America, they brought foods, flavors, and cooking techniques, which they combined with locally available foods. Several cuisines developed from those combinations, influenced also by the arrival of other groups. Thus, the Cuban cuisine combined native foods with those of both Spanish and Chinese immigrants, whereas the Puerto Rican cuisine combined native foods with Spanish and African contributions. In Mexico, the Spanish influence mingled with that of local Native American cuisines.

The Mayans, Aztecs, and other populations in Mexico grew corn, beans, and chili peppers; these were the basis of Mexican cuisine. They also grew such fruits as avocados, papayas, and pineapples. By the end of the fifteenth century, wheat, chickpeas, melons, radishes, grapes, and sugar cane had been brought to the New World. Rice, citrus fruits, and some kinds of nuts came soon afterward. The Spanish also introduced beef, lamb, and chicken. Native inhabitants had previously eaten mostly fish and wild game. Spices such as cinnamon, black pepper, cloves, thyme, marjoram, and bay leaves were introduced and became part of the cuisine.

Mexican cuisine today shows regional variety. In southern Mexico, savory sauces and stews and corn tortillas reflect the native heritage. The Gulf states are renowned for delicious seafood dishes prepared with tomatoes, herbs, and olives, whereas Yucatan cuisine follows Mayan tra-

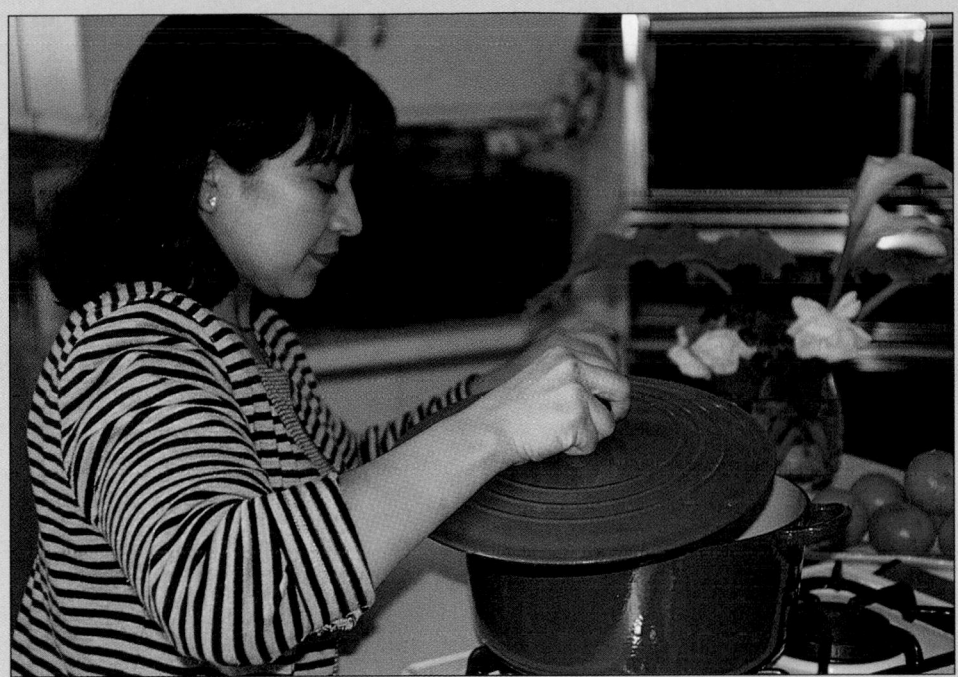

Our cooking habits often reflect our ethnic heritage.

dition, with such specialties as wild turkey and fish flavored with lime juice. Fresh produce adds color, flavor, and nutrition to authentic Mexican dining. Markets in the United States are beginning to offer some of these plant foods, such as chayote, squash, jicama root, plantains, and cactus leaves and fruit. Traditional Mexican cooking is healthful in that it is high in complex carbohydrates, beans, fruits, and vegetables, particularly those rich in vitamins A and C. This pattern is reflected in the Latin American Diet Pyramid issued by Oldways Preservation & Exchange Trust in 1996 (Fig. 2-6). For more information on this and other ethnic diet pyramids, see the web site http://www.oldwayspt.org. Today, true Mexican cooking bears little resemblance to the dishes usually found in "Mexican" restaurants. Usually it is neither oily nor heavy and is based primarily on rice and beans. Restaurant Mexican food tends to use larger portions of meat, as well as adding portions of high-fat sour cream, guacamole, and cheese to many dishes.

NORTHERN EUROPEAN-AMERICANS

Immigrants from Western Europe are responsible for the "meat-and-potatoes" presentation of traditional American home cooking.[13] The first large group of settlers from Europe—the English, French, and Germans—brought their traditional foodways with them. As all cooks and cultures must do, these immigrants adapted to the foods available in the regions in which they settled. Native Americans shared foods, which are now staples of the American diet: corn and corn products, such as popcorn and hominy; some kinds of squash; and tomatoes.

However, because the immigrants often settled in regions of the "new land" that most closely resembled their homes in Europe, they were able to grow many familiar foods and retain many of their traditional foodways. One of these foodways involved the way food is presented.

A sizable portion of meat arranged with vegetables and potatoes in separate portions on a plate is the European pattern, compared with other cuisines in which a mixture of starch, vegetables, and a much smaller portion of protein (such as a stir-fry) is more typical. The meat on the "American" dinner plate may be, for example, sausage or roast beef, the potatoes may be boiled or mashed, and the vegetable may be sauerkraut or green peas. Whatever the choices, the Western European pattern is still followed by many in this country.

This traditional pattern provides abundant protein and nutrients from dairy and meat products. However, the protein also contains saturated fat, and the large portions of protein and starch may mean that insufficient amounts of whole grains, vegetables, and fruits are eaten.

■ FIGURE 2-6 The traditional healthy Latin American Diet Pyramid. A variety of diet pyramids have been developed by Old-ways Preservation & Exchange Trust. These pyramids reflect the typical diets of rural peoples in the region—in this case, Latin America. Text accompanying the Latin American Pyramid, as is true for the other Oldways ethnic pyramids, states that alco-hol may be consumed with meals, but con-sumption should be avoided during pregnancy and whenever it would put the individual or others at risk. As you will no-tice throughout this Nutrition Perspective, all pyramids developed by governmental or private organizations always have fruits, vegetables, and grains at the base. The Latin American Diet Pyramid then adds nuts and beans to this base; other pyra-mids also slightly alter the base.

Copyright 1998 Oldways Preservation & Exchange Trust.

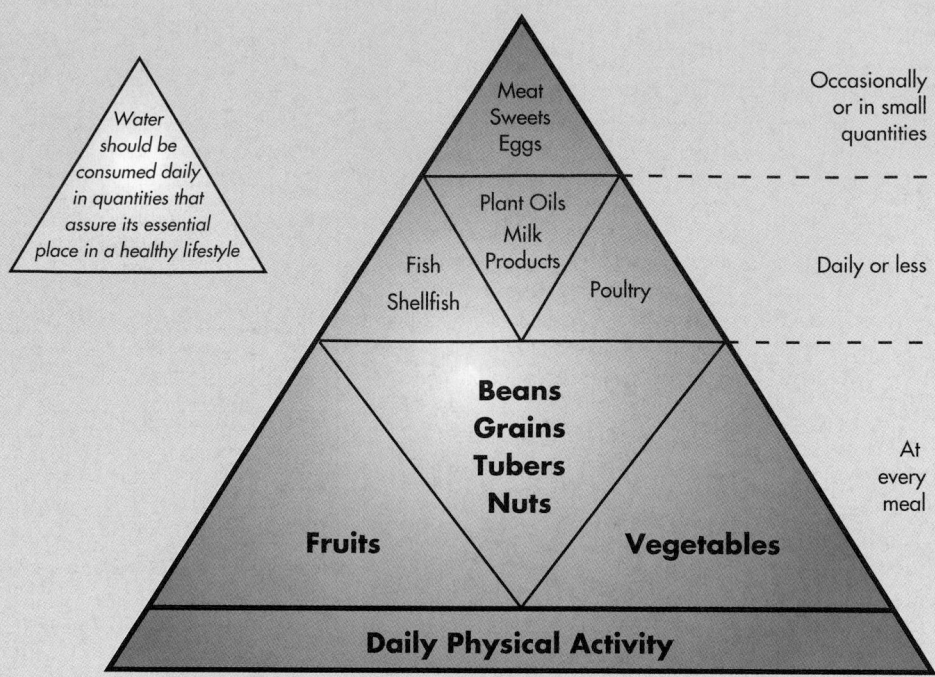

Alcohol may be consumed by adults in moderation and with meals, but consumption should be avoided during pregnancy and whenever it would put the individual or others at risk.

AFRICAN-AMERICANS

Involuntary immigrants to the New World, people from West Africa struggled to survive under harsh conditions. Their ability to adapt familiar foodways to new conditions became a lasting influence on today's American cuisine.

The "soul food" of African-Americans is the basis of the regional cuisines of the American South. Many understand "soul food" to consist mainly of barbecued meat, fried chicken, sweet potatoes, and chitterlings. In fact, true soul food includes a wide range of dishes created by African-American cooks. They used traditional methods and foods brought from Africa, such as yams, okra, and peanuts, as well as what was available in the New World. African-Amer-ican women, cooking for their families, created dishes that they often adapted for the planta-tion owner's table as well, creating the basis of Southern cuisine. The combination of these African-American foodways with Native American, Spanish, and French traditions produced the Cajun and Creole cuisines enjoyed today in Louisiana and throughout the nation.

Pork and corn products were the basis of soul food. The plantation owner ate the better parts of the pig. As with other foods, slaves learned to make the less desirable parts of the pig, such as entrails, feet, ears, and head, palatable. Corn was ground for corn bread. Unrefined yellow cornmeal was mixed with water and lard to make "hoecake," baked on a hoe blade by cooks who had neither ovens nor cooking utensils for their own use. The plantation owner probably ate white cornbread made from refined cornmeal.

Among other dishes still considered soul food staples are greens, usually cooked with a small portion of smoked pork. The greens used include collards, mustard, turnip, or dandelion greens, and kale. Black-eyed peas, first brought to the New World by slaves, are also cooked with pork. Sweet potatoes and yams were and remain basic soul foods; sweet potato pie is the soul food equivalent of pumpkin pie.

Today's traditional African-American cuisine has both nutritional benefits and deficits. The variety of fruits, vegetables, and grain products used provides ample vitamins, minerals, and di-etary fiber. For instance, African-Americans in general consume more cruciferous vegetables, and fruits and vegetables containing vitamins A and C than do Caucasian Americans. However, cured pork products contribute undesirable levels of salt as well as saturated fat. Traditional re-liance on frying, especially with lard, also adds much fat to the diet. Boiling vegetables for long periods depletes water-soluble vitamins. Dairy products may not be used enough, especially by older people who follow traditional dietary customs. This avoidance is based in part on the difficulty many African-American adults experience in digesting lactose; see Chapter 5 for details.

To help guide African-Americans toward a healthy food plan, Hebni Nutrition Consultants has developed a Soul Food Pyramid. It differs from the Food Guide Pyramid primarily by emphasizing lactose-reduced dairy products in the milk, yogurt, and cheese group and placing very-high-fat meats, such as bacon and sausage, in the fats, oils, and sweets category. To obtain a copy of the Soul Food Pyramid, call/Fax 407-345-7999.

ASIAN-AMERICANS

As noted in the Expert Opinion in this chapter, Okinawa, an island southwest of Japan, boasts some of the oldest, healthiest people in the world. Their diet of fresh vegetables, minimal amounts of meat (mainly pork and fish), and moderate fat (lower than American diets but higher than traditional Japanese fare) has influenced the eating habits of Japan and the United States alike. Studies prove that the Okinawan diet of more fresh versus pickled vegetables, more fiber, less salt, and a little more fat than traditional Japanese cuisine has protected them from premature death from problems such as stroke. Since this discovery, the Japanese diet has become more like that of the Okinawans.

This idea of large portions of vegetables and grains, and small portions of meat, is becoming known in the United States, but people are having difficulty complying with this more disciplined way of eating. Also influenced by Japanese cuisine is the growing popularity of soy products, such as tofu, soy milk, and miso, as well as use of flavors such as soy sauce, cilantro, and ginger.

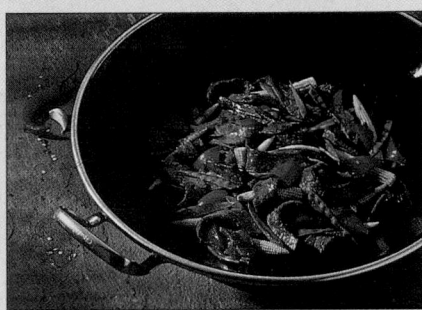

Stir-fry is commonly used in Chinese cooking.

More than 200 different vegetables are used in Chinese cuisine; bok choy and other forms of Chinese cabbage are perhaps the most widely eaten vegetables in the world. In the southeastern coastal region of China, home of the Cantonese cuisine, the number of dishes may be as high as 50,000. Rice is the core of the diet in southern China, whereas, in the temperate North, wheat is used in noodles (China is the original home of pasta), bread, and dumplings. Popular dishes include hot pots (stews containing many ingredients) and stir-fried mixtures of vegetables and small amounts of meat or fish cooked in a lightly oiled, very hot pan.

An Asian Diet Pyramid has been proposed to reflect the Asian dietary pattern (Fig. 2-7). Like the Latin American Diet Pyramid, the bulk of the diet consists of grains, fruits, vegetables, and plant sources of protein, such as legumes, nuts, and seeds.

The Asian Pyramid does fall short in calcium but otherwise can form the basis of a healthy diet. Overall, most attention should be paid to the bottom portion of whichever pyramid you choose, and if dairy products are not included on a daily basis, other rich sources of calcium should be sought (see Chapter 11 for options).

Chinese immigration to America began with the California gold rush in the middle of the nineteenth century. Chinese workers brought with them food-preparation methods that tend to preserve nutrients, as well as a variety of sauces and seasonings, such as gingerroot, garlic, rice wine, scallions, and sesame seeds and oil. Although many of the traditional foodways have been preserved, North American restaurant versions of Chinese cuisine, whether Cantonese, Szechwan, or Mandarin, are usually not authentic. Chinese-American restaurant food is often prepared with far more fat than in true Chinese cooking, which tends to use flavorful but fat-free sauces and seasoning. The restaurant versions of Chinese dishes also contain much larger portions of protein.

*T*wo issues addressed by various ethnic diet pyramids developed by Oldways Preservation & Exchange Trust but not specifically included as part of the Food Guide Pyramid diagram are physical activity and alcohol intake. The ethnic diet pyramids recommend daily physical activity. Alcohol may be consumed by adults in moderation with meals, but consumption should be avoided during pregnancy and whenever it would put the individual or others at risk. The booklet accompanying the Food Guide Pyramid does address alcohol intake, suggesting that adults have no more than one to two drinks per day.

ITALIAN-AMERICANS

Authentic Italian cuisine, like Asian cuisine, is more diverse than most Americans realize. Foods of different regions reflect Italy's varied geography and climate. Northern Italy, the more affluent part of the country, is the principal producer of meat and dairy products, such as butter and cheese. Rice dishes, such as risotto, are popular there. Fish is more important in regions near the sea, and lighter foods, such as fresh vegetables prepared with herbs, garlic, and olive oil,

$\mathcal{S}$ee the August 2000 issue of the *Journal of the American Dietetic Association* for a "pagoda" version of a desirable Asian diet.

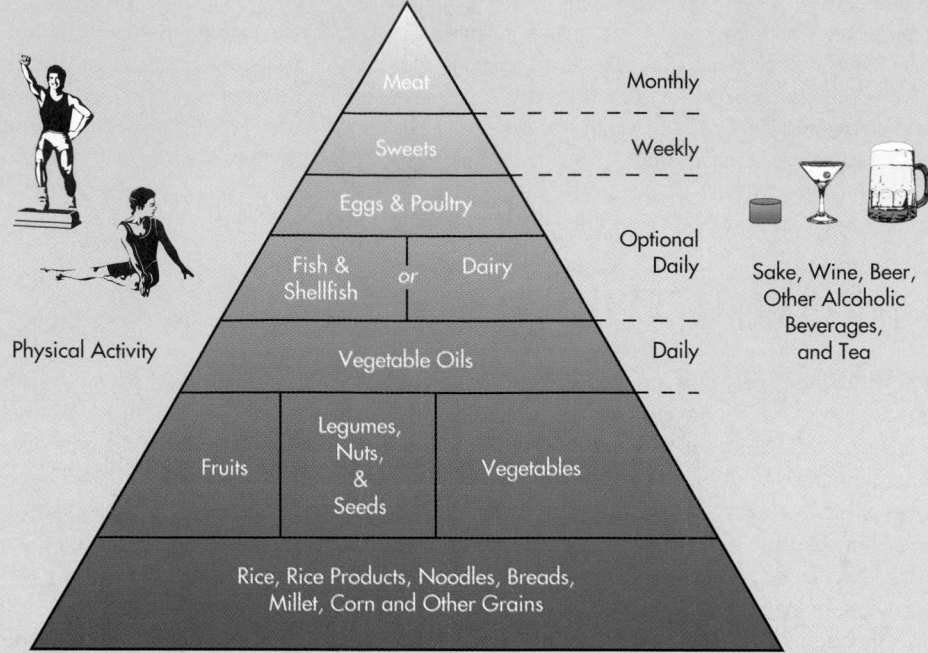

FIGURE 2-7 Asian Diet Pyramid.
Copyright 1997 Oldways Preservation & Exchange Trust.

are characteristic. The poorer regions south of Rome, as well as the island of Sicily, have a diet rich in grains, vegetables, dried beans, and fish, with little meat or oil. Compared with northern Italians of the same class, southern Italians eat less beef, veal, chicken, and butter and more bread, pasta, vegetables, fruit, and fish.

Pasta is the heart of the Italian diet. Italians eat six times more of this simple wheat and water product than do North Americans, although Americans have also learned to enjoy this nutritious dish. Pasta in America, however, often means spaghetti, with a tomato-based sauce that includes meatballs or sausage. In contrast, Italians eat pasta in a variety of shapes and with a variety of sauces, often excluding meat.

Most of the Italian-American cuisine found in restaurants offers foods more common to the north of Italy, including veal, cheese, and cream and pesto sauces for pasta. Pizza, a southern Italian dish, is the exception, and it is fast becoming the most frequently consumed food in the United States. Pizza in this country is served on a variety of flour crusts topped with anything from high-fat meats, such as pepperoni, to vegetables or even fruit, combined with a variety of cheeses, tomatoes, and oregano for seasoning. Purists in Naples, however, insist that classic pizza consists only of a thin crust, tomato, basil, and mozzarella cheese.

Although some components of the Italian diet contain substantial amounts of saturated fat, nutritionists now know that other components, such as pasta, olive oil, and vegetables, contribute to healthy diets. One approach to Italian-American cuisine could be the Mediterranean Diet Pyramid (Fig. 2-8). This is a plan based on food choices like those traditionally found in the simple cuisines of Greece and southern Italy. The Mediterranean Diet Pyramid allows up to 35% of total calories as fat in the diet, compared with the typical recommendation of not more than 30%. However, it recommends consuming the type of fat consumed in the Mediterranean region: olive oil. A cheaper version, which has a similar fat profile and health benefit, is canola oil (see Chapter 6 for details).[8]

ETHNIC DIETS AND PRESENT TRENDS

Only six ethnic diets have been described here; see Table 2-13 for a summary of their advantages and disadvantages. Many other cuisines have also influenced the American diet, and new arrivals continue to bring their traditions and foodways to this country. For example, social upheavals have increased the immigration of Russians and other Eastern European peoples to the United States. On the other side of the world, continuing unrest in Southeast Asia

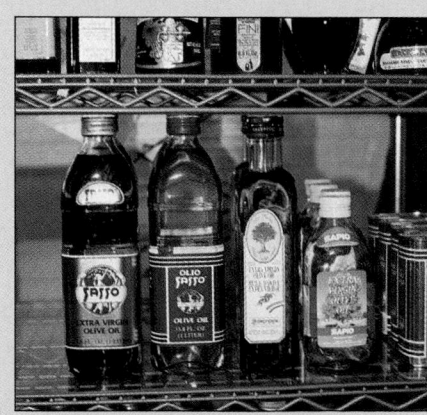

Olive oil is a principal fat source in the Mediterranean diet.

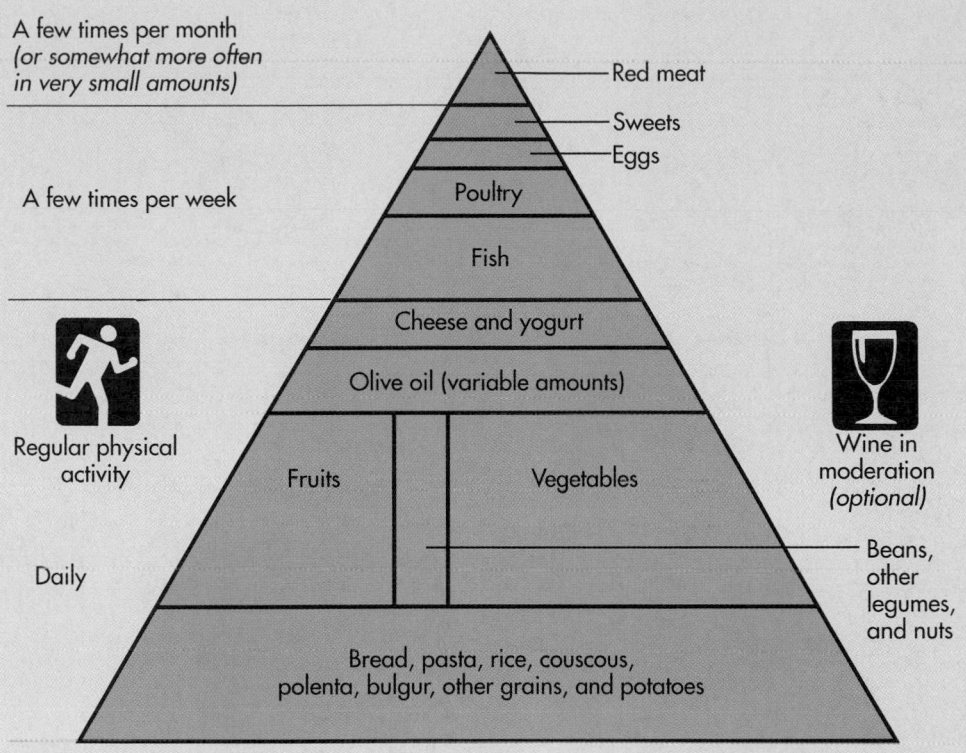

A few times per month
(or somewhat more often
in very small amounts) — Red meat

— Sweets

— Eggs

A few times per week   Poultry

Fish

Cheese and yogurt

Olive oil (variable amounts)

Regular physical
activity

Fruits   Vegetables

Wine in
moderation
(optional)

— Beans,
other
legumes,
and nuts

Daily

Bread, pasta, rice, couscous,
polenta, bulgur, other grains, and potatoes

■ FIGURE 2-8 The traditional healthy Mediterranean Diet Pyramid. This plan is based on long-standing eating habits in southern Italy, Crete, and Greece. The base of the diet is bread and grains, fruits and vegetables, and beans and potatoes. Red meat is consumed sparingly—moderate amounts of fish and poultry are preferred. Wine may be included with meals. Most of the fat in this plan comes from olive oil. Cheese and yogurt supply some fat and calcium. Other low-fat and nonfat milk products also can be included, if desired. Copyright 1994 Oldways Preservation & Exchange Trust.

TABLE 2-13   The World's Fare Has Influenced the American Diet

Diet	Advantages	Shortcomings
Native American; Alaskan Native	Variety of seafood, lean wild game; early Native Americans ate a variety of vegetables, berries, leaves	High fat content of some meat/seafood; low in calcium
Hispanic-American	Excellent variety of vegetables, legumes, fruits; high in dietary fiber	Traditional Hispanic diet may fall short in calcium; Mexican-American restaurants serve much high-fat fare, rich in sour cream, cheese, and guacamole
Northern European-American	Abundant sources of protein, iron, calcium from meat and dairy groups	Less variety from vegetables, fruits, legumes; high in fat
African-American	Good variety of vegetables; high dietary fiber; many variations, including Cajun and Creole dishes	Traditional meals high in fat; may fall short in calcium
Asian-American	Excellent variety of vegetables, grains; cooking methods retain nutrients in foods	Some sauces high in salt and fat; may fall short in calcium
Italian-American	Varies regionally—some regions provide excellent variety of seafood; overall high grain intake, good vegetable and fruit variety	Italian-American restaurants often serve many foods made with high-fat cheese, sauces, and meats, likely low in calcium.

This is a brief summary of healthful attributes and shortcomings of the ethnic diet influences covered in this Nutrition Perspective.

has brought peoples from that area here. Restaurants serving traditional Russian or Thai fare, for instance, are offering new foodways to those willing to experiment.

Based on research also begun many years ago, still other scientists suggest that a healthful diet consists of the inexpensive traditional dishes based on grains, fruits, and vegetables that form the backbone of a number of ethnic cuisines.[5] These are precisely the dishes that people abandon as they become affluent and seek convenience. Simple foods prepared in simple ways have fed most of humanity for virtually its entire existence. As we begin a new century, some Americans are rediscovering the simple foods of their respective pasts, learning to enjoy a variety of cuisines and finding out how each cuisine can contribute to a healthier American diet.

HUMAN PHYSIOLOGIC PROCESSES

chapter 3

*A*ll fundamental activities referred to as nutrition occur within a variety of cells. Although each cell is comprised of the same components, there is enough variety within each cell to provide about 200 distinctive cell types. Each cell performs a specialized task. Groups of cells are organized to form tissues. Tissues unite to form organs. Organs are grouped together to carry out functions in the body and are known as systems.[12]

The integumentary system provides protection from the environment. The skeletal system is the body's structural framework. Movement depends on the muscle system. The circulatory system, composed of the heart and blood vessels, transports blood to all tissues throughout the body in order to deliver essential nutrients and pick up cellular waste. The lymph system is a transport system, but it also provides immunity, the body's defense against foreign invaders. The respiratory system allows the body to exchange gasses with the external environment. The nervous system coordinates activities within the body and detects changes in the internal and external environment. It is responsible for consciousness, learning, and cognition. The endocrine system coordinates activities to preserve homeostasis. The digestive system chemically changes food into absorbable nutrients. The urinary system regulates the composition of the blood and disposes of waste. And the reproductive system provides the sperm or egg, which will develop into a new human. All these systems control our nutritional status, and the nutrients derived from food control all these systems.[4]

KEY CHAPTER CONCEPTS

- The cell is the structural and functional unit of all living organisms. Each cell contains a plasma or cell membrane and organelles, which carry out unique tasks related to the function of the cell.
- Cells join together to make up tissues, tissues unite to form organs, and organs work together as a system.
- The body has 11 organ systems, each controlling one aspect of human nutrition. (There are 12 if the immune and lymphatic systems are counted separately.)
- The integumentary system is the largest system in the body. It provides material (tissues) to cover body surfaces and is a source of vitamin D.
- The muscle and skeletal systems consist of muscles and bones, which permit movement and protection from injury. The skeletal system itself is a storehouse for important nutrients. The muscle system is a significant source of heat.
- The circulatory system delivers oxygen, nutrients, and fluid to all tissues in the body; maintains fluid balance; and removes waste materials, such as carbon dioxide, from the body. Another circulatory system, the lymph, also distributes nutrients and fluids throughout the body and acts as a defense system to protect the body from invading pathogens.
- The immune system coordinates the attack against invading pathogens. There are two types of immunity, specific and nonspecific. The body is exposed to dangerous bacteria, viruses, fungi, and parasites coming in through the skin, mouth (gastrointestinal tract), and respiratory tract. The immune system identifies the microorganisms and destroys them.
- The respiratory system picks up oxygen in the lungs from inhaled air and delivers it to the blood. The lungs recover carbon dioxide from the blood and disposes of it as we exhale.
- The nervous system is composed of cells called neurons, which act as communication links. In order to maintain homeostasis, receptors present throughout the body transmit information about the internal and external environment to the central nervous system (CNS). The CNS, in turn, responds by issuing commands to all the systems that will eventually maintain this homeostasis.
- Located in the body are endocrine glands, which produce chemicals called hormones. Hormones are transported to all parts of the body to help regulate cellular function.
- The gastrointestinal tract digests food and beverages and converts them into absorbable nutrients. This system acts as a barrier against invading pathogens.
- The kidneys filter the blood and remove waste, excess fluid, and substances not needed by the body. The filtrate is urine. Thus, the urinary system constantly maintains the composition of the blood.
- The reproductive system generates new humans. This replaces ones who are dying. Hormones produced by this system control many aspects of nutrition.

REFRESH YOUR MEMORY

As you begin your study of anatomy and physiology in Chapter 3, you may want to review
- The classes of macronutrients in Chapter 1
- Cell structure and the function of various organelles, found from previous coursework in your university-level biology text
- Also from your biology text, each of the body's systems, with special emphasis on how each system may be related to human nutrition

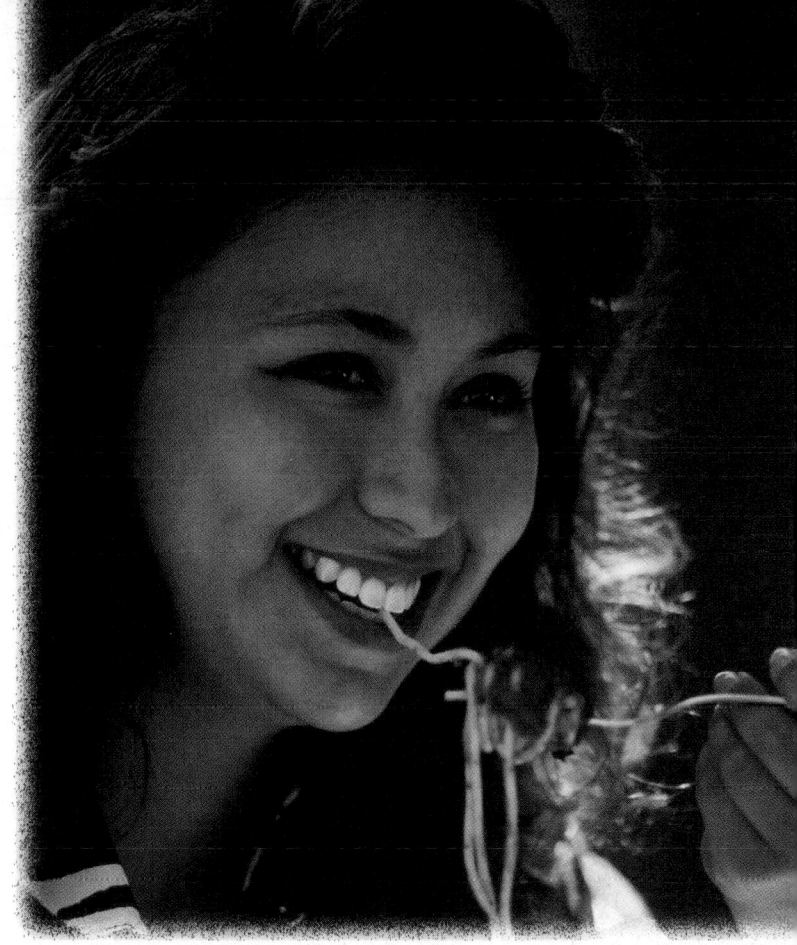

CASE SCENARIO

A fellow student complains to you about a gastrointestinal problem that "just won't go away." She is 20 years old, is very short, and complains of abdominal pain, diarrhea, and joint pain. Her family doctor says it's nothing, just the stress of being a high-achieving university student. She confides in you that she is worried about her health, as she has experienced a sudden weight loss of 5 pounds in the past week. You suggest she visit the Student Health Service immediately.

A barium enema X ray, colonoscopy, and CT scan reveal that the student is suffering from Crohn's disease. What is Crohn's disease? What happens to the intestinal tract when someone has this disease? Are there any treatments to alleviate the symptoms? What, if any, foods should she eat or avoid? Overall, how does she cope with this health problem?

■ HUMAN PHYSIOLOGY

The body is composed of a trillion cells. Each cell is a self-contained, living entity. With the exception of red blood cells, cells of the same type join together, using intercellular substances to form tissues, such as muscle tissue. One, two, or more tissues combine in a particular way to form more complex structures, called organs. All organs contribute to nutritional health, and overall nutrition determines how well each organ functions. At a still higher level of coordination, several organs can cooperate for a common purpose to form a system, such as the digestive system. Overall, the human body is a coordinated unit of many highly structured systems.[13]

Chemical processes (reactions) occur constantly in every living cell: The synthesis of new substances is balanced by the breaking down of older ones, as exemplified by the constant formation and degradation of bone. For this turnover of substances to occur, cells require a continuous supply of energy in the form of dietary carbohydrate, protein, and/or fat. Almost all cells need oxygen to transform the energy in these nutrients to a form of energy the body can use—**adenosine triphosphate,** or **ATP.** Cells also need water, building supplies, especially amino acids and minerals; and chemical regulators, such as the vitamins. All these substances enable the tissues, constituted from individual cells, to function properly.

Getting an adequate supply of all nutrients to the body's cells begins with a healthful diet. To assure optimal use of nutrients, the body's tissues, organs, and systems also must work efficiently.[17]

This chapter covers subject material concerned with the anatomy and physiology of the cell and major systems, especially as they relate to the study of human nutrition. The information you are about to study is limited to the components of the various systems that are specifically influenced by the 45-plus essential nutrients discussed in this text.

adenosine triphosphate (ATP) The main energy currency for cells. ATP energy is used to promote ion pumping, enzyme activity, and muscular contraction.

■ THE CELL: STRUCTURE AND FUNCTION

The cell is the basic structural and functional component of life. Living organisms are made of many different kinds of cells specialized to perform particular functions, and nearly all cells are derived from preexisting cells. In the human body, the 100 trillion cells all have certain basic characteristics that are alike.[18] These components, or cell structures, are designated **organelles,** and each is specialized to perform unique tasks. More than 15 different organelles have been described, with their structure and functions defined. In this introductory nutrition text, only the cell membrane and 10 of these structures will be examined in detail. The following discussion is limited to these structures, which are most closely associated with cellular nutrition (Fig. 3-1).

organelles Compartments, particles, or filaments that perform specialized functions within a cell.

■ Cell (Plasma) Membrane

There is an outside and inside to every cell, as defined by the cell (plasma) membrane.[19] The membrane holds the cellular contents and regulates the direction and flow of substances into and out of the cell, and cell-to-cell communication is by way of this membrane. Some cells can also penetrate and invade other cells.

The membrane is synthesized from lipids (fats), protein, and carbohydrate (see Fig. 3-1). However, 75% of the primary components are **phospholipids,** a type of lipid with a hydrophilic (water-soluble) head and hydrophobic (water-insoluble) tails (see Chapter 6 for details).

This membrane is a bilayer, or double layer, with hydrophilic heads of the phospholipid facing both into the cell proper and outside to the exterior of the cell. Such an arrangement defines an outside (exterior) surface and the inside (interior) surface. The hydrophobic tails then point into the center of the membrane. These phospholipids are highly mobile, so the membrane remains fluid. (*Fluidity* means that lipids

phospholipid Any of a class of fat-related substances that contain phosphorus, fatty acids, and a nitrogen-containing base. Phospholipids are an essential part of every cell.

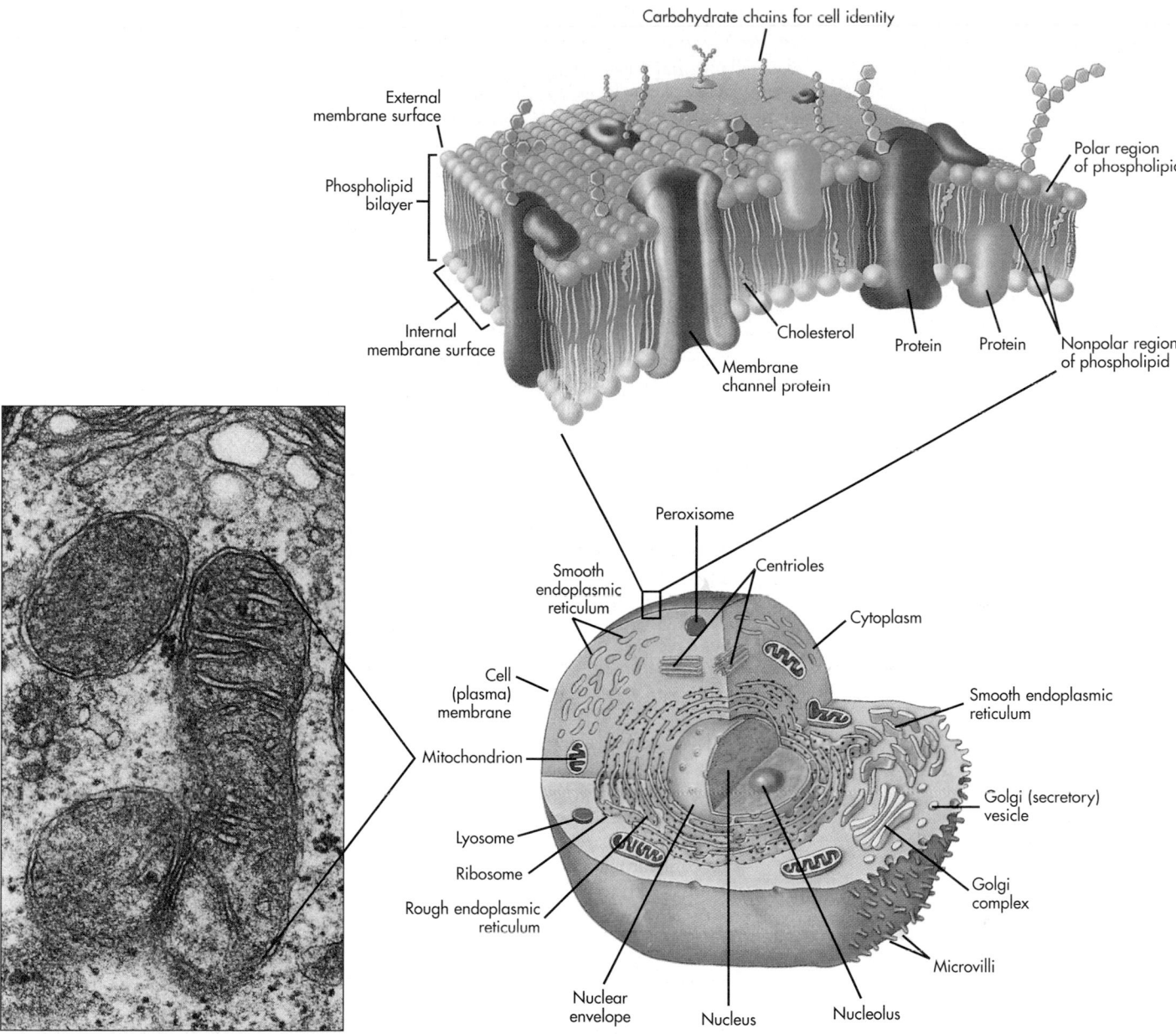

Carbohydrate chains for cell identity

External
membrane surface

Phospholipid
bilayer

Polar region
of phospholipid

Internal
membrane surface

Cholesterol

Protein

Protein

Nonpolar region
of phospholipid

Membrane
channel protein

Peroxisome

Smooth
endoplasmic
reticulum

Centrioles

Cytoplasm

Cell
(plasma)
membrane

Smooth endoplasmic
reticulum

Mitochondrion

Golgi (secretory)
vesicle

Lyosome

Ribosome

Golgi
complex

Rough endoplasmic
reticulum

Microvilli

Nuclear
envelope

Nucleus

Nucleolus

and some proteins can move laterally in the membrane.) The purpose of this phospholipid bilayer arrangement is to erect a barrier between the water-filled compartments found inside and outside the cell. Otherwise, water-soluble substances, such as nutrients and enzymes, could continually move in and out of the cell following their **concentration gradient.**

Every animal cell membrane contains a second type of lipid, cholesterol. Like almost all lipids, cholesterol is water insoluble (hydrophobic), so it is found within in the phospholipid bilayer. Together with phospholipids, cholesterol maintains the permeability of the cell to various fat-soluble substances and contributes to the fluidity of the membrane.

A second component of the cell membrane is protein. Actually, there are a variety of proteins providing structural support and **enzymes** to control chemical reactions within the cell membrane itself. Still other proteins:

1. Act as receptor sites, allowing certain substances to become attached to the membrane.
2. Form open pores or channels in the membrane through which water-soluble materials, and water itself, flow in and out of the cell.

▌ FIGURE **3-1** An animal cell. Almost all human cells contain these various organelles. Shown in greater detail are mitochondria and the cell membrane. Note: Not all cells have microvilli. The nuclear envelope encloses the nucleus. The centrioles participate in cell division.

concentration gradient The gradation in concentration that occurs between two regions having different concentrations.

enzyme A compound that speeds the rate of a chemical process but is not altered by the chemical process. Almost all enzymes are proteins.

3. Act as gates, opening and closing to direct the "flow of traffic."
4. Acts as transport vehicles or pumps and are powered by ATP (the fuel used by the cell). (Chapter 4 discusses ATP in detail.)

These transport vehicles and pumps move various substances from areas of low concentration to areas of high concentration. This is known as moving against a concentration gradient. A lot of our food energy, when converted to ATP, is used to keep these pumps functioning efficiently.

Carbohydrates are attached to the exterior surface of the cell membrane. They are combined with either protein or fat and, so, are respectively known as **glycoproteins** or **glycolipids.** This carbohydrate "coat" is called the **glycocalyx** and identifies the cell as belonging to "one's self." The glycocalyx of one cell communicates with the glycocalyx of an adjacent cell and can attach to or repel an adjacent cell. Some carbohydrates act as receptors for binding hormones in such a way that they initiate a series of events within the cell (see Endocrine System and Hormones). Carbohydrate structures in the cell membrane also participate in immune reactions.

Transport of Molecules Through the Cell Membrane

The cell membrane is a selectively permeable membrane, meaning that ions and molecules of different size are subject to traffic control as they move in and out of the cell. Various mechanisms, such as diffusion, facilitated diffusion, active absorption (transport), endocytosis and exocytosis are used for controlling the transport of substances.[4]

Diffusion is the net movement of molecules or ions from an area of higher concentration to an area of lower concentration. Gasses such as oxygen and carbon dioxide are **nonpolar,** so they can pass easily from one side of the membrane to the other. Oxygen is in high concentration outside the cell and in relatively low concentration inside the cell, so oxygen moves down its concentration gradient to the inside of the cell. The same applies to the gas carbon dioxide, a waste product of metabolism. This gas flows from the higher concentration within the cell to the lower concentration outside the cell (Fig. 3-2). Nonpolar lipid-soluble substances, such as cholesterol, diffuse through the phospholipid layer easily.

Facilitated diffusion works on the same principal as diffusion, except that a carrier (usually a protein) is used to transport a substance across cell membranes. For example, the sugar fructose has a higher concentration outside the cell than within, but it must be escorted into the cell. Fructose is loaded onto a carrier in the membrane and transported into the cell. The purpose of facilitated diffusion is to limit the amount of a substance entering the cell, counteracting the concentration that is always lower in the cell than outside the cell.

Active absorption (transport) involves moving a substance against its concentration gradient. Like riding a bicycle up a steep hill, it takes a lot of energy. In the case of active transport, a carrier (again a protein) acts as a vehicle, and the energy is supplied by ATP. An example of this mechanism involves the movement of sodium and potassium through the cell membrane. Sodium is normally an **extracellular** (outside the cell) ion. It must be constantly pumped out of the cell against its concentration gradient. The sodium is loaded onto a carrier, and the ATP is the fuel used to move the sodium. Simultaneously, potassium, usually an **intracellular** (inside the cell) ion, is constantly pumped back into the cell from outside the cell. The pump uses a carrier and ATP for fuel.

Phagocytosis allows the cell membrane to engulf a substance, so that the cell can "swallow" whole particles. Sometimes this process is called "cell eating." Phagocytosis is a form of "bulk transport" that allows large substances to be moved into a cell from the extracellular environment. White blood cells use this mechanism to swallow whole bacteria and then destroy them by digesting them. **Pinocytosis,** or "cell drinking," allows the cell to swallow a fluid and pull it into the cell. Phagocytosis and pinocytosis are collectively known as **endocytosis.**

Exocytosis is a process by which the cell membrane secretes products out of the cell when they are destined for another site. Products are packaged for export in the

---

glycoproteins Proteins containing a carbohydrate group.

glycolipids Lipids (fats) containing a carbohydrate group.

glycocalyx A hairlike projection on the extracellular surface of the plasma membrane; it consists of short, branched carbohydrate chains.

diffusion The net movement of molecules or ions from regions of higher to regions of lower concentration.

nonpolar A neutral compound; no positive or negative poles are present.

facilitated diffusion The carrier-mediated transport of molecules through the cell membrane along the direction of their concentration gradients. It does not require the expenditure of energy.

active absorption (transport) Absorption using a carrier and expending energy. In this way, the absorptive cell absorbs nutrients, such as glucose, when a high concentration of the nutrient is already present in the absorptive cells.

endocytosis (phagocytosis/pinocytosis) Forms of active absorption in which the absorptive cell forms an indentation in its membrane and particles (phagocytosis) or fluids (pinocytosis) entering the indentation are then engulfed by the cell.

exocytosis The process of cellular secretion in which the secretory products are contained within a membrane-enclosed vesicle. The vesicle fuses with the cell membrane and is open to the extracellular environment.

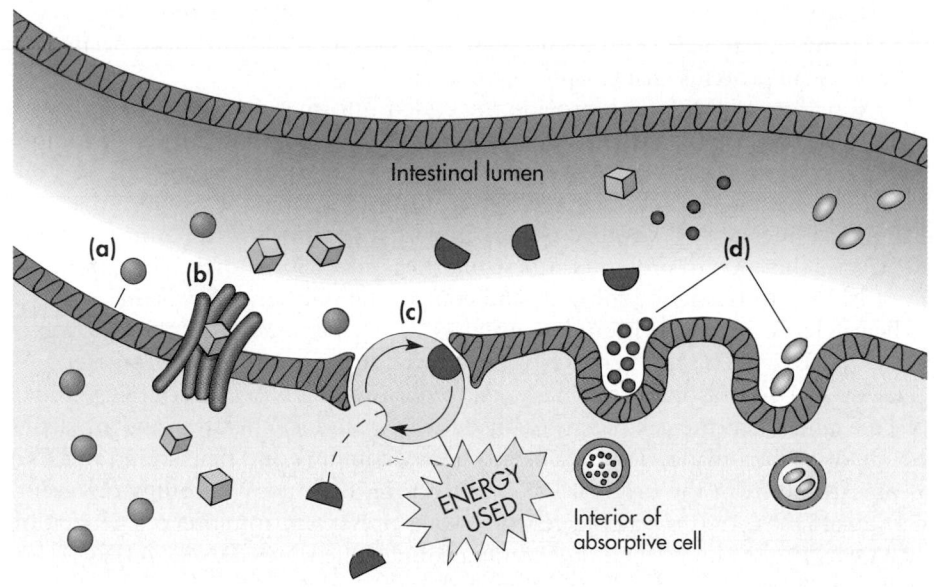

ENERGY USED

Interior of absorptive cell

■ FIGURE **3-2** Nutrient absorption relies on these major forms of absorptive processes. *(a)* Diffusion involves simple diffusion of substances across the cell membrane of absorptive cells. No energy is expended because the substances follow a favorable concentration gradient (from high to low concentrations). Water and fats are absorbed in this manner. *(b)* Facilitated diffusion uses a carrier protein or other process to aid in the absorption of specific substances, such as fructose. No energy is expended; the process is simply aided by the carrier. *(c)* Active absorption (transport) uses a carrier protein and expends energy in the process. The use of energy allows the absorptive cell to absorb nutrients against their concentration gradient (from low to high concentrations). Glucose undergoes active absorption. *(d)* Phagocytosis—"cell eating"—involves cells' taking in substances, including whole particles, by forming an indentation in the cell membrane and then surrounding the particle, with eventual incorporation into the cell. This is an active form of transport of substances. Pinocytosis—"cell drinking"—involves the cellular uptake of liquids in a manner analogous to phagocytosis. Exocytosis (not illustrated) packages products destined for export from the cell. The products are contained within a membrane-enclosed vesicle, which fuses with the plasma membrane, so that the products can be discharged into the extracellular fluid.

Golgi apparatus, and **secretory vesicles** fuse with the cell membrane to release their load into the extracellular environment (see the section on the Golgi complex later in this chapter).

■ Interior Cell Structure

Many of the functions of the cell are achieved within the cell membrane by structures called organelles. Some structures allow the cell to replicate itself, others provide energy, and others destroy the cell when it is worn out. Still other organelles produce and secrete products destined for other cells.[18]

Cytoplasm

The highly organized gel-like material in the cell, including all but the nucleus, is known as cytoplasm. The organelles are positioned in this medium between the cell membrane and the nucleus. The cytosol is the fluid surrounding the organelles.

Within the cytosol are enzymes that produce a small amount of ATP without the participation of oxygen. This ATP production, known as **anaerobic** respiration, is vital to our survival. For a minute or two, we can sustain life without breathing. There will be more about anaerobic metabolism in Chapter 4.

Mitochondria

Almost all the ATP we need is produced by the mitochondria, the power plants of the cell. These organelles are capable of converting the energy in our fuel-yielding nutrients (carbohydrate, protein, and fat) to ATP by chemical transformations, in the process using the oxygen we inhale, water coming either from the diet or that which we make, and enzymes.

With the exception of red blood cells, all cells contain mitochondria; only the size, shape, and numbers vary. The mitochondria have a highly folded inner membrane and an outer membrane, each performing different functions in generating ATP. Mitochondria will be described in more detail in Chapter 4.

The biochemical pathways that operate in the mitochondria are also capable of synthesizing cell components, such as the **carbon skeletons** needed to produce amino acids. These will eventually become cellular protein.

Cell Nucleus

With the exception of the red blood cell, all cells have one or more nuclei. The **cell nucleus** controls actions that occur in the cell, which use the hereditary material

secretory vesicles Membrane-bound vesicles produced by Golgi complex; contains protein to be secreted by the cell.

cytoplasm The fluid and organelles (except the nucleus) in a cell.

anaerobic Not requiring oxygen.

mitochondria The main sites of energy production in a cell. Mitochondria also contain the pathway for oxidizing fat for fuel, among other metabolic pathways.

carbon skeleton An amino acid after the amino group has been removed.

cell nucleus An organelle bound by its own double membrane and containing chromosomes, the genetic information for cell protein synthesis and cell replication.

chromosome A single large DNA molecule and its associated proteins containing many genes: stores and transmits genetic information.

gene The material on chromosomes that makes up DNA. Genes provide the blueprint for the production of cell proteins.

ribonucleic acid (RNA) The single-stranded nucleic acid involved in the transcription of genetic information and translation of that information into protein structure; it contains the sugar ribose and comes in three forms: messenger RNA, ribosomal RNA, and transfer RNA.

ribosomes Cytoplasmic particles that mediate the linking together of amino acids to form proteins; they are attached to the endoplasmic reticulum as bound ribosomes or are suspended in cytoplasm as free ribosomes.

endoplasmic reticulum (ER) An organelle in the cytoplasm composed of a network of canals running through the cytoplasm. Rough ER contains ribosomes. Smooth ER contains no ribosomes.

Golgi complex The cell organelle near the nucleus that processes newly synthesized protein for secretion or distribution to other organelles.

lysosome A cellular organelle that contains digestive enzymes for use inside the cell for turnover of cell parts.

apoptosis A process that occurs over time in which enzymes in a cell set off a series of events that disable numerous cell functions, eventually leading to cell death.

peroxisome A cell organelle that destroys toxic products within the cell.

---

called **DNA.** Long strands of material containing DNA, called **chromosomes,** contain the **genes** for genetic expression. These genes contain the directions needed for synthesizing all proteins (see Chapter 7 for details).

The function of DNA is to provide the coded information for the structure of proteins to be synthesized by the cell. The gene is the sequence of DNA components that codes for a protein. DNA does not leave the nucleus of the cell, so a relative of DNA, **ribonucleic acid (RNA),** must transcribe the code and escape through the nuclear pores to the cytoplasm with a copy of the DNA instructions. RNA carries the code to protein-synthesizing sites called **ribosomes.** Thus, the function of RNA is to transcribe the code and control the synthesis of protein.

The **nucleoli** are areas within the nucleus of the cell containing a combination of protein and RNA. This is where RNA is produced for export to the cytoplasm.

DNA has a second important task, cell replication. DNA is a double-stranded molecule, and when the cell begins to divide each strand is separated, and an identical copy of each is made. Thus, each new DNA contains one new strand of DNA and one strand from the original DNA. Therefore, each copy faithfully represents the original DNA. In this way the genetic code is preserved from one cell generation to the next. Interestingly, the mitochondria contain their own DNA, so they reproduce themselves independently of action in the nucleus.

The transport of proteins, vitamins, and other material from the cytoplasm to the nucleus is through pores in the nuclear membrane. These small molecules serve a variety of functions, including the activation (or inactivation) of certain parts of the DNA chain.

Endoplasmic Reticulum (ER)

The outer membrane of the cell nucleus is continuous with a network of tubes called the **endoplasmic reticulum (ER).** The endoplasmic reticulum comes in two types: rough and smooth. The **rough endoplasmic reticulum (RER)** contains the ribosomes, whereas the smooth does not. The ribosomes on the RER are responsible for reading the coded instructions brought from DNA by RNA and producing proteins. Many of these proteins play a central role in human nutrition. The **smooth ER** is involved in lipid (fat) synthesis, detoxification of toxic substances, and calcium storage and release.

Golgi Complex

The **Golgi complex** consists of sacs within the cytoplasm in which products of the RER are received and "finished" as proteins, separated according to functions and destination, and "packaged" for secretion by the cell. Some carbohydrates are synthesized within these structures. The Golgi complex is like a warehouse and distribution center. The Golgi complex also can convert to secretory vesicles and carry cell products to the cell surface for exocytosis.

Lysosomes

Lysosomes are sacs that contain enzymes for the digestion of foreign material. Sometimes known as "suicide bags," they are responsible for digesting worn-out or damaged cells. They carry out **apoptosis,** or programmed cell death, which occurs naturally or is associated with illness or infections. Cells associated with immunity, called macrophages, contain lots of lysosomes (see Immune System).

Peroxisomes

Peroxisomes contain enzymes that detoxify harmful chemicals. Hydrogen peroxide (H_2O_2) is formed here by enzymes and is important in breaking down poisonous substances within the cell. For students of human nutrition, it is important to note that peroxisomes play a role in metabolizing one possible source of food energy, alcohol. There will be more about alcohol metabolism in Chapter 8. The enzyme catalase, present in the peroxisomes, prevents excessive accumulation of hydrogen peroxide in the cell, which would also damage the cell.

CONCEPT CHECK

*I*n Chapter 1, you learned that fat (lipids), protein, and carbohydrate function as fuels. Now you recognize that these organic nutrients also serve as structural materials in the cell membrane. This is typical of many nutrients; they can carry out multiple functions. The cell receives nutrients and other substances through the cell membrane by using various transport systems.

The basic structural unit in the body is the cell. Within the cell are a variety of organelles with unique functions to perform. Although there is no typical cell, virtually all cells have the same organelles, each performing essential tasks.

■ ORGANIZATION OF THE BODY

When groups of similar cells work together to accomplish a specialized task, the arrangement is referred to as a **tissue.** Tissues are specialized groups of cells with a common structure and function. Humans are composed of four primary types of tissue: **epithelial, connective, muscle,** and **nervous.** Epithelial tissue is composed of cells that cover body surfaces. These secrete important substances, absorb nutrients and excrete waste. Connective tissue supports and protects the body, stores fat, and produces blood cells. Muscle tissue (skeletal, smooth, and cardiac) is designed for movement. Nervous tissue found in the brain and spinal cord is designed for communication.

When groups of tissue work together to perform a variety of actions, this collection is called an **organ.** For example, the liver is an organ that has a variety of tissues, which process nutrients, control the composition of the blood, produce a vital digestive substance, and act as a detoxification center.

Several organs that join together to carry out similar or related functions are called a **system.**[13] We will be particularly concerned in this chapter with the digestive system. The nutrients we consume in food are unavailable until such time as they have been processed by the digestive system using chemical and mechanical means to alter food, so that the nutrients can be released and absorbed into the body for distribution to body tissues. Table 3-1 summarizes the components and functions of the various systems.

Sometimes organs within a system can serve another system. For example, the basic function of the digestive system is to convert the food we eat into absorbable nutrients. At the same time, the digestive system serves the immune system by preventing dangerous pathogens from invading the body and causing illness. As you study nutrition, you will note the multiple roles played by many organs.

The overriding theme of human nutrition is to understand the actions of nutrients as they affect different cells, tissues, organs, and systems. Each type of system is impacted by nutrient intake and simultaneously determines how each nutrient is used.

Our task now is to explore the various systems in the body as they specifically relate to the study of human nutrition. This part of the chapter will set the stage for a more detailed look at the systems in later chapters, as we investigate the various nutrients associated with human nutrition.

■ Integumentary System

The first system to examine in detail is the system we are most familiar with, the **integumentary** system, which is made up of dissimilar elements, such as the skin, hair, various glands, and nails.[18] The largest organ in the body, the skin, consists of two principal layers, the **epidermis** and the **dermis.** The epidermis is the layer of skin composed largely of dead cells, which are used for protection from environmental pathogens, toxins, injury, and water. We don't want to absorb water through the skin, nor do we want water to readily escape the body.

---

tissues Collections of cells adapted to perform a specific function.

epithelial tissue The surface cells that line the outside of the body and all external passages within it.

connective tissue Protein tissue that holds different structures in the body together. Some structures are made up of connective tissue—notably, tendons and cartilages. Connective tissue also forms part of bone and the nonmuscular structures of arteries and veins.

muscle tissue A type of tissue adapted to contract.

nervous tissue Tissue composed of highly branched, elongated cells, which transport nerve impulses from one part of the body to another.

organ A group of tissues designed to perform a specific function—for example, the heart. It contains muscle tissue, nerve tissue, and so on.

system A collection of organs that work together to perform an overall function.

integumentary Having to do with the skin, hair, glands, and nails, the largest organ in the body.

epidermis The outermost layer of the skin, composed of epithelial layers.

dermis The second, or deep, layer of the skin, under the epidermis.

TABLE 3-1   Organ Systems of the Body

System	Major Components	Functions
Integumentary	Skin, hair, nails, and sweat glands	Protects, regulates temperature, prevents water loss, and produces a substance that converts to vitamin D
Skeletal	Bones, associated cartilage, and joints	Protects, supports, and allows body movement; produces blood cells; and stores minerals
Muscular	Smooth, cardiac, and skeletal muscle	Produces body movement, maintains posture, and produces body heat
Nervous	Brain, spinal cord, nerves, and sensory receptors	A major regulatory system: detects sensation, controls movements, and controls physiological and intellectual functions
Endocrine	Endocrine glands, such as the pituitary, thyroid, and adrenal glands	A major regulatory system: participates in the regulation of metabolism, reproduction, and many other functions
Cardiovascular	Heart, blood vessels, and blood	Transports nutrients, waste products, gases, and hormones throughout the body and plays a role in the immune response and the regulation of body temperature
Lymphatic	Lymph vessels, lymph nodes, and other lymph organs	Removes foreign substances from the blood and lymph, combats disease, maintains tissue fluid balance, and aids in fat absorption
Respiratory	Lungs and respiratory passages	Exchanges gases (oxygen and carbon dioxide) between the blood and the air and regulates blood acid-base balance
Digestive	Mouth, esophagus, stomach, intestines, and accessory structures	Performs the mechanical and chemical processes of digestion, absorption of nutrients, and elimination of wastes
Urinary	Kidneys, urinary bladder, and the ducts that carry urine	Removes waste products from the circulatory system and regulates blood acid-base balance, overall chemical balance, and water balance
Reproductive	Gonads, accessory structures, and genitals of males and females	Performs the processes of reproduction and influences sexual functions and behaviors

The cardiovascular and lymphatic organ systems contribute to the circulatory functions. The endocrine and nervous organ systems contribute to the regulatory functions. The digestive, urinary, integumentary, and respiratory organ systems contribute to the excretory functions, while the muscular and skeletal organ systems contribute to storage functions in the body.

decubitus ulcers Chronic ulcers that appear in pressure areas of the skin over a body prominence. These develop when people are confined to bed or immobilized (i.e., bedsores).

CRITICAL THINKING

Molly was excited to read about hair analysis as a "guaranteed" method for determining a person's nutritional status. She is submitting a sample of her hair to learn how healthy she is. She says it is worth the $100 just to know she is eating a well-balanced diet. Why do you think she is wasting her money on such a procedure? What do you tell her when she gets the printout from the hair analysis company with advice to purchase a variety of supplements to cure her nutrient deficiencies?

The dermis is a deeper and thicker layer of skin, with an extensive network of blood vessels, sweat glands, oil-secreting glands, nerve endings, and hair follicles. When people are confined to bed for long periods of time, **decubitus ulcers,** also called bed sores, may develop due to restricted blood flow to the dermis. This lack of blood causes cells to die and open wounds to develop—a potentially life-threatening situation. Adequate protein, vitamin A, vitamin C, and zinc intake may help prevent this problem.

The appearance of the skin, hair, and nails is clinically important, because it can indicate nutritional deficiencies. For instance, hot, dry skin is an obvious sign of dehydration due to inadequate water intake. Other signs and symptoms of nutrient deficiencies, as manifest by the skin, will be described in the following chapters as the function of individual nutrients are explained.

The skin plays a vital role in temperature regulation. Heat produced by the body's metabolic processes, especially the processes that occur in muscle, must be removed before we are "cooked." Heat is removed from the body through the skin. And, when we are cold, we warm ourselves by shivering as muscle contractions generate heat.

An important nutrient, Vitamin D, can be obtained from our diet, but the skin can make it from a substance, cholesterol, located in the skin. There will be more detail about this process in Chapter 9.

The sweat glands produce perspiration, or sweat, which helps evaporate fluids to cool the body and excrete certain wastes. Mammary glands within the breasts are specialized to secrete milk to feed a newborn.

■ Skeletal System

Approximately 206 bones make up the skeletal system; this is the rigid framework to which soft tissues and organs of the body are attached.[18] Each bone is an organ that participates in the overall functioning of the skeleton. Bones that make up the skull and vertebral column protect the brain and spinal cord from injury. Likewise, the rib cage protects the heart, lungs, liver, and spleen from external damage. Bones have attachment sites to most skeletal muscles, ligaments, and tendons. (Bones attached to muscles allows body movement when muscles contract.) Blood cell formation, known as **hemopoiesis,** takes place within the marrow of some bones. It is estimated that we produce 2.5 million red blood cells every second, thanks to the action of bone. Bones also are a storehouse for minerals such as calcium, phosphorus, magnesium, sodium, and fluoride. Rather than being considered dried, dead tissues, bones are metabolically active and constantly adapting to a changing environment.

Long bones, such as those found in the arms and legs, are of two types: cortical and trabecular (Fig. 3-3). Cortical bone is hard and dense. It forms a protective shell on the exterior of the bone. Trabecular bone is found within the cortical bone at the ends of long bones and in the vertebrae. The shaft of the long bones is a cylinder of cortical bone surrounding a central cavity containing the marrow (see Chapter 11).

At the end of the long bone is the **epiphysis,** consisting of trabecular bone covered by cortical bone. The epiphysis is strong and allows for the attachment of tendons and ligaments. Red bone marrow is made of trabecular bone and is the source of red blood cells, as well as white blood cells and platelets. In children, just behind the epiphysis is the **epiphyseal plate.** This area of bone is responsible for linear growth. When linear growth is complete, an **epiphyseal line** replaces the plate.

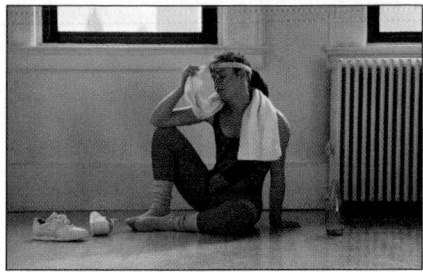

Sweat protects the body from overheating.

hemopoiesis The production of red blood cells.

cortical Tightly packed bone that is superficial to spongy bone, also called dense bone.

trabecular bone Bone tissue with a latticelike structure, also called spongy or cancellous bone.

epiphysis The end of a long bone. The epiphyseal plate—sometimes referred to as the growth plate—is made of cartilage and allows growth of the bone to occur. During childhood, the cartilage cells multiply and absorb calcium, to develop into bone.

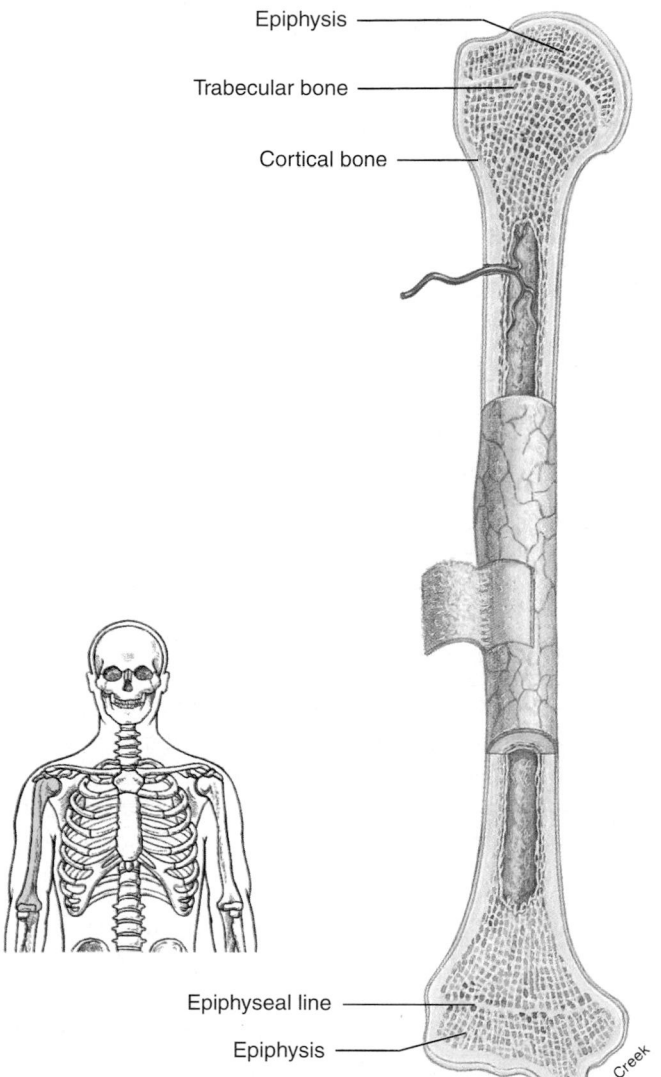

Epiphysis

Trabecular bone

Cortical bone

Epiphyseal line

Epiphysis

Creek

■ FIGURE **3-3** Diagram of a long bone. The epiphysis, consisting of trabecular bone, is surrounded by a layer of cortical bone. The epiphyseal line indicates that the bone has completed growth. The production of red blood cells occurs in the porous chambers of trabecular bone. The collagen material, the structural material of bone, is observed by the open flap. The skeletal system provides a reserve of calcium and phosphorus for day-to-day needs when dietary intake is inadequate.

collagen The major protein of the material that holds together the various structures of the body.

hydroxyapatite A compound, composed primarily of calcium and phosphate, that is deposited into the bone protein matrix to give bone strength and rigidity ($Ca_{10}[PO_4]_6OH_2$).

remodeling The constant building and breakdown of bone throughout life.

resorption The loss of a substance by physiologic or pathologic means.

osteoblasts Cells in bone that secrete mineral and bone matrix (e.g., collagen).

osteoclasts Bone cells that arise originally from a type of white blood cell. Osteoclasts secrete substances that lead to bone erosion. This erosion can set the stage for subsequent bone mineralization.

calcitonin A thyroid gland hormone that inhibits bone resorption.

parathyroid hormone (PTH) A hormone made by the parathyroid glands that increases synthesis of the vitamin D hormone and aids calcium release from bone and calcium uptake by the kidneys, among other functions.

neuron The structural and functional unit of the nervous system, consisting of cell body, dendrites, and axon.

smooth muscle Muscle tissue under involuntary control. Found in the GI tract, artery walls, respiratory passages, the urinary tract, and the reproductive tract.

cardiac muscle Muscle tissue that makes up the walls of the heart. Produces rhythmical involuntary contractions.

skeletal muscle Muscle tissue responsible for voluntary body movements.

myosin A thick filament protein that connects with actin to cause a muscle contraction.

actin A protein in muscle fiber that, together with myosin, is responsible for contraction.

tendon Dense regular connective tissue that attaches a muscle to a bone.

glycogen A carbohydrate made of multiple units of glucose with a highly branched structure; sometimes known as *animal starch*. It is the storage form of glucose in humans and is synthesized (and stored) in the liver and muscles.

Bones are constructed from several types of cells under the influence of a variety of growth factors. These factors stimulate the formation of **collagen,** a type of flexible protein matrix, which forms the basic shape of bone. Minerals—principally, calcium and phosphorus—are embedded in the matrix, which give the bone strength. **Hydroxyapatite,** the name of the calcium phosphorus salt deposited in the protein matrix, constitutes about 85% of minerals in bone and makes it possible for the bone to resist compression and bending.

Ossification (calcification) of bone varies from bone to bone, but most bones are ossified (mature) by ages 17 to 25. However, some bones, such as the sternum (breast bone), may not complete growth until age 30-plus.

Bone is constantly **remodeled** throughout life. Formation and **resorption** of bone occur due to the continual activity of **osteoblasts** and **osteoclasts.** Osteoblasts are bone-building cells and osteoclasts are bone resorbing cells. In the first 20 or so years of life, bone formation is greater than resorption. By age 50 or 60, resorption is greater than deposition and bone diseases are likely to occur.[16] Exercise promotes remodeling, whereas a lack of exercise results in bone loss.

Bone deposition (ossification) and bone resorption (dissolution) also maintain homeostasis of calcium and phosphorus in the blood. Three hormones control the process: the active **vitamin D hormone, calcitonin,** and **parathyroid hormone** (PTH).

There are other hormones involved in bone homeostasis, such as growth hormone; thyroid hormones; sex hormones, especially estrogen; and adrenocorticoid hormones.[2] In addition, vitamins A, K, and C perform important jobs in bone metabolism. There will be more about bones in the chapters covering vitamins, minerals, and exercise, in Chapters 9, 10, 11, and 14.

CONCEPT CHECK

The skin protects the body from toxins, pathogens, and water uptake and loss. It regulates body temperature, so that we are neither too hot nor too cold. The skin contributes to the body's supply of vitamin D.

The skeleton is essential for structural support, protection of underlying soft tissue, strength, mineral storage, and formation of blood cells. Diet, age, hormones, and exercise determine the health of bone.

■ Muscular System

The functions of the muscle system are to provide movement and to generate body heat. Most of the energy released during physical exercise is in the form of heat. Muscle cells called **muscle fibers** respond when stimulated by motor **neurons** (nerve cells).[18, 19] A muscle cell converts the chemical energy in ATP into the mechanical energy of muscle contraction.

There are three types of muscle tissue: **smooth, cardiac,** and **skeletal.** Smooth muscle fibers have a single nucleus and function in involuntary movements within internal organs. Cardiac muscle fiber is **striated** (striped) with a single nucleus. The stripes in muscle fibers are caused by the arrangement of alternating dark and light contractile proteins (**myosin** and **actin**). This type of muscle makes up involuntary rhythmic contractions, such as those found in heart muscle. Skeletal muscle, also containing striated muscle fibers, has several nuclei and is involved in voluntary movements. Skeletal muscle is attached to bone by **tendons.**

Skeletal Muscle

Skeletal muscle fibers are actually long cells with the same organelles as found in other cells. However, unlike most other cells, skeletal muscle cells possess an excellent supply of fuel in the form of **glycogen,** the body's storage form of the sugar glucose.

Skeletal muscles contract when stimulated by motor neurons. Motor neurons can **innervate** several muscle fibers simultaneously. A single muscle fiber is not a very efficient machine. The activation of varying numbers of motor neurons results in increased muscle strength as the number of fibers stimulated by neurons increases.

Muscle Contraction

As previously mentioned, within muscle fibers are the dark and light stripes called striations. Each muscle cell, when viewed in the electron microscope, contains subunits called **myofibrils.** The myofibrils are the source of the light and dark bands or stripes. Viewed at even higher magnification are subsubunits called **filaments.** The importance of these structures is the presence of unique proteins, which make muscles contract and relax. Thick filaments contain the protein myosin. Thin filaments contain the protein actin. The functioning structure of the myofibril makes up a **sarcomere,** the contracting unit.

When a muscle fiber is stimulated by a neuron to contract, one of the first events to occur is the release of large amounts of calcium from storage in the smooth endoplasmic reticulum. This is the "on" switch. The activated site allows the two main proteins, myosin and actin, to get ready to slide into each other and set in motion the **power stroke.** Of course, all this action requires energy to carry out the muscle contraction. Here is where ATP plays the key role (Fig. 3-4).

Another ATP is needed to release the actin form the myosin. This is the end of the contraction. As the muscle moves to the "off" position, the calcium is released and transported back to storage, the muscle fiber relaxes, and it gets ready for another contraction. The reason that muscle action occurs at all is due to the essential nutrient calcium. When the muscle is relaxed, there is very little calcium in the cytoplasm of the muscle cell because calcium is in storage. However, when the muscle is ready to go to work, as directed by the motor neuron, calcium is moved out of storage, which sets in motion the power stroke. And, when the contraction ends, the calcium is released and goes back into storage.

You may wonder what these mechanical activities have to do with the study of human nutrition. First, a lot of energy in the form of ATP must be used to cause the power stroke, and ATP then is also needed for the muscle to relax. The original source of the energy is food in the form of carbohydrates, proteins, and fats. Second, muscle action generates a lot of heat, which the body must remove via the blood; otherwise, the muscle would soon be overheated. And, third, the body will never allow muscles to run out of calcium. The calcium in the muscle is obtained from the calcium "bone bank" found in bones. The "bone bank account" is continually supplied with calcium from the diet. But what happens when the bone bank is overdrawn? There will be much more about "bankruptcy" in Chapter 11, concerning calcium and the disease osteoporosis.

Cardiac and Smooth Muscle

Cardiac muscle and smooth muscle, although similar in many ways to skeletal muscle in their use of calcium as an off/on switch, operate under involuntary control.

In cardiac muscle, the stimulation occurs automatically in a group of heart cells called a **pacemaker.** The pacemaker initiates the heartbeat and the heart rate. Today, many people with an irregular heartbeat have an artificial pacemaker inserted in their chest wall to maintain normal heart rhythm.

Smooth muscles are found in the lungs, blood vessels, and gastrointestinal (GI) tract. In the GI tract, they produce important contractions in a process called **peristalsis** (see later section on digestion). A unique feature of smooth muscle is its ability to stretch. By the end of pregnancy, the smooth muscle in the uterus can be stretched up to eight times its prepregnant length.

■ Circulatory System

The circulatory system is made up of two separate systems: the cardiovascular system and the lymphatic system.[18, 19] The cardiovascular system consists of the heart and

innervate To supply with nerve fibers.

myofibrils A bundle of contractile fibers within a muscle cell.

filaments Parts of a muscle fiber.

sarcomere A portion of a muscle fiber that is considered the functional unit of a myofibril.

power stroke The thick filament pulls alongside the thin filament, causing the muscle contraction.

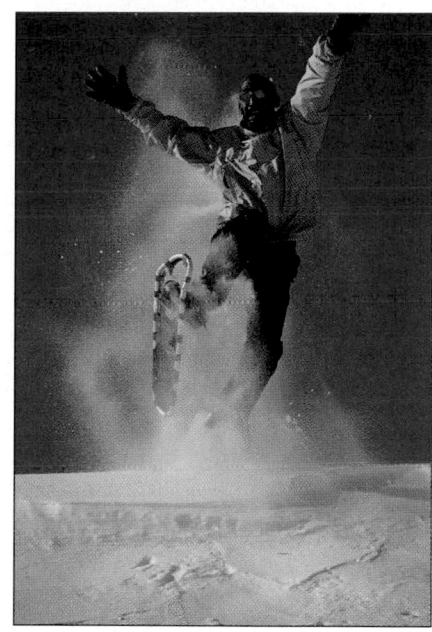

Exercise uses both the skeletal and cardiac muscles.

pacemaker A group of cells in the heart that regulates contractions.

peristalsis A coordinated muscular contraction that is used to propel food down the gastrointestinal tract.

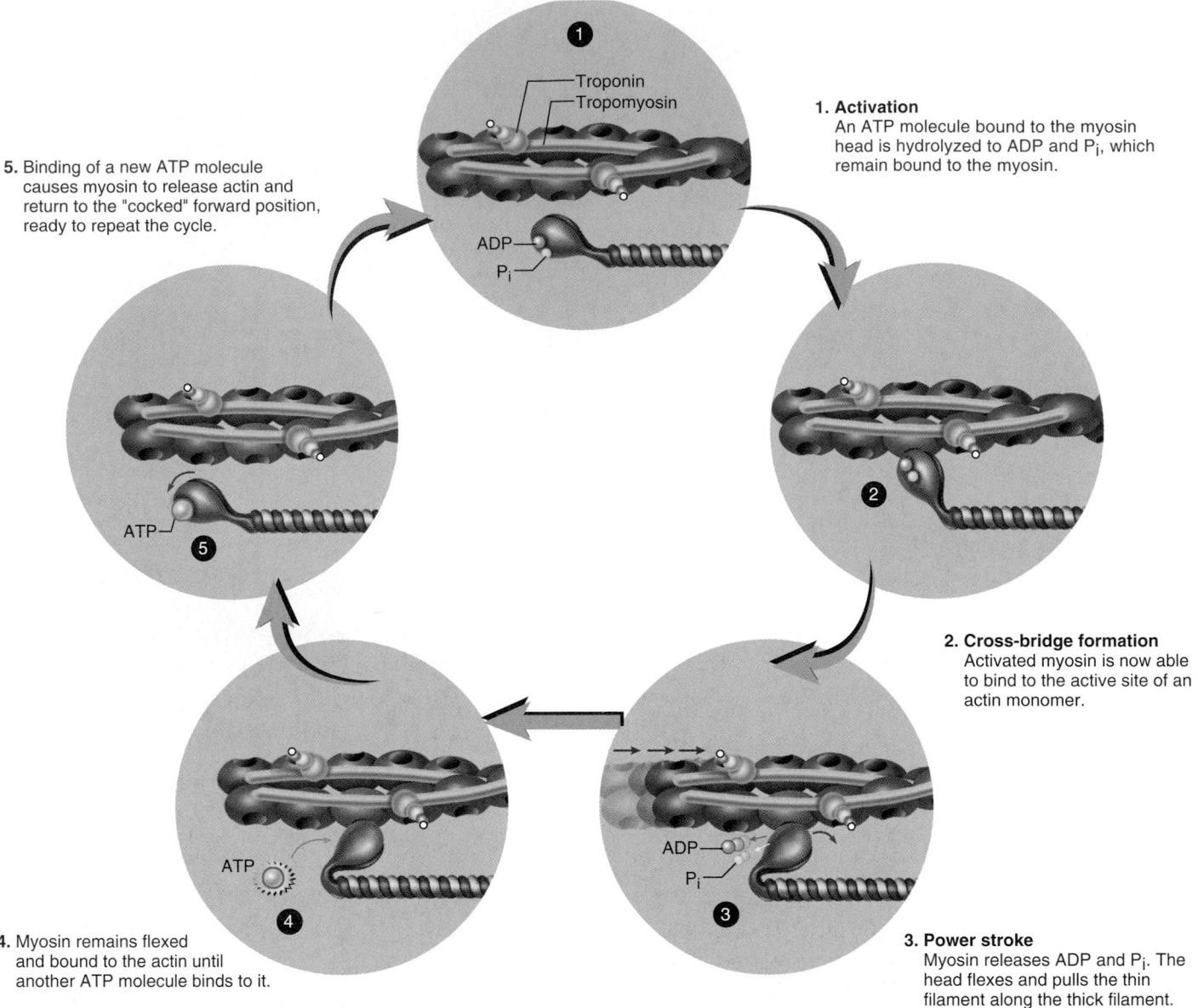

5. Binding of a new ATP molecule causes myosin to release actin and return to the "cocked" forward position, ready to repeat the cycle.

1. Activation
An ATP molecule bound to the myosin head is hydrolyzed to ADP and P$_i$, which remain bound to the myosin.

2. Cross-bridge formation
Activated myosin is now able to bind to the active site of an actin monomer.

3. Power stroke
Myosin releases ADP and P$_i$. The head flexes and pulls the thin filament along the thick filament.

4. Myosin remains flexed and bound to the actin until another ATP molecule binds to it.

■ FIGURE **3-4** Muscle contraction. In Step 1, or activation, an ATP is bound to the myosin head (purple) and is split into ADP and P$_i$. During Step 2, the activated myosin can now bind to the actin (the red beads). In Step 3, the myosin head releases the ADP and P$_i$. The head flexes and pulls the thin filament along the thick filament. This is the *power stroke*. In Step 4, the myosin remains bound to the actin until another ATP binds to the myosin. The new ATP causes the myosin to release the actin, so that it can get ready for another cycle, Step 5. Troponin and tropomyosin are proteins that participate in this process. The white dot in this figure is calcium, a nutrient required for muscle action.

blood vessels. The lymphatic system consists of lymphatic vessels, lymph, and a number of lymph tissues.

One organ vital to our existence is the heart, a four-chambered pump that keeps blood continuously circulating around the body. It takes about 1 minute for blood to leave the heart, circulate to all tissues in the body, and return to the heart. When we are exercising strenuously, the blood can circulate at a rate of six times per minute.

The cells that make up tissues in the body need a constant supply of water, oxygen, and nutrients. In addition, the body needs ATP energy, which in turn comes from the breakdown of energy nutrients within the cells. The blood carries oxygen from the lungs to all organs in the body. The blood also carries nutrients from the digestive tract to all tissues and to storage sites when nutrients are not immediately needed for energy, growth, or repair. Waste materials produced by cells must be removed by way of the skin, lungs, kidneys, and digestive tract. This, too, is a function of the cardiovascular system. The delivery of hormones to their target cells, the maintenance of a constant body temperature, and the distribution of white blood cells to protect against invading pathogens are all performed by the blood and circulatory systems without our ever being aware of any specific action. The circulatory system has chemical means to prevent excessive loss of blood from damaged vessels. It uses the clotting process (see Chapter 9).

Blood Constituents

Red blood cells, known as **erythrocytes,** are carriers of oxygen to all tissues and play a role in the return of carbon dioxide to the lungs. The white blood cells, known as **leukocytes,** function as part of the immune system. They protect the body from invading pathogens. The blood is able to clot because of platelets and other clotting factors. These important components of the blood are known as "formed elements." The liquid part of blood is known as **plasma.**

Heart Structure

The heart has two sides, left and right. The right side is closest to your right arm; likewise, the left side is closest to your left arm. The upper part of the heart has left and right **atria,** which empty simultaneously into the lower part of the heart, the left and right **ventricles.**

Blood travels in blood vessels from the left side of the heart, through the **aorta** to major **arteries.** Arteries become smaller and smaller until they are so tiny they are classified as microscopic **arterioles.** The blood flows from the arterioles into more microscopic, weblike structures called **capillaries.** Capillaries are just one cell layer thick and have pores, which allow oxygen, water, and other nutrients to leave the blood for surrounding cells and which allow waste and other products of cellular metabolism to enter the blood. There are scarcely any cells in the body that aren't close to a capillary. Larger blood vessels are not porous, so blood cannot escape these vessels. Only in the capillaries can the blood discharge and recover substances associated with nearby cells.

As the blood exits the capillaries, it flows into tiny microscopic **venules,** which enlarge and become **veins,** returning the blood to the right side of the heart. The route from the left side of the heart to the capillaries and then back to the right side of the heart is called the **systemic circuit** of blood (Figs. 3-5 and 3-6).

The flow of blood through the circulatory system is measured by pressure in millimeters of mercury. The average arterial (artery) pressure is about 100 mm Hg, whereas the average venous pressure is only 2 mm Hg. To guarantee return flow back to the heart, blood is moved through the veins by the contraction of skeletal muscles. There are also valves in the veins that prevent a backflow of blood.

Flow of Materials Between Capillaries and Cells

As the blood flows from the arterioles into the capillaries, the hydrostatic pressure generated by the force of the heart causes fluid to flow into spaces around the surrounding cells, called the **extracellular fluid (ECF)** (Fig. 3-7). Some of this fluid returns to the capillaries and some enters another nearby vessel called a **lymphatic vessel.**

Oxygen and nutrients leave the capillaries and enter the ECF and are then delivered to cells by one of the mechanisms mentioned earlier: diffusion, active transport, and pinocytosis. Cellular products plus waste substances are collected in the ECF and are either released to the capillaries that connect to the venules or channeled into the lymph vessels. Oxygen travels to the cell by diffusing from the blood into the extracellular fluid and then in through the cell membrane. Carbon dioxide exits the cell and goes to the blood by way of the same mechanism. This is one of two important gas exchange activities in the body and is often referred to as internal respiration.

erythrocyte A mature red blood cell. It has no nucleus and a lifespan of about 120 days; contains hemoglobin, which transports oxygen and carbon dioxide.

atria The two upper chambers of the heart, which receive venous blood.

ventricles The two lower chambers of the heart, which contain blood to be pumped from the heart.

aorta The major blood vessel of the body leaving from the left ventricle.

artery A blood vessel that carries blood away from the heart.

capillary A microscopic blood vessel that connects an arteriole and a venule; the functional unit of the circulatory system.

vein A blood vessel that conveys blood to the heart.

system circuit The part of the circulatory system concerned with the flow of blood from the left ventricle to the body and back to the right atrium.

extracellular fluid (ECF) Fluid present outside the cells; this includes intravascular and interstitial fluids.

lymphatic vessel A vessel that carries lymph.

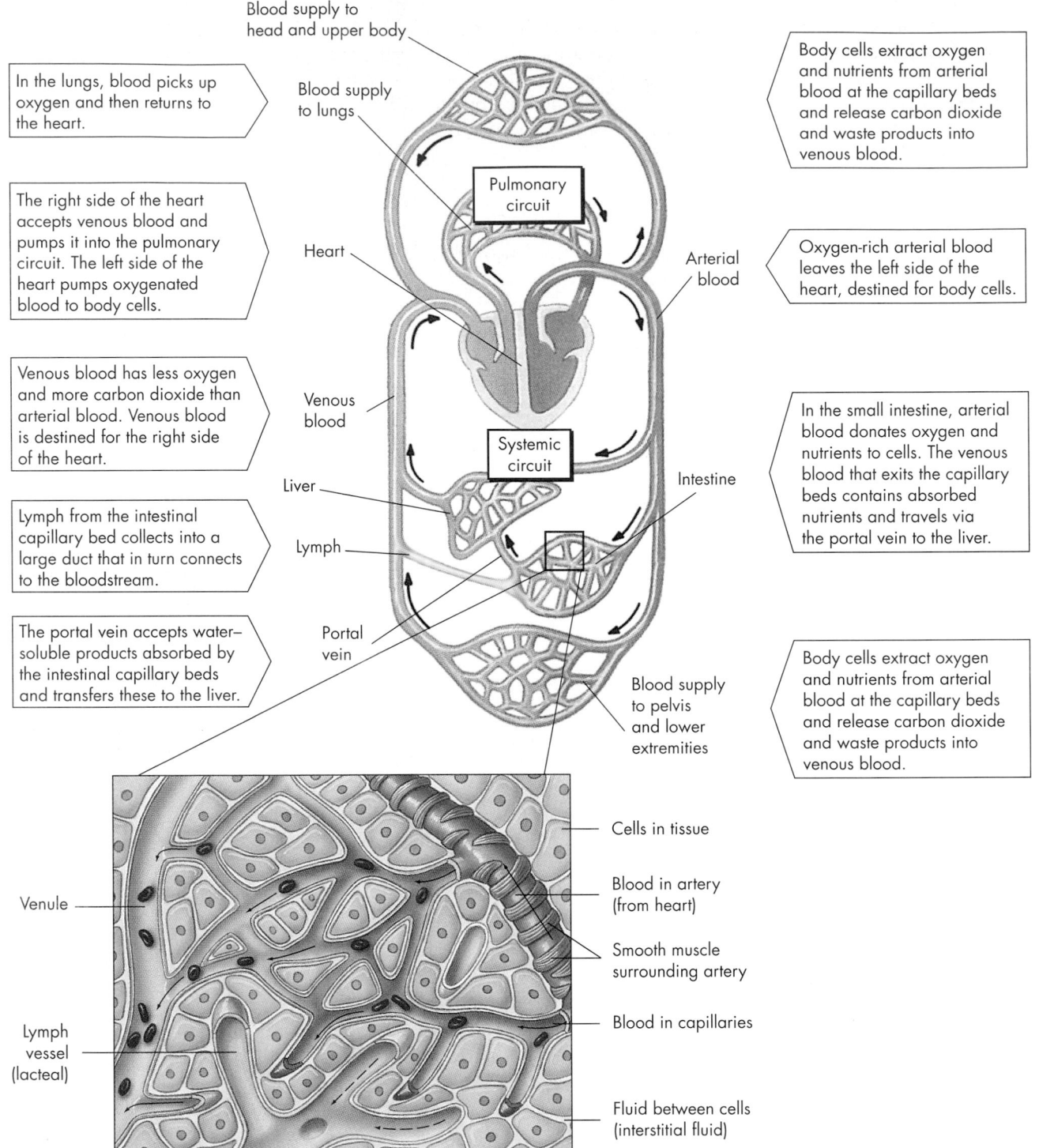

Blood supply to head and upper body

Blood supply to lungs

Pulmonary circuit

Heart

Arterial blood

Venous blood

Systemic circuit

Liver

Intestine

Lymph

Portal vein

Blood supply to pelvis and lower extremities

In the lungs, blood picks up oxygen and then returns to the heart.

The right side of the heart accepts venous blood and pumps it into the pulmonary circuit. The left side of the heart pumps oxygenated blood to body cells.

Venous blood has less oxygen and more carbon dioxide than arterial blood. Venous blood is destined for the right side of the heart.

Lymph from the intestinal capillary bed collects into a large duct that in turn connects to the bloodstream.

The portal vein accepts water-soluble products absorbed by the intestinal capillary beds and transfers these to the liver.

Body cells extract oxygen and nutrients from arterial blood at the capillary beds and release carbon dioxide and waste products into venous blood.

Oxygen-rich arterial blood leaves the left side of the heart, destined for body cells.

In the small intestine, arterial blood donates oxygen and nutrients to cells. The venous blood that exits the capillary beds contains absorbed nutrients and travels via the portal vein to the liver.

Body cells extract oxygen and nutrients from arterial blood at the capillary beds and release carbon dioxide and waste products into venous blood.

Cells in tissue

Blood in artery (from heart)

Smooth muscle surrounding artery

Blood in capillaries

Fluid between cells (interstitial fluid)

Venule

Lymph vessel (lacteal)

FIGURE 3-5 Blood circulation throughout the body. This represents the route blood takes through the two circuits that begin and end at the heart. The red color indicates blood that is richer in oxygen; blue is for blood carrying more carbon dioxide. Oxygen and nutrients are exchanged for carbon dioxide and waste products in the capillaries, the points at which the arteries and veins merge. The bottom box shows a close-up of a capillary bed in the small intestine, including the location of the lymphatic vessels. This second set of circulatory vessels—part of the lymphatic system—picks up the fluid that builds up between cells (interstitial fluid) and large particles, such as some fats. This fluid and the particles become lymph, which travels through further lymph vessels to reach the bloodstream. Lymph vessels in the intestine are also called *lacteals*. Hold the back of this book up to your chest in order to have this figure reflect the true orientation of your heart.

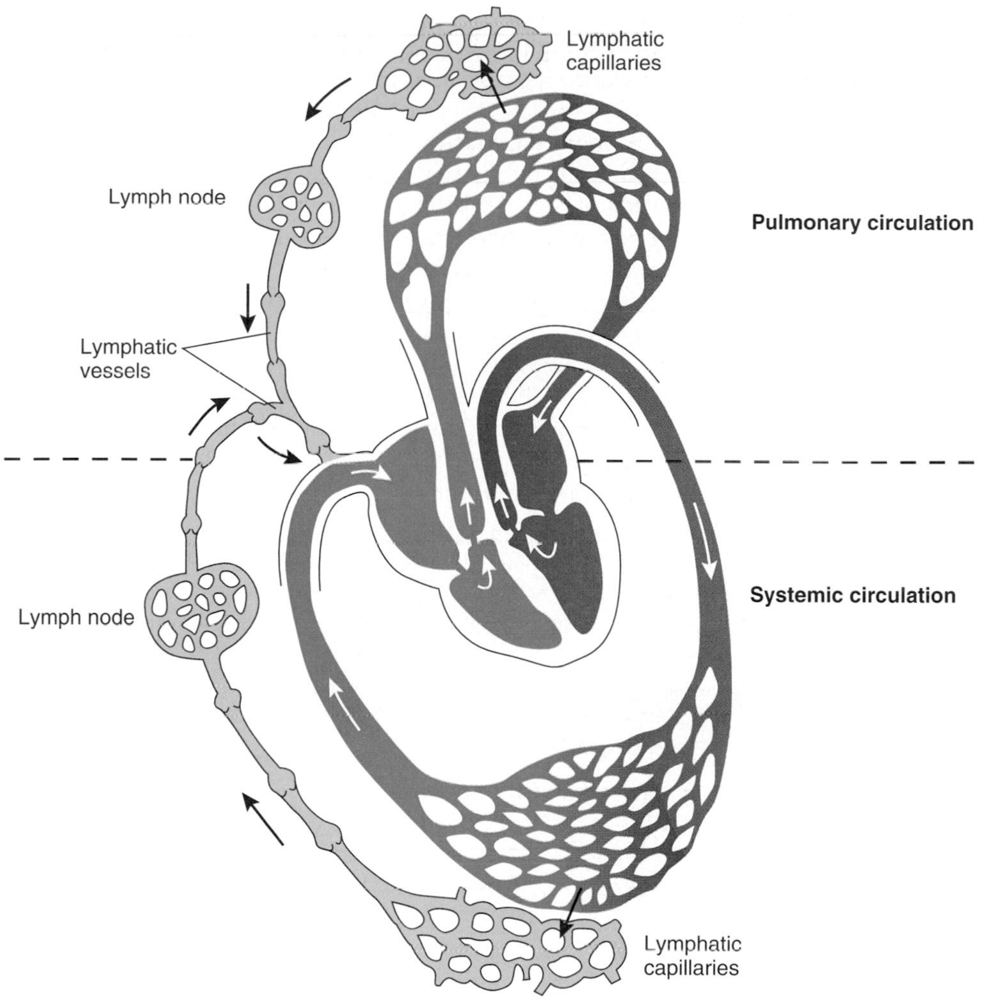

Lymphatic
capillaries

Pulmonary circulation

Lymph node

Lymphatic
vessels

Lymph node

Systemic circulation

Lymphatic
capillaries

■ FIGURE 3-6 Lymph. As lymph moves
through the lymphatic system, it encounters
lymph nodes, containing immune cells,
which destroy invading pathogens. Lymph
also carries dietary fat and fat-soluble nutrients from the digestive tract to the vascular system.

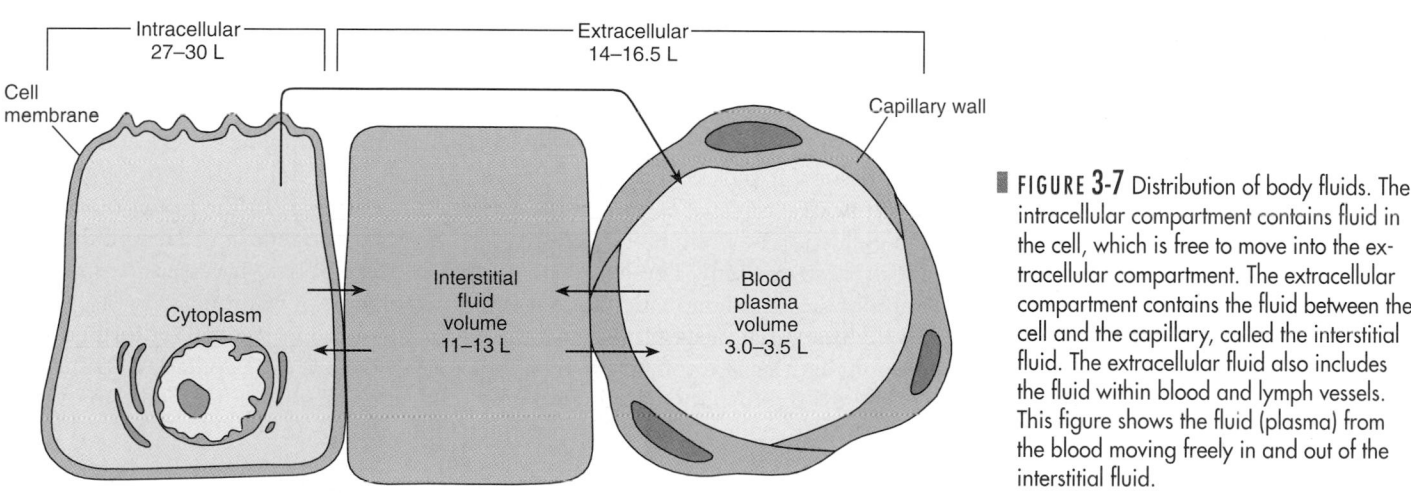

Intracellular 27–30 L	Extracellular 14–16.5 L

Cell
membrane

Capillary wall

Cytoplasm

Interstitial
fluid
volume
11–13 L

Blood
plasma
volume
3.0–3.5 L

■ FIGURE 3-7 Distribution of body fluids. The
intracellular compartment contains fluid in
the cell, which is free to move into the extracellular compartment. The extracellular
compartment contains the fluid between the
cell and the capillary, called the interstitial
fluid. The extracellular fluid also includes
the fluid within blood and lymph vessels.
This figure shows the fluid (plasma) from
the blood moving freely in and out of the
interstitial fluid.

pulmonary circulation The system of blood vessels from the right ventricle of the heart to the lungs and back to the left atrium of the heart.

The right atrium of the heart receives dark red venous blood from the body, which is then pumped into the right ventricle. The right ventricle pumps blood through the pulmonary arteries to the capillaries in the lungs. The lungs then return the freshly oxygenated blood to the left atrium of the heart via the pulmonary veins. This route is known as **pulmonary circulation.**

As the blood moves through the pulmonary capillaries, carbon dioxide is released for expiration, and the inhaled oxygen is taken up by the blood. This is the other site for gas exchange in the body, often referred to as external respiration. The oxygenated blood (now a bright red) in the atrium is pumped to the left ventricle. In the left ventricle, the blood is pumped out again through the aorta to the systemic circuit.

Other Circulatory Systems

hepatic portal system A vein that conveys blood from capillaries in the intestines and portions of the stomach to capillaries in the liver.

One specific capillary bed does not directly return blood to the heart but, rather, directs it toward the liver. This is the **hepatic portal system,** composed of veins, which drain blood from the capillaries in the intestine and stomach. These veins empty into the portal vein, which acts as a direct pipeline to the liver.

The heart also has it own circulatory system. Coronary vessels supply blood to meet cardiac needs. These arteries are particularly susceptible to damage by deposits of cholesterol and other lipids in the artery wall. This accumulation of cholesterol can lead to coronary heart disease. There will be more about this disease in Chapter 6.

CONCEPT CHECK

*M*uscles come in three varieties: skeletal, cardiac, and smooth. Although they all function with the same basic cell parts, they differ in ability to be controlled at will. Skeletal muscle is under voluntary control, whereas the other two types are not. All function with the participation of calcium, and muscle action depends on the production of significant amounts of ATP.

Blood is transported from the heart's right atrium to its right ventricle, to the pulmonary arteries, and to the capillaries in the lungs. Carbon dioxide is removed and oxygen is loaded onto red blood cells. The oxygenated blood returns to the left atrium via the pulmonary vein and into the left ventricle. Here it is pumped into systemic circulation through the aorta. In the capillaries, oxygen is released from the red blood cells and delivered through pores in the capillaries to the surrounding cells. The carbon dioxide is released from the these cells and travels to the blood in the capillaries through the capillary pores.

■ Lymphatic System

lymph node A small structure located along the course of the lymph vessels.

The lymphatic system is closely related to the immune system in that both provide us with defense against pathogenic invaders.[18] As the lymphatic system collects fluid from tissues, it picks up microorganisms as well. The fluid passes through many **lymph nodes** as it makes its way back to the bloodstream. In the nodes is an abundant collection of white blood cells ready to detect pathogens in the lymph fluid and quickly destroy them. The lymphatic system consists of lymph vessels, lymph fluid, lymph nodes, and lymphatic tissue, with its population of immune cells.

The interstitial or extracellular fluid (fluid surrounding the cell) is formed from components that are too large to pass through holes in the capillaries, so they are blocked from returning directly to the bloodstream. Therefore, they take an indirect route back to general circulation, via the lymph system (review Fig. 3-6).

lymphocyte A class of white blood cells involved in the immune system, generally comprising about 25% of all white blood cells. There are several types of lymphocytes with diverse functions, including antibody production, allergic reactions, graft rejections, tumor control, and regulation of the immune system.

Lymph also serves as the passageway by which fat-soluble nutrients are absorbed from the gastrointestinal tract and carried into circulation. Lymph also contains bacteria, viruses, cellular trash, and cancer cells on their way to invade some distant site. Lymph generates immune cells, called **lymphocytes,** which combat these invaders (see next section on the immune system).

At the terminal end of the capillaries, the fluid released from the capillaries into the venules is less than the amount of fluid entering the capillaries from the arterioles. The missing 15% of fluid represents the extracellular fluid that is returned to the vascular system via the lymphatic system. This fluid is subsequently delivered to the lymphatic system by way of specialized capillaries called lymph capillaries. Blood plasma and fluid in the tissues are constantly being interchanged. The fluid, which is now called **lymph,** enters these porous vessels and consists of extracellular fluid and proteins too large to squeeze back into the capillaries.

In addition to microorganisms, the lymph contains absorbed dietary fat. The absorption of fats occurs only in the lymphatic capillaries, **lacteals,** of the small intestine, not the portal vein. From the lacteals, lymph is directed into larger vessels, called **lymph ducts,** and is moved toward the heart with the action of skeletal muscle contractions and other body movements. Eventually, the lymph empties into the thoracic duct and the right lymphatic duct, then into veins that enter the right atrium of the heart, and finally into general circulation (review Fig. 3-6). There will be a further discussion of transport of lipid substances in the lymph system in Chapter 6.

As the lymph makes its way back to the heart, it encounters clusters of lymph nodes containing phagocytic cells, lymphocytes, and mobile **macrophages,** which help destroy invading pathogens and filter the lymph. **T lymphocytes** and **B lymphocytes** are found in these nodes and are major players in immunity (see the section Immune System). When you are ill and seek medical attention, do you ever wonder why your physician checks the lymph glands in your neck for swelling? Swelling means the lymph nodes are in combat against an invading pathogen.

The spleen, thymus gland, and tonsils are considered lymphoid organs. The spleen contains phagocytes, which filter out foreign substances and destroys worn-out red blood cells. The thymus gland is important in immunity during childhood. Tonsils protect against invaders that are inhaled or eaten.

■ Immune System

The cells that carry out immune functions are known collectively as the immune system.[18] Unlike other systems in the body, they do not exist as anatomically connected organs, but rather as separate collections of cells throughout the body. They provide the defense against invading pathogens—microorganisms, or substances capable of producing disease. They recognize "self" from "nonself". They are very sensitive indicators of the body's nutritional status. The most numerous of the immune system cells are the leukocytes.

Our body constantly wages war against disease-producing microorganisms such as bacteria, viruses, fungi, and parasites; or substances capable of producing disease such as toxins from snake venom; or allergens, which trigger allergic reactions; or cancer cells. The most common invaders are bacteria, which are one-cell organisms with a cell wall in addition to a plasma membrane and viruses, which are nucleic acids surrounded by a protein coat. Viruses can't multiply by themselves because they lack ribosomes for protein synthesis, so they survive by taking over a cell and instructing the host to produce the proteins and energy they need for survival.

Leukocytes and Macrophages

The most numerous of the immune system cells are the leukocytes. Leukocytes or white blood cells are produced in the bone marrow and may undergo further development in tissues outside the marrow. They travel via the blood and enter into tissues where they function. They are classified by their structure and the affinity for certain types of dye. For example, the monocyte has a horseshoe-shaped nucleus. Another type of immune cell takes up the red dye eosin, and so is called an eosinophil. There are five general types of leukocytes, which are listed in Table 3-2, along with a brief description of their functions.

Macrophages are found in almost all tissues in the body. They are derived from one kind of leukocyte, the monocyte. When a monocyte leaves the blood and enters

---

*S*ome cancer cells also travel through the lymph. When cancer is found in the body during surgery, the surgeon examines the lymph nodes closest to the site of the cancer to see if it has traveled from the original site to other sites in the body. If cancer cells are found in the lymph nodes, the cancer has probably already spread to other organs in the body.

lymph The clear, plasmalike fluid that flows through lymph vessels.

lacteal A small lymphatic duct within a villus of the small intestine.

lymph duct A large lymphatic vessel, which empties lymph into the circulatory system.

macrophage Any large mononuclear phagocytic cell that is found in the tissues and is derived from a monocyte in the blood. Besides functioning as important phagocytes, macrophages secrete numerous cytokines and act as antigen-presenting cells.

T lymphocyte A type of white blood cell that recognizes intracellular antigens (e.g., viral antigens in infected cells), fragments of which move to the cell surface. T lymphocytes originate in the bone marrow but must mature in the thymus gland.

B lymphocyte A type of white blood cell that recognizes antigens (e.g., bacteria) present in extracellular sites in the body and is responsible for antibody-mediated immunity. B lymphocytes originate and mature in the bone marrow and are released into the blood and lymph.

antigen Any substance that induces a state of sensitivity and/or resistance to microbes or toxic substances after a lag period; substance that stimulates a specific aspect of the immune system.

*I*nflammation is a response to tissue injury, including trauma and infection. Inflammation includes redness, swelling, pain, and heat.

TABLE 3-2   Types and Functions of Leukocytes

Leukocyte	Function
Neutrophil	Phagocytizes bacteria. Forms highly toxic compounds, which destroy bacteria.
Eosinophil	Phagocytizes antigen-antibody complex, allergy-causing antigens, inflammatory chemicals. Attacks parasites, such as worms.
Basophil	Secretes histamine, a vasodilator, thus increasing blood flow to tissues. Secretes heparin, which prevents blood clotting.
Lymphocytes	Natural killer cells attack cells infected with viruses or have turned cancerous. B lymphocytes present antigens and activate other cells of the immune system. Can become plasma cells that secrete antibodies. Serve as memory cells in humoral immunity. T lymphocytes destroy foreign cells, regulate immune response, and serve as memory cells in cellular immunity.
Monocytes	Differentiate into numerous types of macrophages. Macrophages phagocytize pathogens, dead neutrophils, and debris of dead cells. They present antigens and activate other cells of the immune system.

into a tissue it is transformed into a macrophage. At birth, the baby is already supplied with macrophages, which continue to develop throughout life. They are strategically located throughout the body to phagocytize foreign material.

Mast cells are produced in the bone marrow and found in almost all tissues and organs. They release histamine and the other chemicals that are involved in inflammation.

Another participant in the immune system is **cytokines,** a complicated group of protein messengers that are produced by various cells throughout the body. They regulate the host's cells function and growth and are involved in nonspecific and specific immunity.

There are two types of immunity, nonspecific or natural immunity and specific or acquired immunity. The nonspecific immunity protects against foreign invaders without having to recognize specific appearances of the invaders.

Nonspecific Immunity

Nonspecific immunity is an array of mechanisms that are present at birth and do not require any activation. They are barriers such as the skin and the **mucous membranes** of the gastrointestinal tract, reproductive system, urinary tract, and respiratory tract. The **mucus** they produce traps invaders. Internally, other forms of nonspecific immunity include phagocytic cells, which can swallow bacteria and other harmful substances and ultimately destroy them. Acid produced by the stomach (HCl) can destroy ingested pathogens. Inflammation is a local response to infection or injury. The purpose is to destroy or inactivate foreign invaders and begin the process of repair. Fever is also an internal defense mechanism. It seems to aid in the recovery process by reducing the amount of iron in the blood, which in turn reduces bacterial activity. Fever also seems to be associated with an increase in **interferons.** Viral infections are subject to short-term control by this group of proteins, cytokines, released by infected cells. Interferons are receiving a lot of attention today as potent weapons against cancers, hepatitis C, and other diseases.

Specific Immunity

Specific immunity involving the lymphocytes is directed at specific molecules. When nonspecific immunological defenses fail to halt an invasion by pathogens or toxins produced by them, another mechanism comes into action. It is based on the action of antibodies, lymphocytes, and other cells of the immune system. This is known as **antibody-mediated immunity,** or humoral immunity.

Antigens are molecules that are usually large and foreign to the body. (A given molecule can have a number of antigenic determinant sites that stimulate the production of various antibodies.) When we successfully fight off an invader, the chem-

cytokine A protein secreted by a cell that functions to regulate the activity of neighboring cells.

nonspecific immunity Defenses that stop the invasion of pathogens. Requires no previous encounter with a pathogen.

specific immunity The function of lymphocytes directed at specific antigens.

mucous membranes Also called mucosae, line passageways open to the exterior environment.

mucus A thick fluid secreted by glands throughout the body. It contains a compound that has both carbohydrate and protein parts. It acts as a lubricant and means of protection for cells.

interferons A group of proteins released by virus-infected cells that bind to other cells, stimulating synthesis of antiviral proteins that in turn inhibit viral multiplication.

antibody-mediated immunity Immunity provided by B lymphocytes. Also known as humoral immunity.

icals called **antibodies** have been in action. Antibodies are highly specific proteins produced by B lymphocytes in response to antigens. Antigens are detected as dangerous intruders. They are detected because the immune system can identify molecules that are "self"; they belong to *me* personally, from "nonself" molecules; they don't belong to me, an antigen! (Recall that one role of the glycoproteins found on the cell membrane is to identify "self.")

The lymphocytes that produce antibodies, designated B lymphocytes, are produced in the bone marrow. These B lymphocytes wage war against bacterial infections, as well as some viral infections and even a few parasites. B lymphocytes (or B-cells) and antibodies, also known as **immunoglobulins,** come in five major classifications. These bind to the invader, the antigen, and begin a process of attack. This antibody-antigen interaction soon produces **plasma cells,** which results in the production of more antibody proteins to continue the attack. A person can produce as many different antibodies as there are exposures to specific antigens. It is estimated that there are 100 million trillion antibody molecules per person, representing a few million species of antigens. How we are able to produce such a vast defense structure is not completely understood.

Memory cells are then produced by B-cells and provide active immunity. Once you have been exposed to an antigen, you develop active immunity. Obviously, this is the basis of vaccinations; an inactivated pathogen is injected and the body develops immunity to that pathogen.

The antibody-antigen interaction also produces a group of plasma proteins called **complement** proteins. Complement proteins are released into the area of infection and attach to the target pathogen to be destroyed. It is not the antibody-antigen combination that causes the destruction of the pathogenic invader, but this combination of antibody-antigen does identify them, so that they can be attacked by nonspecific immune processes, such as the complement proteins. Complement attaches to the pathogenic invader and drills holes in its membrane, thus leading to its destruction. (The hole in the wall allows water to flow into the cell and causes it to burst.)

T lymphocytes directly attack and destroy specific cells, which are identified by specific antigens on the cell surface. T lymphocytes (or T-cells) produce **cell-mediated immunity** because they actually are in contact with the enemy cell. T cells must be first activated in the thymus gland.

The actual T lymphocytes, T cell, that are killers are known as **cytotoxic T cells.** They recognize the infected cell and attach themselves through a CD8 receptor. There are also **helper T cells.** They attach to an infected cell through the CD4 receptor. They promote phagocytic activity. Together the cytotoxic and helper T cells bind to the infected cell and lead to the cell's destruction. You may have heard of CD4 cells because they are markers for AIDS. When the disease progresses, the CD4 count decreases as the virus attacks T helper cells (and macrophages).

Most of the information concerning the relationship of nutrition to immunity comes from studies in poor countries of the developing world, where children die of infectious diseases secondary to malnutrition. Protein-energy malnutrition, deficiencies of vitamins and minerals, and an inadequate intake of certain fatty acids seriously alter immune function.[10] There will be more information how individual nutrients make it possible to support an immune response in Chapters 9 through 12.

Allergies are types of immune responses. One type of allergic response is almost *immediate.* The symptoms are produced by B lymphocytes exposed to an allergen, as demonstrated by a runny nose, red eyes, and itchy skin (dermatitis). The culprit is **histamine,** an altered form of the common amino acid histadine. This type of immune response can be treated by antihistamine drugs. Allergies will be further discussed with eicosanoids, Chapter 6 and adolescent nutrition Chapter 17.

Delayed hypersensitivity, an abnormal T cell response, can occur as late as 72 hours after exposure. The best known example of this type of immune response is contact dermatitis caused by coming in contact with poison ivy, poison oak, or poison sumac. Hardly anyone is immune to this type of allergic reaction.

antibodies Blood proteins that inactivate foreign proteins found in the body. This helps to prevent and control infections.

immunoglobulins Proteins found in the blood that bind to specific antigens; also called antibodies. The five major classes of immunoglobulin play different roles in antibody-mediate immunity.

plasma cells A form of B lymphocytes that produce about 2000 antibodies proteins per second.

memory cells B lymphocytes that remain after an infection to convey permanent immunity.

complement A series of blood proteins that participate in a complex reaction cascade following stimulation by an antigen-antibody complex or the surface of a bacterial cell. Various activated complement proteins can enhance phagocytosis, contribute to inflammation, and destroy bacteria.

cell-mediated immunity T lymphocytes do not secrete antibodies; they come in actual contact with the invading cells in order to destroy them.

cytotoxic T cells Type of T cells that interact with the infected host cell through special receptor sites on the T cell surface.

helper T cells Type of T cells that interact with macrophages and secrete substances to signal an invading pathogen. Stimulates B lymphocytes to proliferate.

histamine A breakdown product of the amino acid histidine that stimulates acid secretion by the stomach and has other effects on the body, such as contraction of smooth muscles, increased nasal secretions, relaxation of blood vessels, and changes in relaxation of airways. It appears to decrease hunger and food intake.

Another type of immunity is known as autoimmunity. The immune system fails to recognize "self" and thinking a normal cell is an antigen, goes on the attack by activating T lymphocytes and the production of antibodies by B lymphocytes, thus killing the cell. In other words, the defense mechanisms are confused and attack the body rather than invaders. There are at least 40 autoimmune diseases. Some well-known examples include rheumatoid arthritis, type 1 diabetes, and multiple sclerosis.

alveoli, alveolus The basic functional units of the lungs.

pharynx The organ of the digestive tract and respiratory tract located at the back of the oral and nasal cavities.

larynx The structure located between the pharynx and trachea that contains the vocal cords.

trachea The airway leading from the larynx to the bronchi.

bronchial tree The bronchi and the branches on the tree.

bronchioles The smallest division of the lungs.

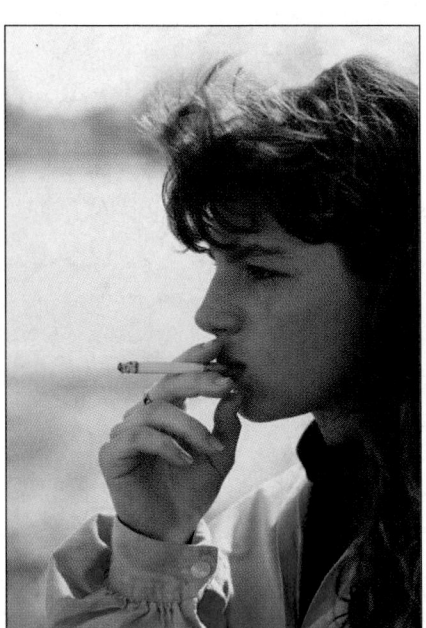

Smoking is especially harmful to the lungs.

Concept Check

The lymph system serves several purposes: the transport of dietary lipids, the absorption of excess interstitial fluid and its return to the bloodstream, and the defense of the body against invading pathogens.

Body defenses are conveyed by the immune system, which depends on the lymph for activation and distribution. Immunity consists of specific and nonspecific immunity. Nonspecific immunity does not require any activation; we are born with this type of immunity. Specific immunity develops after exposure to pathogens. B cells and T cells are agents of specific immunity that attack specific pathogens and contribute to their destruction.

■ Respiratory System

In order to produce sufficient energy to meet body needs, there must be oxygen present to help convert food energy into ATP.[18, 19] When oxygen is supplied to the tissues, carbon dioxide is produced and removed from the body by the combined actions of the cardiovascular and respiratory systems.

The organs of the respiratory system are the nose, pharynx, larynx, trachea, bronchi, and lungs. *Respiration* refers to breathing and the exchange of gases between the blood and other tissues. The respiratory tract features the **alveoli** (plural) in the lungs. These are tiny structures where one form of gas exchange takes place, described previously as external respiration (Fig. 3-8). The **alveolus** (singular), the basic functional unit of respiration, allows oxygen to be recovered from inhaled air and loads it onto red blood cells for transport to target tissues throughout the body. Simultaneously, carbon dioxide in the blood is released into the lungs and ultimately exhaled into the air.

Air reaches the lungs from the nasal cavity and the mouth by first passing through the **pharynx** to the **larynx.** The larynx is open to the trachea during breathing but closes during swallowing. The **trachea** is a tube that connects the larynx to the **bronchial tree.** The bronchial tree is located in the lungs and looks like a tree with branches. The branches on this tree get smaller and smaller the farther out they go from the tree trunk (the trachea) into lung tissue until finally they turn into **bronchioles,** the location of the pulmonary alveoli.

The distance across the aveoli is two cells thick; one cell for the aveoli plus one cell for the pulmonary capillaries. Gas exchange allows CO_2 and O_2 to diffuse easily between the blood and lungs. There is an estimated 300 million aveoli in the lungs, providing a tremendous surface area for the diffusion of gasses.

Another aspect of respiration is the discharge of water through the lungs. This is obvious on a cold day when the breath we exhale turns to ice crystals, and we can see vapor forming around the mouth and nose. Of course, such water loss is much more extensive during hot, humid weather when the body continues to remove heat from the body via the lungs.

Concept Check

Respiration provides oxygen to the tissues and removes the main waste product of the body, carbon dioxide. Air continuously moves in and out of the lungs. Diffusion of oxygen into the blood and carbon dioxide out of the blood occurs in tiny lung sacs called alveoli. Blood transports oxygen to and carbon dioxide from the cells. The oxygen is used to metabolize the food fuels brought into the body by the digestive system.

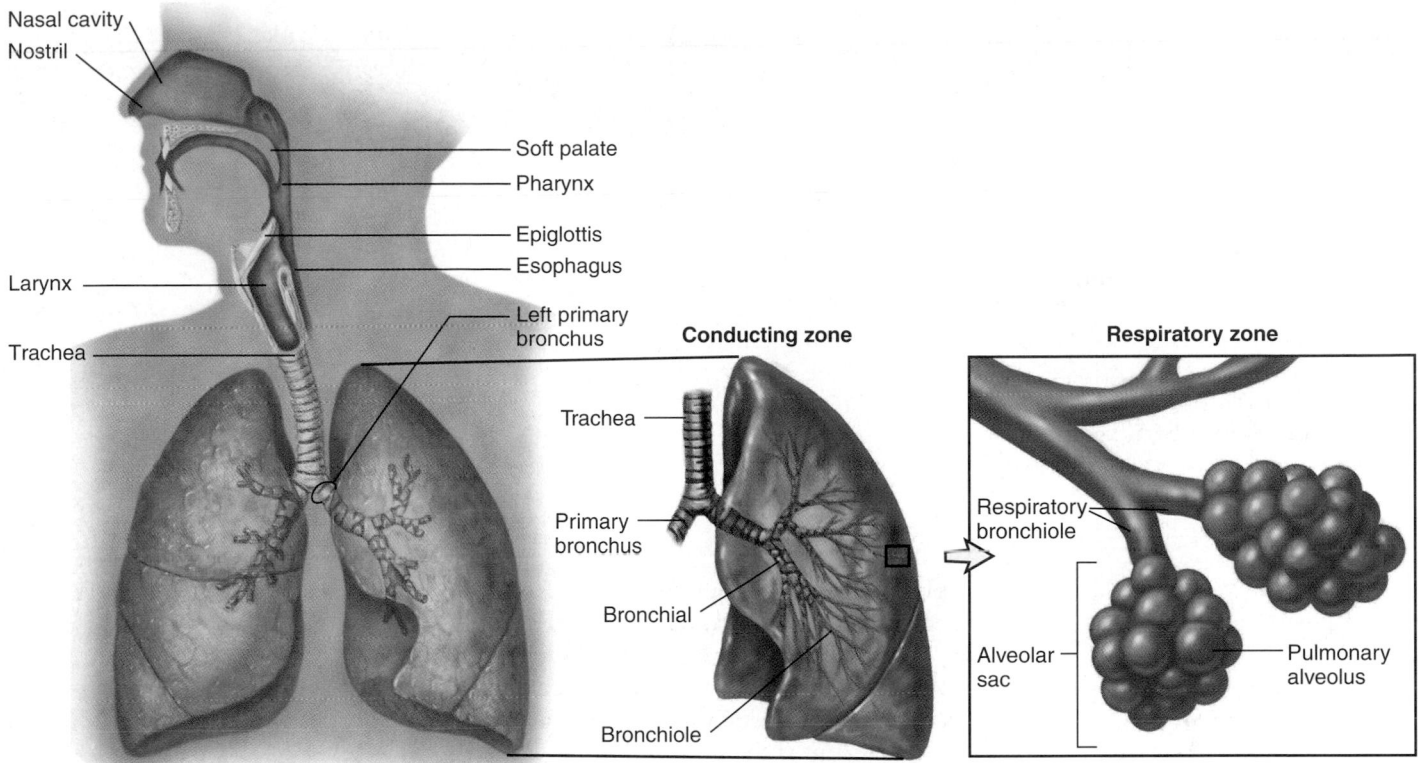

FIGURE 3-8 Anatomy of the respiratory system. Air is conducted through the nose and mouth to the lungs. Air is conducted into bronchioles and gas exchange occurs in the alveoli.

Nervous System

The next system, the nervous system, is a regulatory system controlling a variety of body functions. The nervous system can detect changes occurring in various organs and take corrective action when needed to maintain the constancy of the internal environment, **homeostasis**. The nervous system regulates activities that change almost instantly, such as muscle contractions and perception of danger.

The nervous system consists of the **central nervous system (CNS)** and the **peripheral nervous system (PNS)**.[19] The central nervous system contains the brain and spinal cord. The peripheral nervous system, with its nerves coming from the central nervous system, branch out to all organs of the body.

The basic structural and functional unit of the nervous system is the neuron—a cell that responds to electrical and chemical signals, conducts electrical impulses, and releases chemical regulators (Fig. 3-9). Neurons allow us to perceive what is occurring in our environment, engage in learning, store vital information in memory, and control the body's voluntary actions. Incoming information to the body depends on sensory receptors, such as visual, auditory, smell, and tactile receptors. This information can cause an immediate response—"Ouch, a bee stung me"—or the information can be stored in long-term memory—"The last time I ate at Diamond Herry's Grill, I got very sick to my stomach. I think I'll not eat there again."

Neurons can't produce new cells, although some can regenerate parts of their structures. Loss of nerve tissue causes loss of important functions. A spinal cord injury is likely to cause permanent paralysis, such as that experienced by actor Christopher Reeve following a horseback-riding accident.

Neuroglia (glial cells) protect neurons and aid in their function. They are far more abundant than neurons. For example, one group of neuroglia wraps nerves in a protective sheath, a job associated with vitamin B-12. Another group of neuroglia

homeostasis A series of adjustments that prevent change in the internal environment in the body.

central nervous system (CNS) The brain and spinal cord part of the nervous system.

peripheral nervous system (PNS) The nerves of the central nervous system that lie outside the brain and spinal cord.

neuroglia (glial cells) Specialized support cells of the central nervous system.

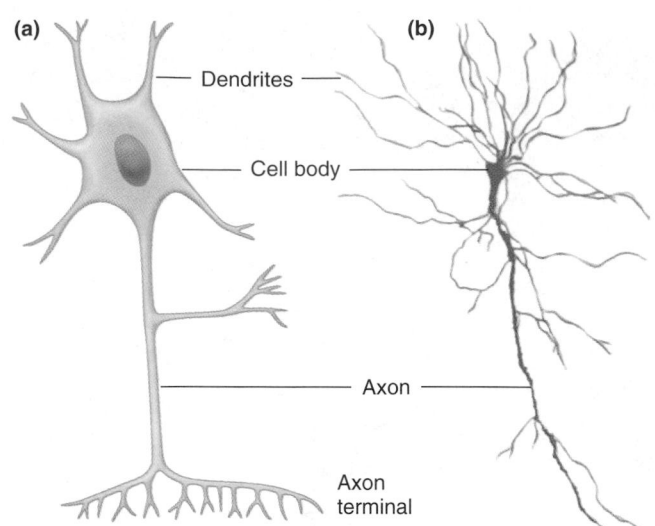

(a)

Dendrites

Cell body

Axon

Axon terminal

(b)

■ FIGURE 3-9 *(a)* An illustration of a neuron or nerve cell, showing the cell body with dendrites and the axon. The axon releases the neurotransmitters. *(b)* How a neuron looks under a light microscope

cell body, dendrites, axon The major structures of a neuron.

nerve A bundle of axons outside the central nervous system.

neurotransmitter A compound made by a nerve cell that allows for communication between it and other cells.

synapse The space between the axon of one neuron and the dendrite of another neuron.

dopamine A neurotransmitter in the CNS.

norepinephrine A neurotransmitter from nerve endings and a hormone from the adrenal gland.

epinephrine A neurotransmitter from nerve endings and also a hormone from the adrenal gland.

acetylcholine A neurotransmitter released from nerve endings.

serotonin A neurotransmitter synthesized from the amino acid tryptophan that appears to both decrease the desire to eat carbohydrates and induce sleep.

monoamine A molecule containing one amide group.

adrenergic The actions of epinephrine and norepinephrine.

cholinergic The actions of acetylcholine.

phagocytize pathogens and dispose of cellular debris in the CNS. Some neuroglia have limited ability to divide (mitosis).

Each neuron contains a **cell body** with a nucleus and rough endoplasmic reticulum, **dendrites,** and an **axon.** Information (electrical or chemical stimuli) enters the cell through the dendrites and/or the cell body, and the output of electrical impulses leave by way of the axon.

By now, you may be wondering about the term *nerve*. A **nerve** is a bundle of axons located outside the CNS. Nerves contain both sensory and motor components.

Axons end close to, or may be in physical contact with, the next neuron. In most cases, however, the electrical signal is converted to a chemical signal at the end of the axon as a chemical called a **neurotransmitter.** This is released into the gap. The transmission from neuron to neuron or from neuron to muscle cell is by way of these neurotransmitters. The space between one neuron and the next is known as a **synapse.** Neurotransmitters that bridge the gap are derived from common nutrients found in foods (see Chapter 11 for more details).

There are a variety of neurotransmitters—**dopamine, norepinephrine, epinephrine, acetylcholine,** and **serotonin,** just to identify a few. Dopamine, epinephrine, norepinephrine, and serotonin are classified as **monoamines.**

The body's fight or flight mechanism—the ability to survive a threat—depends on the **adrenergic** effect provided by andrenergic neurons secreting epinephrine and norepinephrine. The adrenergic effect stimulates the heart to beat faster, constricts blood vessels to raise blood pressure, increases breathing, and promotes the breakdown of glycogen in the liver. This is essential to survival, since it makes it possible to provide plenty of glucose, our basic muscle fuel, instantly, when there is an emergency and muscles need to respond quickly. **Cholinergic** effects usually have the opposite effect of adrenergic neurons.

It is important to recognize that the brain has a tremendous metabolic rate, requiring a constant supply of blood, which accounts for 20% of the total cardiac output. This translates into 750 ml of blood per minute being pumped through the brain, yielding a steady supply of oxygen and glucose. Any interruption in the supply of these two molecules is life-threatening. The brain also generates waste materials, which are promptly removed by this high blood flow rate.

All the various structures that make up the nervous system are related to one's nutritional status. For example, some of the axons of the CNS and PNS are covered by a substance previously mentioned, myelin. Myelin is a lipoprotein that wraps around nerve fibers, acting like insulating material. Vitamin B-12 plays a key role in the formation of myelin.

The transmission of information through the nervous system depends on nutrients obtained from the diet: calcium, sodium, and potassium. The sodium ion (Na^+)

(mostly extracellular) and the potassium ion (K^+) (mostly intracellular) located on either side of the axon membrane exchange places as they flow through ion channels in response to electrical stimulation. This is how an electrical signal is transmitted. They are later pumped back to the previous location.

Other nutrients required for the nervous system are various amino acids. One amino acid we obtain from dietary protein, **tryptophan,** is converted to serotonin by neurons. This neurotransmitter has a variety of behavioral effects. Varying the amount of dietary tryptophan controls the amount of serotonin produced by neurons. The amino acid **tyrosine** can be converted to dopamine, norepinephrine, and epinephrine. Choline (a putative nutrient) is converted to the neurotransmitter acetylcholine.

The calcium ion (Ca^{2+}) plays a central role in nervous system control. Calcium allows the release of neurotransmitters from the axon of a neuron. The neurotransmitter carries the signal to the next neuron as it jumps the synapse. Fortunately, a calcium-deficient diet will never have any effect on nerve transmission. The body can always scrape together enough calcium to keep the nervous system functioning. There are, however, rare instances when a deficiency of calcium causes tetany. (More about tetany appears in Chapter 11.)

Certainly, the most important nutrient for continued efficient brain function is carbohydrate in the form of glucose. Should the diet fail to deliver enough carbohydrate that can form glucose, the body will synthesize it in sufficient amounts to provide for the needs of the brain, or the brain will learn to use an alternative fuel called ketone bodies (see Chapter 4).

It should be noted that the gastrointestinal tract has its own separate nervous system. The sight or smell of food, or one's emotions, can signal muscle cells and glands to prepare the way for food and turn on digestive processes.

■ Endocrine System and Hormones

Endocrine glands secrete regulatory substances, hormones, into the blood for distribution to target tissues or organs.[18] The endocrine gland that secretes a hormone is responding to the need to restore homeostasis. The following section is by no means a complete exploration of all the body's hormones, but it concentrates on those that affect nutrition (Fig. 3-10).

General hormones are classified according to chemical categories: **steroids, glycoproteins, polypeptides,** and **amines.** Hormones control metabolic functions, such as appetite, and the transport of substances through cell membranes. Others control growth, and still others are responsible for sex and reproduction. Some hormones are described as "local," in that they function in the immediate vicinity of their production. There are many interrelationships between hormones and the nervous system. For example, the adrenal gland and the pituitary gland respond to neural stimuli.

Some hormones from the pituitary gland control the secretion of other endocrine glands. And, as mentioned in the previous section, a substance such as norepinephrine secreted as a neurotransmitter, can act as an hormone.

Chemical Classification of Hormones

Steroid hormones are lipid substances synthesized from cholesterol (Table 3-3).[19] The glycoproteins are long chains of amino acids (100 or more) bound to carbohydrate (Table 3-4). Follicle-stimulating hormone (FSH), luteininzing hormone (LH), thyroid-stimulating hormone (TSH), and several other pituitary hormones are such hormones and are referred to as **tropic hormones** because they stimulate the secretion of another hormone and usually stimulate the growth of the associated gland. For example, TSH stimulates the production of the thyroid hormone. Another group of hormones are polypeptide chains made of fewer than 100 amino acids per chain (Table 3-5). Amines are hormones synthesized from the amino acids tyrosine and tryptophan (Table 3-6).

One of the most interesting neurotransmitters is a brain substance called neuropeptide Y, synthesized from another amino acid, glutamic acid. We obtain glutamic acid from dietary protein, or we can make it in the body. Either way, some glutamic acid becomes neuropeptide Y, a powerful stimulant of appetite. Obviously, scientists are searching for a drug that could inhibit the action of neuropeptide Y. For more on appetite and obesity, see Chapter 13.

steroids A group of hormones and related compounds that are derivatives of cholesterol.

polypeptide Fifty to 100 amino acids bonded together.

tropic hormone A hormone that stimulates the secretion of another secreting gland.

One area of the brain deserves special focus. The structure called the hypothalamus secretes a variety of hormones and has a vital role to play in one's emotional state. This structure regulates cardiovascular function, body temperature, water and electrolyte balance, hunger, satiety, gastrointestinal activity, sleep, and sexual arousal. Important to the study of nutrition are two centers in this structure, the so called feeding center and the satiety center, which tells us when we need to seek food and when we have had enough to eat (satiety). There will be many references to this important brain structure as the various nutrients are discussed.

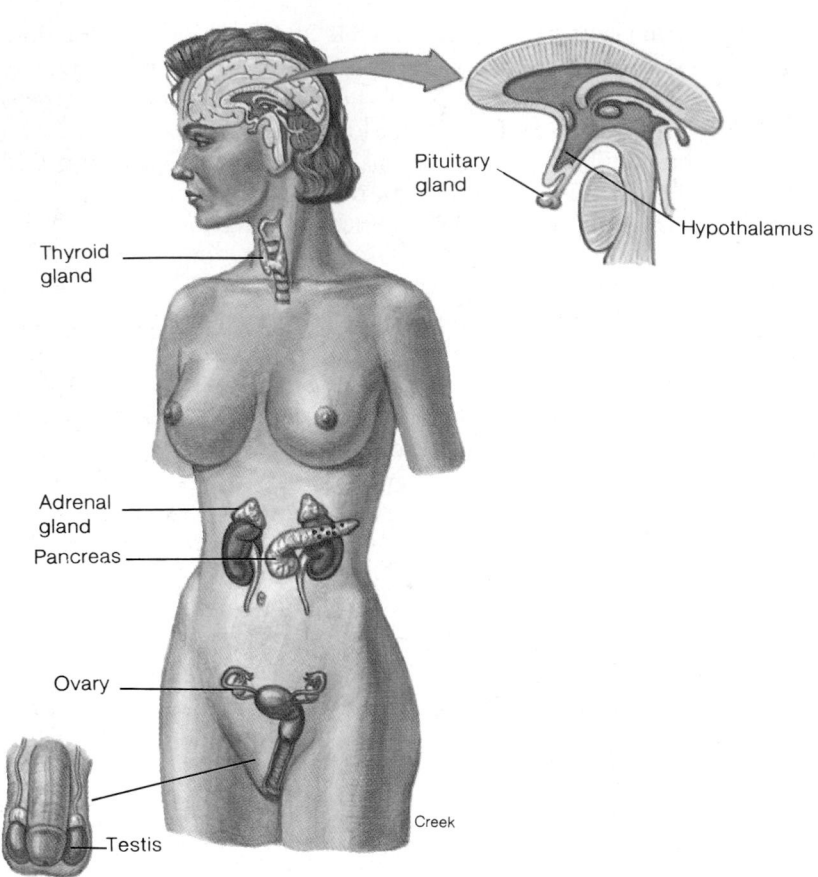

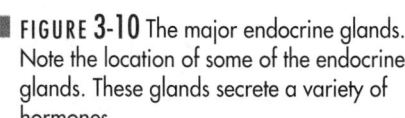
FIGURE 3-10 The major endocrine glands. Note the location of some of the endocrine glands. These glands secrete a variety of hormones.

TABLE 3-3   Steroid Hormones

Hormone	Gland	Target	Effect	Role in Nutrition
Testosterone	Testes, adrenal glands	Reproductive organs	Reproduction, secondary sexual development	Muscle growth
Estrogens, progesterone	Ovaries, adrenal glands	Reproductive organs	Reproduction, secondary sexual characteristics	Maintenance of bone
Cortisol	Adrenal glands	Liver	Glucocorticoid activity	Metabolism of protein, carbohydrate, fat
Aldosterone	Adrenal glands	Kidney	Mineral-corticoid activity	Electrolyte balance

TABLE 3-4   Glycoprotein Hormones

Hormone	Gland	Target	Effect	Role in Nutrition
FSH, LH, TSH	Pituitary gland	Variety of organs	Stimulation of target organ to produce its own hormone	None directly

There are also special hormones that regulate the digestive tract. These will be discussed in the next section on digestion.

Interesting Features of Hormones

The steroid and thyroid hormones can be taken in pill form, since they are not digested in the GI tract; thus, they can be absorbed into the body in their active state. All the other hormones are deactivated when taken by mouth because their biolog-

TABLE 3-5   Polypeptide Hormones

Hormone	Gland	Target	Effect	Role in Nutrition
Antidiuretic hormone	Pituitary gland	Kidney	Water retention, vasoconstriction	Maintenance of proper blood volume
Prolactin (tropic hormone)	Pituitary gland	Mammary gland	Milk production; in males, indirect enhancement of testosterone secretions	Nourishment of newborn
Oxytocin	Pituitary gland	Uterus and mammary glands	Contraction of uterus, mammary secretions	Milk production
Insulin	Pancreas	Fat and muscle cells	Decreased blood glucose concentration	Storage of glucose as glycogen, increased fat storage, increased amino acid uptake by cells
Glucagon	Pancreas	Liver	Increased blood glucose concentration	Release of glucose from liver stores, increased fat mobilization
ACTH (adrenocorticotropic hormone)	Pituitary gland	Adrenal glands	Secretion of glucocorticoids	Secretion of adrenal cortical hormones
Growth hormone (tropic hormone)	Pituitary gland	Most cells	Promotion of amino acid uptake by cells	Promotion of protein synthesis and growth, increased fat utilization for energy
Parathyroid hormone	Parathyroid glands	Intestinal tract, kidneys	Increased blood calcium concentration	Release of calcium from bone into blood
Calitonin	Thyroid gland	Bone	Inhibition of breakdown of bone, stimulation of calcium excretion by kidneys	Reduced blood calcium concentration
Leptin	No gland, just adipose tissue	Hypothalamus	Targeting of satiety center	Decreased appetite

TABLE 3-6   Amine Hormones

Hormone	Gland	Target	Effect	Role in Nutrition
Epinephrine, norepinephrine	Adrenal glands	Heart, blood vessels, brain, lungs	Increased metabolic rate	Release of glucose into the blood, fat mobilization
Thyroid hormones	Thyroid gland	Most organs	Increased oxygen consumption, growth, brain development, development of CNS in fetus	Protein synthesis, increased metabolic rate
Melatonin	Pineal gland	Specific neurons	Maintenance of body (circadian) rhythms, sleep	Scavenging of atoms and molecules that are highly reactive and dangerous

ical activity is destroyed by digestive enzymes. That is why the hormone insulin must be taken by injection to bypass the digestive tract.

Some hormones must undergo chemical changes before they can function. For example, vitamin D synthesized in the skin and/or obtained from food is converted to an active hormone by the kidneys and liver.

In most cases, a single gland secretes a single hormone, but, in a few cases, a single gland secretes more than one hormone. Sometimes a hormone is produced by more than one gland.

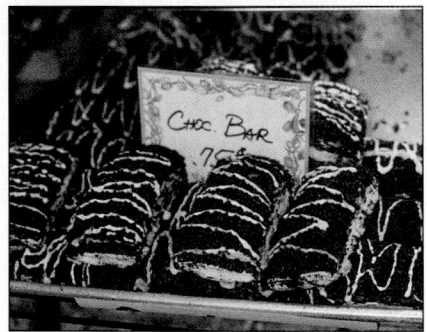

Most of the foods we eat consist of carbohydrates, protein, and fat. Our bodies break down each of these nutrients in a different way.

A sixth taste sensation, called umami, has been proposed. This taste sensation is elicited by monosodium glutamate, a substance often added to Chinese and Japanese foods to enhance flavor. Brothy, meaty, and savory are examples of umami sensations.[20]

Neural and Endocrine Regulation

Whether a chemical is acting as a hormone or a neurotransmitter, the target cell must have a receptor protein to combine with it. This causes a change in the target cell. This also means that there must be a mechanism to turn off the action. Hormones are subject to control by an off switch. For example, when the blood sugar (glucose) concentration has been returned to normal by the action of the hormone insulin, insulin production is turned off. If it were not, the person would experience decreasing glucose concentrations until such time as the concentration drops so low the person goes into shock and dies.

How Hormones Act

Hormones are available to all cells in the body, but only those with the correct receptor protein on the cell membrane can bind the hormone. These binding sites are highly specific. For hormones that pass through the cell membrane, thyroxine and steroid hormones, the receptor protein is within the cytosol of the cell. This receptor guides the hormone into the nucleus of the cell, where the hormone binds to DNA and turns on the production mRNA to produce a specific enzyme.

Hormones that don't penetrate the cell membrane act by another mechanism. The hormone (the messenger) attaches to a receptor protein on the cell surface. This binding site activates a second messenger within the cell to carry out the assigned task, like the activation or inhibition of a specific enzyme. Many hormones activate a form of ATP as the second messenger. Another second messenger is calcium.

In summary, hormones in the blood can act directly with a target cell, can pass its instructions to the cell indirectly with the aid of a second messenger, can be inactivated by a metabolic process, or can be ignored and excreted from the body as they are.

CONCEPT CHECK

The nervous system consists of the central nervous system and the peripheral nervous system. The functional unit of the nervous system is the neuron, or nerve cell.

Hormones are regulatory substances that are produced by glands in response to a change in the internal environment of the body. The gland secretes the hormone into the blood, and the blood delivers it to target cells. The hormone either enters the cell and turns on the production of an enzyme within the cell or attaches to the exterior of the cell and, through the action of a second messenger, causes enzymatic changes within the cell.

▪ Digestive System

The processes of digestion and absorption take place in a long tube, open at both ends, extending from the mouth to the anus. It is essentially part of our exterior environment. With the exception of water, almost all the food and beverages we ingest require some preparation before the nutrients are released and prepared for absorption (Fig. 3-11).[17]

How the Body Reacts to Food

You eat. You are aware of the contents in your mouth because of taste buds located on your tongue.[4] If a food or beverage tastes good, you begin to chew and swallow the food.

There are four types of taste: sweet, sour, salty, and bitter. The salty taste is due to Na^+ enhanced by Cl^-. The sour taste is due to the presence of hydrogen ions (H^+). Bitter and sweet tastes are generated by specific components in the food that interact with membrane receptors on the tongue. Some evidence exists for a fifth sense, water.

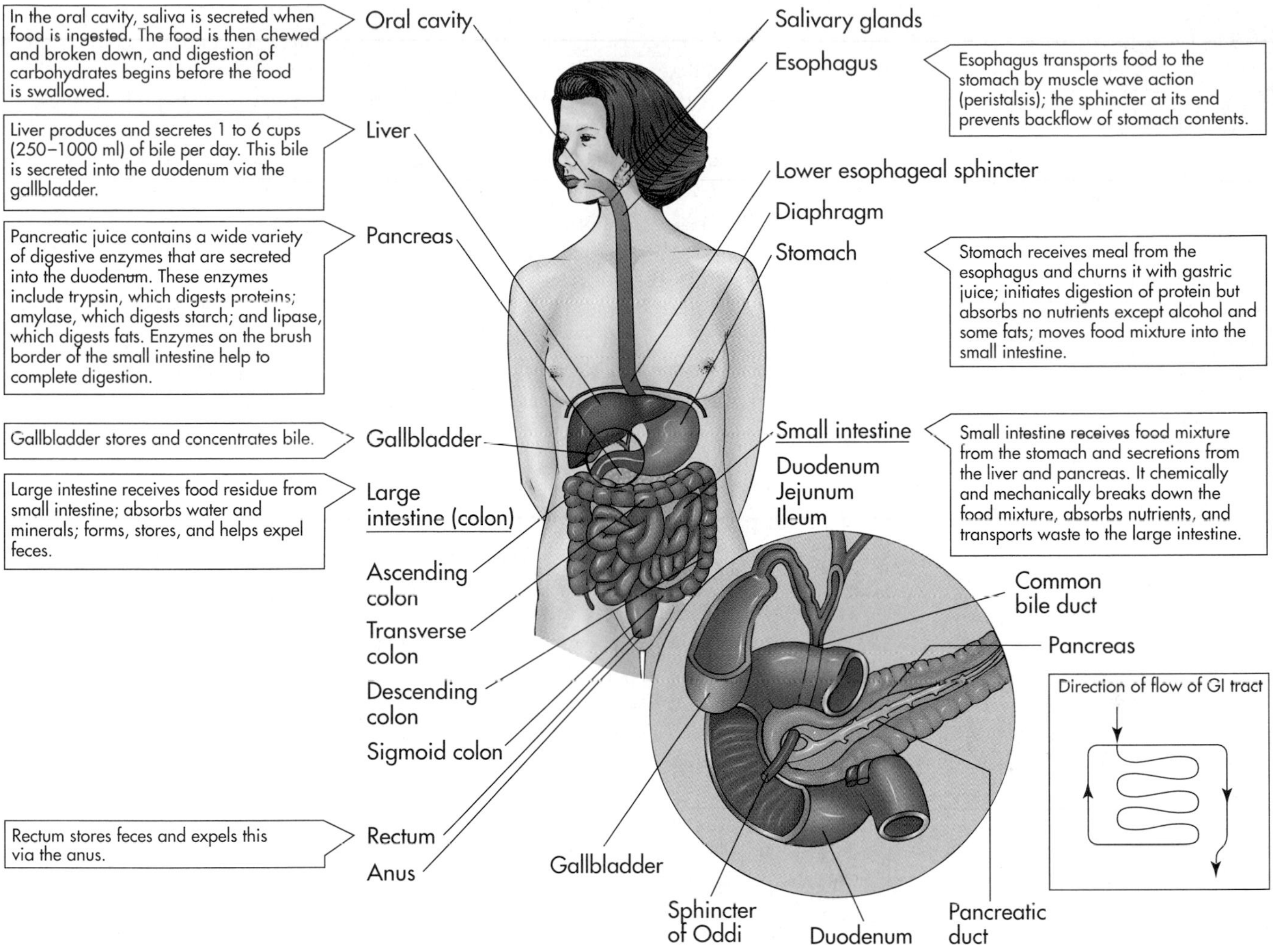

In the oral cavity, saliva is secreted when food is ingested. The food is then chewed and broken down, and digestion of carbohydrates begins before the food is swallowed.

Oral cavity

Salivary glands

Esophagus

Esophagus transports food to the stomach by muscle wave action (peristalsis); the sphincter at its end prevents backflow of stomach contents.

Liver produces and secretes 1 to 6 cups (250–1000 ml) of bile per day. This bile is secreted into the duodenum via the gallbladder.

Liver

Lower esophageal sphincter

Diaphragm

Pancreatic juice contains a wide variety of digestive enzymes that are secreted into the duodenum. These enzymes include trypsin, which digests proteins; amylase, which digests starch; and lipase, which digests fats. Enzymes on the brush border of the small intestine help to complete digestion.

Pancreas

Stomach

Stomach receives meal from the esophagus and churns it with gastric juice; initiates digestion of protein but absorbs no nutrients except alcohol and some fats; moves food mixture into the small intestine.

Small intestine

Small intestine receives food mixture from the stomach and secretions from the liver and pancreas. It chemically and mechanically breaks down the food mixture, absorbs nutrients, and transports waste to the large intestine.

Gallbladder stores and concentrates bile.

Gallbladder

Duodenum
Jejunum
Ileum

Large intestine receives food residue from small intestine; absorbs water and minerals; forms, stores, and helps expel feces.

Large intestine (colon)

Common bile duct

Pancreas

Ascending colon

Transverse colon

Descending colon

Direction of flow of GI tract

Sigmoid colon

Rectum stores feces and expels this via the anus.

Rectum

Anus

Gallbladder

Sphincter of Oddi

Duodenum

Pancreatic duct

FIGURE 3-11 Physiology of the GI tract. Many organs cooperate in a regulated fashion to allow the digestion and subsequent absorption of nutrients.

Detection of the bitter taste is important to health and survival, as many of the most toxic substances taste bitter. Actually, sweet, sour, salty, and bitter are blended together in foods to provide distinctive flavors. Smell, however, contributes even more to flavor than taste does. As we chew a food, chemicals are released that stimulate nasal passages. Aroma, what we call smell, probably has more to do with taste than what we actually have in our mouth. Consider the stuffy nose that accompanies a head cold. When you have a bad cold, the hot, freshly baked apple pie, just out of the oven, can't be appreciated because you can't smell the combined fragrance of cinnamon, nutmeg, and apple. Only with a functioning **olfactory** system do foods taste right. Flavor is also affected by human genetic variation in both taste and olfactory sensations.

Once you have swallowed a mouthful of food, known as a **bolus,** the rest of the digestive and absorptive process is automatic. The digestive system is divided into two functioning units: the gastrointestinal (GI) tract, sometimes known as the alimentary canal, and accessory digestive organs, such as the salivary glands, pancreas, liver, and gallbladder (review Fig. 3-11). The GI tract in an adult is about 15 feet long. The major structures are the mouth, the pharynx, esophagus, stomach, small intestine, large intestine, and rectum.[6]

Lining the surface of the **lumen** of the GI tract from the stomach down to the anus is the epithelium. The epithelium performs secretory activities, as well as acting as a barrier to invaders. Just below the epithelium is a layer of loose connective tissue

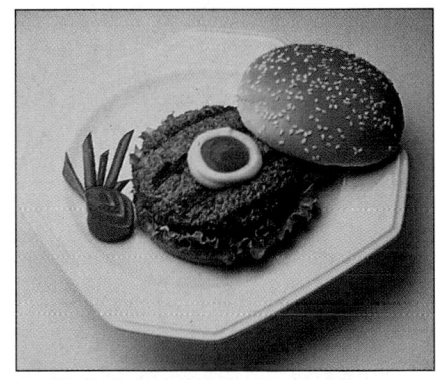

The body digests the foods presented—the order in which foods are eaten plays no role. You can eat a bun and then a burger, or both at the same time.

olfactory Sense of smell.

lumen Space within a tubular structure through which a substance passes.

GI Tract Flow

Mouth
↓
Esophagus
↓

Stomach—4-cup (1-L) capacity. Food remains about 2 to 3 hours. High-fat meals take the longest time to empty.
↓

Small intestine—duodenum (10 in long), jejunum (4 ft long), ileum (5 ft long)—about 10 ft (3.1 m) in total length. Food remains about 3 to 10 hours.
↓

Large intestine (colon)—cecum, ascending colon, transverse colon, descending colon, sigmoid colon—3 1/2 ft (1.1 m) in total length. Food can remain up to 72 hours.

salivary amylase A starch-digesting enzyme produced by salivary glands.

esophagus A tube in the GI tract that connects the pharynx with the stomach.

epiglottis The flap that folds down over the trachea during swallowing.

soft palate The fleshy posterior portion of the roof of the mouth.

uvula The fleshy portion of the soft palate that prevents food from being expelled through the nose during swallowing.

lower esophageal sphincter A circular muscle that constricts the opening of the esophagus to the stomach.

containing blood vessels and immune bodies. The latter protect the GI tract against disease-bearing pathogens. Below this is a layer of smooth muscle. Collectively, these three layers are called mucosa.

The **submucosal** layer under the mucosa contains nerve fibers, blood, and lymph vessels embedded in connective tissue. Below this layer is a third layer (muscularis) with longitudinal and circular muscles, whose contractions mix and stir the contents of the GI tract. These muscular actions occur from the esophagus to the large intestine and are referred to as peristalsis. They move the bolus of food ever onward and downward through the tract, while creating smaller and smaller particles. The fourth layer is composed of the connective tissue that marks the boundary wall.

The lumen of the GI tract is the space within where the food moves along. The lumen is lined with specialized cells which secrete mucus. The absorbed nutrients that have passed through the muscosa enter either the blood or the lymph through the submucosal layer, which has an abundant supply of nerves.

Mouth

In the mouth, salivary glands produce saliva, which functions as a solvent so that dissolved food particles can be separated and tasted, and it contains a starch-digesting enzyme, **salivary amylase** (see Chapter 5). Another component of saliva is mucus, which makes it easy to swallow a bolus of food.

The pharynx connects the mouth and nasal cavity with the esophagus. The pharynx also connects the nasal cavity with the lungs. This dual passageway allows us to inhale air though the mouth and direct that air to the lungs, and it allows us to swallow a bolus of food. One can swallow air (mouth to **esophagus**) and inhale food (mouth to trachea). Of course, the latter is undesirable: No one wants food to enter the lungs. The **epiglottis** closes over the larynx to prevent food from being trapped in the windpipe (trachea) during swallowing (Fig. 3-12). Likewise, when we inhale, a muscle contracts and prevents air from entering the esophagus.

A more detailed look at respiration will help explain how gas exchanges control metabolism. During swallowing, the **soft palate** and **uvula** move to close off the nasal cavity, so that no food or fluid exits the nose. As one swallows either food or fluid, the food is directed by the epiglottis into the esophagus. Only air is allowed into the larynx (the voice box) and eventually the lungs.

The larynx is the connection between the pharynx and the trachea. It produces sound and allows air to enter and exit the lungs. (Should the epiglottis fail to close properly over the larynx during swallowing—a piece of food could become lodged in the opening—the person can suffocate to death.) The trachea connects the larynx to the bronchi. If someone is choking and can't make any noise, you know the situation can be fatal (review Fig. 3-12).

The esophagus is a long tube that connects the pharynx to the stomach. At the end of the esophagus is the **lower esophageal sphincter,** a muscle that constricts after the bolus of food enters the stomach. This sphincter prevents the acidic contents of the stomach from backing up into the esophagus.

■ FIGURE **3-12** The process of swallowing. *(a)* During swallowing, food does not normally enter the trachea because the epiglottis closes over the larynx. *(b)* The arrow shows that the closed epiglottis allows food to proceed down the esophagus. *(c)* When a person chokes, food becomes lodged in the trachea, blocking air flow to the lungs. The food should have moved down the esophagus.
Illustration by William Ober.

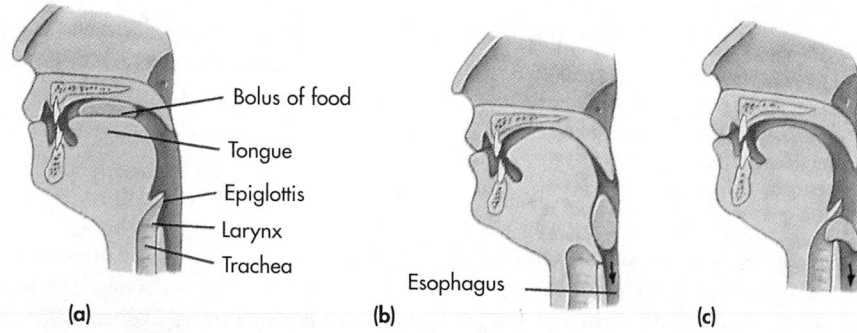

Bolus of food
Tongue
Epiglottis
Larynx
Trachea
Esophagus

(a)   (b)   (c)

Stomach

The stomach is a large tank shaped like the letter J, with the bulky part of the J at the top and the skinny part at the bottom. The capacity of the stomach is about 1 liter, or 4 cups. The stomach empties into the small intestine through the **pyloric sphincter.**

The stomach begins the process of digesting dietary proteins and sterilizes the food using the action of a strong acid, hydrochloric acid (HCl), a component of gastric juice. The mixture of gastric juice and partially-digested food is called **chyme.** The stomach ends at the pyloric sphincter. Like the esophageal sphincter, the pyloric sphincter holds the chyme in the small intestine and prevents it from backing up into the stomach.

The stomach consists of the same four layers as found in other structures of the GI tract, but the muscularis is far more muscular. There is a longitudinal layer, a circular layer and an oblique layer of muscles, which makes it possible to vigorously mix and churn the contents of the stomach. Within the surface of the stomach wall are glands whose cells produce several important substances (Fig. 3-13). See Table 3-7 for a list of cells in these glands and what they produce. The stomach is covered with a thick layer of mucus to protect the epithelium from the harmful effects of acid.

If a person has his or her stomach surgically removed, the digestive processes of the stomach can be carried out by the small intestine, except for one important function—the production of a substance called **intrinsic factor.** This vital material is essential for the absorption of one of the B-vitamins, vitamin B-12 (see Chapter 10).

The HCl in gastric juice maintains the pH of the stomach at less than 2. This strong acidity is important because it:

1. Destroys the biological activity of protein
2. Converts pepsinogen into the active enzyme form, pepsin
3. Partially digests dietary protein
4. Solubilizes dietary minerals, such as calcium, so that they can be absorbed

It is important to recognize that digestion is a chemical process known as **hydrolysis,** in which water is used to split large molecules into smaller ones. The process eventually yields basic molecules, which can be absorbed through the intestinal wall. Enzymes speed up the process by catalyzing the chemical reaction, bringing certain molecules close together and then creating a favorable environment for the intended react (Fig. 3-14).

When the stomach has thoroughly mixed and churned the contents of a meal so that it is a liquid, the chyme is usually ready to leave the stomach within 2 to 4 hours after the food is eaten. As to absorption of food through the stomach, there is virtually none, except for one component of the diet, alcohol. Absorption occurs because alcohol is lipid soluble.

pyloric sphincter The ring of smooth muscle between the stomach and the duodenum.

chyme A mixture of stomach secretions and partially digested food.

intrinsic factor A substance present in gastric juice that enhances vitamin B-12 absorption.

hydrolysis A chemical reaction in which a compound is broken down by the addition of water. One product receives a hydrogen ion (H^+), while the other product receives a hydroxyl ion (OH^-). Hydrolytic enzymes break down compounds using water in the manner just described.

The naming system for enzymes is quite simple. The prefix of the enzyme name usually indicates the target; the suffix is then -ase. For example, lipase is the enzyme that digests certain lipids.

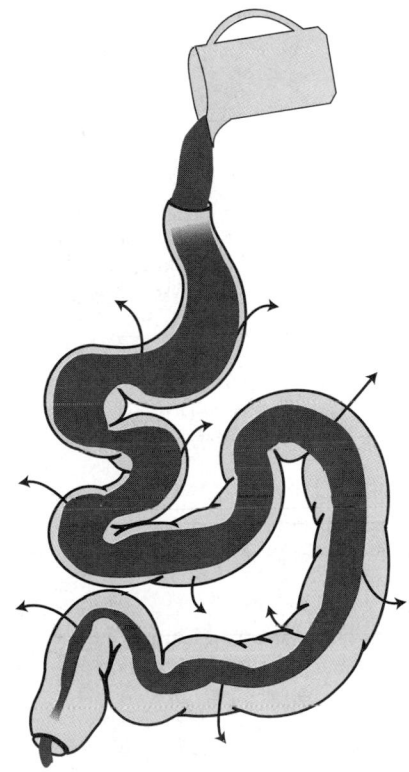

As the intestinal contents pass down the GI tract, nutrients are absorbed from the "hollow tube" into the body.

Cell Types	Secretions
Goblet cells	Mucus
Parietal cells	Hydrochloric acid
Chief cells	Pepsinogen
Enterochromaffin-like cells or ECL	Histamine
G cells	Gastrin
Pepsinogen is the inactive form of the protein-digesting enzyme pepsin.	

TABLE 3-7   Secretions of Stomach Cells

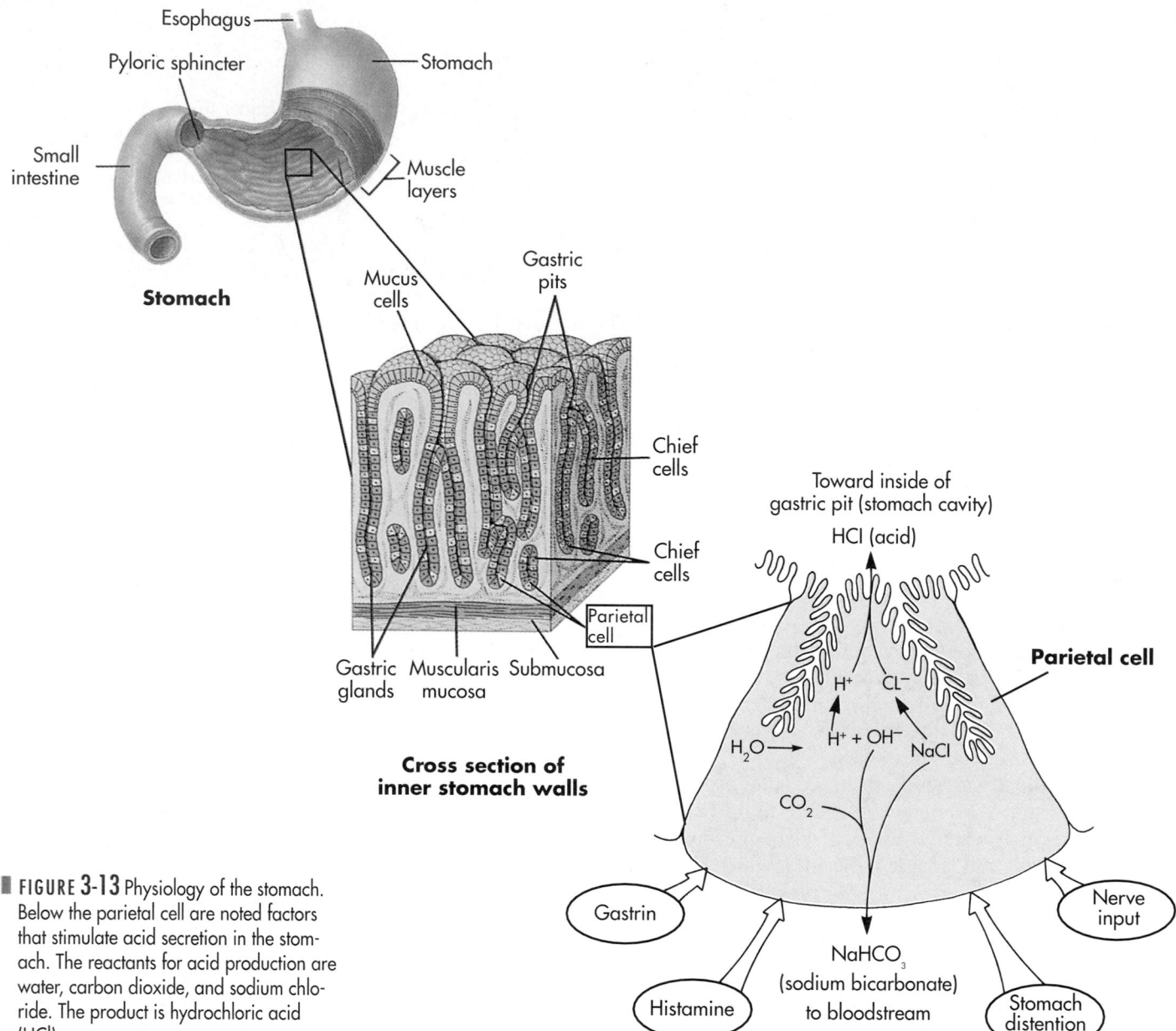

FIGURE 3-13 Physiology of the stomach. Below the parietal cell are noted factors that stimulate acid secretion in the stomach. The reactants for acid production are water, carbon dioxide, and sodium chloride. The product is hydrochloric acid (HCl).

ileocecal sphincter The ring of smooth muscle between the ileum of the small intestine and the colon.

villi The fingerlike protrusions into the small intestine that participate in digestion and absorption of food.

microvilli Microscopic hairlike projections of cell membranes of certain epithelial cells.

Small Intestine

The small intestine is about 1 inch wide and possesses an absorptive surface area of 200 M^2. Its boundaries are the stomach on the "north" and the colon (large intestine) on the "south." The entrance to the colon is through a sphincter, the **ileocecal sphincter,** which prevents the contents of the colon from backing up into the small intestine. The mucosa of the small intestine is covered with fingerlike structures called **villi.** On each villus are tiny projections called **microvilli** (Fig. 3-15). In a light microscope, these projections look like tiny hairs; thus, the surface of the small intestine is sometimes referred to as the brush border. The small intestine serves two purposes: the digestion of food and the absorption of nutrients.

Based on function and the anatomy of the structure, the small intestine is divided into three regions: the **duodenum,** the **jejunum,** and the **ileum.** The duodenum is connected to the stomach at the pyloric sphincter. The duodenum receives bile from the liver via the gallbladder and, in most people, secretions from the pancreas through a common duct. This is where bile and pancreatic juice enter the GI tract

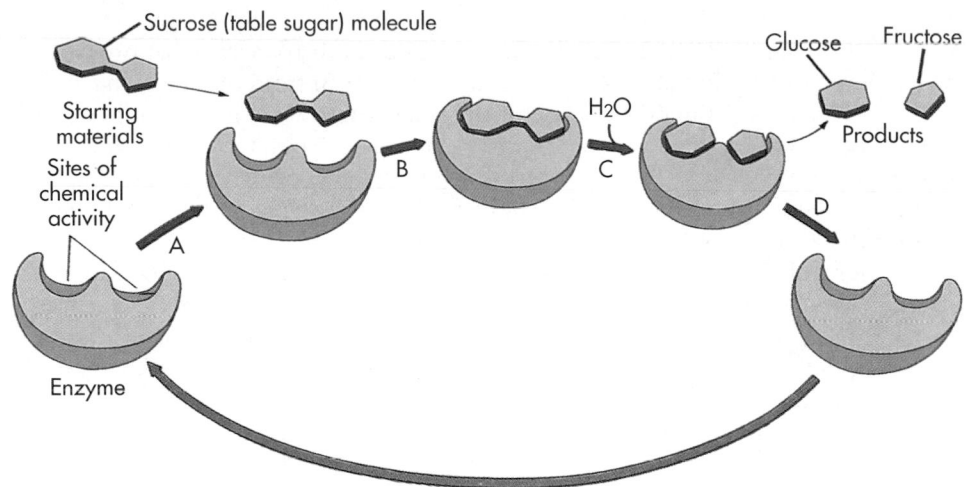

FIGURE 3-14 A model of enzyme action. Enzymes act as catalysts to speed chemical reactions, including those that contribute to the digestion of foodstuffs. In this example, an enzyme is contributing to the breakdown of sucrose (from *A* to *D*) into the smaller sugar forms glucose and fructose. Only these smaller sugar forms are absorbed from the small intestine to enter the bloodstream. Note that, with some enzymes, the reaction can go both ways. In addition, sometimes energy input (ATP) is needed to allow the enzyme to push the reaction along.

Illustration by William Ober.

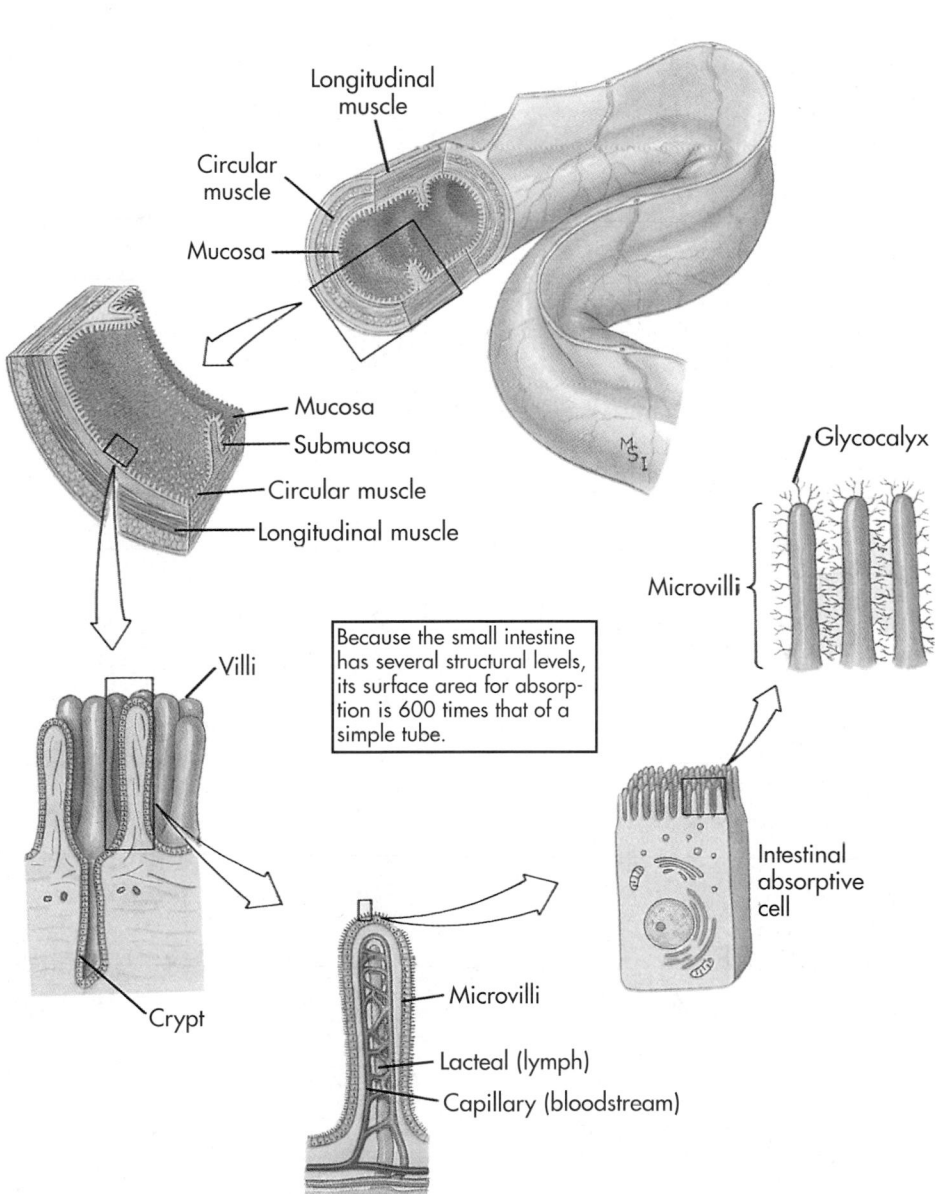

Because the small intestine has several structural levels, its surface area for absorption is 600 times that of a simple tube.

FIGURE 3-15 Organization of the small intestine. The small intestine has several structural levels, which increase the surface area for absorption up to 600 times that of a simple tube.

*P*eople who have pancreatic disease may not produce sufficient enzymes for digestion. In cystic fibrosis, excess production of mucus may block release of enzymes from the pancreas. This results in malabsorption of nutrients and associated discomfort. An affected person can consume replacement enzymes with meals. Some forms are coated to protect against destruction by stomach acid.

through the sphincter of Oddi and are ready to go to work digesting food (review the insert in Fig. 3-11). There are additional glands in the pancreas that produce an alkaline mucus to neutralize the acid chyme as it flows in from the stomach.

The jejunum is the middle portion of the small intestine. It is well supplied with lymph tissues to produce a variety of lymphocytes. The ileum, or terminal end of the small intestine, empties into the **cecum** through the ileocecal sphincter. This segment of the small intestine has abundant lymph tissues and plays a vital role in maintaining the body's immune system.[15]

Nutrient absorption takes place all along the small intestine, but each nutrient has its own site where it can enter the body (Fig. 3-16). The digestion of food takes place in the lumen of the intestine with the aid of bile, digestive enzymes from the pancreas, and digestive enzymes from the wall of the small intestine itself. The microvilli contain digestive enzymes, which complete the digestion of almost any partially digested food and prepare it for **absorption**. A more complete description of the digestive process will be explained in later chapters as each nutrient is introduced.

absorption The process by which nutrient molecules are absorbed by the GI tract and enter the bloodstream or the lymph.

Both the starches and protein in a meal can produce glucose in the body.

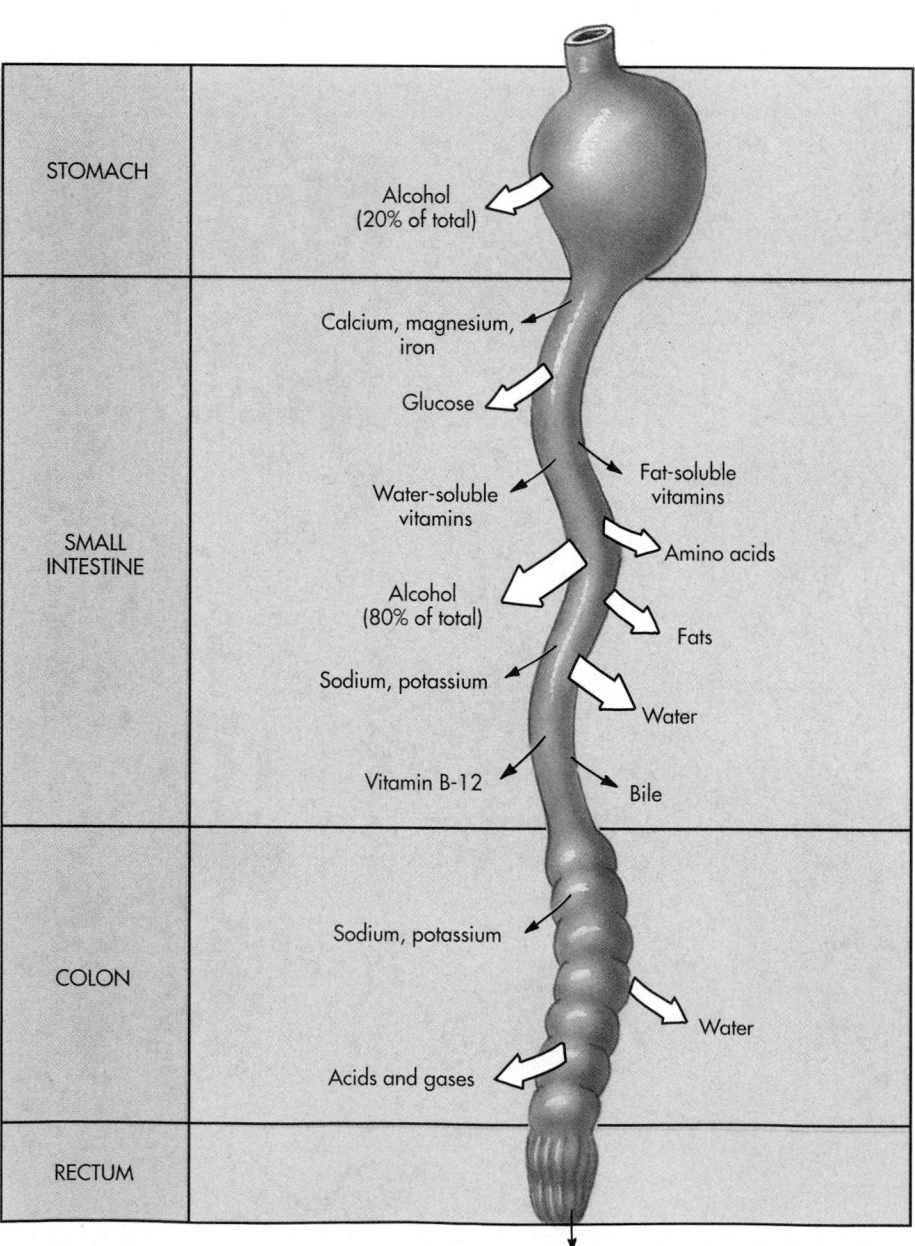

■ FIGURE **3-16** Major sites of absorption along the GI tract. The size of the arrow indicates the relative amount of absorption at that site, notably where there are multiple absorption sites.

STOMACH

Alcohol (20% of total)

SMALL INTESTINE

Calcium, magnesium, iron

Glucose

Water-soluble vitamins

Fat-soluble vitamins

Amino acids

Alcohol (80% of total)

Fats

Sodium, potassium

Water

Vitamin B-12

Bile

COLON

Sodium, potassium

Water

Acids and gases

RECTUM

Feces

Absorption

Each fingerlike villus is covered with **absorptive cells** (enterocytes) and mucus-secreting goblet cells, which are responsible for enzymatic digestion and absorption (review Fig. 3-15). The villus contains blood capillaries and a lacteal. Any water-soluble nutrient entering the villus is immediately picked up by the blood capillaries, whereas the fat-soluble nutrients enter into the lacteals. Blood capillaries empty into a vein serving the villus, which eventually connects to the portal vein. Lacteals empty into lymph vessels. Located in the villus are many lymphocytes, which recognize and destroy any pathogens that have escaped detection and destruction in the GI tract. However, even with the extensive network of immune bodies that reside in the GI tract, some dangerous microorganisms can get through this barrier and into the body.

The cells that cover the surface of the villi have a very short life span—birth to death in less than 6 days. To provide for constant renewal, new goblet and epithelial cells are pushed up from the base of the villi, where they are constantly being synthesized. Is it any wonder why the GI tract is sensitive to nutritional deficiencies? With the incredible wear and tear on the lining, and the need to replace one-fifth of the tract daily, the nutrient demands for this system are incredibly high. Fortunately, many of the old cells can be broken down and the component parts reused.

The contents of the small intestine are propelled along by peristaltic actions, as mentioned before. There is also another type of action, called **segmentation,** which does an excellent job of thoroughly mixing the chyme with the digestive fluids (Fig. 3-17).

Large Intestine

The large intestine, or colon, begins at the ileocecal sphincter and ends at the anus. The contents of the colon move through specific regions, commencing with the cecum at the lower right side of the body; moving up the right side via the ascending colon; continuing across the transverse colon, located just below the liver; moving

absorptive cells A class of cells, also called *enterocytes*, that cover the surface of the villi (fingerlike projections in the small intestine) and participate in nutrient absorption.

segmentation Contractions of the circular muscles in the intestines that lead to dividing and mixing of the intestinal contents. This action aids digestion and absorption of nutrients.

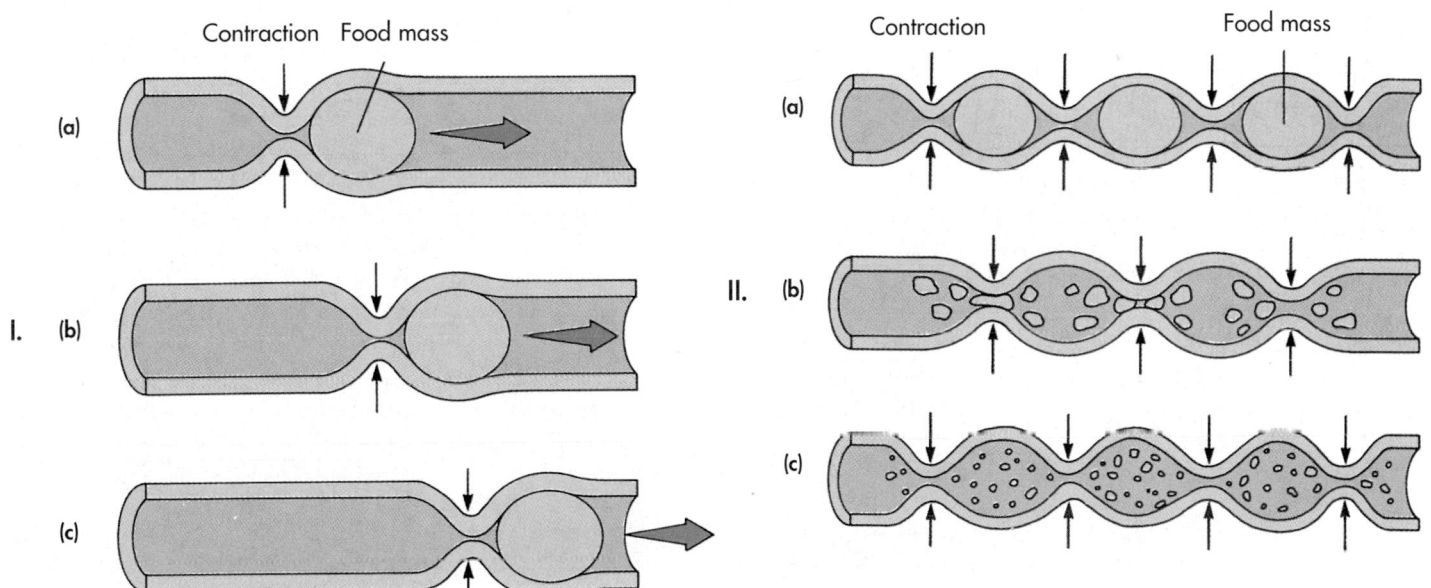

FIGURE 3-17 Peristalsis and segmentation. *I. Peristalsis.* Peristalsis is a progressive movement, propelling material along the GI tract. *(a)* A ring of contraction occurs where the GI wall is stretched, passing the food mass forward. *(b)* The moving food mass triggers a ring of contraction in the next region, which pushes the food mass even farther along. *(c)* The ring of contraction moves like a wave along the GI tract, pushing the food mass forward.

II. Segmentation. Segmentation is the back-and-forth action that breaks apart chunks of the food mass and mixes in digestive juices. *(a)* Ringlike regions of contraction occur at intervals along the GI tract. *(b)* Previously contracted regions relax and adjacent regions contract, effectively chopping the contents of each segment into smaller chunks. *(c)* Contracted regions continue to alternate back-and-forth, chopping and mixing the contents of the GI tract.

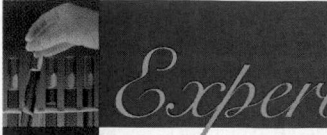

Expert Opinion

PROBIOTICS, PREBIOTICS, AND HUMAN HEALTH

Steve Hertzler, Ph.D., R.D.

The human body consists of over 100 trillion (10^{14}) cells, 90% of which are bacterial. The large intestine (colon) harbors most of these bacteria, containing an amazingly large and diverse population of microorganisms (called microflora) made up of more than 400 species. It is now understood that, because of its microflora, the colon performs many more functions beyond simply the absorption of water and the excretion of waste. The fermentation of undigested carbohydrates by the colonic bacteria produces fatty acids. The fatty acid butyrate helps regulate the growth and development of colon cells. Eventually the fatty acid acetate serves as an energy source for the liver once absorbed into the bloodstream. The normal microflora also participate in the synthesis of vitamins, such as vitamin K, and defend against invading pathogenic microorganisms.

Although we have focused on the beneficial attributes of the colonic microflora thus far, the actions of some types of bacteria can have harmful consequences as well. The enzyme processes found in bacteria such as *Escherichia coli* and the genus *Clostridium* can retoxify drugs and other chemicals that were originally detoxified by the liver and excreted into the small intestine. In addition, these bacteria may be involved in the conversion of bile acids (see discussion in this chapter for details on bile acids) and undigested proteins into toxic substances. The total of these harmful bacterial activities may increase the risk of colon cancer.

PROBIOTICS

There is currently great interest in finding ways to promote the growth or metabolic activity of beneficial bacteria, while inhibiting the harmful bacteria. Probiotics, which means "for life" in Greek, is one approach. The term refers to living microorganisms, which, upon ingestion in certain numbers, exert health benefits beyond inherent general nutrition. Thus, the probiotic approach involves the consumption of live bacterial cells—mainly lactic acid–producing bacteria (e.g., the *Lactobacillus* or *Bifidobacterium* genera)—in foods or as dietary supplements. Numerous studies have shown that the lactic acid produced by these organisms tends to inhibit the growth of less acid-tolerant organisms, such as *E. coli* and the genus *Clostridium*, which are generally regarded as harmful.

Key requirements for the successful use of probiotics are the survival of the probiotic organism as it makes its way through the gastrointestinal tract and the subsequent colonization of the organism in the gut. The hurdles that probiotic bacteria face include destruction by stomach or bile acids and competition with other bacteria in the colon. One method for overcoming this problem is the selection of probiotic bacteria that are highly resistant to stomach and bile acids and that possess the ability to colonize the gastrointestinal tract. This approach requires the meticulous laboratory testing of many bacterial strains, using in vitro systems that can only roughly approximate actual conditions inside the body.

Despite the challenges associated with probiotic survival, the evidence for the health benefits of certain probiotics continues to grow. Yogurt, which is produced using *Lactobacillus bulgaricus* and *Streptococcus thermophilus*, is a common food to which certain probiotic organisms (e.g., *Lactobacillus acidophilus*, bifidobacteria) are often added. Studies have clearly shown that lactose-intolerant individuals can more readily digest the lactose in yogurt than the lactose in milk. This improvement in lactose digestion is due to the presence of the enzyme lactase in the bacterial cells of the starter culture, which is released when the cells encounter bile acids in the small intestine. The active cultures in yogurt also provide other nutritional advantages, including (1) short chains of amino acids formed from milk proteins during yogurt fermentation, which may lower blood pressure; (2) compounds with stimulating effects on the immune system; and (3) a natural inhibitor of the enzyme that synthesizes cholesterol in the body, resulting in the possible lowering of blood lipids. The optimal amount of yogurt to be eaten each day to derive these benefits has yet to be established. Dosage is often expressed in colony forming units (CFU) of bacteria and is generally in the range of 10^8 to 10^{12} CFU per day. (Yogurt with active cultures must have at least 10^8 CFU/ml; an 8-ounce serving of yogurt contains 240 ml.) To date, unrealistically high doses of yogurt (>2 liters/day) have been fed in some of the studies that have shown cholesterol-lowering effects.

Two of the most popular probiotics, *Lactobacillus* GG (Culturelle®) and *Lactobacillus* LC1 (formerly *Lactobacillus acidophilus [johnsonii]* La1) have recently become available as dietary supplements in the United States. *Lactobacillus* GG has been extensively studied and found in animal studies to be safe at doses much higher than the 10^9–10^{10} CFU/day that people would normally consume in fermented foods or supplements (Culturelle® has 10^{10}, or 10 billion, CFU per capsule and costs about $18 for a 1-month supply). *Lactobacillus* GG is effective in the treatment of several types of diarrhea (rotaviral, traveler's, and relapsing *Clostridium difficile*). Studies of the LC1 strain in vitro have shown that it inhibits the growth of *Helicobacter pylori*, the bacteria that are the cause of most cases of peptic ulcer and gastritis. Treatment with LC1 has been shown to reduce the metabolic activity of *Helicobacter pylori* in infected individuals; however, LC1 does not eliminate the infection. Specific medications are needed for that (see the Nutrition Perspective at the end of this chapter).

PREBIOTICS

Because it is so difficult for many probiotic bacteria to survive in and colonize the gastrointestinal tract, a second approach to promoting the growth of healthy bacteria, called prebiotics, has developed. Prebiotics are nondigestible food ingredients that beneficially affect the host by selectively stimulating the growth of one or a limited number of bacteria in the colon. The emphasis in prebiotics is on the provision of an energy source, usually a nondigestible carbohydrate, for the beneficial bacteria that already reside in the colon. The key to a good prebiotic is that it must be used selectively: beneficial bacteria are able to use it, whereas harmful bacteria are not.

The most popular prebiotic carbohydrate is fructooligosaccharide (FOS). The chemical structure of FOS consists of a molecule of glucose joined with two, three, or four fructose units, with the fructose units linked by beta chemical bonds (see Chapter 5 for details on beta chemical bonds in various carbohydrates). Because of its structure, FOS is not digested in the small intestine and becomes available to the colonic bacteria. There it selectively promotes the growth of bifidobacteria in the colon, since bifidobacteria are one of only a few types of bacteria that possess the enzyme necessary to digest FOS. The major brand of FOS in the United States is NutraFlora®. FOS is 30% as sweet as table sugar, contains only 1–2 kcal/g, and does not increase blood glucose, which may make it useful in food products for people with diabetes. FOS has been widely used in Japan for its bifidobacteria-stimulating effect. (The recommended dose is 1–4 g/day and costs about $14/month.) It has recently been included in oral meal-replacement formulas used for hospitalized patients in the United States.

The potential health benefits of FOS include (1) increasing bifidobacteria concentrations in the colon, (2) lowering harmful enzyme activities of other colonic bacteria, (3) increasing calcium absorption from the intestine, (4) lowering blood lipids, and (5) decreasing cariogenicity (does not promote dental caries). Although the ability of FOS to increase bifidobacteria counts has been well documented, additional studies are needed to confirm the results of preliminary work on the other potential health benefits. Current research in my laboratory is evaluating the effect of FOS on colonic bacterial enzyme activities and intestinal gas production.

The increasing threat of antimicrobial-resistant infections around the world, coupled with our new knowledge regarding the colonic microflora in host defense, means that research on prebiotics and probiotics may take on even more importance. In the future, consumers are likely to see many more foods and dietary supplements designed to improve the balance of the intestinal flora.

Dr. Hertzler is an assistant professor of medical dietetics at the Ohio State University. He earned his Ph.D. in human nutrition from the University of Minnesota in 1995 and is actively researching FOS as a prebiotic supplement, as well as the glycemic response to various carbohydrates.

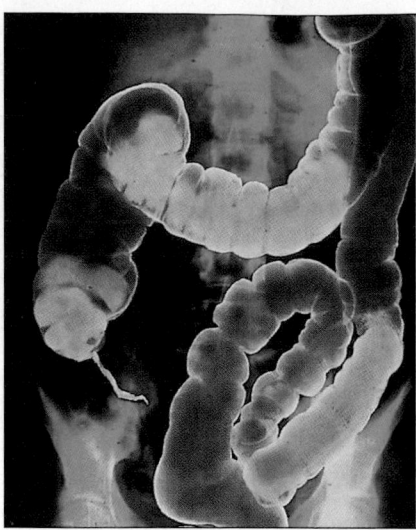

The colon has a large diameter and no villi.

bile A liver secretion that is stored in the gallbladder and released through the common bile duct into the duodenum. It is essential for the absorption of fat.

gallbladder An organ attached to the underside of the liver and in which bile is stored and secreted.

enterohepatic circulation The recycling of compounds between the small intestine and the liver over and over again, as happens with bile acids.

endocrine gland A hormone-producing gland.

exocrine gland A cluster of epithelial cells specialized for secretion. They have ducts, which lead to an epithelial surface.

down the descending colon; curving slightly inward at the sigmoid colon; and concluding its path at the rectum. The rectum is the storage facility for feces. Feces are removed from the body via the anal canal. Two anal sphincters make it possible to remove the feces from the body.

The digestion of food takes place in the small intestine, so the large intestine has little to do with digestion. Thus, there are no villi present. It does however, absorb water, a few vitamins, some fatty acids, and **electrolytes** (e.g. sodium and potassium). Some bacteria residing in the large intestine synthesize vitamins and have other functions, as described by Dr. Hertzler in his Expert Opinion. The extent to which any vitamins are produced and absorbed will be discussed further in Chapter 10.

The muscular action in the large intestine (called haustrations), moves the contents of the colon along, but at a very sluggish rate, compared with peristalsis. Nonetheless, it mixes the colon's contents and divides them into small particles in preparation for elimination from the body.

About 7 to 9 liters of fluid flows through the GI tract every 24 hours. The fluid comes from saliva, the stomach, the pancreas, the liver and gallbladder, and the diet. Actually, about 20% of the fluid is from food and beverages. Of the 7 to 9 liters, only about 0.2 liter is excreted with the feces. The rest is absorbed in the small intestine and colon.

Accessory Digestive Organs

The liver, gallbladder, and pancreas do not directly participate in digestion. They do however, provide digestive fluids that enable the digestive processes to chemically change the food into absorbable components.

Liver and Gallbladder. The water-soluble end products of digestion are absorbed into the blood capillaries of the villi, collected in venules (tiny veins), and finally released into a large vein, the portal vein, which delivers the nutrients to the liver for processing. The portal vein drains fluid from both the large and the small intestines. In turn, capillaries in the liver drain fluid from liver tissues; the fluid is released into the **hepatic veins.** Absorbed nutrients coming in via the portal vein are metabolized by the liver and/or released into the hepatic vein, so that they can eventually enter general circulation.

Bile is produced in the liver and empties into a channel, which funnels it to the **gallbladder** for storage. (See Chapter 6 for more about the actions of bile.) The gallbladder is a sac attached to the underside of the liver. When a signal comes in, saying that the digestive tract needs bile, the gallbladder discharges it into the common bile duct, which carries it to the duodenum.

One interesting aspect of bile transport is that bile can be reabsorbed from the small intestine, returned to the liver via the portal vein, and reused. In this manner, bile (and a lot of other substances) are not wasted. The circuit is known as **enterohepatic circulation.**

In addition to bile, a number of other substances can be released from the liver and travel along with the bile to the gallbladder and into the duodenum. The liver is effectively a cleaning service, removing some unwanted substances from the blood and disposing of them through the duodenum and eventually the feces. For example, certain drugs and hormones can be removed from the body this way.

Besides producing bile, the liver can detoxify dangerous substances and destroy harmful microorganisms. Specialized Kupffer cells produce lymphocytes to carry out phagocytosis on any bacteria that somehow make it through the natural barriers the body erects to keep enemies out.

The liver controls many aspects of carbohydrate, lipid, protein, and alcohol metabolism. The details will be discussed in later chapters.

Pancreas. Glucagon and insulin are hormones produced by the **endocrine glands** of the pancreas. The action of these two hormones will be described in Chapter 5. The pancreas also functions as an **exocrine gland,** secreting pancreatic juice. This digestive juice contains water, bicarbonate, and a variety of digestive enzymes. Both the digestive enzymes from the pancreas and the digestive enzymes produced by the brush border (microvilli) are essential in the digestion of all foods. We can't survive on food alone without a working pancreas and at least 100 cm (40 in) of small intestine.

Regulation of the Digestive System

Although we think of digestion as an automatic process, nerves and hormones are constantly adjusting the actions of the GI tract to respond to the arrival of food and beverages. Just the sight, smell, or thought of food can activate the **vagus nerve** to turn on the digestive system.

vagus nerve The nerve responsible for contractions of the muscles of the GI tract.

Secretions of the gastrointestinal hormones target various structures to carry out their assigned tasks. The gastrointestinal hormones are different from the other hormones in that they are secreted by cells located throughout the gastrointestinal tract; they are not all produced by separate organs. Although some of these hormones are secreted directly into the tract, most reach their targets by way of the bloodstream (Table 3-8).

CONCEPT CHECK

Digestion is a mechanical and chemical process controlled by enzymes and coordinated by hormones and the vagus nerves. The end products of digestion are small molecules of the original food or beverage, small enough to enter into the villi for pickup by either the blood in the capillaries or the lymph fluid in the lacteals. Any dietary component that escapes digestion exits the body in the feces. Whereas swallowing a bolus of food is voluntary, the rest of the digestive process is involuntary. The stomach initiates the process of digestion by mixing food with gastric juice and converting this partially digested food into a liquid called chyme. Absorption takes place mostly in the small intestine. The feces, or undigested material, are expelled from the body.

■ Urinary System

The urinary system is composed of two kidneys located on the back of the abdominal wall, one on each side of the vertebral column (see Fig. 3-18).[18] Each is connected to the urinary bladder by a **ureter.** The bladder is emptied by way of the **urethra.**

ureter A tube that transports urine from the kidney to the urinary bladder.

Each bean-shaped kidney has an outer section called the cortex and an inner section called the medulla. The medulla is composed of cone-shaped pyramids, which

urethra The tube that transports urine from the urinary bladder to the outside of the body.

TABLE 3-8 Gastrointestinal Tract Hormones

Hormone	Stimulus to Secretion	Secreted By	Action
Gastrin	Food in the stomach, especially proteins, caffeine; spices; alcohol	Pyloric region of the stomach and upper duodenum	Stimulates parietal cells to produce HCl, stimulates chief cells to produce pepsinogen, begins digestion of protein
Secretin	Acid chyme, peptones (partially digested protein)	Duodenum, jejunum	Stimulates pancreas to produce bicarbonate and water, neutralizes acid content of small intestine
Cholecystokinin (CCK)	Food, especially fat and proteins in duodenum	Duodenum, jejunum	Stimulates contraction of gallbladder, Secretes pancreatic digestive enzymes, inhibits gastric motility
Gastric inhibitory peptide	Protein and fat in chyme	Small intestine	Inhibits gastric motility, stimulates insulin secretion

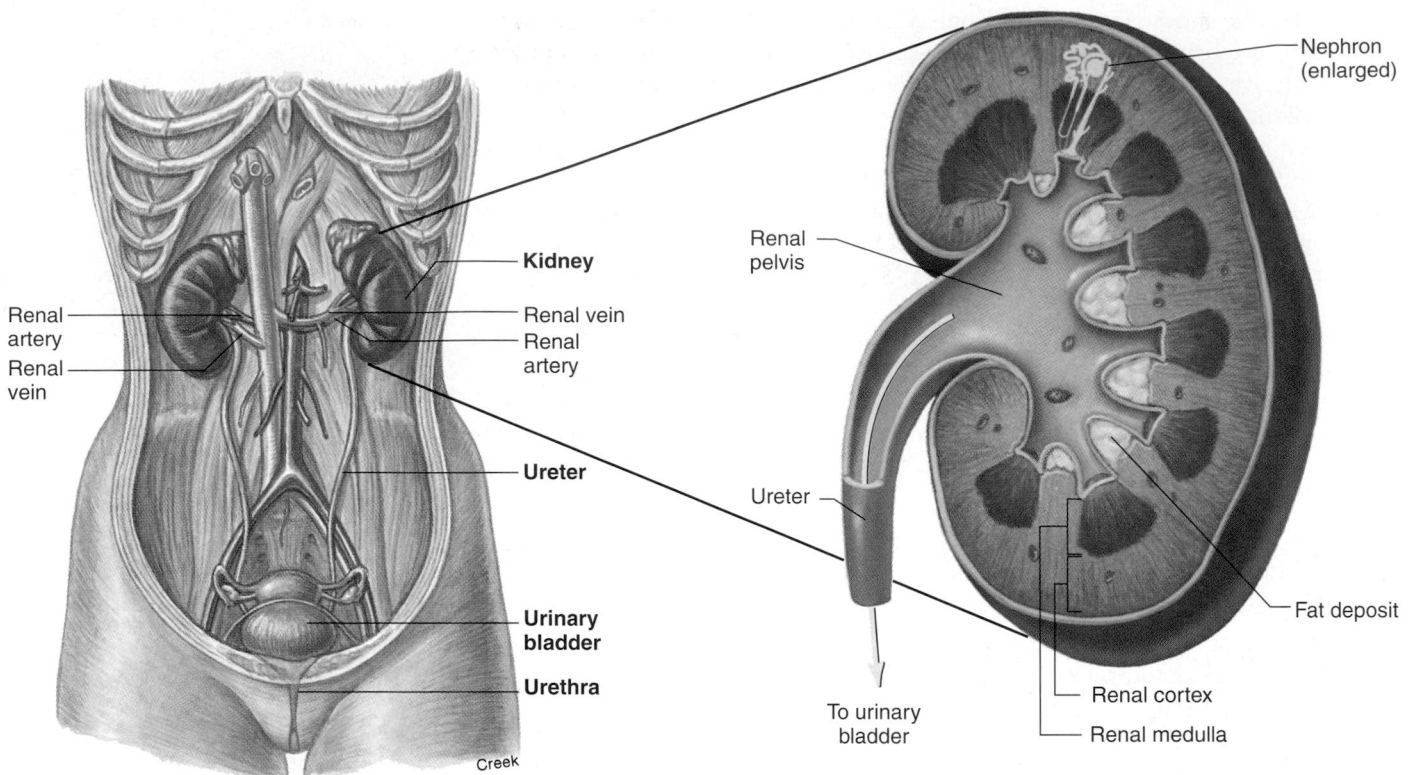

■ FIGURE 3-18 (a and b) Organs of the urinary system. a. The kidneys, bean-shaped organs located on either side of the spinal column, filter waste from the blood, which is then stored in the bladder as urine. The kidneys are connected to the urinary bladder by ureters. The urinary system of the female is shown. The male's urinary system is the same, except that the urethra extends through the penis. b. A Cross section of the kidney. The outer section of the kidney is the cortex, the inner section is the medulla. The functional unit of the kidney, the nephron, loops through the cortex and medulla, and the fluid that flows through these tiny structures is separated so that the waste is removed from the blood into collecting ducts and drains into the renal pelvis. Thus the urine exists by way of the ureter to the bladder. The remaining fluid is returned to the circulatory system to maintain the normal composition of the blood.

empty waste materials into a funnel-shaped tube ending in the ureter. Ureters carry urine from the kidneys to the bladder for temporary storage. Blood flows through the kidneys at a rate of about 120 ml/minute.

Kidney Functions

The kidneys regulate the composition of the blood (plasma) and the interstitial fluid, known together as the extracellular fluid. This regulation is accomplished by filtering the blood and forming urine, which is basically the filtrate. As a result of kidney action and the formation of urine, the volume of blood plasma is controlled, and blood pressure is maintained. The kidneys remove metabolic waste and foreign chemicals from the blood, and they maintain a certain concentration of electrolytes such as Na^+, K^+, and HCO_3^- (bicarbonate) in the plasma. Together with the lungs, the kidneys maintain the pH of the blood. The kidneys constantly monitor the composition of the blood and produce hormones to maintain homeostasis. For example, the kidneys produce the hormone **erythropoietin,** which is responsible for the synthesis of red blood cells. The kidneys convert a form of vitamin D into its active hormone form. During times of fasting, the kidneys can produce glucose from amino acids.

Kidney Structure

Each kidney is enclosed in a fatty, fibrous sack, which protects it from external physical damage. Examined microscopically, the functional unit of the kidney, the

erythropoietin A hormone secreted mostly by the kidneys that enhances red blood cell synthesis and stimulates red blood cell release from bone marrow.

nephron, is disclosed. Nephrons extend through the renal cortex and the renal medulla. There are more than 1 million nephrons per kidney. The nephron consists of small tubules allied with small blood vessels. The tiny capillary filtration unit, the **glomerulus,** is held in a small capsule (Bowman's Capsule). The glomerulus filters large amounts of fluid from the blood, removing the dissolved waste and excess fluid to form urine, which leaves by way of the tubules. The remaining fluid is returned to the blood.

This ingenious mechanism constantly adjusts the composition of the blood. In doing so the essential components are recovered and returned to general circulation, waste products and excess water are removed, and unneeded nutrients (ones where storage compartments are full or there are no storage facilities) are flushed away by the urine.

All the fluid in the body eventually passes through the filtration units (nephrons) in the kidneys, and the waste is removed. The essential nutrients are recovered and returned to the body. The waste—plus some excess nutrients, such as the B-vitamins and vitamin C—are flushed down the toilet.

■ Reproductive System

Reproduction is a fundamental property of all living things.[18, 19] We die, but our genes live on in our progeny. Both ova and sperm, called gametes (sex cells), contain 23 chromosomes. The fertilized egg contains 46 chromosomes (23 from each parent) and is programmed to produce a new human. At conception, the instructions for the developing embryo are all present. Through the actions of the female reproductive organs, supported by hormonal secretions, a human is produced about 38 weeks after conception, providing that essential nutrients are present and no genetic defects are encountered. The most precarious time during pregnancy is during the development of the embryo (the first 13 weeks), when a woman is least likely to know she is pregnant.

The male reproductive organs consist of the scrotum, containing the testis; the penis; the urethra; the seminal vesicles; and the prostate. The female reproductive organs consist of the ovaries, uterus, and vagina.

In addition to reproduction, the sex hormones stimulate bone growth and the closure of the epiphyseal plate, thus causing the cessation of bone growth. Estrogens protect against bone loss. The sex hormone testosterone stimulates protein synthesis, such as muscle growth and bone growth.

Puberty, or the onset of adult sex life, takes place during early adolescence. **Menarche,** the term used to describe the onset of menstruation, occurs usually between the ages of 11 and 16. In the male, sexual maturation occurs somewhat later and is initiated by hormonal secretions from the brain.

The female reproductive system will be discussed in Chapter 15.

CONCEPT CHECK

The urinary system removes the wastes that are produced by the body and most nutrients that are ingested in excess of storage capacity and need. The kidneys maintain the chemical composition of the extracellular fluid and a stable environment within the body. The kidney helps convert vitamin D to its active form. The microscopic unit in the kidney that makes the system work is the nephron, an intricate system of capillaries, tubes, and vessels that fine-tune the system.

The reproductive tract makes it possible to continue the species. Although the reproductive glands and hormones are thought of exclusively as related to sex, their actions have an indirect but powerful effect on nutritional status.

nephron The functional unit of the kidney.

glomerulus The capillaries in the kidney that filter waste material from the blood.

The human body is a vast warehouse of essential components, which are maintained at nearly constant concentrations. The stability of this internal environment is sustained by balancing absorption and excretion. Homeostatic control mechanisms are subject to a hierarchy of importance; thus, homeostasis maintains a certain concentration of water in the body at all times; however, since water can't be stored, the body has evolved with mechanisms that allow adults to exist without water for about 3 days. Other than water, we are able to rely on stored nutrients, allowing us to survive for weeks or months without eating. The human body has the remarkable ability to adapt to continuing changes in the external and internal environments by the 12 systems discussed in this chapter.

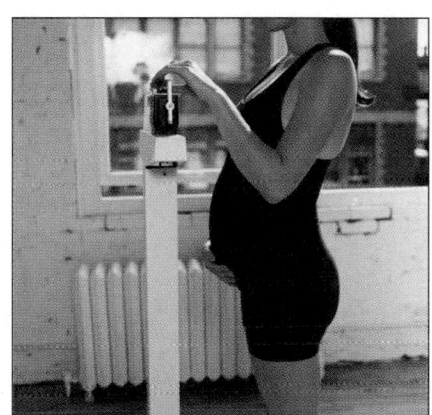

Pregnancy requires all essential nutrients from the moment of conception.

Check out the *Perspectives in Nutrition* web site http://www.mhhe.com/wardlaw for quizzes, flash cards, other activities, and web links designed to further help you learn about issues surrounding human physiologic processes.

SUMMARY

1. The basic structural unit of the human body is the cell. Although almost all cells contain the same collection of organelles (nucleus, mitochondria, endoplasmic reticulum, lysosomes, peroxisomes, and cytoplasm), their structure varies according to the type of job they must perform. In the integumentary system, epithelial cells provide a covering for internal structures, and skin cells provide protection from the environment.

2. A variety of bone cells produce the body's framework and internal support. Blood cells are synthesized within bones.

3. The muscle cells produce movement, as they are elastic. Muscles are classified as skeletal, smooth, or cardiac. Skeletal muscle is under voluntary control. Smooth and cardiac muscle are under involuntary control. Muscle cells generate body heat.

4. Cells that line the aveoli of the lungs make it possible to exchanges gasses (oxygen and carbon dioxide) between the environment and the blood.

5. The cells that make up the nervous system, neurons, are the body's communication network. They control and manage all other systems of the body. Unlike most cells in the body, neurons do not ordinarily regenerate themselves.

6. Cells that make up the endocrine system produce hormones, which chemically regulate almost all other cells.

7. The circulatory system transports nutrients and oxygen to body cells and removes waste materials. This system also distributes products made by the cells to specific sites.

8. The lymph system, like the circulatory system, is a drainage and transport system, but it also functions as part of the body's immune system. Certain immune cells are produced by lymph glands or are found in bones. These cells are responsible for protecting the body from invading pathogens. Immunity is either specific or nonspecific. We are born with some immunity in place, and we activate immunity when we come in contact with a pathogen. T lymphocytes and B lymphocytes are cells associated with specific immunity.

9. The cells that make up the digestive system break down food and convert it to absorbable materials. These cells are an internal passageway from the mouth to the anus. The digestive system is composed of the mouth, esophagus, stomach, small intestine, and colon. The liver, gallbladder, and pancreas make up the accessory organs of the digestive tract.

10. The cells that make up the urinary system are responsible for filtering the blood, removing body wastes, and maintaining the chemical composition of the blood.

11. The female reproductive system produces sex cells (ova), which unite with sperm from the male to produce a human in about 9 months.

12. The male reproductive system produces sex cells (sperm) to deliver to the female's reproductive system.

STUDY QUESTIONS

1. Identify at least one contribution to overall nutrition status provided by each of the 12 systems of the body.

2. Draw and label parts of the cell, and explain the function of each organelle as it relates to human nutrition.

3. All the organs and tissues of the body perform functions that maintain homeostasis: the maintenance of constant or static conditions. How does the digestive system maintain homeostasis?

4. Trace the flow of blood from the right ventricle around the body and back to the right ventricle. How is blood routed through the villi? Which class of nutrients enters the body via the blood? via the lymph?

5. The immune system is divided into specific and nonspecific immunity. Describe how each type of immunity protects us from invading pathogens. Do you think there are any groups of Americans that suffer from a compromised immune system due to a lack of essential nutrients?

6. Identify the four groups of steroid hormones, and explain how they are related to human nutrition.

7. Identify the four basic tastes. Give an example of one food that exemplifies each of these basic taste sensations. Why can't you taste food when you have a cold? What is umami?

8. What is one role of hydrochloric acid in the process of digestion? Where is it secreted? How do the following hormones participate in the digestion of a bolus of food: gastrin, secretin, cholecystokin, GIP?

9. Identify the two accessory organs that empty their contents into the duodenum. How do the digestive substances made by these organs contribute to the digestion of food?

10. In which organ systems would the following substances be found?
Chyme
Erythropoietin
Plasma
Lymph
Urine

■ ANNOTATED REFERENCES

1. Constipation becomes more common with age. *Tufts University Health and Nutrition Letter* 17:7, 1999.

   Normal frequency of bowel movements ranges from three times a day to three times a week. Constipation is an aging problem that can be treated with regular exercise, decreased dosage of medications that cause constipation, increased dietary fiber, more water consumption, and avoidance of laxatives.

2. Ducy P, Schinke T, Karsenty G: The osteoblast: A sophisticated fibroblast under central surveillance. *Science* 289:1501, 2000.

   The hormonal control of bone remodeling is attributed to the sex steroids, PTH, and leptin. The authors predict that other, yet-to-be discovered hormones regulate bone formation.

3. Graham DY and others: Recognizing peptic ulcer disease. *PostGraduate Medicine* 105:113, 1999.

   An algorithm for the clinical evaluation of dyspepsia and the appropriate treatment strategy is explained. Several invasive tests are explained together with the cost of the tests.

4. Guyton AC, Hall JE: *Textbook of medical physiology.* 9th ed. Philadelphia: W. B. Saunders, 1996.

   Although this well-known text is designed for medical students, it still provides the basis for understanding human physiology at the undergraduate level. The chapter concerning the digestive tract explains in detail the processes of converting food into absorbable dietary components.

5. Heartburn, don't ignore it. Mayo Clinic Health Letter. 18:8, 2000.

   The causes of heartburn are explained. The new FDA-approved endoscopic treatments for heartburn are introduced. One treatment is sewing up the lower esophageal sphincter (LES) and the other is burning a scar into the LES that tightens up the sphincter.

6. Klein S and others: The alimentary tract in nutrition: A tutorial. In Shils ME and others (eds.): *Health and disease.* 9th ed. Baltimore MD: Williams & Wilkins, 1999.

   This chapter is a review of the GI tract structure, blood supply, nervous system control, GI tract hormones, nutrient absorption, intestinal microorganisms, and immune system. The response of the GI tract to food is also explained.

7. Levenstein S and others: Stress and peptic ulcer disease. *Journal of the American Medical Association* 282:30, 1999.

   Stress is currently out of favor as a cause of peptic ulcer. But evidence that psychological stress is one of many factors contributing to ulcer disease has come to light in recent years as people report the effects of war, earthquakes, and economic crisis as these events affect the gastrointestinal tract. Several behavioral risk factors have been identified for ulcers—smoking, alcohol abuse, and lack of sleep.

8. Lewis C: Crohn's disease: New drug may help when others fail. *FDA Consumer,* page 26 September/October 1999.

   Provides a description of Crohn's disease and a case study of a patient who has had the disease almost all her adult life. Although the new drug Remicade provided symptomatic relief, it is not a cure. No special diet has proven effective for preventing or treating Crohn's disease.

9. Licht HM: Irritable bowel syndrome. *Postgraduate Medicine* 107:203, 2000.

   IBS is a chronic disorder characterized by abdominal pain and alterations in bowel patterns. There is no identifiable cause. Patient education, counseling, and certain drugs are agents for relief.

10. Nelson DL, Cox MM: *Lehninger principles of biochemistry.* 3rd ed. New York: Worth, 2000.

    This text provides an in-depth explanation of biochemistry as related to the study of human nutrition. The authors provide a detailed look at protein functions, especially the interactions among proteins, the immune system, and immunoglobulins.

11. New treatment alternative for GERD. *Tufts University Health and Nutrition Letter* 18:6, 2000.

    Gastroesophageal Reflux Disease (GERD) is a serious, debilitating disease often leading to cancer. Two new medical procedures allow patients to return to work the following day after such therapy.

12. Nuovo J: Current status of treatment for *H. pylori* infection. *American Family Physician* 62:630, 2000.

    H. pylori infection is difficult to irradicate because the bacteria are acid resistant and hide within the mucus-producing cells of the stomach and small intestine. There are noninvasive tests to determine the presence of the bacteria within the GI tract. Several medications have proven effective treatment. Acquired resistance to two of the medications poses a significant problem.

13. Saladin KS: *Anatomy & physiology: The unity of form and function.* Boston: WCB McGraw-Hill, 1998.

    The body is derived from atoms that form molecules. Molecules are organized into macromolecules, such as DNA. The functioning units of a cell are called organelles, and they house the macromolecules. Cells unite to form tissues; tissues combine to produce organs. A collection of organs produces a system. The organism is built from the interaction of 12 integrated systems.

14. Szarka LA, Locke GR: Practical pointers for grappling with GERD. *Postgraduate Medicine* 105:88, 1999.

    About 18% of the adult U.S. population experiences heartburn at least once a week. The primary cause of symptoms and tissue injury is esophageal exposure to acid and other gastric juices. Treatment includes lifestyle modification, medications such as antacids, H₂ receptor antagonists, and proton pump inhibitors.

15. Takahashi I, Kiyono H: Gut as the largest immunologic tissue. *Journal of Parenteral and Enteral Nutrition* 23:S7, 1999.

    The body is continuously exposed to infectious agents, allergens and toxic substances that enter through the nose and throat. Scattered throughout the cells lining the mucosal surface of the GI are immune cells. This immune system operating within the gastrointestinal tract is highly specialized and both separate and distinct from the systemwide immune system.

16. Teitelbaum SL: Bone resorption by osteoclasts. *Science* 289:1504, 2000.

    The role of osteoclasts in bone resorption is explored with respect to its role in osteoporosis. It is anticipated that new antiresorption drugs will be able to stimulate bone formation.

17. Tso P, Crissinger K: Overview of digestion and absorption. In Stepanuk MH (ed.): *Biochemical and physiological aspects of human nutrition* W. B. Saunders, 2000.

    One chapter in this Human Nutrition textbook identifies the major structures and functions of the digestive tract. Control of absorption and metabolism is explained.

18. Van De Graaff KM, Fox SI: *Concepts of human anatomy & physiology.* 5th ed. Boston: WCB McGraw-Hill, 1999.

    The basis for understanding human nutrition is to comprehend the role of anatomy and physiology as they relate to the foundation for personal health. This text provides the framework for integrating modern biology into the study of scientific nutrition.

19. Vander A and others: *Human physiology: The mechanisms of body function.* 8th ed. Boston: McGraw-Hill, 2000.

    This text provides the fundamentals of physiology for the undergraduate student. Topics include basic cell functions, biological control mechanisms, actions of the various systems, and coordinated body functions.

20. Yamaguchi S, Ninomiya S: Umami and food palatability. *Journal of Nutrition* 130:9321S, 2000.

    Umami is the term used to identify the taste of substances such as glutamate salts and is the main taste in Japanese stock and bouillon.

21. Wong PWK, Kadakia S: How to deal with chronic constipation. *Postgraduate Medicine* 106:199, 1999.

    The authors list the diagnostic criteria used to establish chronic constipation. Treatment includes patient education, bowel habit training, increased fluid and fiber intake, and laxative use.

TAKE ACTION

I. ARE YOU TAKING CARE OF YOUR DIGESTIVE TRACT?

People need to think about the health of their digestive tracts. There are symptoms we need to notice, as well as habits we need to practice in order to protect it. The following assessment is designed to help you examine your habits and symptoms associated with the health of your digestive tract. The Nutrition Perspective explains why these habits are important to examine. Put a Y in the blank to the left of the question to indicate yes and an N to indicate no.

_____ 1. Are you currently experiencing greater than normal stress and tension?

_____ 2. Do you have a family history of digestive tract problems (e.g., ulcers, hemorrhoids, diverticulosis, constipation, lactose intolerance)?

_____ 3. Do you experience pain in your stomach region about 2 hours after you eat?

_____ 4. Do you smoke cigarettes?

_____ 5. Do you take aspirin frequently?

_____ 6. Do you have heartburn at least once per week?

_____ 7. Do you commonly lie down after eating a large meal?

_____ 8. Do you drink alcoholic beverages more than two or three times per day?

_____ 9. Do you experience abdominal pain, bloating, and gas about 30 minutes to 2 hours after consuming milk products?

_____ 10. Do you often have to strain while having a bowel movement?

_____ 11. Do you consume less than 8 cups of a combination of water and other fluids per day?

_____ 12. Do you perform physical activity (e.g., jog, swim, walk briskly, row, stair climb) less than 20 to 30 minutes three times per week?

_____ 13. Do you eat a diet relatively low in dietary fiber (recall that significant dietary fiber is found in whole fruits, vegetables, legumes, nuts and seeds, whole-grain breads, and whole-grain cereals)?

_____ 14. Do you frequently have diarrhea?

_____ 15. Do you frequently use laxatives or antacids?

Interpretation

Add up the number of yes answers you gave and record the total in the blank to the right. _____

If your score is from 8 to 15, your habits and symptoms put you at risk for experiencing future digestive tract problems. Take particular note of the habits to which you answered yes. Consider trying to cooperate more with your digestive tract.

II. OVER-THE-COUNTER MEDICATIONS FOR TREATING COMMON GI TRACT PROBLEMS

After you have read the Nutrition Perspective "When the Digestive Processes Go Awry," visit your local pharmacy and check out the medications on sale for treating indigestion, heartburn, constipation, diarrhea, and hemorrhoids. Select one category and compare four brands for
1. Price/usual daily dose
2. Active ingredients
3. Warning to users
4. Advice as to when to see a physician

Write a critique of your discoveries about these products, and summarize what you would say about the safety and efficacy of these products.

NUTRITION *Perspective*

WHEN THE DIGESTIVE PROCESSES GO AWRY

The fine-tuned organ system we call the *GI tract* can develop problems. Knowing about these common problems can help you avoid them.

ULCERS

Many adults develop ulcers each year. An estimated 25 million Americans develop them during their lifetimes. The principal causes are an acid-resistant bacterial infection *(Helicobacter pylori [H. pylori])*, the heavy use of aspirin and related medications, and disorders that cause excessive acid production in the stomach (Fig. 3-19).[19] *H. pylori* infection has recently been found to be a transmissible disease with a long asymptomatic period. The guess is that the bacteria transfers from animals to humans. And, after being out of favor for some years, stress is now regarded as a predisposing factor, albeit a minor one, for ulcers. As the stomach lining deteriorates and loses its mucus layer protection, the acid erodes the stomach tissue. This specific chain of events results in a gastric ulcer. Acid can also erode the tissue lining of the first part of the small intestine, the duodenum, and result in a duodenal ulcer. *Peptic ulcer* is the general term for both of these two cases.

Most ulcers in young people occur in the duodenum; in older people they occur primarily in the stomach. The typical symptom of an ulcer is pain about 2 hours after eating. Digestive acids acting on a meal irritate the ulcer after most of the meal has moved to the jejunum area of the small intestine.[3]

The primary risk associated with an ulcer is the possibility that it will erode entirely through (perforate) the stomach or intestinal wall. The GI contents could then spill into the body cavities, causing a massive infection, called *peritonitis*. In addition, an ulcer may erode a blood vessel, leading to massive blood loss (hemorrhage). For these reasons, it is important not to ignore the early warning signs of ulcer development. Infected persons have an increased lifetime risk of gastric adenocarcinoma. Accurate, inexpensive, and noninvasive tests are available to diagnose *H. pylori* infection.

In the past, milk and cream therapy—the Sippy diet—was used to help cure ulcers. Clinicians now know that milk and cream are two of the worst foods for an ulcer. The calcium in these foods stimulates stomach acid secretion and actually inhibits ulcer healing.

Today a combination of approaches is used for ulcer therapy. People infected with *H. pylori* are given antibiotics with antacid or bismuth therapy to eradicate *H. pylori*. In many cases, there is a 90% cure rate for *H. pylori* in the first week of this treatment. Recurrence is unlikely if the infection is cured, but an incomplete cure almost certainly leads to repeated ulcer

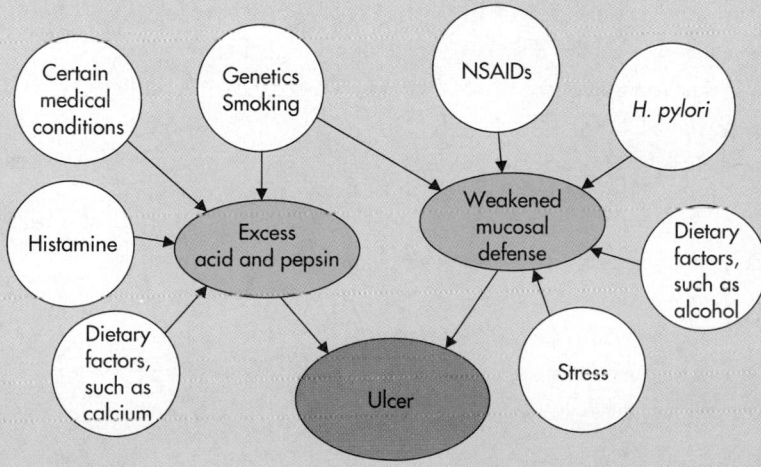

■ FIGURE 3-19 Pathogenesis of peptic ulcer. *H. pylori* bacteria and NSAIDs cause ulcers by impairing mucosal defense. In the same way, smoking, genetics, and stress can impair mucosal defense, as well as cause an increase in the release of pepsin and stomach acid. All of these factors can contribute to ulcers.

H₂ blockers Medications such as cimetidine (Tagamet) that block the increase of stomach acid production caused by histamine.

*A*spirin is part of a class of medications called *nonsteroidal anti-inflammatory drugs* (NSAIDs). Also included are ibuprofen (Motrin or Advil) and naproxen (Aleve).

formation. Unfortunately, many ulcer patients are discovering that *H. pylori* is becoming resistant to many antibiotics.[12] When antibiotic treatment is discontinued before *H. pylori* is completely eradicated, the ulcer reappears. Each time there is a flare up, the antibiotic is less effective. *H. pylori* is mutating fast. Doctors should make patients understand the importance of finishing their course of antibiotic therapy.

Antacid medications may also be part of ulcer care, as is a class of medicines called **H₂ blockers.** These include cimetidine (Tagamet), ranitidine (Zantac), and famotidine (Pepcid), all of which prevent histamine-related acid secretion in the stomach. Some of these medications are now available over the counter in nonprescription doses for cases of indigestion and heartburn (see next section).[14]

Medications that coat the ulcer, such as sucralfate (Carafate), are also commonly used. In addition, medications that reduce acid production by the stomach, such as omeprazole (Prilosec), can be used.

People with ulcers should also refrain from smoking and minimize the use of aspirin and related NSAIDs. Medications that are used to treat arthritis pain, called "Cox-2 inhibitors," are less likely to cause stomach ulcers and, so, have been widely used as a replacement for NSAIDs. They do offer some advantages over NSAIDS, but they may not be totally safe for older patients. These practices reduce the mucus secreted by the stomach. Overall, this combination of lifestyle therapy and medical treatment has so revolutionized ulcer therapy that dietary changes are of minor importance today. Current diet-therapy approaches recommend simply avoiding foods that increase ulcer symptoms (Table 3-9).

Note also that stomach acid is not a problem for those not prone to or currently experiencing ulcers. The acid in the stomach enhances the absorption of iron, calcium, and vitamin B-12. Acid also minimizes bacterial growth in the stomach; the stomach is essentially bacteria free because of its high acid content. Bacteria in food are quickly destroyed, which reduces the risk of these bacteria forming cancer-causing agents or leading to foodborne illness (see Chapter 19). Thus, acid production by the stomach is an important part of the physiology of digestion and absorption. This means that, despite their usual presence alongside the breath mints in a

TABLE 3-9 Recommendations to Prevent Ulcers and Heartburn from Occurring or Recurring

Ulcers

1. Stop smoking, if you are now a smoker.
2. Avoid large doses of aspirin, ibuprofen, and other NSAID compounds unless a physician advises otherwise. For people who must use these medications, FDA has approved an NSAID combined with a prostaglandin-related medication to reduce gastric damage. The prostaglandin medication (misoprostol) reduces gastric acid production and enhances mucus secretion (see Chapter 6 for a discussion of prostaglandins).
3. Limit consumption coffee, tea, and alcohol (especially wine), if this helps.
4. Limit consumption pepper, chili powder, and other strong spices, if this helps.
5. Eat nutritious meals on a regular schedule; include enough dietary fiber (see Chapter 5).
6. Chew foods well.
7. Lose weight if you are currently overweight.

Heartburn

1. Wait about 2 hours after a meal before lying down.
2. Don't overeat at mealtime. Smaller meals that are low in fat are advised.
3. Try elevating the head of the bed (6-in blocks).
4. Observe the recommendations for ulcer prevention.
5. Stop smoking cigarettes.
6. Lose excess weight.

convenience store, antacids should not be used excessively. If an antacid contains magnesium (and many do), magnesium toxicity is another possible result of antacid abuse.

HEARTBURN

Many adults regularly have heartburn. This gnawing pain in the upper chest is caused by the movement of acid from the stomach into the esophagus and, so, the problem is more formally called **gastroesophageal reflux disease (GERD).** Unlike the stomach, the esophagus has very little mucus lining to protect it, so acid quickly erodes the lining of the esophagus, causing pain.[5]

An important dietary measure for avoiding heartburn is to eat smaller meals. Fatty meals remain in the stomach longer than low-fat meals. The large volume of food and secretions that remains in the stomach creates pressure, which can force the stomach contents up into the esophagus.

Several other steps may be taken to prevent heartburn. Cigarette smokers should quit smoking. In addition, it is best not to lie down after eating and to limit foods and other substances that can specifically contribute to heartburn, such as chili powder, onions, garlic, peppermint, caffeine, alcohol, and chocolate. Individuals should discover irritants and tailor their diets accordingly (review Table 3-9.)

Certain physical conditions can lead to heartburn. For example, both pregnancy and obesity result in increased production of estrogen and progesterone. These hormones relax the lower esophageal (cardiac) sphincter, making heartburn more likely. A pregnant woman may find it helpful to eat smaller, more frequent meals. An obese person should slim down to a more healthy weight, so that blood concentrations of these hormones decrease. Adipose tissue turns certain circulating hormones into estrogen; thus, the more adipose tissue, the more estrogen is produced.

Occasional heartburn can be treated medically with antacids, over-the-counter H_2 blockers, and bismuth agents. Over-the-counter H_2 blockers, such as Pepcid, Zantac, and Tagamet, work by reducing the production of acid, whereas other over-the-counter drugs, such as Tums, Alka-Seltzer, and Maalox, neutralize the acid that has already been produced. Proton pump inhibitors, such as Prilosec and Prevacid, are extremely effective acid-suppressing medications and provide successful treatment for GERD with minimal side effects.[12] Another precaution is to drink plenty of water when taking medications, as many are known to irritate the esophagus. And, although it is true that many people suffer occasional heartburn, it is important that this problem not be accepted as a normal part of daily life or self-treated for an extended time. Heartburn that recurs several times a week for at least a month should be investigated by a physician. This heartburn may require aggressive medical therapy because it can lead to alteration in the cells of the esophagus, which increases the risk of a rare form of cancer. There is also a treatment available to surgically attack the problem. The lower esophageal sphincter, the muscle that is at fault in GERD, can be stitched or burned in such a way that narrows the loose valve. This procedure prevents the acid from backing up into the esophagus.[11]

CONSTIPATION AND LAXATIVES

Constipation, which is difficult or infrequent evacuation of the bowels, is commonly reported by adults.[1] Slow movement of fecal material through the large intestine causes constipation. As fluid is increasingly absorbed during the extended time the feces stay in the large intestine, they become dry and hard.

Constipation can result when people regularly inhibit their normal bowel reflexes for long periods. People may ignore normal urges when it is inconvenient to interrupt occupational or social activities. Muscle spasms of an irritated large intestine can also slow the movement of feces and contribute to constipation. Medications such as antacids and calcium and iron supplements can also cause constipation.

The following is a protocol for diagnosing constipation.[21] For at least 12 months patients not taking laxatives report two or more of the following:

gastroesophageal reflux disease (GERD) A disease that results from stomach acid backing up into the esophagus. The acid irritates the lining of the esophagus, causing pain.

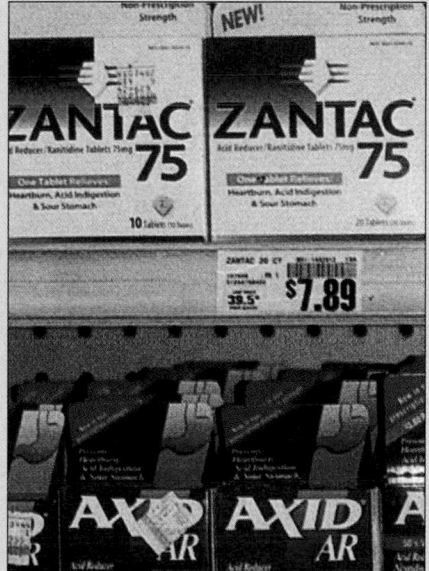

A number of over-the-counter medications are marketed for heartburn. Attention to diet and lifestyle, however, is generally a more important measure to take.

constipation A condition characterized by infrequent bowel movements.

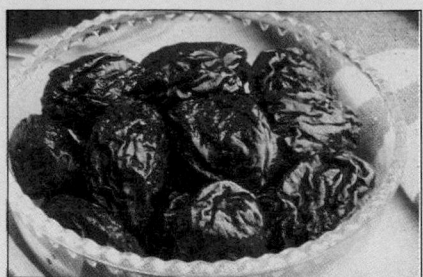

Dried fruits, such as dried plums, aid in treating constipation.

laxative A medication or another substance that stimulates evacuation of the intestinal tract.

*P*erhaps you have heard that taking laxatives after overeating prevents deposition of body fat from the excess energy intake. This erroneous and dangerous premise has gained popularity among followers of numerous fad diets. You may temporarily feel less full after using a laxative because laxatives hasten emptying of the large intestine and increase fluid loss. Most laxatives, however, do not speed the passage of food through the small intestine, where digestion and most nutrient absorption take place. As a result, you can't count on laxatives to prevent fat gain from excess energy intake.

1. Fewer than three bowel movements per week
2. Excessive straining during at least 25% of bowel movements
3. Passage of hard or pelletlike stools during at least 25% of bowel movements
4. A feeling of incomplete evacuation for at least 25% of bowel movements

Or, for at least 12 months, patients have an average of fewer than two bowel movements per week.

Eating foods with plenty of dietary fiber, such as whole-grain breads and cereals, is the best method for treating typical cases of constipation. Dietary fibers stimulate peristalsis by drawing water into the large intestine and helping form a bulky, soft fecal output. People with constipation should also drink more fluids, and eating dried fruits can help stimulate the bowel. In addition, people with constipation may need to develop more regular bowel habits; allowing the same time each day for a bowel movement can help train the large intestine to respond routinely. Finally, relaxation facilitates regular bowel movements, as does regular physical activity.

Laxatives can also lessen constipation. These work by irritating the intestinal nerve junctions to stimulate the peristaltic muscles, or by drawing water into the intestine to enlarge fecal output. The larger output stretches the peristaltic muscles, making them rebound and then constrict. Regular use of laxatives, especially irritating ones, however, can decrease muscle action in the large intestine—in time, causing more constipation. The GI tract can then actually become dependent on laxatives. Thus, it is unwise for anyone to use laxatives routinely, although people in certain circumstances—for example, those who are bedridden or quite elderly—may need periodic help from laxatives to relieve constipation.

HEMORRHOIDS

Hemorrhoids, also called *piles*, are swollen veins of the rectum and anus. The blood vessels in this area are subject to intense pressure, especially during bowel movements. Added stress to the vessels from pregnancy, obesity, prolonged sitting, violent coughing or sneezing, or straining during bowel movements, particularly with constipation, can lead to a hemorrhoid. Hemorrhoids can develop unnoticed until a strained bowel movement precipitates symptoms, which may include pain, itching, and bleeding.

Itching, caused by moisture in the anal canal, swelling, or other irritation, is perhaps the most common symptom. Pain, if present, is usually aching and steady. Bleeding may result from a hemorrhoid and may appear in the toilet as a bright red streak in the feces. The sensation of a mass in the anal canal after a bowel movement is symptomatic of an internal hemorrhoid that protrudes through the anus.

Anyone can develop a hemorrhoid, and about half of adults over age 50 do. Pressure from prolonged sitting or exertion is often enough to bring on symptoms, although diet, lifestyle, and possibly heredity play a role. If you think you have a hemorrhoid, you should consult your physician. Rectal bleeding, although usually caused by hemorrhoids, may also indicate other problems, such as cancer.

A physician may suggest a variety of self-care measures for hemorrhoids. Pain can be lessened by applying warm, soft compresses or sitting in a tub of warm water for 15 to 20 minutes. Dietary recommendations are the same as those for treating constipation, emphasizing the need to consume adequate dietary fiber and fluid. Over-the-counter remedies, such as Preparation H, can also offer relief of symptoms.

IRRITABLE BOWEL SYNDROME

Many adults have irritable bowel syndrome, a combination of cramps, gassiness, bloating, and irregular bowel function (diarrhea, constipation, or alternating episodes of both). It is more common in women than in men.

Symptoms associated with irritable bowel syndrome include visible abdominal distension, pain relief after a bowel movement, increased stool frequency with pain onset, looser stools with pain onset, mucus in stool, and a feeling of incomplete elimination even after a bowel movement.[9]

The cause is thought to be altered intestinal peristalsis, coupled with a decreased pain threshold for abdominal distension. In other words, a minor amount of abdominal bloating causes pain that the average person would not sense. It is also noteworthy that up to 50% of sufferers report a history of verbal or sexual abuse.

Therapy is individualized and can include a trial of high-fiber foods: elimination diets that focus on avoiding dairy products and gas-forming foods, such as legumes and certain vegetables (cabbage, beans, and broccoli) and fruits such as grapes, raisins, cherries, and cantaloupe. The patient should have only moderate caffeine intake or eliminate caffeine-containing foods/beverages altogether. Low-fat and more frequent, small meals may help the patient because large meals can trigger contractions of the large intestine. Other strategies include a reduction in stress, psychological counseling, and certain medications.

Referral to a dietitian can be beneficial, as many patients experience improvement with the elimination of specific problem foods. A good patient/physician relationship is also necessary for the treatment of irritable bowel syndrome; however, before any single treatment is applauded, it is important to note that placebo response alone has been as high as 70% in this population. Although irritable bowel syndrome can be uncomfortable and upsetting, it is harmless; it carries no risk for cancer or other serious digestive problems.

■ CASE SCENARIO
Follow-Up

Crohn's disease is one form of inflammatory bowel disease (IBD) that causes inflammation in the intestinal tract.[8] It has no cure, but there are several promising treatment strategies available. Crohn's disease usually occurs in the ileum, but it can occur in other parts of the GI tract as well. The symptoms include chronic diarrhea, abdominal pain, decreased appetite, weight loss, bleeding, intestinal obstruction, and fistulae (abnormal passages or sores between the intestine and other organs, such as the skin). A blood test may reveal anemia, an increase in white blood cells, and low albumin levels—a sign of inadequate protein status. The cause may be due to an environmental pathogen, such as a bacterium or virus, which triggers the disease. Whatever causes the disease, it produces an overaggressive immune response. It is quite possible that the basis for disease is genetic.

Diagnosis is confirmed with a colonoscopy, along with a biopsy of a tissue specimen. CAT scans show changes in the wall of the entire intestine and intestinal obstruction, abscesses, and fistula formation.

Treatment is with a variety of mediations, including Asacol™ to control inflammation; corticosteriods, such as prednisone, to control inflammation; and methotrexate, an anticancer drug. Growth hormone by injection also shows some promise. A recently approved drug, Remicade, is effective in closing fistulae, but the medication is extraordinarily expensive and generally fails to control a subsequent flare up. Surgery to remove the affected portion of the intestine may be required. Although symptoms-free periods do occur, flare-ups are common.

The word on diet is not good. No special diet has proven effective for either the prevention or treatment of Crohn's disease during an acute attack. Recommendations are for a nutritious diet and no restrictions on any food groups unless some foods in the group cause discomfort, such as may be the case for high fat foods. Then those foods should be limited or omitted. The patient must determine the foods to avoid.

Patients are able to hold jobs and function effectively, but symptoms can occur without warning.

METABOLISM *chapter* 4

*M*etabolism refers to the entire network of chemical processes involved in maintaining life. It encompasses all the sequences of chemical reactions that occur in the body. These biochemical reactions enable us to release and use energy from foods, synthesize one substance from another, and prepare waste products for excretion. More than 1000 kinds of chemical reactions take place in a simple single-cell bacterium.[11]

Studying metabolism can help you comprehend a variety of nutrition concepts. Understanding metabolism clarifies how proteins, carbohydrates, fats, and alcohol are interrelated; how the carbons in proteins become the carbons of glucose; and why the carbons of most fatty acids *cannot* become the carbons of glucose.[8]

Studying metabolic pathways in the cell also sets the stage for examining the roles of vitamins and minerals. Most vitamins function as coenzymes. Many minerals function as cofactors. These compounds, coenzymes and cofactors, contribute to enzyme activity and, thus, are important to metabolic reactions in the cell. Overall, the functions of vitamins and minerals will be easier to understand if you are familiar with the basic metabolic processes in the cell.

■ KEY CHAPTER CONCEPTS

- *Metabolism* refers to the body's chemical processes that maintain life. These processes occur in cells.
- ATP is the major form of energy used for cellular metabolism. This energy is used to pump ions, promote enzyme activity, and contract and later relax muscles.
- In glycolysis, glucose (carbohydrate) is degraded into two pyruvate molecules, yielding NADH + H$^+$ (a form of potential energy) and ATP. Pyruvate can proceed through an aerobic pathway to form carbon dioxide and water. Pyruvate also can react with NADH + H$^+$ in an anaerobic pathway to form lactate.
- Pyruvate enters the mitochondria, in which the remaining energy is eventually extracted from the molecule using the citric acid cycle .
- NADH + H$^+$ and FADH$_2$ produced by citric acid cycle activity then enter the electron transport chain. This is where about 90% of the total possible ATP molecules from glucose are produced, using the combined activity of the citric acid cycle and electron transport chain. Carbon dioxide and water are by-products.
- Fatty acid metabolism is aided by various enzymes and the carrier carnitine. The breakdown products enter the citric acid cycle and electron transport chain to yield ATP, carbon dioxide, and water.
- Incomplete fat metabolism leads to the production of ketone bodies; this can be caused by starvation, uncontrolled type 1 diabetes, and a very low carbohydrate diet.
- Amino acids lose their amino group and become carbon skeletons. These carbon skeletons can be metabolized to other compounds, which enter the citric acid cycle, eventually yielding energy for ATP synthesis. Some carbon skeletons can be converted to glucose. Converting the carbon skeletons of amino acids to glucose is part of a process known as gluconeogenesis. Fatty acids, in general, and alcohol cannot participate in gluconeogenesis.
- Glycolysis occurs in the cytosol of a cell, whereas the citric acid cycle and the electron transport chain occur in the mitochondria. Fatty acid metabolism also occurs in the mitochondria.
- The vitamins thiamin, niacin, riboflavin, biotin, pantothenic acid, and vitamin B-6 and the minerals magnesium, iron, and copper play vital roles in metabolic pathways.

■ REFRESH YOUR MEMORY

As you begin your study of metabolism in Chapter 4, you may want to review

- Various components of the macronutrient classes— carbohydrates, proteins, and lipids—in Chapter 1
- The components of the cell and functions of various organelles in Chapter 3
- Enzyme function and regulation in Chapter 3
- Hormone function in Chapter 3
- Basic chemistry concepts in Appendix B

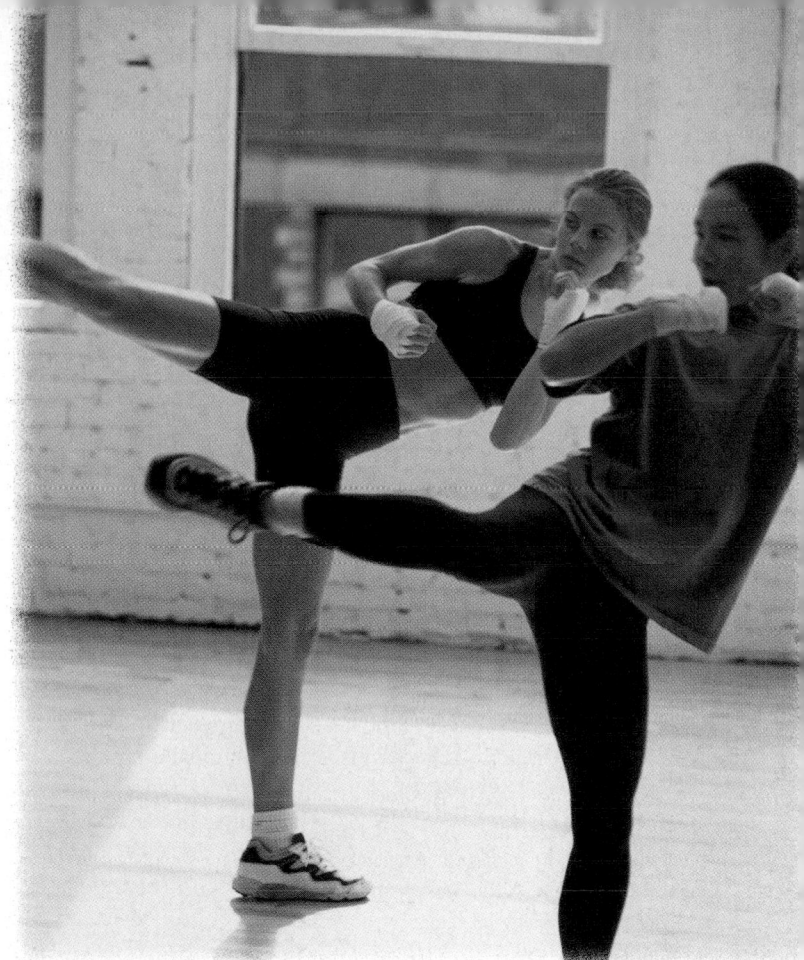

■ CASE SCENARIO

Andrea is a 6-year-old who suffers from epilepsy. Her physicians have tried many combinations of medicines to reduce the number of seizures she experiences. These seizures result from a transient disturbance in brain function due to abnormal nerve cell discharge in the brain. Andrea is not alone in suffering from this disease; it affects approximately 0.5% of the U.S. population. Because her current seizure medication regimens have not been effective, her physicians recommend that she undergo a trial of a very low carbohydrate (ketogenic) diet. The physicians note that it is still not clear why this diet works to control seizures in some people, but research going as far back as the 1920s shows that a rise in ketone bodies in the blood can help.

The main drawback of this ketogenic diet is that it is very low in carbohydrates, amounting to about one-tenth of her usual carbohydrate intake. In place of that carbohydrate, she must consume much more fat than is typical for her. The physicians tell her parents that this will be a very difficult diet to implement, since many of the foods Andrea likes are rich in carbohydrate. However, the physicians feel that, if this diet is effective in reducing her seizures, the restriction in carbohydrate intake will outweigh the inconvenience of following such a plan. In addition, some people find that following this diet for a few years stops the seizures, even when they return to a more normal diet.

What actually are ketone bodies, and why does a very low-carbohydrate diet produce an increase in ketone bodies in the blood? Can you speculate at this time why this is the case? Metabolism of ketone bodies is one theme of this chapter. By developing a greater understanding of this and other aspects of metabolism, you will be able to explain to Andrea's parents why a low carbohydrate diet causes such an effect.

■ METABOLISM—CHEMICAL REACTIONS IN THE BODY

intermediate A chemical compound formed in one of the many steps in a metabolic pathway. For example, citric acid is an intermediate in the citric acid cycle.

monosaccharide A class of simple sugars, such as glucose, that can be absorbed into the body without further chemical alteration.

*A*cids commonly lose a hydrogen ion at the pH found in human cells (pH 7.4). When that ion is lost, the name of the acid is changed by dropping the reference to acid and adding an *ate* ending. Thus, *acetic acid* becomes *acetate.*

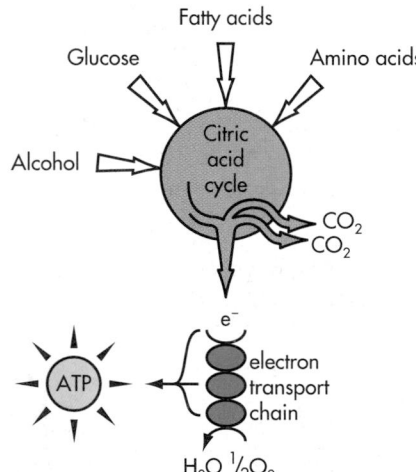

Generation of ATP from fuels during respiration. Dietary carbohydrates are converted mainly to glucose, dietary lipids to fatty acids, and dietary protein to amino acids. The symbol e⁻ represents electrons.

photosynthesis The process by which plants use energy from the sun to produce energy-yielding compounds, such as glucose.

respiration The use of oxygen; in the human organism, the inhalation of oxygen and the exhalation of carbon dioxide; in cells, the oxidation (electron removal) of food molecules, particularly in the citric acid cycle, to obtain energy.

As noted in the chapter overview, *metabolism* refers to the entire network of chemical processes involved in maintaining life and encompasses all of the sequences of chemical reactions that occur in the body. These chemical reactions enable cells to release and use energy from foods, convert one substance into another, and prepare waste products for excretion.

A progression of metabolic chemical reactions from beginning to end is called a *pathway.* Compounds formed as the pathway proceeds are called **intermediates.** Virtually every step in any pathway depends on an enzyme to initiate the necessary chemical reaction (see Chapter 3 for an example).[11] **Anabolic** pathways build compounds. Energy must be expended for anabolic processes to take place. The chemical reactions involving the synthesis of –C–C– bonds (fatty acid synthesis), $-\overset{\overset{\text{O}}{\|}}{\text{C}}-\text{N}-$ bonds (protein synthesis), –C–N– bonds (urea synthesis), and –C–O– bonds (triglyceride synthesis) require such energy input (see Appendix B for details). The chemical elements and compounds used to form the new substances often are called *building blocks.* Conversely, **catabolic** pathways break down compounds into small units. For example, complete catabolism of glucose results in the release of carbon dioxide (CO_2) and water (H_2O). Energy is released in the process; some is trapped for cell use, and the rest is lost as heat.

The production of energy for cell use occurs in three stages. In the first stage, large food molecules, such as proteins, starches, and triglycerides, are broken down during digestion and absorption into smaller units, such as amino acids, **monosaccharides** (simple sugars), and fatty acids. In the second stage, most of these smaller compounds are further degraded to the two-carbon intermediate compound acetic acid $\underset{\text{CH}_3\text{C}-\text{OH}}{\overset{\overset{\text{O}}{\|}}{}}$, the acid found in vinegar.[5] In the third stage, acetic acid (acetate, for short) is degraded to carbon dioxide and water. The electrons and hydrogen ions released during this metabolic process are donated to oxygen atoms to form water. Some of the energy released in this catabolic process drives the synthesis of adenosine triphosphate (ATP). ATP is energy in a form that cells use. Chapter 3 introduced the first stage, digestion and absorption. Let's now examine the last stage.

■ Energy for the Cell

The energy that human cells use comes from chemical bonds found between the atoms in carbohydrate, fat, protein, and alcohol. This energy is originally produced during **photosynthesis,** when plants use solar energy to make glucose and other organic (carbon-containing) compounds. The chemical reactions in photosynthesis form compounds that contain more energy than carbon dioxide and water, the building blocks used (see Chapter 5). Virtually all organisms use the sun—either directly or indirectly, as we do—as their source of energy.

As mentioned in Chapter 1, the body transforms the chemical bond energy trapped in carbohydrate, fat, and protein into other forms of energy:[11]

- Chemical energy, which helps build new compounds, such as glycogen from numerous glucose molecules
- Mechanical energy, which propels muscular movements
- Electrical energy, which promotes nerve transmissions
- Osmotic energy, which maintains ion balance within cells

The by-products of these energy transformations are carbon dioxide, water, and heat. Chemical energy from ingested food that passes through body cells is eventually and irretrievably dissipated to the environment as heat (Fig. 4-1).

Thus, in human **respiration,** the starting materials are energy-yielding compounds, such as glucose, which through an elaborate multistep process are con-

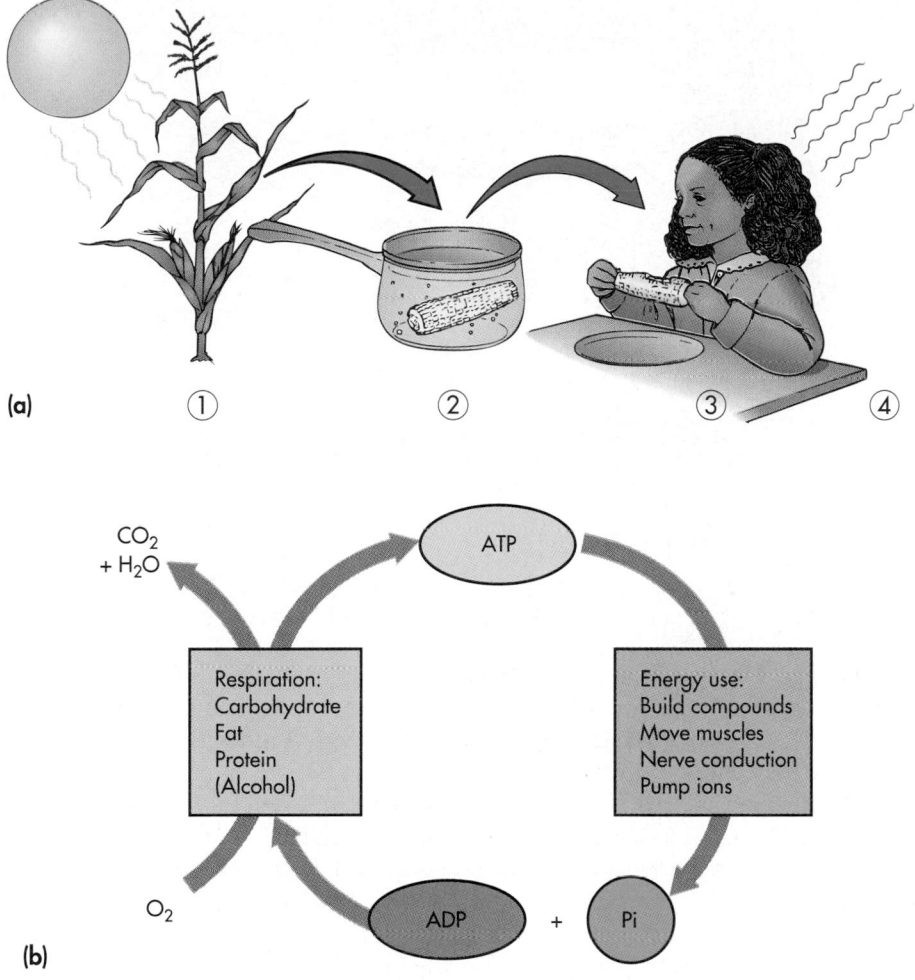

(a)

(b)

FIGURE 4-1 (a) From solar energy to human energy output. (1) The corn plant uses solar energy to synthesize glucose from carbon dioxide and water. (2) We cook and eat the corn, (3) transferring much of the energy in the glucose from the corn to ATP energy for our cells to use. (4) Eventually, this energy leaves our bodies as heat. Some energy may be stored as fat if we overeat, and a small amount is lost in urine and feces.

(b) ATP synthesis and use. Energy from food stuffs is used to synthesize ATP. The ATP provides energy for the cell.

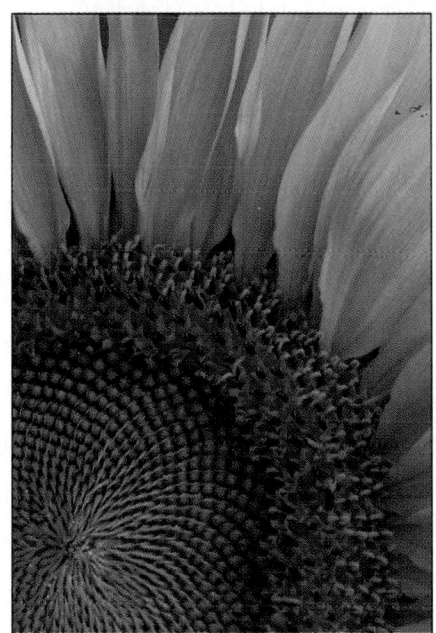

Sunflowers capture solar energy and transfer that into chemical energy in the form of protein carbohydrate, and fat in the sunflower seeds.

verted to end products, such as carbon dioxide and water. This process results in the transfer of energy from food to cells, which in turn allows energy-requiring pathways in cells to function.

Many chemical reactions in the body could not occur without the addition of outside energy supplied by food. Outside energy permits compounds, such as glucose, to be transformed into products such as glycogen, as mentioned earlier. Although glucose molecules themselves contain the energy needed for glycogen synthesis, individual glucose molecules provide neither the right amount of energy for a chemical reaction nor a form of energy that cells can use directly. A glucose molecule contains over 100 times more energy than required to facilitate an individual chemical reaction in a cell. A triglyceride molecule contains about 500 times more energy than is needed. Thus, a cell must have a means of breaking down the glucose and fatty acid molecules to release and then convert the chemical energy trapped in them into smaller, usable energy forms.[11]

Cells Use Adenosine Triphosphate (ATP) as an Energy Source

The form of energy that cells generally use for chemical, mechanical, electrical, and osmotic processes is ATP. To release the energy in ATP, cells split it into adenosine diphosphate (ADP) plus Pi, a free (inorganic) phosphate group (Fig. 4-2). ADP can also be split into adenosine monophosphate (AMP) plus Pi to yield energy, in a reaction muscles are capable of performing during intense exercise when ATP is in short supply (ADP + ADP → ATP + AMP).[4]

Only energy in ATP and its derivatives can be used directly by the cell. Energy released from breaking carbon-hydrogen bonds in a glucose molecule is one of the "fuels" used by body cells to make ATP.

▌ **FIGURE 4-2** ATP stores and yields energy. ATP is the high-energy state; ADP is the lower-energy state. (*a*) When ATP is broken down to ADP plus Pi, energy is released for cell use. (*b*) When energy is trapped by ADP plus Pi, ATP can be formed. Thus, ATP represents a storage form of energy for cell use. Pi is the abbreviaiton for a free phosphate group.

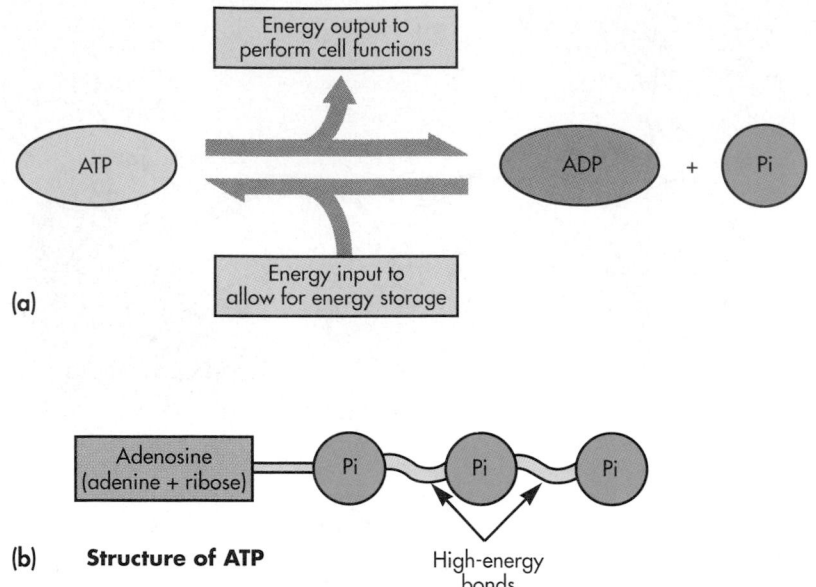

(a)

(b)   **Structure of ATP**

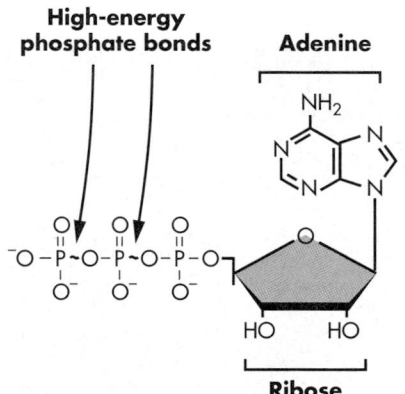

Adenosine triphosphate (ATP).

Metabolic pathways exist in every cell that can combine ADP and Pi to form ATP. An enzyme later can break the ATP bond to release energy needed for metabolic reactions. ATP itself is very stable, so it takes an enzyme to unlock the energy that is stored in the molecule.

During metabolism, a cell is constantly breaking down ATP in one organelle while rebuilding it in another. An exhausted muscle cell has a very high concentration of ADP and a very low concentration of ATP. When this happens, muscle cell activity, such as muscle contraction, may slow down or cease altogether. A low ATP concentration then stimulates metabolic processes that produce ATP. Only by resynthesizing needed ATP can the muscle cell ready itself for future action.

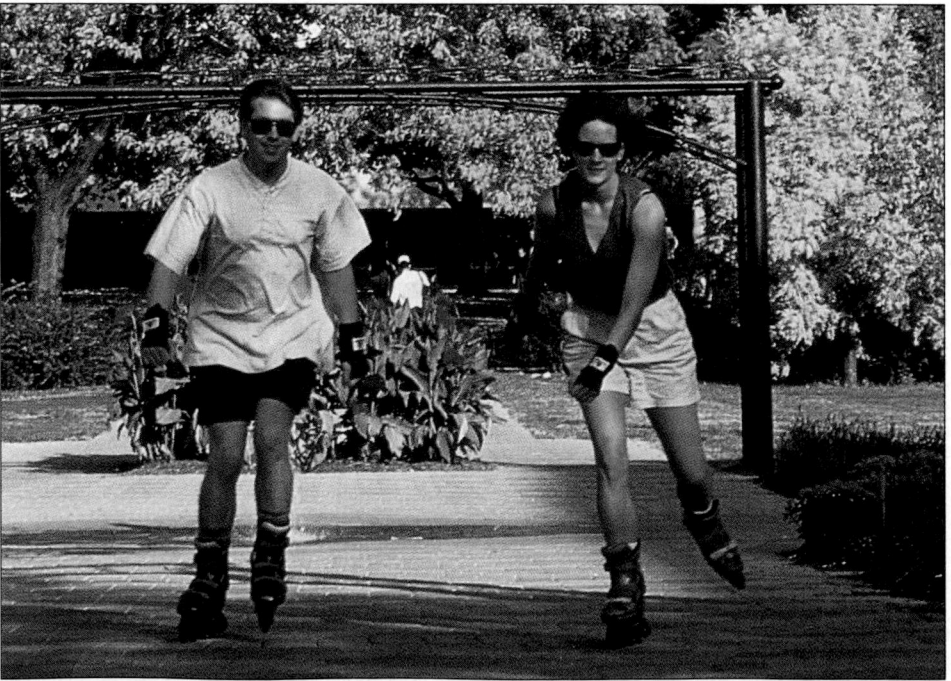

The energy used to perform physical activity is in the form of ATP.

Think about ATP the next time you race for a bus. When you finally sit down, you are exhausted. You breathe hard, and your heart races. Your muscle cells have used up most of their ATP and other high-energy compounds. While you rest, muscle cells begin to use the energy released from the metabolism of food (fuels) to synthesize ATP by fusing together the ADP and Pi released during the breakdown of ATP. If you rest long enough, you can then race to your class using the newly formed ATP.

■ Oxidation-Reduction Reactions—Key Processes in Energy Metabolism

Oxidation-reduction reactions form a vital link between the energy-yielding nutrients and the formation of ATP. The formal meaning of oxidation and reduction can be summarized as:

A substance is *oxidized* when it loses one or more electrons.

A substance is *reduced* when it gains one or more electrons.

Electron flow governs oxidation-reduction processes. If one substance loses electrons (is oxidized), another substance must gain electrons (must be reduced). The two processes go together; one cannot proceed without the other.

Consider the oxidation-reduction reaction between zinc and the copper ion Cu^{2+}:

$$Zn + Cu^{2+} \rightarrow Zn^2 + Cu$$

Here, Zn has lost two electrons (has been oxidized) ($Zn \rightarrow Zn^{2+} + 2e^-$). At the same time, copper has gained two electrons (has been reduced) ($Cu^{2+} + 2e^- \rightarrow Cu$). Another example is the iron in hemoglobin, which can be oxidized from Fe^{2+} to Fe^{3+} and reduced from Fe^{3+} to Fe^{2+}. This occurs during the transport of oxygen to body cells (see Chapter 12).

Oxidation-reduction reactions involving carbon-containing compounds are somewhat more difficult to visualize. A simple rule has been developed to determine oxidation reduction in these compounds. If the compound gains oxygen or loses hydrogen, it has been oxidized. If it loses oxygen or gains hydrogen, the compound has been reduced. The following process illustrates this definition.

This method of determining oxidation and reduction—determining oxygen and hydrogen exchange—is used extensively in nutrition. For example, in the reaction illustrated, pyruvic acid (made from glucose) is reduced to form lactic acid by gaining two hydrogens. This happens during intense exercise (see Chapter 14). Lactic acid is oxidized back to pyruvic acid by losing two hydrogens.

Scientists generally use the terms *oxidation* and *reduction* as verbs or adjectives. As a verb, pyruvic acid is said to be reduced to lactic acid, and lactic acid is oxidized to pyruvic acid. As an adjective, lactic acid is said to be the reduced form of pyruvic acid, while pyruvic acid is the oxidized form of lactic acid.

Oxidation-reduction reactions in the body are controlled by enzymes. One important class of these enzymes, designated *dehydrogenases*, removes hydrogens from energy-yielding nutrients or their breakdown products and donates the hydrogens

*N*ow that you are familiar with oxidation and reduction reactions, we can define the term **antioxidant**. This is typically used to describe a compound that can donate electrons to oxidized compounds, putting them into a more reduced (stable) state. Oxidized compounds tend to be highly reactive; they seek electrons from other compounds to stabilize their chemical configuration. Dietary antioxidants such as vitamin E and vitamin C can donate electrons to these highly reactive compounds, in turn, putting these oxidized compounds into a less reactive state (see Chapters 9 and 10 for details).

coenzyme A compound that combines with an active protein, called an apoenzyme, to form a catalytically active protein, called a holoenzyme. In this manner, coenzymes aid in enzyme function.

to the final acceptor, oxygen, to form water. In the process, large amounts of energy are transferred to ADP plus Pi to make ATP.[11]

Two B vitamins, niacin and riboflavin, assist dehydrogenase enzymes and, in turn, play a role in transferring the hydrogens from glucose to oxygen in the metabolic pathways of the cell. Niacin functions as the **coenzyme** nicotinamide adenine dinucleotide (NAD). This is the oxidized form, which can accept one hydrogen ion and two electrons to become NADH + H$^+$. (The extra hydrogen ion remains free in the cell.) In other words, the oxidized form of niacin, NAD, is reduced to form NADH + H$^+$. Note that NAD is actually NAD$^+$, indicating one less electron than in its complete configuration. By accepting two electrons and one hydrogen ion, NAD$^+$ becomes NADH + H$^+$, with no net charge. (The charge on NAD is ignored to simplify chapter discussions.)

Riboflavin plays a similar role. In its oxidized form, it is known as flavin adenine dinucleotide (FAD). When it is reduced (gains two hydrogens, equivalent to two hydrogen ions and two electrons), it is known as FADH$_2$.

The reduction of oxygen (O) to form water (H$_2$O) provides the driving force for life, as it is vital to the way cells synthesize ATP. Thus, oxidation-reduction reactions are a key to life.

CONCEPT CHECK

*M*etabolism encompasses all of the sequences of chemical reactions in the body. Anabolic pathways build compounds using energy input, whereas catabolic pathways break down compounds into small units, yielding energy. Adenosine triphosphate (ATP) is the form of energy used by a cell. The synthesis of ATP from ADP and Pi involves the transfer of energy from foodstuffs. This uses oxidation-reduction reactions, where electrons (along with hydrogen ions) are transferred from carbohydrates, proteins, fats, and alcohol eventually to oxygen. This reaction forms water and releases much energy, which can be used to produce ATP.

■ CARBOHYDRATE METABOLISM BEGINS WITH GLYCOLYSIS

*A*s each of the subsequent pathways is described, a good way to understand them is to diagram each step as you go. Then compare your figures with those provided throughout the chapter.

Let's now look at how ATP is generated in a human cell. The easiest place to begin studying ATP synthesis is in the metabolism of carbohydrates (Fig. 4-3). Next we'll look at fat and protein metabolism. All of these fuels can be used to synthesize ATP. Note that alcohol metabolism is discussed in detail in Chapter 8.

■ Glycolysis—Glucose to Pyruvate

Glycolysis literally means "breaking down glucose." The glycolysis pathway, found in the cytosol of all cells, has a dual role: It degrades monosaccharides to generate energy, and it provides building blocks for synthesizing needed cell compounds, such as **glycerol** for triglyceride synthesis.[7]

glycolysis The metabolic pathway that converts glucose into 2 molecules of pyruvic acid, with the net gain of 2 ATP and 2 NADH + H$^+$.

glycerol A three-carbon alcohol that provides the backbone to form triglycerides.

Before glycolysis can begin, a cell must obtain glucose. Only a few types of cells, such as liver and kidney cells, can produce their own glucose from amino acids (see later section), and only liver and muscle cells store glucose to a major extent. This glucose is stored as glycogen. Liver and muscle cells break down the glycogen to glucose (or a closely related form). Other body cells must obtain glucose from the bloodstream, so the body needs to maintain a fairly constant concentration of blood glucose to survive (see Chapter 5 for details).

The product of glycolysis is two units of a three-carbon compound called *pyruvic acid (pyruvate)* (Figs. 4-4 and 4-5). Some cells then convert pyruvate to lactic acid (lactate).

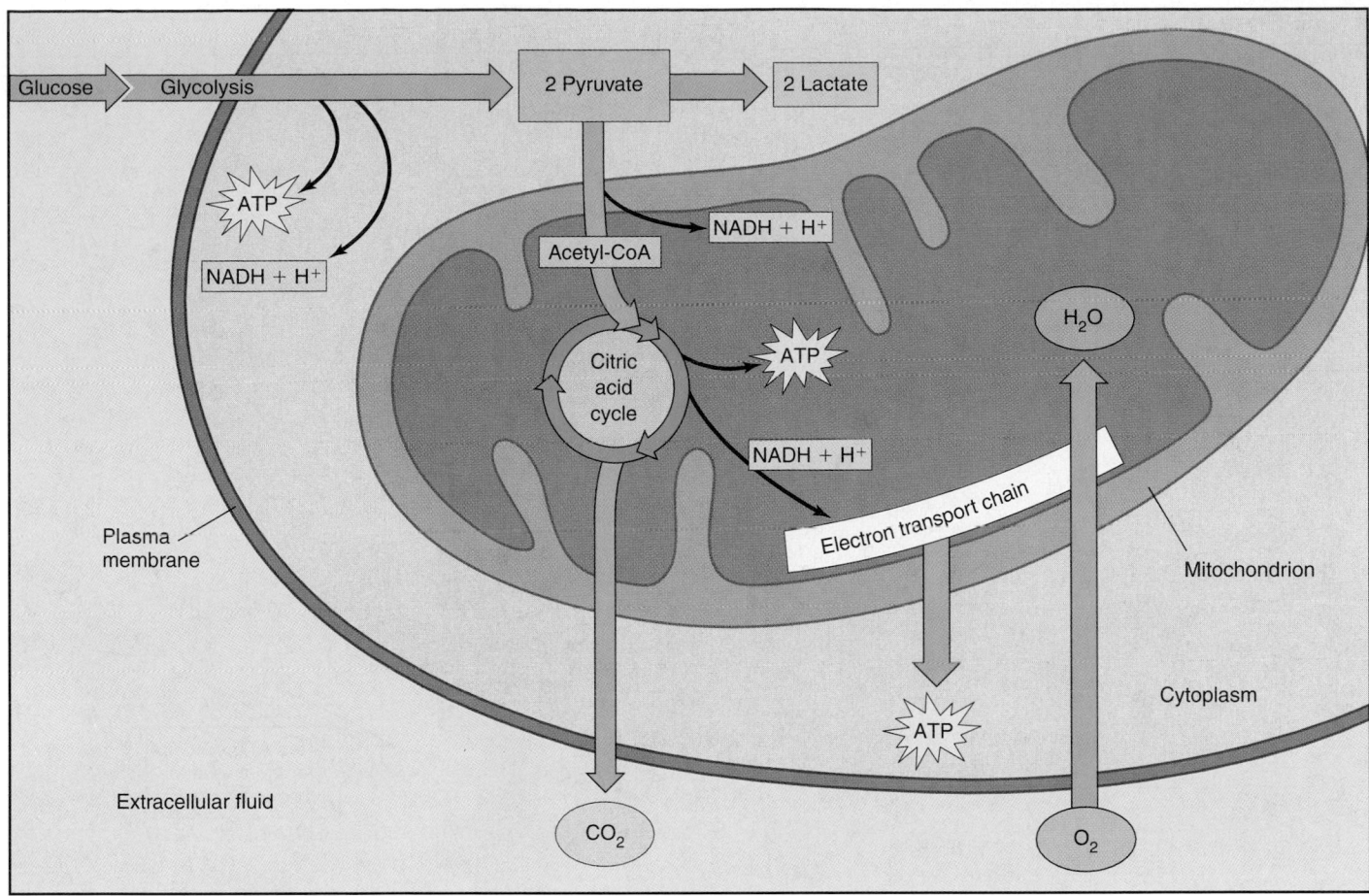

■ FIGURE 4-3 An overview of the cellular respiration of glucose.

To begin glycolysis, a phosphate group is added to glucose, which makes the glucose more reactive. Another phosphate group is added to the newly formed glucose-phosphate compound, which then splits into two three-carbon compounds. These are converted through a series of steps into two molecules of the three-carbon compound pyruvate. Thus, in glycolysis a cell starts with a six-carbon glucose molecule and produces two molecules of the three-carbon compound pyruvate. In the process, four hydrogens (containing a total of four electrons) are removed and four ATP are generated. The electrons and hydrogen ions are picked up by a carrier—in this case, **nicotinamide adenine dinucleotide (NAD).** Each NAD (oxidized form) accepts two electrons and one hydrogen ion, yielding NADH + H+(reduced form). Thus, an end result of glycolysis is also the synthesis of two NADH + H+, with the release of two hydrogen ions.[7]

■ Where Is the ATP?

In glycolysis, the first reaction involves one ATP donating a phosphate group to glucose. In the 3rd step, another ATP is used to add a second phosphate group. Thus, to begin the pathway, a cell uses two ATP. As the two three-carbon molecules are converted to pyruvate, each one generates two ATP, for a total of four ATP. The net energy produced thus far from glycolysis is two ATP, as two ATP prime the system and four ATP are produced. There are more ATP to come; this represents only about 5% of the total ATP production possible from one glucose molecule.[10]

Chemical energy stored in the bonds of NADH can eventually be transferred to ATP. Generally, each NADH + H+ provides enough energy to yield 2.5 ATP.[11] Thus, NADH + H+ is a form of *potential energy for the cell.* A cell eventually uses the energy in NADH + H+ to form ATP. Further discussion later it is described how this happens in the mitochondria.

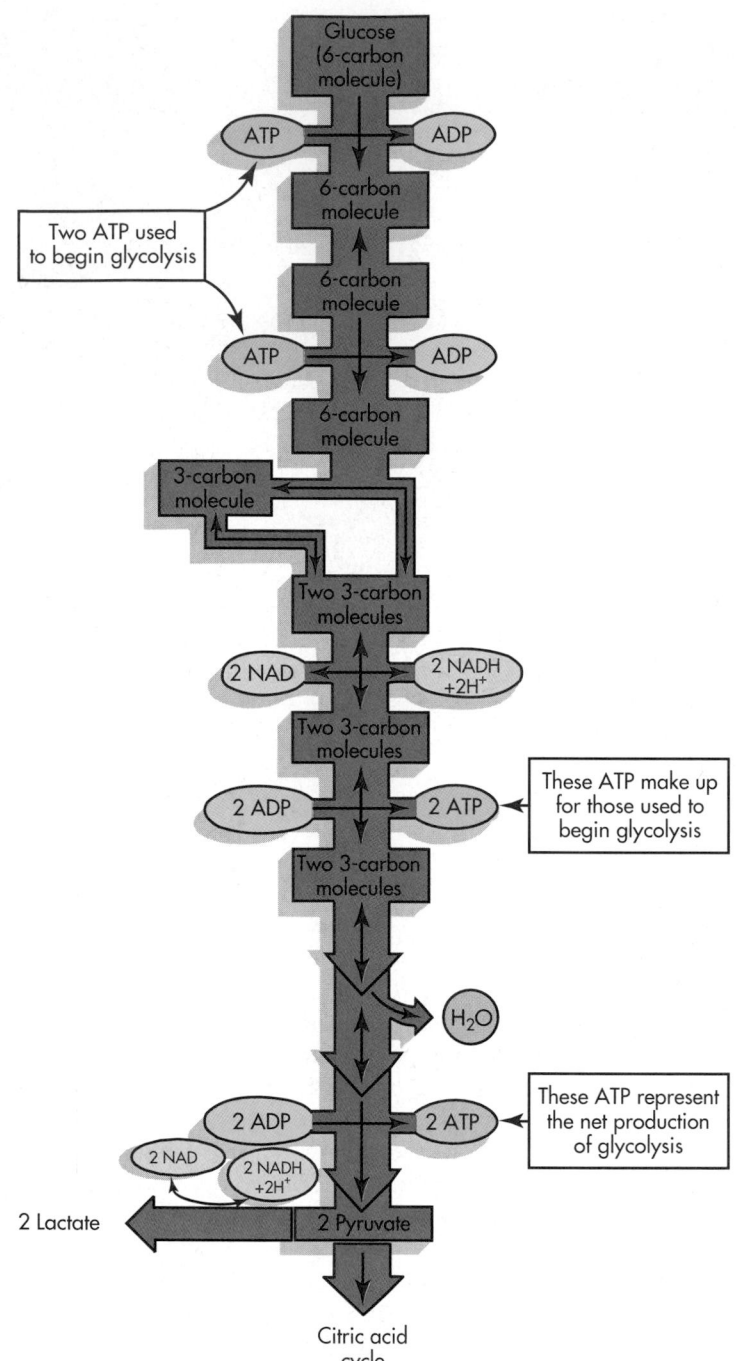

FIGURE 4-4 Glycolysis simplified. The process begins with one glucose ($C_6H_{12}O_6$) and ends with two pyruvates ($C_3H_4O_3$). Some ATP is produced by the process. The four electrons and two of the hydrogen ions released are captured by two NAD. The other two hydrogen ions float free in the cytosol. Pyruvate then can undergo further metabolism in the citric acid cycle, or form lactate under anaerobic conditions.

*R*egenerating NAD by using lactate represents a **fermentation** reaction. Some yeasts produce alcohol (ethanol) instead of lactate to regenerate NAD in anaerobic conditions. This is also a fermentation reaction.

aerobic Requiring oxygen.

The other monosaccharides, fructose and galactose, are converted to intermediate compounds of the glycolytic pathway and follow the same sequence of events as glucose. Pyruvate is eventually formed.

■ Lactate Production Is the Endpoint of Anaerobic Glycolysis

Some cells lack the oxygen-requiring (**aerobic**) pathway needed for using NADH + H$^+$ for ATP synthesis, and in turn they lack the ability to use this process to recycle NADH + H$^+$ back to NAD. The red blood cell is an example. Thus, as a red blood cell converts glucose to pyruvate, NADH + H$^+$ builds up in the cell. Eventually, the NAD concentration falls too low to permit glycolysis to continue, since most of the NAD present is in the form NADH + H$^+$.[7]

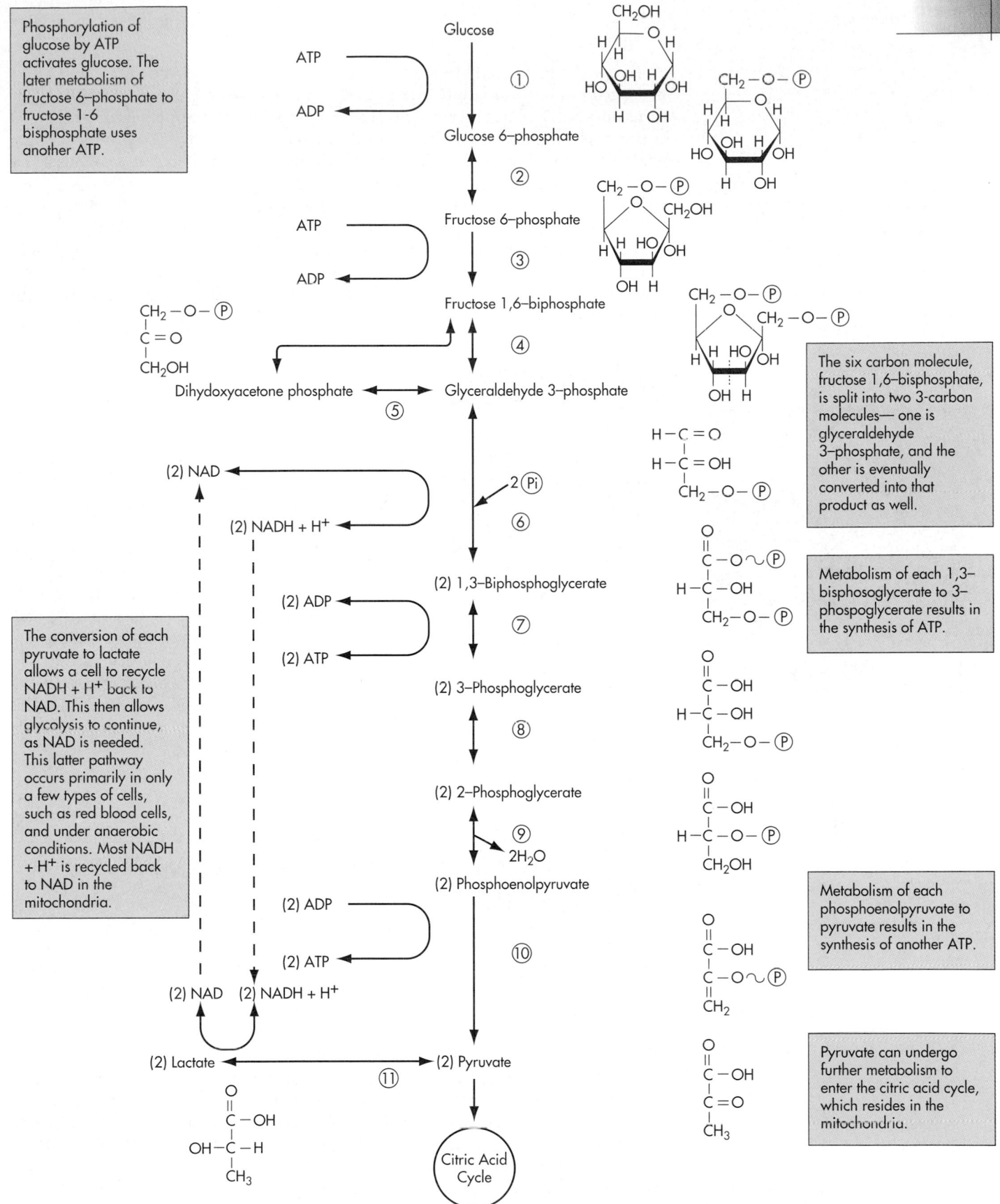

Phosphorylation of glucose by ATP activates glucose. The later metabolism of fructose 6–phosphate to fructose 1-6 bisphosphate uses another ATP.

The six carbon molecule, fructose 1,6–bisphosphate, is split into two 3-carbon molecules— one is glyceraldehyde 3–phosphate, and the other is eventually converted into that product as well.

Metabolism of each 1,3–bisphosoglycerate to 3–phospoglycerate results in the synthesis of ATP.

The conversion of each pyruvate to lactate allows a cell to recycle NADH + H+ back to NAD. This then allows glycolysis to continue, as NAD is needed. This latter pathway occurs primarily in only a few types of cells, such as red blood cells, and under anaerobic conditions. Most NADH + H+ is recycled back to NAD in the mitochondria.

Metabolism of each phosphoenolpyruvate to pyruvate results in the synthesis of another ATP.

Pyruvate can undergo further metabolism to enter the citric acid cycle, which resides in the mitochondria.

■ FIGURE 4-5 The individual chemical reactions that comprise glycolysis—glucose to pyruvate. Glycolysis takes place in the cytosol of the cell. The enzymes in the cytosol that participate at each step are (1) hexokinase, (2) phosphoshexose isomerase, (3) phosphofructokinase, (4) aldolase, (5) phosphotriose isomerase, (6) glyceraldehyde-3-phosphate dehydrogenase, (7) phosphoglycerate kinase, (8) phosphoglycerate mutase, (9) enolase, (10) pyruvate kinase, and sometimes (11) lactate dehydrogenase. Pi represents a phosphate group. The symbol ~ represents a high energy bond.

To compensate, a red blood cell reacts pyruvate with an NADH + H⁺ and a free hydrogen ion to form lactate (see Figs. 4-3 and 4-4). In the process, NADH + H⁺ turns into NAD. This process allows the red blood cell to resupply itself with NAD as these cells do not contain mitochondria. Exercising muscles also produce lactate when they run out of NAD. The increase in lactate in turn contributes to muscle fatigue (see Chapter 14).

The production of lactate by a cell allows **anaerobic** glycolysis to continue, as there remains a steady supply of NAD. Again, this pathway yields only about 5% of the potential ATP per glucose molecule. But, for some cells, such as red blood cells, anaerobic glycolysis is the only available method for making ATP. The lactate is released into the bloodstream, picked up primarily by the liver, and synthesized into glucose.

anaerobic Not requiring oxygen.

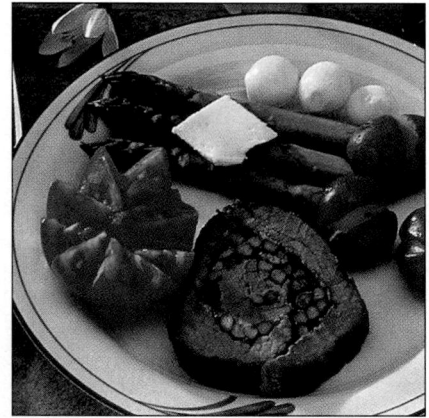

Carbohydrate, protein, fat, and alcohol all contribute chemical energy to the body.

CONCEPT CHECK

To begin glycolysis, 2 phosphate groups from 2 ATP molecules are added to glucose to make the glucose more reactive. This doubly phosphorylated glucose becomes fructose 1, 6 bisphosphate. It eventually splits into 2 molecules of a 3-carbon compound glyceraldehyde 3-phosphate. These molecules go through a series of chemical reactions (steps ⑥ through ⑩) to become the three carbon compound pyruvate. Thus in glycolysis, glucose with 6 carbons and 12 hydrogens and 6 oxygens ($C_6H_{12}O_6$) is converted to 2 molecules of pyruvate containing 3 carbons and 4 hydrogens and 3 oxygens ($C_3H_4O_3$). In the process, 4 hydrogens (containing 4 protons and 4 electrons) are removed and NAD is reduced to form NADH + H⁺. Each NAD accepts 2 electrons and one proton, producing NADH + H⁺ (the extra H⁺ is an unbound proton). Also produced in this phase of glycolysis is 4 ATP (steps ⑦ and ⑩). Pyruvate is either broken down further or converted to lactate. Red blood cells perform the latter reaction, as part of *anaerobic glycolysis*. The conversion of pyruvate to lactate allows the cell to oxidize NADH + H⁺ into NAD. This provides the NAD needed for glycolysis. NADH + H⁺ can also be oxidized to NAD via oxygen-requiring pathways, found in most cells.

▮ THE CITRIC ACID CYCLE COMPLETES GLUCOSE CATABOLISM

The two pyruvate (or lactate) molecules formed at the end of glycolysis still contain much stored energy. Pyruvate passes from the cell cytosol into the mitochondria. A cell then uses pathways found there to extract the remaining energy from pyruvate to form more ATP. One key pathway is called the *citric acid cycle*.

▮ Pyruvate to Acetyl-CoA Is an Irreversible Step

Before the citric acid cycle can begin, pyruvate must lose a carbon dioxide group and eventually form acetyl-CoA. This overall reaction is irreversible, which has important metabolic consequences, as you will see. As pyruvate is converted to acetyl-CoA, another NADH + H⁺ is formed from NAD, so more potential ATP molecules are produced.[6] The conversion of pyruvate to acetyl-CoA requires the B vitamins thiamin, riboflavin, niacin, and pantothenic acid. For this reason, dietary carbohydrates metabolism depends on the presence of these vitamins.

▮ The Citric Acid Cycle

The citric acid cycle is an elegant sequence of chemical reactions used by cells to convert the carbons of acetate to carbon dioxide and to yield energy. Acetyl-CoA

Other names for the citric acid cycle are the tricarboxylic acid cycle (TCA cycle) and the Krebs cycle, named after Sir Hans Krebs, the scientist who first described it.

enters the cycle, and the reactions eventually yield two molecules of carbon dioxide. In the process, the cell produces NADH + H' and other related molecules, which eventually are used to form many ATP.[6]

To begin the citric acid cycle, acetyl-CoA combines with a four-carbon compound, oxaloacetic acid (or oxaloacetate) to form the six carbon compound citric acid (or citrate) (Figure 4-6). In the process, the CoA molecule is released. During one turn of the citric acid cycle, the six-carbon citrate molecule is metabolized to the four-carbon oxaloacetate molecule (steps ② through ⑨ in Figure 4-7) and two carbon dioxide molecules are released (steps ④ and ⑤). The cycle is ready to begin again. Each turn of the cycle yields potential ATP in the form of guanosine triphosphate (GTP) (step ⑥), NADH + H$^+$ and FADH$_2$. FAD is another hydrogen carrier. It can pick up a pair of hydrogens at step ⑦. Each FADH$_2$ provides enough energy to synthesize 1.5 ATP, *one less than* NADH + H$^+$.[11]

To review carbohydrate metabolism so far, the cell started with a six-carbon glucose and eventually produced six carbon dioxide molecules, two at the pyruvate to acetyl CoA step, two each at isocitrate to alpha-ketoglutarate step (step ④) and two each at alpha ketoglutarate to succinyl CoA step (step ⑤). Remember, it takes two turns around the citric acid cycle to process one glucose, since the glucose was split into two 3-carbon fragments as a result of glycolysis. As a result, all the carbons in glucose are released in the form of carbon dioxide. The carbon dioxide eventually leaves the body by way of the lungs. In the process, ATP is synthesized directly using both the glycolysis and citric acid cycle pathways, and NADH + H$^+$ and FADH$_2$ are formed from NAD and FAD (see Fig. 4-3). The NADH +H$^+$ and FADH$_2$ molecules can be used to supply the energy need for ATP synthesis in the electron transport chain (see following discussion).

In this way, some of the energy in the chemical bonds of glucose is transferred to ATP. Thus, some of the energy in food yields a form of energy that cells can use,

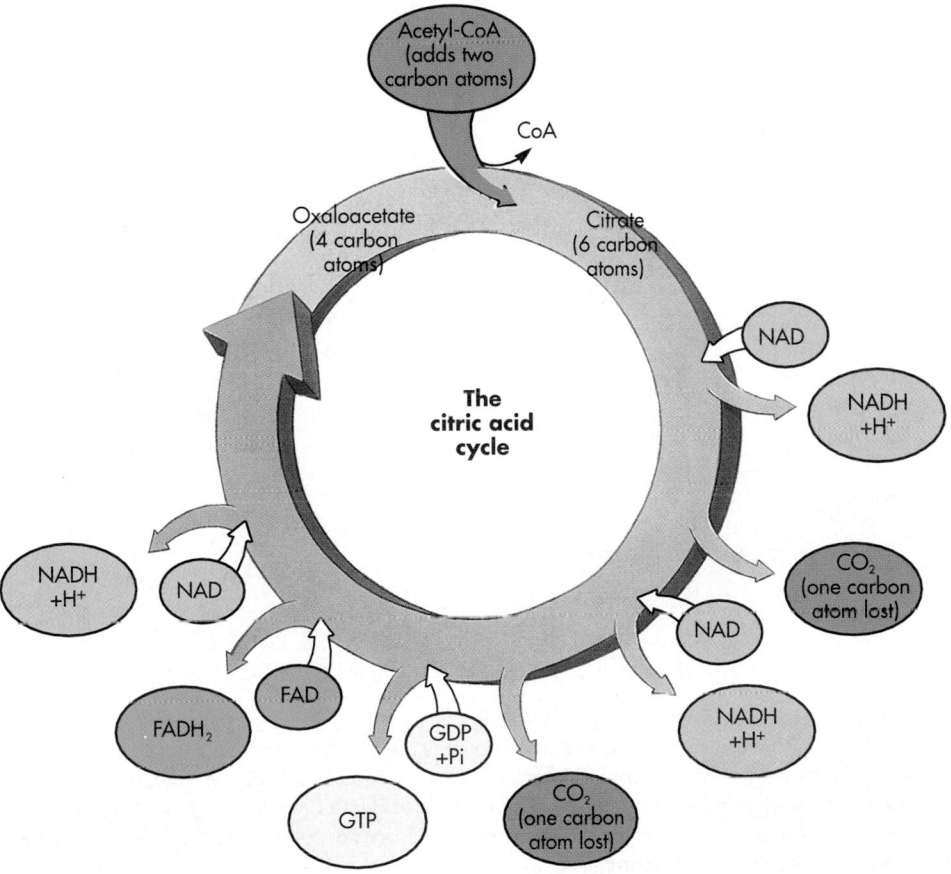

■ FIGURE **4-6** The citric acid cycle simplified. The four carbons from oxaloacetate combine with two carbons from acetyl-CoA to form the six-carbon compound *citric acid,* or citrate. The citrate is ultimately reformed into the original four-carbon oxaloacetate, with a net loss of two carbons as carbon dioxide. The pathway thus begins and ends with the same compound, oxaloacetate, which makes it a cycle. The GTP formed can be used to synthesize ATP.
Illustration by William Ober.

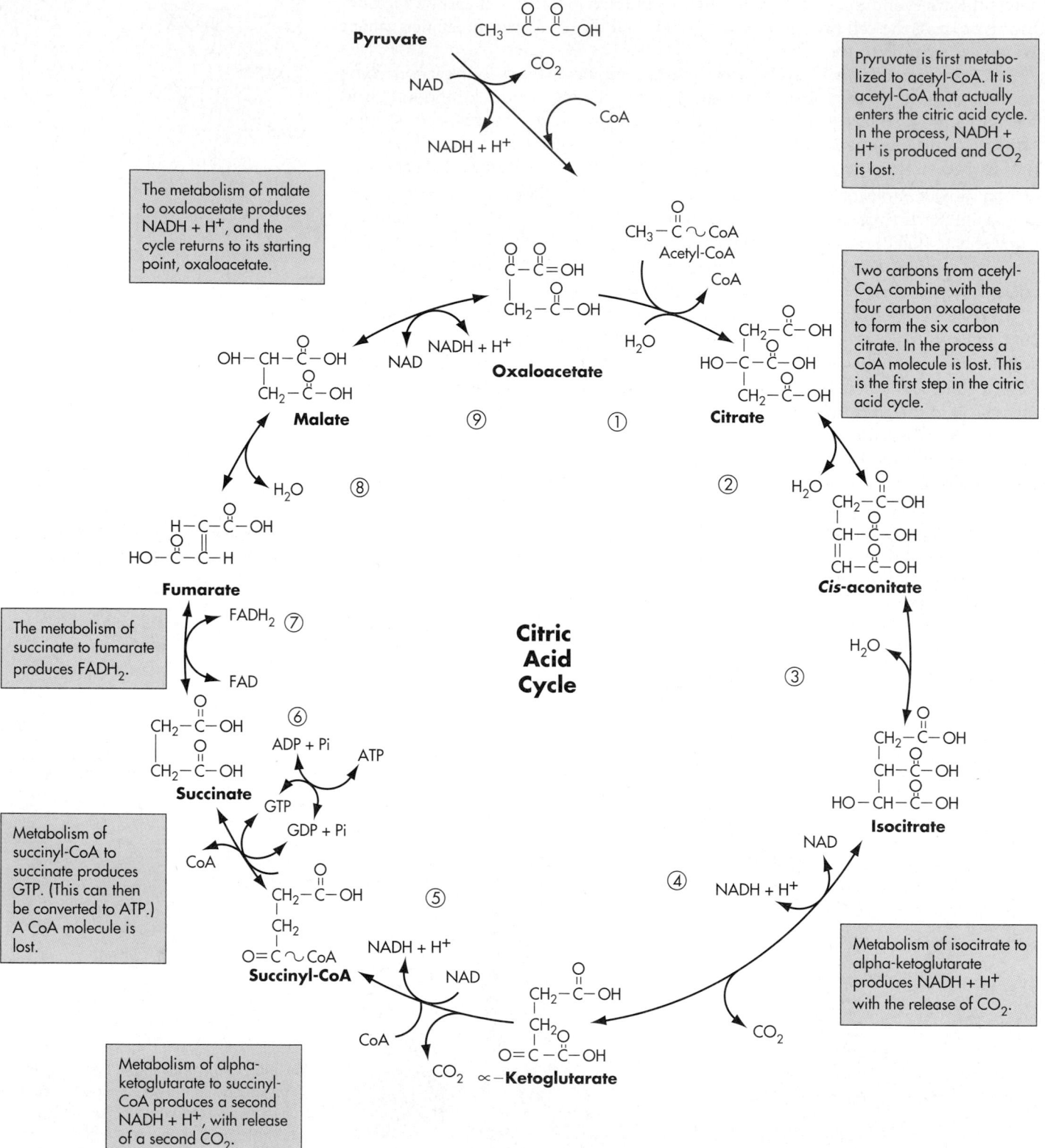

Pyruvate

Pyruvate is first metabolized to acetyl-CoA. It is acetyl-CoA that actually enters the citric acid cycle. In the process, NADH + H+ is produced and CO_2 is lost.

The metabolism of malate to oxaloacetate produces NADH + H+, and the cycle returns to its starting point, oxaloacetate.

Oxaloacetate

Acetyl-CoA

Two carbons from acetyl-CoA combine with the four carbon oxaloacetate to form the six carbon citrate. In the process a CoA molecule is lost. This is the first step in the citric acid cycle.

Malate

Citrate

Cis-aconitate

Citric Acid Cycle

Fumarate

The metabolism of succinate to fumarate produces FADH2.

Isocitrate

Succinate

Metabolism of isocitrate to alpha-ketoglutarate produces NADH + H+ with the release of CO_2.

Metabolism of succinyl-CoA to succinate produces GTP. (This can then be converted to ATP.) A CoA molecule is lost.

Succinyl-CoA

∝-**Ketoglutarate**

Metabolism of alpha-ketoglutarate to succinyl-CoA produces a second NADH + H+, with release of a second CO_2.

FIGURE 4-7 Conversion of pyruvate to acetyl-CoA and the individual chemical reactions of the citric acid cycle. Conversion of pyruvate to acetyl-CoA uses an enzyme complex that includes pyruvate dehydrogenase. The enzymes used in the citric acid cycle are (1) citrate synthase, (2) aconitase, (3) aconitase, (4) isocitrate dehydrogenase, (5) alpha-ketoglutarate dehydrogenase, (6) succinate thiokinase, (7) succinate dehydrogenase, (8) fumararse, and (9) malate dehydrogenase. CoA stands for coenzyme A, which is made from the vitamin pantothenic acid (see Chapter 10 for the chemical structure). Note that the CO_2 molecules lost during one turn of the citric acid cycle are not those from the carbons donated by acetyl-CoA. Instead, the carbons are broken off of the portion of the citrate molecule made up from oxaloacetate.

rather than just being converted to heat, as would have happened if you had ignited the food with a match. In engineering terms, cells capture about 40% of the chemical energy in glucose and transfer it to a useful form when needed—namely, ATP. *This is the main goal of energy metabolism.* The remaining energy (60%) escapes as heat via all the reactions that take place in which ATP, GTP, NADH + H$^+$, or FADH$_2$ is not made. The same 40:60 ratio applies for the energy metabolism of fatty acids and amino acids. That's fairly efficient, compared with an automobile engine, which captures only about 10% of the chemical energy in gasoline.[11]

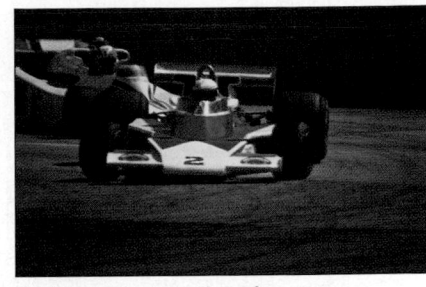

The human body is about four times more efficient than automobiles in extracting energy from carbon-based compounds.

■ THE ELECTRON TRANSPORT CHAIN IS THE PRIMARY SITE FOR ATP SYNTHESIS

During the metabolism of protein, carbohydrate, fat, and alcohol, cells generate NADH + H$^+$ and FADH$_2$. Most cells can use these compounds for ATP synthesis (Fig. 4-8). The pathway that performs this exchange is called the **electron transport chain.** The process, which occurs in the inner membrane of mitochondria, is called *oxidative phosphorylation.* The minerals iron and copper are needed for this process.

In the electron transport chain, NADH donates its chemical energy to an FAD-related compound called *flavin mononucleotide (FMN).* FMN is followed at a junction by Coenzyme Q, which separates the pairs of electrons so they can proceed one electron at a time through the rest of the electron transport chain. Later you will see the hydrogens take another route. (Note that a product called Coenzyme Q-10 is sold as a nutrient supplement in Health Food Stores. However, when the mitochondria needs Coenzyme Q, it makes it. Thus it is not needed in the diet or in the form of a supplement to maintain health.)

The next structures used in the electron transport chain are a group of iron-containing molecules called cytochromes (Fig. 4-9). At the end of the chain of cytochromes is a special cytochrome (called cytochrome a$_3$) whose job it is to donate all the electrons that have moved down the chain to oxygen. The action of the cytochromes is like a bucket brigade, picking up an electron and handing it off to the next cytochrome until finally at the end of the chain there is oxygen waiting to accept the electron. At this final step, the hydrogen ion reunites with the electrons to form hydrogen, which in turn combines with oxygen to form water. Thus although NADH + H$^+$ and FADH$_2$ transfer their hydrogens to the electron transport chain, it should be noted that the hydrogen ions (H$^+$) are not transported with the electrons.

Once the NADH + H$^+$ and FADH$_2$ have transferred their hydrogen to the chain they are again NAD and FAD, and are ready to shuttle more hydrogens to the chain

electron transport chain A series of reactions using oxygen to convert NADH + H$^+$ and FADH$_2$ molecules to free NAD and FAD molecules by the donation of electrons and hydrogen ions to oxygen, yielding water and ATP.

cytochromes Electron-transfer compounds that participate in the electron transport chain.

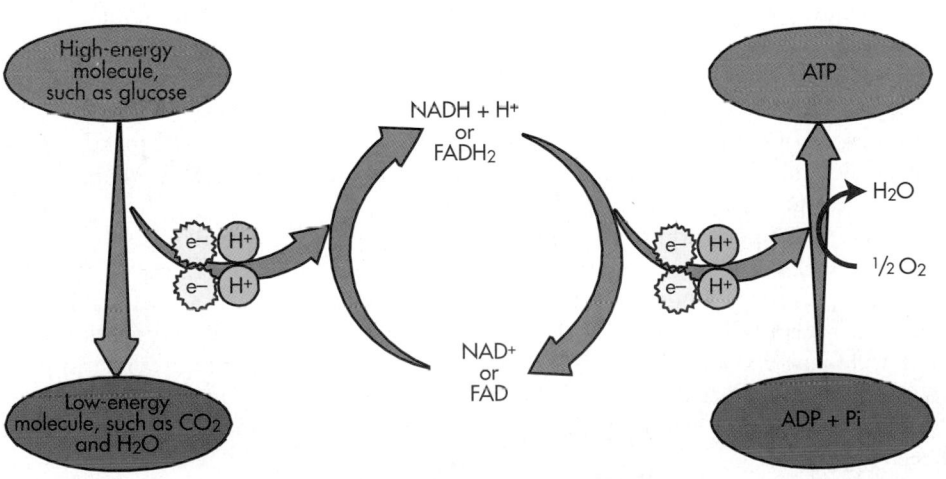

■ FIGURE 4-8 Simplified depiction of electron transfer in energy metabolism. High-energy compounds, such as glucose, give up electrons and hydrogen ions to NAD and FAD. The NADH + H$^+$ and FADH$_2$ that are formed transfer these electrons and hydrogen ions, using specialized electron carriers, to oxygen to form water (H$_2$O). The energy yielded by the entire process is used to generate ATP from ADP and Pi.

Illustration by William Ober.

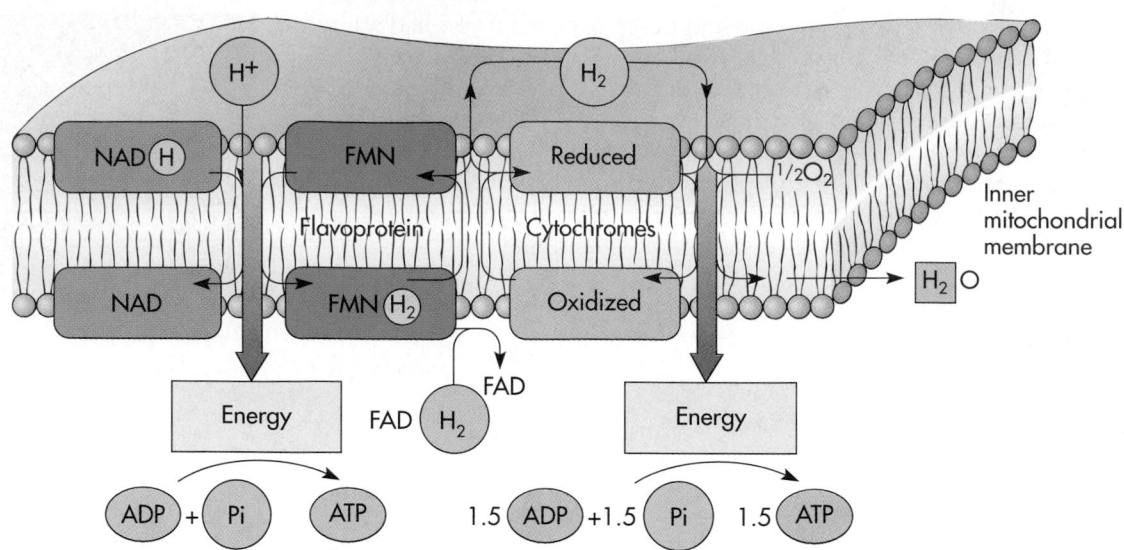

FIGURE 4-9 More detailed depiction of the electron transport chain. NADH and FADH$_2$ transfer their hydrogen ions and electrons to electron carriers located on the inner mitochondrial membrane. Between FMN and the cytochromes sits Coenzyme Q, which separates the pairs of electrons so they can proceed one electron at a time down the electron transport chain. The electrons and hydrogen ions combine with oxygen to form water (H$_2$O). The energy yielded by the entire process is used to generate ATP. The oxygen atoms attract the electrons down the electron transport chain. Each NADH + H$^+$ in the mitochondria releases enough energy to form the equivalent of 2.5 ATP, while each FADH$_2$ releases enough energy to form the equivalent of 1.5 ATP. Of the 30 to 32 ATP yielded by the complete oxidation of glucose, almost 90% are synthesized in the electron transport chain.
Illustration by William Ober.

A n alternative pathway for the metabolism of glucose is the pentose phosphate pathway. This yields ribose and deoxyribose for RNA and DNA synthesis, respectively, as well as a variation of NADH + H$^+$ (NADPH + H$^+$) used in synthetic reactions, such as the synthesis of fatty acids. The pentose phosphate pathway is active in cells that synthesize fatty acids, such as liver cells.

from the citric acid cycle. In Figure 4-9 note that NADH + H$^+$ donates its hydrogen ions and electrons to FMN (flavin mononucleotide). FADH$_2$ donates its pair of hydrogen ions and electrons after FMN to the cytochromes. As the electrons move along the chain they release energy which is used to phosphoralate ADP to ATP. This different placement of FAD and NAD in the chain results in a difference in ATP production. Each NADH + H$^+$ in the mitochondria releases enough energy to form the equivalent of 2.5 ATP, while each FADH$_2$ (which entered lower down the chain) releases enough energy to form the equivalent of 1.5 ATP.[11]

In the meantime, the hydrogen ions are moved between the inner and outer mitochondrial membrane by pumps that deliver the hydrogen ion to the electrons to form hydrogen. The net results of the electron transport chain is the production of ATP and water.

Since oxygen is essential to these processes, the electron transport chain is part of aerobic metabolism. NADH + H$^+$ and FADH$_2$ produced during the citric acid cycle can be regenerated into NAD and FAD only by the eventual transfer of their electrons and hydrogen ions to oxygen. The citric acid cycle has no way to re-form NADH + H$^+$ and FADH$_2$ back to NAD and FAD analogous to the way that anaerobic glycolysis produces lactate. This is ultimately why oxygen is essential to life; a final acceptor of the electrons and hydrogen ions generated from the breakdown of energy-yielding nutrients is needed. Without oxygen, most of our cells are unable to extract enough energy from fuels to sustain life.

This entire description of the metabolism of glucose depicts the essence of metabolism. Cells need to release energy stored in food fuels and then trap as much as possible as ATP. The body cannot afford to lose all energy as heat. Some heat is necessary for warmth, but the body also needs mobilizing energy. Glycolysis, the citric acid cycle, and the electron transport chain accomplish many things. Most important, however, they enable cells to capture the chemical energy in food in the form of ATP, which acts as cellular fuel. In effect, ATP allows cells to get up and do what needs to be done.

GLYCOGEN METABOLISM

Glycogen synthesis uses a form of glucose (glucose 1-phosphate), adding more glucose molecules to an existing glycogen chain. This provides liver and muscle cells with a short-term storage form of glucose.[11] Later, when glucose is needed, glycogen breakdown yields glucose as a glucose-phosphate compound, which eventually begins glycolysis. An enzyme involved in glycogen breakdown uses vitamin B-6.

CRITICAL THINKING

While looking at electron microscopy slides of muscle cells, you observe various organelles. However, the large number of mitochondria you see is remarkable. Your instructor asks you to explain this observation to your classmates. How would you do so?

CONCEPT CHECK

In the citric acid cycle, a two-carbon acetate molecule in the form of acetyl-CoA combines with a four-carbon oxaloacetate molecule to form the six-carbon citrate molecule. Through various chemical reactions, the cycle releases two carbon dioxide molecules and eventually yields another oxaloacetate, the starting material. This new oxaloacetate can combine with another acetyl-CoA molecule to begin the process again. The NADH + H$^+$ and FADH$_2$ produced in the citric acid cycle donate their electrons and hydrogen ions to the electron transport chain, yielding free NAD and FAD, water, and ATP.

LIPOLYSIS: FAT BREAKDOWN

Lipolysis is part of a process of splitting—breaking down—triglycerides into free fatty acids and glycerol. The further breakdown of the fatty acids for energy production is called *fatty acid oxidation*, since the donation of electrons from fatty acids to oxygen is the net reaction in the energy-yielding process. This takes place in the mitochondria and peroxisomes of the cell, but only mitochondria can use the energy released to form ATP.[11]

Fatty acids are liberated from lipid storage in adipose cells by an enzyme called *hormone-sensitive lipase.* The activity of this enzyme is increased by the hormones glucagon, growth hormone, epinephrine, and others and is decreased by the hormone insulin. The fatty acids are taken up from the bloodstream by cells and are shuttled from the cell cytosol into the mitochondria using a carrier called **carnitine.** In healthy people, cells produce the carnitine needed for this process. During acute illness in hospitalized patients, carnitine synthesis may not meet their needs. Thus, it may be added to intravenous nutrition solutions used by these patients.

Almost all fatty acids in nature are composed of an even number of carbons, ranging from 2 to 26. The first step in transferring the energy in a fatty acid to ATP (fatty acid oxidation) is to cleave the carbons, two at a time, and convert the two-carbon fragments to acetyl-CoA. The process of converting a free fatty acid to multiple acetyl-CoA molecules is more specifically called **beta-oxidation,** since the second carbon on a fatty acid (counting after the acid $\left[\begin{smallmatrix} O \\ \parallel \\ -C-OH \end{smallmatrix}\right]$ end) is called the *beta carbon.* This is where the reaction begins. During beta-oxidation, NADH + H$^+$ and FADH$_2$ are produced, so, as with glucose, a fatty acid is eventually degraded into the two-carbon compound acetate, in the form of acetyl-CoA. Some of the chemical energy is transferred to NADH + H$^+$ and FADH$_2$.[11]

The acetyl-CoA enters the citric acid cycle and two carbon dioxides are released, just as with the acetyl-CoA produced from glucose. Thus, the breakdown product of both glucose and fatty acids, acetyl-CoA, uses a common pathway—the citric acid cycle. One big difference, however, is that a 16-carbon fatty acid yields 108 ATP, whereas the 6-carbon glucose yields 30 to 32 ATP. That results in a ratio of about 7 ATP per carbon for fatty acids versus about 5 ATP per carbon for glucose.[11] This difference results from the greater number of C–H bonds per carbon in a fatty acid,

lipolysis The breakdown of triglycerides to glycerol and fatty acids.

carnitine A compound used to shuttle fatty acids from the cytosol of the cell into mitochondria.

beta-oxidation The breakdown of a fatty acid into numerous acetyl-CoA molecules.

compared with glucose. It is the oxidation of these chemical bonds that provides most of the energy to drive ATP synthesis. Note that many of the carbons in glucose are also bonded to hydroxyl groups (–OH), rather than only to hydrogen atoms, as was primarily the case in the fatty acid. Thus, as a whole, the carbons of glucose exist in a more oxidized state. This is why fats yield more kcals/g than carbohydrates—fats are less oxidized (more reduced) than carbohydrates.

No matter how many carbons a fatty acid contains, it is usually broken down into acetyl-CoA. Occasionally, a fatty acid has an odd number of carbons, so the cell forms many acetyl-CoA, plus one three-carbon compound (propionyl-CoA). This enters the citric acid cycle directly, bypassing acetyl-CoA. It can then go on to yield carbon dioxide and other products, even glucose.

■ Carbohydrate Aids Fat Metabolism

In addition to its role in energy production, the citric acid cycle provides compounds that leave the cycle and enter biosynthetic pathways, such as those used to make the red blood cell protein hemoglobin. This means that, even though oxaloacetate is reused in the cycle, a minimum amount of it must still be maintained, because its removal from the citric acid cycle for biosynthetic reactions could prevent the completion of the cycle. One potential source of this additional oxaloacetate is pyruvate. Thus, as fatty acids create acetyl-CoA, carbohydrates, such as glucose, keep the concentration of pyruvate high enough to resupply oxaloacetate to the citric acid cycle. We could say that "fats burn in a fire of carbohydrate," since the entire pathway for fatty acid oxidation works better when carbohydrate is available.[11]

■ Ketogenesis: Producing Ketone Bodies from Fatty Acids

Ketone bodies are products of incomplete fatty acid oxidation. Hormonal imbalances—chiefly, inadequate insulin production to balance glucagon action in the body—allow some metabolic conditions to develop that lead to significant production of ketone bodies called *ketosis*.[9]

1. Fatty acids stored in adipose cells are rapidly released into the bloodstream. A fall in blood insulin is the key reason, as insulin inhibits lipolysis and, instead, favors fat storage. The bulk of the increase in fatty acids in the blood is taken up by the liver.

2. Fatty acid oxidation to acetyl-CoA predominates over fatty acid synthesis in the liver.

3. As the liver takes up the fatty acids and degrades them to acetyl-CoA, the capacity of the citric acid cycle to process the resulting acetyl-CoA molecules decreases. This is mostly because the metabolism of fatty acids to acetyl-CoA yields many ATP, and high amounts of ATP slow citric acid cycle activity in liver cells. Essentially, there is no need to use the citric acid cycle—the main role of which is to transfer energy from fuels for use in ATP synthesis—when the cells have plenty of ATP already.

These metabolic changes encourage the liver cells to form acetyl-CoA and then unite two acetyl-CoA molecules to form a four-carbon compound. This compound is further metabolized and eventually secreted into the bloodstream as the ketone bodies acetoacetic acid and related compounds, beta-hydroxybutyric acid and acetone.

Most ketone bodies are subsequently converted back into acetyl CoA in other body cells, which use the ketone bodies for fuel. The acetyl-CoA is then pushed through the citric acid cycle. One of the ketone bodies formed (acetone) leaves the body via the lungs, giving the breath of a person in ketosis a characteristic, fruity smell.[9]

Ketosis in Semistarvation or Fasting

When a person is in a state of semistarvation or fasting, carbohydrate availability falls, and so insulin production falls. This fall in blood insulin then causes fatty acids to

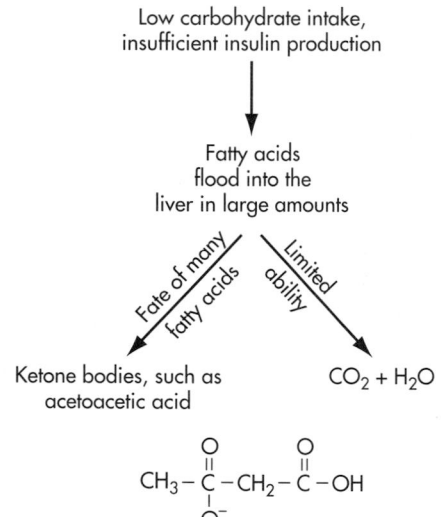

Low carbohydrate intake, insufficient insulin production

↓

Fatty acids flood into the liver in large amounts

Fate of many fatty acids / *Limited ability*

Ketone bodies, such as acetoacetic acid $CO_2 + H_2O$

$$CH_3 - \overset{O}{\underset{\underset{O^-}{|}}{C}} - CH_2 - \overset{O}{C} - OH$$

Acetoacetic acid

Key steps in ketosis.

flood into the bloodstream and eventually form ketone bodies. The heart, muscles, and some parts of the kidneys then use ketones for fuel. After a few days of ketosis, the brain also begins to metabolize ketones for energy.

This is an important adaptive response to semistarvation or fasting. As more body cells begin to use ketone bodies for fuel, the need for glucose as a body fuel diminishes. This then reduces the need for the liver and kidneys to produce glucose from amino acids (and the glycerol released from lipolysis), sparing much body protein from being used as a fuel source. The maintenance of body protein mass is a key to survival in semistarvation or fasting. Death is seen when about half of the body protein is depleted, usually coming after about 50 to 70 days of total fasting. In prolonged fasting, about half of the energy needs are met by the use of ketone bodies; only 5 percent of energy use comes from glucose that was made from amino acids.[9]

Ketosis in Diabetes Can Be Especially Harmful

In type 1 diabetes, little to no insulin is produced. This lack of insulin does not allow for normal carbohydrate and fat metabolism. Without sufficient insulin and the related inability to readily utilize carbohydrate, excess production of ketone bodies occurs, as just noted. If the concentration of ketone bodies rises too high in the blood, the excess spills into the urine, pulling sodium and potassium ions with it. Eventually severe ion imbalances occur in the body. The blood also becomes more acidic because the two major ketone bodies contain acid groups. The resulting condition, known as *diabetic ketoacidosis (DKA)*, can induce coma or death if not treated immediately with insulin, fluids, and electrolytes (see Chapter 5 for more details). The problem usually occurs only in ketosis caused by uncontrolled diabetes; in fasting, blood concentrations of ketone bodies usually do not rise very high.[9]

■ LIPOGENESIS: BUILDING FATTY ACIDS

Lipogenesis is the formation of lipid. The majority of the pathways used are found in the cytoplasm of liver cells. Ingested glucose or protein that the body does not use immediately can be converted into triglycerides and stored as such. Most carbohydrate is stored as glycogen, but the total amount rarely exceeds 350 g. Some protein resides in amino acid pools in the body, but the amount is not significant. Thus, when a lot of glucose and amino acids are left over in the body after a large meal, some of their carbons can be used to synthesize fatty acids. This process requires ATP and the B vitamins biotin, niacin, and pantothenic acid. Since ATP is used, lipogenesis is an energy-losing proposition for a liver cell.

In lipogenesis, the liver begins with carbons from glucose and the carbons from amino acids that are metabolized to acetyl-CoA. Cells in the liver bond the acetate parts of acetyl-CoA molecules (actually in the form of **malonyl-CoA**) together in a series of steps to form a 16-carbon saturated fatty acid, palmitic acid. Insulin increases activity of a key enzyme used in the pathway (fatty acid synthase).[11] This 16-carbon fatty acid can later be lengthened to an 18- or 20-carbon chain, which occurs in the cytosol or mitochondria. Ultimately, the fatty acids are joined to a form of glycerol (produced during glycolysis from glyceraldehyde 3-phosphate) to yield a triglyceride. The triglyceride is later released to the general circulation as a very-low-density lipoprotein, or VLDL (see Chapter 6). Cells that take up fat may use it for ATP production, or it may be stored in fat cells, along with other fats that originate from dietary intake.

The use of a very low carbohydrate diet to induce ketosis for weight loss is covered in Chapters 5 and 13. Note for now that such diets have not been known to be effective in the long term and can lead to many health problems, especially if followed for more than 4 to 6 weeks or by certain individuals, such as children. Another time in which ketosis is dangerous is during pregnancy (see Chapter 16).

lipogenesis The building of fatty acids using derivatives of acetyl-CoA.

malonyl-CoA Building block in fatty acid synthesis: $HO - \overset{O}{\underset{||}{C}} - CH_2 - \overset{O}{\underset{||}{C}} - \text{Coenzyme A}$

CRITICAL THINKING

Stephanie begins a new diet program in which she can eat unlimited amounts of carbohydrate and protein but only very small amounts of fat. Stephanie believes that, if she eats no fat, she can gain no fat. Is this true? How would you explain the body processes that relate to this diet theory?

CASE SCENARIO
Follow-Up

A very-low-carbohydrate diet leads to ketosis because such a diet reduces insulin secretion by the pancreas. This then results in a decrease in the insulin/glucagon ratio, which in turn creates a catabolic state in the body. Triglycerides in the adipose cells break down to yield fatty acids; these flood out of the adipose cells into the bloodstream and are taken up by the liver. The liver metabolizes the fatty acids to ketone bodies and releases these ketone bodies into the bloodstream. Complete metabolism of the fatty acids to CO_2 and H_2O is not possible, as this would yield so much ATP that many enzymes that are part of citric acid cycle activity in the cell would be inhibited. Partial metabolism of fatty acids to ketone bodies yields some ATP for the liver cells, but not so much ATP that such problems arise. Eventually, the blood concentration of ketone bodies then begins to rise. In essence, anything that can lead to a long-term reduction in insulin output causes ketosis. This is seen with very-low-carbohydrate diets (as mentioned), as well as in prolonged fasting and uncontrolled type 1 diabetes.

Glutamic acid

Carbon skeleton (alpha-ketoglutaric acid)

CONCEPT CHECK

Fatty acids are degraded into numerous acetyl-CoA molecules. These molecules participate in the citric acid cycle and electron transport chain to yield carbon dioxide, water, and ATP. To synthesize fat, a cell binds numerous acetate molecules together to form a fatty acid. Three fatty acids can then be joined to glycerol to yield a triglyceride. If acetyl-CoA oxidation in liver cells is limited, such as in cases of long-term fasting, the acetyl-CoA resulting from fatty acid oxidation tends to force the production of ketone bodies. These ketone bodies enter the bloodstream and are eventually metabolized to carbon dioxide and water (after being converted back to acetyl-CoA) by various cells.

■ PROTEIN METABOLISM

Protein metabolism begins after proteins are degraded into amino acids. To use an amino acid for fuel, cells must first split off the amino group ($-NH_2$) (see Chapter 7). These pathways often require vitamin B-6 to function. Removal of the amino group produces carbon skeletons, which mostly enter the citric acid cycle. Some carbon skeletons also yield acetyl-CoA or pyruvate (Fig.4-10).[11]

Amino acid metabolism mostly takes place in the liver. Only branched-chain amino acids—leucine, isoleucine, and valine—are metabolized primarily at other sites—in this case, the muscles. As you will see in future chapters, this knowledge has applications. Branched-chain amino acids are added to some liquid meal replacement supplements given to hospitalized patients. Some fluid replacement formulas marketed to athletes also contain branched-chain amino acids (see Chapter 14).

It is important to note that some carbon skeletons enter the citric acid cycle as acetyl-CoA, whereas others form intermediates of the citric acid cycle or glycolysis. Any part of the carbon skeleton that can bypass acetyl-CoA and enter the citric acid cycle directly or form pyruvate can eventually become part of glucose via gluconeogenesis. Such is true for the amino acids alanine, methionine, arginine, histidine, aspartic acid, and others (see Chapter 7).

■ Gluconeogenesis: Producing New Glucose Molecules from Amino Acids and Other Compounds

The entire gluconeogenesis pathway is present only in liver cells and in certain kidney cells. The starting material for gluconeogenesis is oxaloacetate, which is derived primarily from the carbon skeletons of some amino acids, mostly the amino acid alanine. Pyruvate can also be converted to oxaloacetate (review Fig. 4-10).

The four-carbon oxaloacetate loses one carbon dioxide and converts to a three-carbon compound, which then reverses the path back through glycolysis to glucose. It takes two three-carbon compounds to produce the six-carbon glucose. Some steps in gluconeogenesis are simply a reversal or variation of the glycolysis pathway. This entire process requires ATP as well as coenzyme forms of the B vitamins biotin, riboflavin, niacin, and B-6.

To learn more about gluconeogenesis, let's trace the pathway by converting glutamic acid, an amino acid, to glucose in Figure 4-10. Glutamic acid is first deaminated to form its carbon skeleton, which enters the citric acid cycle directly and is converted by stages to oxaloacetate. Oxaloacetate loses one carbon as carbon dioxide, and the three-carbon compound produced then moves through glycolysis to help form glucose. Eventually, two glutamic acid molecules are needed to form one glucose molecule. Dr. Michael Keenan, in his Expert Opinion, discusses why the same synthesis of glucose is not possible using fatty acids.

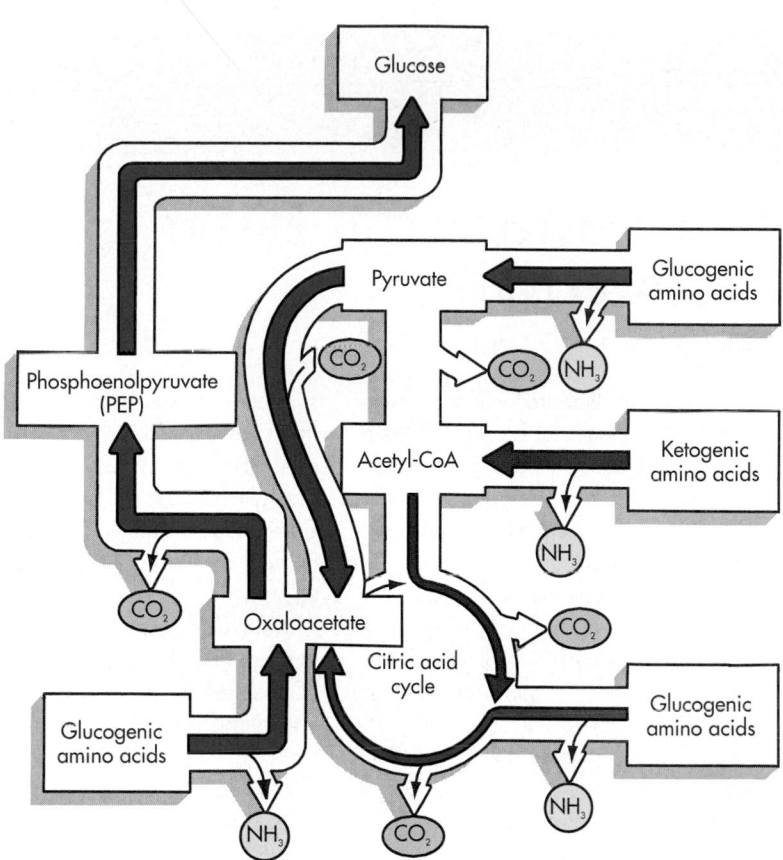

FIGURE 4-10 Gluconeogenesis. Carbon skeletons of amino acids that enter directly into the citric acid cycle (such amino acids include asparagine, arginine, aspartic acid, histidine, glutamic acid, glutamine, isoleucine, methionine, proline, valine, phenylalanine, and tryptophan) or become pyruvate (such as alanine, glycine, cysteine, serine, and threonine) are called *glucogenic amino acids* because these carbons can become the carbons of glucose. Any parts of carbon skeletons that become acetyl-CoA are called *ketogenic* because these carbons cannot become parts of glucose molecules. The deciding factor is whether part or all of the carbon skeleton of the amino acid yields a "new" oxaloacetate molecule during metabolism, two of which are needed to form glucose.

The only part of a triglyceride that can become glucose is the glycerol portion. Propionyl-CoA formed from the metabolism of odd-chain fatty acids can do the same, as mentioned earlier. Glycerol enters into the glycolysis pathway, and propionyl-CoA can directly enter the citric acid cycle at succinyl-CoA. Propionyl-CoA can then flow through the citric acid cycle and through the process of gluconeogenesis to convert to glucose. Glycerol can follow the gluconeogenesis pathway from glyceraldehyde 3-phosphate to glucose. Glucose yield from these compounds is insignificant, however, since the body produces little propionyl-CoA and only about 10% of the molecular weight of a triglyceride is glycerol.[11]

Recall from the earlier discussion on ketosis that, if there is an insufficient amount of carbohydrate in the body to meet ongoing needs, the liver and kidneys are forced to synthesize glucose from body protein to support the energy needs of the brain and red blood cells. Liver and kidney cells primarily begin with carbon skeletons from amino acids that are able to directly enter the citric acid cycle or form pyruvate. These compounds are converted to oxaloacetate, then to a three-carbon intermediate compound, phosphoenolpyruvate, and finally to glucose.[8]

▪ Disposing of Excess Amino Groups from Amino Acid Metabolism

The catabolism of amino acids yields amino groups ($-NH_2$), which then form ammonia (NH_3). The ammonia is excreted because its buildup is toxic to cells. The liver prepares the amino groups for excretion in the urine using the urea cycle. During the urea cycle, two nitrogen groups—one ammonia group and one amino group—react through a series of steps with carbon dioxide molecules to form urea

$(H_2N\overset{O}{\overset{\|}{C}}NH_2)$ and water.[11] Eventually, urea is excreted in the urine (Fig. 4-11). In liver disease, ammonia can build up to toxic concentrations in the blood, whereas in kidney disease the toxic agent is urea. The form of nitrogen in the blood—ammonia or urea—is a diagnostic tool for detecting liver or kidney disease.

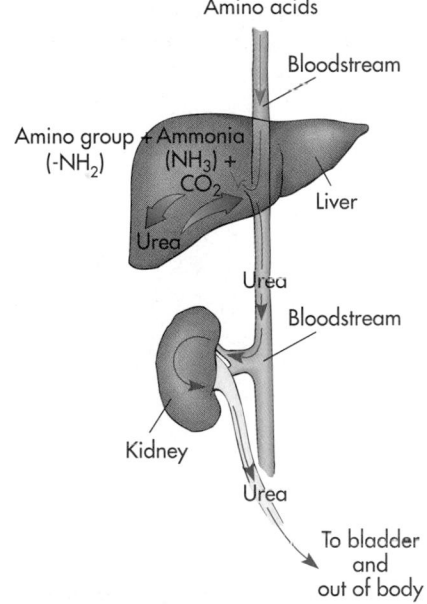

FIGURE 4-11 Disposal of excess amino groups. The nitrogen groups, one as ammonia and the other as an amino group, form part of urea, which is excreted in urine ($H_2N\overset{O}{\overset{\|}{C}}NH_2$). The nitrogen groups originally came from amino acids that went through transamination reactions and ultimately deamination to yield the free nitrogen groups.

Illustration by William Ober.

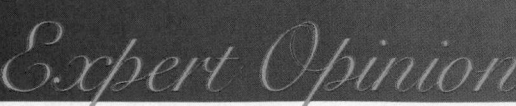

WHY IS AN UNDERSTANDING OF ENERGY METABOLISM IMPORTANT?

Michael Keenan, Ph.D.

An overall understanding of energy metabolism allows you to see the big picture of what happens in your body without getting lost in the details of a myriad of individual chemical reactions.

One of your body's highest priorities is to maintain blood glucose in a normal range, so that the central nervous system (including the brain), retina, kidneys, and smooth muscles have adequate energy. Too little blood glucose (hypoglycemia) results in not enough of an energy supply for these cells. Too much blood glucose (hyperglycemia) for a prolonged period results in too much glucose entering nerve cells and some other tissues, which in the long run can lead to cellular damage.

Except for instances of fasting for several days or so, your brain uses only glucose for energy. Most of your other organs and tissues use a combination of glucose, fatty acids, amino acids, lactic acid, and ketone bodies. Glucose and fatty acid use also spares protein from excessive use for energy needs.

Glucose is the predominant energy source of all tissues for a couple of hours after a meal, called the absorptive phase. In contrast, the major energy source for most tissues between meals, called the post-absorptive phase, is fatty acids. Dietary carbohydrate, if not already absorbed in the form of glucose, is converted under most conditions to glucose in the liver (e.g., fructose as part of sucrose and galactose as part of lactose). In the absorptive phase, glucose is either used immediately for energy or is stored as glycogen (the latter predominantly in the liver and muscle). Small amounts of glucose are also converted to fat for storage; this process especially increases as the carbohydrate content increases in the diet.

During the post-absorptive phase, blood glucose is maintained for use by the brain and other cells mainly by the breakdown of liver glycogen. However, some glucose is produced normally by gluconeogenesis, the predominant source of this glucose being glucogenic amino acids present in body proteins. If the post-ab-

sorptive phase lasts too long (about 16 hours, as when skipping breakfast), or if very little carbohydrate is present in the diet, gluconeogenesis becomes excessive. Thus, adequate amounts of dietary carbohydrate and timely consumption of food will spare body protein.

Fatty acids cannot fully spare protein because they do not provide carbons that can be used for gluconeogenesis. The reason for this is that fatty acids are catabolized to the two-carbon compound acetate. In mammalian cells, acetate cannot be converted to pyruvate or other intermediates of glycolysis, or to any citric acid cycle intermediates, and it is only compounds that are catabolized to these forms that can contribute carbons for glucose synthesis. A good example to test your understanding of metabolism is to answer the following question: How many glucose molecules could be made from a 57-carbon triglyceride? The answer is none. It would actually take two 57-carbon triglycerides to produce one glucose molecule, since it is only the three-carbon

Chapter 8 covers alcohol metabolism in detail.

CONCEPT CHECK

Individual amino acids lose an amino group and become carbon skeletons. Many carbon skeletons can be further metabolized so that they enter either the citric acid cycle or the glycolysis pathway. The carbons can then proceed through gluconeogenesis to form new glucose. If the carbon skeleton forms acetyl-CoA, glucose production is not possible from that part of the amino acid. The amino groups go on to form part of urea, which is excreted from the body in urine.

glycerol backbone of a triglyceride that can enter the glycolysis pathway. This glycerol can be used for gluconeogenesis; two glycerols provide the six carbons needed for one glucose molecule.

In contrast, all carbons from the three fatty acids become part of the two-carbon acetate (acetyl-CoA). This acetate attaches to the four-carbon oxaloacetate to become the six-carbon citric acid; this is the first step in the citric acid cycle. On its way to becoming the four-carbon succinate, citric acid loses two carbons as carbon dioxide.

Another aspect of the big picture of metabolism is that glucose is also used to replace citric acid cycle intermediates when they are removed for the biosynthesis of a variety of compounds in cells. These citric acid cycle intermediates are present in the cell mitochondria only in small (catalytic) amounts.

Keep in mind that the two components of metabolism—catabolism and anabolism—are interwoven. Metabolism could be viewed as a tree. For catabolism, arrows would be drawn downward from branches leading to the trunk, and the trunk includes glycolysis and the citric acid cycle. Anabolism would be represented by having the arrows pointing upward out of the trunk and into the branches.

One final thought to consider is the question of which of the two fuels—glucose or fatty acids—is the primary or major fuel for the body. Often, glucose is given this distinction, but this must always be qualified. Glucose is the primary fuel for the brain and several other organs, as well as for all tissues in the absorptive phase. Fatty acids are the primary fuel for most tissues during the post-absorptive phase, but glucose participates in this use of fatty acids. Glucose is the major overall fuel if you are maintaining your weight and following current dietary recommendations by eating a high-carbohydrate diet. However, if you happen to consume a low-carbohydrate diet that is high in fat, and you are not in positive energy balance, then dietary fat becomes the major overall fuel for energy. The latter condition is apparently occurring when people lose weight when they follow a currently popular diet such as "Dr. Atkin's."

However, a word of caution about some currently popular diets: "Dr. Atkin's" diet is too low in carbohydrate, and some of these low carbohydrate, moderate fat, high protein diets may not discriminate between the type of fat, saturated versus unsaturated. Some researchers currently believe that the fat in such a diet should be high in unsaturated fat, and that the percent fat consumed (30% versus 35% or maybe even 40% of total calories) is not critical as long as the fat is unsaturated and the person is not gaining weight.

Thus, an overall understanding of metabolism helps you clearly see the roles of the energy macronutrients. Carbohydrate is used for maintaining blood glucose and the efficient use of fat, and fatty acids are an important source of energy for most tissues between meals. However, fatty acids cannot completely replace carbohydrate. Protein also can be used for fuel, but its use for energy in most cases is limited by the metabolism of carbohydrate and fat for energy. Finally, carbohydrate is usually our overall primary fuel because it contributes the highest percentage of energy to our diets.

Dr. Keenan is an associate professor in the Division of Human Nutrition and Foods at the Louisiana State University in Baton Rouge, Louisiana. His research interests include the area of obesity in post-menopausal women.

■ WHAT HAPPENS WHERE—A REVIEW

Glycolysis takes place in the cytosol of a cell. The end product of glycolysis, pyruvate, enters the mitochondria, where it is further degraded in the citric acid cycle. The NADH + H⁺ made in the cytosol during glycolysis must be shuttled into the mitochondria if the electron transport chain is to be used to convert NADH + H⁺ back to NAD and simultaneously produce ATP. The type of shuttle determines how many ATP each NADH + H⁺ yields. Generally, 2.5 ATP are formed. One type of shuttle system results in the loss of one potential ATP, so only 1.5 ATP result.

Fatty acid oxidation also occurs in the mitochondria. The product of beta-oxidation, acetyl-CoA, is metabolized by the citric acid cycle in the mitochondria. Fatty acids are synthesized primarily in the cytosol.

"Feasting" encourages

   Glycogen synthesis
   Protein synthesis
   Fat synthesis
   Urea synthesis

"Fasting" encourages

   Glycogen breakdown
   Fat breakdown
   Gluconeogenesis
   Synthesis of ketone bodies

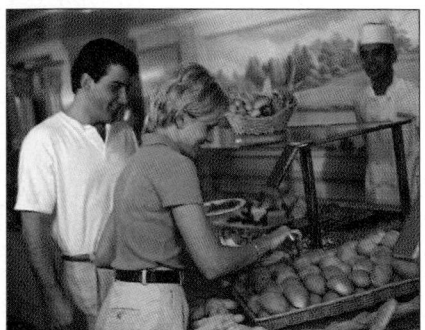

"Feasting" encourages the synthesis of glycogen, protein, and fat.

Gluconeogenesis begins in the mitochondria with the production of oxaloacetate. Oxaloacetate eventually returns to the cytosol, where new glucose is produced. The same is true for the urea cycle; some stages occur in the cytosol and some in the mitochondria (Fig. 4-12).

Since the electron transport chain yields most of the ATP for the cell, the mitochondria are the cell's major energy-producing organelles. Cells that need to make a lot of ATP, such as muscle cells, have thousands of mitochondria, whereas cells that need very little ATP, such as adipose cells, have fewer mitochondria.[11]

Energy metabolism can take many forms in the body. By stringing together the glycolysis pathway and the citric acid cycle, cells can convert carbohydrates into fatty acids, convert carbohydrates into carbon skeletons for synthesis of certain amino acids, and use the energy in carbohydrates to form ATP (see Fig. 4-12). These pathways can also turn carbon skeletons from one amino acid into carbon skeletons of another. Furthermore, they can convert carbon skeletons from amino acids to glucose or have them drive ATP synthesis. Finally, fatty acids can provide energy for ATP synthesis or produce ketones, and the glycerol part of the triglyceride can either be converted into glucose or contribute to ATP synthesis (Table 4-1).

"Feasting," with the resultant increased insulin production by the pancreas, encourages the synthesis of glycogen, protein, and fat. Urea synthesis also increases in response to using some of the protein for fuel. "Fasting," with the resultant fall in insulin production, encourages gluconeogenesis, fat and protein breakdown and production of ketone bodies; however, this is not the only time that production of ketone bodies can occur.

Acetyl-CoA plays a central role in energy metabolism. As noted before, no matter what type of diet you eat—high-carbohydrate, high-protein, or high-fat—almost all pathways that contribute to ATP synthesis include acetyl-CoA at one point.[5]

FIGURE 4-12 A bird's-eye view of cell metabolism. Note that acetyl-CoA forms a crossroads for many pathways and that the citric acid cycle can also be used to help build compounds, such as certain amino acids. Anabolic and catabolic processes may appear to share the same pathways, but generally this is true for only a few steps. Separate enzymes control anabolic and catabolic flow in a pathway. This allows the cell significant control over metabolism, since a specific set of enzymes can be activated to promote either anabolism or catabolism. If the chemical reactions in anabolism and catabolism were catalyzed by the same set of enzymes, the direction of flow of compounds through these pathways would be dictated exclusively by the concentration of the starting materials, rather than by the cell's changing needs for energy or synthesis of needed compounds.
Illustration by William Ober.

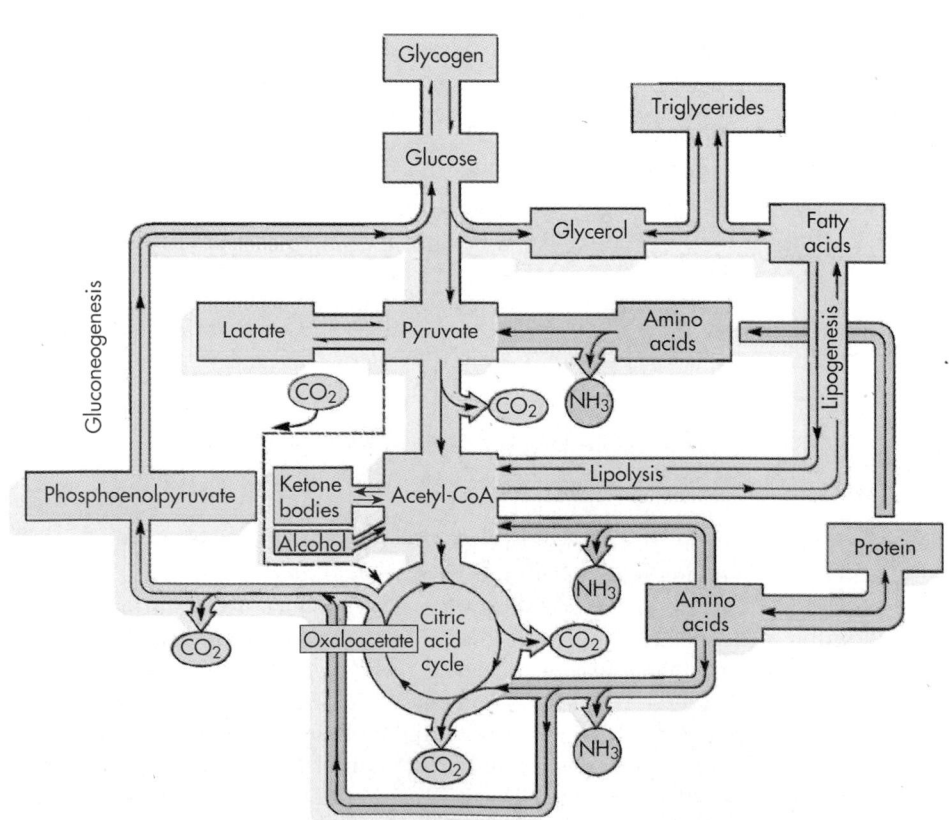

■ REGULATING METABOLISM

Metabolism is regulated by various means. Enzymes are the key regulators for metabolic pathways; both their presence and their rate of activity are critical to chemical reactions in the body. Enzyme synthesis and rates of activity are controlled by cells and by the products of the reactions in which the enzymes participate.[11] For example, diets rich in protein lead to increased synthesis of enzymes associated with amino acid catabolism and gluconeogenesis. Within hours after a shift to a high-carbohydrate diet, synthesis of these enzymes slows.

Hormones, including insulin, glucagon, and epinephrine, also serve as regulators of metabolic processes. Blood glucose concentration is one parameter under their widespread influence.[10]

ATP concentration in a cell regulates metabolism. High ATP concentrations decrease energy-yielding reactions such as glycolysis and promote synthetic reactions such as lipogenesis, which use ATP. High ADP concentrations, on the other hand, stimulate energy-yielding pathways.[4]

A final factor in regulating metabolism is the liver because it contains such a variety of enzymes and because most nutrients pass through it, providing an opportunity for metabolic control (Fig. 4-13).

TABLE 4-1   Summary of energy-yielding nutrient metabolism

Nutrient in Diet	Contributes to Energy Needs	Yields Glucose?	Yields Amino Acids for Body Proteins?	Yields Fat Stores?	Energy Cost of Conversion to Fat Stores
Carbohydrate (glucose)	Yes	Yes	Yes, when amino groups are available, can yield nonessential (dispensable) amino acids	Yes, but not readily	High
Lipid (triglycerides)	Yes	Generally not; the glycerol present provides a minimal amount	No	Yes	Minimal
Protein (amino acids)	Yes, but generally not much	Yes, when sufficient carbohydrate is not available	Yes	Yes	High

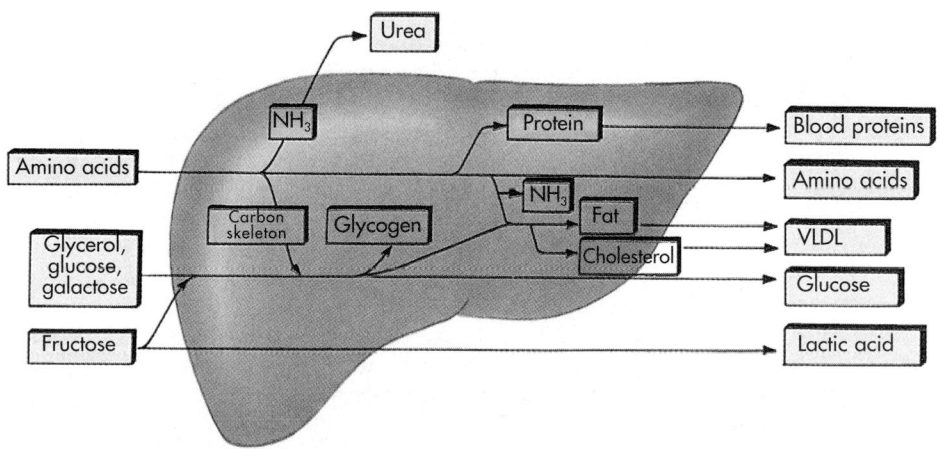

FIGURE 4-13 The liver is the location of many nutrient interconversions. Most nutrients must pass first through the liver after absorption into the body. What leaves the liver is often different from what entered. Key metabolic functions of the liver include monosaccharide conversion, fat and cholesterol synthesis, production of ketone bodies, amino acid metabolism, urea production, and alcohol metabolism. Nutrient storage is an additional liver function. VLDL stands for very-low-density lipoprotein. This carries fat from the liver to other body cells (see Chapter 6 for details).
Illustration by William Ober.

■ EPILOGUE

Figure 4-12 summarized the major pathways you have seen. Don't be surprised if it takes you some time to grasp it thoroughly. It illustrates a complicated system with much activity. Study it part by part. Consider reading this chapter again tomorrow and maybe again in 2 or 3 days until it begins to fit together.

You now know more about what happens in a cell and what vitamins and minerals contribute to these functions. You can see how the B vitamins thiamin, niacin, riboflavin, biotin, pantothenic acid, and vitamin B-6, as well as the minerals magnesium, iron, and copper, play important roles in the metabolic pathways (Fig. 4-14). This introduction sets the stage for Chapters 9 through 12. You can use this knowledge to debunk fad diet claims, such as the touted long-term safety of very-low-carbohydrate diets for weight loss.

Future classes in nutrition, nursing, biology, physiology, biochemistry, pharmacology, and medicine all build on this knowledge of metabolism. This chapter serves as a building block for those later courses.

Check out the *Perspectives in Nutrition* web site
http://www.mhhe.com/wardlaw
for quizzes, flash cards, other activities, and web links designed to further help you learn about metabolism.

CONCEPT CHECK

Glycolysis takes place in the cytosol of the cell; the citric acid cycle and electron transport chain occur in the mitochondria. Fatty acid oxidation occurs in the mitochondria; fatty acids are synthesized mostly in the cytosol. The urea cycle and gluconeogenesis take place in both the mitochondria and the cytosol. Hormone balance, enzyme activity, and the need for ATP all influence the rate at which these metabolic pathways operate. Since many metabolic pathways converge at acetyl-CoA, it is central to energy metabolism.

■ SUMMARY

1. ATP is the major form of energy used for cellular metabolism. As ATP breaks down to ADP plus Pi, energy is released from the broken bond. This energy is used to pump ions, promote enzyme activity, and contract and later relax muscles. All energy available to humans ultimately comes from the sun as solar energy. Plants capture solar energy by way of photosynthesis. In humans, metabolic pathways make it possible to extract energy from food and transform it into ATP; in the process, some energy is lost as heat.

2. In glycolysis, glucose is degraded into two pyruvate molecules, yielding NADH + H+ (a form of potential energy) and ATP. Pyruvate can proceed through other aerobic pathways to form carbon dioxide and water. Pyruvate also can react with NADH + H+ in an anaerobic pathway to form lactate. Both pathways allow NADH + H+ to eventually be re-formed into NAD, which is needed for glycolysis to continue.

3. In the citric acid cycle, acetyl-CoA is formed from pyruvate. A carbon dioxide molecule is released in the process. Acetyl-CoA then undergoes many metabolic conversions, eventually yielding two more carbon dioxide molecules. In this way, the citric acid cycle accepts two carbons from acetyl-CoA and yields two carbons as carbon dioxide. In the process, NADH + H+, FADH$_2$, and a form of energy that can yield ATP directly (GTP) are formed. The NADH + H+ and FADH$_2$ then enter the electron transport chain to yield numerous ATP molecules. Water forms as oxygen combines with the electrons and hydro-

gen ions (released from NADH + H+ and FADH$_2$) in the electron transport chain.

4. In fatty acid oxidation, two-carbon fragments are cleaved from a fatty acid, producing multiple acetyl-CoA molecules. These enter the citric acid cycle and electron transport chain, as did the acetyl-CoA that arose from carbohydrate breakdown, to yield ATP, carbon dioxide, and water. In fat synthesis, acetate molecules in effect are combined to yield a fatty acid, primarily the 16-carbon palmitic acid. These fatty acids can then react with a form of glycerol to produce a triglyceride.

5. During starvation and uncontrolled diabetes, more acetyl-CoA is produced in the liver than can be metabolized to carbon dioxide and water. This excess acetyl-CoA is synthesized into ketone bodies, which flood into the bloodstream and are metabolized by other tissues, such as nervous tissue.

6. Amino acids lose their amino group and become carbon skeletons. These can be metabolized to other compounds that enter the citric acid cycle, eventually yielding energy for ATP synthesis. Some carbon skeletons can be formed into oxaloacetate, an intermediate found in the citric acid cycle, which in turn can be used to form glucose. Converting the carbon skeletons of amino acids to glucose is part of a process known as gluconeogenesis. Acetyl-CoA molecules, and thus fatty acids in general, cannot participate in gluconeogenesis.

7. Glycolysis takes place in the cytosol of a cell, whereas the citric acid cycle and the electron transport chain take place in the

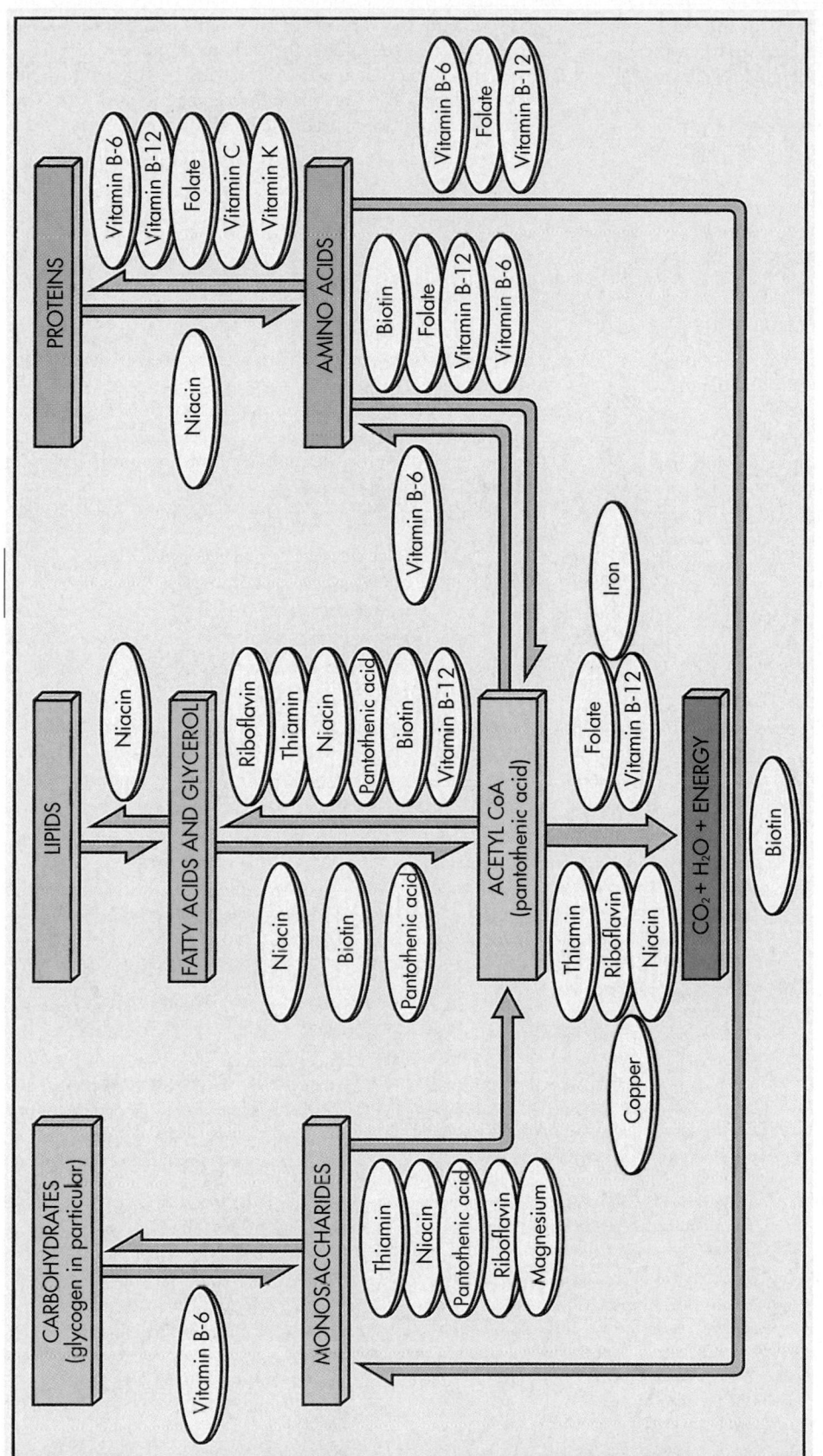

■ **FIGURE 4-14** Many vitamins and minerals participate in the metabolic pathways. Most notable are the B vitamins thiamin, riboflavin, niacin, pantothenic acid, biotin, vitamin B-6, folate, and vitamin B-12, as well as the minerals iron and copper. Many systematic health problems can develop from nutrient deficiencies, since so many metabolic pathways depend on nutrient input.

Illustration by William Ober.

mitochondria. Fatty acid oxidation takes place in the mitochondria, and fatty acids for the most part are synthesized in the cytosol. The synthesis of urea and the pathway for gluconeogenesis both take place partly in the cytosol and partly in the mitochondria. Urea is made in the liver, while glucose is made in the liver and kidneys.

8. Acetyl-CoA is pivotal in cell metabolism because carbohydrates, proteins, amino acids, fatty acids, and alcohol all can yield acetyl-CoA during their metabolism. The coordination of various metabolic pathways for food fuels allows the carbons of glucose to become the carbons of fatty acids and the carbons of some amino acids to become the carbons of glucose.

9. The vitamins thiamin, niacin, riboflavin, biotin, pantothenic acid, and vitamin B-6 and the minerals magnesium, iron, and copper play important roles in the metabolic pathways.

■ STUDY QUESTIONS

1. Many vitamins and minerals are used in energy metabolism. Identify three vitamins and/or minerals and describe their roles in ATP synthesis.
2. For what purposes do cells use ATP energy?
3. Explain how the ATP concentration is maintained in a cell. What is the key stimulus to ATP production?
4. What is the "common denominator" compound of the many pathways of energy metabolism (citric acid cycle, glycolysis, beta-oxidation, etc.)? Why is it considered important in the body's chemical processes?
5. What is lactate and how and where is it formed in the cell? Which tissues produce the most lactate? Why?
6. Trace the steps in gluconeogenesis from body protein to the formation of glucose.
7. What is the meaning of the phrase "fats burn in a fire of carbohydrate"?
8. List the metabolic processes discussed throughout this chapter and their location in the cell.
9. Describe the reason why most fatty acids do not turn into glucose in the body.
10. Explain how physicians can use certain aspects of protein metabolism to diagnose kidney or liver disease.

■ ANNOTATED REFERENCES

1. Giles WH and others: Association between total homocyst(e)ine and the likelihood for a history of acute myocardial infarction by race and ethnicity: Results from the Third National Health and Nutrition Examination Survey. *American Heart Journal* 139:466, 2000.

   There is almost a two-fold increased likelihood of heart attack among people with elevated blood homocysteine. This was seen in people of various races and ethnicity in the United States.

2. Hark L, Deen D: Taking a nutrition history: A practical approach for family physicians. *American Family Physician* 59:1521, 1999.

   In a nutrition history, a person should be asked about the number of meals and snacks eaten in a 24-hour period, dining-out habits, and frequency of consumption of fruits, vegetables, meats, poultry, fish, dairy products, and desserts. Improvements in nutritional status can be measured using body weight, blood pressure, and laboratory test data.

3. Kovacevich DS and others: Nutrition risk classification: A reproducible and valid tool for nurses. *Nutrition in Clinical Practice* 12:20, 1997.

   Factors to consider in nutrition assessment include the presence of current diseases, such as diabetes or kidney disease; evidence of diarrhea, vomiting, or reduced food intake; and recent weight loss. Together, these predict health outcomes in hospitalized patients.

4. Mayes PA: Bioenergetics: The role of ATP. In Murray RK and others (eds.): *Harper's biochemistry*. 25th ed. Stamford, CT: Appleton & Lange, 2000.

   ATP is a high-energy compound due to its chemical structure. The great amount of energy released on breakdown of ATP to ADP and Pi is due to the relief of the repulsion between phosphate groups. ATP acts as the "energy currency" of the cell, transferring energy from substances of higher energy potential to those of lower energy potential.

5. Mayes PA: Overview of intermediary metabolism. In Murray RK and others (eds.): *Harper's biochemistry*. 25th ed. Stamford, CT: Appleton & Lange, 2000.

   In the breakdown of carbohydrate, proteins, and fat for energy needs, all the pathways lead to the production of acetyl-CoA.

6. Mayes PA: The citric acid cycle: The catabolism of acetyl-CoA. In Murray RK and others (eds.): *Harper's biochemistry*. 25th ed. Stamford, CT: Appleton & Lange, 2000.

   The citric acid cycle is a series of reactions in the mitochondria that brings about the catabolism of acetyl-CoA, liberating hydrogen ions. Upon oxidation, these hydrogen ions lead to the release of most of the available energy of tissue fuels and eventual capture as ATP.

7. Mayes PK: Glycolysis and the oxidation of pyruvate. In Murray RK and others (eds.): *Harper's biochemistry*. 25th ed. Stamford, CT: Appleton & Lange, 2000.

   Glycolysis is the pathway found in cells for the metabolism of glucose (or glycogen) to pyruvate or lactate. It can function in regenerating NAD through the coupling of the metabolism of pyruvate to lactate. Thus, lactate is the end product of glycolysis under anaerobic conditions.

8. Mayes PA: Gluconeogenesis and the control of blood glucose. In Murray RK and others (eds.): *Harper's biochemistry*. 25th ed. Stamford, CT: Appleton & Lange, 2000.

   Gluconeogenesis meets the needs of the body for glucose when carbohydrate is not available in sufficient amounts from the diet. A continuous supply of glucose is necessary as a source of energy, especially for the nervous system and the red blood cells. Glucagon, and to a lesser extent epinephrine, stimulates gluconeogenesis in the liver.

9. Mayes PK: Oxidation of fatty acids: Ketogenesis. In Murray RK and others (eds.): *Harper's biochemistry*. 25th ed. Stamford, CT: Appleton & Lange, 2000.

Ketosis does not occur unless there is an increase in the level of circulating free fatty acids in the bloodstream. These free fatty acids are the precursors of ketone bodies made by the liver. Therefore, the factors regulating mobilization of free fatty acids from adipose tissue are important in controlling ketogenesis, such as the insulin/glucagon ratio.

10. McGrane M: Carbohydrate metabolism—Synthesis and oxidation. In Spintanuk MH (ed.): *Biochemical and physiological aspects of human nutrition*. Philadelphia: W. B. Saunders, 2000.

Glycolysis releases energy present in carbohydrates and stores this in the high-energy phosphate bonds of ATP. Glycolysis, however, provides a minor percentage of the ATP produced when compared with a complete oxidation of glucose to CO_2 and H_2O in the citric acid cycle and electron transport chain.

11. Nelson DL, Cox MM: *Lehninger Principles of Biochemistry*. 3rd edition, Worth Publishers, New York, NY 2000.

Principles of Biochemistry is a comprehensive look at the subject. Many of the concepts in this chapter are discussed in greater detail in Principles of Biochemistry. One new concept is the lower yield of ATP from glucose and fatty acid metabolism compared to what was projected in previous editions of the book. For example, classically the ATP yielded from complete metabolism of glucose was thought to be 36 to 38 ATP. Currently a closer estimate is 30 to 32 ATP. The higher numbers could be considered the theoretical maximum, while the lower numbers more consistent with actual experimental results.

12. Schneider SM, Hebuterne X: Use of nutritional scores to predict clinical outcomes in chronic diseases. *Nutrition Reviews* 58(2): 31, 2000.

Factors such as low blood albumin and weight loss are strong predictors of poor health outcomes in hospitalized patients. These are important nutrition assessment parameters to be evaluated along with other, more sophisticated tests.

13. Souba, WW: Nutrition support. *The New England Journal of Medicine* 336:41, 1997.

The simplest way to screen people for malnutrition is to ask them about unintentional weight loss. Low blood albumin at the time of hospitalization also can predict death and length of stay.

14. Stampfer MJ and others: Primary prevention of coronary heart disease in women through diet and lifestyle. *New England Journal of Medicine* 343:16, 2000.

Women who consume a varied diet (one rich in fiber, includes some fish, and is low in fried foods and animal fat), avoid overweight, drink small amounts of alcohol, exercise on a daily basis for about 30 minutes, and avoid smoking reduce their risk of heart disease by over 80%, compared with women without these habits.

15. Willinek WA and others: High–normal serum homocysteine concentrations are associated with an increased risk of early atherosclerotic carotid artery wall lesions in healthy subjects. *Journal of Hypertension* 18:425, 2000.

Moderate increases in blood homocysteine are common in the general population. This has been linked to premature development of heart disease.

TAKE ACTION

I. PUT YOUR KNOWLEDGE OF METABOLISM INTO PRACTICE

A friend is very overweight and describes to you his method of weight loss. He fasted completely for 1 week and then initiated a strict diet of 400 to 600 kcal/day under a physician's supervision. The food energy comes from a liquid formula, which he drinks for breakfast. He skips lunch and eats a small dinner of 3 ounces of protein, 1/2 cup of vegetables, 1 cup of fruit, and two starch items (a small potato, a piece of bread, etc.). He has lost approximately 25 pounds in 12 weeks.

Based on your knowledge of energy metabolism, answer the following questions he poses:

1. During the fasting stage, what were the likely sources of energy for the body's cells? What metabolic processes occurred to provide glucose for red blood cells? brain? kidneys?
2. During the restrictive phase, how did the metabolic processes in the body most likely change from the fasting state?

Possible Answers

1. During fasting, gluconeogenesis supplied the glucose needed for the brain, red blood cells, and kidneys. The carbons used came mostly from body protein, leading to a decrease in lean body mass. Eventually, production of ketone bodies from fatty acid breakdown increased, leading to elevated ketone bodies in the blood and in turn greater use of ketone bodies by many types of body cells. Insulin output fell, leading to glycogen depletion in the liver. Fatty acids from fat stores were dumped into the bloodstream. Thus, fatty acids became the major energy-yielding fuel for the body.
2. During the restrictive phase, insulin output in the body rose as carbohydrate intake increased. This led to a reduction in production of ketone bodies and spared some body protein from being used as a source of carbons for glucose synthesis. The body switched from using primarily fat as fuel to using more of a mixture of fat and carbohydrate.

II. REINFORCE YOUR KNOWLEDGE OF METABOLISM

By this stage in your education, you have likely had a number of exposures to the topic of cell metabolism. Review your textbooks or notes from previous courses that discussed metabolism and see how the following topics were presented from the standpoint of that discipline. For example, coverage of glycolysis might have a different emphasis in a biology class than in a nutrition class.

ATP
Glycolysis
Citric acid cycle
Electron transport chain
Hormones that regulate aspects of metabolism:
    Insulin
    Glucagon
Enzyme activity

A general knowledge of metabolism will benefit you throughout a career in the sciences, whether in the health sciences or the biological sciences. Understanding metabolism especially will help you see how new developments in your field relate to cell function.

ASSESSING NUTRITIONAL HEALTH

Your knowledge of the roles that nutrients play in metabolism, coupled with your appreciation of the various metabolic pathways in cells, has a practical application—assessing nutritional health. For example, determining whether the body has a sufficient amount of certain vitamins and minerals to function efficiently uses the activities of enzymes that participate in particular metabolic pathways in cells. Overall, we ask the question whether a specific enzyme works as quickly as it should. Put another way, is there any evidence that the enzyme lacks the vitamins and mineral input needed to function at peak capacity?

In Chapter 10, you will learn that the thiamin status of the body is measured in part by determining the activity of an enzyme (specifically, transketolase) used in glucose metabolism. It is possible to isolate that enzyme from cells, such as red blood cells, and determine if it can process its starting products quickly enough. To test for this, thiamin is added to the enzyme preparation to see if this speeds the reaction rate by more than 25%. If so, we say that the red blood cells lack sufficient thiamin for the enzyme to function at maximal capacity. Presumably, the body would benefit if maximal capacity was possible.

Such metabolic evidence of nutritional state, however, is only one of many aspects examined when we assess nutritional health. Let's take a closer look at these and other parameters.

STATES OF NUTRITIONAL HEALTH

The body's overall nutritional health is determined by the sum of its **nutritional status** with respect to each needed nutrient. Three general categories of nutritional status are recognized: desirable nutrition, undernutrition, and overnutrition (Table 4-2). The common term **malnutrition** can refer to either overnutrition or undernutrition.

nutritional status The nutritional health of a person as determined by anthropometric measurements (height, weight, circumferences, and so on), biochemical measurements of nutrients or their by-products in blood and urine, a clinical (physical) examination, and a dietary analysis.

T A B L E 4-2 Categories of nutritional status with respect to iron*	
General Conditions	**Condition with Respect to Iron**
Overnutrition: nutrients consumed in excess of body needs (degree of toxicity varies for each nutrient)	Results in toxic damage to liver cells; may contribute to heart disease
Desirable nutrition: nutrients consumed to support body functions and stores of nutrients for times of increased need	Adequate liver stores of iron, adequate blood values for iron-related compounds
Undernutrition: nutrient intake does not meet nutrient needs	Many changes in body functions are associated with a decline in iron status.
Depleted tissue stores	Serum† ferritin, an iron-containing protein in the blood, drops below 12 nanograms per 100 ml (12 ng/dl).‡
Reduced biochemical function (biochemical lesion)	Hemoglobin, an iron-containing pigment in the red blood cells, drops below 11 g/dl.
Clinical signs and symptoms (clinical lesion)	Pale complexion; greatly increased heart rate during activity; "spooning" of the nails in a severe deficiency; poor body temperature regulation, diminished learning capacity in children

*This general scheme can apply to all nutrients. Iron was chosen because you are likely to be familiar with this nutrient.

†Serum is the liquid portion of blood present after the blood clots and is then centrifuged.

‡dl stands for 100 ml; d stands for deci- or 100.

■ Desirable Nutrition

The nutritional status for a particular nutrient is desirable when body tissues have enough of the nutrient to support normal metabolic functions as well as surplus stores that can be mobilized in times of increased need. A desirable nutritional state can be achieved by obtaining essential nutrients from a variety of foods.

■ Undernutrition

When nutrient intake does not meet nutrient needs, stores of nutrients soon become depleted by ongoing body use, some sooner than others. This results in **undernutrition.** The demand for these nutrients exists partly because much of the body is in a constant state of turnover. Cells lining the intestinal tract, for example, are replaced every 2 to 5 days, and red blood cells live only about 120 days. To support this turnover, body stores may be sufficient to compensate for an inadequate diet for a brief time, but serious problems can arise from an inadequate diet in the long run. Some women in the United States, for example, do not consume sufficient iron and eventually deplete their iron stores. Reduced biochemical functions and ultimately clinical signs and clinical symptoms of an iron deficiency can develop (see Table 4-2).

Reduced Biochemical Functions

Once nutrient stores are depleted, a continuing nutritional deficit drains body tissues further. The body can only compensate to a certain point. When tissue concentrations of an essential nutrient fall sufficiently low, the body's metabolic processes eventually slow down or even stop. This response results from a **biochemical lesion,** which develops in response to the nutrient deficiency. Diminished **enzyme** function often is the cause of the slowdown in biochemical function as discussed in the introduction of this Nutrition Perspective. This type of nutrient deficiency is termed **subclinical** because there are no signs or symptoms. At the subclinical stage for poor iron status, low concentrations of hemoglobin (a red blood cell protein) are found in the blood because the synthesis of hemoglobin requires iron.

Clinical Signs and Symptoms

If a biochemical deficit becomes severe, clinical signs and symptoms eventually develop and become outwardly apparent. It is then possible to note **clinical lesions** in the body, perhaps in the skin, hair, nails, tongue, or eyes. In the case of an iron deficiency, the complexion may become very pale in Caucasians, and the heart rate of an affected person can increase greatly during even moderate activity.

■ Overnutrition

Prolonged consumption of more nutrients than the body needs can lead to **overnutrition.** In the short run—for instance, a few weeks or months—overnutrition may cause no signs or symptoms. But keep it up and some nutrients may increase to toxic amounts, espcially in genetically predisposed people. This can lead to serious disease. Iron overload, for example, can result in liver failure, and too much vitamin A can have negative effects, particularly in children and pregnant women. The most common type of overnutrition—excess intake of energy-yielding nutrients—is a principal cause of obesity. Note that this problem is reaching epidemic proportions in the Western world, including in the United States (see Chapter 13). In the long run, obesity can lead to serious diseases, such as type 2 diabetes and various forms of cancer.

For most vitamins and minerals, the gap between desirable intake and overnutrition is wide. Therefore, even if people take a typical multiple vitamin and mineral supplement daily, they probably won't receive a harmful amount of any nutrient. The gap between optimal intake and overnutrition is narrowest for vitamin A and vitamin D, as well as calcium, iron, copper, and other minerals. In very high doses, vitamin B-6 and the vitamin niacin can cause health problems. Thus, if you take nutrient supplements, keep a close eye on your total vitamin and mineral intake both from food and from supplements to avoid toxicity (see Chapter 9 for further advice on the use of nutrient supplements).

---

malnutrition Failing health that results from long-standing dietary practices that do not coincide with nutritional needs.

undernutrition Failing health that results from a long-standing dietary intake that does not meet nutritional needs.

A sign is a feature visible on examination, such as flaky skin. A symptom is a change in body function that is not necessarily apparent to an examiner. An example is stomach pain.

biochemical lesion An indication of reduced biochemical function (e.g., low concentrations of nutrient by-products or enzyme activities in the blood or urine) resulting from a nutritional deficiency.

enzyme A compound that speeds the rate of a chemical reaction but is not altered by the chemical reaction. Almost all enzymes are proteins.

clinical lesion A sign seen on physical examination or a symptom perceived by the patient resulting from a nutritional deficiency.

overnutrition A state in which nutritional intake exceeds the body's needs.

At the beginning of the twentieth century, undernutrition was the main concern of nutrition scientists. Today, the major nutritional problems in the United States and in most developed countries are the result of overnutrition, principally caused by excess intake of energy, saturated and total fat, and sodium. Some people are especially susceptible to ill health when they consume too much saturated fat and sodium. Furthermore, because of the increasing use of vitamin and mineral supplements in recent years, many forms of vitamin and mineral overnutrition have now become a concern.

HOW COULD YOUR NUTRITIONAL STATE BE MEASURED?

To find out how nutritionally fit *you* are, a nutrition assessment—either whole or in part—needs to be performed (Table 4-3).

■ Analyzing Background Factors

Since family history plays an important role in determining nutritional and health status, it must be carefully recorded and critically analyzed as part of a nutrition assessment. Other related background components include (1) a medical history, especially for any disease states or treatments that could impede nutrient absorptive processes or ultimate use, and (2) socioeconomic history, to determine the ability to purchase and prepare appropriate foods needed to maintain health, and (3) amount of education to fine-tune the difficulty of the content presented when teaching dietary concepts.

■ Evaluating the ABCDs

Four components in combination further add to the complete nutritional picture. **Anthropometric** measurements of height, weight, body skinfolds, and body circumferences are an excellent first line of attack. They are easy to obtain and generally reliable.[13] However, an in-depth examination of nutritional health is impossible without the rather expensive process of biochemical assessment. This involves the measurement of specific blood enzyme activities and of the concentration of nutrients and nutrient by-products in the blood, such as was discussed earlier.

A clinical examination would follow, during which a health professional would search for any physical signs and symptoms of diet-related diseases. Last, a diet history, documenting at least the previous few days' intake, is an invaluable tool for insight into possible problem areas.[2] Together these activities form the **ABCDs** of nutritional assessment: **a**nthropometric measurements, **b**iochemical assessment, **c**linical examination, and **d**iet history.

anthropometric Pertaining to the measurement of body weight and the lengths, circumferences, and thicknesses of parts of the body.

TABLE 4-3 Components of a nutrition assessment[2, 3, 12, 13]	
Component	**Example**
Background histories	Medical history, including current diseases, past surgeries, and unintentional weight loss
	Medications history
	Social history (marital status, cooking facilities)
	Family history
	Economic status
	Education attainment
Nutrition parameters	**A**nthropometric assessment: height, weight, skinfold thickness, arm muscle circumference, and other parameters
	Biochemical (laboratory) assessment of blood and urine: enzyme activities; concentrations of nutrients or their by-products
	Clinical assessment (physical examination): general appearance of skin, eyes, and tongue; rapid hair loss; sense of touch; ability to walk
	Diet history: usual intake or record of previous days' meals

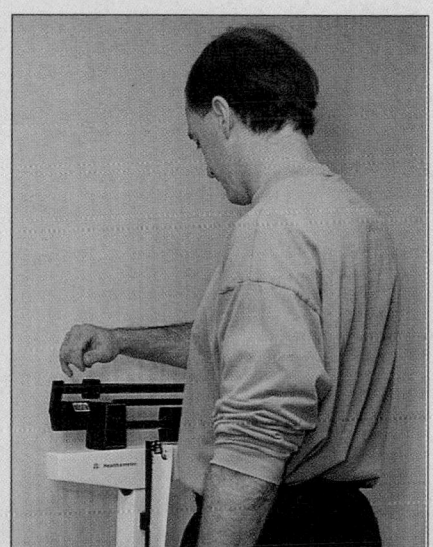

Body weight is a key component of a nutrition assessment.

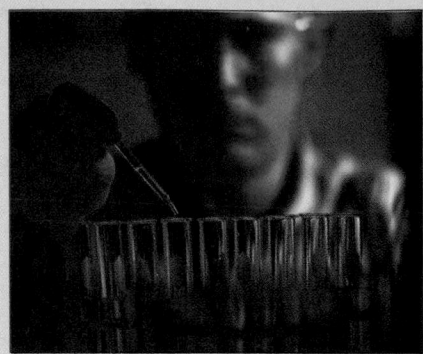

Biochemical analysis of blood and urine is part of a complete nutrition assessment protocol.

heart attack Rapid fall in heart function caused by reduced blood flow through the heart's blood vessels. Often, part of the heart dies in the process (see Chapter 6). Technically called a myocardial infarction.

CRITICAL THINKING

Tom loves to eat hamburgers, fries, and lots of pizza with double amounts of cheese. He rarely eats any vegetables and fruits but, instead, snacks on cookies and ice cream. He insists that he has no problems with his health, is rarely ill, and doesn't see how his diet could cause him any health risks. How would you explain to Tom that, despite his current good health, his diet could predispose him to future health problems?

■ Recognizing the Limitations of Nutrition Assessment

A long time may elapse between the initial development of poor nutritional health and the first clinical evidence of a problem. For example, a diet high in saturated fat often increases blood cholesterol concentration without producing any clinical evidence for years. However, when the blood vessels become sufficiently blocked by cholesterol and other materials, chest pain during physical activity may develop. This buildup of fatty substances also may eventually lead to a **heart attack.** Thus, a person may be on the road to developing a serious disease, but, because it progresses slowly, its effects aren't obvious until quite late—perhaps too late. Much current nutrition research aims to develop better methods for early detection of nutritional problems.

Another example of a delay in signs and symptoms causing serious consequences occurs with calcium deficiency, a particularly relevant issue for adolescent females. Many young women consume well below the recommended amount of calcium but often suffer no ill effects in their younger years. However, women whose bone-density values do not reach full potential during the years of growth are likely to face an increased risk for osteoporosis later in life.

Furthermore, clinical signs and symptoms of nutritional deficiencies are often not very specific. Typical evidence to look for—diarrhea, an irregular walk, facial sores—have many different causes. Long lag times and vague evidence often make it difficult to establish a link between an individual's current diet and nutritional state.

As you study nutrition and learn the importance of nutrients in foods, you may notice people who have very poor diets but show no outward clinical signs and symptoms of poor health. Nonetheless, their health is probably declining in subtle ways. For example, a chronically insufficient intake of iodide encourages development of goiter. Heart disease, strokes, and kidney disease also are related to low intakes of vitamin B-6, folate, and vitamin B-12. An insufficient intake of these vitamins leads to elevated blood concentrations of homocysteine, which in turn likely promotes the development of heart and related circulatory problems.[1, 15] This is a major focus of Chapter 10.

■ Concern about the State of Your Nutritional Health Is Important

Overall, this emphasis in the first few chapters of the text on the importance of nutrition to overall health has merit. In fact, a recent study in *The New England Journal of Medicine* showed that women who ate a varied diet (one that was rich in fiber, that included some fish, and that was low in fried foods and animal fat), avoided overweight, regularly drank a small amount of alcohol daily, exercised on a daily basis for about 30 minutes, and avoided smoking reduced their risk of heart disease by over 80%, compared with women without these habits.[14] The authors concluded that adopting a more healthful lifestyle could prevent a substantial number of heart disease deaths among women. The good news is that this attention to maintaining nutritional health contributes to the goal of achieving a long, vigorous life.

CARBOHYDRATES *chapter 5*

*W*hat did you eat to obtain the energy you are using right now? The next three chapters will examine this question by focusing on the nutrients the human body uses for fuel. These energy-yielding nutrients are mainly carbohydrates (on average, 4 kcal/g) and fats and oils (on average, 9 kcal/g). Little of the other common fuel—protein (on average, 4 kcal/g) is used for that purpose by the body. Most people know that potatoes have carbohydrates and steak has fat and protein, but few people know what those terms signify.

It is likely that you have recently consumed fruits, vegetables, dairy products, cereal, breads, and pasta. All these foods supply carbohydrates.[2] Unfortunately, the benefits of these foods are often misunderstood. Many people think carbohydrate-rich foods are fattening—they are not. Pound for pound, carbohydrates are much less fattening than fats and oils. Furthermore, carbohydrates, especially fiber-rich foods such as fruits, vegetables, whole grains, and legumes, have been promoted by many experts for the important health benefits these foods supply. Some people think sugars cause diabetes or hyperactivity—not so according to well-designed scientific investigations. Almost all carbohydrate-rich foods, except pure sugars, provide essential nutrients and should constitute about 60% of our daily energy intake.[2, 3] Finally, the link between animal fats and cardiovascular disease should prompt us to switch our focus toward carbohydrates.

■ CHAPTER OUTLINE

KEY CHAPTER CONCEPTS

- The simple sugars in our diets are made up primarily of monosaccharides and disaccharides.
- The monosaccharides include glucose, fructose, and galactose. Once absorbed via the small intestine and transported to the liver, much of the fructose and galactose is converted into glucose.
- The major disaccharides are sucrose (glucose plus fructose), maltose (glucose plus glucose), and lactose (glucose plus galactose). When digested, these yield monosaccharide forms: glucose, fructose, and galactose.
- Starches are a more complex form of carbohydrate, containing multiple glucose units chemically-bonded together. Glycogen is an animal form of starch, which acts as a storage form of glucose in the liver and muscles.
- Dietary fibers include the indigestible forms of large carbohydrates—cellulose, hemicelluloses, pectins, gums, and mucilages—as well as the noncarbohydrate lignins. Dietary fiber, especially insoluble varieties, provides mass to the stool, thus easing elimination. Dietary fiber may also reduce the risk of obesity and cardiovascular disease.
- The bulk of carbohydrate digestion and absorption takes place in the small intestine using pancreatic and intestinal enzymes. Some plant fibers are digested by bacteria in the large intestine, and undigested plant fibers exit in the feces.
- Carbohydrates provide energy (on average, 4 kcal/g), protect against needless metabolism of protein for energy, and provide flavor and sweetness to foods. Many carbohydrates can be metabolized to acids by bacteria on teeth. The acid can erode the tooth surface, leading to dental caries.
- A minimal intake of carbohydrate is 50 to 100 grams per day; 60% of total energy intake is a typical recommendation for healthy people.
- Diets should be high in complex carbohydrates, rather than fat. Starches coming from whole grains and pastas, and vegetables—essentially the bottom half of the Food Guide Pyramid— and legumes such as beans should be emphasized.
- The current advice for sugar intake is moderation. Many of us should reexamine our current intakes. The use of alternative sweeteners, such as aspartame, can help in limiting sugar intake.
- Blood glucose is regulated by a system of checks and balances, which includes hormones such as insulin, glucagon, epinephrine, and others. Elevated blood glucose resulting from type 1 diabetes requires insulin therapy, whereas in type 2 diabetes the focus is more on weight control and regular exercise. In both disorders, diet control is important for regulating blood glucose.

REFRESH YOUR MEMORY

As you begin your study of carbohydrates in Chapter 5, you may want to review
- The exchange system in Chapter 2
- The anatomy and physiology of digestion and absorption in Chapter 3
- Hormones that regulate blood glucose in Chapter 3
- The processes of glycolysis, gluconeogenesis, and ketosis in Chapter 4

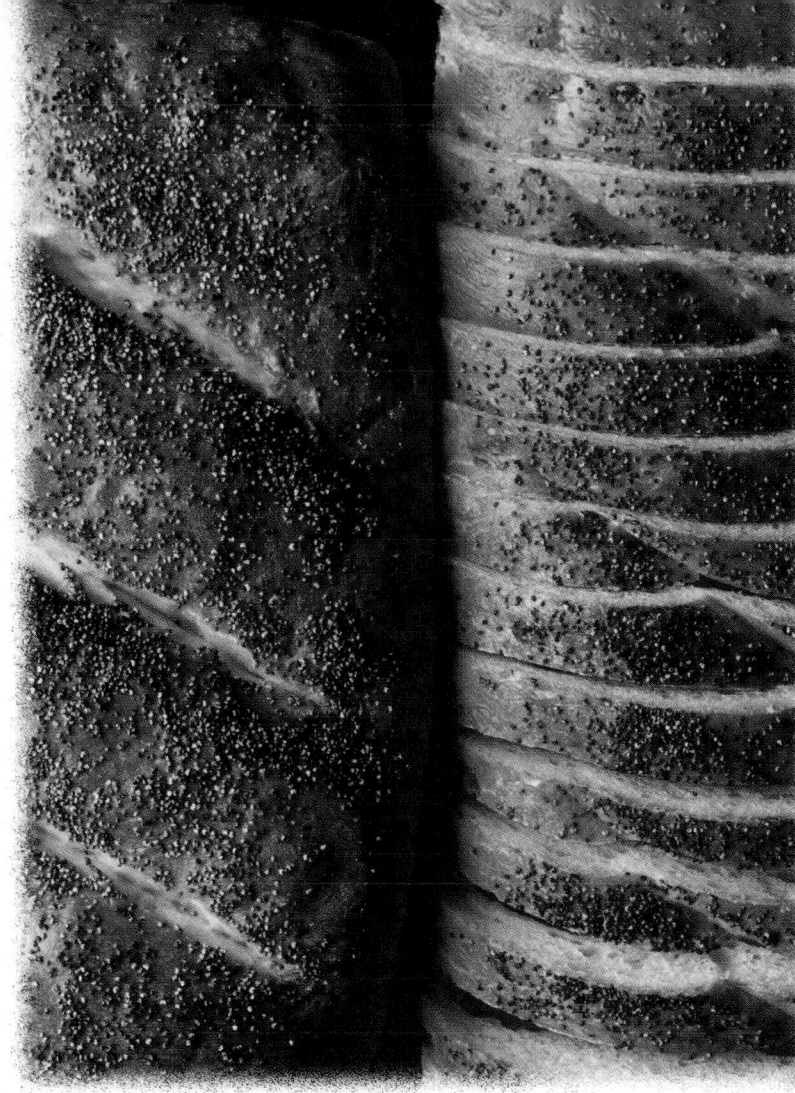

CASE SCENARIO

Myeshia is a 19-year-old African-American female who recently read about the health benefits of calcium and decided to increase her intake of dairy products. To start, she drank 2 cups of 1% milk at lunch. Not long afterward, she experienced bloating, cramping, and increased gas production. She suspected that the culprit of this source of pain was the milk she consumed, especially since her parents and her sister complain of being lactose intolerant (lactose is the chief carbohydrate in milk). As well, the problem first appeared when she added the two servings of milk. She wanted to determine if milk products were, in fact, the cause of her gastrointestinal discomfort, so the next day she again ate two servings of milk products, but this time a cup of yogurt and a glass of milk, for lunch. Subsequently, she did not have any pain. What has Myeshia discovered?

■ CARBOHYDRATES—AN INTRODUCTION

Carbohydrates are a primary fuel source for some cells, such as those in the nervous system and red blood cells. Muscles also rely on a dependable supply of carbohydrate in order to support intense physical activity. Yielding on average 4 kcal/g, carbohydrates are a readily available fuel for all cells in the form of blood glucose and stored in the liver and muscles as glycogen. That stored in the liver can be used to maintain blood glucose availability in times when the diet does not supply enough. Regular intake of carbohydrate is important, because liver glycogen stores are exhausted in about 18 hours if no carbohydrate is consumed. After that point, the body is forced to produce its own carbohydrate from body and food protein; this eventually leads to health problems.[19]

We obtain about 50% of our energy intake from carbohydrate; this percentage is higher in the developing world. We have sensors on our tongues that recognize sweet carbohydrates. Researchers surmise that this sweetness indicated a safe energy source to early humans, and so it became an important energy source. The returning Crusaders brought sugar from the Holy Land to Europe. Columbus introduced sugarcane to the Americas. The French later exploited sugar beets as a source of sugar.

Primarily choosing the healthiest carbohydrate sources, while moderating intake of those that are less healthful, contributes to a well-planned diet. It is difficult to eat so little carbohydrate that body needs are not met, but it is easy to overconsume the carbohydrates that can contribute to health problems. Let's explore this concept further as we look at carbohydrates in detail.

■ STRUCTURES AND FUNCTIONS OF SIMPLE CARBOHYDRATES

Most forms of carbohydrates are composed of carbon, hydrogen, and oxygen in the ratio of 1:2:1, respectively. The general formula is $(CH_2O)n$, where n represents the number of times the ratio is repeated. The chemical formula for glucose is $C_6H_{12}O_6$, or $(CH_2O)_6$. The simpler forms of carbohydrates are called **sugars** and often take the form of single or double sugars, called **monosaccharides** and **disaccharides,** respectively. The more complex forms of carbohydrates are **polysaccharides,** typically either **starches** or **dietary fibers.**

Plants use carbon dioxide, water, and energy (from the sun) to produce the carbohydrates we eat. This complex process is called **photosynthesis.**

■ Monosaccharides: Glucose, Fructose, and Galactose

The common monosaccharides (*mono* meaning "one" and *saccharide* meaning "sugar") are glucose, fructose, and galactose. Glucose is the principal monosaccharide in the body. Other names for glucose are *dextrose* or *blood sugar.* In Figure 5-1, the chemical structure of glucose is shown in both its linear and ring forms. Glucose exists in the body in the ring form. Because it is a six-carbon monosaccharide, glucose is called a **hexose** (*hex* meaning "six," for six carbons; *ose* is the standard word ending for carbohydrates).[19]

Fructose is related to glucose. It is a hexose and can form either a five- or six-member ring (see Fig. 5-1). Fructose, also called levulose, is found in
- Fruit
- Honey (about half fructose, half glucose)
- **High-fructose corn syrup,** which is used in the production of soft drinks, frozen desserts, and confections. The presence of fructose in these products makes it a major sugar in our diets. In most American diets, fructose accounts for about 8 to 10% of total energy intake.

Fructose, after absorption by the small intestine and transport to the liver, is almost all metabolized to glucose. Some fructose is converted to glycogen, **lactic**

---

sugar A simple carbohydrate with the chemical composition $(CH_2O)n$. Most sugars form ringed structures when in solution.

monosaccharide A class of simple sugars, such as glucose, which is not broken down further during digestion.

polysaccharides Carbohydrates containing many glucose units, 3000 or more.

disaccharides A class of sugars formed by the chemical bonding of two monosaccharides.

hexose A general term describing a carbohydrate containing six carbons.

fructose A monosaccharide with six carbons that form a five-membered or six-membered ring with oxygen in the ring; found in fruits and honey.

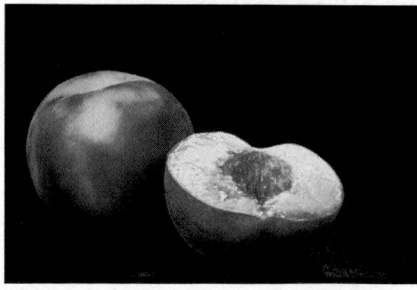

Fruits contain sugars, such as fructose. As fruit ripen, much of the starch content converts to sugars.

acid, or fat, depending on the amount consumed. Synthesis of lactic acid and fat is stimulated by fructose intakes that are two or more times typical intakes.

Galactose is the third major monosaccharide of nutritional importance. Comparison of the structure of this simple sugar with that of glucose shows that the two structures are almost identical, except that the hydrogen (–H) and the hydroxyl group (–OH) on carbon-4 are reversed (see Fig. 5-1). Galactose is not usually found free in nature in large quantities but, rather, combines with glucose to form a disaccharide called *lactose* (present in milk and other dairy products). Once absorbed into the body, galactose is converted into glucose in the liver, which is used to provide immediate energy or is stored as *glycogen.*

Now is a good time to begin emphasizing a key concept in nutrition: the difference between *intake* of a substance and the body's *use* of that substance. The body often does not use all nutrients as such. Some of these substances are broken down and later reassembled into the same or a different substance when and where necessary. For example, galactose in the diet is metabolized to glucose or glycogen. When later required, as in the mammary gland of a lactating female, galactose is resynthesized using a wide variety of compounds in the body.

Another monosaccharide found in nature is **ribose,** a five-carbon sugar (or pentose; *penta* means "five"). This is present in a cell's genetic material. Very little ribose is present in our diet; we produce this sugar from other foods we eat.

Finally, a few sugar alcohols are present in foods and will be discussed later in this chapter, in the section on nutritive sweeteners in foods. Currently, the major sugar alcohol used in the manufacture of edible products is **sorbitol.**[2]

Once you are familiar with the chemical forms of the sugars, it is much easier to understand how they are interrelated, combined, digested, metabolized, and synthesized.

■ Disaccharides: Maltose, Sucrose, and Lactose

Carbohydrates containing 2 to 10 sugar units are called **oligosaccharides.** Within this class are the disaccharides (*di* means "two"). These are formed when two monosaccharides combine. The three most common disaccharides found in nature are **maltose, sucrose,** and **lactose** (Figure 5-2).

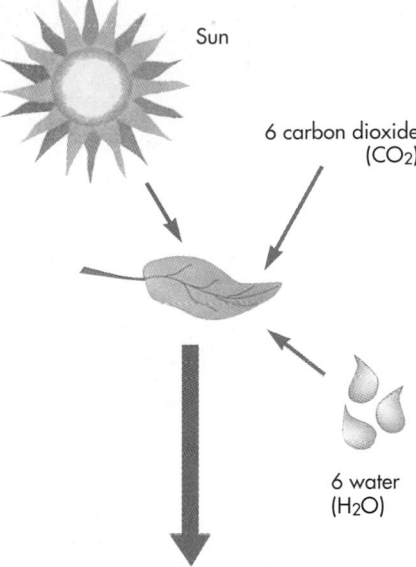

Sun

6 carbon dioxide (CO_2)

6 water (H_2O)

Glucose ($C_6H_{12}O_6$) + 6 oxygen (O_2)

A summary of photosynthesis. Glucose is stored in the leaf but can also undergo further metabolism to form starch and fiber in the plant.

lactic acid A three-carbon acid, also called lactate, that is formed during anaerobic cell metabolism; a partial breakdown product of glucose.

galactose A six-carbon monosaccharide; an isomer of glucose.

sorbitol An alcohol derivative of glucose that yields about 3 kcal/g but is slowly absorbed from the small intestine. It is used in some sugarless gums and dietetic foods.

sucrose Fructose bonded to glucose; table sugar.

lactose A sugar composed of glucose linked to another sugar called galactose.

D – Fructose	D – Glucose	D – Galactose
H	H	H
H – C – OH	C = O	C = O
C = O	H – C – OH	H – C – OH
HO – C – H	HO – C – H	HO – C – H
H – C – OH	H – C – OH	HO – C – H
H – C – OH	H – C – OH	H – C – OH
H – C – OH	H – C – OH	H – C – OH
H	H	H

■ **FIGURE 5-1** Forms of the D-isomer of the six-carbon monosaccharides—fructose, glucose, and galactose—shown in the linear form and in the ring form (predominant form when in solution). Only the D-isomer forms are metabolized by the body (Appendix B reviews the concepts of isomers).

Illustration by William Ober.

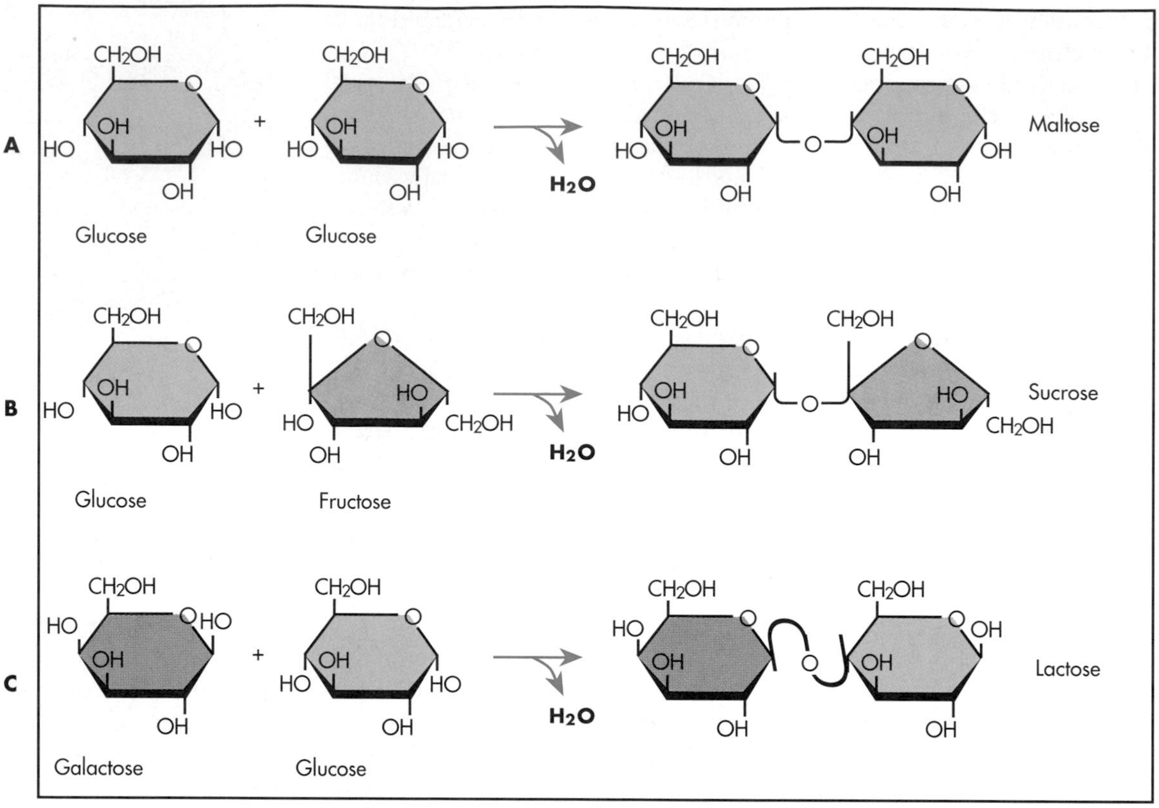

■ FIGURE 5-2 Joining of two monosaccharides forms a disaccharide. (*a*) Maltose is made up of two glucose molecules and is formed in germinating grains. (*b*) Sucrose, or common table sugar, is made up of glucose and fructose. (*c*) Lactose, or milk sugar, is made up of glucose and galactose. Note that lactose contains a different type of bond (beta, or β) from that of maltose and sucrose (alpha, or α), a property that makes lactose difficult to digest for individuals who show a low activity of the enzyme lactase.
Illustration by William Ober.

alpha (α) bond A type of bond that can be digested by human intestinal enzymes; drawn as C⌐O⌐ C.

beta (β) bond A type of bond that cannot be broken by human intestinal enzymes during digestion when it is part of a long chain of glucose molecules; drawn as C ⌐O⌐ C.

fermentation The conversion, without the use of oxygen, of carbohydrates to alcohols, acids, and carbon dioxide.

One carbon on each participating monosaccharide is chemically bound together by oxygen. Two forms of this C—O—C bond exist in nature, called **alpha (α) bonds** and **beta (β) bonds,** and are depicted slightly differently. As shown in Figure 5-2, maltose and sucrose contain the alpha form, whereas lactose contains the beta form. Many carbohydrates contain glucose molecules linked by either alpha or beta bonds. Humans can digest such carbohydrates only if the glucose molecules are linked by alpha bonds.[19] This topic will be covered later in this chapter, when dietary fiber is discussed.

Maltose consists of two glucose molecules joined by an alpha bond. When seeds sprout they produce enzymes that break down the polysaccharides (starch) to sugars such as maltose and glucose. It is this sugar that provides the energy for the plant to initiate growth. In a process called malting, the sprouting process is stopped by heat. This is the first step in the production of alcoholic beverages such as beer. Yeast in the absence of oxygen converts most of the carbohydrates to ethanol (alcohol) and carbon dioxide in a process called **fermentation.** There will more about the production of beer, wine and spirits in Chapter 8. Few other food products and beverages contain maltose. In fact, most maltose that we ultimately digest in the small intestine is produced during the digestion of starch (see a later section of this chapter).

Sucrose, common table sugar, is composed of glucose and fructose linked via an alpha bond. Large amounts of sucrose are found only in plants, such as sugarcane, sugar beets, and maple syrup. The sucrose from these sources may be purified to various degrees. Brown, white, and powdered sugars are common forms of sucrose sold in grocery stores.

Lactose, the primary sugar in milk and milk products, consists of glucose joined to galactose via a beta bond. As discussed in a later section of this chapter, many people are unable to digest large amounts of lactose due to lack of enough of the enzyme lactase that is capable of breaking its beta bond. This can cause intestinal gas, bloating, cramping, and discomfort as the unabsorbed lactose is metabolized into acids and gases by bacteria in the large intestine.[23]

You are likely to encounter many different words referring to the monosaccharides and disaccharides just discussed or products containing these simple sugars. Note that all of the terms listed in Table 5-7 later in the chapter are names for sugars either naturally present in food products or added during their manufacture. These monosaccharides and disaccharides are often referred to as *simple sugars* because they contain only one or two sugar units and, therefore, have a simple chemical structure. Food labels lump all these sugars under one category, listing them as "sugars."

CONCEPT CHECK

Monosaccharides are single sugars. From a nutritional standpoint, important monosaccharides are glucose, fructose, and galactose. Disaccharides are double sugars. The major disaccharides in the diet are sucrose (glucose bonded to fructose), maltose (glucose bonded to glucose), and lactose (glucose bonded to galactose). The disaccharides have either alpha or beta bonds. Our bodies are unable to break down most of the beta bonds. Once absorbed into the body, most carbohydrates are ultimately transformed into glucose by the liver.

■ Larger Oligosaccharides: Raffinose and Stachyose

Larger oligosaccharides contain 3 to about 10 single sugar units (*oligo* means "scant"). Two larger oligosaccharides of nutritional importance are **raffinose** and **stachyose,** which are found in beans and other legumes. These are constructed of typical monosaccharides but are chemically bonded together in such a way that digestive enzymes cannot break them apart. Thus, when we consume beans and other legumes, raffinose and stachyose remain undigested on reaching the large intestine. There, bacteria metabolize them, producing gas and other by-products.[19]

Many people have no trouble digesting beans and other legumes, but others experience unpleasant side effects from intestinal gas. An enzyme preparation called Beano®, which prevents these side effects, can help such people if taken right before a meal. Once consumed, the enzyme preparation breaks down many of the indigestible oligosaccharides in legumes and other vegetables in the gastrointestinal tract before they reach the large intestine. Beano® is made from mold, so persons sensitive to molds may react allergically and should avoid it or use with caution. For more information or free samples, contact the manufacturer (800-257-8650).

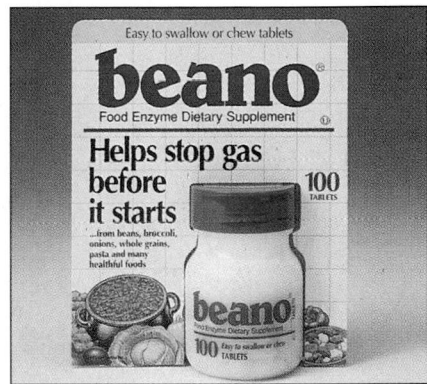

Beano® can be used to reduce intestinal gas produced by bacterial metabolism of oligosaccharides in the intestines.

raffinose An indigestible oligosaccharide made of three monosaccharides (galactose-glucose-fructose).

stachyose An indigestible oligosaccharide made of four monosaccharides (galactose-galactose-glucose-fructose).

Simple
| **Monosaccharides**
| Glucose, fructose, galactose
| **Disaccharides**
| Sucrose, lactose, maltose
| **Polysaccharides**
▼ Amylose, amylopectin, glycogen
More Complex

■ STRUCTURES AND FUNCTIONS OF THE MORE COMPLEX CARBOHYDRATES

The polysaccharides, often referred to as *complex carbohydrates,* include some that are digestible (e.g., starch) and some that are largely indigestible, such as dietary fiber.

amylose A straight-chain type of starch composed of glucose units.

amylopectin A branched-chain type of starch composed of glucose units.

modified food starch A product consisting of chemically linked starch molecules that is more stable than normal, unmodified starches.

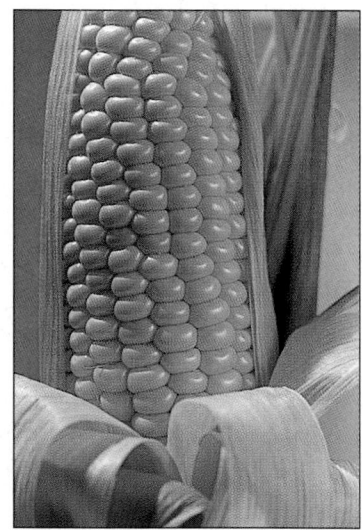

As vegetables age, their sugars are converted to starches.

■ Digestible Polysaccharides: Starch and Glycogen

Polysaccharides are polymers containing many monosaccharide units, 3000 or more. Most polysaccharides of nutritional importance are synthesized from glucose, as when vegetables turn glucose into starch during maturation. This makes peas and corn sweetest when they are young. Starch, the major digestible polysaccharide in our diet, is the storage form of energy in plants. There are two types of plant starch—**amylose** and **amylopectin**—both of which are a source of energy for plants and animals.

Both amylose and amylopectin contain many glucose units linked by alpha (digestible) bonds. The primary difference between the two types of starch is that amylose is a straight-chain polymer, whereas amylopectin is highly branched. Cooking increases the digestibility of these starches by making them more soluble in water and thus more available for attack by digestive enzymes. Amylose and amylopectin are found in potatoes, beans, breads, pasta, rice, and other starchy products, typically in a ratio of about 1:4. Amylopectin raises blood glucose much more readily than amylose, since its numerous branches provide many areas for digestive enzyme activity. The enzymes act only at the ends of the glucose chains. The more numerous the branches of a starch, the more sites (ends) are available for enzyme action (see the discussion of glycemic index in a later section of this chapter).[22]

The branches in amylopectin also allow it to form a very stable starch gel, enabling it to retain water and resist water seepage. Food manufacturers commonly use starches rich in amylopectin in sauces and gravies for frozen foods because they remain stable over a wide temperature range. Manufacturers may also use processes to bond the starch molecules to one another, further increasing their stability. The resulting product, called **modified food starch,** is used in baby foods, salad dressings, and instant puddings.

Glycogen, the storage form of carbohydrate in humans and other animals, is a glucose polymer with alpha bonds and numerous branches. No glycogen is found in meat, however, because it is used up during slaughter and later storage. Overall, the structure of glycogen is similar to that of amylopectin, but the branching patterns are more complicated (Fig. 5-3). As with amylopectin, because glycogen is so highly branched, it is quickly broken down by enzymes in body cells in which it is stored.[19] The liver and muscles are the major storage sites for glycogen. Because only about 120 kcal of glucose are available as such in body fluids, muscle and liver storage sites for carbohydrate energy—amounting to about 1800 kcal—are extremely important. As noted in this chapter's introduction, the 400 kcal of liver glycogen can be turned into blood glucose, while the 1400 kcal of muscle glycogen cannot. Still,

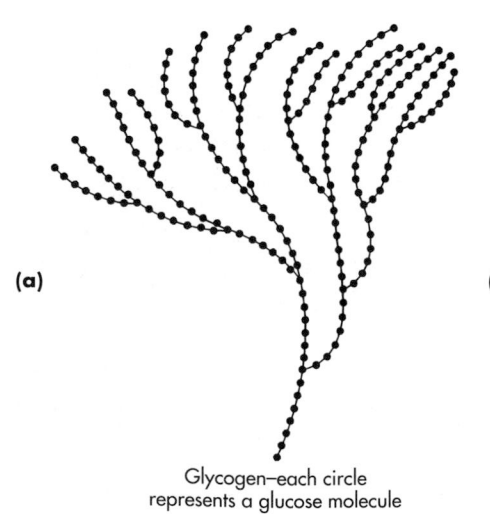

(a)

Glycogen—each circle
represents a glucose molecule

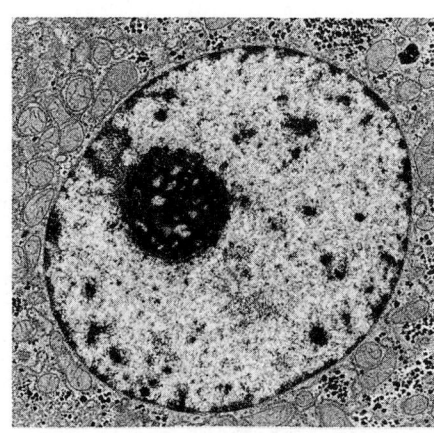

(b)

■ FIGURE 5-3 (*a*) Glycogen structure. (*b*) Glycogen stores as found in the cell.
Illustration by William Ober.

glycogen in muscles supply glucose for muscle use, especially during high-intensity and endurance exercise. (See Chapter 14 for a detailed discussion of carbohydrate use during physical activity.)

■ Indigestible Polysaccharides: Dietary Fiber

Folklore surrounding dietary fiber has been a part of American culture since the 1800s. In the 1820s and 1830s, a minister named Sylvester Graham traveled up and down the East Coast extolling the virtues of fiber. He left us a legacy—the graham cracker. However, today's graham cracker bears little resemblance to the whole-grain product he promoted. The next wave of fiber frenzy crested in the mid-1870s with Dr. John Harvey Kellogg and his brother William, of breakfast cereal fame. Dr. Kellogg became the first person to earn a million dollars from "health foods." One of his patients was Charles W. Post, who followed the Kelloggs' lead and started the Post Toasted Cornflakes Company. In 1901 alone, Post netted $1 million from his Grape-Nuts cereal and other products. As you will see, present-day scientific evidence supports this early promotion of fiber as part of a total diet.

In terms of their chemical composition, dietary fibers are composed primarily of the nonstarch polysaccharides **cellulose, hemicelluloses, pectins, gums,** and **mucilages.** The only noncarbohydrate components of dietary fibers are **lignins,** which includes complex alcohol derivatives (Table 5-1). All forms of dietary fiber come from plants and, as a group, are not digested in the human stomach or small intestine.[19]

Cellulose is a straight-chain glucose polymer similar to amylose; however, unlike amylose, which contains alpha bonds, the glucose units in cellulose are linked by beta bonds. As noted earlier, glucose molecules joined by beta bonds are not broken down by human digestive enzymes. Thus, cellulose is not digestible by humans and is classified as a dietary fiber, not a starch. Because the long glucose chains of cellulose are linear, they can pack closely together, forming fibrous structures of great strength. Overall, cellulose, hemicelluloses, and lignins form the structural part of the plant. A cotton ball is pure cellulose. Bran fiber is rich in hemicelluloses. Since bran layers form the outer covering of all grains, **whole grains** are good sources of this dietary fiber (Fig. 5-4). The woody fibers in broccoli are partly lignins. As a class, these undigestible dietary fibers generally do not dissolve in water and thus are called **insoluble fibers.**

Pectins, gums, and mucilages are found inside and around plant cells. They help "glue" plant cells together (see Fig. 5-4). These dietary fibers either dissolve or swell when put into water and thus are called **soluble fibers.** Some forms of hemicellulose also fall into this soluble-fiber category. Soluble fibers such as gum arabic, guar gum,

cellulose A straight-chain polysaccharide of glucose molecules that is undigestible because of the presence of beta bonds; part of insoluble fiber.

hemicellulose A dietary fiber containing xylose, galactose, glucose, and other monosaccharides bonded together.

pectin A dietary fiber containing chains of galacturonic acid and other monosaccharides; characteristically found between plant cell walls.

gums A dietary fiber containing chains of galactose, glucuronic acid, and other monosaccharides; characteristically found in exudates from plant stems.

mucilages A dietary fiber consisting of chains of galactose, mannose, and other monosaccharides; characteristically found in seaweed.

lignins An insoluble fiber made up of a multiringed alcohol (noncarbohydrate) structure.

whole grains Grains containing the entire seed of the plant, including the bran, germ, and endosperm (starchy interior).

insoluble fibers Fibers that mostly do not dissolve in water and are not metabolized by bacteria in the large intestine. These include cellulose, some hemicelluloses, and lignins.

soluble fibers Fibers that either dissolve or swell in water and are metabolized (fermented) by bacteria in the large intestine. These include pectins, gums, and mucilages.

TABLE 5-1 Classification of Dietary Fibers

Type	Component(s)	Examples	Physiological Effects	Major Food Sources
Insoluble				
Noncarbohydrate	Lignins	Wheat bran	Increases fecal bulk; estrogen-like effects	Whole grains, flax seeds
Carbohydrate	Cellulose Hemicelluloses	Wheat products Brown rice	Increases fecal bulk Decreases intestinal transit time	All plants Wheat, rye, rice, vegetables
Soluble				
Carbohydrate	Pectins, gums, mucilages, some hemi-celluloses	Apples, bananas, oranges, carrots, barley, oats, kidney beans	Delays gastric emptying; slows glucose absorption; can lower blood cholesterol	Citrus fruits, oat products (beta-glucan in particular), beans, thickeners added to foods

Lignins were discussed along with the other phytochemicals in Chapter 2, and in Chapter 18 in the Nutrition Perspective.

*Y*ou may think of wheat bran as pure fiber, but it is actually a mixture of several dietary fibers. It also contains some protein, fat, and trace minerals, as is true of all dietary fiber sources. The age of a plant may also influence its fiber composition; for example, young carrots contain very little lignin, whereas old carrots may contain 10 to 20% of this material.

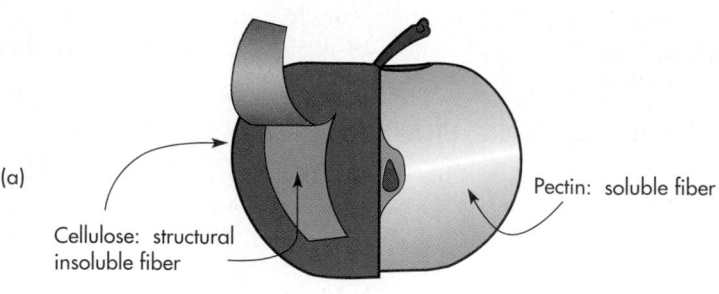

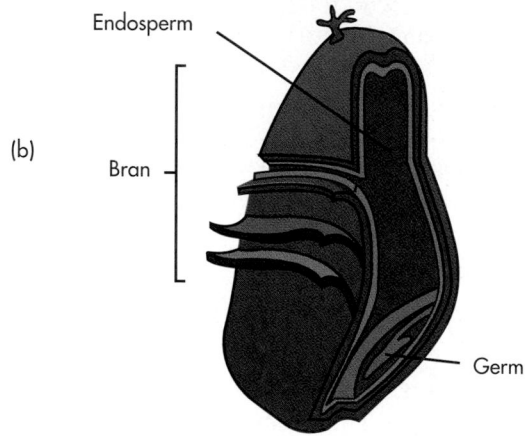

■ FIGURE 5-4 Soluble and insoluble fiber. (*a*) The skin of an apple consists of the insoluble fiber cellulose, which provides structure for the fruit. The soluble fiber pectin "glues" the fruit cells together. (*b*) The outside layer of a wheat kernel is made of layers of bran—insoluble fiber—making this whole grain a good source of fiber. Overall, fruits, vegetables, whole grains, and legumes such as beans are rich in dietary fiber.

psyllium A mostly soluble type of dietary fiber found in the seeds of the plantain plant.

C R I T I C A L   T H I N K I N G

Celia decides to go on a diet and buys over-the-counter pills. You look at the ingredients and note that the pills contain psyllium, a word you recognize from the nutrition course you're taking. What advice can you give Celia about the wisdom of using these diet pills?

locust bean gum, and various pectins are present in numerous food products, especially salad dressings, inexpensive ice creams, jams, and jellies. Other rich sources of soluble fibers include fruits and vegetables in general, soybean fiber, rice bran, and **psyllium** seeds (found in many commercial fiber laxatives).

One workable definition of dietary fiber is the foodstuffs that remain undigested as they enter the large intestine. There is really no common property that characterizes dietary fibers, except their ability to resist digestion in the small intestine. Since some dietary fibers—especially the soluble fibers—are digested by bacteria in the large intestine, it is not accurate to say that dietary fiber is simply that found in the feces.

Bacteria in the large intestine metabolize soluble dietary fibers into products such as short-chain fatty acids (e.g., acetic acid, butyric acid, and propionic acid) and gases, such as hydrogen (H_2) and methane (CH_4). These acids, especially butyric acid, provide fuel for the cells in the large intestine and enhance their health. All these products can also be absorbed into the bloodstream. As a result of bacterial metabolism, soluble dietary fibers yield about 3 kcal/g on average, although the actual value is still in question. Thus, high-fiber foods should not be looked at as calorie free, though they are often lower in calories per serving than low-fiber alternatives.

When intake of dietary fiber is high, its breakdown by bacteria can cause methane and hydrogen to increase in the breath. This is not harmful. In addition, the body tends to adapt over time to a high-fiber intake, producing less gas and adjusting to the increased pressure in the large intestine. Because of this potential for breakdown in the large intestine of some forms of dietary fiber, soluble fibers are also defined as those that are fermentable in the large intestine. If so, insoluble fibers are then defined as those that are nonfermentable.

CONCEPT CHECK

Amylose, amylopectin, and glycogen are all storage forms of glucose, called polysaccharides. Amylose and amylopectin combine in varying proportions to form food starch, such as that found in potatoes and bread. Glycogen is a storage form of glucose in humans. Liver glycogen yields a ready source of blood glucose.

Dietary fiber is essentially the portion of ingested food that remains undigested as it enters the large intestine. Fiber components include cellulose, hemicelluloses, lignins, pectins, gums, and mucilages. There are two general classes of dietary fiber: insoluble and soluble. Insoluble fibers are mostly made up of cellulose, hemicelluloses, and lignins. Soluble fibers are made up mostly of pectins, gums, and mucilages. Both insoluble and soluble fibers are resistant to human digestive enzymes, but bacteria in the large intestine can break down soluble fibers.

■ CARBOHYDRATE DIGESTION AND ABSORPTION

Food preparation can be viewed as the start of carbohydrate digestion because cooking softens tough connective tissues in the fibrous tissue of plants, such as broccoli stalks. When starches are heated, the starch granules swell as they soak up water, making them much easier to digest. All these effects of cooking generally make these foods easier to chew, swallow, and break down during digestion.

■ Carbohydrate Digestion

The enzymatic digestion of starch begins in the mouth, when the saliva, which contains an enzyme called salivary **amylase,** mixes with the starchy products during the mastication of the food. This amylase breaks down starch into many smaller units (e.g., disaccharides, such as maltose) (Fig. 5-5). You can observe this conversion while chewing a saltine cracker. Prolonged chewing of the cracker causes it to taste sweeter as some starch breaks down into the sweeter sugars, such as maltose. Still, food is in the mouth for such a short amount of time that this phase of digestion is negligible. In addition, once the food moves down the esophagus and reaches the stomach, the acidic environment (pH 1-2) inactivates salivary amylase.

After the carbohydrates have reached the small intestine—where the pH of 7 or more is well suited for further carbohydrate digestion—the pancreas releases enzymes, such as pancreatic amylase. The original carbohydrates in a food are present in the small intestine as monosaccharides (mostly any glucose and fructose present as such in food), as well as disaccharides (maltose from starch breakdown, lactose mainly from dairy products, and sucrose from food and that added at the table).

The polysaccharides in the food that were first acted on in the mouth are then digested further by pancreatic amylase. The disaccharides are digested to their monosaccharide units once they reach the wall of the small intestine, where the specialized enzymes on the mucosal cells digest each disaccharide into the monosaccharide components. The enzyme maltase acts on maltose to produce two glucose molecules. Sucrase acts on sucrose to produce glucose and fructose. Lactase acts on lactose to produce glucose and galactose. When considering carbohydrate digestion, you should remember that the key digestive enzymes come from the pancreas and the cells of the intestinal wall.[19]

Intestinal diseases can interfere with the efficient digestion of the sugars maltose, lactose, and sucrose. The portion of these carbohydrates that is not fully digested are not absorbed. When these unabsorbed carbohydrates eventually reach the large intestine, the bacteria there use the sugars to produce acids and gases (review Fig. 5-5). If produced in large amounts, these gases can cause abdominal discomfort. People recovering from intestinal disorders, such as diarrhea or bacterial infections, may

An outmoded term used for dietary fiber is *crude fiber.* This term arose during the early 1900s to reflect the amount of indigestible foodstuff present in animal feed. The animal feed was boiled for 1 hour in acid and for another hour in an alkaline solution. The remains of that chemical digestion was called crude fiber; it consisted mostly of cellulose and lignins. All other types of fiber were destroyed by the chemical action.

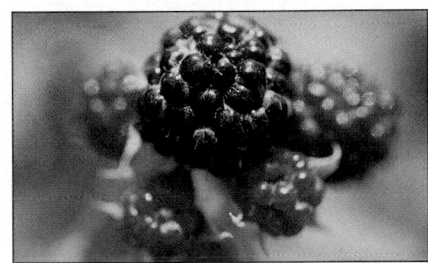

In the search for dietary fiber sources, berries are often overlooked. Just 1 cup of blackberries contains up to 6 g of fiber.

amylase Starch-digesting enzyme from the salivary glands or pancreas.

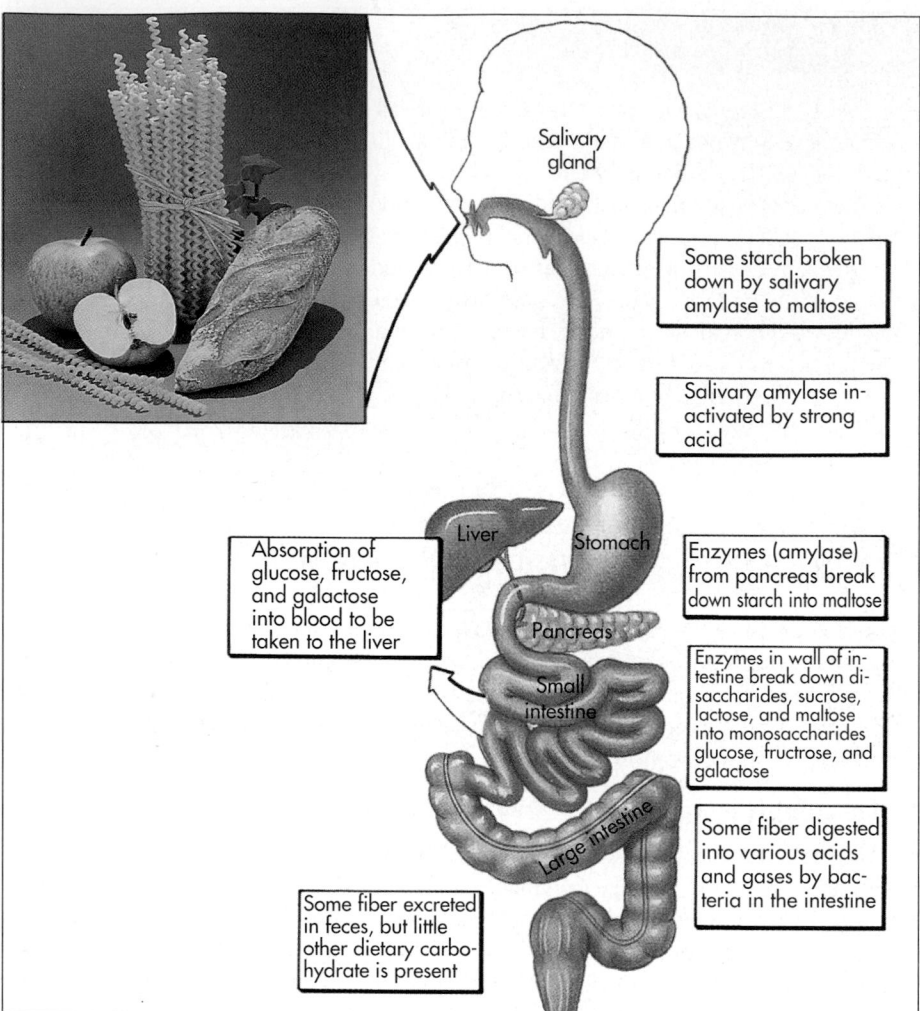

Salivary gland

Some starch broken down by salivary amylase to maltose

Salivary amylase inactivated by strong acid

Liver

Stomach

Enzymes (amylase) from pancreas break down starch into maltose

Pancreas

Absorption of glucose, fructose, and galactose into blood to be taken to the liver

Small intestine

Enzymes in wall of intestine break down disaccharides, sucrose, lactose, and maltose into monosaccharides glucose, fructrose, and galactose

Large intestine

Some fiber digested into various acids and gases by bacteria in the intestine

Some fiber excreted in feces, but little other dietary carbohydrate is present

▌ FIGURE 5-5 A summary of carbohydrate digestion and absorption. Most carbohydrate digestion and absorption takes place in the small intestine. Note that Chapter 3 covered the physiology of digestion and absorption in detail.
Illustration by William Ober.

need to avoid lactose for a few weeks if temporary lactose intolerance is experienced. Two weeks is sufficient time for the small intestine to resume producing enough lactase enzyme to allow for lactose digestion.

▌ Carbohydrate Absorption

Simple sugars found naturally in foods and those formed as by-products of earlier starch digestion in the mouth and small intestine generally follow an active absorption process. Recall from Chapter 3 that this is a process that requires a specific carrier and energy input in order for the substance to be taken up by the absorptive cells in the small intestine. Glucose and its close relative, galactose, undergo active absorption. They are pumped into the absorptive cells along with sodium (Fig. 5-6).[19] The energy used in the process is actually needed to pump the sodium ion back out of the absorptive cell.

Fructose is taken up by the absorptive cells via facilitated diffusion. In this case, a carrier is used, but no energy input is needed. This absorptive process is slower than that seen with glucose or galactose. Thus, large doses of fructose are not readily absorbed and can contribute to diarrhea as they remain in the small intestine and attract water via osmosis. (Chapter 11 will discuss osmosis in detail.)

Once glucose, galactose, and fructose enter the intestinal cells, some fructose is metabolized to glucose. The single sugars in the absorptive cells are then transported via the portal vein to the liver. The liver then exercises its metabolic options—

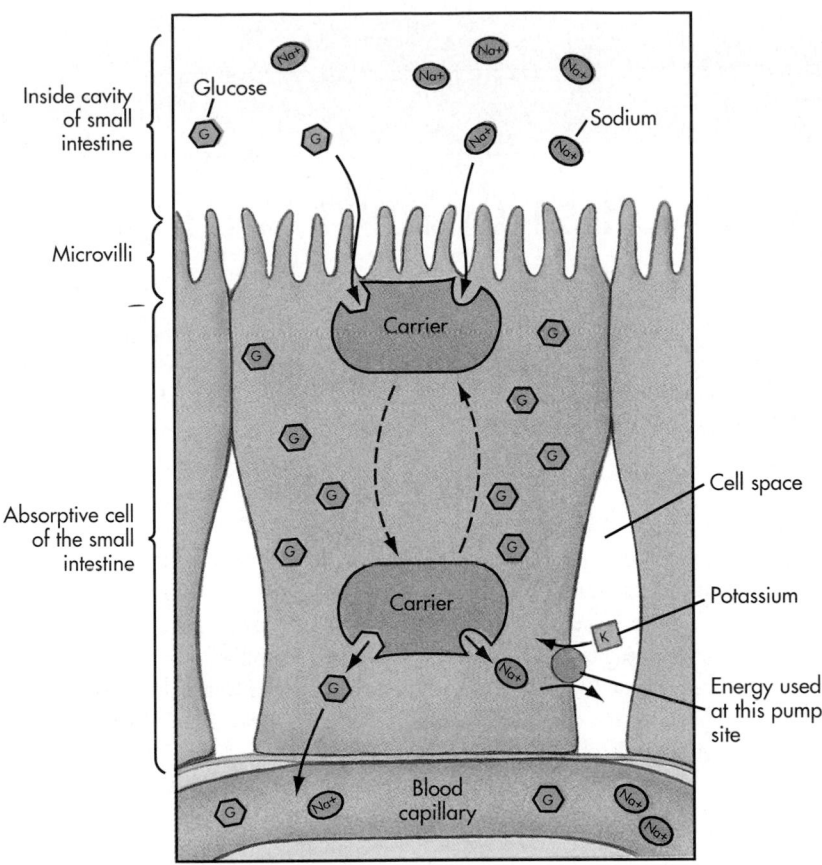

FIGURE 5-6 Active absorption of glucose. Glucose and sodium pass across the cell membrane of the intestinal absorptive cell in a carrier-dependent, energy-requiring process. The energy is used for maintaining a low concentration of sodium in the cell. Once inside the absorptive cell, glucose can exit by facilitated diffusion down its concentration gradient and enter the bloodstream.

transforming the monosaccharides into glucose and releasing it directly into the bloodstream for transport to organs such as the brain, muscles, kidneys, and adipose tissues; producing the storage form of the carbohydrate, glycogen; or producing fat. Of these three options, producing fat is the least likely.

Only a minor amount of starch (about 5%) escapes digestion. This travels down to the large intestine and is fermented there by bacteria. Then some of the starch is absorbed in the form of acids and gases produced by bacterial metabolism, as is true for undigested lactose. As mentioned before, scientists suspect that some of these products actually promote the health of the large intestine by providing a source of energy.

CONCEPT CHECK

Carbohydrate digestion is the process of breaking down larger carbohydrates into their absorbable components. The enzymatic digestion of starches begins in the mouth with salivary amylase. Enzymes made by the pancreas and small intestine complete the digestion of carbohydrates to single sugars in the small intestine. Primarily following an active absorption process, the single sugars (glucose and galactose)—either resulting from the digestive process or present in the meal—are taken up by absorptive cells in the intestine. Fructose undergoes facilitated diffusion; once in the absorptive cell most is metabolized to glucose. All the monosaccharides then enter the portal vein and travel to the liver. The liver finally exercises its metabolic options, primarily producing glucose and glycogen from the monosaccharides.

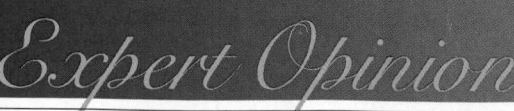

Expert Opinion

THE BENEFITS OF A HIGH-CARBOHYDRATE DIET

William E. Connor, M.D.

The great civilizations of the world developed and flourished consuming high-carbohydrate diets. The classic examples are the Chinese civilization, based on rice; the Egyptian and Babylonian cultures, which consumed wheat; and, in the Americas, the Maya, Inca, and Aztec peoples, whose staples were corn and beans. Except for the affluent countries of the Western world, the majority of the world's population continues to consume a high-carbohydrate diet derived from cereals, legumes, vegetables, and fruits. Indeed, typical amounts of carbohydrates consumed are large, in the range of 400 to 500 g/day, predominantly as starch or other polysaccharides, and constituting from 75 to 80% of the total calories. An example of a culture that my colleagues and I have studied is the Tarahumara Indians of Mexico; they have consumed a high-carbohydrate diet for generations, with the principal foods being corn, beans, and wild plants. Their diet contains ample protein and is nutritionally adequate.

Ecologically, a high-carbohydrate diet makes better use of the world's resources. Cereal crops and legumes require about one-fifth of the resources needed to yield the same energy that beef would require. Thus, the available resources of the world would not be sufficient to produce the high-animal-fat diet of the United States for everyone.

Historically (and today) a high-carbohydrate diet has been based largely on plant foods that contain starch as the carbohydrate source. The only plant exception is fruit, in which the carbohydrates are glucose, fructose, and sucrose, as well as pectin, a fiber. Even nuts, which contain about 50% fat in terms of total calories, also contain a considerable amount of carbohydrate, 20 to 30% of total energy. Foods derived from animals, on the other hand, contain very little or no carbohydrate, instead being composed of protein and fat.

Some hunter-gatherers of the past consumed very little carbohydrate because plant foods were simply not available. The Eskimo of the Arctic are the classic example; most of their calories were derived from seal, fish, whale, caribou, and other land animals. However, for most humans, the only time in life when a high-carbohydrate diet is not consumed is during infancy, when the diet of human milk or infant formulas contains about 50% of the calories from fat and is fairly low in carbohydrate, about 40% of calories. Even in the United States, adults consume 45 to 50% of the total calories as carbohydrate. For children and adults, practical high-carbohydrate diets usually contain from 60 to 65% of total energy, an amount suggested by the Coronary Heart Disease Prevention Group at the Oregon Health Sciences University. Such an alternative diet would contain protein as 15% of energy, fat as 20 to 25% of energy, and cholesterol intake of 100 mg/day or less. This high-carbohydrate diet is designed to prevent not only coronary heart disease but also other diseases associated with an affluent lifestyle, such as cancer.

From the health point of view, a high-carbohydrate diet consisting largely of plant foods is a diet that is rich in fiber, minerals, vitamins, saponins (a phytochemical; see Chapter 2), sitosterol (see Chapter 6 for details), and essential fatty acids. It is thus a diet high in bulk from fiber and, so, weighs considerably more than a low-carbohydrate diet. It is a diet rich in antioxidants, such as vitamin E,

▮ FUNCTIONS OF GLUCOSE AND OTHER SUGARS IN THE BODY

Glucose yields energy, but it has many other functions as well. Since the other sugars can generally be converted to glucose, and more complex carbohydrates (e.g., starches) are broken down to yield glucose, the functions described here apply to most carbohydrates.

▮ Yielding Energy

The main function of glucose is to act as a source of energy to body cells. Certain tissues, such as the red blood cells and most parts of the brain, derive almost all of their

ascorbic acid, and carotenoids, especially lutein and zeaxanthin. These are important in preventing coronary heart disease and cancer and in delaying the aging process. A high-carbohydrate diet is also rich in folic acid; this is sometimes in short supply in the highly purified American diet. Folate helps control abnormal homocysteine levels—an emerging cardiovascular risk factor. Since it comes from plant foods, the high-carbohydrate diet has another advantage in that it is typically low in fat, low in saturated fat, and low in cholesterol content. This means that populations that consume a high-carbohydrate diet have low blood cholesterol and LDL cholesterol, as well as a low incidence of coronary heart disease. A lower-fat diet would reduce the amount of fat in the bloodstream after a meal; this fat contains particles that can contribute to atherosclerosis (see Chapter 6 for details).

Dietary fiber includes several carbohydrates that are largely indigestible by the human gut, such as cellulose, hemicellulose, lignin, pectin, and beta-glucans. Dietary fiber is found only in plants and is common in unprocessed cereals, legumes, vegetables, and fruits. In ruminant animals, dietary fiber is completely digested and is used as a source of energy. In humans, dietary fiber contributes little to the caloric content of the diet but promotes satiety through its bulk and promotes proper functioning of the colon and rectum. Fiber may help prevent certain diseases of the colon and rectum, such as appendicitis, hemorrhoids, and diverticulitis.

Sugar is a conspicuous component of the American diet, perhaps now even increasing from the usual amount of about 20% of total calories. Sugar, of course, includes sucrose, fructose, and glucose. Fruits are natural sources of sugars but would supply only a small amount of sugars vis-à-vis the total energy intake and would contribute valuable nutrients. The addition of large quantities of sucrose to processed food, baked goods, and candies would supply only energy, without the other nutritive benefits of fruit consumption. In the high-carbohydrate diet I recommend, most of the carbohydrate would be supplied by starch. The consumption of sugar would even be reduced from the current 20% of energy to 10 to 15% of energy intake. It would be expected that incidence of dental caries then would be reduced as sugar intake declined.

Another advantage of a high-carbohydrate diet based on plant foods is in the prevention of obesity. There is good evidence that Americans lose weight more easily with a high-carbohydrate diet and are less inclined to gain weight than are those whose carbohydrate intake is lower and fat intake is higher. The energy cost of metabolizing a high starch source of carbohydrate (e.g., corn or beans) is much higher than the energy expenditure necessary to metabolize a dense nutrient, such as meat, or the fat from french fries or even olive oil. Finally, the advantages of a high-carbohydrate, lower-fat diet apply in the control of hypertension.

Given all these benefits, a reexamination of the relative amount of carbohydrate in one's diet is warranted. Much research supports the recommendation to increase complex carbohydrates from vegetables, whole grains, beans, and fruits.

Dr. Connor is a professor of medicine in the Division of Endocrinology, Diabetes, and Clinical Nutrition at the Oregon Health Sciences University, Portland, Oregon. He is a former president of the American Society for Clinical Nutrition and a former member of the Food and Nutrition Board of the National Academy of Sciences.

energy from glucose. In fact, except when the diet contains almost no carbohydrates, the brain and central nervous system use mostly glucose for fuel, about 150g/day. Glucose can also fuel muscle cells and other body cells, but many of these cells usually use fat to meet energy needs.

▪ Sparing Protein from Use as an Energy Source

Glucose is protein sparing. That is, dietary protein can be used to make body tissues and to perform other vital processes only when carbohydrate intake provides enough glucose for body needs. Therefore, if you do not consume enough carbohydrate to yield that glucose, your body is forced to make it from other nutrients, such as proteins found in muscle tissue. This process is termed **gluconeogenesis,** which means "production of new glucose" (review Chapter 4 for details). If the process continues

gluconeogenesis The production of new glucose by metabolic pathways in the cell. Amino acids derived from protein usually provide the carbons for this glucose.

for weeks, these organs can become partially weakened. Generally, Americans consume adequate sources of protein, so sparing protein is not an essential function of carbohydrate in the diet under such conditions. It does become important in some energy-reduced diets and in starvation. (Chapters 7 and 20 discuss specific effects of starvation and famine.)

The life-threatening wasting of protein that occurs during long-term fasting (or starvation) has prompted companies that produce products used for rapid weight loss, such as Optifast, to include enough carbohydrate to supply 100 to 126 g/day. This significantly decreases protein breakdown and thus helps protect vital tissues and organs, including the heart, during rapid weight loss.

■ Preventing Ketosis

An adequate intake of carbohydrates—glucose, other sugars, or both—is necessary for the complete metabolism of fats to carbon dioxide (CO_2) and water (H_2O) in the body. A low carbohydrate intake, with the resulting decline in release of the hormone **insulin,** leads to incomplete breakdown of fatty acids and subsequent formation of **ketone bodies**—acetoacetic acid and its derivatives. (Recall that Chapter 4 discussed metabolism.) Insulin is needed for glucose entry into a few types of cells, including muscle and adipose cells. To get into these cells, glucose needs insulin and glucose transporters. Insulin binds to its receptor on the surface of the target cell. This binding signals release of a glucose transporter from storage. The glucose transporter travels to the plasma membrane and picks up the glucose and transports it into the cytosol and releases it. Without a constant supply of glucose, fat metabolism in these cells is hampered.

We need to eat at least 50 to 100 g of carbohydrates per day to ensure complete fat metabolism. This prevents high accumulation of ketone bodies in the blood and other tissues, a condition called **ketosis,** and the resulting weakness that usually occurs. Note that normally we eat at least twice that much carbohydrate—on average, about 200 to 300 g/day.[2]

In starvation, people do not consume enough carbohydrate, so ketone bodies soon appear in the blood. Again, this is the normal metabolic response to a fuel shortage. Part of the brain and other tissues can use these ketone bodies for fuel. In fact, the use of ketone bodies by the brain and other organs, such as the heart, is an important adaptive mechanism for survival during starvation. If part of the brain could not use ketone bodies, the body would be forced to produce much more glucose from protein to support the brain's energy needs. The resulting self-cannibalization would rapidly break down the muscles, heart, and other organs, severely limiting the body's ability to tolerate starvation.

In untreated **type 1 diabetes,** excessive production of ketone bodies can occur, partly because there is not enough insulin to allow for normal glucose metabolism. In such patients, the resulting ketosis can cause numerous complications (see the Nutrition Perspective at the end of this chapter for further discussion of diabetes).

■ Imparting Flavor and Sweetness to Foods

From birth, humans respond to sugars with a smile. Receptors for tasting sweetness are located on the tip of the tongue. These receptors recognize a variety of sugars and even some noncarbohydrate substances. The sugars vary in sweetness: on a per gram basis, for example, fructose is almost twice as sweet as sucrose under either acid or cold conditions; sucrose is 30% sweeter than glucose; and lactose is less than half as sweet as sucrose (Table 5-2).

Sugars improve the palatability of many foods and thus enhance diets in general. For example, a small amount of sucrose on a grapefruit improves the taste of this sour fruit. Moderation in using sugars is recommended, but there is no need to avoid sugars altogether. Recall from Chapter 2 that the Food Guide Pyramid suggests the following for moderation in sugar intake based on one's energy intake: 1600 kcal, 8 teaspoons; 2200 kcal, 12 teaspoons; 2800 kcal, 18 teaspoons.

insulin A hormone produced by beta cells of the pancreas. Insulin increases the synthesis of glycogen in the liver and the movement of glucose from the bloodstream into muscle and adipose cells, among other processes.

ketone bodies Incomplete breakdown products of fat, containing three or four carbons. Most contain a chemical group called a ketone, hence the name. An example is acetoacetic acid.

ketosis The condition of having high amounts of ketone bodies in the bloodstream and tissues.

type 1 diabetes A form of diabetes in which the person with the disease is prone to ketosis and requires insulin therapy.

Glucose is also used to synthesize the ribose and deoxyribose sugars used in RNA and DNA synthesis, respectively.

TABLE 5-2 The Sweetness of Sugars and Alternative Sweeteners

Type of Sweetener	Relative Sweetness* (Sucrose = 1)	Typical Sources
Sugars		
Lactose	0.2	Dairy products
Maltose	0.4	Sprouted seeds
Glucose	0.7	Corn syrup
Sucrose	1.0	Table sugar, most sweets
Invert sugar†	1.3	Some candies, honey
Fructose	1.2–1.8	Fruit, honey, some soft drinks
Sugar Alcohols		
Sorbitol	0.6	Dietetic candies, sugarless gum
Mannitol	0.7	Dietetic candies
Xylitol	0.9	Sugarless gum
Alternative Sweeteners		
Cyclamate	30	Not currently in use in the United States
Aspartame	180	Diet soft drinks, diet fruit drinks, sugarless gum, powdered diet sweetener
Acesulfame-K	200	Sugarless gum, diet drink mixes, powdered diet sweeteners, puddings, gelatin desserts
Saccharin (sodium salt)	300	Diet soft drinks
Sucralose	600	Diet soft drinks, tabletop use, sugarless gums, jams, frozen desserts

From the American Dietetic Association, 1993, and other sources.

*On a per gram basis

†Sucrose broken down into glucose and fructose

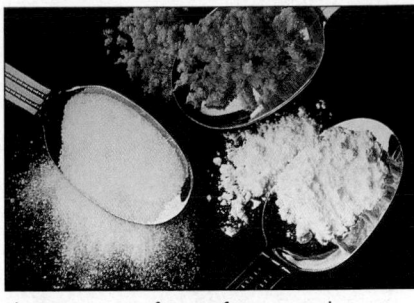

There are many forms of sugar on the market. Used in many foods, together they contribute to our daily intake of approximately 82 g of sugars in our diets.

■ FUNCTIONS OF DIETARY FIBER

Dietary fiber supplies mass to the feces, making elimination much easier. When enough fiber is consumed, the stool is large and soft because many types of plant fibers attract water. The larger size stimulates the intestinal muscles, which aids elimination. Consequently, less pressure is necessary to expel the stool.

When too little dietary fiber is eaten, the opposite can occur: the stool may be small and hard. Constipation may result, which can force one to exert excessive pressure in the large intestine during defecation. This high pressure can force parts of the large intestine (colon) wall out from between the surrounding bands of muscle, forming small pouches called **diverticula.** A person can have many diverticula (Fig. 5-7). **Hemorrhoids** may also result from excessive straining during defecation (see Chapter 3).

Diverticula are asymptomatic in about 80% of affected people; that is, they are not noticeable. The asymptomatic form of this disease is called **diverticulosis.** If the diverticula become filled with food particles, such as hulls and seeds, they may eventually become inflamed, a condition known as **diverticulitis.** Intake of dietary fiber then should be reduced to limit further bacterial activity. Once the inflammation subsides, a high-fiber diet (but free of seeds and hulls) is resumed to ease stool elimination and reduce the risk of a future attack.

Additional health benefits can accrue from the consumption of dietary fiber. A diet high in fiber aids weight control and reduces the risk of developing obesity. The bulky

diverticula Pouches that protrude through the exterior wall of the large intestine.

hemorrhoid A pronounced swelling of a large vein, particularly veins found in the anal region.

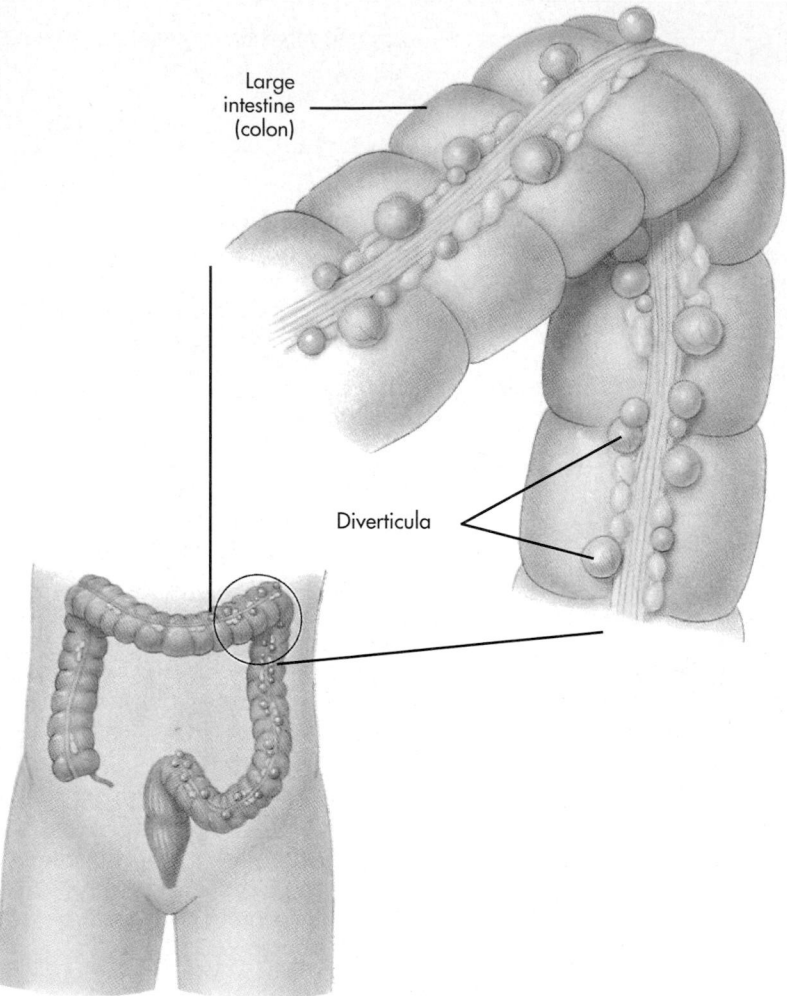

Large intestine (colon)

Diverticula

■ **FIGURE 5-7** Diverticula in the colon. A low-fiber diet increases the risk of developing diverticula.
Illustration by William Ober.

nature of high-fiber foods fills us up without yielding much energy. High-fat foods tend to do just the opposite, contributing to obesity. Increasing intake of foods rich in dietary fiber is one strategy for remaining satisfied after a meal, even if the fat content in a diet is low (review the discussion on energy density in Chapter 2).[27]

Over the past 30 years, many population studies have shown a link between increased dietary fiber intake and a decrease in colon cancer development. However, recent clinical trials have questioned the relationship between intake of dietary fiber and colon cancer development. Currently, most of the research on colon cancer is focusing on the potential preventive effects of vegetable intake; regular exercise; the use of aspirin and related pain medications; estrogen replacement therapy in women; and adequate folate, selenium, and calcium intakes. Smoking, obesity in men, and red meat intake are under study as potential causative factors.[5] Overall, the health benefits to the colon that stem from a high-fiber diet are probably due mostly to the nutrients that are commonly part of high-fiber foods, such as vitamins, minerals, phytochemicals, antioxidants, and in some cases essential fatty acids. Thus it is more advisable to increase fiber intake using fiber-rich foods, rather than mostly relying on fiber supplements.

When consumed in large amounts, soluble dietary fiber somewhat slows glucose absorption from the small intestine. This effect can be helpful in the treatment of diabetes. In fact, women whose main carbohydrate source is low-fiber foods are 2.5 times more likely to develop diabetes than those who have high-fiber diets (see the Nutrition Perspective at the end of this chapter). As well, a recent study found that 50 g of fiber per day improved blood glucose regulation in type 2 diabetes.[6]

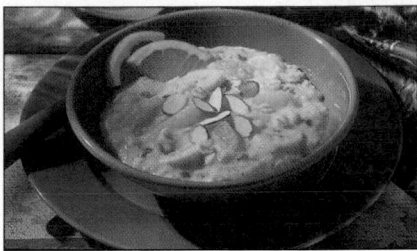

Oatmeal is a rich source of soluble fiber, namely beta-glucan. FDA allows a health claim for the benefits of oatmeal to lower blood cholesterol that arise from the effects of this soluble fiber.

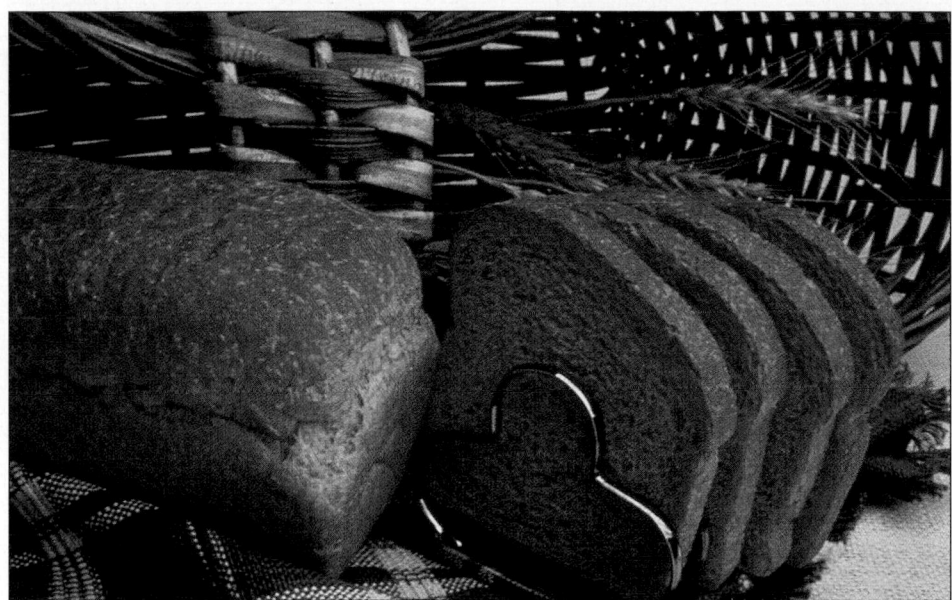

Whole grains are an excellent source of insoluble fiber.

A high intake of soluble dietary fiber also inhibits absorption of cholesterol and bile acid (cholesterol-rich) from the small intestine, thereby reducing blood cholesterol and possibly reducing the risk of developing gallstones. The short-chain fatty acids resulting from bacterial degradation of soluble fiber (e.g., proprionic acid) also probably reduce cholesterol synthesis in the liver. In addition, the reduced glucose absorption that occurs with diets high in soluble fiber is linked to a decrease in insulin release. Since insulin stimulates cholesterol synthesis in the liver, this reduction in insulin may contribute to the ability of soluble dietary fiber to lower blood cholesterol.[28]

One study showed that men who ate more than 25 g of fiber per day had a 36% lower risk of developing coronary heart disease, and those eating 29 g of fiber per day decreased their risk of a heart attack by 41%. A large study of women with a high intake of whole grains (about 2.5 servings per day) showed a 30% decreased risk for coronary heart disease, compared with a low intake of whole grains (less than 1 serving per day).[18] For these reasons, experts are recommending a 10 g/day increase in fiber above the typical 16 g/day intake, especially from grain sources, to prevent coronary heart disease in the average American. Overall, a fiber-rich diet containing fruits, vegetables, beans, and whole grains (including whole-grain breakfast cereals) is advocated as part of a strategy to reduce cardiovascular disease (coronary heart disease and stroke) risk.[31]

CONCEPT CHECK

Carbohydrates provide glucose for the energy needs of red blood cells and parts of the brain and central nervous system. Eating less than 50 to 100 g of carbohydrates per day forces the production of glucose (via gluconeogenesis), using carbons from amino acids. These amino acids are derived from the breakdown of proteins in body organs. An inadequate carbohydrate intake also inhibits efficient fat metabolism, which in turn can lead to ketosis. Sugars also improve the flavor of many foods.

Dietary fiber forms a vital part of the diet by adding mass to the stool, which eases elimination. It also helps in weight control and reduces the risk of developing obesity and cardiovascular disease. Soluble fibers can also be useful for controlling blood glucose in patients with diabetes and in lowering blood cholesterol. Whole grains, vegetables, beans, and fruits are excellent sources of dietary fiber.

*A*dvice from the Dietary Guidelines regarding carbohyrates is

- Choose a variety of grains daily, especially
  whole grains.
- Choose a variety of fruits and vegetables
  daily.
- Choose beverages and foods that limit
  your intake of sugars.

*H*ealthy People 2010 has the
following goals related to carbohydrate
intake:

- Increase the proportion of persons age 2
  years and older who consume at least six
  daily servings of grain products, with at
  least three being whole grains.
- Increase the proportion of persons age 2
  years and older who consume at least two
  daily servings of fruit.
- Increase the proportion of persons age 2
  years and older who consume at least
  three daily servings of vegetables, with at
  least one-third being dark green or orange
  vegetables.

Syndrome X A condition in which the person
has insulin resistance, hypertension,
increased blood triglycerides, and decreased
HDL cholesterol levels. This condition is
usually accompanied by obesity, lack of
physical activity, and a diet high in refined
carbohydrates.

■ RECOMMENDED CARBOHYDRATE INTAKES

No RDA for carbohydrates has been established. A DRI is slated for release in 2001 (check the web site http://www4.nationalacademies.org/IOM/IOMHome.nsf/Pages/Food+and+Nutrition+Board). As discussed before, it is important to consume at least 50 to 100 g of carbohydrates per day to prevent ketosis. It is easy to consume 50 g of carbohydrates. Just three pieces of fruit or three slices of bread or a little more than 3 cups of milk will suffice. In fact, it is difficult to follow a diet that will produce ketosis. As mentioned, the average American eats 200 to 300 g of carbohydrates per day. The top five carbohydrate sources for U.S. adults are white bread, soft drinks, cookies and cakes (including doughnuts), sugars/syrups/jams, and potatoes. Clearly, many Americans (teenagers included) should take a closer look at their main carbohydrate sources and strive to improve these from a nutritional standpoint.[13]

In the United States, carbohydrates supply about 50% of dietary energy intake for adults. Worldwide, however, carbohydrates account for about 70% of all energy consumed. In some countries, carbohydrates account for up to 80% of the energy consumed.

■ How Much Dietary Fiber Do We Need?

A reasonable goal for dietary fiber intake for the average adult is 20 to 35 grams per day (10 to 13 g/1000 kcal). In the United States, the average whole-grain intake is less than one serving per day. This low intake is attributed to the lack of knowledge on the benefits of whole grains, as well as the lack of ability to recognize whole-grain products at the time of purchase. Thus, most of us should increase our dietary fiber intake.[7] (For children over 2, experts recommend a fiber intake of age + 5 g/day.) Eating a high-fiber cereal (≥ 3 grams of fiber per serving) for breakfast is one easy way to increase dietary fiber intake (Fig. 5-8). As mentioned before, whole-food sources such as cereals, not bran supplements, are preferable because foods provide a broader variety of nutrients. This is especially true for many natural high-fiber foods—whole grains, fruits, vegetables, and beans.

As mentioned before, Table 5-3 shows a diet containing 25 to 30 g of dietary fiber but only 1750 kcal. This is an easy diet to follow to meet fiber recommendations if you like whole-wheat bread, fruits, vegetables, and beans. Use Table 5-4 to estimate the fiber content of your diet. What is *your* fiber score?

Currently, recommendations for carbohydrate intake vary widely in the scientific literature and popular press. Aside from the low intakes used to induce ketosis as part of a plan for quick weight loss (note that this diet is not recommended for more than 4 to 6 weeks at a time; see Chapter 13), recommendations vary from 45% of calories in *Syndrome X* diet plan to more than 70% in the *Pritikin Program* and *Eat More, Weigh Less* plan. The Nutrition Facts panel on food labels uses 60% of calories as the standard for recommended carbohydrate intake. This last recommendation has wide support in the scientific community. In addition, one recommendation on which almost all experts agree is that one's carbohydrate intake should be base primarily on fruits, vegetables, whole grains, and beans, not mostly on refined grains and sugar. Dr. Connor discussed this in detail in his Expert Opinion starting on page 172.

Only when a person's blood triglycerides are high is a carbohydrate-rich diet not recommended. (This will be covered further in Chapter 6 with respect to **Syndrome X.**) Actually, the chief culprits in this case are not carbohydrates as a class of nutrients but excessively large meals full of foods both rich in simple sugars and refined starches and low in dietary fiber, coupled with little physical activity.[26] These practices should not form the basis of daily habits, but unfortunately, they do for many adults.[28]

Note that manufacturers list enriched white (refined) flour as wheat flour on food labels. Most people think that if "wheat bread" is on the label, they are buying a

Nutrition Facts (Left Label)

Serving Size 1 cup (55g/2.0 oz.)
Servings Per Container 10

Amount Per Serving	Cereal	Cereal with ½ Cup Vitamins A & D Skim Milk
Calories	170	210
Calories from Fat	10	10
	% Daily Value**	
Total Fat 1.0g*	2%	2%
Sat. Fat 0g	0%	0%
Cholesterol 0mg	0%	0%
Sodium 300mg	13%	15%
Potassium 340mg	10%	16%
Total Carbohydrate 43g	14%	16%
Dietary Fiber 7g	28%	28%
Sugars 16g		
Other Carbohydrate 20g		
Protein 4g		
Vitamin A	15%	20%
Vitamin C	20%	22%
Calcium	2%	15%
Iron	65%	65%
Vitamin D	10%	25%
Thiamin	25%	30%
Riboflavin	25%	35%
Niacin	25%	25%
Vitamin B6	25%	25%
Folate	30%	30%
Vitamin B12	25%	35%
Phosphorus	20%	30%
Magnesium	20%	25%
Zinc	25%	25%
Copper	10%	10%

*Amount in cereal. One half cup skim milk contributes an additional 40 calories, 65mg sodium, 6g total carbohydrate (6g sugars), and 4g protein.
**Percent Daily Values are based on a 2,000 calorie diet. Your daily values may be higher or lower depending on your calorie needs:

	Calories:	2,000	2,500
Total Fat	Less than	65g	80g
Sat Fat	Less than	20g	25g
Cholesterol	Less than	300mg	300mg
Sodium	Less than	2,400mg	2,400mg
Potassium		3,500mg	3,500mg
Total Carbohydrate		300g	375g
Dietary Fiber		25g	30g

Calories per gram:
Fat 9 • Carbohydrate 4 • Protein 4

Ingredients: Wheat bran with other parts of wheat, raisins, sugar, corn syrup, salt, malt flavoring, glycerin, iron, niacinamide, zinc oxide, pyridoxine hydrochloride (vitamin B6), riboflavin (vitamin B2), vitamin A palmitate, thiamin hydrochloride (vitamin B1), folic acid, vitamin B12, and vitamin D.

Nutrition Facts (Right Label)

Serving Size: ¾ Cup (30g)
Servings Per Package: About 17

Amount Per Serving	¾ Cup Cereal	Cereal With ½ Cup Skim Milk
Calories	120	160
Calories from Fat	0	5
	%Daily Value**	
Total Fat 0g*	0%	1%
Saturated Fat 0g	0%	1%
Cholesterol 0mg	0%	1%
Sodium 40mg	2%	4%
Potassium 60mg	2%	8%
Total Carbohydrate 26g	9%	11%
Dietary Fiber 1g	4%	4%
Sugars 15g		
Other Carbohydrate 10g		
Protein 2g		
Vitamin A	25%	30%
Vitamin C	0%	2%
Calcium	0%	15%
Iron	10%	10%
Vitamin D	10%	20%
Thiamin	25%	25%
Riboflavin	25%	35%
Niacin	25%	25%
Vitamin B6	25%	25%
Folate	25%	25%
Vitamin B12	25%	30%
Phosphorus	4%	15%
Magnesium	4%	8%
Zinc	10%	10%
Copper	2%	2%

*Amount in Cereal. One-half cup skim milk contributes an additional 65mg sodium, 6g total carbohydrate (6g sugars), and 4g protein.
**Percent Daily Values are based on a 2000 calorie diet. Your daily values may be higher or lower depending on your calorie needs:

	Calories:	2,000	2,500
Total Fat	Less than	65g	80g
Sat. Fat	Less than	20g	25g
Cholesterol	Less than	300mg	300mg
Sodium	Less than	2,400mg	2,400mg
Potassium		3,500mg	3,500mg
Total Carbohydrate		300g	375g
Dietary Fiber		25g	30g

Calories per gram:
Fat 9 • Carbohydrate 4 • Protein 4

Ingredients: Wheat, Sugar, Corn Syrup, Honey, Caramel Color, Partially Hydrogenated Soybean Oil, Salt, Ferric Phosphate, Niacinamide (Niacin), Zinc Oxide, Vitamin A (Palmitate), Pyridoxine Hydrochloride (Vitamin B6), Riboflavin, Thiamin Mononitrate, Folic Acid (Folate), Vitamin B12 and Vitamin D.

FIGURE 5-8 Reading the Nutrition Facts on food labels helps us choose more nutritious foods. Based on the information from these nutrition labels, which cereal is the better choice for breakfast? Consider the amount of dietary fiber in each cereal, based on the amount per 100 kcal. Do the ingredient lists give you any clues? (Note: Ingredients are always listed in descending order by weight on a label.) When choosing a breakfast cereal, it is generally wise to focus on those that are rich sources of dietary fiber. Simple sugar content can also be used for evaluation. However, sometimes this number does not reflect added sugar but simply the addition of fruits, such as raisins, complicating the evaluation.

whole-wheat product. Not so. If the label does not list "whole-wheat flour" first, then the product is not primarily a whole-wheat bread and thus does not contain as much dietary fiber as it could. Careful reading of labels is important in the search for more dietary fiber—look especially for whole grains.

Keep in mind, however, that any nutrient can lead to health problems when consumed in excess, including carbohydrate and dietary fiber. High carbohydrate, high fiber, and low fat does not mean zero calories. Carbohydrates help moderate energy

TABLE 5-3   Sample 1750 kcal Menu Containing 25 to 30 g of Dietary Fiber*

Menu	Fiber Content (Grams)	Exchanges	Carbohydrate Content (Grams) Based on the Exchange System
Breakfast			
1 cup orange juice (with pulp)	0.5	2 fruit	30
3/4 cup Wheaties	2	1 starch	15
1/2 cup 2% milk	—	½ very-low-fat milk	6
1 slice whole-wheat toast	2	1 starch	15
1 tsp margarine	—	1 fat	0
Coffee	—	Free	0
Lunch			
2 oz lean ham	—	2 lean meat	0
2 slices whole wheat bread	4	2 starch	30
2 tsp mayonnaise	—	2 fat	0
1/4 cup lettuce	0.2	1 vegetable	0
1/3 cup cooked white beans	4	1 starch	15
1 pear (with skin)	4	1 fruit	15
1/2 cup 1% milk	—	½ skim/very-low-fat milk	6
Snack			
1 carrot (as carrot sticks)	2	1 vegetable	5
Dinner			
3 oz broiled chicken (no skin)	—	3 very lean meat	0
1 baked potato (large, with skin)	3	2 starch	30
1 1/2 tsp margarine	—	1½ fat	0
1 cup cooked green beans	4	2 vegetable	10
1/2 tsp margarine	—	½ fat	0
1 cup 1% milk	—	1 skim/very-low-fat milk	12
1 apple (with peel)	3.7	1 fruit	15
Snack			
1 raisin bagel	1.2	2 starch	30
	Total 30.6 grams		Total 234 grams

*The overall diet pattern is based on the Food Guide Pyramid. Breakdown of energy content: carbohydrate, 60%; protein, 20%; fat, 20%.

intake in comparison with fats, but the contribution of high-carbohydrate foods to total energy intake still has to be accounted for.

■ Problems with High-Fiber Diets

Very high intakes of dietary fiber—for example, 60 g/day—can pose some health risks and, so, require close physician supervision if used. A high dietary fiber intake especially requires a high fluid intake. Not consuming enough fluid with the fiber can leave the stool very hard and make it difficult and painful to eliminate. Large amounts of dietary fiber may also bind important minerals, such as calcium, zinc, and iron.

High-fiber diets often contribute to intestinal gas and occasionally to the production of fiber balls, called **phytobezoars,** in the stomach. These have been found in diabetic patients and in elderly people who consume large amounts of dietary fiber. Phytobezoars can lead to blockage of intestinal flow. Dietary fiber may also contribute to blockages in the intestine when intake is high and sufficient fluid is not consumed. Finally, large amounts of dietary fiber may add such an excess of bulk to

phytobezoars Pellets of dietary fiber, characteristically found in the stomach.

TABLE 5-4 Estimate Your Fiber Intake

To roughly estimate your daily fiber consumption, determine the number of servings of each food category listed below that you consumed yesterday. Multiply the serving amount by the value listed and then add up the total amount of fiber. How does your total fiber intake for yesterday compare with the general recommendation of 20 to 35 g of fiber per day?

Food	Servings	Grams
Vegetables (serving size: 1 cup raw leafy greens or 1/2 cup other vegetables)	_____ × 2	
Fruits (serving size: 1 whole fruit; 1/2 grapefruit; 1/2 cup berries or cubed fruit; 1/4 cup dried fruit)	_____ × 2.5	
Beans, lentils, split peas (serving size: 1/2 cup cooked)	_____ × 7	
Nuts, seeds (serving size: 1/4 cup; 2 tbsp peanut butter)	_____ × 2.5	
Whole grains (serving size: 1 slice whole-wheat bread; 1/2 cup whole-wheat pasta, brown rice, or other whole grain; 1/2 each bran or whole-grain muffin)	_____ × 2.5	
Refined grains (serving size: 1 slice bread, 1/2 cup pasta, rice, or other processed grains; and 1/2 each refined bagels or muffins)	_____ × 1	
Breakfast cereals (serving size: check package for serving size and amount of fiber per serving)	_____ × grams fiber per serving	
Total Grams of Fiber =		_____

Adapted from Fiber: Strands of protection. *Consumer Reports on Health*, p. 1, August 1999.

a child's diet that energy intake is reduced; dietary fiber fills the stomach before food intake meets energy needs.

■ Moderating Intake of Simple Sugars Is Important for Many of Us

Nutritionists suggest that simple sugars added to foods should provide no more than about 10% of total energy intake daily. This moderate intake corresponds to a maximum of about 50 g (or 10 teaspoons) of simple sugars per day, based on a 2000 kcal diet. On average, Americans eat about 82 g of added simple sugars daily, amounting to about 16% of energy intake.[2] Table 5-5 suggests ways to reduce intake of simple sugars. For many of us, this would be a healthful practice.[22]

Most of the simple sugars that we eat come from foods and beverages to which sugar has been added during processing and/or manufacture. The major sources are soft drinks, candy, cakes, cookies, pies, fruitades, and dairy desserts, such as ice cream.[13] The rest of the sugar in our diets is present naturally in foods, such as fruits, or comes from the sugar bowl. During food processing, the simple-sugar content is often increased. The more processed the food, generally the higher the simple-sugar content. An apple contains no added sugars, canned apples in heavy syrup contain 10 to 15 g (2 to 3 teaspoons) of added sugars, and one-sixth of a 9-inch apple pie contains 30 g (6 teaspoons) of added sugars. Careful label reading will suggest when a major increase in sugar content has occurred.

*I*t has been mentioned several times that milk and some dairy products contain the milk sugar lactose. This should in no way be construed to mean that milk is a food to avoid in order to limit simple-sugar consumption. In fact, low-fat and nonfat dairy products have an overall high nutrient density and would be one of the last sources of sugars to limit.

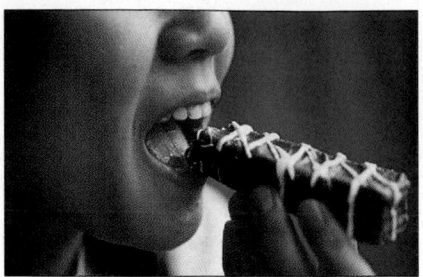

Many foods we enjoy are sweet. These should be eaten in moderation.

TABLE 5-5	Suggestions for Reducing Simple-Sugar Intake

At the Supermarket

- Read ingredient labels. Identify all the added sugars in a product. Select items lower in total sugar when possible.
- Buy fresh fruits or fruits packed in water, juice, or light syrup, rather than those packed in heavy syrup.
- Buy fewer foods that are high in sugar, such as prepared baked goods, candies, sugared cereals, sweet desserts, soft drinks, and fruit-flavored punches. Substitute vanilla wafers, graham crackers, bagels, English muffins, and diet soft drinks, for example.
- Buy reduced-fat microwave popcorn to replace candy for snacks.

In the Kitchen

- Reduce the sugar in foods prepared at home. Try new recipes or adjust your own. Start by reducing the sugar gradually until you've decreased it by one-third or more.
- Experiment with spices such as cinnamon, cardamom, coriander, nutmeg, ginger, and mace to enhance the flavor of foods.
- Use home-prepared items (with less sugar) instead of commercially prepared ones that are higher in sugar.

At the Table

- Use less of all sugars. This includes white and brown sugars, honey, molasses, and syrups.
- Choose fewer foods high in sugar, such as prepared baked goods, candies, and sweet desserts.
- Reach for fresh fruit instead of a sweet for dessert or between-meal snacks.
- Add less sugar to foods—coffee, tea, cereal, and fruit. Get used to using half as much; then see if you can cut back even more.
- Cut back on the number of sugared soft drinks, punches, and fruit juices you drink. Substitute water, diet soft drinks, and whole fruits rather than fruit juice.

Modified from USDA *Home and Garden Bulletin* No. 232-5, 1986.

There is a widespread notion that high sugar intake by children causes hyperactivity, typically part of the syndrome called attention deficit hyperactive disorder (ADHD). However, most researchers find that sucrose may actually have the opposite effect. A high-carbohydrate meal, if also low in protein and fat, has a calming effect and induces sleep; this effect may be linked to changes in the synthesis of certain neurotransmitters in the brain, such as serotonin (see Chapter 13). If there is a problem, it is probably the excitement or tension in situations in which sugar-rich foods are served, such as at birthday parties and on Halloween.

■ Problems with High-Sugar Diets

The main problem with consuming an overabundant amount of sugar is that it provides empty calories; this translates to a decline in the nutritional value of a diet.[2]

Diet Quality

Overcrowding the diet with sweet treats can leave little room for important, nutrient-dense foods, such as fruits and vegetables. Children and teenagers are at the highest risk for overconsuming empty calories in place of nutrients that are essential for growth. Many children and teenagers are drinking an excess of sugared soft drinks and other sugar-containing beverages and much less milk than ever before. Milk contains calcium and vitamin D, both of which are essential for bone health; therefore, this exchange of soft drinks for milk can compromise bone health.[2]

Supersizing beverages is also a growing problem; for example, in the 1950s a typical serving size of soft drink was a 6½ oz bottle, and now a 20 oz plastic bottle is a typical serving. This one change contributes 170 extra kcal to the diet. Filling up on sugared soft drinks in place of foods is not a healthy practice, but enjoying an occasional soft drink or limiting intake to one 12 oz serving a day is generally fine. Switching to diet soft drinks would spare the simple sugar calories, but still lacks in nutritional value, except for the fluid.

The sugar found in cakes, cookies, and ice cream supplies many extra calories that promote weight gain, unless an individual is physically active. Today's low-fat and fat-free snack products usually contain lots of added sugar to produce a product with an acceptable taste. The result is to produce a high calorie food that is equal to or greater in calories than the high-fat food product it was designed to replace. Following the recommendation of having no more than 10% of added sugars is easier if sweet desserts such as cakes, cookies, and ice cream (full and reduced fat), are consumed sparingly.[29]

Dental Caries

Sugars in the diet (and starches that are readily fermented in the mouth, such as crackers and white bread) also increase the risk of developing **dental caries.** Caries are formed when sugars and other carbohydrates are metabolized into acids by bacteria that live in the mouth (Fig. 5-9). These acids dissolve the tooth enamel and underlying structure. Bacteria also use the sugars to make plaque, a sticky substance that both adheres bacteria to teeth and diminishes the acid-neutralizing effect of saliva.[19]

The worst offenders in terms of dental caries are sticky and gummy foods high in sugars, such as caramel, because they stick to the teeth and supply the bacteria with a long-lived carbohydrate source. These long-lived carbohydrates are termed **cariogenic** (*cario* means "cavity"). Although liquid sugar sources (e.g., fruit juices) are not as potent at causing dental caries as sticky and gummy foods, they still warrant consideration. Some experts caution that sports drinks may also lead to dental caries due to their acid content.

Snacking regularly on sugary foods is also likely to cause caries because it gives the bacteria on the teeth a steady source of carbohydrate from which to continually make acid. Sugared gum chewed between meals is a prime example of a poor dental habit. Still, sugar-containing foods are not the only foods that allow acid production by the bacteria in the mouth. As mentioned, if starch-containing foods (e.g., crackers and bread) are held in the mouth for a long time, they can be acted on by enzymes in the mouth that break down the starch to sugars; bacteria can then produce acid from these sugars. Overall, the sugar and starch content of a food and its retentive ability largely determine its cariogenicity.[2]

Fluoridated water and toothpaste have contributed to fewer dental caries in American children over the past 20 years due to the mineral's tooth-strengthening effect (see Chapter 12). Research has also indicated that certain foods—such as cheese, peanuts, and sugar-free chewing gum—can actually help reduce the amount of acid on teeth. In addition, rinsing the mouth after meals and snacks reduces the acidity in the mouth. Certainly, good nutrition, habits that do not present an overwhelming challenge to oral health (e.g., chewing sugar-free gum), and routine visits to the dentist all contribute to improved dental health.

dental caries Erosion in the surface of a tooth caused by acids made by bacteria as they metabolize sugars.

cariogenic Literally, "caries-producing"; a substance, often carbohydrate-rich (such as caramel), that promotes dental caries.

CRITICAL THINKING

John and Mike are identical twins who like the same games, sports, and foods. However, John likes to chew sugar-free gum and Mike doesn't. At their last dental visit, John had no cavities, but Mike had two. Mike wants to know why John, who chews gum after eating, doesn't have cavities and he does. How would you explain this to him?

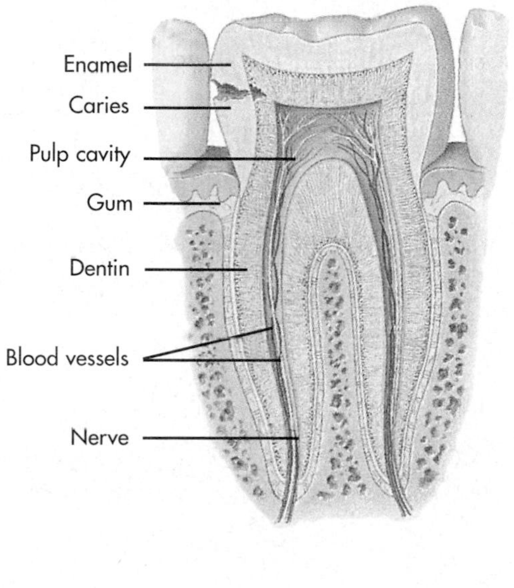

Enamel
Caries
Pulp cavity
Gum
Dentin
Blood vessels
Nerve

■ FIGURE 5-9 Dental caries. Bacteria can collect in various areas on a tooth. Bacteria metabolize simple sugars into acids, which can dissolve tooth enamel, leading to caries. If the caries process progresses and enters the pulp cavity, damage to the nerve may occur. The bacteria also produce plaque to adhere themselves to the tooth's surface.
Illustration by William Ober.

glycemic index (GI) The blood glucose response of a given food, compared to a standard (typically, glucose or white bread). Glycemic index is influenced by starch structure, fiber content, food processing, physical structure, and macronutrients in the meal, such as fat.

low-density lipoprotein (LDL) The lipoprotein in the blood, containing primarily cholesterol; elevated LDL cholesterol is strongly linked to cardiovascular disease risk.

High Glycemic Index

Many foods high in sugar produce a high **glycemic index (GI)** in the body. Glycemic index is defined as the blood glucose response to a given food, compared to a standard (typically, glucose or white bread) (Table 5-6). Glycemic index is influenced by starch structure, fiber content, food processing, physical structure, and macronutrients in the meal, such as fat. Foods with particularly high GI values are baking potatoes (not seen as much with red potatoes, as these are low in amylopectin), mashed potatoes (due to greater surface area exposed), white rice, honey, jelly beans, and vanilla wafers.[22]

Nutritionists are concerned about the effect of high GI carbohydrates on blood glucose because these carbohydrates especially increase insulin output from the pancreas. Chronically high insulin output leads to many deleterious effects on the body: high blood triglycerides; smaller **low-density lipoprotein (LDL)** particles, which are more prone to lead to atherosclerosis and thus cardiovascular disease; increased fat deposition in adipose tissue; increased tendency for blood to clot; increased fat synthesis in the liver; and a more rapid return of hunger after a meal (insulin rapidly lowers the macronutrients in the blood as it stimulates their storage). Over time, this increase in insulin output may actually cause the muscles to become resistant to the action of insulin, creating a state of insulin resistance and eventually type 2 diabetes in some people.[26]

TABLE 5-6   Glycemic Index (GI) of Common Foods

Reference food glucose = 100
Low GI foods—below 55
Intermediate GI foods—between 55 and 70
High GI foods—more than 70

Pastas/Grains		Breads and Muffins	
Brown rice	55	Bagel	72
White, long grain	56	Whole-wheat bread	69
White, short grain	72	White bread	70
Spaghetti	41	Croissant	67

Sugars			
Honey	73		
Sucrose	65		
Fructose	23		
Lactose	46		

Vegetables		Fruits	
Carrots, boiled	49	Apple	38
Sweet corn	55	Banana	55
Potato, baked	85	Grapefruit	25
New (red) potato, boiled	62	Orange	44

Dairy Foods		Beverages	
Milk, whole	27	Apple juice	40
Milk, skim	32	Orange juice	46
Yogurt, low-fat	33	Gatorade	78
Ice cream	61	Coca-Cola	63

Legumes		Snack Foods	
Baked beans	48	Potato chips	54
Kidney beans	27	Vanilla wafers	77
Lentils	30	Chocolate	49
Navy beans	38	Jelly beans	80

Adapted from Brand-Miller J, Wolever T, Colagiuri S, Foster-Powell K: *The glucose revolution—The authoritative guide to the glycemic index.* New York: Marlowe & Company, 1999.

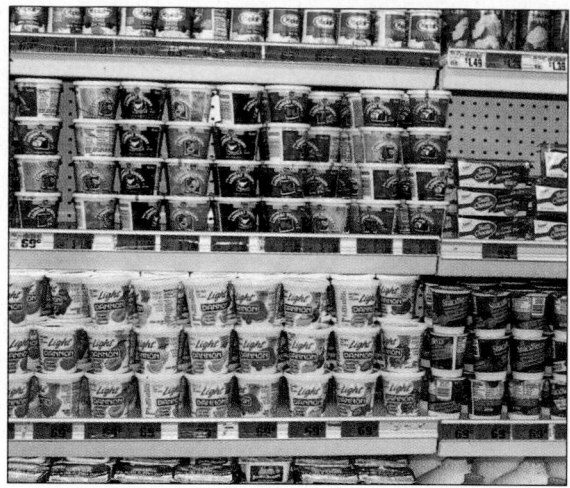

Eating yogurt helps moderately lactose-intolerant individuals meet their calcium needs.

There are many ways to address this problem of high-GI carbohydrates. The most important is to not overeat high-GI carbohydrates at any one meal, especially foods that are rich in added sugars. This greatly minimizes the effects of high-GI foods on blood glucose and the related increased insulin release.[1] Combining a low-GI index food, such as an apple, baked beans, milk, or salad with dressing, with a high-GI index food also reduces the effect on blood glucose. In addition, maintaining a healthy body weight and performing regular physical activity further reduces the effects of a high GI diet.

As you will see in the Nutrition Perspective at the end of the chapter, a focus on low-GI foods helps in the treatment of diabetes; Chapter 14 discusses the use of foods with different GI values in planning diets for athletes.

■ Moderation in Lactose Intake Is Important for Some People

Lactose intolerance (also called lactase nonpersistance) is a normal pattern of physiology that probably develops after early childhood. This *primary* form of lactose intolerance is estimated to be present in about 75% of the world's population, although not all of these individuals experience symptoms.[19] [It is hypothesized that, approximately 3000 to 5000 years ago, a genetic mutation occurred in regions that relied on milk and dairy foods as a main food source, allowing those individuals (mostly in northern Europe, pastoral tribes in Africa, and the Middle East) to retain the ability to maintain high lactase output for their entire lifetime. This was not seen in other populations in the world, and so such tolerance was not retained.] Another form of the problem, *secondary* lactose intolerance, is a temporary condition in which levels of lactase are decreased in response to an underlying disease, such as intestinal diarrhea.

In the United States, approximately 72 million individuals show signs of lactose intolerance, many of whom are Asian Americans, African-Americans, and Hispanic Americans, especially as they age. Still, many of these lactose-intolerant individuals can tolerate moderate amounts of lactose with minimal or no gastrointestinal discomfort, it is unnecessary for them to greatly restrict their intake of lactose-containing foods.[23] These calcium-rich food products are important in preventing osteoporosis. Obtaining enough calcium and vitamin D from the diet is much easier if milk and milk products are included.

Recent studies have shown that nearly all lactose-intolerant individuals can tolerate ½ to 1 cup of milk with meals and that most individuals adapt to intestinal gas production resulting from the colonic fermentation of lactose usually after 4 to 6 months of milk consumption.[24] Combining lactose-containing foods with other foods also helps because certain properties of foods can have positive effects on rates

lactose intolerance (primary and secondary) Primary lactose intolerance occurs when lactase production declines for no apparent reason. Secondary lactose intolerance occurs when a specific cause, such as long-standing diarrhea, results in a decline in lactase production.

of digestion. For example, fat in a meal slows digestion, leaving more time for lactase action. Hard cheese and yogurt also are more easily tolerated than milk. Much of the lactose is lost in the production of cheese, and the active bacteria cultures in yogurt digest the lactose when these bacteria are broken apart in the small intestine and release lactase. In addition, an array of products, such as low-lactose milk and lactase pills, are available to assist lactose-intolerant individuals; still, few people actually need to use these products because their intolerance is moderate.[23, 30]

CASE SCENARIO
Follow-Up

In the case scenario, Myeshia suspected she was sensitive to lactose because, when she consumed two servings of milk during one meal, she developed bloating and gas. She tried to reproduce these symptoms by eating two servings of dairy foods in one meal, but to no avail. However, she inadvertently discovered that yogurt in conjunction with milk during the meal did not produce any symptoms. As you just learned, yogurt is tolerated better than milk by people with lactose intolerance because the bacteria that are present in yogurt digest much of the lactose. Her symptoms likely were also lessened because many people with lactose intolerance can consume moderate amounts of milk products with few or no symptoms.

CONCEPT CHECK

The prevention of ketosis requires consuming 50 to 100 g of carbohydrate per day. The typical American diet provides 200 to 300 g/day. A reasonable goal is to have about half of our energy intake coming from starch and our total carbohydrate intake making up about 60% of our energy intake. This should allow for the recommended intake of 20 to 35 g of fiber/day. High-fiber diets must be accompanied by adequate fluid intakes to avoid constipation and phytobezoars and should be followed under a physician's guidance.

Americans eat about 82 g of simple sugars added to foods each day. Most of these sugars are added to foods and beverages in processing. The rest occurs naturally in foods or is added from the sugar bowl. To reduce consumption of sugars, one must reduce consumption of items with added sugars, such as some baked goods, sweetened beverages, and presweetened breakfast cereals. This is one practice that can help reduce the development of dental caries and likely improve diet quality. Lactose intolerance is a condition that results when cells of the intestine do not make sufficient lactase, the enzyme necessary to digest lactose, resulting in symptoms such as abdominal gas, pain, and diarrhea. Most people with lactose intolerance can tolerate cheeses and yogurt, as well as moderate amounts of milk.

CARBOHYDRATES IN FOODS: FOOD SWEETENERS

In the Exchange System, each milk exchange provides 12 g of carbohydrate; one starch exchange, one other carbohydrate exchange, and one fruit exchange each provides 15 g of carbohydrate; and one vegetable exchange provides 5 g of carbohydrate (review Table 2–9 in Chapter 2).

The foods that yield the highest percentage of energy from carbohydrates are table sugar, honey, jam, jelly, fruit, and plain baked potatoes. These foods are rich sources of carbohydrate; carbohydrates deliver much of their food energy. Corn flakes, rice, bread, and noodles all contain at least 75% of energy as carbohydrates. Foods with moderate amounts of carbohydrate energy are peas, broccoli, oatmeal, dry beans and other legumes, cream pies, french fries, and skim milk. In these foods, the carbohydrate content is diluted either by protein, as in the case of skim milk, or by fat, as in the case of a cream pie. Foods with essentially no carbohydrates include beef, eggs, chicken, fish, vegetable oils, butter, and margarine.

Figure 5-10 shows that, in planning a high-carbohydrate diet, you need to emphasize grains, pasta, fruits, and vegetables. On the other hand, you can't create a diet high in carbohydrate energy from chocolate, potato chips, and french fries because these foods contain too much fat. The percentage of energy from carbohydrate is more important than the total amount of carbohydrate in a food when planning a high-carbohydrate diet.

The various substances that impart sweetness to foods fall into two broad classes: nutritive sweeteners, which can be metabolized to yield energy, and alternative sweeteners, which provide no food energy. As was shown in Table 5-2, the alternative sweeteners are much sweeter on a per-gram basis than the nutritive sweeteners.[15]

■ Nutritive Sweeteners

Both sugars and sugar alcohols provide energy along with sweetness. Sugars are found in many different food products, whereas sugar alcohols have rather limited uses.

Sugars

All of the monosaccharides (glucose, fructose, and galactose) and disaccharides (sucrose, lactose, and maltose) that we discussed earlier are designated *nutritive sweeteners* (Table 5-7). The taste and sweetness of sucrose make it the benchmark against which all other sweeteners are measured. Consumption of table sugar (sucrose) currently ranges from 12 to 48 pounds/year for each person.[2]

A sweetener used today is high-fructose corn syrup, which is 40 to 90% fructose. High-fructose corn syrup is made by treating cornstarch with acid and enzymes. This treatment breaks down much of the starch into glucose. Then some of the glucose is converted by enzymes into fructose. The final syrup is usually as sweet as

TABLE 5-7	Names of Sugars Used in Foods		
Sugar	Invert sugar	Honey	Maple syrup
Sucrose	Glucose	Corn syrup or	Dextrin
Brown sugar	Sorbitol	sweeteners	Dextrose
Confectioner's	Levulose	High-fructose corn	Fructose
sugar (powdered	Polydextrose	syrup	Maltose
sugar)	Lactose	Molasses	Caramel
Turbinado sugar	Mannitol	Date sugar	Fruit sugar

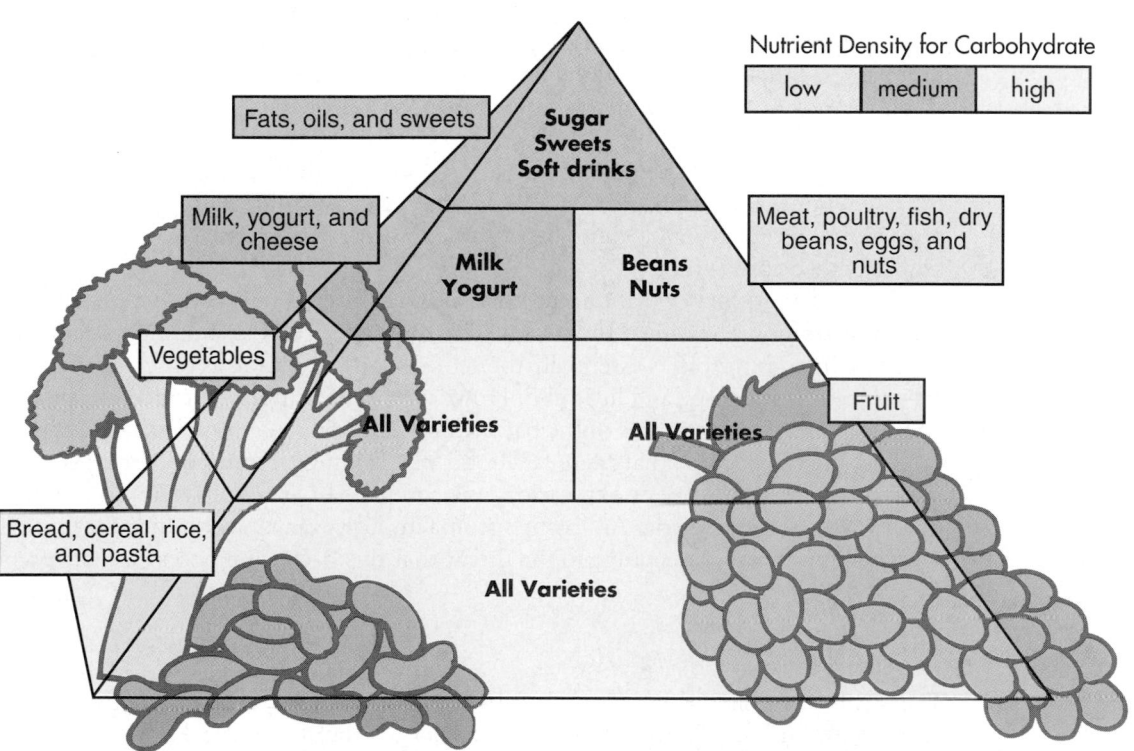

■ **FIGURE 5-10** Sources of carbohydrates from the Food Guide Pyramid. The bread, cereal, rice, and pasta group; fruit group; vegetables group; and milk, yogurt, and cheese group contain many foods rich in carbohydrate. The background color of each group indicates the average nutrient density for carbohydrate in that group.

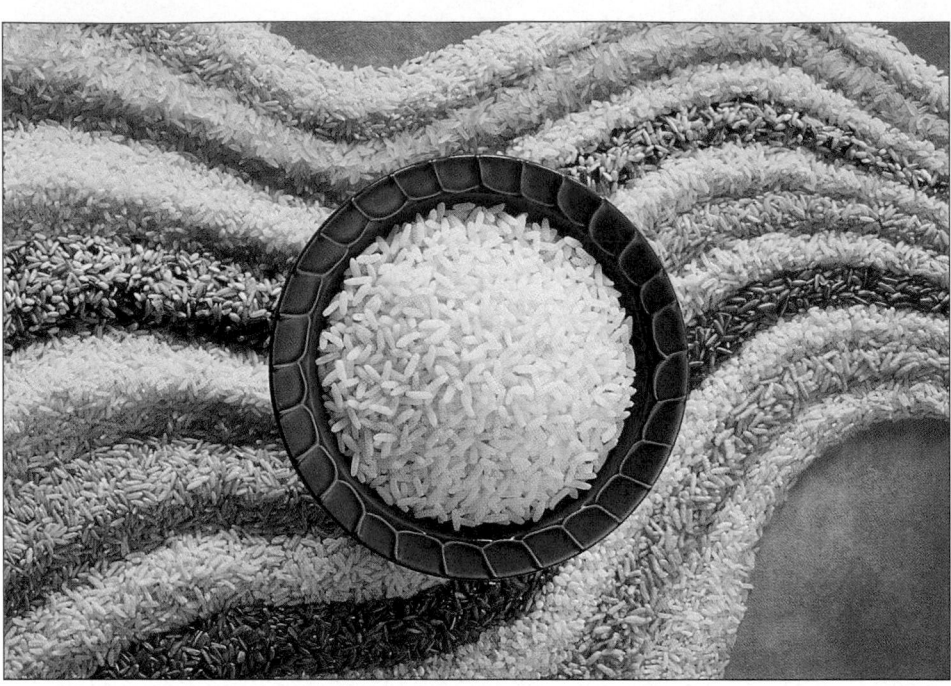

Rice is a rich source of carbohydrate.

sucrose. Its major advantage is that it is cheaper than sucrose. Also, it doesn't form crystals, and it has better freezing properties. High-fructose corn syrups are used in soft drinks, candies, jam, jelly, other fruit products, and desserts (e.g., packaged cookies).

In addition to sucrose and high-fructose corn syrup, brown sugar, turbinado sugar, honey, maple syrup, and other sugars are also added to foods. Turbinado sugar, a partially refined version of raw sucrose, has a slight molasses flavor. Brown sugar is essentially sucrose containing some molasses; either the molasses is not totally removed from the sucrose during processing or it is added to the sucrose crystals.

Maple syrup is made by boiling down and concentrating the sap that runs during the late winter in sugar maple trees. Most pancake syrup sold in supermarkets is not pure maple syrup, which is quite expensive. Instead, it is primarily corn syrup and high-fructose corn syrup.

Honey is a product of plant nectar that has been altered by bee enzymes. The enzymes break down much of the nectar's sucrose into fructose and glucose. As we noted earlier, honey offers essentially the same nutritional value as other simple sugars—a source of energy and little else. However, honey is not safe to feed to infants because it can contain spores of the bacterium *Clostridium botulinum*. These spores can become the bacteria that cause fatal food-borne illness. Honey does not pose the same threat to adults because the acidic environment of an adult's stomach inhibits the growth of the bacteria. An infant's stomach, however, does not produce much acid, making infants susceptible to the threat that this bacterium poses (see Chapters 17 and 19).

Sugar Alcohols

xylitol An alcohol derivative of the five-carbon monosaccharide xylose.

The sugar alcohols sorbitol, mannitol, and **xylitol** are also used as nutritive sweeteners. Although sugar alcohols contribute energy (about 1.5 to 3 kcal/g), they are absorbed and metabolized to glucose more slowly than simple sugars. Still, in large quantities these substances do not provide a significant advantage for people with diabetes because such amounts can cause diarrhea, and they are usually found primarily in diabetic candy and gum. In fact, any products whose foreseeable consumption may result in a daily ingestion of 50 g of sorbitol or mannitol must bear this labeling statement: "Excess consumption may have a laxative effect."

Sugar alcohols must be listed on labels, and if only one sugar alcohol is used in a product it must be distinguished; however, if two or more are used in one product they are grouped together under the heading "sugar alcohols." The actual caloric value is calculated, taking in account each sugar alcohol, so that, when one reads the total amount of calories a product provides, it includes the sugar alcohols in the overall amount.

Sorbitol and xylitol are used in sugarless gum, breath mints, and candy. These are not readily metabolized by bacteria in the mouth and thus do not promote dental caries nearly so readily as simple sugars such as sucrose. Recall from Chapter 2 that such a health claim can be made on these products.

■ Alternative Sweeteners

Often called artificial sweeteners, alternative sweeteners include **saccharin,** cyclamate, **aspartame,** and **acesulfame-K.**[15] From 1971 to 1991, Americans nearly quintupled their intake of low-calorie sweeteners, from 5 pounds per person to 24 pounds. Alternative sweeteners yield little or no energy when consumed in amounts typically used in food products. Four are currently available in the United States: saccharin, aspartame, acesulfame, and **sucralose.** Cyclamate was banned for use in the United States in 1970, although it has never been conclusively proved to cause health problems when used appropriately. Cyclamate is used in Canada as a sweetener in medicines and as a tabletop sweetener.

Saccharin

The oldest alternative sweetener, saccharin, was first produced in 1879 and is currently approved for use in more than 90 countries. It represents about half of the alternative sweetener market in the United States. Saccharin was once thought to pose a risk of bladder cancer based on laboratory animal studies, but it is no longer listed as a potential cause of cancer in humans, due to the failure of population studies to support that assumption.

Aspartame

In 1981, the alternative sweetener aspartame became available. Its trade name is NutraSweet when added to foods and Equal when sold as a powder. Aspartame is in widespread use throughout the world. It has been approved for use by more than 90 countries, and its use has been endorsed by the World Health Organization, the American Medical Association, the American Diabetes Association, and the American Academy of Pediatrics Committee on Nutrition.[2]

The components of aspartame are the amino acids phenylalanine and aspartic acid, along with methanol. Recall that amino acids are the building blocks of proteins, so aspartame is more of a protein than a carbohydrate. Aspartame yields about 4 kcal/g, but it is 180 to 200 times sweeter than sucrose. Thus, only a small amount of aspartame is needed to obtain the desired sweetness, so the amount of energy added is insignificant unless the product is abused. Today aspartame is used in beverages, gelatin desserts, chewing gum, toppings and fillings in precooked bakery goods, and cookies. Aspartame does not cause tooth decay. Like other proteins, however, aspartame is damaged when heated for a long time and thus cannot be widely used in products requiring cooking.

To date, about 7000 complaints have been filed with FDA by people claiming to have had adverse reactions to aspartame: headaches, dizziness, seizures, nausea, and other side effects. It is important for people who are sensitive to aspartame to avoid it. But the percentage of sensitive people is likely to be extremely small. The relatively limited number of complaints about aspartame, considering its wide use in food products, means that most people can use it.[15]

saccharin An alternative sweetener that yields no energy to the body; it is 300 times sweeter than sucrose.

aspartame An alternative sweetener made from two amino acids and methanol; it is 200 times sweeter than sucrose.

acesulfame-K An alternative sweetener that yields no energy to the body; it is 200 times sweeter than sucrose.

sucralose An alternative sweetener that has chlorines in place of some hydroxyl (–OH) groups on sucrose. It is 600 times sweeter than sucrose.

CONTAINS: CARBONATED WATER, ORANGE JUICE, CITRIC ACID, NUTRASWEET* BRAND OF ASPARTAME**, POTASSIUM BENZOATE (A PRESERVATIVE), CITRUS PECTIN, POTASSIUM CITRATE, CAFFEINE, MALTODEXTRIN, GUM ARABIC, NATURAL FLAVORS, BROMINATED VEGETABLE OIL, YELLOW #5 AND ERYTHORBIC ACID (TO PROTECT FLAVOR). *NUTRASWEET® AND THE NUTRASWEET SYMBOL ARE REGISTERED TRADEMARKS OF THE NUTRASWEET COMPANY. PHENYLKETONURICS: CONTAINS PHENYLALANINE.

Note the warning for people with PKU that this diet soft drink with aspartame contains phenylalanine.

INGREDIENTS: SORBITOL, GUM BASE, MANNITOL, GLYCEROL, HYDROGENATED GLUCOSE SYRUP, XYLITOL, ARTIFICIAL AND NATURAL FLAVORS, ASPARTAME, RED 40, YELLOW 6 AND BHT (TO MAINTAIN FRESHNESS). PHENYLKETONURICS: CONTAINS PHENYLALANINE. *NUTRASWEET IS A REGISTERED TRADEMARK OF THE NUTRASWEET CO.

Sugarless Gum

Sugar alcohols can be found in sugarless gum. Note that aspartame is also used to sweeten this product.

One researcher has claimed to have found a link between aspartame and recent increases in brain cancer. Still, most researchers and FDA feel that the findings are invalid due to numerous inconsistencies. For example, the study overlooked the fact that better detection methods for brain cancer were developed during the same time that aspartame was introduced. In addition, the rise in brain cancer cases began before aspartame entered the food supply and have been falling since 1985.

Careful double-blind studies cast doubt on whether aspartame causes headaches and suggest that it generally does not stimulate later food intake, either. However, foods made with aspartame should be used to replace other high-calorie foods, but not used as an excuse to consume greatly larger volumes of food.

The acceptable daily intake of aspartame set by FDA is 50 mg/kg of body weight per day. This is equivalent to about 14 cans of diet soft drink for an adult or about 80 packets of Equal. Aspartame appears to be safe for pregnant women and children, but some scientists suggest cautious use by these groups, especially young children, who need ample food energy to grow.

Persons with a rare disease called phenylketonuria (PKU), which interferes with the metabolism of phenylalanine, should avoid aspartame because of its high phenylalanine content. (PKU is discussed further in Chapter 7.)

Acesulfame-K

The alternative sweetener acesulfame-K (Sunette) was approved by FDA in July 1988. It is approved for use in more than 40 countries and has been in use in Europe since 1983. Acesulfame-K is 200 times sweeter than sucrose. It contributes no energy to the diet because it is not digested by the body, and does not cause dental caries.

Unlike aspartame, acesulfame-K can be used in baking because it does not lose its sweetness when heated. In the United States, it is currently approved for use in chewing gum, powdered drink mixes, gelatins, puddings, baked goods, tabletop sweeteners, candy, throat lozenges, yogurt, and nondairy creamers; additional uses may soon be approved. One recent trend is to combine it with aspartame in soft drinks.

A product called Diabetisweet, uses a combination of acesulfame-K and Isomalt (a sweetener made of sugar alcohols) to produce a product that completely replaces sugar in baking and cooking. This product is a one way for people with diabetes to decrease sugar intake, but it is very expensive in comparison with sugar.

Sucralose

Sucralose (Splenda) is 600 times sweeter than sucrose. It is made by substituting three chlorines (Cl) for three hydroxyl groups (-OH) on sucrose. FDA approved sucralose's use in 1998 as an additive to foods such as soda, gum, baked goods, syrups, gelatins, frozen dairy desserts such as ice cream, jams, and processed fruits and fruit juices and for tabletop use. Sucralose doesn't break down under high heat conditions and can be used in cooking and baking. It is also excreted as such in the feces. The little that is absorbed is excreted in the urine. Because of such recent introduction, it is not clear whether the public will embrace this product. Canadians had access to sucralose before its U.S. introduction.

Other Alternative Sweeteners

Research continues on new forms of alternative sweeteners. Four are under investigation:
- Alitame, which is formed from two amino acids and another small nitrogen group, is 2000 times sweeter than sucrose.
- D-Tagatose, a compound derived from lactose, has the same sweetness as sucrose but yields only half the energy.
- Stevia is a South American shrub that is 100 to 300 times sweeter than sucrose and provides zero calories. This is a natural sweetener that has been used in small amounts by the Japanese since the 1970s. FDA has not approved the use of stevia in foods, due to concerns with toxicity. Stevia can be purchased at health-food stores as a dietary supplement.

- Thaumatins, proteins obtained from the fruit of the West African plant *Thaumatococcus danielii* that are 2000 times sweeter than sucrose, have been available in Japan and Europe for more than 10 years.

Overall, alternative sweeteners enable people with diabetes to enjoy the flavor of sweetness while controlling sugars in their diets; they also provide noncaloric or very-low-calorie sugar substitutes for persons trying to lose (or control) body weight.

CONCEPT CHECK

Foods that are essentially all carbohydrate are sugars, jam, jelly, fruit, and plain baked potatoes. Grains and vegetables are also rich sources of carbohydrate. Most simple sugars are added to foods and beverages during manufacturing or are added from the sugar bowl. To reduce intake of simple sugars, eat fewer items that contain a lot of added sugar, such as some baked goods, certain beverages, and some breakfast cereals. Simple sugars contribute to dental caries and provide few vitamins and minerals, if any. Four major alternative sweeteners are available in America today—saccharin, aspartame, acesulfame-K, and sucralose. These can aid in the goal of reducing simple-sugar intake.

Check out the *Perspectives in Nutrition* web site http://www.mhhe.com/wardlaw for quizzes, flash cards, other activities, and web links designed to further help you learn about carbohydrates.

■ SUMMARY

1. The common monosaccharides are glucose, fructose, and galactose. Once these are absorbed from the small intestine and delivered to the liver, much of the fructose and galactose is converted to glucose.

2. The major disaccharides are sucrose (glucose plus fructose), maltose (glucose plus glucose), and lactose (glucose plus galactose). When digested, these yield their component monosaccharides.

3. One major group of polysaccharides consists of storage forms of glucose: starches in plants and glycogen in humans. In these polymers, the multiple glucose units are linked by alpha bonds, which can be broken by human digestive enzymes, releasing the glucose units. The main plant starches—straight-chain amylose and branched-chain amylopectin—are digested by enzymes in the mouth and small intestine. In humans, glycogen is synthesized in the liver and muscle tissue from glucose. Under the influence of hormones, liver glycogen is readily broken down to glucose, which can enter the bloodstream.

4. Dietary fiber is composed primarily of the polysaccharides cellulose, hemicellulose, pectin, gum, and mucilage, as well as the noncarbohydrate lignins. These substances are not hydrolyzed by human digestive enzymes. However, soluble dietary fibers are metabolized by bacteria in the large intestine.

5. Some starch digestion occurs in the mouth. Carbohydrate digestion is completed in the small intestine. Some plant fibers are digested by the bacteria present in the large intestine; undigested plant fibers become part of the feces. Single sugars mostly follow an active absorption process in the small intestine. They are then transported via the portal vein to the liver.

6. Carbohydrates provide energy (on average, 4 kcal/gram), protect against wasteful breakdown of food and body protein, prevent ketosis, and impart flavor and sweetness to foods. Although no RDA for carbohydrate has been set, a daily intake of at least 50 to 100 g is required to prevent ketosis. If carbohydrate intake is inadequate to supply the body's needs, protein is metabolized to provide glucose (gluconeogenesis) for energy needs. However, the price is loss of body protein, ketosis, and eventually a general body weakening. For this reason, low-carbohydrate diets are not recommended for extended periods (greater than 4 to 6 weeks).

7. Dietary fiber provides mass to the feces, thus easing elimination. In high doses, soluble fibers can help control blood glucose in diabetic people and lower blood cholesterol.

8. Diets high in complex carbohydrates are encouraged as a replacement for high-fat diets. A goal of about half of energy as complex carbohydrates is a good one, with about 60% of total energy coming from carbohydrates in general. Foods to consume are whole-grain cereal products, pasta, legumes, fruits, and vegetables. Many of these foods are rich in dietary fiber.

9. Moderating sugar intake, especially between meals, in turn reduces the risk of dental caries. Other health benefits also occur, such as a reduced glycemic index (GI) for a meal or snack. Alternative sweeteners, such as aspartame, aid in reducing intake of simple sugars.

10. The ability to digest large amounts of lactose often diminishes with age. People in some ethnic groups are especially affected. This condition develops early in childhood and is referred to as *lactose intolerance*. Undigested lactose travels to the large intestine, resulting in such symptoms as abdominal gas, pain, and diarrhea. Most people with lactose intolerance can tolerate cheese and yogurt; tolerance of other dairy products varies among affected individuals.

▮STUDY QUESTIONS

1. Identify the three major disaccharides. Describe how each plays a part in the human diet.
2. How do amylose, amylopectin, and glycogen differ from one another? Why can this be important metabolically and in food processing?
3. What are the possible roles that dietary fiber plays in the diet?
4. Why must we generally limit our dietary fiber intake to no more than 60 g/day? What are the possible effects of a diet too high in fiber (or too low in fluid relative to dietary fiber)?
5. Briefly describe the chemical structure, sweetness, and food uses of alternative sweeteners.
6. Why do we need carbohydrates in the diet? Briefly describe three reasons.

7. Summarize current carbohydrate intake recommendations.
8. Write a list of suggestions for a patient who has been diagnosed with lactose intolerance. Design a 1-day sample menu that provides adequate calcium (1000 mg) for this patient.

After reading the Nutrition Perspective, answer the following questions:

9. How does type 1 diabetes differ from type 2 diabetes in cause and treatment?
10. What treatment is recommended for the typical form of hypoglycemia?

▮ANNOTATED REFERENCES

1. Abbasi F and others: High carbohydrate diets, triglyceride-rich lipoproteins, and coronary heart disease. *American Journal of Cardiology* 85:45, 2000.

   If a high-carbohydrate diet raises blood triglycerides above recommended concentration standards, the person should reduce refined carbohydrate intake and increase monounsaturated fat intake to see if that improves the person's blood lipid profile (see Chapter 6 for details on how to implement such a strategy).

2. ADA Reports: Position of the American Dietetic Association: Use of nutritive and non-nutritive sweeteners. *Journal of the American Dietetic Association* 98:580, 1998.

   Consumers can safely enjoy a range of nutritive and nonnutritive sweeteners when consumed in moderation and within the context of a diet consistent with the Dietary Guidelines for Americans. Nonnutritive sweeteners are safe for use by most persons within recommended intakes.

3. Anderson JW and others: Whole grain foods and heart disease risk. *Journal of the American College of Nutrition* 19:291S, 2000.

   Foods that are rich in dietary fiber, including fruits, vegetables, legumes, and whole-grain cereals, tend to be rich in vitamins, minerals, phytochemicals, antioxidants, and other micronutrients. Each of these components contributes to a reduction in heart disease risk.

4. Brancati FL and others: Incident of type 2 diabetes mellitus in African-American and white adults. *Journal of the American Medical Association* 283:2253, 2000.

   Almost half of the excess risk of type 2 diabetes in African-American women can be reduced by a combination of weight reduction, dietary modifications such as an increased intake of dietary fiber, and regular physical activity. Control of blood pressure is also important in this population.

5. Byers T: Diet, colorectal adenomas, and colorectal cancer. *The New England Journal of Medicine* 342:1206, 2000.

   Nutrients such as folate, selenium, and calcium are associated with a lower risk of colon cancer. Medications such as aspirin and related agents (e.g., celecobix [Celebrex]) also may reduce the risk of this disease. Some studies from around the world also have shown a lower risk of colon cancer among populations with high intakes of fruits and vegetables (especially vegetables).

6. Chandalia AM and others: Beneficial effects of high dietary fiber intake in patients with type 2 diabetes mellitus. *The New England of Medicine* 342:1392, 2000.

   A high intake of dietary fiber, particularly of the soluble type, improves blood glucose control and lowers blood lipids in patients with type 2 diabetes. Intake of fiber in this study was 50 g/day, well above the goal of 20 to 35 g/day currently recommended by the American Diabetes Association.

7. Cleveland LE and others: Dietary intake of whole grains. *Journal of the American College of Nutrition* 19:331S, 2000.

   Consumption of whole grains by U.S. adults, currently only about one serving of whole grains per day, falls well below the recommended amount. A large proportion of the population could benefit from eating more whole grains, and efforts are needed to encourage consumption of these foods.

8. Colberg SR, Swain DP: Exercise and diabetes control. *Physician and Sportsmedicine* 28(4):63, 2000.

   Exercise is a cornerstone of diabetes management and provides many health benefits. It is important for people with diabetes to check their blood glucose before, during, and after activity to make sure it stays within the recommended range. Such persons are especially warned to consume enough food at the right times to avoid hypoglycemia and related problems.

9. Do you know your blood sugar level? *Consumer Reports on Health*, p. 1, July 2000.

   Even just slightly elevated blood glucose can put a person at health risk. People who should especially be tested for elevated blood glucose include those who are overweight, those with relatives with diabetes, non-Caucasians, women who had a baby weighing more than 9 pounds, and those who have hypertension, low HDL, or high blood triglycerides.

10. Flemmer MC, Vinik AI: Evidence-based therapy for type 2 diabetes. *Postgraduate Medicine* 107(5):27, 2000.

    A wide variety of medications can be used to treat type 2 diabetes. Diet therapy is also a cornerstone of treatment. In addition, control of hypertension and elevated blood lipids is important.

11. Gerhard GT and others: Plasma lipid and lipoprotein responsiveness to dietary fat and cholesterol in premenopausal African American and white women. *American Journal of Clinical Nutrition* 72:56, 2000.

    Diets low in total fat, saturated fat, and cholesterol and high in fiber may reduce the risk of heart disease in African-American and White women by lowering LDL cholesterol and reducing the rise in blood triglycerides after fat-rich meals.

12. Goldstein DE: Diabetes screening. *Nutrition & the M.D.*, p. 1, February 2000.

    As many as 16 million people in the United States have diabetes, and almost 50% of affected individuals are currently undiagnosed. Large-scale studies such as the Diabetes Control and Complications Trial (DCCT) show that keeping blood glucose in the recommended range reduces the risk of many diseases linked to diabetes. Currently, a fasting blood glucose of ≥ 126 mg/dl is considered too high and requires treatment. Other indications for treatment are a blood glucose of ≥ 200 mg/dl taken on a random (nonfasting) basis or 2 hours after a meal.

13. Guthrie JF, Morton JF: Food sources of added sweeteners in the diets of Americans. *Journal of the American Dietetic Association* 100:43, 2000.

    Americans older than 2 years consume the equivalent of 82 g of carbohydrate per day from added sweeteners. This accounts for 16% of total energy intake. Adolescent males consume the most added sweeteners, averaging 20% of total energy intake. The biggest source of added sweeteners are regular soft drinks, which account for one-third of intake. Other sources are table sugars, syrups, and cakes and other sweets.

14. Havas S: Educational guidelines for achieving tight control and minimizing complications of type 1 diabetes. *American Family Physician* 60:1985, 1999.

    Tight blood glucose control in patients with type 1 diabetes can delay onset and slow the progression of many diabetes-related diseases. A variety of forms of insulin are available. Besides careful management of insulin therapy, eating a healthy diet; performing regular exercise; and learning the signs, symptoms, and management of hypoglycemia are important for people with type 1 diabetes.

15. Henkel J: Sugar substitutes: Americans opt for sweetness and lite. *FDA Consumer*, p. 12, November/December 1999.

    FDA has approved four sugar substitutes—saccharin, aspartame, acesulfame-K, and sucralose. At least three other sweeteners are under FDA review but have not been approved at this time. FDA stands behind its approval of current sugar substitutes.

16. Howard BV: Insulin resistance and lipid metabolism. *American Journal of Cardiology* 84:28J, 1999.

    Weight loss in insulin-resistant persons can significantly improve insulin action, decrease blood triglycerides, increase HDL cholesterol, and produce other beneficial effects. Exercise also works to do the same things. Certain medications can be added to further improve blood glucose control in people with insulin resistance.

17. Hu FB and others: Walking compared with vigorous physical activity and risk of type 2 diabetes in women. *Journal of the American Medical Association* 282:1433, 1999.

    Physical activity of moderate intensity and duration, such as brisk walking, is associated with a substantial reduction in the risk of type 2 diabetes.

18. Jacobs DR and others: Fiber from whole grains, but not refined grains, is inversely associated with all-cause mortality in older women: The Iowa women's health study. *Journal of the American College of Nutrition* 19:326S, 2000.

    Women who consume whole grains on a regular basis and limited servings of refined grains show lower mortality than women who consume primarily refined grains. Whole grains are nutrient rich and confer many health benefits.

19. Levin RJ: Carbohydrates. *Modern Nutrition in Health and Disease*. 9th ed. In Shils ME and others (eds.): Baltimore: Williams & Wilkins, 1999.

    The chemical structures, history, and metabolism of carbohydrates are reviewed, including the relationship between carbohydrates and diabetes. In addition, some rare carbohydrate metabolic disorders are discussed, such as fructose intolerance and various forms of glycogen storage disease.

20. Meyer KA and others: Carbohydrates, dietary fiber, and incident type 2 diabetes in older women. *American Journal of Clinical Nutrition* 71:921, 2000.

    Grains, especially whole grains, and dietary magnesium are associated with a reduction in the development of diabetes in older women. These factors reduce risk even if the person remains overweight.

21. Morey SS: ADA examines cardiovascular problems in diabetes. *American Family Physician* 61:561, 2000.

    Cardiovascular disease is a common problem in diabetes. Recommendations to minimize risk include smoking cessation, control of blood pressure, control of blood glucose, regular physical activity, weight management, and use of some medications, such as angiotensin converting enzyme (ACE) inhibitors.

22. Morris KL, Zemel MB: Glycemic index, cardiovascular disease, and obesity. *Nutrition Reviews* 57:273, 1999.

    The glycemic index of food is influenced by starch structure (amylose vs. amylopectin), fiber content, food processing, physical structure of the food, and other macronutrients in a meal. Low-glycemic-index diets have been reported to lower blood glucose after a meal and insulin release, to improve blood lipids, and to increase insulin sensitivity.

23. Overview of lactose maldigestion (lactase nonpersistence). *Journal of the American Dietetic Association* 99:481, 1999.

    Recent evidence strongly suggests that people with lactose maldigestion can include the recommended numbers of servings of milk and milk products in their diets without experiencing much gastrointestinal discomfort. Use of such products over time may actually improve tolerance. When milk products are avoided, calcium intake may be compromised.

24. Pribila BA and others: Improved lactose digestion and intolerance among African-American adolescent girls fed a dairy-rich diet. *Journal of the American Dietetic Association* 100:524, 2000.

    Lactose maldigestion should not be a restricting factor in achieving adequate calcium intakes for African-American adolescent girls. They are able to tolerate the amount of lactose that accompanies sufficient milk products to meet calcium recommendations.

25. Rendell M: Dietary treatment of diabetes mellitus. *The New England Journal of Medicine* 342:1440, 2000.

    Combining a high-fiber diet with the use of foods with a low glycemic index effectively lowers blood glucose concentrations. The decrease in blood glucose achieved by a high-fiber diet is similar to that seen with the use of various oral diabetes medications.

26. Roberts K and others: Syndrome X: Medical nutrition therapy. *Nutrition Reviews* 58:154, 2000.

    Lifestyle factors such as overeating and physical inactivity play a pivotal role in Syndrome X. The typical Western diet, which is high in refined carbohydrates, low in fiber, and high in saturated fat, is associated with an increased risk of obesity, leading to insulin resistance and Syndrome X.

27. Roberts SB: High-glycemic index foods, hunger, and obesity: Is there any connection? *Nutrition Reviews* 58:163, 2000.

    Consumption of high-glycemic-index foods may increase hunger and promote overeating in comparison to consumption of foods with lower glycemic index. Based on current knowledge, consumption of whole grains and low-glycemic-index cereals instead of highly refined cereals is a recommended dietary change.

28. Should you be eating more fat and fewer carbohydrates? *Tufts University Health & Nutrition Letter*, p. 1, February 1999.

    Some people find that their blood triglycerides rise beyond desirable amounts when they consume simple carbohydrates. This problem can be avoided by not overeating, engaging in regular physical activity, and losing weight if overweight. Substituting some monounsaturated fat calories for simple carbohydrates calories also helps.

29. Sugar: What's the harm? *Consumer Reports on Health*, p. 1, May 1999.

    Sugar provides only calories with no other nutrients and can crowd out important nutrients in the diet. Many of us consume too much sugar and should cut back on our intake. This is especially important for people who show evidence of insulin resistance or diabetes.

30. Vesa TH and others: Lactose intolerance. *Journal of the American College of Nutrition* 19:165S 2000.

    Many lactose maldigestors tolerate small to moderate amounts of lactose without remarkable discomfort. Lactose-hydrolysed milk products and fermented milk products also can help people exhibiting lactose intolerance.

31. Wolk A and others: Long-term intake of dietary fiber and decreased risk of coronary heart disease among women. *Journal of the American Medical Association* 281:1998, 1999.

    High fiber intakes, particularly from cereal sources, reduce the risk of coronary heart disease in women. This provides further reason to replace refined forms of starch with whole-grain products.

TAKE ACTION

I. HOW DOES YOUR DIET RATE FOR CARBOHYDRATE AND DIETARY FIBER?

Let's reevaluate the nutritional assessment you completed at the end of Chapter 2. Here are your tasks:

1. Look at your analysis and find the total number of grams of carbohydrate you ate.

    TOTAL GRAMS OF CARBOHYDRATE _____

    A. Did you consume more than the minimum amount to avoid ketosis, 50 to 100 g?

    B. Now calculate the percentage of energy in your diet from carbohydrate. You will need the total grams of carbohydrate from your assessment, as well as the total kcals you ate. Use this formula to calculate it:

    $$\frac{\text{Total grams of carbohydrate} \times 4}{\text{Total kcals consumed}} \times 100 = \% \text{ of energy intake from carbohydrate}$$

    ANSWER: _____

    Was about 60% or more of your total energy intake from carbohydrate? Yes _____ No _____

    If not, list several ways you could increase your carbohydrate intake.

    _____

    _____

    _____

2. Look again at the list of foods you ate, including the amounts, and determine the total amount of dietary fiber you consumed. If you have a computer analysis of your diet, your dietary fiber intake is listed in the printout. Otherwise, look up the dietary fiber content of each food you ate in the food composition table in Appendix A; then calculate your total intake, taking into account the amount of each food you ate.

    TOTAL AMOUNT OF DIETARY FIBER CONSUMED _____ grams

    A. Did you eat the 20 to 35 g suggested in this chapter?

    B. If not, what could you do to increase your dietary fiber intake? What foods could you substitute for some of the foods you ate?

    _____

    _____

    _____

3. Finally, use Table 5-5 as a guide, if you need to reduce your intake of sugars, especially if you need to watch your total energy intake to maintain an appropriate weight. What three foods might you, in fact, limit in the future?

    _____

    _____

    _____

TAKE ACTION

II. CAN YOU CHOOSE THE SANDWICH WITH THE MOST DIETARY FIBER?

Assume the sandwiches on the blackboard below are available at your local deli and sandwich shop. All of the sandwiches provide about 350 kcal. The dietary fiber content ranges from about 1 g to about 7.5 g. Rank the sandwiches from highest amount of dietary fiber to lowest amount; then check your answers at the bottom of the page.

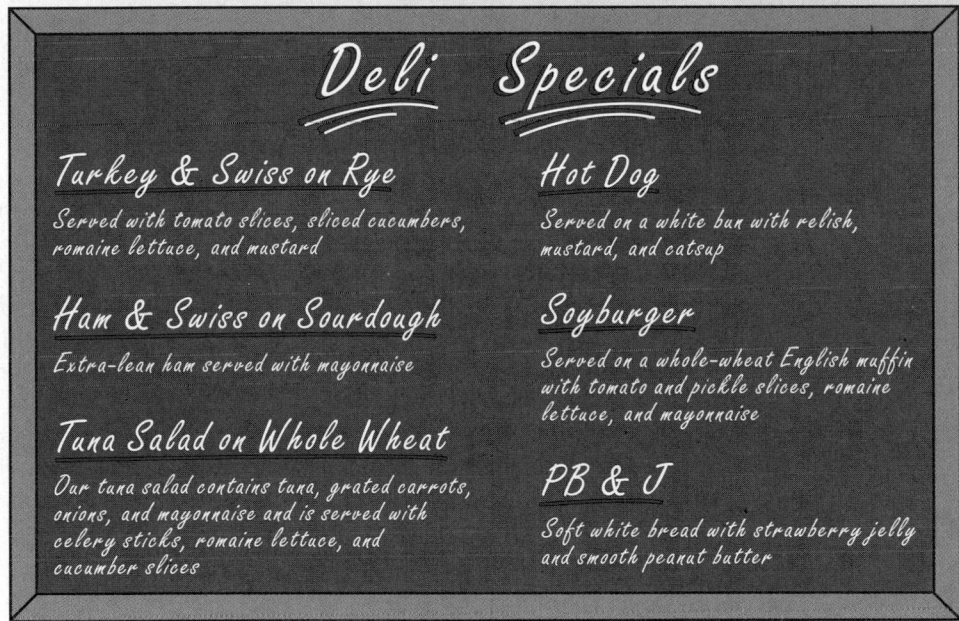

Deli Specials

Turkey & Swiss on Rye

Served with tomato slices, sliced cucumbers, romaine lettuce, and mustard

Ham & Swiss on Sourdough

Extra-lean ham served with mayonnaise

Tuna Salad on Whole Wheat

Our tuna salad contains tuna, grated carrots, onions, and mayonnaise and is served with celery sticks, romaine lettuce, and cucumber slices

Hot Dog

Served on a white bun with relish, mustard, and catsup

Soyburger

Served on a whole-wheat English muffin with tomato and pickle slices, romaine lettuce, and mayonnaise

PB & J

Soft white bread with strawberry jelly and smooth peanut butter

Answer Key: 1. Soyburger: 7.5 g, 2. Tuna Salad on Whole Wheat: 7 g, 3. Turkey & Swiss on Rye: 4 g, 4. PB&J: 3 g, 5. Ham & Swiss on Sourdough: 1.5 g, 6. Hot dog: 1g.

WHEN BLOOD GLUCOSE REGULATION FAILS

Improper regulation of blood glucose results in either hyperglycemia (high blood glucose) or hypoglycemia (low blood glucose). High blood glucose is most commonly associated with diabetes (technically, *diabetes mellitus*), a disease that affects about 16 million Americans, corresponding to 7% of the U.S. population. Of these, it is estimated ⅓ to ½ of these people do not know that they have the disease. Diabetes leads to 180,000 deaths each year in the United States. New recommendations promote testing fasting blood glucose in adults over age 45 every 3 years to help diagnose these missed cases.[10] In contrast, low blood glucose is a much rarer condition.

REGULATION OF BLOOD GLUCOSE

Under normal circumstances, blood glucose usually varies between about 70 and 110 mg/dl (dl represents 100 ml [deciliter]) of blood in the fasting state, which is normally established a few hours after a meal is eaten. If blood glucose rises above 170 mg/dl, glucose begins to spill over into the urine. This leads to hunger and thirst, and eventually to weight loss. If blood glucose falls below 40 to 50 mg/dl, a person begins to feel nervous, irritable, and hungry and may develop a headache. Having high blood glucose is called **hyperglycemia.** Having low blood glucose is called **hypoglycemia.** It is not too surprising that a headache then results, because the brain is fueled almost entirely by glucose.

The liver is the main organ for controlling the amount of glucose that is eventually found in the bloodstream. Since it is the first organ to screen the sugars absorbed from the small intestine, the liver serves as a guard, helping control the amount of glucose that enters the bloodstream after a meal (review Fig. 5-5).[19]

The pancreas is another important site of blood glucose control. Small amounts of insulin are released by the pancreas as soon as a person starts to eat. Once much of the dietary glucose enters the bloodstream, the pancreas releases large amounts of insulin. Insulin affects blood glucose in a variety of ways. It promotes increased glycogen synthesis and thus glucose storage in the liver, as well as increased glucose uptake by muscle cells, adipose cells, and some other cells. Both of these actions of insulin lower blood glucose and help return it to the normal fasting range within a few hours after a person eats. In addition, insulin reduces gluconeogenesis by the liver.

Other hormones counteract the effects of insulin. When a person has not eaten carbohydrates for a few hours, blood glucose begins to fall below the normal fasting range. It can be restored by the hormone glucagon, which is also released from the pancreas. This hormone prompts the breakdown of glycogen in the liver, resulting in the release of glucose to the bloodstream. Glucagon also enhances gluconeogenesis. In these ways, glucagon helps restore blood glucose to normal concentrations (Fig. 5-11).

At the same time, the hormones epinephrine (adrenaline) and norepinephrine are released from the adrenal glands and nearby nerve endings. These hormones trigger the breakdown of glycogen in the liver; the resulting glucose is released into the bloodstream. These hormones are responsible for the "fight or flight" reaction. They are released in large amounts in response to a perceived threat, such as a car approaching head-on. The resulting rapid release of glucose into the bloodstream promotes quick mental and physical reactions. Other hormones, such as cortisol and growth hormone, also help regulate blood glucose (Table 5-8).

In essence, the actions of insulin on blood glucose are balanced by the actions of glucagon, epinephrine, norepinephrine, cortisol, and other hormones. If hormonal balance is not maintained, such as during overproduction or underproduction of insulin or glucagon, major changes in blood glucose concentrations occur. This system of checks and balances for blood glucose regulation is typical of how the body maintains blood and other tissue concentrations of its key constituents within fairly narrow ranges.

hyperglycemia High blood glucose, above 125 mg/dl of blood on a fasting basis.

hypoglycemia Low blood glucose, below 40 to 50 mg/dl of blood.

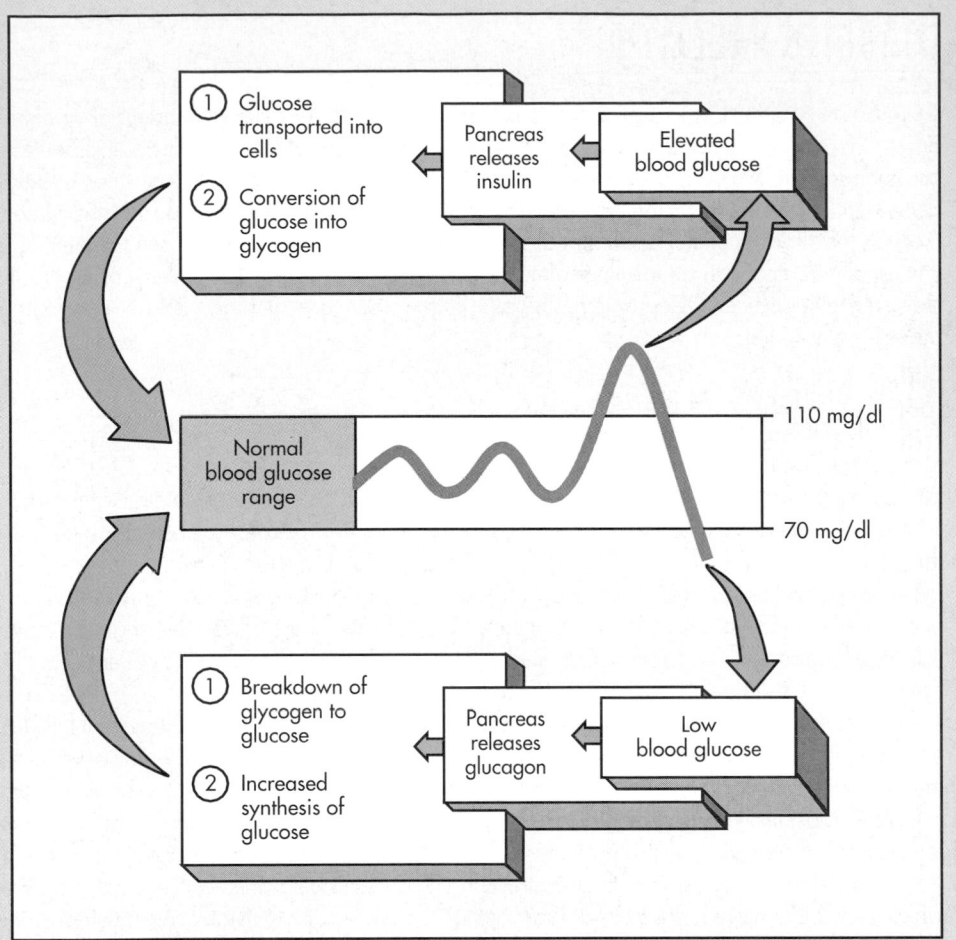

① Glucose transported into cells

② Conversion of glucose into glycogen

Pancreas releases insulin

Elevated blood glucose

Normal blood glucose range

110 mg/dl

70 mg/dl

① Breakdown of glycogen to glucose

② Increased synthesis of glucose

Pancreas releases glucagon

Low blood glucose

■ FIGURE 5-11 Regulation of blood glucose. Insulin and glucagon are key factors in controlling blood glucose. Other hormones, such as epinephrine, norepinephrine, cortisol, and growth hormone, also contribute to blood glucose regulation (see Table 5-8 for details).

Illustration by William Ober.

TABLE 5-8 Role of Various Hormones in the Regulation of Blood Glucose

Hormone	Source	Target Organ or Tissue	Overall Effect on Organ or Tissue	Effect on Blood Glucose
Insulin	Pancreas	Liver, muscle, adipose tissue	Increases glucose uptake by muscles and adipose tissue, increases glycogen synthesis, suppresses gluconeogenesis	Decrease
Glucagon	Pancreas	Liver	Increases glycogen breakdown, with release of glucose by the liver; increases gluconeogenesis	Increase
Epinephrine and norepinephrine	Adrenal glands and nerve endings	Liver, muscle	Increase glycogen breakdown, with release of glucose by the liver; increase gluconeogenesis	Increase
Cortisol	Adrenal glands	Liver, muscle	Increases gluconeogenesis by the liver, decreases glucose use by muscles and other organs	Increase
Growth hormone	Adrenal glands	Liver, muscle, adipose tissue	Decreases glucose uptake by muscles, increases fat mobilization and utilization, increases glucose output by the liver	Increase

DIABETES MELLITUS

There are two major forms of diabetes: type 1 (formerly called insulin-dependent or juvenile-onset diabetes), and **type 2** (formerly called **non–insulin-dependent** or adult-onset **diabetes**). The change in names to type 1 and type 2 diabetes stems from the fact that many "non–insulin-dependent" diabetics eventually have to also rely on insulin injections as a part of their treatment. A third form, called gestational diabetes, occurs in pregnant women (see Chapter 16). It is usually treated with an insulin regimen and diet, and resolves after delivery of the baby. However, evidence of this problem suggests that women are at high risk for developing diabetes later in life.

■ Type 1 Diabetes

Type 1 diabetes often begins in late childhood, around the age of 8 to 12 years, but can occur at any age. The disease runs in certain families, indicating a clear genetic link. Children usually are admitted to the hospital with abnormally high blood glucose after eating, with ketosis.

The onset of type 1 diabetes is generally associated with decreased release of insulin from the pancreas. As insulin in the blood declines, blood glucose increases, especially after eating. When blood glucose exceeds the kidney's threshold, excess glucose spills over into the urine—hence the term *diabetes mellitus,* which means "flow of much urine" (*diabetes*) that is "sweet" (*mellitus*). Figure 5-12 shows a typical glucose tolerance curve observed in a patient with this form of diabetes, following a test load of 75 g (15 teaspoons) of glucose.

An exciting finding regarding the cause of type 1 diabetes may help physicians treat this disease or even prevent its onset in the future. Most cases of type 1 diabetes begin with an immunological disorder, which causes destruction of the insulin-producing beta cells in the pancreas. Most likely, a virus or protein foreign to the body sets off the destruction. Cow's milk is suspected of supplying such a protein, so its introduction before 1 year of age is not advised (see Chapter 17). In response to their destruction, the affected beta cells release other proteins, which stimulate a more furious attack. Eventually, the pancreas loses its ability to synthesize insulin, and the clinical stage of the disease begins. Because of this immunological process, which destroys beta cells, pancreas transplants have proven very difficult in these patients, as this process may destroy the new beta cells. Consequently, early treatment to stop the immune-linked destruction in children may be important. Research on this is continuing.

type 2 (non–insulin-dependent) diabetes A form of diabetes in which ketosis is not commonly seen. Insulin therapy can be used but is often not required. This form of the disease is often associated with obesity.

*T*raditional symptoms of diabetes, known as the three polys, are polyuria (excessive urination), polydipsia (excessive thirst), and polyphagia (excessive hunger). No one symptom is diagnostic of diabetes, and other symptoms—such as unexplained weight loss, exhaustion, blurred vision, tingling in hands and feet, frequent infections, poor wound healing, and impotence—often accompany traditional symptoms.[9]

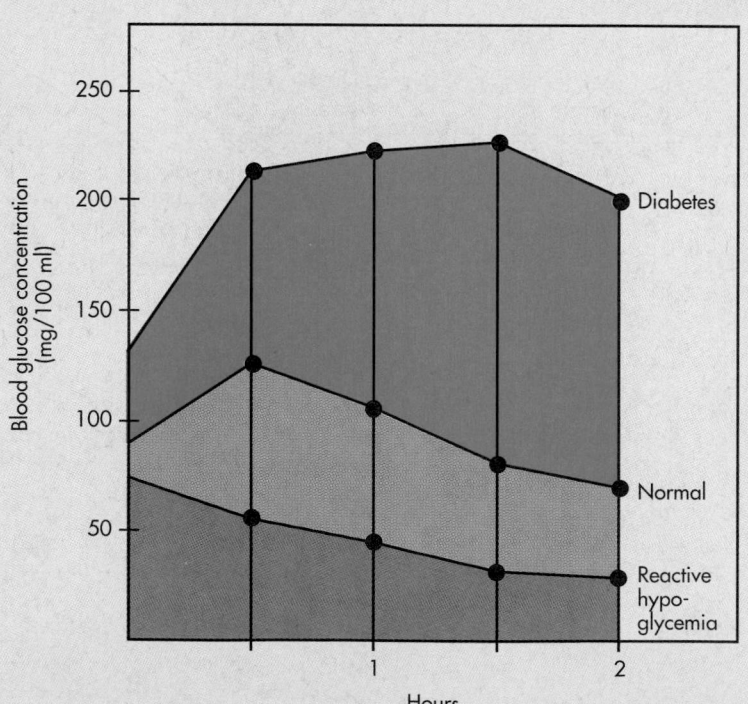

■ **FIGURE 5-12** Glucose tolerance test. These are typical responses seen after consumption of 75 g (15 teaspoons) of glucose by a healthy person and by a person with uncontrolled diabetes or reactive hypoglycemia. Blood glucose concentration is determined during fasting and then at regular intervals after the person consumes the glucose test load. The depiction of reactive hypoglycemia is theoretical; the actual existence of this syndrome is in question. In any case, true hypoglycemia is rare.
Illustration by William Ober.

Before 1921, if a person had type 1 diabetes, a high fat, low-calorie diet was recommended. This approach was found to be the best way to control blood glucose. It was somewhat effective but resulted in poor growth in childhood and was difficult to implement. In the early part of the 1900s, a clinician could walk into a diabetes ward in a hospital and see scores of young, emaciated children. The isolation of insulin by Banting and Best in 1921 and the first use of it soon after in children opened a new door in diabetes care.

Today, type 1 diabetes is treated primarily by insulin therapy, either with injections two to six times a day or with an insulin pump. The pump dispenses insulin at a steady rate into the body, with greater amounts delivered after each meal. Dietary measures include three regular meals and one or more snacks (including one at bedtime), having a regulated carbohydrate:protein:fat ratio to maximize insulin action and minimize swings in blood glucose. If one does not eat often enough, the injected insulin can cause severe hypoglycemia, since it acts on whatever little glucose is available. The diet should be rich in complex carbohydrates, include ample dietary fiber, and supply an amount of energy in balance with energy needs.[14] Typically, an angiotensin converging enzyme (ACE) inhibitor is added to the medication regime, as this reduces the risk of kidney disease in people with diabetes (see Chapter 11 for details on ACE inhibitors). Diabetes, especially if not treated adequately, often leads to eventual kidney disease.[21]

Type 1 patients often make excellent candidates for **carbohydrate counting**, a method that focuses on the amount of carbohydrates in each food choice. Type 1 patients are often very familiar with the exchange system and are motivated enough to learn how to use it to count carbohydrate intake. This method results in improved blood glucose control with a wider selection of foods.

If a high carbohydrate intake raises triglyceride and cholesterol in the blood beyond desired ranges, carbohydrate intake can be reduced and replaced with unsaturated fat. This change tends to reduce blood triglycerides and cholesterol.[1] Chapter 6 discusses how to implement such a diet. Moderate consumption of sugars with meals is fine, as long as blood glucose regulation is preserved and the sugars replace other carbohydrates in the meal, so that undesirable weight gain does not take place.

Because people with diabetes are at a high risk for heart disease and related heart attacks, they should take an aspirin each day if their physicians find no reason not to do so. As discussed in Chapter 6, this practice reduces the risk of heart attack.

The hormone imbalances that occur in people with untreated type 1 diabetes lead to mobilization of body fat, which is released into liver cells. Ketosis is the result because the fat is mostly converted to ketone bodies. Ketone bodies can rise excessively in the blood, eventually forcing ketone bodies into the urine. These pull sodium and potassium ions with them into the urine. This series of events can contribute to a chain reaction, which eventually leads to dehydration, ion imbalance, coma, and even death, especially in patients with poorly controlled type 1 diabetes. Treatment includes insulin, fluids, and electrolytes (e.g., sodium, potassium).

Other complications of diabetes can be degenerative conditions, such as blindness, heart disease and kidney disease; all are caused by poor blood glucose regulation. Nerves can also deteriorate, resulting in many changes that decrease proper nerve stimulation. When this occurs in the intestinal tract, intermittent diarrhea and constipation result. Because of nerve deterioration in the extremities, many people with diabetes lose the sensation of pain associated with injuries or infections. Not having as much pain, they often delay treatment of hand or foot problems. This delay, combined with a rich environment for bacterial growth (bacteria thrive on glucose) sets the stage for complications in the extremities, such as the need for amputation of feet and legs. High blood glucose also contributes to a rapid buildup of fats in blood vessel walls, which eventually chokes off the blood supply to nearby organs such as the heart. See Chapter 6 for details.

Current research, such as the Diabetes Control and Complications Trail (DCCT), has shown that the development of blood vessel and nerve complications of diabetes can be slowed with aggressive treatment directed at keeping blood glucose within the normal range. The therapy poses some risks of its own, such as hypoglycemia, so it must be implemented under the close supervision of a physician.

In both type 1 and type 2 diabetes, control of blood pressure and blood lipids are keys to long term health (see Chapters 6 and 11 for strategies).

carbohydrate counting A diet method that assigns a certain number of food exchanges or carbohydrate grams to each meal and snack. Insulin is matched to carbohydrate intake (i.e., 1 unit of insulin per 10-15 g of carbohydrates), and carbohydrate grams can come from several combinations of exchanges.

A common clinical method to determine a person's success in controlling blood glucose is to measure glycated hemoglobin (hemoglobin A1c). Over time, blood glucose attaches to (glycates) hemoglobin in red blood cells, and more so when blood glucose remains elevated. A hemoglobin A1c value of over 7% indicates poor blood glucose control. An acceptable value is 6% or less.

A person with diabetes generally must work closely with a physician and dietitian to make the correct alterations in diet and medications and to perform physical activity safely. Physical activity enhances glucose uptake by muscles independent of insulin action, which in turn can lower blood glucose. This outcome is beneficial, but people with diabetes need to be aware of their own blood glucose response to physical activity and compensate appropriately.[8]

■ Type 2 DIABETES

Type 2 diabetes usually begins after age 40. This is the most common type of diabetes, accounting for about 90% of the cases diagnosed in the United States. The number of people affected is on the rise, primarily because of widespread inactivity and obesity in our population. In fact, recently there has been a substantial increase in type 2 diabetes in children, due mostly to an increase in overweight in this population (coupled with limited physical activity). This type of diabetes is also genetically linked, but the initial problem is not with the beta cells of the pancreas. Instead, it arises with the insulin receptors on the cell surfaces of certain body tissues, especially muscle tissue. In this case, blood glucose is not readily transferred into cells, so the patient develops hyperglycemia as a result of the glucose's remaining in the bloodstream. The pancreas attempts to increase insulin output to compensate, but there is a limit to its ability to do this. Thus, rather than insufficient insulin production, there is an abundance of insulin, particularly during the onset of the disease. As the disease develops, pancreatic function can fail, leading to reduced insulin output. Because of the genetic link for type 2 diabetes, those who have a family history should be careful to avoid risk factors such as obesity, a diet rich in high-glycemic-index (GI) foods, and inactivity, and should be tested regularly for hyperglycemia.[20, 22]

Many cases of type 2 diabetes (about 80%) are associated with obesity (especially fat located in the abdominal region), but the hyperglycemia is not directly caused by the obesity. In fact, some lean people also develop this type of diabetes. Obesity associated with oversized fat cells simply increases the risk for insulin resistance by the body.

Type 2 diabetes linked to obesity often disappears if the obesity is corrected. Achieving a healthy weight should be a primary goal of treatment, but even limited weight loss can lead to better blood glucose regulation.[4, 16] Oral medications can also help. Some examples are medications that reduce glucose production by the liver (metformin [Glucophage]), increase the ability of the pancreas to release insulin (glipizide [Glucotrol]), and increase the body's response to its own insulin (rosiglitazone [Avandia]). Another class of oral agents used works by delaying carbohydrate digestion and glucose absorption (acarbose [Precose]). A tablet is taken with the first bite of each meal and may be combined with other therapy.[10]

Sometimes it may be necessary to provide insulin injections in type 2 diabetes because nothing else is able to control the disease. (This eventually becomes the case in about half of all cases of type 2 diabetes.) Regular physical activity also helps the muscles take up more glucose.[17] And regular meal patterns, with an emphasis on control of energy intake, consumption of low-glycemic-index complex carbohydrates, with ample dietary fiber, is important therapy.[12] Moderate intake of sugars is fine with meals, but again these must be substituted for other carbohydrates, not simply added to the meal plan. Distributing carbohydrates throughout the day is also important, as this helps minimize the high and low swings in blood glucose concentrations. Moderate alcohol use is fine (one serving per day). One recent study showed that this practice substantially reduced heart attack risk in people with type 2 diabetes. Still, the person must be warned that alcohol can lead to hypoglycemia and that the person must test him- or herself regularly for this possibility.

People with type 2 diabetes who have high blood triglycerides should moderate their carbohydrate intake and increase their intake of unsaturated fat and dietary fiber, as noted earlier for people with type 1 diabetes.[1, 25]

Although many cases of type 2 diabetes can be relieved by reducing excess fat stores, many people are not able to lose weight. They remain affected with diabetes and may experience the degenerative complications seen in the type 1 form of the disease. Ketosis, however, is not usually seen in type 2 diabetes.

*P*reviously, a fasting blood glucose of 140 mg/dl was required to diagnose diabetes. Recently, though, amounts in the 120 mg/dl range have been found to cause tissue damage. For this reason, the diagnostic trigger for diabetes using fasting blood glucose has been decreased to 126 mg/dl. The corresponding cut-off value taken 2 hours after a 75 g glucose load is 200 mg/dl.

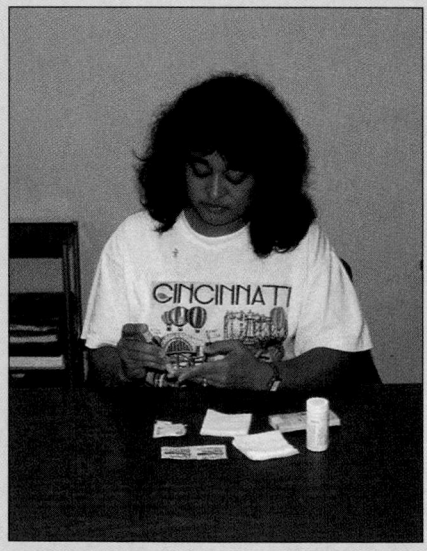

Regularly checking blood glucose is part of diabetes therapy today.

*F*or more information on diabetes, consult the following web sites: http://www.diabetes.org and http://ndep.nih.gov

HYPOGLYCEMIA

As noted earlier, diabetic people who are taking insulin sometimes have hypoglycemia if they don't eat frequently enough. Hypoglycemia can also develop in nondiabetic individuals. The two common forms of nondiabetic hypoglycemia are termed *reactive* and *fasting*.

Reactive hypoglycemia (also called postprandial hypoglycemia) is described as irritability, nervousness, headache, sweating, and confusion 2 to 4 hours after eating a meal, especially a meal high in simple sugars. The cause of reactive hypoglycemia is unclear, but it may be overproduction of insulin by the pancreas in response to rising blood glucose. Some researchers are unwilling even to acknowledge the existence of reactive hypoglycemia, pointing out that the symptoms are more likely tied to recent, intense exercise, psychological stress, medication use, or excess alcohol consumption. **Fasting hypoglycemia** usually is caused by pancreatic cancer, which may lead to excessive insulin secretion. In this case, blood glucose falls to low concentrations after fasting for about 8 hours to 1 day. This form of hypoglycemia is rare.

The diagnosis of hypoglycemia requires the simultaneous presence of low blood glucose and the typical hypoglycemic symptoms. Blood glucose of 40 to 50 mg/100 ml is suggestive, but just having low blood glucose after eating is not enough evidence to make the diagnosis of hypoglycemia. Although many people think they have hypoglycemia, few actually do.

It is normal for healthy people to have some hypoglycemic symptoms, such as irritability, headache, and shakiness, if they have not eaten for a prolonged period of time. Although not diagnostic of hypoglycemia, if you sometimes have symptoms of hypoglycemia, the standard nutrition therapy is one we all could follow. You need to eat regular meals, make sure you have some protein and fat in each meal, and eat complex carbohydrates with ample soluble fiber. Avoid meals or snacks that contain little more than simple carbohydrates. If symptoms continue, try small protein-containing snacks between meals or fruits and juice. Fat, protein, and soluble fiber in the diet tend to moderate swings in blood glucose. Last, moderate caffeine and alcohol intake.

reactive hypoglycemia Low blood glucose that follows a meal high in simple sugars, with corresponding symptoms of irritability, headache, nervousness, sweating, and confusion; also called *postprandial hypoglycemia.*

fasting hypoglycemia Low blood glucose that follows about a day of fasting.

LIPIDS

chapter 6

Your doctor informs you that your "triglycerides are too high." Your bill from a medical laboratory reads "Blood lipid profile—$55." A health-food advertisement suggests using cholestin, a dietary supplement, to lower blood cholesterol. Advertisers plug foods "lowest in saturated fat." All of these substances—triglycerides, saturated fat, and cholesterol—are lipids, a collective term referring to fats and oils.

Lipids contain more than twice the energy per gram (on average, 9 kcal) as proteins and carbohydrates (on average, 4 kcal each). Consumption of common saturated fatty acids also contributes to the risk of cardiovascular disease (CVD).[11] For this reason, some concern about lipids is warranted, but lipids also play vital roles both in the body and in foods. Their presence in the diet is essential to good health.[1, 10]

Let's look at lipids in detail—their forms, functions, metabolism, and food sources. This chapter will then conclude with a look at the link between lipid intake and the major "killer" disease in the United States, cardiovascular disease which involves both the coronary arteries (coronary heart disease) and other arteries in the body.

KEY CHAPTER CONCEPTS

- Lipids are a group of compounds that don't readily dissolve in water and include fatty acids, triglycerides, glycerol, phospholipids, and sterols.
- Fatty acids are part of most lipids and can be grouped according to the type of bonds between the carbons: saturated fatty acids contain no double bonds, monounsaturated fatty acids contain one double bond, and polyunsaturated fatty acids contain two or more double bonds.
- Certain polyunsaturated fatty acids are essential parts of our diet because our bodies need them but don't produce them. We can obtain these essential fatty acids by consuming polyunsaturated vegetable oils and fish on a regular basis.
- Triglycerides are the major form of fat in food and in our bodies. Besides supplying certain essential polyunsaturated fatty acids to the body, triglycerides supply energy, allow efficient energy storage, insulate and protect the body, and transport fat-soluble vitamins.
- Phospholipids are another class of lipids. They are derived from triglycerides. Phospholipids form important parts of cell membranes. Cholesterol is in the class of lipids called *sterols*. It forms part of vital compounds, such as cell membranes, some hormones, and bile acids.
- Fat digestion begins in the stomach, using the enzymes lingual and gastric lipase. Most, however, enter the small intestine. The enzyme pancreatic lipase digests the fat into monoglycerides (glycerol backbone with a single fatty acid attached) and fatty acids. These breakdown products are absorbed by the small intestine and then resynthesized into triglycerides and combined with cholesterol, protein, and other substances to yield a chylomicron. The chylomicron is eventually transported through the bloodstream to body cells.
- Fats are carried in the bloodstream by various lipoproteins: besides chylomicrons, these include very-low-density lipoproteins (VLDL), low-density lipoproteins (LDL), and high-density lipoproteins (HDL).
- Fats provide flavor, texture, and satiety to food. Hydrogenation is a process in which liquid oils are transformed into solid fats by the addition of hydrogen. This increases fat stability but also trans fatty acid content, which is not desirable.
- At this time, there is no RDA for fat. Still, we need to meet essential fatty acid needs.
- Major contributors of fat to our diets include animal foods, whole milk, and pastries. Fat in food is not always obvious.
- Cardiovascular disease, which includes coronary heart disease, is the number one cause of death in the United States. This stems from an array of risk factors, including genetics, hypertension, diabetes, physical inactivity, smoking, and a diet high in saturated fat, cholesterol, and trans fatty acids, as well as from a diet low in fruits and vegetables, omega-3 fatty acids, and dietary fiber.

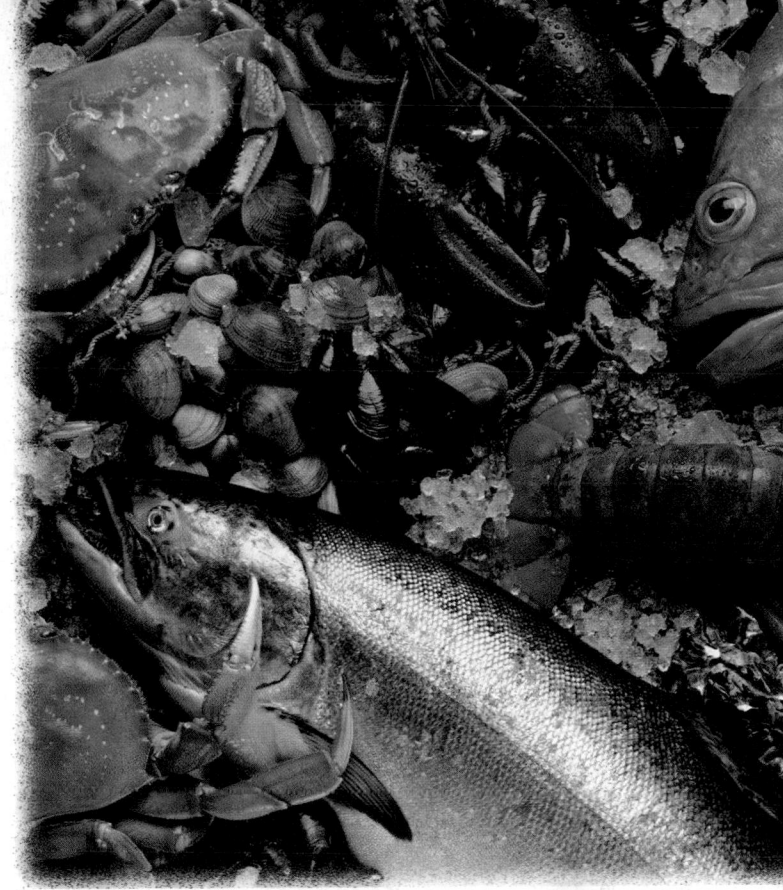

CASE SCENARIO

Jackie is a 21-year-old health-conscious individual, in her third year of nursing school. She recently learned that a diet high in saturated fat can contribute to high blood cholesterol and that exercise is beneficial for the heart. Jackie now takes a brisk 30-minute walk each morning before going to class, and she has started to cut as much fat out of her diet as she can, replacing it mostly with carbohydrates. A typical daily intake for Jackie now might begin with a breakfast of a bowl of Fruity Pebbles with 1 cup of skim milk and 1/2 cup of apple juice. For lunch, she might pack a turkey sandwich on white bread with lettuce, tomato, and mustard; a small package of fat-free pretzels; and a handful of fat-reduced vanilla wafers. Dinner could be a large portion of pasta with some olive oil and garlic mixed in, and a small iceberg lettuce salad with lemon juice squeezed over it. Her snacks are usually baked chips, low-fat cookies, fat-free frozen yogurt, or the fat-free pretzels. She drinks diet soft drinks throughout the day as her main beverage.

Do you think this is a healthy way for Jackie to reduce fat in her diet? Point out some positive practices. What would you suggest changing in her diet to make it more heart healthy?

REFRESH YOUR MEMORY

As you begin your study of lipids in Chapter 6, you may want to review

- Legal definitions for various labeled descriptors, such as low-fat and nonfat in Chapter 2
- The concept of energy density in Chapter 2
- The Mediterranean Diet Pyramid in Chapter 2
- The process of digestion and absorption and gastrointestinal hormones in Chapter 3
- The glycemic index of foods in Chapter 5

■ LIPIDS: COMMON PROPERTIES AND MAIN TYPES

Lipids are a diverse group of chemical compounds. They share one main characteristic: They do not readily dissolve in water but do so in organic solvents, such as chloroform, benzene, and ether. Think of an oil and vinegar salad dressing. The oil is not soluble in the water-based vinegar; on standing, the two separate into distinct layers, with oil on top and vinegar on the bottom.

The diversity of lipids is evident when you compare the structures of two common examples: a **fatty acid** versus cholesterol, shown in Figure 6-1. Triglycerides are the most common type of lipid found in the body and in foods. Each triglyceride molecule consists of a **glycerol** with three fatty acids attached to it. **Phospholipids** and **sterols** are also classified as lipids, although their structures can be quite different from the structure of triglycerides (see Fig. 6-1). All these lipid compounds are described in this chapter.

As noted in Chapter 1, lipids that are solid at room temperature are called *fats*, and lipids that are liquid are called *oils*. Most people use the word *fat* to refer to all lipids because they don't realize there is a difference. As already covered, however, *lipid* is a generic term that includes triglycerides and many other substances. To simplify our discussion, this chapter primarily uses the term *fat*; however, as you will see later, not all the substances we call fats truly are fats. When necessary for clarity, the name of a specific lipid, such as cholesterol, will be used. This word usage is consistent with the way many people use these terms in health-care settings.

■ Fatty Acids: The Simplest Form of Lipids

The fatty acid is common to most lipids, both those in the body and in foods. It is basically a long chain of carbons linked together and flanked by hydrogens. At one end of the molecule, designated the *alpha end*, is an acid (specifically a carboxyl $[-\overset{\overset{O}{\|}}{C}-OH]$) group. At the other end, called the *omega (ω) end*, is a methyl group ($-CH_3$) (Fig. 6-1A). In the Greek alphabet, *alpha* is the first letter and *omega* is the last.

Fats in foods are not composed of a single type or category of fatty acid. Rather, each dietary fat is a complex mixture of different fatty acids. Butterfat, for example, contains numerous different fatty acids.

fatty acid A chain of carbons chemically-bonded together and surrounded by hydrogen molecules. These hydrocarbons are found in lipids and contain a carboxyl (acid group) $(-\overset{\overset{O}{\|}}{C}-OH)$ at one end and a methyl group ($-CH_3$) at the other.

glycerol A three-carbon alcohol used to form triglycerides.

sterol A compound containing a multiring (steroid) structure and a hydroxyl group (–OH).

*I*n some cases *n* is used rather than omega (ω). Thus, you may see n-3 or ω-3 fatty acids as the term used.

Olive and canola oils are rich in monounsaturated fat; olive oil has been awarded much attention in recent years. Canola oil, however, is a much less expensive choice for consumers.

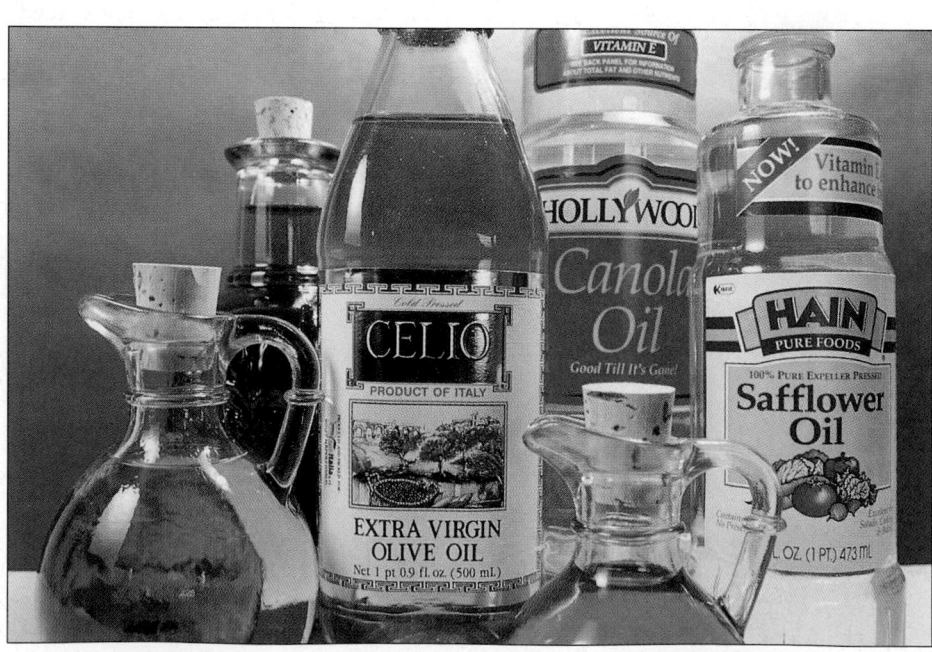

If all the chemical bonds between the carbons are single connections and the carbons are filled with hydrogens, a fatty acid is said to be **saturated** (Fig. 6-1A). To understand this concept, picture a sponge saturated (full) with water.

As noted earlier, most fats high in saturated fatty acids, such as animal fats, remain solid at room temperature. A good example is the solid fat surrounding a piece of uncooked steak at room temperature. Chicken fat, semisolid at room temperature, contains less saturated fat. In some foods, such as whole milk, saturated fats are suspended in liquid, so the solid nature of these fats at room temperature is less apparent. Milk actually contains a combination of liquid and solid fats, as will be discussed shortly.

If a fatty acid is unsaturated, hydrogens are missing from the carbon chain—specifically, at the area of the carbon-carbon double bonds. If a fatty acid has one double bond between the carbons, it is **monounsaturated** (Fig. 6-1B). Canola and olive oils contain a high percentage of monounsaturated fatty acids. If two or more

saturated fatty acid A fatty acid with no carbon-carbon double bonds.

monounsaturated fatty acid A fatty acid containing one carbon-carbon double bond.

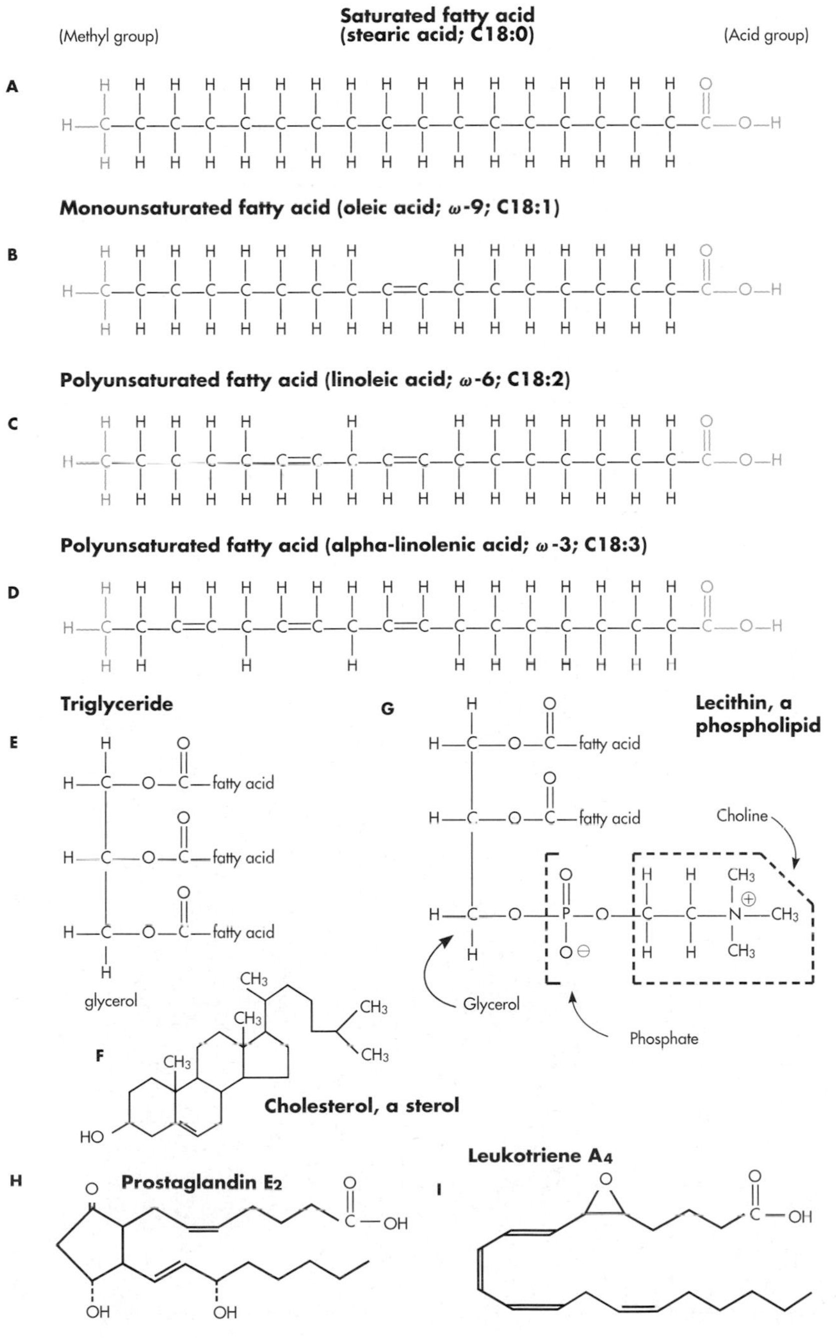

FIGURE 6-1 The families of lipids and some metabolic products (the eicosanoids). For simplicity's sake, the last three structures have most of the carbons and hydrogens deleted. Wherever there is a corner, it represents a carbon with two hydrogens, since a carbon atom must form four bonds for a stable structure. Note also the shorthand notation used to describe fatty acids. The first number indicates the number of carbons; the second number lists the number of double bonds. Thus, stearic acid (structure A) is C18:0.

polyunsaturated fatty acid A fatty acid containing two or more carbon-carbon double bonds.

long-chain fatty acids Fatty acids that contain 12 or more carbons.

omega-3 (ω-3) fatty acid An unsaturated fatty acid with the first double bond on the third carbon from the methyl end (–CH₃).

omega-6 (ω-6) fatty acid An unsaturated fatty acid with the first double bond on the sixth carbon from the methyl end (–CH₃).

bonds between the carbons are double bonds, the fatty acid is **polyunsaturated** and thus even less saturated with hydrogens (Fig. 6-1C, D). Corn, soybean, sunflower, and safflower oils are rich in polyunsaturated fatty acids.

Saturated fatty acids are linear, allowing them to pack tightly together. In contrast, unsaturated fatty acids have a kinked shape and thus pack together only loosely (this is depicted later in the chapter in Fig. 6-11). The loose organization of unsaturated fats is more easily disrupted by heat than is the more ordered organization of saturated fats. Thus, dietary fats high in unsaturated fatty acids melt at a lower temperature than fats high in saturated fatty acids (especially **long-chain** ones [12 carbons or longer]).

Overall, a fat or an oil is classified as saturated, monounsaturated, or polyunsaturated based on the nature of the fatty acids present in the greatest concentration (Fig. 6-2).

Triglycerides that contain primarily saturated fatty acids are solid at room temperature, especially if the fatty acids have a long chain. **Medium-chain** saturated fatty acids (6 to 10 carbons long), such as those in coconut oil, produce liquid oils at room temperature. This remains true even though coconut oil consists primarily of saturated fatty acids, because the shorter chain length overrides the effect of saturation. **Short-chain** saturated fatty acids (less than 6 carbons long) also form liquid oils at room temperature. Dairy fats are sources of these short-chain fatty acids. Triglycerides containing primarily polyunsaturated or monounsaturated fatty acids are also usually liquid at room temperature. These are not affected by chain length.

■ Essential Fatty Acids

The actual location of the carbon-carbon double bonds in the carbon chain of a polyunsaturated fatty acid makes a big difference in how the body metabolizes it. If the first double bond is located three carbons from the methyl (omega) end of the fatty acid, it is an **omega-3 (ω-3) fatty acid** (see Fig. 6-1D). If the first double bond is located six carbons from the methyl end of the fatty acid, it is an **omega-6 (ω-6) fatty acid** (see Fig. 6-1C). Following the same scheme, an omega-9 fatty acid has

CRITICAL THINKING

Advertisements often claim that fats are bad. Your classmate Mike asks, "If fats are so bad for us, why do we need to have any in our diets?" How would you answer him?

Dietary fat	Cholesterol (mg/tbsp)	Breakdown of fatty-acid content (normalized to 100%)			
Canola oil	0	6%	22%	10%	62%
Safflower oil	0	10%	77%	Trace	13%
Sunflower oil	0	11%	69%		20%
Corn oil	0	13%	61%		25%
Olive oil	0	14%	8%	1%	77%
Soybean oil	0	15%	54%	7%	24%
Margarine	0	17%	32%	2%	49%
Peanut oil	0	18%	33%		49%
Vegetable shortening	0	28%	26%	2%	44%
Palm oil	0	45%	12%	1%	37%
Palm kernel oil	0	52%	10%	1%	11%
Coconut oil	0	92%		2%	6%
Lard	12	41%	11%	1%	47%
Beef fat	14	52%	3%	1%	44%
Butter fat	33	66%	2%	2%	30%

Polyunsaturated fat

Saturated fatty acid · Linoleic acid · Alpha-linolenic acid · Monounsaturated fatty acid

■ **FIGURE 6-2** Comparison of dietary fats in terms of saturated fatty acids, the most common unsaturated fatty acids, and cholesterol content.

the first double bond nine carbons from the methyl end of the fatty acid. In foods, **alpha-linolenic acid** is the major omega-3 fatty acid; **linoleic acid** is the major omega-6 fatty acid; and **oleic acid** is the major omega-9 fatty acid.

Because we must obtain linoleic acid (ω-6) and alpha-linolenic acid (ω-3) from foods in order to maintain health, they are called **essential fatty acids.** These omega-3 and omega-6 fatty acids form parts of vital body structures, perform important roles in immune system function and vision, help form cell membranes, and produce hormonelike compounds called **eicosanoids** (see Fig. 6-1H, I).[1, 10] This dietary necessity arises because cells in the human body can produce carbon-carbon double bonds in a fatty acid only after the ninth carbon numbered from the methyl end. In other words, human cells do not have the enzyme to place double bonds between the methyl end and the ninth carbon. On the other hand, omega-9 fatty acids can be synthesized in the body because the double bond falls after the ninth carbon.

Essential fatty acid (EFA) family. All are available from dietary sources; linoleic acid and alpha-linolenic acid must be consumed as body synthesis does not take place. These are the essential fatty acids. The other fatty acids in this figure can be synthesized from the essential fatty acids.

Still, we need to consume only about 1 to 2% of our total energy intake from essential fatty acids. On a 2500 kcal diet, that corresponds to 1 tablespoon of plant oil each day. We easily get that much—via mayonnaise, salad dressings, margarine, and other foods—without even noticing. Barring these foods, regular consumption of whole grains and vegetables can also supply enough essential fatty acids.

Current research also suggests that we should specifically include a regular intake of alpha-linolenic acid or one of its related omega-3 fatty acids, **eicosapentaenoic acid (EPA)** and **docosahexaenoic acid (DHA).** This would almost certainly require twice weekly consumption of fatty fish, such as salmon, tuna, or sardines; regular intake of canola or soybean oil; or consumption of walnuts or flax seeds.[23] All are sources of omega-3 fatty acids. The importance of omega-3 fatty acid intake will be explored further in the next few pages.

CONCEPT CHECK

ipids are a group of compounds that dissolve in organic solvents but do not dissolve readily in water. They include fatty acids, triglycerides, phospholipids, and sterols. Fatty acids differ from one another mainly in the number and location of the double bonds between carbons in the carbon chain. Saturated fatty acids contain no carbon-carbon double bonds; that is, they are fully saturated with hydrogens. Monounsaturated fatty acids contain one carbon-carbon double bond, and polyunsaturated fatty acids contain two or more carbon-carbon double bonds.

Length of the carbon chain in fatty acids affects the consistency of triglycerides at room temperature. Specifically, long-chain saturated fatty acids (greater than or equal to 12 carbons) form solid varieties at room temperature, whereas medium-chain (6 to 10 carbons) and short-chain (less than 6 carbons) saturated fatty acids form liquid varieties at room temperature, as do triglycerides composed of monounsaturated polyunsaturated fatty acids.

If a double bond first occurs at the third carbon from the methyl (–CH₃) end of the carbon chain, the fatty acid is an omega-3 fatty acid. If a double bond first occurs at the sixth carbon, it is an omega-6 fatty acid. Because humans can't synthesize omega-3 and omega-6 fatty acids, which perform vital functions in the body, they are designated *essential fatty acids,* indicating that they must be included in the diet to maintain health.

---

alpha-linolenic acid An essential omega-3 fatty acid with 18 carbons and three double bonds (C18:3, ω-3).

linoleic acid An essential omega-6 fatty acid with 18 carbons and two double bonds (C18:2, ω-6).

oleic acid An omega-9 fatty acid with 18 carbons and one double bond (C18:1, ω-9).

essential fatty acids Fatty acids that must be supplied by the diet to maintain health. Currently, only linoleic acid and alpha-linolenic acid are classified as essential.

eicosanoids Hormonelike compounds synthesized from polyunsaturated fatty acids, such as arachidonic acid. Within this class of compounds are prostaglandins, thromboxanes, and leukotrienes.

eicosapentaenoic acid (EPA) An omega-3 fatty acid with 20 carbons and five carbon-carbon double bonds (C20:5, ω-3). It is present in large amounts in fish oils and is synthesized in the body from alpha-linolenic acid. EPA is metabolized to eicosandoids.

docosahexaenoic acid (DHA) An omega-3 fatty acid with 22 carbons and six carbon-carbon double bonds (C22:6, ω-3). It is present in large amounts in fish oils and is synthesized in the body from alpha-linolenic acid. DHA is especially present in the retina and brain.

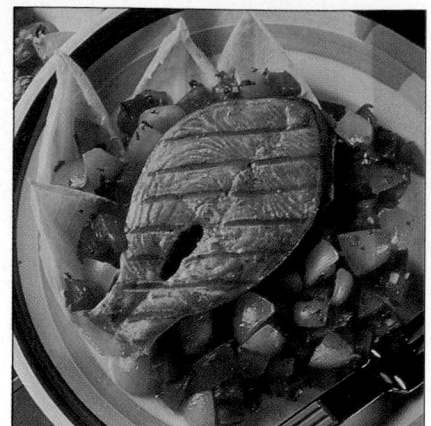

Eating fatty fish, such as salmon, twice a week makes a healthy contribution to a diet and helps meet omega-3 fatty acid needs.

dihomo-gamma-linolenic acid An omega-6 fatty acid with 20 carbons and 3 double bonds; precursor to some eicosanoids.

arachidonic acid An omega-6 fatty acid with 20 carbons and 4 carbon-carbon double bonds (C20:4, ω-6); precursor to some eicosanoids.

oxygenase Enzyme that incorporates oxygen directly into a molecule.

cyclooxygenase Oxygenase enzyme used to synthesize prostaglandins, thromboxanes, and other eicosanoids.

lipoxygenase Oxygenase enzyme used to synthesize leukotrienes and lipoxins, two types of eicosanoids.

prostaglandin (PG) One of several potent hormonelike compounds made of polyunsaturated fatty acids that produce diverse effects in the body.

prostacyclin (PGI) Eiscosanoid made by the blood vessel walls that is a potent inhibitor of blood clotting (PGI$_2$).

*T*he conversion of alpha-linolenic acid (omega-3) to EPA and DHA appears to be relatively inefficient, especially in people who consume the usual amounts of linoleic acid. Because of the important biological effects of the eicosanoids made from EPA and DHA, some scientists believe that these long-chain omega-3 fatty acids should also be considered essential nutrients.

Metabolism and the Role of Essential Fatty Acids in the Body

Omega-3 and omega-6 fatty acids are further metabolized by cells so they can contribute to the synthesis of some biologically active substances called eicosanoids. The essential fatty acids, alpha-linolenic and linoleic, are precursors of the eicosanoids.

Eicosanoids are 20-carbon molecules with hormone-like activity. They are referred to as local hormones because they act in the immediate vicinity of production, and are not carried by the blood to some distant site like typical hormones. Eicosanoids are synthesized from fatty acids recovered from phospholipids in the cell membrane, plus free fatty acids and lipoproteins within the cell. The eicosanoids then bind to receptors on the cell membrane surface, or to adjacent cell membrane surfaces, to initiate a response. (The receptors are just now being identified.) Eicosanoids have a wide variety of actions (100 and counting), some of which will be discussed below.[22]

Eicosanoids fall into separate groups. One group is derived from **dihomo-gamma-linolenic acid,** an omega-6 fatty acid with 3 double bonds. Another group is derived from **arachidonic acid,** an omega-6 fatty acid with four double bonds. A third group is derived from eicosapentaenoic acid, the omega-3 fatty acid with 5 double bonds discussed earlier.

To produce the parent fatty acids, linoleic acid can be lengthened to 20 carbons and undergo desaturation, in which hydrogens are removed and additional carbon to carbon bonds added. This first reaction yields dihomo-gamma-linolenic acid.

$$\text{Linoleic acid} \xrightarrow[\text{2H}]{\text{2C}} \text{Dihomo-gamma-linolenic acid}$$
$$(\text{C18:2, }\omega\text{-6}) \qquad\qquad (\text{C20:3, }\omega\text{-6})$$

This can be further desaturated to form arachidonic acid.

$$\text{Dihomo-gamma-linolenic acid} \xrightarrow[\text{2H}]{} \text{Arachidonic acid}$$
$$(\text{C20:3, }\omega\text{-6}) \qquad\qquad (\text{C20:4, }\omega\text{-6})$$

Alpha-linolenic acid can be elongated to 20 carbons and have two more carbon-carbon double bonds added to produce eicosapentaenoic acid.

$$\text{alpha-linolenic acid} \xrightarrow[\text{4H}]{\text{2C}} \text{Eicosapentaenoic acid}$$
$$(\text{C18:3, }\omega\text{-3}) \qquad\qquad (\text{C20:5, }\omega\text{-3})$$

Eicosapentaenoic acid can also be elongated to 22 carbons and have one more carbon-carbon double bond added to produce docosahexaenoic acid. However, this compound does not form eicosanoids.

$$\text{Eicosapentaenoic acid} \xrightarrow[\text{2H}]{\text{2C}} \text{Docosahexaenoic acid}$$
$$(\text{C20:5, }\omega\text{-3}) \qquad\qquad (\text{C22:6, }\omega\text{-3})$$

Each of the parent fatty acids produces a particular set of eicosanoids. As the eicosanoids are synthesized they take up oxygen by one of two **oxygenase** enzyme systems: **cyclooxygenase** and **lipoxygenase,** forming distinct groups of eicosanoids. (Cyclooxygenase is the enzyme that aspirin and ibuprofen inhibit.) Dihomo-gamma-linolenic is the precursor of the 1 series of eicosanoids, arachidonic acid is the precursor of the 2 series of eicosanoids , and eicosapentaenoic acid is the precursor of the 3 series of eicosanoids (Fig. 6-3).

The functioning eicosanoids include the **Prostaglandins (PG), Prostacyclins (PGI), Thromboxanes (TX), Leukotrienes (LT),** and the **Lipoxins (LX).** In addition to the two-letter designation, the eicosanoids have a third letter following the

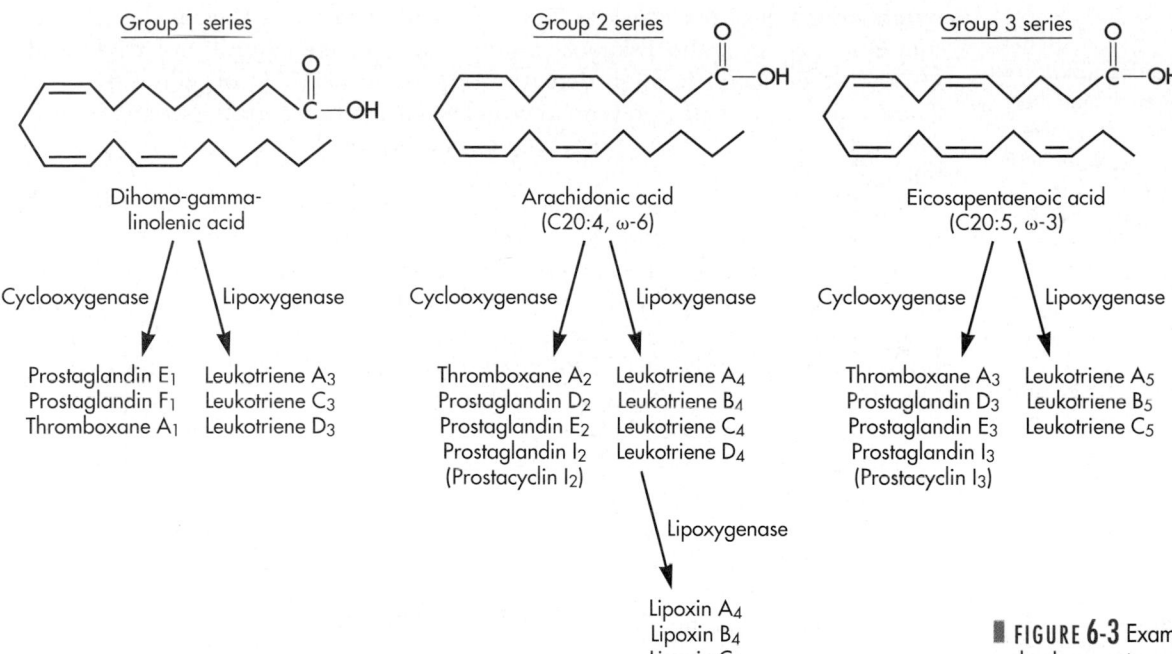

■ **FIGURE 6-3** Examples of eicosanoids from the three major groups. The parent fatty acid produces profound difference in how eicosanoids across the three groups act in the body (e.g., Thromboxane A_1 vs A_2 vs A_3).

first two letters with a subscript designating the number of double bonds in the structure. For example PGE_1 is from a group of prostaglandins (PG) that have one double bond and is of the unique chemical composition specified by E. Some of these eicosanoids are more biologically active than others. The action of the eicosanoids depends on the tissue in which they are produced; not all eicosanoids are formed in all tissues.

Upon stimulation by hormones or other agents, arachidonic acid, eicosapentaenoic acid, and dihomo-gamma-linolenic acid are made available to be converted to eicosanoids. These eicosanoids are important and potent regulators of vital body functions, such as blood pressure, labor, blood clotting, immune response, inflammation, and secretions of the stomach, just to name a few.[1, 23]

A Closer Look at Omega-3 Fatty Acids

The thromboxanes (TX) derived from the cyclooxygenase pathway have a significant effect on blood platelet function. TXA_2 stimulates an action called "platelet aggregation" or blood clotting, and is a potent vasoconstrictor (causes blood vessels to constrict). Both are critical events when someone is bleeding profusely (hemorrhaging). Overproduction of TXA_2 *may* be an important factor in development of a heart attack and the related formation of clots in the coronary arteries. (The name thromboxane comes from its function, forming a thrombus or clot.). Like many of the eicosanoids, TXA_2 has a short half life, about 30 seconds.[22]

PGI_2, one of the prostacyclins, is produced by **endothelial cells** lining blood vessel walls, and are important inhibitors of platelet aggregation. Thus the thromboxanes and the prostacyclins are antagonists. PGI_2 has a half life of a few minutes. Its job is to maintain blood flow free of clots.

These eicosanoid actions were discovered many years ago in studies of Greenland Eskimos. Eskimos have a low incidence of coronary heart disease. They exhibit diminished clotting ability and prolonged clotting time. Their diet is very high in fish oils containing EPA, which gives rise to the series 3 of prostaglandins and thromboxane. TXA_3 and PGI_3 prevent the release of arachidonic acid from the phospholipids in cell membranes, so the PGI_2 and TXA_2 don't form. PGI_3 also is as

thromboxane (TX) A stimulant of blood clotting made in the blood from polyunsaturated fatty acids.

leukotriene (LT) An important mediator of many diseases involving inflammatory or hypersensitivity reactions, such as asthma; it is derived from fatty acids.

lipoxin (LX) Eicosanoids made by white blood cells that are involved in immune and allergic responses.

endothelial cells A layer of flat cells lining the blood and lymphatic vessels and the chambers of the heart.

spirin and other nonsteroidal antiinflammatory drugs can inhibit the platelet cyclooxygenase action involved in the formation of TXA$_2$. This is the reason why many people at risk for heart attack and stroke are taking aspirin, so they can decrease the risk of blood clotting. Still this must be done under a physician supervision since with long-term use bleeding in the gastrointestinal tract is a distinct possibility. Aspirin has other effects on the body—from lowering body temperature and inhibiting blood clotting to easing muscle pain—because it blocks the synthesis of other eicosanoids, such as PGE$_2$.

high-density lipoprotein (HDL) Lipoprotein, synthesized in part by the liver and intestine, that picks up cholesterol from dying cells and other sources and transfers it to the other lipoproteins in the bloodstream, as well as directly to the liver.

hemorrhagic stroke Damage to part of the brain resulting from rupture of a blood vessel and subsequent bleeding within or over the internal surface of the brain.

rancid Containing products of decomposed fatty acids; they yield unpleasant flavors and odors.

potent an inhibitor of clotting as PGI$_2$. All in all, the balance sheet is shifted toward non-clotting. Also, the Eskimos' blood is low in cholesterol and triglycerides. On the other hand, the **high density lipoprotein (HDL)** concentration is high. These are all factors that prevent atherosclerosis and heart attack (see the Nutrition Perspective). As well, their genetic factors, combine with their dietary patterns to influence their development of heart disease.[22]

Some studies show that people who eat fish about twice a week (total weekly intake: 8 ounces [240 g]) run lower risks for heart attack than do people who rarely eat fish. In these cases, the omega-3 fatty acids in fish oil are probably acting to reduce blood clotting. As noted above, blood clots are part of the heart attack process. In addition, these omega-3 fatty acids have a favorable effect on heart rhythm. Consequently, the risk of heart attack decreases, especially for people already at high risk.

We need to remember, however, that blood clotting is a normal body process. Certain groups of people, such as Eskimos in Greenland, eat so much seafood that their blood-clotting ability can be impaired. An excess of omega-3 fatty acid intake can allow uncontrolled bleeding and may cause **hemorrhagic stroke.** However, the risk of stroke has not been seen in studies using moderate amounts of omega-3 fatty acids. In addition, the increased risk of hemorrhagic stroke could be due to the alcoholism that is common in the Greenland Eskimo population.

Studies also have shown that large amounts of omega-3 fatty acids from fish (3 to 4 g/day; one 3 oz serving of fatty fish has about 1.6 g) can lower blood triglycerides in people with high triglyceride concentrations. In addition, these omega-3 fatty acids are suspected to be helpful in managing the pain of inflammation associated with rheumatoid arthritis (by suppressing immune system responses) and may help with certain behavioral disorders and depression.

In some instances, fish oil capsules can be safely substituted (under a physician's guidance) for fish consumption if a person does not like fish. Generally, about 900 mg of omega-3 fatty acids (about three capsules) from fish oil per day is required to enjoy the benefits of reduced risk of cardiovascular disease that are associated with fish consumption twice a week.[16] However, individuals who have bleeding disorders, are taking anticoagulant medications, are anticipating surgery, or have uncontrolled hypertension should not be taking fish oil capsules because of the increased risk of hemorrhagic stroke.

Flax seeds are getting attention today because they are a rich vegetable source of the omega-3 alpha-linolenic acid. About 2 tablespoons per day is typically recommended if used as an omega-3 fatty acid source. Flax seeds can be purchased in many natural food stores rather inexpensively. These need to be chewed thoroughly or they will pass through the gastrointestinal tract undigested. Many people find it easier to grind them first in a coffee grinder. If so, the flax seeds should be consumed soon after, since they turn **rancid** very quickly. Flax seed oil is also available, but (like the seeds) it too turns rancid very quickly.

Other Actions of Eicosanoids

The leukotrienes (LT) and lipoxins (LX) are the metabolic end products of the lipoxygenase reactions. Leukotrienes produced through the lipoxygenase pathway have a fairly long half life, some up to 4 hours. They cause slowly evolving, but prolonged contractions of smooth muscles in airways (and the gastrointestinal tract). LTC$_4$ is converted to LTD$_4$ which is slowly converted to LTE$_4$. These three eicosanoids are part of the response to allergens, which cause tissue damage (inflammation).[22] In an allergic reaction an allergen can instigate the release of leukotrienes in minutes, which are the immediate mediators of the allergic response. The leukotrienes mentioned are made from arachidonic acid, and are released from various white blood cells (eosinophils). They are the cause of contraction of smooth muscle in the bronchii, producing the coughing, wheezing, and breathing problems common to allergies and asthma. They also cause the inflammation and related edema. Epidemiological, clinical, and biochemical studies show the effects of dietary omega-3 fatty acids in reducing risks of inflammatory diseases are due in part to the reduction in the tissue levels of arachiodonic acid.

The prostaglandins PGD_2 and PGE_2 are major metabolites produced in the brain that regulate sleep and wake cycles and body temperature. PGE_2 also enhances the perception of pain. It induces labor, as does PGF_2. In some tissues PGE_2 is a vasodilator, while in others it is a vasoconstrictor. PGE_2 also is believed to be the factor that allows the baby to breathe just after birth. And some other prostaglandins may be involved in ovulation, premature labor, and painful menstrual cramps.

Why are these eicosanoids so confusing? It is because the same eicosanoid can have different effects in different tissues. For example, the PGE series could cause smooth muscle to relax in the bladder and intestines, but the same molecule could cause the smooth muscle in blood vessels to contract. In summary, the eicosanoids are produced by a variety of different organs. They usually regulate the organ in which they are produced. Genetic as well as dietary factors determine how these local hormones react.

■ Effects of a Deficiency of Essential Fatty Acids

If humans fail to consume enough essential fatty acids, their skin becomes flaky and itchy, and diarrhea and other symptoms such as infections often are seen. Growth and wound healing may be retarded, and anemia can develop. These signs of deficiency have been seen in people fed **total parenteral nutrition** solutions containing little or no fat for 2 to 3 weeks, as well as in infants receiving formulas low in fat. However, because our bodies need the equivalent of only about 1 tablespoon of plant oils a day, even a low-fat diet will provide enough essential fatty acids if it follows a balanced plan such as the Food Guide Pyramid and includes a serving of fish twice a week.

total parenteral nutrition The intravenous provision of all necessary nutrients, including the most basic forms of protein, carbohydrates, lipids, vitamins, minerals, and electrolytes. This solution is generally infused for 12 to 24 hours a day in a volume of about 2–3 L.

CONCEPT CHECK

Omega-6 fatty acids are metabolized into arachidonic acid in the body. Omega-3 fatty acids are metabolized into EPA and DHA in the body. Arachidonic acid and EPA are further metabolized into hormonelike compounds called eicosanoids. Arachidonic acid forms eicosanoids with different characteristics than the eicosanoids formed from EPA. In general, eicosanoids made from EPA (omega-3) decrease blood clotting and inflammatory responses in the body, whereas eicosanoids made from arachidonic acid (omega-6) increase blood clotting and inflammatory responses. A serving of fish should be consumed twice a week to obtain adequate amounts of omega-3 fatty acids. This, in turn, is thought to decrease cardiovascular disease risk by decreasing blood clotting and improving heart rhythm. Fish oil supplementation (about 900 mg/day of the related ω-3 fatty acids) is generally acceptable under a physician's guidance if a person does not like fish; however, people with certain medical conditions (e.g., taking anticoagulant medications) should not take fish oil supplements due to increased risk of hemorrhagic stroke. Essential fatty acid deficiency can occur after 2 to 3 weeks if fat is omitted from total parenteral nutrition solutions, which in turn can lead to skin disorders, diarrhea, and anemia.

When patients in the hospital are receiving total parenteral nutrition solutions, essential fatty acids are added daily to the solutions in the form of triglycerides from plant oils. Another option is to provide the essential fatty acids, again in the form of triglycerides from plant oils, in two separate intravenous doses each week.

■ TRIGLYCERIDES

Fats and oils in foods are mostly in the form of triglycerides. The same is true for fats found in body structures. Some fatty acids are found attached to proteins in the bloodstream as they are being transported, but most fatty acids do not exist in the body as such. Instead, they form into triglycerides.

$$H-\underset{\underset{H}{|}}{\overset{|}{C}}-OH \quad HO-\overset{\overset{O}{\|}}{C}-R$$

Ester bond

Glycerol + 3 fatty acids   **Triglyceride + 3 H₂O**

FIGURE 6-4 Forming a triglyceride via esterification. This process yields water as a by-product as ester bonds are formed. The *R* represents the fatty acids.
Illustration by William Ober.

esterification The process of attaching fatty acids to a glycerol molecule, creating an ester bond and releasing water. Removing a fatty acid is called deesterification; reattaching a fatty acid is called reesterification.

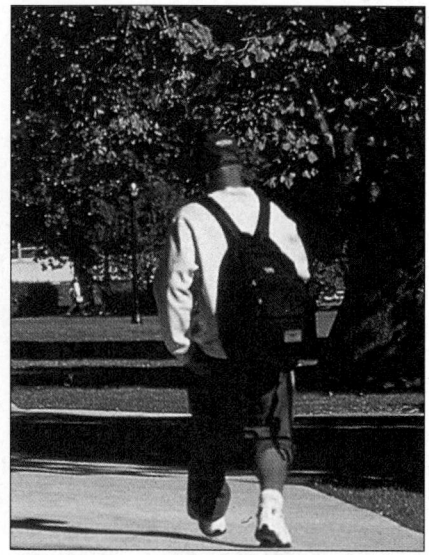

When at rest or during light activity, the body uses mostly fatty acids for fuel. Note also that brisk walking about 30 minutes per day has been shown to reduce coronary heart disease risk.

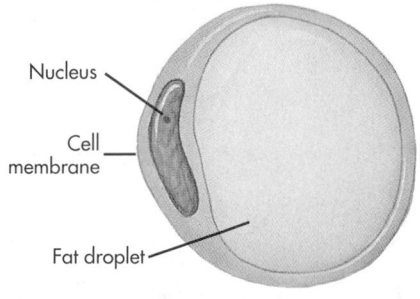

Nucleus

Cell membrane

Fat droplet

Adipose cell

Triglycerides contain a simple three-carbon alcohol, glycerol, which serves as a backbone for the three attached fatty acids. A fatty acid is attached to each of the three hydroxyl groups (–OH) of glycerol. Three water molecules are released in the process of bonding three fatty acids to glycerol (Fig. 6-4). Note that triacylglyceride is the chemical name of the molecule, as *acyl* refers to a fatty acid that has lost its hydroxyl group, and a hydroxyl group is lost when each fatty acid attaches to glycerol.

The bonds between glycerol and each fatty acid are called *ester bonds.* The process of chemically attaching fatty acids to glycerol is called **esterification.** The release of fatty acids from glycerol is called *deesterification.*

By breaking off (deesterifying) one of the fatty acids of a triglyceride molecule, a diglyceride (glycerol with two attached fatty acids) is formed. The deesterification of two of the fatty acids on a triglyceride produces a **monoglyceride** (glycerol with one attached fatty acid). Free fatty acids, monoglycerides, and glycerol—but not triglycerides—can cross cell membranes.

During digestion, enzymes in the small intestine eventually break down the triglycerides in the foods to free fatty acids and monoglycerides; only a small portion of dietary triglycerides is broken down completely to free fatty acids and glycerol. After the free fatty acids, monoglycerides, and any free glycerol enter the intestinal cells, most of these components are rebuilt into new triglycerides (see later section on fat digestion and absorption). The reattachment of fatty acids to glycerol is called *reesterification.* Every time a triglyceride enters or leaves a cell, it must also be deesterified; after entering a cell, the free fatty acids are reesterified into triglycerides. Thus, the body must continually break down and rebuild triglycerides.

Many key functions of fat in the body use triglycerides. These contribute to energy storage, insulation, and transportation of fat-soluble vitamins.

Providing Energy for the Body

Triglycerides both contained in the diet and stored in adipose tissue are the main fuel for muscles while at rest and during light activity. Only in endurance exercise, such as long-distance running and cycling, or in short bursts of intense activity, such as a 200-meter run, do muscles oxidize a lot of carbohydrate in addition to fatty acids supplied by triglycerides. Other body tissues also use fatty acids for energy. Overall, about half of the energy used by the entire body at rest and during light activity comes from fatty acids. On a whole-body basis, the use of fatty acids by skeletal and cardiac muscle is balanced by the use of glucose by the nervous system and red blood cells. Recall from Chapter 4 that cells also need carbohydrate to efficiently process fatty acids for fuel.

Storing Energy for Later Use

We store energy mainly in the form of triglycerides. The body's ability to store fat is essentially limitless. Its fat storage sites, adipose cells, can increase about 50 times in weight. If the amount of fat to be stored exceeds the ability of the cells to expand, the body can form new adipose cells. (This is discussed further in Chapter 13.)

An important advantage of using triglycerides to store energy in the body is that they are energy dense. Recall that these yield, on average, 9 kcal/g, whereas proteins and carbohydrates yield only about half that much. In addition, triglycerides are chemically very stable, so they are not likely to react with other cell constituents, making them a safe form for storing energy. Finally, when we store triglycerides in adipose cells, we store little else; adipose cells contain about 80% lipid and only 20% water and protein. In contrast, imagine if we were to store energy as muscle tissue, which is about 73% water. Body weight linked to energy storage would increase dramatically.

■ Insulating and Protecting the Body

The insulating layer of fat just beneath the skin is made mostly of triglycerides. Fat tissue also surrounds and protects some organs—kidneys, for example—from injury. We usually don't notice the important insulating function of fat tissue, because we wear clothes and add more as needed. But a layer of insulating fat is quite apparent in animals, particularly those in cold climates. Polar bears, walruses, and whales all build a thick layer of fat tissue around themselves to insulate against cold-weather environments. The extra fat also provides energy storage for times when food is scarce.

People with **anorexia nervosa** often lose 25% or more of body weight and become about as fat free as is biologically possible. In turn, they lose the insulating property of fat storage. This poses many other health risks, such as bone loss linked to cessation of menstrual periods (see Chapter 15). In place of the layer of fat tissue under the skin, people with anorexia nervosa often develop downy hair, called **lanugo,** all over the body. These hairs insulate the body by standing up and trapping air.

■ Transporting Fat-Soluble Vitamins

Triglycerides and other fats in food carry fat-soluble vitamins to the small intestine and aid their absorption. If the small intestine is diseased, however, it may not be able to adequately digest and absorb fat from foods. When this happens, the unabsorbed fat carries the fat-soluble vitamins—A, D, E, and K—into the large intestine. From there, they are eliminated in the feces, and the body loses the benefits of the vitamins. If the disease doesn't resolve quickly, medical attention is necessary.

People who absorb fat poorly, such as those with the disease cystic fibrosis, are also at risk for deficiencies of fat-soluble vitamins, especially vitamin K. A similar risk accrues from taking mineral oil as a laxative at mealtimes. Because the body cannot digest or absorb mineral oil, the undigested oil carries the fat-soluble vitamins from the meal into the feces, where they are eliminated.

■ PHOSPHOLIPIDS

Phospholipids are another class of lipid. Like triglycerides, they are built on a backbone of glycerol. However, at least one fatty acid is replaced with a compound containing phosphorus (and often other elements, such as nitrogen). Many types of phospholipids exist in the body, especially in the brain. They form important parts of cell membranes. The various forms of **lecithins** are common examples of phospholipids (Fig. 6-1G). These are found in body cells, where they participate in fat digestion in the intestine. Egg yolks contain lecithins in abundance, as do liver, wheat germ, and peanuts. It is not necessary to consume phospholipids, such as lecithins, in the diet because the body can synthesize them and use them when and where they are needed.

Cell membranes are composed primarily of phospholipids. A cell membrane looks much like a sea of phospholipids with protein "islands" (see Fig. 3-1). Among their

anorexia nervosa An eating disorder involving a psychological loss or denial of appetite and self-starvation, related in part to a distorted body image and to various social pressures commonly associated with puberty.

lanugo Downlike hair that appears after a person has lost much body fat through semistarvation. The hair stands erect and traps air, acting as insulation for the body to compensate for the relative lack of body fat, which usually functions as insulation.

*U*nabsorbed fatty acids can bind minerals, such as calcium and magnesium, and draw them into the stool for elimination. This can harm mineral status (see Chapter 11).

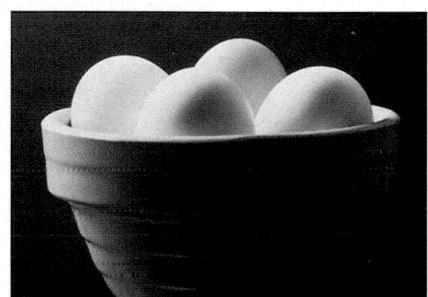

Lecithins are found in abundance in egg yolks. This phospholipid acts as an emulsifier.

lecithins A group of phospholipids containing two fatty acids, a phosphate group, and a choline molecule. Lecithins are a group of compounds, since they can differ based on the types of fatty acids found on each lecithin molecule.

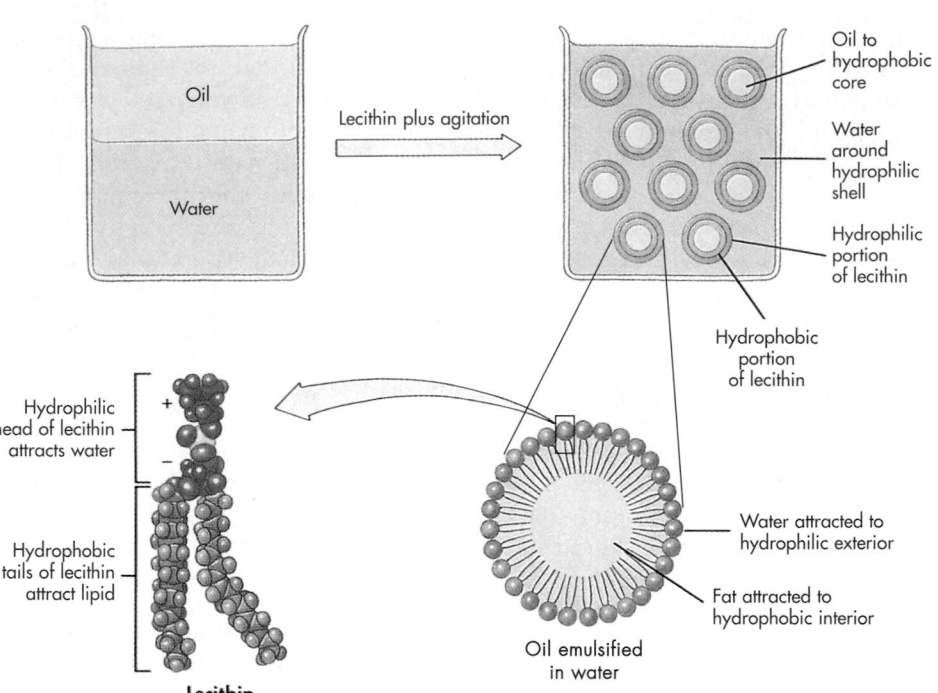

FIGURE 6-5 Emulsification and emulsifiers. Emulsifiers organize oil and water into droplets of oil surrounded by shells of water. The emulsifier molecules form a bridge between the oil and water molecules, isolating one from the other. In the droplet, oil enters the central core, while water surrounds the core. The emulsifier molecules are sandwiched between the two. Formation of such emulsions is a key step in digestion of dietary fat and is important in the manufacture of certain food products, such as mayonnaise and cakes.
Illustration by William Ober.

emulsifier A compound that can suspend fat in water by isolating individual fat droplets, using a shell of water molecules or other substances to prevent the fat from coalescing.

bile acids Emulsifiers synthesized by the liver and released by the gallbladder during digestion.

micelles Water-soluble, spherical structures, formed by lecithin and bile acids, in which the hydrophobic parts of the molecules face inward and the hydrophilic parts face outward. Lipids enclosed within micelles do not separate into an oily layer, as they normally do when mixed with water.

many roles, the proteins form receptors for hormones, function as enzymes, and act as transporters for nutrients. About 5% to 15% of cell membrane fatty acids is made up of aracidonic acid. This serves as a source for eicosanoid synthesis described earlier. Some cholesterol is also present in the membrane.

Some phospholipids, such as the family of compounds mentioned earlier called *lecithins,* function as **emulsifiers.** These allow fat and water to mix. By breaking fat globules into small droplets, emulsifiers enable a fat to be suspended in water. Here's how the process works: The fatty acid ends of lecithins attract fat. The phosphorus and nitrogen at the other end of lecithins form an area containing positive and negative charges. This area attracts water. Since water is attracted to the charges on lecithin, this part of lecithin is called hydrophilic, which means "loving water." The parts with fatty acids are called hydrophobic, since they don't attract (they "fear") water.

When an emulsifier is mixed with oil and water in the proper proportions, it forms spherical structures, in which the hydrophobic parts of the emulsifier molecules are oriented toward the interior and the hydrophilic parts toward the exterior (Fig. 6-5). In this way, the emulsifier acts as a bridge between the oil and water by forming tiny oil droplets surrounded by thin shells of water.

The body's main emulsifiers are the lecithins and **bile acids,** which are produced by the liver and released into the small intestine via the gallbladder during digestion. By breaking up the fat globules, the emulsifiers create more fat surface for fat-digesting enzymes to act on. These very stable emulsified products are called **micelles** (see later section on fat digestion).

■ STEROLS

Sterols are the last class of lipids this chapter covers. Their characteristic multiringed structure makes them different from the other lipids already discussed. Consider the sterol cholesterol. This waxy substance doesn't look like a triglyceride—it doesn't have a glycerol backbone or any fatty acids. Still, because it doesn't readily dissolve in water, it is a lipid. The main building block for the synthesis of cholesterol in the body is acetyl-CoA, a derivative of **acetic acid,** the smallest fatty acid. (Synthesis of longer fatty acids, triglycerides, and phospholipids also makes use of acetyl-CoA.)

Cholesterol forms part of some important hormones, such as the **corticosteroids,** the estrogens, testosterone, and a form of the active vitamin D hormone—namely, $1,25(OH_2)D$. Cholesterol is also the precursor of bile acids, which are needed for fat digestion. Finally, cholesterol is an essential structural component of cell membranes and the particles that transport lipids in the blood, as discussed in the next section. The cholesterol content of the heart, liver, kidney, and brain is quite high, reflecting its critical role in these organs.

Cholesterol is made by body cells (two-thirds of total daily body exposure) and is consumed in the diet (about one-third of total daily body exposure). Each day, our cells produce approximately 700 mg of cholesterol.[22] About 10% of this cholesterol is produced by the liver. Note, however, that this small amount of cholesterol production by the liver is very important in the regulation of blood cholesterol (see the Nutrition Perspective at the end of this chapter). Of this 700 mg, about 400 mg is used to make new bile acids to replenish those lost in the feces, and about 50 mg is used to make steroid hormones. With respect to diet, we consume about 200 to 400 mg of cholesterol per day from animal-derived food products (Table 6-1). Of that, we absorb about 40 to 65%. There is no need to consume cholesterol per se, as body cells can make all that they need.

Some plants have related sterols, such as ergosterol, that can form a type of vitamin D. However, the plant-based foods we eat do not contain cholesterol per se unless animal products have been added.

acetic acid A two-compound fatty acid that is used in the synthesis of lipids.

corticosteroid A steroid produced by the adrenal gland; an example is cortisol.

Cholesterol

Testosterone

Illustration by William Ober.

CONCEPT CHECK

*T*riglycerides are the major form of fat in the body and in food. They are used for and stored as energy, they insulate and protect body organs, and they transport fat-soluble vitamins. Phospholipids have both hydrophilic and hydrophobic parts and, so, are effective emulsifiers—compounds that can suspend fat in water. Phospholipids also form parts of cell membranes and various compounds in the body. Cells produce all the phospholipids the body needs. Cholesterol, a sterol, forms part of cell membranes, hormones, and bile acids; it is essential to the body. Cholesterol is found in animal products and is synthesized by body cells; if sufficient amounts are not ingested, the body makes what it needs.

TABLE 6-1 Cholesterol Content of Selected Foods in Ascending Order

Food	Amount	Cholesterol in Milligrams	Food	Amount	Cholesterol in Milligrams
Skim milk	1 cup	4	Oysters, salmon	3 oz	40
Mayonnaise	1 tbsp	10	Clams, halibut, tuna	3 oz	55
Butter	1 pat	11	Chicken, turkey* (white meat)	3 oz	70
Lard	1 tbsp	12	Beef,* pork	3 oz	75
Cottage cheese	½ cup	15	Lamb, crab	3 oz	85
Low-fat milk (2%)	1 cup	22	Shrimp, lobster	3 oz	110
Half-and-half	¼ cup	23	Heart, beef	3 oz	165
Hot dog*	1	29	Egg (egg yolk)*†	1	210
Ice cream, ~10% fat	½ cup	30	Liver, beef	3 oz	410
Cheese, cheddar	1 oz	30	Kidney	3 oz	540
Whole milk*	1 cup	34	Brains	3 oz	2640

*Leading contributors of cholesterol to the U.S. diet.

†Egg whites are cholesterol-free

■ FAT DIGESTION AND ABSORPTION

Given the right conditions, about 95% of fat consumed is absorbed.

■ Fat Digestion

Fat digestion begins in the stomach, using the enzymes lingual and gastric lipase. These enzymes break down triglycerides containing short- and medium-chain fatty acids into free fatty acids and diglycerides. Since fat may remain in the stomach for up to 2 to 4 hours, there is an opportunity to digest some of these triglycerides and to absorb the fatty acids released through the stomach wall. The short- and medium-chain fatty acids then enter the portal vein. In contrast, long-chain fatty acids are not acted on until they reach the small intestine (Fig. 6-6).[21]

Once the fat reaches the small intestine, the hormone cholesystokinin (CCK) is released from the duodenal cells. This hormone stimulates the release of bile from the gallbladder and lipase enzyme from the pancreas. The bile contains bile acids, lecithin, and cholesterol. The lipase released travels through the pancreatic duct to be mixed with bile in the common bile duct; finally, both enter together into the small intestine. In the small intestine, pancreatic lipase contributes to fat digestion by digesting (specifically hydrolyzing) the triglycerides into monoglycerides and fatty acids. The amount of pancreatic lipase released is much greater than what is needed in most circumstances to digest the fat in a meal. This "overkill" makes fat digestion very rapid and thorough in the right circumstances, which include the presence of bile acids and lecithin from the gallbladder and a protein called colipase. Colipase is

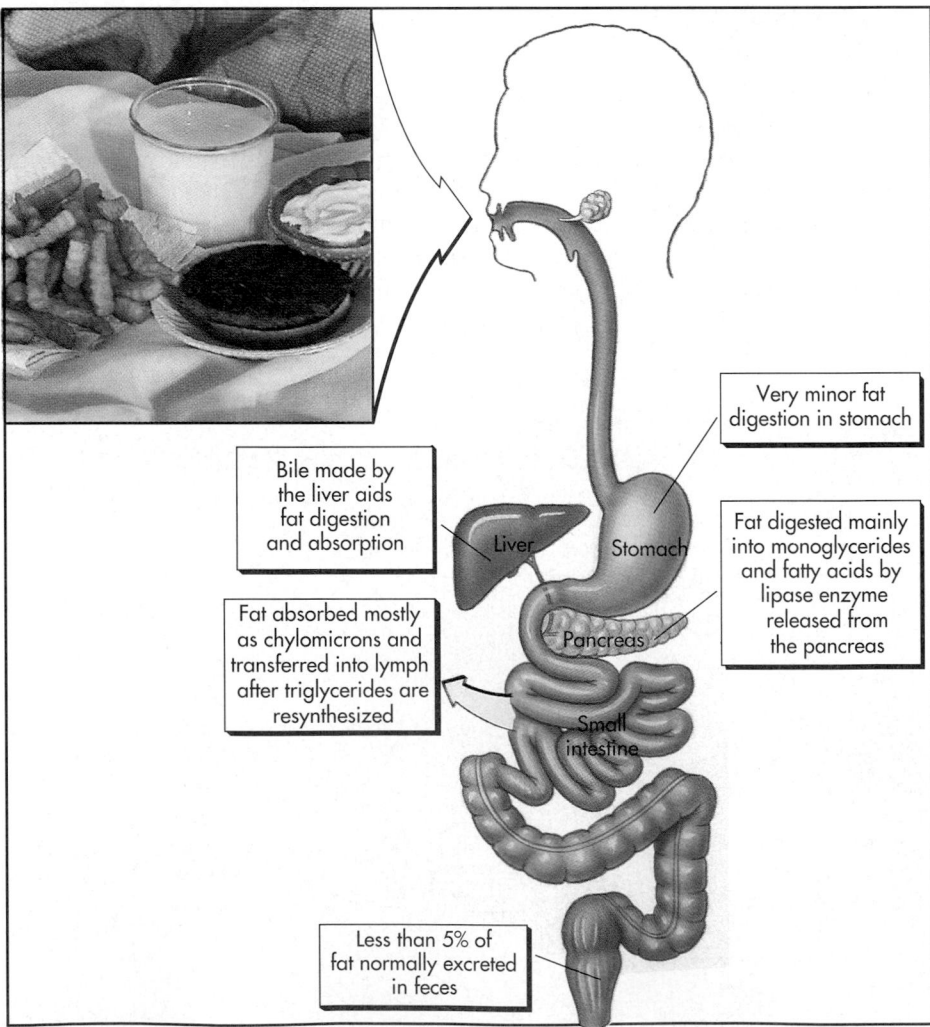

■ FIGURE 6-6 A summary of fat digestion and absorption.

Illustration by William Ober.

found in pancreatic secretions, and it functions by ensuring the attachment of lipase to the lipid droplet.

Since fat is hydrophobic, it needs a medium that will carry it throughout the intestinal tract. Bile acids help do this by emulsifying the fatty substances in the small intestine into micelles, as previously discussed. Emulsification improves digestion and absorption because, as large fat globules are broken down into smaller ones, the total surface area for lipase action increases (Fig. 6-7).

With regard to phospholipid and cholesterol digestion, phospholipase enzymes from the pancreas and glandular cells in the wall of the small intestine digest phospholipids. The eventual products are glycerol, fatty acids, phosphoric acid, and remaining constituents such as choline. Cholesterol esters (cholesterol with a fatty acid attached) are broken down to free cholesterol and fatty acids.

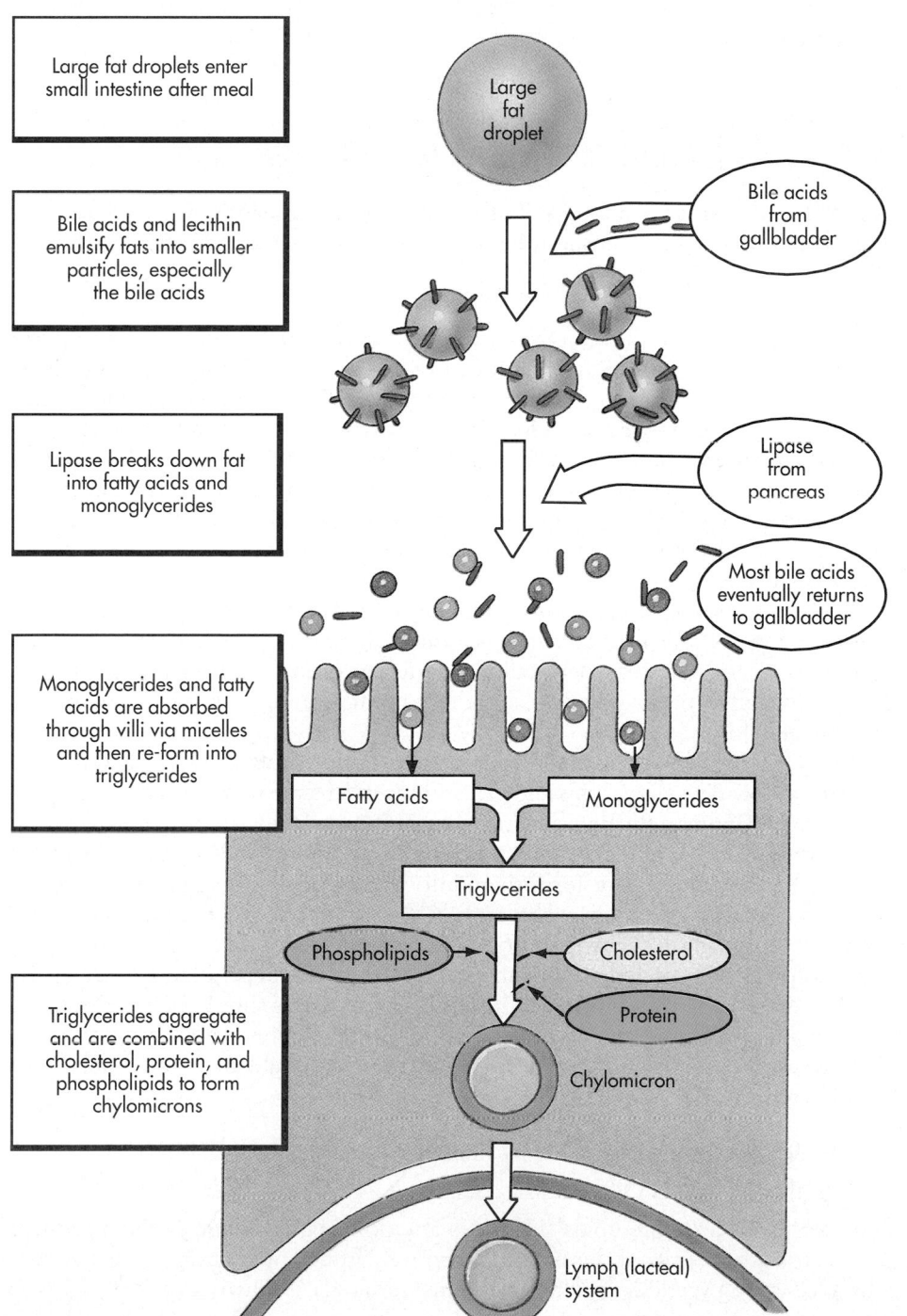

FIGURE 6-7 A simplified look at absorption of triglycerides made up of long-chain fatty acids. These primarily form monoglycerides and free fatty acids. These are absorbed using bile acids and then re-formed into triglycerides in the absorptive cells. The triglycerides are then formed into chylomicrons and enter the lymphatic system. Note that short- and medium-chain fatty acids for the most part pass directly into the portal circulation (not depicted). About 95% of dietary fat is absorbed under normal conditions.

■ Fat Absorption

The lipid content of the micelles is absorbed into the brush border of the absorptive cells lining the duodenum and jejunum. The carbon chain length of fatty acids and monoglycerides then affects their fate after absorption. If a fatty acid is a short- or medium-chain variety (less than 12 carbons), it is water soluble and probably travels out of the absorptive cell (enterocyte) and through the portal vein to the liver. If the fatty acid is a long-chain variety (more than 12 carbons), it is first re-formed into a triglyceride molecule in the absorptive cell. After further packaging (described in the next section), it eventually enters circulation via the lymphatic system, carrying with it fat-soluble vitamins and absorbed cholesterol (see Fig. 6-7).[21] The leftover bile acids (and some of the cholesterol released in the bile) are reabsorbed in the ileum and returned to the liver (by the portal vein) to be used again in fat digestion (about 98% of bile acids are recycled, only 1 to 2% are eliminated in the feces). Recall from Chapter 3 that this recycling is termed enterohepatic circulation.

■ FATS CARRIED IN THE BLOODSTREAM

As noted earlier, fat and water don't mix easily. This incompatibility presents a challenge in transporting fats through the watery media of blood and lymph systems.

■ Carrying Dietary Fats Utilizes Chylomicrons

As just reviewed, once the various dietary fats are digested and absorbed into the small intestine cells, most of the byproducts of digestion—glycerol, monoglycerides, and fatty acids—are re-formed into triglycerides. They are then packaged into **lipoprotein** particles—large droplets of lipid surrounded by a thin shell of phospholipid cholesterol and protein (Fig. 6-8). The lipoprotein particles produced by intestinal cells are called **chylomicrons.** The shell around a chylomicron allows the lipid it is carrying to float freely in the water-based blood. Some of the proteins present—namely, **apolipoproteins**—also help other cells identify this particle as a chylomicron.[22]

After being assembled in intestinal cells, chylomicrons enter the lymphatic system and travel to the thoracic duct, which is located along the spinal column. This duct opens into a large vein in the neck called the subclavian vein. Chylomicrons enter the general circulation of the bloodstream at that point (see Fig. 3-6 for a view of lymphatic circulation).

Once chylomicrons enter the bloodstream, the triglycerides in the chylomicrons are broken down into fatty acids and glycerol by an enzyme on the inside wall of the blood vessel, **lipoprotein lipase.** Muscle cells, adipose cells, and other cells in the vicinity then absorb most of the fatty acids. Cells can immediately use absorbed fatty acids for fuel, or they can re-form them into triglycerides and store them as such. Muscle cells tend to metabolize fatty acids, whereas adipose cells tend to store them.

After eating a meal, the whole process of clearing chylomicrons from the blood via lipoprotein lipase activity takes about 2 to 10 hours, depending in part on fat content. After 12 to 14 hours of fasting, the chylomicrons should be totally absent from the bloodstream. People should fast for 12 to 14 hours before having certain blood tests to assure that chylomicrons, whose presence could affect the results, have been cleared.

■ Transporting Lipids Mostly Made by the Body Uses Very-Low-Density Lipoproteins

The liver produces more lipids than does any other body organ. It also produces cholesterol. The source of the needed carbon, hydrogen, and energy to make such substances as triglycerides and cholesterol includes the carbohydrate and protein the

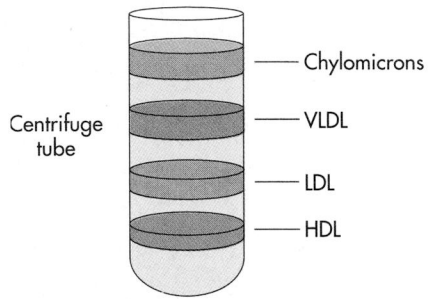

Centrifuge tube — Chylomicrons — VLDL — LDL — HDL

One way to measure the amount of chylomicrons, VLDL, LDL, and HDL is to centrifuge the serum at high speed for about 24 hours in a sucrose-rich solution. The lipoproteins settle out in the centrifuge tube based on their density, with chylomicrons at the top and HDL at the bottom.

lipoprotein A compound found in the bloodstream containing a core of lipids with a shell composed of protein, phospholipid, and cholesterol.

chylomicron Lipoprotein made of dietary fats surrounded by a shell of cholesterol, phospholipids, and protein. Chylomicrons are formed in the absorptive cells (enterocytes) of the small intestine after fat absorption and travel through the lymphatic system to the bloodstream.

apolipoprotein A protein attached to the surface of a lipoprotein or embedded in its outer shell. Apolipoproteins can help enzymes function, act as a lipid-transfer protein, or assist in the binding of a lipoprotein to a cell-surface receptor.

lipoprotein lipase An enzyme attached to the outside endothelial cells that line the capillaries in the blood vessels; it breaks down triglycerides into free fatty acids and glycerol.

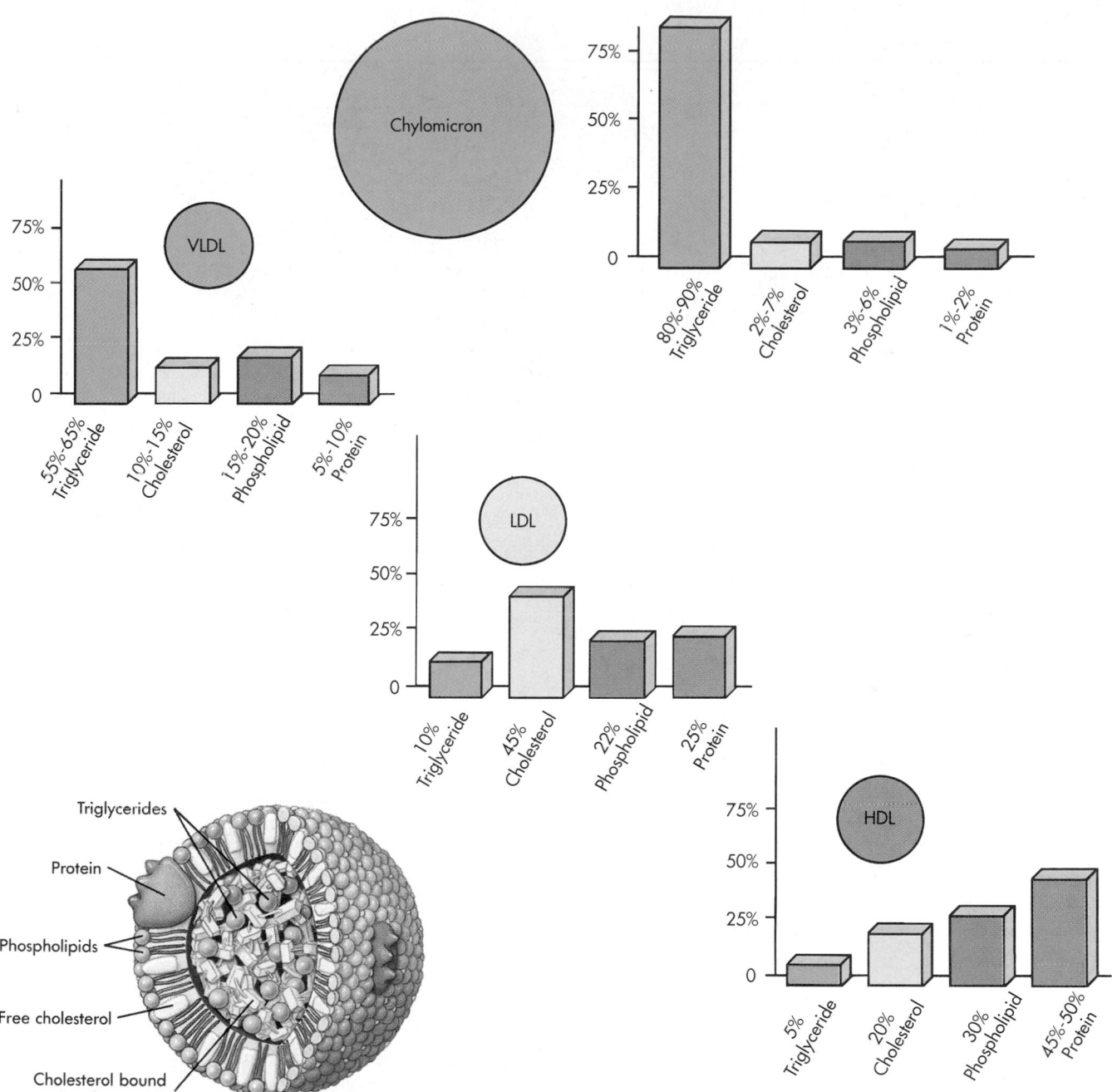

FIGURE 6-8 Structure and composition of lipoproteins. This lipoprotein structure allows fats to circulate in the bloodstream. Note that, for each class of lipoprotein, there are various subclasses of slightly different composition. For our purposes, we will ignore this observation.

liver takes up from the bloodstream. Any alcohol consumed can also be used for lipid synthesis. The liver coats the cholesterol and triglycerides that collect, including some taken up from the bloodstream, with a shell of protein and lipids. This process produces what is called a **very-low-density lipoprotein (VLDL)** fraction (Fig. 6-9).

When the VLDL leaves the liver, the enzyme lipoprotein lipase on the blood vessels breaks down the triglyceride in the VLDL into fatty acids and glycerol. Again, fatty acids and glycerol are released into the bloodstream and are taken up by the body cells. Because fats are less dense than water, the VLDL becomes much

very-low-density lipoprotein (VLDL) The lipoprotein created in the liver that carries cholesterol and lipids newly synthesized by the liver.

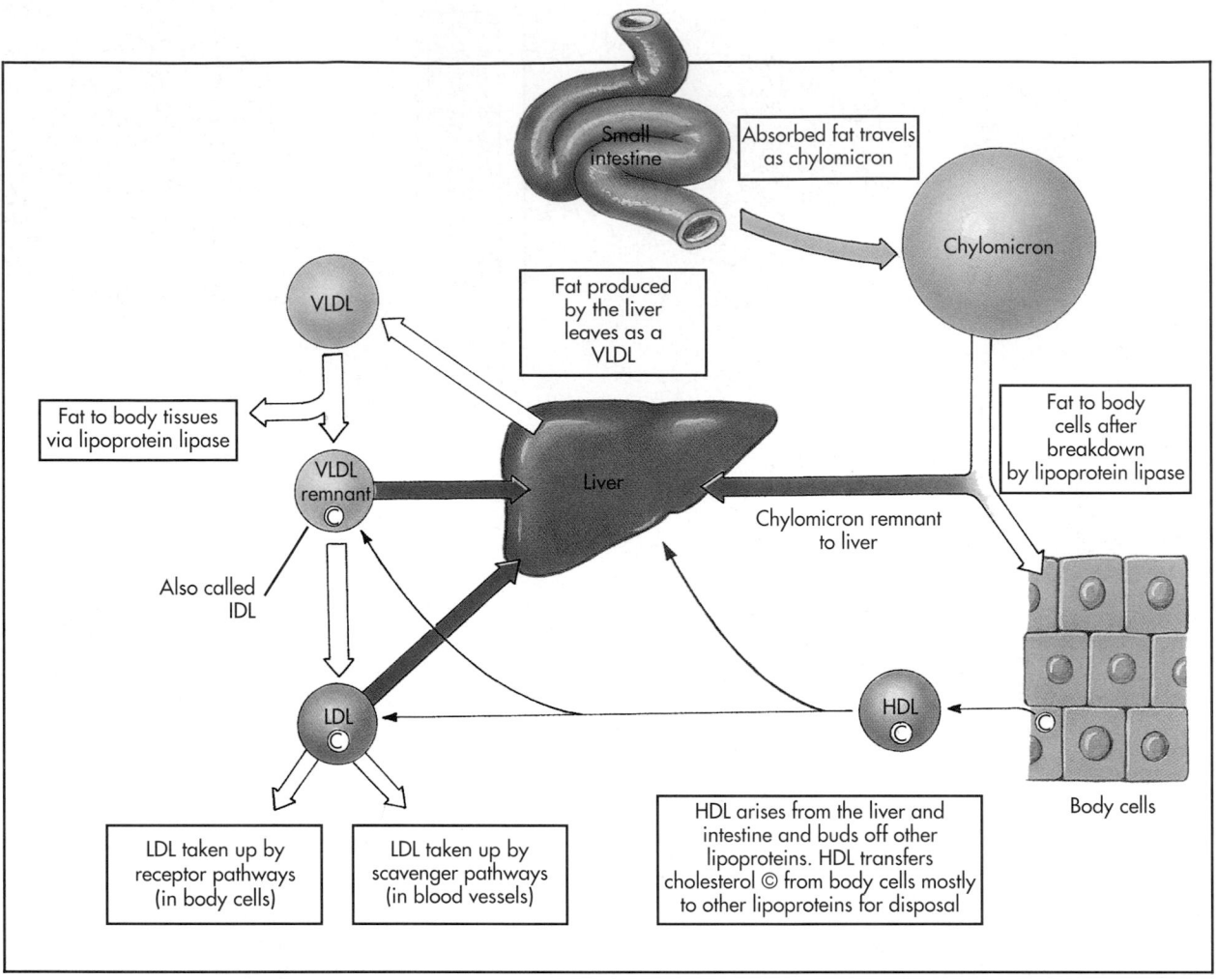

Small intestine

Absorbed fat travels as chylomicron

Chylomicron

VLDL

Fat produced by the liver leaves as a VLDL

Fat to body tissues via lipoprotein lipase

VLDL remnant

Liver

Fat to body cells after breakdown by lipoprotein lipase

Also called IDL

Chylomicron remnant to liver

LDL

HDL

Body cells

LDL taken up by receptor pathways (in body cells)

LDL taken up by scavenger pathways (in blood vessels)

HDL arises from the liver and intestine and buds off other lipoproteins. HDL transfers cholesterol © from body cells mostly to other lipoproteins for disposal

■ **FIGURE 6-9** Lipoprotein interactions. Chylomicrons carry absorbed fat to body cells. VLDL carries fat from the liver to body cells. LDL arises from VLDL and carries mostly cholesterol to cells. HDL arises from body cells, mostly in the liver and intestine, as well as from particles that bud off the other lipoproteins. HDL carries cholesterol from cells to other lipoproteins and to the liver for excretion.
Illustration by William Ober.

receptor pathway for cholesterol uptake
A process by which LDL is bound by cell receptors and incorporated into the cell.

scavenger pathway for cholesterol uptake
A process by which LDL is taken up by scavenger cells embedded in the blood vessels.

heavier—proportionately denser—as triglyceride is released. Much of what eventually remains of the VLDL fraction becomes particles called low-density lipoprotein (LDL) fraction. LDL is composed primarily of cholesterol.

LDL particles are absorbed from the bloodstream by receptors on cells, internalized, and broken down. Most LDL is taken up by receptors on liver cells. Diets low in saturated fat and cholesterol encourage this process, whereas diets high in those lipids can reduce LDL uptake by the liver (see the Nutrition Perspective at the end of this chapter). The cholesterol and protein parts absorbed then are transported throughout the cell. By this process, called the **receptor pathway for cholesterol uptake,** cells take up some of the building blocks necessary for cell growth and development (Fig. 6-10).

A second process, called the **scavenger pathway for cholesterol uptake,** can also remove LDL from the circulation. This pathway is carried out by certain "scavenger" white blood cells, which leave the bloodstream and bury themselves in blood vessels. These scavenger cells detect, alter (oxidize), engulf, and digest the extra circulating LDL. Once within the scavenger cells, the oxidized LDL is prevented from reentering the bloodstream. Over time, cholesterol builds up in the scavenger cells, especially when the amount of LDL in the bloodstream is excessive.[3]

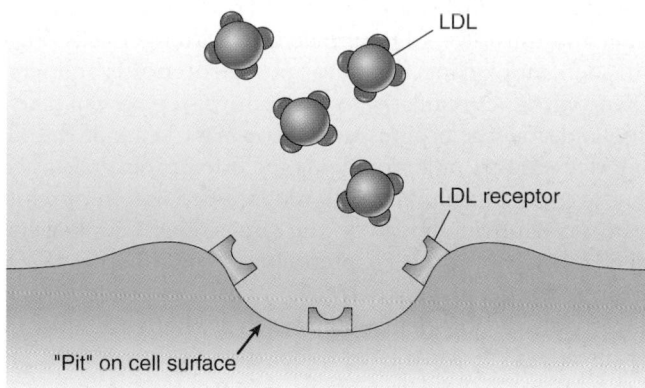

"Pit" on cell surface

Cells have pits on the surface, which contain LDL receptors.

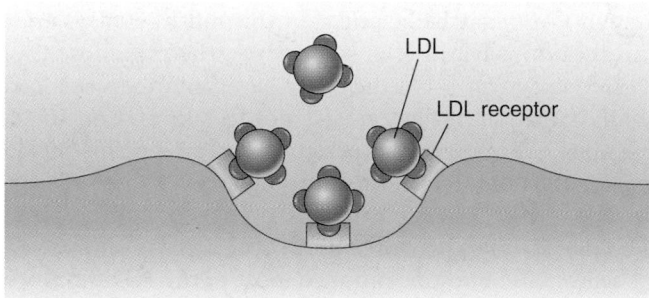

LDL binds to the LDL receptors in the pits.

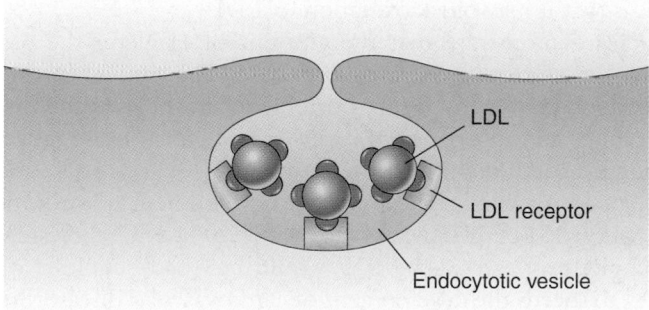

The LDL, bound to LDL receptors, is taken into the cell by endocytosis.

FIGURE 6-10 Transport of LDL into cells. LDL receptors capture circulating LDL and release it inside the cell to be metabolized. Once free of their load, LDL receptors return to the cell surface to await new LDL.

When scavenger cells have collected and deposited cholesterol for many years at a heavy pace, cholesterol builds up on the inner blood vessel walls—especially in arteries—and **plaque** develops (see Fig. 6-14 in the Nutrition Perspective at the end of this chapter). The plaque eventually mixes with connective tissue (collagen) and is then covered with a cap of smooth muscle cells and calcium. Atherosclerosis, also referred to as *hardening of the arteries*, develops as plaque grows in the vessel. This eventually chokes off the blood supply to organs, setting the stage for a heart attack and other problems, or it breaks apart and leads to clot formation in this or another artery. Plaque is probably first deposited to repair damage to the cells lining the arteries (called endothelial cells). The damage that starts plaque formation can be caused by smoking, diabetes, hypertension, homocysteine, and LDL itself. Viral and bacterial infections are also implicated as well as ongoing blood vessel inflammation.[26, 27, 29] Note also that these plaques can develop in arteries throughout the body, not just the coronary arteries. This explains our use of the term cardiovascular disease to describe the general condition.

plaque A cholesterol-rich substance deposited in the blood vessels; it contains various white blood cells, smooth muscle cells, connective tissue (collagen), cholesterol and other lipids, and eventually calcium.

carotenoids Plant pigments, some of which can yield vitamin A.

Some nutrients have antioxidant properties. These likely reduce LDL oxidation in the bloodstream and thus slow LDL uptake into scavenger cells. Fruits and vegetables are rich in such antioxidants as the various **carotenoids** and vitamins C and E. Eating fruits and vegetables regularly is one positive step we can take to reduce cholesterol buildup and slow the progression of coronary heart disease. Fruits and vegetables that are rich sources of antioxidants include prunes, raisins, various berries, plums, oranges, grapes, spinach, broccoli, red bell peppers, and onions. Consuming megadoses of antioxidant vitamins to do the same thing is controversial. The Nutrition Perspective at the end of this chapter, along with Chapters 9 and 10, will discuss this controversy in detail. Currently, the American Heart Association does not support the use of antioxidant supplements, such as vitamin E, in an effort to reduce cardiovascular disease risk.[16] Most large-scale studies of people with existing cardiovascular disease have generally shown no benefit from megadose vitamin E therapy (400–800 IU/day).[7] Other studies are ongoing, using people with cardiovascular disease and those with no evidence of such disease. Still, some experts suggest that megadose vitamin E use may be helpful, but this must be taken under a physician's guidance. This caution is because, in some cases, the megadose use of antioxidant supplements can cause harm.[33] On the other hand, an excessive intake of iron probably speeds LDL oxidation, making it wise not to take an iron supplement unless a physician prescribes it. People who experience iron storage disease and men in general should pay special attention to this warning (see Chapter 12).

A final critical participant in this extensive process of fat transport is high-density lipoprotein (HDL). Its high proportion of protein makes it the heaviest (densest) lipoprotein. The liver and intestine produce most of the HDL in the blood. It roams the bloodstream, picking up cholesterol from dying cells and other sources. HDL donates the cholesterol primarily to other lipoproteins for transport back to the liver to be excreted. Some HDL travels directly back to the liver. Another beneficial function of HDL is that it may block oxidation of LDL.

menopause The cessation of menses in women, usually beginning at about age 50.

Many studies demonstrate that the amount of HDL in the bloodstream can closely predict the risk for cardiovascular disease. The risk increases with low HDL because little blood cholesterol is transported back to the liver and excreted. Women tend to have high amounts of HDL, especially before **menopause,** whereas low amounts are more common in men.

Because high amounts of HDL slows the development of cardiovascular disease, any cholesterol carried by HDL can be considered "good" cholesterol. By convention, then, cholesterol carried by LDL would be "bad" cholesterol because high amounts of LDL speeds the development of cardiovascular disease. Still, LDL is only a problem when it is too high in the bloodstream; low amounts are needed as part of routine body functions.[22]

CONCEPT CHECK

In the stomach, gastric and lingual lipase break down short- and medium-chain triglycerides into smaller components, some of which are absorbed through the stomach wall. All end up in the portal vein and are transported to the liver. In the small intestine, the enzyme pancreatic lipase digests long-chain triglycerides into monoglycerides and free fatty acids. These breakdown products diffuse into the absorptive cells of the small intestine and are mostly resynthesized into triglycerides. The bloodstream carries absorbed dietary fat as chylomicrons.

Lipid synthesized by the liver is carried in the bloodstream as very-low-density lipoprotein (VLDL). Once a VLDL has most triglycerides removed by lipoprotein lipase, it eventually becomes low-density lipoprotein (LDL), which is rich in cholesterol. LDL is picked up by receptors on body cells, especially liver cells. Scavenger cells in the arteries may do the same, speeding the development of atherosclerosis. High-density lipoprotein (HDL) picks up cholesterol from cells and transports it primarily to other lipoproteins for eventual transport back to the liver. HDL may also decrease LDL oxidation, thereby reducing LDL uptake into atherosclerotic plaque. Elevated amounts of LDL in the bloodstream is one major risk factor associated with cardiovascular disease, as is low amounts of HDL.

ANOTHER DIMENSION OF FAT— PROPERTIES IN FOOD

Various fats play important roles in foods. Much ingenuity must go into the production of fat-reduced products to preserve flavor and texture. In some cases, "fat-free" also means tasteless.

Fat in Food Provides Satiety and Flavor

Eating a meal leads to a state of **satiety.** Each macronutrient in the diet contributes to this feeling of being satisfied. The influence of each is dependent on the amount of time it remains in the GI tract. Protein and fat remain in the stomach for longer periods of time, in comparison with carbohydrate. Therefore, eating a mixed meal that contains fat, protein, and carbohydrate would impart more satiety than if the meal were to consist solely of carbohydrate. Fat and protein stimulate the release of the hormone gastric inhibitory peptide (GIP) from the walls of the upper portion of the small intestine (see Chapter 3). GIP slows the release of stomach contents into the small intestine. In addition, the hormones secretin, gastrin, and cholecystokinin (CCK) help keep the stomach from overwhelming the small intestine with acid chyme by slowing the emptying process.[21] This explains why fat and protein in a meal cause a feeling of fullness: The chyme remains in the stomach longer, so we feel full longer. Adding to this hormonal input are receptors in the duodenum, which monitor the concentration of chyme.

Many people who want to lose weight cut much of the fat from their diet. However, if dieters cut too much fat, they lose its *satiety* value and get hungry more quickly. Thus, reducing fat intake below about 20% of total energy intake can actually be self-defeating, unless high-fiber foods are added to contribute bulk, which also makes us feel full (see Chapter 13 for further discussion). Having some low-fat snacks around at times of intense hunger is also a good idea. Fruit is an excellent choice.

Fat components in foods provide important textures and carry flavors. If you've ever eaten a high-fat yellow cheese or cream cheese, you probably agree that fat melting on the tongue feels good. The fat in reduced-fat and whole milk also gives body, which nonfat milk lacks, and the most tender cuts of meat are high in fat, visible as the marbling of meat. In addition, many flavorings dissolve in fat. Heating spices in oil intensifies the flavors of an Indian curry or a Mexican dish by carrying the flavors to the sensory cells in the mouth that discriminate taste and smell. For these reasons, a person who has been following a typical American diet will probably need some time to adjust to a lower-fat diet. For example, if one changes from the regular use of whole milk to 1% low-fat milk but then after a few weeks switches back to the whole milk, it will taste more like cream than milk. One has thus adjusted to the flavor of the low-fat milk and will likely now find the whole milk to be not as palatable. Emphasizing flavorful fruits, vegetables, and whole grains also helps one to adapt to a low-fat diet. Thus, it is certainly possible to make the change from a higher-fat diet to a lower-fat diet, but it takes some effort.

satiety A state in which there is no longer a desire to eat; a feeling of satisfaction.

CRITICAL THINKING

In a class discussion, the topic of "diets" comes up. One of the most frustrating feelings dieters have, the students remark, is "being hungry all the time." Many dieters not only reduce their energy intake but also eliminate much of the fat from their diets. As a nutrition student, you suggest that some fat should be included in meals, even on a weight-reduction diet. How would you justify this advice? What other diet changes could you suggest to help compensate for the reduced fat content in the meal?

■ Hydrogenation of Fatty Acids Aids in Food Formulation but Increases Trans Fatty Acid Content

As previously mentioned, fats with long-chain saturated fatty acids are solid at room temperature, and those with unsaturated fatty acids are liquid at room temperature. In some kinds of food production, solid fats work better than liquid oils. In pie crust, for example, solid fats yield a flaky product, whereas crusts made with liquid oils tend to be greasy and more crumbly. If they are used to replace solid fats, oils with unsaturated fatty acids often must become more saturated (with hydrogen), as this solidifies the vegetable oils into shortenings and margarines. Hydrogen is added by bubbling hydrogen gas into liquid vegetable oils in a process called **hydrogenation.**

In their original form, monounsaturated and polyunsaturated fatty acids are in the *cis* form (Fig. 6-11). By definition, the hydrogens are on the same side of the carbon-carbon double bond. During hydrogenation, some hydrogens are transferred to opposite sides of the carbon-carbon double bond, creating the *trans* form, or a **trans fatty acid.** As seen in Figure 6-11, the *cis* bond causes the fatty acid backbone to bend, whereas the *trans* bond allows the backbone to remain straighter. This makes it identical to the shape of a saturated fatty acid. This may be the mechanism whereby trans fatty acids raise LDL. Trans fatty acids also lower HDL. Thus, people with elevated LDL should limit intake of hydrogenated fat.[18] It is less clear that this is important for the average person, as long as trans fatty acid intake is not excessive and the diet is adequate in polyunsaturated fat. However, since these fatty acids serve no particular role in maintaining the body health, many experts concur with the latest Dietary Guidelines and advice from the American Heart Association that recommend minimal trans fatty acid intake.

As public pressure has persuaded manufacturers to eliminate the tropical oils rich in saturated fat (palm, palm olein, and coconut) from food processing, partially hydrogenated soybean oil—rich in trans fatty acids—has become the major replacement. Currently, trans fatty acid intake in the United States is estimated to contribute about 3% of total calories, amounting to on average about 10 g/day.

FDA is in the process of requiring the labeling of trans fatty acid content in foods. Currently no such labeling is present. The agency hopes to make consumers more aware of trans fatty acid intake, and as well as the negative health consequences associated with high intakes of trans fatty acids. Companies are already responding to this issue before labeling is in place by creating products that are free of trans fatty acids. For example, Promise, Smart Beat, and some Fleischmann's margarines are now trans fatty acid–free products (less than 0.5 g per serving). The new labeling requirements will likely combine grams of saturated fat and trans fatty acids into one category, with an asterisk after the total number, referring to a footnote at the base of the Nutrition Facts label detailing the exact amount of trans fatty acids.

hydrogenation The addition of hydrogen to a carbon-carbon double bond, producing a single bond. Because hydrogenation of unsaturated fatty acids in a vegetable oil increases its hardness, this process is used to convert liquid oils into more solid fats, which are used in making margarine and shortening. Trans fatty acids are a by-product of hydrogenation of vegetable oils.

trans fatty acid A form of an unsaturated fatty acid, usually a monounsaturated one when found in food, in which the hydrogens on both carbons forming the double bond lie on opposite sides of that bond. A *cis* fatty acid has the hydrogens lying on the same side of the carbon-carbon double bond.

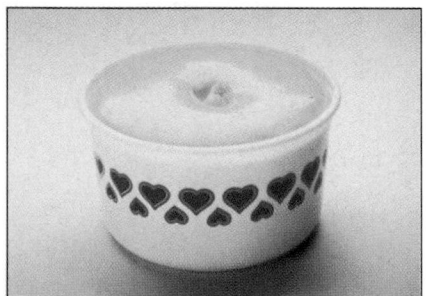

Tub margarine is much lower in trans fatty acids than stick margarine or shortenings (9%, 14%, and 26% of fatty acids respectively).

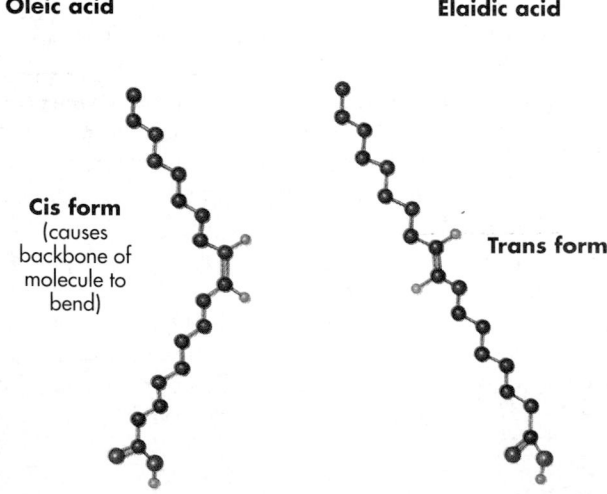

Oleic acid   **Elaidic acid**

Cis form
(causes backbone of molecule to bend)

Trans form

■ **FIGURE 6-11** *Cis* and *trans* isomers of fatty acids. Cis fatty acids are more common in foods than trans fatty acids. The latter are primarily found in foods containing hydrogenated fats—notably, stick margarine, shortening, and deep fat–fried foods. Trans fatty acids raise LDL and lower HDL, so a generous intake is discouraged.
Illustration by William Ober.

This addition of trans fatty acids to labels will help consumers at the grocery store, but, when dining out, consumers are left in the dark as to which foods contain trans fatty acids. Currently, restaurant foods are rich not only in saturated fatty acids but also in trans fatty acids (Table 6-2). Knowing which foods are low in trans fatty acids when ordering at a restaurant is extremely difficult because the information on how these foods are prepared or the precise fat composition is typically not available. You can follow this tip when ordering to limit trans fatty acids: Limit fried (especially deep-fat fried) food items and any pastries or flaky bread products (such as piecrusts and biscuits).

Until FDA approves and enforces the labeling of trans fatty acids, we can also make educated guesses on the trans fatty acid content of foods that have a Nutrition Facts label. The best way to estimate is to add up the amount of saturated fat, monounsaturated fat, and polyunsaturated fat and then subtract that number from the total fat grams listed. In most cases, the difference can be attributed to trans fatty acid content (occasionally, the difference may be due to rounding errors). For example, if a stick margarine has per tablespoon 11 g total fat, 3 g saturated fat, 2 g polyunsaturated fat, and 3 g monounsaturated fat, the difference between total fat and the individual fatty acids is 3 g. This is the approximate amount of trans fatty acids in the product.

Looking at the ingredients on the label is another way to estimate the amount of trans fatty acids in a product. If partially hydrogenated vegetable oil is one of the first three ingredients, you can assume there is a significant amount of trans fatty acids in the product. Unfortunately, partially hydrogenated vegetable oil is a broad term that does not indicate the extent of hydrogenation. Although currently unavailable, this information would be helpful because, the more hydrogenated a product is, the more trans fatty acids it contains.

Limiting trans fatty acids at home is a much easier task. Most important, use little or no stick margarine or shortening; instead, substitute vegetable oils and softer tub margarines (whose labels list vegetable oil or water as the first ingredient). Avoid deep-fat frying any food in shortening. Substitute baking, pan-frying, broiling, steaming, grilling, or deep fat-frying in unhydrogenated vegetable oils. Replace nondairy creamers with reduced-fat or nonfat milk, since most nondairy creamers are rich in hydrogenated vegetable oils. Last, read all food ingredients labels, using the tips listed above on calculating trans fatty acid content. Dr. Holub discusses why this is important in his Expert Opinion.

TABLE 6-2 Trans Fatty Acids in Restaurant Foods

Fried Foods	Calories	Total Fat (g)	Trans Fat (g)
Onion Rings (8 rings—6 oz)	650	47	7
Burger King french fries (king-size—6 oz)	540	24	7
McDonald's chicken nuggets (9)	510	29	3
McDonald's french fries (large—5 oz)	470	19	4
Fried mozzarella sticks (4 sticks—4 oz)	370	23	3
Fried fish (6 oz)	350	16	3
Miscellaneous Foods			
Prime rib, untrimmed (6 oz precooked weight)	480	35	3
Hamburger (5 oz)	470	26	2
Chicken pot pie (7 oz)	370	20	3
KFC biscuit (2 oz)	210	12	4
Pastries and Desserts			
Cinnabon Cinnabun (8 oz)	670	34	6
Apple pie (3.5 oz)	236	12	3

Adapted from *Nutrition Action Health Letter,* June 1999.

Expert Opinion

TRANS FATTY ACIDS

Bruce Holub, Ph.D.

*T*rans fatty acids (TFA) are an increasing health concern, since the amounts in a typical North American diet have increased markedly during the past decade. Unlike naturally occurring monounsaturated and polyunsaturated fatty acids, as found in many liquid non-hydrogenated vegetable oils, TFA have trans double bonds at unsaturation sites within the fat/fatty acid molecule. This imparts a higher melting point and a more solid fat, approaching that for saturated fatty acids. Chemical hydrogenation by the commercial processing of unsaturated liquid vegetable oils containing cis double bonds—with no TFA—results in the transformation of liquid oils into more solid partially hydrogenated oils, including vegetable shortenings.

Partially hydrogenated vegetable oils and vegetable shortenings are used extensively in assorted processed foods and fast foods. While imparting the desired solidity, there is also greater resilience to oxidation/rancidity, providing longer shelf-lives. Products rich in TFA also currently can use labeling/marketing terms including *cholesterol-free, low in saturated fat,* and *free of animal fat,* which are of perceptive appeal to consumers. A considerable portion of the so-called monounsaturates in a North American diet are now represented by TFA (trans-monounsaturates) in addition to the natural cis monounsaturates. Dietary TFA are present mostly as monounsaturated rather than as polyunsaturated fatty acid structures.

ORIGINS, INTAKES, AND FOOD SOURCES

Approximately 90% of the TFA consumed per person daily is derived from vegetable/plant–derived primary food sources, often from processed and fast-food products. Animal sources/fats contribute approximately 10% to the total TFA intake in the form of milk, beef, and butter, where TFA represent approximately 2 to 5% of the total fat. Natural bio-hydrogenation by microorganisms in the stomach of ruminant animals (dairy cows, beef cattle) produce some TFA from the unsaturated dietary fat consumed. Margarines contribute nearly 20% of the total TFA intake in the North American diet, with the remaining majority coming from numerous other foods, including crackers, croissants, cookies, potato chips, and so on; these often contain up to 50% of the total fat as TFA. Other rich TFA sources in many but not all brand-name products include cake/pancake mixes, frozen breakfast waffles, and fast foods including donuts, french fries, and breaded meats such as fish fillets. Approximately 3–5 g of TFA can be found in a single serving of many processed and fast-food products. Recently, my laboratory has determined that many foods directed toward infants and young children (baby biscuits, selected infant cereals, etc.) have a substantial portion of the total fat represented by TFA due to the inclusion of vegetable shortening and partially hydrogenated vegetable oil in these formulated products.

Estimates on the per capita (adult) intake of total TFA in the North American diet have ranged from an average of 6.0 up to 15.0 g/person/day. A recent Canadian assessment indicated the average TFA-monounsaturated intake to be 8.4 g/person/day, or 3.7% of the total dietary energy for Canadian adults, with the highest intakes occurring among the younger population. For example, young male adults (18–34 years) had mean TFA-monounsaturated intakes of 12.5 g/person/day (with ranges up to 38.9 g/person/day or 11.7% of total energy). Unfortunately, one of the highest dietary sources of TFA in the North American food supply is mothers' breast milk; these high physiological levels relate directly to the high maternal dietary intake of TFA. The mean total TFA content was found to be 7.2% of the total milk fatty acids, with the TFA ranging up to 17.2% (corresponding to mean intakes of lactating women of 10.6 g/person/day, with intakes as high as 20.3 g/person/day in some women).

EFFECTS ON HUMAN HEALTH AND CARDIOVASCULAR DISEASE RISK

Epidemiological/population studies have indicated that dietary TFA represent a major dietary risk factors for cardiovascular disease (CVD) in the population. A prospective study on 80,082 women followed for 14 years indicated that the relative risk for developing CVD was approximately doubled for every 2%

increase in energy intake from TFA (i.e., increasing from 1 to 3% of total energy intake). These findings are very disturbing when considered in the context of the aforementioned intakes of TFA in the North American population. Furthermore, when compared on an equal intake basis, dietary TFA was an even greater dietary risk factor for CVD than saturated fats. For example, each 5% of energy intake as saturates increased the risk by 17%, where each 2% increase in energy from TFA increased the risk by 93%.

Controlled intervention studies have indicated that both saturated fatty acids and TFA increase total and LDL-cholesterol in the circulation, thereby increasing the risk of CVD. However, TFA also lower the HDL-cholesterol, whereas saturated fats do not; lowering of HDL-cholesterol has been associated with an increased risk of CVD. In addition, TFA, but not saturates, tend to increase the levels of the highly atherogenic lipoprotein known as lipoprotein(a), which further increases the risk for CVD. Overall, TFA has been determined to increase the risk of CVD to a much greater degree as compared with equivalent amounts of saturated fatty acids based also on the effects on blood lipids/lipoproteins.

High TFA intakes also interfere with the conversion and metabolism of omega-3 fatty acids, which are physiologically important for functioning in the brain and eye. There is also evidence in the scientific literature indicating the potentially deleterious effects of high TFA intakes during pregnancy in terms of the growth and development of infants during the neonatal period.

PENDING FOOD LABELING AND REGULATORY POLICIES

Despite considerable scientific evidence for serious health concerns regarding the high intake of TFA in numerous foods and in the overall North American diet, food regulations and labeling requirements to date have focused on cholesterol and saturated fat without corresponding labeling or control being directed toward TFA. Furthermore, labeling and marketing terms such as *cholesterol-free* and *low in saturated fats*, when allowed by regulatory agencies, imply to many in the public sector that somehow these products have been deemed to be of benefit with respect to the prevention and/or management of CVD. Unfortunately, many of these products so marketed contain substantial amounts of TFA, which could potentially promote rather than prevent the development of CVD via their deleterious effects on risk factors such as LDL-cholesterol, HDL-cholesterol, and lipoprotein(a). There are also concerns regarding excessive intakes of TFA during pregnancy and lactation, resulting in the overexposure of infants to these fatty acids, as well as by adult health-conscious consumers who are not provided information on the TFA content of the foods consumed. Various groups have established maximal intakes of TFA during pregnancy and lactation, as well as for the general public. These are well below current intakes in the North American population. Numerous academic/medical leaders in the field of nutrition-CVD research, as well as expert groups, have long recommended the mandatory declaration of TFA contents on food products in view of their potential hazard to human health. It is both indefensible and potentially misleading to the health-conscious public to list the amounts of cholesterol (and saturated fatty acid) on food labels and to allow claims such as *cholesterol-free* and *low in saturated fat* on products that contain substantial amounts of TFA. Furthermore, public information on the TFA contents of various fast foods are also critical to protect the health of consumers in all categories, but particularly the younger population, who are becoming major users of such food products.

The Food and Drug Administration is planning to institute TFA labeling in the near future. The time for such is long overdue. Such labeling would ideally provide separate quantitative listings for the amount of TFA per serving—preferably in "mg" amounts, as is now done for cholesterol, or in "g" quantities if cholesterol amounts are shifted toward labeling in the same units.

Dr. Holub is professor, Department of Human Biology & Nutritional Sciences at the University of Guelph. He has served as president, Nutrition Society of Canada, and chair, Nutrition Task Force (Heart & Stroke Foundation of Ontario). He has authored more than 200 papers in scientific journals (medical, nutrition, and others) in addition to various book chapters and conference proceedings. His research program is focused on dietary omega-3 fatty acids from fish and fish oils and the health risks associated with foods containing trans fatty acids.

■ Fat Rancidity Limits Shelf Life of Foods

Decomposing oils emit a disagreeable odor and taste sour and stale. Stale potato chips are a good example. As double bonds in fatty acids break down, rancid by-products appear. Ultraviolet rays of light, oxygen, and certain procedures can break double bonds and in turn destroy the structure of polyunsaturated fatty acids. Saturated fats can much more readily resist these effects. Why?

Rancidity is not a major problem for consumers because, although eating rancid oils can cause sickness, the odor and taste generally discourage us from eating enough to become sick. However, rancidity is a problem for manufacturers because it reduces a product's shelf life. For this reason, manufacturers often add hydrogenated plant oils to products to increase shelf life. Foods most likely to become rancid are deep-fried foods and foods with a large amount of exposed surface (such as powdered eggs or powdered milk). The fat in fish is also very susceptible to rancidity because it is highly polyunsaturated.

Vitamin E helps protect foods against rancidity because it acts as an antioxidant. It guards against the fat breakdown caused by various agents, such as metals found as impurities in vegetable oils. The vitamin E in plant oils reduces the breakdown of double bonds in fatty acids. (In Chapter 9, the role of vitamin E is explained more fully.) When food manufacturers want to prevent rancidity in polyunsaturated fats, they often add **BHA** and **BHT**. (Chapter 19 discusses the safety of these and other food additives.) Look for these food additives in salad dressings, cake mixes, and other products that contain fat. They can even be added to a food's paper packaging. Vitamin C may also be added for the same reason. Manufacturers also tightly seal products and use other methods to reduce oxygen levels inside packages.

BHA, BHT Butylated hydroxyanisol and butylated hydroxytoluene—two common synthetic antioxidants added to foods.

■ Fats Act as Emulsifiers

Food manufacturers add emulsifiers in the preparation of many food products, primarily to improve texture. For example, lecithins, polysorbate 60, and other emulsifiers are added to salad dressings to keep the vegetable oil suspended in water. Eggs added to cake batters likewise emulsify the fat with the milk. Monoglycerides and related compounds are also good emulsifiers and, for that reason, are sometimes used in cake mixes and salad dressings. Over the next few days, examine the labels of salad dressings and cake mixes, and see how many emulsifiers are listed.

CONCEPT CHECK

Fat has a variety of roles in foods, including that of contributing to flavor, texture, and satiety. Fat also provides the pleasurable mouth feel of many of our favorite foods, intensifies the taste of many spices, and tenderizes many popular cuts of meat. In addition, fat in the diet allows for a feeling of fullness.

Hydrogenation of unsaturated fatty acids consists of adding hydrogen to carbon-carbon double bonds to produce single bonds; some trans fatty acids are also created. Hydrogenation changes vegetable oil to solid fat. It is wise to monitor trans fatty acid intake, as this form of fat raises LDL and lowers HDL.

The carbon-carbon double bonds in polyunsaturated fatty acids are easily broken, yielding products responsible for rancidity. The presence of antioxidants, such as vitamin E in oils, naturally protects unsaturated fatty acids against oxidative destruction. Manufacturers can use hydrogenated fats and add synthetic antioxidants to reduce the likelihood of rancidity.

Manufacturers of commercial salad dressings find practical use for emulsification. Emulsifiers, such as lecithins, polysorbate 60, and monoglycerides, are added to salad dressings and other fat-rich products to keep the vegetable oils and other fats suspended in the water.

■ RECOMMENDATIONS FOR FAT INTAKE

There is currently no RDA for fat. A DRI for dietary fat and individual fatty acids (omega-3 and omega-6 fatty acids), phospholipids and cholesterol, is under development and should be published in late 2001 (see the web site http://www4. nationalacademies.org/IOM/IOMHome.nsf/Pages/Food+and+Nutrition+Board) . To obtain the essential fatty acids, adults should consume about 4% of total energy intake from plant oils incorporated into foods and eat fish twice a week. The typical American diet derives about 7% of energy content from polyunsaturated fatty acids. An upper limit of 10% of energy intake as polyunsaturated fatty acids is often recommended, in part because the breakdown (oxidation) of those present in lipoproteins is linked to increased cholesterol deposition in the arteries, as previously discussed. Depression of immune function is also suspected to be caused by an excessive intake of polyunsaturated fats.

Current recommendations for the percentage of total calories from fat range widely:

- About 10% for people with existing cardiovascular disease who want to follow the Dr. Dean Ornish **vegan** diet plan to reverse cholesterol-laden plaques in the arteries
- No more than 30% of calories if you follow the Dietary Guidelines
- Up to 35% of calories if you follow the Mediterranean Pyramid (see Chapter 2)
- Up to 40% of calories if a person has Syndrome X and wants to follow the Syndrome X Diet (see the Nutrition Perspective at the end of this chapter for details)

In all cases, watching total calories is also important.

General consensus among nutrition experts suggests that we should limit saturated fat and trans fatty acid intake and that the diet needs to contain some omega-3 and omega-6 fatty acids. Furthermore, if fat intake exceeds 30% of calories, the extra fat should come from monounsaturated fat. No expert suggests that a diet be dominated by saturated fat or trans fatty acids.

Dietary fat supplies about 33% of Americans' total energy intake, in which the major sources are animal flesh, whole milk, pastries, cheese, margarine, and mayonnaise. In contrast, the major sources of fat in the Mediterranean Pyramid diet include liberal amounts of olive oil and the fat found in the small amount of animal flesh and dairy products allowed on the diet. The main sources of fat in Dr. Dean Ornish's vegan diet plan are a scant amount of vegetable oil used in cooking and the negligible amount found in various plant foods.[6]

Because many Americans are at risk for developing cardiovascular disease, the American Heart Association (AHA) promotes dietary and lifestyle goals aimed at reducing this risk. One set of recommendations is made for the general public. (Table 6-3).[16] Then a more detailed list of recommendations is made for those at high risk or who currently have heart disease. (Table 6-4). For high risk individuals the AHA recommendation that total fat intake should not exceed 20 to 30% of total energy intake, with no more than 7 to 10% of total energy intake from saturated fat. The intake of saturated fats currently averages about 13% of energy intake. Table 6-5 shows a diet that follows those AHA guidelines.

Current research shows that our palates can adapt to a lower fat intake over time, so we miss it less. Reducing fat intake also allows us to include more healthful foods—fruits, vegetables, and whole grains—in our diets. A good start for this type of diet is a low-fat breakfast: One option is a high-fiber cereal, reduced-fat or nonfat milk, and fruit juice.

Monitoring by a physician is important when fat is restricted to 20% of calories, as the resulting increase in carbohydrate intake can increase blood triglycerides in some people, which is not a healthful change. Over time, however, this problem of high blood triglycerides on a low-fat diet may self-correct, as has been shown in

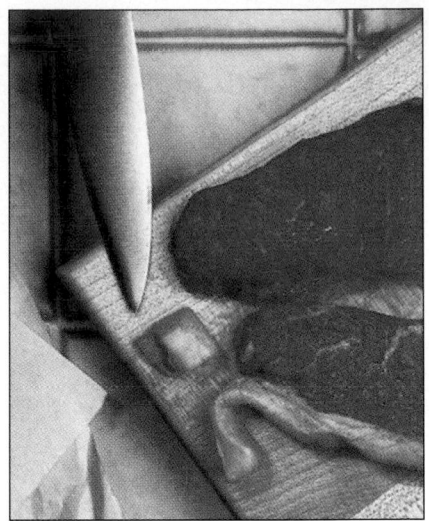

Trim meats before cooking to reduce intake of saturated fat, the major dietary fat that increases blood cholesterol.

vegan A person who eats only plant foods.

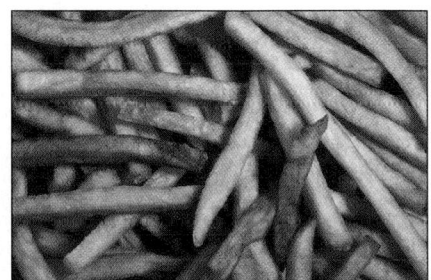

French fries are a common source of fat and trans fatty acids for many adults. For regular consumers, a small serving size is recommended if blood lipids or weight control is a problem.

TABLE 6-3	Current Dietary Guidance for the General Population (2 Years of Age and Older) from the American Heart Association.[16]
Population Goals	**Major guidelines**
Overall Healthy Eating Pattern	Include a variety of fruits, vegetables, grains, low-fat or nonfat dairy products, fish, legumes, poultry, lean meats.
Appropriate Body Weight	Match energy intake to overall energy needs, with appropriate changes to achieve weight loss when indicated.
Desirable Blood Cholesterol Profile	Limit foods high in saturated fat and cholesterol; and substitute unsaturated fat from vegetables, fish, legumes, nuts.
Desirable Blood Pressure	Limit salt and alcohol; maintain a healthy body weight and a diet with emphasis on vegetables, fruits, and low-fat or nonfat dairy products.

TABLE 6-4	Specific Dietary Recommendations from American Heart Association, Especially for Those People at High Risk or Currently Have Cardiovascular Disease.[16]
Diet	**Consume at least:**
	5 servings of fruits and vegetables each day. Up to 9 servings per day is advised if the person has hypertension.
	6 servings of grains, including some whole grains, each day.
	2 servings of fish per week (or 900 mg of a combination of EPA and DHA from fish oil supplements per day).
	25 g of dietary fiber each day, including some sources of soluble fiber.
	Consume no more than:
	30% of calories from total fat or 20% if blood lipids are still too high.
	10% of calories as saturated fat, or 7% if blood lipids are still too high. As well, limit trans fatty acid intake (combine with saturated fat gram allowance).
	300 mg of cholesterol per day (on average), or 200 mg per day if blood lipids are still too high or the person has diabetes or cardiovascular disease.
	6 g of salt each day (6 g equals 2400 mg of sodium).
	2 alcoholic drinks per day for men and one drink for women.
	Additional advice includes:
	Specifically meeting vitamin B-6, folate, vitamin B-12, and potassium needs, limiting sugar intake, and possible use of soy protein and stanol/sterol ester-containing margarines. Megadose vitamin E supplements are not recommended at this time, and vitamin C and beta-carotene supplements provide no benefit.
Body weight	Maintain a body mass index between 18.5 and 25. Waist circumference should not exceed 40 inches (102 cm) in men or 35 inches (88 cm) in women (see Chapter 13 for details).
Physical activity	30 to 60 minutes of brisk activity on most if not all days of the week.

These specific recommendations apply to individuals 2 years of age and older.

TABLE 6-5 Daily Menus Containing 2000 kcal and Various Percentages of Fat

	30% of Energy as Fat Teaspoons of Fat		20% of Energy as Fat Teaspoons of Fat
Breakfast			
Orange juice, 1 cup	0	Same	0
Shredded wheat, ¾ cup	⅕	Shredded wheat cereal, 1 cup	⅕
Bagel, toasted	⅕	Same	⅕
Margarine, 2 tsp	1¾	Margarine, 1 tsp	⅞
1% low-fat milk, 1 cup	½	Nonfat milk, 1 cup	1/10
Lunch			
Whole-wheat bread, 2 slices	½	Same	½
Roast beef, 2 oz	2	Ham, extra lean, 3 oz	1
Mayonnaise, 2 tsp	1½	Mayonnaise, 1 tsp	¾
Lettuce	0	Same	0
Tomato, sliced	0	Same	0
Animal crackers, 8	½	Animal crackers, 10	⅔
Snack			
Apple	⅙	Same	⅙
Dinner			
Chicken parmigiana frozen dinner	4	Healthy Choice chicken parmigiana frozen dinner	⅔
Dinner roll, 1	½	Dinner roll, 2	1
Banana, 1	1/10	Margarine, 2 tsp	1¾
1% low-fat milk, 1 cup	½	Nonfat milk, 1 cup	1/10
Snack			
Raisins, 2 tbsp	0	Raisins, 1/4 cup	0
Popcorn, air-popped, 6 cups	½	Same	½
with 2 tsp margarine	1¾	with 1 tsp margarine	⅞
TOTALS	14⅔		9⅓

people following the Dr. Dean Ornish vegan diet for a year or more. Their blood triglycerides increased initially on the diet but, within a year, fell to normal values.[6]

The National Cholesterol Education Program, established in 1985, also recommends reducing saturated fatty acids to 7% of total energy intake if elevated LDL does not respond to the reduction in saturated fat intake of closer to 10% of energy intake. Cholesterol intake in this regard should be limited to 300 mg per day, with a reduction to 200 mg per day if LDL remains elevated when following a fat-restricted diet containing the higher amount of cholesterol. Recall that adults consume an average of about 200 to 400 mg of cholesterol per day, with men generally consuming the higher amount.

Unfortunately, exceeding 30% of energy intake of fat is all too easy. For example, a bologna and cheese sandwich with mayonnaise contains about 39 g of fat, or about 60% of the fat allowance for a 2000-kcal diet. A half-cup of premium ice cream contains about 18 g of fat, and a slice of apple pie contains about 19 g of fat, almost all of which is in the crust. A super-sized order of fries has 24 g or more of fat, and about a third of that is trans fatty acids.

Most people probably have no idea how much of the energy in their diets comes from fat. You've already tracked your food intake for one day. A Take Action exercise at the end of the chapter asks you to compare your fat intake with current guide-

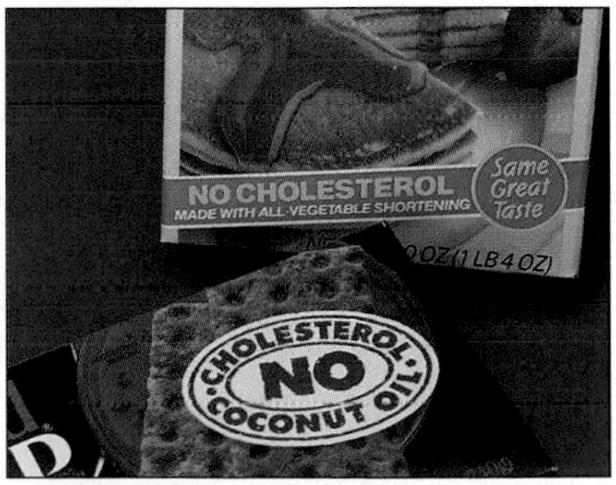

Manufacturers offer a variety of low-cholesterol foods. The general recommendation is to consume ≤300 mg/day of cholesterol.

*R*ecommendations for fat intake are stated as percentages of total energy intake—usually 20 to 30%. The following table shows how many grams of fat per day are allowed with diets ranging from 1000 to 3900 kcal.

Energy Intake (kcal)	Fat Intake Grams	
	30% of Energy	20% of Energy
1000	33	22
1200	40	27
1500	50	33
1800	60	40
2100	70	47
2400	80	53
2700	90	60
3000	100	67
3600	120	80
3900	130	87

lines. Using the information on food labels and recording and analyzing daily food intake also allow you to track fat intake.

The advice to consume 20 to 30% of energy as fat does not apply to infants and toddlers below the age of 2 years. These youngsters are forming new tissue, especially in the brain, so their intake of fat and cholesterol should not be greatly restricted. After that age, children should gradually adopt a diet that contains no more than 30% of energy from fat and 300 mg of cholesterol per day (see Chapter 17 for details). As children begin to consume less fat, they should replace the missing energy with more whole-grain products, fruits, vegetables, and reduced-fat milk products.

■ FATS IN FOOD

Table 6-5 provided an example of the amount of fat in foods in a day's menu. In the Exchange System, foods from both the vegetable and fruit lists are essentially fat free. On the milk list, the amount of fat per cup varies with food choice: skim/very-low-fat milk has a trace (1–3 g); reduced-fat milk has 5 g; and whole milk has 8 g. Most exchanges from both the starch and other carbohydrates lists contain only small amounts of fat, so this is ignored. However, read the label carefully, as some gourmet breads, snack crackers, and cereals can surprise you. On the meat list, the amount of fat per ounce also varies with food choice: very lean meat has a trace (0–1 g); lean meat has 3 g; medium-fat meat has 5 g; and high-fat meat has 8 g. Foods on the fat list have 5 g of fat per serving.

The foods with the highest energy density for fat are salad oils, butter, margarine, and mayonnaise (Fig. 6-12). All contain close to 100% of energy as fat. In fat-reduced margarines, water replaces some of the fat. Typical margarines are 80% fat by weight (11 g per tablespoon). Some fat-reduced margarines are as low as 30% fat by weight (4 g per tablespoon). The extra water added to these margarines can cause texture and volume changes when used in recipes. Cookbooks can provide guidance for appropriate use of these products by suggesting alterations in recipes to compensate. You may be surprised to note that some margarines are even advertised as being fat free. Close inspection of the label shows that these products are made up of monoglycerides and diglycerides. These are not considered to be fats for labeling purposes, as they are not triglycerides, but, of course, they are still fats and energy dense.

Walnuts, bologna, avocados, and bacon have about 80% of energy as fat. Peanut butter and cheddar cheese have about 75%. Marbled steak and hamburgers (ground chuck) have about 60%, and chocolate bars, ice cream, doughnuts, and whole milk have about 50% of energy as fat. Eggs, pumpkin pie, and cupcakes have 35%, as do lean cuts of meat, such as top round (and ground round) and sirloin. Bread contains about 15%. Cornflakes, sugar, and nonfat milk have essentially no fat. Careful label reading is necessary to determine the true fat content of food—these are only rough guidelines.

Animal fats, which contain about 40 to 60% of total fat as saturated fatty acids, are the chief contributors of saturated fatty acids to the American diet. Saturated fatty acids with 12, 14, and 16 carbons (lauric acid, myristic acid, and palmitic acid, respectively) are the primary contributors to elevated LDL. Of these, the 14-carbon myristic acid is mainly responsible for elevating LDL.[3] Dairy fats are rich sources of myristic acid. The 16-carbon palmitic acid also increases LDL, primarily when there is more than 200 to 300 mg of cholesterol in the diet and LDL is already elevated. The saturated fatty acids with 12, 14, or 16 carbons generally constitute about 25 to 50% of the total fat in animal foods. In general, dairy fats and meat are rich in the fatty acids that raise LDL. In some plant oils, these saturated fatty acids also make up a notable percentage of the total fat—for example, cottonseed oil (27%) and coconut oil (89%). Stearic acid is the saturated fatty acid with 18 carbons. It was thought to be

Nutrient Density for Fat

| low | medium | high |

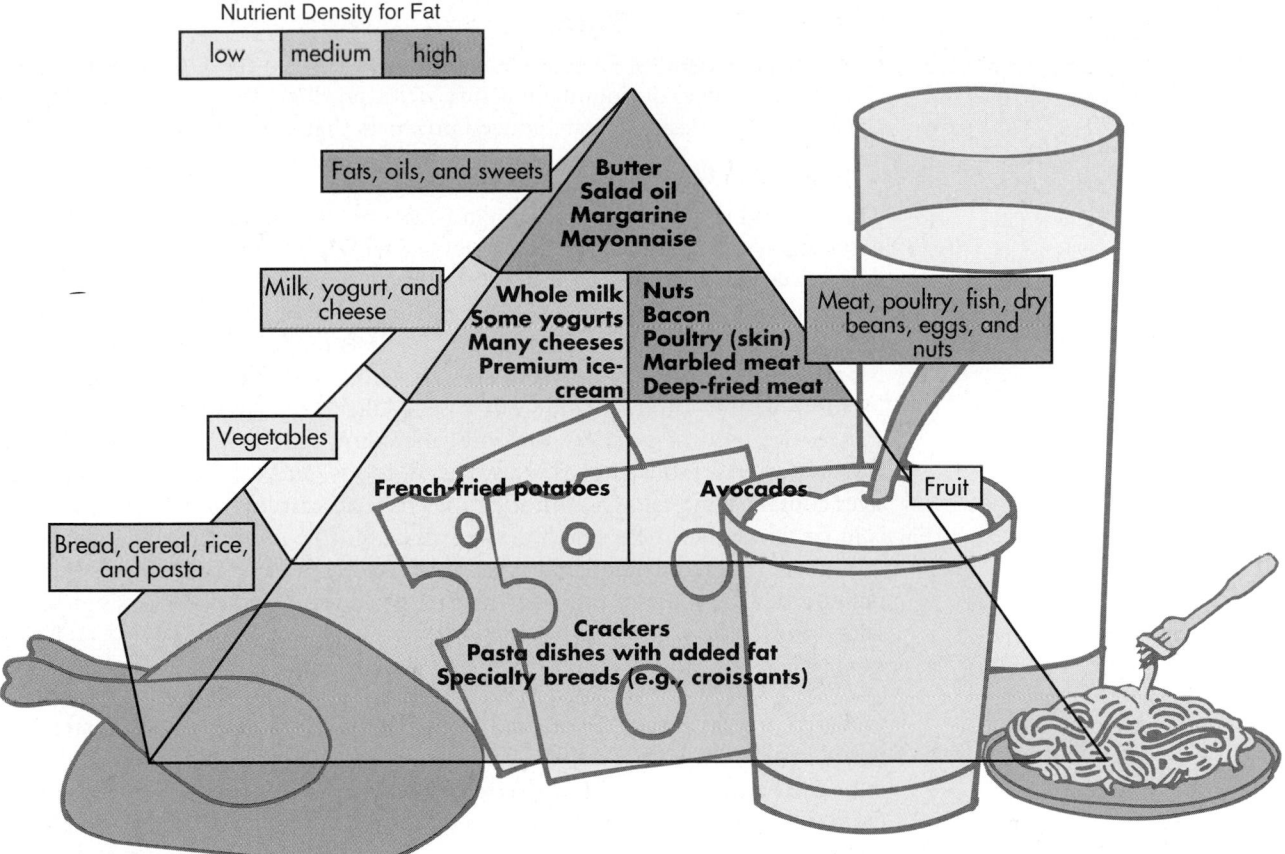

Fats, oils, and sweets

**Butter
Salad oil
Margarine
Mayonnaise**

Milk, yogurt, and cheese

**Whole milk
Some yogurts
Many cheeses
Premium ice-cream**

**Nuts
Bacon
Poultry (skin)
Marbled meat
Deep-fried meat**

Meat, poultry, fish, dry beans, eggs, and nuts

Vegetables

French-fried potatoes

Avocados

Fruit

Bread, cereal, rice, and pasta

**Crackers
Pasta dishes with added fat
Specialty breads (e.g., croissants)**

▌ FIGURE 6-12 Sources of fats in foods from the Food Guide Pyramid. The background color of each group indicates the average nutrient density for fat in that food group. The fruit group and vegetable group are generally low in fat. In the other groups, both high-fat and low-fat choices are available. Careful food label reading can lead you along the low-fat path. In general, any type of frying adds significant amounts of fat to a product, as with french fries and fried chicken.

neutral in cardiovascular disease development because of its conversion to monounsaturated oleic acid once it reached the liver. However, recent studies have revealed that stearic acid may increase the risk of cardiovascular disease. The negative effect on the heart is probably due in part to a reduction in HDL in the blood and an increase in blood clotting prior to conversion to oleic acid in the liver.[11] It constitutes about 20% of saturated fats in meats (see Appendix F).

Plant oils contain mostly unsaturated fatty acids, ranging from 73 to 94% of total fat. Canola oil, olive oil, and peanut oil contain moderate to high amounts of total fat as monounsaturated fatty acids (49% to 77%). Some animal fats are also good sources of monounsaturated fatty acids (30 to 47%) (see Fig. 6-2). Corn, cottonseed, sunflower, soybean, and safflower oils contain mostly polyunsaturated fatty acids (54 to 77%) in terms of total fat. These plant oils supply the majority of the linoleic acid and alpha-linolenic acid in the U.S. food supply. Note that plant oils vary in their content of polyunsaturated fatty acids. Oils that are similar in appearance still may vary significantly in fatty acid composition.

Cholesterol is found only in the animal foods we eat (review Table 6-1). An egg yolk contains about 210 mg of cholesterol. This is our main dietary source of cholesterol, along with meats and whole milk. Some plants contain related sterols, but none we typically eat contains cholesterol. Manufacturers who advertise peanut butter, vegetable shortening, margarines, and vegetable oils as containing no cholesterol are taking advantage of uninformed consumers. Peanut butter and margarine never contain cholesterol—it's not naturally present.

■ Fat Replacement Strategies

Currently, five types of fat replacements are available in the United States. Addition of these substances during manufacture yields products that, to varying degrees, satisfy consumers' desire for fat-reduced products that are still tasty.

Water, Starch Derivatives, and Gums

The first and simplest fat replacement is water. The addition of water yields a product, such as diet margarine, with less fat per serving than the normal product. Starch derivatives that bind water form a second type of fat replacement. The resulting gel replaces some of the mouth feel lost by the removal of fat. Z-trim, the newest starch derivative, was recently created by USDA. It is made from the hulls of oats, soybeans, peas, and rice or bran from corn or wheat. Other derivatives commonly used by food manufacturers include cellulose, Maltrin, Stellar, and Oatrim. These substances are used in a variety of foods, including luncheon meats, salad dressings, frozen desserts, table spreads, dips, baked goods, and candies. Most starch derivatives contain some calories, although they have at least less than half the amount that is in fat. Note that these starch derivatives cannot be used in fried foods.

Gums extracted from plants can also be used to replace fat. They thicken a product and replace some of the body that fat provides. Diet salad dressings have gums added for this reason.

Protein-Derived Fat Replacements

One type of fat replacement on the market consists of proteins that have been treated to produce microscopic, mistlike protein globules. Both egg and milk proteins can be used. When these substances replace fat in a food product, they feel like fat in the mouth, although the product does not contain any fatty acids. Simplesse is a currently used fat replacement of this type. Since it contains protein, Simplesse yields some energy—but only about 1 to 2 kcal/g, much less than the 9 kcal/g supplied by regular fats. Simplesse has this low energy value primarily for two reasons: Proteins contain only 4 kcal/g and the product has a high water content.

Simplesse is used primarily in frozen desserts. It reduces the energy content of these products by about one-half and the fat content to a negligible amount. However, these products tend to develop a grainy texture on refreezing. This is one reason for their limited acceptance to date. Simplesse can also replace fat in mayonnaise, salad dressing, yogurt, sour cream, cheese, and other dairy products. Because high temperatures alter the structure of Simplesse so much that it no longer resembles fat, it cannot be used for cooking or frying. Note also that people who are allergic to milk or egg proteins should not consume Simplesse.

Dairy-Lo is a modified whey protein concentrate that has fatlike properties. It is used in milk and other dairy products, baked goods, frostings, salad dressings, and mayonnaise-type products.

Engineered Fats and Related Products

The fifth form of fat replacement is the engineered fat. This type of product is synthesized in the laboratory from various food constituents. Olestra (Olean) is a good example. It is made by chemically linking fatty acids to sucrose (table sugar). The resulting product cannot be digested by either human digestive enzymes or bacteria that live in the intestine. Therefore, olestra yields no energy to the body.

Olestra can replace much of the fat in salad dressings and cakes and is the first fat replacement that can be used in fried foods. After almost 200 animal and human studies over a 25-year period, olestra was approved by FDA in 1996 for use in fried snack foods. It underwent such strict scrutiny because it did not exist as such in nature or arise from typical cooking procedures, as is the case for the other products mentioned.

Some problems are associated with the use of olestra. It binds the fat-soluble vitamins A, D, E, and K, thus reducing absorption. To compensate, the manufacturer adds these vitamins to olestra. Olestra also may cause abdominal cramping and loose

Olestra, a sucrose polyester (with the maximum number of fatty acids attached).

stools in some people, because, even though it is not absorbed in the small intestine, it still may influence intestinal function. The problem is seen mostly with intakes of 20 g at a meal. In comparison, a 1-ounce bag of chips has about 10 g of olestra and has little effect.[28] Those who experience such symptoms as a result of eating olestra should limit or avoid using products that contain this fat replacement.

The following statement is required on all products made with olestra: "This product contains olestra. Olestra may cause abdominal cramping and loose stools. Olestra inhibits the absorption of some vitamins and other nutrients. Vitamins A, D, E, and K have been added." As a condition of approval, the manufacturer must conduct studies to monitor olestra consumption and its long-term effects. FDA recently reviewed the safety of olestra and did not find enough evidence that it causes severe gastrointestinal problems. Still, the FDA committee was not convinced that consumers are knowledgeable enough about olestra to warrant taking the warnings off the products made with olestra. Canada has turned down the use of olestra in food products; this decision makes the United States the sole country that permits the use of this fat substitute in foods.

One final problem linked to olestra is its ability to bind carotenoids, the yellow, orange, or red pigments found in many fruits and vegetables. Recall from Chapter 2 the discussion of phytochemicals and their proposed contribution to overall health; one class of phytochemicals is carotenoids. Population studies have linked fruits and vegetables containing carotenoids to a reduced risk of cardiovascular disease, some forms of cancer, and certain eye disorders. There is no planned attempt to add carotenoids to olestra. This effect of olestra is most important when it is consumed in large amounts with meals rich in carotenoids. Typical projected intakes of 10 to 20 g don't have much of an effect. Nevertheless, this ability to bind carotenoids has caused some experts to recommend that we not consume olestra. At the very least, organizations such as the American Heart Association recommend moderate intake until we know more about its long-term effects.

Food manufacturers are working on still other types of engineered fats, which either wholly or partially escape absorption by the body. One example is salatrim, which is marketed under the name Benefat and yields only about 5 kcal/g. It is generally composed of stearic acid, which the body absorbs poorly, and short-chain fatty acids. This product is currently used in reduced-fat chocolate. Another product is Appetize, which blends animal fats stripped of cholesterol with plant oils. This produces a stable frying fat low in trans fatty acid content, and is found in some margarines.

■ Hidden Fat

Some fat discussed so far is obvious: butter on bread, mayonnaise in potato salad, and marbling in raw meat. Fat is harder to detect in other foods that also contribute much fat to our diets. Fat is hidden in whole milk, pastries, cookies, cake, cheese, hot dogs, crackers, french fries, and ice cream. When we try to cut down on fat intake, hidden fats need to be exposed and controlled, along with the more obvious sources.

A place to begin searching for hidden fat is on the Nutrition Facts labels of foods you buy in the supermarket. Some signals that can alert you to the presence of fat are chocolate; animal fats, such as bacon, beef, ham, lamb, pork, chicken, and turkey fats; lard; vegetable oils; nuts; dairy fats, such as butter and cream; egg and egg-yolk solids; and hydrogenated shortening or vegetable oil. Conveniently, the label lists ingredients by order of weight in the product. If fat is one of the first ingredients listed, you are probably looking at a high-fat product. Use food labels to learn more about the fat content of the foods you eat (Fig. 6-13). Table 2-8 in Chapter 2 listed the definitions for various fat descriptors on food labels, such as "low-fat," "fat-free," and "reduced-fat." Recall that "low-fat" signifies in most cases that a product contains no more than 3 g of fat per serving. Products claimed to be fat free must have less than ½ g of fat per serving. A claim of "reduced-fat" means the product has at least 25% less fat than is usually found in that food.

When there is no Nutrition Facts label to inspect, moderating portion size is a good way to keep fat intake down. Table 6-6 lists many ways you can avoid eating

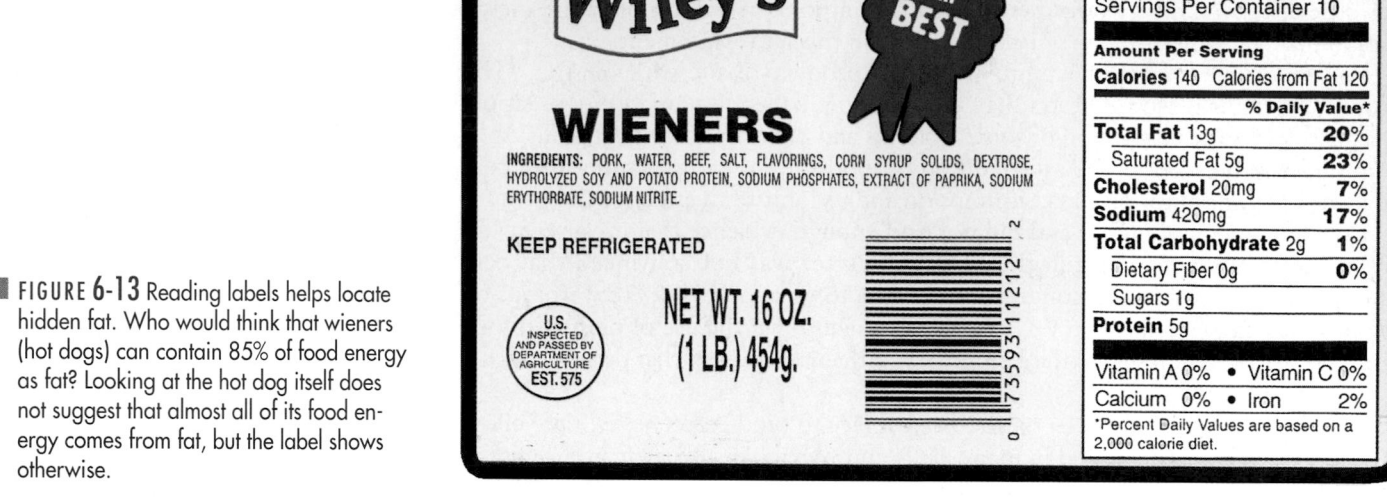

Nutrition Facts		
Serving Size 1 Link (45g)		
Servings Per Container 10		
Amount Per Serving		
Calories 140 Calories from Fat 120		
		% Daily Value*
Total Fat 13g		**20%**
Saturated Fat 5g		**23%**
Cholesterol 20mg		**7%**
Sodium 420mg		**17%**
Total Carbohydrate 2g		**1%**
Dietary Fiber 0g		**0%**
Sugars 1g		
Protein 5g		
Vitamin A 0% •	Vitamin C 0%	
Calcium 0% •	Iron	2%
*Percent Daily Values are based on a 2,000 calorie diet.		

Wiley's

Our BEST

WIENERS

INGREDIENTS: PORK, WATER, BEEF, SALT, FLAVORINGS, CORN SYRUP SOLIDS, DEXTROSE, HYDROLYZED SOY AND POTATO PROTEIN, SODIUM PHOSPHATES, EXTRACT OF PAPRIKA, SODIUM ERYTHORBATE, SODIUM NITRITE.

KEEP REFRIGERATED

U.S. INSPECTED AND PASSED BY DEPARTMENT OF AGRICULTURE EST. 575

NET WT. 16 OZ. (1 LB.) 454g.

■ FIGURE 6-13 Reading labels helps locate hidden fat. Who would think that wieners (hot dogs) can contain 85% of food energy as fat? Looking at the hot dog itself does not suggest that almost all of its food energy comes from fat, but the label shows otherwise.

CASE SCENARIO
Follow-Up

Jackie's approach to lowering blood cholesterol does not incorporate the best choices; she has excluded a great deal of fat in her diet by merely replacing it with refined carbohydrates. To make a shift to a more heart-healthy diet, Jackie would need to include at least two fruit and three vegetable servings a day, along with more whole-grain products (such as whole-wheat bread and a breakfast cereal that has at least 3 g of fiber per serving). Lowering fat as drastically as she has is not really necessary, especially for a 21-year-old female who is physically active. Jackie could allow a more liberal amount of fat in her diet by including more monounsaturated fats (canola oil and olive oil, as well as fats found in nuts and avocados). These do not increase blood cholesterol. In addition to allowing more liberal fat intake from monounsaturated oils and including more fruits, vegetables, and whole grains, Jackie would benefit from including good sources of omega-3 fatty acids (fatty fish, flaxseeds, or soybean and canola oil). One option is to use a canola oil-and-vinegar dressing on her salad, rather than lemon juice.

too much total fat and saturated fat. Whether or not to choose a fat-rich food should depend on how you intend to use it: as a staple item, as an occasional treat, or as a garnish for other foods.

■ Wise Use of Reduced-Fat Foods

In recent years, manufacturers have introduced reduced-fat versions of numerous food products. The fat content of these alternatives ranges from 0% in fat-free Fig Newtons to about 75% of the original fat content in other products. However, the total energy content of most fat-reduced products is not substantially lower than that of their conventional versions. Generally, when fat is removed from a product, something must be added—commonly, sugars—in its place. It is very difficult to reduce both the fat and sugar content of a product at the same time. For this reason, many fat-reduced products (for example, cakes, cookies, and yogurt) are still very energy dense. Similarly, some cookbooks are modifying recipes to make them lower in fat. This is accomplished by replacing the fat with applesauce or other fruit purees. Keep in mind that these carbohydrate replacements still contain calories, but not as much as the fat that is left out. As noted in Chapter 5, don't be fooled into thinking you can eat substantially more of such foods just because some or all of the fat has been removed. "Reduced-fat" is not a license to overeat. Use the Nutrition Facts label to guide the portion size you choose.

CONCEPT CHECK

There is currently no RDA for fat. We need about 4% of total energy intake from plant oils to obtain the needed essential fatty acids. Eating fish at least twice a week is also advised to supply omega-3 fatty acids. Many health-related agencies recommend a diet containing no more than 30% of energy intake as fat, with no more than 10% of energy intake as a combination of saturated fat and trans fatty acids for the general public. The current American diet contains about 33% of energy content as fat, with about 13% of energy content as saturated fat and about 3% as trans fatty acids. Fat-dense foods—those with more

TABLE 6-6 Tips for Avoiding Too Much Fat, Saturated Fat, and Trans Fatty Acids.

1. Steam, boil, or bake vegetables. For a change, stir-fry in a small amount of vegetable oil. Consider buying an insert for a pot, so you can easily steam your vegetables.
2. Season vegetables with herbs and spices, rather than with sauces, butter, or margarine.
3. Try lemon juice on salad or use limited amounts of oil-based salad dressing.
4. To reduce saturated fat, use vegetable oils and tub margarine instead of butter, stick margarine, or hydrogenated shortenings in baked products.
5. Limit baked goods made with large amounts of fat, especially croissants, doughnuts, muffins, biscuits, and butter rolls.
6. Try whole-grain flours to enhance flavors when baking goods with less fat. Use applesauce and other fruit purees in place of fat when possible, such as in quick breads.
7. Replace whole milk with nonfat or reduced-fat milk in puddings, soups, and baked products and for use as a beverage.
8. Substitute plain low-fat yogurt, blender-whipped low-fat cottage cheese, or buttermilk in recipes that call for sour cream or mayonnaise.
9. Choose lean cuts of meat. Limit bacon, ribs, and meat loaf.
10. Trim fat from meat before and after cooking.
11. Roast, bake, or broil meat, poultry, and fish, so that fat drains away as the food cooks.
12. Remove skin from poultry before cooking. This eliminates the temptation to eat it along with the meat.
13. Use a nonstick pan for cooking, so that added fat will be unnecessary; use a vegetable spray for frying.
14. Chill meat or poultry broth until the fat solidifies. Spoon off the fat before using the broth.
15. Eat a vegetarian main dish at least once a week. Include fish (cooked without much added fat) in the diet two times or more a week. Think about this when you make choices in a restaurant.
16. Choose fat-reduced ice cream, low-fat frozen yogurt, sorbet, and popsicles as substitutes for regular ice cream.
17. Try angelfood cake, fig bars, and gingersnaps as substitutes for commercially baked goods high in saturated fat.
18. Limit high-fat cheese intake.
19. Read labels on commercially prepared foods to find out what type of fat or how much saturated fat they contain.
20. Use jam, jelly, or marmalade on bread and toast instead of butter or margarine.
21. Buy whole-grain breads and rolls. They have more flavor and do not need butter or margarine to taste good. The dietary fiber present is an added bonus.
22. Think about the balance of fats in the menu. If a meal contains whole milk, cheese, ice cream, a higher-fat meat, or poultry with skin, use tub margarine and unsaturated vegetable oils for your spreads and dressings. Small amounts of butter, sour cream, or cream cheese can be included if other menu items are low in saturated fat.

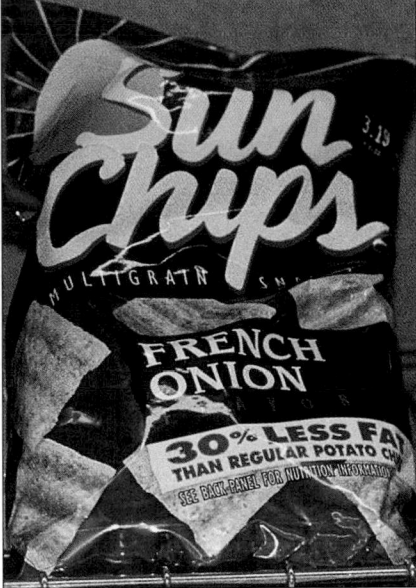

Many manufacturers are trying to devise products that are lower in fat. However, these help reduce calorie intake only if calorie content is also considered.

When many Americans think of a low-fat diet, they include reduced-fat versions of pastries, cookies, and cakes. When health professionals refer to a low-fat diet, they often have a very different plan in mind: replacing high-fat snacks with fruits, vegetables, and whole grains. Most Americans could benefit from this paradigm shift.

than 60% of total energy as fat—include plant oils, butter, margarine, mayonnaise, walnuts, bacon, avocados, peanut butter, cheddar cheese, steak, and hamburger. Of the foods we typically eat, cholesterol is found naturally only in those of animal origin, with eggs being a primary source. Fat is often hidden in foods such as whole milk, pastries, cookies, cake, cheese, hot dogs, crackers, french fries, ice cream, and quick-service foods. Fat free doesn't mean calorie free; moderation in the use of fat-reduced products is still important.

Check out the *Perspectives in Nutrition* Online Learning Center http://www.mhhe.com/wardlaw for quizzes, flash cards, other activities, and web links designed to further help you learn about dietary lipids.

▮ SUMMARY

1. Compared with carbohydrates and proteins, lipids are a group of relatively oxygen-poor compounds that dissolve in organic solvents, such as chloroform, benzene, and ether. Saturated fatty acids contain no carbon-carbon double bonds, monounsaturated fatty acids contain one carbon-carbon double bond, and polyunsaturated fatty acids contain two or more carbon-carbon double bonds in the carbon chain. Triglycerides rich in long-chain saturated fatty acids tend to be solid at room temperature, whereas those rich in polyunsaturated fatty acids are liquid at room temperature.

2. In omega-3 polyunsaturated fatty acids, the first of the carbon-carbon double bonds is located three carbons from the methyl end of the carbon chain. In omega-6 polyunsaturated fatty acids, the first carbon-carbon double bond counting from the methyl end occurs at the sixth carbon. Both omega-3 and omega-6 fatty acids are essential fatty acids; these must be included in the diet to maintain health.

3. Body cells can synthesize hormone compounds called eicosanoids from both omega-3 and omega-6 fatty acids. The eicosanoids produced from omega-3 fatty acids tend to reduce blood clotting, blood pressure, and inflammatory responses in the body. Those produced from omega-6 fatty acids tend to increase blood clotting.

4. Triglycerides are formed from a glycerol backbone with three fatty acids. Triglyceride is the major form of fat in both food and the body. It allows for efficient energy storage, protects certain organs, transports fat-soluble vitamins, and helps insulate the body. Phospholipids are derivatives of triglycerides. Phospholipids are important parts of cell membranes, and some act as efficient emulsifiers.

5. Cholesterol forms vital biological compounds, such as hormones, components of cell membranes, and bile acids. Cells in the body make cholesterol whether we eat it or not. It is not a necessary part of an adult's diet.

6. Fat digestion takes place primarily in the small intestine. Lipase enzyme released from the pancreas digests the long-chain triglycerides into smaller breakdown products—namely, monoglycerides (glycerol backbones with single fatty acids attached) and fatty acids. The breakdown products are then absorbed by the absorptive cells of the small intestine. These products are mostly resynthesized into triglycerides and combined with cholesterol, protein, and other substances to yield a chylomicron. Chylomicrons enter the lymphatic system, in turn passing into the bloodstream.

7. Lipids are carried in the bloodstream by various lipoproteins, which are particles consisting of a central triglyceride core encased in a shell of protein, cholesterol, and phospholipid. Chylomicrons are released from intestinal cells and carry lipids arising from dietary intake. Very-low-density lipoprotein (VLDL) and low-density lipoprotein (LDL) carry lipids synthesized in the liver. High-density lipoprotein (HDL) picks up cholesterol from cells and acts in allowing transport of it back to the liver.

8. In the blood, elevated amounts of LDL and low amounts of HDL are strong predictors of the risk for cardiovascular disease.

9. Fat adds flavor and texture to foods and increases satiety after meals. Hydrogenation is the process of converting carbon-carbon double bonds into single bonds by adding hydrogen at the point of unsaturation. Hydrogenation of fatty acids in vegetable oils changes the oils to solid fats and helps reduce rancidity, which results from the breakdown of fatty acids. Hydrogenation also increases the trans fatty acid content. High amounts of trans fatty acids in the diet are discouraged, as these increase LDL and reduce HDL. When fatty acids break down, food becomes rancid, emitting a foul odor and flavor. Some fats are used in food as emulsifiers. These suspend fat in water.

10. There is currently no RDA for fat. We need about 4% of total energy intake from plant oils to obtain the needed essential fatty acids. Fish is a good source of omega-3 fatty acids and should be consumed at least twice a week.

11. The typical American diet contains about 33% of total energy as fat. Many health agencies and scientific groups suggest reducing fat intake to no more than 30% of energy intake. Some health experts advocate an even further reduction to 20% of energy intake for some people, but such a diet requires professional guidance. If fat intake exceeds 30% of total calories, the diet should emphasize monounsaturated fat.

12. Fat-reduced products aid in the goal of reducing fat intake, but they still must be eaten in moderate amounts to maintain control of total energy intake.

■ STUDY QUESTIONS

1. Describe the chemical structures of saturated and polyunsaturated fatty acids and their different effects in both food and the human body.
2. Relate the need for omega-3 fatty acids in the diet to the recommendation to consume fish twice a week.
3. Describe the structures, origins, and roles of the four major blood lipoproteins.
4. What are the recommendations of health-care professionals regarding fat intake? What does this mean in terms of actual food choices?
5. What are two important attributes of fat in food? How are these different from the general functions of lipids in the human body?
6. What are the significance of and possible uses for reduced-fat foods?

7. Does the total cholesterol concentration in the bloodstream tell the whole story with respect to cardiovascular disease risk?

Read the Nutrition Perspective before answering the following questions:

8. List five risk factors for the development of cardiovascular disease.
9. What lifestyle factors were found to decrease the risk of cardiovascular disease development in the Nurses Health Study?
10. When are medications most effective in cardiovascular disease therapy, and how in general do the various classes of medications operate to reduce risk?

■ ANNOTATED REFERENCES

1. Conner WE: Importance of n-3 fatty acids in health and disease. *American Journal of Clinical Nutrition* 71(suppl):171S, 2000.

   n-3 fatty acids (also called omega-3 fatty acids) favorably affect atherosclerosis, cardiovascular disease, inflammatory disease, and perhaps even behavioral disorders. The antiarrhythmic effect of omega-3 fatty acids is a discovery that also has great relevance to the prevention of sudden death from cardiovascular disease.

2. de Lorgeril M and others: Mediterranean Diet: Traditional risk factors and the rate of cardiovascular complications after myocardial infarction. *Circulation* 99:779, 1999.

   People who had already suffered a heart attack and followed a Mediterranean Diet enjoyed a significantly reduced risk from suffering another heart attack. The majority of the subjects instructed on the Mediterranean diet were compliant, suggesting that implementing this dietary style with instructions from trained individuals is not as difficult as one might think.

3. Grundy SM: Nutrition and diet in the management of hyperlipidemia and atherosclerosis. In Shills ME and others (eds.): *Modern nutrition in health and disease.* 9th ed. Williams & Wilkins, 1999.

   Creeping weight gain in adulthood is a common cause of increased blood cholesterol, which occurs as we get older. This overweight status stands in the way of achieving a desirable blood cholesterol concentration for many persons.

4. Hambreacht R and others: Effect of exercise on coronary endothelial function in patients with coronary artery disease. *The New England Journal of Medicine* 342:454, 2000.

   Patients with coronary heart disease showed improved heart function after 4 weeks of vigorous exercise training. This finding emphasizes the importance of exercise therapy in the treatment regimen of patients who are diagnosed with this disease.

5. He J and others: Dietary sodium intake and subsequent risk of cardiovascular disease in overweight adults. *Journal of the American Medical Association* 282:2027, 1999.

   High sodium consumption was found to significantly increase risk for cardiovascular disease, stroke, and all-cause mortality in overweight individuals. Lowering sodium intake in the diet of overweight individuals is especially important to reduce these risks.

6. Healing broken hearts. *Nutrition Action Health Letter,* p. 1, June 1999.

   Dr. Dean Ornish reviews his diet solution to reversing atherosclerosis in people with obvious disease. The vegan diet used includes about 10% of calories from fat. Yoga, exercise, and stress-management sessions are additional lifestyle changes.

7. Heart Outcomes Prevention Evaluation Study Investigators: Vitamin E supplementation and cardiovascular events in high-risk patients. *The New England Journal of Medicine* 342:154, 2000.

   Vitamin E has antioxidant properties; however, its role in cardiovascular disease prevention is still questioned. This study examined the role of vitamin E on such events in high-risk adults and found that it did not have any effect.

8. Heber D and others: Cholesterol-lowering effects of a proprietary Chinese red-yeast-rice dietary supplement. *American Journal of Clinical Nutrition* 69:231, 1999.

   A proprietary Chinese red-yeast-rice supplement significantly lowered total blood cholesterol, LDL cholesterol, and triglycerides in men an women with high blood cholesterol.

9. Hodgson JM and others: Acute effects of ingestion of black and green tea on lipoprotein oxidation. *American Journal of Clinical Nutrition* 71:1103, 2000.

   Black tea has a mild effect on reducing lipoprotein oxidation in the body; green tea showed similar results but was not as potent.

10. Hu FB and others: Dietary intake of a-linolenic acid and risk of fatal ischemic heart disease among women. *American Journal of Clinical Nutrition* 69:890, 1999.

    A regular intake of alpha-linolenic acid is protective against coronary heart disease in women. The use of oils rich in alpha-linolenic acid in salad dressings, such as soybean and canola oils, is one way to increase intake of this essential fatty acid. Nuts are another source.

11. Hu FB and others: Dietary saturated fats and their food sources in relation to the risk of coronary heart disease in women. *American Journal of Clinical Nutrition* 70:1001, 1999.

    Along with other saturated fatty acids, stearic acid was found in this study to be associated with increased coronary heart disease risk. Since saturated fats are usually found together in foods, there is no need to differentiate between them in the diet (e.g., mystric acid vs. stearic acid).

12. Hu FB and others: A prospective study of egg consumption and risk of cardiovascular disease in men and women. *Journal of the American Medical Association* 281:1387, 1999.

With respect to cardiovascular disease risk, most healthy individuals can safely consume up to one egg per day; however, individuals with diabetes who consume one egg per day are at increased risk.

13. Jacobs DR and others: Whole-grain intake may reduce the risk of ischemic heart disease death in postmenopausal women: The Iowa women's health study. *American Journal of Clinical Nutrition* 68:248, 1998.

    There is a clear association between a generous whole-grain intake and reduced risk of coronary heart disease in women. The constituents of the whole grains that may be responsible for this reduced risk include phytochemicals, fiber, and antioxidants.

14. Jee SH and others: Smoking and atherosclerotic cardiovascular disease in men with low levels of serum cholesterol. *Journal of the American Medical Association* 282:2149, 1999.

    Smoking is a major risk factor for cardiovascular disease, and low blood cholesterol is not protective against smoking-related cardiovascular damage.

15. Knopp R: Drug treatment of lipid disorders. *The New England Journal of Medicine* 341:498, 1999.

    This article provides an excellent overview of the mechanisms of atherogenesis, target blood lipoprotein concentrations, and dietary treatment of hyperlipidemia, as well as a review of the various blood cholesterol-lowering drugs.

16. Krauss RM and others: AHA Dietary Guidelines: Revision 2000: A Statement for Healthcare Professionals From the Nutrition Committee of the American Heart Association. *Circulation* 102:2284, 2000.

    This report contains the latest advice for the public regarding diet and cardiovascular disease from the American Heart Association. The revised guidelines place an increased emphasis on the need for weight control and heart-healthy diet.

17. LaRosa J, He J, Vupputuri S: Effect of statins on risk of coronary disease—a meta analysis of randomized controlled trials. *The Journal of the American Medical Association* 282:2340, 1999.

    The blood cholesterol-lowering effect of statin medications in both men and women and younger and older persons reduced risk 31% with respect to major coronary heart disease events. It is of interest that these results were true for both women and men, as well as younger and older individuals.

18. Lichtenstein AH and others: Effects of different forms of dietary hydrogenated fats on serum lipid and cholesterol levels. *The New England Journal of Medicine* 340:1933, 1999.

    Oil that has not been hydrogenated was found to have the most favorable results on total blood cholesterol and LDL-cholesterol, whereas margarine that was high in trans fatty acids produced more negative blood cholesterol profiles.

19. Liu S and others: A prospective study of dietary glycemic load, carbohydrate intake, and risk of coronary heart disease in U.S. women. *American Journal of Clinical Nutrition* 71:1455, 2000.

    A high dietary glycemic load from refined carbohydrates increases the risk of coronary heart disease, independent of known heart disease risk factors. Such a diet is especially harmful in people with high degrees of insulin resistance and glucose intolerance.

20. MacMahon S: Blood pressure and the risk of cardiovascular disease. *The New England Journal of Medicine* 342:50, 2000.

    Reducing blood pressure is beneficial for people at high risk for major cardiovascular disease events. Aggressive blood pressure reduction in people with diabetes using either an angiotensin-converting enzyme (ACE) inhibitor or a beta-blocker allowed more protection from cardiovascular disease than less aggressive blood pressure reduction therapy.

21. Mayes PA: Digestion and absorption. In Murray RK and others (eds.): 25th ed. *Harper's biochemistry.* Stamford, CT: Appleton & Lange, 2000.

    Fat digestion primarily takes place in the small intestine with the participation of the enzyme lipase, bile acids, and lecithin. Most absorbed fat is in the form of monoglycerides. These reform into triglycerides and exit the absorptive cell as chylomicrons.

22. Mayes PA: Lipid storage and transport. In Murray RK and others (eds.): *Harper's biochemistry.* Stamford, CT: Appleton & Lange, 2000.

    This chapter provides an excellent review of lipoprotein metabolism. The following chapter in the book, on cholesterol synthesis, transport, and excretion, is also very informative. Both document the role of statin drugs in reducing cholesterol synthesis in the liver; the roles of other medications to reduce lipid synthesis in the liver are also discussed. Finally, an additional chapter on eicosanoids by this author (Chapter 25) is quite informative.

23. Nester PJ: Fish oil and cardiovascular disease: Lipids and arterial function. *American Journal of Clinical Nutrition* 71:228S, 2000.

    The benefits of fish oils include improved endothelial cell function and better arterial elasticity. The actual minimum effective amount that provides long-term benefits still needs to be established with more research studies.

24. Nguyen TT: The cholesterol lowering action of plant stanol esters. *Journal of Nutrition* 129:2109, 1999.

    Plant stanols lower total and LDL-cholesterol by interfering with the reabsorption of dietary and biliary cholesterol from the intestinal tract. Plant stanols have the ability to reduce blood cholesterol by 10 to 15% without side effects.

25. Pearce KA and others: Update on vitamin supplements for the prevention of coronary disease and stroke, *American Family Physician* 62:1359, 2000.

    A heart-healthy diet emphasizing fruits and vegetables containing antioxidants and B vitamins may be the best advice in the end for preventing coronary heart disease and stroke. Vitamin E at a dose of 100 to 800 IU per day may be useful for secondary prevention of such diseases, but the results to date from clinical trials are inconsistent.

26. Ridker PM and others: C-reactive protein and other markers of inflammation in the prediction of cardiovascular disease in women. *The New England Journal of Medicine* 342:836, 2000.

    Inflammation in the body is a main hypothesis on the cause of cardiovascular disease development. hs-C-reactive protein, a test that measures inflammation in the body, was found in this study to be an effective method for identifying women at risk for such events.

27. Ross R: Atherosclerosis—an inflammatory disease. *The New England Journal of Medicine* 340:115, 1999.

    High blood cholesterol is important in approximately 50% of patients with cardiovascular disease. Other factors also need to be taken into consideration, such as a chronic inflammatory process in the arteries. Work needs to establish whether reducing this inflammation can in turn reduce the risk of heart disease.

28. Sandler RS and others: Gastrointestinal symptoms in 3181 volunteers ingesting snack foods containing Olestra or triglycerides—a six week randomized, placebo-controlled trial. *Annals of Internal Medicine* 130:253, 1999.

    People who consumed olestra reported more frequent bowel movements than the control group; however, most of the subjects reported that the GI symptoms did not disrupt their normal daily activities.

29. Shor A, Phillips J: Chlamydia pneumoniae and atherosclerosis. *Journal of the American Medical Association* 282:2071, 1999.

    It is suspected that chlamydia pneumoniae, as well as other bacteria, play a role in the development of atherosclerosis. Some studies have reviewed the effect of antibiotic therapy to treat such an infection, but the results have not been convincing and the studies have been small.

30. Stampfer M and others: Primary prevention of coronary heart disease in women through diet and lifestyle. *The New England Journal of Medicine* 343:16, 2000.

Following a set of specific lifestyle factors, including a balanced diet with a small amount of wine each day, exercise, and abstinence from smoking, can help protect women from coronary heart disease.

31. Stefanik ML and others: Effects of diet and exercise in men and postmenopausal women with low levels of HDL cholesterol and high levels of LDL cholesterol. *The New England Journal of Medicine* 339:12, 1998.

This study investigated the effects of exercise and a low-fat, low-cholesterol diet on the LDL-cholesterol and HDL-cholesterol of men and women with already low HDL-cholesterol and moderately increased LDL-cholesterol. The results enforced the importance of exercise in conjunction with such a diet; those who did not include aerobic exercise failed to lower LDL-cholesterol.

32. Syndrome X—the risks of high insulin. *Nutrition Action Health Letter*, p. 1, March 2000

An interview with Dr. Gerald Reaven provides an overview of Syndrome X and how to treat this condition. The article also compares the protein, saturated fat, mono- and polyunsaturated fat, carbohydrate, and cholesterol content of the Syndrome X diet to those of four other popular diets.

33. Tibble DL: Antioxidant consumption and risk of coronary heart disease: Emphasis on vitamin C, vitamin E, and beta-carotene. *Circulation* 99:591, 1999.

It is hypothesized that antioxidants help prevent free radical oxidation—and that free radicals influence the development of coronary heart disease. Epidemiological evidence shows that a high antioxidant intake in one's diet is associated with lower disease risk. Currently, there is no convincing evidence to support supplementation with antioxidants in an effort to prevent heart disease.

34. Wannamethee SG, Shaper AG: Type of alcoholic drink and risk of major coronary heart disease events and all-cause mortality. *American Journal of Public Health* 89:685, 1999.

A moderate amount of alcohol helps prevent coronary heart disease. Wine, in particular, was found to be protective, more so than beer and spirits.

35. Wood MJ, Cox JL: HRT to prevent cardiovascular disease, *Postgraduate Medicine* 108 (3):59, 2000.

Based on the results of current clinical trials, use of hormone replacement therapy (HRT) for prevention of further cardiovascular disease in women who have existing disease cannot be recommended at present. For primary prevention of cardiovascular disease we will have to wait for results of the ongoing Women's Health Initiative to answer questions about safety and effectiveness of hormone replacement therapy.

TAKE ACTION

I. ARE YOU EATING A DIET THAT INCLUDES MANY SATURATED-FAT AND TRANS FATTY ACID SOURCES?

Instructions:
Check the food you would typically select from the two choices given.

1. ____ Bacon and eggs   ____ Ready-to-eat whole-grain breakfast cereal
2. ____ Doughnut or sweet roll   ____ Whole-wheat (or white) roll, bagel, or bread, no margarine
3. ____ Breakfast sausage   ____ Fruit
4. ____ Whole milk   ____ Low-fat or nonfat milk
5. ____ Cheeseburger   ____ Turkey sandwich, no cheese
6. ____ French fries   ____ Plain baked potato with minimal added fat or salad with low-cal or fat-free dressing
7. ____ Meal including fried hamburger or fatty beef   ____ Meal including broiled lean hamburger (ground round), chicken, or fish
8. ____ Creamed soup   ____ Clear soup (could contain some meat or vegetables)
9. ____ Potato salad   ____ Baked potato, limited added fat
10. ____ Cream/fruit pie   ____ Graham crackers
11. ____ Ice cream   ____ Frozen yogurt, sherbet, or fat-reduced ice cream
12. ____ Butter or stick margarine   ____ Vegetable oils or soft margarine in a tub

Interpretation

The foods listed on the left tend to be high in saturated fat, trans fatty acids, cholesterol, and total fat. Those on the right generally are low. If you want to help reduce the risk of heart disease, choose the foods on the right more often than the foods on the left.

TAKEACTION

II. WHAT IS YOUR CURRENT FAT AND CHOLESTEROL INTAKE?

How do your food practices compare with general guidelines suggested for fat, saturated fat, and cholesterol intake? Refer to the nutritional assessment you completed at the end of Chapter 2, and compare it with the following guidelines, issued by the American Heart Association and the National Cholesterol Education Program for people at high risk for development of cardiovascular disease.

- Limit or reduce total fat intake to 20 to 30% or less of total energy intake.
- Reduce saturated fat intake to 7 to 10% of energy intake or less.
- Limit cholesterol to 200 to 300 mg/day.

To compare your nutritional assessment with these guidelines, first fill in the values for your intakes of the following:

TOTAL ENERGY: _____ **TOTAL FAT:** _____ **SATURATED FAT:** _____ **CHOLESTEROL:** _____

Now complete the following steps:

1. Multiply your total grams of fat by 9 (kcal/g of fat). Then divide the result by your total energy intake. Next multiply this number by 100. This will give you the percentage of energy you consumed from fat.

    % OF ENERGY FROM FAT _____ IS IT 30% OR LESS OF TOTAL ENERGY?   YES _____ NO _____

2. Multiply your grams of saturated fat by 9 (kcal/g of fat). Divide the result by your total energy intake. Now multiply this number by 100. This will give you the percentage of energy you consumed from saturated fat.

    % OF ENERGY FROM SATURATED FAT _____

    IS IT 10% OF ENERGY OR LESS?   YES _____ NO _____

3. Look at your milligrams of cholesterol.

    IS YOUR INTAKE LESS THAN 300 mg?   YES _____ NO _____

4. Look back at the foods you ate and notice the foods that contributed the most fat, saturated fat, and cholesterol. If you didn't meet one or more of the guidelines and had elevated LDL, how could you change what you ate that day to improve your diet?

5. Now take the next step. Do you know your HDL and LDL values? If not, have them checked soon. All adults should know whether these values are in the abnormal ranges.

6. Finally, fill in the following assessment of your risk for developing cardiovascular disease. Decide today how you could modify your diet and lifestyle, if necessary, to reduce your risk.

Do you have	YES	NO		YES	NO
A history of smoking?	_____	_____	Diabetes?	_____	_____
Hypertension?	_____	_____	A history of physical inactivity?	_____	_____
High LDL?	_____	_____	A family history of premature heart disease (before age 60 years)?	_____	_____
Low HDL?	_____	_____	A history of obesity?	_____	_____
			A diet that lacks sufficient B vitamins, such as B-6, folate, and B-12?	_____	_____

Other factors also could be considered, as discussed in the Nutrition Perspective, but this provides a good start for assessing your risk.

CARDIOVASCULAR DISEASE

Heart disease typically involves the coronary arteries and thus is frequently termed coronary heart disease (CHD) or coronary artery disease (CAD). Since the buildup of atherosclerosis slows blood flow in the arteries, the disease is also called **ischemic** heart disease (IHD). Ischemia represents an obstruction of blood flow. The general term for this obstruction is **stenosis.**

A heart attack can strike with the sudden force of a sledgehammer, with pain radiating up the neck or down the arm. It can also sneak up at night, masquerading as indigestion, with slight pain or pressure in the chest. Many times, the symptoms are so subtle in women that it often is too late once she or the health professional realizes that a heart attack is taking place. If there is any suspicion at all that a heart attack is taking place, the person should first chew an aspirin (325 mg) thoroughly and then call 911. Aspirin helps reduce the blood clotting that precipitates a heart attack. Typical warning signs are

- Intense, prolonged chest pain or pressure, sometimes radiating to other parts of the upper body (men and women)
- Shortness of breath (men and women)
- Sweating (men and women)
- Nausea and vomiting (especially women)
- Dizziness (especially women)
- Weakness (men and women)
- Jaw, neck, and shoulder pain (especially women)
- Irregular heartbeat (men and women)

Cardiovascular disease (CVD)—is the major killer of Americans. Each year about 500,000 people die of coronary heart disease in the United States, about 60% more than die of cancer. The figure rises to almost 1 million if strokes and other circulatory diseases are included in the global term *cardiovascular disease.* About 1.5 million people each year have a heart attack. The overall male-to-female ratio for heart disease is about 2:1. Women generally lag about 10 years behind men in developing the disease. Still, it eventually kills more women than any other disease—twice as many as cancer. And, for each person in America who dies of cardiovascular disease, 20 more (over 13 million people) have symptoms of the disease.

Healthy People 2010 has set a goal of reducing death from coronary heart disease by 30%, compared with today's incidence.

Worldwide, the highest incidence of cardiovascular disease occurs in the Russian Federation; in contrast, the lowest incidence occurs in Japan. The U.S. numbers are midway between these two countries. This highlights the powerful influence of environment and lifestyle factors on its development.

DEVELOPMENT OF CORONARY HEART DISEASE

The symptoms of cardiovascular disease develop over many years and often do not become obvious until old age. Nonetheless, autopsies of young adults under 20 years of age have shown that many of them had atherosclerotic plaque in their arteries. This finding indicates that plaque buildup can begin in childhood and continue throughout life, although it usually goes undetected for quite some time.

Preventing premature cardiovascular disease—that which appears before age 60 years—deserves everyone's consideration. Heart attacks at ages 40 through 60 are closely linked to the risk factors discussed later in this feature. Most people at risk can greatly improve their chance to avoid premature cardiovascular disease by making some long-term lifestyle changes, as has been clearly demonstrated in women.[30] (See Chapter 18 for further discussion of the premature appearance of disease in adulthood and how to work to prevent it.)

Coronary heart disease and strokes are associated with inadequate blood circulation in the heart and brain. Blood supplies the heart muscle and brain—and other body organs—with oxygen and nutrients. When blood flow via the coronary arteries surrounding the heart is interrupted, the heart muscle can be damaged. A heart attack, or **myocardial infarction,** may result (Fig. 6-14). This may cause the heart to beat irregularly or to stop altogether. About 25% of people do not survive their first heart attack. If blood flow to parts of the brain is interrupted long enough, part of the brain dies, causing a cerebrovascular accident, or stroke. When a stroke causes loss of muscle control, death may occur.

myocardial infarction Death of part of the heart muscle.

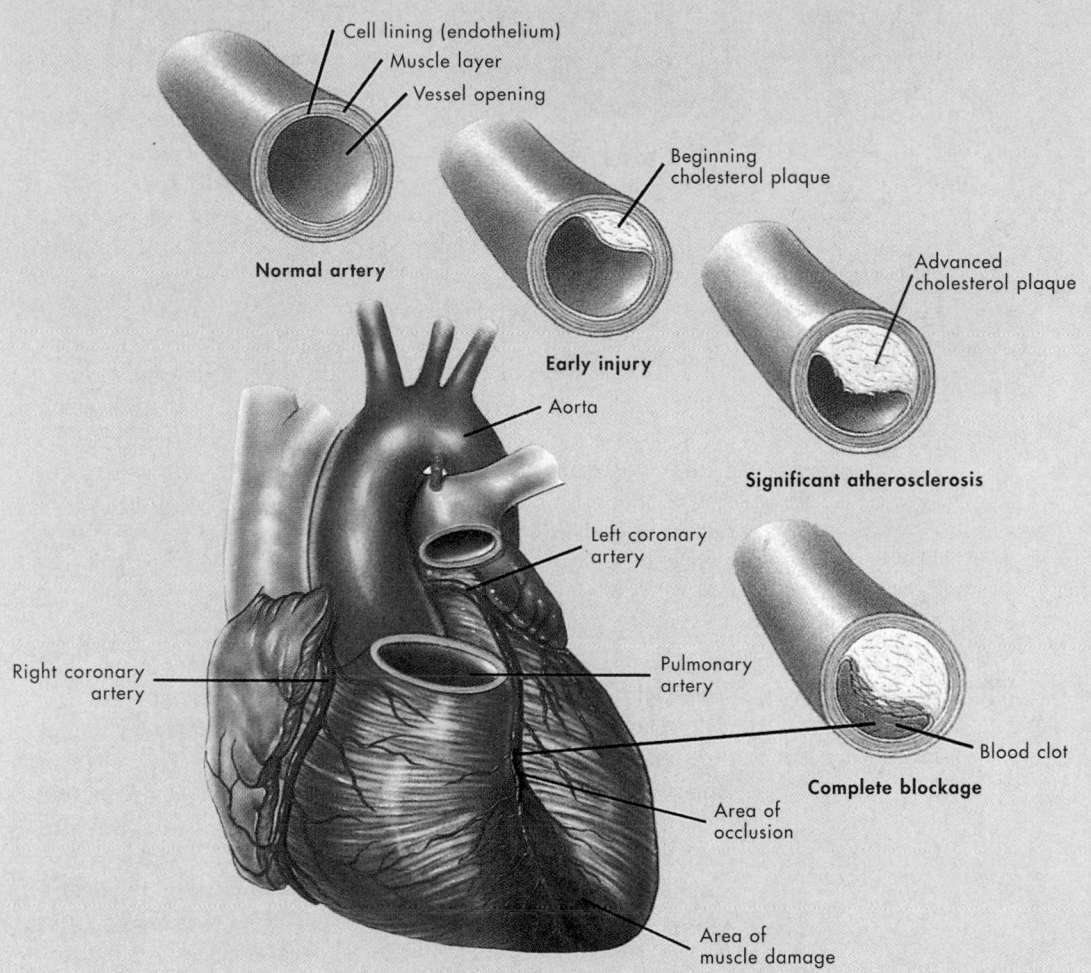

Cell lining (endothelium)
Muscle layer
Vessel opening

Normal artery

Beginning cholesterol plaque

Early injury

Advanced cholesterol plaque

Significant atherosclerosis

Aorta

Left coronary artery

Right coronary artery

Pulmonary artery

Blood clot

Complete blockage

Area of occlusion

Area of muscle damage

▌ FIGURE **6-14** The road to a heart attack. Injury to an artery wall begins the process. This is followed by a progressive buildup of plaque in the artery walls. The heart attack represents the terminal phase of the process. Blockage of the left coronary artery by a blood clot is evident. The heart muscle that is served by the portion of the coronary artery beyond the point of blockage lacks oxygen and nutrients and is damaged and may die. This can lead to a significant drop in heart function and often total heart failure.
Illustration by William Ober.

More than 95% of all heart attacks are caused by blood clots that stop blood flow to the heart or brain. Clots form more readily where atherosclerotic plaque has built up in the arteries that serve the heart (coronary arteries) or brain (carotid arteries) (Fig. 6-15). Actually, the most dangerous lesions aren't the large, advanced ones but the smaller, unstable lesions covered by a thin fibrous cap. In essence, heart attacks generally are caused not by total blockage of the coronary arteries by plaque but by disruption of a partial blockage, leading to eventual clot formation.[27]

As mentioned earlier in this chapter, plaque is probably first deposited to repair injuries in a vessel lining. It develops especially at points where an artery branches into two arteries. Much stress is placed on an artery at these points from the changes in blood flow that occur at the branch point. The *athero* in *atherosclerosis* comes from the Greek and means "gruel or paste." This process of damage repair is part of the initiation phase of atherosclerosis. The rate of further plaque deposition in the next phase, called the progression phase, partly depends on the amount of LDL in the blood. The plaque thickens as layers of cholesterol (part of LDL),

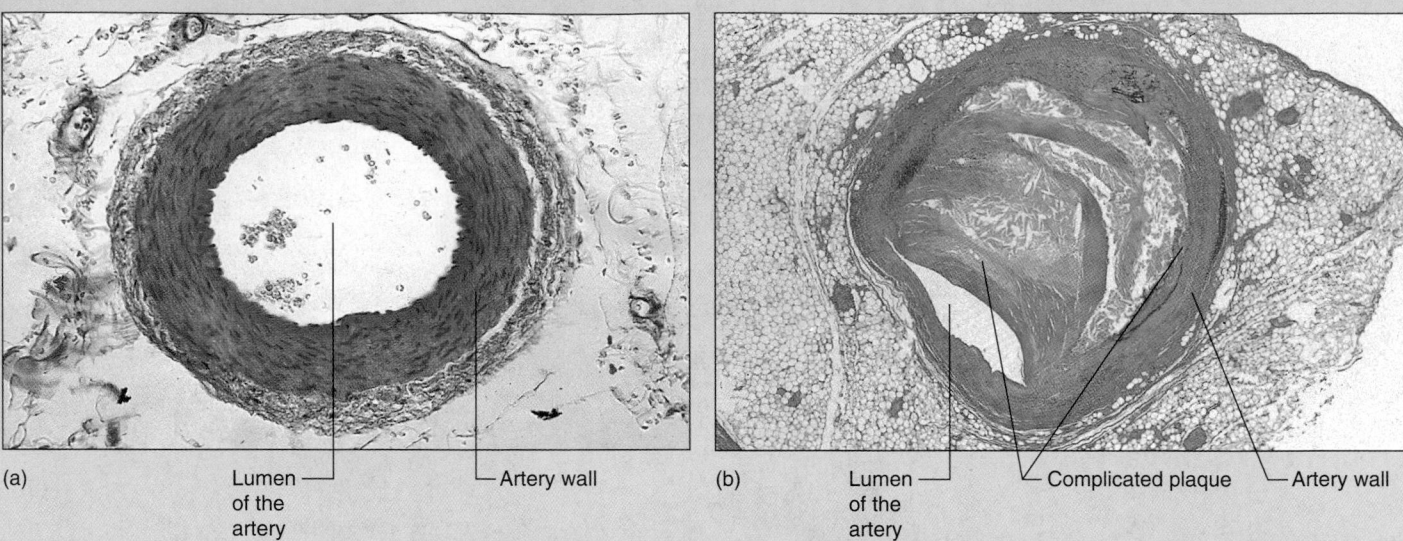

(a)   Lumen — of the artery   — Artery wall   (b)   Lumen — of the artery   — Complicated plaque   — Artery wall

■ FIGURE 6-15 Atherosclerosis. *(a)* Cross section of a healthy coronary artery. *(b)* Cross section of a coronary artery with advanced atherosclerosis. The greatly reduced lumen in the diseased artery can easily be blocked by a blood clot or portion of plaque that breaks off another site and lodges in the narrowed portion of the artery. The latest research indicates, however, that these large plaques pose less of a risk than smaller plaques with a thinner fibrous cap, as the latter rupture very readily. This then leads to blood clots.

connective tissue (collagen), smooth muscle, and calcium are deposited. Arteries harden and narrow as plaque builds up, making them less elastic. They are thus unable to expand to accommodate alterations in blood pressure.

Affected arteries become further damaged as blood pumps through them and pressure increases. Finally, in the terminal phase, a clot or spasm in a plaque-clogged artery leads to a myocardial infarction.

Factors that typically bring on a heart attack in a person at risk include dehydration, acute emotional stress (such as firing an employee), strenuous physical activity when not otherwise physically fit (shoveling snow, for example), waking during the night or getting up in the morning (linked to an abrupt increase in stress), and consuming high-fat meals (increases blood clotting).

RISK FACTORS FOR CARDIOVASCULAR DISEASE

*W*hen 28-year-old gold medallist Sergei Grinkov died suddenly of a heart attack while ice skating, researchers investigated the case and discovered a protein abnormality in his blood. This abnormal protein caused Grinkov's blood to clot more easily than normal. Grinkov was otherwise healthy, with a total cholesterol of 195 mg/dl, HDL of 45 mg/dl, and normal blood triglycerides and LDL. The main risk factor he had was that his father died of heart disease at the age of 52. It is thought that up to 25% of Americans have this same protein abnormality and that the only sign is a family history of heart-related death under age 60. For this reason, it is wise for all adult Americans to have a careful evaluation of cardiovascular disease risks conducted by a physician.

Many of us are free of the risk factors that contribute to rapid development of atherosclerosis. If so, the advice of health experts is to simply consume a balanced diet, perform regular physical activity, and reevaluate risk factors every 5 years.

People who face the highest risk for premature cardiovascular disease have a rare genetic defect, which substantially blocks the clearance of chylomicrons and triglycerides from the blood, reduces LDL uptake by the liver, limits synthesis of HDL, or enhances blood clotting. Other medical conditions, such as certain forms of liver and kidney disease, low concentrations of thyroid hormone, and use of certain medications to treat hypertension, can increase LDL and thus increase the risk for heart disease.

For most people, however, the most likely risk factors are
- Total cholesterol over 200 mg/dl of blood especially when it is at or over 240 mg/dl and coupled with LDL-cholesterol over 130 to 160 mg/dl. We use the term LDL-cholesterol (and HDL-cholesterol) when expressing the serum concentration since it is the cholesterol content of these lipoproteins that is actually measured. The reference standard for expressing blood lipid concentrations also generally refers to the serum concentration. Recall that serum concentration is what remains after blood clots; blood is then centrifuged to remove all red and white blood cells. Although *blood cholesterol* is a common term, the value actually refers to the concentration in the serum portion of the blood.
- HDL-cholesterol under 35 mg/dl, especially when the ratio of total cholesterol to HDL-cholesterol is greater than 4:1. Women often have high values for HDL-cholesterol and therefore it is important for

this to be measured in women to establish cardiovascular disease risk. A value ≥60 mg/dl is especially protective.

- Age. Men over 45 years and women over 55 years.
- Family history of premature cardiovascular disease, especially before age 60
- Smoking. This generally negates the female advantage of later presentation of the disease and is the main cause of about 20% of cardiovascular disease deaths. A combination of smoking and oral contraceptive use worsens matters even more. Smoking greatly increases the ultimate expression of a person's genetically linked risk for cardiovascular disease and even increases risk if one's blood lipids are low.[14] Smoking also makes blood more likely to clot. Even secondhand smoke has been implicated.
- Hypertension. **Systolic blood pressure** over 140 (millimeters of mercury) and **diastolic blood pressure** over 90 indicate hypertension. Ideal blood pressure values are <120 and <80, respectively.[20] (Treatment of hypertension is reviewed in Chapter 11.)
- Diabetes. This disease negates the female advantage. Insulin increases cholesterol synthesis in the liver, in turn increasing LDL release into the bloodstream.[3]
- Obesity (especially fat accumulation in the waist). Typical weight gain seen in adults is a chief contributor to the increase in LDL-cholesterol seen with aging. Obesity also leads to insulin resistance in many people, creating a diabetes-like risk, as discussed.[3]
- Inactivity. Exercise conditions the arteries to adapt to physical stress. Regular exercise also improves insulin action in the body. The corresponding reduction in insulin output leads to a reduction in lipoprotein synthesis in the liver. Both regular aerobic exercise and resistance exercise are recommended. A person with existing cardiovascular disease should seek physician approval before starting such a program, as should older adults (see Chapter 14).[4]

Table 6-7 outlines some blood cholesterol profiles. If any of your blood cholesterol values fall in the column labeled "Requires Treatment," consult your physician because you may be at risk for cardiovascular disease. According to the National Heart, Lung, and Blood Institute, about 50% of all American adults have elevated blood cholesterol. The combined or individual risk factors of high LDL and high triglycerides are all referred to as hyperlipidemia.

Researchers are currently trying to unravel and quantify numerous other factors that may be linked to premature cardiovascular disease, such as an inadequate intake of vitamin B-6, folate, and vitamin B-12 and increased homocysteine in the blood. Homocysteine damages the cells lining the blood vessels, in turn promoting atherosclerosis. It is likely the cause in about 10% of cases (see Chapter 10 for a detailed discussion of homocysteine).

The term *risk factor* is not intended to mean causality; nevertheless, the more of these risk factors one has, the greater the chances of ultimately developing cardiovascular disease. However, common sense suggests that we should initially focus on the three most common contributors: smoking, hypertension, and high LDL-cholesterol. Premature cardiovascular disease is rare in populations who have low LDL-cholesterol, have normal blood pressure, and do not smoke. By minimizing these three risk factors, along with following the Food Guide Pyramid and staying physically active, one will most likely reduce many of the other, less common controllable risk factors as well. In other words, develop and follow a total lifestyle plan. In

Most commonly, LDL-cholesterol is not actually measured in a serum sample but is calculated using the following equation: LDL-cholesterol = total cholesterol − HDL-cholesterol − (triglycerides/5). This formula cannot be used, however, if blood triglycerides are >400 mg/dl. Recently laboratories have also implemented a test that measures LDL-cholesterol directly (without the use of this formula). Refer to Table 6-7 for typical LDL-cholesterol cut-off values.

Healthy People 2010 has set a goal of reducing total blood cholesterol among adults from an average of 206 mg/dl to 199 mg/dl, as well as a reduction in the percentage of adults with high blood cholesterol from 21 to 17%.

TABLE 6-7   Fasting Blood Cholesterol Profile

	Ideal	Borderline	Requires Treatment
Total cholesterol	<200 mg/dl	200–239 mg/dl	≥240 mg/dl
LDL-cholesterol	<130 mg/dl (≤100 mg/dl if person has cardiovascular disease)	130–159 mg/dl*	≥160 mg/dl
HDL-cholesterol	≥60 mg/dl	35–59 mg/dl	<35 mg/dl
Triglycerides	<200 mg/dl**	200–399 mg/dl	≥400 mg/dl

*Treatment is indicated if one or more risk factors for cardiovascular disease is present.

**Many physicians would like to see fasting triglycerides of less than 100 mg/dl because some studies have shown that, for every 100 mg/dl increase in triglycerides, there is a 40% increase in risk for heart attack. Triglyceride values about 150 mg/dl are especially problematic for women and people with diabetes. In addition, elevated triglycerides are often accompanied by other lipoprotein abnormalities.

CRITICAL THINKING

As part of his annual health checkup, Juan has a blood sample drawn for the measurement of cholesterol values. The results of the test indicate that his total cholesterol is 210 mg/dl, HDL cholesterol is 65 mg/dl, and triglycerides are 100 mg/dl. Juan has read that total cholesterol should be less than 200 mg/dl to minimize cardiovascular problems. However, he is happy with the results of the blood test. How would Juan explain his satisfaction to his parents?

addition, cardiovascular disease expert Dr. Richard Havel recommends that, if a person has a history of premature cardiovascular disease in the family but the usual risk factors aren't present, a rarer defect might be the cause. In this case, he advises having a detailed physical examination for other potential causes because only about 50% of one's risk for cardiovascular disease can be accounted for by the main risk factors just discussed. (Table 6-8).

The National Institutes of Health encourage all people over age 20 to have their total cholesterol and HDL-cholesterol measured. Children over 2 years of age with a family history of cardiovascular heart disease deserve similar scrutiny. Experts also recommend having the fasting triglyceride concentration measured, as this is used to calculate LDL-cholesterol and is likely a risk factor in and of itself.

LOWERING LDL-CHOLESTEROL BY DIET CHANGES

If your LDL-cholesterol is high, the first step should be a detailed examination by a physician. Some diseases (for example, a form of kidney disease) raise LDL-cholesterol, and treating the disease may remedy the LDL problem as well. If no such disease is present, diet change is advised.

Nutrition experts recommend several approaches for lowering LDL-cholesterol. Because changes that work for one person may be ineffective for another, values should be rechecked a month or so after any of the changes discussed here are implemented.

■ Reducing dietary saturated fat and cholesterol intake

Reducing saturated-fat intake can lower elevated LDL. Although high total cholesterol in the blood indicates that an individual is at risk for cardiovascular disease, the most potent dietary factor associated with a high LDL-cholesterol value is overconsumption of saturated fat, not of cholesterol.

Almost everyone who minimizes saturated-fat intake can lower elevated LDL-cholesterol by about 15 to 20%, especially if the person has been eating lots of foods that are high in saturated fat. About 10% of the population has trouble decreasing LDL-cholesterol by dietary means. Genetic defects are one reason. On the other hand, about 10% can expect an even bigger drop.[3]

About 20% of the population who eat a diet low in saturated fat find that reducing dietary cholesterol lowers LDL-cholesterol even more. Some people can eat six eggs a day for a month without having their fasting LDL-cholesterol increase, most likely because of a genetic propensity of the liver to compensate by making less cholesterol. Still, most authorities encourage limiting cholesterol intake to less than 200 to 300 mg/day, especially for people with diabetes.[12] Reducing cholesterol intake minimizes the cholesterol content of the chylomicrons that arise right after eating. Deposition of cholesterol from circulating chylomicrons probably contributes to atherosclerosis. In addition, as noted in this chapter, the tendency for palmitic acid—one of the main saturated fatty acids in our diets—to raise LDL-cholesterol is especially prominent when dietary cholesterol intake exceeds 200 to 300 mg/day and blood cholesterol is elevated.

To determine if you are part of the 20% of the population that is especially affected by dietary cholesterol, have your blood lipid profile checked every 5 years. If your LDL-cholesterol is higher than 130 mg/dl, you should restrict dietary cholesterol ≤200–300 mg/day and then see if this improves your cholesterol profile.

High intakes of saturated fat affect the liver's ability to clear LDL from the bloodstream, leading to increased LDL-cholesterol values. It appears that saturated fatty acids promote an increase in the amount of free cholesterol (not attached to fatty acids) in the liver, whereas unsaturated fatty acids do the opposite. As free cholesterol in the liver increases, it causes the liver to reduce cholesterol uptake from the bloodstream, contributing to elevated LDL-cholesterol. (Trans fatty acids are thought to act in the same ways as saturated fatty acids.)

The contribution of dietary saturated fat to elevated LDL-cholesterol can be minimized by eating no more than 7 to 10% of total energy as saturated fats. Finding substitutes for foods rich in animal fat, such as butter, and shortening and hydrogenated (solid) fats (trans fatty acids) is a must. Routinely reading food labels is also important, as saturated fats are often hidden in foods.

TABLE 6-8   Possible Factors Related to Cardiovascular Disease That Are Currently Under Evaluation by Researchers[3, 9, 13, 16, 19, 24, 25, 27, 32, 34]

Factor	Probable Mechanism
LDL particle size	Small LDL particles appear to enter atherosclerotic lesions more readily than larger LDL particles. Genetics influences the size of LDL made by each of us. High blood triglycerides are associated with these small LDL particles.
Lipoprotein patterns that develop after eating (postprandial)	Remnants of chylomicron and VLDL metabolism appear to contribute to atherosclerosis and blood clotting, especially after a high-fat meal is consumed.
Certain forms of apolipoproteins	Certain apolipoproteins of the E class (apoprotein E_4) delay lipoprotein clearance from the bloodstream, thus enhancing atherosclerosis. On the other hand, certain apolipoproteins of the A class are associated with a significant reduction in cardiovascular disease risk.
Loneliness and stress	Social isolation and stress have been linked to an increased risk of myocardial infarction, especially if cardiovascular disease is already present. Increased blood clotting is one likely mechanism.
Coffee preparation	Boiled coffee as served in Scandinavia and French-pressed coffee is associated with increased LDL-cholesterol, linked to specific compounds in the coffee bean. These in turn may influence liver metabolism of lipoproteins.
Excess iron absorption	Iron likely speeds oxidation of LDL, which makes LDL more atherogenic. The degree to which this takes place in the body is a subject of debate. The effect is especially prominent in people with elevated LDL-cholesterol.
Nonnutrient substances in plants (see Chapter 2)	Quercetin, found in plants, and related substances found in tea may reduce oxidation of LDL and thus reduce atherosclerosis development.
Nitric oxide	Nitric oxide is made by cells and causes muscles controlling the arteries to relax. The amino acid arginine is used to produce nitric oxide; plants are rich sources of arginine in comparison with animal products.
Various blood-clotting factors	People with high concentrations of various clotting factors in their blood show higher risks of heart attack.
Dietary calcium intake	Some studies show a fall in LDL-cholesterol when calcium intake increases from about 400 mg/day to 1200 mg/day or more. At the higher intake, calcium is likely binding fatty acids in the intestine, in turn reducing fat absorption.
Tocotrienols	These compounds in the vitamin E class likely reduce cholesterol synthesis in the liver.
Soy compounds	Phytosterols and dietary fiber present in soy products likely reduce cholesterol absorption from the intestine, while the protein present may affect cholesterol metabolism in the body.
Pharmacologic intake of antioxidants	Work is ongoing to see if intake of antioxidants well above that generally available from a diet reduces cardiovascular disease. Current protocols use about 10 to 25 times or more the RDA for vitamin E and 5 to 10 times the RDA for vitamin C (see Chapters 9 and 10 for details).
Lipoprotein(a)	Lipoprotein(a) [Lp(a)] appears to lead to atherosclerosis and increased blood clotting. It consists of LDL with a large protein attached that is related to a blood-clotting factor. Estrogen therapy in women lowers Lp(a), whereas trans fatty acids increase Lp(a).
Syndrome X	Syndrome X, which includes high insulin values, hypertension, high blood triglycerides, and low HDL-cholesterol, is linked to increased cardiovascular disease risk. The best way to treat this problem is to lose weight, become physically active, and make a few minor adjustments to the diet, especially concentrating on reducing refined carbohydrates and including more whole-grain products, fruits, and vegetables. Fat intake up to 40% of calories, with most of the percentage coming from monounsaturated sources, is also recommended.
Red wine	Phenolic substances in red wine may act as antioxidants and reduce LDL oxidation.
Glycemic index	A diet rich in high-glycemic-index foods (primarily, sugars, refined carbohydrates, and white potatoes) increases risk for cardiovascular disease (see Chapter 5 for a review of glycemic index values for foods). The mechanism is primarily the increase in insulin output caused by these foods, which in turn increases lipoprotein synthesis in the liver.

Only animal and fish products contain cholesterol (review Table 6-1). Although egg whites contain no cholesterol, a single egg yolk contains about 210 mg of cholesterol. Thus, to meet the recommendation for cholesterol intake of no more than 300 mg/day, intake of egg yolks must be limited to no more than 1 per day. A reduction to 200 mg/day would essentially mean consuming egg yolks only occasionally. Many egg-containing foods (for example, pancakes, French toast, cookies, and cakes) can be prepared using egg whites rather than whole eggs. Cholesterol-free egg substitutes are also available in the grocery store. Most of these are egg whites colored yellow, to which a small amount of fat has been added to improve the flavor. Trimming the fat before and after cooking a 3- to 4-ounce serving of chicken, beef, or pork leaves roughly one-third to one-half the cholesterol content of an egg. A 10-ounce portion of meat can contain 260 mg of cholesterol, slightly more than the amount of one egg. If meats have a reputation for being high in cholesterol, it is mainly because of an overly generous portion size.

■ Increasing monounsaturated and polyunsaturated fat intake

Until recently, polyunsaturated fatty acids, but not monounsaturated fatty acids, were recommended as a substitute for saturated fatty acids in the diet to lower LDL-cholesterol. However, recent studies show that both monounsaturated and polyunsaturated fatty acids have this effect. In fact, monounsaturated fatty acids may be more beneficial, since LDLs containing these fatty acids are less likely to be oxidized. Recall that oxidized LDL probably contributes more to plaque formation in the arteries than does LDL itself. The key here is to replace saturated fat with monounsaturated fat, not simply to add it to the diet. This may also be beneficial for both blood triglycerides and HDL, because diets that are very low in fat and very high in carbohydrate tend to raise triglycerides and decrease HDL-cholesterol. This can be avoided by replacing saturated fat in the diet with mostly monounsaturated fat.

However, increasing intake of monounsaturated fat is difficult for the typical American. Foods and meals rich in monounsaturated fats are not widely available in the United States, nor are they a big part of our cuisine. If you do much of your own cooking, using canola oil, canola oil blended with other vegetable oils, and olive oil on a regular basis will increase your intake of monounsaturated fats. A further emphasis on monounsaturated fat would probably require the counsel of a registered dietitian to design a specific meal pattern. One approach could be the Mediterranean Pyramid discussed in Chapter 2.[2]

■ Increasing dietary fiber intake

Another dietary means of reducing LDL-cholesterol is increasing intake of soluble fibers, as discussed in Chapter 5. These bind bile acids and, so, reduce their reabsorption. The liver must pull cholesterol out of the bloodstream to make new bile acids. This then lowers LDL in the bloodstream. Although large amounts of fiber must be eaten to have a significant effect, any amount helps—and has other health benefits.[13] Diets with an overall fiber content of 25 to 35 g/day, especially those that emphasize soluble fiber, are most effective. Most people would have to change their diets extensively to achieve high intakes of soluble fiber. Instead, the focus could simply be on high-fiber foods—fruits, vegetables, beans, and whole grains. Use of the psyllium fiber found in some laxatives also helps meet this goal. Since a dietary fiber intake above 35 g/day may cause binding of dietary minerals, one should consult a physician if considering a high-fiber diet exceeding this amount.

LOWERING BLOOD TRIGLYCERIDES

Blood triglycerides are the most diet-responsive blood lipid. Not overeating, limiting alcohol and simple-sugar intake, spreading meals throughout the day (not just one or two), and including some fish in the diet all help. Controlling diabetes, if present, also is important, as are losing excess weight and performing regular physical activity.

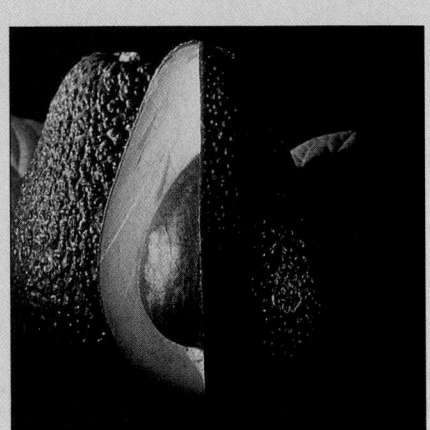

Most fruits and vegetables are low in fat; however, avocados are an exception. Still, most of this fat is monounsaturated and, so, is heart healthy.

RAISING HDL-CHOLESTEROL: A DIFFICULT TASK

Physical activity is one way to raise HDL-cholesterol. Exercising for at least 45 minutes four times a week can raise it by about 5 mg/dl. Sedentary people, in particular, should focus on increasing physical activity because this has other heart-healthy benefits as well.[4] Losing excess weight (especially around the waist), avoiding smoking, and using estrogen replacement in women also help maintain or raise HDL-cholesterol.

In addition, eating regularly (three or more balanced meals daily), balancing the amount of energy eaten with that expended, and eating less total fat often raise HDL-cholesterol because these practices lower blood triglycerides. This in turn is associated with higher HDL-cholesterol. The reason for this is not clear. Certain medications, such as high doses of nicotinic acid and the medications gemfibrozil (Lopid) and simvistatin (Zocar), also lower blood triglycerides, thereby indirectly increasing HDL-cholesterol.

Consumption of alcohol is also associated with higher HDL-cholesterol and reduced blood clotting—two factors that reduce the risk of heart attack. However, excessive consumption of alcohol has many negative effects. The Dietary Guidelines indicate that most people can consume one to two drinks daily (no more) without negative health consequences. But, for people at risk for alcoholism, any alcohol may be too much (see Chapter 8).

It is unfortunate that raising HDL-cholesterol is difficult. Lowering LDL-cholesterol is much easier. Sometimes, as LDL-cholesterol falls, so does HDL-cholesterol. This often occurs with very-low-fat diets. However, if LDL-cholesterol drops to about 100 mg/dl, the fall in HDL-cholesterol is not of much concern. Researchers note that the main problem with low HDL-cholesterol is for people who have high LDL-cholesterol. In this case, the HDL fraction has not increased to compensate for the high LDL-cholesterol value. Researchers also note that people in rural Asia who eat low-fat diets generally have low LDL-cholesterol and HDL-cholesterol, but they also show low risk for cardiovascular disease.[6]

PRIMARY PREVENTION VERSUS SECONDARY PREVENTION OF CARDIOVASCULAR DISEASE

The diet and lifestyle strategies discussed so far to reduce cardiovascular disease risk are appropriate for both **primary prevention** (where a heart attack has not yet taken place but the person has risk factors or where clinical symptoms are evident) and **secondary prevention** (after a heart attack has taken place). However, some people need even more aggressive therapy added to their regimen. The clearest indication for this more aggressive approach is in secondary prevention, but its use in primary prevention in cases of very abnormal blood lipoprotein patterns also deserves consideration.

Medications are the cornerstone of this more aggressive therapy.[15] Currently, medications work to lower LDL-cholesterol in one of two ways. Statins (e.g., fluvastatin [Lescol], lovastatin [Mevacor], simvistatin [Zocor]), and atorvistatin [Lipitor] reduce cholesterol synthesis in the liver by inhibiting the enzyme HMG-CoA reductase. This then reduces the cholesterol content in the liver cells. The cells respond by increasing LDL receptor activity in order to pull cholesterol from the bloodstream to make up for the loss. Recall that LDL is 50% cholesterol. Usually, the first line of defense in secondary prevention, statins can reduce LDL-cholesterol up to as much as 60%, depending on the drug used and the prescribed dosage.[17] The cost of being on one of the statin drugs ranges from $1000–$1800 per year, depending on the dose needed.

A second group of medications binds bile acids in the small intestine, as does soluble fiber, and leads to their elimination, forcing the liver to synthesize new bile acids. The liver removes LDL from the blood to do this. For this reason, these drugs are called bile acid sequestrants or resins (e.g., cholestyramine [Questran] and colestipol [Colestid]). These medications taste gritty and therefore are not very popular with patients. Generally, the resins are not used alone in adults because of this unpleasant texture. The use of one or both of these classes of

*A*s noted in the chapter, aspirin in small doses reduces blood clotting by reducing Thromboxane A_2 production, it is often used under a physician's guidance to treat people at risk for heart attack or stroke, especially if one has already occurred. Studies show this with 325 mg of aspirin per day. Some clinicians suggest that only 80–160 mg/day may be needed for benefits. This lower amount would decrease the side effects of the aspirin, such as risk for ulcers (see Chapter 3).

A person taking a statin medication could experiment with consuming some grapefruit or grapefruit juice at the same time. A compound in grapefruit can increase potency of the medication, possibly allowing for a reduction in the daily dose. Working with one's physician is advised if this strategy is implemented.

M edicare is funding the Dr. Dean Ornish vegan plan for elderly Americans who suffer from severe coronary heart disease to see if that plan can reverse arterial blockage and can be an alternative to surgery.[6]

medications should ideally drive LDL-cholesterol down to about 100 mg/dl—the current therapeutic goal for secondary prevention.

A third group of drugs can be used to lower blood triglycerides by decreasing the triglyceride production of the liver. As mentioned, these include gemfibrozil (Lopid) and megadoses of the vitamin nicotinic acid. The use of nicotinic acid does result in pesky side effects, however, but these are typically manageable.

One trial studied the effect of vitamin E and angiotension-converting enzymes (ACE inhibitors, such as ramipril) on reducing cardiovascular disease death in people with the disease. Vitamin E was not found to be successful; however, ACE inhibitors were found to be successful.[7] It is suspected that the mechanism of cardiovascular disease protection from ACE inhibitors is due to its ability to stabilize plaque deposits; relax blood vessels, in turn reducing blood pressure; and inhibit blood clotting (see Chapter 11 for more on ACE inhibitors).

Estrogen replacement therapy may be helpful for reducing cardiovascular disease risk in postmenopausal women, as it tends to reduce LDL-cholesterol and increase HDL-cholesterol values. Currently researchers are unsure about the overall benefit of this therapy since studies that show a reduced risk of cardiovascular disease may have done so because the women in the studies were healthier and better educated than average women. As well, short term intervention trials using women with existing cardiovascular disease have not shown a benefit from such therapy. A large-scale trial to answer the question concerning safety and effectiveness of estrogen replacement therapy for the prevention of cardiovascular disease (and other diseases) is ongoing. The results are due out in 2005 (see the Expert Opinion in Chapter 11 for a discussion of the pros and cons of estrogen therapy for postmenopausal women).[35]

It is troubling to note that, currently, many U.S. adults with evidence of cardiovascular disease quit risk-reducing therapy within the first year of diagnosis. Part of this is due to the cost and side effects of some of the medications typically used. Overall, mortality from cardiovascular disease is reduced when treatment to lower elevated LDL-cholesterol in people who are at high risk for such disease or who have had a heart attack is followed for a few years or more by a physician. Furthermore, new research shows that plaque even regresses in arteries when high LDL-cholesterol is treated aggressively. It is suspected that these aggressive therapies to lower LDL-cholesterol stabilize the development of atherosclerotic plaque, thereby lowering the risk of rupture and reducing the chance of myocardial infarction caused by clot formation.[15]

OTHER MEDICAL THERAPIES FOR CARDIOVASCULAR DISEASE

Cholestin comes from a strain of Chinese red yeast that has been used as a natural flavoring agent and food coloring in Chinese cooking for many years. Cholestin has an active component called lovastatin, which is in the prescription drug Mevacor (a cholesterol-lowering drug approved by FDA). Cholestin has been successful in reducing blood cholesterol in numerous studies.[8] However, currently FDA does not regulate this product based on the limitation put on FDA by Congress with regard to dietary supplements (see the Nutrition Perspective in Chapter 18). Cholestin is labeled as a dietary supplement and can be purchased in many stores. However, to self-prescribe cholestin as a drug in the treatment of high blood cholesterol is not recommended by many physicians, due to lack of regulation by FDA. The lack of FDA oversight means that consumers cannot be sure the dietary supplement contains the active ingredient or the amount specified on the bottle. Cholestin is also very expensive. Overall, high blood cholesterol is a serious disease that requires medical supervision. In addition, if a physician does not follow a person, how will the person know that cholestin is actually lowering blood cholesterol? For this reason, cholestin should be used in conjunction with a physician's supervision.

FDA has approved two margarines that have positive effects on blood cholesterol levels—Benecol and Take Control. These margarines contain plant stanol/sterol esters, which have been researched since the 1950s for their cholesterol-lowering effects. However, it wasn't until the mid-1990s that researchers modified the plant stanols to be fat soluble and found a suitable medium for consumption. The plant stanol/sterol esters work by competing with cholesterol for incorporation into the micelle in the small intestine, thus causing decreased absorption of dietary cholesterol and lower return of biliary cholesterol to the liver through enterohepatic circulation.[24] The liver responds by increasing the clearance of cholesterol from the blood. The studies done on the cholesterol-lowering effect of these margarines have found that 2 to 5 g of plant stanol/sterol esters per day reduces total blood cholesterol by 8 to 10% and LDL-cholesterol by 9 to 14% (similar to what is seen with some cholesterol-lowering drugs).

Benecol is made from plant stanol esters called sitostanols, which are extracted from wood pulp trees. This product is sold as margarine and has been added to salad dressings. Take Control is made from plant sterol esters called sitosterols, which are isolated from soybeans. The recommended serving size for both is about 2 to 3 tablespoons per day. Use would cost about $1.00 per day.

In people who have borderline high total blood cholesterol (between 200 and 239 mg/dl), these margarines can be helpful in avoiding future drug therapy. Even though these products exhibit significant results, it is still important to follow a balanced diet low in saturated fat and trans fatty acids, as well as to exercise on a regular basis. People with high total blood cholesterol (>240 mg/dl) who plan to consume these margarines should inform their physicians because, if they are currently on cholesterol-lowering drug therapy, their doctors may be able to decrease the dosage. For healthy individuals with total blood cholesterol within normal limits, the use of these margarines is unnecessary, especially because their cholesterol-lowering effect is not needed and they are expensive.

In summary, individuals with elevated LDL-cholesterol in consultation with their physicians, are best suited to determine their desire and ability to make lifestyle changes, supplemented with medications, plant stanol/sterol margarines, and possibly cholestin supplements to lower cardiovascular disease risk. Some physicians also recommend caution about initiating aggressive LDL-lowering treatment in persons over 65 to 70 years of age because of concern about the safety and cost-effectiveness of such interventions in older people (see Chapter 18).

GENERAL STRATEGY FOR REDUCING CARDIOVASCULAR DISEASE RISK

Table 6-9 outlines a comprehensive strategy for lowering LDL-cholesterol and preventing cardiovascular disease development. Of particular interest with regard to dietary strategies is the results obtained from a Harvard study done on nurses.[30] This study revealed that women who used a group of lifestyle factors had a greater than 80% lower risk for cardiovascular disease than those who did not include these advantageous lifestyle factors in their lives. The lifestyle factors that translated into such a drop in risk are a healthy body weight, moderate to vigorous activity (e.g., brisk walking) for at least 1/2 hour per day, nonsmoking or quitting smoking, an average of ½ drink of alcohol per day, and a score in the highest intakes of the following categories on a food intake questionnaire: cereal fiber, omega-3 fatty acids, and the vitamin folate. In addition, these women had a higher intake of polyunsaturated fatty acid with low-saturated and trans-fatty-acids intake and consumed a low-glycemic-index load. This study shows that combining several lifestyle factors are highly effective in protecting against cardiovascular disease in women. The bottom line for almost anyone is to combine these lifestyle factors as a comprehensive approach to reduce cardiovascular disease risk.

LATEST TECHNOLOGY IN CARDIOVASCULAR DISEASE DETECTION

An up-and-coming way to detect cardiovascular disease risk is a test called high sensitivity C reactive protein (hs-CRP). This test measures a protein that is made in the liver in response to inflammation in the body; it has been shown to be reliable in detecting cardiovascular disease risk in women. This test has yet to be adopted by many physicians simply due to a lack of

The two most popular surgical treatments for coronary artery blockage are percutaneous transluminal coronary angioplasty (PTCA) and coronary artery bypass graft (CABG). PTCA involves the insertion of a balloon catheter into an artery in the arm or groin. Once it is advanced to the area of the lesion, the balloon is expanded to crush the lesion. This method works best when only one vessel is blocked, and it may need to be repeated within weeks or months. CABG involves the removal of a saphenous vein or use of a mammary artery. The saphenous vein is sewn to the main heart vessel (aorta) and then used to bypass the blocked artery, as is the mammary artery. The procedure usually remains effective for 5 to 10 years and can be performed on one to five blockages. Related therapy is used to keep LDL-cholesterol to about 100 mg/dl.

For more information on cardiovascular disease, see the web site of the American Heart Association at http://www.americanheart.org or the heart disease section of Healthfinder at http://www.healthfinder.gov/tours/heart.htm. This is a site created by the U.S. government for consumers. In addition, visit the web site http://www.nhlbi.nih.gov/chd.

TABLE 6-9   General Diet-Related Strategies for Reducing the Risk of Cardiovascular Disease and Heart Attack.[4, 5, 9, 13, 19, 31, 34]

Action	Rationale
Consume less saturated fat and trans fatty acids, while replacing this decreased amount of fat with monounsaturated fat and omega-3 and omega-6 fatty acids.	These unsaturated fatty acids have positive effects on blood cholesterol, whereas saturated fats and trans fatty acids exhibit negative effects.
Eat fish rich in omega-3 fatty acids at least twice a week and include plant sources that are rich in omega-3 fatty acids in your diet.	Omega-3 fatty acids decrease blood clotting and have a favorable effect on heart rhythm.
Eat plenty of fruits and vegetables and include some soy on a regular basis.	The dietary fiber, antioxidants, and other phytochemicals present in these foods can reduce risk of cardiovascular disease.
Eat more whole grains and less refined carbohydrates.	Whole grains are rich in dietary fiber, vitamins, and minerals and have been shown to decrease blood cholesterol, whereas refined carbohydrates provide little if any heart benefits
Eat at least three regularly spaced meals, while combining any high-glycemic-index foods with low-glycemic-index foods.	The frequency of meals affects blood triglycerides. Studies show that increasing meal frequency while controlling portion size (from three to nine per day or so) can help reduce LDL production (see Chapter 5 for glycemic index values of various foods).
Consume moderate amounts of alcohol with food, if you can control this practice and your physician gives approval based on your age and current health.	Consumption of red wine, in particular, has been noted to reduce cardiovascular disease, but it is speculated that small amounts of any form of alcohol may have the same effect. Reducing blood clotting is just one mechanism that is suspected of having protective effects.
Moderate coffee intake, and replace some use with tea.	Heavy coffee use, especially unfiltered coffee (espresso and French press types), increases LDL. Moderate intake of filtered coffee appears to be fine for most healthy individuals. And instead of drinking coffee exclusively, consider switching to some black or green tea—they contain many flavonoids and antioxidants that counteract free radicals, which are involved in cardiovascular disease development.
Moderate salt intake	High intakes of salt in overweight people have been found to cause a higher risk of death from cardiovascular disease. It is a good idea for all individuals to moderate salt in the diet, since it can cause some people's blood pressure to rise too high.

knowledge of what exactly the test measures and how to interpret the results. The hs-CRP test is generally inexpensive and is especially useful for someone who exhibits normal to slightly abnormal blood cholesterol values. A positive test could give that person the motivation to make improved lifestyle choices to deter cardiovascular disease.

PROTEINS

chapter 7

onsuming enough protein is vital for maintaining health. Proteins form important structures in the body, make up a key part of the blood, help regulate many body functions, and can fuel body cells.[13]

Americans eat a lot of protein—generally more than is needed to maintain health. Our daily protein intake comes mostly from meat, poultry, fish, eggs, milk, and cheese.[24] In contrast, our Stone Age ancestors obtained a greater percentage of their protein from vegetables. They primarily picked and gathered their dietary protein, rather than hunted it. Not until *Homo erectus,* our immediate ancestors, emerged about 2.5 million years ago did meat displace other foods in a primarily vegetarian diet. Diets that are mostly vegetarian still predominate in much of Asia and areas of Africa.

Few of us wish to exchange our comfortable modern lifestyles with those of our Stone-Age ancestors, yet we could benefit from eating more plant sources of proteins. It is possible—and desirable—to incorporate the most nutritious practices of both eras and enjoy the benefits of animal and plant protein.[19] Let's see why this is worth your attention.

■| CHAPTER OUTLINE

■ KEY CHAPTER CONCEPTS

- The building blocks of proteins, amino acids, contain a very usable form of nitrogen,
- Of the 20 or so types of amino acids found in food, 9 are essential and must be obtained in the diet. The other amino acids can be synthesized by the body.
- High-quality, or *complete,* protein foods contain ample amounts of all nine essential amino acids. This is typical of animal protein foods. Lower-quality, or *incomplete,* protein foods lack sufficient amounts of one or more of the essential amino acids. This is typical of many plant foods.
- A variety of plant foods eaten together generally complement one another's essential amino acid deficits, yielding a high-quality protein content for the meal.
- Individual amino acids link together to form proteins. The sequential order of amino acids determines the protein's ultimate form and function. DNA in the nucleus directs this order.
- Protein digestion begins in the stomach, splitting the proteins into breakdown products containing shorter chains of amino acids. In the small intestine, these shorter protein chains are further digested into amino acids. These individual amino acids travel via the portal vein to the liver.
- Important body components—such as muscles, connective tissue, transport proteins, visual pigments, enzymes, some hormones, and immune bodies—are made of proteins. In addition, proteins help maintain fluid and acid-base balance and provide some energy for the body. Cells are constantly degrading these body proteins and creating new proteins.
- The RDA for protein for a 70-kg (156-lb) person is 56 g, and that for a 55-kg (120-lb) person is 44 g. American men consume about 95 g of protein daily, and women consume closer to 65 g. Thus, the American diet generally supplies plenty of protein.
- Some research has linked the long-term intake of high-protein diets to increased calcium loss in the urine, as well as high intakes of red meat to certain forms of cancer, such as colon cancer.
- Plant proteins are important constituents of the diet. Foods such as nuts and legumes add many nutrients and dietary fiber to the diet.
- Protein-energy malnutrition occurs when a person consumes extremely limited amounts of protein and energy. Kwashiorkor occurs when the diet has little protein compared with total energy content. Marasmus is the wasting away of the body that occurs over time with minimal energy and protein intake.
- Anyone considering vegetarianism should realize that a healthful diet does not occur automatically. It takes careful planning, especially for children and pregnant women. Consuming a wide variety of foods is especially important.

■ REFRESH YOUR MEMORY

As you begin your study of proteins, you may want to review

- The anatomy and physiology of digestion and absorption in Chapter 3
- The immune system in Chapter 3
- Amino acid use in energy metabolism in Chapter 4
- The processes of gluconeogensis and ketosis in Chapter 4

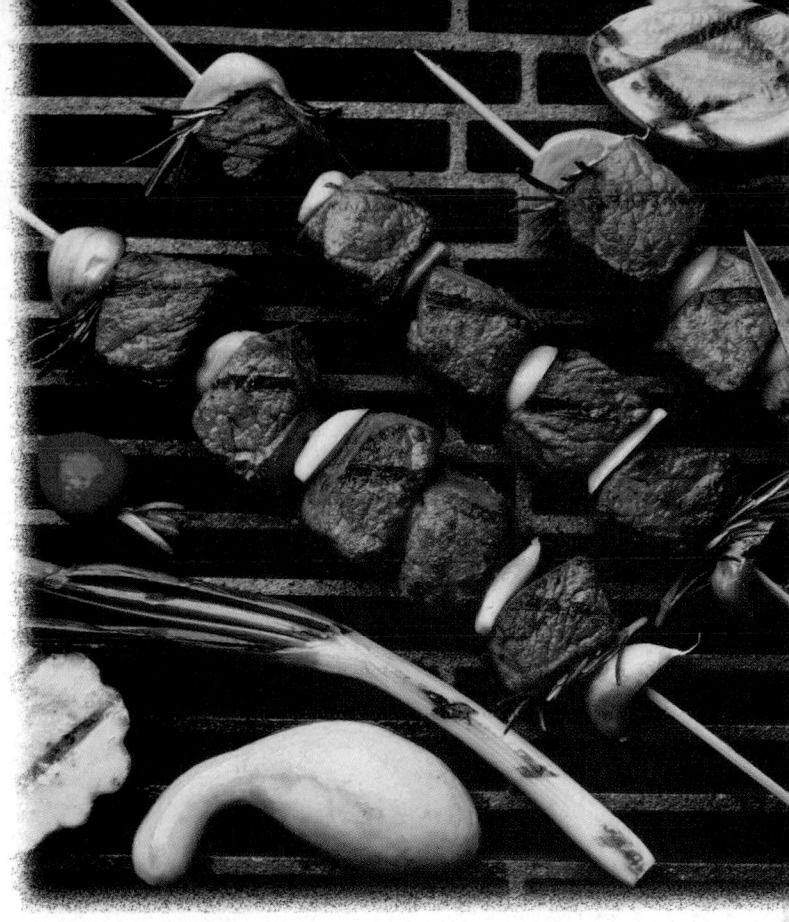

■ CASE SCENARIO

Shannon is a freshman in college. She lives in a campus dorm and is an aerobics instructor in the afternoon. She eats two or three meals a day at the dorm cafeteria and snacks between meals. Shannon and her roommate both decided to become vegetarians because they recently read a magazine article describing the health benefits of a vegetarian diet. Yesterday her vegetarian diet consisted of a pop tart for breakfast and a tomato-pasta dish (no meat) with pretzels and a diet soft drink for lunch. In the afternoon, after her aerobic class, she had a few cookies. At dinnertime, she had a vegetarian sub sandwich with two glasses of fruit punch. In the evening, she had a bowl of popcorn.

What type of vegetarian is she? How could she improve her new diet to meet her nutritional needs?

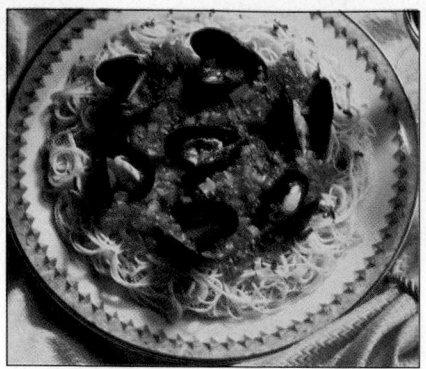

Small amounts of animal protein in a meal easily add up to meet daily protein needs.

■ PROTEIN—AN INTRODUCTION

The term *protein* comes from the Greek word *protos,* which means "to come first." In the developing world, such a primary focus on protein in diet planning is important because diets in those areas of the world can be deficient in protein. In contrast, diets in the developed world are generally rich in protein, and therefore a specific focus on eating enough protein is not needed.[24]

High protein diets have come and gone over the past 30 years. Recently, these have risen again as weight-loss diets, such as the Atkins Diet. As discussed in Chapter 13, these are hardly a magic bullet for weight loss and are even dangerous if followed for more than 4 to 6 weeks, or at all, by some people. The more moderate Zone Diet plans recommend 30% of calories coming from proteins; this is two to three times more than nutrition experts generally recommend. There is no support in the nutrition literature for such a high protein intake, including for athletes (see Chapter 14).

Thus, although proteins were given a primary focus in diet planning in ancient times, most of us today need not focus specifically on protein intake. Protein is available from a wide variety of foods and is ample in Western diets.[8]

■ PROTEINS—VITAL TO LIFE

Thousands of substances in the body are made of **proteins.** Aside from water, proteins form the major part of lean body tissue, totaling about 17% of body weight. Amino acids—the building blocks for proteins—contain a special form of nitrogen: essentially, carbon linked to nitrogen. Plants combine nitrogen from soil and air with carbon and other elements to form amino acids. They then link these amino acids together to make proteins. We get the nitrogen we need by consuming dietary proteins. Proteins are thus very important because they supply nitrogen in a form we can readily use—namely, amino acids. Directly using simpler forms of nitrogen is, for the most part, impossible for humans.[13]

Proteins are crucial to the regulation and maintenance of the body. Body functions such as blood clotting, fluid balance, hormone and enzyme production, visual processes, and cell repair require specific proteins. The body generates proteins in many configurations and sizes, so that they can serve these greatly varied functions. All these proteins use the amino acids in the protein-containing foods we eat, plus some arising from cell synthesis. Proteins can also supply energy for the body—on average, 4 kcal per gram.

If you fail to consume an adequate amount of protein for weeks at a time, many metabolic processes slow down. This is because the body does not have enough amino acids available to build the proteins it needs. For example, the immune system no longer functions efficiently when it lacks key proteins, thereby increasing the risk of infections, disease, and eventually death.[26]

Amino acids contain carbon, hydrogen, oxygen, and nitrogen, and some contain sulfur. Body protein is made using 20 amino acids, each with different metabolic fates in the body (e.g., some can be made into glucose or hormones) and varying composition. Each amino acid is composed of a central carbon bonded to four groups. The first three of these groups are a nitrogen group ($-NH_2$), called an amino group (or amine group), an acid group ($-\overset{\overset{O}{\|}}{C}-OH$) , and a hydrogen ($-H$). The fourth group, often signified by *R*, completes the amino acid. In the margin is the basic model of an amino acid and structures of two amino acids, glycine and alanine. The chemical structures of the rest of the amino acids are shown in Appendix B.

$$R-\underset{\underset{H}{|}}{\overset{\overset{NH_2}{|}}{C}}-\overset{\overset{O}{\|}}{C}-OH$$

"Generic" amino acid

$$H-\underset{\underset{H}{|}}{\overset{\overset{NH_2}{|}}{C}}-\overset{\overset{O}{\|}}{C}-OH$$

Glycine

$$CH_3-\underset{\underset{H}{|}}{\overset{\overset{NH_2}{|}}{C}}-\overset{\overset{O}{\|}}{C}-OH$$

L-alanine

The L isomer is the form of amino acid used by the body for protein synthesis.

■ Amino Acid Form Determines Function

The form that the R portion of the amino acid assumes determines the type name of the amino acid. If R is a hydrogen, the amino acid is glycine, if R is a methyl group

$(-CH_3)$, the amino acid is alanine, and so on. Some amino acids have chemically similar R portions. These related amino acids form special classes, such as acidic amino acids, basic amino acids, or branched-chain amino acids.[13] This distinction with regard to classes of amino acids has important practical implications. For instance, branched-chain amino acids are used for fuel by the muscles, especially during injury and other related forms of trauma. Liquid formulas used to feed hospitalized patients may be enriched in branched-chain amino acids in order to provide ample amounts of these amino acids. The same holds true for some fluid replacement drinks marketed to athletes (see Chapter 14).

The body needs to use 20 different forms of amino acids to function. Although they are all important, 11 of these amino acids are considered **nonessential** (also dispensable)—it isn't essential to consume them because our bodies make them using other amino acids we consume (Table 7-1) The 9 amino acids the body cannot make are known as **essential** (also called indispensable)—they must be obtained from foods. This is because body cells cannot make the needed carbon backbone (also called carbon skeleton) of the amino acid, cannot put a nitrogen group on the needed carbon backbone, or just cannot do the whole process fast enough to meet body needs. The first estimates of these amino acid requirements of humans were made by Rose and his colleagues in the 1940s.

Two amino acids—cysteine and tyrosine—are synthesized in the body from methionine and phenylalanine, respectively. Both methionine and phenylalanine are essential amino acids. Cysteine and tyrosine must be made from their essential amino acid counterparts unless they are consumed in the diet. If cysteine and tyrosine are consumed, the body can synthesize protein from them directly. Thus, consumption of cysteine and tyrosine then frees the essential amino acids methionine and phenylalanine to contribute directly to protein synthesis. Therefore, cysteine and tyrosine are classed as semiessential (also called *conditionally dispensable*) amino acids.[13]

Both nonessential and essential amino acids are present in foods that contain protein. If you don't consume enough food to yield a sufficient supply of essential amino acids, your body first struggles to conserve what essential amino acids it can. However, eventually your body progressively slows production of new proteins until at some point you will break down protein faster than you can make it. When this happens, as noted, health deteriorates. Therefore, the two main functions of proteins

nonessential amino acids Amino acids that can be synthesized by a healthy body in sufficient amounts; there are 11 nonessential amino acids. These are also termed *dispensable amino acids*.

essential amino acids The amino acids that cannot be synthesized by humans in sufficient amounts and therefore must be included in the diet; there are nine essential amino acids. These are also called *indispensable amino acids*.

TABLE 7-1 Classification of Amino Acids	
Essential (Indispensable) Amino Acids	**Nonessential (Dispensable) Amino Acids**
Histidine	Alanine
Isoleucine*	Arginine
Leucine*	Asparagine
Lysine	Aspartic acid
Methionine	Cysteine†
Phenylalanine	(Cystine)
Threonine	Glutamic acid
Tryptophan	Glutamine
Valine*	Glycine
	Proline
	Serine
	Tyrosine†

*A branched-chain amino acid

†These amino acids are also classed as semiessential. This means they must be made from essential amino acids if insufficient amounts are eaten. When that occurs, the body's supply of certain essential amino acids is depleted. Researchers now suggest that some other nonessential amino acids assume a more essential status when the body cannot readily generate them. This occurs during some illnesses. Glutamine may assume an essential status in traumatic injury, especially in the period after intestinal surgery, and arginine is essential for infants and children.

*B*ecause two cysteine molecules can bind to form a new amino acid called cystine, the number of nonessential amino acids is sometimes listed as 12. If this form of cysteine is not counted as a unique form, then there are 11 nonessential amino acids. Our discussion will not count cystine and thus use the figure of 20 amino acids in foods— 9 essential and 11 nonessential.

in our diets are (1) to provide the nine essential amino acids needed by our bodies and (2) to provide either the nonessential amino acids our bodies use or nitrogen from an amino acid, which in turn can be used to make the nonessential amino acids.

◼ Transamination and Deamination

A common metabolic process for synthesizing nonessential amino acids is called **transamination.** This process requires vitamin B-6.[15] Figure 7-1 illustrates transamination: Pyruvic acid (this is not an amino acid) accepts the amino group ($-NH_2$) from the amino acid glutamic acid and becomes the amino acid alanine.

Some amino acids, such as glutamic acid, can simply lose their amino group without transferring it to another carbon skeleton. This process is called **deamination.** The amino group, in the form of ammonia, is incorporated into **urea** in the liver. The urea is then transferred through the bloodstream to the kidneys and is mostly excreted in the urine. Once an amino acid breaks down to its amino-free carbon skeleton, the carbon skeleton can be used for fuel or synthesized into other compounds, such as fatty acids (see Chapter 4).

◼ Essential and Nonessential Amino Acids in Perspective

Eating a balanced diet can supply us with both the essential and nonessential amino-acid building blocks needed to maintain good health. Let's now take a more detailed look at this concept of essential amino acids, especially in relation to nonessential amino acids.

Physiological Aspects

The disease phenylketonuria (PKU) illustrates the importance of one essential amino acid. Recall from Chapter 5 that a person with PKU has a limited ability to metabolize the essential amino acid phenylalanine. Normally, the body uses an enzyme to convert much of our dietary phenylalanine intake into the nonessential amino acid tyrosine by adding a hydoxyl group ($-OH$):

$$\text{phenylalanine} \xrightarrow[\text{phenylalanine hydroxylase}]{} \text{tyrosine}$$

In PKU-diagnosed persons, the enzyme activity may be grossly or mildly insufficient in processing phenylalanine to tyrosine. When the enzymes cannot synthesize enough tyrosine, both amino acids must be derived from foods. The key point here

transamination The transfer of an amino group from an amino acid to a carbon skeleton to form a new amino acid.

deamination The removal of an amino group from an amino acid.

urea nitrogenous waste product of protein metabolism; The major source of nitrogen in the urine; chemically $NH_2-\overset{O}{\underset{}{C}}-NH_2$.

CRITICAL THINKING

Rina is 7 months pregnant and has read about various tests that her baby will undergo when he or she is born. How can you explain to Rina the purpose and significance of one of those tests, the one that screens for PKU?

◼ FIGURE 7-1 Transamination. This pathway allows cells to synthesize nonessential amino acids. In this example, pyruvic acid gains an amino group to form the amino acid alanine. By looking only at the bottom half of the reaction, deamination is seen when glutamic acid loses its amino group. The enzymes used in these reactions are called aminotransferases.

is that both amino acids become *essential* in terms of dietary needs because the body can't produce enough tryrosine. In the treatment of PKU, consumption of phenylalanine must also be controlled using a special diet (ideally throughout life) because phenylalanine and its by-products, such as phenylpyruvic acid, can rise to toxic concentrations in the body. These are thought to cause the severe mental retardation seen in untreated PKU cases.

Dietary Considerations

Animal and plant proteins can differ greatly in proportions of essential and nonessential amino acids. Animal proteins contain ample amounts of all nine essential amino acids. (Gelatin—made from the animal protein collagen—is an exception because it loses one essential amino acid during processing and is low in other essential amino acids.) With the exception of soybeans, plant proteins don't match our need for essential amino acids as precisely as animal proteins. Many plant proteins, especially those found in grains, are low in one or more of the nine essential amino acids.[11]

As you might expect, human tissue composition resembles animal tissue more than it does plant tissue. The similarities enable us to use proteins from single animal sources more efficiently to support human growth and maintenance than we do those from single plant sources. For this reason, animal proteins, except gelatin, are considered **high-quality** (also called **complete**) **proteins**—they contain all the amino acids we need in sufficient amounts. Individual plant sources of proteins are considered **lower-quality** (also called **incomplete**) **proteins** because their amino-acid patterns can be quite different from ours. A single plant protein, such as corn alone, cannot easily support body growth and maintenance. To obtain a sufficient amount of amino acids, a variety of plant proteins need to be consumed because each protein lacks adequate amounts of one or more essential amino acids.

When only lower-quality protein foods are consumed, enough of the essential amino acids needed for protein synthesis may not be obtained. Therefore, a greater amount of this type of protein is needed to meet the needs of protein synthesis. Moreover, once any of the nine essential amino acids in the plant protein were used up, further protein synthesis would be impossible. The remaining amino acids would be used for energy or converted to fat or carbohydrate and stored as such. Because the depletion of just one of the essential amino acids prevents protein synthesis, the process illustrates the *all-or-none principle:* Either all essential amino acids are available or none can be used. The essential amino acid in smallest supply in a food or diet in relation to body needs becomes the limiting factor (called the **limiting amino acid**) because it limits the amount of protein the body can synthesize.[13]

For example, assume the letters of the alphabet represent the 20 or so different amino acids we consume. If *A* represents an essential amino acid, we need four of these letters to spell the hypothetical protein *ALABAMA*. If the body had an *L*, a *B*, and an *M*, but only three *A*s, the "synthesis" of *ALABAMA* would not be possible. *A* would then be seen as the limiting amino acid.

When two or more proteins combine to compensate for deficiencies in essential amino acid content in each protein, the proteins are called **complementary proteins** (Table 7-2).[11] Mixed diets generally provide high-quality protein because a complementary protein pattern results. Therefore, healthy adults should have little concern about balancing foods to yield the proteins needed to obtain enough of all nine essential amino acids. Even on plant-based diets, complementing proteins need not be consumed at the same meal by adults. Meeting amino acid needs over the course of a day is a reasonable goal for adults because there is a ready supply of amino acids from those present in body cells and in the blood (see Figure 7-3 on page 266). In addition, adults need only about 11% of their total protein requirement to be supplied by essential amino acids. Typical diets supply an average of 50% of protein as essential amino acids.

The estimated needs for essential amino acids for infants and preschool children are 30% of total protein intake; however, in later childhood the number drops to

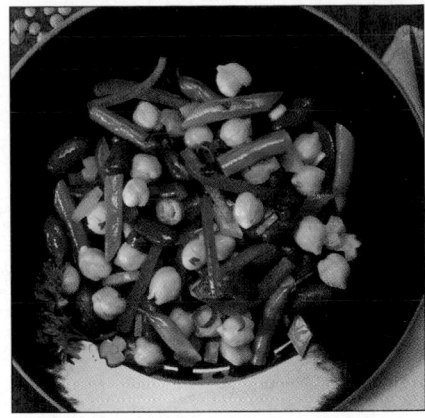

Amino acids in vegetables are best used when a combination of vegetable protein sources is consumed.

high-quality (complete) proteins Dietary proteins that contain ample amounts of all nine essential amino acids.

lower-quality (incomplete) proteins Dietary proteins that are low in or lack one or more essential amino acids.

CRITICAL THINKING

Leon, a vegetarian, has heard of the "all-or-none principle" of protein synthesis but doesn't understand how this law applies to protein synthesis in the body. He asks you, "How important is this nutritional concept for diet planning?" How would you answer his question?

limiting amino acid The essential amino acid in lowest concentration in a food or diet relative to body needs.

complementary proteins Two food protein sources that make up for each other's inadequate supply of specific essential amino acids; together they yield a sufficient amount of all nine and, so, provide high-quality (complete) protein for the diet.

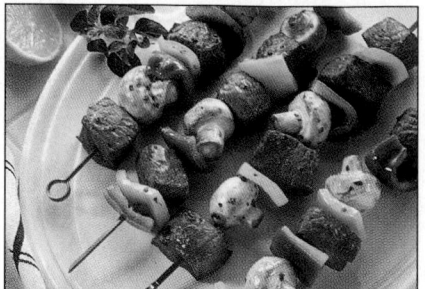

When combined with vegetables, high-protein foods such as meats, help balance the amino acid content of the diet.

TABLE 7-2   Limiting Amino Acids in Plant Foods

Food	Limiting Amino Acids	Good Plant Source of the Limiting Amino Acids*	Traditional Uses in Which the Proteins Complement Each Other in a Meal
Beans (legumes)	Methionine	Grains, nuts, seeds	Red beans and rice
Grains	Lysine, threonine	Legumes	Rice and red beans, lentil curry, and rice
Nuts and seeds	Lysine	Legumes	Soybeans and ground sesame seeds (miso); peanuts, rice, and black-eyed peas; green peas and sunflower seeds
Vegetables	Methionine	Grains, nuts, seeds	Green beans and almonds
Corn	Tryptophan, lysine	Legumes	Corn tortillas and beans

Note: As you might suspect from the information in this table, the amino acids most likely to be low in a diet are lysine, methionine, threonine, and tryptophan. If a diet is low in an amino acid, nutrition experts recommend finding a good food source to supply it. Finding the right combinations of amino acids, such as a dish of rice and beans, is recommended.[18] Forget about amino acid supplements—they can lead to problems, such as decreased absorption of other, similar amino acids. Amino acids as such also have a disagreeable odor and flavor.

*Animal products in the diet serve the same purpose, such as when fish is consumed with rice.

20%.[13] Consequently, diets for young children must be carefully planned to make sure enough proteins are present to yield high-quality protein intake. Including some animal products in the diet, such as human milk, infant formula, or cow's milk, helps ensure this. Otherwise, complementary amino acids from plant proteins should be consumed in each meal or within two subsequent meals. A major health risk for children occurs in famine situations in which only one type of cereal grain is available, increasing the probability that one or more of the nine essential amino acids are lacking in the total diet. This is discussed further in a later section in the chapter.

CONCEPT CHECK

The human body uses 20 different amino acids from protein-containing foods. Because a healthy body can synthesize 11 of the amino acids, it is not necessary to get all amino acids from foods—only 9 of these must be obtained from the diet and are therefore termed *essential (indispensable) amino acids.* Foods that contain all 9 essential amino acids in about the proportions we need are considered high-quality (complete) protein foods. Those low in one or more essential amino acids are lower-quality (incomplete) protein foods. When different lower-quality protein foods are eaten together, the total intake of amino acids generally makes up for the individual foods' shortcomings to yield a high-quality protein meal.

■ PROTEINS—AMINO ACIDS JOINED TOGETHER

One way of classifying proteins is based on the number of amino acids present. Two amino acids chemically bonded together form a dipeptide, and three amino acids form a tripeptide. An oligopeptide has more than 3 but fewer than 50 amino acids. A polypeptide has 50 to 100 amino acids, and a protein has a minimum of 100 amino acids. Most foods contain proteins of more than 100 amino acids. However, specialized liquid meal replacement supplements used in hospitals often contain various peptides, as these show enhanced absorption, compared with larger, intact proteins (see a later section in this chapter).

Amino acids are joined by a strong, covalent **peptide bond.** An amino group $(-NH_2)$ reacts with a carboxyl group $(-\overset{\overset{O}{\|}}{C}-OH)$, and a water molecule is split off in an enzyme-catalyzed reaction. The body can synthesize many different proteins by joining the 20 types of amino acids with peptide bonds.

peptide bond A chemical bond formed to link amino acids in a protein.

■ Protein Synthesis

Since the human genome was deciphered in 2000, interest in human genetics and the role it plays in disease has increased. We discussed that in Chapter 1. What wasn't covered in detail in that chapter is how cells use the genome to make body proteins.

We need to begin with the composition of DNA, present in the nucleus of the cell. Recall from Chapter 3 that DNA is a double stranded molecule in a helical form. Each strand of DNA is composed of four nucleotides: adenine (A), guanine (G), cytosine (C), and thymine (T). Each of the nucleotides is complementary to (binds to) another nucleotide; A and T are complementary, as are C and G. Soon you will see why that is important.

DNA contains coded instructions for protein synthesis that exists in a sequence of three nucleotides per unit of instruction (i.e., which specific amino acid are to be placed in a protein).[6] These nucleotide units (e.g., GAG) are called codons. Each DNA codon represents a specific amino acid. For example, the codon CTC represents the amino acid glutamic acid. Some amino acids have only one possible codon, whereas others have as many as six. The amino acid glutamic acid actually has two codons: CTC and CTT. Having the correct codons in the DNA is critical for producing the correct protein, since the order of the codons in the DNA indicates the order of the specific amino acids needed to synthesize a particular protein. This is important, since mistakes in the order or types of amino acids in a protein can result in profound health consequences (see the discussion of sickle cell disease in a later section of this chapter).

Protein synthesis in a cell takes place in the cytosol, not in the nucleus. Thus, the DNA code used for synthesis of a specific protein must be transferred to the cytosol to allow for such synthesis. That is the job of messenger RNA (mRNA). To produce mRNA, the DNA in the nucleus unwinds from its supercoiled state. Enzymes read the code on the DNA and transcribe that into a complementary single-stranded mRNA, called the primary transcript (Fig. 7-2). This is the transcription phase of protein synthesis. The segment that is read is the gene. In this process, A becomes uricil (U) C becomes G, T becomes A, and G becomes C. You might wonder why A did not become T, as A and T are complementary. It turns out that mRNA uses uricil (U) instead of thymine (T) in its code. Thus, the DNA code ACTGAT yields an mRNA of UGACUA. The actual DNA codons are ACT and GAT:

$$
\begin{array}{cccccc}
A & C & T & G & A & T \\
\downarrow & \downarrow & \downarrow & \downarrow & \downarrow & \downarrow \\
U & G & A & C & U & A
\end{array}
$$

The primary transcript mRNA undergoes processing in the nucleus to remove any parts of the DNA code that do not code for protein synthesis, called introns (these actually make up much of the DNA). (The portions of the DNA that code for protein synthesis are called exons.) Some additional processing then takes place and the final (mature) mRNA transcript is ready to leave the nucleus.

The mRNA travels to the ribosomes in the cytosol, present on the rough endoplasmic reticulum. The ribosomes read the codons on the mRNA and translate those instructions in order to produce a specific protein. This is the translation phase of protein synthesis. Amino acids are added one at a time to the polypeptide chain as directed by the instructions on the mRNA. Energy input from ATP is needed to add

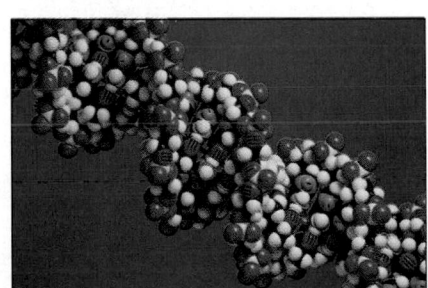

Genes are present on DNA—a double-helix. The cell nucleus contains most of the DNA in the body.

■ **FIGURE 7-2** Protein synthesis (simplified). *(a)* DNA present in the nucleus of the cell is composed of four nucleotides: adenine (A), guanine (G), cytosine (C), and thymine (T). The DNA code is read, three nucleotides at a time, called codons. Each DNA codon represents a specific amino acid. The DNA unwinds from its supercoiled state and the code embedded in the order of the nucleotides is transcribed into a complementary messenger RNA (mRNA; labeled as the primary RNA transcript). The mRNA is processed in the nucleus and then is ready to leave the nucleus. The mRNA travels to the cytosol, where the ribosomes then read the codons on the mRNA and translate those instructions in order to produce a specific protein (see Figure 7-2b). *(b)* Protein synthesis at the ribosomes begins at a specific starting point, indicated by AUG. Protein synthesis then continues by adding one amino acid at a time to the growing polypeptide chain until a specific ending (stop) codon is reached, such as UAA, UAG, or UGA. Transfer RNA (tRNA) units bring amino acids to the ribosomes as needed during protein synthesis. The tRNA carriers have a complementary code to the mRNA—such that, if an arginine were needed during synthesis, the AGA on the mRNA would correspond to UCU on the tRNA. Numerous tRNA carriers are present during protein synthesis to continually supply the ribosomes with needed amino acids. ATP is used to supply the energy needed to activate tRNA in order to form each new peptide bond. The polypeptide is then released from the ribosome. Appendix B contains the abbreviations used for the amino acids in this figure, such as "met" for "methionine."

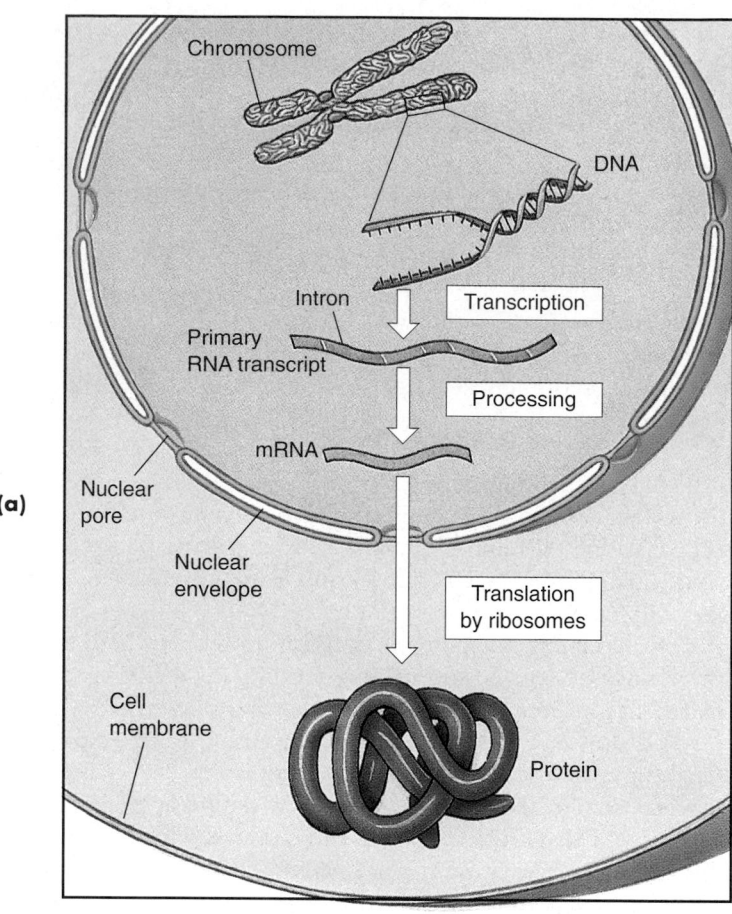

(a)

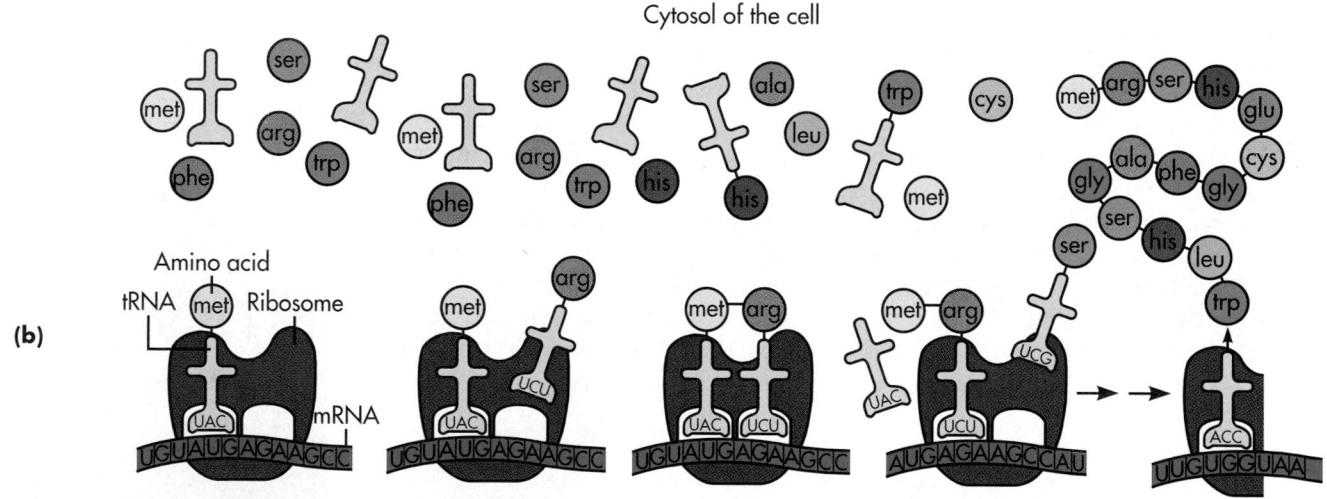

(b)

The initiation complex forms when the ribosomal subunits and the first tRNA molecule lock into a strand of mRNA at the start codon (AUG).

A tRNA carrying the amino acid specified second in the mRNA sequence plugs into the complex.

A peptide bond forms between the adjacent amino acids.

As the first tRNA detaches from the mRNA template, the second moves over, trailing its small amino acid chain. A third tRNA sits down at the vacated site, which is now situated over the next codon in the sequence.

each amino acid to the growing polypeptide chain, making protein synthesis very "costly" to the body in terms of energy use. Many ribosomes can combine to simultaneously translate a large mRNA.

Protein synthesis begins at a specific starting point on the mRNA, indicated by AUG. It then continues until a specific ending (stop) codon is reached, such as UAA, UAG, or UGA.

One key participant in protein synthesis in the cytosol is transfer RNA (tRNA). These units bring amino acids to the ribosomes as needed during protein synthesis (see Fig. 7-2). The tRNA carriers have a complementary code to the mRNA—such that, if an arginine were needed during synthesis, the AGA on the mRNA would correspond to UCU on the transfer RNA. Numerous tRNA carriers are present during protein synthesis to continually supply the ribosomes with needed amino acids.

Once synthesis of the polypeptide is completed, indicated by the ending codon, it is released from the ribosomes, as is the mRNA. The polypeptide may then undergo further metabolism in the cell, such as is true for the hormone insulin, or be functional as such. Generally, if synthesis of a particular protein needs to be increased in a cell, more mRNA for that protein is made.

The important message in this discussion is the relationship between DNA and the ultimate proteins produced by a cell. If the DNA contains errors, an incorrect mRNA will be produced. The ribosomes will then read this incorrect message and produce an incorrect polypeptide chain. As discussed in Chapter 1, ultimately we may be able to correct gene defects such that the correct DNA code can be placed in the nucleus, so that the correct protein can be made by the ribosomes.

■ Protein Turnover

Cell proteins are constantly undergoing degradation (breakdown) and synthesis. This process, called protein turnover, allows cells to adapt to changing circumstances. For example, when we eat more protein, the liver needs to make more enzymes to process the waste product of some the resulting amino acid metabolism—ammonia—into urea. The amino acids needed to make the enzymes can come from the diet and from amino acids released from the breakdown of other proteins in cells. For example, the GI tract lining is constantly **sloughed** off. The digestive tract treats sloughed cells just like food particles and absorbs the amino acids released during their digestion. In fact, most protein breakdown products—amino acids—released throughout the body can be recycled and are added to the pool of amino acids available for future protein synthesis. Overall, protein turnover is a process by which a cell can respond to its changing environment and produce needed proteins while reducing the content of proteins not currently needed (Figure 7-3).[15]

During any day, an adult makes and degrades about 300 g of protein; many of the amino acids are recycled. By comparing 300 g with the 65–95 g or more of protein typically consumed by adults, you can see the importance of recycling amino acids in the body when possible.[15]

Hormones that increase protein synthesis are insulin and growth hormone. In contrast, the hormone cortisol increases protein breakdown (see Chapter 4).

A practical example of the concept of protein turnover occurs in untreated AIDS, as is seen in the developing world (see Chapter 20). Rates of protein synthesis are similar in healthy people and those with untreated or untreatable cases of AIDS, but the rates of protein degradation are much higher due to the effects of the disease. Over time, this results in much protein wasting in such people with AIDS.

■ Protein Organization

The sequential order of the amino acids in the polypeptide chain, called *primary structure,* determines a protein's shape. The key point is that only correctly positioned amino acids can interact and fold properly to form the intended shape for the

---

A Synopsis of the Steps in Protein Synthesis
Part of DNA code (gene) is transcribed to mRNA in the nucleus.

↓

mRNA leaves the nucleus and travels to cytosol.

↓

Ribosomes in the cytosol and rough endoplasmic reticulum read the mRNA code and translate that into directions for a specific order of amino acids in a polypeptide chain

↓

To produce the polypeptide, tRNA brings the appropriate amino acid to the ribosome as dictated by the mRNA code. The amino acid is added to the existing amino acid chain, which begins with the amino acid methionine.

↓

When synthesis of the polypeptide is complete, it is released from the ribosome.

↓

Often the polypeptide will undergo further cell metabolism in order to function as a specific body protein—once it folds into its active form.

sloughed Shed or cast off.

*S*ulfur-containing amino acids stabilize many compounds, such as the hormone insulin. Sulfur atoms can bond together ($-S-S-$), creating a bridge between two protein strands or two parts of the same strand. This stabilizes the structure of the molecule and is also part of what is called *secondary structure.*

▌FIGURE 7-3 Amino acid metabolism. The amino acid pool in a cell can be used to yield body proteins, as well as a variety of other possible products—from fat and glucose to urea. The urea is a waste product made from the nitrogen-containing ammonia (NH_3) released during amino acid breakdown.

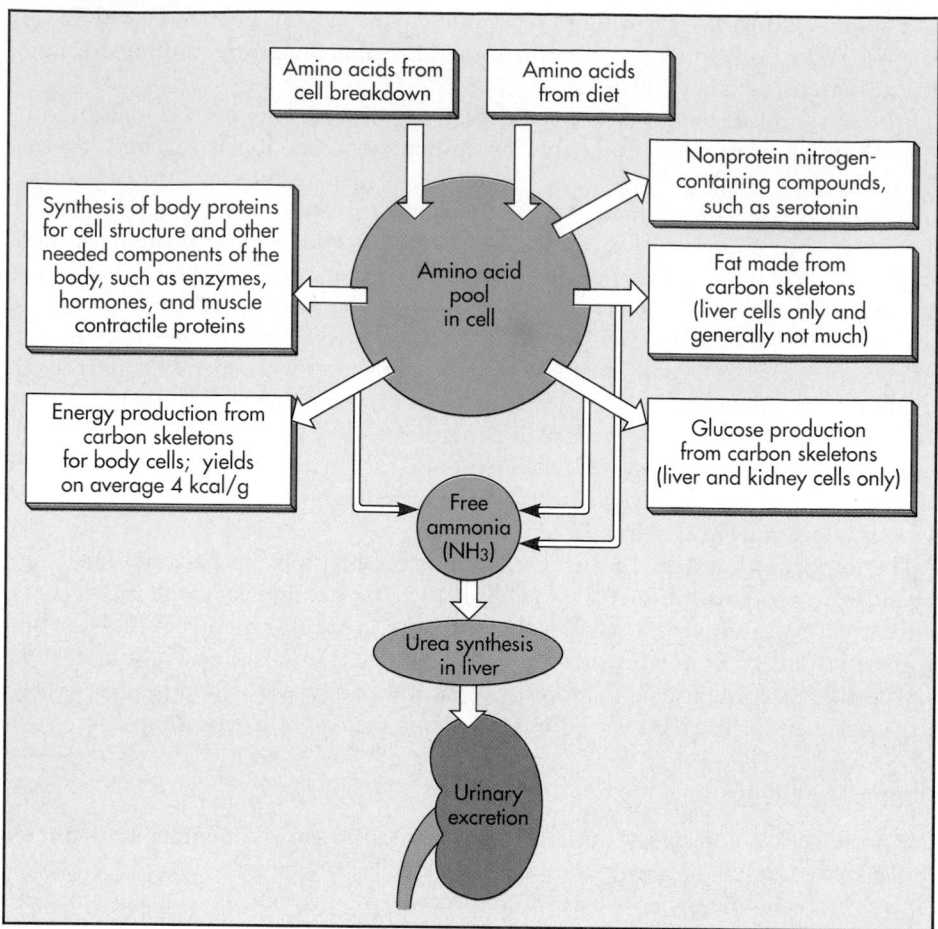

protein and, in turn, allow for the chemical attractions to form between amino acids that are needed to stabilize the structure, such as hydrogen bonds (see Appendix B for details). This is part of what is called *secondary structure*. The resulting unique three-dimensional form, called *tertiary structure,* dictates the function of each protein. If it lacks the appropriate configuration, a protein cannot function.[13]

In some cases, two or more separate protein units interact to form an even larger new protein form, termed a *quaternary structure* (Fig. 7-4). This organization becomes significant when it is important to have a protein active only at certain times. A protein may be active when the units are joined but inactive when the units are separate.

Sickle cell disease (also called **sickle cell anemia**) illustrates what happens when amino acids are out of order in the primary structure of a particular protein. African-Americans (about 3 cases per 1000 births) are especially prone to this genetic disease.[10] It originates from a mutation in the genetic sequence and results in defective production of the protein chains of hemoglobin, a compound found in red blood cells. In two of its four protein chains, a slight error in the amino acid order occurs. This small error produces a profound change in hemoglobin structure: It can no longer form the shape needed to carry oxygen efficiently inside the red blood cell. Instead of forming normal biconcave disks, the red blood cells collapse into crescent shapes (Fig. 7-5). Health deteriorates, and eventually episodes of severe bone and joint pain, abdominal pain, headache, convulsions, and paralysis may occur. This is because the sickled cells clump in the capillary beds, hampering blood flow to the target tissue. Treatment for this disease includes blood transfusions and possibly medications (e.g., hydroxyurea) to increase red blood cell synthesis.

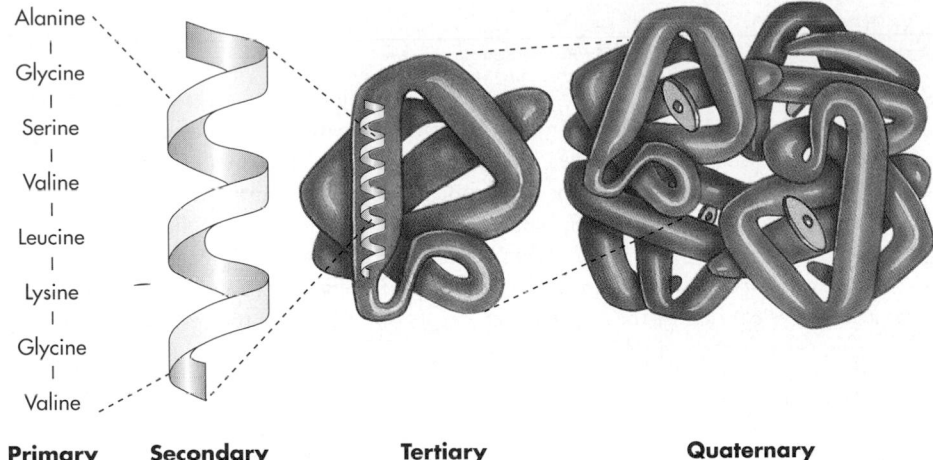

Alanine
|
Glycine
|
Serine
|
Valine
|
Leucine
|
Lysine
|
Glycine
|
Valine

Primary   Secondary   Tertiary   Quaternary

FIGURE **7-4** Levels of protein structure. Four different levels of structure are found in proteins. The primary structure of a protein is the linear sequence of amino acids in the polypeptide chain. Secondary structure consists of areas in the polypeptide chain which have a specific shape stabilized by hydrogen and other bonds. The total three-dimensional shape of entire proteins is called tertiary structure. Some proteins also show quarternary structure where two or more protein units join together to form a larger protein, such as hemoglobin depicted in the figure.

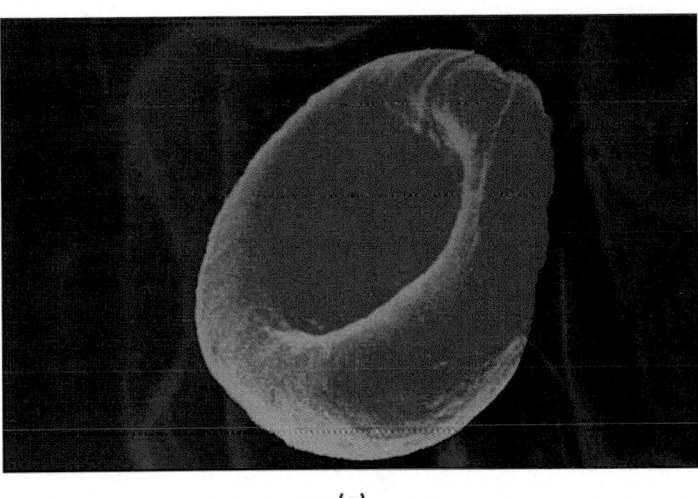

(a)

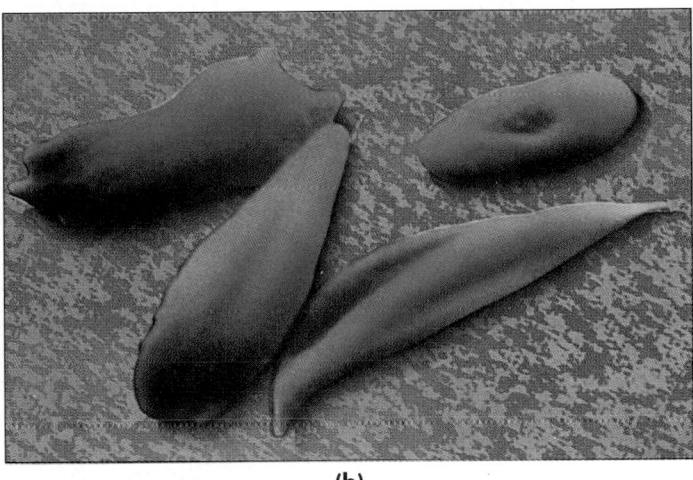

(b)

FIGURE **7-5** Sickle cell disease from the perspective of the red blood cell. (a) Normal red cell, (b) blood from a person with sickle cell disease. Note the abnormal crescent (sicklelike) shape of the red blood cell near the center.

■ Denaturation of Proteins

Treatment with acid or alkaline substances, heat, or agitation can alter a protein's structure, leaving it in a **denatured** state. The protein can no longer perform its function. For example, once the bacteria in yogurt have synthesized enough acid and enzymes to precipitate some of the milk protein, the product solidifies irreversibly. Note that denaturation does not affect the primary structure.

Unraveling a protein's shape often destroys its normal functioning, such that it loses its biological activity. That characteristic is useful for some body processes, such as digestion. The secretion of stomach acid denatures some bacteria, plant hormones, many active enzymes, and other forms of proteins in foods. The heat produced during cooking likewise denatures proteins. Both processes make foods safer to eat. Digestion is also enhanced because the unraveling increases exposure of the food to digestive enzymes. Denaturing proteins in some foods can also reduce their tendencies to cause allergic reactions.

Recall that we need proteins in the diet to supply essential amino acids—not the active proteins themselves. We dismantle the dietary proteins and use the amino acids to assemble proteins we need.[15]

denaturation Alteration of a protein's three-dimensional structure, usually because of treatment by heat, enzymes, acid or alkaline solutions, or agitation.

CRITICAL THINKING

Samantha's mother's blood concentration of urea is high. From a health status point of view, what might this indicate?

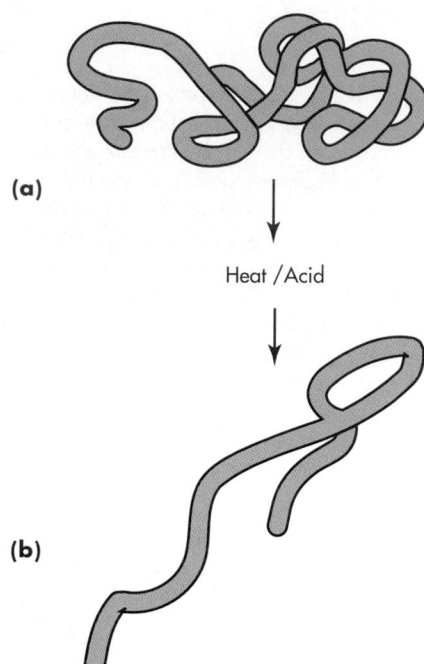

(a)

Heat /Acid

(b)

(a) Protein showing a typical coiled state. (b) Protein is now partly uncoiled, exhibiting a denatured state. This uncoiling typically reduces protein function.

pepsin A protein-digesting enzyme produced by the stomach.

gastrin A hormone that stimulates enzyme and acid secretion by the stomach.

trypsin A protein-digesting enzyme secreted by the pancreas to act in the small intestine.

CONCEPT CHECK

Amino acids are linked together in specific sequences to form distinct proteins. Proteins in cells are in a constant state of turnover. The degradation of existing proteins and synthesis of new proteins takes place on a minute-by-minute basis, amounting to a turnover about 300 g a day for the entire human body. DNA provide the directions for synthesizing these new proteins. Specifically, DNA directs the order of the amino acids on the protein. The amino acid order within a protein determines its ultimate shape and function. Destroying the shape of a protein denatures it. Acid conditions present during the body's digestive processes, heat, and other factors can denature proteins, causing them to lose their biological activity.

■ PROTEIN DIGESTION AND ABSORPTION

As with carbohydrates, cooking food can be viewed as a first step in protein digestion. Cooking unfolds (denatures) proteins and softens tough connective tissue in meat. Cooking also makes many protein-rich foods easier to chew, swallow, and break down during later digestion and absorption. As you will see in Chapter 19, cooking also makes many protein-rich foods, such as meats, eggs, fish, and poultry, much safer to eat.

■ Protein Digestion

The enzymatic digestion of protein begins in the stomach.[14] When proteins are denatured by stomach acid, **pepsin,** a major enzyme for proteins, goes to work (Fig. 7-6). Pepsin attacks the polypeptide chains and breaks them down into shorter chains of amino acids. Pepsin does not completely separate proteins into amino acids because it can break only a few of the many peptide bonds found in these large molecules. The reaction that takes place is a hydrolysis reaction, since water is used to break down the bond.

Pepsinogen, the inactive form of pepsin, lies in the chief cells of the stomach. In proximity are acid-forming cells (called *parietal cells*) and mucus-forming cells (called *goblet cells*) in gastric pits in the stomach (review Fig. 3-13). If pepsin were not stored as an inactive enzyme, it would digest the stomach glands while waiting to be secreted from the pits. Once pepsinogen enters the stomach's acidic environment (pH between 1 and 2), part of the enzyme is split off, forming the active enzyme pepsin.

The release of pepsin is controlled by the hormone **gastrin** (review Table 3-8). Thinking about food or chewing food stimulates gastrin-producing cells in the terminus of the stomach to release the hormone. Gastrin also strongly stimulates the stomach's parietal cells to produce acid.

The partially digested proteins move with the rest of the nutrients and other substances in a meal (chyme) from the stomach into the duodenum, the first part of the small intestine. Once in the small intestine, the polypeptide units (and any fats accompanying them) trigger the release of the hormone cholecystokinin (CCK) from the walls of the small intestine. CCK, in turn, travels through the bloodstream to its target organs, the pancreas and gallbladder. This causes the pancreas to release the protein-splitting enzymes **trypsin,** chymotrypsin, and carboxypeptidase, which are released into the small intestine in their inactive forms and then activated by digestive secretions. Together, these digestive enzymes divide the polypeptides into short peptides and amino acids. Eventually, digestion of all peptides into amino acids occurs, using other enzymes secreted into the intestinal lumen by glands located in the small intestine, as well as enzymes inside the absorptive cells of the small intestine.

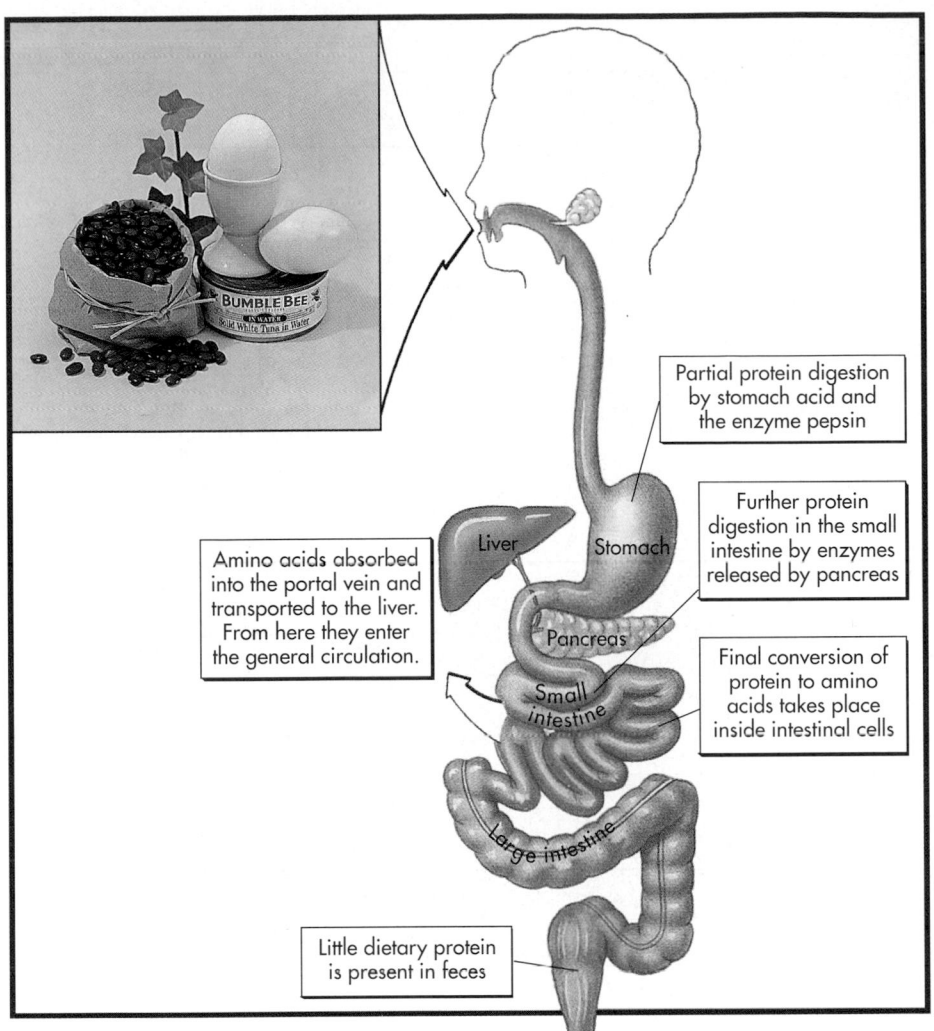

Partial protein digestion by stomach acid and the enzyme pepsin

Further protein digestion in the small intestine by enzymes released by pancreas

Amino acids absorbed into the portal vein and transported to the liver. From here they enter the general circulation.

Final conversion of protein to amino acids takes place inside intestinal cells

Liver

Stomach

Pancreas

Small intestine

Large intestine

Little dietary protein is present in feces

■ FIGURE **7-6** A summary of protein digestion and absorption. Enzymatic protein digestion begins in the stomach and ends in the absorptive cells of the small intestine, where the last peptides are broken down into single amino acids. Stomach acid and enzymes contribute to protein digestion. Absorption from the intestinal lumen into the absorptive cells requires energy input.
Illustration by William Ober.

■ Amino Acid Absorption

The small peptides and amino acids in the lumen of the small intestine are actively absorbed into the cells of the small intestine (Fig. 7-7). Eleven or so different amino acid transport mechanisms in the intestinal tract have been described.[14] Few whole proteins are absorbed. The only time that this is not true is during infancy (up to 4 to 5 months of age). Until that time, whole proteins can be absorbed by the intestines of infants. This is particularly harmful if infants are fed cow's milk or egg whites, as these may predispose the infant to food allergies (see Chapter 17 for details).

The absorbed small peptides, then, are eventually broken down to individual amino acids inside the intestinal cells. The amino acids travel via the portal vein to the liver, where they are combined into protein, converted to glucose or fat, used for energy needs, or released into the bloodstream.

CONCEPT CHECK

Enzymatic protein digestion begins in the stomach. In the small intestine, protein breakdown products formed in the stomach separate into dipeptides and tripeptides and finally into amino acids, as these further breakdown products enter the absorptive cells of the small intestine. The amino acids then travel via the portal vein to the liver.

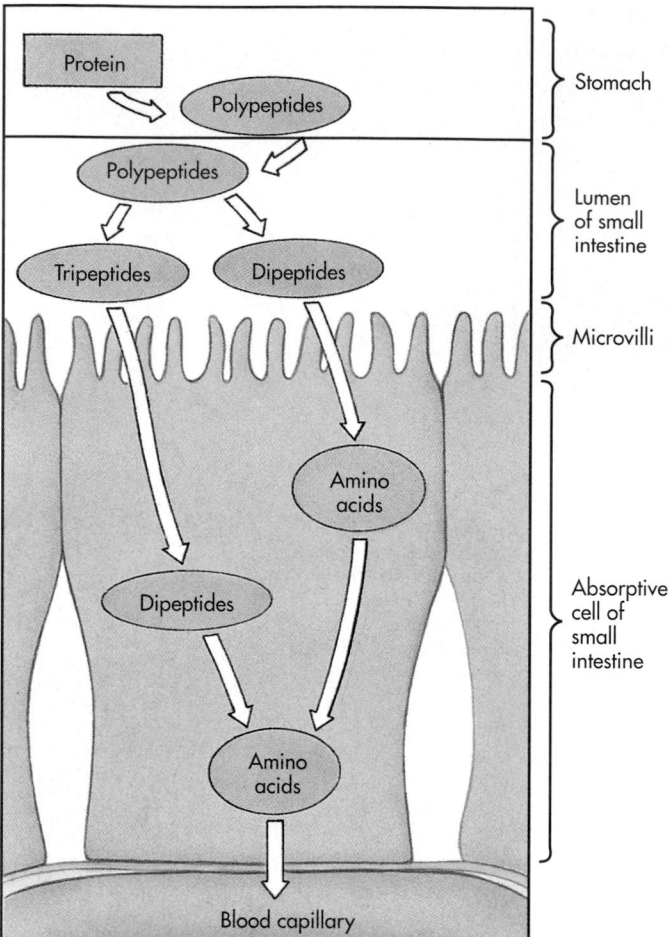

■ FIGURE 7-7 Protein digestion and amino acid absorption. This takes place in the stomach, lumen of the small intestine, and the absorptive cells of the small intestine. In a sodium-dependent, energy-requiring process (active absorption) much like glucose absorption, all of the end products of protein digestion are broken down at the microvilli surface and within the absorptive cell to amino acids. These free amino acids are released into the bloodstream. The enzymes used come from the stomach, pancreas, and absorptive and glandular cells that line the small intestine.

Illustration by William Ober.

■ FUNCTIONS OF PROTEINS

As you have learned, proteins function in many crucial ways in human metabolism and the formation of body structures (review Figure 7-3). We rely on foods to supply the amino acids needed to form these proteins. Note, however, that only when we also eat enough carbohydrate and fat can food proteins be used most efficiently. If we don't consume enough energy to meet energy needs, some amino acids from proteins are broken down to produce needed energy, rather than used to make needed body proteins.

■ Producing Vital Body Constituents

Every cell contains protein. Muscles, connective tissue, mucus, blood-clotting factors, blood-transport proteins, lipoproteins, enzymes, immune bodies, some hormones, visual pigments, and the support structure inside bones are mainly made of protein. Half of body protein is made up of the structural proteins collagen, actin, and myosin, as well as the oxygen-transporting protein hemoglobin.[13] This structural role is the primary function of protein in the body. Measurements of the amounts of certain body proteins, particularly some of those in the blood, are used as indicators of health or disease. Excess protein in the diet doesn't necessarily enhance the synthesis of body components, but eating too little can impede it.

As mentioned before, most vital body proteins are in a constant state of breakdown, rebuilding, and repair, especially in the bone marrow and the intestine. If a person habitually doesn't eat enough protein, the rebuilding and repairing process

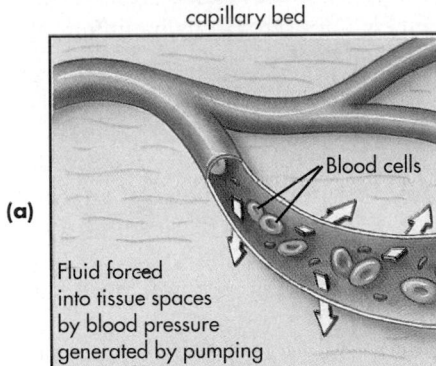
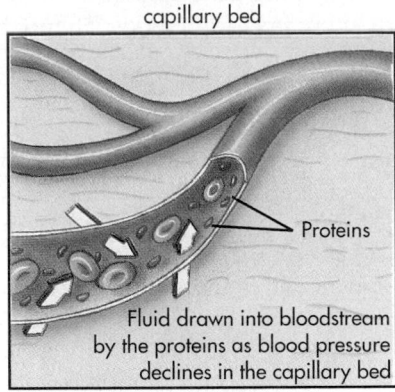

Arterial end of
capillary bed

Venous end of
capillary bed

(a)

Blood cells

Proteins

Fluid forced
into tissue spaces
by blood pressure
generated by pumping
action of heart

Fluid drawn into bloodstream
by the proteins as blood pressure
declines in the capillary bed

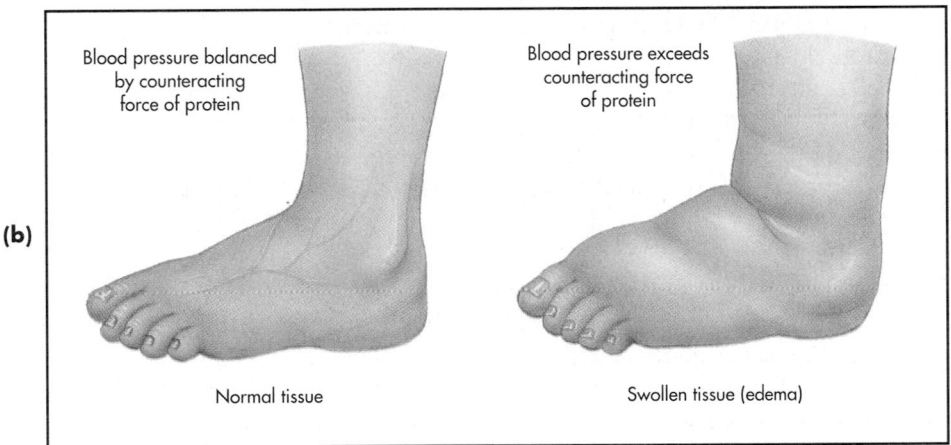

(b)

Blood pressure balanced
by counteracting
force of protein

Blood pressure exceeds
counteracting force
of protein

Normal tissue

Swollen tissue (edema)

■ FIGURE **7-8** Blood proteins in relation to fluid balance. (*a*) Blood proteins are important for maintaining the body's fluid balance, since they draw fluid back into the capillary bed. (*b*) Without sufficient protein in the bloodstream, edema develops because the counteracting force to blood pressure provided by blood proteins declines.

Illustration by William Ober.

slows. Eventually, skeletal muscles, heart, liver, blood proteins, and other organs decrease in size or volume. Only the brain resists protein breakdown.

■ Maintaining Fluid Balance

Blood proteins—albumins and globulins—maintain body fluid balance. Blood pressure in the arteries forces blood into capillary beds. The blood fluid then enters from the **capillary beds** into the spaces between nearby cells (**extracellular spaces**) to provide nutrients to those cells (Fig. 7-8). Proteins in the bloodstream are too large to move out of the capillary beds into the tissues. The presence of these proteins in the capillary beds attracts the fluid back to the blood, partially counteracting the force of blood pressure. This is especially true in the areas of the capillary beds right next to their venous connections.

Unless enough protein is consumed, the concentration of proteins eventually decreases in the bloodstream. Excessive fluid then builds up in the surrounding tissues because the counteracting force produced by the smaller amount of blood proteins is too weak to pull much of the fluid back from the tissues into the bloodstream. As fluids pool in the tissues, the tissues swell, causing clinical **edema.** Because edema sometimes leads to serious medical problems, the cause must be identified. An important step in diagnosing the cause is to measure the concentration of blood proteins, although many other medical problems cause edema.

■ Contributing to Acid-Base Balance

Proteins help regulate the **pH**—the acid-base balance—in the blood. Proteins located in cell membranes pump chemical ions in and out of cells. The pumping action, among other factors, keeps the blood slightly alkaline. **Buffers**—compounds that maintain acid-base conditions within a narrow range—are another means

*F*igure 3-5 in Chapter 3 provides a detailed view of a capillary bed.

capillary bed Minute vessels one cell thick that create a junction between arterial and venous circulation. It is here that gas and nutrient exchange occurs between body cells and the blood.

extracellular space The space outside cells.

edema The buildup of excess fluid in extracellular spaces.

pH A measure of relative acidity or alkalinity of a solution. The pH scale is 0–14. A pH below 7 is acidic; a pH above 7 is alkaline.

buffers Compounds that cause a solution to resist changes in acid-base balance.

of regulating acid-base balance in the blood. Some blood proteins are especially good buffers for the body. Hemoglobin is extremely important in maintaining normal blood pH.

■ Forming Hormones and Enzymes

Amino acids are required for the synthesis of many hormones—our internal body messengers. Some hormones, such as the thyroid hormones, are made from only one amino acid, tyrosine. Insulin, on the other hand, is composed of 48 amino acids. These and other hormones classified as proteins perform important regulatory functions in the body, such as controlling the metabolic rate and amount of glucose taken up from the bloodstream.

Almost all enzymes are proteins or have a protein component. Enzymes are compounds that speed chemical reactions. Occasionally, a cell lacks the correct genetic information to make needed enzymes. For example, an infant who has the disease **galactosemia** can't make an enzyme needed to metabolize the single sugar galactose. If the infant is not started on a galactose-free diet soon after birth—which in practical terms means no cow's milk, human milk, liver, and certain other foods—its growth and mental development will be depressed. A special infant formula must be used. The galactose-free diet is then continued, ideally throughout life. This example underscores the crucial roles that enzymes, and thus proteins, play in cell function.

■ Contributing to Immune Function

Proteins compose key parts of the cells used by the immune system. Also, the antibodies produced by one type of immune cell (β-lymphocytes) are proteins. These antibodies can bind to foreign proteins in the body, an important step in removing invaders from the body (recall from Chapter 3 how the immune system works). Without sufficient dietary protein, the immune system lacks the cells and other tools needed to function properly. Thus, immune incompetence—**anergy**—and a protein-deficient diet often appear together. Anergy can turn measles into a fatal disease for a malnourished child. It also can encourage unusual infections, such as widespread yeast *(Candida)* growth in the mouth and throat of a hospitalized adult.

■ Forming Glucose

In Chapter 5 you learned that the body must maintain a fairly constant concentration of blood glucose to supply energy for red blood cells and nervous tissue. At rest, the brain uses about 19% of the body's energy requirements, and it gets most of that energy from glucose. If you don't consume enough carbohydrate to supply the glucose, your liver (and kidneys, to a lesser extent) will be forced to make glucose from amino acids (review Fig. 7-3). Recall from Chapter 4 that the process is called gluconeogenesis (review Figure 4-10).

Making some glucose from amino acids is normal. For example, when you skip breakfast and haven't eaten since 7 P.M. the preceding evening, glucose must be manufactured. Taken to an extreme, however, such as occurs in starvation, the conversion of amino acids into glucose wastes much muscle tissue and can produce edema.

■ Providing Energy

Proteins supply very little of the energy to the body, except during prolonged exercise (see Chapter 14 for information about the use of amino acids for energy during exercise). Under most conditions, cells use primarily carbohydrates and fats for energy. Proteins and carbohydrates contain the same amount of usable energy—on average, 4 kcal/g. However, proteins are a very costly source of energy, considering the amount of metabolism and processing the liver and kidneys must perform to use this energy source. The monetary cost of protein-rich foods is also a consideration.

Neurotransmitters, released by nerve endings, are often derivatives of amino acids. This is true for dopamine (synthesized from tyrosine), norepinephrine (synthesized from tyrosine), and serotonin (synthesized from tryptophan). The way in which diet influences the synthesis of some of these neurotransmitters is currently under study. For example, high-carbohydrate meals can induce sleepiness as a result of increased serotonin synthesis in the brain.

anergy Lack of an immune response to foreign compounds entering the body.

The vitamin niacin can be made from the amino acid tryptophan, illustrating another role of proteins.

CONCEPT CHECK

*V*ital body constituents—such as muscle, connective tissue, blood transport proteins, enzymes, hormones, buffers, and immune factors—are mainly proteins. Proteins can also provide fuel for the body and be used for glucose production.

■ PROTEIN NEEDS

How much protein (actually, amino acids) do we need to eat each day? People who aren't growing need to eat only enough protein to match whatever they lose daily from protein breakdown products found in urine, feces, skin, hair, nails, and so on. In short, people need to balance protein intake with such losses. This maintains a state of protein equilibrium (Fig. 7-9).[14]

When a body is growing or recovering from an illness, it needs a positive protein balance to supply the raw materials required to build new tissues. To achieve this, a person must eat more protein daily than he or she loses. In addition, the hormones insulin, growth hormone, and testosterone all stimulate positive protein balance. Merely eating more protein does not produce additional body tissue unless the right hormonal condition exists. Resistance exercise (weight training) also enhances positive balance.[17]

For healthy people, the amount of dietary protein needed to maintain protein equilibrium (wherein intake equals losses) can be determined by increasing protein intake until it just equals losses. Energy needs must be met so that amino acids are not diverted for energy use. To determine this balance between protein gain and loss by the body, researchers actually calculate nitrogen balance; only the nitrogen from

*T*he RDA for protein translates into about 8 to 10% of calories. Many experts recommend up to 15% of calories to provide more flexibility in diet planning, in turn allowing for the variety of protein-rich foods North Americans typically consume. This amount generally provides enough protein for the active

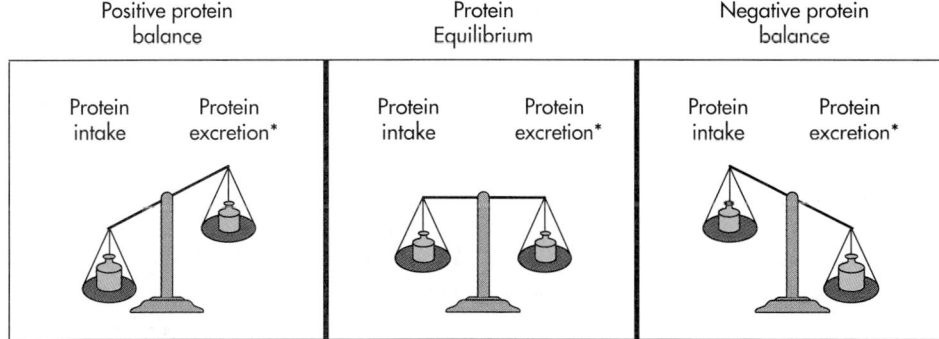

Situations in which protein balance is positive:

Growth
Pregnancy
Recovery stage after illness
Athletic training**
Increased secretion of hormones, such as insulin, growth hormone, and testosterone

Situations in which protein balance is negative:

Inadequate intake of protein (fasting, intestinal tract diseases)
Inadequate energy intake
Conditions such as fevers, burns, and infections
Bed rest (for several days)
Deficiency of essential amino acids
Increased protein loss (as in some forms of kidney disease)
Increased secretion of certain hormones, such as thyroid hormone and cortisol

*Based on losses of urea and other nitrogen-containing compounds in the urine, as well as protein as such from hair, nails, skin, and other sources.
**Only when additional lean body mass is being gained. Nevertheless, the athlete is probably already eating enough protein to support this extra protein synthesis; protein supplements are not needed.

■ FIGURE 7-9 Protein balance in practical terms. Determining this balance requires measuring nitrogen intake and loss.

weight of a protein, so nitrogen intake or output divided by 0.16 yields a rough estimate of protein intake or output. One can also multiply by the reciprocal of 0.16, which is 6.25:

$$\text{nitrogen (grams)} \times 6.25 = \text{protein (grams)}$$

As an example of the measurement of nitrogen balance, first a person's protein intake is monitored: This includes protein that comes in the form of fluids and foods. The grams of protein consumed is divided by 6.25 to yield the approximate grams of nitrogen (N) consumed. This value is then compared with the amount of nitrogen lost from the body. To do this, urine output for the same 24-hour period is collected and analyzed for urea nitrogen content. This value is then put into one of various formulas available to estimate total nitrogen loss from the body. Since most of the nitrogen lost from the body is in the form of urea (urinary urea N), this approach is fairly accurate. The other factors in a specific formula account for nitrogen loss in the urine that is not in the form of urea (e.g., 0.2 × urinary urea), as well as nitrogen loss from all other body sources, such as hair, skin, feces, and other nonurine sources (e.g., 2 g).

$$\text{nitrogen balance} = \frac{\text{protein intake}}{6.25 \text{ g}} - \text{urinary urea N} - (0.2 \times \text{g urinary urea N}) - 2 \text{ g}$$

For example, suppose a person consumes 70 g of protein in a 24-hour period; during that time he excreted 7 g of nitrogen as urea. His state of nitrogen balance is 0.8, based on the following calculation:

$$\text{nitrogen balance} = \frac{70}{6.25} - 7 - (0.2 \times 7) - 2$$
$$= 0.8$$

Since this is a positive number, the person is in slight positive nitrogen balance. Due to measurement error, he could also simply be in nitrogen equilibrium.

Today the best estimate for the amount of protein required for nearly all adults to maintain protein equilibrium is 0.8 g of protein per kilogram (kg) of healthy body weight. This is the current RDA for protein. The amount approximately doubles during infancy. (Specific values for infants and children are discussed in Chapter 17 and the concept of healthy weight in Chapter 13). Healthy weight is used as a baseline because excess fat storage doesn't contribute much to protein needs. This RDA works out to about 56 g of protein daily for a typical 70-kg (154-lb) man and about 44 g of protein daily for a typical 55-kg (120-lb) woman.

$$\text{Convert weight from pounds to kg:} \quad \frac{154 \text{ pounds}}{2.2 \text{ pounds/kg}} = 70 \text{ kg}$$

$$\frac{120 \text{ pounds}}{2.2 \text{ pounds/kg}} = 55 \text{ kg}$$

$$\text{Calculate RDA:} \quad 70 \text{ kg} \times \frac{0.8 \text{ grams protein}}{\text{kg body weight}} = 56 \text{ g}$$

$$55 \text{ kg} \times \frac{0.8 \text{ grams protein}}{\text{kg body weight}} = 44 \text{ g}$$

Approximate protein needs based on the 1989 RDA publication are listed in the inside cover of this textbook. A new DRI for protein will be published in 2001 (see the website http://www4.nationalacademies.org/IOM/IOMHome.nsf/Pages/Food+and+Nutrition+Board). It is easy to consume the amount of protein currently suggested each day to meet body needs (Table 7-3). American men typically consume about 95 g of protein daily, whereas women typically consume 65 g daily.

TABLE 7-3 The Protein Content of a 1200 kcal Diet and a 2400 kcal Diet*			
1200 kcal Diet	**Protein (Grams)**	**2400 kcal Diet**	**Protein (Grams)**
Breakfast			
Nonfat milk, 1 cup	8	2% reduced-fat milk, 1 cup	8
Cheerios, 1 cup	2	Cheerios, 1 cup	2
Orange	1	Eggs, soft cooked, 2	12
		Orange	1
Lunch			
Whole-wheat bread, 2 slices	5	Whole-wheat bread, 2 slices	5
Chicken breast, 2 oz	17	Chicken breast, 2 oz	17
Mayonnaise, 1 tsp	—	Provolone cheese, 2 oz	15
Tomato slices, 2	—	Tomato slices, 2	—
Carrot sticks, 1 cup	1	Mayonnaise, 1 tsp	—
Fig, 1 large	0.5	Oatmeal-raisin cookies, 2	2
Diet soda	—	Figs, 2	1
		Diet soda	—
Dinner			
Mixed green salad, ½ cup	—	Mixed green salad, ½ cup	—
Italian dressing, 2 tsp	—	Italian dressing, 2 tsp	—
Beef tenderloin, 2 oz	14	Beef tenderloin, 4 oz	28
Spinach pasta, 1 cup, with garlic butter, 1 tsp	7	Spinach pasta, 1 cup, with garlic butter, 1 tsp	7
Zucchini, ½ cup, sauteed in oil, 1 tsp	0.5	Zucchini, ½ cup, sauteed in oil, 1 tsp	0.5
Nonfat milk, 1 cup	8	Carrot sticks, ½ cup	0.5
Bagel, toasted, ½ of a 3 ½" bagel	4		
Jam, 2 tsp	—	**Snack**	
		2% reduced-fat milk, 1 cup	8
		Bagel, toasted, ½ of 3½" bagel	4
		Jam, 2 tsp	—
		Fruited yogurt, 1 cup	10
TOTAL	70		122

*This table illustrates how little energy need be consumed while still meeting the RDA for protein. It also shows how much protein we eat when we consume typical energy intakes. The amounts work out to be about 25% of calories as protein, quite a generous amount.

Recall that an RDA is an allowance, not a requirement. Some people need less than that amount of protein. Most of us, however, get much more because we like many high-protein foods and can afford to buy them. Excess protein eaten cannot be stored as such, so it is turned into glucose or fat and then either stored or metabolized for energy needs (review Fig. 7-3). Pregnancy raises protein needs by about 10 to 15 g per day averaged over the 9 months and totaling 60 g/day in all for the diet. However, mental stress, physical labor, and routine weekend sports activities do not require an increase in the protein RDA.

To support the training needs of endurance and highly trained athletes, the protein allowance can be increased to about 1.5 to 2 times the RDA. There is no clear, demonstrated advantage however in exceeding 1.8 to 2 g of protein per kg of healthy body weight per day.[17] Many Americans, especially men, eat close to that much protein already. In addition, athletes do not need individual amino acid supplements. All of us, athletes included, can meet our protein needs using basic foods.

Surveys show that only older women as a group fail to eat enough protein to meet the RDA, and the deficiency is very slight. Older adults may also have slightly higher protein needs than those established by the RDA. Some researchers advocate an intake up to 1.2 g of protein/kg of healthy body weight.

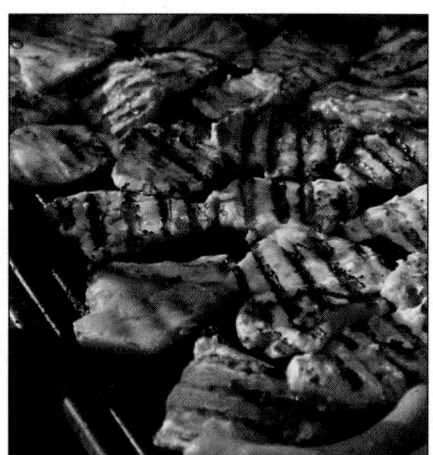

Animal protein foods are typically our favorite sources of amino acids.

■ DOES EATING A HIGH-PROTEIN DIET HARM YOU?

People frequently ask whether the high protein intake of adults in America is harmful. The extra vitamin B-6, iron, and zinc that accompany protein foods are often beneficial. However, high-protein diets typically are low in plant foods and, so, low in fiber, some vitamins (e.g., folate), some minerals (e.g., magnesium), and phytochemicals. As well, these diets are typically rich in saturated fat. As a consequence, consumption of animal protein (if not well trimmed of fat) has been linked to cardiovascular disease in humans, likely due to this saturated fat content.[4]

High-protein diets can increase calcium loss in urine.[5] Certain types of amino acids—especially some of those rich in animal proteins—cause this effect. Based on the research to date, it is reasonable to assume that individuals who have inadequate calcium intakes are further compromising bone health by consuming excessive amounts of protein. People meeting their calcium needs should not be concerned about this effect of dietary protein.

Excessive intake of red meat is linked to colon cancer in population studies. This link could be attributable to the protein or fat in the food products or to substances that form during cooking of red meat at high temperatures (heterocyclic amines; see the Nutrition Perspecive in Chapter 10).[22] Excessive fat intake associated with diets rich in red meat, or low dietary fiber intake, may also be a contributing factor. More research on this topic is needed before red meat can be singled out as a causative factor in colon cancer (cancer is discussed further in Chapter 10).

Some researchers have also expressed the concern that a high protein intake may unduly burden the kidneys by forcing them to excrete the resulting excess nitrogen as urea. Low-protein diets marginally slow the decline in kidney function in humans if begun early in the course of developing kidney disease, and laboratory animal studies show that protein intakes that just meet nutritional needs preserve kidney function over time better than high-protein diets. Preserving kidney function is especially important for people with diabetes, for people who show signs of kidney disease, and for people who have only one functioning kidney. High-protein diets are discouraged in these cases.[23] For people without diabetes or kidney disease, the risk of suffering kidney failure is very low; thus, the risk of a high-protein diet's contributing to kidney disease in later life is also low.

Generally speaking, most experts recommend that not more than twice the RDA for protein be consumed on a regular basis. Reducing intake to approximately RDA amounts may benefit some of us, as pointed out earlier, but the research is still too incomplete to permit a firm conclusion.

The amino acids most likely to cause toxicity when consumed in large amounts are methionine and tyrosine. The potential for amino acid imbalances and toxicities is too great to recommend that any be taken individually as supplements. As emphasized earlier, the body is designed to handle whole proteins as a dietary source of amino acids. When individual amino acid supplements are taken, they can overwhelm the absorptive mechanism in the small intestine, triggering amino acid imbalances in the body. These imbalances occur because groups of chemically similar amino acids compete for absorption sites in the absorptive cells. An excess of one can hamper other amino acids from being absorbed. Overall, every amino acid taken in excess can be harmful. Stick to whole foods as your source for amino acids.

Infants' diets must be limited in protein because their kidneys have difficulty excreting large amounts of urea and minerals, which remain after protein metabolism. Thus, regular cow's milk must not be used for feeding young infants—it is too high in protein and other nutrients (see Chapter 17 for details).

■ PROTEIN IN FOODS

The Exchange System provides an easy way to estimate the protein content of a food. The fruit and fat lists contain no protein; the vegetable list yields 2 g of protein; the starch list yields 3 g of protein; the meat list yields 7 g of protein; and the milk list yields 8 g of protein. The most nutrient-dense source of protein is water-packed tuna, which has over 80% of its energy as protein. Based on the typical foods

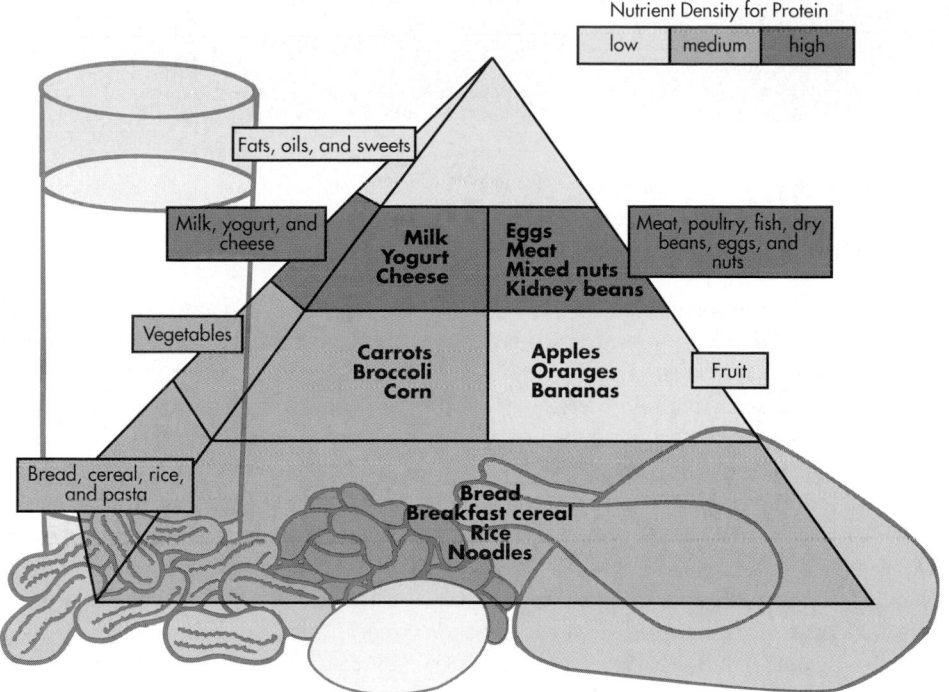

Nutrient Density for Protein

low	medium	high

Fats, oils, and sweets

Milk, yogurt, and cheese

Milk Yogurt Cheese

Eggs Meat Mixed nuts Kidney beans

Meat, poultry, fish, dry beans, eggs, and nuts

Vegetables

Carrots Broccoli Corn

Apples Oranges Bananas

Fruit

Bread, cereal, rice, and pasta

Bread Breakfast cereal Rice Noodles

■ FIGURE 7-10 Sources of protein in foods from the Food Guide Pyramid. The fruit group; vegetable group; and fats, oils, and sweets group contain few foods rich in protein, whereas the other groups contain foods with moderate to high amounts. The background color of each group indicates the average nutrient density for protein in that group.

we eat, about 69% of protein comes from animal sources (Fig. 7-10).[24] In the United States, meat, poultry, and fish consumption amounts to about 145 pounds (weight without bones) per person per year. Worldwide, 35% of protein comes from animal sources. In Africa and East Asia, about 20% of the protein eaten comes from animal sources.

■ The Value of Plant Protein

Vegetable sources of proteins deserve more attention from Americans. Many plant foods—in proportion to the amount of energy they supply—provide not only much protein but also ample magnesium and dietary fiber, along with other benefits.[20] The protein is used somewhat less efficiently by the body than are animal proteins (10 to 20% less), but this drop is not significant enough to influence diet planning when a variety of foods is used. The vegetable proteins we eat also contain no cholesterol and little saturated fat, unless these are added during processing. Regular use of plant foods high in protein makes a valuable addition to a diet because these supply a variety of other nutrients. Soy sources of proteins are receiving much attention today.[7] Dr. Mark Messina discusses why in his Expert Opinion.

Nuts are often overlooked as a source of plant protein. Recent studies have linked consumption of nuts to decreased blood cholesterol, heart disease, and blood pressure. The protective action of nuts probably stems from their lack of cholesterol and abundance of unsaturated fatty acids.[21, 27] These unsaturated fats do not raise total cholesterol like saturated fat. Of course, this benefit occurs only if nuts are used to replace saturated fats in the diet. Phytochemicals in nuts, such as flavonoids, are also thought to provide health benefits. For these reasons, a 30 g (1 oz) serving of nuts per day or 2 tbsp of peanut butter provide a rich source of protein. Nuts also contain vitamin E, magnesium, calcium, and fiber. However, it is important to keep in mind that nuts are very energy dense.

Legumes are a plant family with pods that contain a single row of seeds: garden and black-eyed peas; green, black, red, great northern, lima, kidney, pinto, and garbanzo beans; lentils; and soybeans. Dried varieties of the mature seeds—what we know as beans—also make an impressive contribution to the protein, vitamin, mineral, and dietary fiber content of a meal (Fig. 7-11). Regularly consuming these legume protein sources can add substantial amounts of nutrients to a diet.[12] More-

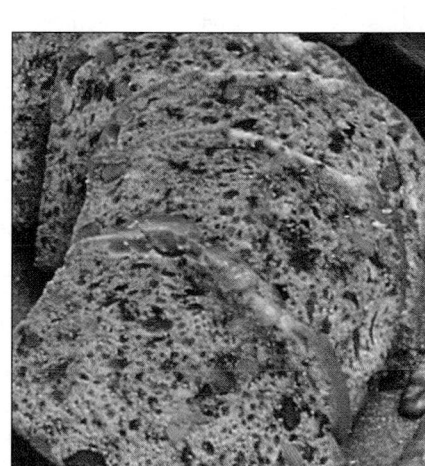

Nuts, like walnuts, can be incorporated into one's diet in numerous ways, such as adding them to banana bread.

*R*ecall from Chapter 5 that consumption of the oligosaccharides in beans can lead to intestinal gas and that a preparation called Beano® can greatly lessen symptoms if taken right before the meal.

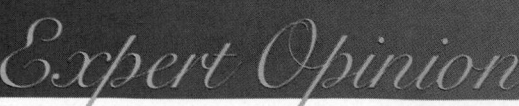
Expert Opinion

A CLOSE LOOK AT SOYBEANS

Mark Messina, Ph.D.

The reported health effects of soy have created a marked increase in consumer demand for soyfoods. The food industry has responded with a vast array of new soy products, prompted in part by an FDA decision to approve a health claim for the cholesterol-lowering effects of soy protein (see Chapter 2). Initial interest in soy during the early 1990s focused primarily on cancer prevention, but interest has expanded to include areas such as osteoporosis, heart disease, and relief of menopausal symptoms. Consequently, soy is being considered as a possible alternative to hormone replacement therapy for postmenopausal women. Like all plant foods, soy is a complex chemical mixture, but much of the focus on soy is because it is a unique dietary source of a group of phytochemicals called isoflavones.

SOY NUTRITION

Although soy protein was once considered inferior to animal protein, data now clearly indicate that soy protein is similar in quality to animal protein. As a result, the USDA now allows soy protein to totally replace (previous limitation was 30%) animal protein in the Federal School Lunch Program. Soybeans are relatively high in fat (40% of calories), with the predominant fatty acid being linoleic acid. The omega-3 fatty acid, α-linolenic acid, comprises about 7 to 8% of the total fat content. This makes soybeans one of the few good plant sources of this essential fatty

acid, an important attribute, since dietary data indicate that Americans do not consume enough of the omega-3 fatty acids.

Soybeans are also a relatively good source of calcium and—despite being high in oxalic acid and phytic acid, two factors that inhibit calcium absorption—calcium absorption from soy is similar to that from dairy milk. However, tofu (unless coagulated with calcium salts) and soymilk (unless calcium fortified) are not good sources of this calcium. Furthermore, calcium from fortified soymilk is absorbed only about 75% as well as from dairy milk.

ISOFLAVONES

As previously mentioned, soybeans are a unique dietary source of a group of phytochemicals called isoflavones (1 to 3 mg/g protein), with a typical serving containing about 25 to 40 mg. The two primary isoflavones are genistein and daidzein. Isoflavones are referred to as phytoestrogens (plant-estrogens) because they bind to estrogen receptors, although they possess only 1/100 to 1/1000 the activity of 17β-estradiol (one form of estrogen in the body). Despite their low potency, isoflavones can be expected to exert physiological effects, since serum isoflavone levels in people consuming soyfoods are 1000 to 10,000 times higher than endogenous estrogen levels.

Furthermore, recent work indicates that genistein binds to the newly identified estrogen receptor (estrogen receptor-beta, ERβ) with almost as much affinity as does

estrogen. This suggests that previous estimates have likely underestimated the relative estrogenic potency of isoflavones. And isoflavones may have tissue-selective effects, since ERβ and ERα (the original estrogen receptor) have different tissue distributions. That is, like the drugs tamoxifen and raloxifene, isoflavones (soy) may have estrogenic effects in some tissues but either no effects or antiestrogenic effects in other tissues. Thus, isoflavones are viewed by some as selective estrogen receptor modulators (SERMs). See Chapter 11 for details on the use of SERMs in osteoporosis. Finally, isoflavones are antioxidants, influence the activities of key enzymes involved in cell growth, and affect other biological processes. Thus, the physiological effects of isoflavones are by no means limited to those associated with binding to the estrogen receptor.

SOY AND CORONARY HEART DISEASE

Products that provide at least 6.25 g of soy protein per serving can include on their food labels a health claim for the cholesterol-lowering effects of soy protein. This figure is based on the premise that 25 g of soy protein per day will lower blood cholesterol and that the consumption of four servings of soy per day is reasonable. This blood cholesterol reduction depends largely on initial blood cholesterol levels; however, on average, for those with total serum cholesterol levels between 200 and 240 mg/dl, a decrease in LDL of 2 to 5% can be expected. Although such decreases pale in comparison with those of cholesterol-lowering drugs, they are not clinically unimportant.

Beyond blood cholesterol reduction, isoflavones may reduce coronary heart disease risk by directly affecting blood vessels, such as by increasing arterial flexibility, by inhibiting LDL oxidation, and by inhibiting smooth muscle cell proliferation. These effects may prove to be more important than blood cholesterol reduction, especially since there are many effective ways to reduce blood cholesterol.

SOYFOODS AND BONE HEALTH

Even prior to the publication of experimental data, because of isoflavones' weak estrogenic activity and their similarity in chemical structure to the osteoporosis drug ipriflavone (a synthetic isoflavone), there was speculation that isoflavones would promote bone health. Studies in rodents that have had their ovaries removed so that their estrogen output is reduced clearly support this hypothesis, as do several, but not all, small studies in pre-, peri-, and postmenopausal women. Thus far, however, effects have been observed primarily only at the spine. Long-term human studies evaluating the effects of soy/isoflavones on bone mineral density and fracture rates are needed before definitive conclusions can be drawn. Beyond isoflavones, soy protein—when substituted for animal protein—decreases calcium loss from the bones and should, therefore, improve bone health.

CANCER PREVENTION AND TREATMENT

Genistein inhibits the growth of a wide range of both hormone-dependent and hormone-independent cancer cells, including breast and prostate cancer cells. In vitro anticancer effects are likely due to the effects of genistein on enzymes involved in cell regulation, as previously noted. Somewhat surprisingly, given the low breast cancer mortality rates in Asian countries, adult soy consumption is generally not associated with a reduced risk of postmenopausal breast cancer risk in epidemiologic studies. In contrast, animal studies generally show that soy inhibits mammary tumor development, whereas findings from human studies examining markers of breast cancer risk are mixed. Interestingly, animal data and very limited human data suggest that soy consumption early in life (childhood) markedly protects against breast cancer later in life.

Several epidemiologic studies suggest that consuming just one to two servings of soyfoods may reduce prostate cancer risk by 70%. Obviously, this relationship is speculative, but several studies have found that isoflavones markedly inhibit tumor development in mice implanted with prostate cancer cells.

SOY IN FOODS

Soy can be consumed in a variety of forms and with the rise in consumer demand comes easier access to more soy products. Most stores now carry many traditional soyfoods, such as soymilk and tofu. Increasingly, though, soy is found in the form of user-friendly products made with soy isolate (90% protein) and soy concentrates (70% protein), such as energy bars, breakfast cereals, breads, and pasta. Furthermore, there are more than 100 companies selling isoflavone supplements.

There is a divergence of opinion on the relative merits of consuming pills versus soyfoods. It is unlikely that pills lower serum cholesterol, but many of the other effects of soy are attributed directly to isoflavones. Soyfoods are the preferred way to incorporate soy into the diet; however, for those unable to consume sufficient soyfoods to derive the hypothesized benefits, pills remain a possible alternative.

Some concerns have been raised about the possible adverse effects of soy consumption, especially those related to breast cancer risk (specifically for women with estrogen-receptor-positive breast cancer), thyroid function, mineral balance, and cognitive function. All of these areas warrant additional research, especially given the likelihood that soy will play an increasingly larger role in the American diet. However, the available data indicate that, for the vast majority of healthy adults consuming a well-balanced diet, any possible adverse consequences resulting from the consumption of soy in amounts equal to or somewhat above those typical in Asia are minimal and are far outweighed by substantial potential benefit.

Dr. Messina is a former program director in the Diet and Cancer Branch of the National Cancer Institute. He now devotes his time to the study of the attributes of soyfoods; is president of Nutrition Matters, Inc.; and is an adjunct associate professor of nutrition at Loma Linda University.

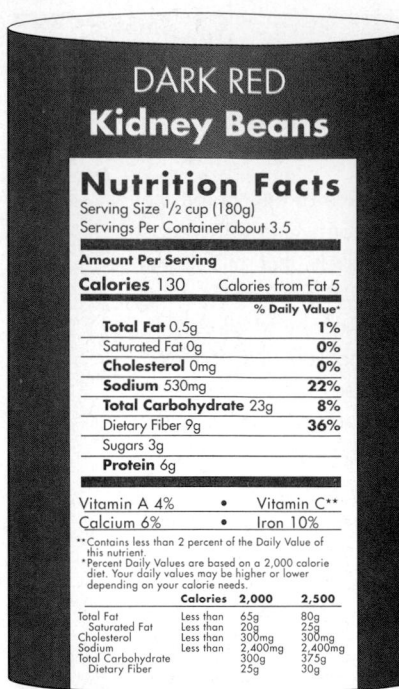

FIGURE 7-11 Legumes are rich sources of protein. One-half cup meets about 10% of protein needs, and at a cost of only about 5% of energy needs.

$$BV = \frac{g \text{ nitrogen retained}}{g \text{ nitrogen absorbed}}$$

*T*he concept of biological value has clinical importance whenever protein intake must be limited. This is because we want what little protein that is consumed to be used efficiently by the body. For example, protein intake during liver disease and kidney disease may need to be controlled in order to lessen the effects of the disease. In these cases, most of the protein consumed should come from high biological value sources, such as eggs, milk, and meat.

$$PER = \frac{g \text{ weight gain}}{g \text{ protein consumed}}$$

over, as discussed in Chapter 5, legumes contain soluble fiber, which can help lower blood cholesterol. In addition, the soluble fiber moderates the swings in blood glucose that occur after eating.

■ Evaluation of Protein Quality

A final consideration with regard to proteins in foods is protein quality, which is the ability of a food protein to support body growth and maintenance. Methods exist to both measure and estimate protein quality.[13] Each has its uses and limitations. Keep in mind, also, that the concept of protein quality applies only under conditions in which the amount of protein consumed is equal to or less than the amount of protein required to meet the need for essential amino acids. When protein intake exceeds this amount, efficiency of protein use declines, regardless of the balance of amino acids present. This occurs even with the highest-quality proteins because, after the need for essential amino acids has been met, the remaining essential and nonessential amino acids cannot be stored on a long-term basis and will primarily be degraded and used as a source of energy.

Biological Value

The **biological value (BV)** of a protein is a measure of how efficiently food protein, once absorbed from the GI tract, can be turned into body tissues. If a food possesses enough of all nine essential amino acids, it should allow a person to efficiently incorporate the food protein into body proteins. The biological value of a food, then, depends on how closely its amino acid pattern reflects the amino acid pattern in body tissues. The better the match, the more completely food protein turns into body protein. We actually measure protein retention by measuring nitrogen retention in the body. Both humans and laboratory animals are used to generate data for determining biological value of food proteins.

If the amino acid pattern in a food is quite unlike tissue amino acid patterns, many amino acids in the food will not become body protein. They simply become "leftovers." Their nitrogen groups are removed and excreted in the urine as urea (review Fig. 7-3). Since not much of the nitrogen is retained, the ratio of retained nitrogen to absorbed nitrogen, and the consequent biological value, is low.

Egg-white protein has a biological value of 100, the highest biological value of any single food protein. In other words, essentially all nitrogen that is absorbed from egg protein can be retained. Milk and meat proteins also have high biological values. This makes sense because humans and other animals have similar tissue amino acid compositions. Plant amino acid patterns differ greatly from those of humans. For example, corn has only a moderate biological value of 70; it is high enough to support body maintenance, but not growth. Peanuts consumed as the only source of protein show a low biological value of about 40.

Protein Efficiency Ratio

The **protein efficiency ratio (PER)** is another means of measuring a food's protein quality. FDA uses this method to set standards for labeling of foods intended for infants. The PER compares the amount of weight (in grams) gained by a growing rat after 10 days or more of eating a standard amount of protein (9.09% of its energy intake) from a single protein source to the grams of protein consumed. The PER of a food reflects its biological value, since both basically measure protein retention by body tissues. Plant proteins, because of their incomplete nature, generally yield low PER values, whereas the values for animal proteins are higher, often above 2.0.

Chemical Score of Protein

Protein quality of a food can be estimated by its chemical score. To calculate a food's **chemical score,** the amount of each essential amino acid provided by a gram of the food's protein is divided by an "ideal" amount for that essential amino acid per gram of food protein. The "ideal" protein pattern is based on the minimal amount (in milligrams) of each of the nine essential amino acids that is needed per gram of food protein. The amino acid needs of young children is the standard typically used. The lowest amino acid ratio calculated for any essential amino is the chemical score. Scores vary from 0 to 1.0.

Protein Digestibility Corrected Amino Acid Score (PDCAAS)

The most widely used measure of protein quality is the **Protein Digestibility Corrected Amino Acid Score (PDCAAS).** This is used in place of PER evaluations for foods intended for children over 1 year of age and for nonpregnant adults. To calculate the PDCAAS of a protein, its chemical score is determined. For example, wheat has a chemical score of 0.47. The score is then multiplied by the digestibility of the protein (generally, 0.9 to 1.0), in turn yielding the PDCAAS. The PDCAAS for wheat is about 0.47×0.90, which equals about 0.40. The maximum value is 1.0, which is the value of milk, eggs, and soy protein. A protein totally lacking any of the nine essential amino acids has a PDCAAS of 0, since its chemical score is 0. For labeling purposes, protein content when listed as % Daily Value is reduced if the PDCAAS is less than 1. For example, if the protein content of ½ cup of spaghetti noodles is 3 g, only 1.2 g will be counted when calculating % Daily Value, since the PDCAAS of wheat is 0.40 ($3 \text{ g} \times 0.40 = 1.2$). Other PDCAAS values are egg white, 1.0; soy protein, 0.92 to 0.99; beef, 0.92; and black beans, 0.53. Currently the Nutrition Facts panel rarely contains the % Daily Value for protein because the manufacturers do not want to spend the money needed to determine the PDCAAS.

$$\text{Chemical score} = \frac{\text{actual mg of each essential amino acid per g of protein}}{\text{Required mg needs of that essential amino acid per g of protein}}$$

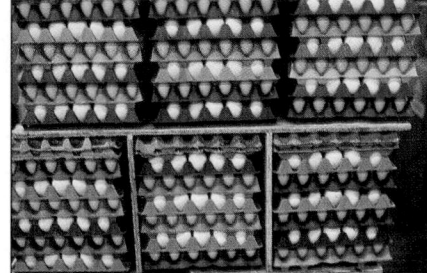

Egg-white protein has the highest biological value of any single food protein.

CONCEPT CHECK

*T*he Recommended Dietary Allowance (RDA) for adults is 0.8 g of protein per kg of healthy body weight. This is approximately 56 g of protein daily for a 70-kg (156-lb) person. The average American man consumes about 95 g of protein daily, and a woman consumes about 65 g. Thus, typically we eat more than enough protein to meet our needs. Diets high in protein can increase calcium loss in the urine, compromise kidney health in people with diabetes and those with kidney disease, and animal protein sources likely increase cardiovascular disease risk.

Most protein in the American diet comes from meat. Plant protein sources can play an important role in the diet. *Protein quality* refers to the ability of a protein to contribute to protein needs. Using any of the methods available for testing, individual foods with ample amounts of all nine essential amino acids show high protein quality.

■ PROTEIN-ENERGY MALNUTRITION

Rarely an isolated condition, protein deficiency usually accompanies a deficiency of dietary energy and other nutrients resulting from insufficient food intake. In developing areas of the world, people often have diets low in energy and as a result protein. This state of undernutrition stunts the growth of children and makes them more susceptible to disease throughout life.[26] (Note that undernutrition is a main focus of Chapter 20). People who consume too little protein and food energy can go on to develop **protein-energy malnutrition (PEM),** also referred to as *protein-calorie malnutrition (PCM)*. In its milder form, it is difficult to tell if a person with PEM is consuming too little energy or protein, or both. But if the nutrient deficiency—especially for energy—is quite severe, a deficiency disease called **marasmus** can result. When an inadequate intake of nutrients, including protein, is combined with an already existing disease, a form of malnutrition called **kwashiorkor** can develop. These two conditions form the tip of the iceberg with respect to states of undernutrition, and symptoms of these two conditions even can be present in the same person (Fig. 7-12).

protein-energy malnutrition A condition resulting from regularly consuming insufficient amounts of energy and protein. The deficiency eventually results in body wasting, primarily of lean tissue, and an increased susceptibility to infections.

marasmus A disease that results from consuming a grossly insufficient amount of protein and energy; one of the diseases classed as protein-energy malnutrition. Victims have little or no fat stores, little muscle mass, and poor strength. Death from infections is common.

kwashiorkor A disease occurring primarily in young children who have an existing disease and consume a marginal amount of energy and considerably insufficient protein in relation to needs. The child generally suffers from infections and exhibits edema, poor growth, weakness, and an increased susceptibility to further illness.

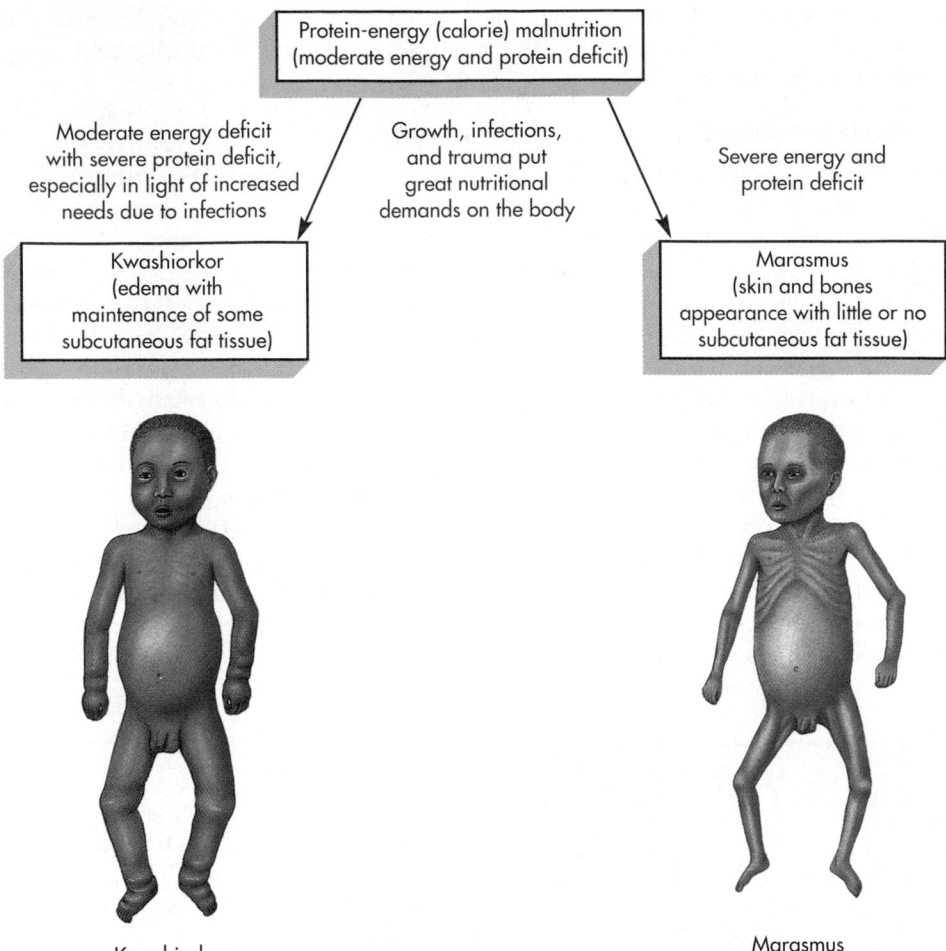

■ **FIGURE 7-12** Schema for classifying undernutrition. The presence of subcutaneous fat (directly underneath the skin) is a diagnostic key for distinguishing kwashiorkor from marasmus.
Illustration by William Ober.

As many as 2 million people worldwide die each year from tuberculosis, as this disease reemerges as the world's leading fatal infectious disease. In fact, up to one-third of the world population may be infected with the dreaded disease. A protein deficiency may lead to susceptibility to tuberculosis, and an improved diet may help delay fatalities. Unfortunately, as covered in Chapter 20, improving the diets for protein-malnourished people around the world remains an overwhelming task and will not likely be solved soon.

■ Kwashiorkor

Kwashiorkor is a word from Ghana that means "the disease that the first child gets when the new child comes." From birth, an infant is usually breastfed. Typically, it is believed that, by the time the child reaches 1 to 1.5 years of age, the mother is usually pregnant or has already given birth again, and breastfeeding is no longer possible for the first child. This child's diet abruptly changes from nutritious human milk to native starchy roots and gruels. These foods have low protein densities, compared with total energy. Additionally, the foods are usually full of plant fibers, which are often bulky, making it difficult for the child to consume enough to meet energy needs. The child may also have infections and parasites, which acutely raise energy and protein needs. For these reasons, energy needs of these children are met marginally, at best, and their protein needs are not met, especially when needs are greatly increased by infections and marginal energy intakes. Usually, many vitamin and mineral requirements are also far from being fulfilled. Famine victims face similar problems.

The major symptoms of kwashiorkor are apathy, listlessness, failure to grow and gain weight, and withdrawal from the environment. These symptoms complicate other diseases present and can make conditions such as measles, a disease that normally makes a healthy child ill for only a week or so, severely debilitating and even fatal. Further signs and symptoms of the disease are changes in hair color, potassium deficiency, flaky skin, fatty infiltration in the liver, reduced muscle mass, and massive edema in the abdomen and legs. The presence of edema in a child who has some subcutaneous fat still present is the hallmark of kwashiorkor (see Fig. 7-12). In addition, these children hardly move. If you pick them up, they don't cry. When you hold them, you feel the plumpness of edema, not muscle and fat tissue.

Many symptoms of kwashiorkor can be explained based on what we know about proteins. Proteins play important roles in fluid balance, lipoprotein transport, immune function, and production of tissues, such as skin and hair. We should not expect children with an insufficient protein intake to grow and mature normally. And they don't.

If children with kwashiorkor are helped in time—if infections are treated and a diet ample in protein, energy, and other essential nutrients is provided—the disease process reverses. They begin to grow again and may even show no signs of their previous condition, except perhaps shortness of stature. Unfortunately, by the time many of these children reach a hospital or care center, they already have severe infections. In spite of the best care, they still die. Or, if they survive, they return home only to repeat the cycle.

■ Marasmus

Marasmus typically occurs as an infant slowly starves to death. It is caused by diets containing greatly insufficient amounts of protein, energy, and other nutrients. As previously noted, the condition is also commonly referred to as *protein-energy malnutrition,* especially when experienced by older children and adults. Typically, it occurs in infants who are slowly starving to death. The word *marasmus* means "to waste away." Victims have a "skin and bones" appearance, with little or no subcutaneous fat (see Fig. 7-12).

Marasmus commonly develops in infants who either are not breastfed or have stopped breastfeeding in the early months. Often the weaning formula used is improperly prepared because of unsafe water and because the parents cannot afford sufficient infant formula for the child's needs. The latter problem may lead the parents to dilute the formula to provide more feedings, not realizing that this provides only more water for the infant.

Marasmus in infants commonly occurs in the large cities of poverty-stricken countries. In the cities, bottle-feeding is often necessary because the infant must be cared for by others when the mother is working or away from home. When people are poor and sanitation is lacking, bottle-feeding often leads to marasmus. An infant with marasmus requires large amounts of energy and protein—like a preterm infant—and, unless the child receives them, full recovery from the disease may never occur. The majority of brain growth occurs between conception and the child's first birthday. In fact, the brain is growing at its highest rate at birth. If the diet does not support brain growth during the first months of life, the brain may not grow to its full adult size. This reduced or retarded brain growth may lead to diminished intellectual function. Both kwashiorkor and marasmus wreak havoc on infants and children; mortality rates in developing countries are often 10 to 20 times higher than in the United States.

■ Kwashiorkor and Marasmus Malnutrition in the Hospital

Kwashiorkor can result when a hospitalized patient is fed glucose intravenously for many days, such as when a slow recovery from surgery prevents normal food consumption. Or a person may feel too sick to eat, in spite of the increased nutrient needs caused by his or her disease. Intravenous glucose feeding can meet energy needs to some extent but provides no protein. As a result, the person develops edema, and often the immune function is diminished, leaving the patient at great risk for infections. One of the best markers for kwashiorkor is a person's albumin concentration in the blood. When the value falls below the normal range (generally 3.5 to 5.5 g/dl of blood), the person is at a very high risk for infections and disease.

Studies have demonstrated that a hospital patient with low body weight, low albumin, and a low white blood cell (especially lymphocyte) count is at a four to six times greater risk of complications and death than a patient with normal values for those three factors. In response, nutrition support teams have been formed in hospitals. One of their missions is to ensure that patients receive enough oral or balanced intravenous nutrition support to meet their needs for energy, protein, carbohydrate, and other nutrients.

Marasmus occurs in a hospitalized patient who simply does not receive enough energy and other nutrients. This can be caused by anorexia nervosa, cancer, AIDS, and some intestinal disorders. The person either does not eat enough food or does not absorb enough nutrients from the intestinal tract to meet nutritional needs. Muscle, vital organ tissue, and fat stores waste away, and the person eventually looks like "skin and bones." Skinfold measurements of the arm can be used as an indication of marasmus. (Chapter 13 reviews this technique.) However, appearance alone is often enough to indicate the disease. Death from starvation or heart failure can result. A hospitalized person may also have mixed kwashiorkor-marasmus. This is characterized by edema in a person with greatly diminished fat stores.

CONCEPT CHECK

Most undernutrition consists of mild deficits in energy, protein, and often other nutrients. If a person needs more nutrients because of disease and infection but does not consume enough energy and protein, a condition known as kwashiorkor can develop. The person suffers from edema and weakness. Children around age 2 are especially susceptible to kwashiorkor, particularly if they already have other diseases. Famine situations in which only starchy root products are available to eat contribute to this problem. Marasmus is a condition wherein people—infants, especially—starve to death. Symptoms include muscle wasting, absence of fat stores, and weakness. Both an adequate diet and the treatment of concurrent diseases must be promoted to maintain nutritional health. This also is true in an adult suffering from anorexia nervosa, cancer, or AIDS. The symptoms of marasmus, especially, are seen in these situations.

Check out the Perspectives in Nutrition *Online Learning Center* http://www.mhhe.com/wardlaw *for quizzes, flash cards, other activities, and web links designed to further help you learn about proteins.*

SUMMARY

1. Amino acids, the building blocks of proteins, contain a very usable form of nitrogen for humans. Of the 20 types of amino acids found in food, 9 must be consumed as food and the rest can be synthesized by the body.

2. High-quality, also called complete, protein foods contain ample amounts of all nine essential amino acids. Furthermore, foods derived from an animal source provide high biological value protein. Lower-quality, also called incomplete, protein foods lack sufficient amounts of one or more essential amino acids. This is typical of plant foods, especially cereal grains. Different types of plant foods eaten together often complement each other's amino acid deficits, thereby providing high-quality protein in the diet.

3. Individual amino acids are linked together to form proteins. The sequential order of amino acids determines the protein's ultimate shape and function. This order is directed by DNA in the cell nucleus. Diseases such as sickle cell anemia can occur if the amino acids are incorrect on a polypeptide chain. When the three-dimensional shape of the protein is unfolded—denatured—by treatment with heat, acid or alkaline solutions, or other processes, the protein also loses its biological activity.

4. Protein digestion begins in the stomach, dividing the proteins into breakdown products containing shorter chains of amino acids. In the small intestine, these polypeptide chains eventually separate into amino acids. These free amino acids are absorbed by the enterocytes and travel via the portal vein to the liver.

5. Important body components—such as muscles, connective tissue, transport proteins, visual pigments, enzymes, some hormones, and immune bodies—are made of proteins. These proteins are in a state of constant turnover. Proteins also provide carbons, which can be used to synthesize glucose when necessary.

6. The protein RDA for adults is 0.8 g per kg of healthy body weight. For a typical 70-kg (156-lb) person, this corresponds to 56 g of protein daily; for a 55-kg (120-lb) person, this corresponds to 44 g/day. The North American diet generally supplies plenty of protein: Men typically consume about 95 g of protein daily, and women consume closer to 65 g. The combined protein intake is also of sufficient quality to support body functions.

7. Almost all animal products are nutrient-dense sources of protein. The high quality of these proteins means that they can be

easily converted into body proteins. Plant foods generally contain less than 20% of their energy content as protein; however, legumes are an excellent source of high-quality protein if eaten with grains or animal products.

8. Protein quality can be measured by determining the extent to which the body can retain the nitrogen contained in the protein absorbed; this is called biological value. In addition, the balance of essential amino acids in a food can be compared with an ideal pattern. The comparison with the ideal pattern is referred to as the chemical score. When multiplied by the degree of digestibility, the chemical score yields the Protein Digestibility Corrected Amino Acid Score (PDCAAS).

9. Undernutrition can lead to protein-energy malnutrition in the form of kwashiorkor or marasmus. Kwashiorkor results primarily from an inadequate energy and protein intake in comparison with body needs, which often increase with concurrent disease and infection. Kwashiorkor often occurs when a child is weaned from human milk and fed mostly starchy gruels. Marasmus results primarily from extreme starvation—a negligible intake of both protein and energy. Marasmus commonly occurs during famine, especially in infants. Variations of these diseases appear in some hospitalized Americans.

■ STUDY QUESTIONS

1. Discuss the relative importance of essential and nonessential amino acids in the diet. Why is it important for essential amino acids lost from the body to be replaced in the diet?
2. Explain the process for synthesizing nonessential amino acids. When an amino acid loses its amino group without transferring it to another carbon skeleton the chemical reaction is called _____.
3. What is a limiting amino acid? Explain why this concept is a concern in a vegetarian diet. How can a vegetarian compensate for limiting amino acids in specific foods?
4. Briefly describe the organization of proteins (i.e., primary structure, etc.). How can this organization be altered or damaged? What might be a result of damaged protein organization?
5. Describe four functions of proteins? Provide an example of how the structure of a protein relates to its function.
6. How are DNA and protein synthesis related?
7. What would be one health benefit of preventing protein-energy malnutrition in children?
8. What characteristics of vegetable proteins could improve the American diet? What foods would you include to provide a diet that has ample protein from both plant and animal sources but is moderate in fat?
9. Outline the major differences between kwashiorkor and marasmus.
10. What are the possible long-term effects of an inadequate intake of dietary protein among children between the ages of 6 months and 4 years?

■ ANNOTATED REFERENCES

1. Alexander H and others: Risk factors for cardiovascular disease and diabetes in two groups of Hispanic Americans with differing dietary habits. *Journal of the American College of Nutrition* 18:127, 1999.

   Lactovegetarians exhibit a more favorable blood lipid profile, lower blood pressure, and lower risk for type 2 diabetes than do people with a similar Hispanic background who do not consume a primarily plant-based diet.

2. Americans and red meat: A love-hate relationship. *Harvard Health Letter*, p. 1, July 1998.

   People who consume red meat on a regular basis should focus on lean cuts of such meat. A typical recommendation is to limit red meat to one to two 3-ounce servings per week. The fat in meat, when exposed to high temperature, is altered in such a way that it increases the risk for colon cancer.

3. Aulikki T and others: Dietary intake of vitamin D in premenopausal, healthy vegans was insufficient to maintain concentrations of serum 25-hydroxy vitamin D and intact parathyroid hormone within normal ranges during the winter in Finland. *Journal of the American Dietetic Association* 100:434, 2000.

   Increasing vitamin D intake should be recommended for vegans in winter months if adequate sun exposure is not possible. Selections of foods fortified with vitamin D or supplements should be emphasized.

4. Davidson MH and others: Comparison of the effects of lean red meat vs. lean white meat on serum lipid levels among free-living persons with hypercholesterolemia: A long-term, randomized clinical trial. *Archives of Internal Medicine* 159:1331, 1999.

   A fat-controlled diet containing lean red meats produces reductions in blood cholesterol similar to those for lean white meats. Red meats can be part of a diet designed to lower blood cholesterol as long as they are lean varieties and trimmed of visible fat.

5. Giannini S and others: Acute affects of moderate dietary proteins restriction in patients with idiopathic hypercalciuria and calcium nephrolithiasis. *American Journal of Clinical Nutrition* 69:267, 1999.

   A moderate protein restriction decreases urinary calcium excretion in people who generally overexcrete calcium in the urine. Control of protein intake will likely reduce the risk of kidney stones in such people.

6. Granner DK: Protein synthesis and the genetic code. In Murray RK and others (eds.): 25th ed. *Harper's biochemistry*. Stamford, CT: Appleton & Lange, 2000.

Protein synthesis is a complex process utilizing numerous cell components. DNA, mRNA, tRNA, amino acids, and ribosomes all participate. The discussion in your textbook only begins to describe the process.

7. Henkel J: Soy: Health claims for soy proteins, questions about other components. *FDA Consumer*, p. 13, June 2000.

   In October 1999, FDA gave food manufacturers permission to put labels on products indicating that soy proteins in these foods may help lower heart disease risk. There is less evidence to support the consumption of other components of soy, especially when consumed as concentrated supplements.

8. How much protein is enough? *Consumer Reports on Health*, p. 8, February 2001.

   It is particularly important for pregnant women, breastfeeding women, young children, and older adults to meet protein needs. A daily intake of about 15% of total calorie intake is adequate to meet the protein needs of most people.

9. Hunt JR and others: Zinc absorption, mineral balance, and blood lipids in women consuming controlled lactoovovegetarian diets for 8 wk. *American Journal of Clinical Nutrition* 67:421, 1998.

   Inclusion of whole grains and legumes in a lactoovovegetarian diet contributes much zinc and helps maintain zinc balance in such vegetarians.

10. JAMA patient page: Facts about sickle cell anemia. *Journal of the American Medical Association* 281:176, 1999.

    Sickle cell anemia is particularly common among people whose ancestry is from sub-Saharan Africa, South and Central America, Cuba, Saudi Arabia, India, Greece, and Italy. Early diagnosis of sickle cell anemia is important, so that children who have the disorder can receive proper treatment. Antibiotics, blood transfusions, and some medications may be helpful during flare-ups of the disease.

11. Johnston TK: Nutritional implications of vegetarian diets. In Shils ME and others (eds.): *Modern nutrition in health and disease.* 9th ed. Baltimore: Williams & Wilkins, 1999.

    Vegetarian diets have a long history. There are many positive aspects of a primarily plant-based diet, including ample consumption of fruits and vegetables. Many typical diseases, such as heart disease, hypertension, and osteoporosis, are less common in vegetarians than in people consuming animal protein–rich diets. These findings are discussed in detail.

12. Liebman B, Hurley J: Beans: No longer a bore. *Nutrition Action Health Letter*, p. 13, May 1999.

    If one hasn't consumed beans on a regular basis, it is best to start with small portions and increase this gradually over a few weeks, so one's GI tract has a chance to adjust. Use of the product Beano® can also help reduce intestinal gas-related discomfort.

13. Matthews DE: Proteins and amino acids. In Shils ME and others (eds.): *Modern nutrition in health and disease.* 9th ed. Baltimore: Williams & Wilkins, 1999.

    Proteins in the body are not static; proteins are constantly broken down and then resynthesized. This chapter reviews in detail amino acid metabolism, measures of protein turnover and balance, assessment of protein needs, and evaluation of the quality of specific proteins.

14. Mayes PA: Digestion and absorption. In Murray RK and others (eds.): 25th ed. *Harper's biochemistry.* Stamford, CT: Appleton & Lange, 2000.

    The enzymatic digestion of protein begins in the stomach. Pepsin splits proteins into large polypeptides. Enzymes in the small intestine such as trypsin and aminopeptidases complete the digestion process, yielding amino acids. A multiplicity of carriers are then used to transport the amino acids into the absorptive cells.

15. McNurlan MA, Garlick PJ: Protein synthesis and degradation. In Stipanuk MH (ed.): *Biochemical and physiological aspects of human nutrition.* Philadelphia: W.B. Saunders, 2000.

    Cells are constantly degrading existing proteins and synthesizing new proteins. DNA in the cell is transcribed to mRNA. This mRNA is translated by ribosomes in the cytosol to the new protein. Total protein turnover in the body is about 300 g degraded and 300 g synthesized each day.

16. Milea D and others: Blindness in a strict vegan. *The New England Journal of Medicine* 342:897, 2000.

    Vitamin B-12 supplementation is essential in persons who are strict vegetarians. Not doing so can result in vitamin B-12 deficiency, leading to severe, irreversible damage to the optic nerve.

17. Metges CC, Barth CA: Metabolic consequences of a high dietary-protein intake in adulthood: Assessment of the available evidence. *Journal of Nutrition* 130:886, 2000.

    In a healthy population, there is no need to increase protein intake above that habitually consumed by well-nourished populations in technically advanced nations (above 2 g per kg of body weight per day). Physical activity does not increase protein needs significantly because it has a positive effect on nitrogen retention, as long as energy needs are met.

18. Messina V: Purely vegetarian. *Today's Dietitian*, p. 40, August 1999.

    Planning optimal menus for vegetarians is somewhat more complex than simply replacing meat with a plant source of protein. It is important for the person to base this diet on whole grains, fruits, and vegetables; to include moderate amounts of beans and nuts; to consume some vegetable oils; to use calcium supplements if necessary; and to consume a good source of vitamin B-12 daily (fortified foods or supplements).

19. Moving towards a plant-based diet. American Institute for Cancer Research, Washington, DC 1998.

    There is convincing evidence that a diet rich in vegetables and fruits reduces the risk of many forms of cancer. Consuming an abundance of vegetables, fruits, and other plant foods may also protect against heart disease, osteoporosis, type 2 diabetes, hypertension, and certain birth defects. Purchasing a vegetarian cookbook can ease the transition to a more plant-based diet.

20. Pszczola DE: Health and functionality in a nutshell. *Food Technology* 54(2):54, 2000.

    Nuts are a good source of magnesium, copper, and fiber. Including some nuts each day in a diet is common recommendation for improving diet quality.

21. Raloff J: High-fat and the healthful: Scientists offer a nutty recipe for hale hearts and slim physiques. *Science News* 154:328, 1998.

    Nuts are rich in monounsaturated fats. A variety of studies have shown that replacing nuts for sources of saturated fat reduces blood cholesterol. One has to be careful to moderate nut consumption, as these are very energy dense.

22. Red meat and cancer risk. *American Institute of Cancer Research Newsletter*, p. 4, Summer 1999.

    Cooking meat at high temperatures creates compounds that cause cancer in laboratory animals, and it is likely they have similar effects in humans. People need not cut out all meat from their diets. It would be better to look at meat as something to be added to dishes mostly made up of vegetables and grains, rather than as the dominant part of the meal.

23. Russell RM: The impact of disease states as a modifying factor for nutrition toxicity. *Nutrition Reviews* 55:50, 1997.

High-protein diets increase blood flow and blood pressure in the kidneys, which can result in injury to the kidneys over time. It is important to control protein intake to RDA amounts when there is evidence of ongoing kidney disease.

24. Smit E and others: Estimates of animal and plant protein intake in US adults: Results from the third National Health and Nutrition Examination Survey, 1988–1991. *Journal of the American Dietetic Association* 99:813, 1999.

The main source of protein in the American diet is animal protein (69%). Meat, fish, and poultry protein contributes most of the animal protein. Women tend to consume a lower percentage of red meat and a higher percentage of proteins from chicken, dairy, fruits, and vegetables.

25. Spiller GA, Bruce B: Vegan diets and cardiovascular health. *Journal of the American College of Nutrition* 17:407, 1998.

The consumption of a diet consisting of whole grains, fruits, vegetables, and nuts and seeds has been associated with a more favorable lipoprotein profile than a diet based more on animal proteins. Vegan diets pose a risk for vitamin B-12 deficiency, but this can be easily prevented, given minimal knowledge. There appears to be a clear message for moving toward a vegan diet, or at least a diet based more on plant foods.

26. Torun B, Chew F: Protein-energy malnutrition. In Shils ME and others (eds.): *Modern nutrition in health and disease.* 9th ed. Baltimore: Williams & Wilkins, 1999.

Protein-energy malnutrition can affect all age groups, but is more frequent among infants and young children. This is because ongoing growth increases nutritional requirements. In addition, they often cannot obtain food by their own means. Infants who are weaned prematurely from the breast or who are breastfed for a prolonged time without adequate complementary feeding become malnourished from a lack of adequate energy and protein intake. Older children usually have milder forms of protein-energy malnutrition because they can cope better with social and food availability limitations.

27. Zambon D and others: Substituting walnuts for monounsaturated fat improves the serum lipid profile of hypercholesterolemic men and women: A randomized, crossover trial. *Annals of Internal Medicine* 132:538, 2000.

The replacement of some of the fat in a Mediterranean-type diet with nuts provides some benefit in lowering blood lipids. Overall, both approaches contribute to lower blood lipids.

TAKE ACTION

I. IS YOUR PROTEIN INTAKE SUFFICIENT TO MEET YOUR NEEDS?

1.   How much protein do you eat in a typical day? Look at the nutrition assessment you completed at the end of Chapter 2. Review it closely. Find the figure indicating the amount of protein you consumed on that day, and write it in the space below:

TOTAL PROTEIN _____

Compare your protein intake with your RDA for protein. Find your healthy weight for height in pounds using Figure 13-8 in Chapter 13. Choose a midrange value. Divide this number by 2.2 to reveal your healthy weight in kilograms. Next, multiply by 0.8 per kilogram of this weight or your current body weight if the numbers are close. This will indicate the RDA for protein for your weight and gender. Write it in the space below:

RDA FOR PROTEIN _____

How does your consumption compare with your RDA?

_____

_____

_____

If you consumed either more or less than the RDA, what foods could you add, delete, or eat more or less of? (Look at the foods you ate.)

_____

_____

_____

_____

Was most of your protein from animal or plant sources?

_____

_____

If your protein intake was primarily from plants, did this come from a wide variety to encourage protein complementarity for the day?

_____

_____

_____

TAKE ACTION

II. PROTEIN AND THE VEGETARIAN.

Alania is excited about all the health benefits that might accompany a vegetarian diet. However, she is concerned that she will not consume enough protein to meet her needs. She is also concerned about possible vitamin and mineral deficiencies. Use your nutrition software to see if her concerns are valid.

Protein Grams

Breakfast

Calcium fortified orange juice, 1 cup
Soybean milk, 1 cup
Fortified bran flakes, 1 cup
Banana, medium

Snack

Calcium-enriched granola bar

Lunch

GardenBurger, 4 oz
Whole-wheat bun
Mustard, 1 tbsp
Soy cheese, 1 oz
Apple, medium
Green leaf lettuce, 1½ cups
Peanuts, 1 oz
Sunflower seeds, ¼ cup
Tomato slices, 2
Mushrooms, 3
Vinaigrette salad dressing, 2 tbsp
Iced Tea

Dinner

Kidney beans, ½ cup
White rice, ¾ cup
Fortified margarine, 2 tbsp
Mixed vegetables, ¼ cup
Hot Tea

Dessert

Strawberries, ½ cup
Angel food cake, 1 small slice
Soy milk, ½ cup

TOTAL PROTEIN GRAMS _____

Alana's diet contained 2150 kcal, with _____ g (you fill in) of protein (plenty for her), 360 g of carbohydrate, 57 g of total dietary fat (only 9 g of which came from saturated fat), and 50 g of fiber. Her vitamin and mineral intake with respect to those of concern in vegetarians—vitamin B-12, vitamin D, calcium, iron, and zinc—met her needs.

VEGETARIAN DIETS

Vegetarianism has evolved over the centuries from a necessity into an option. Historically, vegetarianism was linked with specific philosophies and religions or with science. In the sixth century B.C., Pythagoras advocated a meatless diet for its physical health, ecological, religious, and philosophical benefits.

Today, there are about 12 million vegetarians in the United States, about double the number in 1985. Over the past two decades, vegetarian diets have gone from dull to delicious, with the inclusion of such new products as soy-based sloppy joes, chili, tacos, burgers, and more. In addition, cookbooks that feature the use of a variety of fruits, vegetables, and seasonings are enhancing food selection for vegetarians of all degrees.

Vegetarianism is popular among college students. Fifteen percent of college students in one survey said they select vegetarian options at lunch or dinner on any given day. In response, dining services offer vegetarian options at every meal, the most common being pastas with meatless sauce and pizza. Many teenagers are also turning to vegetarianism out of respect for animals. And a survey by the National Restaurant Association found that 20% of their customers want a vegetarian option when they eat out. Many customers cite health and taste as reasons for choosing vegetarian fare.

As nutrition science has grown, new information has enabled the design of adequate vegetarian diets. It is important for vegetarians to take advantage of this information because a diet of only plants can lead to various nutrient deficiencies and a substantial growth retardation in infants and children. People who choose a vegetarian diet can meet their nutritional needs by following a few basic rules and knowledgeably planning their diets[11] (Fig. 7-13).

Studies show that death rates from some chronic diseases, such as certain forms of heart disease, cancer, and type 2 diabetes, and obesity, are lower for vegetarians than for nonvegetarians.[1] Healthful lifestyles (not smoking, abstaining from alcohol and drugs, and increasing physical activity) and social class bias probably partially account for these findings.

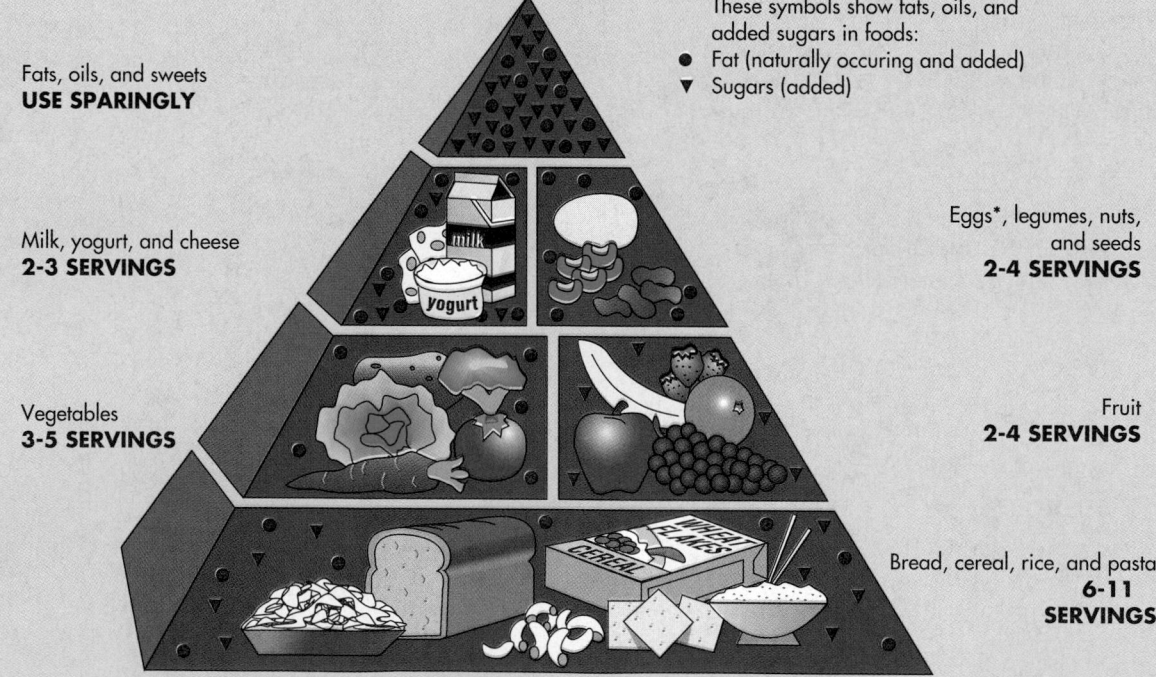

These symbols show fats, oils, and added sugars in foods:
● Fat (naturally occuring and added)
▼ Sugars (added)

Fats, oils, and sweets
USE SPARINGLY

Milk, yogurt, and cheese
2-3 SERVINGS

Eggs*, legumes, nuts, and seeds
2-4 SERVINGS

Vegetables
3-5 SERVINGS

Fruit
2-4 SERVINGS

Bread, cereal, rice, and pasta
6-11 SERVINGS

FIGURE 7-13 Food Guide Pyramid for lactoovovegetarian. Base serving size on Food Guide Pyramid in Chapter 2.
*Lactovegetarians would omit eggs as a choice.

WHY DO PEOPLE PRACTICE VEGETARIANISM?

People choose vegetarianism for a variety of reasons. Some believe that killing animals for food is unethical. Hindus and Trappist monks eat vegetarian meals as a practice of their religion. In the United States, many Seventh Day Adventists base their practice of vegetarianism on biblical texts and believe it is a more healthful way to live. Some people might pursue vegetarianism because meat is expensive.

People might choose vegetarianism after realizing that animals are not efficient protein factories. Animals actually use much of the protein they eat just to maintain themselves rather than to synthesize new muscle tissue. Note that 40% of the world's grain production is used to breed meat-producing animals. Animals that humans eat sometimes eat grasses that humans cannot digest. Many, however, also eat grains humans can eat.

People might also practice vegetarianism because it encourages a high intake of carbohydrates; vitamins A, E, and C; carotenoids; magnesium; and dietary fiber while limiting saturated-fat and cholesterol intake.[25] This produces a diet closely resembling that suggested in the Dietary Guidelines for Americans, covered in Chapter 2.

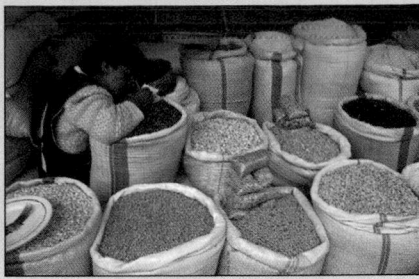

Primarily vegetarian diets are typical among rural peoples throughout the world.

FOOD PLANNING FOR VEGETARIANS

There are a variety of vegetarian styles. **Vegans** eat only plant foods. **Fruitarians** primarily eat fruits, nuts, honey, and vegetable oils. This plan is not recommended because it can lead to nutrient deficiencies in people of all ages. **Lactovegetarians** modify vegetarianism a bit—they include dairy products and plant foods. **Lactoovovegetarians** modify the diet even further and eat dairy products and eggs, as well as plant foods. Including these animal products makes food planning easier because they are rich in some nutrients that are missing or present in low amounts in plants. The more variety in the diet, the easier it is to meet nutritional needs. Thus, the practice of eating no animal sources of food significantly separates the vegans and fruitarians from all other semivegetarian styles.

It has been suggested that "almost vegetarians" (those who allow dairy and regular fish intake) are the healthiest group of all vegetarians. Perhaps this is due to the health benefits of a high fruit and vegetable diet, rather than the complete exclusion of all animal products.[11]

Most people who call themselves vegetarians consume at least some dairy products, if not all dairy products and eggs. A food-group plan has been developed for lactovegetarians and vegans (Table 7-4). This plan includes servings of nuts, grains, legumes, and seeds to help meet protein needs. There is also a vegetable group, a fruit group, and a milk group.

This plan differs a little from the Food Guide Pyramid for **omnivores.** Figure 7-13 shows how the Food Guide Pyramid could be adapted for lacto- or lactoovovegetarians. The key to this plan is seeking foods other than meat that supply the nutrients contained in meat. It's not nutritionally sound simply to stop eating meat without making sure the body's needs are still met. Good-quality plant sources of nutrients, such as nuts, grains, legumes, and seeds, should be eaten to supply nutrients that normally come from meat in the diet. By following such a food plan, a lactovegetarian should be able to have an adequate diet.[9, 11]

THE VEGAN

A vegan diet requires some creative planning. A real effort must be made to use grains and legumes to yield high-quality protein and other key nutrients in meals, especially when used with infants and children. Then, if energy needs are satisfied, protein needs should also be met. Including a wide variety of protein sources should provide all amino acids needed for a high-quality protein diet. The essential amino acids deficient from one food protein are supplied by those of another protein in the same meal or in the next. For example, many legumes do not provide enough of the essential amino acid methionine, and cereals are limited in lysine. When

vegan A person who eats only plant foods.

fruitarian A person who primarily eats fruits, nuts, honey, and vegetable oils.

lactovegetarian A person who consumes plant products and dairy products.

lactoovovegetarian A person who consumes plant products, dairy products, and eggs.

omnivore A person who consumes both plant and animal food sources.

*O*ldways Preservation & Exchange Trust has published a Vegetarian Pyramid. The base consists of fruits, vegetables, whole grains, and legumes (at every meal). The middle tier is nuts, seeds, egg whites, soy milks, dairy products, and plant oils (daily). Eggs and sweets form the tip (small quantities). Alcohol intake is optional, and daily physical activity is recommended. See its site for further information (htpp://www.oldwayspt.org).

*T*able 7-2, earlier in this chapter, lists traditional dishes in which vegetable proteins combine to provide high-quality (complete) protein in the meal.

Chapter 6 noted that a vegan diet coupled with regular exercise and other lifestyle changes can lead to a reversal of atherosclerotic plaque in the coronary arteries.

TABLE 7-4   Food-Group Plan for Lactovegetarians and Vegans§

	Servings		
Group†	Lactovegetarian‡	Vegan§‖	Key Nutrients Supplied
Grains¶	6–11	8–11	Protein, thiamin, niacin, folate, vitamin E, zinc, magnesium, iron, and dietary fiber
Legumes	1–2	2	Protein, vitamin B-6, zinc, magnesium, and dietary fiber
Nuts, seeds	1–2	2	Protein, vitamin E, and magnesium
Vegetables	3–5 (include one dark green or leafy variety daily)	4–6 (include one dark green or leafy variety daily)	Vitamin A, vitamin C, and folate
Fruits	2–4	4	Vitamin A, vitamin C, and folate
Milk	2–3	—	Protein, riboflavin, vitamin D, vitamin B-12, and calcium

†Base serving size on those listed for the Food Guide Pyramid (see Chapter 2). This plan yields about 1600 to 1800 kcal. Increase the number of servings, or add other foods to meet higher energy needs.

‡Contains about 75 g of protein in 1650 kcal.

§A calcium-fortified food, such as orange juice or soy milk, is needed unless a calcium supplement is used. In addition, use of a vitamin B-12 supplement or foods fortified with vitamin B-12 is a must. Overall, fortified soy milk makes a valuable contribution to a vegan diet.

‖Contains about 79 g of protein in 1800 kcal.

¶One serving of vitamin- and mineral-enriched breakfast cereal is recommended.

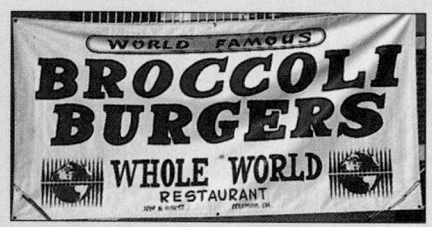

Vegetarian adaptations of traditional foods is a growing trend in our society.

Fish oil supplements (about 900 mg/day of the ω-3 fatty acids) may be beneficial for the vegan to provide a concentrated source of long-chain ω-3 fatty acids (see Chapter 6 for details). In addition, regular use of canola oil, soybean oil, flax seeds, or walnuts is advised to obtain alpha-linolenic acid, another ω-3 fatty acid.

a combination of these two foods is eaten, the body is supplied with adequate amounts of both amino acids, so cereals and legumes complement each other.

Purchasing some vegetarian cookbooks will simplify the task of menu planning. They provide numerous ideas for imaginative and nutritious ways to use plant foods.

The vegan diet must also include good sources of riboflavin, vitamins D and B-12, calcium, iron, and zinc.[3, 11] A fortified breakfast cereal provides a good start in meeting those needs. Riboflavin can be obtained from green leafy vegetables, whole grains, yeast, and legumes, part of most vegan diets. A major source of riboflavin in the typical American diet is milk, which is omitted from the vegan diet. Vitamin D can be obtained through regular sun exposure and fortified margarine. Otherwise, a supplement containing vitamin D should be considered (see Chapter 9).

The vegan should find a reliable source of vitamin B-12, such as fortified soybean milk or fortified breakfast cereals and special yeast grown on media rich in vitamin B-12. Use of a balanced vitamin and mineral supplement is another option. Vitamin B-12 occurs naturally only in animal foods, although plants can contain soil or microbial contamination that provides at most a trace amount of vitamin B-12. Because the body can store enough vitamin B-12 for about 4 years, a deficiency can take a long time to develop after animal foods are removed from the diet. If a deficiency develops, nerves can be damaged irreversibly and brain function can decrease. Evidence of a vitamin B-12 deficiency has been noted in vegetarian mothers and their infants. The milk produced by the vegetarian mothers is low in vitamin B-12. The earliest sign of a vitamin B-12 deficiency is mental dysfunction; a prolonged deficiency can lead to irreversible nerve damage.[16] Excess blood concentration of homocysteine has also been noted to vegans who underconsume vitamin B-12. This can lead to other health problems. Therefore, vegans need to be careful to prevent a vitamin B-12 deficiency (see Chapter 10).

To obtain calcium, the vegan can drink fortified soy milk or fortified orange juice and consume calcium-rich tofu (check the label) or other calcium-fortified foods, such as certain breakfast cereals and snacks. Green leafy vegetables and nuts also contain calcium, but the calcium is either not well absorbed or not very plentiful. Calcium supplements are another option (see Chapter 11).

For iron, the vegan can consume whole grains, dried fruits and nuts, and legumes. The iron in these foods is not absorbed as well as that found in animal foods, but a good source of vitamin C taken with these foods modestly enhances iron absorption. Thus, a recommended strategy is to consume vitamin C with every meal that contains adequate iron-rich plant foods. Cooking in iron pots and skillets can also add iron to the diet (see Chapter 12).

The vegan can find zinc in whole grains, nuts, and legumes, but phytic acid and other substances in these foods limit zinc absorption. Grains are most nutritious when leavened, as in bread, because this process reduces the influence of phytic acid.

Of all these nutrients, calcium and iron are the most difficult to consume in sufficient quantities. Special diet planning is required.

Veganism during childhood can pose problems. The most common nutritional concerns are deficiencies of iron, calcium, vitamin D, and vitamin B-12. Iron deficiency anemia is a frequent occurrence during childhood, however it can be avoided by supplementing the diet with iron-fortified cereals, and other iron-fortified foods. A vitamin B-12 supplement may be needed for children who exclude all animal products from their diets. Vitamin D supplements are recommended for children who do not get much sunlight exposure and who do not have any dietary source of vitamin D. Calcium can be obtained in the diet through dairy products or calcium-enriched products, such as tofu and orange juice. Finally, the fiber content of a child's diet may need to be decreased with high fiber sources replaced with some refined grain products, fruit juices, and peeled fruit. Overall, vegan children need concentrated sources of energy to help avoid these problems. Examples include fortified soy milk, nuts, dried fruits, avocados, cookies made with vegetable oils or tub margarine, and fruit juices.

Soy milk, soy yogurt, and soy cheese are excellent choices for vegan children (and vegan adults). When fortified with calcium and vitamin B-12, these substitutes can provide many of the key nutrients found in milk.

Finding excellent iron and zinc sources is important in planing vegan diets, especially for infants and children. Pregnancy also deserves special attention. Overall, both infancy and childhood are life stages in which vegetarianism is appropriate, but it must be implemented with knowledge and, ideally, professional guidance.[11] An especially informative website is http:// www.ivu.org, supported by the International Vegetarian Union.

CASE SCENARIO
Follow-Up

Shannon is a vegan if she had no cheese on the sub sandwich, and a lactovegetarian if she did have cheese. This diet plan is not healthy, as it does not come close to following the recommendations in the Nutrition Perspective. Where are the whole grains, nuts, soy products, beans, two to four fruits, and three to five vegetables, that form the base of such diets? The diet is also low in the many phytochemicals under study. Overall, she is not benefiting as she had hoped to from her vegetarian diet, since so little care has gone in to following a healthy pattern.

ALCOHOL

chapter 8

A lcohol use is an issue requiring careful attention by health professionals, law enforcement officials, the courts, elected officials, the entertainment industry, university professors, parents, students, and those engaged in the production and distribution of alcoholic beverages. Although not a nutrient per se, alcohol is an energy source for many adults. We also know that moderate consumption of alcohol has some benefits.[1, 3, 25] But when it leads to excessive consumption, many unfortunate consequences are almost inevitable. By far the most commonly abused drug, alcohol can destroy families and friendships; spur deadly behaviors such as suicide, rape and violence; and fill jails and prisons. Its abuse costs American society more than 20,000 lives each year, with about 16,000 of them from highway deaths.[12] Alcohol accounts for as much as $75 billion per year in health-care expenditures.

About 15 million Americans are currently classified as alcoholics, and another 31.9 million engage in binge drinking. Approximately 11 million of the current drinkers are under the age of 21. From early adulthood through later years in life, excess alcohol intake has damaging effects on one's nutritional status and overall health.[16]

The American Medical Association defines alcoholism as an illness characterized by significant impairment directly related to persistent and excessive use of alcohol. Impairment can involve physiological and social dysfunction, and for psychological, social, and genetic reasons some people are more vulnerable to this disorder than others.[9] It is important to examine the biochemical and physiological aspects of alcohol consumption in order to understand the causes and treatment of alcohol abuse.

KEY CHAPTER CONCEPTS

- Unlike carbohydrate, fat, or protein, alcohol requires no digestion and provides no essential nutrients. Alcohol metabolism takes precedence over metabolism of the other energy nutrients.
- Alcohol is metabolized in the liver and other tissues. Metabolism of alcohol depends on a number of factors, such as gender, race, and body composition. The benefits of alcohol use are associated with low to moderate alcohol consumption. These benefits include the pleasurable and social aspects of alcohol use, as well as a reduction in cardiovascular disease risks in some people.
- When alcohol is consumed, it should be only by people of legal drinking age, in moderation, and with meals. Women are advised to limit consumption to no more than one drink per day; men should stop at two.
- Alcohol use also creates many health risks. Excessive consumption of alcohol contributes significantly to 5 of the 10 leading causes of death in the United States. Alcohol increases the risk of developing certain forms of heart disease, inflammation of the pancreas, gastrointestinal tract damage, vitamin and mineral deficiencies, hepatitis, cirrhosis of the liver, a variety of cancers, hypertension, stroke, and irreversible brain damage—to name a few.
- Early detection of alcoholism is key in successful treatment, as well as in the reduction of health-care costs. The CAGE questionnaire and other self-assessment tools can help a person determine whether he or she has an alcohol problem.
- There are several methods available to treat alcoholism. Alcoholics Anonymous, the medications ReVia and Antabuse, medical detoxification, and behavioral conditioning have varying success rates. All treatment regimens focus on the importance of treating the whole person: individually, socially, psychologically, and medically.
- Binge drinking is a widespread problem but is especially acute on college campuses. As this behavior has gained popularity, it has tended to become a norm. Students who are over 21 tend to drink more often, but underage drinkers are more likely to be the binge drinkers.

REFRESH YOUR MEMORY

As you begin your study of alcohol, you may want to review

- The role of the GI tract, liver, and pancreas in digestion and absorption in Chapter 3
- Oxidation and reduction reactions in Chapter 4
- Glycolysis, the citric acid cycle, and electron transport chain in Chapter 4
- Fermentation reactions in Chapter 4
- Forms of carbohydrates in Chapter 5
- Protein-energy malnutrition in Chapter 7

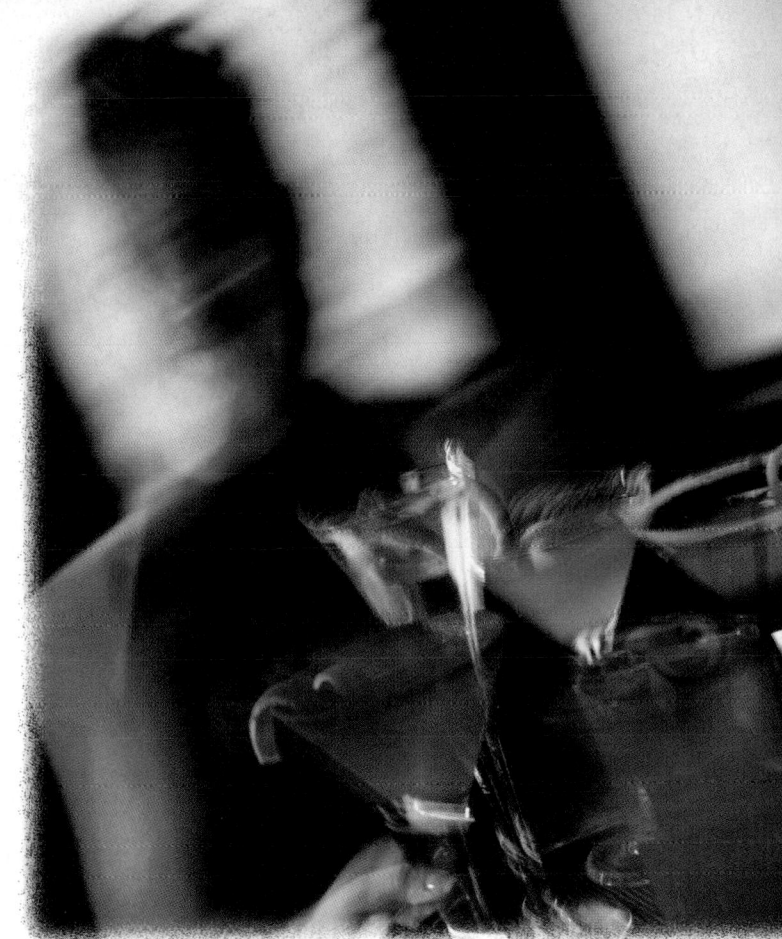

CASE SCENARIO

Todd is a college junior. He was a very serious student in high school and achieved excellent grades, but as a college student he has begun binge drinking. As a result, his grades have fallen sharply and he is becoming socially isolated. He has been arrested once for drunk driving.

Last night, he had eight beers and three shots of whiskey at an off-campus party he attended with his girlfriend, Alyssa. Unfortunately, everyone who knows Todd says he tends to get angry and says things he doesn't mean when he drinks too much. He often becomes cruel and destructive to those he cares for and respects. He has been involved in several fights.

As the party began to die down, Alyssa tried to get Todd to leave. He responded rudely and forcefully grabbed her arm. She became frightened with his aggressive behavior and left without him.

The next morning, Alyssa awoke early, still thinking about the hurtful events of the previous night. Having known of one student who died from an overdose of alcohol (he drank 23 shots of whiskey on his 21st birthday) Alyssa decided to e-mail Todd, expressing her anxiety about his alcohol abuse. She did not want to see everything he had worked so hard for ruined by alcohol.

What should Alyssa say in the e-mail about alcohol and how it affects various organs in the body? What long-term problems are associated with such alcohol abuse? Is Alyssa correct in taking the initiative in communicating to Todd her concerns about his drinking problem?

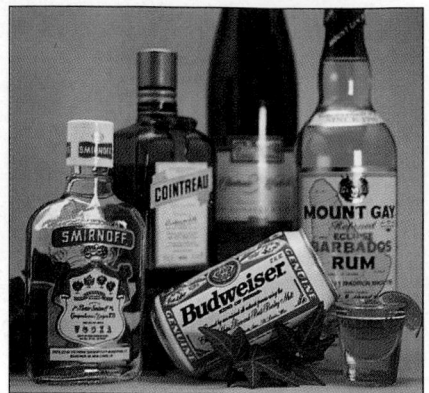

The following servings of each type of alcoholic beverage provide the same amount of alcohol: wine—5 ounces, hard liquor—1.5 ounces, beer or wine cooler—12 ounces.

fermented/fermentation Enzymatically controlled changes that occur in foods and beverages by the action of anaerobic microorganisms; method of preservation by chemical means producing alcohol, acids, and carbon dioxide.

■ ALCOHOL—AN INTRODUCTION

Given the wide spectrum of alcohol use and abuse, knowledge of alcohol consumption and its relationship to overall health is essential information to the study of nutrition. Alcohol, chemically known as ethanol, has played many roles throughout history. It can be considered a food, primarily because it contributes energy to the diet (7 kcal/g) (Table 8-1). It is also a social stimulant because it takes away inhibitions, it is a thirst quencher when used as a safe alternative to polluted water, it is an analgesic to treat aches and pain, and it is a "remedy" for all kinds of ailments.

Alcohol requires no digestion. It is absorbed rapidly by simple diffusion—no specific transport mechanisms are required for ethanol to enter a cell—so it is the most efficiently absorbed of all energy sources. Different parts of the gastrointestinal tract absorb alcohol at different rates. The duodenum and jejunum absorb alcohol fastest, but it depends on how quickly the stomach empties, which in turn depends on the kinds of foods consumed along with the alcohol.[7]

Alcohol acts on various organs but has no cellular receptors per se, as do other compounds that affect the body, such as insulin, vitamin A, or thyroid hormones.

■ HOW ALCOHOLIC BEVERAGES ARE PRODUCED

Any number of natural foods can be **fermented,** but production temperatures and composition of the food itself determine the characteristics of the final product. High-carbohydrate foods encourage the growth of yeast, the microorganism responsible for alcohol production. Brewer's yeast is one source of the enzyme that is necessary to make alcohol production possible.[23]

During glycolysis, glucose is converted to pyruvate. Yeast cells then convert pyruvate to alcohol and carbon dioxide in a simple, two-step process. In the first step, the

TABLE 8-1	Energy, Carbohydrate, and Alcohol Content of Alcoholic Beverages*			
Beverage	**Amount (fluid ounce)**	**Alcohol (grams)**	**Carbohydrates (grams)**	**Energy (kcal)**
Beer				
Regular	12.0	13	13	146
Light	12.0	11	5	99
Distilled Spirits				
Gin, rum, vodka, bourbon, whiskey (80 proof)	1.5	14	—	105
Brandy, cognac	1.0	9	—	64
Wine				
Red	3.5	10	2	74
White	3.5	10	1	70
Dessert, sweet	3.5	16	12	158
Rosé	3.5	10	1	73
Mixed Drinks				
Manhattan	3.0	26	3	191
Martini	3.0	27	—	189
Bourbon and soda	3.0	11	—	78
Whiskey sour	3.0	15	5	122

Source: USDA.

*There is little to no fat or protein contribution to energy content.

3-carbon pyruvate is converted to the 2 carbon acetaldehyde in an irreversible reaction with the release of CO_2. In the second step, another enzyme donates a pair of hydrogens to acetaldehyde to form ethanol. This enzyme uses the B-vitamin niacin in the form of the coenzyme $NADH + H^+$ (see Chapter 4 for details). Ethanol and CO_2 are the end products of the process.

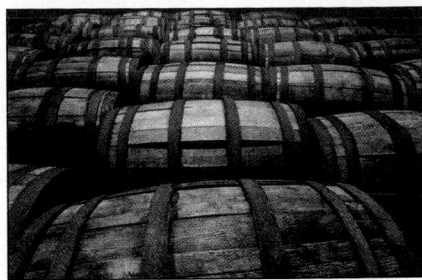

1. Glucose $\longrightarrow$ Pyruvate $\longrightarrow$ CO_2 / Acetaldehyde

2. Acetaldehyde $\xrightarrow{\quad NADH + H^+ \quad NAD \quad}$ Ethanol

The overall reaction is

$$C_6H_{12}O_6 + 2ADP + 2\,P_i \longrightarrow 2\,C_2H_5OH + 2\,CO_2 + 2ATP + 2\,H_2O$$
Glucose   Ethanol

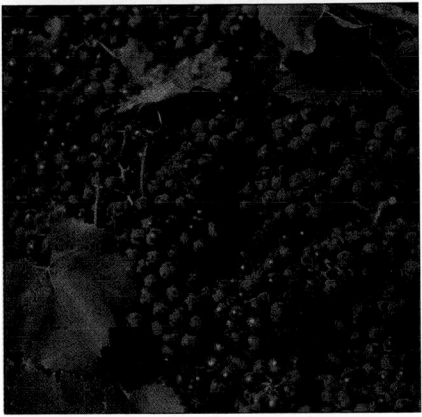

Wine is a historic beverage. It has been produced and consumed for more than 10,000 years.

Thus, under anaerobic conditions, two pyruvates are fermented by yeast to two ethanol and two carbon dioxide molecules.

The carbohydrate must be either a disaccharide or a monosaccharide, such as maltose or glucose, in order for the yeast to use it as food. If the carbohydrate is a starch, such as the polysaccharides found in cereal grains, it must be broken down to these smaller forms, or "malted." During malting, the cereal grain seeds are allowed to sprout to produce the hydrolytic enzymes that break down the polysaccharides to simple sugars (e.g., amylases). The sprouting is stopped by heating. The yeast cells and water are then added to the malt. The yeast grows aerobically, using the sugars for energy. When the oxygen in the vat (the mixture of water, yeast, and malt) is used up, the yeast switches to anaerobic metabolism and ferments the remaining sugar to produce ethanol and CO_2. After fermentation has ceased, the product is finished in a variety of ways. In some cases, the ethanol itself is recovered from the product.

Beer is made from malted cereal grain, such as barley; it is flavored with hops and brewed by slow fermentation. The carbon dioxide released is collected and used to carbonate the beer, thus producing the desirable fizz associated with a quality beverage.

Wine is the fermented juice of grapes. Climate, geographic region, and variety of grape determine the quality of the wine. After fermentation, wines are aged in oak barrels to decrease the acidity and remove undesirable impurities.

distillation A physical method used to separate liquids based on their boiling points.

Distilled spirits are made from the **distillation** of the ethanol after fermentation. Any number of fruits, vegetables, and grains can be fermented and the resulting mash distilled. The difference between the boiling point of water and the boiling point of ethanol allows these two liquids to be separated by distillation and the ethanol to be recovered. Some distilled spirits are marketed "unaged." Vodka and gin are examples of unaged beverages. Other spirits, such as whiskeys, rums, and brandies, are aged in oak barrels. Spirits are also allowed to mature, some more than 20 years.

Government standards for each nation determine the kinds of alcoholic beverages allowed to be produced and sold. For instance, single malt scotch whiskey produced in Scotland for export to the United States must meet Bureau of Alcohol, Tobacco, and Firearms standards before it can be shipped from Scotland to the United States.

■ HISTORY OF ALCOHOL USE

For thousands of years, many important foods have been produced by fermentation. Bread is the product of fermentation by bakers' yeast, milk is transformed into cheese by microorganisms, meat is aged, cabbage is made into sauerkraut, soy sauce is made from soybeans, and alcoholic beverages have been produced from just about every plant material that can be fermented.[23]

The process of production and consumption of alcohol has been a part of almost all modern cultures. It is known to be absent only from polar societies and Australian aborigines. Based on the earliest records, alcohol has provided a release from the drudgery of everyday life. A recipe for beer, dating from 4000 years ago, was found on a clay tablet in Mesopotamia. It is estimated that alcohol was probably known as early as the Stone Age, 10,000 years ago.

Throughout history, alcohol has been a valued beverage as an alternative to contaminated drinking water. A long ocean voyage, such as that planned by Christopher Columbus, was made possible by the wine carried on board.

In some early cultures, the production of alcohol fell under the domain of priests and clergy. Production of alcohol is still to be found in some European monasteries. In England, the wine trade profession is ranked as highly by people as are the professions of medicine and law.

If one consults ancient literature, drinking water was seldom mentioned, whereas wine and beer were identified as thirst quenchers.[31] Certainly, populations in the West evolved with the ability to metabolize alcohol. People in the East, on the other hand, had the practice of boiling water to make tea. This created a potable water supply, so evolutionary forces did not produce the ability to metabolize very much alcohol.

■ ALCOHOL METABOLISM

After a person drinks an alcoholic beverage, his or her blood concentration of alcohol rises rapidly. Alcohol is readily absorbed into the blood from different segments of the gastrointestinal tract by simple diffusion.[7] You've probably been warned, with good reason, not to drink on an empty stomach. Alcohol absorption depends partly on the rate of stomach emptying. Food slows the stomach's emptying rate and stimulates secretions, such as gastric acid, which dilute the alcohol and slow its absorption into the bloodstream. Certain drugs also control gastric-emptying time and thus overall absorption. The type of beverage consumed also determines alcohol absorption. The alcohol in beer is absorbed more slowly than the alcohol in whiskey, which is slower than wine. Pure alcohol is absorbed fastest of all but, of course, such a beverage is not for sale.

Alcohol is readily distributed in the fluid compartments within the body because alcohol is found wherever water is distributed in the body. Alcohol moves easily through the cell membranes; however, as it does, it damages proteins in the membranes by the process of denaturation. Most of alcohol's damaging effects are concentrated in the liver because this is the first organ that is exposed to alcohol after absorption, and the liver is the chief site for alcohol oxidation.[7] Although it is true that gastrointestinal cells are in contact with alcohol, they are constantly being replaced because of their naturally short life span. Thus, they are not subject to the same damage as liver cells, which have a much longer life span.

Metabolism of alcohol is dependent on numerous factors, such as gender, race, size, physical condition, what is eaten, the alcohol content of the beverage, and even how much sleep one has had. The ability to produce the enzyme **alcohol dehydrogenase (ADH)** is the key to alcohol metabolism. Women absorb and metabolize alcohol differently than men do. A woman cannot metabolize much alcohol in the cells that line her stomach because of low activity of the enzyme ADH. When a man and woman of similar size drink equal amounts of alcohol, a larger proportion of the alcohol reaches the woman's bloodstream.[7] Alcohol is initially metabolized by alcohol dehydrogenase from gastric juice. Men metabolize about 30% of the alcohol

alcohol dehydrogenase (ADH) An enzyme used in alcohol (ethanol) breakdown—metabolism; the major enzyme used in the liver when alcohol is in low concentration.

ingested, but women metabolize only 10%, since they produce smaller amounts of the enzyme. Thus, women develop alcohol-related ailments, such as **cirrhosis** of the liver, more rapidly than men do with the same alcohol-consumption habits. Also, certain histamine-blocking drugs used to treat ulcers and heartburn inhibit ADH activity, as does chronic alcohol abuse and aging.[7]

Most of the alcohol consumed is metabolized in the liver. Only a small percentage is excreted directly through the lungs, urine, and sweat. The alcohol content of expired air exhibits a constant relationship to the blood alcohol concentration in the lungs. This is the basis of the breathalyzer test. As one continues to drink, one's blood alcohol concentration (BAC) continues to rise (Table 8-2). A social drinker who weighs 150 pounds and has normal liver function metabolizes about 7 to 14 g of alcohol per hour (100 to 200 mg/kg of body weight per hour). This is about 8 to 12 ounces of beer or half an ordinary-sized drink. When the rate of alcohol consumption exceeds the liver's metabolic capacity, blood alcohol rises and symptoms of intoxication appear as the brain begins to be exposed to alcohol.

Because alcohol cannot be stored in the body, it has absolute priority in metabolism as a fuel source. The liver and stomach are the major sites for alcohol metabolism. The liver contains 3 pathways: alcohol dehydrogenase (ADH) pathway, the **microsomal ethanol oxidizing system** (MEOS), and **catalase.** Each pathway produces acetaldehyde.[16]

■ Alcohol Dehydrogenase Pathway

During the first step, alcohol at low to moderate quantity is converted to acetaldehyde by the action of alcohol dehydrogenase and the coenzyme NAD. NAD (oxidized coenzyme form) picks up two hydrogens from the alcohol to form NADH + H$^+$ (reduced form) and produces the intermediate acetaldehyde (Fig. 8-1).

$$\text{Ethanol} \xrightarrow[\text{NAD} \quad \text{NADH + H}^+]{} \text{Acetaldehyde}$$

TABLE 8-2 Blood Alcohol Concentration and Symptoms

Concentration*	Sporadic Drinker	Chronic Drinker	Hours for Alcohol to Be Metabolized
50 (party high) (0.05%)	Congenial euphoria; decreased tension	No observable effect	2–3
75 (0.075%)	Gregarious	Often no effect	
100 (0.1%)	Uncoordinated; 0.1% is legally drunk (as in drunk driving) in most states; note that 0.08% is legal drunkenness in a growing number of areas in the United States†	Minimal signs	4–6
125–150 (0.125–0.15%)	Unrestrained behavior; episodic uncontrolled behavior; legally drunk at 0.15% in all states	Pleasurable euphoria or beginning of uncoordination	6–10
200–250 (0.2–0.25%)	Alertness lost; lethargic	Effort is required to maintain emotional and motor control.	10–24
300–350 (0.3–0.35%)	Stupor to coma	Drowsy and slow	
>500 (>0.5%)	Some will die.	Coma	>24

Modified from Wyngaarder JB, Smith LH: *Cecil Textbook of Medicine,* fourth edition, Philadelphia, 1988, WB Saunders. Used with permission.

*Milligrams of alcohol per 100 milliliters of blood.

†Commencing in 2004, all states will need to use 0.08% as the definition of legally drunk to attain federal highway funds. On an empty stomach, a man reaches this state with 4 drinks within one hour, while a women reaches this state with one less drink.

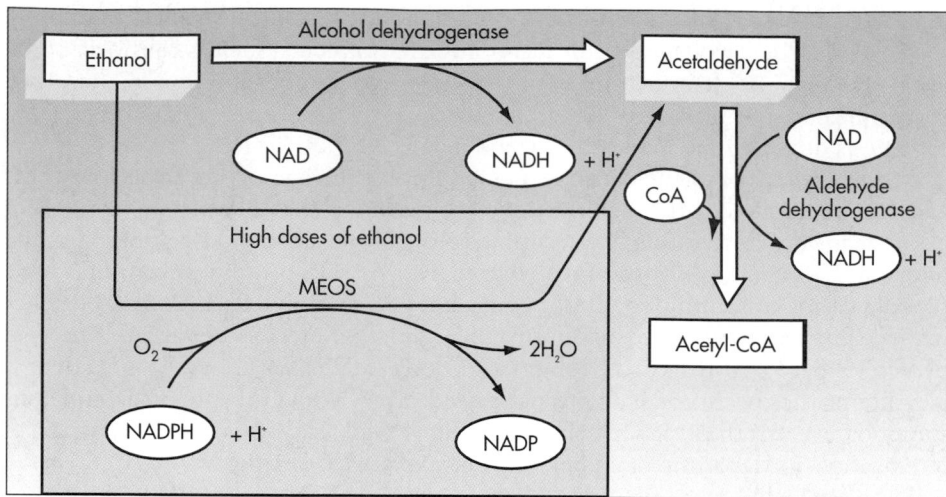

FIGURE 8-1 Alcohol metabolism. At low alcohol intake, the alcohol dehydrogenase pathway in the cytosol is used. At high alcohol intake, the microsomal ethanol oxidizing system (MEOS) in the cytosol also is used. The MEOS uses rather than yields energy.
Illustration by William Ober.

Distinctly different forms of alcohol dehydrogenase are found in the liver and the stomach. Each varies in its rate of alcohol metabolism. This enzyme requires the mineral zinc for activity.

The acetaldehyde formed is then converted to acetyl-CoA, again yielding NADH + H$^+$ with the aid of aldehyde dehydrogenase and Coenzyme A.

$$\text{Acetaldehyde} \xrightarrow[\text{NAD} \quad \text{NADH} + \text{H}^+]{} \text{Acetic acid} \xrightarrow[\text{Coenzyme A}]{} \text{Acetyl-CoA}$$

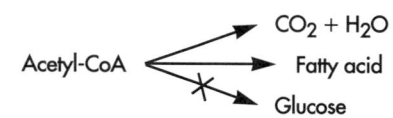

Metabolic fates of acetyl-CoA.

The increase in NADH + H$^+$ may promote fatty acid synthesis, with accumulation of body fat.[17] The acetyl-CoA enters the citric acid cycle, and the NADH + H$^+$, FADH$_2$, and GTP molecules produced in the citric acid cycle can then be used to synthesize ATP via the electron transport chain (see Chapter 4).

Structurally, ethanol with its hydroxyl group (-OH) resembles a carbohydrate. However, since it is converted directly into acetyl-CoA, alcohol carbons cannot support glucose production. Thus, alcohol is metabolized more like a fatty acid than a carbohydrate and is considered fat in metabolic terms.

■ Microsomal Ethanol Oxidizing System

When a person drinks moderate to excessive amounts of alcohol, the enzyme alcohol dehydrogenase cannot keep up with the demand to metabolize all of the alcohol into acetaldehyde. For this and other reasons, another enzyme system exists to metabolize alcohol. This system is called the **microsomal ethanol oxidizing system (MEOS).** The MEOS system is not found in the stomach.

The liver uses the MEOS to metabolize drugs and other foreign substances. When the liver is overwhelmed with excess amounts of alcohol, it treats the excess as a foreign substance and activates the MEOS. This system uses oxygen—another niacin coenzyme (NADP)—and produces water and acetaldehyde. Once the MEOS is active, alcohol tolerance increases because the rate of alcohol metabolism increases.[7]

$$\text{Ethanol} \xrightarrow[\text{NADPH} + \text{H}^+ \quad \text{NADP}]{\text{O}_2} \text{Acetaldehyde} + 2\,\text{H}_2\text{O}$$

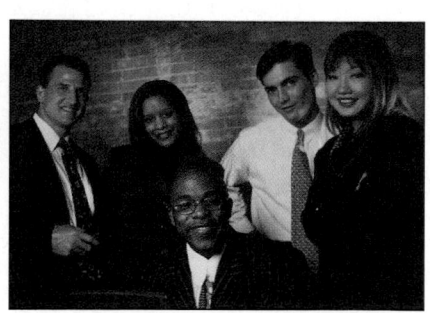

Compared with Caucasians, some Asians and Native Americans make relatively little aldehyde dehydrogenase.

There are two interesting aspects of the body's reliance on MEOS. First, rather than forming the niacin-containing coenzyme, NADH + H$^+$ with alcohol dehydrogenase, the MEOS uses the niacin-containing coenzyme NADPH + H⁺, a compound analogous to NADH + H⁺. Rather than yielding "potential" ATP molecules from the first step in alcohol metabolism, the MEOS *uses* "potential" ATP energy in the form of NADPH + H⁺. NADPH + H⁺ is converted to NADP. This partly explains why alcoholics do not gain as much weight as might be expected from the amount of alcohol-derived energy they consume.[7] The liver inefficiently uses excessive amounts of alcohol because it requires energy for the initial metabolic step in metabolism. A person with alcoholism wastes some energy by inducing this alternate metabolic pathway. Liver damage from alcohol, such that other metabolic pathways are hampered, also is implicated in the reduced energy yield associated with high alcohol consumption. In addition, alcohol slightly increases the metabolic rate of the body.[13]

Use of the MEOS also increases the potential for a drug overdose. While the MEOS is metabolizing alcohol, its capacity for metabolizing other drugs, such as many sedatives (barbiturates), is reduced, since both substrates are competing for the same enzymes. If large amounts of alcohol and sedatives are consumed simultaneously, the alcohol gets preferential treatment. Since this means the liver is not able to metabolize the sedatives fast enough, the user may lapse into a coma and even die. This is due to a lack of enzymes to convert the sedatives to harmless substances. Alcohol itself is toxic in high quantities. Mixed with sedatives, it creates an extremely lethal combination.

■ Catalase

The catalase system found in the liver, but not in the stomach, is a minor pathway for metabolizing alcohol. It is located in the cell organelle, the peroxisomes.[7]

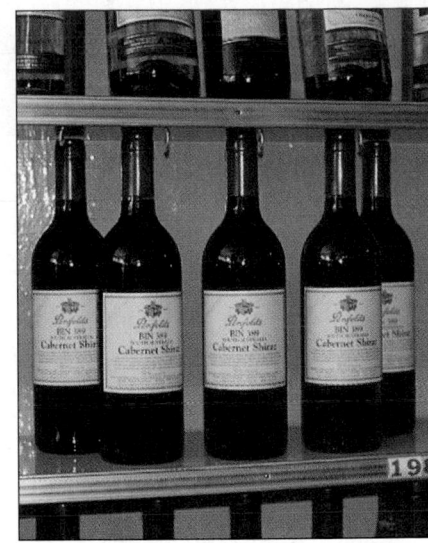

Of all the alcohol sources, red wine is often singled out as the best choice because of the added bonus of the many phytochemicals present. These were leached out from the grape skins as the red wine was fermented. Still, the American Heart Association recently stated that use of red wine does not substitute for controlling the other cardiovascular risk factors discussed in Chapter 6.

■ BENEFITS OF ALCOHOL USE

The benefits of alcohol use are linked to specific intakes of about one drink a day for men and slightly less than one for women.[24] One standard drink is universally defined as one 12-ounce bottle of beer or wine cooler, one 5-ounce glass of wine, 3 ounces of sherry or liqueur, or 1.5 ounces of 80-proof distilled spirits. Note that beer ranges considerably in its alcohol content, with malt liquor being higher in alcohol than most other forms of beer.

The benefit of moderate alcohol use begins with the many pleasurable and social aspects of its use. People enjoy meeting a friend over a beer or settling down to a glass of wine in the evening with dinner. These behaviors are not considered excessive, as long as they are practiced by people of legal drinking age, remain under control, and cause no obvious harm. Coronary heart disease (CHD) and **ischemic stroke** risk is decreased in moderate drinkers as opposed to those who abstain from alcoholic beverages.[3, 11, 32] Dr. Klatsky discusses this and other potential benefits of alcohol in his Expert Opinion.

Many of the benefits of moderate alcohol use are effective only in the short term. Previous consumers of alcohol no longer experience the benefits of alcohol when consumption ceases.[29]

ischemic stroke A stroke caused by the absence of blood flow to a part of the brain.

Alcohol can protect individuals against harmful bacteria in the stomach. In vivo as well as in vitro, research has shown that ethanol can kill bacteria such as *Helicobacter pylori*.[4] This bacterium, implicated in heartburn, peptic ulcer, and stomach cancer, is most common in nondrinkers and decreases as daily alcohol intake increases. It must be kept in mind, however, that other microorganisms are helpful to our digestive systems. If these are decreased, alcohol may produce detrimental effects on gastrointestinal function.

CONCEPT CHECK

Alcohol is not an essential nutrient. It requires no digestion, and alcohol metabolism takes precedence over metabolism of the other energy-yielding nutrients. Alcohol is metabolized in the liver and other tissues. Metabolism mostly depends on the enzyme alcohol dehydrogenase. A number of individual factors, such as gender, race, and body composition, determine how a person reacts to alcohol. The microsomal ethanol oxidizing

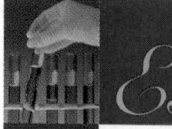

Expert Opinion

SENSIBLE, SAFE, AND BENEFICIAL ALCOHOL DRINKING

Arthur L. Klatsky, M.D.

In a speech to a temperance society more than 100 years ago, Abraham Lincoln said, "It is true that many were injured by intoxicating drink, but none seemed to think the injury arose from the use of a bad thing, but from the abuse of a very good thing." It is unlikely, of course, that Mr. Lincoln knew about the medical benefits of lighter drinking; he simply liked his whiskey and drank for pleasure. Most adults, in fact, are light to moderate drinkers who drink for nonmedical reasons and for whom any harm or benefit is incidental, yet they justifiably demand expert advice about the risks of drinking.

DETERMINING A SAFE LIMIT

The health risks of heavier drinking and the relative safety of lighter drinking have always been evident. Of the many attempts to define a safe limit, perhaps the most often quoted since the 1860s has been "Anstie's rule." Presumably intended to apply primarily to adult men, this rule advised an upper limit of about three standard drinks daily. Sir Francis Edmund Anstie was a distinguished British neurologist and public health advocate who defended the safety of moderate drinking but also emphasized individual differences in the ability to handle alcohol. These differences are related to age, sex, and individual risk/benefit considerations and should be an important focus in any discussion of safe or sensible limits. For example, women seem to merit a lower limit for safe drinking because of their smaller size, greater proportion of body fat, and slower metabolism of alcohol in the stomach.

DEFINING LIGHT, MODERATE, AND HEAVY DRINKING

Although all definitions are arbitrary, my definitions of light, moderate, and heavy drinking are based on the level of drinking above which increased health risks are usually seen. Thus, "light," "lighter," or "moderate" drinking means less than three drinks per day, and "heavy" or "heavier" drinking means three or more drinks per day. A steady drinking pattern, rather than a binge pattern, is assumed. These limits, based on large population studies, correspond closely to Anstie's commonsense observation. Keep in mind, however, that in data based on population surveys, systematic "underestimation" (lying) by survey participants probably makes the threshold for harmful effects seem lower than it actually is because some heavier drinkers appear to be lighter imbibers.

The amount of alcohol in a standard-size drink of wine (about 5 oz), liquor (about 1.5 oz), and beer (about 12 oz) is approximately the same; each contains about 0.4 oz of ethyl alcohol (ethanol). Since people think in terms of the number of drinks, rather than milliliters or grams of alcohol, alcohol intake is usually described as a given number of drinks consumed per day or week. In determining your own safe level of intake, it is important to observe these serving sizes.

RISKS OF HEAVY DRINKING

Research has produced compelling evidence of the increased medical risks faced by heavy drinkers, who are at the highest overall risk of morbidity (i.e., illness) and mortality, compared with abstainers and light to moderate drinkers. Heavy drinking is associated with health problems, including liver cirrhosis, inflammation of the pancreas or stomach, certain types of cancer, hypertension, cardiomyopathy (disease of the heart muscle), heart rhythm disturbances, hemorrhagic stroke, and an increased incidence of accidents and suicide.

system (MEOS) is used whenever the liver detects more alcohol than can be processed by the alcohol dehydrogenase enzymes. Once the MEOS is active, alcohol tolerance increases because alcohol is being metabolized more rapidly.

The benefits of alcohol use are realized with moderate consumption. Under the correct circumstances, alcohol can be pleasurable, add to social occasions, and decrease the risk of coronary heart disease and ischemic stroke. Mortality risk is somewhat greater in those who abstain from alcohol, and the risk appears to be decreased in those consuming up to two drinks per day; furthermore, the protective effect of alcohol is somewhat less in women, and overall mortality risk increases in both sexes above these amounts.

BENEFITS AND RISKS OF LIGHT DRINKING

Light drinking, compared with abstinence, is associated with a lower risk of certain serious health problems, including coronary heart disease (CHD), the most common cause of death among Americans. Light drinkers are also less likely to suffer ischemic stroke, an important cause of morbidity but a less common cause of death. Finally, gallstones are less common among light drinkers than among abstainers.

Light drinking, however, is not without risk. The most obvious risk is that of addiction, which is clearly increased by a family history of alcoholism. In addition, there are concerns about the link between light to moderate drinking and the risk of female breast cancer, harm to the fetus in pregnant women, and colon cancer in both sexes.

MAKING PUBLIC HEALTH RECOMMENDATIONS

The evidence that moderate drinking lowers the risk of CHD has been recognized in the text of the 2000 Dietary Guidelines for Americans (discussed in Chapter 2), which contains this statement: "Drinking in moderation may lower risk for coronary heart disease, mainly among men over age 45 and women over age 55. However, there are other factors that reduce the risk of heart disease, including a healthy diet, physical activity, avoidance of smoking, and maintenance of a healthy weight. Moderate consumption provides little, if any, health benefit for younger people." The text concludes with this advice: "If you drink alcoholic beverages, do so in moderation....Limit intake to one drink per day for women or two per day for men, and take with meals to slow alcohol absorption. Avoid drinking before or when driving, or whenever it puts you or others at risk." The most recent United Kingdom Department of Health report, "Sensible Drinking," goes even further, suggesting that the "maximum health advantage" can be achieved with one or two daily units (small drinks) and that people in age groups with substantial CHD risk should "consider the possible benefits of lighter drinking."

Not surprisingly, these statements are very controversial. When making public health recommendations for alcohol use, the serious health problems caused by heavy drinking remain of paramount concern. The increased medical risks that predominate among heavy drinkers greatly outweigh any potential CHD benefit. All heavy drinkers should reduce their alcohol intake or abstain.

Although concern about the risks of drinking makes it inappropriate to advise all nondrinkers to drink for health benefit, individual exceptions can be made based on age, sex, personal and family history of problem drinking, and risk of CHD, certain types of cancer (mostly notably, breast cancer), and other medical problems. Such exceptions require the advising health professional to have personal knowledge about his or her client. And, for CHD prevention, lighter drinking is, of course, only part of the picture—not smoking, following a proper diet, staying physically active, and taking other measures must be emphasized (see Chapter 6 for a further discussion).

It is hoped that we have entered an age in which our historical view of alcohol, current governmental guidelines, and sound scientific evidence have converged in a balanced view of moderate drinking and a reasonable, rational concept of sensible limits for individuals.

Dr. Klatsky is a senior consultant in cardiology at Kaiser-Permanente Medical Center in Oakland, California. His research interest is the effect of alcohol consumption on health, and he has published articles on this topic in The New England Journal of Medicine, the Annals of Internal Medicine, the British Medical Journal, and other prestigious periodicals.

■ PROBLEMS OF ALCOHOL USE

Despite the few benefits of regular, moderate alcohol use, the risks of abuse are more numerous and harmful. Alcoholism, in and of itself, is one of the most preventable health problems in the United States. Excessive consumption of alcohol contributes significantly to 5 of the 10 leading causes of death in the United States—heart disease, certain forms of cancer, cirrhosis of the liver, motor vehicle and other accidents, and suicides. Tobacco, often used simultaneously, interacts with alcohol in a way that reinforces its effects and causes esophageal and oral cancer. In addition, excessive alcohol drinking increases the risk of some types of heart disease, nutritional deficiencies, fetal damage, obesity, colorectal cancer, and many other disorders (Fig. 8-2).[2, 10, 14] Alcohol ingestion also reduces fat oxidation and promotes a positive energy balance.[13]

Alcohol has little nutritional value. The protein and vitamin content is extremely low, except in beer, where it is marginal. Iron content varies from drink to drink, with red wine ranking especially high in iron. Excess use of some alcoholic beverages can lead to iron toxicity, as well as that from lead or cobalt.

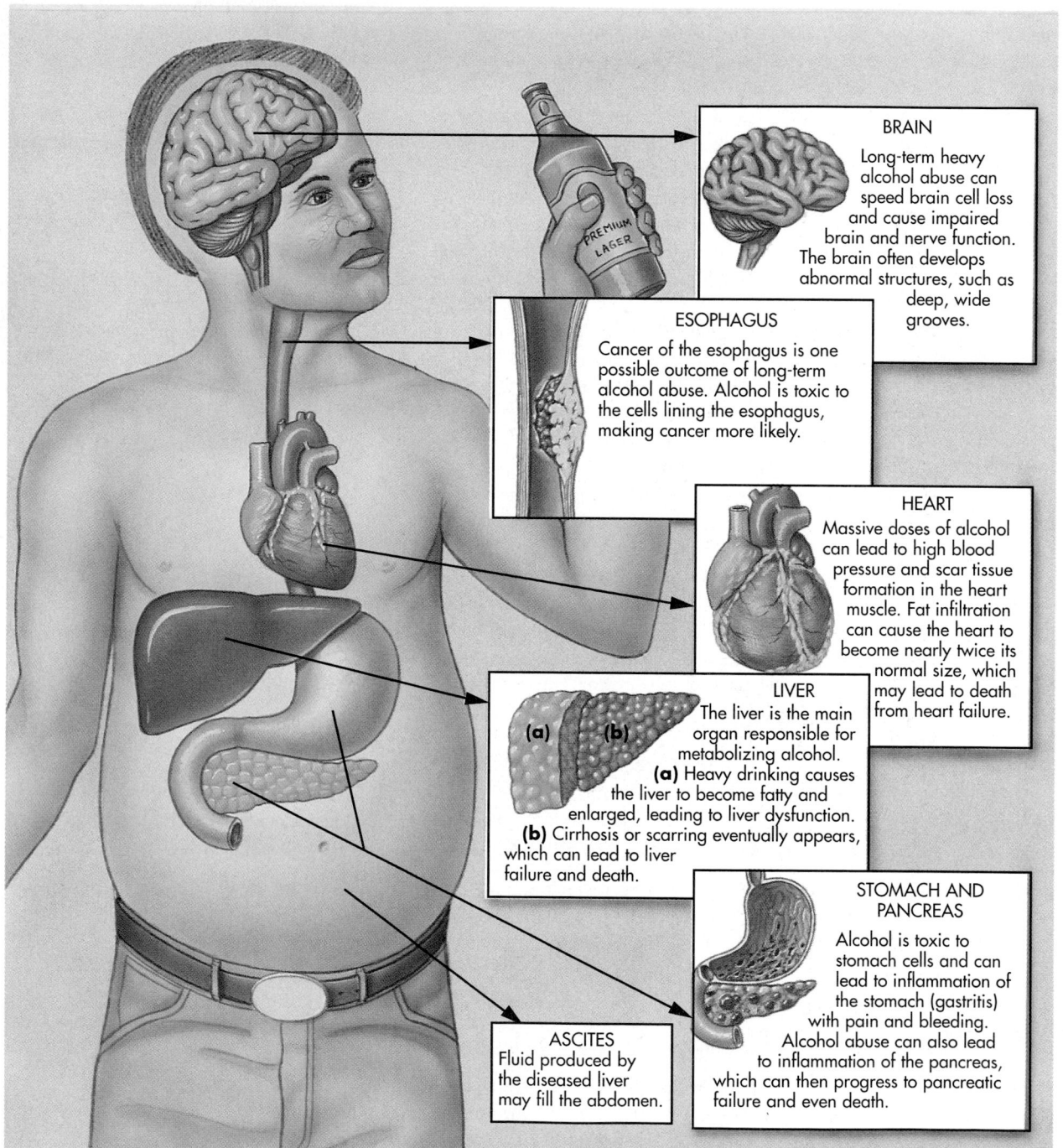

BRAIN
Long-term heavy alcohol abuse can speed brain cell loss and cause impaired brain and nerve function. The brain often develops abnormal structures, such as deep, wide grooves.

ESOPHAGUS
Cancer of the esophagus is one possible outcome of long-term alcohol abuse. Alcohol is toxic to the cells lining the esophagus, making cancer more likely.

HEART
Massive doses of alcohol can lead to high blood pressure and scar tissue formation in the heart muscle. Fat infiltration can cause the heart to become nearly twice its normal size, which may lead to death from heart failure.

LIVER
The liver is the main organ responsible for metabolizing alcohol.
(a) Heavy drinking causes the liver to become fatty and enlarged, leading to liver dysfunction.
(b) Cirrhosis or scarring eventually appears, which can lead to liver failure and death.

STOMACH AND PANCREAS
Alcohol is toxic to stomach cells and can lead to inflammation of the stomach (gastritis) with pain and bleeding. Alcohol abuse can also lead to inflammation of the pancreas, which can then progress to pancreatic failure and even death.

ASCITES
Fluid produced by the diseased liver may fill the abdomen.

FIGURE 8-2 Effects of alcohol abuse on the body. The mind-altering effects of alcohol begin soon after it enters the bloodstream. Within minutes, alcohol inhibits nerve cells in the brain. The heart muscle strains to cope with alcohol's depressive action. If drinking continues, rising blood alcohol causes impaired speech, vision, balance, and judgment. With an extremely high blood alcohol content, respiratory failure is possible. Over time, alcohol abuse increases the risk of liver and pancreas failure and certain forms of heart damage and cancer.
Illustration by William Ober.

■ Gastrointestinal Tract Damage

Excess alcohol intake damages the gastrointestinal tract, causing many associated problems. The damage to the GI tract also promotes iron absorption and may result in iron overload disease (see Chapter 12). Malabsorption, diarrhea, and steatorrhea (the formation of fatty, foamy, greasy stools) can also result. Alcohol-related inflammation of the gall bladder and pancreas often occurs from abuse. Reduced enzyme output by the pancreas and decreased bile production by the liver makes the digestion and absorption of nutrients difficult. In such cases, many patients also find food intake is limited by abdominal pain, nausea, and vomiting. These patients are often nutritionally depleted by inadequate food intake due to abdominal pain accompanied by years of poor digestion.[7]

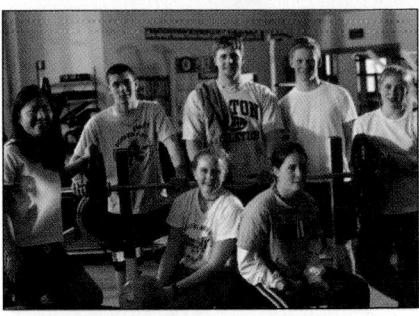

Young people benefit most from diet and exercise to decrease future risk of cardiovascular disease. There is no related benefit at this age for alcohol use.

■ Compromised Vitamin and Mineral Status

Alcohol use can interfere with nutrient intake, especially in cases of alcoholism, when alcohol replaces some or all of the food in the diet. Nutritional problems are common among alcoholics. Protein-energy malnutrition results when a person relies on alcohol for most, if not all, of his or her energy needs. The symptoms are the same as those seen in children with marasmus (see Chapter 7). Besides potential protein and energy deficiencies, deficiencies of a variety of nutrients are possible. Vitamin and mineral status is especially compromised by excessive consumption of alcohol.[16]

If a person were to use beer as a nutrient source, he or she would need to consume
- *15–20 liters daily to meet protein requirements*
- *25 liters for thiamin needs*
- *1 liter for nicotinic acid requirements*

Water-Soluble Vitamins

Thiamin deficiency can be caused by decreased thiamin absorption or decreased liver activity, which converts thiamin to its active coenzyme form. An extreme deficiency is considered a medical emergency, and patients are given thiamin injections when admitted to the hospital emergency room in a coma or stupor. Typical symptoms of thiamin deficiency, such as **polyneuropathy,** are frequently diagnosed in alcoholics. Some alcoholics exhibit nervous system problems similar to those seen in the most severe thiamin deficiency, **Wernicke-Korsakoff syndrome** (see Chapter 10 for details). Assessment of thiamin deficiency is sometimes difficult, so routine thiamin replacement is often used.

polyneuropathy A disease process involving a number of peripheral nerves.

Wernicke-Korsakoff syndrome A thiamin deficiency disease caused by excessive alcohol consumption. Symptoms include eye problems, difficulty walking, and deranged mental functions.

Niacin deficiency and the resulting classical deficiency disease pellagra are caused by a diet deficient in this B-vitamin, along with an overall poor protein intake. Alcohol also uses large amounts of niacin as NAD and NADP during metabolism, limiting the amount available for other metabolic activities.

Vitamin B-6 deficiency generally stems from a deficient intake of the vitamin and possibly increased breakdown of vitamin B-6 in its coenzyme form. Acetaldehyde pulls the vitamin B-6 coenzyme out of its orientation with its enzyme, causing increased destruction of the vitamin. This leads to decreased red blood cell production and causes a form of anemia in alcoholics.

Vitamin B-12 deficiency results from alcohol's interference with absorption. A decrease in the output of the digestive enzyme trypsin by the pancreas can reduce vitamin B-12 absorption. Trypsin is needed to release vitamin B-12 from food, so that it can be absorbed (see Chapter 10).

Folate deficiency can be caused by an inadequate intake of folate-rich foods and reduced nutrient absorption due to damage of the **mucosa.** The liver cannot retain as much folate and the kidneys increase excretion. A folate deficiency inevitably leads to a decreased number of villi, which decreases the absorption of almost all nutrients. A folate deficiency also results in increased homocysteine in the blood, which you saw in Chapter 6 is linked to cardiovascular disease. Certain forms of anemia are more common in folate-depleted patients who consume excess alcohol (see Chapter 10).

mucosa Mucous membrane consisting of cells and supporting connective tissue. It lines cavities that open to the outside of the body such as the stomach and intestine and generally contains glands that secrete mucus.

Vitamin C deficiency may result primarily from a decrease in dietary intake or altered liver metabolism, or both, and eventually leads to scurvy. When alcohol intake exceeds 30% of total calories, vitamin C intake is usually less than the RDA. Daily supplementation may be required for weeks to months to restore blood and urinary vitamin C concentrations to normal amounts.

*V*itamin A toxicity is also a potential problem in alcoholism. Excess vitamin A contributes to liver cell destruction, as does alcohol. Thus, any use of vitamin A supplements in the treatment of alcoholism should not contain greater than twice the Daily Value listed on the Nutrition Supplement Facts label.[15]

Fat-Soluble Vitamins

Vitamin A deficiency may be caused by deficient diet or inability of the liver to produce the protein that delivers the vitamin to all parts of the body (see Chapter 9). Vitamin A stores in alcoholism are diminished whether dietary vitamin A intake is low, adequate, or high. In addition, the chemical-detoxifying systems in the liver induced by chronic alcohol consumption may hasten the degradation of vitamin A. Vitamin A concentrations are especially low in cases of cirrhosis. Since alcohol can reduce pancreatic enzyme output, the enzymes needed to digest fat are low and this ultimately reduces vitamin A absorption. The conversion of one form of vitamin A (beta-carotene) to the form the body uses (retinoids) is impaired by alcoholism. Many alcoholics have trouble seeing in the dark (night blindness) due to an alcohol-induced vitamin A deficiency (see Chapter 9). Beta-carotene, by contrast, a precursor of vitamin A, interacts with alcohol and this interferes with its conversion to vitamin A. Smokers who consume alcohol and β-carotene supplements are at great risk for developing lung cancer.

Vitamin D deficiency is usually due to inadequate intake of the vitamin or lack of exposure to sunlight. Dietary vitamin D may not be absorbed because the alcohol-damaged pancreas can't produce enough fat-digesting enzymes to facilitate fat absorption, which in turn inhibits vitamin D absorption. If the liver is damaged by alcohol, the capacity to convert vitamin D to its biologically active form may be impossible. Alcoholism may cause bone cell dysfunction, which diminishes bone formation and reduces bone mineralization, leading to osteoporosis. With alcohol intoxication, the chances of falling and fracturing a bone increase. Vitamin D deficiency compromises calcium and phosphorus metabolism as well.

Vitamin K deficiency results from decreased absorption due to a lack of fat-digesting enzymes. It also occurs because alcohol-damaged intestinal bacteria are less able to synthesize the vitamin (see Chapter 9).

Vitamin E deficiency is probably due to the same reasons that vitamin A, D, and K are low in alcoholics—reduced pancreatic enzyme output. In order to absorb the fat-soluble vitamins, the fat-digesting enzymes must be produced. Anything that interferes with fat digestion, and that includes decreased bile production by the liver, reduces the amount of fat-soluble vitamins that finally are absorbed into the body.

Mineral Deficiencies

Magnesium deficiency may develop with severe alcohol abuse. Large doses of alcohol, such as consumed by binge drinkers, promotes magnesium loss via the urine, as evidenced by low blood concentrations of magnesium. This can cause **tetany**—muscle twitches, cramps, and carpopedal spasms and seizures. Impairment of the central nervous system also results. Magnesium deficiency is partly responsible for the hallucinations experienced by people withdrawing from alcohol intoxication.

tetany A state marked by the sharp contraction of muscles, with a failure to relax afterward; usually caused by abnormal calcium metabolism.

Zinc deficiency results from decreased absorption and increased urinary excretion. The consequences of zinc deficiency in conjunction with chronic alcoholism is associated with a change in taste and smell, anorexia, trouble seeing at night, and impaired wound healing.

Iron deficiency and iron overload disease are both possible in alcoholics. The iron deficiency may be due to injuries that develop in the gastrointestinal tract, which cause bleeding. If a patient has existing liver disease, alcohol increases the uptake and storage of iron in the liver.

Overall, clinicians may not be aware of the many nutritional effects of excess alcohol consumption.

*T*he overt signs of liver failure associated with cirrhosis are jaundice (the whites of the eyes and the skin turn yellow), ascites (fluid produced by the liver accumulates in the abdomen), and significant enlargement of the veins in the neck.

■ Cirrhosis

Long-term alcohol use causes fatty liver, alcoholic hepatitis, and eventually cirrhosis. Cirrhosis is a chronic and usually relentlessly progressive disease characterized by fatty infiltration of the liver. Fatty liver occurs in response to increased liver synthesis of fat from accelerated acetyl-CoA production.[7] There is good evidence that the increased production of fat in the liver is also associated with a decrease in the activities of enzymes associated with the citric acid cycle resulting from liver damage. These enzymes would be used to metabolize fat. Eventually, the enlarged fat deposits choke off the blood supply, depriving the liver cells of oxygen and nutrients. Liver cells can accumulate so much fat that they burst and die and are replaced by connective (scar) tissue. This scarring process is called *cirrhosis.* When too many liver cells die, the liver dies, and the alcoholic patient dies. In North America, most cases of cirrhosis are caused by alcohol consumption. Cirrhosis develops in about 15 to 20% of cases of alcoholism. In addition to the amount and duration of alcohol consumption, genetic factors and individual differences determine one's risk for the disease, such as obesity, exposure to hepatotoxins (e.g., acetaminophen [Tylenol]), and infections with hepatitis C. Once a person has cirrhosis, there is a 50% chance of death within 4 years, a far worse prognosis than many forms of cancer. Most of the deaths from alcoholic cirrhosis occur in people between the ages of 40 and 65 years.

A number of possible mechanisms underlie the liver damage from alcohol abuse. In chronic alcoholism, acetaldehyde concentration also increases in the liver, and is thought to be the underlying cause of the toxic effects of alcohol. Another cause is the production of **free radicals,** highly reactive molecules that destroy cell membranes and DNA. Alcohol inhibits the body's natural defenses against free radical damage. A by-product of free radical damage is inflammation, a process that can destroy healthy liver tissue.[18]

No specific amount of alcohol consumption guarantees cirrhosis. One perceptible pattern is that cirrhosis commonly results from a 15-year consumption of approximately 80 g of alcohol (the equivalent of seven beers) per day. Some evidence suggests that damage is caused by a dose as low as 40 g/day for men and 20 g/day for women. Early stages of alcoholic liver injury are reversible, but advanced stages usually are not. If a person is terminally ill, a liver transplant is necessary for survival.

A nutritious diet helps prevent some complications associated with alcoholism, but usually alcoholism brings about serious destruction of vital tissues regardless of the quality of the food consumed. Laboratory animal studies show clearly that, even when a nutritious diet is fed, alcohol abuse can lead to cirrhosis. Still, deficient nutritional status compounds the problem of cirrhosis, as it makes the liver more vulnerable to toxic substances by depleting supplies of antioxidants, such as vitamins E and C. If present in adequate amounts, these two vitamins reduce free radical damage to the liver.[7]

■ Toxicity to the Fetus

Alcohol consumption during pregnancy can result in **fetal alcohol syndrome (FAS)** and **fetal alcohol effect (FAE).** These diseases are discussed in detail in Chapter 15. Note that FAS and FAE are completely avoidable and are the most preventable birth defects in the United States. Alcohol reaches the fetus because alcohol passes freely through the cell membranes of the **placenta;** it then deprives the fetal brain of oxygen and essential nutrients. The full syndrome is found in babies whose mothers drank four to five drinks a day or engaged in binge drinking while pregnant. Some mothers who drank less than four drinks a day still have produced babies with FAS.

No safe level of alcohol consumption has been determined for the pregnant woman. The best choice is complete abstinence from alcohol during pregnancy or when one could become pregnant. A warning for pregnant women posted in restaurants, in bars, and on alcohol containers reads "Women should not drink alcoholic beverages during pregnancy because of the risk of birth defects." The 2000 Dietary Guidelines strengthen the language concerning pregnant women by saying "Women who may become pregnant or who are pregnant" should not drink.[14] When a pregnant women drinks alcohol, so does the fetus. However, the fetus metabolizes alcohol more slowly than the mother, leading to higher levels of blood alcohol than in an adult. Binge drinking, especially in the early weeks of pregnancy, puts the fetus at risk (see the Nutrition Perspective for more on binge drinking).

Because it reduces the secretion of the body's antidiuretic hormone, alcohol increases urination. It also causes the blood vessels to dilate, releasing body heat.

free radicals Short-lived forms of compounds that exist with an unpaired electron in the outer electron shell, causing it to seek an electron from another compound. Free radicals are strong oxidizing agents and can be very destructive to electron-dense cell components, such as the DNA and cell membranes.

Alcohol use is generally not recommended while a woman is breast-feeding her infant, since alcohol consumed by the mother passes into the breast milk. An exception is if a mother uses a breast pump to extract the breast milk for the child and then consumes a moderate amount of alcohol.

fetal alcohol syndrome (FAS) A group of irreversible physical and mental abnormalities in the infant that result from the mother's consuming alcohol during pregnancy.

fetal alcohol effect (FAE) Hyperactivity, attention deficit disorder, poor judgment, sleep disorders, and delayed learning as a result of being prenatally exposed to alcohol.

placenta An organ, formed only during pregnancy, that secretes hormones to maintain the pregnant state and makes possible the transfer of oxygen and nutrients from the mother's blood to the fetus, as well as removal of fetal wastes.

ventricles Four interconnecting cavities in the brain.

white matter Brain tissue composed of myelin-coated nerve cell fibers, which carry information between nerve cells in the brain and spinal cord.

dopamine A type of neurotransmitter in the central nervous system that leads to feelings of euphoria, among other functions; it is also the precursor of norepinephrine, another neuro-transmitter molecule.

carcinogenic Having the potential to cause cancer.

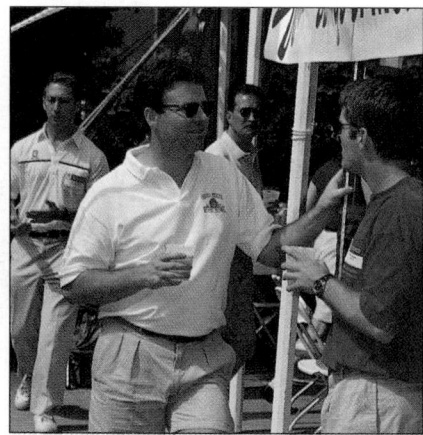
Alcohol intake encourages fat deposition, especially in the abdominal region.

myocardial depression Decrease activity of the heart muscle.

arrhythmias Abnormal heart rhythms, which may be too slow, too early, too rapid, or too irregular.

cardiomyopathy A primary heart-muscle disease of unknown origin.

■ Brain Damage

Long-term use of alcohol can lead to brain damage, accompanied by cognitive dysfunction and motor nerve deficits. Imaging technology has shown that in alcoholism the brain is shrunken, the **ventricles** are larger, and there is less **white matter.** Physical brain damage results from reduced delivery of oxygen and nutrients to the brain. These changes may be partially reversed with later abstinence from alcohol.

Alcohol affects the brain more than any other organ. Acting as a sedative, alcohol tends to relieve the drinker's anxiety, to cause slurred speech, to reduce coordination in walking, to impair judgment, and to encourage uninhibited behavior. The mechanism for these effects is thought to be linked to changes in the synthesis of neurotransmitters, such as **dopamine,** and altered cell membrane fluidity in the brain. Because alcohol lowers inhibition, it appears to act as a stimulant, but, in fact, it is a powerful depressant. As William Shakespeare wrote, "It stirs up desire, but takes away the performance."

■ Cancer

There is evidence to suggest that acetaldehyde, the chemical that promotes the hangover after a night of heavy drinking, also causes cancer. In particular, it damages the building blocks (nucleotides) that are incorporated into DNA. Prolonged alcohol intake beyond the liver's capacity to detoxify acetaldehyde especially increases cancer risk. People who lack the gene responsible for producing the enzyme aldehyde dehydrogenase are especially prone to cancer, and heavy drinking greatly increases acetaldehyde production.[27] Overall, acetaldehyde is a **carcinogenic** compound. Because of this, alcohol consumption is linked to a variety of cancers.

Common gastrointestinal tract cancers realted to alcohol use include cancers of the mouth, pharynx, larynx, esophagus, liver, colon, and rectum.[2] Although not GI tract–related, breast cancer incidence is also affected by alcohol consumption. An increased breast cancer risk is seen with alcohol consumption of greater than one to two drinks per day, especially in women who underconsume the vitamin folate. Breast cancer researchers suggest that, if a woman has a family history of breast cancer, an early onset of menstruation, or benign breast disease, alcohol should be avoided completely. A woman who has no strong risk for breast cancer may safely consume up to one drink per day (providing she is not pregnant or considering pregnancy).

■ Hypertension and Stroke

Heavy consumption of alcohol, greater than 45 g of alcohol per day, is a major cause of hypertension. Hemorrhagic strokes also are related to alcohol consumption. As mentioned, excess alcohol consumption decreases oxygen and nutrient supply to the brain.

■ Other Organ Damage

The heart eventually can be damaged by alcohol use as well. Hearts of alcoholics can double in size due to fat accumulation. Increased homocysteine concentration in the blood results from a high-protein diet, and the malabsorption of vitamins increases the risk for this problem. Severe thiamin deficiency also can result in a form of heart disease. **Myocardial depression;** frequent **arrhythmias;** and, as mentioned, hypertension are also common among alcoholics. Diseases of the heart muscle, known as **cardiomyopathy,** can also result.[10] Alcohol abuse can lead to impaired left ventricle emptying at rest. Fortunately, this effect is minimized by exercise, but the lifestyles of many alcoholics do not include exercise.

The blood and bone marrow can also be affected. Inadequate production of white and red blood cells is often caused by alcohol-related vitamin B-6 deficiency. Platelet function can also be impaired. The effect of alcohol on blood cells is not caused by identifiable nutritional deficiencies. Consequently, an adequate diet or nutrient supplementation cannot protect blood cells.

■ OTHER PROBLEMS ASSOCIATED WITH ALCOHOL ABUSE

Many social problems accompany the medical problems associated with alcohol abuse.

■ Problem Drinking in the Workplace

Problem drinking can result in decreased job performance, an increased number of sick days, interference with regular sleep at home, and increased sleeping on the job.[19] Rather than ignoring the issue, it is important that these alcohol-related problems be addressed. We all know people who dislike their jobs or a specific coworker. Because we spend about one-third of our lives working, the job environment can have a strong effect on quality of life. Workplace alienation can lead to drinking. Some workplace cultures accept and encourage alcohol consumption, whereas others forbid or discourage this behavior. Alcohol availability is strongly linked to consumption in the workplace. Sometimes it is very easy to bring alcohol onto the job site. Employer-sponsored health promotion programs may help reduce employee drinking and increase awareness of these issues.

■ Operation of Motor Vehicles and Related Equipment

It is extremely dangerous to mix drinking with activities requiring sound judgment and responsibility.[21, 33] Driving, boating, athletics, and water sports are all activities where alcohol does not belong. Consuming alcohol prior to or during these and many other activities increases the risk of injury to oneself and others. Note the warning label on alcoholic beverages.

■ Sexually Transmitted Diseases

Due to the inhibition-reducing effect of alcohol, drinking increases the incidence of high-risk sexual activity and infection by a **sexually transmitted disease (STD).** Unplanned and unprotected sexual intercourse often results from overconsumption of alcohol. Multiple sex partners also increase the risk for contracting an STD, as well as hepatitis C and AIDS.

■ Unplanned Pregnancy

Along with STDs, an unplanned pregnancy can be the result of unprotected sex while under the influence of alcohol. And, if the drinking continues during the first month of pregnancy, the chances of delivering an infant with fetal alcohol syndrome increase.

■ Children of Alcoholics

Alcoholism affects the entire family. Children of alcoholics have a hard time developing in a normal way. Living with an alcoholic family member causes stress for everyone, and, for a child, this dysfunction reduces the chances of becoming intellectually, culturally, and socially independent. Almost one in five Americans have grown up with an alcoholic in the family, and this environment influences children's perception of alcohol use, especially when it comes to their own decisions about this issue. Children of alcoholics often have long-lasting emotional problems, which carry over into adulthood.

*S*ome people even have food-related allergic and asthmatic reactions to alcohol. Accidents, violence, suicide, and workplace problems are often caused in part by the misuse of alcohol.

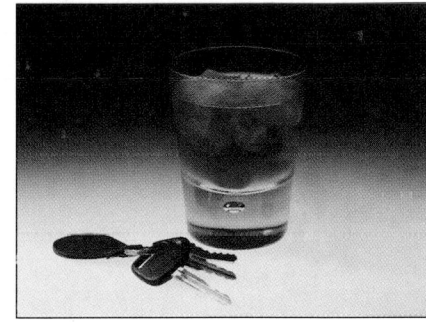

Drinking and driving should never be combined. The consequences are dangerous and possibly deadly.

sexually transmitted disease (STD) A contagious disease usually acquired by sexual intercourse or genital contact. Common examples include AIDS, gonorrhea, and syphilis. Also called venereal disease.

CRITICAL THINKING

Often when people consume alcohol, they do things they would not normally do. Unplanned sexual activity, the damaging of property, and other harmful events can occur. For many people, drinking and smoking go hand-in-hand. What risks and diseases could correlate with the combination of these behaviors with alcohol abuse?

CONCEPT CHECK

*E*xcessive alcohol use can result in an array of medical problems. It increases the risk of developing hypertension, certain forms of strokes and heart disease, birth defects, inflammation of the pancreas, damage to the brain and heart, malnutrition, and osteoporosis, to name a few. Furthermore, alcoholism interferes with all aspects of family, professional, and social life.

Healthy People 2010 set an important goal regarding alcohol use: Reduce by 25% the proportion of adults who exceed the guidelines for appropriate alcohol use (currently, 73% of those who consume alcohol).

RECOMMENDATIONS FOR ALCOHOL USE

Neither the surgeon general's office, the National Academy of Science, nor the USDA/DHHS recommends drinking alcohol. All groups caution that, if adults do consume alcohol, they should (1) drink alcohol only in moderation with meals (no more than two drinks a day for men and one for women or anyone over age 65 years); (2) avoid drinking any alcohol before or while driving, operating machinery, taking medications, or engaging in any other activity requiring sound judgment; and (3) avoid drinking alcohol while pregnant.

There is no recommendation for a nondrinker to start consuming alcohol for the health benefits. In fact, the health benefits of alcohol use do not take effect until the later years of life. Exercising, eating right, practicing healthful behaviors, and improving all areas of wellness are just a few of many ways to protect oneself from disease. People who have a drink or so a day and are not prone to abuse should know that there's nothing wrong with moderate drinking, as long as they are not putting themselves or others at risk.

The federal labels currently added to some wine bottles convey a noncommittal message. They state the positive and negative aspects of drinking wine, so that consumers are aware of both sides of the issue and can make up their own minds. These labels do not endorse drinking but refer consumers to other informative venues. It is unfortunate that the wine industry has become increasingly aggressive in promoting wine as a means of reducing the risk of heart disease. Producers and distributors have latched onto the 2000 Dietary Guidelines for Americans as a means of marketing their product. Alcoholic beverages account for more than $50 billion in annual sales in the United States.

Currently, about 32% of all Americans have three drinks or less each week, about 22% have two drinks or less a day, and only about 11% have more than two drinks a day.

ALCOHOL DEPENDENCY AND ABUSE

Many factors determine a person's chances of becoming alcohol dependent.[9] Studies have shown links tying gender, genetics, ethnicity, parental influence, nurture, and depression to alcohol dependency and abuse. For some people, alcohol can be addictive and dangerous.

Some studies suggest that 40 to 60% of a person's risk for alcoholism comes from genetic factors, although the gene, or genes, have not been identified.[27] The genetic influence on alcohol dependency and abuse has been indicated by a number of studies, including twin and adoption research. Twins and first-degree relatives share a tendency toward alcohol addiction. Children of alcoholics have a fourfold-increased risk of developing alcoholism, even when adopted by a family with no history of alcoholism. This suggests that individuals with a family history of alcoholism need to be especially alert for evidence of the early signs of alcohol dependence.

It is suggested that children with a family history of alcoholism be warned of the dangers of drinking by the age of 10. At this age, they are old enough to understand the consequences of alcoholism but are not yet under the strong influence of their peers. Children as young as 10 may begin experimenting with alcohol to feel grown up, to fit in and belong to a group, to relax and feel good, to take risks and rebel against authority, and simply to satisfy curiosity. When there are alcoholic beverages available in the home, it is easy for a child to sample a variety of drinks and to share them with friends.

A low threshold of response to alcohol may be genetic. If this is the case, it requires greater amounts of alcohol to produce the desired effect. Other studies question the importance of the genetic component. Any one of us can become addicted if we drink long enough and consume ever increasing quantities of alcohol.

Ability to "hold one's liquor" is a strong indicator of genetic risk.

Gender plays a key role in alcohol metabolism, dependency, and, surprisingly, treatment. The male:female ratio of alcohol dependency is 4:1, but there is evidence that women delay seeking treatment for alcohol abuse. As previously noted, the recommended limit for alcohol use is also different for men and women. Women's bodies have more fat and less muscle tissue than men's do. Alcohol can be diluted by water-holding muscle tissue, but not by fat tissue. Therefore, alcohol is diluted more quickly in men than in women. In addition, women cannot metabolize alcohol as quickly as men and, so, it remains in their blood longer.[20] Higher BAC's make women more susceptible to alcoholic liver disease, heart muscle damage, and brain injury. As previously mentioned, lower acetaldehyde dehydrogenase activity in a woman's stomach results in a larger proportion of ingested alcohol reaching the blood.

Many ethnic distinctions play an important role in the probability of alcohol dependency and abuse. Compared with Caucasians, Asians and Native Americans synthesize relatively little acetaldehyde dehydrogenase. For example, 40% of Japanese are unable to produce much of this enzyme and thus are very susceptible to the damaging effects of alcohol.[27] The major cause of death among North American Indians and Alaskan natives is unintentional injuries related to alcohol use, especially high rates of motor vehicle accidents. Other alcohol-related mortality statistics confronting Native Americans are suicide, homicide, domestic abuse, and fetal alcohol syndrome. Among African-Americans, it is known that long-term alcohol dependency endangers the immune system. African-American alcoholics are at greater risk than other racial groups for tuberculosis, hepatitis C, AIDS, and other infectious diseases.

Depression and alcohol abuse often go hand-in-hand. Researchers have discovered that the risk for heavy drinking is higher among women with a history of depression than among women with no such history. This finding holds up even when other factors that increase the risk of heavy drinking, such as age, family history of drinking, and personality disorder, are accounted for. The more symptoms of depression women report, the more likely they are to drink heavily. There may be several reasons for this association. One reason is self-medication to relieve the symptoms of depression. Research has shown that, although alcohol may alleviate depression in the short term, it tends to increase it over time. A second reason is that women who are more depressed may not pay attention to their drinking and may not be concerned about the effects it can have on their health and behavior. More research is needed to determine if there is a genetic or environmental factor that links depression and heavy drinking.[9]

The majority of suicides and interfamily homicides are alcohol-related. Clinicians need to be careful when dealing with depressed alcoholic patients to determine the psychological reasons for their drinking and how these behaviors might cause the death of the alcoholic or a family member. Alcohol consumption appears to be associated with youth suicide. The younger the drinker, the more likely he or she is to commit suicide, often via traffic accidents.

Alcohol dependence is the most common psychiatric disorder, affecting 13% of the population. Overall, about $116 billion is spent annually in terms of lost productivity, premature deaths, direct treatment expenses, and legal fees associated with alcoholism. A liver transplant costs about $150,000 and is needed in cases of excessive alcohol use. On the positive side, it costs only about $5000 to treat a person who is abusing alcohol. Identifying alcoholism early can be a way to control and decrease health-care costs.[5]

■ Alcoholism Diagnosis

Alcoholism is often considered a two-phase problem.[22] Initially, it begins as problem drinking. This includes the repetitive use of alcohol, often to alleviate anxiety or solve other emotional problems. Alcohol addiction, the second phase, is defined as a true addiction following the repeated use of alcohol.

The diagnosis of alcoholism is based on a list of major criteria. These criteria do not fit every individual but are commonly seen in cases of alcoholism:

CRITICAL THINKING

Jose is a well-liked 17-year-old. It always seems as if everything is going his way— an A on a test, a scholarship to his dream school, you name it. Lately, however, Jose has experienced some disappointments. His grandfather has just passed away, and he and his girlfriend of 6 months have broken up. When he arrived home late with the smell of alcohol on his breath, his parents started to worry. They talked to his school counselor, who suggested they look for certain signs that could indicate depression and/or alcohol dependence. What might those signs be?

Alcohol addiction is seen in high incidence among homeless individuals.

- Physiologic dependence manifested by evidence of withdrawal symptoms when intake is interrupted
- Tolerance to the effects of alcohol, prompting greater alcohol intake to achieve the desired effect
- Evidence of alcohol-associated illnesses such as alcoholic liver disease or irreversible brain damage exhibited by memory loss, inability to concentrate, and decline in intellectual functions
- Continued drinking in defiance of strong medical and social contraindications and disruptions in normal life
- Depression and blackouts, as well as impairment in social and occupational functioning

facies The appearance of the face of an alcoholic when blood vessels break near the surface, causing a blushed look.

ecchymoses The discoloration of an area of the skin or mucous membrane caused by blood seeping into the tissue due to fragility of the vessel walls.

Other signs of alcoholism include the basic alcohol stigmas: alcohol odor on the breath, alcoholic **facies,** flushed face, tremor, **ecchymoses,** and peripheral neuropathy. Unexplained work absences, frequent accidents, and falls or injuries of vague origin may all lead a clinician to consider a possible diagnosis of alcoholism.

Laboratory tests are helpful alternatives to these somewhat subjective criteria. These tests include elevated values for liver function enzymes (these leak from the diseased liver cells into the blood), mean corpuscular volume (MCV) of the red blood cells (related to a folate deficiency), blood uric acid, and triglycerides.[7]

■ Do You Have a Problem with Alcohol?

Asking a person about the quantity and frequency of alcohol consumption is an important means of detecting abuse and dependence. The following questionnaire (CAGE) is commonly used in routine health care (Table 8-3).[5]

Other questions to ask along with the CAGE questionnaire are:

1. Have you had memory lapses or blackouts due to drinking?
2. Do you continue to drink even though you have health problems caused by alcohol?
3. Do you get withdrawal symptoms, such as headaches, chills, shakes, and a strong craving for alcohol, and, as a result, drink more to get rid of these symptoms?
4. Do you take part in high-risk behaviors, such as having unsafe sex in a non-monogamous relationship or driving a boat or car when under the influence of alcohol?
5. Has drinking caused trouble at home, at work, or in relationships with others?
6. Do you have to drink alcohol for any of the following reasons?
   a. To get through the day or unwind at the end of the day
   b. To cope with stressful life events
   c. To escape from ongoing problems

Answering yes to any of these questions should prompt the respondent to consult a family physician or a certified counselor for help.

TABLE 8-3 CAGE Questionnaire to Screen for Alcohol Abuse

C: Have you every felt you ought to *cut* down on drinking?
A: Have people *annoyed* you by criticizing your drinking?
G: Have you ever felt bad or *guilty* about your drinking?
E: Have you ever had a drink first thing in the morning to steady your nerves or get rid of a hangover (*eye-opener*)?

More than one positive response to the CAGE questionnaire suggests an alcohol problem. Another key point to probe is tolerance. Does it take more to make you inebriated than it did in the past?

Source: See reference no. 5

■ TREATMENT OF ALCOHOLISM

Once a diagnosis of alcohol abuse or dependence is established, one should seek the guidance of a physician to arrange appropriate treatment and counseling for the person and family. An important goal of counseling is to identify ways to compensate for the loss of pleasure from drinking. This helps the drinker confront the immediate problem of how to stop drinking. Total abstinence must be the ultimate objective. For alcoholics, there is no such thing as controlled drinking. A problem drinker cannot return safely to social drinking.

The person should enter an Alcoholics Anonymous (AA) 12-step program, or another reputable therapy program for people with alcoholism. For more information, one can check with a local mental health treatment center for programs available in the community or call 800-245-4656. Substance Abuse and Mental Health Services can be reached at 800-729-6686 or http:\\www.health.org for alcohol and drug information. In addition, one may visit the Alcoholics Anonymous web page at http://www.alcoholics-anonymous.org or contact AA at

AA World Services, Inc.
P.O. Box 459
New York, NY 10163
212-870-3400

According to AA's literature, "AA is a fellowship of men and women who share their experience, strength, and hope with each other that they may solve their common problem and help others recover from alcoholism." As an informal society chartered in 1935, Alcoholics Anonymous includes more than 2 million recovered alcoholics. The only requirement for membership is to desire to stop drinking. There are no rules, regulations, dues, or fees. In addition, the group is not a political or formal organization.

It is helpful for the spouse to join the treatment program as well. AA has two types of meetings—open and closed. Alcoholics and their families and friends are invited to the open meetings, whereas the closed meetings are reserved for alcoholics only.

Current research does not support the generally negative public opinion about the prognosis for alcoholism. In most job-related alcoholism treatment programs, where workers are socially stable and—because of the risk to jobs and pensions—well motivated, recovery rates reach 60% or more. This remarkably high cure rate is probably accounted for by early detection. Once a person moves from problem drinking to an advanced stage of alcoholism, success rates seldom exceed 50%. Early identification and intervention remain the most important steps in the treatment of alcoholism. Success is usually proportionate to participation in AA, other social agencies' programs, and religious counseling. About 2 years of treatment should be expected.

Social aspects of the treatment of alcoholism are important. The use of a variety of services such as Alcoholics Anonymous (Al-Anon for the spouse) or religious counseling is necessary because the person needs a lot of support.[21] The person needs to feel he or she is being supervised, not under surveillance. The person must develop new habits to manage anger, resolve conflicts, and find ways to have fun while sober. Everyone heals differently and at his or her own rate.

New medications have been approved for the treatment of alcoholism. Inpatient hospital treatment may be necessary for the alcoholic to go through detoxification. It is important that the patient be given a physical examination and that the physician frequently checks the laboratory tests related to alcoholism discussed previously.

Two medications are available to treat alcoholism. The medication naltrexone (ReVia) blocks the craving for alcohol and the pleasure of intoxication.[8, 30] Disulfiram (Antabuse) causes physical reactions, such as vomiting, when drinking alcohol. Detoxification drugs are also important in treating alcoholism, and using some form of psychotherapy is stressed.

For more than 10 years, ReVia has been available to treat opiate addiction, which has been found to be similar to alcohol abuse. It was first approved for use in treating alcoholism in 1994. Opiates and alcohol share similar pleasurable effects, and these can be blocked with ReVia. It is thus used to decrease alcohol cravings and cause drinking to be less enjoyable. By blocking the opioid receptors in the brain, it prevents the euphoric feeling one gets after consuming alcohol (Fig. 8-3). This drug can stop the vicious cycle of alcohol addiction, in which one drink almost always leads to a full-blown relapse.

ReVia is considered generally safe and well tolerated. When used with psychological support, it is found to be particularly helpful in decreasing alcohol relapse rates in compliant subjects. As seen with most medications, ReVia has some side effects, including nausea, dizziness, headache, and weight loss. The drug can be taken with meals or at bedtime to control nausea. Another concern is that ReVia may worsen the liver damage that has already occurred from alcoholism. Research is looking at the more liver-friendly cousin of ReVia, nalmefene.

The medication disulfiram (Antabuse) produces a severe hypersensitivity to alcohol, which may persuade the alcoholic to stop drinking. It works by inhibiting acetaldehyde metabolism, producing a series of symptoms, which lasts from 30 minutes to several hours. These symptoms include drowsiness, headache, restlessness, and a variety of other side effects. This treatment must be avoided if the patient has been consuming alcohol, since the symptoms are acute and can cause unconsciousness, seizures, and death. For this reason, Antabuse is infrequently used. It is also contraindicated in patients with medical problems such as diabetes, goiter, epilepsy, heart disease, cirrhosis, nephritis, and suicidal tendencies and psychosis. Use of Antabuse can result in the inflammation of the liver, so use must be closely monitored. Like ReVia, it is emphasized that Antabuse is not a total treatment of alcoholism but, rather, only an element of the comprehensive treatment program.

The effects of Antabuse may last for 1 to 2 weeks after discontinuing use of the medication. This is important to note because, if the alcoholic decides to discontinue

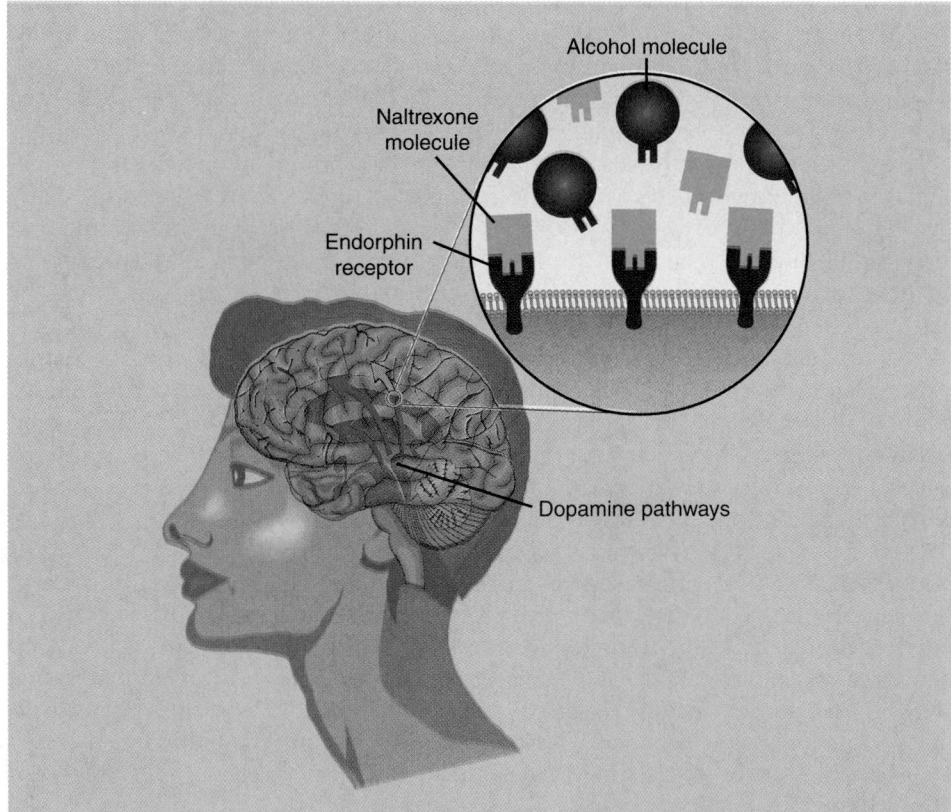

■ FIGURE **8-3** The euphoria that arises from alcohol use involves alcohol binding to specific receptors in the brain. It is likely that this binding, in turn, causes a release of the neurotransmitter dopamine. The increase in dopamine in the brain is thought to cause the characteristic high associated with alcohol use. Naltrexone (ReVia) works by blocking alcohol's ability to bind to brain receptors. This, then, reduces dopamine release and blocks the pleasant feelings elicited by alcohol use.

use of Antabuse, especially with the intention of returning to old drinking habits, the effects of the medication will still be in place. The ill effects may cause the person to resume drinking.

Medical detoxification is often used for treating alcohol and other drug abuse.[22] Medications to reduce the patient's **withdrawal** symptoms are accompanied by psychological support. Withdrawal begins within hours after the patient's last drink and peaks 48 to 72 hours later. Early signs include anxiety, nausea, vomiting, and headache; these can progress through more serious symptoms, culminating in hallucinations and delirium. The treatment plan is initiated on patient assessment, which includes medical, nursing, dietetic, psychological, and psychiatric evaluation.

This treatment includes limiting the use of inappropriate medications to moderate amounts and eliminating the withdrawal symptoms the person experiences when he or she stops using an addictive substance. Medical detoxification can help initiate rehabilitation because it is useful in eliminating medically dangerous withdrawal symptoms and decreasing the associated physical discomfort. This method is often performed on an outpatient basis but requires daily visits with the physician. In addition, a support person is needed to help monitor the patient's progress.

Another possible treatment for alcoholism is known as aversion therapy. Using the approaches of behavioral conditioning, aversion therapy is frequently successful. For example, a patient may be given a shot of whiskey followed by a shot of apomorphine. This will make the patient violently ill and he or she will vomit. This therapy is repeated until the connection between alcohol and vomiting is made and understood.

From a psychological standpoint, the clinician should keep a nonjudgmental attitude. The clinician must also be prepared to deal with denial presented by the patient.

withdrawal A state that ranges from anxiety, decreased cognition, tremulousness, increased irritability, and hyperreactivity to full-blown delirium tremors. Symptoms can begin about 8 hours after the last drink and usually pass by the third day.

New and improved future treatments for alcoholism are currently being researched. One example is a nutritional supplement called polyunsaturated lecithin (PUL). It is a mixture of fatty acids extracted from soybeans. PUL is used to protect against scarring of the liver. This may be helpful in treating alcoholism in the near future.[18]

CONCEPT CHECK

Treatment of alcoholism often includes the use of medicine, psychotherapy, and social support. The clinicians involved must treat the entire person. Alcoholics Anonymous and other support groups are very helpful. Naltrexone can be prescribed to decrease alcohol cravings. Another option is disulfiram, which produces a violently ill feeling when the patient consumes both the medicine and alcohol. With all of the treatments for alcoholism, it is important to find the one that works best for the individual with alcoholism.

Check out the *Perspectives in Nutrition* Online Learning Center http://www.mhhe.com/wardlaw for quizzes, flash cards, other activities, and web links designed to further help you learn about issues surrounding alcohol use and abuse.

■ CASE SCENARIO
Follow-Up

Alcohol is a central nervous system depressant that affects both respiration and heart rate. In large quantities, alcohol can depress both systems to the point of terminating respiration and cardiac function. Obviously, this is fatal. Alcohol abuse is a common problem, and continued alcohol abuse can lead to dependence problems, although alcohol abuse and dependence are different.

As a close friend, Alyssa has a responsibility to hold Todd accountable for his actions. Sometimes it is difficult to realize that one has a drinking problem, although it may be obvious to others. Alyssa should talk privately to Todd when he is sober and calm about the most recent incident. It is important to deal with situations such as these very carefully, as the problem drinker will probably respond defensively. She could explain how his drinking is causing problems for both of them, she could tell him about the harmful consequences of his drinking, and she could refuse to go with him to any alcohol-related events, but she must be prepared to carry out the threat. Alyssa could talk with a counselor, who may help her learn ways to approach Todd effectively. Offering to go with Todd to a treatment program or an AA meeting and get help is one idea. There is strength in numbers, so other members of Todd's family or close friends also should be enlisted to help, under the guidance of a therapist trained in treating alcoholics.

■ SUMMARY

1. Alcohol use is a complex issue because it involves psychological, social, economic, health, legal, and family issues.
2. Since the Stone Age 10,000 years ago, alcohol has provided an alternative to unsafe drinking water and a pleasurable stimulant to social interaction.
3. Alcohol is metabolized in the liver and other tissues. Metabolism depends on the enzyme alcohol dehydrogenase. A number of factors, such as gender, race, and body composition, determine how a person reacts to alcohol.
4. The body uses the microsomal ethanol oxidizing system (MEOS) whenever the liver detects more alcohol than can be processed by the alcohol dehydrogenase enzymes. Once the MEOS is active, alcohol tolerance increases because alcohol is being metabolized more rapidly.
5. The benefits of alcohol use are associated with low to moderate alcohol consumption. These benefits include the pleasurable and social aspects of alcohol use, a reduction in coronary heart disease and ischemic stroke risks, and protection against harmful stomach bacteria, such as *Helicobacter pylori*.
6. Alcohol use also creates many health risks. Excessive consumption of alcohol contributes significantly to 5 of the 10 leading causes of death in the United States. Alcohol increases the risk of developing certain forms of heart damage, inflammation of the pancreas, gastrointestinal tract damage, vitamin and mineral deficiencies, cirrhosis of the liver, certain forms of cancer, hypertension, and hemmorhagic stroke—to name a few.
7. If alcohol is consumed, it should be consumed in moderation with meals. Women are advised to drink no more than one drink per day; men are advised to limit intake to two drinks a day.
8. Gender, genetics, ethnic background, and ongoing depression all determine a person's chances of becoming alcohol dependent.
9. Early detection of alcoholism is key to successful treatment and a reduction of health-care costs. The CAGE questionnaire can help a person determine whether or not he or she has an alcohol problem.
10. Many methods are available to treat alcoholism. Alcoholics Anonymous, ReVia, Antabuse, medical detoxification, and behavioral conditioning approaches have been successful. All treatments place importance on treating the entire person socially, psychologically, and medically.

■ STUDY QUESTIONS

1. Where in the body does most of the metabolism of alcohol take place? What are the by-products of alcohol metabolism?
2. Why does it take a woman longer than a man to metabolize alcohol?
3. List two benefits of alcohol use.
4. List four problems associated with alcohol abuse.
5. Which nutrient deficiency remains an alcohol-related problem, despite whether intake of the nutrient is low, adequate, or excessive? Why?
6. Define the term *one drink*. How much alcohol use is considered to be moderate for men? for women?
7. Why can some ethnic groups hold their liquor better than others can?
8. Name four criteria that might indicate someone has a problem with alcohol. What is this group of criteria checklist called?
9. Describe four methods used in treating alcoholism. List a pro and con of each method.
10. After reading the Nutrition Perspective, answer the following. What is binge drinking? With which segment of the population is this increasing in popularity?

■ ANNOTATED REFERENCES

1. Albert CM and others: Moderate alcohol consumption and the risk of sudden cardiac death among US male physicians. *American Family Physician* 61:944, 1999.

   Moderate alcohol intake decreases the risk of sudden cardiac death.

2. American Institute for Cancer Research: Alcohol: Healthy living and lower cancer risk. *Facts on Preventing Cancer* 1998.

   Alcoholic drinks increase the risk of cancers of the mouth, pharynx, larynx, and esophagus. Alcohol also increases risk of liver cancer and probably increases the risk for colon, rectal, and breast cancers.

3. Berger K and others: Light-to-moderate alcohol consumption and the risk of stroke among U.S. male physicians. *The New England Journal of Medicine* 341:1557, 1999.

   One to four drinks per week reduced the risks of total stroke and of ischemic stroke in a group of healthy, predominantly White physicians. The authors suggest, however, that any public health recommendation that emphasizes the positive aspects of alcohol would likely do more harm than good.

4. Brenner H and others: Alcohol consumption and *Helicobacter pylori* infection: Results from the German national health and nutrition survey. *Epidemiology* 10:214, 1999.

   Infections with Helicobacter pylori—*a bacterium implicated in heartburn, peptic ulcer, and stomach cancer—may be reduced by moderate alcohol consumption. It is the alcohol, not the beverage, that accounts for the effect.*

5. Epperly TD, Moore KE: Health issues in men: Part II Common psychosocial disorders. *American Family Physician* 62:117, 2000.

   During screening examinations, physicians should be alert for signs and symptoms of common psychosocial disorders in men, including alcohol abuse. The article includes both the CAGE questionnaire and the Michigan Alcoholism screening test.

6. Evans C: "I don't like Mondays"—day of the week of coronary heart disease deaths in Scotland: Study of routinely collected data. *British Medical Journal* 320:218, 2000.

   Binge drinking over the weekend may explain why men and women under 50 are the most likely to die from coronary heart disease on a Monday.

7. Feinman L, Lieber CS: Nutrition and diet in alcoholism. In Shills ME and others (eds.): *Modern nutrition in health and disease.* 9th ed. Baltimore, MD: Williams & Wilkens, 1999.

   This chapter offers a detailed discussion of the concepts described in this chapter of this textbook.

8. Garbutt JC and others: Pharmacological treatment of alcohol dependence, a review of the evidence. *Journal of the American Medical Association* 281:1318, 1999.

   Authors emphasize that preliminary evidence tends to support the use of naltrexone but additional study is required.

9. Gordis E: Research on alcohol problems. *Phi Kappa Phi Journal National Forum* 79(4):24, 1999.

   Some people are more vulnerable to alcohol problems than others. There are effective ways to prevent and treat alcohol abuse and alcoholism.

10. Hillbom M and others: Recent heavy drinking of alcohol and embolic stroke. *Stroke* 30:2307, 1999.

    Heavy drinking including binge drinking may cause cardiogenic brain embolism. Alcohol seems to be cardiotoxic and causes cardiomyopathy.

11. Hommel M, Jaillard A: Alcohol for stroke prevention? *The New England Journal of Medicine* 341:1605, 1999.

    The higher a patient's baseline cardiovascular risk, the more likely that alcohol may be protective. Thus, alcohol may have a particular benefit in secondary prevention after ischemic stroke or myocardial infarction. Any recommendations about alcohol intake must take into consideration the risks that come with alcohol use.

12. JAMA patient page: Driving safely by avoiding alcohol. *Journal of the American Medical Association* 283:2340, 2000.

    Safe driving requires that one have total mental focus, physical coordination, and sound judgment. Many things can impair one's mental and physical processes, making driving dangerous. This includes the adverse effects of alcohol.

13. Jequire F: Alcohol intake and body weight: A paradox. *American Journal of Clinical Nutrition* 69:173, 1999.

    Energy intake from ethanol plays a role in energy balance regulation. Further study on alcohol intake and body weight regulation is needed, but we know calories from alcohol do count.

14. Johnson RK, Kennedy E: The 2000 dietary guidelines for Americans: What are the changes and why were they made? *Journal of the American Dietetic Association* 100:769, 2000.

    The 2000 year guideline on alcohol strengthens the language concerning pregnant women by saying "women who may become pregnant or who are pregnant" should not drink.

15. Leo MA, Lieber CS: Alcohol, vitamin A and beta-carotene: Adverse interactions, including hepatotoxicity and carcinogenicity. *American Journal of Clinical Nutrition* 69:1071, 1999.

    There is a narrow therapeutic window between the depletion of vitamin A and vitamin A toxicity. High doses of vitamin A are very toxic when the liver shows damage, such as from alcohol intake.

16. Lieber CS: Alcohol: Metabolism and interaction with nutrients. Annual Review of Nutrition 20:325, 2000.

    Alcohol alters the metabolism of many vitamins and minerals.

17. Mayes, PA: Lipid transport and storage in R.K. Murray and others (eds.) *Harper's biochemistry:* 25th ed., Appleton & Lange, 2000.

    Metabolism of alcohol promotes formation of fatty acids and fat deposition.

18. National Institute on Alcohol Abuse and Alcoholism: Alcohol and the liver: Research update. *Alcohol Alert* 42:1, 1998.

    During the past 5 years, research has significantly increased our understanding of the mechanisms by which alcohol consumption damages the liver. The major offending agents are acetaldehyde and free radicals. This update highlights recent research on the mechanisms and treatment of alcohol-induced liver disease.

19. National Institute on Alcohol Abuse and Alcoholism: Alcohol and the workplace. *Alcohol Alert* 44:1, 1999.

    Drinking among U.S. workers can threaten public safety, impair job performance, and result in costly medical, social, and other problems affecting employees and employers alike.

20. National Institute on Alcohol Abuse and Alcoholism: Are women more vulnerable to alcohol's effects? *Alcohol Alert* 46:1, 1999.

    When women and men drink at the same rate, women are at higher risk than are men for certain serious medical consequences of alcohol use, including liver, brain, and heart damage.

21. National Institute on Alcohol Abuse and Alcoholism National Institutes of Health: What you don't know can harm you. NIH Publication 99-4324, 1999.

    The complications of alcohol abuse include drunk driving, interpersonal problems, alcohol-related birth defects, and long-term health problems. Also included in this pamphlet is a listing of support groups and the types and amounts of alcohol considered to be one serving.

22. Prater CD and others: Outpatient detoxification of the addicted or alcoholic patient. *American Family Physician* 60:1175, 1999.

    The stages of alcohol withdrawal are Stage I—shaking, elevated pulse, increased blood pressure, and agitation; Stage II—all of Stage I symptoms plus hallucinations with insight; and Stage III—all of the Stage I symptoms plus a temperature above 38.3°C (101°F) and hallucinations without insight.

23. Prescott and others: Microbiology of food in: *Microbiology* 4th ed., McGraw-Hill, 1999.

    The production of foods and beverages by fermentation prevents spoilage, improves taste/texture and may significantly increase energy value of the product.

24. Rehm JT and others: Alcohol consumption and coronary heart disease morbidity and mortality. *American Journal of Epidemiology* 146:495, 1997.

    There is a definite gender difference in the relationship between alcohol use and coronary heart disease risk reduction. Females obtained maximum benefit on less than one drink per week and the least benefit with levels greater than four drinks per day. In contrast, heavy drinking, greater than four drinks per day, did not increase coronary heart disease risk in men.

25. Renaud SC and others: Wine, beer, and mortality in middle-aged men from eastern France. *Archives of Internal Medicine* 158:1865, 1999.

    In eastern France, moderate wine consumption was associated with a lower all-cause mortality; drinking both wine and beer reduced the risk of cardiovascular death.

26. Saitz R and others: Alcohol abuse and dependence in Latinos living in the United States. *Archives of Internal Medicine* 159:718, 1999.

    There is a high prevalence of alcohol abuse by Latinos in a primary-care practice. The CAGE is useful in detecting current alcohol abuse.

27. Schuckit MA: New findings in the genetics of alcoholism. *Journal of the American Medical Association* 281:1875, 1999.

    A number of combined genetic factors appear to explain approximately half of the alcoholism risk, and the search for genes that have an effect on risk has important implications. The range of potential causes seen in genetic studies implies that there is not a single definitive treatment that will work for everyone.

28. Schwenk TL: Alcohol use in adolescents, *The Physician and Sportsmedicine* 28(6):71, 2000.

TAKE ACTION

I. COULD YOU OR SOMEONE YOU KNOW HAVE A PROBLEM WITH ALCOHOL?

Problem drinking often has its seeds in the teen years. Significant health consequences of this typically arise in adulthood. A prominent contributor to 5 of the 10 leading causes of death in the United States, misuse of alcohol is one of our most preventable health problems. The social consequences of alcohol dependency include divorce, unemployment, and poverty. The following questionnaire was developed by the National Council on Alcoholism. With this assessment, you can determine whether you or someone you know might need help. Answer the following questions by placing an "X" in the appropriate blank.

	Yes	No
1. Do you occasionally drink heavily after disappointment, after a quarrel, or when someone gives you a hard time?	____	____
2. When you have trouble or feel under pressure, do you drink more heavily than usual?	____	____
3. Have you ever noticed that you're able to handle liquor better than you did when you first started drinking?	____	____
4. Do you ever wake up the morning after you've been drinking and discover that you can't remember part of the evening before, even though your friends tell you that you didn't pass out?	____	____
5. When drinking with other people, do you try to have a few extra drinks when others won't know it?	____	____
6. Are there certain occasions when you feel uncomfortable if alcohol isn't available?	____	____
7. Have you recently noticed that, when you begin drinking, you're in more of a hurry to get the first drink than you used to be?	____	____
8. Do you sometimes feel a little guilty about your drinking?	____	____
9. Are you secretly irritated when your family or friends discuss your drinking?	____	____
10. Have you recently noticed an increase in the frequency of memory blackouts?	____	____
11. Do you often find that you wish to continue drinking after your friends say they've had enough?	____	____
12. Do you usually have a reason for the occasions when you drink heavily?	____	____
13. When you're sober, do you often regret things you have done or said while drinking?	____	____
14. Have you tried switching brands or following different plans to control your drinking?	____	____
15. Have you often failed to keep promises you've made to yourself about controlling or stopping your drinking?	____	____
16. Have you ever tried to control your drinking by changing jobs or moving to a new location?	____	____
17. Do you try to avoid family or close friends while you're drinking?	____	____

Alcohol use by high school and college athletes receives little attention, compared with the use of other illicit drugs. Given the nature and magnitude of the problem, it deserves close attention and intervention, where possible, by parents, physicians, trainers, mental health specialists, coaches, and athletic directors.

29. Suter PM, Vetter W: Alcohol and ischemic stroke. *Nutrition Reviews* 57:310, 1999.

    The potential benefit of alcohol use in reducing ischemic stroke risk disappears rapidly when alcohol intake is above two drinks per day.

30. Swift RM: Drug therapy for alcohol dependence. *The New England Journal of Medicine* 340:1828, 1999.

    Naltrexone shows efficacy in the treatment of alcoholism. Any drug therapy should be com-

bined with psychotherapy or group therapy to help address the social and psychological aspects of alcohol dependence. Patients with psychiatric disorders, such as depression and anxiety, should be treated with drugs that are effective for the psychiatric condition.

31. Vallee BL: Alcohol in the Western world. *Scientific American* 278 (June):80, 1998.

    The role of alcohol in Western civilization began 10 millennia ago. It has been the most popular and most common daily beverage to dispense calories, fluid, and social stimulation in almost every culture. Early Hebrews, Greeks, and Romans cautioned about the dangers of drunkenness.

32. Valmadrid CT and others: Alcohol, heart disease, and type 2 diabetes. *Journal of the*

American Medical Association 281:239, 1999.

Coronary heart disease is the leading cause of death in persons with type 2 diabetes. Moderate alcohol use reduces death from coronary heart disease in type 2 diabetes.

33. Zador PL and others: Alcohol-related relative risk of driver fatalities and driver involvement in fatal crashes in relation to driver age and gender. *Journal of Studies on Alcohol* 61:387, 2000.

    The results of this study clearly show that even drivers with a BAC under 0.10% pose highly elevated risk both to themselves and to other road users.

TAKE ACTION

	Yes	No
18. Are you having an increasing number of financial and work problems?	____	____
19. Do more people seem to be treating you unfairly without good reason?	____	____
20. Do you eat very little or irregularly when you're drinking?	____	____
21. Do you sometimes have the "shakes" in the morning and find that it helps to have a little drink?	____	____
22. Have you recently noticed that you can't drink as much as you once did?	____	____
23. Do you sometimes stay drunk for several days at a time?	____	____
24. Do you sometimes feel very depressed and wonder whether life is worth living?	____	____
25. Sometimes after periods of drinking do you see or hear things that aren't there?	____	____
26. Do you get terribly frightened after you have been drinking heavily?	____	____

INTERPRETATION

These are all symptoms that may indicate alcoholism. "Yes" answers to several of the questions indicate the following stages of alcoholism:

Questions 1–8:   Potential drinking problem
Questions 9–21:   Drinking problem likely
Questions 22–26: Definite drinking problem

It is vital that people assess themselves honestly. If you or someone you know demonstrates some or a number of these symptoms, it is important that help be pursued. If there is even a question in your mind, go talk to a professional about it. Alcohol abuse is one of many problems adults, including older people, face.

II. INVESTIGATE ALCOHOL USE WITH THE CAGE QUESTIONNAIRE

Have a few of your friends complete the CAGE questionnaire in Table 8-3. What observations have you made? Alcoholism often has its seeds in young adulthood. Do you see evidence of that in you or your friends?

NUTRITION *Perspective*

BINGE DRINKING

acute alcohol intoxication A temporary deterioration in mental function, accompanied by muscular incoordination and partial paralysis as a result of drinking alcoholic beverages too rapidly.

A college student on the diving team became so intoxicated he dove head first into the shallow end of a neighbor's swimming pool. He is lucky to be alive but is paralyzed from the neck down. Still other students have drowned while intoxicated, even though they knew how to swim.

*H*ealthy People 2010 recommends an important goal regarding binge drinking: Reduce by at least one-half the number of high school and college students engaging in binge drinking (currently estimated at 32% and 40%, respectively).

College students are drinking more heavily and more frequently than ever before. Excessive alcohol consumption is an even bigger problem than illicit drug use on college campuses today. Binge drinking is common among college students. Young athletes are more likely to abuse alcohol than their nonathlete peers. Drunken athletes are more likely to drive while drinking, fight, experience memory loss, and be in academic trouble.[28] Bingeing is defined as four or more drinks for women and five or more for men per occasion. **Acute alcohol intoxication** is a major cause of suicide, hazing deaths, and academic failure. About 40% of college students practice binge drinking. Each year, this leads to death in otherwise healthy young adults. For example, in 2000 a student at the University of Michigan rapidly drank 20 shots to celebrate his 21st birthday and died shortly after with a blood alcohol concentration of 0.39 percent.

Binge drinking has a variety of contraindications. It can lead to unplanned sexual activity, damaged property, injury to oneself or others, and death. Death due to alcohol misuse can result, for example, from inhalation of vomit. In other cases, the body systems slowly shut down due to alcohol's overpowering depressant effect (Table 8-4). Other injuries can occur, resulting in paralysis or other lifelong medical problems.

Many problems associated with binge drinking can affect all aspects of life. Binge drinkers are more likely to miss class, damage property, and experience impaired academic performance than are students who are light drinkers. They often do not think they have a problem because binge drinking has become so acceptable on college campuses. Recent research suggests that binge drinking over a weekend may explain why men and women under 50 were the most likely to die on a Monday from coronary heart disease.[6]

According to U.S. law, one must be 21 years old to drink in all 50 states. However, alcohol use often begins in adolescence. For example, 31% of 12th-graders reported frequent drinking during 1999. Premature alcohol use is often seen in conjunction with athletics, as older, highly visible role models advertise products or are seen consuming alcohol. Peer pressure at school and on sports teams can cause many adolescents to drink. These habits become dangerous when young adults choose to drive drunk or ride with friends who are intoxicated. They are also creating habits that may continue and worsen throughout their lives. Education and prevention strategies should focus on behavioral and psychosocial consequences because athletic performance typically does not suffer yet.

Overall, it is important that binge drinkers be aware that these habits can cause lifelong problems, especially when drinking becomes habitual.

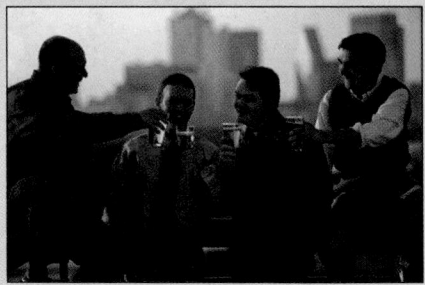

Alcohol use often begins in young adulthood and is carried into later years.

TABLE 8-4   Signs and Symptoms of Alcohol Poisoning

Being aware of the warning signs and dangers of alcohol poisoning is important. It could help save the life of someone you love. The warning signs and symptoms include the following:

• Semiconsciousness or unconscious

• Slow respiration of eight or fewer breaths per minute or lapses between breaths of more than 8 seconds

• Cold, clammy, pale, or bluish skin

• Strong odor of alcohol, which usually accompanies these symptoms

Note: Although these are obvious warning signs of alcohol poisoning, the list is certainly not all inclusive.

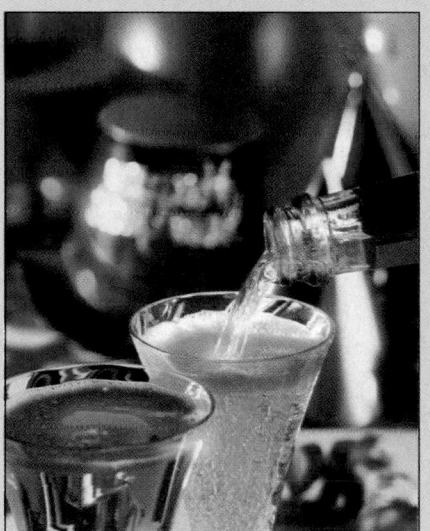

Know your limit when you party: 2 drinks for men and 1 drink for women.

What is your alcohol tolerance? The body can metabolize 0.1–0.2 g of alcohol per kg of body weight per hour. A 12-ounce can of beer contains 13 g of alcohol. How much beer can you safely drink?

CRITICAL THINKING

Imagine you are president of your college or university where there is a tradition of the "fourth-year fifth", a long-standing practice of seniors to consume a fifth of liquor during the last quarter/semester prior to graduation. Every weekend between 3 and 10 students arrive in the local emergency room with alcohol poisoning or alcohol-related injuries, and there are several alcohol-related deaths each year. As the head of this institution, how do you and the Board of Trustees tackle this problem?

PART THREE THE VITAMINS AND MINERALS

THE FAT-SOLUBLE VITAMINS

chapter 9

When it comes to vitamins, we often hear "If a little is good, then more must be better." Some people believe that consuming vitamins far in excess of their needs provides them with extra energy, protection from disease, and prolonged youth. Americans are spending about $14 billion annually on supplements. About 40% of Americans take vitamin and/or mineral supplements, some at unsafe levels. Non-Hispanic White women are most likely to take supplements.[1]

In stark contrast, our total vitamin needs to prevent deficiency signs and symptoms are really quite small. In general, humans require a total of about 1 oz (28 g) of vitamins for every 150 lb (70 kg) of food consumed. Vitamins are found in plants and animals. Plants synthesize all the vitamins they need. Animals vary in their ability to synthesize vitamins. For example, guinea pigs and humans are two of the very few organisms that are unable to synthesize their own supply of vitamin C.[4]

This chapter first briefly reviews some general properties of the vitamins. These vital nutrients are divided into two groups: the fat-soluble vitamins and the water-soluble vitamins. Attention then focuses on the functions and sources of the fat-soluble vitamins and human requirements for them. The water-soluble vitamins are described in detail in the next chapter.

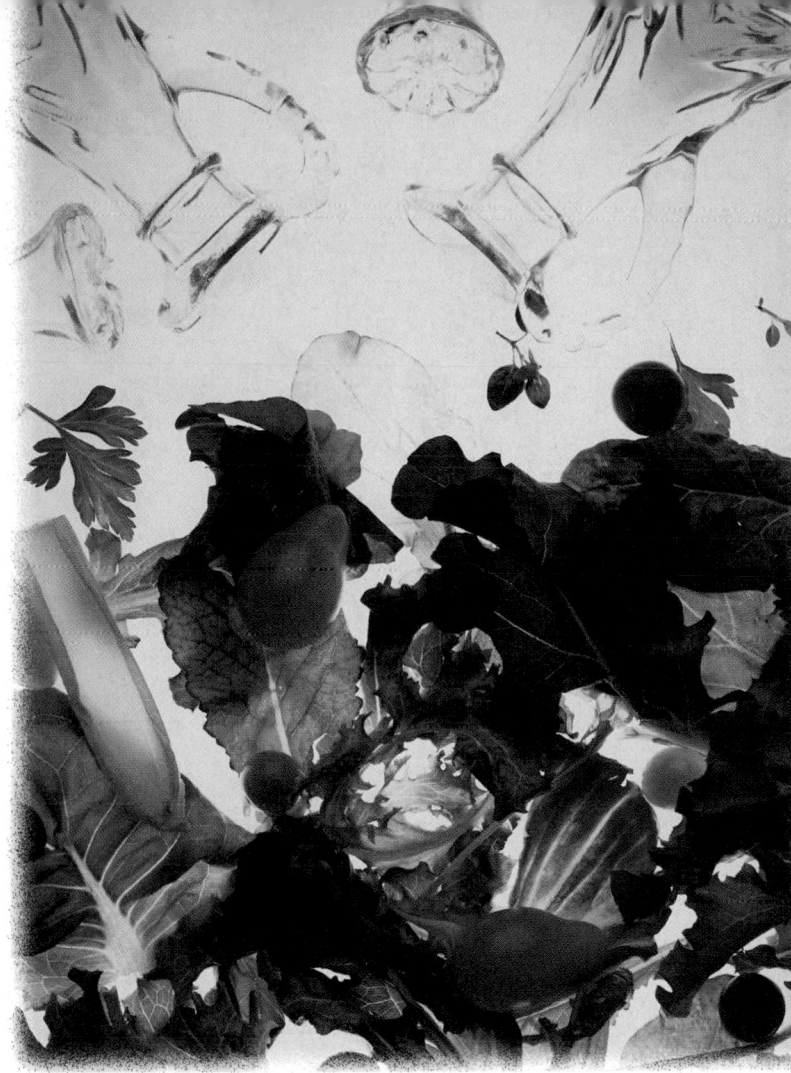

KEY CHAPTER CONCEPTS

- Although vitamins provide no energy to the body, they aid in many energy-yielding reactions. In this way, vitamins promote growth, development, and maintenance of body tissues.
- Vitamins A, D, E, and K are fat soluble and are not readily excreted from the body. The B-vitamins and vitamin C are water soluble and are more easily excreted.
- When taken as supplements in doses greatly exceeding human needs, vitamins A and D are especially toxic.
- Fat-soluble vitamins are absorbed along with dietary fat and reach the bloodstream via the lymphatic system. People with fat malabsorption diseases often have trouble absorbing these vitamins, particularly vitamins E and K.
- Vitamin A is found preformed in animal foods and in its provitamin form, beta-carotene and other carotenoids, in plant foods. Vitamin A helps maintain vision, cell development, and immune function. Beta-carotene and related carotenoids may protect the body from oxidizing agents; some carotenoids can be transformed into vitamin A when needed.
- Among its many functions, vitamin D contributes to calcium absorption and bone function. It can be synthesized in the body with adequate sun exposure.
- Vitamin E functions as an antioxidant, and an important food source is plant oils. Consuming megadoses of vitamin E is controversial because the body already has an array of defense mechanisms against free radicals, and as well most scientific studies have failed to prove any significant health benefits. More research trials are underway.
- Vitamin K is readily available from a variety of green leafy vegetables and vegetable oils, and some is synthesized by intestinal bacteria. There is no evidence that a deficiency is likely to occur, except possibly in some older people. Vitamin K participates in the formation of blood-clotting factors and the production of bone proteins.
- Some segments of the population, such as women during their childbearing years, pregnant women, strict vegans, those on low-calorie diets, and older adults, likely benefit from a multivitamin and mineral supplement.
- Supplements are very loosely regulated by FDA, but those labeled USP (United States Pharmacopia)-approved are generally safe if taken in quantities up to the Daily Value listed on the label. Any use of supplements beyond that, especially in excess of any Upper Level set, should be carefully considered, and all use should be made known to your physician.

REFRESH YOUR MEMORY

As you study this chapter on fat-soluble vitamins, you may want to review

- The integumentary system concerning the skin and vitamin D production, the skeletal system with respect to bone formation, the gastrointestinal system for the digestion and absorption of fat-soluble nutrients, and the urinary system for vitamin D activation in Chapter 3
- Oxidation and reduction reactions in Chapter 4
- The digestion and absorption of dietary lipids and the formation of lipoproteins in Chapter 6
- Amino acid metabolism, protein synthesis, and protein-energy malnutrition in Chapter 7

CASE SCENARIO

Josh, a 71-year-old retired auto mechanic, has experienced "eye problems" during the past 5 years, and now his vision is seriously impaired. He has treated the condition with massive doses of vitamin A, since he read that vitamin A is the vision vitamin. Because he developed bone and joint pain; headaches; and dry, itchy skin, he decided to consult a physician. A physical examination revealed advanced cataracts in both eyes and evidence of vitamin A poisoning. Surgery was scheduled to replace the cloudy lenses with artificial lenses to restore his vision. It may take much longer for his body to dispose of the excess stores of vitamin A, providing he avoids any more vitamin pills.

What is the message here?

■ VITAMINS: VITAL DIETARY COMPONENTS

By definition, vitamins are essential organic (carbon-containing) substances needed in small amounts in the diet for the normal function, growth, and maintenance of body tissues. Although vitamins themselves provide no energy to the body, they often facilitate energy-yielding chemical reactions. Vitamins A, D, E, and K dissolve in organic solvents, whereas the B-vitamins and vitamin C dissolve in water. Obviously, the body does not contain ether or benzene to dissolve the fat-soluble vitamins, so they are digested, absorbed, and transported in such a way that they can exist in a polar environment. In addition, the B-vitamins and vitamin K function as parts of coenzymes (i.e., molecules that facilitate enzyme function).

Vitamins are generally indispensable in human diets because they can't be synthesized in sufficient quantities to meet individual need, or synthesis is curtailed by environmental factors, or they can't be synthesized at all. Vitamins such as niacin and vitamin D can be synthesized by the body, and vitamin K and biotin are synthesized to some extent by bacteria in the intestinal tract.

To be designated a vitamin, the substance must be organic and must carry out one or more biochemical or physiological reactions in the body. Also, if the vitamin intake is insufficient to meet needs, a deficiency occurs, accompanied by a measurable decline in health. If the deficiency is not too far advanced, the symptoms disappear when the vitamin is restored to the body.

In addition to their use in correcting deficiency diseases, a few vitamins have also proved useful as pharmacological agents in treating a limited number of non-deficiency diseases. These medical applications often require the administration of **megadoses**, well above the typical human needs for the vitamin. For example, megadoses of niacin are used as part of blood cholesterol-lowering treatment for appropriately selected individuals (see the Nutrition Perspective in Chapter 6). Another example is the use of vitamin D **analogs** for psoriasis. Nevertheless, at this time any claimed benefits for the use of vitamin supplements, especially intakes in excess of the Upper Limit (if set) should be viewed critically because many unproved claims have been, and are continually, made.[4, 5]

Both plant and animal foods supply vitamins in the human diet. Whether isolated from foods or synthesized in the laboratory, vitamins are the same chemical compounds and generally work equally well in the body. Contrary to claims in the health-food literature, "natural" vitamins isolated from foods are for the most part no more healthful than those synthesized in a laboratory, but there are exceptions. Vitamin E is two times as potent in its natural form as its synthetic form (see the Expert Opinion in this chapter), while folic acid, the synthetic form of the vitamin added to cereals, is more potent than the natural form, folate. Some vitamins exist in several related forms that differ in chemical or physical properties. These forms exist both in nature and in synthesized vitamin supplements. It is important to have enough of the specific vitamin forms that the body can use; the various forms will be identified throughout the next two chapters.

■ Historical Perspective on the Vitamins

Long before any vitamins had been identified, certain foods were known to cure illnesses brought on by what we now recognize to be vitamin deficiencies. The ancient Egyptians, for example, treated night blindness with topical applications of juice extracted from liver, a rich source of vitamin A. As you'll see, vitamin A plays a critical role in vision. During the fifteenth and sixteenth centuries, British sailing ships did not carry sufficient amounts of fresh fruits and vegetables with them for long sea voyages. This resulted in a tremendous loss of life. In one expedition, 1000 men set out from England for the Pacific but only 145 returned. The rest had died from the disease known as scurvy. Scientists eventually discovered that lime juice cured scurvy; after lemons and limes were included as a routine part of British sailors' rations, cases

megadose Intake of a nutrient in excess of 10 times of human needs.

analog A chemical compound that differs slightly from another naturally occurring compound. Analogs generally contain extra or altered chemical groups and may have similar or opposite metabolic effects, compared with the native compound.

of scurvy declined greatly. We now know that this disease, marked by weakness, anemia, and open sores in the mouth, results from a deficiency of vitamin C.

As scientists began to identify various vitamins, related deficiencies such as scurvy, beriberi, pellagra, and rickets were dramatically cured. For the most part, as the vitamins were discovered, they were named alphabetically: A, B, C, D, E, and so on. Later, many substances originally classified as vitamins were found not to be essential for humans and were dropped from the list. This explains the many gaps in alphabetical listing. Other vitamins thought at first to have a single chemical form turned out to exist in many forms, so "vitamin B" now comprises eight separate entities.

It took some time to uncover the true nature of the various vitamins. For example, when scientists realized that both protein foods and nicotinic acid (a form of the vitamin niacin) can cure pellagra, they eventually went on to discover that the amino acid tryptophan can be synthesized into niacin. Finally, as mentioned, it was determined that some vitamins (such as biotin and vitamins D and K) can be synthesized by the body or bacteria present in the intestinal tract.

Although some researchers still hope to discover one or more additional vitamins, we can be relatively confident that the vitamins needed by humans have been discovered. The ability of total parenteral nutrition (TPN) to support human life for years strongly supports this view. With TPN, the patient receives intravenously a carefully formulated preparation containing all necessary nutrients. The gastrointestinal tract is completely bypassed, as no food or beverages are consumed. Those who receive protein, carbohydrate, fat, and all known vitamins and essential minerals in this manner may continue not only to live but also to build body tissue, have a baby, heal wounds, and combat existing diseases. Although a difficult way to meet nutrient needs, it is a lifesaver for those who need it.

■ Storage of Vitamins in the Body

Except for vitamin K, the fat-soluble vitamins are not readily excreted from the body. In contrast, the water-soluble vitamins are generally lost from the body quite rapidly, partly because the water in cells dissolves these vitamins and flushes them out of the body via the kidneys. One exception is vitamin B-12, which is stored much more readily than both the other water-soluble vitamins and fat-soluble vitamin K. Because of the limited storage of many vitamins, they should be consumed in the diet daily, although an occasional lapse in the intake of even water-soluble vitamins generally causes no harm. An average person, for example, must consume no thiamin for 10 days or no vitamin C for 20 to 40 days before developing the first signs and symptoms of a related deficiency. The signs and symptoms of a vitamin deficiency occur only when that vitamin is lacking in the diet and body stores are essentially exhausted.

■ Vitamin Toxicity

Because fat-soluble vitamins are not readily excreted, some can easily accumulate in the body and cause toxic effects. And, although a toxic effect from an excessive intake of any vitamin is theoretically possible, toxicities of the fat-soluble vitamins A and D are the most frequently observed. Vitamin E and the water-soluble vitamins niacin, vitamin B-6, and vitamin C can also cause toxic effects, but only when consumed in very large amounts (15 to 100 times human needs or more). These six vitamins are unlikely to cause toxic effects unless taken in supplement (pill) form. Vitamins A and D can cause toxicity with long-term intake beginning at just 3 times human needs.

Because regular use of a "once-a-day" type of multivitamin/mineral supplement usually contains less than two times the Daily Values of the components, this practice is unlikely to cause toxic effects in nonpregnant adults. But consuming many vitamin pills, especially highly potent sources of vitamin A and vitamin D, can cause

Evidence suggests that health declines when choline, a substance the body makes, is not included in a diet during some life stages, such as growth spurts. Thus, one day choline may be added to the list of known vitamins. Currently, an Adequate Intake (AI) has been established. This is discussed later in more detail in Chapter 10.

problems. In the 1930s, consumption of cod liver oil and other fish oils, which contain high concentrations of vitamin A and vitamin D, was quite common and often led to toxicity symptoms. Today, concentrated vitamin A and vitamin D supplements are widely available in grocery, drug, and health-food stores and still pose risks for toxicity when used inappropriately. See the Nutrition Perspective at the end of this chapter to find out whether you should take a vitamin and mineral supplement and, if so, how to do it safely.

■ Malabsorption of Vitamins

Vitamins consumed in foods must be absorbed efficiently from the intestine to meet body needs. If absorption of a vitamin is defective, a person must consume larger amounts of it or he or she is likely to develop deficiency symptoms. As discussed in a following section, fat malabsorption resulting from various diseases is associated with malabsorption of the fat-soluble vitamins. Alcohol and certain intestinal diseases also can lead to malabsorption of some B-vitamins (e.g., folate).

■ Preservation of Vitamins in Foods

Substantial amounts of vitamins in foods can be lost from the time a fruit or vegetable is picked until it is eaten. The water-soluble vitamins—particularly thiamin, vitamin C, and folate—can be destroyed with improper storage and excessive cooking. Heat, light, exposure to the air, cooking in water, and alkalinity are all factors that can destroy vitamins. The sooner a food is eaten, the less chance of nutrient loss.

In general, if the food is not eaten within a few days, freezing is the best method to retain nutrients. In fact, frozen vegetables and fruits are often as nutrient-rich as supermarket-fresh ones. Frozen foods are often processed immediately after harvesting. As part of the freezing process, vegetables are quickly blanched in boiling water. This destroys the enzymes that would otherwise degrade the vitamins. Table 9-1 provides some tips to aid in preserving the vitamins in food.

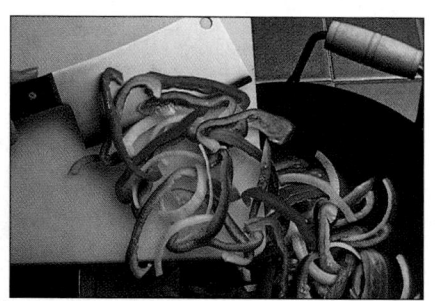

The rapid cooking of vegetables in minimal fluids aids in preserving vitamin content. Stir-frying is one possible method.

TABLE 9-1   Tips for Preserving the Vitamin Content of Foods

What to Do	Why
Keep fruits and vegetables cool.	Enzymes in food begin to degrade vitamins once the fruit or vegetable is picked. Chilling reduces this process. Refrigerate fresh produce (except for potatoes and onions) until they are consumed.
Refrigerate foods in moisture-proof containers.	Nutrients keep best at temperatures near freezing, at high humidity, and away from exposure to air.
Avoid trimming and cutting fruits and vegetables into small pieces as much as possible.	The more surface exposed, the faster oxygen breaks down vitamins. Keep in mind the outer leaves of lettuce and other greens have higher values of vitamins and minerals than the inner, tender leaves or stems. Potato skins and apple skins are higher in vitamins and minerals than the inner parts.
To retain the maximum amounts of nutrients in vegetables, microwave cooking, steaming, or using a pan or wok with very small amounts of fat and a tight-fitting lid is best.	The less contact with water and the shorter the cooking time, the more nutrients are retained. Whenever possible, cook fruits or vegetables in their skins.
Minimize reheating food.	Prolonged reheating reduces vitamin content.
Do not add fats to vegetables during cooking if you plan to discard the liquid.	Discarding fat can lead to loss of fat-soluble vitamins in the liquid. Add fats to vegetables after they are fully cooked and drained.
Don't add baking soda to vegetables to enhance the green color.	Alkalinity destroys much vitamin D, thiamin, and other vitamins.
Store canned goods in a cool place.	To get maximal nutritive value from the canned goods, serve any liquid packed with the food whenever possible. Canned foods vary in the amount of nutrients lost, largely because of differences in storage time and temperatures in the canning process.

■ Absorption of the Fat-Soluble Vitamins

The discussion of the individual fat-soluble vitamins—A, D, E, and K—begins by looking at how they are absorbed (Fig. 9-1). You can see from the chemical structures at the beginning of each vitamin section that these vitamins are lipidlike molecules. Because these vitamins are absorbed along with dietary fat, adequate absorption of the fat-soluble vitamins depends on efficient fat absorption. This, in turn, depends on fat digestion mediated by bile salts and the enzyme lipase in the small intestine, as well as adequate absorptive capacity from a healthy intestinal wall. Under these conditions, about 40 to 90% of the fat-soluble vitamins consumed are absorbed when they are taken in typical amounts. Absorption efficiency generally falls with intakes greatly in excess of human needs.

Once absorbed, fat-soluble vitamins are packaged and delivered to target cells throughout the body in a manner similar to that used for dietary fats—namely, by way of chylomicrons and other lipoproteins. Recall from Chapter 6 that, as a chylomicron circulates in the bloodstream, much of its triglyceride content is removed by body cells. What remains—the remnant—is taken up by the liver. This remnant contains the fat-soluble vitamins absorbed from the diet. The liver can "repackage" fat-soluble vitamins with blood proteins for transport in the general circulation, or they can be stored in the liver for future use.

People with **cystic fibrosis, celiac disease, Crohn's disease,** or any other disease that hampers fat absorption also absorb fat-soluble vitamins poorly. Some medications, such as the weight-loss drug orlistat (Xenical), also interfere with fat absorp-

cystic fibrosis A disease that often leads to overproduction of mucus. Mucus can invade the pancreas, decreasing enzyme output.

celiac disease An immunological or allergic reaction to the protein gluten in certain cereals, such as wheat or rye. The effect is to destroy the intestinal enterocytes, resulting in a much reduced surface area due to flattening of the villi. The elimination of wheat, rye, and certain other grains from the diet restores the intestinal surface.

Crohn's disease An inflammatory disease of the gastrointestinal tract, but generally more pronounced in the terminal ileum. A family history is a major risk factor. The disease limits the absorptive capacity of the small intestine.

■ FIGURE 9-1 An overview of the digestion and absorption of vitamins. Key participants in the process include bile, pancreatic enzymes, intestinal enzymes, and a healthy small intestine absorptive surface. Adequate fat digestion and absorption are critical for the ultimate absorption of fat-soluble vitamins. Carotenoids are absorbed mainly in the duodenum in conjunction with dietary fat.

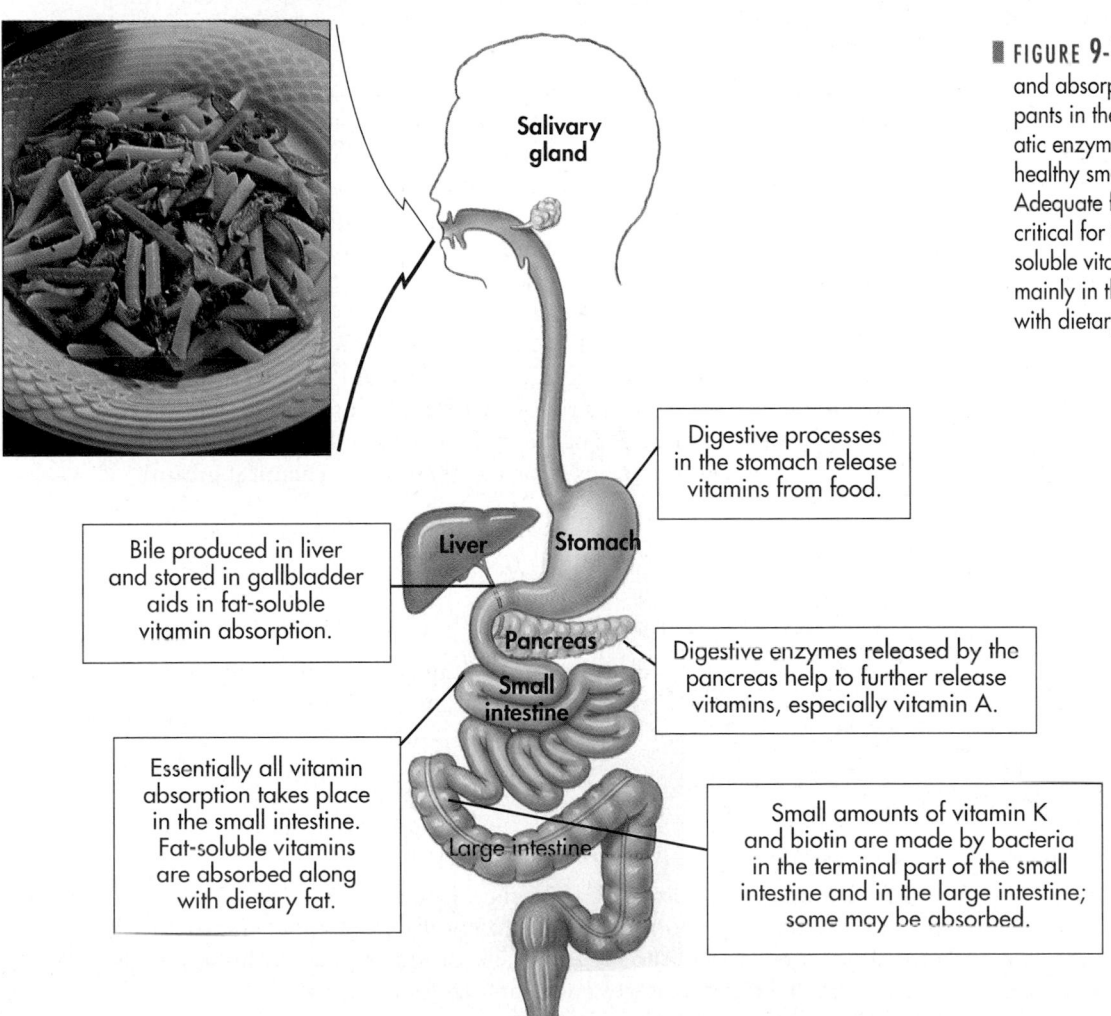

Salivary gland

Digestive processes in the stomach release vitamins from food.

Bile produced in liver and stored in gallbladder aids in fat-soluble vitamin absorption.

Liver   Stomach

Pancreas

Small intestine

Digestive enzymes released by the pancreas help to further release vitamins, especially vitamin A.

Essentially all vitamin absorption takes place in the small intestine. Fat-soluble vitamins are absorbed along with dietary fat.

Large intestine

Small amounts of vitamin K and biotin are made by bacteria in the terminal part of the small intestine and in the large intestine; some may be absorbed.

tion. Unabsorbed fat carries these vitamins to the large intestine, where they are incorporated into the feces and excreted. People with such conditions are especially susceptible to vitamin K deficiency because body stores of vitamin K are lower than those of the other fat-soluble vitamins. Vitamin supplements, taken under a physician's guidance, are part of the treatment for preventing the vitamin deficiency associated with fat malabsorption (Chapter 13 discusses orlistat use in detail).

CONCEPT CHECK

In general, the fat-soluble vitamins—A, D, E, and K—are less readily excreted than are the water-soluble B-vitamins and vitamin C. When a person ingests a vitamin-free diet, the first deficiency signs will be due to a lack of thiamin and will appear after about 10 days. This shows that even water-soluble vitamins persist to some extent in the body, so an occasional inadequate daily consumption is of no health concern. It is important, however, to regularly consume foods rich in both water-soluble and fat-soluble vitamins. The fat-soluble vitamins A and D, when taken in supplement form, pose the greatest risk of toxicity. The water-soluble vitamins known to show toxic effects when taken in supplement form are niacin, vitamin B-6, and vitamin C. Vitamins obtained from food for the most part pose no health threat.

β-carotene

2 molecules of retinal (vitamin A)

Retinol

Retinoic acid

Vitamin A family.

*S*ee Appendix B to review cis and trans isomers

retinoids Collective term for the biologically active forms of vitamin A including retinol, retinal, and retinoic acid.

carotenoids Pigment materials in fruits and vegetables that range in color from yellow to orange to red.

■ VITAMIN A

Americans are at little risk of developing a deficiency of vitamin A, since this vitamin is abundant in our food supply.[16] But vitamin A deficiency constitutes one of the major public health problems in developing countries. Worldwide, vitamin A deficiency is the leading cause of nonaccidental blindness. Children from impoverished nations in Africa, Asia, and South America are especially susceptible because their inadequate intake and diminished stores of vitamin A fail to meet the increased needs associated with rapid growth. Among the world's most destitute nations, hundreds of thousands of children become blind each year because they lack vitamin A. Currently, vitamin A deficiency is estimated to result in 250,000 to 500,000 such cases.[5]

Vitamin A refers to provitamin A **carotenoids** and the preformed **retinoids,** plus their metabolites. Vitamin A is a ring structure with a fatty acid tail. As preformed vitamin A, it exists in three forms: retinol (an alcohol), retinal (an aldehyde), and retinoic acid. The tail terminates in one of these three chemical groups.

$$
\begin{array}{ccc}
\text{H} & & \\
| & \text{H} & \text{O} \\
-\text{C}-\text{OH} & | & || \\
| & -\text{C}=\text{O} & -\text{C}-\text{O}-\text{H} \\
\text{H} & & \\
\text{Retinol} & \text{Retinal} & \text{Retinoic acid}
\end{array}
$$

The tail can vary from cis to trans configuration. This orientation influences the function of the specific retinoid (see Functions of Vitamin A).

$$
\begin{array}{cc}
\text{H H} & \text{H} \\
| \ | & | \\
-\text{C}=\text{C}- & -\text{C}=\text{C}- \\
& | \\
& \text{H} \\
Cis & \text{Trans}
\end{array}
$$

Provitamin A or carotenoids are dietary precursors of retinol. Retinol can be oxidized to retinal and retinoic acid. Carotenoids can be enzymatically split to form retinal or retinol within the intestinal cells or in liver cells within the body.

Preformed vitamin A is present in animal foods as retinol, the alcohol form, and retinyl ester-compounds that have a fatty acid attached to retinol. The retinyl esters don't exhibit vitamin A activity but are hydrolyzed to retinol in the intestinal tract. The most common forms of carotenoids in the North American diet include alpha-carotene, lycopene, lutein, zeaxanthin, beta-carotene, and beta-cryptoxanthin. Alpha-carotene, beta-carotene, and beta-cryptoxanthin can be converted to retinol.[5] These are the provitamin A carotenoids. (The yellow-orange pigment in fruits and vegetables is due to provitamin A beta-carotene.) The other carotenoids do not have vitamin A activity.

■ Digestion, Absorption, Transport, Storage, and Excretion of Vitamin A

The release of vitamin A from food requires bile, digestive enzymes from the pancreas and the intestinal tract, and integration into micelles. Preformed vitamin A (retinoids) can be absorbed up to 90%. Retinoic acid is absorbed via the portal vein bound to the protein albumin. Vitamin A is retinyl esters are absorbed into the lymph via chylomicrons. Provitamin A (carotenoids) is much less likely to be absorbed, perhaps as little as 3%.[24] Absorption via the lymph is utilized. Bile salts are crucial to carotenoid absorption. Overall, absorption depends on the amount of fat in the diet. Within the intestinal wall, some of the carotenoids can be converted to the retinoid form. Both forms of vitamin A are transported via chylomicrons and released to the liver as chylomicron remnants. When vitamin A as a retinoid is released from the liver into general circulation, it is bound to a protein carrier called retinol-binding protein. When carotenoids are released from the liver, they are carried by the lipoprotein VLDL.

Retinoids are stored in the liver. Carotenoids are stored in both the liver and adipose tissue. When needed, stored carotenoids are released from adipose tissue and returned to the liver, where they undergo conversion (cleavage) to retinoids. Under normal circumstances, the liver contains more than 90% of vitamin A in the body.[5] The normal reserve in the liver is adequate for several months, so signs and symptoms of vitamin A deficiency in adults take a long time to develop. It is not readily excreted by the body. Some is lost in the urine. Kidney disease increases the risk of vitamin A toxicity if this route of excretion is compromised.

■ Cellular Retinoid-Binding Proteins

Retinoids are bound to specific retinoid-binding proteins in the blood plasma, within intercellular spaces and within cells. In cells that take up retinoids, there is a family of cellular-binding proteins (CRBP) that hold retinoids and direct them to functional sites within the cell. Nearly all cells contain one or more of these binding proteins, which seem to have a variety of roles and affect different tissues. Besides transport, these binding proteins protect the vitamin from oxidation and enzymatic reactions.

■ Nuclear-Retinoid Receptors

There are two main families of nuclear-retinoid receptors, **RAR** and **RXR.** These receptors within the cell nucleus bind specific retinoids (retinoic acid) in the nucleus of the cell and then bind to DNA to regulate the activity of retinoid-responsive genes on DNA. The binding to RAR or RXR permits the interaction of the vitamin with a specific area of DNA, thus regulating the formation of mRNA and the subsequent production of body proteins (and body processes). Actually, the event can activate or inhibit specific **gene expression** (Fig. 9-2).

■ Functions of Vitamin A

Each of the three active forms of vitamin A—retinol, retinal, and retinoic acid—performs important functions. Their biochemical or physiologic actions include vision; the growth and differentiation of epithelial, nervous, bone, and other tissue; and immunity.

The first fat-soluble vitamin was recognized as A in 1916.

During protein-energy malnutrition, synthesis of retinol-binding protein and prealbumin is reduced by the lack of amino acids and energy. These proteins are used as clinical indicators of protein synthesis in a person because decreased concentrations in the blood suggests inadequate protein intake.

RXR, RAR The abbreviations for retinoid X receptor and retinoic acid receptor. These two subfamilies of retinoid receptors interact with retinoic acid and bind with specific sites on DNA. This allows for cell differentiation.

gene expression The activation of a specific site on DNA, which results in either the activation or the inhibition of the gene.

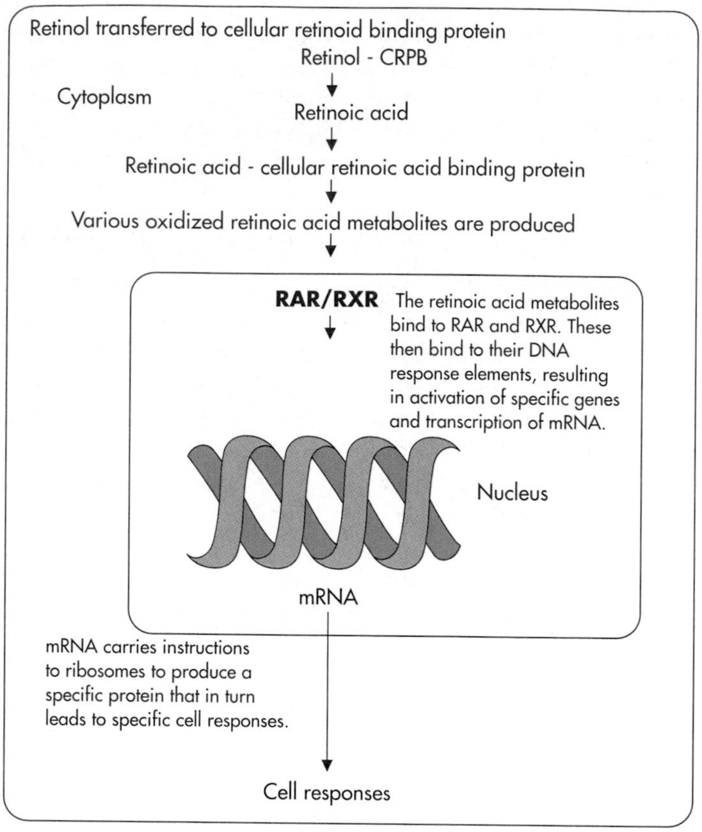

FIGURE 9-2 Nuclear retinoid receptors, RAR and RXR, bind retinoic acid metabolites and then bind to DNA activating gene transcription. The resulting messenger RNA (mRNA) has the code for the protein that ultimately produces the cellular responses (see Chapter 7 for details on protein synthesis using mRNA). Nearly all cells have at least one member of the RAR and RXR families.

rhodopsin A photoreceptor in the rod cells composed of 11-cis retinal and opsin.

photon A unit of light intensity at the retina having the brightness of one candle.

photoisomerization The molecular isomerization of a compound by the energy of light.

bleaching process The process by which light depletes the rhodopsin concentration in the eye. This fall in rhodopsin concentration allows the eye to become adapted to bright light.

Vision

Vitamin A is needed both as retinal in the retina of the eye, to turn visual light into nerve signals to the brain, and as retinoic acid, to maintain normal differentiation of the cells that make up the various structural components of the eye, such as the cones and rod cells (Fig. 9-3).[16]

The sensory elements of the retina consist of specialized cells known as rods and cones. The rods are responsible for the visual processes that occur in dim light, translating objects into black-and-white images and detecting motion. The cones are responsible for the visual processes occurring under bright light, translating objects into color images.

In the rods, 11-cis-retinal binds to a protein called opsin to form the visual pigment called **rhodopsin** (visual purple). The absorption of a **photon** of light catalyzes the **photoisomerization** of 11-cis-retinal to all-trans retinal, causing opsin to separate from all-trans retinal. This isomerization event leads to a cascade of biochemical events, which trigger a change in ion permeability (hyperpolarization) of the photoreceptor cells. This, in turn, initiates a signal to the neuronal (nerve) cells that communicate with the brain's visual cortex. Actually, thousands of rod cells containing millions of molecules of rhodopsin are triggered simultaneously.

In order to keep the visual processes functioning, the 11-cis-retinal in the rod cells must be regenerated in the pigment containing cells in the eye. All-trans retinal is converted to retinol, then to 11-cis-retinol, and finally back to 11-cis-retinal. This is a slow process. The 11-cis-retinal then moves back to the photoreceptor site, where it recombines with opsin and is ready for another cycle. This process takes several minutes.

The release of 11-cis-retinal from opsin is designated a **bleaching process.** During exposure to bright light, the rods' rhodopsin is completely activated and cannot respond to more light until it returns to its resting state. Enzymes regenerate the ini-

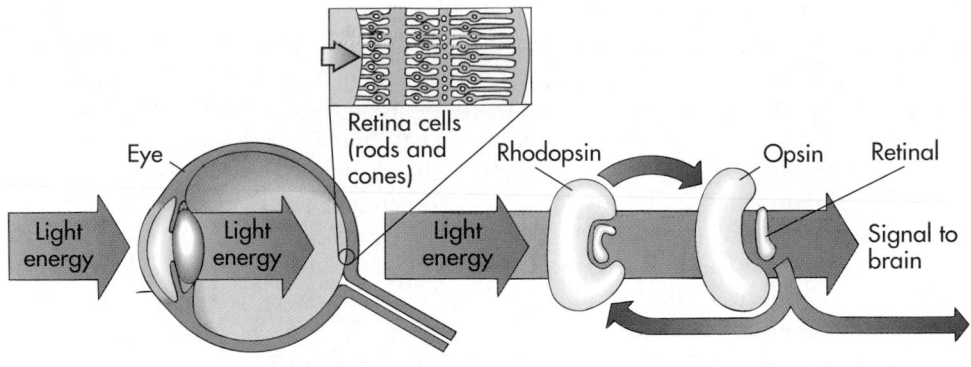

Light causes a change in retinal and retinal is in turn released (*trans* form). This change in rhodopsin to opsin and *trans* retinal in turn initiates a signal to the brain.

Rhodopsin is then rebuilt after forming retinal back into its original shape (*cis* form).

Some retinal is lost from cycle. This must be replaced by retinol from the bloodstream. It is converted to retinal in the eye.

■ FIGURE 9-3 Vitamin A participates in the visual cycle as retinal. Rhodopsin, 11-cis-retinal and the protein opsin, absorb a photon of light after which the retinal changes shape to all-trans retinal and separates from the opsin. This event changes ion permeability of the photoreceptor cell, which signals "light" to the visual cortex of the brain.

tial form of rhodopsin, so that it can respond to light again. If there is a limited amount of rhodopsin in the rod cells, it is difficult to adapt to seeing in dim light (night blindness).[16]

Not all retinal is reused, so there is a pool of retinyl esters in the eye to keep a supply of vitamin A on hand. Should the pool of vitamin A be low, the process of **dark adaptation** is slowed down. Children are more likely to experience a lack of vitamin A because they haven't had time to build up body stores.

Cones are less sensitive to light than rods are, but cones provide color vision and much greater visual acuity. During daylight, light bleaches out the rods, allowing the cones to provide acute color vision. Color vision is due to the activation of three types of cones, each containing retinal and proteins called iodopsins. The protein is unique for each of the three cone pigments and responds to different wavelengths of light. The three types of cones are blue, green, and red. Color vision depends on which combination of cone cells is stimulated by any given wavelength of visible light.

Various cell types in the retina, cornea, and **epithelium** of the eye depend on the presence of retinoic acid for maintaining structural integrity. Vitamin A is delivered to the target sites by tears. More about cellular action of vitamin A appears in the next section.

dark adaptation The process by which the rhodopsin concentration in the eye increases in dark conditions. This, in turn, allows improved vision in the dark.

epithelium The covering in internal and external surfaces of the body, including the lining of vessels and other small cavities. It consists of epithelial cells joined by a small amount of cementing material.

Cellular Growth and Differentiation

The fundamental function of retinoic acid is **cell differentiation.** The retinoic acid receptors, RAR and RXR, are part of a very large family of steroid and thyroid hormone nuclear transcription factors. Two forms of vitamin A, all-trans retinoic acid and 9-cis-retinoic acid, regulate finely tuned gene expression through the activation of RAR and RXR. RAR and RXR express themselves in "time and location-specific patterns." They code for a variety of structural proteins, such as enzymes and those in epithelial cells (skin keratins). The two forms of retinoic acid (all-trans retinoic acid and 9-cis-retinoic acid) are bound to RXR and RAR, which in turn bind to specific DNA gene sequences. This event results in gene expression (review Fig. 9-2). Cell differentiation is often accompanied by inhibition of **cell proliferation.** It is hypothesized that differentiation, inhibition of proliferation, and apoptosis (programmed cell death) are related to the actions of retinoids.[16]

Retinoic acid is necessary for the production, the structure, and the normal function of epithelial cells in the lungs, trachea, skin, gastrointestinal tract, and many other systems. It is also essential in the formation and maintenance of mucus-forming cells in these organs.

cell differentiation The process of transforming an unspecialized cell into a specialized cell.

cell proliferation The continuous development of cells in tissue formation.

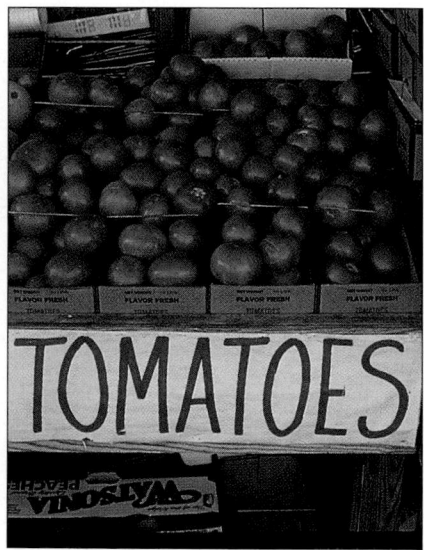

Tomatoes are a rich source of the carotenoid lycopene, especially after cooking, as this releases the lycopene from cells. Lycopene may reduce prostate cancer risk in men and the risk of various cancers associated with the digestive tract.

CRITICAL THINKING

Check out the ready-to-eat breakfast cereals at your local supermarket. Which ones have beta-carotene added? Why do you think the manufacturers are pursuing this kind of fortification?

conjunctiva The mucous membrane covering the anterior surface of the eyeball and the posterior surface of the eyelids.

Vitamin A as retinoic acid affects growth and development. Studies of rodents and primates reveal that retinoids control the embryonic development of the central nervous system, limbs, cardiovascular system, and eyes. In a study of vitamin A-deficient children (6 to 48 months old), supplementation improved linear growth modestly. The older children and nonbreastfed children benefited most in linear growth with supplementation than did the younger children and breastfed children. Supplementation had its biggest effect on the children with the lowest levels of serum vitamin A. This study showed that breastfeeding protects young children from linear growth failure when there is a lack of vitamin A-rich foods.[6] It is important to note, however, that vitamin A deficiency is rarely, if ever, diagnosed in either the United States or Canada.

Another function of vitamin A is in cell-to-cell communication. One cell membrane constituent, glycoproteins, are important in cell interaction, cell recognition, and cell aggregation. Vitamin A controls the production of glycoproteins.[16]

Immunity

As early as the 1920s, researchers recognized that vitamin A deficiency is associated with decreased resistance to infections. Immunity to pathogens is highly specific, and the type of response that occurs depends on the host. The severity of some infections, such as measles and diarrhea, is reduced by vitamin A supplementation. Vitamin A seems to function through cell-mediated and antibody-mediated responses, such as macrophage and natural killer cell activity, and growth and differentiation of B-lymphocytes. In addition, nonspecific immunity, the maintenance of epithelial tissues, and mucus production all act as powerful deterrents to invading pathogens. Overall, vitamin A contributes to a variety of immune processes.[16]

Carotenoid Actions

In vitro, carotenoids appear to function as antioxidants—they trap free radicals. Beta-carotene and lycopene interact with singlet oxygen radicals, and beta-carotene can trap peroxyl radicals. (See the Vitamin E section for a discussion of free radicals.) Whether these actions occur in humans is not yet known. Currently, the only established function of provitamin A carotenoids is to act as a source of vitamin A, but other benefits are suspected.[4]

Carotenoids may decrease the risk of cataracts and macular degeneration in the eye, decrease the risk of some cancers, and decrease the risk of some cardiovascular diseases. Research suggests that deterioration of the retina is more likely to take place when a person's diet is low in carotenoids, such as lutein and zeaxanthin, over an extended period of time.[2] Still, clinical trials have not clearly shown carotenoids to be responsible for any specific reduction in disease risk. It could be some other components found in fruits and vegetables or certain lifestyle choices, and not carotenoids, that convey good health.[25] And, as of now, there are no established clinical effects of consuming a diet low in carotenoids as long as one's diet is adequate in preformed vitamin A. In fact, beta-carotene in pill form can be harmful for certain people, including smokers and former smokers. The excess beta-carotene may interfere with the absorption of other carotenoids.[23]

■ Vitamin A Deficiency

When the retinol in blood plasma is insufficient to replace the retinal lost during the visual cycle, the rod cells in the eye recover from flashes of light more slowly. The resulting night blindness is a common early symptom of vitamin A deficiency.

Without vitamin A, mucus-forming cells deteriorate and are no longer able to synthesize mucus, the essential lubricant used throughout the body. The eye, especially the cornea, is adversely affected by the loss of mucus, which keeps the eye surface moist and washes away dirt and other particles that settle on the eye. Deterioration of the eye results from bacterial invasion, because vitamin A plays an important role in resistance to infection. Conjunctival xerosis (abnormal dryness of the **conjunctiva** of the eye) and Bitot's spots (drying out of the eye and appearance of hardened epithelial cells) appears as vitamin A deficiency worsens. The corneal ulceration and keratomatacia (softening of the cornea) result in scarring (Fig. 9-4). The ultimate scarring may be barely detectable, or it could lead to loss of sight. This sequence of changes in the eye—collectively known as **xerophthalmia**—causes irreversible blindness in millions of people worldwide, as mentioned before.[5]

Vitamin A deficiency also produces skin changes referred to as **follicular hyperkeratosis.** Keratin, the normal component of the outer layers of skin, protects the inner layers and reduces water loss through the skin. During severe vitamin A deficiency, kertinized cells normally present only in the outer layers replace the normal epithelial cells in the underlying skin layers. Hair follicles become plugged with keratin, giving a bumpy appearance and rough texture to the skin, and the skin is very dry.

In areas of the world where vitamin A deficiency causes a decrease in appetite, poor growth follows. If liver vitamin A stores are established after an infant is weaned, they can supply retinol for several months or even longer. Vitamin A deficiency in children occurs most often during the postweaning period. Giving supplements of 15,000 to 60,000 µg to young children at risk may protect them for up to 6 months.[6] Finding a suitable food to improve intake is a must for a long-term solution to vitamin A deficiency. The problem is that most children do not like the vegetables that are the richest source of provitamin A, and insufficient dietary fat inhibits the absorption of what little vitamin A there is in the diet.

■ Cancer Prevention and Treatment

Although many animal studies using natural and synthetic retinoids have shown a reduction in various cancers, such effects with long-term use in humans has not been demonstrated. If there is any mechanism that works to prevent cancer, it is probably through the fundamental role of retinoids in cell differentiation, inhibition of proliferation, and perhaps induction of programmed cell death (apoptosis). In contrast, beta-carotene in supplement form has not been shown to prevent any type of cancer.[15]

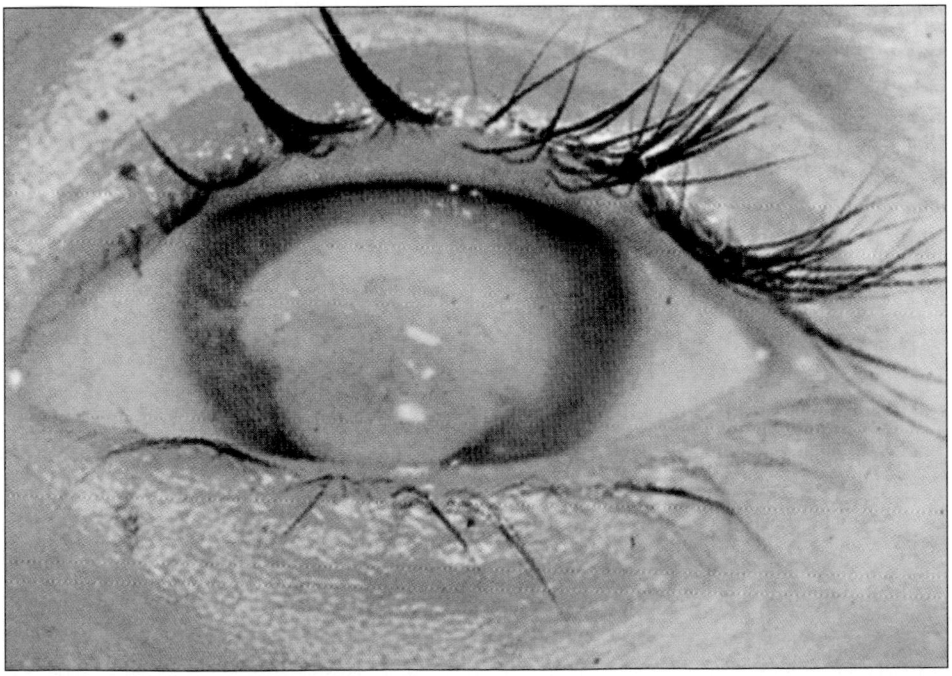

xerophthalmia A condition, marked by dryness of the cornea and eye membranes, that results from vitamin A deficiency and can lead to blindness. The specific cause is a lack of mucus production by the eye, which then leaves it more vulnerable to surface dirt and bacterial infections.

follicular hyperkeratosis A condition in which keratin, a protein, accumulates around hair follicles.

Fortification of food with vitamin A is being examined as a possible solution to widespread vitamin A deficiency in many developing countries. Guatemala already fortifies sugar with vitamin A, and countries such as the Philippines and Indonesia are considering the fortification of MSG. Technical expertise and funding often stand in the way of such fortification.

■ FIGURE **9-4** A Vitamin A deficiency can eventually lead to blindness. Note the severe effects on this eye. This problem is commonly seen today in southeast Asia. In contrast, the leading cause of blindness in North America is accidents in children and diabetes in adults.

When the word *carotenoids* is mentioned, most people think of carrots. Perhaps our minds should jump first to tomatoes; the familiar vegetable (actually, it's a fruit) contains 14 carotenoids (including lycopene). Carrots contain only 3.

reactive oxygen species Several oxygen derivatives produced during the formation of ATP. Formed constantly in the human body and shown to kill bacteria and inactivate proteins, they are implicated in a number of diseases. They have been linked to inflammatory processes and cancer development.

epithelial cells Cells that cover the surface of the body and line all body cavities.

sebum A substance secreted by sebaceous consisting of fat, keratin, and cellular material.

Prostate cancer is one of the most common cancers among American men. The dietary carotenoid lycopene (the red pigment found in tomatoes, watermelon, and several other fruits) seems to protect against this type of cancer. The proposed biological role of lycopene may be that of an antioxidant against singlet oxygen, a **reactive oxygen species.** As of now, the association between lycopene intake and protection from prostate cancer is weak and inconsistent.[13] Some food companies (e.g., Campbell Soup Company) however, have been advertising their tomato-based products as important sources of lycopene.

■ Cardiovascular Disease Prevention

Carotenoids in general may play a role in preventing cardiovascular disease in persons at high risk, possibly linked to carotenoids' antioxidant capability (see Chapter 6). Until definitive studies are complete, many scientists recommend that we consume a total of at least five servings of a combination of fruits and vegetables per day as a part of an overall effort to reduce the risk of cardiovascular disease.[4]

■ Eyesight

Age-related macular degeneration is a leading cause of legal blindness among American adults over the age of 65. The disease is associated with changes in the central region of the macula, the area of the eye that provides the most detailed vision. Age, smoking, and genetics seem to be risk factors. The macula contains the carotenoids lutein and zeaxanthin in high enough concentrations to impart a yellow color. In one notable study of 876 subjects, the higher the total number of dietary carotenoids (beta-carotene, lutein, and zeaxanthin) consumed, the lower was the risk for age-related macular degeneration. This is an interesting hypothesis, but as already mentioned, it may be that other factors, such as fruit and vegetable intake, may affect the risk rather than the intake of these specific carotenoids. Note that the manufacturers of Centrum Silver™ and other similar supplements are adding a source of lutein to their products.

■ Pharmacologic Use of Vitamin A

Natural and synthetic retinoids control **epithelial cell** proliferation and differentiation of the epidermis. Various forms of vitamin A have been used successfully to treat acne, psoriasis, and certain skin cancers. Both systemic and topical agents are used to bring about and regulate the expression of skin growth factors. They can decrease **sebum** secretion. 13-cis-retinoic acid (Accutane) is an oral drug used to treat severe acne. It is a potent suppresser of sebocyte proliferation and sebum production. Retin-A (tretinoin) is applied topically for less aggressive treatment of acne.[17] Acitretin is used to treat severe psoriasis. These medications can produce toxic symptoms and birth defects if used during pregnancy.

High doses of all-trans retinoic acid have been used to induce remission of a form of leukemia, but a significant percentage of patients experienced severe side effects and quite a few developed kidney failure, which was fatal. Thus it can be used for only a short period of time. All vitamin A analogs must be administered under the strict supervision of a physician.

■ Dietary Sources of Vitamin A and Carotenoids

Preformed vitamin A is found in liver, fish, fish oils, fortified milk, and eggs. Margarine is fortified with vitamin A. Provitamin A carotenoids are mainly found in dark green and yellow-orange vegetables and some fruits. Carrots, spinach and other greens, winter squash, sweet potatoes, broccoli, mangoes, cantaloupe, peaches, and apricots are examples of such sources. About 65 to 75% of the vitamin A in the typical North American diet comes from animal (preformed vitamin A) sources, whereas provitamin A predominates in the diet among poor people in other parts of the world (Fig. 9-5).

Among common foods, those having the highest nutrient density for vitamin A (μg/kcal) are carrots, liver, spinach and other greens, sweet potatoes, winter squash, romaine lettuce, broccoli, apricots, and nonfat and low-fat milk. Many of the vegetables listed are good sources of alpha-carotene and beta-carotene. Fruits such as apricots and peaches contain beta-cryptoxanthin. Though rarely consumed in the United States, the oils from the livers of saltwater fish and marine mammals are extremely rich sources of vitamin A. Consumption of large amounts of such foods can even lead to symptoms of vitamin A toxicity.

Beta-carotene accounts for some of the orange color of carrots. In vegetables such as broccoli, this yellow-orange color is masked by dark-green chlorophyll pigments. Still, green vegetables contain provitamin A. Consuming a varied diet rich in green vegetables and carrots ensures sufficient sources for meeting vitamin A needs.[5] Green, leafy vegetables, such as spinach and kale, have a high concentration of lutein and zeaxanthin. Tomato juice and other tomato products, such as pizza sauce, contain significant amounts of lycopene.[13] Since these tomato products have undergone heat processing, the lycopene is more bioavailable.

■ Retinol Activity Equivalent (RAE)

At one time, the amounts of most nutrients in foods were expressed in **international units (IUs)**, a crude measure of vitamin activity. Today we can directly measure very small quantities of nutrients more precisely; consequently, milligrams

Dietary Sources of Vitamin A

Food Item	Amount	Vitamin A (RAE)*
Fried Beef Liver	1 oz	3042
Baked Sweet Potato	½ cup	958
Cooked Spinach	⅔ cup	494
Fresh Mango	⅖ lb	398
Cooked Acorn Squash	⅔ cup	244
Cooked Kale	½ cup	206
Cooked Broccoli	1 cup	138
Skim Milk	½ cup	74
Margarine	1 pat	50
Scallions	1 Tbsp	32
Parmesan Cheese	1 Tbsp	12

*Retinol Activity Equivalents

international unit (IU) A crude measure of vitamin activity, often based on the growth rate of animals. Today these units often have been replaced by precise measurements of actual quantities in milligrams or micrograms.

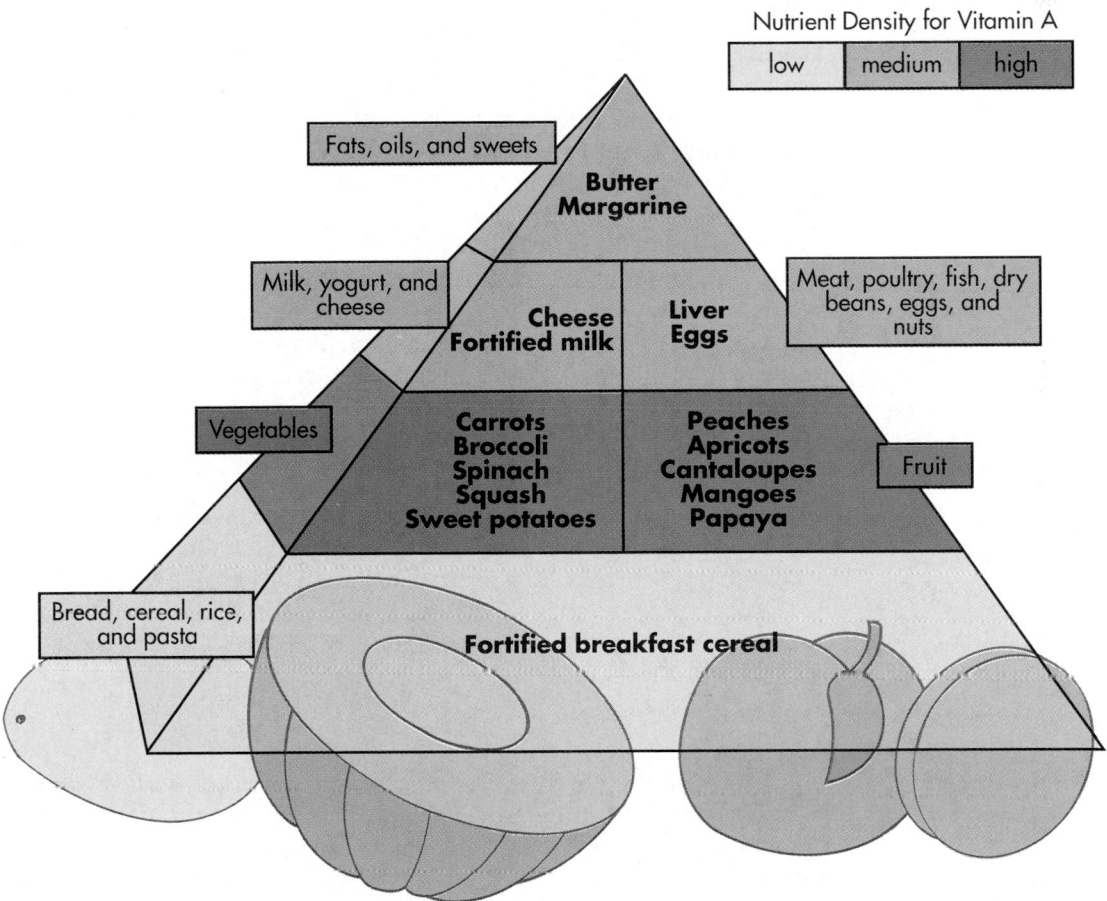

FIGURE 9-5 Food sources of vitamin A from the Food Guide Pyramid. The fruit and vegetable groups supply abundant carotenoids if they have an intense yellow-orange or green color. Some of these carotenoids yield vitamin A. Liver is the richest source of preformed vitamin A, because that is the major site of vitamin A storage in animals. Milk is often fortified with vitamin A. The background color of each food group indicates the average nutrient density for vitamin A in that group.

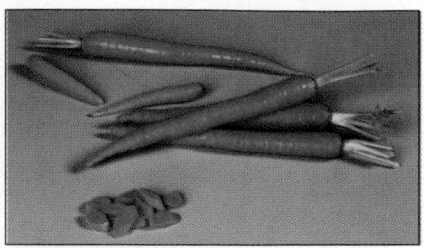

Carrots are rich in provitamin A carotenoids.

*A*n older unit for vitamin A was the retinol equivalent (RE). This RE assumed that there was a greater contribution to vitamin A needs from carotenoids than we assume today. Food composition tables and nutrient databases still contain this older RE standard, as is the case for Appendix A in this text. RAE and RE units are equal for preformed vitamin A, but RAE units are only about half the RE value listed for provitamin A sources. It will take some time for food composition tables to be updated with RAE values.

*I*t is important to ensure adequate vitamin A intake among people who are on iron supplements. Supplementation with iron may increase the severity of new infections or may exacerbate existing infections. Adequate vitamin A status is thought to protect the immune system from these potential effects of iron supplementation.

hypervitaminosis A condition resulting from the intake of excessive amounts of one or more vitamins.

teratogenic Tending to produce physical defects in a developing fetus.

(1/1000 of a gram) and micrograms (1/1,000,000 of a gram) have generally replaced international units as customary units of measure, although vitamin supplements may still display the older IU values.

For vitamin A, the current unit of measurement is the retinol activity equivalent (RAE), which is basically 1 µg of retinol. In this system, it is assumed that 12 µg of beta-carotene yield 1 µg of vitamin A activity and that 24 µg of the other two provitamin A carotenoids (alpha carotene and beta-cryptoxanthin) yield 1 µg of vitamin A activity. The total RAE value for a food is calculated by adding the actual weight of retinol and the adjusted equivalent weights of the provitamin A carotenoids present in the food. For example, a diet that contains 500 µg retinol, 1,800 µg beta-carotene and 2,400 µg alpha-carotene supplies 750 µg RAE (500 + (1,800 ÷ 12) + (2,400 ÷ 24) = 750 µg RAE).[5]

Table 9-2 is a handy tool for converting amounts of vitamin A and carotenes expressed in one unit of measure into another unit of measure.

TABLE 9-2 Conversion Values for Retinol Activity Equivalents[5]	
1 retinol activity equivalent (RAE)	1 IU Vitamin A activity
= 1 µg of all-*trans*-retinol	= 0.3 µg of all-*trans*-retinol
= 12 µg of dietary all-*trans*-beta-carotene	= 3.6 µg of dietary all-*trans*-beta-carotene
= 24 µg of other dietary provitamin A carotenoids	= 7.2 µg other dietary provitamin A carotenoids

■ RDA for Vitamin A

The Estimated Average Requirement for vitamin A is 625 µg Retinol Activity Equivalents for men 19 to 70+ and 500 µg Retinol Activity Equivalents for women 19 to 70+. At this intake, adequate body stores of vitamin A are maintained. Increasing this amount by 40% to account for variation in individual needs yields an RDA of 900 µg Rentinol Activity Equivalents for men and 700 µg Retinol Activity Equivalents for women. Average intakes for adult men and women in the United States meet the RDAs.

Most adults in the United States have liver reserves of vitamin A that are three to five times greater than needed to provide good health. Thus, the use of vitamin A supplements by most people is unnecessary. At present, there is no separate RDA for beta-carotene or any of the other provitamin A carotenoids.[4]

■ North Americans at Risk for Vitamin A Deficiency

Deficient vitamin A status may be seen in preschool children who do not eat enough vegetables. The urban poor, older adults, and people with alcoholism or liver disease (which limits vitamin A storage) can also show diminished vitamin A status, especially with respect to stores. Finally, children and adults with severe fat-malabsorption syndromes, as in cases of celiac disease, chronic diarrhea, pancreatic insufficiency, Crohn's disease, cystic fibrosis, HIV and AIDS, may also experience vitamin A deficiency.

■ Vitamin A Toxicity

Signs and symptoms of toxicity from excessive vitamin A—called **hypervitaminosis A**—can appear with long-term supplement use at 3 times the RDA for preformed vitamin A (Fig. 9-6). Three kinds of vitamin A toxicity exist: acute, chronic, and **teratogenic.** Acute toxicity is caused by the ingestion of one very large dose of vitamin A or several large doses taken over several days (about 100 times the RDA). The effects of acute toxicity are largely gastrointestinal upset, headache, blurred vision, and muscular incoordination.[18] Once the dosing is stopped, these signs disappear. Extraordinarily large doses, about 12 g (13,000 times the RDA), however, can be fatal.

In chronic toxicity, infants and adults show a wide range of signs and symptoms: bone and muscle pain, loss of appetite, various skin disorders, headache, dry skin, hair loss, liver damage, double vision, hemorrhage, vomiting, and coma. Toxicity of vitamin A probably causes instability in retinoid-sensitive membranes and the inappropriate expression of certain genes. The treatment is simply to discontinue the supplement. Effects then decrease over the next few weeks to a month as blood concentrations fall to within a normal range. Permanent damage to the liver, bones, and eyes, as well as recurrent joint and muscle pain, however, can occur with chronic ingestion of excessive amounts of the vitamin. The Upper Level for vitamin A intake is established at 3000 µg preformed vitamin A for men and women ages 19 to 70+. This amount is based on the presence of birth defects occurring during pregnancy and liver toxicity in general with intakes above this amount.

The most serious and tragic effects of hypervitaminosis A are teratogenic—most notably, birth defects just mentioned. Vitamin A and its related analog forms, all-*trans*-retinoic acid (topical tretinoin to reduce wrinkling and acne) and 13-*cis*-retinoic acid (oral isotretinoin, or Accutane, used to treat acne), have been subjects of concern for years. Accutane causes spontaneous abortion and birth defects in experimental animals. The risk is significant for pregnant women taking large doses of Accutane for acne. Their offspring show congenital malformations of the head, probably because neural crest cells, which are important in the development of the head and brain, are known to be very sensitive to excess amounts of vitamin A. Women who expect to become pregnant are advised not to take the medicinal forms of vitamin A that produce these effects. There appears to be no clear relationship between birth defects and excessive use of vitamin A as topical tretinoin.

Vitamin A is particularly harmful in early pregnancy, a time when many women do not know that they are pregnant. Hypervitaminosis A may cause a spontaneous abortion or birth defects.

It is even possible for women to get too much vitamin A from food if they consume high-vitamin A foods, such as liver and fortified breakfast cereals. For this reason, it is recommended that pregnant women limit their intake of these foods, and,

People in developing countries typically pose an exception to the rule that moderately large doses of vitamin A can cause toxicity. Because of their minimal storage of vitamin A, these people can tolerate intermittent large doses of the vitamin.

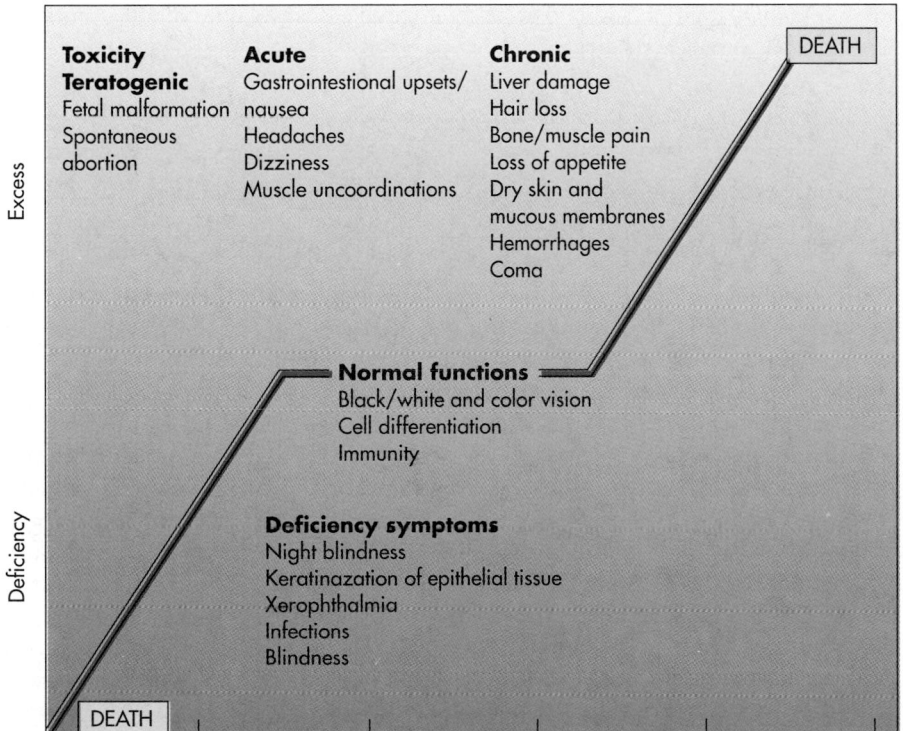

■ **FIGURE 9-6** Consuming the right amount of vitamin A is critical to overall health. A very low (deficient) or a very high (toxic) vitamin A intake can produce damaging signs and symptoms and even lead to death. The severity of effects and the intake range vary among individuals.

Increasing vitamin A intake

CASE SCENARIO
Follow-Up

Josh was suffering from chronic vitamin A toxicity. Self-diagnosis and self-treatment are a risky form of medicine. When serious health symptoms occur and over-the-counter medications and vitamins don't promptly alleviate the problem, it is time to seek professional medical help.

hypercarotenemia Elevated amounts of carotenoids in the bloodstream, usually caused by consuming a diet high in carrots or squash or by taking beta-carotene supplements.

Cholecalciferol
(vitamin D₃)

CH₃

Action by liver and kidney to yield the final product

CH₂

OH

HO

1,25 (OH)₂ vitamin D₃

HO   OH

Vitamin D family.

rickets A disease characterized by softening of the bones caused by poor calcium deposition. This deficiency disease arises in infants and children with poor vitamin D status.

osteomalacia The softening of the bones that occurs in adults as a result of bone decalcification linked to inadequate vitamin D status.

if using supplements, they should check that much of the vitamin A is in the form of beta-carotene. FDA recommends that women of childbearing years limit their intake of preformed vitamin A to about 100% of the Daily Value listed on food labels.

Consuming carotenoids in huge amounts from foods does not readily result in toxicity in most people. The carotenoids' rate of conversion into vitamin A (retinol), when possible, is relatively slow. In addition, the efficiency of carotenoid absorption from the small intestine decreases markedly as the oral intake increases.

If someone consumes large amounts of carrots (e.g., in the form of carrot juice) or if an infant eats a lot of winter squash, the resulting high carotenoid concentrations in the body can turn skin a yellow-orange color. The result is termed **hyper-carotenemia,** or just carotenemia. (Recall that *hyper* means "high" and *emia* means "in the bloodstream.") The person appears to have jaundice; however, unlike a true jaundice, the sclerae (whites of the eyes) are white (rather than yellow) and the liver is not enlarged. This carotenemia is generally thought to be harmless. Lycopeno-dermia results from excessive intake of foods rich in lycopene; food such as tomatoes. A deep orange discoloration of the skin is evident.

CONCEPT CHECK

*V*itamin A has diverse functions, many of which are yet to be fully understood. Accumulating evidence suggests that the binding of vitamin A (retinoic acid) to DNA can influence cell growth and differentiation through regulation of gene expression. Vitamin A is important for maintaining vision and epithelial tissues reproduction, growth, and ensuring proper function of the immune system. Vitamin A in the diet comes in two forms: retinoids (preformed vitamin A) and certain carotenoids (provitamin A). At present, there is no definitive answer as to whether retinoids and carotenoids have specific anticancer properties. However, a diet that meets the RDA for vitamin A and contains plenty of carotenoid-containing fruits and vegetables is considered sound nutrition. Major food sources of vitamin A include liver, carrots, eggs, tomatoes, milk, and many vegetables. Americans most at risk for poor vitamin A status are preschool children and alcoholics. Large doses of vitamin A can be toxic, even at chronic dosages only about 3 times the RDA, especially during early pregnancy.

■ VITAMIN D

The status of vitamin D as a vitamin is ambiguous because, in the presence of sunlight, skin cells are capable of synthesizing a sufficient supply of the vitamin from a derivative of cholesterol. Since a dietary source is not required in this case, the vitamin is more correctly classified as a **prohormone** (i.e., a precursor of an active hormone). The prohormone form of vitamin D, whether synthesized in the body or obtained from the diet, is converted to the active form by enzymes in the liver and kidneys. The active form then is delivered to target organs, where it exerts its biological effects (Fig. 9-7). *Vitamin D* is a generic term for both the provitamin (prohormone) and the active vitamin form. Vitamin D achieves vitamin status because the diseases **rickets** and **osteomalacia** can be prevented and, to some extent, treated by the consumption of vitamin D-rich foods.

The amount of sun exposure individuals need to produce vitamin D depends on skin color, age, time of day, season of the year, and geographic location. Experts recommend that people expose their hands, face, and arms two to three times a week to 30 to 50% of the amount of sun needed to cause a sunburn. In other words, for a person who would sunburn in just a half-hour, 10 to 15 minutes of exposure is

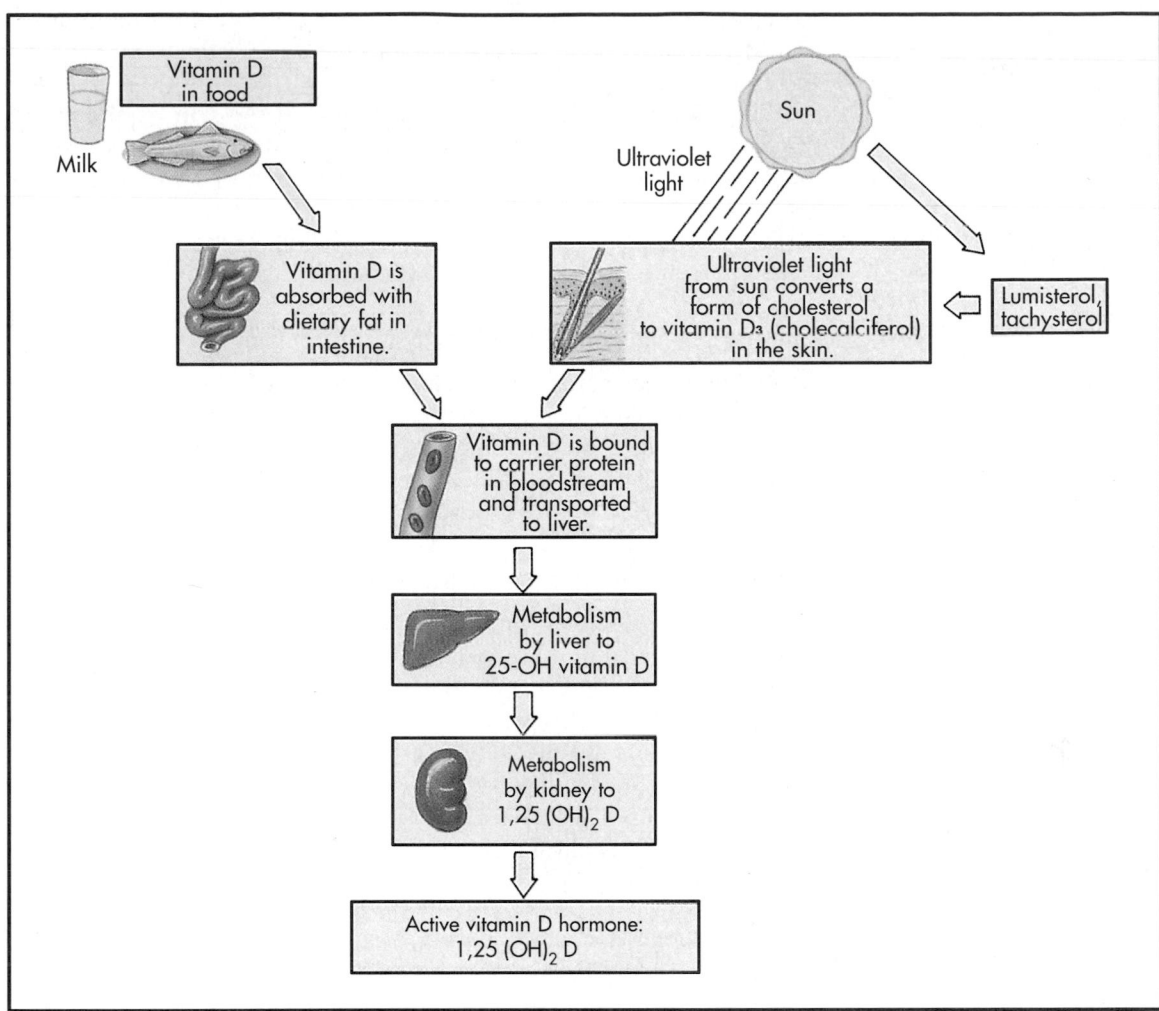

■ **FIGURE 9-7** The many facets of vitamin D metabolism. Whether synthesized in the body or obtained from foods, vitamin D ultimately functions as a hormone. During exposure to sunlight, some of the epidermal reservoir of 7-dehydrocholesterol is converted to previtamin D_3. Lumisterol and tachysterol in the skin can also be converted to previtamin D_3 with the action of sunlight.

recommended. This sun exposure is effective for vitamin D synthesis only if done between about 8 A.M. and 4 P.M. in all areas of the country. It is not effective at all in the winter in northern climates. Some people may be able to use the vitamin D that was stored from summer months in their fat cells, but most people in northern climates should find alternate vitamin D sources in the winter months. Overall, anyone who does not receive enough sunshine to synthesize an adequate amount of vitamin D (the most reliable source) must have a dietary source of the vitamin (Fig. 9-7).

■ Vitamin D Formation in the Skin

Synthesis of vitamin D begins with provitamin D (7-dehydrocholesterol), located in the skin. During exposure to sunlight, one ring on the molecule breaks open creating **previtamin D_3.** Over the next few hours, previtamin D_3 undergoes a transformation aided by body heat to form vitamin D_3. This change allows D_3 to enter the bloodstream; bound to a protein, it is now on its way to becoming a hormone.

In Boston, Massachusetts (42° N), production of previtamin D_3 in the skin is adequate to meet needs from March through October. From November through February, the UV light is too low on the horizon to produce previtamin D_3. In Los

previtamin D_3 The precursor of vitamin D_3, formed as a result of sunlight opening a ring on 7-dehydrocholesterol in the skin.

The solar radiation that causes wrinkles in the skin and skin cancer is the same radiation that produces vitamin D₃. Sunscreens that protect the skin can diminish or completely prevent vitamin D₃ production. Children and adolescents are not particularly careful about applying sunscreens before going outdoors, so their production of vitamin D in the skin is equal to taking 50 to 125 µg (10,000 to 25,000 IU) of vitamin D by mouth. Older people are much more likely to apply sunscreens prior to sun exposure. The amount of 25-OH-D—the precurrsor form of the vitamin D hormone in the bloodstream—is substantially lower in this population group, indicating the possibility of vitamin D deficiency. Because aging decreases the ability to produce D and older people are likely to use sunscreens, low blood levels of 25-OH-D should be investigated by a physician.[8]

Angeles (34° N), production of previtamin D₃ occurs throughout the year. Prolonged exposure doesn't increase the production of vitamin D₃ beyond needs, since any excess is rapidly degraded.

Aging decreases production of vitamin D in the skin by about 75% when one reaches the age of 70.[7] Older people are advised to get sun exposure during early morning and late afternoon to receive the benefit of vitamin D synthesis without also increasing skin cancer risk.

The more pigment in the skin, the less vitamin D₃ is made. Melanin acts as a natural sunscreen.

■ Absorption and Formation of Vitamin D from Food

Following the consumption of vitamin D-containing foods, about 80% of vitamin D is incorporated into micelles in the small intestine and then absorbed and transported to the liver by chylomicrons through the lymphatic system. Patients with chronic fat-malabsorption syndromes (e.g., cystic fibrosis, Crohn's disease, and celiac disease) have trouble absorbing vitamin D and may develop a deficiency.

■ Metabolism, Transport, and Storage of Vitamin D

When vitamin D (either synthesized in the skin or consumed from food or supplements) enters general circulation, it is bound to a protein. The formation of the hormone form of vitamin D from its precursor occurs in the liver and kidneys. In the liver, the vitamin is hydroxylated on carbon 25, converting it to 25-OH-D. This inactive form circulates in the blood for weeks. The next stop is the kidney, the principal site for the production $1,25(OH)_2D$, also known as calcitriol or the hormone form of the vitamin, and is active for about 1 day. Patients with chronic kidney failure have very low concentrations of circulating $1,25(OH)_2D$. They are routinely treated with $1,25(OH)_2D$. Thus, the kidney is the organ in which activation of vitamin D occurs.

Once vitamin D enters general circulation, it can be stored in fat tissues for later use or converted to 25-OH-D in the liver. When there is a shortage of calcium in the blood, the parathyroid glands increase production of parathyroid hormone (PTH). Parathyroid hormone then increases the production of $1,25(OH)_2D$ in the kidney. Eventual excretion of vitamin D takes place mostly via the bile, with small amounts leaving via the urine.

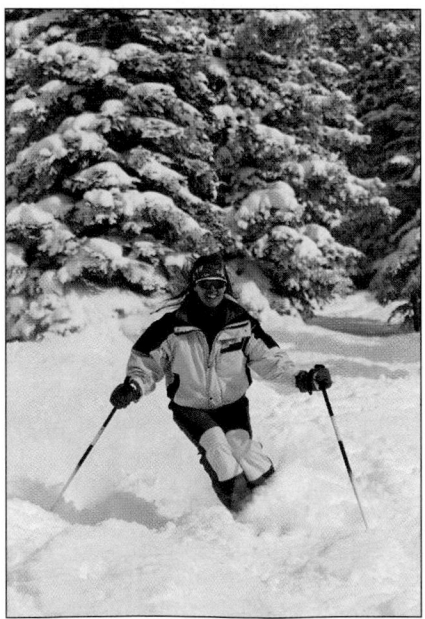

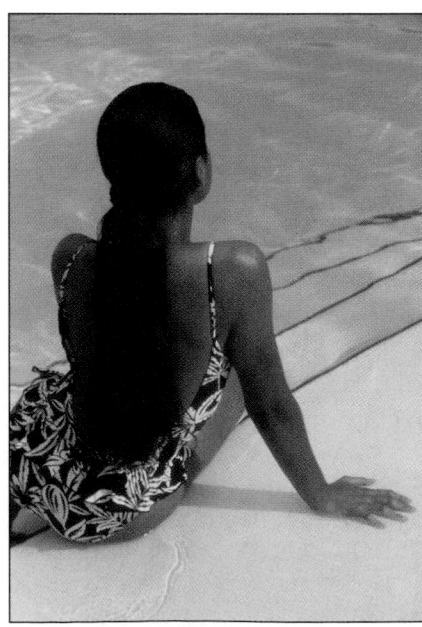

Who is making more vitamin D? Why?

■ Functions of Vitamin D

The principal function of vitamin D is to maintain serum calcium and phosphorus concentration within the range that supports neuromuscular function, bone calcification, and other cellular processes. By helping maintain the blood calcium concentration within the normal range, $1,25(OH)_2D$ plays another vital role: maintaining the function of **neuromuscular junction** (see Chapter 11 for more details). The function of $1,25(OH)_2D$ is fundamentally to control the production and action of several calcium-binding proteins in the small intestine. One protein in particular is activated by $1,25(OH)_2D$ and is responsible for the rate of flow of calcium across the intestinal mucosa. Another function of $1,25(OH)_2D$ is to increase the absorption of phosphorus.

> **neuromuscular junction** A chemical synapse between a motor neuron and a muscle fiber.

The $1,25(OH)_2D$ reacts with a specific receptor in target tissue. (This receptor belongs to the family of putative steroid hormone zinc-finger receptors.) The receptor binds $1,25(OH)_2D$ to a vitamin D receptor and the retinoic acid receptor, RXR (described earlier) to form a complex. This then interacts with specific DNA sequences known as vitamin D-responsive elements. By binding to these vitamin D-responsive elements, $1,25(OH)_2D$ complex either enhances or inhibits the transcription of vitamin D-responsive genes. If the hormone-specific gene is turned on, it can produce the related mRNA transcripts, which are then translated into several different proteins, including the calcium-binding protein.

Following is a summary of vitamin D's biological functions (Fig. 9-8):[22]

- Vitamin D maintains serum calcium levels by mobilizing calcium and phosphorus from bone stores during a time of calcium shortage.
- $1,25(OH)_2D$ induces **stem cell** monocytes to become mature osteoclasts. Osteoclasts are bone-degrading cells, which release calcium into the blood.
- Vitamin D is not needed for bone calcification but is responsible for maintaining extracellular calcium and phosphorus concentrations in a supersaturated state,

> **stem cell** An undifferentiated cell that divides continuously and forms a supply of cells for differentiation into functionally specific cells.

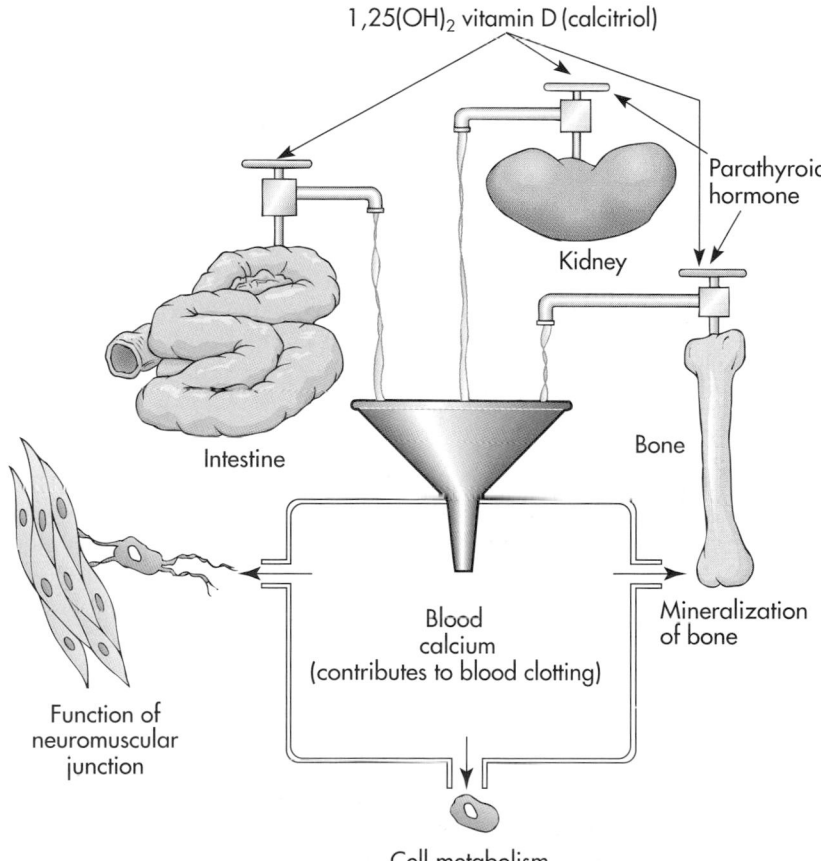

1,25(OH)$_2$ vitamin D (calcitriol)

Parathyroid hormone

Kidney

Intestine

Bone

Function of neuromuscular junction

Blood calcium (contributes to blood clotting)

Mineralization of bone

Cell metabolism

▌ FIGURE **9-8** The active vitamin D hormone—$1,25(OH_2)D$ (calcitriol)—and parathyroid hormone interact to control blood calcium concentration. Normal amounts of calcium in the blood are needed to support bone health, nerve function, muscle action, and other functions. Low blood calcium is a trigger for many hormonal responses. Parathyroid hormone and $1,25(OH_2)D$ mobilize calcium from the bone. The kidney's involvement in calcium reabsorption is in question. $1,25(OH_2)D$ by itself stimulates intestinal calcium absorption. All these responses raise blood calcium. Conversely, when calcium in the blood becomes too high, the hormone calcitonin responds by promoting calcium deposition in the bone (not shown).

The best way to assess a person's vitamin D status is to determine the concentration of 25-OH-D in the blood.

which results in the mineralization of bone. The cells that actually form bone are called osteoblasts.

- Human epidermal cells have nuclear receptors for $1,25(OH)_2D$, so it effects the proliferation and differentiation of skin cells. At present, there are 20 different cell types in the human body that are sensitive to $1,25(OH)_2D$.

Vitamin D is also capable of influencing differentiation in some cancer cells, such as skin, bone, and breast cancer cells. Indeed, adequate vitamin D status has been linked to a reduced risk of developing breast, colon, and prostate cancer. Studies are not yet conclusive, though, and are mainly supported by in vitro experiments.

■ Rickets and Osteomalacia

Without adequate calcium and phosphorus in the blood available for deposition in the bone, the skeleton fails to mineralize properly and bones weaken and bow under pressure.[20] When these effects occur in a child, the disease is called rickets (Fig. 9-9). Signs of rickets include enlarged head, joints, and rib cage; a deformed pelvis; and bowed legs. In the United States today, rickets is most commonly associated with fat malabsorption, such as is seen in children with cystic fibrosis.

Rickets in adults is called osteomalacia, which means "soft bones." It can cause fractures in the hip, spine, and other bones. (Do not confuse this with the disease osteoporosis, which will be discussed in Chapter 11.) Osteomalacia is most likely to occur in people with kidney, stomach, gallbladder, or intestinal disease (especially when most of the intestine has been removed) and in those with cirrhosis of the liver. These diseases affect both vitamin D metabolism and calcium absorption. Combinations of sun exposure and treatment with vitamin D or $1,25(OH)_2D$ can be used to treat osteomalacia.

■ Dietary Sources of Vitamin D

Because some people may not receive enough sun exposure to generate sufficient active vitamin D for the body's needs, they need to pay attention to dietary sources. Actually, few foods contain appreciable amounts of vitamin D.

The most nutrient-dense sources of vitamin D (μg/kcal) are fatty fish (e.g., sardines and salmon), fortified milk, and some fortified breakfast cereals. In the United States, milk is fortified with 10 μg (400 IU) per quart. Although eggs, butter, liver, and a few brands of margarine contain some vitamin D, large servings must be eaten to obtain an appreciable amount of the vitamin; thus, these foods are not considered significant sources.

Foods of animal origin contain vitamin D_3, whereas plants contain a slightly different provitamin D—called ergosterol, or vitamin D_2. Metabolism of vitamin D_2 in the body yields 1,25-dihydroxy ergocalciferol. This compound has vitamin D activity in humans. The usual form of vitamin D in supplements is D_2.[27]

■ Vitamin D Needs

The Food and Nutrition Board has set an Adequate Intake for vitamin D (see Chapter 2 for details about Adequate Intakes and how these standards differ from RDAs). The Adequate Intake for vitamin D is 5 μg/day (200 IU/day) for people under age 51 and increases to 10 μg/day (400 IU/day) for people between 51 and 70 and 15 μg/day (600 IU/day) for older Americans. Young, light-skinned people can produce enough vitamin D from casual sun exposure on just the face and hands. The marker used to determine the Adequate Intake for young adults is the concentration of 25-OH-D in the blood, the precursor to the active form of the vitamin. For older persons indicies of bone maintenance are also used.

Infants are born with a sufficient supply of vitamin D to last about 9 months. At or before that time, a breastfed infant should be regularly exposed to some sunlight or treated with a supplement under a physician's guidance. Pasteurized milk is usually fortified with vitamin D, as are infant formulas.

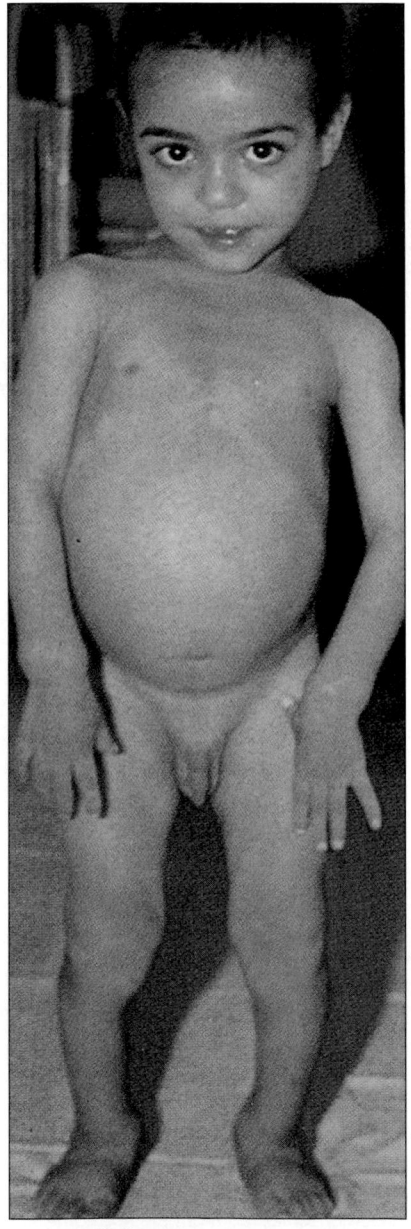

■ FIGURE 9-9 The bowed legs of rickets, a vitamin D-deficiency disease.

North Americans at Risk of Vitamin D Deficiency

Studies suggest older people and anyone else who stays indoors most of the day and ingests little or no vitamin D are at risk for developing a vitamin D deficiency. This is a particularly important concern for older people who live in northern climates or reside in nursing homes. Not only do these people experience little sun exposure, they also can have defective $1,25(OH)_2D$ production from kidney resistance, which decreases conversion to the active form of the hormone. For this reason, it is thought that up to 40% of such patients who are admitted to hospitals with hip fracture may be deficient in vitamin D.[9]

One epidemiological survey of older nursing home residents (free living and hospitalized) who took supplements containing vitamin D or drank two to three glasses of vitamin D-fortified milk per day showed that 80% were still borderline deficient at the end of winter. Thus, it is suggested that the older persons obtain sunlight exposure during spring, summer, and autumn to provide vitamin D for storage in fat tissue for use during winter months.[9] Providing 1250 μg (50,000 IU) once a month is another strategy.

Vitamin D Resistance

Some humans show resistance to the action of certain vitamins, including vitamin D. Resistance to vitamin D can be caused either by a lack of $1,25(OH)_2D$ synthesis in the kidney or by an inability of $1,25(OH)_2D$ to bind to nuclear receptors throughout the body. In both cases, the treatment is a large dose of $1,25(OH)_2D$. This treatment works well in the first case but is not as successful in the second.

Vitamin D Supplements

If a person has a low circulating concentration of 25-OH-D, he or she should take 20 μg (800 IU) of vitamin D each day until the concentration reaches the midnormal range. People who are likely to fall into this category are older people, especially those with osteoporosis, and patients with malabsorption syndromes, liver failure, and kidney disease or failure. After concentrations are normal, 10 μg (400 IU/day) from a multivitamin/mineral supplement should be sufficient. Some sun exposure would also be helpful.

■ Pharmacologic Use of Vitamin D

Normal keratinocytes (skin-producing cells) require 28 to 44 days to move from the basal cell layer of the skin to the surface of the epidermis. Among patients with psoriasis, the movement takes only 4 days. This results in a scaly and embarrassing dermatitis. Today, vitamin D analogs applied to the skin are used as a safe, effective treatment of hyperproliferation epidermal disorders, such as psoriasis.

■ Vitamin D Toxicity

Vitamin D can be a very toxic substance. If consumed regularly, an intake of just 5 times the Adequate Intake can be dangerous, especially during infancy. Adults would likely have to consume 10 times the Adequate Intake for 6 months to a year to experience toxicity. Furthermore, toxicity occurs from excess supplementation, not from sun exposure or milk consumption. Anyone contemplating or using supplements of vitamin D should consider a dosage no higher than 10 to 20 μg/day (400 to 800 IU/day). The Upper Level set for vitamin D is 50 μg/day (2,000 IU/day), based on development of an excess concentration of calcium in the blood. This can lead to eventual calcium deposits in the kidneys, heart, and blood vessels. In addition, excess vitamin D can have effects similar to those of too little vitamin D by causing too much calcium to move from the bones to the blood and then to the urine for excretion. This excess can also be toxic to the liver. Other symptoms of hypercalcemia also occur. Severe vitamin D toxicity in infants causes mental retardation, narrowing of pulmonary arteries and the aorta, and changes in facial characteristics. Calcium deposits in organs cause local cell death. Additional effects then result as a

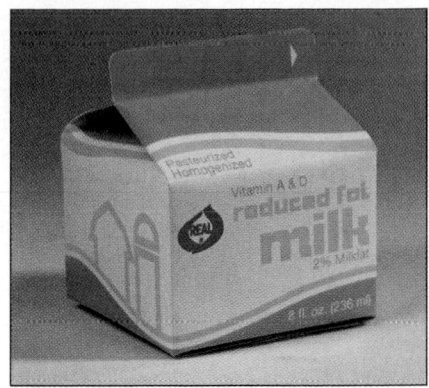

Milk is usually fortified with vitamin D, as well as vitamin A.

*D*ietary Sources of Vitamin D

Food Item and Amount	Vitamin D (IU)	Vitamin D (μg)
Baked herring, 3 oz	1775	44.00
Smoked eel, 1 oz	1021	26.00
Baked salmon, 3 oz	238	6.00
Canned tuna, 3 oz	136	3.50
Skim milk, 8 oz	98	2.50
Sardines, 1 oz	77	2.00
Raisin bran cereal, ¾ cup	42	1.00
Pork sausage, 1 oz	31	0.75
Egg yolk, 1	25	0.66

*I*n areas of the world where a strict Muslim dress code is enforced and foods are not fortified with vitamin D, women experience high blood concentrations of parathyroid hormone (PTH), along with low concentrations of vitamin D. These are the symptoms of osteomalacia. An additional group that is at risk for deficiency of vitamin D is breastfed infants of mothers who have had multiple births.

large number of cells die. Vitamin D can be a very toxic substance if consumed at amounts above 250 µg/day (10,000 IU/day). That is over 16 o 50 times the Adequate Intake set for adults of various ages. It is especially toxic to infants.

CONCEPT CHECK

itamin D is a vitamin only for people who fail to produce enough from exposure to sunlight. Most people can synthesize adequate vitamin D by the action of sunlight on the skin. Older people and breastfed infants are at risk of a vitamin D deficiency. Vitamin D_3 is later activated by the liver and kidneys to form the active hormone $1,25(OH)_2D$. This hormone increases calcium absorption in the intestine and works with other hormones to maintain proper blood calcium concentrations and calcium metabolism in bones and other organs in the body. The hormone $1,25(OH)_2D$ is also an important regulator of cell differentiation in many tissues of the body. Fish oils and fortified milk are significant food sources of vitamin D. An excess of vitamin D is quite toxic, especially during infancy; continuous intakes greater than 50 µg/day should be consumed only with a physician's guidance. Sun exposure poses no risk of vitamin D toxicity.

■ VITAMIN E

Health-food literature attests to many benefits of vitamin E, including prevention of arthritis, cataracts, stroke, diabetes, cancer, and heart disease; increased immune function; delayed symptoms of Alzheimer's disease; relief of asthma; and protection of the skin from pollution. Though only some of these benefits are actually supported by reliable scientific investigations, Americans are spending more than $300 million on vitamin E supplements each year. The following section attempts to sort out fact from fiction in the debate over this high-profile vitamin.

A vitamin E deficiency in laboratory animals can result in muscular dystrophy, inability to produce viable offspring, and impotence. The link between vitamin E deficiency and inability to reproduce in rats, first noted in 1922, gave vitamin E its chemical name tocopherol (*toco* means "related to childbirth"). Although vitamin E is able to cure at least one human medical problem (excessive breakdown of red blood cell membranes), there is no scientific evidence that links a deficiency in this vitamin with muscular dystrophy, infertility, or impotence, notwithstanding what some health-food literature claims.

What we call vitamin E is actually a family of eight naturally occurring compounds—four **tocopherols** (alpha, beta, gamma, delta) and four **tocotrienols** (alpha, beta, gamma, delta)—with widely varying degrees of biological activity. The most active form of the vitamin is the RRR isomer of alpha-tocopherol. This is the form found in nature, and in varying amounts in many vitamin supplements. However, recent research shows that other forms, such as gama-tocopherol, may also be important to the body.[4] Dr. Taber discusses the activity of various isomers of vitamin E in her Expert Opinion.

■ Absorption, Transport, Storage, and Excretion of Vitamin E

The degree of absorption of vitamin E depends on the total absorption of dietary fat. Like the other fat-soluble nutrients, vitamin E must be incorporated into micelles within the lumen of the small intestine, which in turn is dependent on bile and pancreatic enzymes. Once taken up by the enterocytes, vitamin E is incorporated into chylomicrons for transport by the lymph to tissues and the liver. The precise degree of absorption is not known.

The chylomicron remnants release the vitamin E to the liver, which can then deliver the vitamin to VLDL, LDL, and HDL. Vitamin E can be stored in the liver and

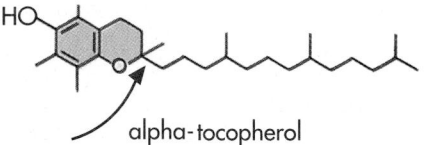
alpha-tocopherol
Site of recognition for alpha-tocopherol transfer protein

Vitamin E. The carbon chain attached to the ringed structure is called the phytal tail.

tocopherols A group of four structurally similar compounds that have vitamin E activity. The "d" isomer of alpha-tocopherol is the most active form.

tocotrienols A group of four compounds with the same basic chemical structure as the tocopherols but containing slightly altered side chains. They exhibit much less vitamin E activity than the corresponding tocopherols.

in adipose tissues and skeletal muscle. Eventually, vitamin E positions itself in cell membranes, where is it associated with phospholipids.

Excretion of vitamin E is via the urine and bile. Because of the limited absorption of vitamin E from the intestinal tract, there is a significant amount in the feces.

■ Functions of Vitamin E

Most, if not all, functions of vitamin E are related to its role as an antioxidant. It functions as a chain-breaking antioxidant that prevents the propagation of **free radicals.**[21] The vitamin acts as a **peroxyl radical** scavenger and protects polyunsaturated fatty acids within cell membrane phospholipids and in plasma lipoproteins from oxidative damage. The fatty acid tail of vitamin E can insert itself into the lipid-like interior of the cell membrane, mitochondrial membrane, and other cellular membranes (Fig. 9-10). An antioxidant protects other substances from oxidation by being oxidized itself. Antioxidants are more properly termed **redox agents.** By donating electrons to electron-seeking compounds, called **oxidizing agents,** antioxidants protect other molecules or parts of a cell from attack. As an example, the peroxyl radical designated ROO• reacts with vitamin E as vitamin E-OH, yielding ROOH and vitamin E-O•.

$$ROO^\bullet + \text{vitamin E-OH} \rightarrow ROOH + \text{vitamin E-O}^\bullet$$

The vitamin E radical, vitamin E-O• can be changed—reduced in the chemical sense—by other antioxidants, or react with other vitamin E radicals to form nonreactive, harmless products. Or it could become a prooxidant, albeit not a very reactive one, and oxidize other lipids.[4]

If vitamin E is not available to do its job, an electron-seeking compound can pull electrons from cell membranes, from DNA, and other electron-dense cell components, which alters the cell's DNA and could cause the cell to die. Cell membranes that are subject to high risk of oxidation are found in the lungs, brain, and red blood cells because they are exposed to high levels of oxygen. People subject to components of air pollution (ozone) and smokers experience a lot of oxidative damage in

free radical The short-lived form of a compound that has an unpaired electron, causing it to seek an electron from another compound. Free radicals are strong oxidizing agents and can be very destructive to electron-dense cell components, such as the DNA and cell membranes.

peroxyl radical A compound containing −O−O− are peroxides. The radical has one unpaired electron, designated ROO•.

redox agents Chemicals that can readily undergo both oxidation (loss of an electron) and reduction (gain of an electron).

oxidizing agent In one sense, a substance capable of capturing an electron from another compound. A compound is oxidized when it loses an electron.

A dietary antioxidant is defined as a substance in food that significantly decreases the adverse effect of reactive species, such as reactive oxygen and reactive nitrogen, on normal physiological functions in humans.

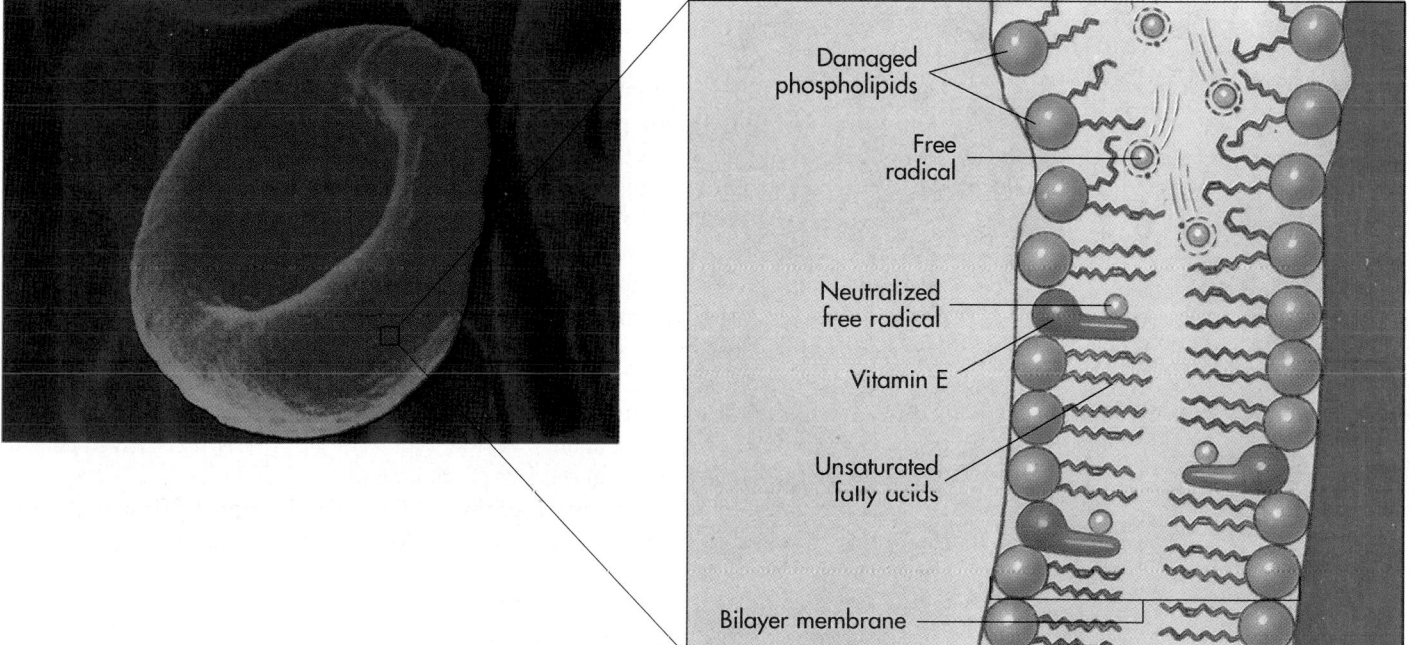

Damaged phospholipids

Free radical

Neutralized free radical

Vitamin E

Unsaturated fatty acids

Bilayer membrane

■ **FIGURE 9-10** Vitamin E protects unsaturated fatty acid components of cell membranes from free-radical attack by itself becoming oxidized. If not interrupted, these free-radical chain reactions cause extensive oxidative damage to cells and premature cell death.

*O*xidizing agents that cells encounter include highly reactive oxygen species such as singlet oxygen ($^1O_2$), hydrogen peroxide (H_2O_2), hydroxyl radical ($^•OH$), superoxide ($O_2^{•-}$), ozone (O_3) and nitrogen-oxygen combinations that are typical of air pollutants ($NO^•$).

*L*ipid peroxidation of polyunsaturated fatty acids (oxidation) causes fats and oils to become rancid (spoiled), and it also damages cell membranes.

lipid peroxidation A process initiated by an environmental component that induces the formation of an organic free radical, $R^•$.

glutathione peroxidase A selenium-containing enzyme that can destroy peroxides. It acts in conjunction with vitamin E to reduce free radical damage to cells.

superoxide dismutase Enzymes containing manganese, copper, or zinc that destroy superoxide.

*O*ne way to assess the vitamin E status of a person is to incubate a sample of his or her red blood cells with peroxide for 3 hours and then measure the extent of red blood cell destruction. A newer method uses the same procedure but measures the amount of a breakdown product of polyunsaturated fatty acids.[11] These tests can be used in addition to measuring vitamin E in the blood.

the lungs, but smokers consuming even 160 times the adult RDA of vitamin E still show lower vitamin E concentration in lung tissue. Thus, the safest way to protect the lungs from significant oxidative damage is not to smoke.

As part of the immune system's arsenal against invading pathogens, white blood cells (leukocytes) generate free radicals to destroy the agents that cause infections. Overall, exposure to oxidizing agents is part of life, and for the most part essential, but the body must be able to regulate this exposure and avoid the undesirable effects, a task assigned to antioxidants.

Stopping Free Radical Chain Reactions

The group of electron-seeking compounds found in cells, free radicals, are highly reactive molecules containing an unpaired electron. Many free radicals are derived from oxygen and are generated in the cell by the cleavage of covalent chemical bonds, with each breakdown product taking an electron from the original pair. This action produces two molecules (or atoms), each having one unpaired electron. Free radicals seek electrons by attacking other compounds—most notably, polyunsaturated fatty acids in the phospholipids that constitute the cell membrane.

Free radicals cause cell damage in part because they can set off a chain reaction where a single free radical can generate thousands in just a few minutes. A flood of free radicals can lead to **lipid peroxidation,** with subsequent destruction of cell membranes. Overall, vitamin E is the body's primary means of interrupting free radical chain reactions. In the following section, other antioxidant systems, and free radical scavengers within cells will be identified, ones that quench free radicals.

Other Antioxidant Systems and Vitamin E

In addition to vitamin E, the body has various other mechanisms for protecting itself from oxidative damage. Earlier you saw that carotenoids, like vitamin E, likely have antioxidant capability in humans. The body also contains numerous enzymes that convert reactive oxidizing agents to less reactive compounds. These enzymes include **glutathione peroxidase, superoxide dismutase,** and catalase.

Glutathione peroxidase catalyzes the breakdown of peroxidized fatty acids, converting them to less harmful substances. Peroxidized fatty acids, and peroxides in general, tend to form free radicals. As the amounts of these in a cell decrease, the rate of formation of free radicals in the cell likewise decreases. Consequently the need for vitamin E decreases because fewer free radicals will be formed. Glutathione peroxidase thus aids vitamin E in reducing oxidative damage to cells (Fig. 9-11). The activity of glutathione peroxidase depends on the mineral selenium, the functional part of this enzyme. An adequate dietary intake of selenium reduces the need for vitamin E, whereas an inadequate intake of selenium increases the need.

The enzymes superoxide dismutase and catalase react directly with reactive oxygen species or peroxides to reduce their reactivity and thereby help protect cells from oxidative damage. Various forms of superoxide dismutase contain zinc, copper, and manganese. Still other systems and substances present in the body, such as bilirubin, interfere with oxidizing processes. In addition, certain cellular proteins and blood proteins are able to bind metals, such as iron and copper, preventing the metals from catalyzing free radical production. Thus, cells do not rely exclusively on vitamin E for protection from oxidizing agents (review Fig. 9-11). Systems also exist in cells to repair molecules that have been oxidatively damaged, such as DNA.

This discussion raises the question of the relative role of vitamin E in oxidant protection in the body. It is unknown whether taking vitamin E supplements confers any additional protection against cardiovascular disease and cancer than that achieved by improving one's diet, performing regular physical activity, not smoking, and controlling body weight. In fact, a 4.5-year study of patients at high risk for cardiovascular disease showed no positive effect of vitamin E supplementation.[28] This finding is in agreement with three other such studies of high risk patients (and one in healthy people), but conflicts with one from Great Britain which showed a positive effect.[4, 10] Other experts suggested that maybe longer trials are needed to

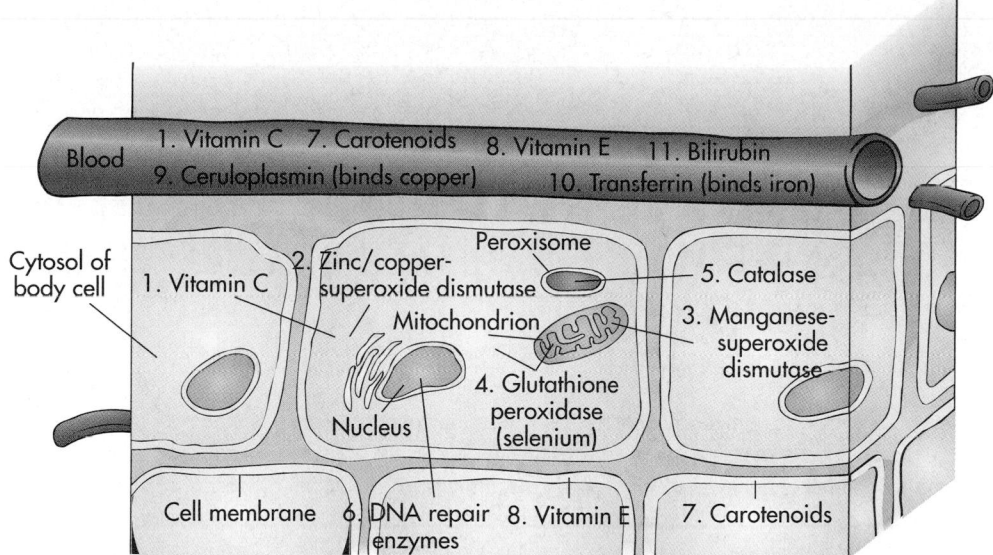

■ FIGURE **9-11** Numerous antioxidant systems and compounds are at work in a cell at any one time. These provide protection against free radicals and other destructive compounds. The variety of defense mechanisms are able to function because of vitamins and minerals obtained from the diet.

1. Vitamin C present in the blood and cytosol of the cell may act as an antioxidant, in part, to regenerate some of the oxidized vitamin E to its active form.

2. Zinc/copper superoxide dismutase in the mitochondrion metabolizes superoxide to oxygen and water.

    $$2O_2^{\bullet-} + 2H^+ \rightarrow O_2 + H_2O$$

3. Manganese superoxide dismutase found in mitochondrion and cytosol performs the same reaction as the zinc/copper dismutase.

    $$2O_2^{\bullet-} + 2H^+ \rightarrow O_2 + H_2O$$

4. Glutahione peroxidase (contains the trace mineral selenium) in mitochondrion metabolizes peroxides to water.

    $$H_2O_2 + 2GSH \quad \rightarrow \quad GSSG + 2H_2O$$
    reduced glutathione   oxidized glutathione

5. Catalase found in peroxismones metabolizes peroxides to water and oxygen.

    $$2H_2O_2 \rightarrow 2H_2O + O_2$$

6. DNA repair enzymes reverse effects of oxidative damage on DNA.

7. Carotenoids in blood and cell membranes likely reduce activity of certain reactive oxygen species (ROS), such as singlet oxygen.

8. Vitamin E in cell membranes, including red blood cells, protects polyunsaturated fatty acids in phospholipids from free radical damage.

9. Ceruloplasmin in blood binds copper, so that it won't generate free radicals.

10. Transferrin in blood binds iron, an important prooxidant, so it can't produce reactive oxygen species.

11. Bilirubin acts as an antioxidant in the blood.

determine if vitamin E is useful in reducing cardiovascular disease risk.[11] As recently as October, 2000, The American Heart Association has stated that it is premature to recommend vitamin E supplements to the general populations, based on current knowledge (see Chapter 6). This conclusion is in agreement with latest report on vitamin E by the Food and Nutrition Board.[4]

Other Roles for Vitamin E

Vitamin E helps protect the carbon-carbon double bonds in dietary saturated fatty acids and other lipid-soluble nutrients, such as vitamin A. In addition, vitamin E is needed for iron metabolism in the cell and for the maintenance of nervous tissues and immune function.

A large number of studies have been carried out in the past decade that directly or indirectly address the relationship between vitamin E intake and chronic diseases.

*B*ecause vitamin E is only one of a group of antioxidants, it is likely that a combination of antioxidants is more effective than vitamin E alone. You can diversify your antioxidant intake by planning a diet with variety. For example, a salad can be improved by the addition of red or green peppers for vitamin C and carotenoids, and sunflower seeds and plant oils for vitamin E.

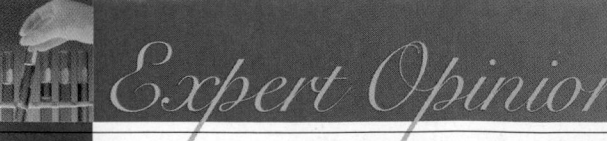

VITAMIN E: AN EXCEPTION TO THE RULE THAT SYNTHETIC AND NATURAL FORMS OF VITAMINS ARE IDENTICAL

Maret G. Traber, Ph.D.

Over 50 years ago, the first reports were published, demonstrating that natural alpha-tocopherol is more potent than synthetic alpha-tocopherol. This phenomenon was reflected in the definition of the IU (international unit), which is still displayed on the label of products containing vitamin E. The IU definition is based on a rat assay. A female, vitamin E–deficient rat is made pregnant, and the amount of vitamin E required to allow her to carry her fetuses for the full duration of the pregnancy is measured. This test is based on the observations published in the 1930s by Evans, the discoverer of vitamin E. Evans showed that vitamin E is required for successful pregnancy in rats, in order to prevent fetuses from being resorbed—hence the test name "fetal resorption assay."

It was recognized early in vitamin E history that various compounds with vitamin E antioxidant activities have very different abilities to maintain rat pregnancies. The most potent form of vitamin E in the fetal resorption assay was alpha-tocopherol; other forms, such as gamma tocopherol and the tocotrienols, were much less effective. As part of the ongoing DRI revisions, The Institute of Medicine, National Academy of Science, has recently proposed that the definition of vitamin E activity be revised based only on studies carried out in humans.

Commercially available vitamin E usually contains alpha-tocopherol that is derived by one of two different processes. Preparations labeled "dl" contain alpha-tocopherol that is entirely chemically synthesized, whereas preparations labeled "d" contain tocopherols isolated from vegetable oil and chemically converted to alpha-tocopherol. These latter preparations are labeled "natural" or "natural source." For purposes of commerce, the IU was defined as 1 mg of dl alpha-tocopheryl acetate or 0.74 mg of d alpha-tocopheryl acetate.

Since "d" and "dl" alpha-tocopherols are prepared differently, they are labeled differently. But they also have different potencies because of differences in chemical structures. The prefixes "d" and "dl" even indicate a misconception about the structure—"d" implies the compound rotates light only to the right, whereas "dl" suggests that the mixture contains equal proportions of compounds that rotate light either to the left or to the right. However, it is now known that alpha-tocopherol has three *chiral centers* (carbons to which are attached four different chemical groups; see Appendix B for a discussion of chiral centers and related terms.) Each center can be right or left and is labeled "*R*" or "*S*" ("d" and "l" can be used only if there is one chiral center). Therefore, the chemically synthesized dl alpha-tocopherol contains eight stereoisomers ($2 \times 2 \times 2$ equals 8). In contrast, the naturally occurring alpha-tocopherol contains only one stereoisomer. The correct terminology for the d alpha-tocopherol is *RRR*-alpha-tocopherol, whereas dl is a mixture of all the possible isomers (called a *racemic* [abbreviated *rac*] mixture). Thus, *all rac*-alpha-tocopherol contains a mixture of equal amounts of *RRR, RSR, RRS, RSS, SSS, SRS, SSR,* and *SRR*-alpha tocopherols.

Numerous scientific studies of the biological basis of the differences between

Vitamin E from supplements has been shown to inhibit LDL oxidation, both in vitro and in vivo. Vitamin E inhibits protein kinase C activity, which in turn is involved in cell proliferation and cell differentiation in smooth muscle cells, platelets, and monocytes. Vitamin E decreases the adhesion of blood cell components to the endothelial cells that line blood vessels. Vitamin E enhances the release of prostacyclin (PGI_2), a potent vasodilator and inhibitor of platelet aggregation in humans. (Vasodilation is enlargement of blood vessels. Platelet aggregation is the clumping of platelets so that the blood forms clots.)[4] And vitamin E may influence the inflammatory responses of certain immune cells.[26] Check out Table 9-3 for a summary of vitamin E functions: real, suspected, or not supported by current research. But remember, a specific role for vitamin E in a required metabolic reaction is yet to be found. As of now, it is just a nonspecific chain-breaking antioxidant.

"d" and "dl" alpha-tocopherols have been carried out in humans. In these, it was apparent that the differences in chemical structures between the forms are important for establishing potencies. When *RRR* and *all rac*-alpha tocopherols were administered to humans in a 1 to 1 ratio, both *RRR*- and *all rac*-alpha-tocopherols were absorbed, but only half the *all rac*-alpha-tocopherols were maintained in the blood. In contrast, not only was the *RRR* form maintained in the blood but also it was maintained in the tissues at double the concentration of the *all rac*-alpha-tocopherol.

This preference is a result of a liver protein, the alpha-tocopherol transfer protein, which selectively regulates alpha-tocopherol concentrations in the bloodstream. The alpha-tocopherol transfer protein is essential for this function; humans with a genetic defect in the protein become vitamin E deficient. The protein recognizes the state of only one of the three chiral centers in alpha-tocopherol—namely, the first site on the phytal tail (see vitamin E structure on page 344). This must be in the R form (called the 2-*R* form). Thus, the four forms *RRR, RSR, RRS,* and *RSS* in *all rac*-alpha-tocopherol provide alpha-tocopherol activity and are important for its alpha-tocopherol potency.

The human vitamin E requirements in the recently published DRIs were defined and limited to alpha-tocopherol because only alpha-tocopherol, of the various chemical compounds having vitamin E antioxidant activity, has been shown to reverse human vitamin E–deficiency symptoms. The RDA, or the amount required daily by humans, was set at 15 mg alpha-tocopherol, based on studies of experimental vitamin E deficiency in humans.

The differences in potency between *RRR*- and *all rac*-alpha-tocopherols were specifically cited in the new human vitamin E requirements. The definition of potency was limited to only the 2-*R* forms of alpha-tocopherol because these are the forms that are maintained in the blood by the alpha-tocopherol transfer protein. Therefore, the present definition for IUs, where "d" is set as only one-third more active than "dl," do not reflect human needs. The new values show that *RRR*- is twice as active as the *all rac*-alpha-tocopherol forms (the "d" forms are therefore twice as active as the "dl" forms).

The Upper Level for vitamin E was also set in the DRI publication. Recall from Chapter 2 that this value is an amount, when consumed daily, that should not cause adverse effects in 99% of the population. Here the absorption of the various forms of vitamin E, rather than their potency, was taken into account. The report emphasizes that all forms of vitamin E are absorbed and therefore may contribute to potential adverse effects. Thus, the Upper Level was set at 1000 mg alpha-tocopherol. Using the old definitions for IUs, 1000 mg alpha-tocopherol is contained in 1500 IU of "d" (*RRR*) or 1100 IU "dl" (*all rac*).

There is currently tremendous interest in vitamin E with regard to its potential health benefits. The new requirement for vitamin E in the DRI publication emphasizes that the data available show that vitamin E is required by humans but that there is insufficient evidence to set amounts that may be beneficial in preventing or ameliorating certain chronic diseases. Further research is required to delineate whether vitamin E supplements are beneficial. For now, we know that the form of vitamin E consumed is an important consideration when evaluating intake and needs.

Dr. Maret G. Traber is an associate professor in the Department of Nutrition and Food Management and an investigator in the Linus Pauling Institute, Oregon State University, Corvallis, OR, 97331-6512. Her research has focused on mechanisms by which vitamin E is absorbed, transported, and delivered to tissues.

■ Dietary Sources of Vitamin E

The most nutrient-dense food source of vitamin E (mg/kcal) are plant oils (e.g., corn, soybean, safflower, sunflower, cottonseed, and wheat germ oil), wheat germ, asparagus, and peanuts. Products made from the plant oils—margarine, shortenings, and salad dressing—are good sources. Finfish and shellfish add vitamin E to the diet. Also, grain meals, such as oatmeal; nuts (e.g., almonds); and seeds (e.g., sunflower seeds) are other good sources (Fig. 9-12). In milling whole grains, most of the vitamin E is lost and not restored. Animal fats have practically no vitamin E. A tablespoon of plant oil consumed daily is effective in meeting one's needs for vitamin E.

An advantage of obtaining vitamin E and other natural antioxidants from food is that this produces a balance of the various antioxidants. There is concern that taking

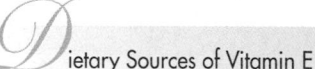

*D*ietary Sources of Vitamin E

Food Item and Amount	Vitamin E (mg)
Sunflower seeds, 1 oz	14.0
Sunflower oil, 1 tbsp	7.0
Almonds, 1 oz	7.0
Safflower oil, 1 tbsp	6.0
Wheat germ, ¼ cup	5.0
Peanut butter, 2 tbsp	3.0
Italian dressing, 2 tbsp	3.0
Avocado, 1	2.7
Mango, 1	2.0
Mayonnaise, 1 tbsp	0.5

TABLE 9-3 Functions and Possible Functions of Vitamin E[4]

In Vivo Function	In Vitro Function or Animal Studies	No benefit, Conflicting Results or Minor Action
Chain-breaking antioxidant that prevents propagation of free radical reactions	Decrease monocyte adhesion to endothelial cells, decrease monocyte superoxide production	Possibly decreases central nervous system disorders: Parkinson's disease* Alzheimer's disease[†] Down syndrome*
Peroxyl radical scavenger; protects poly-unsaturated fatty acids within cell membrane phospholipids and in blood lipoproteins	Inhibits protein kinase C activity, which is involved in cell proliferation and differentiation in smooth muscle cells, platelets, and monocytes	Possibly decreases cardiovascular disease[†]
Exerts inhibition of LDL oxidation	Enhances release of prostacyclin (PGI_2), a potent vasodilator and inhibitor of platelet aggregation in humans	Possibly decreases complications of diabetes[†]
	Inhibits plasma release of thrombin	Possibly enhances immune function in the elderly[†] Possibly reduces risk of prostate cancer[†] Reduces cataracts*

*No benefits
[†]Conflicting results
[‡]Minor action

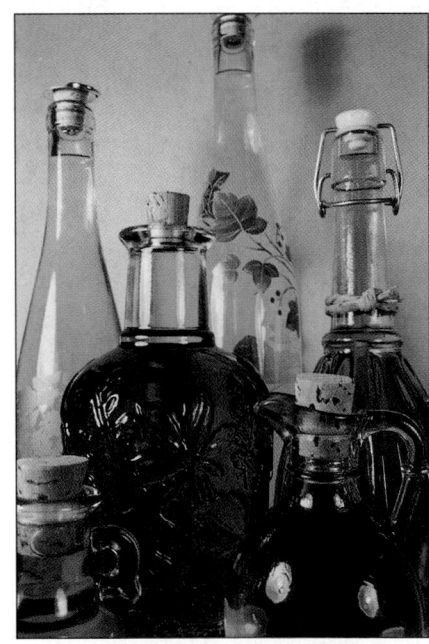

Plant oils are rich sources of vitamin E.

hemolysis The destruction of red blood cells, caused by the breakdown of the red blood cell membrane. This allows the cell contents to leak into the fluid portion (plasma) of the blood.

megadoses of one antioxidant might disrupt the metabolism of other antioxidants. Overall, the entire symphony of antioxidant processes in the body is quite complex. Some scientists warn against tinkering with these processes beyond simply consuming a varied diet. Most of what we know about the benefits of antioxidants has come from studies of people who consume diets rich in fruits and vegetables. That may be why FDA currently only allows claims for fruits and vegetables as part of a low-fat diet in an effort to reduce risks for cancer and cardiovascular disease. No equivalent claim is permitted by FDA for the supplemental use of vitamin E.

The actual vitamin E content of a food depends on harvesting, processing, storage, and cooking because vitamin E is highly susceptible to destruction by oxygen, metals, light, and deep-fat frying. In any case, a varied diet supplies the vitamin E needed for good health. Synthetic antioxidants, such as BHA and BHT, also add to the cellular protection provided by vitamin E. (See Chapter 19 for more on BHA and BHT.)

▪ Vitamin E Needs

The committee assigned by the Food and Nutrition Board to reevaluate the RDA for vitamin E was reluctant to use the most contemporary research data because this came mostly from in vitro studies.[4] Rather, the committee relied on older data from human studies, which showed only one discernible deficiency symptom, **hemolysis** of red blood cells. When there is a shortage of vitamin E, the red blood cell membrane is subject to attack by free radicals, leading to disintegration of the membrane and loss of the cell contents—hemoglobin—into surrounding plasma. Hemolysis of red blood cells was prevented at an intake of 12 mg per day. This amount was used to establish the Estimated Average Requirement. To establish the RDA, the Estimated Average Requirement was increased by 20% to account for individual variability, yielding an RDA of 15 mg for both men and women. This is equivalent to 22 IU of natural source of vitamin E or 33 IU of the synthetic form.

The RDA is set using mg d-alpha-tocopherol. To determine the number of mg of d-alpha-tocopherol from a synthetic source in a multivitamin supplement, convert

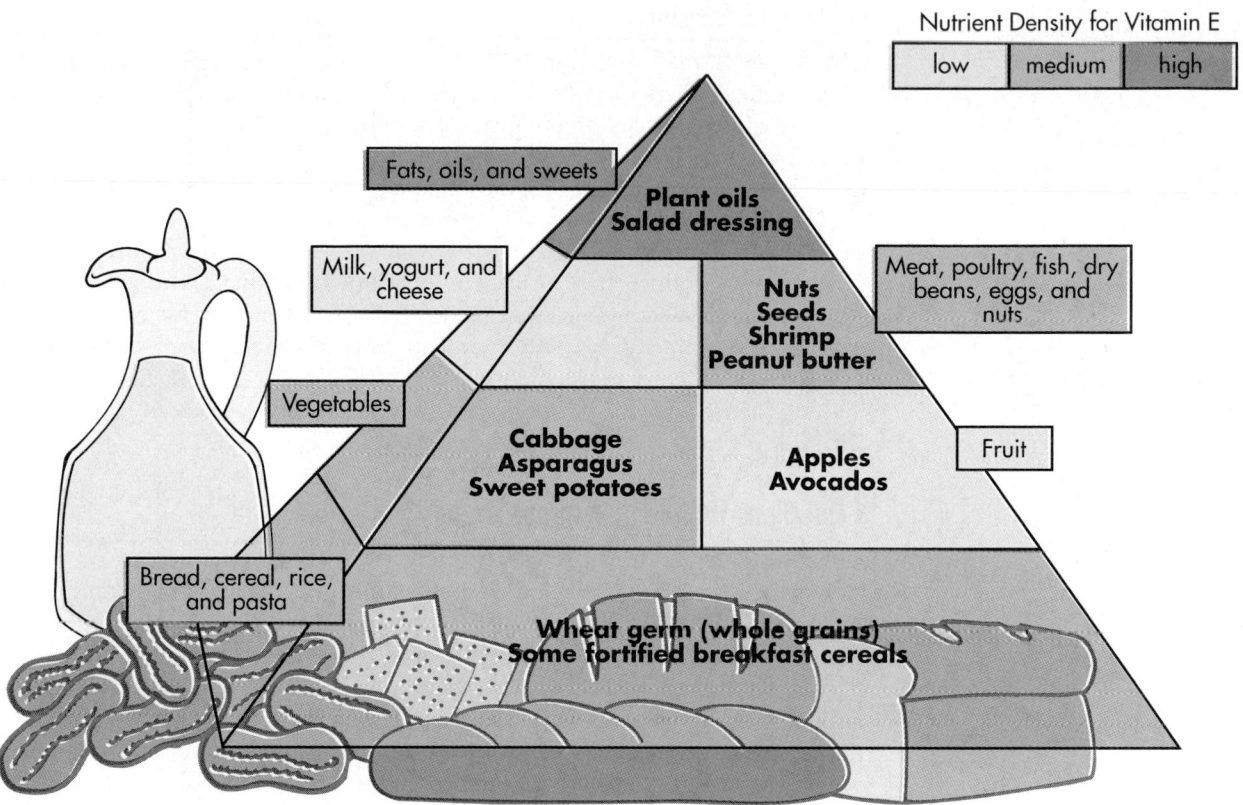

Nutrient Density for Vitamin E

| low | medium | high |

FIGURE 9-12 Food sources of vitamin E from the Food Guide Pyramid. Vitamin E is concentrated in plant oils, nuts, seeds, and some vegetables. The background color of each food group indicates the average nutrient density for vitamin E in that group.

the older IU units by multiplying by 0.45 (400 IU of synthetic [dl] vitamin E provides 180 mg). If the vitamin is derived from natural sources the d-alpha-tocopherol value is the IU multiplied by 0.67. This shows that the natural form has a greater amount of the active vitamin than the synthetic form. Incidentally, the natural form is more expensive and has a shorter shelf life.

Current studies using vitamin E are at the extremes of intake. The highest dose studies are between 400 and 800 IU per day. The lowest dosage amount is 30 mg (45 IU). Experts note that more studies with different-size dose/response levels are needed to fill in the wide gap of information concerning optimal vitamin E intakes.[4]

Medical Problems Associated with Vitamin E Deficiency

The medical condition that may be caused by a deficiency of vitamin E is hemolytic anemia, a disease characterized by the breakdown of red blood cells (hemolysis). Preterm infants are particularly susceptible to the hemolysis of red blood cells, since they are born with limited tissue stores of vitamin E and are inefficient in absorbing vitamin E from the intestinal tract. Second, the rapid growth of preterm infants exhausts what little vitamin E stores exist. To prevent hemolytic anemia, special formulas and supplements for preterm infants are prescribed to prevent vitamin E-related disorders of preterm births.

Maldigestion of lipids, such as found in cystic fibrosis, celiac disease, liver disease, and insufficient bile production, can compromise vitamin E status. Vitamin E deficiency is rare in healthy humans. Deficiency occurs only as a result of a genetic abnormality, or the previously mentioned fat-malabsorption syndromes. The primary vitamin E deficiency symptom is a peripheral neuropathy, characterized by degeneration of sensory neurons.

The latest nutrition surveys show that adults only consume about two-thirds of the RDA for vitamin E. Daily use of nuts, a ready-to-eat breakfast cereal containing extra vitamin E, or a multivitamin and mineral supplement would close this nutrient gap.

■ Vitamin E Toxicity

The Upper Level for vitamin E is based on hemorrhagic effects in adults. It applies to all eight isomers of alpha-tocopherol. For adults ages 19 and older the Upper Level is 1,000 mg/day of any form of supplementary alpha-tocopherol. In international units, the Upper Level is 1500 IU for vitamin E isolated from natural sources and 1100 IU for synthetic vitamin E. The lower IU value for the synthetic form reflects the greater number of isomers present in the synthetic product, some of which do not contribute to vitamin E activity in cells but are still absorbed. This Upper Level also is confined to a healthy population. Individuals who are vitamin K-deficient or who are taking anticoagulants are especially at risk for hemorrhaging from megadose vitamin E use.[4] The Food and Nutrition Board confined their discussion of adverse effects to supplements, food fortification, and pharmacological agents. The synthetic forms of vitamin E are used almost exclusively in supplements, food fortification and pharmacological agents.

■ Questions That Remain About Vitamin E

The RDA for children ages 1 through 18 is extrapolated from the adult RDA. Large-scale studies are needed to assess more specifically their vitamin E requirements. Because calories are frequently underreported in population studies, as is the case with dietary fat, the form of vitamin E and quantity of vitamin E intake are underestimated. What is needed are better methods for estimating intake. Little is known about the intake of vitamin E intake and tissue levels of the vitamin. In addition, do large doses of vitamin E that protect LDL against oxidation also protect tissues against peroxidation or the actions of other reactive oxygen species? This information could help determine the relationship between oxidative stress and vitamin E status.

There is a great deal of circumstantial evidence suggesting that vitamin E confers a variety of health benefits. Clinical trials are needed to determine if vitamin E can reduce the risk or prevent a whole range of chronic diseases. We especially need to determine if amounts greater than that which can be found in a balanced diet outweigh the expense (about 7 cents/day) and possible risk of taking vitamin E supplements. And there is certainly a need for more information about the biological actions of the seven other naturally occurring forms of vitamin E.

CONCEPT CHECK

Enzymes and other body mechanisms scavenge and minimize the formation of free radicals and other oxidative compounds, but they are not 100% effective. Hence, diet-derived antioxidants may be critical in diminishing cumulative oxidative damage and helping us to stay healthy. Vitamin E is one such nutrient that functions primarily as an antioxidant. It can donate electrons to electron-seeking compounds, such as free radicals. By quenching free radicals, vitamin E helps prevent oxidative damage, especially of cell membranes. The best sources of vitamin E are plant oils. When more plant oils are consumed, more vitamin E is needed to protect the double bonds found in plant oils from oxidation. However, the vitamin E content in plant oils is usually high. Because of their poor vitamin E status, preterm infants are particularly susceptible to oxidative breakdown of their red blood cell membranes (hemolysis). Among adults, people who smoke or show long-term fat malabsorption run the biggest risk of vitamin E deficiency. In the former case, the best therapy is to stop smoking. At present, there is insufficient evidence to conclude that taking large amounts of vitamin E in supplement form approaching or exceeding the Upper Level over a long period of time is safe or provides any special health benefits; research is ongoing.

■ VITAMIN K

Vitamin K is essential for blood clotting. A Danish researcher first noted the relationship between vitamin K and blood clotting and named the fat-soluble vitamin "K" after *koagulation*, the Danish spelling for *coagulation*.

The family of compounds known as vitamin K includes **phylloquinone** (vitamin K_1) from plants and the menaquinones (vitamin K_2) found in fish oils and meats. The menaquinones are also synthesized by bacteria in the human intestine.

■ Absorption, Transport, Storage, and Excretion of Vitamin K

It appears that up to 80% of dietary vitamin K as phylloquinone and menaquinone is taken up by **enterocytes** and are incorporated into chylomicrons. The process requires bile and pancreatic juice. The menaquinones synthesized by bacteria in the colon are absorbed, but the amount absorbed is still unknown.[5] Some vitamin K is stored in the liver, some is inactivated, and some is incorporated in VLDL, LDL, and HDL for transport throughout the body. It is found in the spleen and bone. Mineral oil and other non absorbable lipids interfere with vitamin K absorption, so their use close to meals should be discouraged. Most vitamin K excretion occurs via the bile, with a small amount of excretion via the urine.

■ Functions of Vitamin K

Vitamin K contributes to the synthesis of seven blood-clotting factors (Fig. 9-13). These clotting factors are produced in the liver from precursor proteins. Vitamin K is required for the conversion of some precursor proteins to the active clotting factors. In this reaction, carbon dioxide (CO_2) is added to a glutamic acid in the precursor protein, yielding the active factor containing the unique amino acid gamma-carboxyl glutamic acid. One example of this process is the conversion of a precursor protein to **prothrombin,** one of the participants in the blood-clotting cascade. All these vitamin K-dependent proteins depend on calcium interaction with gamma-carboxyl glutamic acid in order to participate in the clotting reaction.[14]

In the body, vitamin K is converted to an inactive form once it has acted. This must be reactivated for its biological action to persist. Drugs such as warfarin, which strongly inhibit this reactivation process, act as powerful anticoagulants. People taking oral anticoagulants, such as warfarin, to lessen blood clotting should not consume vitamin K supplements or foods rich in vitamin K. These reduce the effect of drugs that reduce the recycling of vitamin K, because active vitamin K would be continually available from the diet.

Vitamin K functions as a **cofactor** for the enzyme that catalyzes the conversion of protein-bound glutamate residues to gamma-carboxyglutamate residues and the synthesis of two bone proteins. The first protein is a "Gla" protein, or **osteocalcin,** secreted by the osteoblasts. Recall that osteoblasts are bone-building cells. The second bone protein, called "matrix Gla protein," is found in the organic matrix of bone. Both these proteins depend on vitamin K for the gamma-carboxylation reaction involving glutamic acid. Low concentrations of circulating vitamin K have been associated with low bone mineral density. It may be that inadequate intake of vitamin K increases the risk of hip fracture in women, but more research is needed to support this hypothesis.[3, 5]

A deficiency of vitamin K most likely occurs when a person takes antibiotics or has impaired fat absorption. Antibiotics destroy the bacteria in the intestines that normally account for some of the vitamin K absorbed. Before performing surgery, a surgeon generally establishes, via a blood test, that the patient does not have a vitamin K deficiency, which could lead to excessive bleeding.

The most reliable clinical evidence of vitamin K deficiency is an increase in clotting time, which is a measure of how quickly prothrombin in the blood can form a clot. The actual vitamin K and prothrombin concentration in the blood can also be measured.

Phylloquinone (K_1)

Vitamin K.

phylloquinone A form of vitamin K that comes from plants; also called vitamin K_1.

cofactor An organic or inorganic substance that binds to a specific region on an enzyme and is necessary for the enzyme's activity.

enterocytes Villi are lined with these epithelial cells, which are highly specialized for digestion and absorption.

prothrombin One of the numerous proteins that participate in the formation of blood clots. Conversion of its precursor protein to the active blood-clotting factor in the liver requires vitamin K.

osteocalcin A protein produced in bone that is thought to bind calcium; the synthesis of osteocalcin is aided by vitamin K.

CRITICAL THINKING

Tim was diagnosed as having blood clots in his leg and has been using anticoagulant medications for 2 months. On examination, the doctor is surprised to find that the clots he expected to have dissolved are still there. What is a possible nutritional explanation for this finding?

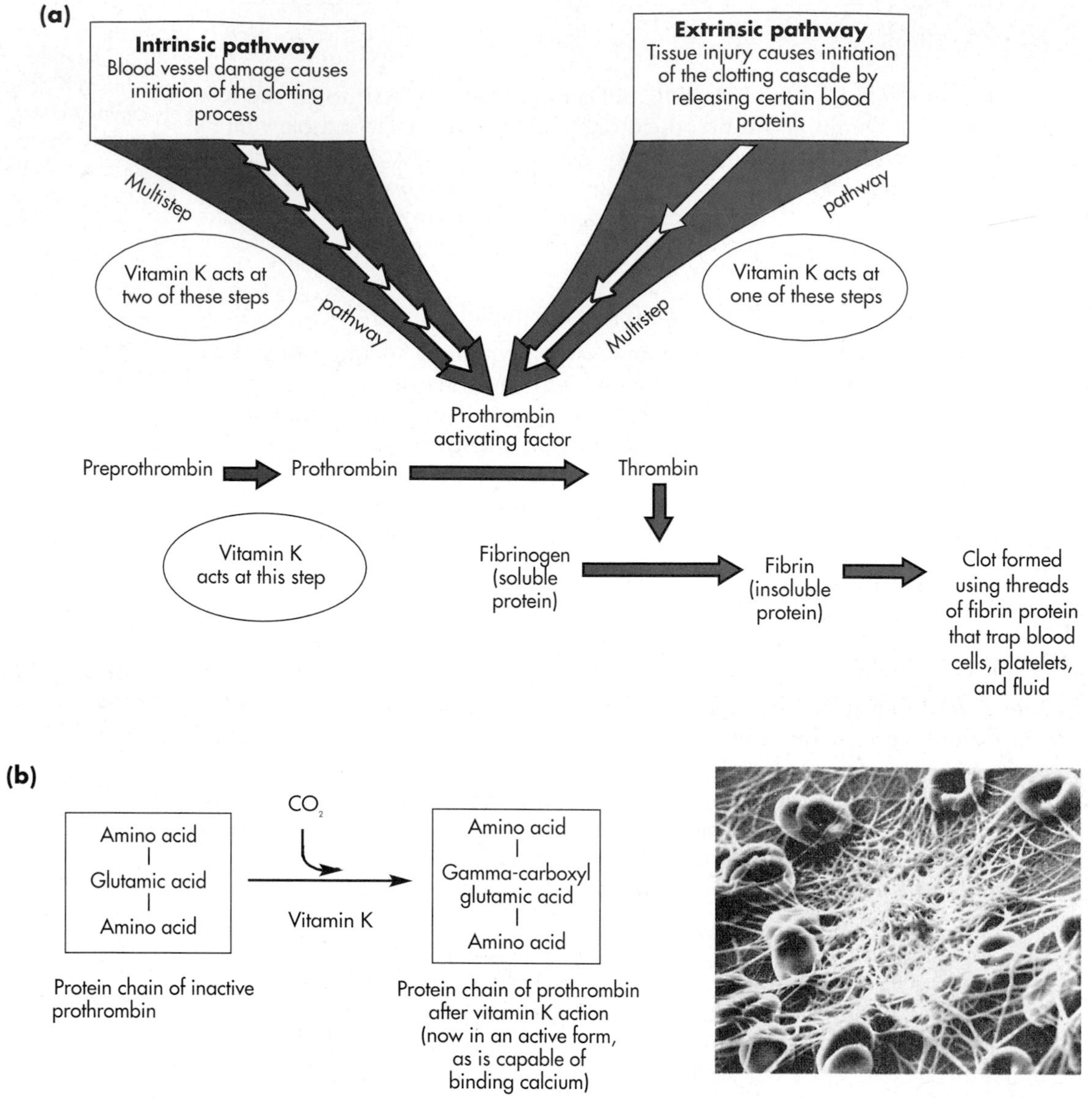

(a)

Intrinsic pathway
Blood vessel damage causes initiation of the clotting process

Extrinsic pathway
Tissue injury causes initiation of the clotting cascade by releasing certain blood proteins

Multistep
pathway

Multistep
pathway

Vitamin K acts at two of these steps

Vitamin K acts at one of these steps

Prothrombin activating factor

Preprothrombin → Prothrombin → Thrombin

Vitamin K acts at this step

Fibrinogen (soluble protein) → Fibrin (insoluble protein) → Clot formed using threads of fibrin protein that trap blood cells, platelets, and fluid

(b)

Amino acid
|
Glutamic acid
|
Amino acid

Protein chain of inactive prothrombin

CO_2
Vitamin K

Amino acid
|
Gamma-carboxyl glutamic acid
|
Amino acid

Protein chain of prothrombin after vitamin K action (now in an active form, as is capable of binding calcium)

FIGURE 9-13 Vitamin K metabolism. (*a*) Forming a blood clot requires the participation of vitamin K in both the intrinsic and extrinsic blood-clotting pathways. Note that, although the two pathways are activated by different events, there is some overlap in the pathways, but for simplicity we have not shown that. (*b*) Vitamin K specifically adds a carbon dioxide to glutamic acid in a precursor protein to yield gamma-carboxyl glutamate in that protein. This change imparts calcium-binding capacity to the protein, as in the conversion of a precursor protein to prothrombin, an active clotting factor.

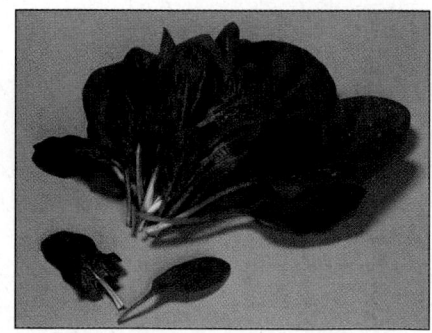

Spinach is a nutrient-dense source of vitamin K.

Dietary Sources of Vitamin K

The most nutrient-dense food sources of vitamin K (mg/kcal) are liver, green leafy vegetables (e.g., kale, turnip greens, salad greens, cabbage, and spinach), broccoli, peas, and green beans. One reason to consume a diet rich in green vegetables is to obtain sufficient vitamin K. Other common sources are vegetable oils, such as soy and canola. Most vitamin K consumed in a day disappears from the body by the next day. Nevertheless, vitamin K is abundant in the diet, and a deficiency is uncommon. Vitamin K is quite resistant to cooking losses.

Vitamin K Needs

The Adequate Intake set for vitamin K is based on the amount consumed by apparently healthy populations. For women 19 to 70+ the amount is 90 μg/day and for men 19 to 70+ the amount is 120 μg/day. Laboratory animal studies have shown that excessive amounts of vitamins A and E are known to antagonize the actions of vitamin K.[5] Vitamin A is thought to interfere with the absorption of vitamin K from the intestine. Large doses of vitamin E can lead to a decrease in vitamin K-dependent clotting factors and increased bleeding tendency. In either case, megadose supplements of these vitamins may pose a risk to vitamin K status.

Vitamin K deficiency can occur in newborns because they lack the gastrointestinal bacteria that synthesize vitamin K. Neither is there much vitamin K in human milk. Thus, at birth, infants run the risk of defective blood clotting and eventual hemorrhage because of a lack of vitamin K. To prevent this possible vitamin K deficiency, physicians routinely provide vitamin K by injections within 6 hours of delivery. This protection is intended to last until infants' intestinal bacteria begin to synthesize vitamin K. Older people may also be at risk due to poor green vegetable intake.

Toxicity from vitamin K is unlikely because, although fat soluble, it is readily excreted by the body. However, one medicinal form of vitamin K, water-soluble menadione, can lead to toxic signs and symptoms, including jaundice and hemolytic anemia, in infants. No Upper Level for vitamin K has been set.

The fat-soluble vitamins are reviewed in Table 9-4.

*D*ietary Sources of Vitamin K

Food Item and Amount	Vitamin K (µg)
Cooked kale, ½ cup	650
Cooked collard greens, ½ cup	375
Spinach, ½ cup	324
Cooked brussels sprouts, ½ cup	225
Raw turnip greens, 1 cup	200
Cooked broccoli, ½ cup	88
Canola oil, 1 tbsp	27
Soybean oil, 1 tbsp	27
Cooked green beans, ½ cup	14
Fat-free milk, 1 cup	9

CONCEPT CHECK

*V*itamin K is important for blood clotting because it stimulates the conversion of precursor proteins to active clotting factors, such as prothrombin. This conversion involves the addition of carbon dioxide to glutamic acid in the precursor protein, yielding gamma-carboxy glutamate, which in turn can bind calcium. Some of the vitamin K we absorb every day comes from bacterial synthesis in the intestines, but most comes from the diet. The amount in the diet alone generally meets our needs. Thus, except for newborns and possibly some older people, a deficiency of vitamin K is unlikely, even though it is readily excreted from the body.

*C*heck out the *Perspectives in Nutrition* Online Learning Center http://www.mhhe.com/wardlaw for quizzes, flash cards, other activities, and web links designed to further help you learn about the fat-soluble vitamins.

TABLE 9-4   Summary of the Fat-Soluble Vitamins: Their Functions, Deficiency Conditions, and Food Sources

Major Vitamin	Functions	Deficiency Symptoms	People at Risk	Sources	RDA or Adequate Intake	Toxicity Symptoms*
Vitamin A Preformed retinoids and provitamin A carotenoids	Vision in dim light and color vision, cell differentiation and growth, immunity	Poor growth, night blindness, blindness, keratinization of epithelium, xerophthalmia	Rare in United States but common in preschool children living in poverty in developing countries, alcoholics	**Preformed vitamin A:** liver, fortified milk, fish liver oils **Provitamin A:** red, orange, dark green, and yellow vegetables; orange fruits	700-900 µg RAE	Headache, vomiting, double vision, hair loss, dry mucous membranes, bone and joint pain, liver damage, hemorrhage, coma, teratogenic effects: spontaneous abortions, birth defects
Vitamin D Cholecalciferol Ergocalciferol	Maintenance of intracellular and extracellular calcium concentrations and epidermal tissue	Rickets in children, osteomalacia in older adults	Older adults, breastfed infants from vitamin D-deficient mother	Vitamin D-fortified milk, fish oils	5–10 µg (200-400 IU) 15 µg > 70 yrs	Calcification of soft tissues, growth retardation, excess calcium excretion via the kidney
Vitamin E Tocopherols Tocotrienols	Antioxidant, prevention of propagation of free radicals	Hemolysis of red blood cells, degeneration of sensory neurons	Patients with fat-malabsorption syndromes (deficiency is rare)	Plant oils, seeds, nuts, products, made from oils	15 mg alpha tocopherol for men and women (22-33 IU)	Few side effects, effects of lifetime exposure to excess vitamin E unknown
Vitamin K Phylloquinone Menaquinone	Synthesis of blood-clotting factors and bone proteins	Hemorrhage, fractures	Those taking antibiotics for a long period of time (still quite rare)	Green vegetables, liver, synthesis by intestinal microorganisms	90-120 µg	Seen only with medicinal forms

*Toxicity is seen only with supplement use; foods pose no threat.

SUMMARY

1. Vitamins are essential organic (carbon-containing) compounds needed for important metabolic reactions in the body. They are not a source of energy. Instead, they promote many energy-yielding and other reactions in the body, thereby promoting the growth, development, and maintenance of various body tissues. Vitamins A, D, E, and K are fat soluble, whereas the B-vitamins and vitamin C are water soluble. Fat-soluble vitamins are excreted less readily from the body and are less susceptible to cooking loss than are water-soluble vitamins.

2. Some fat-soluble vitamins pose a potential threat for toxicity. Vitamins A and D can readily accumulate in the body to toxic concentrations. The water-soluble vitamins niacin, vitamin B-6, and vitamin C can also induce toxic signs and symptoms, but only at doses much higher than their RDAs.

3. Fat-soluble vitamins are absorbed along with dietary fat. They travel by way of the lymphatic system into general circulation, carried by chylomicrons, one type of lipoprotein. In disease states in which fat digestion is limited, fat-soluble vitamin status may be compromised, especially with vitamins A, E, and K.

4. Vitamin A consists of a family of retinoid compounds: retinal, retinol, and retinoic acid. A plant derivative known as beta-carotene, along with some other carotenoids, yields vitamin A after metabolism by the intestine or liver. Vitamin A contributes to the maintenance of vision, the proper development of cells (especially mucus-forming cells), and immune function. Vitamin A is found in foods of animal origin, such as liver, fish oils, and fortified milk. Carotenoids are obtained from plants and are especially plentiful in dark green and orange vegetables and in some fruits. These likely contribute to protection from oxidizing agents for the body.

5. Americans at risk for poor vitamin A status are people exhibiting limited fat absorption and alcoholics. Vitamin A can be quite toxic when taken at 3 times or more the RDA, but only with preformed vitamin A. Use is especially dangerous during pregnancy because it can lead to fetal malformations.

6. For most people, vitamin D is more correctly viewed as a hormone rather than a vitamin because sufficient amounts of it can be produced by the body. Provitamin D is synthesized in the skin from a derivative of cholesterol in a process that depends on ultraviolet light. With adequate sun exposure, no dietary intake of vitamin D is needed. The provitamin, whether produced in the skin or obtained from the diet, is metabolized in the liver and kidneys to yield $1,25(OH)_2D$ (or calcitriol), the active hormonal form of vitamin D. $1,25(OH)_2D$ is important for calcium absorption from the intestine and, with other hormones, it helps regulate bone metabolism. Vitamin D is found in fish oils and fortified milk. Vitamin D can be very toxic when taken in supplement form, especially in infancy, when an intake just three times or more than the Adequate Intake can be toxic. Anyone who feels a need to use a vitamin D supplement containing more than two times the Adequate Intake, such as an older person, should consult a physician first.

7. Vitamin E functions as an antioxidant. By donating electrons to electron-seeking compounds (oxidizing agents), it neutralizes their action. One group of electron-seeking compounds, known as free radicals, can cause widespread destruction, both to cell membranes and to DNA. Vitamin E is one of several components in the body's defense system against oxidizing agents, which reduces damage to cells. Vitamin E is plentiful in plant oils. The more plant oils one consumes, the more vitamin E one needs, but this need is usually met by the same plant oils. To date, the use of megadose supplements of vitamin E by healthy adults to limit cardiovascular disease and cancer risk in people at high risk has not shown to be effective in most major trials.

8. Vitamin K contributes to the body's blood-clotting ability by facilitating the conversion of precursor proteins to active clotting factors, such as prothrombin, which promotes blood coagulation. Vitamin K also plays a role in bone metabolism. Some of the vitamin K absorbed each day likely comes from bacterial synthesis in the intestine; most comes from foods, primarily green leafy vegetables and vegetable oils. Vitamin K is readily excreted in the body, but the usual daily intake from diet alone meets one's needs.

STUDY QUESTIONS

1. Describe two forms of vitamin A that are available in common foods.
2. Explain how retinal functions in black-and-white and color vision.
3. Describe how retinoic acid participates in protein synthesis.
4. What factors determine whether a person needs a dietary source of vitamin D or can rely on self-synthesis?
5. Describe how vitamin D, parathyroid hormone, and calcitonin regulate the concentration of calcium and phosphorus in the blood.
6. Define a free radical and explain how vitamin E controls free radical damage.
7. List several important dietary sources for each of the fat-soluble vitamins. Identify the Adequate Intake or RDA and the Upper Level for each of the fat-soluble vitamins.
8. Identify the two primary functions of vitamin K in the body.
9. What properties of the fat-soluble vitamins make them a greater risk for toxicity than the water-soluble vitamins?
10. Identify the Americans most at risk for fat-soluble vitamin deficiencies.

■ ANNOTATED REFERENCES

1. ADA Reports: Position of the American Dietetic Association: Food fortification and dietary supplements. *Journal of the American Dietetic Association* 101:115:2001.

   The best nutritional strategy for promoting optimal health and reducing the risk of chronic disease is to wisely choose a wide variety of foods. Additional vitamins and minerals from fortified foods and/or supplements can help some people meet their nutritional needs.

2. Chasan-Taber L and others: A prospective study of carotenoid and vitamin A intakes and risk of cataract extraction in US women. *American Journal of Clinical Nutrition* 70:509, 1999.

   After age, smoking, and other potential cataract risk factors were controlled for, the intake of lutein and zeaxanthin resulted in a 22% decreased risk for cataracts. Vitamin A and other carotenoids were not associated with protection. Spinach and kale are rich sources of lutein.

3. Feskanich D and others: Vitamin K intake and hip fractures in women: A prospective study. *American Journal of Clinical Nutrition* 69:74, 1999.

   Low concentrations of circulating vitamin K have been associated with low bone mineral density and bone fractures. Vitamin K mediates the carboxylation of glutamate residues on several bone proteins, notably, osteocalcin.

4. Food and Nutrition Board, Institute of Medicine. *Dietary reference intakes for vitamin C, vitamin E, selenium and carotenoids.* Washington, D.C.: National Academy Press, 2000.

   This is a report from the panel evaluating dietary antioxidants and related compounds used to establish the current DRIs.

5. Food and Nutrition Board, Institute of Medicine: *Dietary reference intakes for vitamin A, vitamin K, arsenic, boron chromium, copper, iodine, iron, manganese, molybdenum, nickel, silicon, vanadium, and zinc.* Washington, DC: National Academy Press, 2001.

   Dietary Reference Intakes have recently been set for vitamin A and vitamin K. The rationale used to set the RDA or Adequate Intake and Upper Level for these nutrients is discussed in detail.

6. Hadi H and others: Vitamin A supplementation selectively improves the linear growth of Indonesian preschool children: Results from a randomized controlled trial. *American Journal of Clinical Nutrition* 71:507, 2000.

   High doses of vitamin A modestly improved linear growth in children who were deficient in vitamin A. The best response was among the most deficient children. Breastfeeding of children up to 24 months of age protects children from linear growth deficit due to vitamin A deficiency.

7. Harris S and others: Plasma 25-hydroxyvitamin D responses to younger and older men to three weeks of supplementation with 1800 IU/day of vitamin D. *Journal of the American College of Nutrition* 18:470, 1999.

   There is an age-related decline in the absorption, transport, or liver hydroxylation of orally consumed vitamin D. This suggests there may be an age-related decline in circulating 25-OH-D due to a reduced response to orally consumed vitamin D.

8. Holick MF: Vitamin D. In Shils ME and others (eds.): *Modern nutrition in health and disease.* 9th ed. Baltimore, MD: Williams & Wilkins, 1999.

   Author provides information about history, photobiology, absorption, metabolism, functions, assays (use and interpretation), and recommendations for intake of vitamin D.

9. LeBoff MS and others: Occult vitamin D deficiency in postmenopausal US women with acute hip fracture. *Journal of the American Medical Association* 281:1505, 1999.

   Older women who are deficient in vitamin D could be at increased risk for hip fractures. Vitamin D deficiency was associated with elevated parathyroid hormone levels. The correction of vitamin D deficiency with supplements or sun exposure may lead to the reduction of hip fractures in aged women.

10. Meagher EA and others: Effects of vitamin E on lipid peroxidation in healthy persons. *Journal of the American Medical Association* 285: 1178, 2001.

    Doses of vitamin E ranging from 200 to 2000 IU/day had no effect on markers of lipid peroxidation in healthy people in this 8 week study.

11. Meydani, M: Vitamin E and prevention of heart disease in high-risk patients, *Nutrition Reviews* 58: 278, 2000.

    Current supplementation trials using vitamin in various population groups will help answer the question of whether intakes above which are provided by a balanced diet confer additional health benefits. To date, most clinical trials in high risk cardiovascular patients have not shown a clear benefit.

12. Multivitamins: Do you need one? Mayo Clinic Health letter, p. 4, April 2001.

    Multivitamins usually provide the RDA of most vitamins. Some contain the RDA of select minerals. Still, it is important to check the label to make sure one is not getting too much of any nutrient. In some cases an excess may be harmful.

13. Nguyen ML and SJ Schwartz: Lycopene: Chemical and biological properties. *Food Technology* 53:38, 1999.

    Lycopene acts an antioxidant and scavenger of free radicals, which are often associated with carcinogenesis. Even with overwhelming laboratory evidence linking lycopene to various health benefits, the epidemiological data regarding disease prevention are inconsistent. Perhaps lycopene is just a marker for good dietary habits and a healthy lifestyle.

14. Olson R: Vitamin K. In Shils ME and others (eds.): *Modern nutrition in health and disease.* 9th ed. Baltimore, MD: Williams & Wilkins, 1999.

    This chapter presents the history, chemistry, nomenclature, absorption, distribution, metabolism, functions, deficiency, evaluation of nutritional statues, requirements, allowances, and toxicity of vitamin K.

15. Pryor WA and others: Beta carotene: From biochemistry to clinical trials. *Nutrition Reviews* 58:39, 2000.

    The large-scale clinical trials testing the effects of supplemental beta-carotene on the risk for chronic diseases showed no protection against lung cancer. Supplements produced an even higher risk. The association between eating fruits and vegetables and reduced risk for a number of diseases is consistent. Studies suggest a need for further research to gain a clearer understanding of the relationship of beta-carotene to important public health problems.

16. Ross C: Vitamin A and retinoids. In Shils ME and others (eds.): *Modern nutrition in health and disease.* 9th ed. Baltimore, MD: Williams & Wilkins, 1999.

    Author provides the history, chemistry, metabolism, functions, pharmacological use, deficiency, toxicity, and methods to assess vitamin A status.

17. Russell JJ: Topical therapy for acne. *American Family Physician* 61:357, 2000.

    Topical retinoids such as tretinoin (Retin-A) and other topical creams are effective in many patients with acne.

18. Russell RM: The vitamin A spectrum: From deficiency to toxicity. *American Journal of Clinical Nutrition* 71:878, 2000.

    Vitamin A toxicity is more common among the elderly than young adults. The longer a person overdoses on the vitamin, the greater the potential for toxicity.

19. Stahl P: The antioxidant conundrums: Two recent studies point in different directions. *Journal of the American Dietetic Association* 100:510, 2000.

    A conflicting recommendation by registered dietitians as to cancer patient use of antioxidant supplements is explored. Dietitians should be cautious about recommending supplements to cancer patients. They should encourage obtaining micronutrients from food.

20. Thacher TD and others: A comparison of calcium, vitamin D, or both for nutritional rickets in Nigerian children. *The New England Journal of Medicine* 341:563, 1999.

Nigerian children with rickets had a low calcium intake. Supplementation with calcium or a combination of calcium and vitamin D healed the rickets. Vitamin D deficiency alone was not an important cause of rickets in these children.

21. Traber M: Vitamin E. In Shils ME and others (eds.): *Modern nutrition in health and disease.* 9th ed. Baltimore, MD: Williams & Wilkins, 1999.

Author presents the history, structure, nomenclature, sources, absorption, transport, distribution, metabolism, excretion, causes and pathology of deficiency, requirements, and recommended intake of vitamin E.

22. Van De Graff KM, and Fox SI: *Concepts of human anatomy and physiology.* 5th ed. Boston: McGraw-Hill, 1999.

Authors explain interactions of 1,25(OH)₂D parathyroid hormone, and calcitonin in bone deposition and bone resorption and how they maintain calcium and phosphate concentrations in the blood.

23. Van den Berg H: Carotenoid interactions. *Nutrition Reviews* 57:1, 1999.

Perhaps supplementation with high doses of beta-carotene reduce the absorption and blood concentrations of all the other carotenoids.

24. van het Hof K and others: Dietary factors that affect the bioavailability of carotenoids. *Journal of Nutrition* 130:503, 2000.

This is a review of absorption of various carotenoids as related to the type of food matrix in which they are located. The amount of dietary fat required seems to be low, but depends on the characteristics of the carotenoid ingested. Vegetables vary in their bioavailability of various carotenoids present.

25. van het Hof K and others: Bioavailability of lutein from vegetables is 5 times higher than that of β-carotene. *American Journal of Clinical Nutrition* 70:261, 1999.

Vegetable consumption promotes a more moderate increase of beta-carotene in blood than does purified beta-carotene. Increased vegetable consumption enhanced blood concentrations of vitamin C and carotenoids such as lutein substantially.

26. Van Tits LJ and others: Alpha-tocopherol supplementation decreases production of superoxide and cytokines by leukocytes ex vivo in both normolipidemic and hypertriglyceridemic individuals. *American Journal of Clinical Nutrition* 71:458, 2000.

Alpha-tocopherol may influence the inflammatory responses of immune cells infiltrating subendothelial spaces. Vitamin E may be related to chronic inflammatory processes, such as seen in atherogenesis.

27. Vitamin D Differences in response to sunlight and forms of supplementation. *Nutrition and the M.D.,* p. 6, August 1999.

Vitamin D₂ and Vitamin D₃ should not be considered nutritionally equivalent. D₃ is 70% more efficient in increasing serum 25-OH-D. The usual form of vitamin D supplement is D₂, derived from irradiation of yeast lipid (irradiated ergosterol).

28. Yusuf S: Vitamin E supplementation and cardiovascular events in high-risk patients. *The New England Journal of Medicine* 342:254, 2000.

In patients at high risk for cardiovascular events, treatment with 400 IU vitamin E per day for 4.5 years had no apparent effect on cardiovascular outcomes.

T A K E A C T I O N

I. MEASURING YOUR VITAMIN INTAKE AGAINST THE RDAS

This activity requires you to reexamine the nutritional assessment you did for Chapters 1 and 2. You recorded all the foods and drinks you consumed for 1 day and their quantities. Then you assessed your intake by recording the total amounts of nutrients you consumed. You were then asked to compare your nutrient intake with established standards. Take your completed assessment and look at your intakes of vitamins A, E, C, B-6, and B-12, and thiamin, riboflavin, niacin, and folate. Record these numbers in the following table. Next, record the RDA for each of these nutrients from your assessment. Then, record the percentage of the RDA you consumed for each vitamin. Lastly, place +, -, or = in the space provided, reflecting an intake higher than, lower than, or equal to the RDA.

Vitamin	Intake	RDA	% of RDA	+, -, =
A				
E				
C				
Thiamin				
Riboflavin				
Niacin				
B-6				
Folate				
B-12				

Analysis

1. Which of your vitamin intakes equaled or exceeded the RDA?

   _____

2. Which of your vitamin intakes were below the RDA?

   _____

3. What foods could you eat to improve your dietary intake of vitamins in low amounts in your diet? (Review sources of certain vitamins in this chapter and the next.)

   _____

   _____

TAKE ACTION

II. A CLOSER LOOK AT SUPPLEMENT USE

With the current popularity of vitamin and mineral supplements, it is more important than ever to understand how to evaluate a supplement. Study the accompanying label and then answer the following questions. Then, by way of comparison, go to a store and examine a general multivitamin/mineral supplement. When you have done that, answer the set of questions again. How do the answers change? Which of the two do you think would be safer to take on a regular basis?

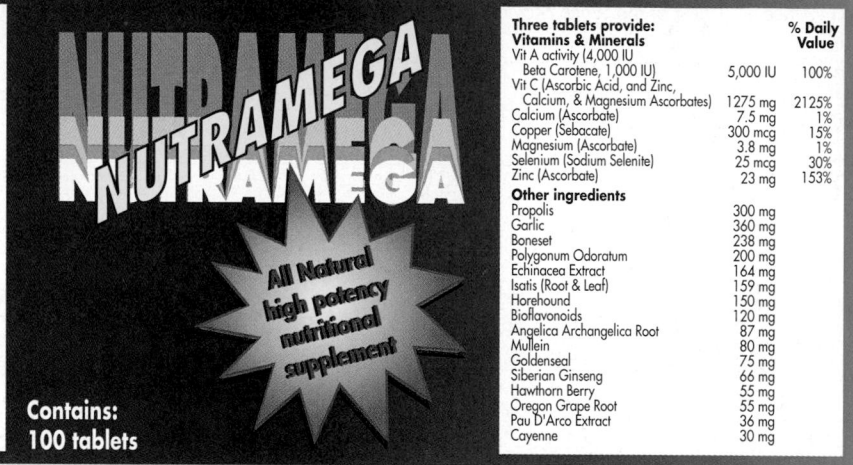

Our protective formula has been extensively researched to bring you the best answer to problems associated with changing seasons.

Suggested use: For best results, begin taking *Nutramega* tablets at the very first signs of imbalances in your well-being. During imbalances, take 2 to 3 tablets every three hours. For daily maintenance, take 1 or 2 tablets a day. Or, take as recommended by your health care professional.

WARNING: Not for use by pregnant or nursing women.

KEEP OUT OF THE REACH OF CHILDREN.

Contains: 100 tablets

Three tablets provide: Vitamins & Minerals		% Daily Value
Vit A activity (4,000 IU)		
Beta Carotene, 1,000 IU)	5,000 IU	100%
Vit C (Ascorbic Acid, and Zinc,		
Calcium, & Magnesium Ascorbates)	1275 mg	2125%
Calcium (Ascorbate)	7.5 mg	1%
Copper (Sebacate)	300 mcg	15%
Magnesium (Ascorbate)	3.8 mg	1%
Selenium (Sodium Selenite)	25 mcg	30%
Zinc (Ascorbate)	23 mg	153%
Other ingredients		
Propolis	300 mg	
Garlic	360 mg	
Boneset	238 mg	
Polygonum Odoratum	200 mg	
Echinacea Extract	164 mg	
Isatis (Root & Leaf)	159 mg	
Horehound	150 mg	
Bioflavonoids	120 mg	
Angelica Archangelica Root	87 mg	
Mullein	80 mg	
Goldenseal	75 mg	
Siberian Ginseng	66 mg	
Hawthorn Berry	55 mg	
Oregon Grape Root	55 mg	
Pau D'Arco Extract	36 mg	
Cayenne	30 mg	

1. What is the recommended dosage of this supplement? _____

2. Based on the recommended dosage, are there any individual vitamins for which the intake would be greater than 100% of the Daily Value? List these vitamins. _____

3. Are any suggested intakes above the Upper Level for the nutrient? _____

4. Are there any superfluous ingredients, such as herbs or flavors, in the supplement? You can often tell this because these ingredients do not have a percent of Daily Value. _____

5. Does at least 50% of the vitamin A in the product come from beta-carotene or other provitamin A carotenoids (to reduce risk of preformed vitamin A toxicity)? _____

6. Are there any warnings on the label as to populations who should not consume this product? _____

7. Are there any other signs that tip you off that this may not be a safe product? _____

NUTRIENT SUPPLEMENTS: WHO NEEDS THEM?

Today, supplements are marketed as good for anything that ails you. This cure-all approach is promoted by the supplement industry and countless health-food stores, pharmacies, and supermarkets.

According to the Dietary Supplement Health and Education Act of 1994, a supplement is a product intended to supplement the diet that bears or contains one of more of the following dietary ingredients:

- A vitamin
- A mineral
- An herb or another botanical
- An amino acid
- A dietary substance to supplement the diet, which could be an extract or a combination of the first four ingredients in this list

The definition is very broad and covers a wide variety of nutritional substances.

The use of supplements to the diet is a common practice among Americans and generates about $14 billion annually for the industry.[1] In spite of the explosive growth of the industry, there is very little the public can do protect itself from dangerous or worthless products. The supplement makers can make broad claims about their products under the "structure function" provision of the law, allowing the product onto the market without testing for safety or efficacy. The products, however, cannot claim to prevent, treat, or cure a disease. (See the Nutrition Perspective in Chapter 18 for more details.) Since pregnancy, menopause, and aging are not diseases per se, products alleging to treat these conditions can be marketed without FDA approval. For example, a product that claims to treat morning sickness can be sold without any testing to prove that the product actually works, but a product that claims to decrease the risk of heart disease by reducing blood cholesterol must have scientific studies that justify the claim.

Why do people take supplements? Reasons that are frequently given include the following:

- To reduce susceptibility to health problems (e.g., colds)
- To prevent heart attacks
- To prevent cancer
- To reduce stress
- To increase "energy"

Should you take a supplement? The answer is a qualified yes. Currently opinions vary about the wisdom and safety of supplement use even among knowledgeable scientists. Typically, nutrition scientists have recommended that supplement use is needed only by a few groups of our population at large. However, over the last few years some reputable nutrition scientists have recommended supplementation of specific nutrients for many or all adults.

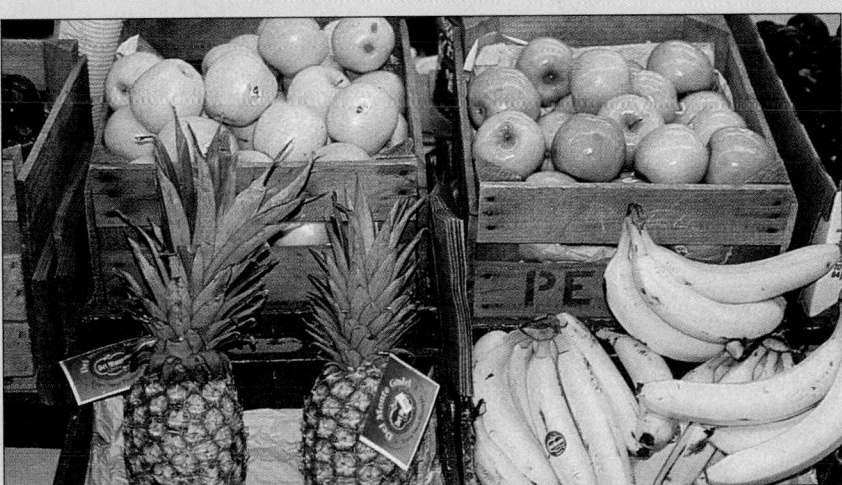

Focus first on foods for meeting nutrient needs.

*B*ecause research on a variety of nutrient supplements has revealed a lack of product quality, the USP (United States Pharmacopeia) designation is being extended to an increasing number of nutrient supplements. The USP standards designate strength, quality, purity, packaging, labeling, speed of dissolution, and acceptable length of storage of ingredients for drugs. The purpose of applying them to vitamin and mineral supplements is to establish professionally accepted standards for these products. Consumers who buy nutrient supplements should look for a USP label when comparing similar products, such as calcium supplements. If no USP label is present, the next best approach is to purchase nationally-advertised brands.

*V*itamin and mineral supplements should generally be taken with or just after meals to maximize absorption.

This change in philosophy has arisen primarily because Americans have been unwilling to change their food habits, such as including ample fruits and vegetables. This gap leaves many diets low in the vitamin folate. Adequate folate status when a woman is pregnant reduces the risk of certain birth defects in her offspring (400 µg/day of synthetic folate is recommended). Folate also limits homocysteine in the blood, a risk factor for cardiovascular disease that can affect all of us. In addition, the committee appointed by the Food and Nutrition Board that set current nutrient standards for vitamin B-12 suggested that adults over age 50 consume vitamin B-12 in a synthetic form, such as that added to breakfast cereals or present in supplements. Synthetic vitamin B-12 is more easily absorbed than that found in food; this helps compensate for the fall in vitamin B-12 absorption typically seen as we age into our later years (see Chapter 10 for details). This latter observation has caused nutrition experts at Tufts University to add a recommendation for vitamin B-12 supplements to the Food Guide Pyramid they developed for older persons. The Tufts scientists also include calcium and vitamin D supplements, as these nutrients can be deficient in the diets of older persons (see Chapter 16).

Another example of this change in philosophy is an editorial in the April 9, 1998 issue of *The New England Journal of Medicine* entitled "Eat Right and Take a Multivitamin." Note that "eat right" is part of the recommendation. All the health-promoting effects of foods cannot be found in a bottle; recall the discussion of phytochemicals in Chapter 2. Few or no phytochemicals are present in supplements.[12]

Overall, supplement use cannot fix a poor diet in all respects. Uninformed megadose supplement use also can lead to harm. Thus, we are advised to first take a good look at our dietary habits and then improve them as possible, as outlined in Chapter 2. Finally, find out which nutrient gaps remain, and identify food sources that can help. Examples could be ready-to-eat breakfast cereals to increase folate and vitamin B-6 intake and provide highly absorbable forms of vitamin B-12 (many currently contain the RDA amounts or more per serving), calcium-fortified orange juice to increase calcium intake, or milk to increase vitamin D and calcium intake. Only after that should we worry about the need to take supplements.[1] Recall as well from Table 2-8 in Chapter 2 that a well-planned diet containing just 1800 kcals can meet all known nutrient needs.

If supplement use is desired, one should discuss this practice with a physician, as some supplements can interfere with certain medicines. For example, vitamin B-6 can offset the action of L-dopa (used in treating Parkinson's disease), and high intakes of vitamin K or vitamin E alter the action of oral anticoagulants. Large doses of vitamin C can interfere with certain chemotherapy regimens.[19] Remember, you can get too much of a good thing.

Some research is also pointing to the advantages for some of us taking specific supplements in amounts not possible to achieve by diet alone. Three examples are vitamin D (15 µg day or 600 IU/day), and vitamin B-12 (up to 25 µg/day) for older adults, and possibly vitamin E (50 to 800 IU) for adults in general. To meet the recommendations arising from this research, one would need to take supplements. Vitamin B-12 supplement use has a low potential for toxicity and is inexpensive. Some multivitamins sold in grocery stores and drugstores (costing about $0.08 per day) already contain the intended amounts. Vitamin E supplement use is fairly nontoxic for most adults and inexpensive (again about $0.07 per day). Still, as noted in the chapter, we do not have solid information that supports widespread megadose vitamin E supplementation. Vitamin D needs could be met with the amount found in a typical multivitamin coupled with 2 servings of milk. Otherwise a separate supplement could be added.

PEOPLE MOST LIKELY TO NEED SUPPLEMENTS

Various medical and health-related organizations suggest that the following vitamin and mineral supplementation can be important for certain groups of healthy people:
- Women in their childbearing years may need extra synthetic folate.
- Women with excessive bleeding during menstruation may need extra iron.
- Women who are pregnant or breastfeeding may need extra iron, folate, and calcium.
- People with very low energy intakes (less than about 1200 kcal per day) need a range of vitamins and minerals. This is true of some women and many older people.

- Strict vegans may need extra calcium, iron, zinc, and vitamin B-12.
- Newborns, under the direction of a physician, need a single dose of vitamin K.
- People with limited milk intake and sunlight exposure may need extra vitamin D.
- People with lactose intolerance or allergies to dairy products may need extra calcium.
- Adults over age 50 may need a synthetic source of vitamin B-12.
- People on very low fat diets may need some extra vitamin E.

Individuals with certain medical conditions (e.g., vitamin-resistance diseases or long-standing fat malabsorption) and those who use certain medications also may require supplementation with specific vitamins and minerals. Finally, smokers and alcohol abusers may benefit from supplementation, but cessation of these two activities is far more beneficial than any supplementation. Still, a physician should guide all of this therapy.[12]

■ Which Supplement Should You Choose?

If you decide to take a vitamin and/or mineral supplement, which one should you choose? As a start, choose a national brand from a supermarket or pharmacy that generally contains no more than the Upper Level for each vitamin and mineral. (See the inside cover of this textbook for Upper Levels.) Men should use a product that is low in iron or iron free to avoid possible iron overload (see Chapter 12 for details), and older people may want to seek a product that is fortified with extra vitamin B-12 (as discussed). One should read the label carefully to be sure of what is being taken.

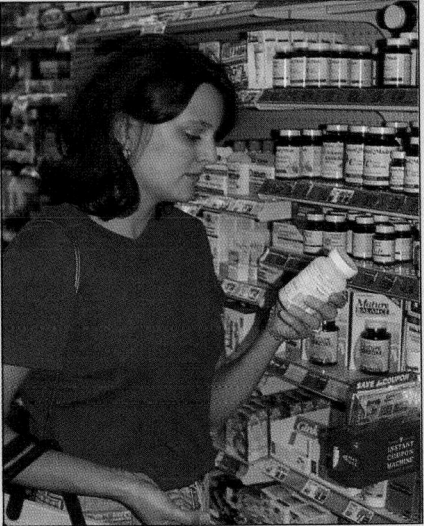

Long-term intake of just three or more times the Daily Value for some fat-soluble vitamins—particularly vitamins A and D— can cause toxic effects. Read supplement labels carefully for amounts of these vitamins.

Overall, any supplementation should make nutrition sense in terms of nutrient gaps in a diet and a balanced formulation (based on approximately equal % Daily Value quantities) in a supplement is important. Balance will minimize the chance of vitamin and mineral competition as well as possible accompanying toxicity problems, such as the following:

- Excessive intake of vitamin C can cause overabsorption of iron and can contribute to iron toxicity in susceptible people, as well as decrease the ability of certain diagnostic tests to asses the development of diseases.
- Excessive zinc intake can inhibit iron and copper absorption.
- Large amounts of folate can mask signs and symptoms of a vitamin B-12 deficiency (see Chapter 10).

Another consideration in choosing a supplement is avoiding superfluous ingredients, such as para-amino benzoic acid (PABA), hesperidin complex, inositol, bee pollen, and lecithins. These are not needed in our diets. They are especially common in expensive supplements sold in health-food stores and by mail. In addition, use of l-tryptophan and high doses of beta-carotene or fish oils are discouraged.

Would the overall health of the nation be improved if our citizens routinely took supplements? Or would this additional intake lead to an unbalanced nutrient state and, in turn, untoward effects? There is no consensus on this question. Consuming a healthy, balanced diet is still the overriding theme, whether supplements are advocated in addition or not at all. In addition, many foods are already fortified with vitamins and minerals, so check out the breakfast cereals, orange and other juices, and dairy products consumed for their contributions of essential nutrients via fortification. As well, this list of fortified foods gets longer each year. Thus, it is unnecessary for many of us to spend money on supplements, since many foods we eat each day are rich sources of natural or added nutrients. Monitor your food intake for the next few days and note how many of these foods are fortified with vitamins and minerals. The number may surprise you.

Five web sites to help you evaluate ongoing claims and evaluate safety of supplements are:

http://www.acsh.org

http://www.quackwatch.com

http://www.ncahf.org

http://dietary-supplements.info.nih.gov

http://www.consumerlabs.com

The sites are maintained by groups or individuals committed to providing reasoned and authoritative nutrition and health advice to consumers.

CRITICAL THINKING

Many vitamin supplements supply nutrients in amounts that exceed the Daily Values listed on the label. Miguel believes that "more is better." How can you explain to him that the supplement he is about to start taking is "worse," since it contains amounts that exceed the Daily Values by 10 times for many nutrients, including vitamin A and vitamin D?

The Water-Soluble Vitamins

chapter 10

As defined in Chapter 9, vitamins are essential organic substances needed in very small amounts in the diet to support the metabolism, growth, and maintenance of body cells.

The water-soluble vitamins discussed in this chapter include eight B-vitamins, vitamin C, and a newcomer to the list of essential nutrients, a dietary component called choline.[4, 21] The B vitamins form coenzymes—organic compounds that enable certain enzymes to function. As a group, the B-vitamins are necessary for converting solar energy into cellular energy, transforming nutrients into characteristic cell structures, and creating various proteins, lipids, and carbohydrates. Vitamin C also participates in a wide variety of metabolic processes, although not in the form of a coenzyme. Choline is needed to form lecithin and other compounds.

The end of the chapter briefly describes some "vitamin-like" compounds, which some people may require in their diets under atypical circumstances. These compounds currently are not classified as true vitamins because a healthy person does not require a dietary source of them and no specific deficiency disease results when they are absent from the diet.

- Thiamin is crucial for carbohydrate metabolism. Because nervous tissue is fueled by carbohydrate, nervous system dysfunctions occur in thiamin deficiency. Thiamin deficiency is most likely to occur in alcoholics. Pork, dried beans, and enriched grains are excellent sources of thiamin.
- Riboflavin takes part in the metabolism of all energy-yielding nutrients. Riboflavin deficiency, if it occurs, likely does so in conjunction with other B-vitamin deficiencies. Dairy products and enriched grains are good sources of riboflavin.
- Niacin is also used for the metabolism of energy-yielding nutrients. Severe skin lesions, dementia, diarrhea, and eventually death can be seen in niacin deficiency; this deficiency usually occurs only in alcoholics. Niacin is found in high-protein foods and can also be synthesized from the amino acid tryptophan.
- Pantothenic acid participates in many aspects of cell metabolism and is found in a wide variety of foods. Deficiency is unlikely.
- Biotin takes part in glucose and fatty acid synthesis, and ushers the carbon skeletons of certain amino acids into the energy-producing pathways. A deficiency results in skin changes. Biotin can be found in eggs, cheese, and peanuts and is synthesized in the intestine to some degree by bacteria.
- Vitamin B-6 participates in amino acid metabolism, neurotransmitter synthesis, and other metabolic functions. A deficiency may result in headaches, anemia, nausea, and vomiting, whereas megadoses may result in the destruction of nervous system tissues. Vitamin B-6 is found in animal protein foods, cauliflower, and broccoli.
- Folate is essential for DNA synthesis. Deficiency can result in defective red blood cell division, inflammation of the tongue, diarrhea, and poor growth. Such deficiency symptoms are most likely to occur with alcoholism. Because folate needs increase with pregnancy and folate likely prevents a type of birth defect, the government is currently requiring grain fortification with a synthetic form (folic acid). Folate can be found in green leafy vegetables, organ meats, legumes, and fortified cereals.
- Vitamin B-12 is needed for metabolizing folate and maintaining normal nerve function. A deficiency results in nerve destruction and a form of anemia. Vitamin B-12 is widely available in animal foods; deficient status may be found in older adults, vegans, and people with AIDS.
- Vitamin C aids in the formation of connective tissue, enhances iron absorption, and is needed for the synthesis of several hormones and neurotransmitters. Deficiency leads to scurvy, which is evidenced by fatigue, poor wound healing, pinpoint hemorrhages in the skin, and bleeding gums. Fresh fruits and vegetables, especially citrus fruits, are good sources. Too much vitamin C can lead to diarrhea and other gastrointestinal problems in some people.
- Choline forms part of lecithin, and has other functions in the body. Choline is widely distributed in foods and synthesized in the body, but apparently not in sufficient quantities to meet the needs in all stages of human life.
- A variety of vitamin-like compounds are found in the body. Cells synthesize them using common building blocks, such as amino acids and glucose. In disease states, synthesis may not meet needs, making dietary intake more critical.
- Cancer develops through three stages: initiation, promotion, and progression. Throughout these stages, diet plays a part in both the prevention and facilitation of the disease. Eating fruits, vegetables, whole grains, fish, and low-fat or fat-free dairy products and avoiding excess fat, alcohol, and energy intake currently form the best dietary advice for preventing cancer.

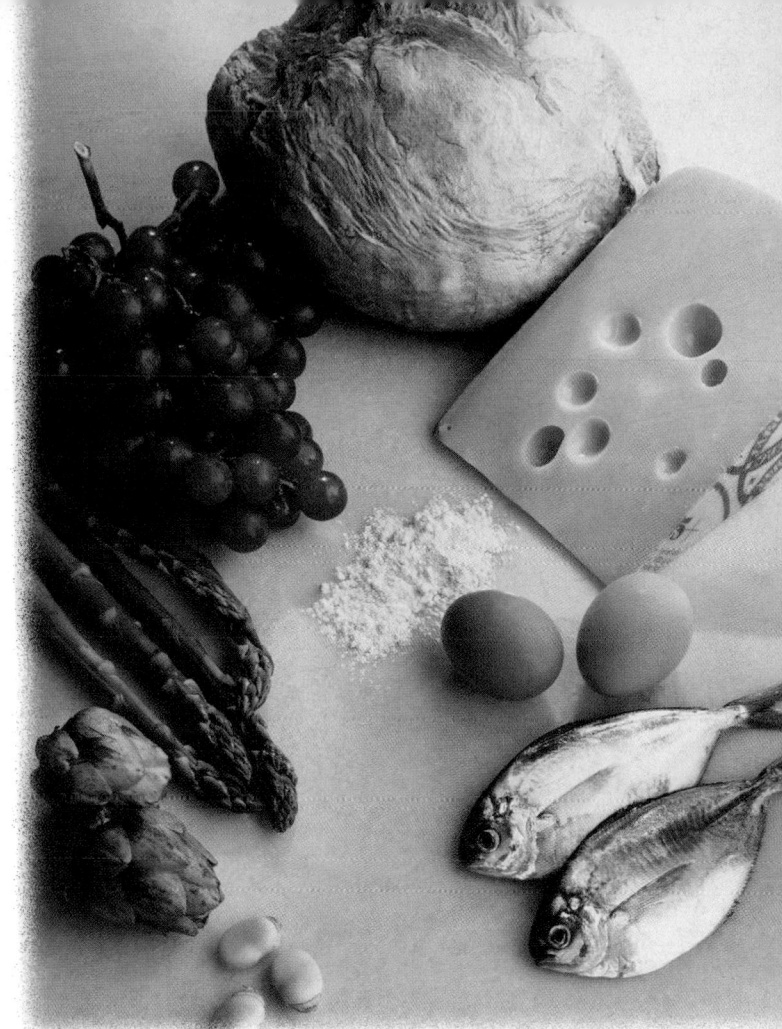

CASE SCENARIO

Suzanne and Ted are expecting their first child. Prior to conception, Ted (who completed one university-level nutrition course) has been trying to persuade Suzanne to eat a folate-rich breakfast cereal or take a multivitamin-mineral supplement every morning. Ted is concerned because Suzanne's sister gave birth to a child with spina bifida last year. Suzanne doesn't like to be hassled about her eating habits but admits her diet is "awful." Breakfast is usually a sweet pastry and coffee, lunch is whatever snack is available from a vending machine, and dinner is frequently eaten at a fast-food restaurant. She consumes no more than one or two servings of fruits and vegetables per day.

Her first visit to the obstetrician has her worried about the health of her fetus. Should she and Ted be concerned?

REFRESH YOUR MEMORY

As you begin your study of the water-soluble vitamins, you will want to review

- Energy metabolism, especially glycolysis, the citric acid cycle, and the electron transport chain in Chapter 4
- Oxidation-reduction reactions in Chapter 4
- The metabolism of carbohydrates in Chapter 5
- Amino acid metabolism with respect to deamination and transamination, as well as the link between DNA and protein synthesis in Chapter 7

GENERAL PROPERTIES OF THE WATER-SOLUBLE VITAMINS

For most of human history, diseases such as scurvy, beriberi, pellagra, and pernicious anemia caused enormous suffering and death. Early in the twentieth century, scientists began to recognize that these illnesses were caused by the absence of certain vital substances from the diet—now called the B-vitamins and vitamin C. It was soon discovered that restoring these vitamins to the diet dramatically reverses these deficiency diseases if done before significant deterioration of the body takes place.

The second vitamin to be discovered was designated vitamin B, according to the letter convention discussed in Chapter 9. This water-soluble substance, which can cure **beriberi,** was initially thought to be a single chemical compound. When subsequent research showed that this substance actually consists of several compounds, named the B-vitamins, numbers were added to the letter B to distinguish them. Of the eight B-vitamins, only two are still commonly referred to by letter and number: vitamins B-6 and B-12. The others now are usually referred to by the following names: thiamin (previously B-1), riboflavin (previously B-2), niacin (previously B-3), pantothenic acid, biotin, and folate. The older designations are sometimes used on vitamin supplement labels.

In their coenzyme forms, B-vitamins serve as carriers of specific ions or chemical groups, in turn allowing highly coordinated metabolic pathways in a cell to proceed (Fig. 10-1). All the eight B-vitamins participate in energy metabolism; some also have other roles in the chemical reactions that take place within cells. Although vitamin C does not function as a coenzyme, it plays a role in the synthesis of several important compounds in cells.

The B-vitamins are present in foods in their coenzyme forms bound to specific proteins. After ingestion, the bound vitamin coenzymes are released in the stomach and small intestine. The free vitamins are then absorbed in the small intestine.

Typically, about 50 to 90% of the B-vitamins in the diet are absorbed. Once inside cells, the coenzyme forms of the vitamins are resynthesized. Health-food stores sell the coenzyme forms of some vitamins, although they have no specific benefits to the consumer, since vitamins are not absorbed in this form.

Because they are water soluble, many of the B-vitamins and vitamin C are more easily excreted from the body than the fat-soluble vitamins. Moreover, some of the water-soluble vitamins are rather easily destroyed during cooking due to heat or alkalinity; all are subject to leaching into the cooking water. Retention of the B-vitamins and vitamin C is greatest in foods that are prepared by steaming, stir-frying, microwaving, or simmering in minimal moisture (see Table 9-1 in Chapter 9).

B-VITAMIN AND VITAMIN C STATUS OF NORTH AMERICANS

The nutritional status of most North Americans with respect to the B-vitamins and vitamin C is generally good. Typical diets in the United States contain plentiful and varied natural sources of these vitamins (Table 10-1). In addition, many common foods are fortified with one or more of the water-soluble vitamins. In some developing countries, however, deficiencies of the water-soluble vitamins are more common, and the resulting deficiency diseases pose significant public health problems. (A detailed discussion of nutritional deficiencies worldwide is presented in Chapter 20.)

Despite the generally good B-vitamin and vitamin C status of North Americans, marginal deficiencies of the water-soluble vitamins may occur among some North Americans and others in the Western world, especially older adults. The long-term

beriberi The thiamin-deficiency disorder characterized by muscle weakness, loss of appetite, nerve degeneration, and sometimes edema.

*A*nother group susceptible to B-vitamin deficiencies is alcoholics. The extremely unbalanced diets of some people with alcoholism, in combination with alcohol-induced alteration of vitamin absorption and metabolism, create a significant risk. Chapter 8 covered this topic in detail.

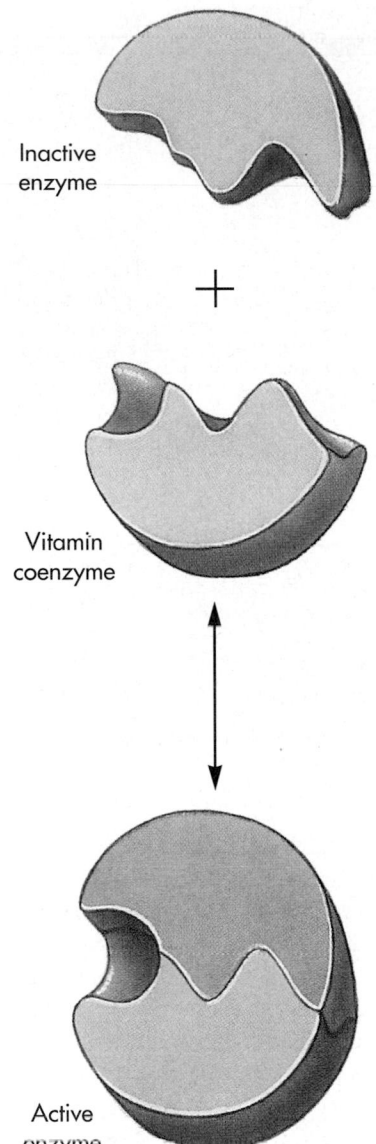

Inactive
enzyme

+

Vitamin
coenzyme

Active
enzyme

▋ **FIGURE 10-1** The Enzyme-coenzyme interaction. The B-vitamins form coenzymes,
which are compounds that enable specific
enzymes to function.
Illustration by William Ober.

effects of such marginal deficiencies are as yet unknown, but increased risk of heart disease, cancer, and cataracts of the eye is suspected. However, in the short run, in most people such a marginal deficiency likely leads only to fatigue or other bothersome and unspecific signs and symptoms.

▋ ENRICHMENT AND FORTIFICATION OF FOODS WITH B-VITAMINS

In the milling of grains, the seeds are crushed and the germ, bran, and husk layers are removed. This process leaves just the starch-containing endosperm, which is used to make flour, bread, and cereal products. Since the discarded fractions are rich in many nutrients, the time-honored milling process leads to loss of vitamins and minerals.

To counteract this nutrient loss, bread and cereal products made from milled grains are enriched with four B-vitamins—thiamin, riboflavin, niacin, and folate—and with the mineral iron. This enrichment program, which began in the 1940s in

---

TABLE 10-1   Sample Meal Plan That Meets B-Vitamin and Vitamin C Needs

Breakfast
Hard-cooked egg, 1
Low-fat toasted oat cereal, 1 cup
Nonfat milk, ¾ cup
Orange juice, 1 cup

Snack
Granola bar, 1

Lunch
Bagel sandwich
   Whole-wheat bagel, 1
   Ham, 2 slices
   Lettuce, 1 leaf
   Mustard, 2 tsp
Celery, 3 stalks
Peanut butter, 3 tbsp
Pretzels, ½ oz
Apple, 1
Nonfat milk, 1 cup

Snack
Cheese, 2 oz and crackers, 6
Low-fat yogurt, ½ cup

Dinner
Hamburger
   Hamburger bun
   Ground beef patty, 3 oz
   Ketchup, 2 tsp
   Mustard, 2 tsp
French fries, 3 oz
Salad
   Lettuce, 1 cup
   Shredded carrots, 2 tbsp
   Cauliflower, ¼ cup
   Broccoli, ¼ cup
   Low-calorie Italian dressing, 2 tbsp

Snack
Fat-free pudding snack, 1

This sample plan provides approximately 2200 kcal, roughly the minimum amount of energy needed for an active college student.

---

the United States with all the nutrients listed except folate, has helped protect North Americans from the common deficiency diseases associated with a dietary lack of the added nutrients. (Folate fortification began in 1998.) This process, however, still leaves the products with less vitamin B-6, vitamin E, magnesium, and zinc than that present in the whole grains. This is one reason nutrition experts advocate the regular consumption of whole-grain products, such as whole-wheat bread, rather than just consuming enriched grain products.

THIAMIN

Thiamin consists of a central carbon, to which is attached a six-member nitrogen-containing ring and a five-member sulfur-containing ring. The name comes from *thio*, meaning "sulfur," and *amine*, referring to the nitrogen groups in the molecule. In modern spelling, the *e* is dropped from the word.

The chemical bond between each ring and the central carbon in thiamin is easily broken by prolonged exposure to heat (overcooked foods), thus destroying the functions of the vitamin. This is also true if food is cooked in alkaline solutions (pH > 8.0). Sometimes baking soda is added to the water in which fresh green beans are cooked to retain their bright green color; this practice is not recommended.

■ Absorption, Transport, Metabolism, and Excretion of Thiamin

Thiamin is absorbed mainly in the jejunum by a carrier-mediated system, requiring the phosphorylation of the vitamin, and by passive diffusion at higher concentrations. It is transported in the blood and by red blood cells. Since storage is poor, any excess is promptly excreted in the urine.

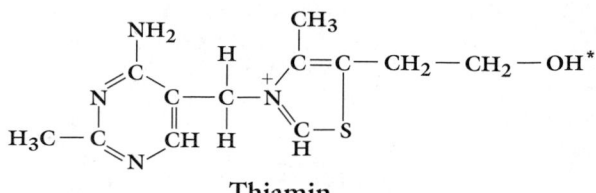

Thiamin

Thiamin has two phosphate groups added here (red asterisk) to form the coenzyme thiamin pyrophosphate (TPP).

■ Functions of Thiamin

Thiamin functions as the coenzyme thiamin pyrophosphate (TPP) in the metabolism of carbohydrates and branched-chain amino acids (leucine, isoleucine, and valine) (Fig. 10-2). In its coenzyme form, thiamin is the biologically active part of several enzyme systems. It functions in oxidative **decarboxylation** of **alpha keto acids** and in the action of the enzyme **transketolase**. The decarboxylation reaction removes a carboxyl group ($-\overset{\overset{\text{O}}{\|}}{\text{C}}-\text{OH}$) from a substrate and releases it as carbon dioxide. Several amino acids can undergo oxidative decarboxylation with the aid of TPP. The conversion of pyruvate to acetyl-CoA is one example; this is a critical step in the aerobic metabolism of glucose.[25]

decarboxylation The action of removing one molecule of carbon dioxide from a carboxylic acid.

alpha keto acids The breakdown product of several amino acids.

transketolase An enzyme whose functional component is TPP (thiamin pyrophosphate); it converts glucose to pentose sugars.

Thiamin as TPP

$$\text{Glucose} \longrightarrow \text{Pyruvate} \xrightarrow[\hspace{1cm}\text{CO}_2\hspace{1cm}]{\overset{\text{CoA} \quad \text{NAD} \quad \text{NADH + H}^+}{}} \text{Acetyl-CoA} \longrightarrow \begin{array}{c}\text{Citric}\\\text{acid cycle}\end{array}$$

In addition to thiamin, the other coenzymes that participate in this step are all B-vitamins; pantothenic acid (CoA), niacin (nicotinamide adenine dinucleotide), and riboflavin. This step will deliver acetyl-CoA to the citric acid cycle.

In the citric acid cycle, TPP converts the intermediate compound, alpha-ketoglutarate, to succinyl CoA in a second oxidative decarboxylation step.

Thiamin as TPP

$$\text{Alpha-ketoglutarate} \xrightarrow[\hspace{1cm}\text{CO}_2\hspace{1cm}]{\overset{\text{CoA} \quad \text{NAD} \quad \text{NADH + H}^+}{}} \text{Succinyl-CoA}$$

*I*n November 1996, the United States began to experience a shortage of multivitamins for total parenteral nutrition feedings. Patients who did not receive adequate thiamin for more than 7 days developed lactic acidosis, as pyruvate could not be converted to acetyl-CoA. Instead, the pyruvate was turned into lactate.

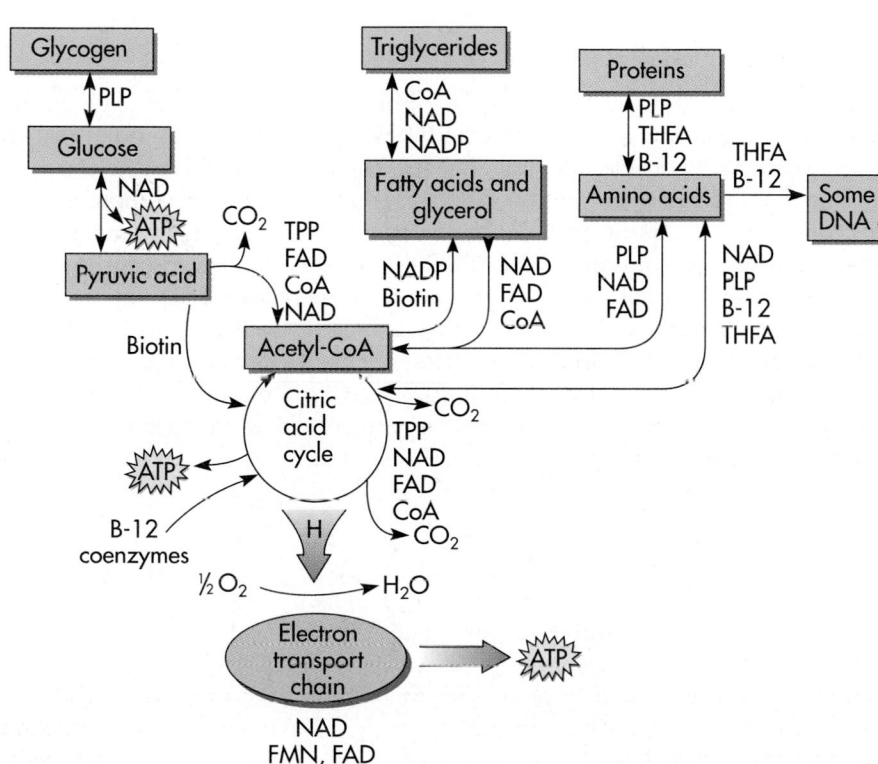

■ FIGURE 10-2 Many metabolic pathways, including those involved in energy metabolism, use coenzyme forms of the B-vitamins: thiamin as Thiamin Pyrophosphate TPP; riboflavin as Flavin Adenine Dinucleotide (FAD) and Flavin Mononucleotide (FMN); niacin as Nicotinamide Adenine Dinucleotide (NAD) and Nicotinamide Adenine Dinucleotide Phosphate (NADP); pantothenic acid as Coenzyme A; Vitamin B-6 as pyridoxal phosphate (PLP); and folate as Tetrahydrofolic Acid (THF). Vitamin B-12 exists in two coenzyme forms. Biotin exists as a cofactor. Other, minor pathways associated with energy metabolism also exist but are not depicted in this figure.

Several amino acids also can undergo oxidative decarboxylation with the aid of TPP.

Transketolase is the TPP-dependant enzyme responsible for the formation of the five-carbon sugar components of RNA and DNA from the six-carbon glucose using a series of reactions called the pentose phosphate pathway. The amount of transketolase activity in the red blood cell is a functional test for thiamin status. TPP also plays a role in nerve function. It may aid in the synthesis of neurotransmitters and participate in the conduction of nerve impulses. It seems to be involved in impulse conduction related to peripheral nerves.

■ Thiamin-Deficiency Diseases

The classic thiamin-deficiency disease, beriberi, has afflicted rice-eating populations for centuries. If little besides polished rice is eaten for weeks at a time, the disease develops.

Beriberi

In Sinhalese, the language spoken by the inhabitants of Sri Lanka, the word *beriberi* means "I can't, I can't." This is because thiamin-deficient individuals are very weak due to impaired function of the cardiovascular, muscular, nervous, and gastrointestinal systems.

The clinical signs of thiamin deficiency include anorexia, weight loss, apathy, loss of short-term memory, confusion, irritability, **peripheral neuropathy** and muscle weakness. There are two distinct types of beriberi: wet and dry. In wet beriberi, in addition to peripheral neuropathy, edema occurs along with an enlarged heart and congestive heart failure. In dry beriberi, there is also peripheral neuropathy, plus extreme muscle wasting. In infants, the disease presents as cardiac failure, which may occur very suddenly. In countries such as the United States and Canada, thiamin deficiency is associated with alcoholism.

Functions that are associated with the central nervous system are often quick to exhibits signs of thiamin deficiency. This is because neurons (nerve cells) rely primarily on glucose for energy, and the ultimate conversion of pyruvate to CO_2 and H_2O, yielding ATP, is dependant on thiamin. The clinical signs can be observed in only 7 days on a thiamin-free diet.

Wernicke-Korsakoff Syndrome

The thiamin-deficiency disease found primarily in Western countries such as the United States and Canada among people with heavy alcohol consumption is called Wernicke-Korsakoff syndrome. Alcoholics have a triple problem related to thiamin. Alcohol diminishes thiamin absorption, alcohol increases thiamin excretion, and alcoholics consume such a poor quality diet that there may be few, if any, vitamins in the foods and beverages consumed. Since the vitamin is not readily stored, the symptoms can occur rapidly. Ocular motor signs; **ataxia**, a staggering gait; and deranged mental functions characterize it. The ocular signs include double vision, cross eyes, and **nystagmus.** The disorientation, listlessness, memory loss, and other symptoms, including alcohol withdrawal, are due to lesions in the brain. Not all alcoholics experience Wernicke-Korsakoff syndrome, so it is assumed that there must be a genetic predisposition to the disease.

■ Thiamin in Foods

Thiamin is found in a wide variety of foods, although generally in a small amount. Major individual contributors of thiamin to our diets are white bread and rolls, crackers, pork, hot dogs, luncheon meats, ready-to-eat cereals, and orange juice. White bread, bakery products, and cereals are usually enriched with thiamin.

Foods with a very high nutrient density for thiamin (mg/kcal) are pork products, sunflower seeds, legumes, wheat germ, and watermelon. Whole grains and enriched grains, green beans, asparagus, organ meats (such as liver), peanuts and other seeds,

When physicians see a person suffering from unexplained delirium in the emergency room, they must consider whether it may be caused by a thiamin deficiency related to alcoholism. The treatment is an injection of thiamin. Dietary supplementation will not suffice because thiamin is absorbed slowly, especially in a person with alcoholism.

peripheral neuropathy Impaired sensory, motor, and reflex functions, affecting arms and legs and causing calf muscle tenderness and difficulty in rising from a squatting position.

ataxia An inability to coordinate muscle activity during voluntary movement; incoordination.

nystagmus Involuntary, rapid rhythmic movement of the eyeball.

and mushrooms also are good sources. Overall, enriched, fortified, and whole-grain products make the greatest contribution of thiamin to the diet of the U.S. adult population.

Many foods—especially meat (except pork), milk and milk products, seafood, and most fruits—contain very little thiamin. Some fish and shellfish contain an enzyme called thiaminase, which destroys thiamin. Fortunately, cooking destroys the thiaminase. Eating a variety of foods in line with the Food Guide Pyramid is the most reliable way to obtain sufficient thiamin from a diet (Fig. 10-3).

■ Thiamin Needs

The activity of transketolase in red blood cells is regarded as the best test for thiamin status.[21] For this reason, it has been used to establish the RDA, along with urinary excretion of the vitamin. The Estimated Average Requirement is 1.0 mg/day for men and 0.9 mg/day for women. Increasing this by 20% to account for individual variability sets the RDA. The RDA for thiamin for men and women 19 to 70+ years is approximately 1.2 mg/day and 1.1 mg/day, respectively (refer to the inside cover of this text for vitamin recommendations for other age groups).

Recent national surveys indicate that the average daily intake for thiamin in the United States for young men is close to 2 mg per day. For young women, it is approximately 1.2 mg/day. Canadian studies show a slightly lower intake.

There appears to be no adverse effects with excess intake of thiamin from food or supplements. Thus, there is no Upper Level for this nutrient.

Dietary Sources of Thiamin

Food Item and Amount	Thiamin (mg)
Pork chop, 4 oz	0.9
Soy milk, 8 oz	0.7
Brewer's yeast, 2 tbsp	0.6
Wheat germ, ¼ cup	0.5
Ham slices, 2 oz	0.5
Canadian bacon, 2 oz	0.5
Baked acorn squash, 1 cup	0.4
Peanuts, ¼ cup	0.3
Orange juice, 8 oz	0.2
Vegetarian baked beans, ½ cup	0.2

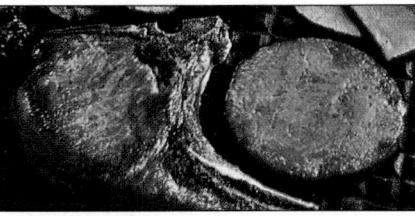

Pork is a nutrient-dense source of thiamin.

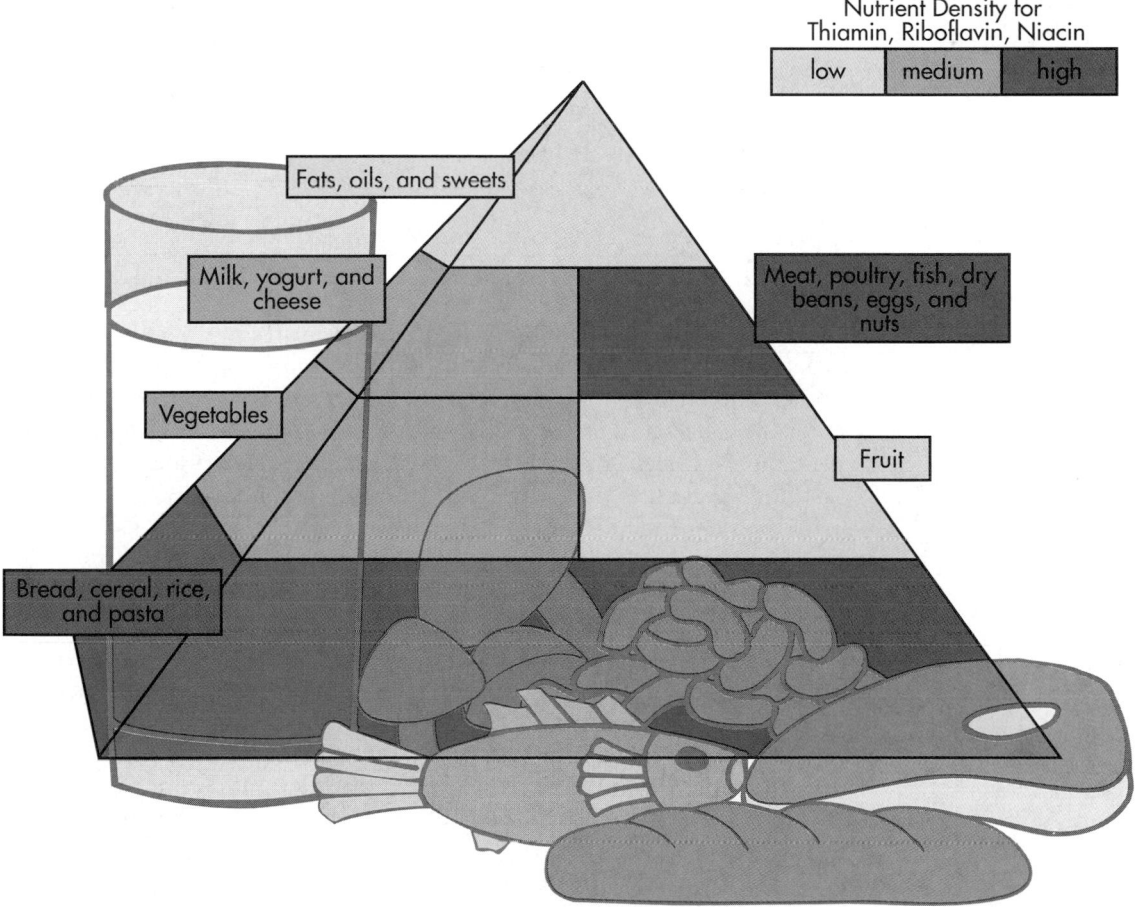

Nutrient Density for Thiamin, Riboflavin, Niacin

| low | medium | high |

Fats, oils, and sweets

Milk, yogurt, and cheese

Meat, poultry, fish, dry beans, eggs, and nuts

Vegetables

Fruit

Bread, cereal, rice, and pasta

■ **FIGURE 10-3** Food sources of thiamin, riboflavin, and niacin from the Food Guide Pyramid. The meat, poultry, fish, dry beans, eggs, and nuts group and the bread, cereal, rice, and pasta group are especially rich sources of these nutrients. The milk, yogurt, and cheese group is especially rich in riboflavin. The background color of each food group indicates the average nutrient density for the nutrients in that group.

CRITICAL THINKING

Gary suffers from alcoholism and pays no attention to his diet. In addition to the detrimental effects on the liver, excess alcohol consumption can cause deficiencies in certain B-vitamins. Explain why this can occur.

■ North Americans at Risk for Thiamin Deficiency

Some groups of people, such as the poor and older adults, barely meet their need for thiamin. Otherwise, very few North Americans are at risk for thiamin deficiency. Thiamin deficiency is mainly found in association with chronic alcoholism.

■ RIBOFLAVIN

Riboflavin contains three linked six-membered rings, with a sugar alcohol attached to the middle ring. The name comes from its yellow color (*flavin* means "yellow" in Latin). Riboflavin is a component of two coenzymes: flavin mononucleotide (FMN) and flavin adenine dinucleotide (FAD). The coenzyme forms are present in many foods; the free vitamin is found in milk and enriched grain products. All these forms can be used to meet the body's needs for riboflavin.[14]

■ Absorption, Transport, Metabolism, and Excretion of Riboflavin

In the stomach, HCl releases riboflavin from its bound forms. Absorption is via active or facilitated transport in the small intestine. At very high intakes, it is absorbed passively. The degree of absorption increases with intake. In the blood, riboflavin is transported by protein carriers. Riboflavin is converted to its coenzyme forms, FMN and FAD, in most tissues, but mainly in the small intestine, liver, heart, and kidney. A small amount of riboflavin is stored in the liver; any excess is excreted in the urine. For people who take excessive amounts in supplement form, riboflavin imparts a bright yellow color to the urine.

■ Functions of Riboflavin

The enzyme succinate dehydrogenase is an FAD-containing enzyme that accepts hydrogens from succinate to form fumarate during the citric acid cycle. The hydrogens are then passed on to the electron transport chain.

$$\text{Succinate} \xrightarrow{\quad FAD \quad\quad FADH_2 \quad} \text{Fumarate}$$

Another FAD-containing coenzyme participates in the breakdown of fatty acids (beta oxidation) to acetyl-CoA, the entry compound for the citric acid cycle. The other riboflavin-containing coenzyme, FMN, shuttles hydrogen ions and electrons into the electron transport chain. Still other FAD-containing enzymes help form the vitamin B-6 coenzyme and convert the amino acid tryptophan to the B-vitamin niacin. Metabolism of the oxidized form of glutathione (GSSG) to the reduced form (GSH) is dependent on the FAD-requiring enzyme glutathione reductase. (See Fig. 9-11 in Chapter 9). This reaction is used to assess riboflavin status.

■ Riboflavin Deficiency

The signs and symptoms associated with a pure riboflavin deficiency (technically, called **ariboflavinosis**) include inflammation of the tongue (glossitis), cracking of tissue around the corners of the mouth (cheilosis), seborrheic dermatitis (a disease of the sebaceous glands of the skin), inflammation of the mouth (stomatitis) and throat, various eye and nervous system disorders, and confusion (Fig. 10-4). The first evidence of a deficiency is inflammation of the mouth and tongue. The complete picture of a deficiency develops after approximately 2 months on a riboflavin-deficient diet (consuming one-fourth of the RDA). Diseases such as cancer, cardiac disease, and diabetes also are known to precipitate or worsen riboflavin deficiency. However, a deficiency disease associated with an isolated lack of dietary riboflavin is rarely seen in otherwise healthy people. Because riboflavin functions along with

Riboflavin (oxidized)

Riboflavin (reduced)

For riboflavin, the italicized *R* denotes H in the free vitamin; phosphate in FMN; and an adenine dinucleotide in FAD. In the reduced form of riboflavin, the hydrogens are shown in red in this figure.

other B-vitamins (e.g., vitamin B-6, niacin, thiamin, and folate) in numerous metabolic pathways, some symptoms ascribed to riboflavin deficiency are actually caused by the failure of metabolic pathways associated with a lack of other nutrients. And, as already noted, this assortment of B-vitamins, such as riboflavin, thiamin, and niacin, is often found in the same foods.

■ Riboflavin in Foods

One-quarter of the riboflavin in our diets comes from milk products. The milk, yogurt, and cheese group of the Food Guide Pyramid is the major contributor of riboflavin to the diet. The rest of our riboflavin intake typically comes from enriched white bread, rolls, and crackers, as well as eggs and meat (review Fig. 10-3).[21] The most nutrient-dense sources of riboflavin (mg/kcal) are liver, mushrooms, spinach and other green leafy vegetables, broccoli, asparagus, low-fat and nonfat milk, and cottage cheese.

Exposure to light (ultraviolet radiation) causes riboflavin to break down rapidly. To prevent this light-induced breakdown, paper and plastic cartons—not glass—are used in packaging riboflavin-rich foods, such as milk, milk products, and cereals.

■ Riboflavin Needs

The most commonly used method for assessing riboflavin status involves the determination of erythrocyte (red blood cell) glutathione reductase activity and urinary riboflavin excretion. These data are used to establish the Estimated Average Requirement of 1.1 mg/day for men and 0.9 mg/day for women 19 and older. The RDA is set by increasing this amount by 20% to account for individual variability. Therefore, the RDA for men is 1.3 mg/day and for women 1.1 mg/day. Based on recent survey data, Canadians and Americans have an intake of approximately 2.1 mg/day for men and 1.5 mg/day for women.[21]

There appears to be no adverse effects from consuming large amounts of riboflavin due to limited absorption and rapid excretion via the urine and, so, there is no Upper Level.

■ North Americans at Risk for Riboflavin Deficiency

Although riboflavin deficiencies are rare, some people consume amounts that are barely adequate. Marginal intakes are most likely seen in those who do not consume milk or milk products. Such people would be wise to search for another plentiful dietary source of riboflavin, such as enriched breads and breakfast cereals. Alcoholics risk a riboflavin deficiency because they often eat a very nutrient-deficient diet. Long-term use of phenobarbital may also compromise riboflavin status, as this drug produces metabolic changes in the liver that increase the breakdown of the vitamin.

Dietary Sources of Riboflavin

Food Item and Amount	Riboflavin (mg)
Fried beef liver, 1 oz	1.2
Steamed oysters, 10	1.1
Brewer's yeast, 2 tbsp	0.7
Low-fat yogurt, 1 cup	0.5
Braunschweiger sausage, 1	0.4
Milk, 8 oz	0.4
Buttermilk, 8 oz	0.4
Cooked spinach, 1 cup	0.3
Raw mushrooms, 1 cup	0.3
Hard cooked egg, 1	0.3

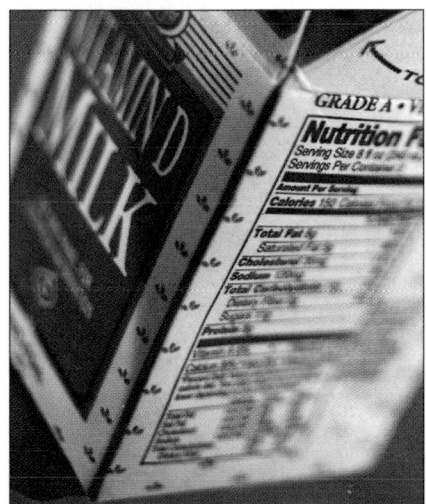

Milk is a good source of many vitamins, including riboflavin.

■ NIACIN

The B-vitamin niacin actually exists in two forms—nicotinic acid (niacin) and nicotinamide (niacinamide). In the body, both forms of the vitamin perform the functions attributed to niacin. The two coenzyme forms of niacin are nicotinamide adenine dinucleotide (NAD) and nicotinamide adenine dinucleotide phosphate (NADP).[3]

■ Absorption, Transport, Storage, and Excretion of Niacin

Nicotinic acid and nicotinamide are readily absorbed from the stomach and the intestine by active transport and passive diffusion, so that almost all niacin consumed is absorbed. Niacin is transported from the liver to all tissues, where it is converted to its coenzyme forms, NAD and NADP. These forms can be stored in the liver. Any excess niacin is excreted as a variety of metabolic products.

Nicotinic acid

Oxidized

Reduced

Coenzyme forms using nicotinamide

The two coenzyme forms of niacin, NAD and NADP, contain nicotinamide linked to adenine dinucleotide or adenine dinucleotide phosphate, indicated by the italicized *R*. Both coenzymes undergo oxidation and reduction by loss or addition of an electron and a hydrogen (red) in this figure.

■ Functions of Niacin

Like the coenzyme forms of riboflavin, the coenzyme forms of niacin, NAD and NADP, are active participants in oxidation-reduction reactions. The niacin coenzymes function in at least 200 reactions in cellular metabolic pathways, especially those used to produce ATP. NAD participates in catabolic reactions, acting as an electron and hydrogen ion acceptor in glycolysis (the conversion of glucose to pyruvate) and the citric acid cycle. Under anaerobic conditions, the resulting reduced form, NADH + H^+, is used in converting pyruvate to lactate, thereby regenerating NAD.

Glucose to Pyruvate

$$\text{Glucose} \xrightarrow{\quad 2\,ADP \quad 2\,Pi \quad 2NAD \quad 2NADH + H^+ \quad} 2\ \text{Pyruvate}$$

2 ATP

The Citric Acid Cycle

$$\text{Isocitrate} \xrightarrow{\quad NAD \quad NADH + H^+ \quad} \text{Alpha-ketoglutarate}$$

$$\text{Alpha-ketogluterate} \xrightarrow{\quad NAD \quad NADH + H^+ \quad} \text{Succinyl CoA}$$

$$\text{Malate} \xrightarrow{\quad NAD \quad NADH + H^+ \quad} \text{Oxaloacetate}$$

Pyruvate to Lactate

$$\text{Pyruvate} \xrightarrow{\quad NAD \quad NADH + H^+ \quad} \text{Lactate}$$

Under aerobic conditions, NADH also donates an electron and hydrogen to other acceptor molecules in the electron-transport chain.

Electron-Transport Chain

$$\text{NADH} + H^+ \quad NAD$$
$$2\ H^+ + 2e^- + \tfrac{1}{2}\,O_2 \longrightarrow H_2O$$

Alcohol dehydrogenase also uses NAD to convert alcohol to acetaldehyde (see Chapter 8).

Synthetic pathways in the cell—those that make new compounds—use NADPH + H^+. This coenzyme is important in the biochemical pathway for fatty-acid synthesis. Cells that synthesize a lot of fatty acids (e.g., those in the liver and female mammary glands) have higher concentrations of NADPH + H^+ than cells not involved in fatty-acid synthesis (e.g., muscle cells).

■ Niacin Deficiency: Pellagra

The first official record of the niacin-deficiency disease, pellagra, was made by Spanish physician Casal in 1735. It was named *mal de la rosa*, or "red sickness." The typical red rash appears in areas exposed to sunlight, especially around the neck, which is today called "Casal's necklace." Later the disease was renamed *pellagra* (from Italian *pelle*, meaning "skin," and *agra*, meaning "rough.")

Since almost every metabolic pathway uses either NAD or NADP, it is not surprising that a niacin deficiency causes widespread damage in the body. The effects of pellagra are known as the three *D*s—dementia, diarrhea, and dermatitis (Fig. 10-5). If the disease is not successfully treated, death (the fourth D) follows. Clinical

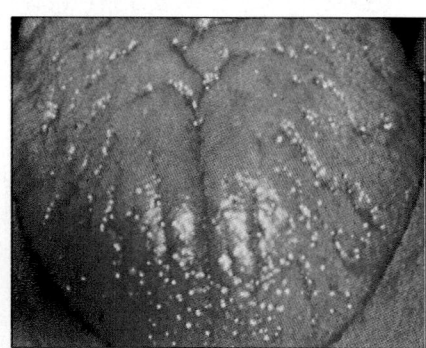

FIGURE 10-4 A painful, inflamed tongue (glossitis) can signal a deficiency of niacin, vitamin B-6, riboflavin, folate, or vitamin B-12. Often more than one deficiency is the cause. Since other medical conditions can also cause glossitis, further evaluation is needed before a nutrient deficiency can be diagnosed.

evidence of pellagra develops 50 to 60 days after instituting a niacin-deficient diet. Early symptoms include diminished appetite, weight loss, and weakness.

Pellagra is the only dietary deficiency disease ever to reach epidemic proportions in the United States. During the early 1900s, cases of pellagra increased dramatically in the southeastern region of the country, where corn—a poor source of naturally available niacin and the amino acid tryptophan—was being increasingly used as a primary component of the diet. More than 10,000 Americans died of pellagra in 1915. From the end of World War I until the end of World War II, an estimated 200,000 Americans suffered from the disease. So many had such severe dementia that they were forced to live out their lives in mental institutions.

Two discoveries were crucial to breaking the epidemic: In the 1920s, high-protein diets were found to prevent pellagra, and, in the 1930s, insufficient niacin intake was shown to cause the disease. The introduction of niacin-enriched grains in 1941 and improved intake of dietary protein resulting from wartime prosperity led to the rapid disappearance of pellagra in the United States. The ability of high-protein diets to cure pellagra was finally explained in 1948, when researchers demonstrated that the amino acid tryptophan was converted into niacin in the body. Pellagra is still found today throughout Southeast Asia and Africa among populations whose diets lack sufficient protein and niacin.

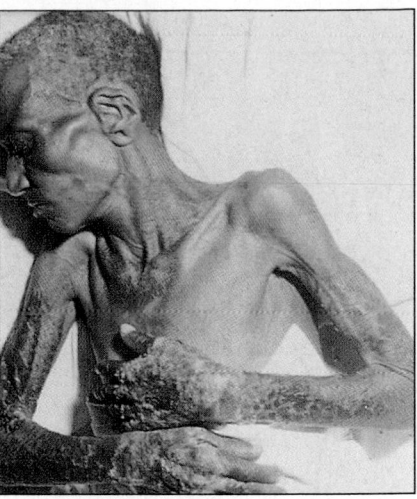

◼ FIGURE 10-5 The dermatitis of pellegra. Dermatitis on both sides of the body (bilateral) is a typical symptom of pellagra. Sun exposure worsens the condition.

◼ Niacin in Foods

About 25% of the preformed niacin in U.S. diets comes from mixed dishes that include meat, fish, and poultry and from poultry alone. Another 11% comes from bread and bread products. In the United States, milled grain products have been fortified with niacin in a form that is much more bioavailable than the natural form. If on a high-tryptophan intake, a greater proportion of the tryptophan is available for conversion to niacin, since needs for protein synthesis are met. For most people, about half or more of niacin needs are supplied by the body's synthesis of niacin from tryptophan, but there is substantial individual differences in conversion efficiency. The number of milligrams of niacin supplied by dietary protein can be estimated by dividing dietary protein intake (in grams) by 6. For example, if one consumes 90 grams of protein, the body will synthesize about 15 mg of niacin. Coffee and tea contribute a little niacin to the diet. Unlike some other water-soluble vitamins, niacin is very heat stable, and little is lost in cooking. The most nutrient-dense sources of niacin (mg/kcal) are mushrooms, wheat bran, tuna (as well as other fish), chicken, turkey, asparagus, and peanuts (review Fig. 10-3).

Animal proteins (except gelatin) are especially rich in tryptophan. Since food composition tables list only preformed niacin, they can underestimate the total niacin supplied by protein foods. For example, although eggs and milk lack niacin, they contain abundant tryptophan and thus indirectly contribute substantial amounts of niacin.

Considering the link between corn as a staple food and pellagra, you might be surprised to learn that the niacin content of corn is similar to that of rice and considerably higher than that of most other vegetables. However, the niacin in corn is marginally absorbed because it is tightly bound by a protein. Soaking corn in an alkaline solution, such as lime water (calcium hydroxide dissolved in water), releases bound niacin, rendering it more usable by the body. Look for evidence of this form of processing on the label when you buy corn-meal products, such as tortillas. Because this practice was common among native peoples of Mexico and Central and South America, they did not suffer from pellagra. Early Spanish explorers of the New World took corn—a crop native to the Americas—back to Europe, but they were unaware of the importance of soaking corn in lime water. Thus, as the use of corn as a staple spread in Europe, pellagra became widespread during the 1700s. In contrast, Spanish settlers in Latin America learned from the native populations to soak corn meal in lime water before using it in cooking. The Hispanic populations descended from these settlers continued this practice and rarely suffered from pellagra, whereas other Americans who used untreated corn as a staple often did.

A niacin deficiency also can result from deficiencies of other nutrients involved in the synthesis of niacin from tryptophan, such as riboflavin and vitamin B-6.

*D*ietary Sources of Niacin

Food Item and Amount	Niacin (NE mg)
Steak, 4 oz	5.6
Roast turkey, 3 oz	4.9
Roast chicken, 3 oz	4.8
Ground beef patty, 3 oz	4.5
Broiled halibut, 3 oz	4.2
Canned tuna, 3 oz	4.1
Salmon, 3 oz	4.0
Peanuts, ½ cup	3.1
Fried beef liver, 1 oz	1.8
Peanut butter, 2 tbsp	1.3

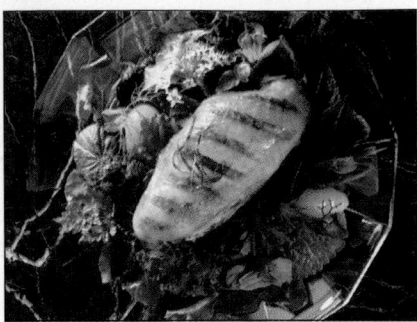

Chicken is a rich source of niacin. The tryptophan present can also be metabolized to niacin.

Niacin Needs

The RDA for niacin is expressed as niacin equivalents (NE) to account for niacin received preformed from the diet, as well as that synthesized from tryptophan. For adult men of all ages, the RDA is 16 mg of NE/day, and for adult women of all ages it is 14 mg of NE/day. The RDA was derived from an Estimated Average Requirement of 12 mg of NE/day for men and 11 mg of NE/day for women, increasing this by 30% to account for individual variability.[21] The primary criterion used to establish the RDA for niacin is the urinary excretion of N-methyl nicotinamide, a niacin metabolite, and other metabolites.

A recent study showed that the average intake of preformed niacin from food in the U.S. diet is approximately 28 mg for men and 18 mg for women. A combination of both food and typical supplement use totals 40 to 70 mg of NE/day, depending on age. In Canadian studies, the average intake of preformed niacin was approximately 41 mg for men and 28 mg for women.

As long as one follows a varied diet, developing a niacin deficiency is highly unlikely. About the only population groups to exhibit a niacin deficiency are people with rare disorders of tryptophan metabolism (e.g., Hartnup's disease), alcoholics, and those with diseases that greatly impair food intake.

Pharmacologic Use and Toxicity of Niacin

In 1955, it was discovered that very large doses of nicotinic acid reduce blood cholesterol. Consuming 1.5 to 2 g of nicotinic acid per day—about 75 to 100 times the RDA—can decrease LDL-cholesterol and increase HDL-cholesterol. When combined with diet, exercise, and other cholesterol-lowering drugs, megadoses of niacin can slow and even reverse the progression of atherosclerosis. Unfortunately, such megadose therapy may have adverse effects, including flushing of the skin (the initial adverse effect), itching, gastrointestinal upsets (such as nausea and vomiting), and liver damage. These effects (gastrointestinal disturbances and liver damage) have been observed at 3 g/day of nicotinamide and 1.5 g nicotinic acid per day. Some people experience symptoms at dosages as low as 50 mg/day. Because of the potential for side effects, megadose use must be supervised by a physician. The use of various medicinal forms of nicotonic acid and other medications can lessen the side effects. For example, premedication with aspirin reduces the flushing reactions.

Flushing from excess niacin intake was considered the most appropriate effect on which to base the Upper Level. For adults, this is 35 mg/day.

CONCEPT CHECK

The B-vitamins thiamin, niacin, and riboflavin function in various biochemical pathways used for the metabolism of glucose, amino acids, and fatty acids. Enriched grains are adequate sources of all three vitamins. Otherwise, pork is an excellent source of thiamin; milk is an excellent source of riboflavin; and protein foods in general are excellent sources of niacin. Deficiencies of all three vitamins can occur with alcoholism; of the three, a thiamin deficiency is the most likely. Only niacin leads to toxic effects when consumed in high doses.

PANTOTHENIC ACID

Pantothenic acid is part of coenzyme A (CoA). This coenzyme is formed when the vitamin combines with ADP and the amino acid cysteine. Cysteine provides the sulfur atom, which is the functional end of the coenzyme.

■ Functions of Pantothenic Acid

Coenzyme A is essential for the metabolism of carbohydrate, protein, alcohol, and fat. The formation of acetyl-CoA from the acetate that arises from their metabolism allows the two-carbon acetate to then enter the citric acid cycle. In another series of reactions, acetyl-CoA condenses with carbon dioxide to begin the synthesis of fatty acids:

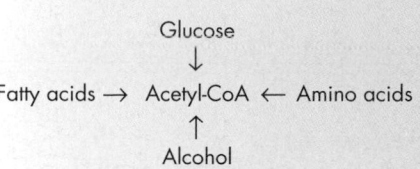

$$\text{Glucose}$$
$$\downarrow$$
$$\text{Fatty acids} \rightarrow \text{Acetyl-CoA} \leftarrow \text{Amino acids}$$
$$\uparrow$$
$$\text{Alcohol}$$

$$CO_2$$

Acetyl-CoA- - - - - - → Malonyl-CoA - - - - - → Fatty acid
2 carbons   3 carbons

Pantothenic acid also forms part of a compound called the *acyl carrier protein*. This protein attaches to fatty acids and shuttles them through the pathway designed to increase their chain length. Finally, pantothenic acid as coenzyme A also donates fatty acids to proteins in a process that can determine their location and function within a cell.[17, 21]

$$HO-CH_2-\underset{\underset{CH_3}{|}}{\overset{\overset{CH_3}{|}}{C}}-\overset{\overset{OH}{|}}{CH}-\overset{\overset{O}{||}}{C}-NH-CH_2-CH_2-\overset{\overset{O}{||}}{C}-OH$$

Pantothenic acid

$$RO-CH_2-\underset{\underset{CH_3}{|}}{\overset{\overset{CH_3}{|}}{C}}-\overset{\overset{OH}{|}}{CH}-\overset{\overset{O}{||}}{C}-NH-CH_2-CH_2-\overset{\overset{O}{||}}{C}\underset{\text{[}}{\underline{}}NH-CH_2-CH_2-SH$$

Coenzyme A (CoA)

Pantothenic acid is converted to coenzyme A by combining with a part of the amino acid cysteine (box) and with a derivative of adenosine diphosphate (ADP), indicated by the italicized R.

Pantothenic acid is so widely distributed in foods a naturally occurring deficiency has never been reported. The only way to induce a dietary deficiency is to consume a semisynthetic diet without the vitamin or to consume a pantothenic acid anti-vitamin.

■ Pantothenic Acid in Foods

The Greek word *pantothen*, meaning "from every side," reflects the ample supply of pantothenic acid in foods. Common sources include meat, milk, and many vegetables. Nutrient-dense sources of pantothenic acid (mg/kcal) are mushrooms, liver, peanuts, eggs, yeast, broccoli, and milk.

■ Pantothenic Acid Needs

For adults, the Adequate Intake set for pantothenic acid is 5 mg/day. (Recall that an Adequate Intake is an acceptable intake established by the Food and Nutrition Board for some nutrients for which insufficient data are available to set RDAs). There is no national representative estimate of intake of pantothenic acid from either food or supplements. The primary criterion used to estimate an Adequate Intake is the amount needed to replace urinary excretion.

A deficiency of pantothenic acid might occur in cases of alcoholism in which a very-nutrient-deficient diet is consumed. However, the effects would probably be hidden among deficiencies of thiamin, riboflavin, vitamin B-6, and folate, so the pantothenic acid deficiency might go unrecognized. There is no known toxicity for pantothenic acid, and so there is no Upper Limit.

*D*ietary Sources of Pantothenic Acid

Food Item and Amount	Pantothenic Acid (mg)
Sunflower seeds, 1/4 cup	2.3
Fried beef liver, 1 oz	1.7
Raw mushrooms, 1 cup	1.5
Brewer's yeast, 2 tbsp	1.4
Peanuts, 1/2 cup	1.3
Yogurt, 1 cup	1.2
Baked acorn squash, 1 cup	1.2
Roast chicken, 3 oz	0.8
Cooked broccoli, 1 cup	0.8
Milk, 8 oz	0.8

■ BIOTIN

Biotin is commonly found in two forms in foods: the free vitamin and the protein-bound coenzyme form, called biocytin. In the formation of biocytin, biotin forms a bond with the amino acid lysine in a protein. Biotin is absorbed from the small

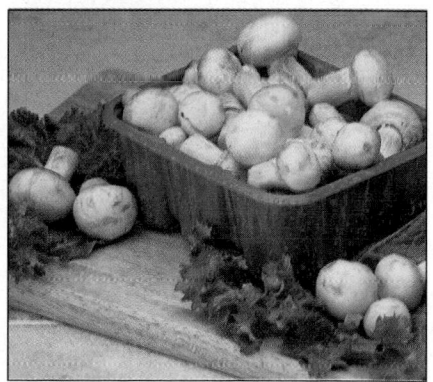

Mushrooms are a nutrient-dense source of pantothenic acid in the diet.

O
||
C
HN   NH
| |
HC——CH   O
| | ||
H₂C   C——CH₂—CH₂—CH₂—CH₂—C—OH
\   /   *
S   H

Biotin

The vitamin biotin attaches to a protein by formation of a bond between its carboxyl group (red asterisk) and lysine in a protein, yielding the bound cofactor form called biocytin.

intestine, whereas the biocytin form is not. The enzyme biotinidase, which is present in the small intestine, cleaves the bond linking biotin to a protein, releasing the free vitamin.[15]

About 1 in 60,000 infants is born with a genetic defect that leaves the infant with very low amounts of the enzyme biotinidase. Because the infant cannot break down biocytin to the absorbable free form, a biotin deficiency is likely to develop. If a deficiency is suspected, the infant is treated with 100 μg of biotin, which is about three times to our typical biotin needs.

■ Functions of Biotin

Biotin functions as an essential cofactor for four carboxylase enzymes, which covalently bind to biotin. Carboxylases add carbon dioxide to a substance. One biotin carboxylase catalyzes the carboxylation of acetyl-CoA to form malonyl-CoA (see the section on pantothenic acid for reaction). This reaction is the first step in the elongation of the carbon chain to form a fatty acid. Another biotin carboxylase reaction involves the addition of carbon dioxide to the three-carbon pyruvate to yield the 4-carbon oxaloacetate, an intermediate in the citric acid cycle. This reaction replenishes any lost oxaloacetate and, so, helps keep the citric acid cycle functioning. In the liver and kidney, oxaloacetate also can be converted to glucose when glucose supplies are running low, an initial step in gluconeogenesis.

$$ATP \quad CO_2$$

Pyruvate - - ➤ - - ➤ - - - ➤ Oxaloacetate - ┬ - - - - ➤ Glucose
3 carbons   4 carbons   └ - - ➤ Citric acid cycle
                    ADP + Pi

If biotin were missing, the citric acid cycle could not run effectively, resulting in a buildup of lactate, the anaerobic by-product of glycolysis. This event would be accompanied by a decrease in aerobic metabolism.

A third biotin-dependent carboxylase catalyzes the breakdown of the amino acid leucine, and a fourth allows the essential amino acids threonine, methionine, and isoleucine to be oxidized for energy via the citric acid cycle. Clearly, biotin is required for the metabolism of carbohydrates, amino acids, and fatty acids.

■ Sources of Biotin: Food and Microbial Synthesis

Biotin content of food has been determined for only a small number of foods, so foods containing biotin are not included in most food composition tables. Biotin is widely distributed in food but concentration varies considerably. For instance, liver contains approximately 100 μg of biotin/100 grams, whereas fruits and most meats contain only about 1 μg/100 grams.

It is likely that the intestinal synthesis of biotin by bacteria supplies at least part of our needs, as evidenced by the rather rare incidence of biotin deficiency. In fact, we excrete more biotin than we consume. However, questions remain about the actual bioavailability of the biotin synthesized by the intestinal bacteria, since this production takes place mostly in the large intestine, whereas biotin is most efficiently absorbed from the small intestine.

A protein called **avidin** in raw egg whites binds biotin and inhibits its absorption. Feeding many raw egg whites to animals leads to the classic "egg-white injury" deficiency disease. An occasional raw egg in eggnog is of no concern for this problem because it would take a regular daily consumption of 12 to 24 raw eggs to produce a biotin deficiency. Biotin deficiency resulting from consuming raw eggs has been reported, however, in people with alcoholism who eat as few as three raw eggs a day. These people probably exist on very deficient diets. The main concern about eating

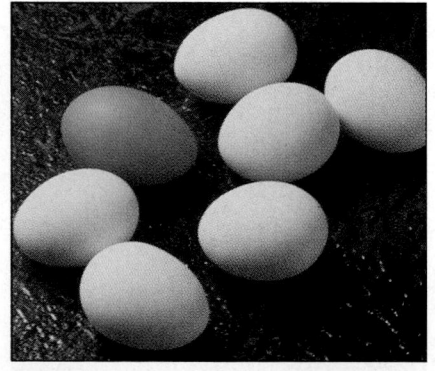

Egg yolks are one of the most nutrient-dense sources of biotin.

avidin A protein found in raw egg whites that can bind biotin and inhibit absorption; cooking destroys avidin.

raw eggs for healthy people is the risk of foodborne illness caused by *Salmonella* bacteria, which may contaminate eggs (see Chapter 19).

■ Biotin Needs

The Adequate Intake for biotin for adults of 30 µg/day is extrapolated from the intake seen in exclusively breastfed infants. The results of such an extrapolation likely overestimates the amount needed for adults because adults require biotin only for maintenance, not for growth.[21] One U.S. study of biotin intake estimated average intake in young women at 39 µg/day.[21] A similar Canadian study showed an estimated dietary intake of 62 µg/day.

There is no Upper Level for biotin.

■ North Americans at Risk for Biotin Deficiency

If undetected, a lack of biotinidase activity leads to a severe biotin deficiency in infants. Signs and symptoms may appear within a few months of life, beginning with a skin rash and hair loss. Other signs and symptoms include convulsions, other neurological disorders, and impaired growth. The only other well-documented cases of biotin deficiency have occurred with total parental nutrition, when the biotin was omitted from the formula. Overall, a biotin deficiency is rare. However, a diet low in biotin and high in raw egg whites can cause clinical symptoms such as neurological damage, dermatitis, and hair loss.

There are many gaps in the knowledge about biotin, especially its bioavailability in common foods.

■ VITAMIN B-6

Vitamin B-6 is actually a family of three compounds: pyridoxal, pyridoxine, and pyridoxamine.[10] All three forms can be phosphorylated to the active vitamin B-6 coenzymes, the primary one being pyridoxal phosphate (PLP). The generic name for the vitamin is B-6.

■ Absorption, Metabolism, Excretion, and Storage of Vitamin B-6

Both the phosphorylated and nonphosphorylated forms of vitamin B-6 can be absorbed by passive means. Vitamin B-6 as such is transported to the liver via the portal blood, where ultimately the three forms of the vitamin are phosphorylated. From the liver the phosphorylated forms (mainly PLP) are released to general circulation bound to a blood protein (albumin) for transport. When the liver's capacity to hold phosphorylated B-6 is reached, the excess is released into general circulation as the nonphosphorylated form, pyridoxal. The main storehouse of vitamin B-6 in the body is muscle tissue. At very high intakes, much of the vitamin B-6 is excreted in the urine.

■ Functions of Vitamin B-6

Vitamin B-6 as PLP plays a coenzyme role in more than 100 enzymatic reactions.

Amino Acid Metabolism

PLP functions as a decarboxylase, an enzyme that removes CO_2 from amino acids. It also participates in transamination reactions, the conversion of amino acids to keto acids, and the transfer of the amino group to another keto acid to form a nonessential amino acid. (If we didn't have the services of PLP, every amino acid would be essential and would have to be supplied by the diet.) Any remaining keto acid—also called the carbon skeleton—can enter the citric acid cycle to produce ATP. The keto acid also can be converted to glucose (through gluconeogenesis) or fat.

**Vitamin B-6
(represented by pyridoxal)**

Pyridoxal, one form of vitamin B-6, is converted to an active coenzyme—pyridoxal phosphate (PLP)—by the addition of a phosphate group to the hydroxyl group, indicated in this figure by the red asterisk.

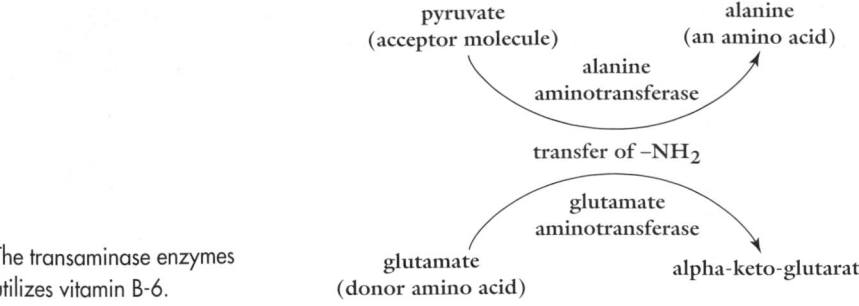

The transaminase enzymes utilizes vitamin B-6.

racemase A group of enzymes that catalyzes reactions involving structural rearrangement of a molecule (e.g., conversion of D-alanine isomer to L-alanine isomer).

PLP is responsible for the interconversion of D- and L-amino acids—it acts as a **racemase.** Recall from Chapter 7 that humans only use the L form of amino acids for protein synthesis. PLP can also move sulfur groups from one amino acid to another. This is particularly important in the conversion of homocysteine to cysteine, which occurs during methionine (an amino acid) metabolism.

Blood Cell Synthesis and Function

In the red blood cell, PLP catalyzes the first step in the synthesis of heme, the iron-containing protein in hemoglobin. Heme is the oxygen-carrying constituent of red blood cells. Vitamin B-6 as pyridoxal also participates in binding oxygen to hemoglobin, whereas PLP lowers the O_2-binding capacity.[10] This allows hemoglobin to pick up oxygen in the lungs and to release it to target tissues throughout the body. PLP is also necessary for the synthesis of lymphocytes, a type of white blood cell that is an essential component in the immune response.

Carbohydrate Metabolism

In addition to providing carbon skeletons to produce glucose by gluconeogenesis, PLP is part of the enzyme that releases glucose from glycogen during glycogen breakdown, glycogenolysis. Therefore, vitamin B-6 helps maintain blood glucose concentrations.

Lipid Metabolism

PLP is needed in the synthesis of the fatty acid arachidonic acid from the essential fatty acid linoleic acid. PLP also participates in the formation of myelin, the lipidlike sheath that covers nerves.

Neurotransmitter Synthesis

Of considerable interest is the role that PLP plays in the synthesis of the neurotransmitters serotonin from tryptophan, dopamine (DOPA) and norepinephrine from tyrosine, histamine from histadine, and gama-aminobutyric acid (GABA) from glutamic acid. These biochemical actions have led many physicians to prescribe megadoses of vitamin B-6 to patients with various "psychological problems." At this time, it is unclear whether this therapy is effective.

In the early 1950s, some infants were accidentally fed a commercial formula in which vitamin B-6 had been destroyed by oversterilization. The infants developed abnormal electroencephalogram (EEG) readings and experienced convulsions. The reason was probably associated with a lack of neurotransmitter synthesis in the brain. The situation was successfully treated with vitamin B-6.

Vitamin Formation

PLP participates in the conversion of the amino acid tryptophan to the B-vitamin niacin.

*O*ne study showed that healthy people with the highest vitamin B-6 concentrations in the blood score highest on cognitive tests of memory. In addition, those with the highest homocysteine concentrations score as low on such tests as people with mild Alzheimer's disease. Although this is only one study, it is possible that there are yet undiscovered functions of vitamin B-6. Still, RDA amounts in the diet suffice to maintain cognitive health.

■ Vitamin B-6 Deficiency

The symptoms of Vitamin B-6 deficiency include seborrheic dermatitis, **microcytic hypochromic anemia,** convulsion, depression, and confusion. The anemia reflects a decline in heme synthesis due to an inadequate amount of PLP; the accumulation of abnormal metabolites of tryptophan in the brain or a lack of neurotransmitters may cause the convulsions. Because vitamin B-6 is essential for the formation of lymphocytes, a deficiency is associated with diminished immune function.

microcytic hypochromic anemia An anemia characterized by small, pale red blood cells that lack sufficient hemoglobin and thus have reduced oxygen-carrying ability. It often also is caused by an iron deficiency.

■ Vitamin B-6 in Foods

Vitamin B-6 is stored in the muscle tissues of animals, and thus meat, fish, and poultry are some of the best sources of this vitamin (Fig. 10-6). Although vitamin B-6 in animal foods is often more readily absorbed than that in plant foods, whole grains also are good sources of vitamin B-6. However, vitamin B-6 is lost during the refining of grains, and this is not one of the vitamins added during enrichment. Some of the most nutrient-dense sources of vitamin B-6 (mg/kcal) are whole-wheat bread, peanut butter, garbanzo beans, raw carrots, cooked potatoes, chicken breast, water-packed tuna, bananas, and avocados. Ready-to-eat breakfast cereals and mixed dishes containing meat, poultry, or fish account for 20% of the U.S. intake of vitamin B-6.

Vitamin B-6 is not stable under heat or alkaline conditions. Heat processing and other destructive processing technologies can reduce the vitamin B-6 content of a food by 10 to 50%. The bioavailability of vitamin B-6 is about 75% based on a mixed diet.

𝒟ietary Sources of Vitamin B-6

Food Item and Amount	Vitamin B-6 (mg)
Brewer's yeast, 2 tbsp	0.81
Salmon, 3 oz	0.80
Banana, 1	0.68
Avocado, 1	0.56
Roast turkey, 3 oz	0.48
Roast chicken, 3 oz	0.48
Baked potato, 1	0.47
Fried beef liver, 1 oz	0.41
Watermelon, 1 1/2 cup	0.33
Sunflower seeds, 1/4 cup	0.26

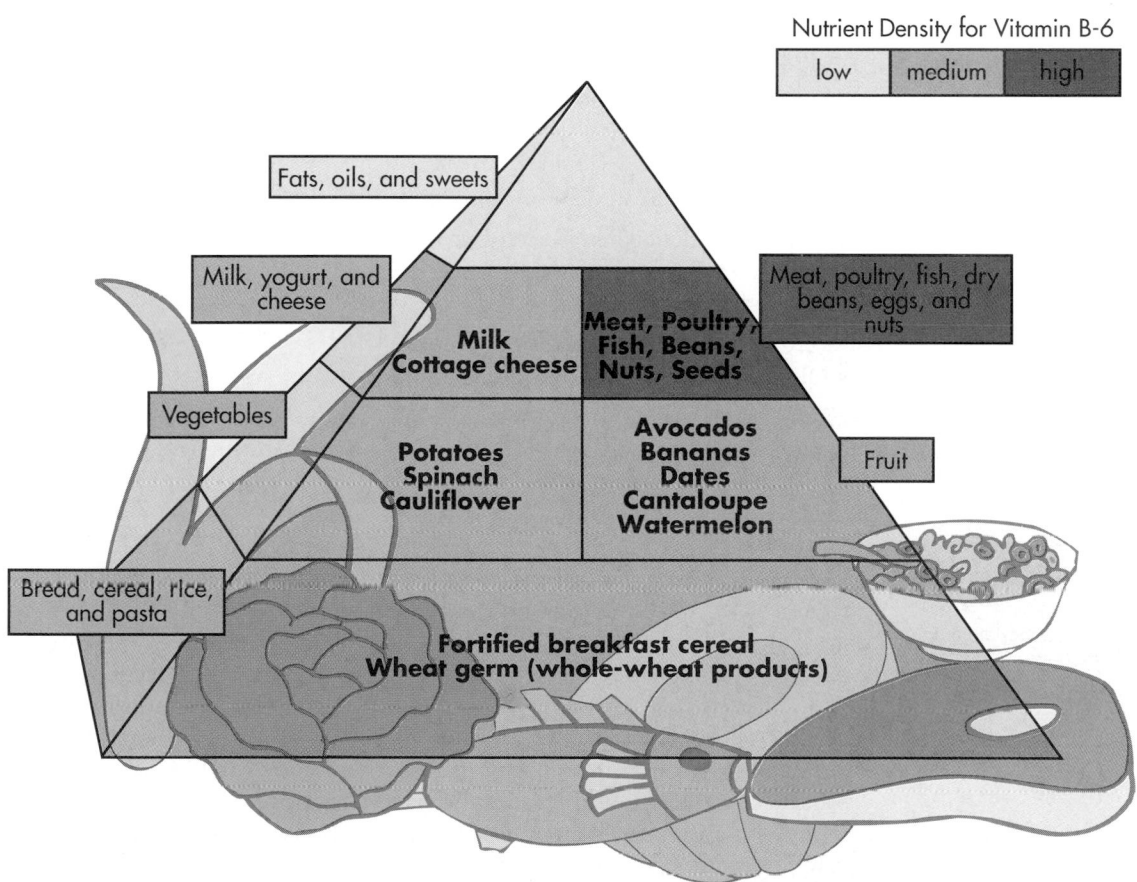

■ FIGURE 10-6 Food sources of vitamin B-6 from the Food Guide Pyramid. The meat, poultry, fish, dry beans, eggs, and nuts group is an especially rich source of this nutrient. The background color of each food group indicates the average nutrient density for vitamin B-6 in that group.

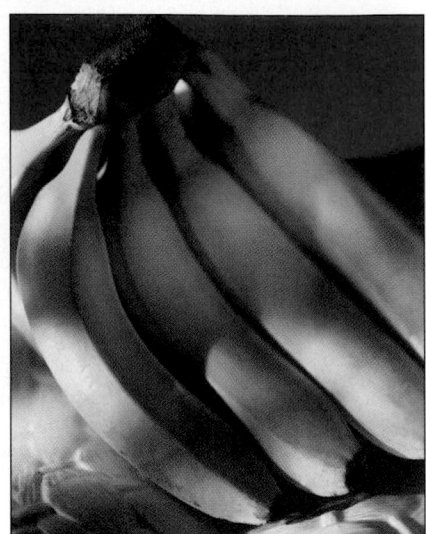

Bananas are a rich plant source of vitamin B-6.

preeclampsia Part of the disease pregnancy-induced hypertension. This serious disorder can include high blood pressure, kidney failure, convulsions, and even death of the mother and fetus. Mild cases are known as preeclampsia: more severe cases are called eclampsia—or, more correctly, toxemia.

premenstrual syndrome (PMS) A disorder found in some women a few days before a menstrual period begins. It is characterized by depression, anxiety, headache, bloating, and mood swings. Severe cases are currently termed premenstrual dysphoric disorder (PDD).

■ Vitamin B-6 Needs

Various studies have established an Estimated Average Requirement of 1.1 mg/day for men and women ages 19 to 50.[21] To establish the RDA for vitamin B-6, the Estimated Average Requirement is increased by 20% to account for individual variability. The RDA is then 1.3 mg of vitamin B-6 per day. For men over 50, the RDA is 1.7 mg/day and 1.5 mg/day for women over 50. By comparison, the Daily Value use on food labels is 2 mg. The indicator used to estimate needs is the amount of vitamin B-6 needed to maintain an adequate PLP concentration in the blood.

The average intake of vitamin B-6 from food in the United States is approximately 2 mg/day for men and 1.4 mg/day for women. Vitamin B-6 intake from food and supplements combined brings the U.S. intake up to 6 to 10 mg/day. In one Canadian population study, the intake was approximately 1.8 mg/day for men and 1.3 mg/day for women.

■ Factors That Affect Vitamin B-6 Requirement

Dietary protein intake was once thought to influence vitamin B-6 requirements, but a number of studies in young and elderly men and women have failed to demonstrate this link.

A number of medications—especially L-DOPA, used to treat Parkinson's disease, and isoniazid, a common antituberculosis medication—reduce blood concentrations of PLP. Patients should be advised to obtain extra vitamin B-6 when taking these medications, under a physician's guidance.

When alcohol is metabolized in the body, an intermediate, acetaldehyde, is produced. Acetaldehyde decreases the formation of PLP by cells and perhaps competes with PLP for protein-binding sites.

Pregnant women with **preeclampsia** have lower blood concentrations of PLP and proteinuria, but further studies are needed to determine if a supplement with vitamin B-6 prevents this serious disorder.

■ North Americans at Risk for Vitamin B-6 Deficiency

Vitamin B-6 deficiency is rare, but some older people have been found to exhibit signs of a deficiency, such as reduced immune function and a high concentration of homocysteine in the blood.

■ Pharmacologic Use of Vitamin B-6 and Toxicity

Carpal tunnel syndrome, a nerve disorder in the wrist, has been treated with large daily doses of vitamin B-6. However, because of defects in the design of trials, and insufficient convincing evidence of its effectiveness, vitamin B-6 is not recommended for this condition.

Studies of vitamin B-6 and **premenstrual syndrome (PMS)** indicate that the evidence is so shaky that it is unwise to make a definitive recommendation for taking vitamin B-6. Since there are no laboratory tests for PMS, and the cause of symptoms has not yet been elucidated, well-controlled trials are needed to clarify the possible benefits and side effects of vitamin B-6 in the treatment of PMS.

Intakes of 2 to 6 g of vitamin B-6 per day for 2 or more months can lead to irreversible nerve damage, as can long-term intakes of greater than 200 mg/day. Body builders and women attempting to treat themselves for PMS have sustained symptoms such as walking difficulties and hand and foot numbness. Some nerve damage in individual sensory neurons is probably reversible, but damage to ganglia (where many nerve fibers converge) is probably permanent. The Upper Level for adults is set at 100 mg of vitamin B-6 per day, based on such damage.

CONCEPT CHECK

*P*antothenic acid and biotin both participate in metabolism of carbohydrate, protein, and fat. A deficiency of either vitamin is unlikely because pantothenic acid is found in a wide variety of foods and our need for biotin is partially met by synthesis from intestinal bacteria. Vitamin B-6 is important for protein metabolism, neurotransmitter synthesis, and other key metabolic functions. Headache, anemia, nausea, and vomiting can result from a vitamin B-6 deficiency. Animal protein sources and plant foods such as broccoli, spinach, and bananas are good sources of vitamin B-6. Doses of vitamin B-6 in excess of approximately 1500 times the RDA for a few months or 150 times the RDA for long-term use can cause nerve destruction.

■ FOLATE

Two of the B-vitamins, folate and vitamin B-12, produce a number of identical deficiency signs and symptoms when omitted from the diet.[5] These two water-soluble vitamins share a close relationship because of their biochemical interactions. For example, both folate and vitamin B-12 are responsible for DNA synthesis. Folate will be explored first.

What we call folate today was known earlier as either folic acid or folacin. Today, the term **folate** is preferred because it encompasses the various forms of the vitamin found in foods. Only a few food forms are in the folic acid configuration, but vitamin supplements often contain this form. It is also the form used to fortify foods.

Folic acid

Pteridine · Para-aminobenzoic acid · Glutamate

Folic acid, also called folate monoglutamate, is the form absorbed in the intestine. This is the form found in fortified foods and supplements. Most of the folate naturally found in foods contains additional glutamate molecules linked to the carboxyl group, indicated in this figure by the red asterisk.

Folate consists of three parts: pteridine, para-aminobenzoic acid (PABA), and one or more molecules of the amino acid glutamic acid, or glutamate. If only one glutamate molecule is present, it is designated folic acid (folate monoglutamate). In food, about 90% of the folate molecules have three or more glutamates attached and are known as polyglutamates.

■ Metabolism, Absorption, Storage, and Excretion of Folate

To be absorbed, folate polyglutamates must be broken down (hydrolyzed) to the monoglutamate form in the gastrointestinal tract. Enzymes, folate **conjugases,** located in the enterocytes accomplish the removal of the excess glutamates. The monoglutamate form is actively transported across the intestinal wall. When very large doses of folic acid from supplements are consumed, they are also absorbed by passive diffusion. When synthetic folic acid is consumed as a supplement and without food, it is nearly 100% bioavailable. Consumed with food, as in fortified cereal grains, its absorption is slightly reduced.

conjugase Enzyme systems in the intestine that enhance folate absorption; they remove glutamate molecules from polyglutamate forms of folate.

The portal blood delivers the monoglutamate form of folate to the liver, where these are changed back to polyglutamate products and are either stored in the liver or released into the blood or bile. The normal amount of folate stored in the body is from 5 mg to 10 mg, of which about half is in the liver. Most of the urinary excretion of folate exits as metabolic products. Urinary folate represents only a very tiny amount of dietary folate. Biologically active folate is also excreted into the bile and is reabsorbed by enterohepatic circulation. Alcohol interferes with this process, so most alcoholics become folate deficient.

Intestinal bacteria synthesize folate, but probably nearly all is excreted in the feces. Therefore, it has been difficult to determine how much excreted folate comes from the diet and how much is from microbial synthesis.

■ Functions of Folate

In the body's target cells, all forms of folate are readily converted to the basic coenzyme form, called tetrahydrofolic acid (THFA). There are actually five active coenzyme forms of THFA. These participate in metabolic reactions by accepting and donating single-carbon groups.

Metabolic Reactions

THFA transfers the following single-carbon groups: methyl ($-CH_3$), formyl ($-CH=O$), methylene ($-CH_2-$), and methynyl ($-CH=$).

Transfer of these single-carbon units is needed for the synthesis of DNA, the metabolism of various amino acids and their derivatives, cell division, and the maturation of red blood cells and other cells. A crucial reaction requiring THFA is the transfer of a one-carbon methylene group ($-CH_2-$) to uridylate, forming thymidylate, an essential component of DNA and thus cell replication:

$$\text{THFA}(-CH_2-) \qquad \text{THFA (free)}$$

$$\text{uridylate} \dashrightarrow \text{thymidylate} \dashrightarrow \text{DNA}$$

THFA is also needed for the synthesis of adenine and guanine, so DNA synthesis and repair may decline as a result of a folate shortage.

Because THFA is needed for DNA synthesis, folate deficiency may be induced during a common form of cancer therapy. One example is the cancer drug methotrexate. It inhibits a key aspect of folate metabolism. When methotrexate is taken in high doses, it reduces DNA synthesis throughout the body by interfering with folate metabolism. This reduction in DNA synthesis can halt the growth of cancer cells, but it also affects other rapidly proliferating cells, such as intestinal cells and red blood cells. Therefore, the typical side effects of methotrexate therapy are the same as for a folate deficiency (e.g., anemia and diarrhea).

Research is currently underway in the link between folate and cancer protection. Because folate aids in the transfer of methyl groups for DNA synthesis, it is hypothesized that even mild folate deficiency contributes to abnormal DNA integrity, which in turn affects certain cancer-protecting genes. A daily intake of 400 μg (the RDA) is thought to be chemo-preventive.

Methotrexate acting as a folate antagonist is also used to treat rheumatoid arthritis, psoriasis, asthma, alcoholic cirrhosis, and inflammatory bowel disease. Side effects include gastrointestinal distress and severe folate deficiency. When patients are given methotrexate, they need to follow a high-folate diet and/or take folate supplements because this reduces the toxic side effects of the drug. High supplemental doses do not reduce methotrexate's effectiveness.

Another key function of folate is the formation of neurotransmitters in the brain. Supplements of folate can improve the depressed state in some cases of mental illness.

Other Functions

THFA is important in amino acid metabolism, especially the interconversions of amino acids. It accepts one-carbon groups from various amino acids and is responsible for the glycine to serine reaction, the histidine to glutamate reaction, and the important homocysteine to methionine reaction.

Approximately 30 years ago, it became evident that the amino acid homocysteine has the ability to increase the risk of blood vessel injury. The Physicians Health Study, an examination of 15,000 American doctors, found that that those with the highest homocysteine concentration in their blood experienced the highest rate of heart attack. As the amount of homocysteine in the blood increased, there was increased damage to blood vessels, especially veins. The speculation at this time is that thromboses (blood clots) form in arteries and veins in response to elevated homocysteine concentrations and lead to strokes and heart attacks.[2] The B-vitamins folate, vitamin B-6, and vitamin B-12 each plays a role in keeping homocysteine concentration in the blood under control. Although there are many ongoing homocysteine trials to determine if folate therapy is relevant to cardiovascular disease, it is now being recommended that, as part of a program to control homocysteine and, so, improve heart health, adults should:

- Consume plenty of foods containing the three B-vitamins vitamin B-6, folate, and vitamin B-12
- Consider use of a fortified breakfast cereal with 50 to 100% of the Daily Values for vitamin B-6, folate, and vitamin B-12 per serving, or possibly take a multivitamin containing that amount of vitamin B-6, folate, and vitamin B-12.

■ Folate Deficiency

Folate deficiency generally results from a low intake; inadequate absorption, which often is associated with alcoholism; increased requirement, most commonly occurring in pregnancy; compromised utilization, typically associated with vitamin B-12 deficiency; and excessive excretion, linked to long-standing diarrhea.

Megaloblastic Anemia

As mentioned already, a deficiency of folate first affects cell types that are actively synthesizing DNA; such cells have a short life span and rapid turnover rate. Thus, one of the first major folate-deficiency signs to appear is changes in the early phases of red blood cell synthesis, as these cells turn over every 120 days. Without folate, the precursor cells in the bone marrow cannot divide normally to become mature red blood cells because they cannot form new DNA. The cells grow larger because there is continuous formation of RNA, leading to increased synthesis of protein and other cell components to make new cells. Hemoglobin synthesis intensifies. However, when it is time for the cells to divide, they lack sufficient DNA for normal division. The cells thus remain in a large, immature form, known as **megaloblasts** (Fig. 10-7). Unlike normal, mature red blood cells, megaloblasts retain their nuclei.

Since the bone marrow of a folate-deficient person produces mostly large, immature megaloblasts, few normal-size, mature red blood cells (erythrocytes) arrive in the bloodstream. With fewer normal mature red blood cells present, oxygen-carrying capacity decreases, causing anemia. In short, the weakness and tiredness associated with a folate deficiency are caused by a form of anemia called megaloblastic (or **macrocytic**) **anemia.**

Large, immature cells also appear along the entire length of the gastrointestinal tract during chronic folate deficiency. This change contributes to decreased absorptive capacity of the tract and a persistent diarrhea. White blood cell synthesis also is disrupted by a folate deficiency.

Because folate is stored in the body, it takes some time on a folate-free diet for a deficiency to be noticeable. For example, depending on their folate stores, individuals will show changes in red blood cell formation after 7 to 16 weeks on a folate-free diet. The large size of the megaloblasts causes an inevitable increase in mean corpuscular volume (MCV), which is a clinical measure of the average size of red blood cells. Physicians focus primarily on red blood cells in the initial diagnosis of a folate deficiency because they are easy to examine. The need to continually replenish red blood cells leads to a great demand for folate, making anemia the first major

megaloblast A large, nucleated, immature red blood cell, which results from the inability of a precursor cell to divide when it normally should.

macrocytic anemia Anemia characterized by the presence of abnormally large red blood cells.

Steps in Folate Deficiency
1. Decrease in blood folate concentration
2. Decrease in red cell folate
3. Defective DNA synthesis
4. Change in structure of certain white blood cells
5. Increase in blood concentration of homocysteine
6. Megaloblastic changes in bone marrow and other rapidly dividing cells
7. Increase in the size of circulating red blood cells
8. Megaloblastic (macrocytic) anemia

Red blood cell precursor (stem cell)

Folate and vitamin B-12 adequate

Cells divide normally

Folate or vitamin B-12 deficient

Cells are unable to divide

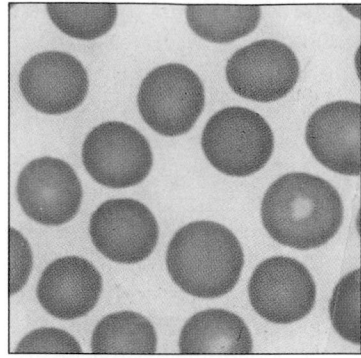

Normal blood cells in the bloodstream. The size, shape, and color of the red blood cells show that they are normal. Mature red blood cells have lost their nuclei.

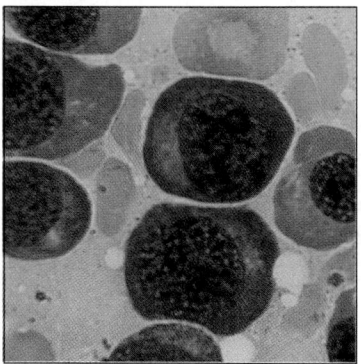

Megaloblastic blood cells seen here in the bone marrow are arrested at an immature stage of development. They still have their nuclei and are slightly larger than normal red blood cells.

■ **FIGURE 10-7** Megaloblastic anemia occurs when blood cells are unable to divide, leaving large, immature red blood cells. Either a folate or vitamin B-12 deficiency may cause this condition. Measurements of serum concentrations of both vitamins are taken to help determine the cause of the anemia.

neural tube defect A defect in the formation of the neural tube occurring during early fetal development. This type of defect results in various nervous system disorders, such as spina bifida. Folate deficiency in the pregnant woman increases the risk that the fetus will develop this disorder.

identifiable symptom of folate deficiency. Other clinical signs and symptoms of folate deficiency include inflammation of the tongue and mouth, abnormal pigmentation of the skin, diarrhea, poor growth, depression and mental confusion, and problems in nerve function.

Neural Tube Defects

A maternal deficiency of folate and a genetic predisposition have been linked to the development of **neural tube defects** in the fetus (Fig. 10-8). These defects include spina bifida (spinal cord or spinal fluid bulge through the back) and anencephaly (absence of a brain). Approximately 2000 infants are so affected annually in the United States. Victims of spina bifida exhibit paralysis, incontinence, hydrocephalus, and learning disabilities. Children born with anencephaly die shortly after birth. Adequate folate nurture is crucial for all women of childbearing years since neural tube closure begins 21 days after conception and is completed by day 28, a time when many women are not even aware that they are pregnant. Perhaps as many as 50% of these defects could be avoided by adequate folate status before conception (see Chapter 16 for details). All research has been done with synthetic folic acid supplementation, and it appears that even women with varied diets may not consume adequate folate to prevent neural tube defects (400 μg/day) unless specific attention to synthetic folic acid sources, such as many breakfast cereals, is given. Earlier it was noted that most grain products are now fortified with folate.

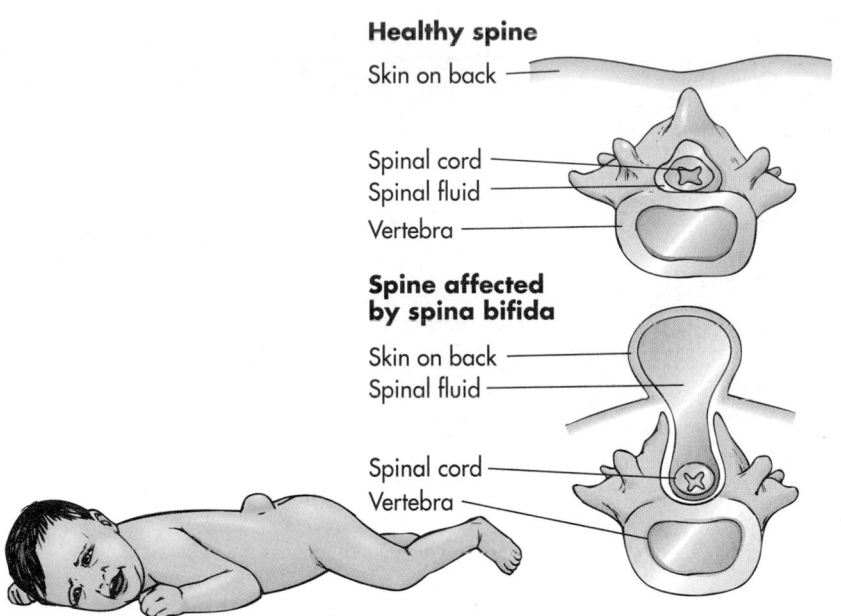

Healthy spine

Skin on back

Spinal cord
Spinal fluid
Vertebra

**Spine affected
by spina bifida**

Skin on back
Spinal fluid

Spinal cord
Vertebra

■ FIGURE 10-8 Neural tube defects result from a developmental failure affecting the spinal cord or brain in the embryo. Very early in fetal development, there is a ridge of neural-like tissue along the back of the embryo. As the fetus develops, this material differentiates into both the spinal cord and body nerves, at the lower end, and into the brain, at the upper end. At the same time, the bones that make up the back gradually surround the spinal cord on all sides. If any part of this sequence goes awry, many defects can appear. The worst is total lack of a brain (anencephaly). Much more common is spina bifida, in which the backbones do not form a complete ring to protect the spinal cord. Deficient folate status in the mother during the beginning of pregnancy increases the risk of neural tube defects.

Because the metabolism and functions of folate and B-12 are linked, regular consumption of large amounts of folate can prevent the appearance of the primary early warning sign of vitamin B-12 deficiency—enlarged red blood cells. To prevent such masking of vitamin B-12 deficiency, it is the goal of FDA to increase the folate intake of women of childbearing years through grain fortification without producing excessive intake by other groups (> 1 mg/day).

■ Folate in Foods

The biological availability of folate varies with the source of the vitamin. The best sources, from the standpoint of amount and availability, are liver, fortified breakfast cereals and other grain products, legumes, and vegetables in general (the term *folate* is derived from the Latin *folium,* meaning "foliage"). Other, less rich sources of folate that contribute this vitamin to our diets include eggs, dried beans, and oranges (Fig. 10-9).

The most nutrient-dense sources of folate (μg/kcal) are spinach and other leafy greens, romaine lettuce, asparagus, broccoli, orange juice, wheat germ, liver, sunflower seeds, cauliflower, and cabbage.

Food processing and preparation can destroy 50 to 90% of the folate in food. Folate is extremely susceptible to destruction by heat, oxidation, and ultraviolet light. Consequently, it is important to eat fresh fruits and lightly cooked (or raw) vegetables on a regular basis. If vegetables must be cooked, this should be done quickly in a minimum amount of water—by steaming, stir-frying, or microwaving. Vitamin C in foods helps protect folate from oxidative destruction.

■ Folate Needs and Dietary Folate Equivalents

Dietary folate equivalents (DFE) are the units used to express folate needs. These units reflect the differences in absorption of food folate and synthetic folic acid. When folic acid is consumed as a supplement, it is nearly 100% bioavailable. Folic acid consumed with food (e.g., fortified cereal grains) is absorbed at a slightly reduced level. Naturally occurring folate is less well absorbed.[21]

To estimate the amount of DFE requires some calculations.[24] First, determine how much of a day's food intake comes from food folate and how much comes from synthetic folate added to foods. When in doubt, assume all folate in a diet is derived from food, except that coming from breakfast cereals and refined grain products.

𝒟ietary Sources of Folate

Food Item and Amount	Folate (μg)
Brewer's yeast, 1 tbsp	280
Cooked asparagus, 1 cup	263
Cooked lentils, ½ cup	179
Romaine lettuce, 1½ cup	114
Orange juice, 8 oz	109
Cooked spinach, ½ cup	103
Cooked broccoli, 1 cup	78
Sunflower seeds, ¼ cup	76
Cooked beets, ½ cup	68
Fried beef liver, 1 oz	62

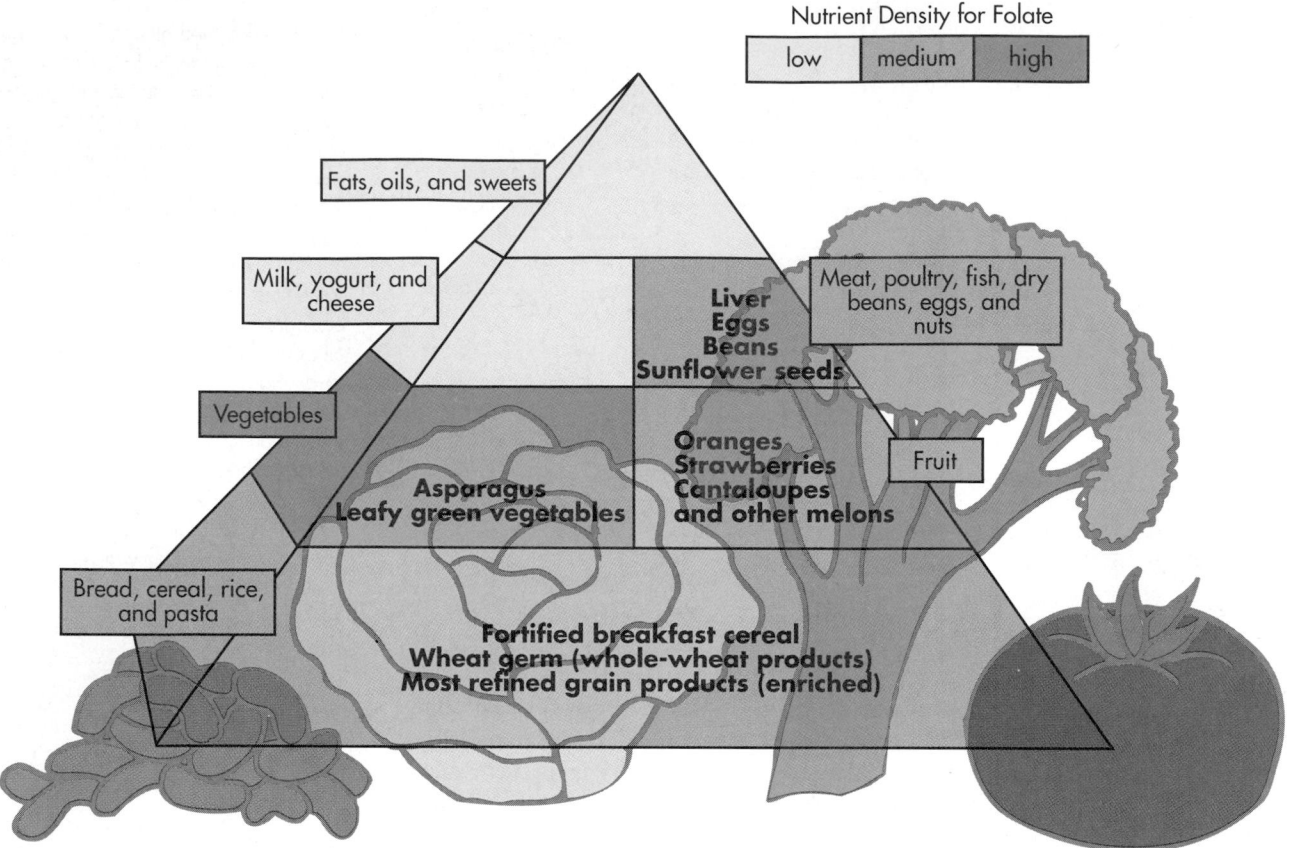

■ FIGURE 10-9 Food sources of folate from the Food Guide Pyramid. The vegetables group is an especially rich source of this nutrient. The background color of each food group indicates the average nutrient density for folate in that group.

CASE SCENARIO
Follow-Up

Suzanne and Ted should remember that spina bifida is caused by a failure of the spinal cord to close during the first 28 days of pregnancy, a time when neither Ted nor Suzanne realized Suzanne was pregnant. The B-vitamin folate must be available at the time of conception to prevent spina bifida and other birth defects. One hopes that Suzanne's prepregnancy diet provided enough synthetic folate; if not, there is a reason to worry. The fact that a close relative of Suzanne's has already produced a child with this birth defect should have been a warning sign.

Also include in this second category any folate consumed as part of dietary supplements. To calculate the DFE for the diet, multiply total synthetic folate intake by 1.7 and add that value to the total food folate. The following is an example. The Daily Value for a serving of ready-to-eat breakfast cereal is listed on the label as 50%, so the amount of folate is 200 µg per serving (Daily Value of 400 µg × 0.50). Since this folate is synthetic folic acid, the 200 µg is multiplied by 1.7, or 340 µg. The person also consumed 300 µg of food folate. To obtain the total folate intake for the day, add the 300 µg to the 340 µg, which equals 640 µg.

The Estimated Average Requirement for adults 19 and older is 320 µg of dietary folate equivalents/day. This is then increased by 20% to account for individual variability, resulting in the RDA of 400 µg/day for both men and women. The Estimated Average Requirement is based on the amount needed to maintain red blood cell folate, control blood homocysteine, and maintain normal blood folate concentrations. Also considered was the intake necessary to prevent neural tube defects for women capable of becoming pregnant.

■ North Americans at Risk for Folate Deficiency

Folate deficiencies sometimes appear in pregnant women. They need extra folate to meet an increased rate of cell division and thus of DNA synthesis in their own bodies and in the developing fetus. Today, prenatal care often includes vitamin and mineral supplements enriched with folate to compensate for the extra needs associated with pregnancy.

Young women in general often register low serum folate values. It is important for them to seek good sources of synthetic folate that they enjoy eating and then to eat those foods regularly. Folate-fortified foods is one option. The use of a balanced vitamin supplement is another option (see the Nutrition Perspective in Chapter 9). As previously mentioned, older adults are also at risk for folate deficiency. Finally, persons suffering from alcohol abuse or taking certain prescription drugs and those who smoke need to recognize that they have increased folate needs. However, more information is needed before higher recommendations are made for smokers than for nonsmokers.

■ Toxicity of Folate

FDA limits the amount of folate in nonprescription vitamin supplements for non-pregnant individuals to 400 µg when no statement of age is listed on the supplement label. When age-related doses are listed, there can be no more than 100 µg for infants, 300 µg for children, and 400 µg for adults. Prenatal supplements sold over-the-counter can contain 800 µg. FDA regulates the potency of folate supplements because of the ability of excessive amounts of folate can mask a vitamin B-12 deficiency. The Upper Level for synthetic folate is 1 mg, based on this observation. However, this does not apply to folate in foods since absorption is limited.

■ VITAMIN B-12

What we call vitamin B-12 includes the free vitamin (cyanocobalamin) and two active coenzymes—methylcobalamin and 5-deoxyadenosylcobalamin. This vitamin has a complex structure containing the mineral cobalt.[26]

All vitamin B-12 compounds are synthesized exclusively by bacteria, fungi, and algae. Animals such as cows and sheep obtain vitamin B-12 either from bacterial synthesis in their multiple stomachs (rumen) or from the soil they ingest while eating and grazing. The only reliable source of the vitamin for humans is animal foods. Plants do not synthesize vitamin B-12. There is minor contamination of vegetable products by bacteria and soil. The process of fermentation also contributes a small amount of vitamin B-12 to a food.

■ Absorption, Transport, and Storage of Vitamin B-12

In the stomach, vitamin B-12 in food is released from proteins by the action of HCl and pepsin in gastric juice. The free B-12 binds to a protein, designated **R-protein,** that originates in the salivary glands in the mouth and is swallowed along with the food. The R-protein/vitamin B-12 complex travels to the small intestine, where it encounters pancreatic proteases (e.g., trypsin), which release the vitamin. Awaiting the free B-12 is **intrinsic factor,** a glycoprotein produced by the parietal cells in the stomach. The intrinsic factor/vitamin B-12 complex travels to the terminal portion of the small intestine, the ileum, where it attaches to special receptor cells on the brush border. Several hours later, cells within the ileum absorb vitamin B-12 and transfer it to a specific transport protein, transcobalamin II. This vitamin-protein complex enters the portal blood and is taken up by the liver, eventually the bone marrow, and red blood cells (Fig. 10-10).

It is assumed that 50% of dietary vitamin B-12 is absorbed by healthy adults with normal gastric function. Vitamin B-12 is continually secreted into the bile, and most of it is reabsorbed by enterohepatic circulation. Failure in any of the links found in the absorptive process reduces absorption to 2% or less of dietary vitamin B-12.

Absorption of vitamin B-12 can be disrupted by numerous defects, including the following:

**Vitamin B-12
(cyanocobalamin)**

The cyanocobalamin form of vitamin B-12 is converted to the active coenzyme forms by replacement of the cyano group (red) with another group, such as a methyl group or a hydroxyl group.

R-protein A protein produced by the salivary glands that enhances absorption of vitamin B-12, possibly by protecting the vitamin during its passage through the stomach.

intrinsic factor A substance present in gastric juice that enhances vitamin B-12 absorption.

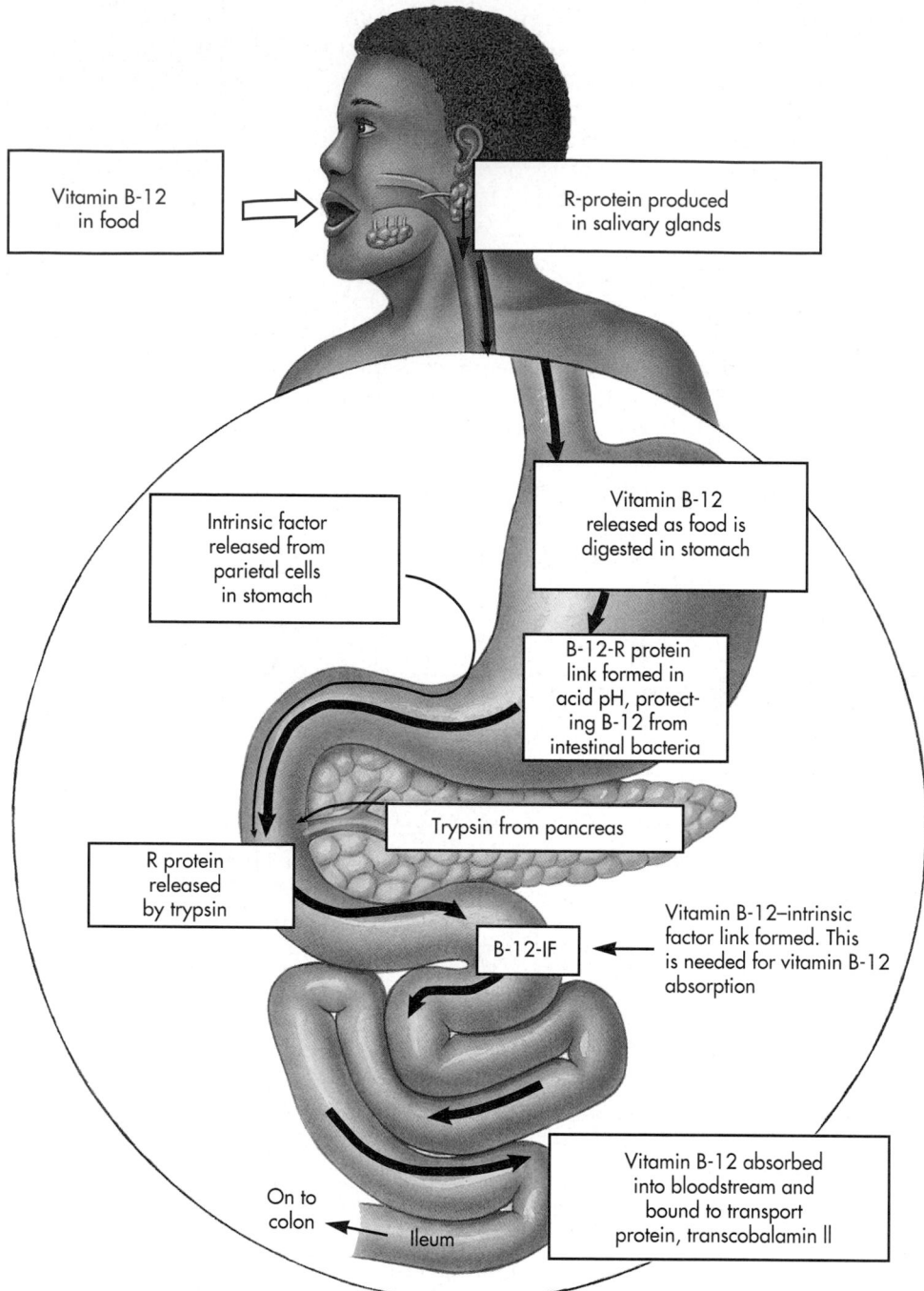

Vitamin B-12 in food

R-protein produced in salivary glands

Intrinsic factor released from parietal cells in stomach

Vitamin B-12 released as food is digested in stomach

B-12-R protein link formed in acid pH, protecting B-12 from intestinal bacteria

Trypsin from pancreas

R protein released by trypsin

B-12-IF

Vitamin B-12–intrinsic factor link formed. This is needed for vitamin B-12 absorption

On to colon

Ileum

Vitamin B-12 absorbed into bloodstream and bound to transport protein, transcobalamin II

■ FIGURE 10-10 Absorption of vitamin B-12. Many factors and sites in the gastrointestinal tract participate. Defects arising in the stomach or small intestine can interfere with vitamin B-12 absorption, in turn causing pernicious anemia.
Illustration by William Ober.

- Absence or defective synthesis of R-protein, pancreatic proteases, or intrinsic factor
- Defective binding of the intrinsic factor/vitamin B-12 complex to receptor cells in the ileum
- Absence (or surgical removal) of much or all of the ileum and stomach
- Bacterial overgrowth of the small intestine
- Tapeworm infestation
- Use of certain antiulcer medications that significantly reduce acid production by the parietal cells (e.g., omeprazole [Prilosec])
- Chronic malabsorption syndromes, as can be seen in AIDS

Three types of therapy are possible for patients diagnosed with a defect in vitamin B-12 absorption: monthly injections of vitamin B-12 to bypass the gastrointestinal tract, use of a vitamin B-12 nasal gel (nasal absorption does not require the intrinsic factor), and weekly ingestion of vitamin B-12 supplements in megadoses (300 times the RDA), which allow absorption by passive diffusion. Ninety-five percent of all cases of vitamin B-12 deficiency among otherwise healthy people in the United States result from a defect in vitamin B-12 absorption, rather than from inadequate intake.

About 50 to 90% of the body's total supply of vitamin B-12 is stored in the liver. Stores range from 5 to 12 mg. In the body, vitamin B-12 is very stable and little is lost—just the small amount that escapes enterohepatic circulation of the bile. Since storage is so great, a single monthly injection of vitamin B-12 is sufficient to prevent a deficiency when absorption of dietary sources is significantly hampered.

In the 1920s, researchers found that a vitamin B-12 deficiency can be cured by consumption of massive amounts of liver or concentrated water extracts of liver. In this case, the deficiency was caused by an absorption defect. If enough of the vitamin is ingested, it can be absorbed by simple diffusion, thereby overcoming the defective R-protein/intrinsic factor system.

■ Functions of Vitamin B-12

Vitamin B-12 is associated with methylmalonyl CoA **mutase,** which requires the coenzyme 5 deoxyadenosyl cobalamin. The methylmalonyl CoA mutase requires vitamin B-12 to convert methylmalonyl CoA to succinyl CoA, an intermediate in the citric acid cycle. This reaction allows three-carbon fatty acids to be oxidized for energy. Methionine synthase requires methylcobalmin as its coenzyme for the transfer of a methyl group from methyltetrahydrofolate to homocysteine to form methionine and tetrahydrofolate (Fig. 10-11). The importance of this reaction is that stores of methionine are maintained and tetrahydrofolate is available to participate in the synthesis of DNA.

Vitamin B-12 is essential for normal red blood cell formation and proper nerve function. In the absence of vitamin B-12, THFA is trapped in the methyl-bound form, and the cell develops a shortage of enough of the folate coenzymes such that it can't meet its metabolic needs. For example, the folate shortage inhibits DNA synthesis. Thus, a vitamin B-12 deficiency contributes to a secondary folate deficiency. And a deficiency of either folate or vitamin B-12 results in the same blood changes, resulting in megaloblastic anemia. Measurement of blood folate and vitamin B-12 concentrations aids in determining which is the cause. The role of vitamin B-12 in nerve function is in maintaining the myelin sheath that insulates nerve fibers. People with vitamin B-12 deficiencies show patchy destruction of the myelin sheath, especially in areas surrounding the nerves in the spinal cord.

mutase An enzyme that rearranges the functional groups on a molecule.

■ Vitamin B-12 Deficiency: Pernicious Anemia

Researches in midnineteenth-century England noted a form of anemia that causes death within 2 to 5 years of initial diagnosis. They called this disease **pernicious anemia** (*pernicious* literally means "leading to death"). Clinically, this disease looks like a folate-deficiency anemia. For patients with either a folate or vitamin B-12 deficiency, many megaloblasts (macrocytes) are seen in the blood. As in folate deficiency, the cause of the anemia is an interference with normal synthesis of DNA.

Infants who are breastfed by vegetarian or vegan mothers can develop vitamin B-12 deficiency, accompanied by anemia and long-term neurological problems, such as diminished brain growth, degeneration of the spinal cord, and poor intellectual development. The problems may have their origins during pregnancy, when the mother is deficient in vitamin B-12. Chapter 7 noted that vegan diets supply little vitamin B-12 unless it is included as part of food choices enriched in vitamin B-12 or supplements are used.

pernicious anemia The anemia that results from the inability to absorb sufficient vitamin B-12; it is associated with nerve degeneration, which can result in eventual paralysis and death.

■ Vitamin B-12 in Foods

Sources of vitamin B-12 include meat, poultry, seafood, and eggs. The most nutrient-dense sources of vitamin B-12 ($\mu g/kcal$) are organ meats (especially liver,

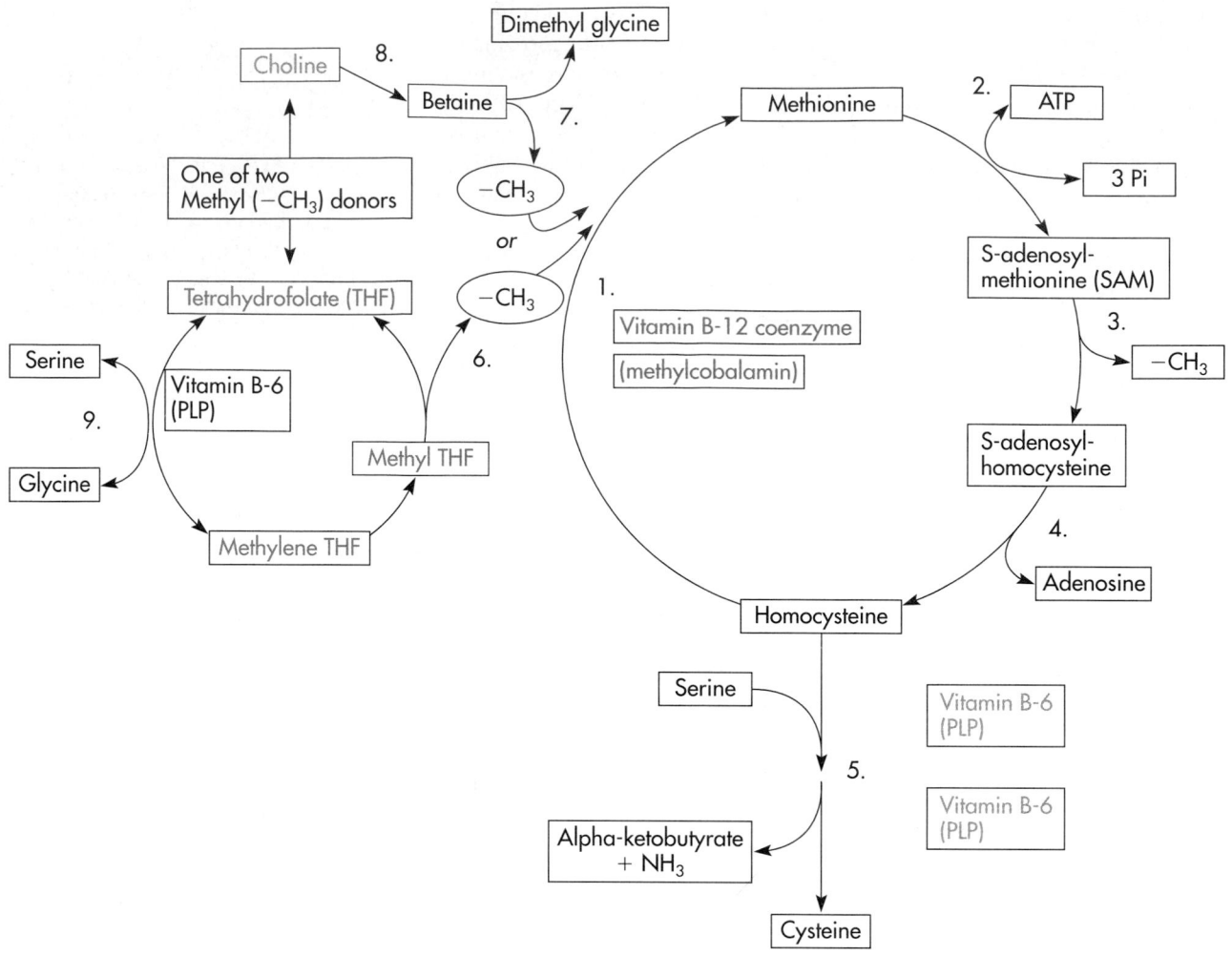

FIGURE 10-11 Detailed diagram of folate, vitamin B-12, vitamin B-6, and choline metabolism.

1. With the aid of the vitamin B-12 coenzyme (methylcobalamine), the methyl group (CH₃) is transferred from the folate coenzyme, methyl THF, to homocysteine to form methionine. Another important function of this reaction is to make the resulting tetrahydrafolate coenzyme available to participate in DNA synthesis.
2. Methionine can be converted to S-Adenosyl-methionine (SAM) with the addition of adenosine from ATP. The three phosphate groups are removed.
3. S-Adenosyl-methionine is converted to S-Adenosyl homocysteine by removal of the CH₃, which is donated to a variety of methyl group acceptors.
4. S-Adenosyl homocysteine is converted back to homocysteine with the removal of adenosine.

Overall, this cycle controls the concentration of homocysteine in the blood.

5. With the aid of vitamin B-6 coenzyme PLP, homocysteine is used to make the nonessential amino acid cysteine. The nonessential amino acid serine contributes its carbon skeleton to homocysteine. This is another pathway that helps control blood homocysteine concentration.

6. Either methyl tetrahydrofolate or
7. Betaine are donors of a methyl group to form methionine.
8. The betaine is derived from choline.
9. Note that the serine-glycine reaction is reversible in conjunction with THF and methylene THF. Here is another example of vitamin B-6 in action as PLP.

In summary, the coenzymes of vitamin B-12, folate, and vitamin B-6, along with choline, work together as a team to control the amount of homocysteine in the blood. Excess homocysteine may lead to cardiovascular disease, stroke, birth defects, and other health problems. That's why it is important to include foods rich in these vitamins. For older adults, a synthetic vitamin B-12 source is recommended.

kidneys, and heart), seafood, beef, eggs, hot dogs (they contain many organ meat scraps), and ham. Another source of vitamin B-12 is milk and milk products.

▪ Vitamin B-12 Needs

The Estimated Average Requirement for vitamin B-12 is based on the amount needed for the maintenance of normal red blood cell status.[21] For adult men and women age 19 to 50, the Estimated Average Requirement is 2 µg/day. To compute the RDA, this is increased by 20% to account for individual variation. Thus, the RDA for men and women is 2.4 µg of vitamin B-12 per day. For men and women 51 years and older, the RDA is also 2.4 µg of vitamin B-12 per day, but this population group is advised to select foods fortified with vitamin B-12 (e.g., ready-to-eat breakfast cereals) and/or take a supplement. This is because absorption of food-borne vitamin B-12 is hampered by the typical fall in gastric acid output seen in aging, called **achlorhydria.**

No adverse effects have been observed with excess vitamin B-12 intake from food or from supplements.

▪ North Americans at Risk for Vitamin B-12 Deficiency

People with malabsorption syndromes of any kind have an increased need for vitamin B-12. These include postgastrectomy patients, postgastric bypass surgery patients, and ileal resection patients, as well as patients with Crohn's disease or any disease involving the terminal ileum. HIV-positive patients with chronic diarrhea may require increased oral or intravenous vitamin B-12. Several other medical conditions, such as reduced secretions of the pancreas (chronic pancreatic disease) and bacterial infections of the intestinal tract, require extra vitamin B-12 because of decreased bioavailability of the vitamin from food. Those with pernicious anemia stemming from a vitamin B-12 deficiency also experience nerve degeneration, which is eventually fatal. The neurological complications produce sensory disturbances in the legs as tingling and numbness, **paresthesia,** which are worse in the lower legs. Walking is difficult and "position sense" is seriously affected. Many mental problems exist as well, such as loss of concentration and memory, disorientation, and dementia. As the condition worsens, bowel and bladder control is lost. Visual disturbances are common. There also are numerous gastrointestinal problems, from sore tongue to constipation.

As noted previously, deficiency of vitamin B-12—and, hence, pernicious anemia—is generally caused by diminished ability to absorb the vitamin. Before the discovery and isolation of the vitamin in 1948, this condition was a death sentence. Today, once pernicious anemia is diagnosed, an injection of vitamin B-12 reverses the defects in red blood cell maturation and in some other clinical signs within 1 to 2 days, if the deficiency is caught in time.

Pernicious anemia and its accompanying nerve destruction most likely occurs after middle age. Up to 20% of older adults may show such a problem. The average age of onset in Caucasians is 68 years; in African-Americans and Hispanics, the disease typically appears about a decade sooner. As the stomach's parietal cells age, they lose their ability to synthesize the intrinsic factor needed for vitamin B-12 absorption. This failure likely arises from an autoimmune reaction; that is, people make white blood cells and other factors that attack their own parietal cells. Thus, the immediate cause of pernicious anemia is vitamin B-12 deficiency, but the root problem is lack of intrinsic factor.

Dietary Sources of Vitamin B-12

Food Item and Amount	Vitamin B-12 (µg)
Fried beef liver, 1 oz	31.8
Baked clams, 1 oz	15.6
Steamed oysters, 2	14.4
Roast beef, 3 oz	2.0
Yogurt, 1 cup	1.4
Fortified soy milk, 8 oz	1.0
Milk, 8 oz	0.9
Beef hot dog, 1	0.9
Boiled egg, 1	0.6
Cooked ham, 3 oz	0.5
Ham lunchmeat, 2 oz	0.4

achlorhydria A decrease in stomach acid primarily due to age-associated loss of acid-producing parietal cells.

paresthesia An abnormal spontaneous sensation such as of burning, prickling, and numbness.

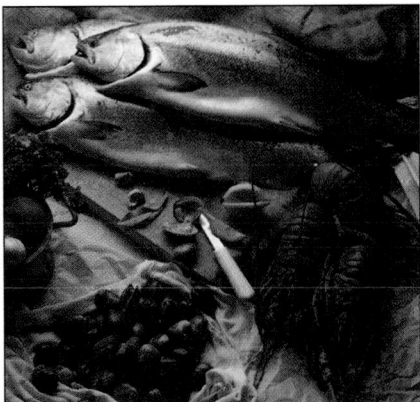

Fish, seafood, and related products are good sources of vitamin B-12.

CONCEPT CHECK

olate is needed for cell division because it is essential for DNA synthesis. A folate deficiency results in macrocytic anemia, as well as diarrhea, inflammation of the tongue, and poor growth—all signs of inadequate cell division. Folate is found in fresh vegetables and organ meats. Folate deficiency is most commonly found in pregnant women, when needs are elevated, and in alcoholics, since alcohol interferes with absorption of folate. Vitamin B-12 is necessary for folate metabolism. Without dietary vitamin B-12, folate deficiency symptoms, such as macrocytic anemia, develop. In addition, vitamin B-12 is necessary for maintaining the nervous system; paralysis can develop from a vitamin B-12 deficiency. Vitamin B-12 is found only in animal foods; meat eaters generally have a 3- to 5-year supply stored in the liver. However, vitamin B-12 absorption may decline in older persons. In this case, a deficiency of vitamin B-12 is generally corrected by monthly injections of the vitamin.

■ CHOLINE

The dietary component choline is the latest addition to the list of essential nutrients.[28]

■ Absorption, Metabolism, and Excretion of Choline

Choline is absorbed from the small intestine by way of transport proteins. Choline is taken up rapidly by the liver from the portal vein. All tissues contain choline. Some choline is excreted in the urine, but most of the excess is converted to **betaine.**

■ Functions of Choline

Choline functions as a precursor for acetylcholine, a neurotransmitter associated with attention, learning and memory, muscle control, and many other functions. It is a precursor of phospholipids, such as phosphatidylcholine (lecithin), the major component of the cell membrane. Liver export of VLDL is also associated with the action of choline. Finally, choline is a precursor for the methyl donor betaine. A significant portion of choline is converted to betaine in the liver and kidney. The methyl group of betaine can be used to form methionine from homocysteine. Review Figure 10-11, which shows how choline, methionine, vitamin B-12, and folate metabolism interact at the point where homocysteine is converted to methionine. Also see the Expert Opinion by Dr. Zeisel on even more possible functions of choline.

■ Choline Deficiency

There has been only one published study examining the effect of inadequate dietary intake of choline in healthy humans. The study of male volunteers showed decreased choline stores and liver damage. When humans were fed choline-deficient total parental nutrition solutions, they developed fatty livers and liver damage. Based on this one study, plus animal studies, choline has been deemed essential.

■ Choline in Foods

Choline is widely distributed in foods, mostly in the form of phosphatidylcholine in membranes. Milk, liver, eggs, and peanuts are rich sources. Lecithins often are added to food during processing, so this is yet another source. There is so much choline available in ordinary foods that it is unlikely that a dietary deficiency exists. Choline also can be synthesized from the nonessential amino acid serine.

betaine An oxidation product of choline metabolism and a methyl (CH_3) donor in methionine metabolism.

Choline

Lecithin

Choline forms part of the natural emulsifiers called *lecithins*.

Choline Needs

The Adequate Intake for choline for men 19 years and older is 550 mg/day; for women 19 years and older, it is 425 mg/day. This is based on the intake of choline required to maintain liver function as assessed by measuring an enzyme (alanine aminotransferase) concentration in the blood.

Few data exist to assess whether a dietary supply is needed at all life stages. Although Adequate Intakes are set for choline, it may be that the choline requirement can be met by body synthesis at some or all stages of life. We consume ample choline from food, at least 700-1000 mg/day.

High doses of choline have been associated with a fishy body odor, vomiting, salivation, sweating, low blood pressure (hypotension), and gastrointestinal effects. The fishy odor is due to the excretion of a choline metabolite. The Upper Level for adults is 3.5 g/day, based on development of a fishy body odor and low blood pressure.

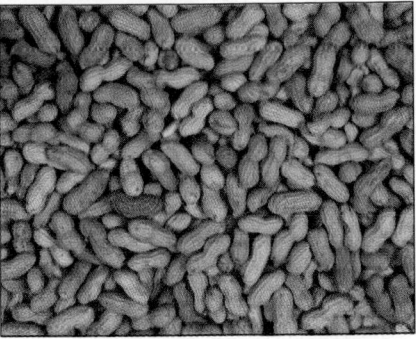

Peanuts are a good source of choline. Body cells also produce choline.

VITAMIN C

Vitamin C is found in all living tissues, and most animals are capable of synthesizing their own supply from glucose.[9] Humans and other primates, guinea pigs, and a few birds, bats, and fish are unable to make their own vitamin C and therefore must obtain it from dietary sources. What is strange is that animals that synthesize vitamin C often make very large amounts. For instance, a hog produces 8 g/day, although we do not know how a hog benefits from this large amount. Incidentally, pork is not a good source of the vitamin, since it is lost in processing. This 8 g amount is more than 80 times the human RDA of 90 mg for men and 75 mg for women. Why some animals make so much vitamin C, whereas a few other animals, including humans, appear to need so little, has fueled much controversy surrounding this vitamin.

Vitamin C refers to its reduced form, called ascorbic acid. The oxidized form is called dehydroascorbic acid. The two forms are interchangeable, and both are biologically active. Hydrolysis of dehydroascorbic acid irreversibly converts it to a product with no vitamin C activity, diketogulonic acid. This is further metabolized to oxalic acid and other compounds.

Absorption, Metabolism, Storage, and Excretion of Vitamin C

Absorption of vitamin C occurs in the small intestine by means of active transport at low gastrointestinal concentrations, and with passive diffusion at higher concentrations. Efficiency of the absorptive mechanism decreases as intake increases. About 70 to 90% of vitamin C is absorbed at daily intakes between 30 and 180 mg, whereas absorption efficiency declines to about 50% or less with increasing doses above 1 g/day. Excretion by the kidneys increases as dietary intake increases. At a very low intake, virtually no vitamin C is excreted.

Within the cell and in blood, vitamin C exists predominantly in the reduced form, ascorbic acid (ascorbate). The amount of vitamin C varies widely by tissue. High concentrations are found in the pituitary and adrenal glands, white blood cells, eyes, and brain. The lowest concentrations are in the blood and saliva. The total amount of vitamin C in the body varies over a wide range. A body pool of less than 300 mg is associated with scurvy. The maximum body pool size seems to be about 2 grams.

Functions of Vitamin C

Vitamin C performs a variety of important cell functions (Table 10-2). It does this primarily by acting as a nonspecific **reducing agent.** A reducing agent is a substance that donates electrons and, in turn, becomes oxidized. For example, vitamin C can donate electrons to metal ions, such as iron and copper. In the oxidized state, ferric iron (Fe^{3+}) can be reduced to ferrous ion (Fe^{2+}), and cupric ion (Cu^{2+}) to cuprous ion (Cu^{+}).

Ascorbic acid (reduced)

Dehydroascorbic acid (oxidized)

Vitamin C undergoes reversible oxidation and reduction by loss or addition of two hydrogens (red).

reducing agent A compound capable of donating electrons (also hydrogens) to another compound.

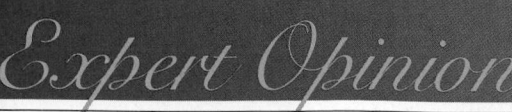

Expert Opinion

IS THERE A NEED FOR CHOLINE IN THE HUMAN DIET?

Steven H. Zeisel, M.D., Ph.D.

Human cells absolutely require choline and die by programmed cell death (apoptosis) when deprived of this nutrient. Choline is needed for the synthesis of the phospholipids in cell membranes, methyl group ($-CH_3$) metabolism, cholinergic neurotransmission, transmembrane signaling, and lipid-cholesterol transport and metabolism. Until the 1998 Dietary Reference Intake report listed Adequate Intakes for choline, there was no recommendation that humans include a source of choline in their diet. Prior to this, the debate as to whether the human diet must contain choline arose because there is a pathway (most active in the liver) for the de novo *(new)* biosynthesis of choline from phosphatidylethanolamine and *S*-adenosylmethionine (Fig. 10-11). The ability to form choline within the body means that some of the demand for choline can, in part, be met by using methyl groups derived from one-carbon metabolism (via methyl-folate and methionine).

Usually, animal feeds include a source of choline because many species of animals, including the baboon, fed a choline-deficient diet deplete choline stores and develop liver dysfunction. Also, animals fed a choline-deficient diet may develop growth retardation, kidney dysfunction and hemorrhage, or bone abnormalities.

Because it was not appreciated that humans, too, might have a requirement for choline, total parenteral nutrition (TPN) solutions did not contain added choline (although lipid emulsions contain a small amount of lecithin [phosphatidylcholine] as an emulsifier). Patients fed intravenously with such solutions devoid of choline, but adequate for methionine and folate, developed fatty liver and liver damage, some of which resolved when a source of dietary choline was provided. Fatty liver occurred because choline is required to make the phosphatidylcholine portion of the VLDL lipoprotein particle that is used to secrete triglyceride from the liver. In the absence of choline, VLDL is not secreted, and lipid accumulates in hepatic cytosol. The liver cell death occurred in choline deficiency because hepatocytes initiate programmed cell death when deprived of choline. Because methyl group supplementation with betaine, methionine, folate, or vitamin B-12 did not prevent apoptotic death induced by choline deficiency in cultured hepatocytes, it must be that the depletion of intracellular choline, rather than the depletion of methyl groups, was the critical parameter in-

volved in induction of apoptosis. The data from TPN studies support the conclusion that the de novo synthesis of choline is not always sufficient to meet human requirements for choline. However, patients who require intravenous feeding are ill and may have abnormal nutrient requirements.

We know little about the variation in dietary choline intake in healthy humans because there is no comprehensive database of foods that contain this nutrient. Most foods contain some choline in the form of choline, phosphocholine, glycerophosphocholine, phosphatidylcholine, or sphingomyelin. Eggs have a high choline content (about 200-300 mg per egg, mostly in the form of phosphatidylcholine), as does milk (about 40 mg per 8 oz). We do not know whether there are populations of humans who are eating a low-choline diet; this awaits the availability of a comprehensive food database. However, we know that choline in breast milk increases after a mother eats a choline-containing meal and that mothers in Ecuador who eat what appears to be a low-choline diet have much less choline in their milk than do mothers in Boston. This suggests that significant dietary variation might exist relative to choline intake.

---

collagen The major protein of the material that holds together the various structures of the body.

connective tissue The material that holds together the various structures of the body. Tendons and cartilage are composed largely of connective tissue. Connective tissue also forms part of bone and the nonmuscular structures of arteries and veins.

Collagen Synthesis

Collagen is the fibrous protein that is a major component of **connective tissue.** Indeed, collagen is found wherever tissues are needed for strength, especially in those tissues with a protective, connective, or structural function. Collagen fibers are critical to the maintenance of bone and blood vessels, and they are essential in wound healing.

A collagen molecule consists of three-polypeptide chains wound together to form a triple helix. The polypeptide chains constituting the basic structure of collagen contain many proline and lysine components. The synthesis of mature collagen depends on hydroxylation (addition of -OH groups) to these two amino acids, which

When healthy men with normal folate and vitamin B-12 status were fed a choline-deficient diet, they developed diminished blood choline and phosphatidylcholine concentrations, as well as evidence of liver damage. For these individuals, the de novo synthesis of choline was not adequate to meet the demand for the nutrient. Studies of choline requirements in women, children, and infants have not been conducted. Thus, we do not know whether choline is needed in the diets of these groups. Female rats are less sensitive to choline deficiency than are male rats, perhaps because estrogen enhances females' capacity to form choline from S-adenosylmethionine. This is likely the case in premenopausal women. Thus, the choline requirements of healthy females may differ from those of males. Studies are underway in my laboratory to characterize these differences in dietary requirements. And, although female rats are resistant to choline deficiency, pregnant rats are as vulnerable to deficiency as are males. During pregnancy, large amounts of choline are delivered to the fetus across the placenta, and this depletes maternal stores of choline. The need for choline is likely to be further increased during lactation because so much choline must be secreted into milk. Thus, there is likely to be an increased dietary choline requirement for women during pregnancy and lactation.

There may be a special and critical requirement for dietary choline during embryogenesis (development of the egg into an embryo). There is a period in rat brain development during which the availability of dietary choline determines whether optimal development occurs in the memory centers in the brain. When higher than normal amounts of dietary choline were supplied to the rat mother during the time that cells in these brain regions of the rat fetus were undergoing cell division and migration, the number of cells populating these memory centers was increased. When lower than normal amounts of choline were supplied, there were fewer cells populating these areas. These structural changes correlated with electrophysiological changes in these brain centers and were associated with memory changes. Choline supplementation during this critical period then elicited a major improvement in memory performance in the mother's offspring. These changes in memory lasted the lifetime of the rat offspring; they were not altered by adding or removing choline in the diet of the adult rats (after the critical period in development had gone by). In the rat, this critical period occurs at days 12-18 of gestation, equivalent to about weeks 20-30 in the human fetus. Are these findings in rats likely to be true in humans? We do not know.

In summary, choline in the diet is important for many reasons. The nutrition community now has a set of recommendations about choline in the diet (see the inside cover of this textbook). In the near future, we should learn more precisely about choline requirements in women. As our understanding of the importance of folate and homocysteine nutrition increases, there should be increased interest in how choline interacts with one-carbon metabolism. During the next few years, it is likely that food composition data will be available for choline, and this will make it possible to examine interactions among choline, folate, and methionine when considering epidemiological data. Recent findings about choline in brain development should stimulate comparable studies in humans. Perhaps when the Dietary Reference Intake recommendations for choline are revised the next time, more information about human requirements for choline will be available.

Dr. Zeisel is professor and chairman of the Department of Nutrition, School of Public Health and School of Medicine, The University of North Carolina at Chapel Hill, Chapel Hill, NC 27599-7400. He is internationally known for his research in choline and for his commitment to furthering nutrition education in the medical school curriculum in general.

yields hydroxyproline and hydroxylysine. Hydroxyproline is necessary for the formation of stable collagen triple helices, and hydroxylysine plays a role in linking these helices together (Fig. 10-12).

The role of vitamin C in **post-translational** hydroxylation of peptide-bound proline and lysine (in intact proteins) is accomplished by changing the iron in the enzyme (Fe^{3+} to Fe^{2+}) that hydroxylates proline to form hydroxyproline and changing the copper in the enzyme (Cu^{2+} to Cu^+) that hydroxylates lysine to hydroxylysine. There is evidence to suggest that vitamin C also plays a role in the biosynthesis of other connective tissue components besides collagen, including **elastin.** Scurvy is associated with the deterioration of elastic tissues.

post-translational Occurring or formed after protein synthesis is completed by the ribosomes.

elastin The rubberband-like connective tissue protein found in lungs and large arteries, where elastic properties are essential.

TABLE 10-2   Functions of Vitamin C: In Vivo, In Vitro, or Controversial[4]

In Vivo Functions	In Vitro or Animal Studies	Association Weak, Conflicting, or Lacking
Antioxidant due to high reducing ability for a variety of biochemical reactions	Regenerates vitamin E	Protection against periodontal disease, some cancers, cardiovascular disease
Provides reduced form of iron for copper metalloenzymes	Increases dietary iron absorption	Protection against asthma and chronic obstructive pulmonary disease
Protective water-soluble antioxidant in intracellular and extracellular environment, as it quenches a variety of reactive oxygen species and reactive nitrogen species	Inhibits oxidation of LDL by metals, free radicals, macrophages	Protection against the common cold or infectious diseases
Tyrosine metabolism; provides stability to a wide variety of hormones	Cofactor for enzymes involved in biosynthesis of collagen, carnitine, epinephrine, norepinephrine, and other nervous system components	Maintenance of memory and cognitive function
Connective tissue biosynthesis		
Scavenger for reactive oxygen species and reactive nitrogen species in white blood cells, lungs, and stomach; protects against lipid peroxidation		
In smokers, helps prevent damage from oxidative stress		

glutathione A reducing agent; it can remove the toxic peroxides that form in the cell during aerobic metabolism.

The vitamin C deficiency disease scurvy was the curse of sailors throughout the nineteenth century. On long sea voyages, a captain often lost more than half of his crew to scurvy. Defective collagen synthesis is at the heart of the problem. From 1550 to 1857, more than 114 scurvy epidemics were reported in Europe. Soldiers in the U.S. Civil War died of scurvy. In 1740, Dr. James Lind, working aboard the HMS *Salisbury,* showed that citrus fruits—two oranges and one lemon a day—can cure scurvy. Fifty years after Lind's discovery, limes were added to the rations for British sailors to prevent scurvy. That is why the British today may be referred to as "limeys."

Antioxidant Activity

Vitamin C can both donate and accept hydrogen atoms readily; it is a reducing agent, or antioxidant, because it can reverse oxidation. Vitamin C works with vitamin E as a pair of free radical scavengers. (Recall that vitamin E is a fat-soluble antioxidant in the cell membrane.) Vitamin C is a water-soluble intracellular and extracellular antioxidant; however, in order for it to continue to function, it must be constantly enzymatically regenerated. There are several agents capable of this task, such as $NADH + H^+$, $NADPH + H^+$, and **glutathione.** Vitamin C is a ready scavenger for reactive oxygen species (ROS). Remember that Reactive Oxygen Species and Reactive Nitrogen Species (RNS) are formed during normal cellular metabolism generate free radicals.

Vitamin C is present in high concentrations in the eye to protect against photolytically generated free radicals. It is also present in high concentrations in white blood cells (e.g., neutrophils) for protection against the ROS produced during phagocytosis. In semen, vitamin C protects DNA in sperm from oxidative damage. However, the results of studies testing the effectiveness of vitamin C on cellular DNA damage are mixed. It is possible that vitamin C may spare or regenerate vitamin E to its active state by donating electrons to the free radical form of vitamin E. Vitamin C in vitro prevents ROS and RNS from attacking LDL, but the evidence is less convincing in vivo. Some studies have shown a reduced risk of cardiovascular disease with vitamin C supplementation (doses of 50 mg/day to 1 g/day), whereas others have shown no association.[4] Currently the American Heart Association does not endorse use of vitamin C supplements to reduce cardiovascular disease risk.

The most dramatic evidence that vitamin C functions as an antioxidant in vivo are studies of smokers who were supplemented with 1 to 2 g/day of vitamin C and showed a significant decrease in oxidative stress. *Oxidative stress* refers to the highly oxidized environment within cells that forces these cells into a highly activated state due to loss of control of their regulatory systems. Smokers have low concentrations

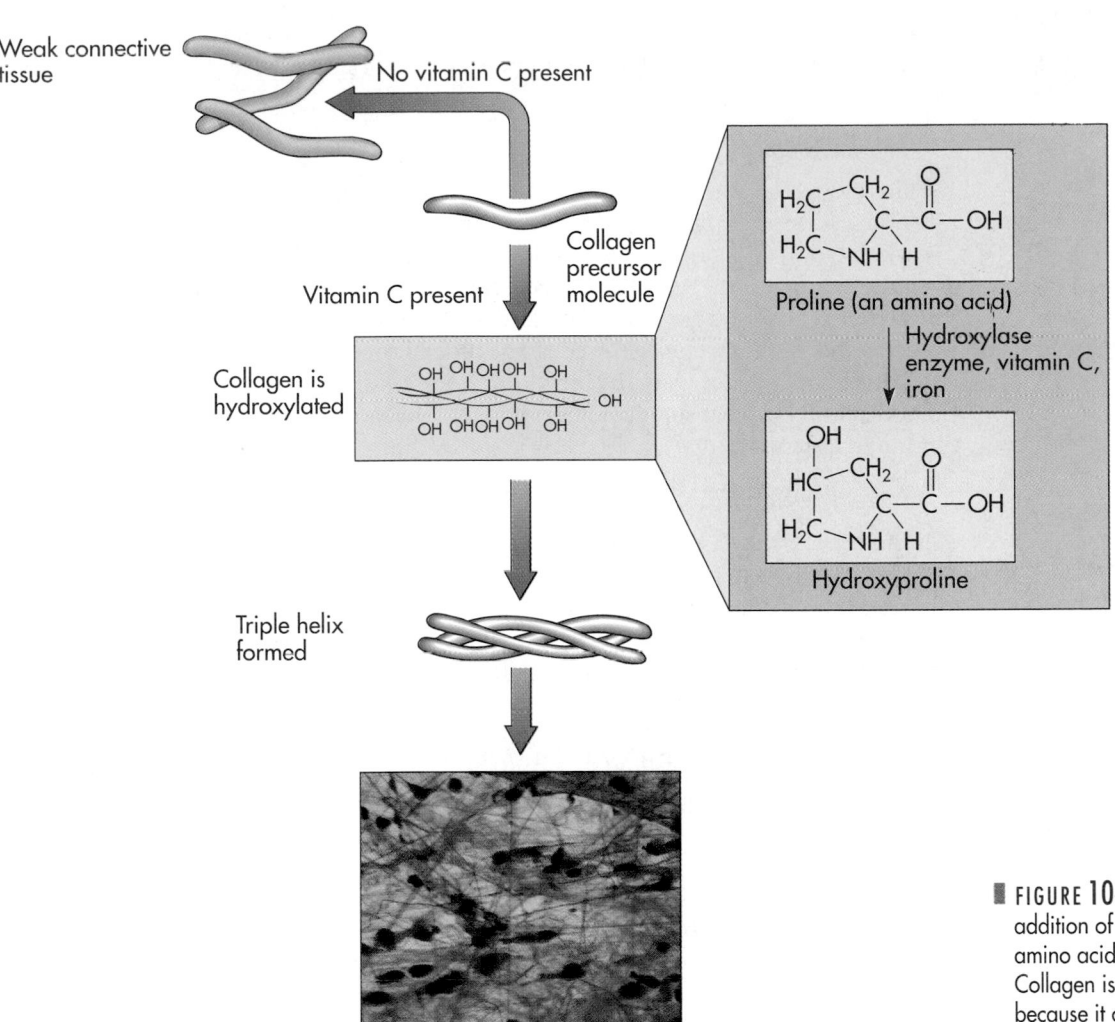

Weak connective tissue

No vitamin C present

Collagen precursor molecule

Vitamin C present

Collagen is hydroxylated

Triple helix formed

Strong connective tissue.

Proline (an amino acid)

Hydroxylase enzyme, vitamin C, iron

Hydroxyproline

■ FIGURE 10-12 Vitamin C is needed for the addition of hydroxyl groups (-OH) to the amino acid proline in collagen molecules. Collagen is unique among body proteins because it contains large amounts of the amino acid hydroxyproline, which is necessary for the formation of stable collagen fibers.

of vitamin C with evidence of increased oxidative stress, which vitamin C appears to correct. Even nonsmokers exposed to secondhand smoke showed a significant decline in vitamin C in the blood and increased lipid peroxidation. Nonsmokers exposed to tobacco smoke are urged to ensure they obtain adequate dietary vitamin C.[4]

Iron Absorption

Vitamin C added to meals facilitates the intestinal absorption of nonheme iron (iron that is not in hemoglobin) due to the conversion of iron in the gastrointestinal tract to ferrous iron (Fe^{2+}). Vitamin C also counters the action of certain food components that inhibit iron absorption. However, studies of vitamin C added to meals over long periods of time have not shown a major improvement of iron status.

Synthesis of Other Vital Cell Compounds

Carnitine is a transport compound that moves fatty acids from the cytoplasm into the mitochondria for energy productions. Vitamin C participates in two separate steps in carnitine biosynthesis. The biosynthesis of norepinephrine and epinephrine depends on vitamin C as an electron donor to maintain the metals in the synthesizing enzymes in a reduced form. The conversion of the essential amino acid tryptophan to the neurotransmitter serotonin requires vitamin C. Vitamin C is necessary for the biosynthesis of thyroxine (the thyroid hormone) and many other nervous

CRITICAL THINKING

Carlos just returned from a local mall and is excited because he saw an advertisement claiming that vitamin C will cure just about everything, from colds to heart disease. How would you explain to him vitamin C's main functions in the human body?

respiration The intracellular oxidation of substances coupled with the production of ATP; may be anaerobic or aerobic.

neutrophil activation A type of white blood cell being prepared for immune response.

*A*lthough the development of scurvy in an otherwise healthy child is rare, it is possible. A 5-year-old boy developed scurvy after eating nothing but Pop-Tarts, cheese pizza, biscuits, and water for 5 months. The boy, who was growing and maturing normally, started to limp; his gums became swollen; and small, purple spots began to appear on his skin. His baffled doctors finally diagnosed the boy as having scurvy and gave him vitamin C, and his condition began to improve within a week.

system components. Vitamin C is also involved in the biosynthesis of corticosteroids and aldosterone, the conversion of cholesterol to bile acids, and tyrosine metabolism.

Immune Function

White blood cells provide immune defenses of the body. These contain the highest vitamin C concentration of all body constituents. A high concentration of vitamin C in white blood cells provides protection against the oxidative damage associated with cellular **respiration.** Reactive oxygen species generated during phagocytosis and **neutrophil activation** are associated with infections and inflammation. The amount of vitamin C in neutrophils is used as the index for establishing the RDA. Vitamin C effectively neutralizes oxidants but doesn't inhibit bactericidal activity by the white blood cells. Note that supplemental vitamin C beyond body needs does not improve immune function.

Cancer Prevention

In the past 25 years, there has been considerable interest in vitamin C as a cancer-preventive nutrient. Varied intake of vitamin C with respect to breast, colorectal, gastric, and bladder cancer has not produced compelling evidence that vitamin C reduces in vivo DNA oxidative damage. Among several studies, when only vitamin C intake was varied, some indicators of DNA damage showed no change, some decreased, and one increased.[4]

■ Vitamin C Deficiency: Scurvy

A deficiency of vitamin C prevents the normal synthesis of collagen, thus causing widespread and significant changes in connective tissues throughout the body. The first signs and symptoms of scurvy, the deficiency disease, appear after about 20 to 40 days on a vitamin C-free diet and include fatigue and pinpoint hemorrhages (petechiae) around hair follicles on the back of the arms and legs (Fig. 10-13). These hemorrhages are the most characteristic sign of scurvy. In addition, there is bleeding in the gums and joints, a classic sign of connective tissue failure. Other effects of scurvy include impaired wound healing, bone pain, fractures, and diarrhea. Psychological problems, such as depression, are common in advanced scurvy.

Worldwide, scurvy is associated with poverty. It is especially common in infants who are fed boiled milk (all forms of milk are poor sources of vitamin C) and are not provided with a good food source of vitamin C or a supplement.

■ Vitamin C in Foods

Citrus fruits, potatoes, and green vegetables in general are good sources of vitamin C (Fig. 10-14). The Food Guide Pyramid guideline of at least 5 servings/day of combined fruits and vegetables provides ample vitamin C. The major contributors of vitamin C to American diets are oranges and orange juice, grapefruit and grapefruit juice, tomatoes and tomato juice, fortified fruit drinks, tangerines, and potatoes. Although the isoascorbate (erythorbate) used as a food preservative in fruits and vegetables has no vitamin C activity, it does act as an antioxidant in the body.

The most nutrient-dense sources of vitamin C (mg/kcal) are green peppers, cauliflower, broccoli, strawberries, papayas, romaine lettuce, oranges, and spinach and other greens.

Vitamin C is easily lost in processing and cooking. Juices are good foods to fortify with vitamin C because their acidity reduces vitamin C destruction. Vitamin C is very unstable when in contact with heat, iron, copper, and oxygen.

■ Vitamin C Needs

The Estimated Average Requirement for vitamin C is based on an intake that maintains near-maximal white blood cell (specifically neutrophil) concentration with minimal urinary excretion of vitamin C.[4] For men, it is 75 mg/day, 60 mg/day for

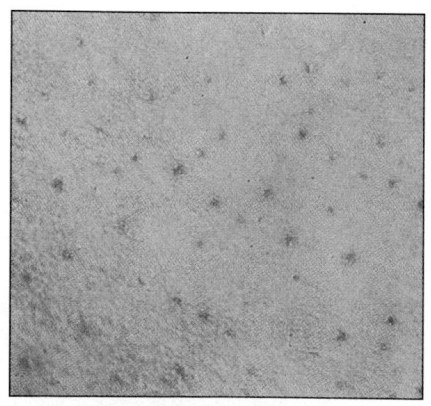

■ FIGURE **10-13** Pinpoint hemorrhages of the skin—an early symptom of scurvy. The spots on the skin are caused by slight bleeding into hair follicles. The person also will often show inadequate wound healing—all signs of defective collagen synthesis.

Nutrient Density for Vitamin C

low	medium	high

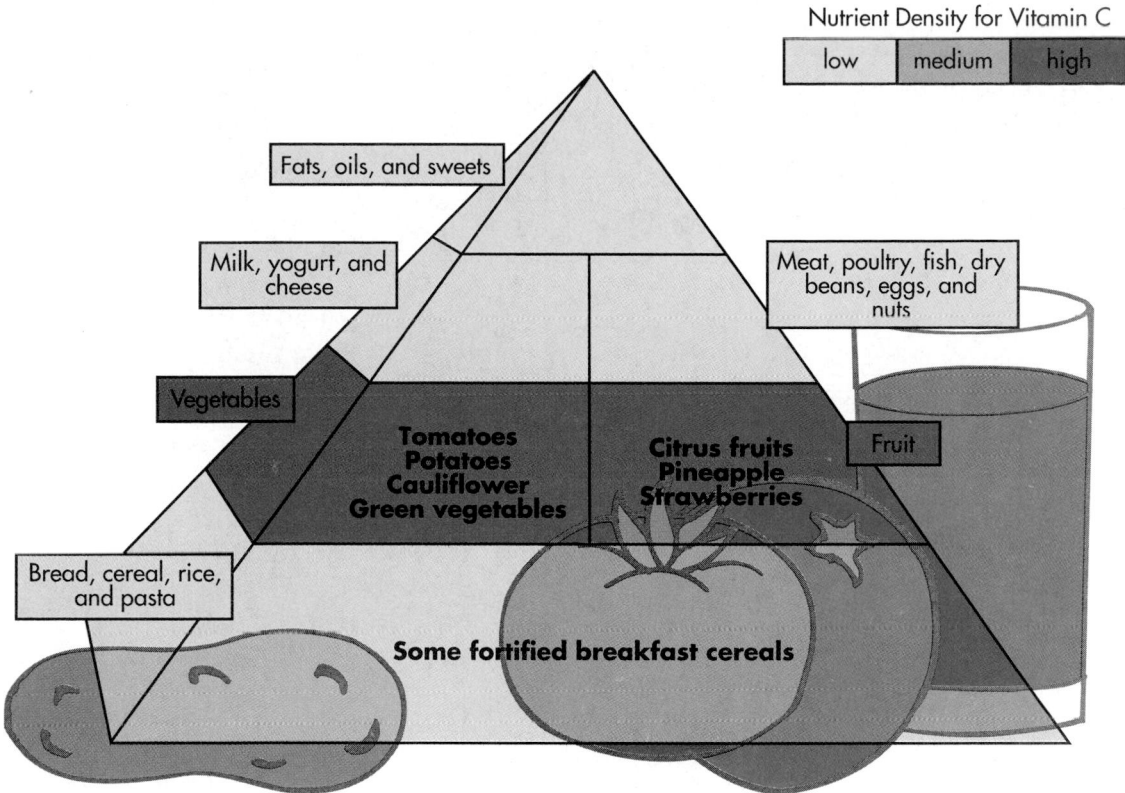

■ FIGURE 10-14 Food sources of vitamin C from the Food Guide Pyramid. The fruit group and the vegetables group are especially rich sources of this nutrient. The background color of each food group indicates the average nutrient density for vitamin C in that group.

women. The RDA is set by increasing this 20% to account for individual variation. The RDA for vitamin C for adult men 19 and older is thus 90 mg/day; for adult women 19 and older, 75 mg/day. Because smoking causes oxidative stress, the requirement for smokers increases by 35 mg/day. An estimate of vitamin C intake for adults in Canada and the United States is 72 mg/day and 102 mg/day, respectively.

■ North Americans at Risk for Vitamin C Deficiency

Today, vitamin C deficiency is most likely to occur in alcoholics and those addicted to other drugs, as they often consume a nutrient-poor diet. Older men who eat very few fruits and vegetables are also susceptible to vitamin C deficiency. Men in general are more at risk of vitamin C deficiency compared with women because they are less apt to consume vitamin supplements. Finally, people exposed to cigarette smoke generally have lower vitamin C status than nonsmokers.

■ Toxicity of Vitamin C

The principal adverse effects associated with a very high intake of vitamin C are gastrointestinal disturbances, including nausea, abdominal cramps, and osmotic diarrhea. There are conflicting data as to whether megadoses of vitamin C cause increased uric acid excretion. The in vivo data do not show a clear causal relationship between megadoses of vitamin C by healthy individuals and kidney stone formation, excess iron absorption, vitamin B-12 deficiency, reduced copper levels, pro-oxidant effects, dental enamel erosion, or allergic response in adults and children. At one time, all these conditions were blamed on excess vitamin C consumption. The Upper Level is 2 g/day, based on osmotic diarrhea and gastrointestinal disturbances.

Table 10-3 summarizes much of what is known about the B-vitamins, choline, and vitamin C.

*D*ietary Sources of Vitamin C

Food Item and Amount	Vitamin C (mg)
Orange juice, fresh, 8 oz	124
Brussels sprouts, cooked, 1 cup	97
Brussels sprouts, raw, 1 cup	74
Papaya, cubed, 1 cup	87
Strawberries, whole, 1 cup	82
Kiwifruit, 1	74
Grapefruit juice, 8 oz	72
Red pepper, ¼ cup	71
Orange, 1	70
Green pepper rings, 5	45
Tomato juice, 8 oz	44
Broccoli, raw ½ cup	41
Cabbage, raw, shredded, 1 cup	23
Cauliflower, raw, ½ cup	23
Spinach, cooked, 1 cup	18
Spinach, raw, 1 cup	8

CRITICAL THINKING

Examine the list of dietary sources of vitamin C. Why do you think cooking doubles the amount of vitamin C in spinach but only slightly increases the amount of vitamin C in brussels sprouts?

T A B L E 10-3   A Summary of Water-Soluble Vitamins

Vitamin	Major Functions	Deficiency Symptoms	People Most at Risk	Dietary Sources	RDA or Adequate Intake	Toxicity*
Thiamin	Coenzyme in carbohydrate and amino acid metabolism: essential to nerve function	Beriberi: anorexia, weight loss, weakness, peripheral neuropathy; Wernicke-Korsakoff syndrome	Alcoholics and people living in poverty	Pork and pork products, enriched and whole-grain cereals, nuts and seeds	Men: 1.2 mg/day; women: 1.1mg/day	None
Riboflavin	Coenzyme in numerous oxidation-reduction reactions	Ariboflavinosis: inflammation of mouth and tongue, cracks at corner of mouth, eye disorders	People taking certain medications if no dairy products consumed	Milk, mushrooms, spinach, liver, enriched grains	Men: 1.3 mg/day; women: 1.1 mg/day	None
Niacin	Coenzyme in numerous oxidation-reduction reactions in energy metabolism, synthesis and breakdown of fatty acids	Pellagra: diarrhea, dermatitis, dementia (death)	Alcoholics and people living in poverty where corn is the dominant food	Meat, poultry, fish, enriched and whole-grain breads and cereals; also from tryptophan conversion to niacin	Men: 16mg NE/day; women: 14 mg NE/day	Flushing of skin: Upper Level for adults: 35 mg/day from supplements
Pantothenic acid	Coenzyme involved in energy metabolism and fatty-acid synthesis	No natural deficiency disease or symptoms	None	Widely distributed in foods	Adequate Intake for adults: 5 mg/day	None
Biotin	Cofactor for four carboxylases	Dermatitis, conjunctivitis, hair loss, nervous system abnormalities	Alcoholics	Widely distributed in foods	Adequate Intake for adults: 30 μg/day	Unknown

Vitamin	Major Functions	Deficiency Symptoms	People Most at Risk	Dietary Sources	RDA or Adequate Intake	Toxicity*
Vitamin B-6	Coenzymes involved in amino acid metabolism, heme synthesis, lipid metabolism; homocysteine metabolism	Dermatitis, anemia, convulsion, depression, confusion	Alcoholics	Animal protein foods, bananas, potatoes, watermelon, avocados	Adults: 19 to 50 1.3 mg/day; men over 50: 1.4 mg/day; women over 50: 1.3 mg/day	None from food but from supplements cause neuropathy and skin lesions; Upper Level: 100 mg/day
Folate	Coenzyme involved in DNA synthesis, homocysteine metabolism	Megaloblastic anemia; birth defects	Alcoholics, pregnant women, people on certain medications	Green vegetables, liver, enriched cereal products, legumes, oranges	400 µg/day of dietary folate equivalents	None; Upper Level for adults set at 1000 µg/day for synthetic folate, exclusive of food folate
Vitamin B-12	Cofactor for two enzymes, control of folate metabolism, homocysteine metabolism	Megaloblastic anemia, paresthesia	Older adults, vegans, HIV-positive patients, patients with malabsorption syndromes	Animal foods and fortified breakfast cereals	Adults 19-50: 2.4 µg/day; adults 51 and older: same, but use fortified foods or supplements	None
Vitamin C	Collagen synthesis, antioxidant, hormone and neurotransmitter synthesis	Scurvy: poor wound healing, pinpoint hemorrhages, bleeding gums	Alcoholics, older men living alone	Fruits and vegetables	Men: 90 mg/day; women: 75 mg/day; + 35 mg/day for smokers	Diarrhea and other gastrointestinal problems; Upper Level: 2 g/day
Choline	Precursor for acetylcholine, phospholipids, and betaine; homocysteine metabolism	No natural deficiency	None	Widely distributed in foods, plus self-synthesis	Adequate Intake for Men: 550 mg/day; women: 425 mg/day	Upper Level: 3.5 g/day

*Toxicity arise only from supplement use.

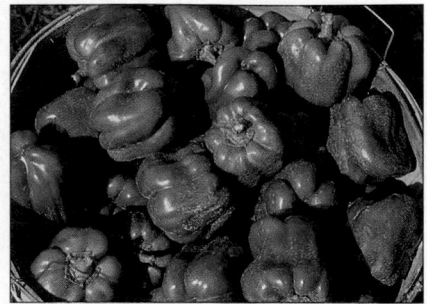

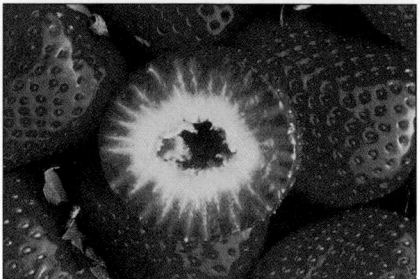

Vegetables such as green peppers are one source of vitamin C, and fruits such as strawberries are another rich source.

CONCEPT CHECK

*O*nly guinea pigs, monkeys, some birds and fish, and humans need dietary vitamin C. It is used mainly in the synthesis of collagen, a major connective tissue protein. A vitamin C deficiency causes scurvy, which is marked by many changes in the skin and gums, such as small hemorrhages, because of reduced collagen synthesis. Vitamin C also modestly improves iron absorption and is involved in the synthesis of certain hormones and neurotransmitters. Citrus fruits, green peppers, cauliflower, broccoli, and strawberries are good sources of vitamin C. As with folate, fresh or lightly cooked foods are the best sources, since loss of vitamin C in cooking can be high. At intakes greater than about 2 g/day, vitamin C can lead to diarrhea and other gastrointestinal upsets.

◼ VITAMIN-LIKE COMPOUNDS

The various vitamin-like compounds—carnitine, inositol, taurine, and lipoic acid— are necessary to maintain normal metabolism in the body. They all can be synthesized by the body, but their biosynthesis often occurs at the expense of other nutrients, such as essential amino acids. The need for these compounds often increases during times of rapid tissue growth, as is the case with the premature infant.

There is no concern that deficiencies of these vitamin-like compounds exist in the average healthy adult. But more research is needed to clarify whether deficiencies might arise in certain disease states and whether the compounds should be included in infant formulas and total parenteral nutrition solutions. Currently, manufacturers often add these vitamin-like compounds to infant formulas.

Carnitine.

◼ Carnitine

Carnitine is a relatively simple compound that can be synthesized in the liver from the amino acids lysine and methionine. Human needs for carnitine are met from both animal foods and biosynthesis. Adults and children who are severely malnourished or on total parenteral nutrition can have lower-than-normal concentrations of carnitine in their blood. An inadequate supply of protein (i.e., a lack of the amino acids needed for making carnitine) leads to abnormal fatty-acid metabolism. There is speculation that people with cirrhosis may need carnitine from the diet to offset inadequate liver production.

Within the cell, carnitine transports fatty acids from the cytosol into the mitochondria, where the fatty acids are then metabolized for energy. Carnitine also aids the mitochondria in removing excess organic acids, products of metabolic pathways.

Myo-inositol.

Meat and dairy products are the main sources of carnitine. We consume about 100 to 300 mg/day. Vegetarian diets are very low in carnitine because it is almost absent from plant foods. However, vegetarians show normal blood concentrations of carnitine. Consequently, it is doubtful that carnitine is necessary in the diets of healthy people. It may be considered a conditionally essential nutrient in times of recovery from disease, serious trauma, kidney dialysis, or preterm birth.

In addition, carnitine has displayed pharmaceutical usefulness in the removal of compounds that can build to toxic amounts in people with inborn errors of metabolism. Dosages approximately 10 times typical dietary intakes have also been shown to improve the condition of persons with progressive muscle disease and heart muscle deterioration.

*C*ontrary to the advertisements, carnitine supplements do not burn fat, nor do they enhance aerobic performance of endurance athletes.

◼ Inositol

Of the nine possible isomers of inositol, only one—called myo-inositol—has nutritional implications for humans. The structure of inositol is related to that of glucose, from which it is synthesized in the body.

Much of the inositol in body cells occurs in phosphorylated forms, such as inositol triphosphate (IP_3), which is found free in the cell cytosol. Inositol is also incorporated into the phospholipids located in cell membranes. These inositol phospholipids are important precursors of the eicosanoids, which have numerous hormonelike actions (see Chapter 6). Under certain conditions (e.g., the binding of hormones), enzymes in the cell membrane act on the inositol phospholipids, releasing IP_3. This compound, in turn, mobilizes calcium ions (Ca^{2+}) from stores within cells. The resulting increase in the intracellular calcium concentration then leads to various cell responses in various tissues, such as the recognition and transfer of stimuli by nerve cells. This inositol-dependent function may explain why high concentrations of inositol phospholipids are found in brain tissue.

Both free inositol and inositol phospholipids are present in animal foods. Some plant foods (e.g., wheat bran) also contain inositol, mostly as part of phytic acid, a compound that binds minerals. The average American diet provides about 1 g of inositol per day, and another 4 g/day or more are synthesized in the kidneys.

The metabolism of inositol is altered by several medical conditions. The hyperglycemia associated with diabetes inhibits inositol transport. Abnormal inositol metabolism is also noted in multiple sclerosis, kidney failure, and certain cancers. Overall, it appears that inositol is an essential nutrient only in certain medical conditions.

■ Taurine

Taurine is synthesized from the sulfur-containing amino acids methionine and cysteine. It is abundant in muscle, platelets, and nerve tissue. It is also attached to bile acids. Although its mechanism of action is not well understood, taurine is involved in many vital functions. It is associated with photoreceptor activity in the eye, antioxidant activity in white blood cells, the protection of pulmonary tissue from oxidation, central nervous system function, platelet aggregation, cardiac contraction, insulin action, and cell differentiation and growth.

Taurine is found only in animal foods. Americans consume about 40 to 400 mg/day. No clear cases of taurine deficiencies have been diagnosed in vegans, even though it is not found in plants, suggesting that synthesis by the body meets needs. Thus, it appears that healthy people need not worry about consuming taurine.

Taurine supplementation may be of benefit to children with cystic fibrosis. Some experience increased growth when treated with taurine, perhaps because of increased fat absorption from the action of taurine as part of bile. Preterm infants supplemented with taurine may also exhibit improved fat absorption.

■ Lipoic Acid

Lipoic acid is used in reactions in which a carbon dioxide molecule is lost from a substrate, as when pyruvate is converted into acetyl-CoA. Lipoic acid also works with several antioxidants in the body. Lipoic acid itself is a redox agent, in that it quenches singlet oxygen by donating an electron, especially when lipoic acid is in its reduced form. Reduced lipoic acid, in turn, can recycle vitamin C and glutathione, two other antioxidants. This function of lipoic acid also helps vitamin E stay in its reduced form.

Even though lipoic acid serves such beneficial functions in the body, it is unnecessary to obtain it from outside sources. Rich dietary sources are meats, liver, and yeast.

Inositol in supplement form is promoted as treatment for insomnia. There are a variety of causes for sleep disorders, but probably none are linked to an inositol deficiency.

One web site states that many individuals are deficient in L-taurine. Since taurine is found in the central nervous system the "pill pusher" claims it controls epileptic seizures, motor tics, and facial twitches. It is also promoted as preventing cataracts and certain forms of heart disease. Scientific evidence for these claims is lacking.

Taurine.

Some supplement manufacturers claim the body is unable to manufacture sufficient lipoic acid. They also claim that a deficiency of lipoic acid prevents antioxidants from working properly together. No scientific evidence supports these claims.

Lipoic acid.

■ BOGUS VITAMINS

Health-food enthusiasts promote a variety of compounds as vitamins, even though these substances have no importance in human nutrition. Because some of these so-called vitamins may cause increased growth in lower organisms, some vitamin marketers try to promote them as important for humans.

The list of these pseudovitamins changes frequently, The following are some of the more persistent pseudos:

- Para-aminobenzoic acid (PABA): Although this compound is part of the vitamin folate, humans can't use it to make folate. Entrepreneurs represent PABA as "a member of the B-complex family," omitting the words "for bacteria" when they sell it as a food supplement. If consumed along with sulfa antibiotics, it can defeat the effect of the antibiotic.

- Laetrile: This cyanide-containing compound, wrongly labeled vitamin B-17, is promoted as a cure for cancer. FDA does not recognize it as a legitimate cancer therapy. Chronic cyanide intoxication from laetrile in the diet has produced cases of slowly progressing nerve damage, resulting in blindness, deafness, and muscle weakness.

- Bioflavonoids: These compounds, wrongly labeled vitamin P, include rutin and hesperidin. They were originally thought to be more effective than vitamin C alone for treating fragile blood vessels in scurvy. Today, no nutritional requirement for these compounds or related flavonoids is recognized, although some may enhance vitamin C absorption, and epidemiological evidence links the consumption of foods rich in flavonoids with decreased risk from some cancers (the phytochemical link was discussed in Chapter 2). Rich sources of rutin and hesperidin are whole grains and the inner rind of lemons and oranges.

- Pangamic acid: This bogus compound, wrongly labeled vitamin B-15, has no link to nutrition and deserves no attention from anyone, including athletes. Its roots are in quackery, pure and simple. It is illegal to distribute this substance in the United States.

Other compounds will surely come and go in the next few years. Again, because people have been maintained for years on intravenous feedings that contain all the known essential nutrients without developing deficiency symptoms, the discovery of any new vitamin is unlikely. You can be sure that, if a new compound has the potential to be a vitamin, the Food and Nutrition Board of the National Academy of Sciences will closely examine it. If it then appears with the rest of the nutrients in related Food and Nutrition Board publications, you can be confident that the compound can be called a vitamin and merits your attention.

CONCEPT CHECK

A variety of vitamin-like compounds are found in the body. They can be synthesized by cells using common building blocks, such as amino acids and glucose. Sometimes in disease states synthesis may not meet body needs, and therefore dietary intake can be crucial. The needs for dietary carnitine and taurine in certain conditions (e.g., in preterm infants or in total parenteral nutrition) are current areas of research. Supplement manufacturers promote a variety of other compounds they call vitamins, even though they do not meet the criteria necessary to be a vitamin.

Check out the *Perspectives in Nutrition* Online Learning Center http://www.mhhe.com/wardlaw for quizzes, flash cards, other activities, and web links designed to further help you learn about the water-soluble vitamins.

SUMMARY

1. Thiamin in its functional form as TPP serves as a coenzyme in decarboxylation and transketolase reactions of carbohydrates. It is involved in neurotransmission and nerve conduction. About the only North American population that could be deficient in thiamin are alcoholics. Pork, pork products, and enriched grains are reliable sources of thiamin.

2. Riboflavin in functional form, FAD and FMN, participates in a wide variety of oxidation-reduction reactions in numerous metabolic pathways that produce energy. A pure riboflavin deficiency is unlikely but could accompany other B-vitamin deficiencies. Dairy products and enriched grains are good dietary sources.

3. Niacin as NAD and NADP are coenzymes. NAD is important in oxidation-reduction reactions that yield energy. A deficiency of the vitamin produces the disease pellagra. Alcoholism can lead to a deficiency. Food sources of niacin are enriched cereal grains and protein foods. The body is able to synthesize the vitamin from the amino acid tryptophan. Megadoses of niacin produce a variety of toxic symptoms.

4. Pantothenic acid in coenzyme form (CoA) shuttles two carbon fragments from the metabolism of glucose, amino acids, fatty acids, and alcohol into the citric acid cycle during energy metabolism. A deficiency of pantothenic acid is unlikely, since it is widely distributed in foods.

5. Biotin functions as a cofactor in four carboxylases, enzymes that add carbon dioxide to a substance. Biotin is widely distributed in foods. No deficiency exists in healthy people. Intestinal bacteria also synthesize biotin.

6. Vitamin B-6 in coenzyme form (PLP) participates in amino acid metabolism, especially the synthesis of nonessential amino acids. It is essential in the synthesis of heme in hemoglobin and the formation of certain neurotransmitters. Anemia, convulsions, and decreased immune response are symptoms of a deficiency. Animal protein foods, vegetables, and whole-grain cereals are good sources of this vitamin. It is not effective in treating PMS or carpal tunnel syndrome. Toxic effects include nerve damage.

7. Folate in one of its many coenzyme forms (tetrahydrofolic acid) accepts one-carbon groups from various donors and serves up one-carbon groups to a variety of metabolic pathways. The most notable job performed by folate is DNA synthesis. A dietary lack of the vitamin produces megaloblastic anemia and spina bifida and is one cause of heart disease (through the homocysteine link). Deficiency is common among alcoholics. Folate is found in green vegetables, legumes, liver, and fortified cereal grains. Folate is destroyed by high cooking temperatures.

8. Vitamin B-12 in two coenzyme forms allows three-carbon fatty acids to be oxidized for energy and promotes normal red blood cell formation. Because of its interaction with folate, a deficiency of vitamin B-12 results in the same type of megaloblastic anemia, as well as excess homocysteine in the blood. Defective absorption of vitamin B-12 is the cause of the deficiency disease pernicious anemia, which frequently occurs in older adults. In such cases, megadose supplements or injection of the vitamin is necessary. Vitamin B-12 occurs in animal foods but not in plant foods. Vegans need to look for foods fortified with the vitamin or take a supplement. Normally, the liver has a 5-year supply of vitamin B-12 in storage.

9. Choline is a dietary component that is available from a wide variety of foods and is synthesized in the body. No natural deficiency of choline has been reported. The amino acid methionine, vitamin B-6, vitamin B-12, and folate, along with choline, are intricately involved in the metabolism of the amino acid homocysteine. Elevated homocysteine in the blood is considered a risk factor for atherosclerosis.

10. Vitamin C does not function as a coenzyme, like the B-vitamins. One of its many roles is in the synthesis of collagen, the protein used to form connective tissue. A deficiency of vitamin C causes the disease scurvy. Fresh fruits and vegetable are reliable sources of this vitamin. Like folate, vitamin C is destroyed by heat. Among North Americans, alcoholics and older men who don't eat fresh produce are most likely to develop a deficiency. Megadoses of the vitamin causes gastrointestinal upsets but little else.

11. Carnitine, inositol, taurine, and lipoic acid, while participating in many important biochemical reactions in the body, are not true vitamins because they can be synthesized in the body from readily available precursors, or obtained from the diet.

STUDY QUESTIONS

1. Define and explain the terms *coenzyme* and *cofactor*. Identify the vitamins that function as coenzymes and those that function as cofactors.

2. Which vitamins can be synthesized in the body, and how are they synthesized?

3. Explain why individual B-vitamin deficiencies are rare in the United States and Canada. Which B-vitamins are added to cereal grains as part of the enrichment program?

4. Homocysteine is of great health concern today. Why?

5. Define Upper Level and explain why certain vitamins have this designation.

6. Some vitamins have an Adequate Intake designation rather than an RDA. Why?

7. Draw a map of the energy-transformation pathways in the cell and identify the biochemical reactions where B-vitamins participate in energy metabolism (Hint: review Fig. 10-2).

8. Name the vitamins that have been used as pharmacologic agents, and identify the medical conditions for which they are used as therapy. Don't forget the fat-soluble vitamins.

9. Draw the Food Guide Pyramid and place the various B-vitamins and vitamin C into the food groups where they are most likely to be found.

10. Suppose you read in the newspaper or hear on TV news that a "new" vitamin has been discovered. What criteria will have to be met in order for this substance to be a true vitamin?

■ ANNOTATED REFERENCES

1. Ahmad N, Mukhtar H: Green tea polyphenols and cancer: Biologic mechanisms and practical implications. *Nutrition Reviews* 57:78, 1999.

   Polyphenolic antioxidants in green tea seems to possess cancer chemopreventive properties. It might be the prevention of mutagenicity and genotoxicity, the inhibition of biochemical markers of tumor initiation and promotion, detoxification enzymes, or antioxidant free radical scavengers, but there is still much speculation as to the actions of green tea.

2. Brattström L, Wilcker DEL: Homocysteine and cardiovascular disease: Cause or effect? *American Journal of Clinical Nutrition* 72:315, 2000.

   Hypertension and atherosclerosis lead to kidney damage and a decline in kidney function, which in turn cause elevated blood homocysteine. Low folate and low vitamin B-12 may cause elevated homocysteine. Elevated homocysteine may be the cause of heart attack and stroke.

3. Cervantes-Laurean D and others: Niacin. In Shils ME and others (eds.): *Modern nutrition in health and disease.* 9th ed. Baltimore, MD: Williams & Wilkins, 1999.

   The history, chemistry, and terminology associated with niacin and nicotinamide are described. Niacin, nicotinamide, and tryptophan are precursors of NAD and NADP. They function in a variety of oxidation-reduction reactions. The disease pellagra and the use of niacin as a pharmacologic agent are explored.

4. Food and Nutrition Board, Institute of Medicine: *Dietary Reference Intakes for vitamin C, vitamin E, selenium, and carotenoids.* Washington, D.C.: National Academy Press, 2000.

   The functions of antioxidant nutrients; how RDA and related standards were determined; and deficiency and toxicity symptoms are explained. This is the definitive report by the panel of experts on nutrient needs for dietary antioxidants.

5. Herbert V: Folic acid. In Shils ME and others (eds.): *Modern nutrition in health and disease.* 9th ed. Baltimore, MD: Williams & Wilkins, 1999.

   The metabolic functions of folate, together with its interrelationship with vitamin B-12, is described. Absorption, storage, and excretion are explained. Various deficiency states and symptoms are described.

6. Holmes M and others: Association of dietary intake of fat and fatty acids with risk of breast cancer. *Journal of the American Medical Association* 281:914, 1999.

   High intake of dietary fat has been postulated to increase the risk of breast cancer, based on animal studies. Report of the Nurses' Health Study found no evidence that lower intake of total fat or specific types of fatty acids is associated with decreased risk of breast cancer.

7. Holt PR: Dairy foods and prevention of colon cancer: Human studies. *Journal of the American College of Nutrition,* 18:379S, 1999.

   Combined data from several studies suggest that daily consumption of 850 mg of calcium per day is accompanied by a reduced incidence of adenomatous colon polyps. Low-fat dairy foods or supplemental calcium may reduce colon cancer incidence.

8. Huffman GB: Level of alcohol intake and risk of breast cancer. *American Family Physician* 58:224, 1998.

   There is a positive association between invasive breast cancer in women and alcohol consumption. The higher risk occurred when women drank 2.3 to 4.5 bottles of beer, 2.8 to 5.6 glasses of wine, or 2 to 4 drinks of liquor per day.

9. Jacob RA: Vitamin C. In Shils ME and others (eds.): *Modern nutrition in health and disease.* 9th ed. Baltimore, MD: Williams & Wilkins, 1999.

   The history of the discovery of vitamin C is reported. The chemistry of ascorbic acid and dehydroascorbic acid is explained, and the major biochemical functions are elucidated. Deficiency and toxicity symptoms are described. The effects of smoking as related to vitamin C requirements are explained.

10. Leklem JE: Vitamin B$_6$. In Shils ME and others (eds.): *Modern nutrition in health and disease.* 9th ed. Baltimore, MD: Williams & Wilkins, 1999.

    This chapter explains the chemistry of vitamin B-6 in foods and in humans. Its functions are briefly described, along with the signs and symptoms of deficiency. Vitamin B-6 used as a drug to treat a variety of medical conditions has generally been a failure, and toxic side effects have occurred from pharmacologic doses.

11. Lichtenstein P and others: Environmental and heritable factors in the causation of cancer—Analyses of cohorts of twins from Sweden, Denmark, and Finland. *The New England Journal of Medicine* 343:78, 2000.

    Inherited genetic factors make only a minor contribution to susceptibility to most types of cancers. Environmental factors, such as smoking, infections, and diet, play the principal role in causing cancer.

12. Lieberman DA and others: Use of colonoscopy to screen asymptomatic adults for colorectal cancer. *The New England Journal of Medicine* 343:62, 2000.

    Colonoscopy screening can detect cancers in asymptomatic adults that would not be detected with sigmoidoscopy. Colonoscopy should become the standard method of detecting colon cancer.

13. Understanding your cancer diagnosis. *Mayo Clinic Health Letter* 17:1, 1999.

    This article provides definitions of common words associated with cancer. The information is suitable for the lay public.

14. McCormick D: Riboflavin. In Shils ME and others (eds.): *Modern nutrition in health and disease.* 9th ed. Baltimore, MD: Williams & Wilkins, 1999.

    The history, biochemistry, and functions of riboflavin are explained. A pure riboflavin deficiency is probably never encountered in humans but is part of an overall vitamin-deficiency state.

15. Mock DM: Biotin. In Shils ME and others (eds.): *Modern nutrition in health and disease.* 9th ed. Baltimore, MD: Williams & Wilkins, 1999.

    The sources, absorption, functions, and deficiency symptoms of biotin are explained. There are only two documented situations leading to a deficiency, eating raw egg whites and using intravenous feedings without biotin supplementation.

16. Breast cancer. *Nutrition Action Healthletter,* December 6, 1999.

    A growing number of studies relate excess weight gain with risk of breast cancer in postmenopausal women. Women who drink alcoholic beverages have a slightly elevated risk of breast cancer.

17. Plesofsky-Vig, N: Pantothenic acid. In Shils ME and others (eds.): *Modern nutrition in health and disease.* 9th ed. Baltimore, MD: Williams & Wilkins, 1999.

    The food sources and function of pantothenic acid are explored, along with the chemistry and metabolism of this B-vitamin. Pantothenic acid deficiency in humans is rare.

18. Rebouche CJ: Carnitine In Shils ME and others (eds.): *Modern nutrition in health and disease.* 9th ed. Baltimore, MD: Williams & Wilkins, 1999.

    The biochemical functions in long-chain fatty-acid oxidation are explained. Carnitine is derived in the human body from the essential amino acids lysine and methionine. Carnitine is abundant in foods.

19. Savage PD: Molecular basis of human neoplasm. In Shils ME and others (eds.): *Modern nutrition in health and disease.* 9th ed. Baltimore, MD: Williams & Wilkins, 1999.

    This is a tutorial describing the crucial steps in changing the normal cell to a cancer cell. An analogy of the automobile gas pedal (oncogenes) and brake pedal (tumor suppressor genes) explains the progression of cell changes.

TAKE ACTION

I. SPOTTING FRAUDULENT CLAIMS ON THE INTERNET.

Using the World Wide Web, search for vitamins and vitamin-like substances that are sold over the Internet. Then write a report concerning any claims made on behalf of these products that you consider fraudulent or misleading. Are these web sites really selling vitamins, or are they actually a cover for selling something else? Compare the price of the vitamins from these sites with the price you would pay at the local supermarket. Do any of these sites display any disclaimers or warnings about the products?

II. SPOTTING FRAUDULENT CLAIMS IN POPULAR BOOKS FOR SALE AT HEALTH FOOD STORES AND BOOK STORES.

Visit a health-food store in order to examine the books that are for sale. How many books represent sound nutrition, and how many are mostly filled with nutrition quackery? Visit your campus book store. Identify the books (and authors) that represent sound nutrition and the ones that are mostly filled with nutrition quackery. Consult last Sunday's edition of the *New York Times* best-seller list. How many books represent sound nutrition, and how many are nutrition quackery? Write a report comparing these three sources of nutrition information.

20. SEER Cancer Statistic Review 1973-1997 National Cancer Institute/National Institutes of Health: Annual report shows continuing decline in U.S. cancer incidence and death rates; special section focuses on colorectal cancer. *National Cancer Institute Press Release*, May 14, 2000. http://rex.nci.gov/massmedia/pressreleases/cancer_decline.html

    This report provides information about incidence, mortality, and survival statistics from 1973 through 1997. Information is available for about 26 cancers for all races and major ethnic groups.

21. Standing Committee on the Scientific Evaluation of Dietary Reference Intakes: Dietary Reference Intakes for thiamin, riboflavin, niacin, vitamin B-6, folate, vitamin B-12, pantothenic acid, biotin, and choline. Washington, D.C.: National Academy Press, 1998.

    Explanation as to how the DRI were established for the B-vitamins and choline, with specific reference to establishing RDA and related standards. The functions of each of the B-vitamins are explained.

22. Stipanuk MH: Homocysteine, cysteine, and taurine. In Shils ME and others (eds.): *Modern nutrition in health and disease.* 9th ed. Baltimore, MD: Williams & Wilkins, 1999.

    This chapter describes the interactions involving homocysteine, methionine, vitamin B-12, choline, and folate. In the past decade, the role of plasma homocysteine concentrations and the development of vascular disease and neural tube defects has gained attention.

23. Sugimura T, Wakabayashi K: Carcinogens in foods. In Shils ME and others (eds.): *Modern nutrition in health and disease.* 9th ed. Baltimore, MD: Williams & Wilkins, 1999.

    This summary article is about genotoxic carcinogens (i.e., mutagens/carcinogens) in foods. The author describes four separate groups: the first group is about the naturally occurring mycotoxins, second group concerns the plant-origin carcinogens, third group are the nitrosamines, and the fourth group deals with the carcinogens in cooked foods.

24. Suitor CW, Bailey LB: Dietary folate equivalents: Interpretation and application. *Journal of the American Dietetic Association* 100:88, 2000.

    The authors explain the new DFEs, which account for differences in the absorption of naturally occurring and synthetic folate. Synthetic folic acid is more bioavailable than the food form of folate.

25. Tanphaichitr V: Thiamin. In Shils ME and others (eds.): *Modern nutrition in health and disease.* 9th ed. Baltimore, MD: Williams & Wilkins, 1999.

    The history and chemistry of thiamin are discussed, along with the biochemical functions of TPP. The two forms of adult beriberi (wet and dry) and infantile beriberi are described. Wernicke-Korsakoff syndrome, which results from a severe thiamin deficiency due to alcoholism, is described.

26. Weir DG, Scott JM: Vitamin B-12 "Cobalamin." In Shils ME and others (eds.): *Modern nutrition in health and disease.* 9th ed. Baltimore, MD: Williams & Wilkins, 1999.

    The history, definitions, chemistry, and functions of vitamin B-12 are explained. The interacting roles of vitamin B-12 and folate are described, along with the signs and symptoms of pernicious anemia. Almost all B-12 deficiency cases are due to absorption problems.

27. Willett WC: Diet, nutrition, and the prevention of cancer. In Shils ME and others (eds.): *Modern nutrition in health and disease.* 9th ed. Baltimore, MD: Williams & Wilkins, 1999.

    Excessive energy intake increases risk of human cancer. The author recommends consuming more fruits and vegetables, avoiding excess intake of red meat and animal fat, and limiting alcohol intake.

28. Zeisel SH: Choline and phosphatidylcholine. In Shils ME and others (eds.): *Modern nutrition in health and disease.* 9th ed. Baltimore, MD: Williams & Wilkins, 1999.

    Explanations are provided as to why choline has been designated an essential nutrient. The functions of choline and phosphatidylcholine are described. Choline can be synthesized in the body. A deficiency probably never occurs, except in rare cases such as during infancy, during pregnancy, and among liver patients fed via total parenteral nutrition.

NUTRITION AND CANCER

Cancer is currently the second leading cause of death for American adults.[20] The good news is that new cancer cases and cancer deaths for all cancers (except lung cancer in women), has declined between 1990 and 1997 in the United States. The number of new cases per 100,000 persons declined an average of 0.8% each year between 1990 and 1997. The number of new cases each year peaked in 1992 and has been declining since. The decrease has been greater among men, who have a higher number of cases than women.

Lung, prostate, breast, and colorectal cancers account for slightly over half of all cancers and were (through 1997) the leading cause of cancer death for every racial and ethnic group. Cases are declining for prostate cancer incidence and mortality. The incidence of breast cancer remains unchanged, but deaths have dropped since 1995. Overall deaths from lung cancer continue to decrease for men since 1990, but for women it is up. Colorectal cancer has been decreasing since 1985.

The only cancer that is increasing significantly is non-Hodgkin's lymphoma, but deaths rate have leveled off since 1989, due to improved treatment.

WHAT IS CANCER?

Cancer is not a single disease but exists in at least 100 different forms (Fig. 10-15). The factors that cause skin cancer are different from those leading to breast cancer, and treatments for the different types of cancer vary with the type of cancer itself. Cancer is essentially abnormal and uncontrollable cell division. If untreatable or not treated, it leads to death. Most cancers take the form of tumors, although not all tumors are cancers. A tumor is spontaneous new tissue growth that serves no physiological purpose. Tumors can be **benign,** such as a wart that doesn't spread, or **malignant,** such as lung cancer that spreads to surrounding tissues and organs. A malignant **neoplasm** means the same thing as malignant tumor.

Most cancers fall into one of three groups: **carcinomas** comprise 80 to 90% of all cancers; they develop from cells that cover the body. They affect secretory organs, such as the breast. **Sarcomas** are cancers of connective tissues, such as in bone. Leukemias and lymphomas form the third group. **Leukemias** are malignant neoplasms of the blood-forming tissues, the bone

benign Noncancerous; describes tumors that do not spread.

malignant Essentially, malicious; in reference to a tumor, the property of spreading locally and to distant sites.

neoplasm A new and abnormal growth of tissues, which may be benign or cancerous.

carcinoma An invasive malignant tumor derived from the epithelial tissues that cover the body.

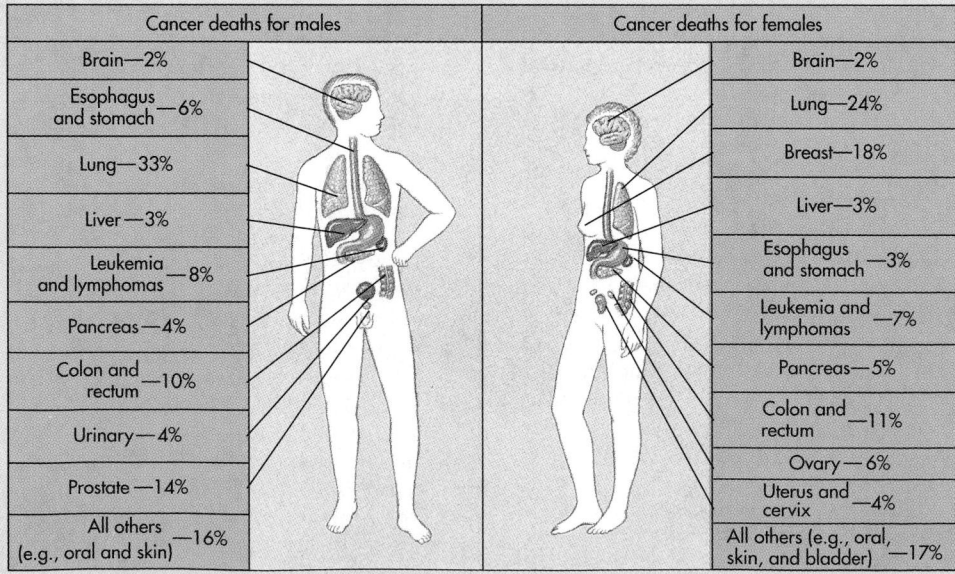

Cancer deaths for males		Cancer deaths for females	
Brain—2%		Brain—2%	
Esophagus and stomach —6%		Lung—24%	
Lung—33%		Breast—18%	
Liver—3%		Liver—3%	
Leukemia and lymphomas —8%		Esophagus and stomach —3%	
Pancreas—4%		Leukemia and lymphomas —7%	
Colon and rectum —10%		Pancreas—5%	
Urinary—4%		Colon and rectum —11%	
Prostate —14%		Ovary —6%	
		Uterus and cervix —4%	
All others (e.g., oral and skin) —16%		All others (e.g., oral, skin, and bladder) —17%	

FIGURE 10-15 Cancer is actually many diseases. Numerous types of cells and organs are its target. Note that about one-third of all cancers arise from smoking.
Illustration by William Ober.

410

marrow. **Lymphomas** are various malignant tumors that are in the lymph nodes or lymphoid tissues.

Benign tumors are enclosed in a membrane that prevents them from spreading. They are dangerous only if they interfere with normal function. For instance, a benign brain tumor can cause illness and death if it blocks blood flow in the brain. Malignant tumors, on the other hand, are capable of invading surrounding structures, including blood vessels, the lymph system, and nerve tissue. They can **metastasize** to distant sites via the blood or lymph, thereby producing invasive tumors in almost any part of the body (Fig. 10-16).

A cancer such as leukemia, a cancer found in white blood cells (leukocytes) does not produce a mass, so it isn't classified as a tumor; however, exhibits the fundamental property of rapid and inappropriate growth. It is still malignant and therefore represents a form of cancer.

Mechanisms of Carcinogenesis

Most cells exist in a homeostatic state; there is a balance between the turning-on and turning-off of cellular replication. Regulation of the cell cycle exists between the gene products that spur replication and gene products that deter replication.[19]

■ Oncogenes and Other Genes

Genes that produce products that cause a resting cell to divide are referred to as **protooncogenes,** and genes that prevent cells from dividing are known as **tumor suppressor genes.** Cancer often results from a lack of suppressor genes or too much action by the protooncogenes. The cancer gene, or **oncogene,** is the protooncogene out of control; it is making dozens or hundreds of copies of itself, and there are no mechanisms to overcome the process. In the final analysis, all cancer is genetic, in that defects in specific genes lead to the proliferative growth.

The tumor suppressor genes are the braking mechanisms within a cell, preventing uncontrolled growth. When something goes wrong with these tumor suppressor genes, the oncogenes

metastasize Spreading disease from one part of the body to another, even to parts of the body that are remote from the site of the original tumor. Cancer cells can spread via blood vessels, the lymphatic system, or direct growth of the tumor.

protooncogenes Genes that cause a resting cell to divide.

tumor suppressor genes Genes that prevent cells from dividing.

oncogene A protooncogene out of control.

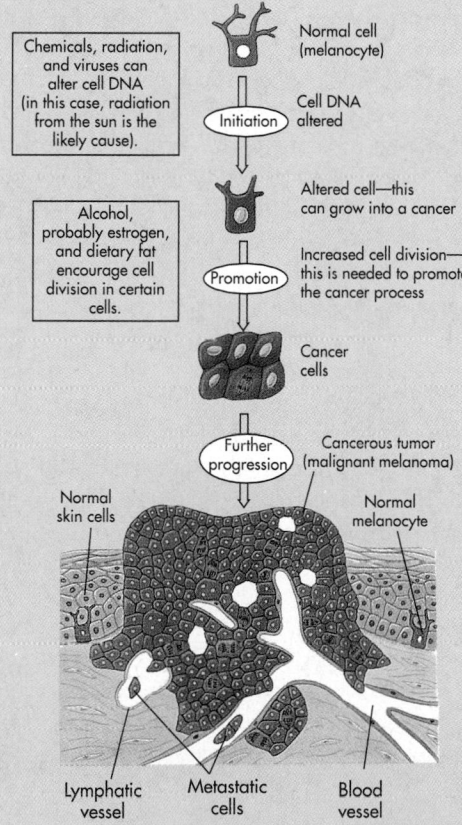

Chemicals, radiation, and viruses can alter cell DNA (in this case, radiation from the sun is the likely cause).

Normal cell (melanocyte)

Initiation — Cell DNA altered

Alcohol, probably estrogen, and dietary fat encourage cell division in certain cells.

Altered cell—this can grow into a cancer

Promotion — Increased cell division—this is needed to promote the cancer process

Cancer cells

Further progression — Cancerous tumor (malignant melanoma)

Normal skin cells   Normal melanocyte

Lymphatic vessel   Metastatic cells   Blood vessel

■ FIGURE 10-16 Progression from a normal skin cell to skin cancer through the initiation, promotion, and progression stages. The ball of cells is a developing tumor. As the mass of cells grows, it can invade surrounding tissues, eventually penetrating into both lymph and blood vessels. These vessels carry spreading (metastatic) cancer cells throughout the body, where they can form new cancer sites.

Illustration by William Ober.

p53 gene A tumor-suppressor gene that can prevent inappropriate cell division.

telomeres Caps at the end of chromosomes.

telomerase An enzyme that maintains length and completeness of chromosomes.

cancer initiation The stage in the process of cancer development that begins with alterations in DNA, the genetic material in a cell. This may cause the cell to no longer respond to normal physiological controls.

cancer promotion The stage in the cancer process when cell division increases, in turn decreasing the time available for repair enzymes to act on altered DNA and encouraging cells with altered DNA to develop and grow.

cancer progression The final stage in the cancer process, during which the cancer cells proliferate, forming a mass large enough to significantly affect body functions.

genotoxic carcinogen A compound that directly alters DNA or is converted in cells to metabolites that alter DNA, thereby providing the potential for cancer to develop.

mutation A change in the chemistry of a gene, which is perpetuated in subsequent divisions of the cell in which it occurred; a change in the sequence of the DNA base pairs.

are free to promote rapid cell growth. One tumor suppressor gene, known as **p53 gene,** can prevent the abnormal growth associated with tumors. Alteration in this gene has been discovered to cause cancers of the ovary, breast, lung, and colon.

There are repair mechanisms within a cell that constantly look for errors in DNA replication and make corrections. Sometimes the repair mechanisms fail, which results in an inherited defect for cancer, such as hereditary colon cancer. Early defects in DNA replication that aren't caught and repaired are likely to predispose the cell to even more errors, thus leading to cancer.

Other agents that play a part in the cell replication process are **telomeres,** caps at the ends of chromosomes. An enzyme called a **telomerase** maintains their length and completeness. Each time a cell divides, the telomeres of the daughter cells are slightly shorter, and telomerase activity within the cell decreases. At some point, telomeres becomes so short that the genes at the ends of the chromosome can no longer function, and the cell undergoes apoptosis (see Chapter 9 for a discussion of apoptosis). That is, the cell is no longer able to function normally and it dies. In malignant tumor cells, the telomerase activity increases, and the length of the telomere is longer, resulting in a cell that can live indefinitely. There seems to be a difference in telomerase activity between normal tissue and cancer tissue. Much more is to be learned about conditions that promote abnormal telomerase activity and whether this enzyme can become a target in cancer therapy.

■ Cancer Initiation, Promotion, and Progression

Carcinogenesis, the development of cancer in a body, is a multiple-step event, starting with the exposure of a cell to a carcinogen, which triggers **cancer initiation.** Subsequently, it is followed by **cancer promotion** and finally **cancer progression** (review Fig. 10-16). Initiation can develop spontaneously or can be induced by agent's known as **genotoxic carcinogens.** The affected cells can then dictate their own rate of division. Agents that are responsible for carcinogenesis include tobacco, alcohol, radiation, occupational toxins, infections, diet, and drugs. (See Table 10-4.)

A mechanism that can prevent cancer initiation is cytochrome P450 in liver and intestinal cells. Cytochrome P450 is an iron-containing compound that participates in a process that converts numerous endogenous compounds, and toxins from external sources, into harmless water-soluble metabolites. Eventually, these products are excreted from the body. That makes cytochrome P450 a first line of defense against carcinogens when they try to lodge themselves in the intestinal wall. The p53 gene, already identified as a tumor suppressor gene, is another way to prevent abnormal growth associated with tumors, as it can postpone cell division. This allows time for damage repair. Enzymes can travel up and down the DNA double helix, repairing broken components and correcting defects. About 99% of the time, the repair enzymes find the damage and correct it before the cell divides again and thus undergoes **mutation.**

The initiation stage of carcinogenesis, during which time DNA is altered, is relatively short. It could be minutes or days. The promotion state may last for months or years. During this period, the damage is "locked" into the genetic material in cells. Compounds that increase cell division are called promoters or epigenetic carcinogens. These are thought to promote cancer either by decreasing the time available for repair enzymes to act or by encouraging cells with altered DNA to develop and grow. Some putative promoters are estrogen, alcohol, and possibly a high intake of dietary fat. Bacterial infections in the stomach are also suspected agents. For example, infection with *Helicobacter pylori,* which cause ulcers, may ultimately promote stomach cancer.

The final stage in carcinogenesis, cancer progression, begins with the appearance of cells that grow autonomously (out of control). During the progression phase, these malignant cells proliferate, invade surrounding tissue, and metastasize to other sites. Early in this stage, the immune system may find the altered cells and destroy them, or the cancer cells may be so defective that their own DNA limits their ability to grow, and they die. If nothing impedes cancer cell growth, one or more tumors eventually develop that are large enough to affect body functions, and the signs and symptoms of cancer appear (review Table 10-4).

TABLE 10-4   The Cancer Development Process

Cancer Initiation

Process: DNA alteration occurs in this relatively short phase (minutes to days).
Causes:
   Radiation: e.g., sun overexposure
      Cross-links double strands of DNA or breaks them into fragments
   Chemicals: e.g., aflatoxin (mold from peanuts and cereal grains), benzo(a)pyrene (smoke
      from charbroiled meat fat). These agents are transformed to highly reactive cancer initiators
      by cytochrome P450, an enzyme system that detoxifies foreign compounds in the body. These
      metabolites are then able to cause mutations in DNA, RNA, and proteins.
   Biological agents: e.g., viruses
      Promote uncontrolled growth of cells by inserting viral DNA or RNA into normal cells, which
      alters the cell's genes

Cancer Promotion

Process: DNA alterations are "locked" into the genetic material of cells over a period of months to
   more than 10 years.
Causes:
   Excess estrogen exposure
   Excess alcohol
   Excess dietary fat (controversial)
   Bacterial infections: e.g., *Helicobacter pylori*

Cancer Progression

Process: Cells that can grow autonomously appear. These cells spread to surrounding tissue and
   other sites.
Causes:
   Excess energy intake
   Lack of early detection
   Development of blood supply to the tumor
      The tumor uses newly formed capillaries to grow and spread cancer cells to remote sites in the
      body.

Anything that increases the rate of cell division decreases the chance that the repair enzymes will find the altered part of the DNA in
time to do their work. Once a cell multiplies and incorporates its newly altered DNA into its genetic instructions, the repair enzymes
can no longer detect the changes in DNA.

IS CANCER ENVIRONMENTAL OR HEREDITARY?

Inherited mutations cannot account for the dramatic differences in cancer rates around the
world. In poorer countries, cancers of the stomach, liver, mouth, esophagus, and uterus are
most common, whereas, in affluent countries, cancers of the lung, colon-rectum, breast, and
prostate predominate. Our best source of cancer information comes from studies of twins, the
standard for distinguishing between genetics and environmental factors.[11] In a recently published study of 44,788 twins, the researchers concluded that inherited genetic factors make
only a minor contribution to the susceptibility to most types of cancer. The environment has the
principal role in causing sporadic cancer. For nearly all body sites, the twin of a person with
cancer has only a moderate risk of developing cancer at the same site. The researchers found
that risk factors in the environment shared by a family can include human papillomavirus infection for cervical cancer, smoking (passive and active) for lung cancer, diet for colon cancer,
and *Helicobacter pylori* for stomach cancer. There were, however, heritable factors detected in
this study for colorectal, breast, and prostate cancer. This was in agreement with other population-based studies. For colorectal cancer, 35% could be explained by heritable factors; for
breast cancer, 27%; and, for prostate cancer, 42%. The impact of heredity on the other cancers
was so small that inherited genetic factors accounted for 1 to 15% of all the cancers.

DIET AND CANCER

Oxidative damage to DNA is likely to cause mutations and can be enhanced by some dietary factors or reduced by enzymes such as those that incorporate the trace mineral selenium. There is evidence that intake of selenium above the RDA has an anticancer effect in humans, but there aren't enough data at this time to make a recommendation as to the extra amount needed.

Excessive energy intake in relation to need increases the risk of human cancer.[16] Animal studies have shown that energy restriction during periods of rapid growth is protective against cancer. No doubt obesity increases the risk of cancers of the uterus, breast, kidney, and possibly the prostate, colon, and gallbladder. Excess body fat may affect sex hormone production, which increases cancer risk, or cancer cells may grow more easily when fuel is plentiful.

However, no link has been found between a low fat diet and the development of breast cancer,[16] but excess body weight increases the risk. Perhaps certain fatty acids, such as monounsaturated and polyunsaturated fatty acids in fish and olive oil, are beneficial. Certainly, more research is needed in the area of body fat and the types of dietary fats consumed.

High intakes of vegetables and fruits have been associated with lower risks of many cancers. The constituents that are protective against cancer have not been identified, but the evidence supports the B-vitamin folate. Studies of colorectal cancer show an inverse relationship between folate status and the rate of cancer. An inadequate intake of folate could also influence the risk of mutation.

The data for vitamin C and protection from various cancers are either inconsistent or not specific enough to make a recommendation for intake.

High intake of meat and protein products has been associated with an increased risk of prostate cancer, which might be related to the saturated fat content of the food. Again, one should be cautious about concluding that all meat causes cancer, since there are so many types of meat consumed.

In addition, there is no question that excess alcohol consumption increases the risks of upper gastrointestinal tract cancers.[8] Even moderate alcohol intake seems to increase the risk of cancers of the breast and colon.

Meat cooked at high temperatures over an open flame, such as in charcoal broiling, produces polyaromatic hydrocarbons, one being benzo-[a]pyrene. In generating benzo-[a]pyrene, this cooking method produces a by-product, which binds to DNA and produces tumors, such as in the colon.

Nitrosamines are carcinogenic. Nitrosamines are formed from nitrite. Nitrite exists in various foods and is produced endogenously from nitrate in vegetables. Nitrosamine compounds are found in cooked bacon, sausage, hot dogs, beer, cheese, and some nitrite-preserved foods.[23]

Mycotoxins are toxins produced by fungi. Among the many examples is aflatoxin B_1, a component of many moldy foods, such as moldy grain and peanuts. It is classified as a human carcinogen and is thought to cause liver cancer. Drought conditions in Asian and African countries have resulted in the widespread contamination of foods by aflatoxins. Even in the United States, corn has been found with increased carcinogen levels from aflatoxin B_1 due to changing weather conditions, but grain elevators and FDA monitor grains for unsafe amounts. Current studies are focusing on various antioxidants that may protect us from environmental carcinogens, such as aflatoxins.

The National Academy of Sciences' 1980 review of *Diet, Nutrition, and Cancer* recommended a fat intake of no more than 30% of calories, primarily to reduce the incidence of cancer. More recent evidence raises questions about this recommendation. The association between fat intake and cancer rates has come from large international differences in rates of breast, colon, prostate, and endometrial cancer. These international differences are assumed to be due to the effect of animal fats, but the type of fat has remained controversial. Moreover, there are still more recent surveys that fail to find a correlation between fat intake and cancer. Certainly, there are wide gaps in the knowledge linking fat and cancer. A long-standing excess energy intake is likely a more important cause of cancer than fat per se.

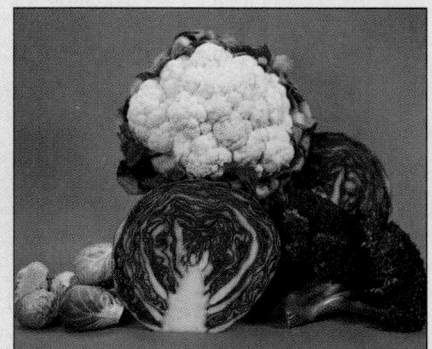

Cruciferous vegetables are rich in cancer-preventing phytochemicals.

Another recent discovery resulting from attempts to find dietary prevention of cancer suggests that calcium and vitamin D (or moderate sun exposure) may be part of the answer.[7] Calcium intake is inversely related to cancer, especially colon cancer. It may be that calcium binds free fatty acid and bile acids in the colon, so that they are less likely to interact with certain types of intestinal cells, which in turn become cancer.

The hormone form of vitamin D—1,25(OH)$_2$D—has been shown to inhibit the progression of human colorectal cells from cancerous polyps in vitro. Vitamin D also has been shown to inhibit rapid colon/rectal cell growth in patients with ulcerative colitis. These combined data suggest a chemopreventive action of vitamin D against colon neoplasms. This may be the beneficial effect of vitamin D-fortified dairy foods.

Based on our current knowledge of diet and cancer risk, the following guidelines are about all that can be recommended at this time:[27] Remain physically active, avoid obesity, engage in physical training that promotes the formation of lean muscle, consume an abundance of fruits and vegetables and whole grains, consume plenty of low-fat and nonfat dairy products, avoid a high intake of red meat and animal fat, and avoid excessive use of alcohol (Tables 10-5 and 10-6).

CANCER WARNING SIGNS

Remember also that, if a cancer is left untreated, it can spread quickly throughout the body. When this happens, it is much more likely to lead to death. Thus, early detection is critical. Aids to early detection include the following warning signs:

- Unexplained weight loss
- A change in bowel or bladder habits
- A sore that does not heal
- Unusual bleeding or discharge
- A thickening or lump in the breast or elsewhere
- Indigestion or difficulty in swallowing
- An obvious change in a wart or mole
- A nagging cough or hoarseness

There are still other ways to detect cancer early. Colonoscopy examinations for middle-age and older adults,[12] PSA (prostate-specific antigen) tests for men over age 50, and Papanicolaou tests (Pap smears) and regular breast examinations (and mammograms starting about age 40 to 50) for women are recommended. Finally, to learn still more about cancer, review these sources of credible cancer information on the Internet:

http://www.cancer.org   American Cancer Society

http://www.icic.nci.nih.gov   CancerNet

http://cancer.med.upenn.edu   Oncolink

TABLE 10-5   Some Food Constituents Suspected of Having a Role in Cancer[1,7,8,23,27]

Constituents	Dietary Sources	Action
Possibly Protective		
Calcium	Low-fat dairy foods, supplements, fortified foods such as orange juice	Inhibits colon cell proliferation
Phytoestrogens (isoflavonoids and lignans)	Soy-rich foods, flax	Inhibits growth of hormone-dependent cells (e.g., lowers breast cancer risk).
Folate,	Many fruits, vegetables, fortified foods, especially breakfast cereals	Lowers risk of pancreatic and breast cancer.
Indoles and phenols	Broccoli and other cruciferous vegetables	Sulforaphane inhibits carcinogenesis.
Flavanoids	Tea	EGCG (a primary catechin in green tea) acts as an antioxidant. Decreases mutagenicity and genotoxicity and offers other chemopreventive effects.
Possible Carcinogens		
Mycotoxins: aflatoxin B_1	Moldy peanuts and grains	Increases risk for liver cancer.
Nitrates, Nitrites	Salted or smoked meats, such as ham and smoked fish; other foods preserved with sodium nitrate	Under high temperatures, bind to amino acid derivatives to form nitrosamines, potent carcinogens.
Benzo(a)pyrene	Meat cooked at high temperatures over an open flame—e.g., charcoal broiling	Produces potent mutagens.
Total fat	Animal fats, especially in red meats	Promotes prostate cancer.
Alcohol	Beer, wine, distilled spirits	Promotes cancers of mouth, pharynx, larynx, esophagus, liver, colon, rectum, breast.

TABLE 10-6 **Example of a Diet Intended to Limit the Risk for Cancer—Low in Fat and High in Fruits and Vegetables and Provides Plenty of Calcium**

Breakfast

6 oz orange juice
1 cup ready-to-eat breakfast cereal
1 cup 1% fat milk
1 banana
1 slice whole-wheat toast, jelly, butter, or margarine
Hot tea

Lunch

Sandwich:
¾ cup chicken salad served on
    bagel or 2 slices of whole-wheat bread
Assorted raw vegetables: carrots, celery, broccoli, chopped lettuce
1½ cups 1% fat milk
Fresh fruit in season: strawberries, melon, grapes, apple
Cookies

Dinner

3 oz baked fish (e.g., cod, white fish, salmon)
Baked potato topped with shredded mozzarella cheese
Roasted corn on the cob, butter or margarine
Fresh garden salad with Italian dressing
1 whole-wheat dinner roll
1 scoop lemon ice or orange sherbet
Hot tea

Snack

12-oz can diet cola
2 cups popcorn
⅓ cup mixed nuts

WATER AND THE MAJOR MINERALS

chapter 11

ater—the most versatile medium for a variety of chemical reactions—constitutes the major portion of the human body. Without water, biological processes necessary to life would cease in a matter of days. We operate on about 2 quarts (2 L) of water daily and must replenish it regularly because the body does not store water per se.[1,2] We experience this constant demand for water as thirst. Many nutrients, including minerals, exist in the body dissolved in water. Because the functioning of minerals is related to the characteristics of water, water and its roles in the body are explored first in this chapter.

Many minerals, like water, are vital to health. They are considered inorganic because they are typically not bonded to carbon atoms. Minerals are key participants in body metabolism, muscle movement, body growth, and water balance, among other wide-ranging processes. Some of the minerals found in our bodies—for example, vanadium and arsenic—may not be necessary to sustain human life. Nevertheless, we know that some mineral deficiencies can cause severe health problems.[6] For this reason, the study of minerals is critical to understanding human nutrition.

KEY CHAPTER CONCEPTS

- Water constitutes 50 to 70% of the human body. It serves as a medium for chemical reactions, temperature regulation, and lubrication. For adults, daily water needs are estimated at 1 ml/kcal expended. Sources include all beverages and many nonbeverage foods.
- Many minerals are vital for sustaining life. For humans, animal products are the most bioavailable sources for most minerals. Supplements of minerals exceeding any Upper Level (UL) should be taken only under a physician's supervision, because toxicity and nutrient interactions are a likely possibility.
- Sodium is the major positive ion (Na^+) found outside cells. The typical American's diet provides abundant sodium; about 10 to 15% of adults are at risk for developing hypertension if they consume too much sodium.
- Potassium is the major positive ion found inside cells. Milk, fruits, and vegetables are good sources.
- Chloride, which is part of table salt (NaCl), is the major negative ion found outside cells.
- Calcium forms a major part of bone structure and is essential for blood clotting, muscle contraction, nerve transmission, and cell metabolism. Low calcium intakes are one of the many factors that increase risk for developing osteoporosis. Dairy products are important calcium sources. Women are particularly at risk for inadequate calcium intake.
- Phosphorus aids function of many enzymes and forms part of key metabolic compounds, cell membranes, and bone. Good food sources are dairy products, bakery products, and meats.
- Magnesium is important for nerve and heart function and as a cofactor for many enzymes. Whole grains (such as bran), vegetables, nuts, seeds, milk, and meats are good food sources.
- Currently, one out of four American adults (and one out of two older adults) suffers from hypertension. Controlling weight, salt, and alcohol intake, performing regular physical activity, and consuming adequate potassium, magnesium, and calcium also play a part in decreasing hypertension risk.

REFRESH YOUR MEMORY

As you begin your study of water and the major minerals in Chapter 11, you may want to review
- Intracellular and extracellular fluid compartments in Chapter 3
- The muscular and skeletal systems in Chapter 3
- The health risk of high-protein diets in Chapter 7
- The functions of vitamin D and vitamin K related to calcium and bone health in Chapter 9
- The role of vitamin C in collagen synthesis in Chapter 10

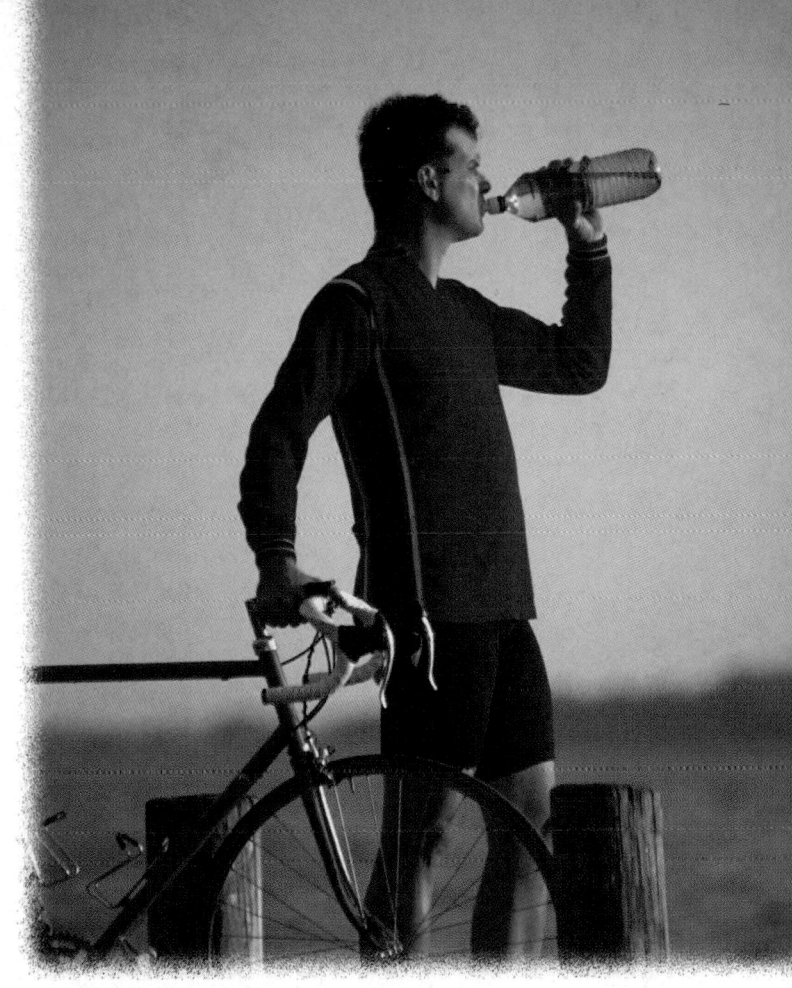

CASE SCENARIO

Jana, a sophomore in high school, recently became a vegan. Her mother is concerned about her diet, because she is not a vegan herself, and worries about Jana's health. One of her primary concerns is osteoporosis, particularly because she knows that 95% of bone growth occurs by ages 16-17. Jana needs an adequate source of calcium in her diet to aid with her rapid bone development. Jana also recently started smoking, and her only physical activity is choir practice.

Jana's diet on a recent day consisted of the following items. For breakfast, she had oatmeal made with water, a banana, and a cup of fruit juice. At midmorning, she bought a snack cake from the vending machine. At lunch, she had vegetable pasta, bread with olive oil, a side salad, one ounce of mixed nuts, and a soft drink. For dinner, she had a soy burger along with mixed vegetables and rice. As an evening snack, she had some cookies and another soft drink.

What factors place Jana at risk for osteoporosis in the future? Suggest any necessary changes to her current diet.

■ WATER

To appreciate how minerals operate in the body, it helps to understand the nature and general chemical properties of water, as well as specific nutrient-related functions. Water is the largest component of the human body, making up 50 to 70% of the body's weight (about 10 gallons, or 40 liters). Lean muscle tissue contains about 73% water. Adipose tissue is about 20% water. Thus, as fat content increases (and the percentage of lean tissue decreases) in the body, total body water decreases toward 50%.

Depending on how much fat has been stored, an adult can survive for about 8 weeks without eating food but only a few days without drinking water. This occurs not because water is more important than carbohydrate, fat, protein, vitamins, or minerals but, rather, because there is no storage site for water.

Looking at a molecular level, water is highly polar, as the positive charges tend to be located near the hydrogens and the negative charges near the oxygen.

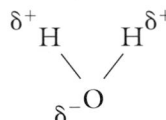

$$\delta^+ H \qquad H \delta^+$$
$$\delta^- O$$

δ denotes partial charge

Because of this, water can dissolve most substances, and, in doing so, it enables minerals and other chemicals to undergo biological reactions in the body (see Appendix B for details).

■ Water in the Body—Intracellular and Extracellular Fluid

Water flows in and out of body cells through cell membranes. Water inside cells forms part of the **intracellular fluid**—fluid within the cells. When water is outside cells or in the bloodstream, it is part of the **extracellular fluid**—fluid outside cells (review Figure 3-7 in Chapter 3). Extracellular fluid is further divided into **interstitial fluid**—water between cells—and **intravascular fluid**—water in the bloodstream and lymph. Interstitial fluid forms a transport link between tissue cells and the blood.

Because cell membranes are permeable to water, water shifts freely in and out of cells. For example, if blood volume decreases, water can move from the areas inside and around cells to the bloodstream to increase blood volume.

The body controls the amount of water in each compartment mainly by controlling the electrolyte concentrations in each compartment. In solution, electrolytes dissociate into charged particles called ions. Water is attracted to ions, such as sodium, potassium, chloride, phosphate, magnesium, and calcium. By controlling the movements of ions in and out of the cellular compartments, the body maintains the appropriate amount of water in each compartment. Where ions go, water follows.[24]

Osmosis

Much of the movement of body water results from water's tendency to move across a semipermeable membrane so as to equalize the total particle concentration in the compartments on each side of the membrane. A semipermeable membrane is one through which water, but not particles, can pass. In the body, the particles are primarily electrolytes, and the membranes are cell membranes. This passage of water (or other solvent), called **osmosis,** results in the movement of water from a less concentrated to a more concentrated solution. The specific concentration is expressed as **osmolality,** representing the number of particles per kg of solvent.

Figure 11-1 illustrates how osmosis works. When particles are added to the compartment on one side of a semipermeable membrane, this makes that compartment

intracellular fluid Fluid contained within a cell represents about two-thirds of all body fluid.

extracellular fluid Fluid present outside the cells; it includes intravascular and interstitial fluids; represents about one-third of all body fluid.

interstitial fluid Fluid between cells.

intravascular fluid Fluid within the bloodstream (that is, in the arteries, veins, and capillaries and lymph vessels).

osmosis The passage of a solvent (water) through a semipermeable membrane from a less concentrated compartment to a more concentrated compartment.

osmolality A measure of the total concentration of a solution; the number of particles of solute per kg of solvent.

more concentrated than the other compartment. Since particles can't pass easily across the membrane, water moves by diffusion from the diluted compartment to the more concentrated compartment until their particle concentrations become identical. The term **osmotic pressure** refers to the amount of force needed to prevent dilution of the compartment containing the higher particle concentration. Examples of osmosis are sugar pulling fluid from strawberries, a salty salad dressing wilting lettuce, and red blood cells swelling or shrinking when put into solutions of different salt concentrations. Adding water—instead of particles—to a compartment dilutes its particle concentration, so the compartment tends to donate water by the action of osmosis to more concentrated compartments nearby. This happens when you drink water. Some water absorbed by the body moves from the bloodstream into body cells, which in turn equalizes the particle concentration in the cells with that in the various nearby body sites.

Water and Ions in the Body—a Balancing Act

The movement of water across the membrane, depicted in Figure 11-1 occurs by simple diffusion. Little of this actually occurs across cell membranes because of their high lipid content. Rather, certain proteins in cell membranes act as channels through which water can move. In addition, cell membranes possess an extremely sophisticated gatekeeping system, which makes them selectively permeable to many electrolytes as well as other compounds. For example, a specific protein located in the membrane can pump potassium ions into and sodium ions out of a cell (Fig. 11-2). Energy is used by this sodium-potassium pump to move each of these ions against its concentration gradient. By the use of such mechanisms in addition to osmotic processes, cells maintain their intracellular water volume and electrolyte concentrations within quite narrow ranges.

Positive ions (cations), such as sodium and potassium, pair with negative ions (anions), such as phosphate and chloride. Intracellular water volume depends primarily on intracellular potassium and phosphate concentration. Extracellular water volume depends primarily on the extracellular sodium and chloride concentration.[24]

Besides balancing the ion concentrations between the inside and outside of cells, body cells must also balance ion charges. If a negative ion enters a cell, a positive ion must also enter the cell, or another negative electrolyte must leave it.

■ Functions of Water

Because of its unique chemical and physical characteristics, water plays several key roles in metabolic processes. Water functions in several ways in the body's chemical reactions: Because it is polar, it serves as a solvent for many chemical compounds, it provides a medium in which many chemical reactions occur, and it actively participates as a reactant or becomes a product in some reactions, such as in the citric acid cycle. It also is the transport medium of the body.

osmotic pressure The exerted pressure needed to keep particles in a solution from drawing liquid toward them across a semipermeable membrane.

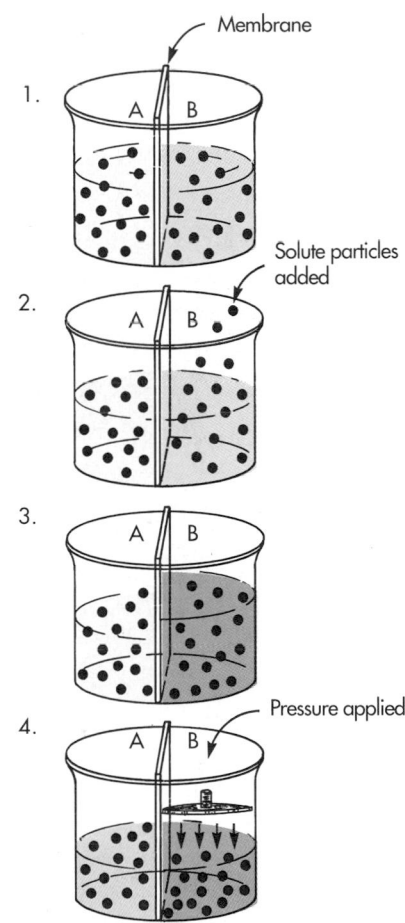

■ **FIGURE 11-1** A graphic representation of osmosis and osmotic pressure. *1.* An equal number of particles on each side allows equal amounts of water. *2.* Now additional particles are added to side B, but the particles cannot flow across the membrane. *3.* Water can flow across the membrane, so it flows to side B, causing the particle concentration on sides A and B to again become equal. *4.* If physical pressure (such as a pump) were to compress the fluid on side B to restore its original volume, the pressure would equal the osmotic pressure exerted by the added particles.

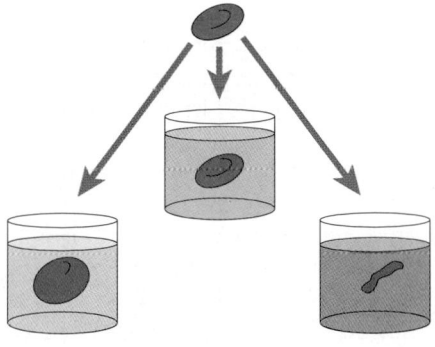

The effects of osmosis are easily demonstrated with red blood cells. When water is added to the fluid surrounding the cells, thereby diluting the fluid, water moves into the cells, causing them to expand. Conversely, when particles (e.g., ions) are added to the fluid, thereby concentrating it, water moves out of the cells, causing them to shrink.

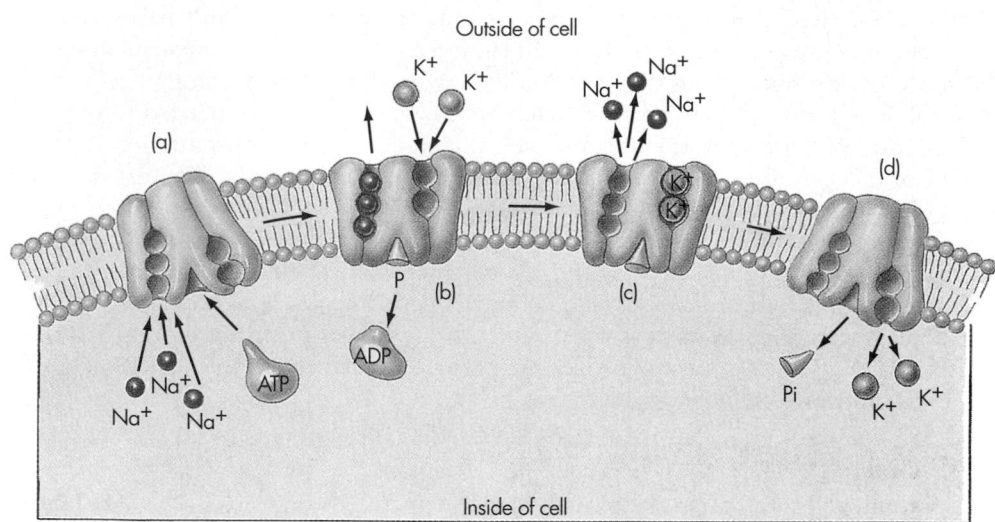

FIGURE 11-2 Schematic diagram of the sodium (Na⁺) and potassium (K⁺) pump cycle. (*a*) Three Na⁺ ions bind from inside the cell. (*b*) The Na⁺/K⁺ pump is activated by ATP. (*c*) Activation causes a change of the protein form. This results in a decrease in the affinity of Na⁺-binding sites and an increase in affinity of K⁺-binding sites. The three Na⁺ ions are then released to the outside of the cell. (*d*) Two K⁺ ions occupy the K⁺-binding sites, and the pump protein releases the phosphate donated from ATP and returns to its original conformation. The affinity of the K⁺-binding sites decreases, and that of the Na⁺ sites increases. The K⁺ ions are released to the cell. The pump is now ready to bind three Na⁺ ions, and the cycle starts again. This Na-K pump uses about 20 to 40% of the energy expended by the body at rest.

Illustration by William Ober.

Water Contributes to Temperature Regulation

Water changes temperature slowly because it has a great ability to hold heat. It takes much more energy to heat water than it does to heat fat. Compare the time it takes to melt ice cubes with the time it takes to melt frozen butter in a microwave oven. Foods with high water content heat up and cool down slowly. Because water requires so much energy to change states—for example, from a liquid to a gas—it forms an ideal medium for removing heat from the body. Water has this high heat capacity (**specific heat**) because water molecules are strongly attracted to each other. In contrast, the molecules in fat are not strongly attracted to each other, and fats thus exhibit lower specific heat values than water.

As the amount of heat energy contained within the body increases, water in the surrounding tissues absorbs any excess heat energy. The body then secretes fluids in the form of perspiration, which evaporates through skin pores. To evaporate water, heat energy is required, so, as perspiration evaporates, heat energy is taken from the skin, cooling it in the process. Each quart (liter) of perspiration evaporated represents approximately 600 kcal of energy lost from the skin and surrounding tissues. For this reason, fever increases one's need for energy.

Recall from Chapter 4 that about 60% of the chemical energy in food is turned directly into body heat. Only about 40% is converted to ATP energy, and almost all of that energy eventually leaves the body in the form of heat. If this heat could not be dissipated, the body temperature would rise enough to prevent enzyme systems from functioning efficiently. Perspiration is the primary way to prevent this rise in body temperature.

However, to cool efficiently, perspiration must be allowed to evaporate. If it simply rolls off the skin or soaks into clothing, perspiration doesn't cool us much. Evaporation of perspiration occurs readily when humidity is low. This is why humans often tolerate hot, dry climates far better than they do hot, humid climates.

specific heat The amount of heat required to raise the temperature of any substance 1°C compared with the heat required to raise the temperature of the same volume of water 1°C. Water has a high specific heat, meaning that a relatively large amount of heat is required to raise its temperature; therefore, it tends to resist large temperature fluctuations.

Water Helps Remove Waste Products

As discussed in Chapter 3, water is an important vehicle for ridding the body of waste products. Most unwanted substances in the body are water soluble and can leave the body via the urine. In addition, liver metabolism converts some fat-soluble compounds into water-soluble compounds, so that they, too, can be excreted in the urine, such as some fat-soluble medications and potential cancer-causing substances.

A major body waste product is urea. This by-product of protein metabolism contains nitrogen. The more protein we eat in excess of needs, the more nitrogen we excrete—in the form of urea—in the urine. Likewise, the more sodium we consume, the more sodium we excrete in the urine. Overall, the amount of urine a person needs to produce is determined primarily by excess protein and sodium chloride (salt) intake. By limiting excess protein and salt intakes, it is possible to limit urine output—a useful practice, for example, in space flights. This type of diet is also used to treat some kidney diseases in which the ability to produce urine output is hampered.

A typical urine volume is about 1 to 2 liters (1 to 2 quarts) per day, depending mostly on the amount of fluid, protein, and sodium intake. Somewhat more urine output than that is fine, but less—especially less than 600 ml (2½ cups)—forces the kidneys to form a very concentrated urine. The heavy ion concentration increases the risk of kidney stone formation in susceptible people, generally men. Kidney stones are simply minerals and other substances that have precipitated out of the urine and accumulated in kidney tissues.

Other Functions of Water

Water is incompressible, so it helps form the lubricants found in knees and other joints of the body. It is the basis for saliva, bile, and **amniotic fluid.** Amniotic fluid acts as an important shock absorber surrounding the growing fetus. Electrolyte concentrations vary in each fluid compartment to accommodate specific needs, such as maintenance of a specific range in pH.

amniotic fluid The fluid contained in a sac within the uterus. This surrounds and protects the fetus during its development.

■ Water Needs

Adults need roughly 1 ml of water per kcal expended. We consume about 1 liter (1 quart) of water a day in various liquids, such as fruit juice, coffee, tea, soft drinks, and water itself (Fig. 11-3). Foods supply another liter of fluid; many fruits, vegetables, and beverages are more than 80% water (Table 11-1). Water as a by-product of metabolism provides approximately 350 ml (1½ cups) of additional water. All these

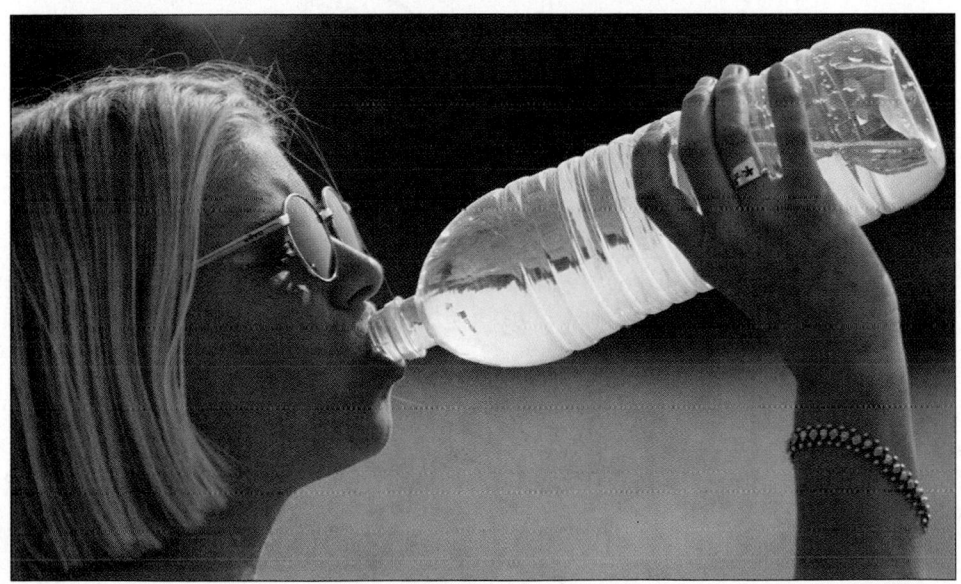

Regular intake of water is essential to replace daily fluid losses. A recent trend in America is to carry this water with us.

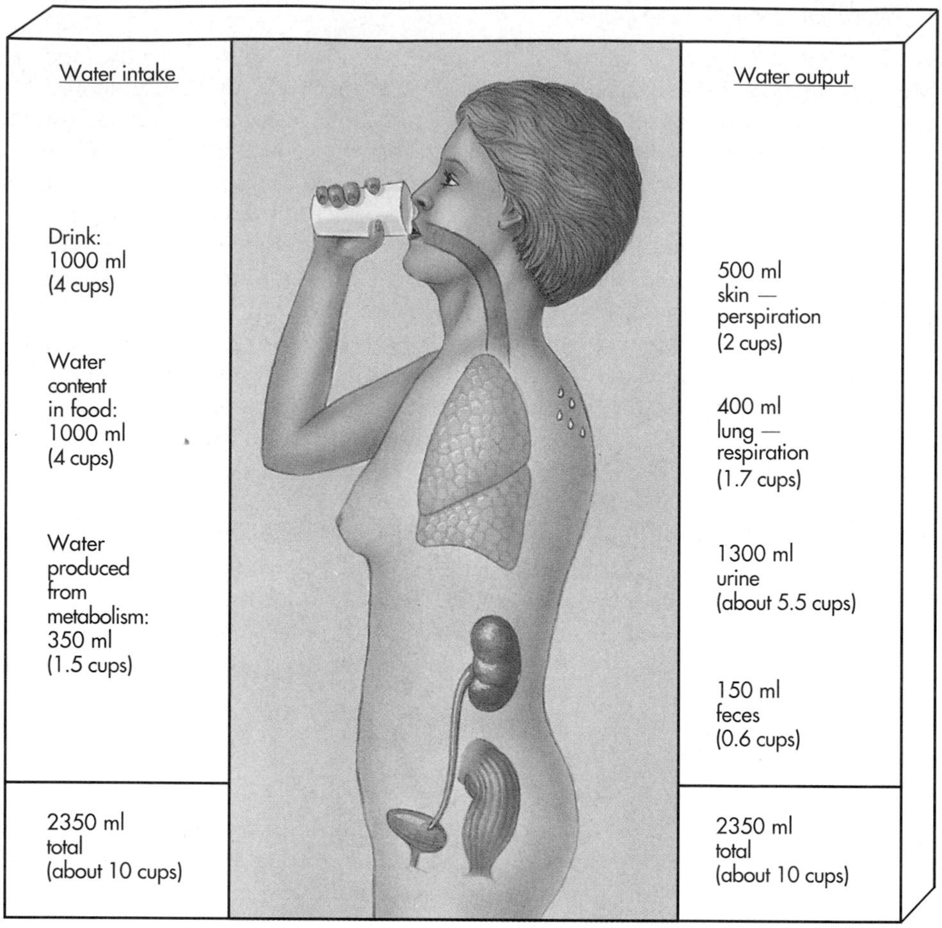

Illustration by William Ober.

FIGURE 11-3 Water balance—intake versus output. We maintain body fluids at an optimum amount by adjusting water intake and output. Most water comes from the liquids we consume. Some comes from the moisture in more solid foods, and the remainder is manufactured during metabolism. Water output includes that lost via lungs, kidneys, skin, and bowels.

insensible In this case, not perceived by the person, such as water lost with each breath.

sources together yield a total of about 2.4 liters (10 cups) of water for a 2400-kcal diet, or about 1 ml per kcal expended.

Of the 2.4 liters of water needed, about 1.4 liters is used to produce urine. The rest, about 1 liter, compensates for typical water losses through the lungs (400 ml), feces (150 ml), and skin (500 ml) (see Fig. 11-3). We are not normally aware of these **insensible** water losses. Note also that, when we consider the large amount of water used to facilitate gastrointestinal (GI) tract function, the loss of only 150 ml of water a day through the feces is remarkable. About 8000 ml of water enters the GI tract daily via secretions from the mouth, stomach, intestine, pancreas, and other organs. The diet supplies an additional 2000 ml or more. The kidneys also conserve water, reabsorbing about 97% of the water filtered from waste products.[24]

Water Deficiency

If you don't drink enough water, your body generally lets you know by signaling thirst. Your brain is communicating the need to drink. This thirst mechanism is not always reliable, however, especially during athletic practices and events, in infancy, during illness, and in one's older years.[12] For this reason, athletes should weigh themselves before and after training sessions to determine their rate of water loss and thus their water needs. Replacing at least 75% of this weight loss is advised, especially as weight loss approaches 2 to 3%. Two cups (½ liter) of water weigh about a pound (about half a kilogram) (see Chapter 14 for details on fluid use in athletics). Sick youngsters—especially those with fever, vomiting, diarrhea, and increased perspiration—and older persons often need to be reminded to drink plenty of fluids. As Chapter 17 discusses in further detail, infants easily become dehydrated. Long air-

TABLE 11-1   Water Content of a Typical Day's Food Intake

Meal	Fluid Ounces
Breakfast	
8 fl oz orange juice	7.2
½ cup skim milk	3.6
½ cup strawberries	2.7
1 cup Cheerios	0.4
Midmorning Snack	
1 cup of water	8.0
1 banana	3.0
Lunch	
2 oz water-packed tuna	2.2
2 slices whole-wheat bread	0.9
1 large tomato	5.0
8 oz low-fat yogurt	6.8
1 cup water	8.0
1 kiwi fruit	2.6
Dinner	
2 oz baked skinless chicken	1.3
2 cups romaine lettuce	4.0
2 oz sliced red peppers	1.8
1 slice bread	1.0
1 baked potato	3.5
1 cup skim milk	7.0
1 tbsp oil-and-vinegar dressing	0.0
1 cup of tea	8.0
Total	77 fluid ounces (9.6 cups)

plane flights are another situation that demands extra fluid intake: A traveler can lose about 6 cups (1.5 liters) of water during a 3-hour flight. The dehumidified air in an airplane is so dry that it induces excessive insensible perspiration and evaporation.

What If the Thirst Message Is Ignored?

Once the body registers an increase in blood concentration, it increases fluid conservation. The pituitary gland releases **antidiuretic hormone (ADH)** to force the kidneys to conserve water. The kidneys respond by reducing urine flow. At the same time, as fluid volume decreases in the bloodstream, blood pressure falls. This fall initiates a sequence of events beginning in the kidneys. Signaled by highly sensitive pressure receptors, the kidneys release an enzyme called **renin.** Renin, in turn, activates a circulating blood protein called angiotensinogen to form angiotensin I. Angiotensin I is converted to **angiotensin II,** which, among other effects, triggers the adrenal glands to release the hormone **aldosterone.** This hormone, in turn, signals the kidneys to retain more sodium and chloride, and, therefore, more water (Fig. 11-4). Remember that water always follows electrolytes. Thus, low blood pressure, through this roundabout measure using the kidneys, causes increased water conservation in the body.

However, despite these mechanisms to conserve water, fluid is still constantly lost via the insensible routes—feces, skin, and lungs. Those losses must be replaced. In addition, there is a limit to how concentrated urine can become. Eventually, if fluid is not consumed, the body becomes dehydrated and suffers ill effects.

antidiuretic hormone (ADH) A hormone that is secreted by the pituitary gland and acts on the kidneys to cause a decrease in water excretion. It is also called arginine vasopressin (AVP).

renin An enzyme formed in the kidneys in response to low blood pressure; it acts on a blood protein to produce angiotensin I.

angiotensin II A compound, produced from angiotensin I, that increases blood vessel constriction and triggers production of the hormone aldosterone.

aldosterone A hormone produced in the adrenal glands that acts on the kidneys, causing them to retain sodium and, therefore, water.

Alcohol inhibits the action of ADH. One reason people feel so weak the day after heavy drinking is that they are very dehydrated. Even though they may have consumed a lot of liquid in their drinks, they have lost even more liquid because alcohol has inhibited ADH. Caffeine also produces a diuretic effect on the body.

CRITICAL THINKING

Stacy has been working in the yard with her brother Tom. They have been busy mowing the lawn and pulling weeds since noon. Tom tells Stacy that he is feeling weak and has a headache. Stacy is concerned that her brother might be somewhat dehydrated. How can his symptoms be explained? How could Tom's risk of dehydration have been decreased?

By the time a person loses 1 to 2% of body weight in fluids, he or she will be thirsty. This loss of body weight contributes to fatigue, as well as impaired physiological and performance responses.[12] At a 4% loss of body weight, muscles lose significant strength and endurance. By the time body weight is reduced by 10 to 12%, heat tolerance is decreased and weakness results. At a 20% reduction, coma and death may soon follow (Fig. 11-5).

■ Water in Foods

It is important to achieve an adequate water intake, either through drinking water or by adding water-rich foods to your diet. Dark yellow instead of pale urine is a typical sign of insufficient water intake.

Water can be found in abundance in fruits and vegetables. Foods that are highest in water content include fruits and vegetables, particularly romaine lettuce, tomatoes, watercress, zucchini, asparagus, cantaloupe, grapefruit, and honeydew; orange juice; cottage cheese; tofu; water-packed tuna; and milk. Other sources that fall between 75 and 50% water are potatoes, corn, rice, hard-cooked eggs, bananas, beans, skinless chicken, part-skim mozzarella cheese, pasta, ice cream, baked salmon, and cod. The foods that are less than 35% water include breads, other cheeses, dry cereals, popcorn, and sugar.

■ Water Safety: How Safe Is the Water We Consume?

These days, it is common to see 5-gallon bottles of water being delivered to homes. Grocery store shelves are now stocked with many kinds of bottled waters—ranging from simple plastic jugs containing "pure spring water" to fancier, imported varieties of mineral water in glass bottles. In Europe, bottled water is an institution, as popular as soft drinks are in the United States.

Currently, it is quite fashionable to order a bottle of Evian at a restaurant or bar. Not only are people looking for alternatives to alcoholic beverages and soft drinks, but they are also attracted to the perceived health value or taste of bottled water. Is this practice of bottled water use worth the effort and expense?

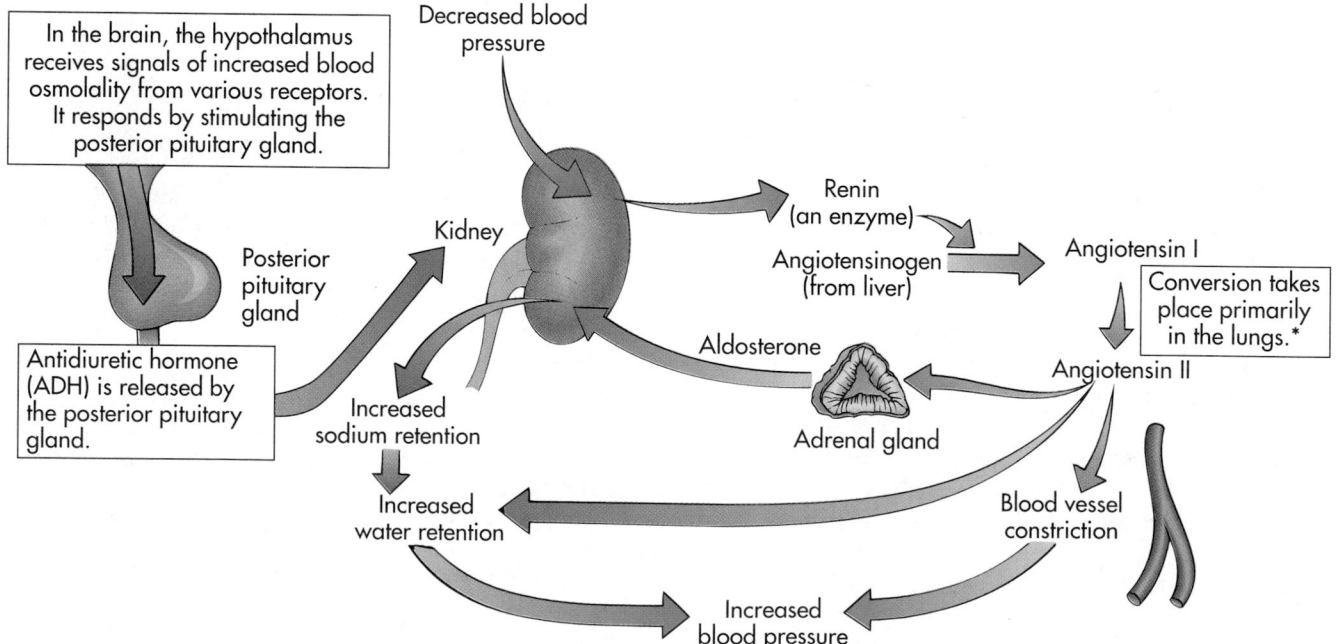

■ FIGURE 11-4 The renin-angiotensin system is one regulator of blood pressure. It functions with antidiuretic hormone to control blood pressure.

*The angiotensin converting enzyme (ACE) inhibitors use to treat hypertension and other disorders act at this site.

Most people in the United States enjoy very safe tap water. The Environmental Protection Agency (EPA) and local municipalities pay careful attention to possible contaminants that can appear in tap water, and 90% of public water facilities have been found to be in compliance with current regulations.[26] Local municipalities also are required by law to inform customers of any dangerous amounts of contaminants and indicate specific actions to take, such as the need to boil water. These agencies also have to provide a yearly report of ongoing water quality evaluations.

Currently, it is estimated that 10 million people in the United States are at risk for consuming tap water that does not meet EPA guidelines. These individuals are primarily in rural communities, where agricultural runoff from farmlands can pollute both ground water used for wells and streams and rivers used as a water source. These individuals may have their water tested to see if a water purifier or bottled water is indicated. Testing is available through the local health department or county extension agencies. The cost for this testing is minimal.

Another threat to water safety comes from a parasite called *Cryptosporidium*. **Cryptosporidiosis** is an intestinal disease that can spread from hand to mouth by having direct contact with infected human or animal feces, by swallowing the parasite via tap water or swimming pool water, or by consuming undercooked contaminated food.

As noted in Chapter 20, scarcity of clean water is a growing problem in many developing countries.

cryptosporidiosis An intestinal disease, characterized by diarrhea, that originates from a protozoan parasite of the genus *Cryptosporidium*.

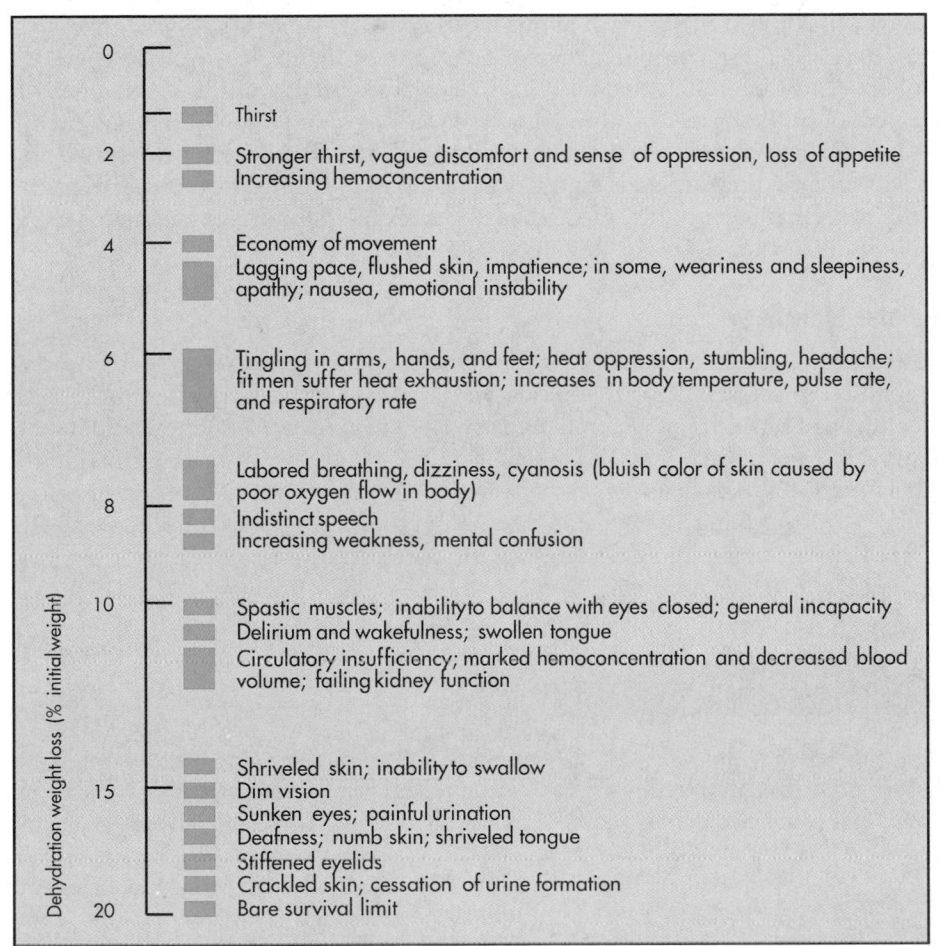

NORMAL WEIGHT

Dehydration weight loss (% initial weight)

- 0 — Thirst
- 2 — Stronger thirst, vague discomfort and sense of oppression, loss of appetite
  Increasing hemoconcentration
- 4 — Economy of movement
  Lagging pace, flushed skin, impatience; in some, weariness and sleepiness, apathy; nausea, emotional instability
- 6 — Tingling in arms, hands, and feet; heat oppression, stumbling, headache; fit men suffer heat exhaustion; increases in body temperature, pulse rate, and respiratory rate
- Labored breathing, dizziness, cyanosis (bluish color of skin caused by poor oxygen flow in body)
- 8 — Indistinct speech
  Increasing weakness, mental confusion
- 10 — Spastic muscles; inability to balance with eyes closed; general incapacity
  Delirium and wakefulness; swollen tongue
  Circulatory insufficiency; marked hemoconcentration and decreased blood volume; failing kidney function
- Shriveled skin; inability to swallow
- 15 — Dim vision
  Sunken eyes; painful urination
  Deafness; numb skin; shriveled tongue
  Stiffened eyelids
  Crackled skin; cessation of urine formation
- 20 — Bare survival limit

DEATH

FIGURE 11-5 The effects of dehydration range from thirst to death, depending on the extent of body weight loss.

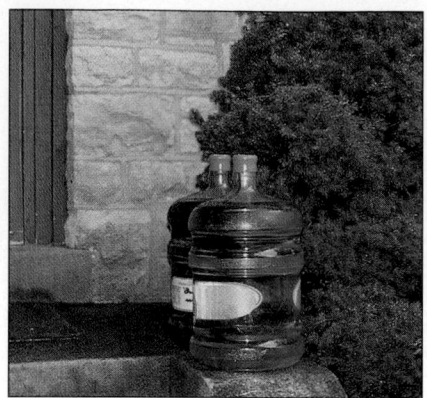

Concern over tap water quality has led some Americans to purchase bottled water. This concern has merit, especially in rural communities.

*A*s bottled water becomes more and more popular, the industry now generates more than $3 billion per year. In 1996, FDA instituted definitions for the various types of bottled water on the market; FDA also tests products for microbial and chemical content. For a list of manufacturers that meet federal guidelines, contact the International Bottled Water Association at 1-800-928-3711 or http://www.nsf.org. Some experts recommend that children not be given bottled water exclusively, as it does not contain an adequate fluoride supply to protect against dental caries. For adults, bottled water is typically an unnecessary expense, as it is often very similar to tap water.

In 1993, 400,000 people in Milwaukee became ill and 100 died from water contaminated with *Cryptosporidium*. Another recent attack happened in Sydney, Australia. This parasite poses little risk to healthy people—other than a case of diarrhea—but this is not true for people who have HIV/AIDS or other diseases that compromise function of the immune system (such as some forms of cancer therapy or organ transplant therapy). Recently, these high-risk patients have, in fact, been advised to boil for 1 minute tap water they use for cooking or drinking to ensure the parasite is destroyed. Alternatively, one can purchase a water filter that screens out *Cryptosporidium* (the National Sanitation Foundation at 800-673-8010 can provide a list of manufacturers) or use bottled water that is certified to be free of this parasite (contact the supplier if in doubt). Generally, distilled water or that which has undergone reverse osmosis is free of *Cryptosporidium*.

As a safeguard against microbial contamination, chlorine and ammonia are added to water to kill bacteria (although such chlorination does not kill *Cryptosporidium*). The addition of such chemicals has raised concern that drinking water may increase rectal and bladder cancer risk, although there is currently no conclusive proof of such risk. If chlorine in tap water does increase cancer risk, the risk is extremely small (perhaps two cases of cancer in 1 million people).

If you find the taste of chlorinated tap water unpleasant or are concerned about the slight cancer risk, you can remove the chlorine from tap water by boiling it or by letting a large container filled with water stand uncovered overnight. In both cases, the chlorine will evaporate, taking its characteristic flavor with it. Alternatively, you can install a filter on the household spigot from which you obtain your water. It should be designed to remove trihalomethanes, common chlorine by-products.

Overall, if you are concerned about the safety of your tap water, you can ask the municipal water department for the most current test results, or, if you have well water (or are just interested), you can have the water tested yourself. Compared with the cost of bottled water or water filters, the testing fee is insignificant. As noted in Chapter 19, letting cold water run for a minute or so before taking a drink or before using it in meal preparation is a good way to limit possible lead exposure, especially if the water has been off for more than an hour. In addition, for the same reason, avoid using hot tap water for food preparation.

■ Water Toxicity

Too much water—whatever amount the kidneys are unable to excrete—can also lead to serious side effects. Water intoxication is most likely to occur if water intake is not accompanied by sufficient electrolytes. However, an excessive amount would have to approach many quarts (liters) each day. Very few people are at risk of drinking too much water, but problems do accompany some disease states and mental disorders. When excessive water overwhelms the kidneys' capacity to excrete it, headache, blurred vision, cramps, convulsions, and ultimately death may occur.

CONCEPT CHECK

*B*ecause the body can not store water, we can survive only a few days without it. Water dissolves substances, serves as a medium for chemical reactions and as a lubricant, and aids in temperature regulation. Water accounts for 50 to 70% of body weight and distributes itself throughout the body: among lean and other tissues (in both intracellular and extracellular fluids) and in urine and other body fluids. Adults need about 1 ml of water or other fluids for each kcal expended. Thirst is the body's first sign of dehydration. If this thirst mechanism is faulty, as it may be during illness or vigorous exercise, hormonal mechanisms also help conserve water by reducing urine output. Overall, the U.S. water supply is generally safe; thus, bottled water and home water purification is unnecessary in most communities. Excess fluid intake can be hazardous to a person's health.

■ MINERALS

Minerals are divided into major minerals and trace minerals, depending on the amount we need per day. Generally speaking, if we require 100 mg (1/50 of a teaspoon) or more per day of a mineral, it is considered a **major mineral;** otherwise, it is considered a **trace mineral.** Using these criteria, calcium and phosphorus are major minerals, and iron and zinc are trace minerals.

The functions and nutritional significance of the major minerals are discussed in this chapter, and the trace minerals in Chapter 12. But, before examining the properties of the individual major minerals, let's consider some topics relevant to all the nutrients.

■ Absorption, Transport, and Excretion of Minerals

A significant factor determining the degree to which a mineral may be absorbed is the physiological need for that mineral at the time of consumption. Other factors are discussed in the following paragraphs.

Many minerals have similar molecular weights and charges (valences). Magnesium, calcium, iron, and copper can exist in the 2^+ valence state. Having similar size and the same charge causes some of these minerals to compete with each other for absorption mechanisms, thereby affecting each other's **bioavailability** and metabolism. Because of this, people should avoid taking individual mineral supplements unless a medical condition specifically warrants it. This is because an excess of one mineral influences the absorption and metabolism of other minerals. For example, the presence of a large amount of zinc in the diet decreases copper absorption.

Some vitamins improve mineral absorption. Vitamin C improves iron absorption when the two are consumed in the same meal. The vitamin D hormone $1,25 (OH)_2$ D improves calcium, phosphorus, and magnesium absorption.[6]

Mineral bioavailability can be greatly influenced by nonmineral substances in the diet. Foods contain and supply us with many minerals, but the body varies in its capacity to absorb and use available minerals. Although minerals may be present in foods, they are not bioavailable unless the body can absorb them. The ability to absorb minerals from a diet depends on many factors. The amount of a mineral listed in a food composition table does not necessarily reflect the amount that can be actually absorbed.

Components of fiber, especially phytic acid (phytate) in wheat grain fiber, can limit the absorption of some minerals by chemically binding to it and preventing it from being released during digestion. An intake above the recommendation of 20 to 35 g of dietary fiber per day can cause problems with mineral status of the body (see Chapter 5 for details). However, if grains are leavened with yeast, as they are in bread, enzymes produced by the yeast can break some of the chemical bonds between phytic acid and minerals. This in some cases reduces the effect of phytates on mineral absorption. The zinc deficiencies found among some Middle Eastern populations are attributed partly to their consumption of unleavened breads, resulting in low bioavailability of dietary zinc. This is discussed in detail in Chapter 12.

Oxalic acid, or **oxalate,** is another substance in plants that binds minerals and makes them less available to the body. Spinach, for example, contains plenty of calcium, but only about 5% of it can be absorbed because of the vegetable's high concentration of oxalic acid. On average, about 25% of dietary calcium is absorbed by adults, with the highest percentage coming from dairy products.[6]

Once absorbed, minerals travel in the blood either in a free form or bound to proteins. For example, calcium ions can be found in the blood as such, as well as bound to the blood protein albumin. Many of the trace minerals have specific binding proteins, which transport them in the bloodstream. Trace minerals in their free from are often highly reactive and, so, would be toxic if not so bound. You will see, as well, in Chapter 12 that many trace minerals also are bound by specific cellular proteins once taken up by cells.

major mineral A mineral vital to health that is required in the diet in amounts greater than 100 mg/day.

trace mineral A mineral vital to health that is required in the diet in amounts less than 100 mg/day.

bioavailability The degree to which the amount of an ingested nutrient is absorbed and is available to the body.

oxalic acid (oxalate) An organic acid that is found in spinach, rhubarb, and other leafy green vegetables and that can depress the absorption of certain minerals present in the food, such as calcium.

Mineral excretion takes place primarily through the urine. When kidney function fails, mineral intake must be controlled in order to avoid mineral toxicity, such as with phosphorus and magnesium. Some minerals are discharged through the bile into the intestinal tract and then excreted through the feces. Gallbladder disease can then cause mineral toxicity, especially for copper and manganese because they can't be readily eliminated. Intake needs to be closely monitored in these cases, such as when gallbladder disease develops in preterm infants.

■ Functions of Minerals

The metabolic roles of minerals and the amounts of them in the body vary considerably (Fig. 11-6). Some minerals, such as copper and selenium, function as cofactors, enabling enzymes to carry out a chemical reaction. Minerals also are components of many body compounds. For example, iron is a component of hemoglobin in red blood cells. Sodium, potassium, and calcium aid in the transmission of nerve impulses throughout the body. Body growth and development also depend on certain minerals, such as calcium and phosphorus. Water balance requires sodium, potassium, calcium, and phosphorus. At all levels—cellular, tissue, organ, and whole body—minerals clearly play important roles in maintaining body functions.

■ Food Sources of Minerals

Minerals in the average American's diet come from both plant and animal sources. Overall, minerals from animal products are more easily absorbed because various binders, such as phytates in dietary fiber, are not present to hinder absorption. In addition, as an animal eats plants year after year, minerals from the plants concentrate in the animal's body tissues. A human's diet free of animal products is very likely to be marginal in the major mineral calcium and in some trace minerals, such as iron and zinc. A key exception is magnesium, which is far more plentiful in plant than in animal foods. Otherwise, some plant foods are good, but not excellent, sources of many minerals. Vegans need to be aware of this and regularly choose good plant sources of minerals, such as iron and zinc (see Chapter 7). Furthermore, generally the more refined a plant food—as in the case of white flour—the lower its mineral

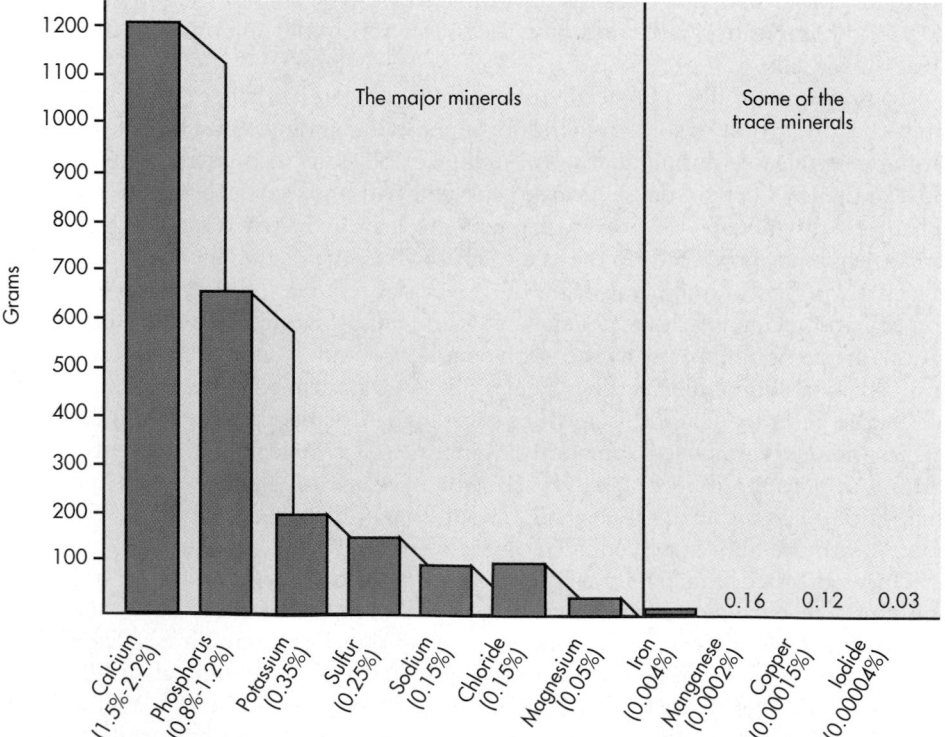

■ FIGURE 11-6 Approximate amounts of various minerals present in the average human body. The percent values in parentheses indicate the amounts as percentages of body weight. Other trace minerals of nutritional importance not listed include chromium, fluoride, molybdenum, selenium, and zinc.

content. The enrichment process for grains adds only the mineral iron. The selenium, zinc, copper, and other minerals lost when grains are refined are not replaced. This is just one more reason to consume whole grains on a regular basis.

■ North Americans at Risk for Mineral Deficiencies

Typically, the major mineral at risk for being deficient in adult diets is calcium. Currently, most North Americans do not meet the recommended intake for calcium.[22] For trace minerals, iron and zinc are most likely to be deficient in diets; these minerals are discussed in Chapter 12.

■ Toxicity of Minerals

Excess mineral intake can lead to toxic results, especially with the trace minerals, such as iron and copper. This potential for toxicity is yet another reason to consider carefully the use of mineral supplements. Every year, people poison themselves using mineral supplements, even though their intent is to maximize health. Many trace minerals are quite toxic at doses not much above typical needs. Thus, doses of mineral supplements exceeding the Upper Tolerable Intake Level (Upper Level or UL) should be taken only under a physician's supervision because toxicity and nutrient interactions are possible (see the inside cover of this text for Upper Levels for minerals).

CONCEPT CHECK

Minerals are vital to the functioning of many body processes. Their bioavailability depends on many factors, including a mineral's interaction with dietary fiber, vitamins, and other minerals. Animal products often yield better mineral absorption than do plants. Still, both animal and plant sources help us meet our mineral needs. Taking large amounts of an individual mineral supplement can greatly diminish the absorption and metabolism of other minerals. In addition, some minerals are potentially toxic at intakes not much in excess of human needs. These are two good reasons to consider carefully any use of mineral supplements.

■ SODIUM (NA)

Health professionals issuing dietary recommendations generally suggest North Americans limit intake of sodium.[11] Salt contributes almost all the sodium to our diets. Salt is 40% sodium and 60% chloride. Typical recommended intakes are about half of what North Americans currently consume. Still, as reviewed in the Nutrition Perspective at the end of this chapter, salt intake is not the major cause of the epidemic of hypertension in North America (obesity and inactivity are more important).[17]

Absorption, Transport, Storage, and Excretion of Sodium

The human body absorbs almost all sodium that is consumed. In fact, about 95% of ingested sodium is absorbed. Sodium is very soluble and easily absorbed from the stomach, small intestine, and colon. Some sodium in the bloodstream is filtered by the kidneys, where the excess is removed by the urine. The rest is returned to the blood to maintain an appropriate concentration. Excretion of sodium is maintained by a mechanism involving glomerular filtration, the renin-angiotensin system, parts of the nervous system circulating catecholamines (e.g., norepinephrine), and blood pressure (review Fig. 11-4).[24]

Only about 10% of the sodium consumed in the average diet is needed by the body; the rest is eliminated through three routes: the kidneys, skin, and GI tract. The major route of excretion is through the kidneys. Some sodium, however, is stored in the bones.

The importance of salt to human health has been recognized since antiquity. Salt was a commodity in the classical world. Indeed, the Latin word *salary* reflects the way a soldier's wages were paid.

To assess the sodium, potassium, chloride, magnesium, or phosphorus status of a person, blood concentrations can be measured. Other methods, often more sensitive ones, when appropriate, will be noted in this chapter.

Mrs. Massa has recently seen and heard a lot about the amount of salt (sodium) in foods. She has been surprised by the number of articles that advise the public to decrease the amount of salt in their food. If sodium is such a bad thing, Mrs. Massa wonders, why do you need to have any at all? How would you explain this need for some sodium to her?

Many commercially prepared condiments, sauces, and seasonings are high in sodium. Examples include onion, celery, garlic, seasoned, and sea salts; baking powder; salad dressings; pickles; soy, steak, barbecue, chili, and Worcestershire sauces; meat tenderizer; baking soda; salt pork; brine; catsup; mustard; bouillon; monosodium glutamate (MSG); and relish.

Functions of Sodium

Sodium is the major positive ion (cation) in extracellular fluid and a key factor in retaining body fluids. Sodium balance is regulated by the hormone aldosterone. Sodium also helps regulate the fluid balance of the body both within and outside the cells. The high blood levels of sodium contribute to its osmolality and, in turn, the regulation of fluid volume of the extracellular and intracellular compartments.

As both potassium and sodium shift across the cell membrane, they create an electrical potential charge, which allows muscles to contract and nerve impulses to be conducted. Sodium also participates in the absorption of other nutrients (e.g., glucose) in the small intestine.

Sodium Deficiency

A low-sodium diet—coupled with excessive perspiration, persistent vomiting, or diarrhea—can deplete the body of sodium. This state can lead to muscle cramps, nausea, vomiting, dizziness, and later shock and coma. The likelihood of this happening, however, is minimal because early kidney responses to low sodium status eventually trigger the body to conserve sodium.[24] In addition, people generally eat a lot of sodium.

Sodium in Foods

About one-third to one-half the sodium we consume is added during cooking or at the table. Most of the rest is added during food manufacturing (Table 11-2). Many health authorities are calling for manufacturers to use less salt, so that our total sodium intakes fall. To some extent, this is taking place (e.g., low-sodium soups and crackers). Almost all foods naturally contain a little sodium; the higher amount found in milk (about 120 mg/cup) is one exception. The more home cooking a person does, the more sodium control that person has.

TABLE 11-2   Increase in Sodium Content of Foods During Processing*

Food Category	Sodium (mg)
Dairy Products	
Fruited yogurt, ¾ cup	107
2% milk, 1½ cups	182
Cheddar cheese, 1¾ oz	307
American cheese food, 2 oz	548
Meats	
Beef roast, 1 oz	17
Beef jerky, ⅔ oz	540
Pork loin, 1 oz	22
Bacon, 2 pieces	202
Ham, 1½ oz	564
Vegetables	
Fresh peas, 1 cup	5
Frozen peas, 1 cup	139
Frozen peas in cheese sauce, ⅔ cup	205
Canned peas, 1 cup	372
Grain Products	
Flour, ⅓ cup	1
Bread, 2 slices	286
Saltine crackers, 12	486

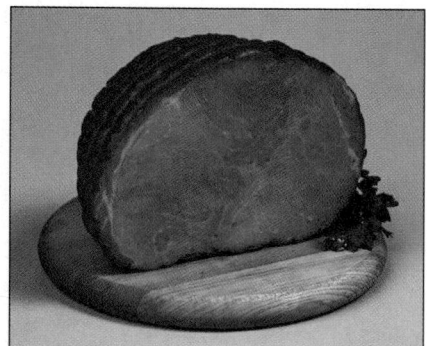

Cured meats, such as ham, are very high in sodium.

*All examples in a particular group contain the same amount of food energy.

Major contributors of sodium in the adult diet are white bread and rolls, hot dogs and lunch meats, cheese, soups, and spaghetti with tomato sauce, partly because these foods are eaten so often. Other foods that generally are especially high in sodium include salted snack foods, French fries and potato chips, and sauces and gravies. (If we were to eat only unprocessed foods and add no salt, we would consume about 500 mg of sodium per day, or about 1/10 of current intakes.)[17] And, in cases where sodium intake must be very limited, even contributions from tap water (especially from softened water, which contains more sodium), as well as medicines that contain sodium, must be considered.

As discussed in Chapter 2, nutrition labels list a food's sodium content. In addition, various descriptive terms, such as sodium-free, salt-free, and low-sodium, may appear elsewhere on labels (review Table 2-8 in Chapter 2). When dietary sodium must be severely restricted, these labels are very helpful.

Sodium Needs

The body needs only about 100 mg of sodium a day. The 1989 RDA publication set 500 mg/day as a minimum requirement for health. Under FDA food-labeling rules, the Daily Value for sodium is 2400 mg. FDA established this value because it is consistent with the government reports that encourage reduced sodium intakes. The American Heart Association also recently supported this recommendation. Typical sodium intakes of adults are generally two or more times this amount (4-7 g/day).

How Much Sodium Do You Consume? You can evaluate your sodium consumption habits by completing the questionnaire in Table 11-3. The more checks in the "often" or "regularly" column, the higher your dietary sodium intake. However, not all the habits in the table contribute the same amount of sodium. For example, many natural cheeses are relatively moderate in sodium, whereas processed cheeses and cottage cheese are much higher. You can choose to reduce your sodium intake by cutting back on those items for which you checked "often" or "regularly." You needn't suddenly eliminate foods from your diet. Rather, to moderate sodium intake, choose lower-sodium foods from each food group more often and balance high-sodium food choices with low-sodium ones.[14] It is also important to pay attention to the sodium values listed on food labels and to taste foods before adding salt. In addition, when eating out, avoiding foods commonly prepared with lots of

---

TABLE 11-3   Questionnaire for Evaluating Your Sodium Habits with Respect to Typically Rich Sources

How Often Do You . . .	Rarely	Occasionally	Often	Regularly (Daily)
1. Eat cured or processed meats, such as ham, bacon, sausage, frankfurters, and other luncheon meats?	☐	☐	☐	☐
2. Choose canned or frozen vegetables with sauce?	☐	☐	☐	☐
3. Use commercially prepared meals, main dishes, or canned or dehydrated soups?	☐	☐	☐	☐
4. Eat cheese, especially processed cheese?	☐	☐	☐	☐
5. Eat salted nuts, popcorn, pretzels, corn chips, or potato chips?	☐	☐	☐	☐
6. Add salt to cooking water for vegetables, rice, or pasta?	☐	☐	☐	☐
7. Add salt, seasoning mixes, salad dressings, or condiments—such as soy sauce, steak sauce, catsup, and mustard—to foods during preparation or at the table?	☐	☐	☐	☐
8. Salt your food before tasting it?	☐	☐	☐	☐
9. Ignore labels for sodium content when buying foods?	☐	☐	☐	☐
10. When dining out, choose foods with sauces, or foods that are obviously salty?	☐	☐	☐	☐

The more checks you have in the last two columns, the higher your dietary sodium intake.

Adapted from *USDA Home and Garden Bulletin* No. 232-6, April 1986.

sodium and asking to have sauces served on the side and then using only small amounts are two other ideas.

It is also a good idea to have your blood pressure checked regularly. If you have hypertension due to salt sensitivity, you should try to reduce your sodium intake as part of a comprehensive plan to treat this disease and see if this helps the problem.[17]

Adapting to a Lower Sodium Intake. Should you be advised by a physician or simply choose to consume less sodium, you can eventually adapt to a low-sodium diet. At first, foods will taste quite flat, but eventually you will perceive more flavor as the tongue's salt receptors become more sensitive to the natural salt content of foods. By slowly reducing dietary salt and substituting garlic, oregano, lemon juice, and other herbs and spices, you can eventually become accustomed to a diet containing less sodium. Many new cookbooks offer tested recipes for flavorful low-sodium foods. Except when baking breads with yeast, omitting salt from food preparation can still yield many excellent products.

North Americans at Risk for a Sodium Deficiency

Only when weight loss from perspiration exceeds 2 to 3% of total body weight (or about 5 to 6 lb) should sodium losses be of concern.[24] Even then, merely salting foods is sufficient to restore body sodium for most people. Endurance athletes, however, may need to consume sports drinks during competition to avoid depletion of sodium (see Chapter 14). Note also that, although perspiration tastes salty on the skin, sodium is not highly concentrated in perspiration. Rather, water evaporating from the skin leaves concentrated sodium behind. Perspiration contains about two-thirds the sodium concentration found in blood.

Toxicity of Sodium

A sodium intake > 2 g/day also increases calcium loss in the urine. This is especially a problem for people who consume much salt and little calcium.

Most humans can adapt to various dietary sodium intakes, although it can contribute to hypertension in some people. A very high intake also can be toxic, especially when the kidneys cannot excrete the excess in the urine. Sodium is also toxic when a high intake is accompanied by a lack of water. An Upper Level for sodium has yet to be set.

CONCEPT CHECK

Sodium is the major positive ion in the extracellular fluid. It is important for maintaining fluid balance and conducting nerve impulses. In the North American diet, sodium is provided predominantly through processed foods and salt added in cooking and at the table. The more foods prepared at home, the more control one has over sodium intake. For adults, the minimum sodium requirement for health is 500 mg/day. Many scientific groups suggest that, for all adults, sodium intake should be limited to about 2.4 g/day, but there is not universal support for this recommendation. This amount is about half of what an average adult consumes. About 10 to 15% of North Americans are sensitive to dietary sodium and may develop hypertension as a result of high salt intakes. Sodium depletion is unlikely, since North American diets have abundant sources, and most sodium consumed is absorbed.

■ POTASSIUM (K)

Like sodium, potassium is a primary electrolyte in body fluids. Unlike sodium, potassium is associated with lower, rather than higher, blood pressure values.

Absorption, Transport, and Excretion of Potassium

The body absorbs about 90% of the potassium consumed. As with sodium, potassium balance is achieved primarily through the kidneys, with aldosterone being the major regulatory hormone.[24]

Functions of Potassium and the Effects of a Deficiency

Potassium performs many of the same functions as sodium, such as fluid balance and nerve-impulse transmission. It also influences the contractility of smooth, skeletal, and cardiac muscle. Potassium is the major cation inside the cell. Intracellular fluids contain 95% of the potassium in the body.

Low blood potassium is a life-threatening problem. Symptoms often include a loss of appetite, muscle cramps, confusion, and constipation. Eventually, the heart beats irregularly, decreasing its capacity to pump blood.

Potassium in Foods

Unlike sodium, potassium is not generally added to foods. Overall, fresh fruits and vegetables are the most nutrient-dense (mg/kcal) sources of potassium. Milk, whole grains, dried beans, and meats are also sources. Major contributors of potassium to the adult diet include milk, potatoes, coffee, tomatoes, and orange juice (Fig. 11-7).

Potassium Needs

The adult minimum potassium requirement for health set by the 1989 RDA is 2000 mg per day. Typically, adults meet potassium needs by eating a wide variety of foods. North Americans average 2 to 3 g/day. The Daily Value for potassium used for food labels is 3500 mg. Information about a food's potassium content is required on the Nutrition Facts panel only if the food contains added potassium as a nutrient or if claims about this nutrient appear on the label. In all other cases, it is voluntary.

North Americans at Risk for a Potassium Deficiency

Some diuretics used to treat hypertension deplete the body's potassium. People who take potassium-wasting diuretics need to monitor their potassium intakes carefully. For these people, high-potassium foods—such as fruits, fruit juices, and vegetables—

Food Sources of Potassium

Food Item and Amount	Potassium (mg)
Baked winter squash, ¾ cup	780
Cooked kidney beans, 1 cup	710
Baked potato, 1	610
Cantaloupe, 1 cup	490
Orange juice, 1 cup	470
Banana, 1	470
Steamed zucchini, 1 cup	450
Cooked lima beans, ½ cup	370
Raisins, ¼ cup	300
Cooked asparagus, 1 cup	290

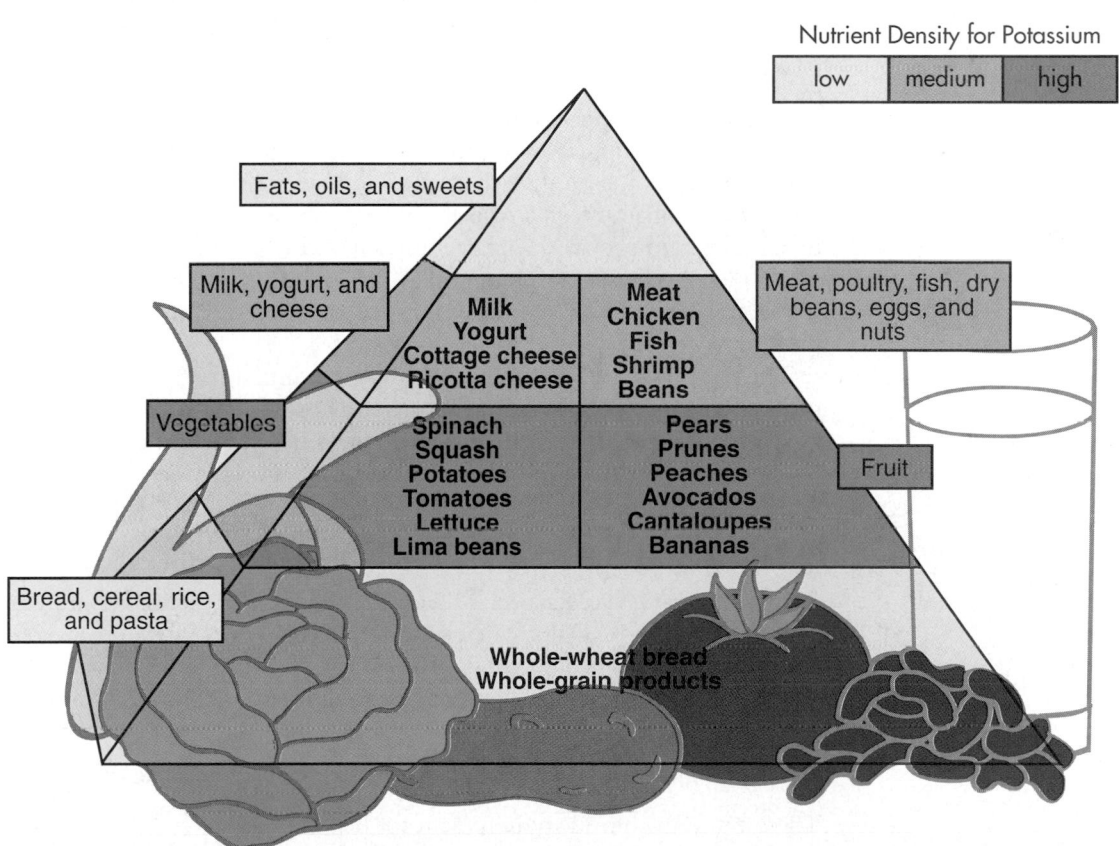

■ FIGURE 11-7 Food sources of potassium from the Food Guide Pyramid. The fruit group and the vegetables group are the best dietary sources of this nutrient, but it is widely distributed in foods. The background color of each food group indicates the average nutrient density for potassium in that group.

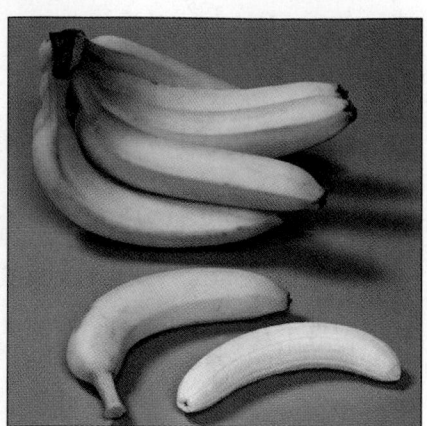

Bananas are a rich source of potassium.

are good additions to the diet, and, if recommended by a physician, so are potassium chloride supplements.

A continual deficient food intake, as may be the case in alcoholism, can also result in potassium deficiency. This also can be true for people with anorexia nervosa and bulimia nervosa, whose diets are poor and whose bodies can be depleted of nutrients because of vomiting (see Chapter 15). People on very low-calorie diets are also at risk, as well as athletes who exercise heavily. As covered in Chapters 13 and 14, all of these people should compensate for potentially low body potassium by consuming potassium-rich foods.

Toxicity of Potassium

Potassium in supplement form is harmless if the kidneys function normally; however, taken in excessive amounts, it causes a gastrointestinal upset. When the kidneys function poorly, potassium builds up in the blood, creating a condition called hyperkalemia.[24] This inhibits heart function, causing slowed heartbeat. If untreated, this can be fatal, as the heart eventually stops beating. Consequently, in cases of reduced kidney function, close control of potassium intake is critical. An Upper Level for potassium has yet to be set.

■ CHLORIDE (CL)

Chlorine is an element, but humans need the chloride ion (Cl^-).

Absorption, Transport, and Excretion of Chloride

Chloride is almost completely absorbed in the small intestine and colon. As is the case with sodium, excretion of chloride occurs through three routes: the kidneys, skin, and GI tract. The major route of excretion is through the kidneys.

Functions of Chloride and the Effects of a Deficiency

Chlorine is a very poisonous gas. In our bodies, chloride—the anion form of chlorine—forms an important negative ion for the extracellular fluid. Chloride's negative charge balances the positive charges on sodium ions and is therefore of great importance in the maintenance of electrolyte balance. Chloride is a component of hydrochloric acid produced in the stomach and is used during immune responses as white blood cells attack foreign cells. Chloride aids in the transport of carbon dioxide from cells to the lungs, as well as the disposal of carbon dioxide by way of exhaled air.[24]

During the late 1970s, a chloride-deficient infant formula was manufactured and sold. The infant formula caused severe convulsions and other health problems, such as retarded growth, in the infants who consumed it. This incident showed what can happen when the need for a nutrient normally abundant in our diet is not given adequate attention.

Chloride in Foods

Seaweed, olives, rye, lettuce, a few fruits, and some vegetables are naturally good sources of chloride. Chlorinated water is also a source. However, we consume most chloride as salt added to foods. Knowing a food's salt content, one can predict closely its chloride content; recall that salt is 60% chloride. Naturally occurring sodium or chloride won't significantly affect the prediction.

Chloride Needs

The minimum chloride requirement for health in adults set by the 1989 RDA is 700 mg/day. Assuming that the average adult consumes at least 7.5 g of salt daily, that supplies 4.5 g (4500 mg) of chloride, an abundance of this ion.

North Americans at Risk for a Chloride Deficiency

A chloride deficiency is unlikely because our dietary sodium chloride (salt) intake is so high. Frequent and lengthy bouts of vomiting—if coupled with a nutrient-poor diet—can contribute to a deficiency because stomach secretions contain much chloride.

Chloride Toxicity

Dietary chloride has been implicated in the blood pressure-raising ability of sodium chloride. Still, as one lowers sodium intake as part of hypertension therapy, chloride intake automatically falls as well. Large chloride intakes, above 15 g/day, may cause fluid retention.

CONCEPT CHECK

Potassium performs functions similar to those of sodium, except that it is the main positive ion (cation) found inside, not outside, cells. Potassium is vital to fluid balance and nerve transmission. A potassium deficiency—caused by an inadequate intake of potassium, persistent vomiting, or use of some diuretics—can lead to loss of appetite, muscle cramps, confusion, and heartbeat irregularities. Fruits and vegetables are generally rich sources of potassium. Potassium intake can be toxic if a person's kidneys do not function properly. Chloride is the major negative ion (anion) of extracellular fluid. Chloride also functions in digestion as part of hydrochloric acid and in immune and nervous system responses. Deficiencies of chloride are highly unlikely because we eat so much sodium chloride (salt), the major source.

■ CALCIUM (CA)

All cells need calcium, but more than 99% of the calcium in the body is used as a structural component of bones and teeth. This calcium represents 40% of all the minerals present in the body and equals about 2.5 lb (1200 g). As calcium circulates in the bloodstream, it supplies the calcium needs of body cells.

Absorption, Transport, Storage, and Excretion of Calcium

Unlike sodium, potassium, and chloride, the amount of calcium in the body depends on the amount absorbed from the diet.

Absorption. Calcium absorption occurs primarily in the upper part of the small intestine (duodenum) because calcium requires a pH below 6 to stay in solution in an ionic state (Ca^{2+}). By the time the acidic stomach contents reach the duodenum, they have been partially neutralized by bicarbonate released from the pancreas but are still slightly acidic. This provides a suitable environment for calcium absorption. In addition, calcium absorption within the upper small intestine depends greatly on the active vitamin D hormone 1,25 $(OH)_2$ D. Because the intestinal contents become more alkaline as they pass down the gastrointestinal tract, calcium absorption decreases at the terminal end of the small intestine and colon, although some still occurs via passive absorption.[6]

Humans absorb about 25% of the calcium in the foods eaten; however, when the body needs extra calcium—such as during infancy and pregnancy—absorption might reach as high as 60%. Young people tend to absorb calcium better than do older people, especially those older than 70. Postmenopausal women generally absorb the least calcium, unless they receive supplements of the hormone estrogen. Estrogen therapy is associated with an increased synthesis of 1,25 $(OH)_2$ D, which aids calcium absorption.

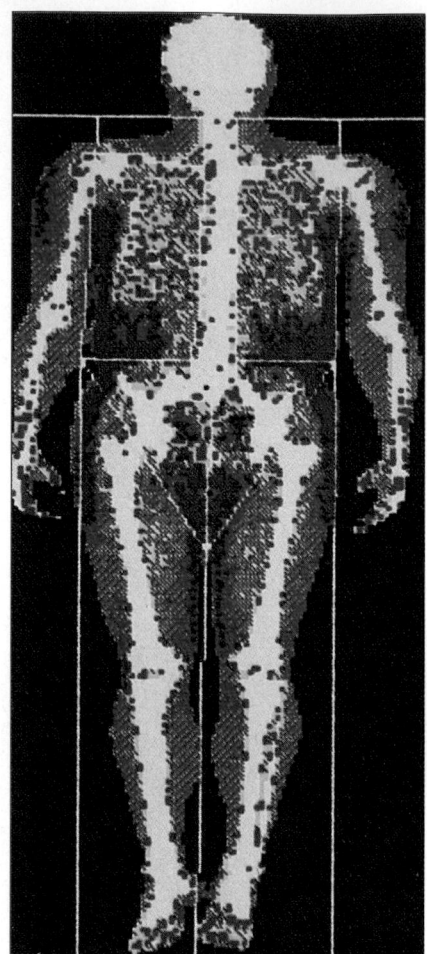

Ninety-nine percent of calcium in the body is in bones.

Other factors that enhance the absorption of calcium include parathyroid hormone; dietary glucose and lactose; and normal intestinal motility (flow). Factors limiting calcium absorption include large amounts of phytic acid in dietary fiber from wheat bran; excessive amounts of dietary phosphorus; polyphenols (tannins) in tea; a vitamin D deficiency; and diarrhea.

Transport, Storage, and Excretion. Each cell has a critical need for calcium. This is probably the reason humans have such excellent hormonal systems to control blood calcium. Normal blood calcium can be maintained despite an inadequate calcium intake, as much is stored in bones. (The bones, however, pay the price.) This makes blood calcium a poor measure of calcium status.[6]

As discussed in Chapter 9, when blood calcium falls, the parathyroid gland releases parathyroid hormone. This hormone, working with $1,25 (OH)_2$ vitamin D, increases the kidneys' retrieval of calcium before it is excreted in the urine (review Fig. 9-9 in Chapter 9). Parathyroid hormone also helps increase calcium absorption indirectly by increasing the synthesis of $1,25 (OH)_2$ D. In addition, parathyroid hormone, often working in conjunction with $1,25 (OH)_2$ vitamin D, causes increased calcium release from bones by stimulating the activity of osteoclasts (bone-resorbing cells). In all these ways, then, parathyroid hormone increases blood calcium.

When blood calcium is too high, the release of parathyroid hormone falls. Then calcium loss from the kidneys increases. Synthesis of $1,25 (OH)_2$ D also decreases; thus, calcium absorption decreases. In addition, the thyroid gland secretes the hormone calcitonin, which decreases calcium loss from bones. All these metabolic changes cause blood calcium to remain within the normal range.

Other routes for calcium loss include the skin and the feces losses that result from intestinal secretions into the intestinal lumen.

Functions of Calcium

Forming and maintaining bones are calcium's major roles in the body.

Bone Development and Maintenance. Despite its "dead" appearance, bone is very active metabolically. Bone contains two types of cells—osteoblasts and osteoclasts—which are integral to maintaining bones. As covered in Chapter 3, osteoblasts secrete a collagen protein matrix, which forms the support structure of bone. They mature to osteocytes and then secrete bone mineral, which causes bone mineralization. This mineral matures and eventually approaches the composition of $Ca_{10}(PO_4)_6OH_2$, called hydroxyapatite. In contrast, osteoclasts continually break down bone in areas where bone is not needed. Osteoclast activity is stimulated by parathyroid hormone, often in conjunction with $1,25 (OH)_2$ D. These bone cells are very active when a diet is deficient in calcium; their action releases calcium from the bone so it can enter the blood. Remember, a supply of calcium is vital to all cells, not just to bone cells.[22]

Recall also from Chapter 3 that bone turnover (**bone remodeling**) is a cycle of bone breakdown by osteoclasts, followed by bone rebuilding by osteoblasts. In this way, bone is re-formed when necessary to respond to the physical demands placed on it. Before new bone can be built, the old bone in that area must be partially broken down.

During human growth, total osteoblast activity exceeds osteoclast activity, so we make more bone than we break down, with more bone being built in areas put under high stress. A right-handed tennis player, for example, builds more bone in that arm than in the left arm. In older years, osteoclast activity generally becomes more dominant. Most bone is built from infancy through the late adolescent years.[1] Small increases in **bone mass** continue between 20 and 30 years of age. Genes control up to 80% of the variation in the peak bone mass ultimately built.

Bone loss begins in midadulthood and increases significantly at menopause in women. By age 65 to 70, the rate of bone loss falls to about the same rate as before menopause. In men, bone loss is slow and steady from around age 30. Overall, this bone loss in both genders progresses without signs or symptom. During their life-

bone remodeling A process by which bone is first resorbed by osteoclasts and then re-formed by osteoblasts. This process allows the body to form bone where needed, such as in areas of high mechanical stress.

bone mass The total mineral substance (such as calcium or phosphorus) in a cross section of bone, generally expressed as grams per centimeter of length. In contrast, bone mineral density is the total mineral content of bone at a specific bone site divided by the width of the bone at that site, generally expressed as grams per cubic centimeter.

times, about one-third to one-half of all women go on to experience fractures associated with low bone mass. This is especially true of women who live beyond age 75. In addition, some women have much more bone than others. They probably built more bone when they were young, so they are able to endure greater bone loss without experiencing more fractures. Actually, the reason for such variations in bone mass and fracture risk in women of any age still needs more research. However, researchers have identified numerous factors—including physical activity and body weight—associated with higher bone mass (Table 11-4). Even more factors are associated with low bone mass: slim figure; family history of hip fracture or osteoporosis; vitamin D receptor activity in the intestine; irregular menstruation; premature menopause; use of certain medications (such as corticosteroids); excess dietary protein and caffeine (which increase calcium loss in the urine); and prolonged bed rest.[31]

Visual observation of the cross sections of a bone reveals two primary bone structural types in the body: cortical (also called compact) bone and trabecular (also called cancellous or spongy) bone. These in turn interact within each bone to form quite an engineering marvel of strength (Fig. 11-8).The entire outer surface of all bones is composed of cortical bone, which is very dense. The shafts of long bones, such as those of the arm, are almost entirely cortical bone. Trabecular bone is found in the ends of the long bones, inside the spinal vertebrae, and inside the flat bones of the pelvis. Trabecular bone forms an internal scaffolding network for a bone. It supports the outer cortical shell of the bone, especially in heavily stressed areas, such as joints.

Bone strength especially depends on a person's bone mineral density (bone mass/bone width). The more densely packed the bone crystals, the stronger the bone structure. Another important element of bone strength is the trabecular bone support network inside a bone (review Fig. 11-8).

Blood Clotting. Calcium ions participate in several reactions in the cascade that leads to the formation of fibrin, the main protein component of a blood clot (review Fig. 9-13 in Chapter 9). For example, the conversion of prothrombin to thrombin requires the calcium ion.

The tooth consists of a hard, yellowish tissue called dentin, which is covered with enamel in the crown and cementum in the root. When dentin and cementum are damaged, they can repair themselves. Damaged enamel cannot be naturally repaired because enamel is a secretion produced before the tooth erupts, and it does not have a blood supply like the other two tissues. To repair broken or damaged enamel requires the skills of a dentist. In contrast, bone is well supplied with blood vessels, so a fracture can be repaired (healed) by the body given time.

TABLE 11-4   Diet and Lifestyle Factors Associated with Bone Status and Related Action Plans to Implement.[1, 4, 16, 23, 30]

Diet and lifestyle factors	Action plans to implement
Adequate diet containing a sufficient amount of protein, calcium, phosphorus, magnesium, potassium, vitamin A, vitamin C, vitamin D, vitamin K, zinc, copper, fluoride, and manganese (and boron ?)	Follow a diet plan such as the Food Guide Pyramid with special emphasis on adequate amounts of fruits and vegetables. Consider use of fortified foods (or supplements) to make up for specific nutrient shortfalls, such as vitamin D calcium.
Healthy body weight	Be aware that low body weight (slender figure) increases the risk for low bone mass.
Normal menses	During childbearing years, seek medical advice if menses cease (such as in cases of anorexia nervosa or extreme athletic training). Women at menopause and beyond should consider use of current medical therapies to reduce bone loss linked to the fall in estrogen output.
Weight-bearing physical activity	Peform weight-bearing activity as this contributes to bone maintenance, whereas bed rest and a sedentary lifestyle lead to bone loss. Strength training is especially helpful to bone maintenance.
Excessive intake of protein, phosphorus, sodium, caffeine, wheat bran, and alcohol	Moderate intake of these dietary constituents is recommended. Problems primarily arise if adequate calcium is not consumed. Excessive soft drink consumption is especially discouraged.
Smoking	Since smoking lowers estrogen output in women, smoking cessation is advised.
Use of certain medications, such as corticosteroids	Corticosteroids lead to bone loss, and so medical therapy to counteract the bone loss should be instituted if use is long term.

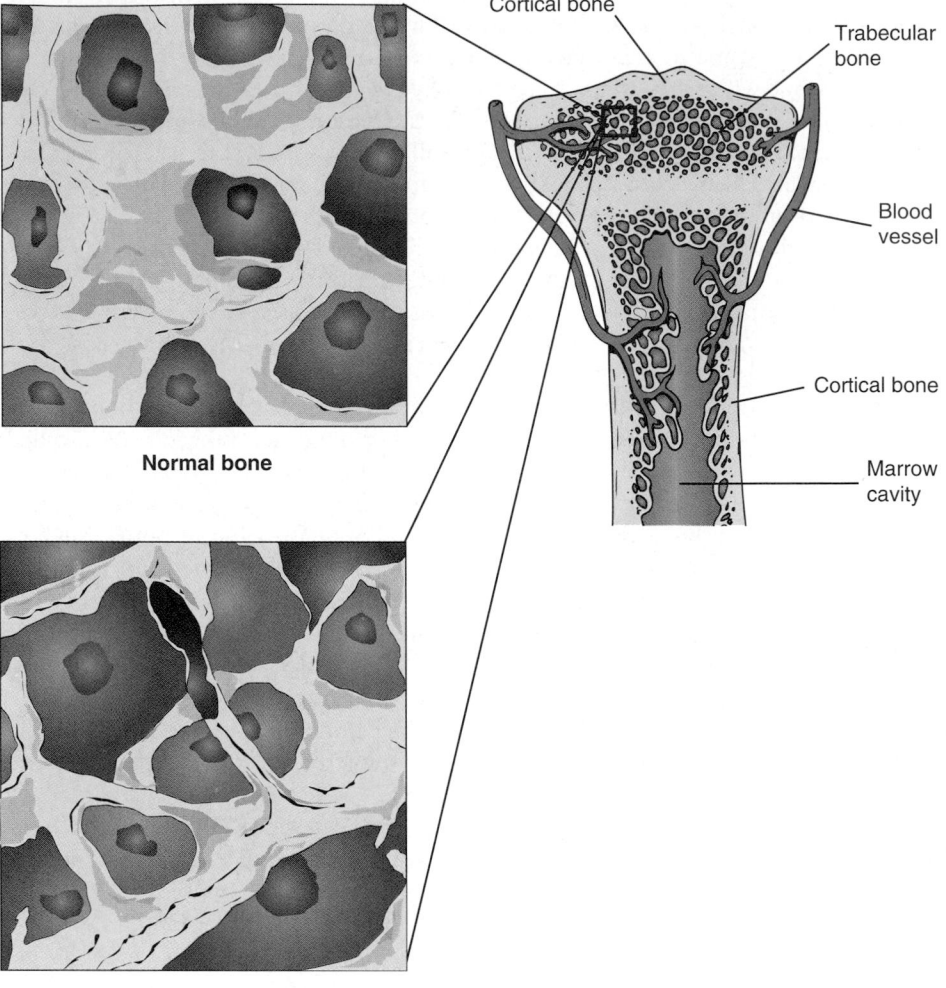

■ FIGURE 11-8 Cortical and trabecular bone. Cortical bone forms the shafts of bones and the outer mineral covering. Trabecular bone supports the outer shell of cortical bone in various bones of the body, as in the bone pictured. Note in the lower picture how there is much less trabecular bone. It is especially critical for the horizontal trabeculae to extend continuously—without breaks—between the areas of vertical trabeculae. Any break in either the horizontal or more vertical trabecular beams weakens the support system of a bone and increases the risk for bone fracture. And, once these beams are broken, there is currently no way to rebuild them. This is why it is so important to limit bone loss as people age.

tetany A body condition marked by sharp contraction of muscles and failure to relax afterward; usually caused by abnormal calcium metabolism.

hypocalcemia Low blood calcium, typically arising from inadequate parathyroid hormone release or action.

Transmission of Nerve Impulses to Target Cells. When a nerve impulse reaches its target site—such as a muscle, other nerve cells, or a gland—the impulse is transmitted across the junction between the nerve and its target cells. In many nerves, the arrival of the impulse at the target site stimulates an influx of calcium ions into the nerve from the extracellular medium. The rise in intracellular calcium ions then triggers the release of neurotransmitters from synaptic vesicles, which are responsible for storing the neurotransmitter until needed. The released neurotransmitter then carries impulses to the target cells (Fig. 11-9).

In an entirely different process, nerve impulses develop spontaneously if insufficient calcium is available, leading to what is called hypocalcemic **tetany.** This condition is characterized by muscle spasms, as the muscles receive continual nerve stimulation. Inadequate parathyroid hormone release or action is the typical cause of **hypocalcemia.**

Muscle Contraction. The critical role of calcium in muscle contraction is most easily understood in the case of skeletal muscles. When a skeletal muscle is stimulated by a nerve impulse from the brain, calcium ions are released from intracellular stores within the muscle cells. The resulting increase in the concentration of calcium ions in a muscle cell is one factor, along with ATP, that permits the contractile proteins actin and myosin to slide into each other. This leads to muscle contraction. Then, to allow for subsequent relaxation, the calcium ions are returned to intracellular stores, and the actin and myosin proteins slide apart (review Fig. 3-4 in Chapter 3).

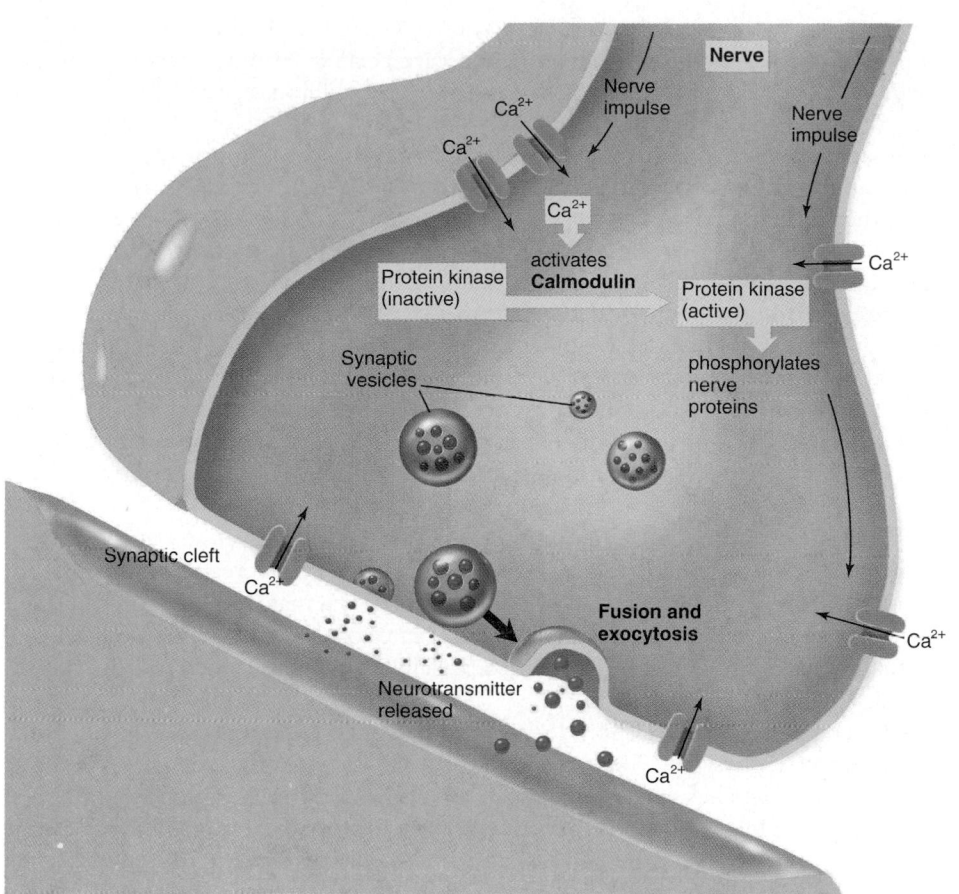

■ FIGURE 11-9 The release of a neurotransmitter. Nerve impulses, by opening Ca^{2+} channels, stimulate the fusion of synaptic vesicles with the cell membrane of the nerve terminals. This leads to exocytosis and the release of a neurotransmitter. The activation of protein kinase (an enzyme that adds a phosphate group to a molecule) by Ca^{2+} may also contribute to this process.

Cell Metabolism. Calcium ions help regulate metabolism in the cell by participating in the **calmodulin** system. When calcium enters a cell (often because of hormone action) and binds to the protein calmodulin, the resulting protein-calcium complex can regulate the activity for various enzymes, including one that breaks down glycogen to many units of glucose 1-phosphate (Fig. 11-10).

Other Attributes of a Diet Rich in Calcium. As discussed in the Nutrition Perspective at the end of this chapter, calcium may contribute to lower blood pressure values in some people. Calcium may also reduce the risk of colon cancer by binding bile acids and free fatty acids in the lumen of the colon; these stimulate colon cells, likely leading to colon cancer. There is also speculation that calcium may reduce the symptoms associated with premenstrual syndrome. A few studies have shown that calcium may even lower blood cholesterol by binding saturated fatty acids in the small intestine, reducing absorption. Finally, in some people, calcium may reduce the risk of kidney stones, but a person should be under medical care if he or she has a history of such stones and wants to experiment with higher calcium intakes. Overall, there are many reasons to meet calcium needs on a regular basis.[22]

Calcium Deficiency

The most common calcium-related disease is osteoporosis. Failure to maintain adequate bone mass in the body eventually leads to a state of **osteopenia.** Osteopenia can be caused by the vitamin D deficiency disease osteomalacia, the use of certain medications, and cancer.[31] If these or similar causes are not present, the diagnosis is osteoporosis, especially when the bone loss is quite marked. People who develop more bone by early adulthood can sustain greater age-related bone loss with less fracture risk than those with who have less bone. Thus, osteoporosis is considered to be a "pediatric disease" with geriatic consequences.

calmodulin A cell protein that binds calcium ions. The resulting calmodulin-Ca^{2+} complex influences the activity of some enzymes in the cell.

osteopenia Decreased bone mass caused by cancer, hyperthyroidism, or other reasons.

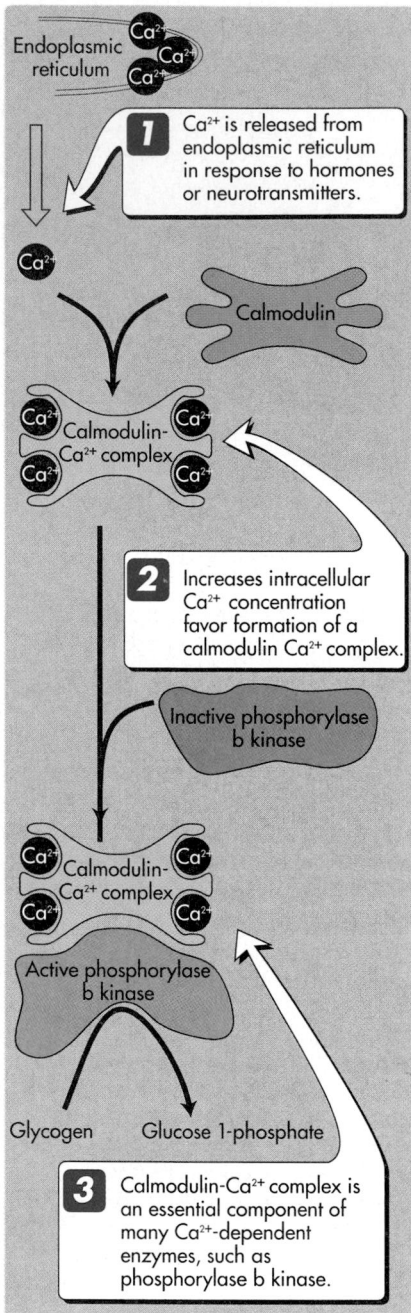

Endoplasmic reticulum Ca²⁺

1 Ca²⁺ is released from endoplasmic reticulum in response to hormones or neurotransmitters.

Ca²⁺

Calmodulin

Ca²⁺ Calmodulin-Ca²⁺ complex Ca²⁺

2 Increases intracellular Ca²⁺ concentration favor formation of a calmodulin Ca²⁺ complex.

Inactive phosphorylase b kinase

Ca²⁺ Calmodulin-Ca²⁺ complex Ca²⁺

Active phosphorylase b kinase

Glycogen   Glucose 1-phosphate

3 Calmodulin-Ca²⁺ complex is an essential component of many Ca²⁺-dependent enzymes, such as phosphorylase b kinase.

▌ FIGURE 11-10 Calmodulin mediates many of the effects of intracellular calcium—in this case, the regulation of the break down of glycogen to many units of glucose 1-phosphate.

Osteoporosis currently leads to approximately 1.5 million fractures per year, resulting in over $14 billion in direct health-care costs.[21] About 10 million women have osteoporosis in the United States, and about 18 million other women show low values for bone mass.[18]

As women mature, different strategies for preventing osteoporosis are needed, based on the risk factors present.[16] Young women should meet calcium, vitamin D, and other nutrient needs, as well as see a physician with any sign of irregular menstruation. In young women, regular menstruation is a main contributor to bone maintenance, as evidenced by low bone mass in some nonmenstruating female athletes and other women with irregular menstruation (e.g., anorexia nervosa). An active lifestyle that includes weight-bearing physical activity is also important (to build and maintain muscle mass). Greater muscle mass linked to physical activity is associated with greater bone mass, as muscle keeps tension on bone.[1] Still, physical activity cannot prevent the bone loss associated with irregular menstruation. Thus, female athletes with irregular menstruation should be closely monitored by a physician.

Smoking and excessive alcohol intake decrease bone mass at any age. Smoking lowers the estrogen concentration in the blood in women, increasing bone loss. Alcohol is toxic to bone cells, and alcoholism is probably a major undiagnosed and unrecognized cause of osteoporosis. Moderation in phosphorus, caffeine, sodium, and protein intake is also advised. These are especially problematic when insufficient calcium is consumed.[8]

At menopause, women should discuss estrogen replacement and other related therapies with a physician. They also need to accurately track their height. A decrease of more than 1½ inches from premenopausal values is a sign that significant bone loss is taking place (Fig. 11-11). Currently, there are four medical therapies that can be used to slow bone loss at menopause in women.[2] Some can even be used in men who develop low bone mass. The approved drugs are estrogen (various forms are available; some contain added progestins); bisphosphonates (alendronate [Fosamax]), selective estrogen receptor modulators (SERMs) (raloxifene [Evista]); and calcitonin (nasal form is Miacalcin).[2] Estrogen and SERMs blunt bone turnover by binding to receptors on bone; bisphophonates blunt bone resorption by binding to bone mineral; and calcitonon inhibits osteoclast activity and, so, bone resorption. All these medications have side effects, so use needs to be tailored to a person's current health status (see the Expert Opinion by Dr. Rebecca Jackson). Any use of these medications also benefits from meeting calcium and vitamin D needs.[23]

Older men and women need to stay physically active—including some weight-bearing and resistance activities—and they should meet the Adequate Intake for calcium set for their particular age. This physical activity and calcium intake are most likely to limit bone loss in some areas of the body, such as the hip. Older people also need to minimize the risk for falls, especially by limiting their use of medications and alcohol, which might disturb coordination, and they should take corrective measures if visual function is impaired. Regular sun exposure and the consumption of food sources of vitamin D are very important. Supplements containing about 10 to 20 μg (400 to 800 IU) are also appropriate (see Chapter 9). To find out more about osteoporosis, check out the web site of the National Osteoporosis Foundation (http://www.nof.org) or call (800) 464-6700. Another helpful web site is that of the National Dairy Council (http://www.nationaldairycouncil.org).

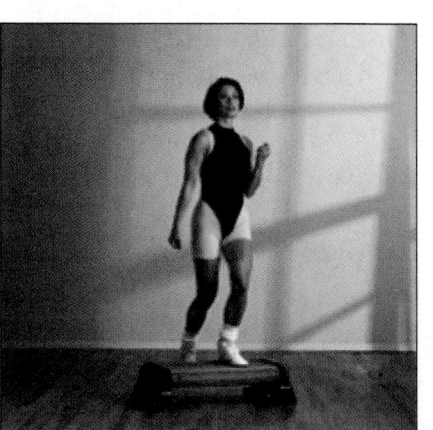

Regular moderate physical activity contributes to bone health.

Calcium in Foods

Dairy products, such as milk and cheese, provide about 75% of the calcium in American diets. The exception is cottage cheese, because most calcium is lost during production. White bread, rolls, crackers, and other foods made with milk products are secondary contributors. Foods with the highest nutrient density of calcium are leafy greens (such as spinach), broccoli, nonfat milk, romano cheese, Swiss cheese, sardines, and canned salmon. However, much of the calcium in some leafy green vegetables, notably spinach, is not absorbed because of the presence of oxalic acid. This effect is not as significant, however, in kale, collard, turnip, and mustard greens. Overall, nonfat milk is the most nutrient-dense source of calcium because of its high bioavailability and low energy value, with some of the vegetables just noted following close behind (Fig. 11-12). The calcium-fortified versions of orange juice, cranberry juice, and other beverages, as well as calcium-fortified cottage cheese, yogurt, breakfast cereals, breakfast bars, bread, chocolate candies, and snacks also provide almost as much calcium as milk. Another source of calcium is soybean curd (tofu), if it is made with calcium carbonate (check the label). Note that it is the bones in canned fish, such as salmon and sardines, that supply the calcium.

One reason the Food Guide Pyramid contains a milk, yogurt, and cheese group is to supply calcium to the diet.[22] People who do not like milk can use products made with milk, such as chocolate milk, yogurt, cheese, and ice cream. All forms of milk, yogurt, and cheese allow about the same degree of calcium absorption. Information about calcium is mandatory on food labels.

Calcium Supplements

Calcium supplements can be used by people who don't like milk or who can't incorporate enough milk products or calcium-fortified foods into their diet. Calcium carbonate, the form found in calcium-containing antacids, has the highest

Research is also ongoing in the area of phytoestrogens, plant compounds that have hormonelike effects in the body. Phytoestrogens can come in the form of isoflavones from soy products or lignans from grains (flaxseed), fruits, and vegetables. It is hoped that these phytoestrogens will act like synthetic estrogen therapy, such as in bone and heart protection. If soy is used to help reduce bone loss, intakes of about 40 g/day of soy protein is needed. Experts currently do not recommend the use of soy isoflavone supplements.[3] More information is needed to discover the full potential of these food-borne substances.

Food Sources of Calcium

Food Item and Amount	Calcium (mg)
Parmesan cheese, 2 oz	670
Romano cheese, 2 oz	600
Swiss cheese, 2 oz	550
Low-fat yogurt, 1 cup	450
Milk, 1 cup	300
Buttermilk, 1 cup	280
Cooked spinach, 1 cup	280
Canned sardines, 2 oz	220
Cooked turnip greens, 1 cup	200
Canned salmon (with bone), 3 oz	180

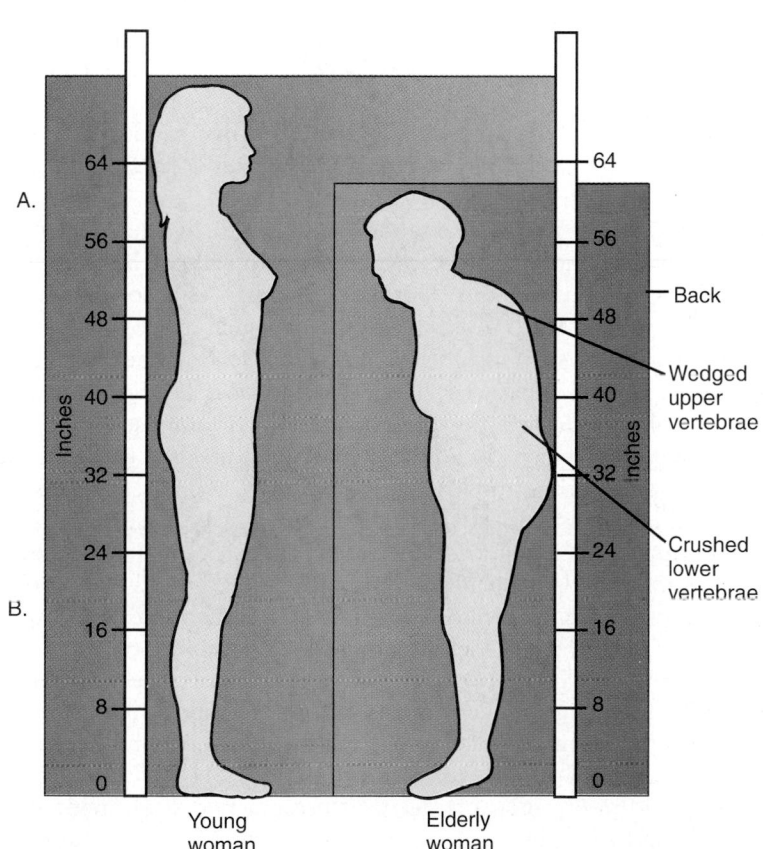

■ FIGURE 11-11 A loss of height and a distorted body shape are common signs of osteoporosis. Monitor your adult height changes to detect early osteoporosis. All women 65 years and older should be screened for this disease. Medicare covers the cost of the needed DEXA (dual energy, x-ray absorptiometry) bone scan. It measures bone mass and bone density in the spine, hip, and total body, using a small amount of x-ray radiation. The ability of a bone to block the path of the radiation is used as a measure of bone mass and bone density at that bone site. Younger women are advised to have the same test at menopause if they have associated risk factors or if the results of the screening would help them decide what treatment plan is appropriate. A less accurate measure uses ultrasound evaluation of the foot.[27]

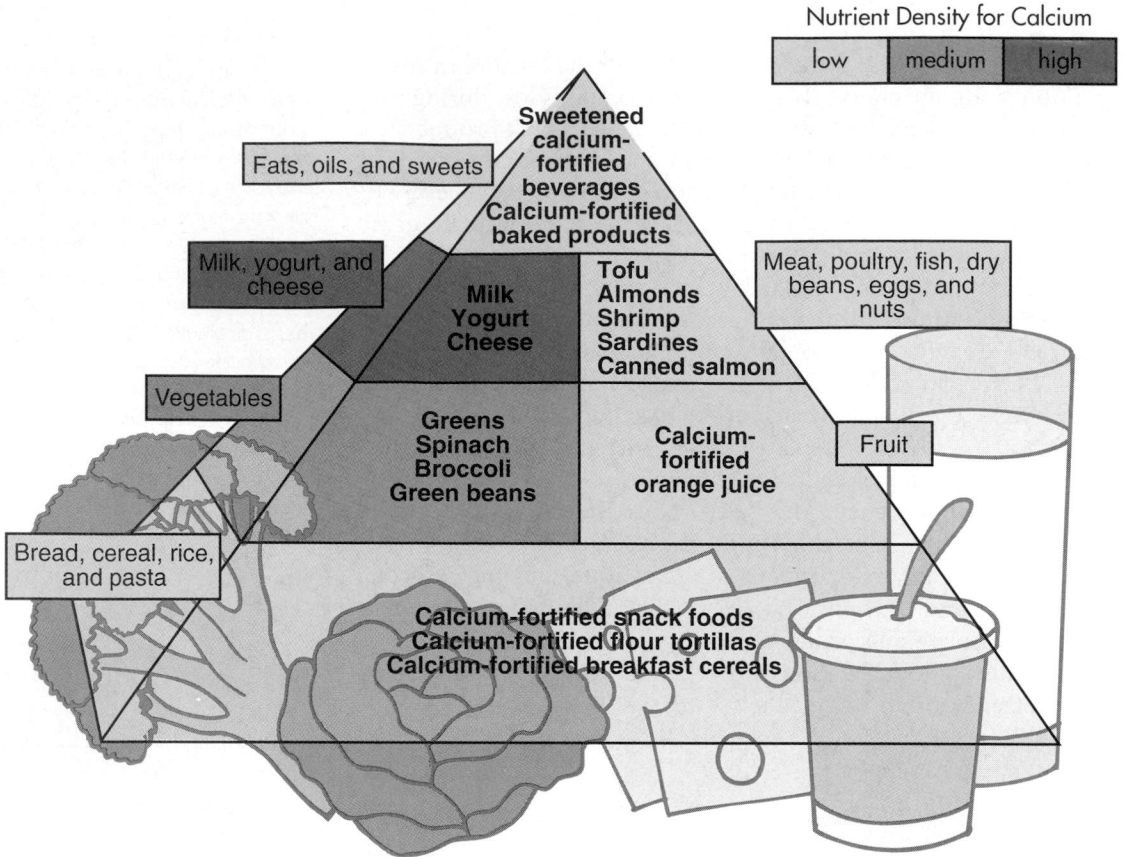

Nutrient Density for Calcium

| low | medium | high |

FIGURE 11-12 Food sources of calcium from the Food Guide Pyramid. The milk, yogurt, and cheese group includes the best dietary sources of this nutrient. The background color of each food group indicates the average nutrient density for calcium in that group. Additional calcium-fortified foods appear in stores each year and, thus, add to the food sources currently listed for various groups.

CRITICAL THINKING

Manuela is a vegan. She stopped eating meat and dairy products when she was 12 years old and is now in her midtwenties. She wants to start a family but is concerned about whether she can obtain enough calcium from her diet to ensure her baby's health. She is also concerned that she may be at risk for osteoporosis. How can she consume enough calcium to meet her own and her baby's needs?

Some calcium supplements are poorly digested, because they do not readily dissolve. To test for solubility, put a supplement in 6 oz of cider vinegar. Stir every 5 minutes. It should dissolve within 30 minutes.

concentration of calcium by weight (40%). Calcium citrate has 21% calcium, and calcium phosphate has 8% calcium by weight. Other forms of calcium in supplements include calcium gluconate and calcium lactate.

Calcium carbonate is the most common supplement used. People with ample output of gastric acid should generally take this supplement between meals or at bedtime in doses of about 500 mg. This practice enhances absorption and limits its negative impact on absorption of other minerals, such as iron. People with low gastric acid production, such as older persons, should take the calcium carbonate supplement with meals, so that what little acid is produced during digestion can aid absorption. People with low gastric acid production also can use a supplement containing calcium citrate, which is acidic itself, between meals. The lower percentage of calcium in calcium citrate, however, requires using a greater number or size of pills or consuming it in a tablet form that is designed to be dissolved first in water.

Some calcium supplements pose a risk for lead toxicity. Currently, FDA has no standards for lead in food supplements, but in the future it does plan to regulate the lead content of supplements, including calcium. Until then, it is important to avoid bonemeal, the worst offender when it comes to lead. Tablet or liquid calcium supplements with the USP (United States Pharmacopeia) seal of approval are less likely than others to contain high concentrations of lead or other contaminants.

Overall, taking 1000 mg of calcium daily in divided doses of 500 mg each in the form of calcium carbonate or calcium citrate is probably safe, but people using a supplement should notify their physician of the practice. Still, many people have difficulty adhering to a supplement regimen. In contrast, regular food habits can be integrated easily into a routine. In addition, it is difficult to consume an excess amount of calcium in foods. All this points to focusing first on improving diet when addressing calcium needs.[22]

Calcium Needs

The Adequate Intake for calcium for adults ranges from 1000 to 1200 mg/day. For adolescents between the ages of 9 and 18, the Adequate Intake is set higher at 1300 mg/day to contribute to building a higher bone mass.[4] The Adequate Intake for adults is based on the amount of calcium needed each day to offset calcium losses in urine, feces and other routes.[6] The Adequate Intake for young people includes an additional amount to allow for increases in bone mass during growth and development.

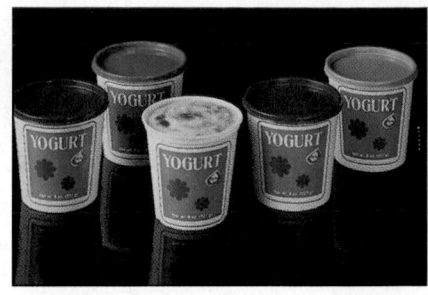

Dairy products, such as yogurt, are common sources of calcium in the American diet.

North Americans at Risk for a Calcium Deficiency

In the United States, average calcium intakes range from approximately 600 to 800 mg/day for women and 800 to 1000 mg/day for men About 25% of women consume only about 300 mg/day.[22] Thus, dietary intakes of calcium by many women, especially young women, are well below the Adequate Intake amount, whereas intakes by most men are roughly equivalent to it. The greater food consumption by men, to support their higher energy outputs, accounts for part of the difference. An easy way for women to increase calcium intake is to increase their physical activity and, in turn, their food consumption. It is very important for vegetarians to focus on eating good plant sources of calcium as well as on the total amount of calcium ingested. Those at highest risk for inadequate calcium intake are adolescents and older adults.

Calcium Toxicity

Normally, the small intestine prevents excess calcium from being absorbed. If, at this level of control, the system breaks down, the calcium concentration in the blood may rise and lead to calcification of the kidneys and other organs, irritability, headache, kidney failure, kidney stones in some people, possibly prostate cancer, and decreased absorption of other minerals.[6] Ordinarily, calcium in food does not pose a health threat because it is present in relatively modest amounts. Calcium toxicity is reported to occur only among individuals using excessive amount of supplemental calcium. The Upper Level for calcium is 2500 mg/day, based on the risk of developing kidney stones.

CASE SCENARIO Follow-Up

Jana is increasing her chances of developing osteoporosis later in life because of her current high-risk lifestyle. Many factors contributing to her potential risk include physical inactivity, smoking, and poor dietary intake of calcium and other important minerals. If Jana remains a vegan, she especially needs to find some reliable sources of calcium. These could include calcium-fortified juices, calcium-fortified bread and snack bars, and calcium-fortified chocolate candies. Tofu (made with calcium) is another potential source, as well as calcium-fortified soy milk. Meeting the Adequate Intake of 1300 mg/day for her age would not be that hard if she were to make a conscious effort to use these calcium-rich foods and/or find other rich sources.

CONCEPT CHECK

About 99% of calcium in the body is found in the bones. Calcium requires a slightly acid pH and the vitamin D hormone for efficient absorption. Factors that reduce calcium absorption include large amounts of dietary fiber (especially wheat bran), decreased estrogen production, and a great excess of phosphorus in the diet. Blood calcium is regulated primarily by hormones and does not closely reflect daily intake. Aside from its critical role in bone, calcium also functions in blood clotting, muscle contraction, nerve-impulse transmission, and cell metabolism. A person can decrease risk for osteoporosis by consuming adequate calcium and vitamin D; exercising, (weight-bearing exercise); considering estrogen replacement or other medications that decrease bone loss, if a postmenopausal female; and moderating sodium, alcohol, and caffeine intake. Dairy products are rich food sources of calcium. Certain calcium-fortified foods, such as beverages, are rich sources as well. Supplemental forms, such as calcium carbonate, are well absorbed by most people. However, overzealous supplementation can result in the development of kidney stones and other health problems.

To estimate your calcium intake, use the rule of 300s. Give yourself 300 mg for calcium provided by a typical diet of moderate energy intake. Add to that another 300 mg for every 8 oz of milk or yogurt or 1.5 ounces of cheese. If you eat a lot of tofu, almonds, or sardines or drink calcium-fortified beverages, use Table 11-5 or food consumption tables to obtain a more accurate account of your calcium intake.

ASSESSING THE RISKS AND BENEFITS OF ESTROGEN REPLACEMENT THERAPY

Rebecca D. Jackson, M.D.

Menopause (a women's final menstrual period) is a major change in a woman's life. The hallmark of menopause is the reduction in estrogen secretion by the ovaries that predisposes a woman to a number of health concerns. In the United States, the average age at menopause is approximately 51 years, and, by the age of 55, more than 90% of women have experienced menopause. In the next two decades, nearly 40 million American women will become menopausal. Although the age at menopause has remained relatively constant for years, the life expectancy of women has increased by more than 20 years over the past decade. Thus, a woman is now expected to spend nearly one-third of her life in postmenopause. Estrogen replacement therapy (ERT) has been shown to alleviate some symptoms and potentially prevent several diseases in the aging woman. However, making an informed decision regarding the benefits and risks of ERT is a complex and often confusing health decision for the postmenopausal woman, and new alternatives to ERT offer options to reduce some of the health risks or symptoms of menopause for some women.

Menopause may be associated with symptoms that affect the quality of life of women. Up to 90% of women experience hot flashes, sweats, mild mood depression, irritability, anxiety, or sleep disturbances. These can range from a minor inconvenience to intense discomfort. Vaginal dryness, bladder irritability, and incontinence are also common. It is well accepted that the short-term use of ERT around the time of menopause can alleviate the symptoms experienced during the menopause transition and is the most universally agreed upon use for estrogen replacement. What remains more controversial is the role of long-term use of ERT for the prevention of the diseases of advancing age.

Osteoporosis is a systemic skeletal disease defined as a reduction in bone mass associated with an impairment in bone architecture (structure), leading to an increased risk for fracture. It has been estimated that more than 25 million postmenopausal women have low bone mass or osteoporosis. Osteoporosis results in 1.5 million fractures per year, including almost 300,000 hip fractures. One in two white women will suffer an osteoporotic fracture at some time in her lifetime. Women are predisposed to the development of osteoporosis, in part due to rapid rates of bone loss during the menopause transition. ERT is effective at maintaining bone mass at both cortical (compact) and trabecular (cancellous) skeletal sites in 90% of female patients. Prospective clinical trials have confirmed that ERT is effective in reducing spine fractures. Epidemiological data also suggest that ERT reduces hip fracture by 50%, but no prospective studies have confirmed this observation. The benefits of ERT on bone mass require continued use of estrogen: When ERT is discontinued, bone loss rapidly recurs at a rate more rapidly than normally predicted for a woman at that particular age. Within 10 years after discontinuation, the benefits of ERT use for the prevention and treatment of osteoporosis are no longer apparent.

Estrogen may also play a role in the prevention of cardiovascular disease (CVD). This is the leading cause of death in women, accounting for 45% of total mortality. The prevalence of CVD is markedly lower in women than men under the age of 50, but, within 10 years after menopause, the incidence of and complications from CVD in women dramatically rise. ERT may impact favorably on mechanisms that contribute to an increased risk for CVD. ERT has been shown to favorably reduce total-cholesterol and LDL-cholesterol by 10 to 15% and increase HDL-cholesterol. However, it also increases triglycerides, an independent risk factor for CVD in women. It lowers homocysteine and significantly decreases lipoprotein(a), two other factors that contribute to CVD risk. It may substantially decrease the formation of the atherosclerotic lesions by reducing the overgrowth of muscle and endothelium layers in the blood vessels in response to injury in the arterial wall. ERT may reduce the risk for a heart attack by lowering the ability to form thrombus (clot) at an atherosclerotic lesion. Finally, it can improve blood flow by decreasing blood vessel constriction.

Observational studies have shown a 35 to 50% reduction of fatal and nonfatal heart attacks with ERT use in postmenopausal women. The greatest benefit in these observational studies appears to be in women with pre-existing heart disease. However, the Heart and Estrogen-progestin Replacement Study, a recent randomized clinical trial of the effect of ERT (with progestin) in postmenopausal women with pre-existing CVD, showed no benefit of ERT in reducing the number of heart attacks. In fact, this study suggested that the initiation of ERT results in an early increase in the number of heart attacks during the first year of treatment. More recently, this finding of an early increase in risk for CVD events was also extended to women with no prior history of heart disease. Thus, the long-term impact of ERT in preventing or reducing CVD is not yet known.

ERT may also reduce the risk for a number of other diseases that affect older women. Alzheimer's disease (AD) is the most common cause of dementia in older people, and women are 1.5- to 3-fold more likely than men to develop AD. Studies have shown that women who use ERT have a 50% reduction in the risk for dementia, compared with nonusers. A number of plausible mechanisms support a possible beneficial effect of ERT on memory, but further study is needed. A large case-control study also has suggested that ERT use is associated with a 75% decrease in the risk for macular degeneration, an age-related cause of loss of vision and blindness experienced by many women. Recent studies also suggest a possible impact on colorectal cancer incidence, the third leading cause of cancer in women.

The use of any medication can be associated with some adverse effects, [and the potential risks of ERT have clearly] had an impact on a woman's decision to use this treatment. The use of estrogen alone in a woman who has not undergone a hysterectomy (surgical removal of the uterus) stimulates growth of the endometrium (the lining of the uterus). If this overgrowth continues, endometrial hyperplasia develops, which can later lead to uterine cancer. The addition of a progestin (synthetic form of progesterone) to the ERT to counteract this effect completely blocks this risk, and combined estrogen-progestin is now the drug regime of choice for women who have not had a hysterectomy. This progestin, however, may reduce any lipid benefits, and thus the potential degree of CVD benefit with ERT. There are insufficient data to know the impact this addition of progestin may have on other potential benefits of ERT.

ERT may be associated with a number of symptoms, including breast tenderness, bloating, and headache in 5 to 10% of women. Most symptoms are mild and do not require the discontinuation of ERT. ERT also increases the risk of blood clots in the legs or lungs and gallbladder disease. The greatest concern of women regarding ERT is the controversy surrounding the relationship of ERT to breast cancer. Some studies have shown an increased risk for breast cancer with estrogen use, whereas others have not. Overall, statistical analysis of all these studies would suggest that the risk increases with long duration of use. There is no excess risk with less than 5 years of use, increasing to a 36% excess risk after 10 or more years. However, mortality studies have shown a lower mortality for tumors that developed while women were taking ERT. The impact of progestin on breast cancer risk remains an issue of intense debate.

In summary, ERT clearly alleviates the symptoms associated with estrogen deficiency. In addition, there are many plausible mechanisms to suggest that the long-term use of ERT may reduce the relative risk for osteoporotic fracture, CVD, and cognitive changes with aging in postmenopausal women. Their promise however, awaits confirmation by the results of prospective, randomized, controlled clinical trials addressing the primary and secondary prevention of these diseases and the relative risks of long-term use, particularly in regard to the risk for breast cancer. Until the results of trials such as the National Institutes of Health-sponsored Women's Health Initiative are known in 2005, a recommendation for the general use of ERT for the prevention and treatment of diseases associated with aging should not be offered.

The options available for women's health, however, do not end at ERT: Women now have alternatives to reduce some of the symptoms and health risks associated with menopause. Plant-based estrogens, such as soy and black cohash, have been shown to reduce the symptoms of menopause and reduce total-cholesterol and LDL-cholesterol without any evidence of increased risk for breast cancer. A new class of drugs, the selective estrogen receptor modulators (SERMs), act as estrogen-like compounds at some tissues (e.g., the heart and bone) and as estrogen antagonists at other sites (uterus and breast). The first of these drugs, raloxifene, is similar to ERT in that it is effective at preventing bone loss at the spine and hip, reducing the incidence of spine fractures in women with osteoporosis and reducing the total-cholesterol and LDL-cholesterol (although it does not increase HDL). However, unlike ERT, it will not reduce the symptoms of menopause, but it will also not stimulate the uterine lining or breast tissue, thus reducing the potential risk for endometrial and breast cancer that may occur with ERT. There are preliminary data to suggest that raloxifene might also play a role in the prevention of breast cancer in women at high risk. The use of other specific drugs to reduce the risk for osteoporosis (such as the bisphosphonates and calcitonin for prevention of hip fracture) or to improve lipid levels to reduce the risk for CVD (statins, niacin, or bile acid sequestrants) is also an option for certain women. Finally, lifestyle changes, including modifications of diet, exercise, and smoking cessation, can impact a woman's risk for disease.

Thus, the decision to initiate treatment for each woman in menopause should reflect a careful analysis of her risk factors for diseases that might be amenable to estrogen or estrogen-progestin replacement therapy or one of the many alternative treatment strategies. Today, by individualizing therapy directed at each women's health profile, we can provide women with the best alternatives as they age.

Dr. Jackson is an associate professor of internal medicine and physical medicine at The Ohio State University. She is a principal investigator at the OSU Clinical Center of the Women's Health Initiative Clinical Trial and Observational Study.

T A B L E 11-5   A Tool for Estimating Current Calcium Intake

For all of the following foods, write the number of servings eaten in a day. Total the number of servings in each category and then multiply the totals by the milligrams of calcium for each category. Finally, add the total milligrams to estimate calcium intake for that day.

Food	Serving Size	Number of Servings	Calcium (mg)	Total Calcium (mg)
Plain low-fat yogurt	1 cup	_____		
Nonfat dry milk powder	½ cup	_____		
	Total servings	_____	× 400	= _____ mg
Canned sardines (with bones)	3 oz	_____		
Fruit flavored yogurt	1 cup	_____		
Skim or low-fat milk, buttermilk	1 cup	_____		
Whole milk, chocolate milk	1 cup	_____		
Parmesan cheese (grated)	¼ cup	_____		
Swiss cheese	1 oz	_____		
	Total servings	_____	× 300	= _____ mg
Cheese (all other hard cheese)	1 oz	_____		
Pancakes	3	_____		
	Total servings	_____	× 200	= _____ mg
Canned pink salmon	3 oz	_____		
Tofu (processed with calcium)	4 oz	_____		
	Total servings	_____	× 150	= _____ mg
Collards or turnip greens, cooked	½ cup	_____		
Ice cream or ice milk	½ cup	_____		
Almonds	1 oz	_____		
	Total servings	_____	× 75	= _____ mg
Chard, cooked	½ cup	_____		
Cottage cheese	½ cup	_____		
Corn tortilla	1 med	_____		
Orange	1 med	_____		
	Total servings	_____	× 50	= _____ mg
Kidney, lima, or navy beans, cooked	½ cup	_____		
Broccoli	½ cup	_____		
Carrot, raw	1 med	_____		
Dates or raisins	¼ cup	_____		
Egg	1 large	_____		
Whole-wheat bread	1 slice	_____		
Peanut butter	2 tbsp	_____		
	Total servings	_____	× 25	= _____ mg
Calcium-fortified orange juice	6 oz	_____		
Calcium-fortified snack bars	1 each	_____		
Calcium-fortified breakfast bars	½ bar	_____		
	Total servings	_____	× 200	= _____ mg
Calcium supplements	1 each	_____	× 500	= _____ mg
		Total calcium intake		= _____ mg

Other calcium sources to consider include many breakfast cereals (100 to 250 mg per cup) and some vitamins/mineral supplements (up to 500 mg per tablet).

Reprinted with permission from *Topics in Clinical Nutrition*, "Putting Calcium into Perspective for Your Clients," G. Wardlaw and N. Weese; 11:1, p. 29. © 1995 Aspen Publishers, Inc.

■ PHOSPHORUS (P)

Efficient absorption plus the wide availability in food makes phosphorus a much less important major mineral than calcium in diet planning.

Absorption and Excretion of Phosphorus

The body absorbs phosphorus quite efficiently, up to about 70% of dietary intake in adults and 90% of dietary intake in infants and children. The active vitamin D hormone 1,25 $(OH)_2$ D enhances phosphorus absorption, as it does for calcium, but most absorption occurs by passive absorption based on the phosphorus concentration in the lumen of the small intestine and colon. Excretion of phosphorus is achieved via the kidneys.[6]

Urinary loss of phosphorus increases as blood phosphorus concentration increases. This kidney excretion is the primary mechanism by which blood phosphorus is regulated. This mechanism differs from that of calcium, in which changes in absorption are a more significant factor.

Functions of Phosphorus and the Effects of a Deficiency

Phosphorus plays many roles in the body. It is one of the most essential elements and is found in abundance in body tissues. Approximately 80% is found in bones and teeth in the form of calcium phosphate. The remainder of phosphate is found in every cell in the body and in the extracellular fluid, as PO_4^{3-}. It is a component of many enzyme systems, adenosine triphosphate (ATP), DNA and RNA, and the phospholipids in cell membranes. It also participates in acid-base balance.

A chronic deficiency of phosphorus can contribute to bone loss, decreased growth, and poor tooth development. Symptoms of rickets may occur in phosphorus-deficient children. Furthermore, symptoms of a deficiency include anorexia, weight loss, weakness, irritability, stiff joints, and bone pain.[6]

Phosphorus in Foods

Milk, cheese, yogurt, bakery products, and meat provide most of the phosphorus in the adult diet. Cereals, bran, eggs, nuts, and fish are also good sources. About 20 to 30% of dietary phosphorus comes from food additives, especially in baked goods, cheeses, processed meats, and many soft drinks (about 75 mg per 12-oz [⅓ liter] serving of soft drinks). Next time you have a soft drink, look for a listing of phosphoric acid on the label.

Phosphorus Needs

Phosphorus needs are based on the amount that maintains an adequate blood concentration, which corresponds to an Estimated Average Requirement of 580 mg/day for men and women 19 years of age and older. The Estimated Average Requirement is increased by 20% to account for individual variation, resulting in an RDA of 700 mg/day.[6] Adults consume about 1000 to 1600 mg or more of phosphorus per day. Thus, a phosphorus deficiency is unlikely in healthy adults, especially because it is so efficiently absorbed. The Daily Value used for food labeling is 1000 mg.

North Americans at Risk for a Phosphorus Deficiency

Marginal phosphorus status can be found in premature infants, vegans, alcoholics, elderly people on nutrient-poor diets, people experiencing long-term bouts of diarrhea and weight loss, and people who use aluminum-containing antacids daily (in the small intestine these bind to phosphorus).

People who have experienced weight loss and long-standing poor nutrient intake are at risk of low blood phosphorus and a related condition called refeeding syndrome.[13] If these individuals are aggressively refed, such as in a hospital or in a famine relief setting (in the developing world), much of the small amount of phosphorus in the bloodstream shifts into cells in order to participate in essential metabolic pathways. This reduces phosphorus in the blood even further; it can cause blood phosphorus to be so low that respiratory failure and other critical health conditions may result. To avoid this problem, clinicians generally check blood phosphorus before feeding such a person, so as to correct a phosphorus deficiency if present. Under such circumstances, people then are gradually refed and blood phosphorus is monitored to make sure it remains within the normal range.

Food Sources of Phosphorus

Food Item and Amount	Phosphorus (mg)
Sardines, 3 oz	420
Swiss cheese, 2 oz	340
Dried almonds, ½ cup	340
Milk, 8 oz	240
Broiled salmon fillet, 3 oz	220
Roast beef, 3 oz	210
Roasted turkey, 3 oz	180
Roasted chicken, 3 oz	170
American cheese, 1 slice	160
Fried beef liver, 1 oz	130

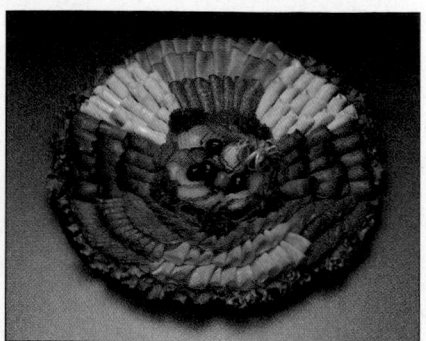

Meats are rich in phosphorus.

Toxicity of Phosphorus

Typical phosphorus intakes in and of themselves do not appear to be toxic for healthy adults, but large amounts can lead to problems in patients with certain kidney diseases. In this case, reduced excretion by the kidneys leads to high blood concentrations, which in turn can cause calcium-phosphorus precipitates to form in body tissues, as well as contribute to bone loss by inducing the release of parathyroid hormone (see Chapter 9 to review the relationship between blood phosphorus and parathyroid hormone).

A chronic imbalance in the calcium-to-phosphorus ratio in the diet, resulting from a high phosphorus intake coupled with a low calcium intake, can also contribute to bone loss. This situation most likely arises when calcium needs are not met, as can occur in adolescents and adults who regularly substitute soft drinks for milk or otherwise underconsume calcium. The Upper Level for phosphorus in adulthood is 3-4 g/day, based on the risk of developing impaired kidney function.[6]

■ MAGNESIUM (MG)

Magnesium, like calcium, is a divalent cation. Because magnesium is found in chlorophyll, green leafy vegetables are rich sources.

Absorption, Transport, Storage, and Excretion of Magnesium

We normally absorb about 40 to 60% of the magnesium in our diets, but absorption efficiency can increase up to about 80% if intakes are low. Both passive and active absorption in the small intestine is used. The active vitamin D hormone 1,25 $(OH)_2$ D enhances magnesium absorption to a limited extent. The kidneys primarily regulate the blood concentration of magnesium and are able to increase magnesium reabsorption from the filtrate when blood magnesium is low. Alcohol increases magnesium loss in the urine. Some magnesium is stored in bones; a small amount is stored in other tissues, such as muscles.

Functions of Magnesium and the Effects of a Deficiency

Magnesium has a vital role in a varying range of biochemical and physiological processes.[28] More than 300 enzyme-catalyzed reactions require magnesium, and many energy-yielding compounds in cells require magnesium to function properly. Magnesium ions bind to ATP to form active ATP. In this form, a magnesium ion bridges between the second and the last phosphate groups on the ATP molecule. Magnesium also contributes to DNA and RNA synthesis during cell proliferation and potassium and calcium metabolism, in turn contributing to bone structure. It is also important for nerve and heart function, as well as insulin release from the pancreas and ultimate insulin action on cells. Other possible benefits of magnesium include decreasing blood pressure, by dilating arteries, and preventing heart rhythm abnormalities.[6]

Animals deficient in magnesium become very irritable and, with severe deficiency, eventually suffer convulsions and often die. In humans a magnesium deficiency causes a rapid heartbeat, sometimes accompanied by weakness, muscle spasms, disorientation, nausea and vomiting, and seizures. Currently, an intravenous dose of magnesium is being investigated as part of the treatment during the early phases of a heart attack. A fall in blood calcium is also seen in magnesium deficiency, as well as resistance to 1,25 $(OH)_2$. It is possible that a chronically deficient intake of magnesium then may increase the risk of osteoporosis. Note that a magnesium deficiency develops very slowly because our bodies store it readily.[28]

Magnesium in Foods

The richest sources of magnesium are plant products, such as whole grains (such as wheat bran), broccoli, squash, green leafy vegetables, beans, nuts, seeds, and chocolate. Animal products, such as milk and meats, supply some magnesium, although less than the foods in the previous list (Fig. 11-13). Another source of magnesium is hard tap water, which contains a high mineral content (hard water also contains calcium). About 45% of dietary magnesium comes from vegetables, fruits, grains, and nuts, whereas about 30% comes from milk, meat, and eggs. Refined foods generally are low in magnesium.

Magnesium Needs

Magnesium needs are based on a daily intake that equals daily losses. This amount corresponds to an Estimated Average Requirement of 330 mg/day for men 19 to 30 years of age and 255 mg/day for women 19 to 30 years of age. The Estimated Average Requirement is increased by 20% to account for individual variation, resulting in an RDA of 400 mg/day for men 19 to 30 years of age and 310 mg/day for women 19 to 30 years of age.[6] Magnesium needs increase slightly (an additional 10 mg/day) beyond this age for men and women. The Daily Value used for food labeling is 400 mg.

Adult men consume an average of 325 mg/day, whereas women consume closer to 225 mg/day. Women particularly should find some good food sources of magnesium that they like and eat them regularly.

Food Sources of Magnesium

Food Item and Amount	Magnesium (mg)
Cooked spinach, 1 cup	130
Baked acorn squash, 1 cup	105
Toasted wheat germ, ¼ cup	90
Tofu (soybean curd), 3 oz	88
Cashews, ¼ cup	85
Cooked blackeyed peas, ½ cup	45
Sunflower seeds, ¼ cup	40
Cooked kidney beans, ½ cup	40
Cooked broccoli, 1 cup	37
Whole-wheat bread, 1 slice	25

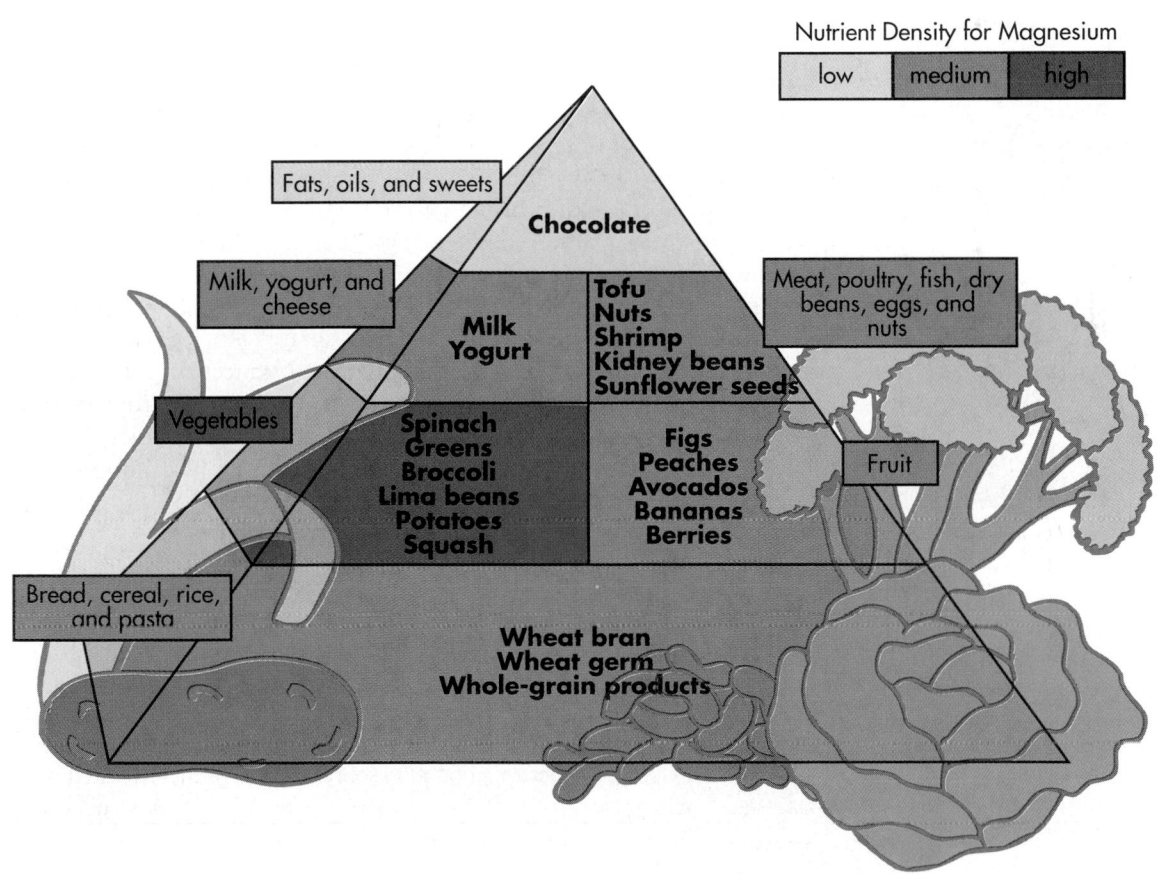

FIGURE 11-13 Food sources of magnesium from the Food Guide Pyramid. The vegetable group and whole-grain choices in the bread, cereal, rice, and pasta group are the best dietary sources of this nutrient. The background color of each food group indicates the average nutrient density for magnesium in that group.

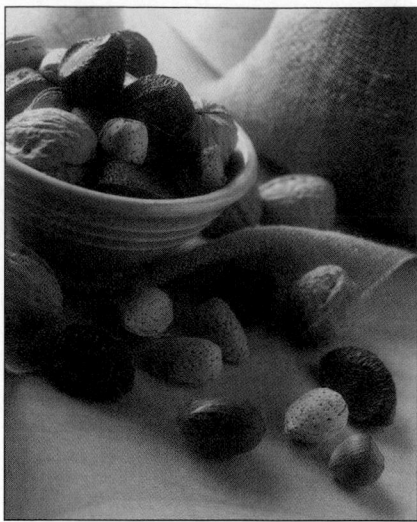

Nuts are a rich source of magnesium.

North Americans at Risk for a Magnesium Deficiency

Poor magnesium status is primarily found among users of certain diuretics, which increase magnesium excretion in the urine. In addition, heavy perspiration for weeks in hot climates and bouts of long-standing diarrhea or vomiting cause significant magnesium loss. Alcoholism also increases the risk of a deficiency because dietary intake may be poor and because, as noted earlier, alcohol increases magnesium excretion in the urine. The disorientation and weakness associated with alcoholism closely resemble the behavior of people with low blood magnesium. People with diabetes may also show poor magnesium status. However, currently there is no test for magnesium deficiency that is both sufficiently accurate and available for use in routine clinical practice.[28]

Toxicity of Magnesium

Magnesium toxicity does not occur in healthy people who eat typical foods. The Upper Level of 350 mg refers to supplement and other nonfood sources only, such as certain laxatives and antacids.[6] Resulting intakes above this amount can lead to diarrhea. Toxicity also can be seen in kidney failure because the kidneys primarily regulate blood magnesium. In this case, high blood magnesium leads to weakness, nausea, slowed breathing, eventual malaise, coma, and death. Older people in general are at particular risk of magnesium toxicity, as kidney function may be compromised.

■ SULFUR (S)

The minerals discussed so far function in the body primarily in the form of charged ions. In contrast, much of the sulfur in the body occurs in nonionic forms as an integral component of organic compounds, such as the vitamins biotin and thiamin. Because the amino acids methionine and cysteine both contain sulfur, it also is present in proteins. Disulfide bridges form when the sulfur atoms in two cysteine residues bind to each other; these bridges stabilize the structure of many protein molecules (see Chapter 7). For example, this is necessary for the formation of collagen, the protein found in connective tissue, and for keratin, which is found in nails, skin, and hair. Ionic forms of sulfur, such as sulfate (SO_4^{2-}), participate in the acid-base balance in the body, are present in many substances found in the extracellular fluid, and play an important role in some drug-detoxifying pathways in the body.

We actually do not need to consume sulfur as such in our diets because proteins supply the sulfur we need. Sulfur is naturally a part of a healthful diet. Sulfur compounds are also used to preserve foods (see Chapter 19).

Table 11-6 provides a summary of the major minerals.

Protein-rich foods supply sulfur in the diet.

*C*heck out the *Perspectives in Nutrition* Online Learning Center http://www.mhhe.com/wardlaw for quizzes, flash cards, other activities, and web links designed to further help you learn about issues surrounding water and the major minerals.

CONCEPT CHECK

*M*agnesium is a mineral found mostly in plants. It is important for nerve and heart function and as an activator for many enzymes. Whole grains (bran portion), vegetables, nuts, seeds, milk, and meats are good food sources. Sulfur is incorporated into certain vitamins and amino acids. Its ability to bond with other sulfur atoms enables it to stabilize protein structure.

TABLE 11-6   A Summary of the Major Minerals

Name	Major Functions	Deficiency Symptoms	People Most at Risk	RDA, Adequate Intake, or Minimum Requirement	Nutrient-Dense Dietary Sources	Results of Toxicity
Sodium	Functions as a major cation of the extracellular fluid; aids nerve impulse transmission; water balance.	Muscle cramps	People who severely restrict sodium to lower blood pressure (250–500 mg/day); excessive sweating	500 mg	Table salt, processed foods, condiments, sauces, soups, chips	Contributes to hypertension in susceptible individuals: leads to increased calcium loss in urine.
Potassium	Functions as a major cation of intracellular fluid; aids nerve impulse transmission; water balance.	Irregular heart beat, loss of appetite, muscle cramps	People who use potassium-wasting diuretics or have poor diets, as seen in poverty and alcoholism	2000 mg	Spinach, squash, bananas, orange juice, other vegetables and fruits, milk, meat, legumes, whole grains	Slowing of the heartbeat, as seen in kidney failure.
Chloride	Functions as a major anion of the extracellular fluid; participates in acid production in stomach; aids nerve transmission; water balance.	Convulsions in infants	No one	750 mg	Table salt, some vegetables, processed foods	Linked to hypertension in susceptible people when combined with sodium.
Calcium	Provides bone and tooth structure, blood clotting; aids nerve-impulse transmission; required for muscle contractions; contributes to cell permeability.	Increases the risk for osteoporosis.	Women, especially those who consume few dairy products	1000-1200 mg (age > 18 years) 1300 mg (age 9-18 years)	Dairy products, canned fish, leafy vegetables, tofu, fortified orange juice (and other fortified foods)	Intakes > 2.5 g/day (Upper Level) may cause kidney stones and other problems in susceptible people; poor mineral absorption in general.
Phosphorus	Required for bone and tooth strength; serves as part of various metabolic compounds; functions as major ion of intracellular fluid, acid-base balance.	Probably none; poor bone maintenance is a possibility.	Older people consuming very-nutrient-poor diets; possibly vegans and people with alcoholism	700 mg (age > 18 years) 1250 mg (age 9-18 years)	Dairy products, processed foods, fish, soft drinks, bakery products, meats	Impairs bone health in people with kidney failure; results in poor bone mineralization if calcium intakes are low. Upper Level is 3–4 g/day.
Magnesium	Provides bone strength; aids enzyme function; aids nerve and heart function.	Weakness, muscle pain, poor heart function	Women and patients on thiazide diuretics	Men: 420 mg Women: 350 mg	Wheat bran, green vegetables, nuts, chocolate, legumes	Causes diarrhea, as well as weakness in people with kidney failure. Upper Level of 350 mg/day refers to supplements only.
Sulfur	Comprises part of vitamins and amino acids; aids drug detoxification; participates in acid-base balance.	None have been described.	No one, as long as protein needs are met	None	Protein foods	None are likely.

■ SUMMARY

1. Water constitutes 50 to 70% of the human body. Its unique chemical properties enable it to dissolve substances as well as serve as a medium for chemical reactions, temperature regulation, and lubrication. Water also helps regulate the acid-base balance in the body. For adults, daily water needs are estimated at 1 ml/kcal expended.

2. Many minerals are vital for sustaining life. For humans, animal products are the most bioavailable sources of most minerals. Supplements of minerals exceeding the Upper Level should be taken only under a physician's supervision because toxicity and nutrient interactions are a likely possibility.

3. Sodium, the major positive ion (cation) found outside cells, is vital in fluid balance and nerve impulse transmission. The American diet provides abundant sodium through processed foods and table salt.

4. Potassium, the major positive ion (cation) found inside cells, has a similar function as sodium. Milk, fruits, and vegetables are good sources. Chloride is the major negative ion (anion) found outside cells. It is important in digestion as part of gastric hydrochloric acid and in immune and nerve functions. Table salt supplies most of the chloride in our diets.

5. Calcium forms a vital part of bone structure and is very important in blood clotting, muscle contraction, nerve transmission, and cell metabolism. Calcium absorption is enhanced by stomach acid and the active vitamin D hormone. Dairy products are rich calcium sources. Women are particularly at risk for not meeting calcium needs. They are also typically at risk of developing osteoporosis as they age. Numerous lifestyle and medical options help reduce this risk.

6. Phosphorus aids function of some enzymes and forms part of key metabolic compounds, cell membranes, and bone. It is efficiently absorbed, and deficiencies are rare. Typical food sources are dairy products, bakery products, and meats.

7. Magnesium is a mineral found mostly in plants. It is important for nerve and heart function and as an activator for many enzymes. Whole grains (bran portion), vegetables, nuts, seeds, milk, and meats are typical food sources. Sulfur is incorporated into certain vitamins and amino acids. Its ability to bond with other sulfur atoms enables it to stabilize protein structure.

■ STUDY QUESTIONS

1. Approximately how much water does one need each day to stay healthy? Identify at least two situations that increase the need for water. Then list three sources of water in the average person's diet.

2. Why are most minerals present in higher concentrations in animal foods than in plant foods?

3. How is water eliminated from the body? What physiological forces regulate this output?

4. What is the main physiological difference between teeth and bones?

5. Identify four factors that influence the bioavailability of minerals from food.

6. What is the relationship between sodium and water balance, and how is that relationship monitored as well as maintained in the body?

7. Within what physiological system do potassium, chloride, and calcium interact? What are the individual roles of these minerals in this system?

8. What might you tell a 12-year-old child about the importance of consuming sufficient calcium?

9. In terms of total amounts in the body, calcium and phosphorus are the first and second most abundant minerals, respectively. Name two ways in which phosphorus and calcium are alike and two ways in which they differ.

10. Describe the relationship between magnesium and the function/health of the heart.

■ ANNOTATED REFERENCES

1. Anderson JJB: The important role of physical activity in skeletal development: How exercise may counter low calcium intake. *American Journal of Clinical Nutrition* 71:1384, 2000.

A greater bone mass gained early in life is now considered a critical factor in protecting against osteoporotic fractures later in life. The critical years for skeletal growth and accumulation of bone mass are in the prepubertal and pubertal decades. These years are a particularly good time for regular physical activity, as it, along with adequate diet, increases bone mass.

2. Beck BR, Shoemaker RM: Osteoporosis: Understanding key risk factors and therapeutic options. *The Physician and Sportsmedicine* 28(2):69, 2000.

Pharmacologic options for treating osteoporosis include calcium, vitamin D, estrogen, biphosphonates, selective estrogen receptor modulaters, and calcitonin. Any such medication should be taken in conjunction with exercise and fall precautions.

3. Burke GL and others: Soybean isoflavones as an alternative to traditional hormone replacement therapy: Are we there yet? *Journal of Nutrition* 130:664S, 2000.

Soy isoflavones should not at this time be viewed as a viable alternative to traditional hormone replacement therapy for perimenopausal women. The use of isoflavone supplements is premature, but a healthful diet could include one to two servings of soy per day for women in this age group.

4. Byrant RJ and others: The new Dietary Reference Intakes for calcium: Implications for osteoporosis. *Journal of the American College of Nutrition* 18:406S, 1999.

The DRI recommendations for calcium are being promoted to ensure that adequate intakes are met to prevent osteoporosis and related bone disease. These guidelines of 1000-1200 mg/day in adulthood establish intakes to aid in the maintenance of bone and overall nutritional status.

5. Cooper RS and others: The puzzle of hypertension in African Americans. *Scientific American*, p. 56, February 1999.

About 35% of African-Americans suffer from hypertension. Environmental factors are probably very important causes because black adults in Africa do not show nearly the same prevalence of the disease. Widespread obesity among African-Americans could be one of these environmental causes.

6. Food and Nutrition Board, Institute of Medicine: Dietary Reference Intakes for calcium, phosphorus, magnesium, vitamin D, and fluoride. Washington, DC: National Academy Press, 1997.

The DRIs for major minerals are discussed in detail. A major change in setting these new estimates of human needs is the use of a specific biological marker that shows adequacy, such as the use of measuring the balance between calcium intake and excretion as a method for determining calcium needs in adults.

7. Harsha DW and others: Dietary approaches to stop hypertension: A summary of study results. *Journal of the American Dietetic Association* 99(Suppl):S35, 1999.

Dietary recommendations to increase fruits, vegetables, and low-fat dairy foods complement the variety of behavioral changes currently available to persons who need to lower their blood pressure. These other behavioral changes include reducing salt intake, increasing physical activity, limiting alcohol intake, and reducing excess weight.

8. Heaney RP: Calcium, dairy products and osteoporosis. *Journal of the American College of Nutrition* 19(2):83S, 2000.

The results of several studies have shown that there is no single intervention, whether nutritional, hormonal, or pharmacologic, that can solve the problem of osteoporosis. Instead, what is needed is a combination of approaches, such as adequate calcium intake for women on hormone replacement therapy.

9. Ignall TJ: Preventing ischemic stroke. *Postgraduate Medicine* 107(6):34, 2000.

The treatment of hypertension is the most important intervention for decreasing the risk of ischemic stroke. Other risk factors related to the development of stroke in general include alcohol abuse, stress, and smoking.

10. Joshipura KJ and others: Fruit and vegetable intake in relation to risk of ischemic stroke. *Journal of the American Medical Association* 282:1233, 1999.

Numerous studies have shown a protective relationship between the consumption of fruits and vegetables and reduced risk of ischemic stroke. This study highlighted the effects of cruciferous vegetables (e.g., broccoli, cauliflower, kale), green leafy vegetables, and citrus fruit and juice in showing a reduced risk for this health problem.

11. Kaplan NM: The dietary guideline for sodium: Should we shake it up? No. *American Journal of Clinical Nutrition* 71:1020, 2000.

The U.S. Dietary Guideline for sodium (2400 mg/day) may not be set low enough to prevent the development of hypertension in some people. In order to reduce sodium intake, certain interventions can be accomplished: promoting consumer label reading, targeting fast-food chains to offer alternative choices, and encouraging less salt added to processed foods.

12. Kleiner SM: Water: An essential but overlooked nutrient. *Journal of the American Dietetic Association* 99:200, 1999.

Dehydration of as little as a 2% loss of body weight results in decreased physiological responses. New research indicates that fluid consumption in general and water consumption in particular can reduce the risk of kidney stones, certain cancers, obesity, and mitral valve prolapse. Adequate fluid intake is especially important for the overall health of older adults.

13. Knochel JP: Phosphorus. In Shils ME and others (eds.): *Modern nutrition in health and disease.* 9th ed. Baltimore, MD: Williams & Wilkins, 1999.

A dietary deficiency as the causal factor in phosphorus deficiency is rare because of the abundance of phosphorus in almost all foods. It is also avidly retained by the kidneys. Conditions that can result in a phosphorus deficiency include chronic alcoholism and certain medical conditions, such as rapid refeeding of a previously undernourished hospital patient.

14. Korhonen MH and others: Effects of a salt-restricted diet on the intake of other nutrients. *American Journal of Clinical Nutrition* 72:414, 2000.

For a sodium-restricted diet, emphasis should be placed on lowering the amount of salt added to foods, in addition to limiting foods rich in salt. Such diets can be undertaken by hypertensive subjects without any untoward changes in the intake of other nutrients.

15. Kurtzweil P: Lessening the pressure. *FDA Consumer*, p. 18, July-August 1999.

Individuals particularly at risk for high blood pressure are African-Americans, people with a family history of high blood pressure, people who drink alcoholic beverages excessively, and people who are physically inactive. In addition, as many as 65% of people with diabetes have high blood pressure. High blood pressure produces numerous health problems and, so, needs to be treated.

16. Lambing CL: Osteoporosis prevention, detection, and treatment. *Postgraduate Medicine* 107(7):37, 2000.

The goal of osteoporosis management is to prevent fractures by achieving the highest possible peak bone mass, preventing further bone loss, and minimizing chances for falls. The use of glucocorticoids that are often part of treatment for asthma, lung disease, and inflammatory bowel disease needs more attention by physicians because currently about 25% of patients receiving long-term glucocorticoid therapy develop osteoporosis.

17. Liebman B: High blood pressure: The end of an epidemic? *Nutrition Action Health Letter*, p.1, December 2000.

The DASH-Sodium trial included intakes of 3300 mg/day, 2400 mg/day, or 1500 mg/day of sodium in addition to the standard DASH diet plan. Each reduction in sodium intake resulted in a further fall in both systolic and diastolic blood pressure. Thus, people with hypertension should consider following the basic DASH diet and lowering sodium intake as much as possible.

18. Marwick C: Consensus panel considers osteoporosis. *Journal of American Medical Association* 283:2093, 2000.

An estimated 18 million people in the United States have low bone mass, which places them at a higher risk for fractures. One in five people who sustain a hip fracture are no longer alive after one year, making this a very serious health problem that needs more attention by the medical community.

19. McCarron DA: The dietary guideline for sodium: Should we shake it up? Yes. *American Journal of Clinical Nutrition* 71:1013, 2000.

Some experts have concluded that current sodium intakes in the majority of the U.S. population have only minimal effects on blood pressure. These experts feel that sodium restrictions are beneficial only to those in the older population group who have an established diagnosis of hypertension.

20. McCarron DA, Reusser BA: Finding consensus in the dietary calcium-blood pressure debate. *Journal of the American College of Nutrition* 18:398S, 1999.

 The ability of calcium to lower blood pressure is mostly in persons consuming low amounts of dietary calcium. Adequate dietary calcium intake is critical to optimum blood pressure regulation.

21. McGarry KA, Kiel DP: Postmenopausal osteoporosis. *Postgraduate Medicine* 108:79, 2000.

 An estimated 1.5 million Americans develop osteoporotic fractures each year. The annual cost of osteoporotic fractures in the U.S. is $14 billion per year. Numerous medications have been approved by FDA for the prevention of osteoporosis and related bone loss.

22. Miller GD and others: The role of calcium in prevention of chronic disease. *Journal of the American College of Nutrition* 18:371S, 1999.

 Calcium is essential to our health, and it has many roles in the body, including structural support, muscle contraction, and blood coagulation. It is also responsible for reducing the risk of several chronic diseases, such as osteoporosis, hypertension, colon cancer, kidney stones, and lead toxicity.

23. NIH Consensus Development Panel on Osteoporosis Prevention, Diagnosis, and Treatment; Osteoporosis prevention, diagnosis, and treatment, *Journal of the American Medical Association* 285:785, 2001.

 Optimal treatment of osteoporosis with any drug therapy also requires calcium and vitamin D intake meeting recommended levels. The preferred source of calcium is dietary. Calcium supplements need to be absorbable and should have United States Pharmacopeia designation.

24. Oh MS, Uribarri J: Electrolytes, water, and acid-base balance. In Shils ME and others (eds.): *Modern nutrition in health and disease.* 9th ed. Baltimore, MD: Williams & Wilkins, 1999.

 Regulation of fluid balance in the body depends on the hormone renin, various forms of angiotensin, and aldosterone and the resulting effects these factors have on the kidneys and blood vessels. Antidiuretic hormone also contributes to fluid balance in the body.

25. Perry HM and others: Effect of treating isolated systolic hypertension on the risk of developing various types and subtypes of stroke. *Journal of the American Medical Association* 284:465, 2000.

 Greater attention today is being paid to the control of systolic as well as diastolic blood pressure in reducing hemorrhagic and ischemic stroke risk. Controlling systolic blood pressure is especially important in reducing these health problems.

26. Schardt D: Water, water, everywhere. *Nutrition Action Health Letter,* 41, June 2000.

 On the whole, people in the United States can feel confident about the quality of their drinking water. Almost 90% of public water systems in the United States report no violations of EPA limits for drinking water contaminants. The main individuals at risk from contaminated drinking water are those with compromised immune systems and possibly people in rural communities. The former persons should take the extra precaution to boil tap water for at least 1 minute, whereas the latter may consider having their tap water tested to see if it meets current EPA standards.

27. Schnirring L: Osteoporosis management: What's on the cutting edge? *The Physician and Sportsmedicine* 28(3):15, 2000.

 The gold standard used for diagnosing osteoporosis is the Dual-energy x-ray absorptiometry (DEXA). Ultrasound appears to be adequate for a screening tool; however, it is not a good choice for monitoring response to drug therapy.

28. Shils ME: Magnesium. In Shils ME and others (eds.): *Modern nutrition in health and disease.* 9th ed. Baltimore, MD: Williams & Wilkins, 1999.

 Magnesium is involved in more than 300 essential metabolic reactions. Health problems that can lead to magnesium deficiency include alcoholism, diabetes, and long-term use of certain diuretics.

29. Sorrentino MJ: Turning up the heat on hypertension. *Postgraduate Medicine* 105(5):82, 1999.

 People who already have coronary heart disease, cerebrovascular disease, peripheral vascular disease, kidney disease, and retinal disease are at the greatest risk for complications regarding high blood pressure. Currently, only about one-fourth of people who have high blood pressure are being adequately treated for the problem.

30. Teegarden D and others: Dietary calcium, protein, and phosphorus are related to bone mineral density and content in young women. *American Journal of Clinical Nutrition* 68:749, 1998.

 Body weight and lean body mass are the most powerful predictors of bone mass. Adequate calcium intake is also important, as this offsets the urinary and fecal losses associated with typical protein and phosphorus intakes.

31. Ullom-Minnich P: Prevention of osteoporosis and fractures. *American Family Physician* 60:194, 1999.

 Osteoporosis is a problem that is not likely to go away. About 30% of persons over 60 years of age have osteoporosis, and about 66% have some evidence of osteopenia. The use of caffeine, tobacco, and corticosteroids is associated with a decrease in bone mass, whereas calcium and vitamin D contribute to bone maintenance.

32. Whelton PK and others: Sodium reduction and weight loss in the treatment of hypertension in older persons. *Journal of the American Medical Association* 279:839, 1998.

 Reduced sodium intake and weight loss constitute a feasible, effective, and safe nonpharmacologic therapy for hypertension in older persons. This lifestyle therapy can reduce the need for antihypertensive medication.

TAKE ACTION

I. HOW DOES YOUR MINERAL INTAKE MEASURE UP?

To complete this activity, reexamine your nutritional assessment from Chapter 2. Compare your intake of selective minerals with the RDA, Adequate Intake (AI), or other established standard. Use your completed nutritional assessment to complete the following table. For each mineral, record your intake, the intake recommended, the percentage of that intake you consumed, and a +, −, or = to indicate an intake higher, lower, or equal to that intake. Note that, for sodium, chloride, and potassium, minimum requirements for health are designated and already recorded in the table (these can also be found on the inside front cover of this book).

Mineral	Intake	RDA/AI	% of Needs	+/−/=
Calcium				
Phosphorus				
Sodium		500 mg		
Potassium		2000 mg		
Chloride		750 mg		
Magnesium				

Analysis

1. Which of your mineral intakes equaled or exceeded the RDA (or other standard set)? Do the nutrients for which you exceeded the desired amounts pose a likely risk for toxicity, based on the total amount consumed?

    _____

2. Which of your intakes were below the RDA (or other standard)?

    _____

3. What foods and cooking practices could be emphasized or deemphasized to modify your deficient intakes? Indicate for each food the specific amount of the missing nutrient(s) supplied.

    _____

    _____

    _____

    _____

TAKEACTION

II. WORKING FOR DENSER BONES

Osteoporosis and related low bone mass affect more than 25 million people in the United States. One-third of all women experience fractures because of this disease, amounting to about 1.5 million bone fractures per year. Given the rise in the number of older people in the United States, osteoporosis-related illness and death are anticipated to increase dramatically in coming years.

   This is a disease you can do something about. Some risk factors can't be changed, but others can. To what degree are you doing the things that can help prevent this debilitating disease? Answer yes or no to the following questions by placing an X in the appropriate blank.

	Yes	No
1. Do you average at least 10 to 20 minutes of sun exposure per day to at least your hands and face to get vitamin D, or do you drink vitamin D-fortified milk regularly?	___	___
2. Do you engage in weight-bearing physical activity (jogging, brisk walking, etc.) for at least 30 minutes on most or all days of the week?	___	___
3. If you are a woman, do you experience regular menstruation?	___	___
4. Do you avoid smoking cigarettes?	___	___
5. Do you avoid regular consumption of large amounts (greater than one to two drinks per day) of alcohol?	___	___
6. Do you consume milk and other dairy products regularly or substitute other sources to meet at least the Adequate Intake for calcium for your age?	___	___
7. Do you regularly meet the Food Guide Pyramid recommendations for fruit and vegetable intake?	___	___
8. Do you moderate your intake of phosphorus, sodium, protein, and caffeine?	___	___

The more *yes* answers you have, the more you are actively preserving your bone density for the future. Also, remember that this is not just a consideration for women, because if men plan to live well into their 80s and 90s, they are at risk for osteoporosis. In fact, about 14% of all spine fractures and 25% of all hip fractures linked to osteoporosis occur in men.

MINERALS AND HYPERTENSION

An estimated 50 million American adults have hypertension, as does one out of two of those over age 65.[17] Blood pressure is expressed by two numbers. The higher number represents systolic blood pressure, which is the pressure in the arteries when the heart actively pumps blood. The second value is for diastolic blood pressure, which is the artery pressure when the heart is relaxed. Optimal systolic blood pressure is less than 120 mm of mercury (mm Hg). Optimal diastolic blood pressure is less than 80 mm Hg. A high diastolic pressure shows a strong relationship to various diseases (especially **strokes**),[9, 25] as does a high systolic pressure.

Hypertension is defined as sustained systolic pressure exceeding 140 mm Hg or diastolic blood pressure exceeding 90 mm Hg (Table 11-6). Most cases of hypertension (about 95% of cases) have no clear-cut cause. It is described as primary, or essential, in nature (e.g., essential hypertension). Kidney disease, sleep-disordered breathing (sleep apnea), and other causes often lead to the other 5% of cases, known as secondary hypertension. African-Americans are more likely than Caucasians to develop hypertension and to do so earlier in life.[5] As a result, they also experience more from hypertension-related diseases and, so, are particularly advised to have their blood pressure checked regularly and to have any evidence of hypertension treated aggressively.

Unless blood pressure is measured periodically, the development of hypertension is easily overlooked. Thus, it's described as a silent disorder, because it usually does not cause symptoms. A physician usually does not treat hypertension with medication until the diastolic blood pressure measures at least 90 mm Hg and/or the systolic blood pressure reaches 140 mm Hg on three or more occasions.

WHY CONTROL BLOOD PRESSURE?

Blood pressure needs to be controlled mainly to prevent heart disease, kidney disease, strokes and related declines in brain function, poor blood circulation in the legs, problems with vision, and sudden death. All these conditions are much more likely to be found in individuals with hypertension than in people with normal blood pressure. Smoking and elevated blood lipoproteins make these diseases even more likely. Individuals with hypertension need to be diagnosed and treated as soon as possible, as the condition generally progresses to a more serious stage over time and even resists therapy if it persists for years.[17]

stroke Damage to the brain tissue caused by an interruption of blood flow. This can result from blockage (ischemic stroke) or hemorrhage (hemorrhagic stroke) in the arteries in the brain. Also known as a cerebrovascular accident (CVA).

Symptoms of Stroke
Individuals experiencing any of the following symptoms of stroke should seek immediate treatment. This is because physicians can administer drugs that can reduce the extent of the damage caused by most strokes (i.e., ischemic strokes). Currently about 750,000 Americans suffer strokes each year.

- Sudden disturbances in sight, speech, and steadiness
- Sudden sleepiness or severe headache
- Sudden temporary blindness in one eye or other visual effects
- Sudden numbness, weakness, or paralysis of an arm, a leg, or an entire side of the body
- Sudden difficulty with speech or the ability to swallow
- Coma or convulsions

TABLE 11-6	Classification of Blood Pressure for Adults Age 18 Years and Older in Millimeters of Mercury*		
Category	**Systolic**		**Diastolic**
Optimal	< 120	and	< 80
Normal	< 130	and	< 85
High-normal†	130-139	or	85-89
Hypertension			
Stage 1	140-159	or	90-99
Stage 2	160-179	or	100-109
Stage 3	≥ 180	or	≥ 110

*Not taking high blood pressure drugs and not acutely ill

†People with diabetes or kidney or heart disease should be treated at this stage.

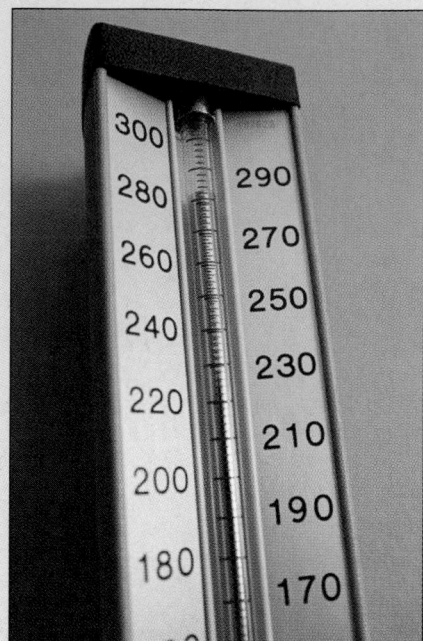

High blood pressure is harmful to many organs in the body. Maintenance of healthy systolic and diastolic blood pressure is a key to disease prevention throughout life.

CAUSES OF HYPERTENSION

Blood pressure usually increases as a person ages. Some increase is caused by atherosclerosis. As plaque builds up in the arteries, the arteries become less flexible and cannot expand. When vessels remain rigid, blood pressure remains high. Eventually, the plaque begins to choke off the blood supply to the kidneys, decreasing their ability to control blood volume and, in turn, blood pressure.

The enzyme renin (secreted by the kidneys) and some hormonelike compounds affect blood pressure. Medications are available to reduce their effect on the renin-angiotensin system.

Obesity is often associated with high blood pressure, especially in women. In fact, overweight people have six times greater risk of having hypertension than lean people. Overall, obesity is considered the number 1 lifestyle factor related to hypertension. The increase in fat mass increases the need for blood circulation. The extra miles of associated blood vessels increases work by the heart and increase blood pressure. Elevated blood insulin concentration associated with insulin-resistant adipose cells is another reason for this link to obesity. Insulin increases sodium retention in the body and accelerates atherosclerosis. Additionally, an estimated 65% of people with diabetes also have hypertension.[15]

A weight loss of as little as 10 to 15 pounds often can help treat hypertension.[29, 32] This, then, can decrease the need for hypertension drugs, which, by themselves may cause headache, impotence, reduced exercise tolerance, persistent cough, and other side effects.[17] The sleep apnea linked to hypertension also typically improves with weight loss.

Inactivity also is associated with hypertension. It is considered the number 2 lifestyle factor related to hypertension. If an obese person can engage in regular physical activity (at least five days per week for 30 to 45 minutes per session) and lose weight, blood pressure often returns to normal.

Excess alcohol intake is responsible for about 10% of all cases of hypertension, especially in middle-aged males and among African-Americans in general. It is considered the number 3 lifestyle factor related to hypertension. When hypertension is caused by excessive alcohol intake, it is usually reversible. A sensible intake for people with hypertension is two or fewer drinks per day for men and one or no drinks per day for women, the same recommendation given to healthy adults.[17] As discussed in Chapter 8, some studies suggest that such a low alcohol intake may reduce the risk of ischemic stroke. These data, however, should not be used to encourage alcohol use in nonconsumers.

Preliminary studies show a link between bone lead concentrations and increased risk of hypertension. More information is needed, but it is suspected that even small amounts of lead stored over decades may damage the kidneys and eventually result in hypertension. This is just one of the deleterious effects of lead exposure (see Chapter 19 for more information on lead).

SALT AND BLOOD PRESSURE

Excess salt intake tends to increase blood pressure, particularly in African-Americans, older persons, and people in general who are susceptible to developing a problem regulating sodium concentration in the body.[11] It is not clear whether the sodium ion or the chloride ion is most responsible for the effect. Still, as reviewed in this chapter, if one reduces sodium intake, chloride intake naturally falls; the opposite is also true. For the most part, when nutrition recommendations suggest consuming less sodium, that is equivalent to saying consume less salt. Since only some Americans are very susceptible to increases in blood pressure from salt intake, it is likely only the number 4 lifestyle factor related to hypertension.[19] Thus, it is unfortunate that salt intake receives the major portion of public attention with regard to hypertension; obesity and inactivity should be given much more attention.

The latest dietary advice from the Dietary Guidelines for Americans and the American Heart Association suggests that adults consume no more than the Daily Value for sodium (2400 mg). Currently, Americans consume daily, on average, almost double that amount (4-7 g). Both sets of recommendations note that there is no risk in reducing sodium intake to that amount.

The exact mechanism whereby sodium increases blood pressure is not clear. Studies suggest that there is a genetically influenced ability that determines the ease at which the body can excrete sodium. In salt-sensitive individuals, the kidneys require a higher blood pressure in order to excrete sodium from the body, compared with salt-resistant people. This causes salt-sensitive individuals to retain more sodium. This sodium retention in the body then leads to fluid retention. Ultimately, the fluid retention leads to increased blood volume and, in turn, the increased blood pressure needed to maintain sodium excretion.

Physicians usually resort to a combination of antihypertensive medications, such as diuretics (to increase urine output) and moderate sodium restriction (3-4 g/day) as an initial form of therapy. This reduces blood volume and, therefore, is often effective in controlling blood pressure.[11]

OTHER MINERALS AND BLOOD PRESSURE

Minerals such as calcium, potassium, and magnesium also deserve attention when it comes to prevention and treatment of hypertension. People often register slightly lower blood pressures—especially the systolic component—when they consume at least the 1000 mg of calcium per day, as compared with one-third to one-half that amount. It is reasonable for a person with hypertension to experiment, in consultation with a physician, with increasing calcium intake to see if that produces the desired effect.[20] So far, FDA has found the evidence linking calcium to a decrease in blood pressure too inconsistent to approve a health claim regarding hypertension and calcium-containing products.

Potassium supplementation in the range of 2 to 4 g/day also has been shown to moderately decrease blood pressure in people currently consuming far below this amount. FDA recently approved the following health claim for potassium and a reduction in blood pressure: "Diets containing foods that are good sources of potassium and low in sodium may reduce the risk of high blood pressure and stroke." This health claim will be allowed on foods that contain at least 350 mg of potassium (10 percent of the Daily Value) and 140 mg or less of sodium. In addition, qualifying foods must have less than 3 g of fat, 1 g or less of saturated fat, and 20 mg or less of cholesterol. Some studies indicate that magnesium also is capable of lowering blood pressure at intakes of about twice the RDA.

Recent studies show that a diet rich in calcium, potassium, and magnesium and low in sodium can lead to a decrease in blood pressure within days of beginning a specific diet, especially among African-Americans.[17] The response is even similar to that seen with commonly used medications. The diet, called the DASH diet, closely follows the Food Guide Pyramid, with a few modifications (Table 11-7). The DASH diet is seen as a total dietary approach to treating hypertension.[7] It is not clear which of the many factors contributed by this diet are responsible for the fall in blood pressure. An additional attribute of the DASH diet is that the participants in the study also experienced a fall in blood homocysteine, which should contribute to a lower risk of cardiovascular disease and stroke. Other studies also show a reduction in stroke risk among people who consume a diet rich in fruits, vegetables, and vitamin C (recall that fruits and vegetables are rich sources).[10] Overall, a diet rich in low-fat and nonfat dairy products, fruits, vegetables, whole grains, and some nuts can substantially reduce blood pressure and stroke risk in many people. The current challenge is to find a way to convince North Americans to follow such a diet.

PREVENTION OF HYPERTENSION

Many of these and other risk factors for hypertension and stroke are controllable, and appropriate lifestyle changes can reduce a person's risk (Table 11-8). Experts typically recommend that those with hypertension in the high-normal and Stage 1 categories attempt to lower blood pressure through diet and lifestyle changes before resorting to blood pressure medications. Such a focus on diet and lifestyle is important because many people discontinue their blood pressure medications because of expense and side effects. Currently, physicians have a long way to go in establishing good blood pressure control among people with hypertension.[29]

TABLE 11-7 The DASH Diet—a Sample Menu (Provides Approximately 2000 Calories)

Breakfast

Shredded Wheat, 1 cup	2 grains
1% low-fat milk, 8 oz	1 milk
Sugar, 1 tsp	
Banana, 1 medium	1 fruit
Grapefruit juice, 4 oz	1 fruit

Snack

Bread sticks, ¾ oz	1 grain
Diet soft drink, 12 oz	

Lunch

Chicken salad, ¾ cup	1 meat
(made with reduced-fat	1 fat
mayonnaise)	
Whole-wheat bread, 2 slices	2 grains
Carrots, 5 baby	1 vegetable
Low-fat yogurt, 1 cup	1 milk
(with artificial sweetener)	
Applesauce, ½ cup	1 fruit

Snack

Mixed nuts, ¾ oz	1 nut
Grape juice, 4 oz	1 fruit

Dinner

Baked orange roughy, 3 oz	1 meat
Rice, 1 cup	2 grains
Steamed broccoli, 1 cup	2 vegetables
Mixed greens salad, 2 cups	1 vegetable
(made with vegetables)	
Light Italian dressing, 1 tbsp	½ fat
Whole-wheat roll, 1 small	1 grain
Margarine, 1 tsp	1 fat
1% low-fat milk, 8 oz	1 milk

Snack

Watermelon, 1¼ cup	1 fruit

The Dietary Approaches to Stop Hypertension (DASH) diet was found to decrease systolic blood pressure by 5.5 mm Hg and diastolic blood pressure by 3.0 mm Hg more than the control diet. Overall, this diet provides approximately 18% of energy as protein, 55% as carbohydrate, and 27% as fat, with 6% from saturated fat. The diet contains more fruit and vegetable servings than the Food Guide Pyramid, contains less fat, and includes a serving of nuts. All DASH participants consumed no more than 3 g of sodium and one to two alcoholic drinks per week. Researchers estimate that if Americans were to follow the DASH diet, there would be a 15% decrease in heart disease and 27% fewer strokes.

A DASH 2 diet trial tested three daily sodium intakes (3300 mg, 2400 mg, and 1500 mg). People showed a steady decline in blood pressure on the DASH diet as sodium intake declined (see Sacks FM and others: Effects on blood pressure of reduced dietary sodium and the dietary approaches to stop hypertension (DASH) diet. *The New England Journal of Medicine* 344: 3, 2001).

MEDICATIONS TO TREAT HYPERTENSION

Potassium-wasting diuretics, such as thiazides (chlorothiazide [Diuril]) are commonly used for drug therapy to treat hypertension. People need to monitor their potassium intakes carefully when on these drugs. Other typical medications to treat hypertension include angiotensin-converting enzyme (ACE) inhibitors (captopril [Capoten], beta-blockers (atenolol [Tenormin]), and calcium channel blockers (amlodipine [Norvasc]).[15, 29] A combination of two or more drugs is commonly used. The beta-blockers act to slow heart rate and cause some vasodilation, whereas the calcium channel blockers lead to general vasodilation.

TABLE 11-8 A Nutritional Plan to Minimize Hypertension and Stroke Risk*

1. Follow the Food Guide Pyramid. Also consider going beyond this to include more fruit, vegetables, and some nuts (e.g., DASH diet), especially if one has hypertension.

2. Make sure to meet nutrient recommendations for calcium, potassium, and magnesium listed in this chapter.

3. Attain and maintain a healthy body weight.

4. Incorporate regular physical activity (at least five times per week for 30 to 45 minutes per session).

5. Consume alcoholic beverages in moderation, if at all (two drinks per day maximum for men and one drink per day maximum for women).

6. Consume moderate amounts of sodium (salt) and see if this helps. The Daily Value is a reasonable limit (2400 mg sodium or 6 g salt [1¼ tsp]).

7. Don't smoke.

8. Maintain blood lipoproteins in the normal range (see Chapter 6).

*In addition, make sure to have blood pressure measured on a regular basis (i.e., yearly physician checkups).

TRACE MINERALS

chapter *12*

Trace minerals constitute less than 1% of all minerals in the body. A trace mineral is defined as a mineral for which our daily nutritional need is less than 100 mg. Grouping them together this way, however, is too simplistic because the functions, mechanisms of absorption, and metabolism of the various trace minerals vary considerably. For example, the body carefully regulates the absorption of iron, copper, and zinc, but not of selenium and iodide,[4, 23] so selenium and iodide concentrations in the body depend more on the mineral content of foods consumed than on the percentage absorbed through the intestinal wall. The trace minerals are also very interactive; the abundance of one mineral in the diet and in the body can affect the absorption and metabolism of several other minerals.[22]

Information about trace minerals is perhaps the most rapidly expanding area of nutrition science. With the exception of iron and iodide, the importance of trace minerals to humans has been recognized only within the last 50 years. Let's examine some of these new findings.

- Trace minerals are present in the body in amounts that are smaller than the amounts of the major minerals. Because it is sometimes difficult to gauge the clinical signs or symptoms of a deficiency, establishing the actual need for a trace mineral is difficult. It is possible that some minerals found in body tissues play no biological role whatsoever; they are there by accident and provide no threat or benefit to a person.

- Iron is found in several heme proteins, hemoglobin being just one. Infants and premenopausal women are at the greatest risk for developing iron deficiency. A severe form of the disease is iron deficiency anemia. Iron absorption is carefully controlled by the body's need for iron. This is advantageous, since iron is not readily excreted from the body. Except for milk, animal protein foods provide the most bioavailable form of iron.

- Zinc is present in almost every cell in the body and is part of nearly 100 enzyme systems. Zinc is especially needed for normal growth and development during childhood, adolescence, and pregnancy. It is also essential for function of the immune system, and it is needed for wound healing and sense of taste.

- Selenium is found in one of the antioxidant enzyme systems, which breaks down peroxides before they form free radicals. Selenium works with vitamin E to protect the cell from oxidative damage.

- Iodide in the body is found in the thyroid gland, where it is used to make the hormone thyroxine. A lack of dietary iodide causes an enlargement of the thyroid gland, or a goiter. Although this deficiency disease was once common in parts of the United States, the addition of iodine to table salt has virtually eliminated the problem in North America.

- Like zinc and selenium, copper is the active part of several enzyme systems. Copper is fundamentally involved in iron metabolism. It also plays a part in the synthesis of the protein collagen.

- Fluoride is obtained from drinking water, either naturally or as added by a municipal water department. Regular fluoride exposure makes teeth decay-resistant.

- Other minerals that provide health benefits are manganese, chromium, and molybdenum. The needs for arsenic, boron, nickel, silicon, and vanadium are still under study.

REFRESH YOUR MEMORY

As you begin your study of trace minerals in Chapter 12, you may want to review

- Respiration, the muscle and skeletal systems, cell structure and function, digestion, absorption and transport, immunity, and the endocrine system in Chapter 3
- The electron transport chain in Chapter 4
- Vitamins in Chapters 9 and 10
- Calcium in Chapter 11

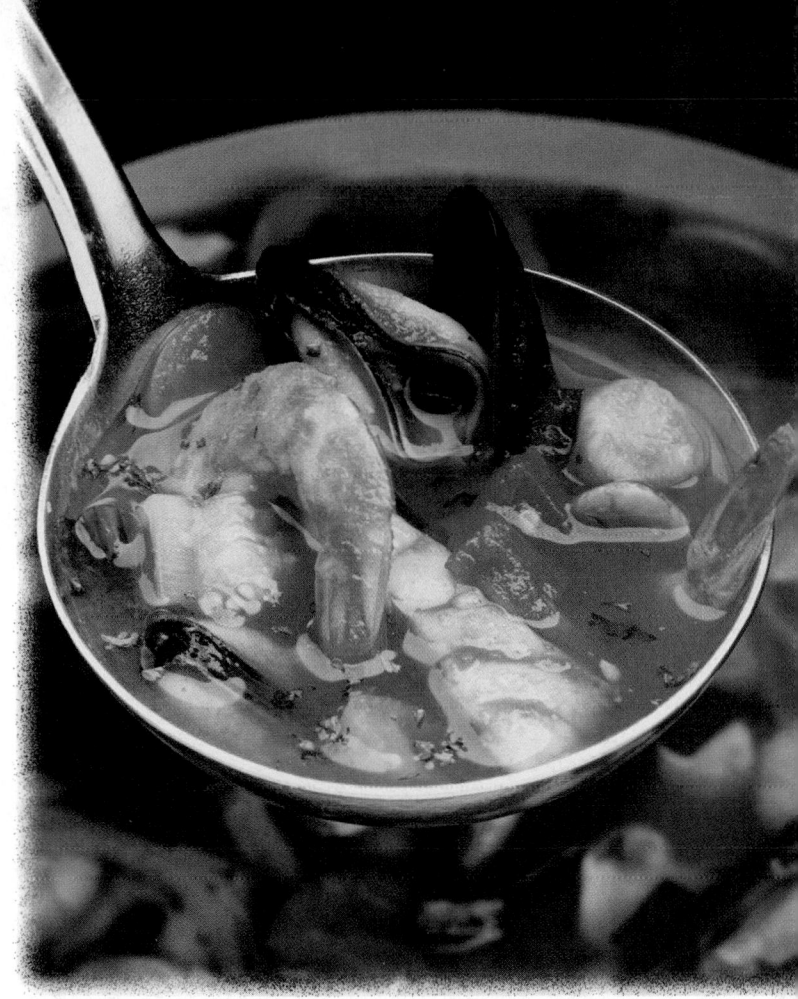

CASE SCENARIO

Gina has a history of colon cancer in her family. She has done a lot of reading on the web about cancer and has come across a number of references to the potential importance of an intake of 200 μg/day of the trace mineral selenium in prevention of this disease. She went to her local supermarket and found that a bottle of 100 supplements containing 200 μg each of selenium costs $7.50. This seemed like cheap 'insurance' against developing colon cancer, and so she began daily supplementation with 200 μg.

Why might selenium reduce the risk of colon cancer? What other forms of cancer have been prevented in certain people consuming such a dose? Is Gina's practice harmful? Should we all follow her example?

TRACE MINERALS—AN INTRODUCTION

The terms *trace mineral* and *micromineral* are somewhat imprecise, since there are several definitions of these terms that have evolved over time. Originally, the terms were used to describe minerals that are not easily quantified by existing analytical methods, but today we have precise techniques for determining the concentration of tiny amounts of minerals in tissues and in foods. Thus, we will use the terms trace mineral and micromineral as related to "a daily nutritional need of less than 100 mg." These minerals are dietary essentials, in that they have specified biological functions, and a dietary deficiency produces physiological or structural abnormalities.

Discovering the importance of these trace minerals to humans has a fairly recent history, although the use of dietary iron to treat the effects of blood loss can be traced back to ancient civilizations. In 1961, scientists linked dwarfism in villagers in the Middle East to a zinc deficiency. Other researchers later recognized that an obscure form of heart disease in an isolated area of China was linked to a selenium deficiency. In the United States, deficiencies of some trace minerals were first observed in the late 1960s to early 1970s, when these nutrients were omitted in the preparation of synthetic formulas used in total parenteral nutrition.[25] Because research on trace minerals in humans is still in its infancy, the current understanding of trace mineral metabolism relies heavily on the knowledge gained from studies with farm and laboratory animals.

RESEARCH ON TRACE MINERALS

Not only are trace minerals needed in much smaller amounts than the major minerals, but the actual need for some trace minerals is still debatable. In Table 1–3 nine essential trace minerals and some possible entries were listed. Demonstrating the essential nature of this latter group of nutrients is hampered by difficulty in measuring their amounts and by the rarity of naturally occurring deficiencies. Before looking at each of the trace minerals, let's look at why research in this area is so complex.

■ Difficulties in Studying Trace Minerals

Determining trace mineral needs is difficult because the body requires only minute amounts, and highly sophisticated technology is needed to measure such small amounts in both food and body tissues. Rigorous protocols often are required to produce a deficiency in animals. (All animal research referred to in this discussion was conducted with farm and/or laboratory animals.) The animals may need to be raised in ultraclean environments and have their diets carefully formulated from individual essential nutrients to ensure that no mineral contamination occurs. Stainless steel and plastic cages may also be needed, so that the animals do not obtain any trace minerals, such as zinc, from chewing on the cages. Minerals must sometimes even be filtered from the air, and the water must be as free of minerals as possible. In addition, glassware used for chemical analysis may need to be rinsed repeatedly in acid to eliminate trace mineral contamination; sometimes only plastic bottles are appropriate.

In view of the difficulties encountered in experimentally producing most trace mineral deficiencies in laboratory animals, overt human deficiencies are unlikely, considering all the mineral sources in food, air, and water. However, some evidence is available indicating that marginal dietary intakes of certain trace minerals (e.g., iron, zinc, copper, and chromium) do occur, leading to mild, undetected deficiencies in humans.[4, 7, 8, 29] The lack of precise tests to pinpoint these deficiencies is the main reason there is concern but not hard evidence.

Researchers generally like to use blood tests to assess mineral status because of the ease of obtaining blood. Unfortunately, the blood tests currently available for trace minerals are not reliable for every mineral under every circumstance. For instance, blood concentrations of the copper-containing protein **ceruloplasmin** are sometimes used to assess copper status, but these values can also be influenced by other dietary factors.[24] Thus, a researcher can't always tell a person's true mineral status. Indeed, the main factor limiting zinc research today is the lack of a sensitive measure of the zinc status of body tissues and fluids.

■ Nutrient Needs for Trace Minerals

The difficulty in measuring trace mineral nutrition in humans makes setting specific human needs problematic. Most trace minerals have only an Adequate Intake (AI), not a more precise RDA.

The primary method used to set trace mineral nutrient needs is the balance study. The same basic technique used for nitrogen balance studies works for minerals (see Chapter 7). Researchers try to determine the lowest mineral intake that compensates for all mineral losses from urine, feces, hair, skin, perspiration, menses, and so on. These studies are very expensive to perform. In addition, a balance study tells only the amount of dietary intake needed to maintain a specific **pool** of the mineral in the body, but this pool does not necessarily represent the amount needed to maintain good health.

There are further problems in establishing nutrient needs for trace minerals. Clinical signs and symptoms often appear only with severe deficiencies. We lack knowledge of the subtle physiological changes associated with most trace mineral deficiencies, so we cannot always detect people who are experiencing related ill health. They may consume just enough of a mineral to prevent obvious signs and symptoms from being expressed.

A final complication is that trace minerals interact with each other. An overabundance of copper or iron in the digestive tract can interfere with the absorption of the other minerals, such as zinc. Thus, to set human dietary needs for zinc, nutrition scientists must estimate the amounts of copper and other minerals that will be consumed to predict how much zinc the body will actually absorb. Overall, quite a lot of scientific judgment must go into setting desired intakes for trace minerals.

■ Trace Minerals in Foods

As mentioned in Chapter 11, the mineral content of plants depends primarily on the mineral concentration in the soil. Animal foods are generally better sources of trace minerals because animals eat a variety of plant products; in addition, some animals (especially cattle) are shipped from one area to another during their lifetimes. Thus, they generally consume foods grown under multiple soil conditions.

The bioavailability of trace minerals is another issue in planning diets. Even if a food is high in a particular mineral, it will not supply much to the body unless the mineral is absorbed well in the small intestine. Many factors found in foods inhibit mineral absorption. Mineral absorption from some plant sources can amount to only 3 to 6% of the total present.[12] In general, animal sources of minerals are superior to plant sources because they show more efficient absorption. Animal sources also often contain factors that enhance mineral absorption, even for those trace minerals supplied by plant foods in a meal.

This book repeatedly recommended eating a variety of foods. By doing so, you can eat plants and animals that have derived nutrients from a variety of soils and, thus, maximize your chances of consuming adequate amounts of trace minerals. In addition, with regard to most trace minerals, it is best to consume as many minimally processed foods as possible. Generally, the more refined a food, the lower its content of trace minerals. For example, during the refining of wheat into white flour, the trace minerals iron, selenium, zinc, and copper are lost. The enrichment of white flour restores iron but not the other minerals.

ceruloplasmin A blue copper-containing protein in the blood that can remove an electron from Fe^{2+} (ferrous form) to yield Fe^{3+} (the ferric form). The Fe^{3+} form of iron can then bind with iron transport and storage proteins, such as transferrin.

pool The amount of a mineral or other substance stored within the body that can be easily mobilized when needed.

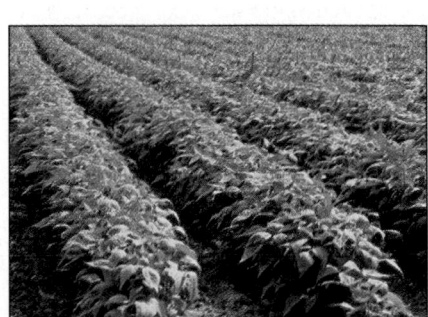

The trace mineral content of plant foods reflects the trace mineral concentration in the soil in which they were grown.

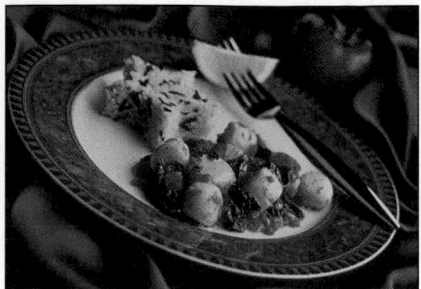

Seafood, such as scallops, is a rich source of many trace minerals.

■ IRON (FE)

Iron is found in every living cell; total body content is about 5 g (about 1 teaspoon). But there is a substantial sex difference, as menstruating women average 40 mg/kg, whereas men average 50 mg/kg of body weight. The importance of iron for the maintenance of health has been recognized for centuries. In 4000 B.C., Persian physician Melampus gave iron supplements to sailors to compensate for the iron lost from bleeding during battles. Today, iron deficiency and iron deficiency anemia are common worldwide, affecting an estimated 1 billion or more people in developing and developed countries.[5] In most developing nations, about two-thirds of all children and women of childbearing age experience iron deficiency; many of them have the more severe form of the disorder, iron deficiency anemia.

■ Absorption, Transport, Storage, and Excretion of Iron

The body uses several mechanisms to regulate iron absorption. Controlling absorption is important because the body cannot easily eliminate excess iron once absorbed. Iron absorption from foods typically is about 15% in healthy people. The extent of iron absorption depends on a variety of factors, the most important of which is to replace the amount of body iron lost each day by absorbing a similar amount of iron from dietary sources. (See Table 12-1).[10]

Iron in foods occurs in several forms, which differ in their absorption by the body. Iron that is part of the **hemoglobin** and **myoglobin** molecules in animal flesh (about 40% of total iron present), called **heme iron,** is absorbed more than twice as efficiently as simple elemental iron, known as **nonheme iron.** Nonheme iron is also present in animal flesh, eggs, and milk, as well as in vegetables, grains, and other plant foods. Overall, the difference in absorption of heme and nonheme iron makes animal flesh (e.g., red meat, seafood, and pork) a rich source of dietary iron, considering both its iron content and the increased efficiency of absorption of the heme iron present. Greater body needs are associated with greater absorption of iron in general.

Consuming heme iron and nonheme iron together increases nonheme iron absorption. A protein factor in meat, fish, and poultry also facilitates nonheme iron absorption. Eating meat with vegetables and grain products generally improves the absorption of the nonheme iron present in the meat.

Organic acids, such as vitamin C, modestly increase nonheme iron absorption by adding an electron to Fe^{3+} (the ferric form), yielding Fe^{2+} (the ferrous form). Vitamin C then forms a complex, called a **chelate,** with Fe^{2+}, thereby enhancing absorption. For vegetarians, or those who limit intake of animal flesh, combining vitamin C–rich foods with plant foods is a useful strategy.

hemoglobin The iron-containing protein in red blood cells that transports oxygen to the body tissues and some carbon dioxide away from the tissues. It is also responsible for the red color of blood.

myoglobin The iron-containing protein that controls the rate of diffusion of oxygen (O_2) from red blood cells to muscle cells.

heme iron Iron provided from animal tissues primarily as a component of hemoglobin and myoglobin. Approximately 40% of the iron in meat is heme iron; it is readily absorbed.

nonheme iron Iron provided from plant sources and elemental iron components of animal tissues. Nonheme iron is less efficiently absorbed than heme iron, and absorption is also more closely dependent on body needs.

chelates Complexes formed between metal ions and substances with polar groups, such as proteins. The polar groups form two or more attachments with the metal ions, forming a ringed structure. The metal ion is then firmly bound and sequestered.

TABLE 12-1   Factors That Affect Iron Absorption

Increase Absorption	Decrease Absorption
Gastric acid	Phytic acid (in dietary fiber)
Heme iron in food	Oxalic acid in leafy vegetables
High body demand for red blood cells (blood loss, high altitude, physical training, pregnancy)	Polyphenols in tea, as well as in coffee, red wine, and other foods
Low body stores of iron	Full body stores of iron
Meat protein factor (MPF)	Excess of other minerals (Zn, Mn, Ca)*
Vitamin C	Reduced gastric acid output
	Some antacids

*Especially when taken as supplements

Ferrous iron (Fe^{2+}) is absorbed better than ferric iron (Fe^{3+}) because it crosses the mucous layer of the small intestine more readily to reach the brush border of intestinal absorptive cells. There, Fe^{2+} must then have an electron removed, oxidizing it to Fe^{3+}, before it enters the absorptive cells. At the cell membrane of the brush border, Fe^{3+} binds to a receptor protein, called membrane iron-binding protein, which finally transfers iron into the absorptive cell.

Although no iron absorption occurs in the mouth, esophagus, or stomach, gastric acid plays an important role in iron absorption by promoting the conversion of Fe^{3+} to Fe^{2+} and by solubilizing nonheme iron. The decreased production of gastric acid experienced by many older people can lower their iron absorption and ultimately body stores of iron. Once acted on by acid in the stomach, iron absorption then occurs primarily in the duodenum and upper jejunum.

Heme iron follows a different absorptive process. It is likely absorbed directly into the absorptive cells after the globin (protein) fraction has been removed. Once inside the absorptive cells, the iron is released from the heme portion.

Several dietary factors interfere with our ability to absorb iron. Phytic acid and other factors in grain fibers and oxalic acid in vegetables can all bind iron, reducing its absorption. A long-term concern about increasing dietary fiber intake above 35 g/day is the tendency for fiber components to bind iron (and other trace minerals), in turn decreasing absorption. Polyphenols, such as tannins found in tea and related substances found in coffee, also reduce iron absorption.[12] People trying to rebuild iron stores are advised to reduce coffee and tea consumption, particularly at meal times. Finally, although several studies have shown that calcium interferes with dietary iron absorption, recent studies show that most use of calcium supplements (e.g. calcium carbonate) does appear to inhibit iron absorption at first but that the body seems to be able to adapt over time and maintain stored iron levels.[21] Still, experts on calcium and iron interactions recommend that individuals with high iron requirements avoid taking calcium supplements at meals that contain most of the dietary iron. They should also consider taking calcium supplements at bedtime to avoid calcium-iron interactions.[16]

Because of the various influences on iron absorption, it is difficult to estimate the amount of iron actually absorbed from individual foods. Rather, it is the overall composition of a meal and the needs of the person that largely determine the degree of absorption and ultimately the amount of iron delivered to the body.

Depending on body needs, some iron in the intestinal absorptive cells are ushered directly into the bloodstream, where it is bound by the protein **transferrin.** The rest binds to apoferritin in the intestinal cells to form **ferritin.** Ferritin provides a short-term form of iron storage in intestinal cells. Eventually, the iron is either absorbed or sloughed off into the GI tract with the intestinal cell.

The extent of iron stores in the body, principally in the liver, spleen, and bone marrow, is the most important factor influencing iron absorption.[10] When iron stores are adequate, all the iron-binding sites on transferrin are full (saturated) or nearly so. As a result, the transfer of iron (especially nonheme iron) from the intestinal cells to the blood is inhibited, and much of the iron in these cells remains in the intestinal cells in the protein-bound form, ferritin. When intestinal cells are sloughed at the end of the 2- to 5-day life cycle, the iron returns to the GI tract and is excreted in the feces. On the other hand, when iron stores are low, transferrin in the blood readily binds more iron, shifting it directly from the intestinal cells into the blood, or from ferritin stores in the intestinal cells into the blood. By this means—under normal circumstance—iron is absorbed only as needed. This mechanism for resisting absorption of excess iron, primarily that in the nonheme form, is termed a *mucosal block* (Fig. 12-1).

Almost all cells in the body have receptors for transferrin, so they can take up iron from the blood. About 70% of iron in the body is found in hemoglobin molecules in the red blood cells and myoglobin in muscle tissue (Fig. 12-2). Some iron is stored in the bone marrow, and a small portion goes to other body cells or to the spleen

CRITICAL THINKING

Annie, Tom's friend, is taking a nutrition class at her university. She suggested that he consume some extra vitamin C-rich foods every day. Tom is confused by this advice, since his doctor told him to increase the amount of iron in his diet to help treat low blood iron, but not the amount of vitamin C. How can Annie explain her recommendation to him?

transferrin A protein that transports iron in the blood.

ferritin A protein compound that serves as the storage form of iron in the blood and tissues.

*T*he copper-containing blood protein ceruloplasmin removes an electron from Fe^{2+}, yielding Fe^{3+}, the form bound by transferrin. Thus, copper metabolism and iron metabolism are closely linked. Eventually, most of the iron in transferrin is deposited in the liver, forming ferritin.

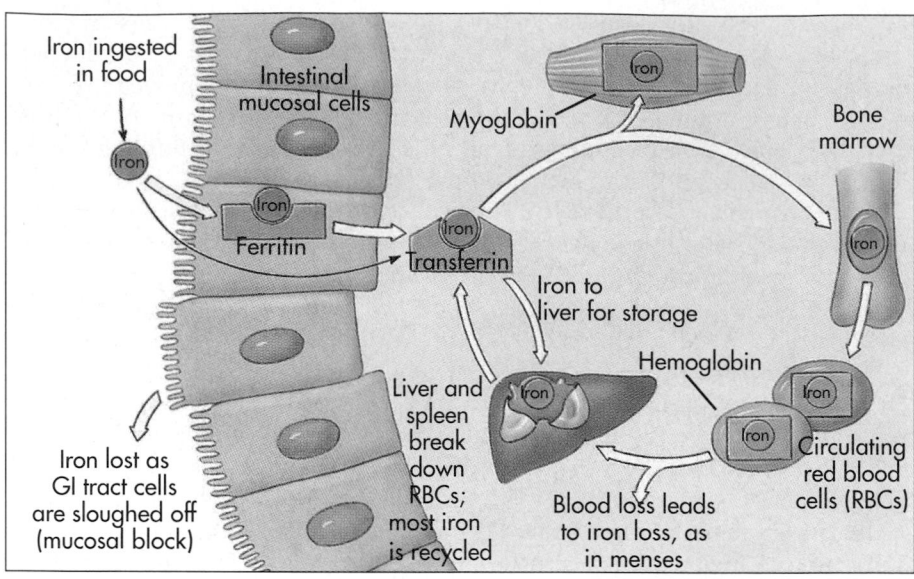

■ **FIGURE 12-1** Iron absorption and distribution. Iron binds with a protein called apoferritin to form ferritin when stored in cells. If the intestinal absorptive cells are sloughed before iron is absorbed from them, the iron is not absorbed into the blood. This allows the body to control the absorption of iron, especially nonheme iron.

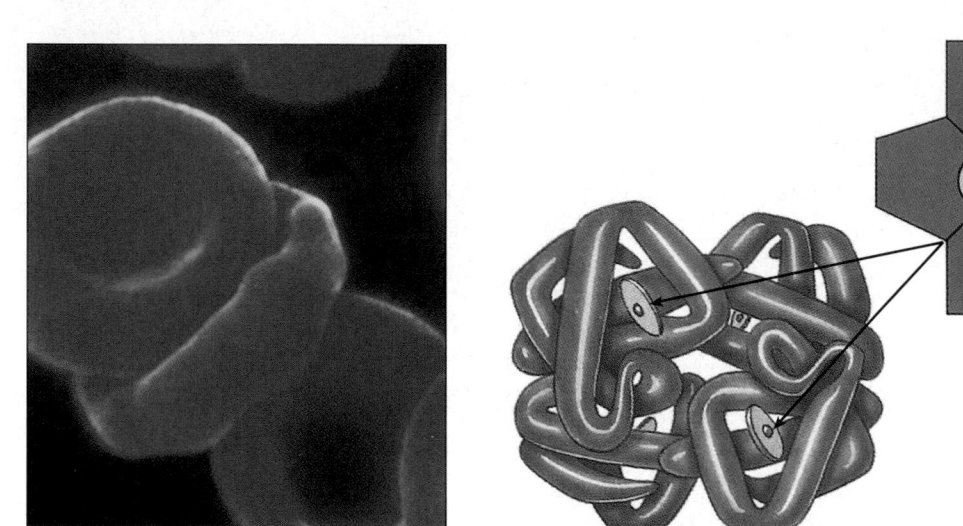

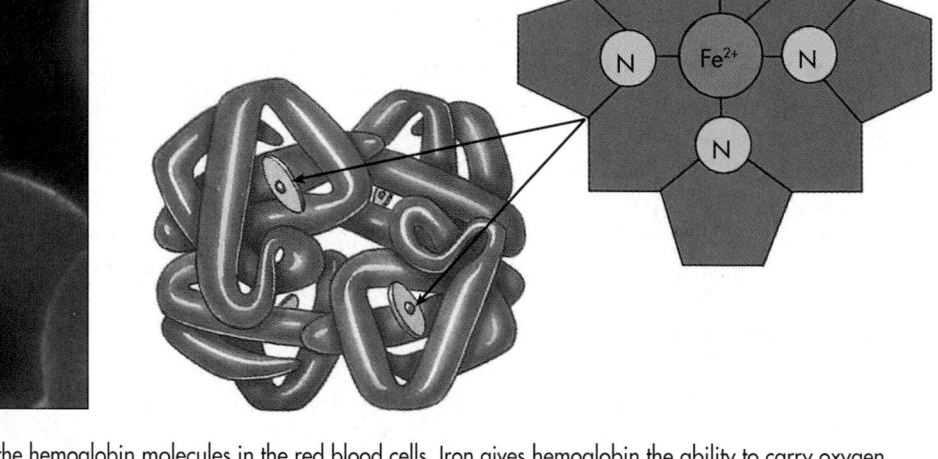

■ **FIGURE 12-2** Most iron in the body is present in the hemoglobin molecules in the red blood cells. Iron gives hemoglobin the ability to carry oxygen.

hemosiderin An insoluble iron-protein compound in the liver. Hemosiderin stores iron when the amount of iron in the body exceeds the storage capacity of ferritin.

and liver for storage in the form of ferritin. Each ferritin molecule can bind up to about 4000 iron atoms. This sequestering of iron is important because free iron atoms are very reactive and could catalyze widespread cell destruction. As the liver concentration of ferritin increases, associated with iron absorption in excess of needs, it is partly broken down by the liver cells. The iron then forms a more insoluble product called **hemosiderin.**

As iron is needed, it can be mobilized from body stores and enter the blood. It is thought that a deficiency of vitamin A may impair the body's ability to release iron from these stores. In addition, if dietary intake of iron is inadequate, eventually these iron stores become depleted. Only then do signs and symptoms of an iron deficiency appear.

Fortunately, the body conserves and reuses iron. As red blood cells die, macrophages in the liver, spleen, and other tissues release the iron from the red blood cells. The iron then attaches to transferrin in the blood and thus again becomes available either for storage as ferritin or ultimately for hemoglobin production. More than 90% of hemoglobin iron is recycled.

Adult men and nonmenstruating women lose about 1 mg of iron per day from the GI tract, urine, and skin. Women lose more iron because of menstrual blood loss. This varies among women, although each woman's menstrual blood loss generally is constant from month to month. When averaged over the entire month, iron losses for women are about 1.5 mg/day, depending on the amount of menstrual blood loss.

▪ Functions of Iron

Iron plays an important role in many parts of the body, including immune function, cognitive development, temperature regulation, energy metabolism, and work performance.[5]

Iron is a component of various proteins, which are involved in the transport and metabolism of oxygen. In hemoglobin, iron is the oxygen carrier of the blood, which transports oxygen from the lungs to all tissues and assists in the transport of some carbon dioxide back to the lungs for expiration. When the oxygen-carrying capacity of the blood begins to decline, the kidneys produce the hormone erythropoietin, which targets the bone marrow, so that more red blood cells will be produced. As a red blood cell matures, its nucleus is expelled, along with DNA (Fig. 12-3). Then the cell cannot replace itself. The red blood cell goes on to have a life span of about 120 days.

In myoglobin, iron provides oxygen to skeletal and cardiac muscle cells. Within the mitochondria, the electron transport chain uses iron as a component of cytochromes that carry electrons from $NADH + H^+$ and $FADH_2$ to molecular oxygen. The first step in the citric acid cycle, the conversion of citrate to isocitrate, requires an iron-containing enzyme. The limitation of these three processes in iron deficiency helps explain why it leads to fatigue. Iron found in cytochrome P450 in the endoplasmic reticulum controls alcohol metabolism, drug detoxification, and carcinogen excretion.

Iron in the peroxidase enzymes helps break down toxic oxygen species, such as hydrogen peroxide (H_2O_2). Peroxidase enzymes are found in leukocytes (white blood cells) and platelets (clotting factors in the blood) and are involved in eicosinoid metabolism (review Chapter 6 for details on eicosinoids). Iron also functions as a cofactor for some enzymes, including those involved in the synthesis of collagen and of various neurotransmitters (e.g., dopamine, epinephrine, norepinephrine, and serotonin).

▪ Iron Deficiency Anemia

If neither the diet nor body stores can supply the iron needed for hemoglobin synthesis, red blood cell synthesis is reduced. Eventually, the number of red blood cells falls so low that the amount of oxygen carried in the blood is decreased. Then a person exhibits anemia, which is characterized by a decreased oxygen-carrying capacity of the blood. Although there are many types of anemia, the major type found worldwide is iron deficiency anemia.[5]

Signs and Symptoms of Iron Deficiency Anemia

In iron deficiency anemia, the percentage of the total blood volume occupied by red blood cells, called the **hematrocrit,** falls below 34 to 37%. The blood hemoglobin concentration also declines to less than 10 to 11 g/100 ml of blood. A variety of diseases can reduce hemoglobin and hematocrit values, but, usually if both are reduced, the diagnosis is iron deficiency anemia. Further evidence of anemia is a decreased volume of each red blood cell.

Keep in mind that many people with mild iron deficiency experience no obvious problems, other than vague symptoms of tiredness, headache, irritability, or depression. These people are iron deficient without showing signs or symptoms of anemia. It takes a long time for iron deficiency anemia to develop. Overall, iron deficiency remains one of the most common and easily preventable nutrient deficiencies. It is im-

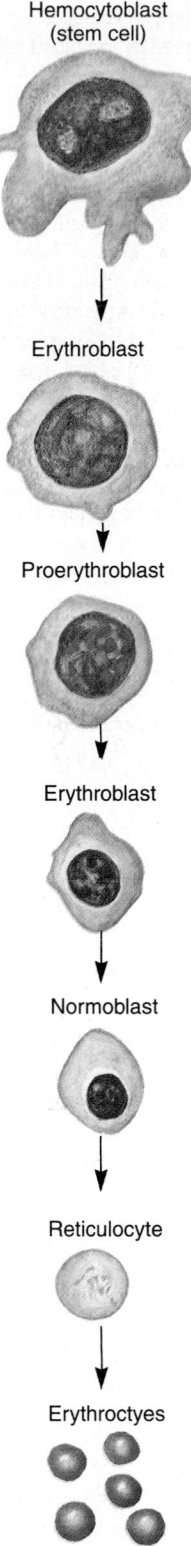

Hemocytoblast
(stem cell)

Erythroblast

Proerythroblast

Erythroblast

Normoblast

Reticulocyte

Erythroctyes

▪ **FIGURE 12-3** The formation of erythrocytes (red blood cells) begins with an undifferentiated stem cell in the bone marrow and proceeds through six steps until a mature cell is ready to be released into circulation. Note that the nucleus of the precursor cell is lost in the process.

hematocrit The percentage of total blood volume occupied by red blood cells.

*C*onsumption of dirt and similar non-food substances may lead to iron deficiency anemia because these can bind much of the iron in the GI tract. The practice of eating nonfood items, termed *pica*, is discussed in Chapter 16. Blood loss caused by intestinal and bloodborne parasite infections is another common cause of anemia among poor populations, especially when people do not wear shoes. Parasites, such as hookworms, can easily penetrate the soles of the feet and legs and enter the bloodstream. Although hookworm disease has been largely eradicated through improved sanitation in the United States and other industrialized nations, it continues to plague more than one-fifth of the world's population, mostly in tropical regions.

free erythrocyte protoporphyrins (FEP) A form of immature red blood cells released from the bone marrow containing suboptimal iron content. An elevated blood FEP reflects a decreased ability to make red blood cells and suggests iron deficiency anemia. Lead poisoning also raises blood FEP.

microcytic Describing red blood cells that are smaller than normal; literally, "small cell."

hypochromic Describing pale red blood cells lacking sufficient hemoglobin as a result of iron deficiency. Hypochromic cells have a reduced oxygen-carrying ability.

portant to identify individuals experiencing the effects of iron deficiency by use of regular physical examinations and to initiate treatment when needed. And, of course, prevention is the best treatment.

Other Causes of Iron Deficiency Anemia

Iron deficiency anemia can be caused by chronic blood loss from heavy menses, ulcers, hemorrhoids, and colon cancer. Iron deficiency anemia in men is usually linked to ulcers, colon cancer, or hemorrhoids.

The donation of 1 pint (0.5 L) of blood represents a loss of 200 to 250 mg of iron. It generally takes several months to replace this iron. Most healthy people can donate blood two to four times a year without harmful consequences; generally, women need the longer interval between donations to rebuild their iron stores. As a precaution, blood banks first screen potential donors' blood for evidence of anemia.

In many developing countries, a primary cause of iron deficiency anemia is the inefficient absorption of iron from vegetable foods. The diets in these countries are largely vegetarian because meat is too expensive for most people to afford. Iron deficiency and anemia eventually affect the majority of individuals in such populations. Recent studies show that cooking vegetables, such as broccoli, cabbage, red and green peppers, and tomatoes, in iron cookware increases the amount of digestible iron. Providing iron skillets and pots for households in less developed countries may be a useful method of decreasing iron deficiency.[1]

Measurement of Iron Status

The most sensitive measure of iron stores in the body currently available in healthcare settings is the concentration of ferritin in the blood. If ferritin is low, iron stores likely are low.

As iron deficiency proceeds, the total iron-binding capacity of blood proteins increases. Many iron-binding sites on the blood proteins become free, leaving more room than usual for extra iron to bind. At the same time, the bone marrow, which synthesizes red blood cells, begins releasing immature red blood cells called **free erythrocyte protoporphyrins (FEP).** As iron deficiency becomes more serious, hemoglobin and hematocrit values fall. The red blood cells are then very small and pale. This blood picture is referred to as a **microcytic** (small cell) **hypochromic** (pale) anemia (Fig. 12-4). Only very severe cases of iron deficiency ever reach this point.

In healthy individuals, serum ferritin is the most sensitive test of iron deficiency, with values of < 12 ng/ml indicating "no body iron stores" (recall that nanogram represents 10^{-9} g). However, serum ferritin does not provide useful information on tissue iron deficiency once iron stores are essentially exhausted. Now there is a new measure of iron status, but this has yet to make it into widespread clinical practice. The test is based on transferrin receptors found in the blood that can detect mild iron deficiency, as well as distinguish a deficiency of iron from other types of anemia. More than two-thirds of the body's iron is incorporated into hemoglobin in both developing precursor and mature red blood cells. The uptake of iron into these precursor cells depends on transferrin receptors, as it does for all other cells that take up iron. Measuring transferrin receptors in the blood then becomes a sensitive index of tissue iron availability, since these receptors increase in concentration continuously in response to a decrease in iron stores. Acute or chronic infections do not affect the results of the test (which is a problem with other iron tests), and the test is not responsive to other types of anemia. Its use is even more important during pregnancy, when other factors concerned with gestation can confuse the results of other tests of iron status.[3]

Treatment of Iron Deficiency Anemia

To speed the cure of iron deficiency anemia, medicinal forms of iron, such as ferrous sulfate, need to be ingested. In adults, 200 to 250 mg/day of iron is usually the

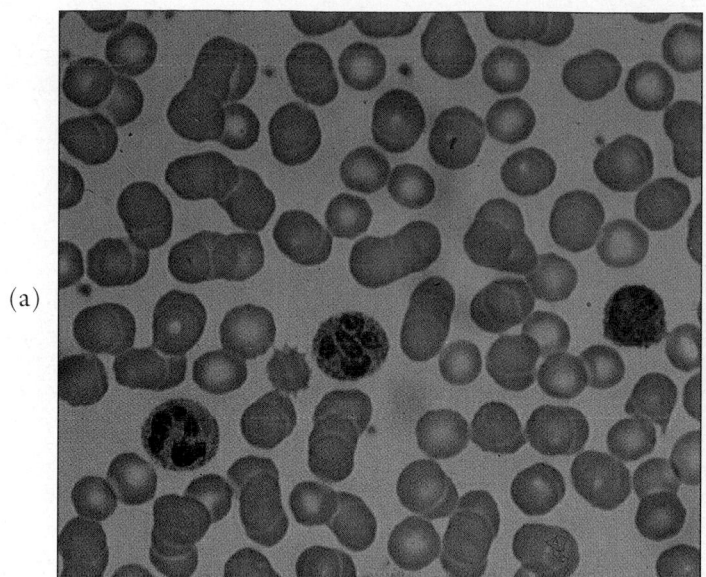
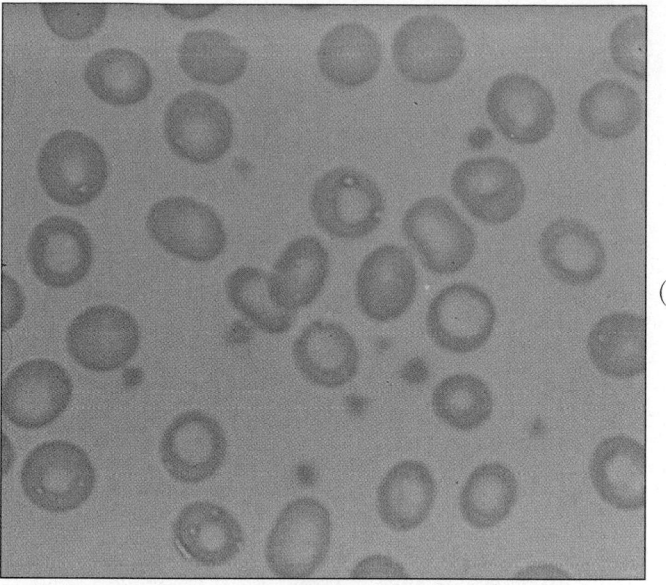

(a)

(b)

■ FIGURE 12-4 Iron deficiency anemia. (a) Normal cells—both cell size and color are normal. (b) Iron-deficient cells—both cell size and color are decreased. The loss of color stems from the lower amount of the pigment hemoglobin. The stages of iron depletion in the body progress from (1) low serum ferritin to (2) low transferrin saturation to (3) an increase in free erythrocyte protoporphyrins to (4) microcytic hypochromic anemia.

initial treatment dose, and 3 mg/kg body weight is usually a starting point for infants. Dosage can be cut in half once the blood hemoglobin concentration rises into the acceptable range. At least 6 months of therapy is needed to rebuild iron stores. A well-balanced diet may prevent iron deficiency anemia, but medicinal iron is a better cure. If oral iron is poorly absorbed, intravenous or intramuscular iron must be used, although the latter is not preferred. Symptoms such as diarrhea, constipation, nausea, and abdominal pain may be experienced by 10 to 20% of patients using oral iron therapy. Such symptoms can be reduced by taking iron supplements with meals, although this does decrease absorption by about half. (Iron absorption is also enhanced when supplements are taken with water or juice rather than tea, coffee, or milk.) Furthermore, a lower dose can be tried, with the time of treatment extended; the dose then can be increased as tolerance increases. Supplemental vitamin A can benefit iron-deficient people who also have marginal vitamin A status. Finally, the physician must find the cause of the anemia, since it is a condition that has more than 100 potential causes. However, treatment can begin before a cause is determined.[4]

■ Iron in Foods

Because much of the iron in animal foods is heme iron, the most bioavailable form, meats are the richest sources of iron. The major iron sources in American diets are animal foods, such as beef steaks, roasts, and hamburger (Fig. 12-5). The next greatest sources are bakery products, including white breads, rolls, and crackers. Most of the iron in these products is elemental forms of iron added to refined flour as part of the enrichment process. Only about 5% of this iron is absorbed.

Relative Bioavailability of Nonheme Iron

Foods providing the highest nutrient density for iron (mg/kcal) are spinach, oyster, liver, peas, legumes, and beef. However, as you've seen already, neither the total iron content nor the nutrient density of individual foods is a totally accurate guide for choosing dietary sources of iron. Rather, the bioavailability of the iron present in a meal, which depends on its form and the presence or absence of factors that influence absorption, and the body's need for iron ultimately determine how much iron actually is delivered to the body.

Dietary Sources of Iron

Food Item, Amount of iron (mg), and Bioavailability (in parentheses)	
Steamed oysters, 3	6.9 (High)
Cooked spinach, 1 cup	6.4 (Low)
Cooked kidney beans, 1 cup	5.2 (Low)
Sirloin steak, 5 oz	4.8 (High)
Pot roast, 4 oz	3.9 (High)
Fried beef liver, 2 oz	3.6 (High)
Prune juice, 8 oz	3.0 (Low)
Braunschweiger sausage, 1	2.7 (High)
Sauerkraut, ½ cup	1.7 (High)
Cooked green peas, ½ cup	1.3 (Low)

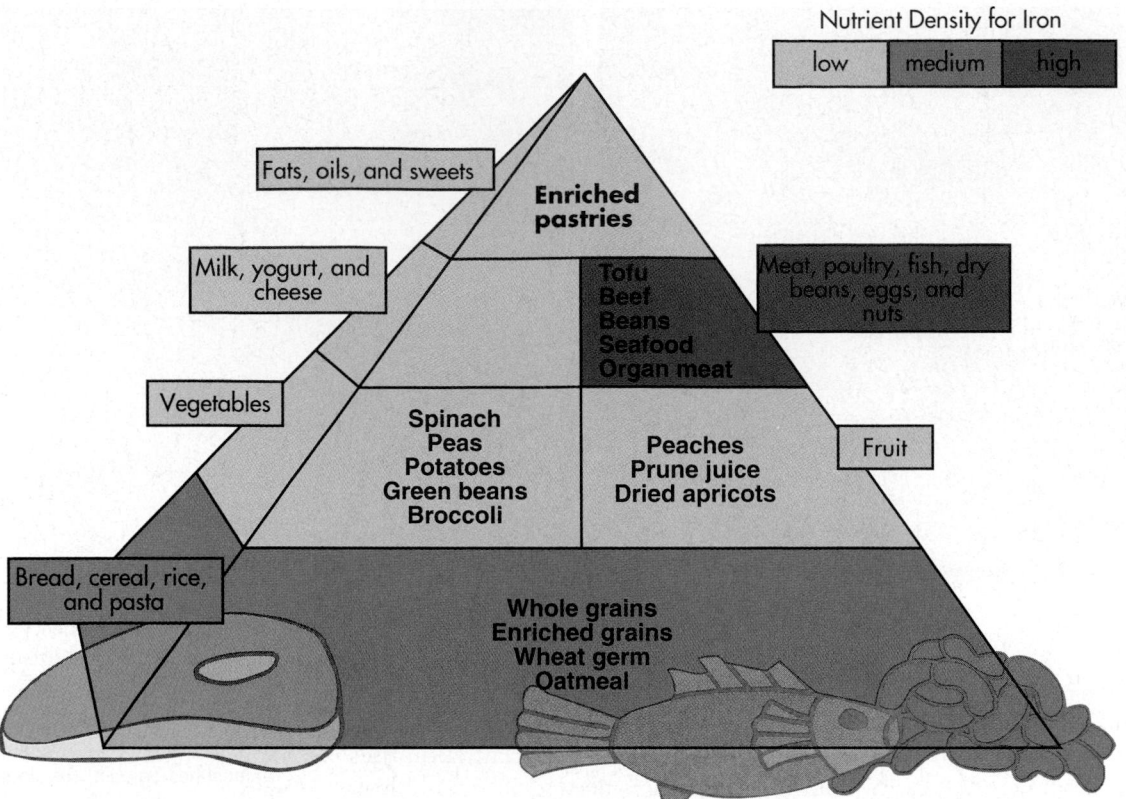

■ FIGURE 12-5 Food sources of iron from the Food Guide Pyramid. The meat, poultry, fish, dry beans, eggs, and nuts group is the best dietary sources of this nutrient. The heme iron in the meat, poultry, and fish group is especially well absorbed. The iron content of a food containing mostly nonheme iron is only an approximate measure of the amount delivered to body cells, as body need greatly influences the absorption of nonheme iron. The background color of each food group indicates the average nutrient density for iron in that group.

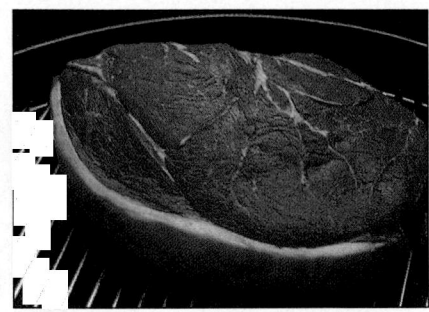

Red meat is a major source of iron in the American diet.

A common cause of iron deficiency anemia in children is an overreliance on milk, a very poor source of iron, and too little meat in their diets. In the United States, a major contributor to decreasing rates of iron deficiency anemia in preschool children has been the use of iron-fortified formulas and cereals in the Special Supplemental Food Program for Women, Infants, and Children (WIC program) (see Chapters 16 and 20).

As previously mentioned, another source of iron is cooking utensils. When acidic foods, such as tomato sauce, are cooked in iron cookware, some iron from the pan is taken up by the food. The replacement of iron cookware with stainless steel and aluminum cookware in recent times likely has decreased the amount of iron in the diet.[1]

■ Iron Needs

The Estimated Average Requirement for iron is 6 mg/day for men 19 and older and women over 50. For girls and women 19 to 50, the Estimated Average Requirement is 8.1 mg/day. The Estimated Average Requirement is based on the amount of iron needed for adequate tissue function without greatly increasing tissue stores. The Estimated Average Requirement is then increased to meet the needs projected for almost all healthy people (97th percentile), yielding the RDA of 8 mg/day for men 19 and older and women over 50, and 18 mg/day for girls and women 11 to 50.[12] (Throughout the rest of this chapter, consult the inside front cover for other age groups). The RDA values for iron are based on the assumption that about 18% of dietary iron is absorbed. If iron absorption exceeds that, less dietary iron is needed. On average, men consume about 17 mg, and women consume about 12 mg of iron per day.

The iron RDA is set higher for women primarily to account for menstrual blood loss. Women who menstruate more heavily and longer than "average" need even more dietary iron; those who have lighter and shorter flows may need less. The variation in menstrual blood loss makes it difficult to set an RDA for iron that is applicable to most women.

People who find out they are not consuming the RDA for iron are advised to make dietary changes, so that they will meet the RDA. Use of a fortified breakfast cereal or multivitamin-mineral supplement with iron would be helpful. Whether persistent intakes below the RDA actually harm health is difficult to determine, as need drives absorption efficiency. Furthermore, despite the availability of very sensitive measures of iron stores in the body, we lack the knowledge to translate this information into predictors of health status.

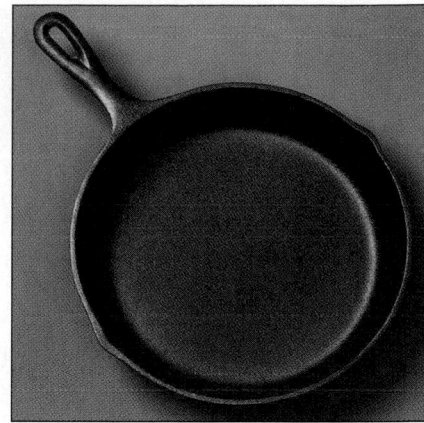

Cooking in an iron skillet adds some iron to the diet.

■ North Americans at Risk for Iron Deficiency and Related Anemia

Iron deficiency is most common when iron needs greatly exceed normal intake— such as during infancy and the preschool years, puberty, and women's childbearing years. Studies show that infants with iron deficiency anemia have decreased mental and motor development. Further, these infants continue to test lower than their peers years later, even after 2 to 3 months of treatment for the iron deficiency. The most common age for iron deficiency anemia is 6 months to 2 years.[4] About 3% of infants and toddlers experience iron deficiency anemia. In early childhood, iron deficiency interferes with longitudinal growth, weight gain, and behavioral development. Behavioral problems associated with childhood anemia are thought to be caused by interruptions in nerve-impulse transmission. Inadequate iron stores can also decrease cognitive development and intellectual performance, work performance, and immune status, even before a person actually becomes anemic.[5]

In the United States, 9 to 11% of adolescent girls and women in their childbearing years have scant or no iron stores and thus are considered to be iron deficient. In most cases, iron-deficient women actually have hemoglobin values that are normal; thus, they do not experience iron deficiency anemia. Such women, however, have no iron stores to draw from in times of illness, injury, or pregnancy. Iron deficiency during pregnancy is especially dangerous because it significantly increases the risk of maternal and infant death, as well as **preterm** birth. Repeated pregnancies pose a special challenge to women to maintain adequate iron stores. During these critical life stages, the risk for iron deficiency anemia is greatest either because growth, which is accompanied by increased blood volume and muscle mass, increases iron needs or because low energy intakes make it difficult to consume enough iron. Female athletes, distance runners, and vegetarian athletes are other groups of individuals who appear to be at risk for developing altered body iron stores. These groups should maintain an adequate consumption of iron from the diet and consider the use of iron supplements under the care of a physician.[6]

The North American diet contains about 5 to 7 mg of iron per 1000 kcal. Thus, men, who commonly have daily energy intakes of 2000 to 3000 kcal, generally meet their RDA for iron and achieve a good iron status. Most women, on the other hand, can't consume 3000 kcal daily and still maintain healthy weight. Thus, they have difficulty consuming 18 mg of iron daily unless they include nutrient-dense forms of iron (e.g., fortified breakfast cereals and red meat) in their diets. If a change in diet does not suffice, a supplement should be used, under a physician's scrutiny. Inadequate iron stores and even iron deficiency anemia are found among all social strata, not just among the poor. Vegans also should pay special attention to their intakes. In addition, athletes may incur a type of anemia called **sports anemia,** as is discussed in Chapter 14. Athletes should have their blood hemoglobin and other indicators of iron status monitored to ensure adequate status.

Iron is the only nutrient for which adult women have a greater RDA than adult men.

preterm Born before 37 weeks of gestation; also known as premature.

sports anemia A decrease in the blood's ability to carry oxygen found in otherwise healthy athletes. It may be caused by iron loss in perspiration and feces, red blood cell destruction due to the impact of the foot striking the ground during exercise, and increased blood volume.

Expert Opinion

IRON OVERLOAD: TOO MUCH OF A GOOD THING

Barbara A. Bowman, Ph.D., and Giuseppina Imperatore, M.D., Ph.D.

Nutritionists consider iron to be the gold standard of micronutrients, because we know more about the dietary intake, metabolism, and nutritional requirements of iron than any other trace element. Despite this extensive knowledge and the array of sophisticated techniques for evaluating iron nutrition, however, more than 1 billion people suffer from iron deficiency, which is the most prevalent micronutrient deficiency in the world.

Iron deficiency is also a significant health problem in the United States, especially in young children and women of childbearing age, particularly pregnant women. Iron deficiency is a special concern for women and children because one of its major side effects is anemia. Anemia, which is defined as a low concentration of hemoglobin in blood, leads to decreased work capacity in adults, developmental delays and behavioral disturbances in children, increased susceptibility to infection, and increased mortality in both children and adults. In the United States, about 3.3 million women of childbearing age and 240,000 children age 1–2 years have iron deficiency anemia, the most severe form of iron deficiency.

Iron overload lies at the opposite end of the spectrum of iron status. If untreated, iron overload disease, like iron deficiency, can lead to illness and even death. Let's examine iron overload in more detail.

ETIOLOGY OF IRON OVERLOAD

What causes iron overload? The major cause of iron overload in the United States is hereditary hemochromatosis, a genetic condition that affects about one person out of every 200 to 500 in the United States. Iron overload can also occur in chronic liver disease due to alcohol abuse, viral infections, and chronic anemias requiring frequent blood transfusions (e.g., thalassemia). The specific genetic lesion in hereditary hemochromatosis was identified in 1996, and two major mutations have been identified. The fundamental defect involves the regulation of iron absorption. In hereditary hemochromatosis, iron absorption is excessive, and iron absorption is not reduced when iron status is normal. The human body does not have a mechanism for eliminating excess iron. Therefore, after many years of absorbing too much iron, excessive amounts of iron can accumulate in the body, leading to

iron overload and tissue injury. If undetected and untreated for many years, iron levels can build up in the liver, heart, pancreas, joints, and pituitary gland and can eventually lead to liver disease, heart disease, diabetes, arthritis, and hypopituitarism with hypogonadism. People at a late stage of iron overload may have skin that turns bronze or gray. The diseases caused by iron overload usually appear by age 40 to 60, although some people are affected earlier and others never become ill. With early detection and treatment, organ damage can be prevented. However, without lifelong treatment, organ damage may be permanent and life-threatening.

Up to 1 million Americans, mostly people of European descent, have the mutation for hemochromatosis. However, far fewer actually develop iron overload. Some people have the mutation but never get iron overload. This is probably because clinical expression of iron overload depends on additional factors, including the severity of the metabolic defect, the amount and type of iron in the diet, other dietary factors that enhance or inhibit iron absorption, environmental factors, and blood loss (menstruation, for example).

■ Toxicity of Iron

The Upper Level for iron is 45 mg/day, based on the ability of larger amounts to cause gastric irritation. Although not as common as iron deficiency, iron overload can be serious because it can easily lead to toxic symptoms. Even a large single dose of iron of this amount or more can be life-threatening to a 1-year-old. Children are frequently victims of iron poisoning because iron pills and vitamin supplements containing iron are tempting targets on kitchen tables and in cabinets. FDA has recently ruled that all iron supplements must carry a warning about its toxicity to children, and supplements with greater than 30 mg/tablet must be individually wrapped. The cause of death in cases of acute iron poisoning is respiratory collapse due to shock.

DIAGNOSIS AND TREATMENT OF IRON OVERLOAD

Early detection and lifelong treatment can prevent the complications of hemochromatosis. The major approach to diagnosis is a series of blood tests to measure the amount of iron in the blood, such as the extent to which transferrin is saturated with iron. The same blood tests are used during treatment to monitor the amount of iron in the body and the response to treatment. Genetic testing is also being studied. However, not everyone with the mutation develops iron overload. Because of concern about the need for privacy and possible discrimination in employment and insurance, genetic screening for hereditary hemochromatosis is not recommended. People who have been diagnosed with hereditary hemochromatosis should tell their family members and urge them to get tested, too.

Treatment of iron overload is straightforward, safe, and effective. After they have been diagnosed, people with iron overload have blood removed regularly, usually a unit or pint of blood, to remove the excess iron that has accumulated. The procedure, which is called phlebotomy, is exactly the same as when you donate blood. The frequency of phlebotomy depends on how much iron has built up.

When iron overload is first diagnosed, phlebotomy may be needed every week or two. When accumulated iron has been reduced to a safe amount, phlebotomy may be needed only a few times a year, but it must be continued. Health-care providers use blood testing to determine when phlebotomy treatment is needed.

People with hemochromatosis must be sure to follow their doctor's advice and get tested regularly to prevent complications from developing. For most, periodic phlebotomy will be needed for the rest of their lives. It is also important for people with hemochromatosis to avoid alcohol and raw shellfish, which can damage the liver. Dietary supplements that contain iron must not be used, and foods highly fortified with iron, should be avoided. The same advice may be given as well for vitamin C supplements. Most people with hereditary hemochromatosis are not aware that they have a predisposition to accumulating excessive amounts of iron. If such a person were to decide to use iron supplements to increase his or her energy or to combat fatigue, for example, iron accumulation and tissue damage could be accelerated and enhanced, increasing the risk of chronic disease. For this reason, iron supplements should not be used indiscriminately but should be used only when iron deficiency has been diagnosed by a health professional and iron therapy is prescribed.

As you can see, with iron more than perhaps any other nutrient, it is critical to meet daily requirements for the proper nutrient intake—not too little, not too much, but just the right amount. Different individuals have different needs. People who don't consume enough iron to meet their needs can develop iron deficiency and eventually anemia. On the other hand, for some people, consuming too much iron every day can lead to serious illness, including death. Hereditary hemochromatosis is one of the first examples of how a gene interacts with nutrition (iron intake) to affect risk of disease. As the public and health professionals become more aware of hereditary hemochromatosis, iron overload can be detected earlier, treated more effectively, and, ultimately, prevented.

Drs. Imperatore and Bowman are epidemiologists at the Centers for Disease Control and Prevention in Atlanta, GA. Dr. Imperatore is a genetic epidemiologist and Dr. Bowman is Chief of the Chronic Disease Nutrition Branch. Both are especially interested in the disease hemochromatosis.

Smaller doses of iron (but still greater than what is needed) over a long period can also cause problems. A form of iron toxicity, for example, has been observed in an African tribe that brews beer in iron pots. Some people of Mediterranean descent have a type of anemia caused by increased destruction of red blood cells; low dose iron therapy used to treat this disease can lead to toxicity symptoms. Repeated blood transfusions also lead to iron toxicity.

In addition, iron toxicity accompanies the genetic disease called hereditary **hemochromatosis.** Dr. Barbara Bowman and Dr. Giuseppina Imperatore discuss this problem in detail in their Expert Opinion.

hemochromatosis A disorder of iron metabolism characterized by increased absorption, saturation of iron-binding proteins, and deposition of hemosiderin in the liver tissue.

Hemosiderosis is the storage of excess iron in the form of hemosiderin. This form of excess iron is not associated with the organ damage of hemochromatosis, as excess iron is stored in areas of normal storage. In hemochromatosis, the iron accumulates in body organs outside normal areas and causes organ deterioration, such as in the liver and heart.

CONCEPT CHECK

Iron absorption depends mostly on its form and the body's need for it. Absorption is affected by a mucosal block, but excess iron intake can override the system, leading to toxicity. Iron absorption increases somewhat in the presence of vitamin C and decreases in the presence of large amounts of some components of grain fiber, such as phytic acid. Iron is most important in synthesizing hemoglobin and myoglobin, in supporting immune function, and in energy metabolism. An iron deficiency can cause decreased red blood cell synthesis, which can lead to a form of anemia. It is particularly important for women of childbearing age to consume adequate iron, primarily to replace that lost in menstrual blood. Sources include red meat, pork, liver, enriched grains and cereals, and oysters. Iron toxicity usually results from a genetic disorder called hemochromatosis. This disease causes the overabsorption and accumulation of iron, which can result in severe liver and heart damage.

ZINC (ZN)

Although zinc has been recognized as an essential nutrient in animals since the early 1900s, zinc deficiency was first recognized in humans in the early 1960s in Egypt and Iran. The deficiency was determined to be the cause of growth retardation and inadequate sexual development in humans. Curiously, the dietary zinc content was fairly high. However, the customary diet contained almost exclusively unleavened bread and little animal protein. Unleavened bread is very high in phytic acid and other factors that decrease zinc bioavailability. Yeast fermentation in the preparation of bread dough reduces the effect of phytic acid by 10-fold. In addition, parasite infestation and the practice of eating dirt also contributed to the these cases of severe zinc deficiency observed in humans.

In the United States, zinc deficiencies were first observed in the early 1970s in hospitalized patients receiving total parenteral nutrition. Originally, zinc was not added to the intravenous solutions, but the protein source in the solutions was based on milk protein or blood fibrin, which are naturally rich in zinc. When the solutions were later changed to include mostly isolated amino acids as the protein source, zinc-deficiency symptoms quickly developed. This isolated amino acid source of protein is very low in zinc.

■ Absorption, Transport, Storage, and Excretion of Zinc

Zinc is absorbed throughout the small intestine, with the jejunum being responsible for most of the absorption. Factors that affect the absorption of zinc include the body's need for zinc and the composition of the meal in which zinc is consumed. The absorption and transport of zinc utilizes a two-step process. The first step is the uptake or membrane binding at the mucosal surface. The second step is the transport of zinc across the mucosal cell and the release into the bloodstream, but the process is not completely understood. After entering the blood, zinc binds to blood proteins, such as albumin, for transport to the liver. The liver releases zinc into general circulation bound to proteins, such as globulins. Absorbed zinc in the body is classified as functional zinc and little, if any, is held in storage.[22] The main organ involved in zinc metabolism is the liver. About one-third of the absorbed zinc enters the liver; the remaining zinc is distributed throughout the body, mainly in muscle and bone.

metallothionein A protein that binds and regulates the release of zinc and copper in intestinal and liver cells.

When zinc is absorbed into intestinal cells, it induces the synthesis of **metallothionein;** a protein that binds zinc in much the same way that ferritin binds iron. Homeostatic regulation of zinc absorption may partly be due to the synthesis of metallothionein, since it hinders the movement of zinc from intestinal cells. If zinc is not transferred to the blood from the intestinal cells within 2 to 5 days, it is sloughed off along with the cell and excreted. Thus, a mucosal block works against the overabsorption of zinc and iron, but much more so in the case of iron (Fig. 12-6). If large doses of zinc are taken, they override the mucosal block. Luckily for overconsumers, zinc is also readily excreted via the pancreas into the intestinal tract and leaves the body by the feces. It is also excreted in small amounts in urine and sweat.

Like iron absorption, zinc absorption is influenced by the types of food ingested. Absorption is more likely when animal protein sources are consumed, when the body's zinc needs are elevated, or when small amounts are consumed. The RDA for zinc is based on absorption of about 40% of intake.

Whereas inadequate dietary intake of zinc may be the cause of poor zinc status in some, inhibitors of zinc absorption are likely the most common causative factor in depleted zinc status. As previously mentioned, phytic acid decreases zinc absorption, as do high intakes of calcium. Studies have found that up to a 50% decrease in zinc absorption occurs when calcium supplements are taken with a meal. For this reason, postmenopausal women and other groups who take calcium supplements may need to increase their zinc intake, as well as avoid use of calcium supplements at meals that are rich in zinc. The interaction of calcium and zinc is not fully understood, and more studies are needed on individual population groups. Certain milk proteins also have been shown to have a negative effect on zinc absorption. Finally, zinc is known to compete with copper and iron for absorption. Although this competition can be harmful if excess zinc is routinely consumed, it can also be advantageous as part of the treatment of disease, such as Wilson's disease, in which there is limited copper excretion (this will be discussed further in a following section on zinc toxicity).

Zinc intakes worldwide are generally low. Toasting cereals also reduces zinc absorption, as it binds with flour constituents. Because most people worldwide rely on cereal grains for their sources of protein, energy, and zinc, finding adequate zinc

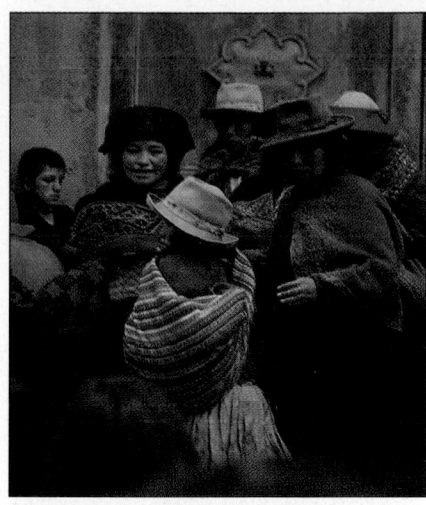

Minimal intakes of protein and zinc limit the growth of people worldwide.

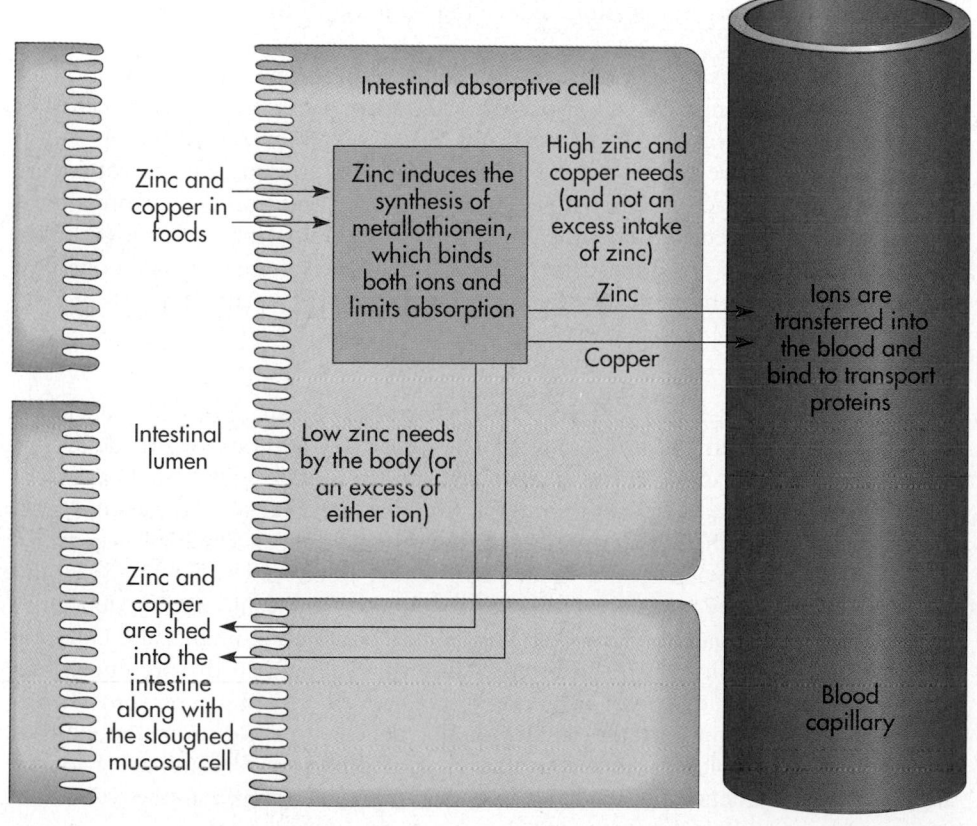

FIGURE 12-6 Zinc and copper absorption. Both minerals influence the absorption of the other. The effect is most obvious with excessive zinc intake, which greatly depresses copper absorption by inducing the synthesis of metallothionein; this protein avidly binds copper. The short life span of the intestinal absorptive cells also influences the absorption of these minerals, since any metallothionein-bound copper or zinc is sloughed off along with the intestinal cell into the intestinal tract.

Many companies are singing the praises of zinc as a cold remedy. Products such as Cold-Eeze are lozenges that contain zinc, and their claims are based largely on a study done at the Cleveland Clinic with 100 participants. The 50 individuals in the experimental group took about 13 mg of zinc via the lozenges every 2 hours for the duration of their symptoms. Cold symptoms subsided after 4 days in the experimental group and 7 days in the control group. Unfortunately, nausea was a common side effect of the zinc lozenges. In addition, out of 10 other similar studies, only half show beneficial results from zinc. This may be due to the bioavailability of various forms of zinc or simply to the more bitter flavor of the lozenges in the experimental versus the control group (placebo effect). In any case, more information is needed before zinc is recognized as a reputable treatment for the common cold.[20]

CRITICAL THINKING

As noted above, zinc lozenges have received much attention as a treatment for the common cold. You tell a classmate that you do not feel that the evidence is convincing enough to recommend this practice to the general public. Your friend would like to know what it would take to convince you that zinc is a reasonable treatment for the common cold.

sources and maintaining adequate zinc intakes is a problem. And, since zinc and iron are most available from the same foods—protein-rich foods—individuals with iron deficiency are also at very high risk for zinc deficiency.

▪ Functions of Zinc

Since zinc is present in every living cell in the body, it has many diverse biological functions, primarily as components of various enzymes. Nearly 100 enzymes require zinc as a cofactor for optimal activity. Adequate zinc intake is necessary to support many body functions, such as:[22]

- Nucleic acid synthesis and function
- Protein metabolism, wound healing, and growth
- Immune function (intakes in excess of the RDA do not provide any extra benefit to immune function)
- Development of sexual organs and mineralization of bone-matrix
- Storage, release, and function of insulin
- Cell membrane structure and function
- Component of superoxide dismutase, an enzyme that aids in the prevention of oxidative damage to cells

Clinicians treating malnourished children observed that weight gain occurs much faster when the children consume zinc supplements containing about three times the RDA. These findings highlight the importance of zinc for growth. Zinc is also important for behavioral development in infants.

Two enzymes that require zinc are carbonic anhydrase and alcohol dehydrogenase. Carbonic anhydrase combines water (H_2O) and carbon dioxide (CO_2) to form carbonic acid (H_2CO_3); this reaction is crucial for maintaining acid-base balance in the blood. Alcohol dehydrogenase converts alcohol to acetaldehyde.

Current areas of zinc research include the potential to decrease diarrhea and malaria among poor people in developing countries, reduce head and neck cancer via a role in apoptosis (programmed cell death), slow the progression of macular degeneration of the eye, and possibly reduce the duration of the common cold. More research is needed in these areas.

Zinc also functions at the gene level. For some time, a nonenzymatic function for zinc in special proteins has been suspected. The term *zinc finger* has been coined to describe the pattern of two amino acids (histidine and cysteine) surrounding zinc in those proteins that are known to bind to DNA in the cell nucleus. These proteins are called transcription factors. They act as a switch turning on or off gene expression at special sites of the gene. It takes the zinc to bind this transcription factor to DNA. Although there is no proof that zinc fingers actually exist, there have been observations that several hormones exert their action through this mechanism.

▪ Zinc Deficiency

Severe zinc deficiency is rare, but many people are at risk for marginal zinc deficiency, which is extremely difficult to diagnose.[12] The signs and symptoms of zinc deficiency are nonspecific and can include inadequate growth, an acnelike rash, diarrhea, lack of appetite, weight loss, a decline in immune function, delayed wound healing, a reduced sense of taste, hair loss, mental confusion, the delivery of low-birth-weight infants by pregnant women, and inadequate sexual development in children and adolescents (Fig. 12-7). Reduced learning ability also may result, as zinc deficiency can be a cause of impaired neuropsychological function among infants and children, as is seen in iron deficiency. A persistent skin rash, especially in the presence of an inadequate diet, should prompt a clinician to evaluate zinc status in a person. The variety of signs and symptoms associated with zinc deficiency is not surprising, considering the diverse biological functions that zinc encompasses. Preliminary evidence suggests that zinc deficiency results in a decreased production of lymphocytes. Zinc deficiency also rapidly decreases antibody (B lymphocyte) and cell-mediated (T lymphocyte) responses in humans.[13]

Zinc in Foods

In general, protein-rich diets are also rich in zinc. Americans get about 70% of their dietary zinc from animal foods. Lean meats—especially beef, other red meats, and shellfish—are among the best zinc sources because zinc from these animal sources is not bound by phytic acid.

Foods with the highest nutrient density for zinc (mg/kcal) are oysters, wheat germ, crab, shrimp, beef and pork, liver, turkey, and legumes (Fig. 12-8). Plant sources of zinc, such as nuts, beans, and whole grains, can also deliver substantial amounts of zinc to body cells. Zinc is not part of the enrichment process, so refined flours are not a good source. Zinc is likely adequate in breast milk until an infant reaches 6 months of age, at which time weaning foods should contain zinc. Although zinc in foods is the preferred source of zinc, zinc in supplement form has shown to be an effective way to maintain zinc status in those at risk of deficiency.

Zinc Needs

The Estimated Average Requirement for zinc is 9.4 mg/day for men and 6.8 mg/day for women. This is based on the amount of dietary zinc needed to replace daily losses in feces, skin, urine, and other routes. The Estimated Average Requirement is increased by 20% to account for individual variability, yielding the adult

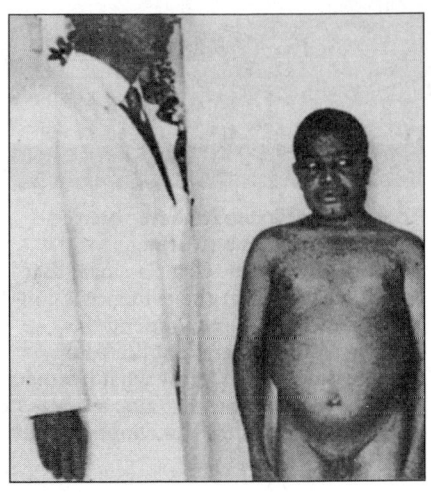

FIGURE 12-7 An example of zinc deficiency. An Egyptian farm boy, age 16 years and 49 inches tall, with dwarfism and inadequate sexual development associated with a zinc deficiency.

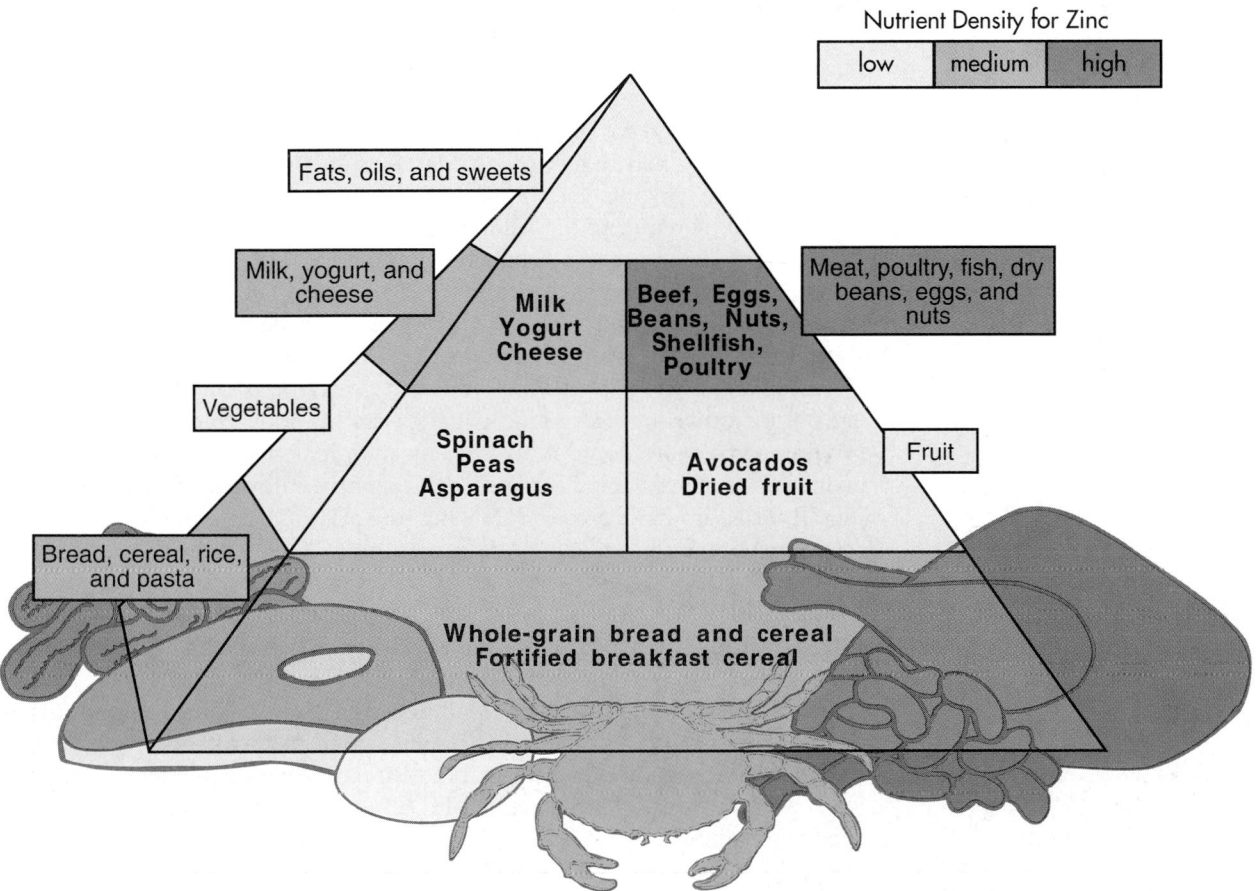

FIGURE 12-8 Food sources of zinc from the Food Guide Pyramid. The meat, poultry, fish, dry beans, eggs, and nuts group includes the best dietary sources of this nutrient. Some zinc is supplied by whole grains and fortified breakfast cereals from the bread, cereal, rice, and pasta group. The background color of each food group indicates the average nutrient density for zinc in that group.

Dietary Sources of Zinc

Food Item and Amount	Zinc (mg)
Steamed oysters, 6	76.4
Sirloin steak, 4 oz	7.4
Pot roast, 3 oz	6.3
Lamb chop, 3 oz	5.2
Canned crab meat, 4 oz	4.6
Wheat germ, ¼ cup	3.5
Fried beef liver, 2 oz	3.1
Roasted turkey, 3 oz	2.6
Cooked blackeyed peas, 1 cup	2.2
Shrimp, 4 oz	1.8
Milk, 1 cup	1.0

A rare disease, acrodermatitis enteropathica, results from an inherited inability to absorb zinc. Signs and symptoms in infants include rash, hair loss, depressed immune response, lack of appetite, and inadequate growth. This disease can be treated with supplements of zinc in amounts of about 30 to 45 mg/day, about 15 to 20 times the needs for infants.

Z inc deficiency in developing countries is becoming a growing concern, because research is showing that zinc deficiency is related not only to decreased growth but also to increased morbidity. Recent studies have shown zinc supplementation to be effective in reducing the morbidity associated with infections in infants and children, possibly by improving immune function.[19] As previously mentioned, adequate zinc status may decrease the duration of diarrhea, a major cause of death in developing countries.

RDA for zinc of 11 mg/day for men and 8 mg/day for women.[12] The average adult intake of zinc is 13 mg and 9 mg daily for men and women, respectively. Although some women may have marginal intakes, there is no evidence of widespread moderate or severe zinc deficiencies among otherwise healthy adult women or men in North America. Homeostatic control of absorption and excretion helps maintain persons in zinc balance even when intakes are somewhat lower than those furnished by typical diets. However, the long-term effects of marginal zinc intakes are not known.

■ North Americans at Risk for Zinc Deficiency

Zinc deficiencies have been recognized in many groups of the population in both less-developed and industrialized countries. Worldwide, protein-energy malnutrition is an important cause of zinc deficiency (see Chapter 20). Zinc deficiencies are also commonly found in hospital patients with severe malabsorption syndromes. Sickle cell disease increases zinc needs by destroying massive numbers of red blood cells, which contain a significant amount of zinc. In addition, children aged 1 to 3 years, adolescent females, pregnant women, vegans, alcoholics, or people with anorexia nervosa or over the age of 70 can be deficient in zinc because of either an inadequate overall nutrient intake or a diet low or lacking in animal foods.[8] Greater zinc intake in these people can sometimes increase their appetite and sense of taste. Older individuals appear to be at particular risk for zinc deficiency because of poorly fitting dentures, poor appetite, decreased consumption of animal products, low income, interaction of zinc with medications, and changing nutrient requirements associated with changes in physiology and metabolism with aging.

In the United States, the symptoms of zinc deficiency have been observed in groups of middle-income and low-income children exhibiting inadequate growth. As mentioned, zinc supplementation can improve growth and appetite, especially if the child is stunted for his or her age. There is also substantial evidence that zinc supplementation may reduce the impact of many diseases, such as sickle cell disease, kidney disease, chronic gastrointestinal disorders, and HIV infection or AIDS (in this last case by reducing the fall in immune system function).

Although many Americans may have a marginal zinc status, there is a lack of sensitive clinical measures for determining zinc status. The available clinical tests register a zinc deficiency only when body stores are very depleted. The assessment of zinc status is difficult because the amount of zinc in the blood does not reflect body stores, and no test using a zinc-containing enzyme is currently accepted.[12] More clinical measures are being studied, such as the body zinc clearance test, and are proving to be more useful in diagnosing marginal zinc deficiency. Although this is promising, further testing is required. Currently, information regarding zinc nutritional status can be obtained only when dietary data are combined with biochemical, anthropometric, and clinical information.[22]

■ Toxicity of Zinc

The Upper Level set for zinc is 40 mg/day, based on the ability of zinc to interfere with copper status as measured by a fall in the activity of the form of superoxide dismutase that contains copper. Zinc does this by stimulating the synthesis of the mineral-binding protein metallothionein, which in turn binds copper in intestinal cells and lessens its transfer into the bloodstream. Zinc supplements at approximately 5 to 20 times the RDA can reduce HDL-cholesterol, perhaps by interfering with copper metabolism. That is disturbing for two reasons. First, it is associated with an increased risk of developing cardiovascular disease (see Chapter 6). Second, it is common for people who take zinc supplements to consume this amount. Again, this shows why mineral supplements should not be consumed in excess of the Upper Level unless under close scrutiny of a physician. Zinc intakes over 100 mg/day also result in diarrhea, cramps, nausea, vomiting, and depressed immune system function, especially if intake exceeds 2 g/day.

■ COPPER (CU)

For many decades, copper has been widely accepted as an essential trace element required for survival by all organisms from bacterial cells to humans. This trace element has a variety of roles in cells and organs, including contributing to the activity of many enzymes and aiding in iron metabolism. Copper homeostasis is maintained primarily by excretion rather than by absorption. Copper, like other essential trace minerals, can be toxic at the cellular, tissue, and organ levels when present in excess.

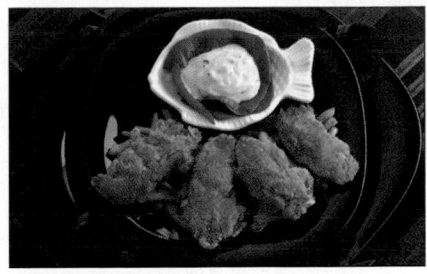

Oysters are an excellent source of iron, zinc, and copper.

■ Absorption, Transport, Storage, and Excretion of Copper

Copper is absorbed primarily in the stomach and duodenum. About 12 to 75% of dietary copper is absorbed, with higher intakes associated with lower absorption. Phytates, dietary fiber, and high dose supplements of vitamin C, zinc, and iron may all interfere with copper absorption. Protein carriers, such as ceruloplasmin, albumin, and transcuperin transport newly absorbed copper to body tissues in two phases. In the first phase, copper is transported from the intestine to the liver and kidney. During the second phase, copper travels from the liver, and perhaps the kidney, to other organs bound to globulins. Copper is also present in and transported by other body fluids, including those bathing the brain and central nervous system.

Most of the copper in the body is found in the liver, brain, blood, skeletal muscle, and skeleton, including the bone marrow. The cellular uptake and intracellular distribution of copper is a precisely orchestrated process. Much of the absorbed copper recycles back and forth daily between certain tissues and the digestive tract. Copper homeostasis is coordinated by several proteins to ensure that it is delivered to specific organs and copper-requiring proteins.[26] This inhibits the release of free copper ions, which could cause damage to cellular components. Bile is the primary route of excretion from the body. Little copper is stored in the body.

■ Functions of Copper

Copper increases iron absorption by helping form the protein ceruloplasmin (also known as ferroxidase I). This compound facilitates the binding of ferric iron (Fe^{3+}) to the protein transferrin in the bloodstream, and so helps iron leave the intestinal cell and enter the bloodstream.

Copper is part of an enzyme that forms cross-links in collagen and elastin—connective tissue proteins. In laboratory animals with a copper deficiency, blood vessels rupture because collagen is not available to form the important connective tissue network needed to strengthen blood vessels (review Fig. 10–11 in Chapter 10 for a review of collagen metabolism). The terminal enzyme in the electron-transport chain (cytochrome C oxidase) contains copper. This enzyme contributes to the formation of water from hydrogen and oxygen, in turn allowing for the formation of ATP.

Copper is also part of enzymes that convert dopamine to norepinephrine. In addition, copper-containing enzymes are needed in the formation and maintenance of myelin, the insulation material around nerves. One of the body's major scavengers for superoxide free radicals, the enzyme superoxide dismutase, also contains copper and zinc. (This is true for both the intracellular and extracellular forms of the enzyme.) Finally, copper participates in immune system function, red and white blood cell maturation, blood clotting, bone strength, brain development, and cholesterol and glucose metabolism.

■ Copper Deficiency

Clinically-evident copper deficiency, for most population groups, is not believed to be a widespread public health concern. Copper deficiency is usually the consequence of decreased copper stores at birth, inadequate dietary copper intake, poor absorption, elevated requirements induced by rapid growth, or increased copper losses.[7]

Oat Flakes

Nutrition Facts

Serving Size 1 cup (55g)
Servings Per Container About 8

Amount Per Serving	Oatmeal Crisp with Almonds	with ½ cup skim milk
Calories	230	270
Calories from Fat	50	50
	% Daily Value**	
Total Fat 6g*	9%	9%
Saturated Fat 0.5g	3%	4%
Cholesterol 0mg	0%	1%
Sodium 320mg	13%	16%
Potassium 150mg	4%	10%
Total Carbohydrate 38g	13%	15%
Dietary Fiber 3g	12%	12%
Sugars 11g		
Other Carbohydrate 24g		
Protein 6g		
Vitamin A	25%	30%
Vitamin C	30%	30%
Calcium	10%	25%
Iron	45%	45%
Vitamin D	10%	25%
Thiamin	25%	30%
Riboflavin	25%	35%
Niacin	25%	25%
Vitamin B6	25%	25%
Folic Acid	25%	25%
Phosphorus	15%	25%
Magnesium	10%	15%
Zinc	25%	30%
Copper	8%	8%

*Amount in Cereal. A serving of cereal plus skim milk provides 6g fat (1g saturated), less than 5mg cholesterol, 380mg sodium, 360mg potassium, 45g carbohydrate (17g sugars), and 10g protein.
**Percent Daily Values are based on a 2,000 calorie diet. Your daily values may be higher or lower depending on your calorie needs:

	Calories:	2,000	2,500
Total Fat	Less than	65g	80g
Sat Fat	Less than	20g	25g
Cholesterol	Less than	300mg	300mg
Sodium	Less than	2,400mg	2,400mg
Total Carbohydrate		300g	375g
Dietary Fiber		25g	30g

FIGURE 12-9 Breakfast cereals generally are better sources of iron and zinc than of copper. This is because adding copper would speed fat breakdown in the product.

Copper deficiency has been seen when copper is omitted from total parenteral nutrition formulas. Signs and symptoms of copper deficiency include a form of normocytic, hypochromic anemia, decreased numbers of white blood cells (specifically, the neutrophils), bone loss, and inadequate growth. Copper stores are extremely important during fetal development. Studies have shown that fetal copper stores accumulate primarily during the last trimester of pregnancy. Therefore, inadequate copper stores predispose preterm infants to the risk of copper deficiency.

Menkes syndrome is an example of a naturally occurring human copper deficiency. Defects in a gene inhibit the adequate absorption of copper from the gastrointestinal tract. In Menkes syndrome, the failure to absorb and transport copper occurs mainly in the transfer from mother to fetus. Results often lead to severe mental retardation; connective tissue abnormalities; steely, white, brittle hair; and, ultimately, death by the age of 3 years. Supplemental copper is given in an attempt to partially reverse this condition, although patients are often nonresponsive.

Recent studies have linked various forms of heart disease and osteoporosis to marginal copper deficiencies.[12] However, despite increased understanding of the physiologic roles of copper, the diagnosis of marginal copper deficiency has yet to be perfected. This creates problems for clinicians looking for evidence of marginal copper deficiency.

■ Copper in Foods

Copper is primarily found in organ meats (liver), seafood, cocoa, mushrooms, legumes, nuts, seeds, and whole-grain breads and cereals. It is not added in significant amounts to breakfast cereals, since it speeds fat breakdown in the product (Fig. 12-9). Milk is also very low in copper, as was the case for iron.

Foods with the highest nutrient density for copper (mg/kcal) are oysters, lobster, liver, sunflower seeds, and various nuts. Food composition tables often list few values for copper, and even those values may not be reliable because soil conditions greatly affect the copper content of plant foods. In addition, water may supply 13 to 50% of copper needs, depending on the copper content of the local soil.

■ Copper Needs

The Estimated Average Requirement for copper is 0.7 mg/day for adults. This is based on the amount of copper needed to maintain adequate concentration of copper ceruloplasmin in the blood, as well as maintain superoxide dismutase activity in red blood cells. The Estimated Average Requirement is increased by 30% to yield an RDA of 0.9 mg for adult men and women. Our average intake is about 1.1 to 1.6 mg daily. Women generally have the lower intakes. Overall, the copper status of adults in North America appears to be fine. As with zinc, though, the absence of sensitive measures for copper status may result in many cases of marginal deficiencies being overlooked. Regular use of a typical multivitamin-mineral supplement would fill any gap between daily intake and need in people at risk of deficiency.

■ North Americans at Risk for Copper Deficiency

Among those at the greatest risk for a copper deficiency are preterm infants; infants recovering from undernutrition on a diet dominated by milk, which is an inadequate source of copper; people recovering from intestinal surgery, which reduces copper absorption; and people on long-term total parenteral nutrition if there is insufficient copper in the formula. Kidney patients undergoing dialysis may experience excessive losses of copper via the dialysis procedure. Excessive losses of copper may also occur through the skin in burn patients.[7]

A copper deficiency can result from the overzealous supplementation of zinc, as noted earlier, since excess zinc can hamper copper absorption (review Fig. 12-6). Zinc increases the synthesis of the protein metallothionein, which binds both minerals—but particularly copper—in the intestinal cells, reducing the future transfer of copper into the bloodstream. The use of large doses of antacids also may bind enough copper in the intestine to cause a deficiency.

■ Toxicity of Copper

The Upper Level for copper is 10 mg/day, based on the risk of liver damage. Generally, copper toxicity in humans is not very common because intakes are usually low and because our bodies can regulate copper storage through excretion via the bile. At single supplemental doses of 10 to 15 mg, though, copper provided in aqueous forms also tends to cause vomiting.

Another inherited copper-related disease called Wilson's disease results in the accumulation of copper in the liver, brain, kidneys, and cornea of the eye. People with this disease can't incorporate copper into ceruloplasmin, as well as experience a decreased ability to excrete copper in the bile. Wilson's disease is present at birth but usually is not detected until later in childhood, adolescence, or young adulthood. The disease can be very difficult to diagnose, because up to 15% of patients have normal ceruloplasmin concentration, an indicator of copper status. Some of the wide range of symptoms includes hepatic, neurological, and psychiatric disorders, as well as kidney abnormalities. If caught early, lifelong treatment with agents that bind copper, such as penicillamine, can prevent tissue damage and reduce the mental degeneration commonly seen in Wilson's disease. Otherwise, these people die prematurely.

CONCEPT CHECK

Similar to iron absorption, zinc absorption is partly regulated by a mucosal block. Animal protein sources, increased body needs, and small intakes lead to increased zinc absorption. Zinc functions as a cofactor for many enzymes and is important for growth, immune function, and sense of taste. Beef, seafood, and whole grains are rich food sources of zinc. Copper functions mainly as part of enzymes and other compounds involved in iron metabolism, cross-linking of collagen, myelination of nerve cells, and neurotransmitter synthesis. A copper deficiency can result in a form of anemia and impaired immune function. Food sources of copper are liver, seafood, legumes, nuts, and whole grains.

■ SELENIUM (SE)

Selenium first attracted the attention of scientists in the 1930s, when it was found to cause a chronic poisoning of livestock. This resulted from the animals' consuming plants that were grown on high-selenium soils. The significance of selenium in human nutrition became evident in the late 1980s, when Chinese scientists reported that selenium supplementation prevents the development of Keshan disease, which causes a form of heart disease. The known biological roles of selenium are diverse. It is vital for normal development, growth, and metabolism.

■ Absorption, Transport, Storage, and Excretion of Selenium

Selenium enters the body in many ionic forms. Most selenium in foods is bound to derivatives of the amino acids methionine and cysteine. Therefore, the two major forms of selenium that enter the body are as selenomethionine, derived ultimately from plants, and selenocysteine, from animals.[28] Because these substances are readily absorbed, the bioavailability of selenium is considerably higher than that of iron and zinc. About 50 to 100% of dietary selenium intake is absorbed, and it is not affected by selenium nutritional status.[9] Since no physiological mechanism appears to control selenium absorption, selenium has a definite potential for toxicity.

Not much is known about the transport of selenium. What is known is that selenium is made available for use when the particular amino acid it is bound to is

Dietary Sources of Copper

Food Item and Amount	Copper (mg)
Steamed oysters, 3	2.0
Steamed lobster, 3 oz	1.7
Fried beef liver, 1 oz	1.3
Brazil nuts, ½ cup	1.2
Brewer's yeast, 3 tbsp	0.8
Walnuts, ½ cup	0.7
Sunflower seeds, ¼ cup	0.6
Cooked kidney beans, 1 cup	0.4
Molasses, 3 tbsp	0.3
Wheat germ, ¼ cup	0.2

You have now seen that the absence of many nutrients from the diet can lead to anemia:

- Vitamin E deficiency can lead to hemolytic anemia (see Chapter 9).
- Vitamin K deficiency, especially coupled with use of antibiotics, can lead to blood loss and thus to hemorrhagic anemia (see Chapter 9).
- Vitamin B-6 deficiency can lead to microcytic anemia (see Chapter 10).
- Folate deficiency can lead to megaloblastic anemia (see Chapter 10).
- Vitamin B-12 malabsorption can lead to megaloblastic anemia (see Chapter 10).
- An iron deficiency can lead to microcytic hypochromic anemia.
- A copper deficiency can lead, although rarely, to a secondary iron deficiency anemia, as copper aids in iron metabolism.

catabolized. The selenium can then be incorporated into macromolecules, transported to various organs, or excreted. Homeostasis of selenium in the body is achieved through excretion, mainly via the urine and feces. Studies show that the urinary excretion of selenium increases as dietary intake increases.[9] Storage of selenium primarily is found bound to the amino acid methionine and as part of glutathione peroxide enzyme. Both are found throughout the body.

■ Functions of Selenium

Currently, the best understood role for selenium is as a cofactor for a major form of the enzyme glutathione peroxidase. Selenium also plays a role in thyroid hormone metabolism and likely has other metabolic functions, which have yet to be clearly established.[18]

Glutathione peroxidase participates in a process that metabolizes peroxides into less toxic alcohol derivatives and water. In Chapter 9, you saw that peroxides tend to become free radicals, which in turn can attack and break down cell membranes, causing cell damage. As a cofactor for glutathione peroxidase, selenium is important for protecting heart cells and other cells against oxidative damage. Selenium also may aid immune function via activity of glutathione peroxidase.

Recall that vitamin E also functions to prevent attacks on cell membranes by free radicals. Thus, vitamin E and selenium work together. Selenium participates in an enzyme system that prevents free radical production by reducing peroxide concentration in the cell, and vitamin E can stop the action of free radicals once they are produced. Thus, an adequate selenium intake spares some of the body's need for vitamin E, as it reduces the peroxide load in a cell (Fig. 12-10).

Chapter 10 discussed how electron-seeking compounds, especially free radicals, can alter DNA. Alterations in DNA are known to cause cancer. Because of selenium's ability to reduce free radical production, adequate intake of this mineral may be important in preventing cancer. In fact, recently, people with a history of skin cancer (basal cell or squamous cell carcinomas) were treated with an oral supplement of

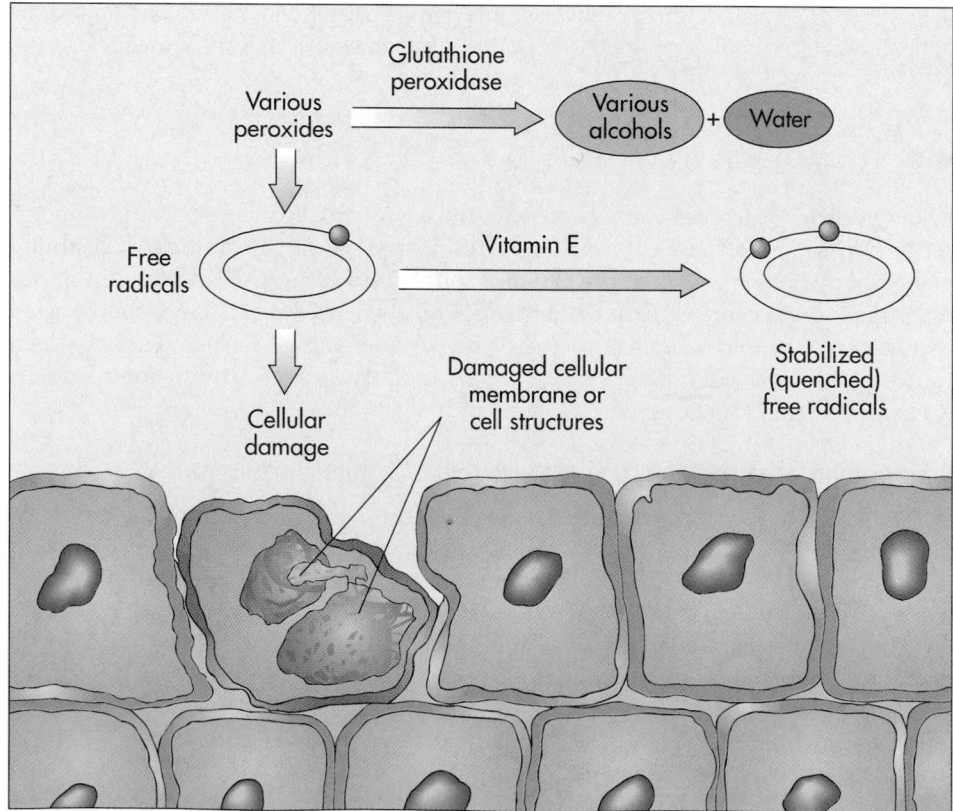

■ FIGURE 12-10 Selenium is part of the glutathione peroxidase system, which breaks down perioxides, such as H_2O_2 to water (H_2O), before they can form free radicals. This, in turn, spares some of the need for vitamin E, which is a major free radical scavenger.

200 µg of selenium/day or a placebo. There was no effect on the further development of cancer of the skin; however, there was a significant reduction in development of other cancers, such as lung, colon, rectal, and prostate. This study has peaked interest in selenium in cancer prevention and also has prompted follow-up studies. Another study using selenium (and vitamin E) supplements in men who have an enlarged prostate gland is in the planning stages. The dose of selenium will be 200 µg/day and 400 mg/day for vitamin E. Vitamin E is part of the protocol, since some supplement trials have hinted at a protective effect against prostate cancer.

■ Selenium Deficiency

The signs and symptoms of a selenium deficiency in animals and humans include muscle pain, muscle wasting, and cardiomyopathy, a form of heart disease resulting from heart muscle damage. These same signs and symptoms are noted when there is insufficient selenium in total parenteral nutrition solutions. Farm animals in areas with low soil concentrations of selenium (e.g., New Zealand and Finland) and humans in some areas of China develop characteristic heart disorders associated with an inadequate selenium intake.

Keshan disease, a deficiency state that results in varying degrees of heart deterioration in children, is associated with inadequate selenium intake. This disease occurs when the soil is almost devoid of selenium. Note that, although selenium is protective against development of the disease, selenium cannot correct the heart disorders once they have occurred. A selenium deficiency can also result in an accumulation of fatty acid peroxides in the heart, which leads to the formation of substances that enhance blood clot formation. Additional studies have associated low blood selenium with both the incidence of myocardial infarctions and an increased death rate from cardiovascular disease. Studies have also reported a relationship between kidney disease and depressed selenium status.[9] Further studies will be identifying the effects of supplementation and its application in the prevention of certain chronic diseases.

■ Selenium in Foods

Fish, meat (especially organ meats), eggs, milk, and shellfish are good animal sources of selenium. Grains and sources of nuts and seeds grown in soils containing selenium are good plant sources.

Foods providing the highest nutrient density for selenium (µg/kcal) are tuna, whole-wheat bread, ham, eggs, oatmeal, white bread and related flour-based products, beef, and chicken.

■ Selenium Needs

The Estimated Average Requirement for selenium is 45 µg/day for men and women ages 19 to 70 years. This is based on the amount of selenium needed to maximize glutathione peroxidase activity. The Estimated Average Requirement is increased by 20% to account for individual variability to yield an RDA for both men and women ages 19 to 70 years of 55 µg/day. There is no indication of average intakes below the RDA in either the United States or Canada; in fact, average intakes are about 105 µg/day from food.

■ North Americans at Risk for Selenium Deficiency

Since North Americans, on average, consume twice the RDA for selenium, deficiencies are rare. The RDA is easily achieved by eating a mixed diet. Those who should be most concerned about a possible selenium deficiency are kidney patients, especially those who are receiving dialysis treatments. People with AIDS may also show evidence of deficiency.[9]

■ Toxicity of Selenium

Excess selenium can be toxic. The Upper Level is 400 µg/day for adults 19 years and older, based on overt signs of selenium toxicity, such as hair loss and high blood

CRITICAL THINKING

Tammy read an article about antioxidants and their role in preventing free radical damage to cells. When Tammy went to the drug store to take a closer look at such supplements, she saw that selenium was one of the antioxidants in the supplements. Why does selenium deserve consideration as an antioxidant?

Dietary Sources of Selenium

Food Item and Amount	Selenium (µg)
Canned tuna, 3 oz	68.1
Sirloin steak, 5 oz	47.6
Shrimp, 4 oz	45.0
Cooked egg noodles, 1 cup	35.0
Roasted ham, 3 oz	30.0
Roasted chicken, 3 oz	24.0
Boiled egg, 1	11.0
Whole-wheat bread, 1 slice	10.0
Oatmeal, ½ cup	10.0
White bread, 1 slice	8.0

concentrations. Daily intakes as low as 1 to 3 mg can cause toxicity symptoms if taken for many months. These signs and symptoms besides hair loss, include a garlicky odor of the breath, nausea, diarrhea, fatigue, and changes in fingernails and toenails. Rashes and cirrhosis of the liver may also develop.

■ CASE SCENARIO
Follow-Up

Selenium is a component of the enzyme glutathione peroxidase. This enzyme breaks down hydrogen peroxide and other peroxides, and so helps reduce oxidative damage in cells. Such oxidative damage could increase the risk of cancer by damaging the DNA and other cell constituents. One study has shown that people with a history of skin cancer were less likely to develop other forms of cancer, such as lung, colon, rectal, and prostate when they consumed 200 µg of supplement of selenium per day compared to people on placebo. This finding has caused the federal government to sponsor studies to see if selenium supplements can reduce the risk of cancer in other groups of people, such as those with an enlarged prostate gland. The dose of selenium that Gina has chosen is half of the Upper Level of 400 µg/day, so this is likely a safe practice. However, we need much more research before we suggest that otherwise healthy people such as Gina take this step to reduce cancer risk. More important habits to consider were discussed in the Nutrition Perspective in Chapter 10.

■ IODIDE (I)

*I*odine (I_2), which is quite poisonous, can be used in a water solution as a topical anti-infective agent. The iodide ion (I^-) is the form of this trace mineral that is an essential nutrient. The term *iodine* is sometimes used in nutrition instead of iodide; to avoid confusion with this poisonous form, the term *iodide* will be used exclusively.

Iodine (I_2), present in food as iodide (I^-) and other nonelemental forms, was linked to the presence of an enlarged thyroid gland (goiter) during World War I. Men drafted from the Pacific Northwest and the Great Lakes region of the United States had a much higher rate of goiter than men from other areas of the country. The soil in these areas is very low in iodide. During the 1920s, researchers in Ohio found that goiter can be prevented in children by feeding them low doses of iodide for an extended period. Following the lead of the Swiss, American companies began adding iodide to table salt. Use of iodized salt is the major method for correcting iodide deficiencies.

Today, many nations, such as Canada, require iodide fortification of salt. In the United States, salt can be purchased either fortified or plain. Check for this on the label of a package of salt next time you are in a grocery store. By law, the label on a salt container sold in the United States must clearly state if iodide is present or not. Some areas of Europe, such as northern Italy, have very low iodide concentrations in the soil but have yet to adopt the practice of fortifying salt with iodide. People in these areas, especially women, still suffer from goiter, as do people in areas of Latin America, the Indian subcontinent, Southeast Asia, and Africa. About 250 million people worldwide are at risk of iodide deficiency, and approximately 20% of these people have goiter.[17]

■ Absorption, Transport, Storage, and Excretion of Iodide

Iodide is efficiently absorbed along the gastrointestinal tract in its inorganic form, the most common form of dietary iodine. Iodide is also easily absorbed in other forms, such as the iodate (IO_3^-) form that is added to bread. After iodide is absorbed into the bloodstream, it is transported as free ions and bound to proteins, including thyroid-binding globulin and albumin. The transported iodide is then distributed throughout the body's extracellular compartments.[14]

About three-quarters of the iodide found in the adult human body is found in the thyroid gland. The thyroid gland actively accumulates and traps iodide from the bloodstream to support thyroid hormone synthesis. The thyroid hormones thyroxine (T_4) and triiodothyronine (T_3) are synthesized from the amino acid tyrosine and

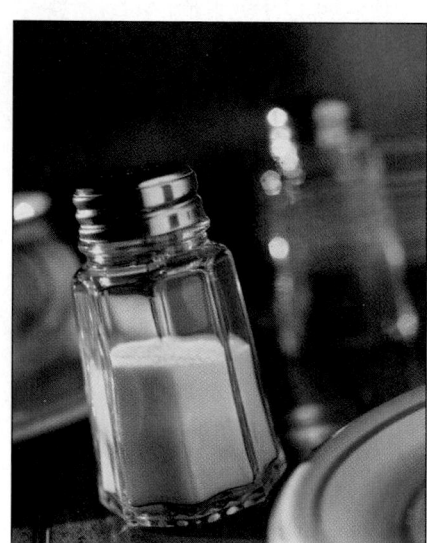

Iodized salt is the predominant source of dietary iodine in Canadian and American diets.

iodide. If a person's iodide intake is insufficient, the thyroid gland enlarges as it attempts to take up more iodide from the blood. Iodide also accumulates in other tissues, such as the salivary glands, but in much smaller amounts. When iodide intake is low, the body is able to recycle it by removing iodide from the thyroid hormones in the liver and then releasing the iodide into the bloodstream for reabsorption by the thyroid gland.

The kidneys are the principal route for iodide excretion. The amount of iodide found in urine is an adequate measurement of the status of iodide intake, along with current blood concentration of iodide. Other paths for excretion occur via feces, sweat, and breast milk in lactating women.

Structure of thyroxine (T_4). Note that triiodothyronine (T_3) lacks one iodide (I), indicated in this figure with a red asterisk.

■ Functions of Iodide

The major function of iodide is the synthesis of thyroxine (T_4). The control of T_4 production is under the influence of the **thyroid-stimulating hormone (TSH)** from the pituitary gland.[14] The thyroid gland also secretes T_4 in response to TSH secretion from the pituitary gland. Almost all organs in the body are targets for T_4, but T_4 is actually considered a prehormone. Within the target cell, T_4 is converted to T_3, the active form of the hormone (Fig. 12-11). T_3 controls the rate of cell metabolism (called the **basal metabolism**). Hyperthyroidism results in an abnormally high basal metabolism, while hypothyroidism causes the opposite effect. T_3 also contributes to human growth and development, particularly during fetal development.

T_3 stimulates mRNA and protein synthesis, which is especially important for development of the central nervous system. During periods of rapid growth (the first 6 months in utero), T_3 is essential to normal brain development. If T_3 is lacking, the development of the brain is seriously impaired. Under normal circumstances, T_3 also increases glucose utilization and protein synthesis.

thyroid-stimulating hormone (TSH) The hormone that regulates the uptake of iodide by the thyroid gland and release of the thyroid hormone, TSH is secreted in response to a low blood concentration of circulating thyroxine.

basal metabolism The minimal energy the body requires to support itself when resting and awake in a warm, quiet environment. It amounts to roughly 1 kcal/minute, or about 1400 kcal/day, the values are often referred to as basal metabolic rate.

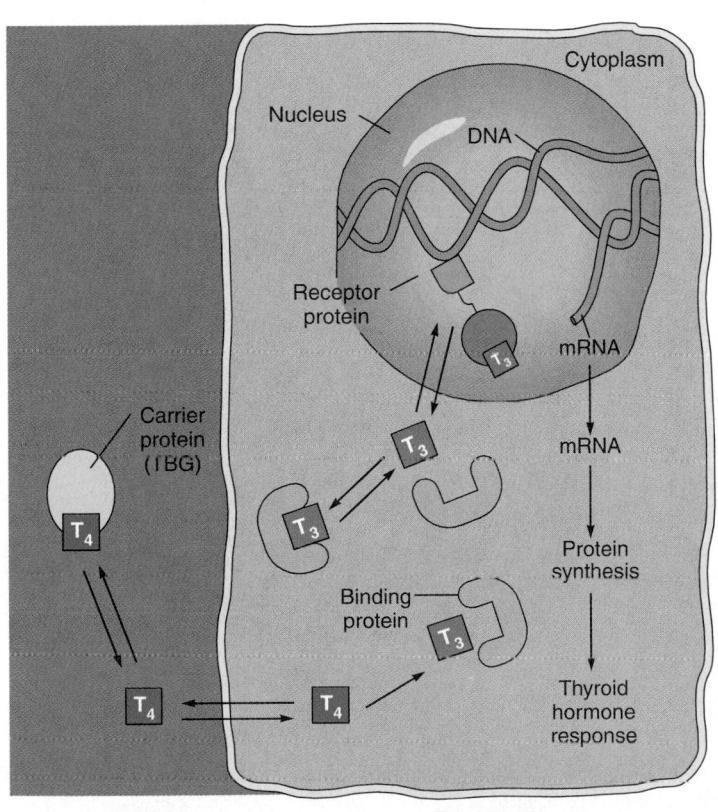

■ FIGURE 12-11 The mechanism of the action of thyroid hormones on the target cell. T_4 is carried by a thyroid binding globulin in the blood. Upon release T_4 enters the target cell and is converted into T_3 in the cytoplasm. T_3 enters the nucleus and binds to its nuclear receptor. The hormone-receptor complex can then bind to a specific area of DNA to activate specific genes and produce the hormone response. T_4 binding can lead to the same response, but it is 10 times weaker than that of T_3.

▪ Iodide Deficiency

In an iodide deficiency, insufficient T_4 is produced to shut off the synthesis of thyroid-stimulating hormone. The constant release of TSH by the pituitary gland causes continual growth of the gland, eventually producing a greatly enlarged gland, or goiter. A fall in metabolic rate and an increase in blood cholesterol are two other symptoms of thyroid hormone deficiency.

Simple goiter is a painless condition, but if uncorrected it can lead to pressure on the trachea (windpipe), which may cause difficulty in breathing. Treatment with iodide can result in a slow reduction in the size of the thyroid gland, although surgical removal of part of the gland may be required in severe cases.

An iodide-deficient diet poses a major threat to pregnant women and the fetus, especially during the latter two-thirds of pregnancy.[30] Some of the harmful documented effects include stillbirth, low birth weight, increased infant mortality, goiter, impaired mental function, and retarded development. Increasing the mother's intake of iodide prior to the 4th month of pregnancy, but preferably sooner, can prevent these abnormalities. The World Health Organization estimates that at least 30 million people in the world suffer from varying degrees of preventable brain damage due to the effects of iodide deficiency on fetal brain development.[15] The resulting retarded body growth is referred to as **cretinism.** Cretinism was common in certain areas of the United States before the program to fortify salt with iodide. Today, cretinism still appears in parts of Europe, Africa, Latin America and Asia (Fig. 12-12). In these areas, iodinated vegetable oil given orally or by injection is being used in an attempt to decrease iodide deficiency, in addition to the fortification of salt with iodide. The eradication of iodide deficiency is a goal of many health-related and service organizations worldwide. Iodide deficiency is common and poses a major threat to public health in many countries. An estimated 1.5 billion people are at risk of iodide deficiency disease.

cretinism The stunting of body growth and mental development during fetal and later development that results from inadequate maternal intake of iodide during pregnancy.

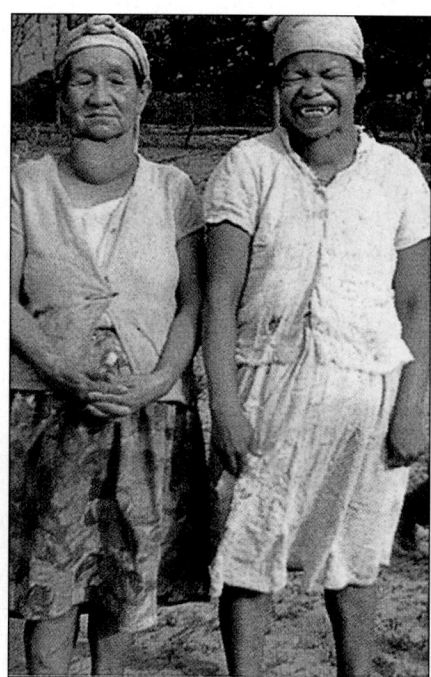
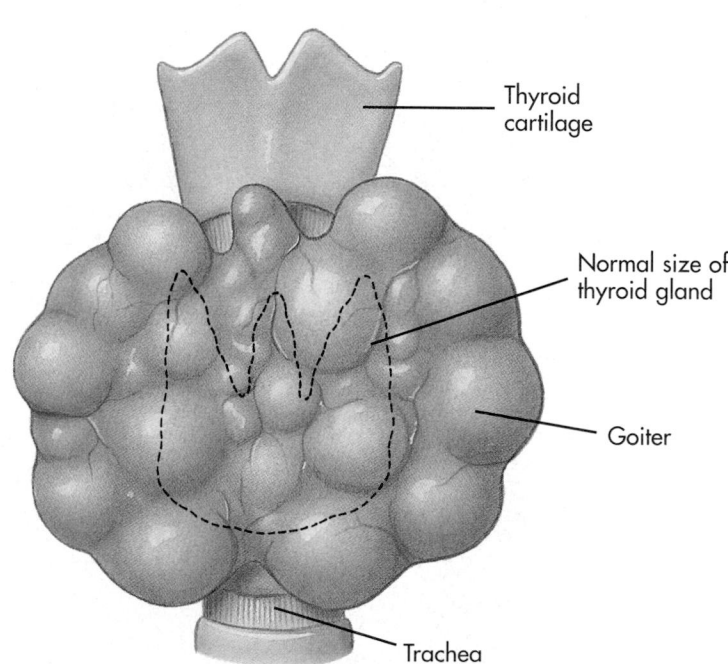

Thyroid cartilage

Normal size of thyroid gland

Goiter

Trachea

▪ **FIGURE 12-12** Goiter and cretinism in Bolivia. The mother on the left is goitrous but otherwise normal. The daughter is goitrous, mentally retarded, deaf, and mute. Both mother and daughter exhibit characteristics typical of iodide deficiency.
Illustration by William Ober.

■ Iodide in Foods

Saltwater fish, seafood, iodized salt, molasses, and some plants contain various forms of iodide, especially the leaves of plants grown near the sea. Sea salt found in health-food stores, however, is not a good source because the iodide is lost during processing. A half teaspoon (about 2 g) of iodide-fortified salt supplies the adult RDA for iodide. The actual amount of fortification in the United States is 76 μg of iodide per gram of salt.

The ocean is the source of some iodide naturally present in our diets. As ocean mist blows onto nearby land, iodide becomes part of the soil. Plants grown in that soil accumulate the iodide.

Goiter is also associated with the consumption of **goitrogens.** Large amounts of these substances are found in raw vegetables, such as turnips, cabbage, brussels sprouts, cauliflower, broccoli, rutabagas, and cassava, as well as other plants and even waterborne sources. Goitrogens inhibit iodide metabolism by the thyroid gland and, in turn, inhibit thyroid hormone synthesis. However, goitrogens are not an important cause of goiter in developed countries, since they are destroyed by cooking, and the foods they are found in do not play an important role in the customary diets. They are, however, linked to goiter in less-developed parts of the world.

Dietary Sources of Iodide

Food Item and Amount	Iodide (μg)
Iodized salt, 1/2 tsp	200
Baked haddock, 3 oz	125
Buttermilk, 1 cup	98
Baked cod, 3 oz	87
Cottage cheese, 1/2 cup	49
Mozzarella cheese, 1 oz	34
Shrimp, 3 oz	29
Boiled egg, 1	22
Baked perch, 3 oz	18
Cheddar cheese, 1 oz	14

■ Iodide Needs

The Estimated Average Requirement for iodide for adults is 95 μg/day. This amount of iodide is needed to maintain adequate iodide uptake and turnover by the thyroid gland. The Estimated Average Requirement is increased by 40% to account for individual variability, yielding the RDA for iodide for adults of 150 μg/day. Probably the minimum intake to prevent goiter is 50 μg/day. Most North Americans consume much more iodide than the RDA. Consumption is estimated to be about 190 to 300 μg/day (not including the iodide contributed by the use of iodized salt at the table), with men consuming the higher amounts.

Such intakes of iodide are typical because it is used as a sterilizing agent in dairies and restaurants, as a dough conditioner in bakeries, in food colorants, and in iodized salt.

■ North Americans at Risk of Iodide Deficiency

The North American diet today, for most people, is appropriate for iodide intake and related good health. But recent data show some decline in iodide intake during the past two decades, especially in women of reproductive age. This rather recent reduction of dietary iodide may be due to several factors, including the dairy industry's effort to reduce iodide in milk, the replacement of iodide with bromine salts as the dough conditioner in commercial bread production, the reduced intake of eggs because of concerns over cholesterol content, and the reduced use of table salt because of hypertension concerns. Lack of public awareness of the importance of using iodized salt might also be a contributing factor to the decline of dietary iodide intake in the United States; in Canada, the iodination of salt is mandatory. Therefore, women in the United States, especially during pregnancy, should pay particular attention to their dietary iodide intake (e.g., purchase iodized salt).[23]

■ Toxicity of Iodide

When very high amounts of iodide are consumed, thyroid hormone synthesis is inhibited, as in a deficiency. This is evidenced by a rise in TSH in the blood. The Upper Level of 1.1 mg/day is based on such an effect. A "toxic goiter" eventually results. Toxic goiter can appear in people who eat a lot of seaweed, since some seaweeds contain as much as 1% iodide by weight. Total iodide intake then can add up to 60 to 130 times the RDA.

■ FLUORIDE (F)

Dentists in the early 1900s noticed a lower incidence of dental caries in the south-western United States, where the water naturally contained high concentrations of fluoride. Many people in these areas had small spots on the teeth, called **mottling,** due to deposits of fluoride; although discolored, these mottled teeth contained were virtually free of dental caries. After experiments showed that fluoride in the water does indeed decrease the rate of dental caries, the controlled fluoridation of water in parts of the United States began in 1945 (see Chapter 5 for a review of the development of dental caries).

People who have grown up drinking fluoridated water generally have 40 to 60% fewer dental caries than people who did not drink fluoridated water as children. Dentists can provide fluoride treatments, and schools can provide fluoride tablets, but it is much less expensive and more reliable to simply add fluoride to the community's drinking water. However, not all public or private water sources contain enough fluoride. When in doubt, contact your local water plant or have the water in your home analyzed for fluoride content. If the water doesn't contain the recommended amount—1 part per million parts of water (1 ppm, or 1 mg/L)—talk to your dentist about the best means for obtaining sufficient fluoride. And, although the most important clinical aspect of fluoride is its benefits in the prevention of dental caries, fluoride has also been shown to protect against the demineralization of other calcified tissues.[2]

■ Absorption, Transport, Storage, and Excretion of Fluoride

The absorption of fluoride occurs very rapidly. A significant proportion of dietary fluoride is absorbed in the stomach. Absorption continues to take place throughout the gastrointestinal tract by passive diffusion. Overall, about 80 to 90% is absorbed. Fluoride is then transported throughout the body via the bloodstream in the ionic form.

Calcified tissue deposition and renal excretion are the two major mechanisms by which fluoride is removed from circulation. An estimated 50% of the fluoride absorbed each day is deposited in calcified tissues, bones and teeth. The amount of fluoride deposited depends on the stage of development of the bone, with the developing stages being the most significant. The major path for the excretion of fluoride from the body occurs through the kidneys via the urine.

■ Functions of Fluoride

Although an essential function has not been described for fluoride, it is still recognized as a trace element with the beneficial property of protecting against the demineralization of calcified tissues. The action of fluoride on the erupted teeth of children and adults is due to its effects on the metabolism of bacteria in dental plaque. It also works to reduce dental caries by

- Reducing the acid solubility of the enamel by forming **fluorapatite** crystals, rather than the typical hydroxyapatite crystals
- Promoting the remineralization of enamel lesions
- Increasing the deposition of minerals that retard the development of caries
- Reducing the net rate of transport of minerals from the enamel surface

The fluoride present in bones is constantly released into the blood, and more so if the bone fluoride content is high. This combines with daily fluoride exposure from fluoridated water (if available) and toothpaste (if used). Blood fluoride then contributes to fluoride in the saliva, which in turn bathes the teeth to provide daily fluoride protection. Overall, lifelong fluoride exposure on a daily basis is the most beneficial way to receive the dental caries-preventive function of fluoride.

Due to its ability to increase bone mass, high doses of fluoride (>20 mg/day) are being used experimentally in adults to treat severe osteoporosis, especially that seen

---

mottling The discoloration or marking of the surfaces of teeth from exposure to excessive amounts of fluoride (fluorosis).

*L*ike chlorine, fluorine (F_2) is a poisonous gas. The fluoride ion (F^-) is the form of this trace mineral that contributes to human health.

fluorapatite A fluoride-containing, acid-resistant crystalline substance that is produced during bone and tooth development. Its presence in teeth helps prevent dental caries.

in the spine. Fluoride has the means to stimulate osteoblasts (bone-forming cells) to increase the production of proteins that ultimately undergo rapid mineralization to form new bone.[32] Such high fluoride dosages can cause significant side effects, such as stomach upset and bone pain. Ongoing research is attempting to establish an effective dose and duration of treatment. Sodium fluoride is an appealing treatment option for osteoporosis, due to its low cost and rapid response. A recent study reported that low-dose fluoride therapy increases spine bone mass and reduces vertebral fracture. The question remains as to how strong the treated bone actually will be in the long run.

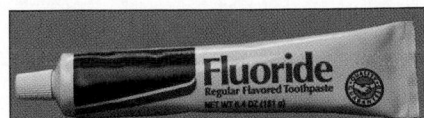

Toothpaste with fluoride is an important source of dietary fluoride.

■ Fluoride in Foods

In the United States, the major source of dietary fluoride is drinking water. Typical fluoridated water contains about 0.2 mg/cup. Tea, seafood (especially marine fish that are consumed with their bones), and seaweed are among the richest dietary sources of fluoride. Estimating fluoride content in food can be difficult, since water sources can vary in amount. Toothpaste, mouth rinses, and fluoride treatments performed by dentists are other sources of fluoride.

■ Fluoride Needs

The Adequate Intake for fluoride is 3.1 mg/day for women and 3.8 mg/day for men. For infants up to 6 months of age, the Adequate Intake is 0.01 mg/day and increases to 0.5 mg/day through age 1. For childhood and adolescence, the fluoride Adequate Intake ranges from 0.7 to 3.2 mg/day. This range of intake provides the benefits of resistance to dental caries without causing mottling of the teeth, which is the basis for setting the Adequate Intake.[11]

■ Toxicity of Fluoride

Although life-threatening cases of acute fluoride toxicity are extremely rare, substantial amounts of fluoride in toothpastes, mouth rinses, or dietary supplements are found in most North American households and should be of special concern for parents with young children. The signs and symptoms of fluoride toxicity can develop very rapidly and include nausea, vomiting, diarrhea, abdominal pain, excessive salivation and tearing, pulmonary disturbances, cardiac insufficiency and weakness, convulsions, sensory disturbances, paralysis, and coma.

A fluoride intake greater than 6 mg/day can mottle teeth during their developmental stage. Children who consume large amounts of fluoridated toothpaste as part of daily tooth care are at greatest risk. Limiting the amount used to "pea" size is the best way to prevent this problem. When fluoride intakes reach 20 mg/day during tooth development, the tooth structure is weakened and can crumble. This is called **fluorosis** and appears in humans and other animals. With this in mind, the Upper Level set for children over 9 years of age and adults is 10 mg/day, based on the risk of skeletal fluorosis. Note that high fluoride intake in adults does not cause mottling of teeth.

fluorosis A condition caused by excessive fluoride intake that is characterized by poor tooth structure and discoloration.

CONCEPT CHECK

Selenium is important for the activity of glutathione peroxidase, an enzyme that reduces the concentration of peroxides, thus lessening the free radical load in the body. In this way, selenium spares some of the need for vitamin E. A deficiency results in muscle and heart disorders. Organ meats, eggs, fish, and grains are good selenium sources; however, the selenium content in plants depends on the selenium concentration in the soil. A high selenium intake is potentially toxic. Iodide is vital in the synthesis of thyroid hormones. A prolonged insufficient intake will cause the thyroid gland to enlarge, resulting in goiter. Insufficient intake in pregnancy can lead to mental retardation in the offspring. The use of iodized salt has virtually eliminated this condition in the United States. Fluoride incorporated into teeth during development makes them resistant to acid and bacterial attack, in turn reducing development of dental caries. Regular fluoride exposure also aids in the remineralization of teeth once decay begins. Most of us receive adequate amounts of fluoride from that added to drinking water and toothpaste. A high fluoride intake during tooth development can lead to spotted, or mottled, teeth.

■ CHROMIUM (CR)

Chromium is an essential trace mineral that is widely distributed in small amounts throughout the food supply. The importance of chromium in human diets has been recognized only in the past 40 years. Although not much is understood about this mineral, many studies suggest that chromium plays an important role in maintaining proper carbohydrate and lipid metabolism, which may help alleviate type 2 diabetes and gestational diabetes in some individuals.

■ Absorption, Transport, Storage, and Excretion of Chromium

Only about 2 to 10% of chromium from food is actually absorbed. However, the bioavailability of chromium in humans is difficult to assess because the concentrations in human tissues are very low. Chromium is transported in the bloodstream primarily by the iron-binding protein transferrin, and it appears to be a bone-seeking element. Chromium accumulates in bone, as well as in the spleen, liver, and kidneys. The excretion of chromium occurs via the feces.[29]

■ Functions of Chromium

The most studied function of chromium in the maintenance of glucose uptake into cells. Our current understanding is that chromium's ability to enhance insulin action occurs when a chromium-binding protein binds to insulin receptors and then boosts receptor activity: Chromium also enhances the conversion of glucose to body fat. This results in more efficient glucose utilization. Dr. Nielsen discusses these and other findings on chromium and human health in the Nutrition Perspective in this chapter.

■ Chromium Deficiency

A chromium deficiency is characterized by impaired glucose tolerance and elevated blood cholesterol and triglycerides. The mechanism by which chromium influences cholesterol metabolism is not known but may involve enzymes that control cholesterol synthesis. Chromium deficiency appears in people maintained on total parenteral nutrition not supplemented with chromium, as well as in children suffering from undernutrition. Since sensitive measures of chromium status are not available, marginal chromium deficiencies may go undetected.

■ Chromium in Foods

As previously mentioned, chromium is widely distributed in small quantities throughout the food supply. Specific data regarding the chromium content of various foods are scant, and most food composition tables do not include values for this trace mineral. Processed meats, organ meats (liver), whole-grain products, egg yolks, mushrooms, broccoli, nuts, some legumes (such as dried beans), and beer are the most reliable sources. Yeast is also a source. Generally speaking, whole grains and cereals contain higher concentrations of chromium than do fruits and vegetables. The amount of chromium in foods is closely tied to the local soil content of chromium. To provide yourself with an adequate chromium intake, regularly choose whole grains in preference to refined grains.

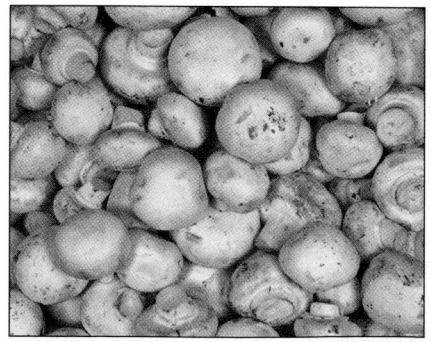
Mushrooms are a good source of chromium.

■ Chromium Needs

The Adequate Intake for chromium is 35 µg/day for men and 25 µg/day for women. This is based on the amount typically found in well balanced diets. The average dietary intake for adults in the United States generally meets the Adequate Intake standards. Some adults may become chromium-deficient as they age, and this may contribute to the increased risk for the development of type 2 diabetes in older persons. A recent study observed that, when yeast chromium was fed to older persons, there was improvement in glucose tolerance. Chromium intakes of less than 20 µg/day may be detrimental to the significant portion of the population that has marginally elevated blood glucose. Regular use of a vitamin-mineral supplement would meet any shortfall in intake.

■ Toxicity of Chromium

Chromium in foods as such has not shown any toxicity, so no Upper Level has been set. Chromium toxicity has been reported in people exposed to chromium in industrial settings and in painters using art supplies with a very high chromium content. Exposure to chromium occurs most frequently from workplace air or food or water from soil near chromium waste sites. Chromium poisoning damages the lungs and causes allergic responses in the skin. Consuming large amounts of chromium supplements can cause stomach upsets, ulcers, convulsions, kidney damage, liver damage, certain forms of cancer, and even death. In addition, the most popular form of chromium in dietary supplements, chromium picolinate, appears to be absorbed in a different fashion than from dietary chromium and can lead to the production of harmful hydroxyl radicals.[31]

■ MANGANESE (MN)

It is easy to confuse the mineral manganese with magnesium (Mg). Their names are similar, and in a few metabolic pathways they can substitute for each other.

Manganese is a cofactor for certain enzymes, including pyruvate carboxylase, an enzyme used in carbohydrate metabolism, and superoxide dismutase, an antioxidant enzyme. Manganese is also important in bone formation. No manganese-deficiency symptoms have been observed in humans. Animals on manganese-deficient diets exhibit changes in brain function, bone formation, and reproduction. If human diets were low in manganese, these problems would probably appear in humans as well. As it happens, our need for manganese is very low, and our diets tend to be adequate in manganese if good food sources, which include nuts, oats and other whole grains, beans, tea, and leafy vegetables, are consumed.

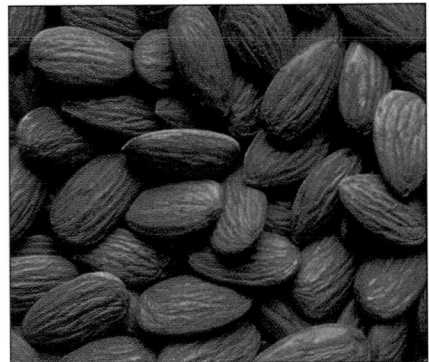

Nuts are a good source of manganese.

The Adequate Intake is 2.3 mg/day for men and 1.8 mg/day for women. Average intakes fall within this amount.[12] Oral toxicity is extremely rare. The Adequate Intake is based on the amount present in typical adult diets in the U.S. Manganese toxicity has been seen in people working in manganese mines and includes severe psychiatric abnormalities, hyperirritability, violence, hallucinations, and impaired control of muscles. The Upper Level is 11 mg/day, based on the development of neurotoxic symptoms.

■ MOLYBDENUM (MO)

Molybdenum is notable for its interactions with iron and copper. In particular, high intakes of molybdenum inhibit copper absorption.

Several enzymes—including **xanthine dehydrogenase** and a related form, xanthine oxidase—require molybdenum. The oxidase form of the enzyme is produced from the dehydrogenase form during tissue injury. No molybdenum deficiency has

xanthine dehydrogenase An enzyme containing molybdenum and iron, which functions in the formation of uric acid and the mobilization of iron from liver ferritin stores.

been observed in people consuming a normal diet, although deficiency signs and symptoms have appeared in people on total parenteral nutrition. These symptoms include increased heart and respiration rates, night blindness, mental confusion, edema, weakness, and coma.[12]

Good food sources of molybdenum include milk and milk products, beans, liver, whole grains, and nuts. The Estimated Average Requirement for molybdenum is 34 μg/day for adults. This is based on the amount needed to balance daily losses. The Estimated Average Requirement is increased by 30% to yield an RDA of 45 μg/day. Typical American intakes are 75 to 110 μg/day, with the higher intakes seen in men.[12] When laboratory animals consume high dosages of molybdenum, they develop evidence of toxicity, including anemia, weight loss, and decreased growth. The Upper Level of 2 mg/day is based on decreased growth and reproduction in laboratory animals.

See Table 12-2 to review the minerals discussed so far in this chapter.

ULTRATRACE MINERALS

There are many elements of the periodic table that occur in microgram/gram amounts in body tissues (Table 12-3). Ultimately, some may be elevated to the status of essential nutrient, but at this time elements such as aluminum, cadmium bromine, germanium, lead, lithium, rubidium, and tin have not been shown to have any beneficial effects in humans. In fact, lead is a danger to young children, as evidenced by toxicity to those children living in older homes that have been contaminated with peeling lead-based paint (see Chapter 19 for more details on lead).

One possibility to consider is that many ultratrace minerals present in tissues are there by accident, and, although they don't provide any health benefits, neither do they represent a threat. All the current knowledge about the minor trace elements has come from animal studies, which may suggest possible benefits for humans, but the evidence is tentative at best. Let's look at the ultratrace minerals most likely to be of benefit to humans.[12]

Boron (B)

Boron has long been known as an important growth factor for plants. In humans, boron may be involved in the metabolism of steroid (cholesterol-containing) hormones, such as the vitamin D hormone and the estrogens. There appears to be a close interrelation among boron, calcium, and magnesium, but more information is needed to understand how each mineral affects the absorption of the others. Several hypotheses suggest that boron acts as a regulator in cell membrane function, such as membrane stability, or acts as the regulator of the movement of cations and anions through the cell membrane. Sources of boron are peanuts, fruits (especially raisins), legumes, potato chips, vegetables, and wine. In a recent survey, coffee and milk, which are low in boron, were two major contributors of boron to the American diet due to the high volume consumed.[27] No Adequate Intake for boron has been established. Adults consume about 0.75 to 1.35 mg/day. The Upper Level for boron is 20 mg/day, based on developmental abnormalities in laboratory animals.

Nickel (N)

No biochemical function has been clearly defined for nickel for humans, but a variety of deficiency signs have been reported for farm animals and rats. Nickel may function as a cofactor in a variety of enzymes. It seems to be involved in the breakdown of the branched-chain amino acids and the odd-chain-length fatty acids. It also may be involved in the metabolism of vitamin B-12 and folic acid during the synthesis of methionine from homocysteine. It is found in chocolate, nuts, legumes, and grains. No Adequate Intake has been set. Americans have an intake of 69 to 162 μg/day. The Upper Level is 1 mg/day, based on poor weight gain in laboratory animals.

TABLE 12-2   A Summary of Key Trace Minerals

Mineral	Major Functions	Deficiency Symptoms	People Most at Risk	RDA or Adequate Intake	Nutrient-Dense Dietary Sources	Results of Toxicity
Iron	Functional component of hemoglobin and other key compounds used in respiration; immune function; cognitive development	Fatigue; small, pale red blood cells; low blood hemoglobin values	Infants, preschool children, adolescents, women in childbearing years	Men: 8 mg Women: 18 mg	Meats, seafood, broccoli, peas, bran, enriched breads	Gastrointestinal upset; toxicity especially seen when children consume many iron pills; toxicity also seen in people with hemochromatosis; Upper Level is 45 mg/day
Zinc	Required for more than nearly 100 enzymes, including enzymes involved in growth, immunity, alcohol metabolism, sexual development, reproduction	Skin rash, diarrhea, decreased appetite and sense of taste, hair loss, poor growth and development, poor wound healing	Vegetarians, elderly people, people with alcoholism	Men: 11 mg Women: 8 mg	Seafoods, meats, greens, whole grains	Supplement use can reduce copper absorption; can cause diarrhea, cramps, depressed immune function; Upper Level is 40 mg/day
Copper	Aids in iron metabolism; works with many antioxidant enzymes, and those involved in protein metabolism and hormone synthesis	Anemia, low white blood cell count, poor growth	Infants recovering from semistarvation, overzealous supplementation of zinc	900 µg	Liver, cocoa, beans, nuts, whole grains, dried fruits	Supplement use can cause vomiting; nervous system disorders; Upper Level is 8–10 mg/day
Selenium	Part of an antioxidant system	Muscle pain, muscle weakness, form of heart disease	Unknown	55 µg	Meats, eggs, fish, seafoods, whole grains	Supplement use can cause nausea, vomiting, hair loss, weakness, liver disease; Upper Level is 400 µg/day
Iodide	Component of thyroid hormones	Goiter; mental retardation, poor growth in infancy when mother is iodide deficient during pregnancy	Few people in North America, because salt is usually fortified	150 µg	Iodized salt, white bread, saltwater fish, dairy products	Inhibition of function of the thyroid gland; Upper Level is 1.1 mg/day
Fluoride	Increases resistance of tooth enamel to dental caries	Increased risk of dental caries	Areas where water is not fluoridated and dental treatments do not make up for a lack of fluoride	Men: 3.8 mg Women: 3.1 mg	Fluoridated water, toothpaste, dental treatments, tea, seaweed	Stomach upset; mottling (staining) of teeth during development; bone pain; Upper Level is 10 mg/day
Chromium	Enhances insulin action	High blood glucose after eating	People on intravenous nutrition, perhaps elderly people with type 2 diabetes	25–35 µg	Egg yolks, whole grains, pork, nuts, mushrooms, beer	Caused by industrial contamination, not dietary excess; no Upper Level set
Manganese	Cofactor of some enzymes, such as those involved in carbohydrate metabolism	None in humans	Unknown	1.8–2.3 mg	Nuts, oats, beans, tea	Nervous system disorders; Upper Level is 11 mg/day
Molybdenum	Aids action of some enzymes	None in healthy humans	Unsupplemented total parenteral nutrition support	45 µg	Beans, grains, nuts	Poor growth in laboratory animals; Upper Level is 2 mg/day

TABLE 12-3   A Summary of Ultratrace Minerals, Some of Which Human Needs Have Not Been Established

Mineral	Proposed Functions	Estimates of Daily Human Needs	Dietary Sources
Boron	Cell membrane function (ion transport), steroid hormone metabolism	1–13 mg	Fruits, leafy vegetables, nuts, beans
Nickel	Amino acid and fatty acid metabolism	25–35 μg	Chocolate, nuts, beans, whole grains
Silicon	Bone formation	25–30 mg	Root vegetables, whole grains
Arsenic	Amino acid metabolism, DNA function	12–25 μg	Fish, grains, cereal products
Vanadium	Mimicry of insulin action	10 μg	Shellfish, mushrooms, black pepper

Deficiency symptoms have been produced mostly in experimental animals. Many trace minerals pose a high risk for toxicity. Any supplement use should not exceed the estimates of human needs listed in this table.

■ Silicon (Si)

In animals such as the chick and rat, silicon is involved the formation of bone. In silicon-deficient animals, the bones and joints are poorly formed, and growth is depressed. Specifically, silicon changes the cartilage composition of bone and promotes calcification. In bone, it is found in areas of active growth associated with the osteoblasts. Plant foods, including unrefined grains of high fiber content, cereals, and root vegetables, are good sources of silicon. It is difficult to set a silicon requirement, since much of dietary silicon is not in an absorbable form. No Adequate Intake has been set. The average daily silicon intakes apparently range from 20 to 50 mg/day. Circumstantial evidence indicates that a severe lack of dietary silicon could adversely effect brain and bone function and composition. No Upper Level for silicon intake has been set.

■ Arsenic (As)

Arsenic has long been associated with plays, movies, and novels about homicide; the most famous being the old comedy *Arsenic and Old Lace*. Obviously, arsenic is a "killer" mineral, but it has also been used over the centuries to treat a variety of medical conditions. It is seldom used today, as it has been replaced by more effective medications. Depending on the form of arsenic consumed, absorption varies from 20 to 90%. It is rapidly excreted in the urine and via the bile. Although not clearly defined, arsenic is probably biologically active in the metabolism of the amino acid methionine and methyl groups. Another possible role is in the regulation of gene expression to produce certain proteins. Also, arsenic seems to enhance DNA synthesis in white blood cells. For this reason arsenic is being used in some cancer chemotherapy regimens. The U.S. intake is about 30 μg/day. Fish, grains, and cereal products contribute the most arsenic to the diet.[25] No Adequate Intake or Upper Level has been set.

■ Vanadium (V)

Vanadium, both in vivo and in vitro, shows pharmacological activity that mimics the actions of insulin, preventing the symptoms of diabetes in diabetic rats; thus, vanadium may have a role in treating human diabetes. Clinical studies with the trace mineral in both type 1 and type 2 diabetes showed some improvement in glucose utilization. Type 2 diabetes patients displayed improved insulin sensitivity. Vanadium is poorly absorbed and is excreted in the urine and bile. Other than vanadium's possible pharmacologic properties in diabetes treatment, a defined biochemical function for humans has not been described. In laboratory animals, it also seems to stimulate the mineralization of bones and teeth and has a variety of in vitro actions. A vanadium deficiency has not been identified in humans. Human diets supply about 6 to 18 µg per day. Vanadium is found in shellfish, mushrooms, parsley, dill, and some prepared foods. No Adequate Intake has been set. The Upper Level is 1.8 mg/day, based on development of kidney toxicity.

CONCEPT CHECK

Chromium may increase the action of the hormone insulin. The amount of chromium found in food depends on soil content. Whole grains, egg yolks, and meat are some of the better sources of chromium. Manganese is a component of bone and many enzymes, including those involved in glucose production. Since our need for it is low, deficiencies are rare. Good food sources of manganese are nuts, oats, tea, and beans. Molybdenum is a component of some enzymes. Deficiencies have appeared only with total parenteral nutrition. Beans, milk and milk products, grains, and nuts are sources of molybdenum. Boron contributes to ion transport across cell membranes, nickel contributes to amino acid metabolism, and silicon contributes to bone metabolism. The roles for some other trace minerals—including arsenic and vanadium—have not been fully established in humans. These minerals are required in such small amounts that diets including a variety of foods and containing some plant protein and whole grains most likely supply adequate amounts.

Check out the *Perspectives in Nutrition* Online Learning Center http://www.mhhe.com/wardlaw for quizzes, flash cards, other activities, and web links designed to further help you learn about issues surrounding the trace minerals.

SUMMARY

1. Six of the trace minerals (iron, zinc, iodide, copper, molybdenum, and selenium) have an RDA. An Adequate Intake has been set for three minerals (manganese, chromium, and fluoride).

2. Some trace minerals are difficult to detect in humans, and it is often hard to determine the exact amount of a trace mineral in food. Deficiencies were first observed in small, geographically isolated groups (e.g., selenium deficiency in an area of China) or people nourished exclusively by total parenteral nutrition that did not contain sufficient trace minerals.

3. Iron is a critical component of hemoglobin, myoglobin, and cytochromes. Iron acts as a cofactor for several enzyme systems. Two-thirds of the body's iron is found in hemoglobin in red blood cells, where its job is to transport oxygen from the lungs to the tissues. A prolonged low intake of iron can lead to decreased production of red blood cells and a lack of oxygen being delivered to the tissues. This condition is called iron deficiency anemia, which results in fatigue and apathy, as well as decreased learning ability in children.

4. The absorption of iron depends on the body's need for the mineral and on the form of iron in food. The body cannot readily excrete excess iron, but the body has evolved a mucosal block, which limits overabsorption. Heme iron from animal foods is better absorbed than nonheme iron obtained primarily from plant sources. The best sources of dietary iron are animal protein, including beef and other dark meats, oysters, liver, and broccoli.

5. Girls and women have a higher RDA for iron than men because of menstrual blood loss. Infants and children who live in poverty are often iron deficient because of a lack of heme iron in diet.

6. Iron toxicity occurs because of a genetic disorder called hemochromatosis, which causes the overabsorption of iron. A common form of poisoning also occurs among toddlers and young children who swallow a large number of iron pills. Death can occur.

7. Zinc functions as a cofactor for more than nearly 100 enzyme systems, which are important for growth, sexual development, immune function, wound healing, and taste. A zinc deficiency results in growth failure, loss of appetite, inadequate mental function, a persistent rash, and decreased immune function. Zinc deficiency in the United States and Canada is rare.

8. Like iron, the best dietary sources of zinc are found in animal foods. Need drives absorption. And like iron, there is a mucosal block in the intestinal cells, which regulates the amount of zinc that can be absorbed. Calcium, copper, and iron in supplement form can interfere with zinc absorption. The richest source of zinc is oysters. Other animal proteins are excellent sources. Plant sources are whole grains, peanuts, and legumes.

9. Copper aids in iron absorption and mobilization from body stores. Copper is responsible for the cross-linking in collagen formation and for nerve cell myelination, and it acts as part of an enzyme that is a scavenger for free radicals. A copper

deficiency can result in a secondary iron deficiency. Copper is found in liver, cocoa, legumes, and whole grains. The copper content of the soil where a plant is grown affects the copper content of the plant food.

10. Selenium acts as a cofactor for the enzyme glutathionine peroxidase, which protects cells against destruction by hydrogen peroxide and free radicals. In some instances, selenium can replace some of the need for vitamin E. Human deficiency is rare in the United States and Canada. The selenium content of the soil where a plant is grown greatly affects the selenium content of the plant food. In a few areas in China where the soil is selenium poor, the inhabitants experience selenium deficiency. Meat, eggs, fish, and shellfish are sources of selenium. Plant sources include grains and plant seeds.

11. Iodide forms part of the thyroid hormones, one being thyroxine. Thyroid hormone controls the basal metabolic rate. A lack of dietary iodide causes an enlarged thyroid gland, known as goiter. The iodide content of the soil where a plant is grown greatly affects the iodide content of the plant food. Iodide deficiency at one time was common in areas around the Great Lakes in North America because the soil is iodide poor. Today, iodide deficiency in Canada and the United States is virtually unknown because of the fortification of table salt with iodide, but there is some concern about iodide status in pregnant women.

12. Fluoride exposure makes the tooth crystal resistant to dental caries, and fluoride in saliva aids in the remineralization of damaged tooth surfaces. Most North Americans receive fluoride from fluoridated drinking water and toothpaste.

13. Chromium contributes to the action of insulin. Chromium is found in meats and whole grains.

14. Manganese functions in several important enzyme systems. Deficiency is rare. Whole grains, legumes, and animal foods are reliable food sources.

15. Molybdenum is found in several enzyme systems. Deficiency is rare. Molybdenum is found in plant foods such as legumes and whole grains.

16. Boron contributes to ion transport in cell membranes. Fruits, leafy vegetables, nuts, and beans are sources.

17. Nickel likely participates in amino acid metabolism. Nickel is found in nuts, beans, and whole grains.

18. Silicon is involved in bone formation. Root vegetables and whole grains are sources.

19. Arsenic likely participates in amino acid and DNA metabolism. Fish, grains and cereal products are sources.

20. Vanadium likely has insulin-like actions in the body. Shellfish and mushrooms are sources.

■ STUDY QUESTIONS

1. What is a balance study, and why is it only a limited tool in evaluating the need for trace minerals?
2. What is anemia? How does a deficiency of vitamins E, K, B-6, and B-12 and the trace minerals iron and copper cause anemia? Describe the signs and symptoms of such anemias.
3. Explain three key functions of iron in the human body.
4. What factors increase the absorption of dietary iron? How might an excess of zinc, manganese, and calcium inhibit iron absorption?
5. What are some tests used to measure iron status? What exactly do these tests measure?
6. Carbonic anhydrase and alcohol dehydrogenase are two enzymes requiring zinc as a cofactor. How do these enzymes function at the cellular level?

7. The fluoridation of drinking water began in the United States in 1945. Today, what percentage of the population consumes fluoridated water? How else do humans obtain fluoride?
8. Describe the chief function in the body of fluoride, copper, chromium, manganese, boron, nickel, and silicon.
9. Why are animal foods a better source of iron, zinc, and selenium than foods of plant origin?
10. Prior to the 1920s, why was goiter such a health problem for people living in the Pacific Northwest and the Great Lakes region of the United States and Canada? How was this deficiency disease controlled?

■ ANNOTATED REFERENCES

1. Abdulaziz A and others: Effect of consumption of food cooked in iron pots on iron status and growth of young children: A randomized trial. *Lancet* 353:712, 1999.

   In less-developed countries, novel strategies are needed to control iron deficiency anemia, the most common form of undernutrition. Ethiopian children fed food from iron pots had lower rates of anemia and better growth than children whose food was cooked in aluminum pots.

2. ADA Reports: Position of the American Dietetic Association: The impact of fluoride on health. *Journal of the American Dietetic Association* 101:126, 2001.

   The American Dietetic Association reaffirms that fluoride is an important element for all mineralized tissues in the body. Appropriate fluoride intake is beneficial to bone and tooth health.

3. Ahluwalia N: Diagnostic utility of serum transferrin receptors measurement in assessing iron status. *Nutrition Reviews* 56(5):133, 1998.

   Recently, attention has turned to a new way of assessing iron status that involves the measurement of transferrin receptors in the serum portion of the blood. Transferrin receptors are a sensitive index of tissue iron availability, which increase progressively in response to iron deficiency and are unaffected by underlying acute or chronic infection. The latter is true of the conventional tests.

4. Andrews NC: Disorders of iron metabolism. *The New England Journal of Medicine* 341:1986, 1999.

   Iron is able to accept and donate electrons, so it is capable of binding oxygen and participating in many enzyme systems. However, iron can damage tissues by causing the conversion of hydrogen peroxide to free radicals. Iron can't be readily excreted from the body; the cells that line the gastrointestinal tract act as a barrier to overabsorption.

5. Baynes RD: Iron. In Stipanuk MH: *Biochemical and physiological aspects of human nutrition.* Philadelphia: W.B. Saunders, 2000.

   Iron is part of a variety of body proteins, particularly those involved in the transport and metabolism of oxygen. Iron deficiency anemia is relatively rare in the United States and Canada but very common in poor nations throughout the world.

6. Beard J, Tobin B: Iron status and exercise. *American Journal of Clinical Nutrition* 72:594S, 2000.

   Female athletes, distance runners, and vegetarian athletes are at greatest risk for developing altered body iron due to increased rates of whole-body iron turnover. These groups should maintain an adequate consumption of iron from the diets and should consider the use of iron supplements under the care of a physician.

7. Beshgetoor D, Hambidge M: Clinical conditions altering copper metabolism in humans. *American Journal of Clinical Nutrition* 67:1017S, 1998.

   Overt copper deficiency is not believed to be a widespread public health concern for most population groups. However, acquired copper deficiency has been documented in conditions predisposing to inadequate copper intakes, in prematurity, in malabsorption syndromes, and in states showing excessive copper losses.

8. Briefel R and others: Zinc intake of the U.S. population: Findings from the third National Health and Nutrition Examination Survey, 1988–1994. *Journal of Nutrition* 130:1367S, 2000.

   Young children age 1–3 years, adolescent females age 12-19 years, and persons age 71 years and older are at the greatest risk of inadequate zinc intakes.

9. Burk R, Levander O: Selenium. In Shils ME and others (eds.): *Modern nutrition in health and disease.* 9th ed. Baltimore: Williams & Wilkins, 1999.

   Because of its role in glutathione peroxidases, selenium affects the antioxidant balance of the cell. The absorption, metabolism, transport, homeostasis, and excretion of selenium are discussed in detail.

10. Eisenstein RS: Iron regulatory proteins and the molecular control of mammalian iron metabolism. *Annual Review of Nutrition* 20:627, 2000.

    Control of iron metabolism is through the action iron regulatory proteins. These proteins control iron homeostasis in the body through the transport, cellular uptake, and metabolism of iron.

11. Food and Nutrition Board, Institute of Medicine: *Dietary Reference Intakes for calcium, phosphorus, magnesium, vitamin D, and fluoride.* Washington, DC: Standing Committee on the Scientific Evaluation of Dietary Reference Intakes National Academy Press, 1997.

    Owing to its ability to inhibit and even reverse dental caries and stimulate new bone formation, fluoride has been elevated to the status of an essential dietary nutrient. An Adequate Intake and a Upper Level have been established for this trace mineral. Most of the fluoride consumed by Canadians and Americans comes from drinking water and toothpaste.

12. Food and Nutrition Board, Institute of Medicine: *Dietary Reference Intakes for vitamin A, vitamin K, arsenic, boron, chromium, copper, iodine, iron, manganese, molybdenum, nickel, silicon, vanadium, and zinc.* Washington, DC: Standing Committee on the Scientific Evaluation of Dietary Reference Intakes National Academy Press, 2001.

    Dietary Reference Intakes have recently been set for many trace minerals. The rationale used to set RDA or Adequate Intakes and Upper Levels for these nutrients is discussed in detail.

13. Fraker P and others: The dynamic link between the integrity of the immune system and zinc status. *Journal of Nutrition* 130:1399S, 2000.

    The results of more than three decades of work indicate that zinc deficiency rapidly diminishes antibody and cell-mediated responses in both humans and animals. There is substantial evidence that zinc supplementation in people who underconsume the nutrient may reduce the impact of many diseases by preventing this dismantling of the immune system.

14. Freake H: Iodine. In Stipanuk MH: *Biochemical and physiological aspects of human nutrition.* Philadelphia: W.B. Saunders, 2000.

    The sole function of iodide in humans and other mammals is the synthesis of the thyroid hormones. However, the multiple actions of the thyroid hormones mean that iodide ends up having an impact on a wide range of metabolic and developmental functions. Further information regarding absorption, transport, metabolism, storage, and excretion of iodide are discussed in detail.

15. Haddow J and others: Maternal thyroid deficiency during pregnancy and subsequent neuropsychological development of the child. *The New England Journal of Medicine* 341:549, 1999.

    Hypothyroidism caused by iodide deficiency during pregnancy results in adverse affects to the fetus's neuropsychological development and may cause mental retardation. Therefore, screening for thyroid deficiency during pregnancy may be warranted.

16. Hallberg L: Does calcium interfere with iron absorption? *American Journal of Clinical Nutrition* 68:3, 1998.

    Some studies have shown that calcium has an adverse effect on the absorption of iron when both are consumed at the same meal. Therefore, practical considerations are that those with high iron requirements (adolescents and menstruating and pregnant women) should try to restrict calcium intake with meals that contain most of the dietary iron and that calcium supplements, when needed, should be taken when going to bed.

17. Hetzel B: Iodine and neuropsychological development. *Journal of Nutrition* 130:493S, 2000.

    The establishment of the essential links among iodine deficiency, thyroid function, and brain development has emerged over the past 20 years. Iodide deficiency is now regarded by the WHO as the most common preventable cause of brain damage in the world today, with at least 30 million suffering from this preventable condition.

18. Holben D, Smith A: The diverse role of selenium within selenoproteins: A review. *Journal of the American Dietetic Association* 99:836, 1999.

    The biological roles of selenium are diverse, including its role as a component of glutathione peroxidase and its role in thyroid hormone metabolism. Selenium is vital for normal development, growth, and metabolism.

19. Huffman G: Zinc can reduce pediatric respiratory infections. *American Family Physician* 58:2127, 1998.

    Zinc supplementation in the RDA amounts has been shown to be effective in reducing the morbidity associated with acute lower respiratory infections in infants and children, possibly by improving immune status.

20. Jackson JL and others: Zinc and the common cold: A meta-analysis revisited. *Journal of Nutrition* 130:1512S, 2000.

    An analysis of current studies using zinc supplements to treat the common cold failed to find evidence of a significant reduction in cold duration. Studies reporting a benefit from zinc therapy have been criticized for poor blinding of the study subjects.

21. Kalkwarf H, Harrast S: Effects of calcium supplementation and lactation on iron status. *American Journal of Clinical Nutrition* 67:1244, 1998.

    The findings from this study suggest that in the long-term calcium supplementation in women does not impair iron stores. Calcium supplementation had no effect on serum ferritin concentrations of the women in this study who were in the postpartum period.

22. King JC, Keen CL: Zinc. In Shils ME and others (eds.): *Modern nutrition in health and disease.* 9th ed. Baltimore: Williams & Wilkins, 1999.

   Zinc is present in many different enzymes. This and other roles of zinc are reviewed in this chapter, as well as signs and symptoms of zinc deficiency and toxicity.

23. Lee K and others: Too much versus too little: The implications of current iodine intake in the United States. *Nutrition Reviews* 57:177, 1999.

   Recent data show a decline in iodide intake during the past two decades, especially in women of reproductive age. The recent reduction in dietary iodide may be owing to several factors, including the dairy industry's effort to reduce iodide in milk, the replacement of iodide with bromine salts as the dough conditioner in bread products, and the reduced intake of eggs for concern over cholesterol content.

24. Milne D: Copper intake and assessment of copper status. *American Journal of Clinical Nutrition* 67:1041 S, 1998.

   The diagnosis of marginal copper deficiency has not been perfected, despite an increased understanding of the physiologic roles of copper. Copper-containing enzymes in blood cells may be better indicators of copper stores than plasma concentrations of copper.

25. Nielsen F: Ultratrace minerals. In Shils ME and others (eds.): *Modern nutrition in health and disease.* 9th ed. Baltimore: Williams & Wilkins, 1999.

   At least 18 elements could be considered ultratrace minerals: aluminum, arsenic, boron, bromine, cadmium, chromium, fluoride, germanium, iodine, lead, lithium, molybdenum, nickel, rubidium, selenium, silicon, tin, and vanadium. The role of each in human and laboratory animal physiological systems is reviewed in this chapter.

26. Pena M and others: A delicate balance: Homeostatic control of copper uptake and distribution. *Journal of Nutrition* 129:1251, 1999.

   It is widely accepted that copper is an essential trace element required for survival by all organisms from bacterial cells to humans. The cellular uptake and intracellular distribution of copper are precisely orchestrated to ensure that it is delivered to copper-requiring proteins without releasing free copper ions, which would otherwise cause damage to cellular components.

27. Rainey C and others: Daily boron intake from the American diet. *Journal of the American Dietetic Association* 99:335, 1999.

   Coffee and milk are low in boron, yet they are the top two contributors of boron to the American diet due to the high volume of consumption. Other sources are peanut butter, raisins, and wine.

28. Schrauzer G: Selenomethionine: A review of its nutritional significance, metabolism and toxicity. *Journal of Nutrition* 130:1653, 2000.

   Although the need for selenium in human and animal nutrition is well recognized, the question concerning the proper form of selenium for supplemental use is still being debated. Since selenomethionine is a major natural food form of selenium it should be given in supplemental form if supplements are required.

29. Stoecker B: Chromium. In Shils ME and others (eds.): *Modern nutrition in health and disease.* 9th ed. Baltimore: Williams & Wilkins, 1999.

   Chromium is widely distributed, albeit in small quantities, throughout the food supply. Chromium is a bone-seeking element, and its uptake in bone appears to be rapid. Several investigators have noted that chromium accumulates in bone, the spleen, the liver, and the kidneys. These findings, along with more on the bioavailability and absorption of chromium, are discussed.

30. Utiger R: Maternal hypothyroidism and fetal development. *The New England Journal of Medicine* 341(8):601, 1999.

   Thyroid deficiency during the latter two-thirds of gestation and the first months after delivery can result in mental retardation and sometimes neurological deficits. These abnormalities can be prevented by increasing the mother's intake of iodide, but it must be increased by the beginning of the third month of pregnancy, if not sooner.

31. Vincent J: The biochemistry of chromium. *Journal of Nutrition* 130:715, 2000.

   Chromium has been known to be an essential micronutrient for mammals for four decades. However, the most popular form of chromium in dietary supplements, chromium picolinate, appears to be absorbed in a different fashion than from dietary chromium and can lead to the production of harmful hydroxyl radicals.

32. Whitford G: Fluoride. In Stipanuk MH: *Biochemical and physiological aspects of human nutrition.* Philadelphia: W.B. Saunders, 2000.

   Based on its ability to increase bone mass, fluoride is being used as an experimental drug in the treatment of osteoporosis. Fluoride stimulates bone-forming cells, osteoblasts, to increase the production of several proteins to form new bone. Although the literature contains conflicting reports, recent studies with a slow-release fluoride formulation have shown positive results.

TAKE ACTION

I. HOW DOES YOUR TRACE MINERAL INTAKE MEASURE UP?

To complete this activity, you must reexamine the nutritional assessment you did for Chapter 2. Based on that analysis of your nutritional intake for 1 day, fill in the values for your intake, the RDA and the percentage of the RDA you consumed for each of the minerals listed in the following table. In the right-hand column, indicate whether your intake was higher than (+), lower than (−), or about equal to (=) the recommended intakes.

Mineral	Intake	RDA	% of RDA	+, −, =
Iron	____	____	____	____
Zinc	____	____	____	____
Selenium	____	____	____	____
Copper	____	____	____	____

Analysis

1. Which of your mineral intakes equaled or exceeded the RDA?

2. Which of your intakes were below this standard for your age and gender?

3. What foods or cooking practices could be emphasized or deemphasized to modify your dietary deficiencies?

II. CHECK OUT YOUR MUNICIPAL WATER SUPPLY

Healthy People 2010 set a goal that 75% of Americans will be served by community water systems that add sufficient fluoride. Today, only about 60% of Americans have access to naturally or artificially fluoridated water. Is your hometown (or college town) water supply fluoridated? To find the answer, check with your local water department. What amount of fluoride is added to drinking water, and how long has this procedure been in operation? You can also check with your family dentist, as he or she will know how much fluoride is added to the water in your hometown. If the water supply is not fluoridated, what procedures does your dentist recommend for obtaining sufficient fluoride?

CHROMIUM—40 YEARS OF NUTRITIONAL CONTROVERSY CONTINUES, FORREST H. NIELSEN PH.D.

Dr. Nielsen, the center director and research nutritionist at the USDA, ARS, Grand Forks Human Nutrition Research Center in Grand Forks, North Dakota, focuses his research efforts on the ultratrace elements. The opinions expressed are those of Forrest H. Nielsen; they do not represent or should not be construed as the official position or policy of the U.S. Department of Agriculture.

In 1959, trivalent chromium was identified as the active component of the "glucose tolerance factor" that alleviated impaired glucose tolerance in rats fed torula yeast-sucrose diets. Since that time, the acceptance of chromium as an essential nutrient and an element of clinical nutrition importance has ebbed and flowed. When one wants to illustrate polarized views, unproven claims and counterclaims, suspicions about commercial bias and conflict of interest in nutrition, chromium can be considered a prime candidate. Forty years after it was first suggested, chromium essentiality is still debated. The situation is similar for the contention that chromium has anti-diabetic properties. Today chromium supplements are still being touted as being able to help build muscle, promote weight loss as fat, prevent cardiovascular disease, and extend life span. In contrast, some scientists are raising alarm about the possibility that some forms of chromium, particularly chromium picolinate, can increase cellular concentrations of this element to amounts that can cause the generation of DNA-damaging hydroxyl radicals. With such uncertainty among scientists, the discussion provided here about the role of chromium in nutrition could change as more research findings are reported.

◼ Is Chromium Essential?

In 1959, the definition of essentiality generally accepted was that a dietary deficiency of a substance had to consistently and adversely change a biological function from optimal, and this change had to be preventable or reversible by nutritional, not pharmacological, intakes of the substance. Thus, when it was reported that chromium was needed for normal glucose tolerance, it was generally accepted as essential. Essentiality of chromium for humans gained acceptance when it was reported in 1977 that a human on long-term total parenteral nutrition containing a low amount of chromium developed impaired glucose tolerance, or hyperglycemia, with glucose spilling into the urine, and a resistance to insulin action; these abnormalities were reversed by chromium supplementation. In the 1980s and 1990s, establishing essentiality on the basis of the above definition began to receive resistance when a large number of elements were suggested to be essential based on some small change in a physiological or biochemical variable. Many of these changes were suggested to be caused by pharmacological or toxicological action, not deficient essential function, in the body. Thus, today if the lack of an element can not be shown to cause death or interrupt the life cycle, many scientists, probably a majority, now do not consider an element essential unless it has a defined biochemical function. With this new definition, the essentiality of chromium became a controversial issue.

Those not accepting chromium as essential stated that a defined biochemical function was needed for this element because nutritional, metabolic, physiological or hormonal stressors generally had to be used to induce experimental animals to respond to chromium deprivation, and the responses were not remarkable. Chromium deprivation did not cause death or interrupt the life cycle. Moreover, it was pointed out that the human cases reportedly supporting chromium essentiality did not ascertain that chromium was specifically needed; that is, it was not ascertained whether supplementation with another element such as copper, manganese, or vanadium would have had a similar effect.

Recently the doubt about chromium essentiality has ebbed because a small peptide that binds four chromic ions called chromodulin has been found in a variety of tissues from several animals. Chromodulin has the ability to potentiate the conversion of glucose into carbon dioxide or lipid though stimulating the action of insulin. This stimulation is directly dependent on the chromium content of chromodulin, and is not induced by any other naturally occurring chromium-containing substance. Although it has been suggested that chromodulin is nothing more than a molecule for the detoxification and excretion of chromium, the preponderance of the biochemical evidence associated with chromodulin, along with the finding that chromium has beneficial effects on glucose and lipid metabolism in animals and humans, supports the contention that chromium is an essential nutrient for humans.

■ Adequate Chromium Intakes

A new Dietary Reference Intake (DRI) for chromium has been formulated: the Adequate Intake is 20–35 µg/day for adults. It should be noted, however, because other substances in the diet influence the absorption of chromium, chromium intake adequacy depends in part on the composition of the diet. For example, vitamin C (ascorbic acid) and aspirin increase absorption, while antacids decrease it.

Data exist that suggest a chromium intake of less than 20 µg/day is inadequate. Based on dietary surveys, a significant number of North Americans may be consuming less than this amount. As a result, it is not surprising that some studies identified some individuals who responded to chromium supplementation. However, a much larger number of individuals in these studies did not respond to chromium supplements. This indicates that when chromium status is adequate, a higher intake or supplementation would have little or no effect on existing glucose or lipid metabolism, and thus have no effect on such things as body composition, weight loss, muscle building, or aging.

■ Chromium as a Therapeutic Agent for Diabetes

In a double-blind randomized study of 180 residents of Beijing, China, some measures selected for high blood glucose, including glycosylated hemoglobin, were improved by 200 µg/day, and reduced to near normal by 1000 µg chromium/day provided as a picolinate supplement. Since 1970, numerous other reports have appeared indicating that chromium can potentiate the action of low amounts of insulin or improve the efficacy of insulin, such that the need for exogenous sources is reduced or eliminated for some type 2 diabetics. Some expert groups assembled to evaluate these reports have concluded that the data are still too sparse and inconclusive to make a recommendation about the use of chromium for diabetics. They feel that large, long-term, placebo-controlled randomized clinical trials in well-characterized at-risk populations are necessary to determine the effects of high chromium supplementation on variables associated with diabetes. Nonetheless, there is a growing body of evidence suggesting that chromium supplementation might be a viable treatment option for some people with diabetes resulting from inadequate synthesis of insulin or with insulin resistance. However, it needs to be emphasized that only a select group of people would be able to use this as a basis for taking high, or pharmacological, doses of chromium, and this would be best done while under the care of a physician.

■ Misleading Claims for Chromium Supplements

The promotion of chromium picolinate as an ergogenic aid or weight loss inducer provides examples of the deceptive use of valid research findings or use of questionable data for the purpose of making an unscrupulous profit. The positive ergogenic and weight loss findings that have come from research supported by the maker of chromium picolinate have failed to be duplicated. Interestingly, the promoters of chromium as a weight loss aid fail to inform potential consumers that in one fairly well-controlled study, chromium picolinate supplementation resulted in a significant weight GAIN in young obese women. In brief, most ergogenic-oriented studies have found chromium supplementation to be ineffective for increasing muscle mass, strength gain and athletic performance, and there are no data from well-designed studies to support the claim that chromium picolinate supplementation is an effective weight loss modality.

■ A Reasonable Approach

Regardless of the uncertainties about chromium, substantial evidence shows that it is an essential nutrient that many individuals are routinely consuming in inadequate amounts, and thus would benefit from an increased intake. The best and most enjoyable way of doing this is by eating a varied diet with good sources of chromium. Processed meats, liver, whole grain products including some ready-to-eat breakfast cereals, legumes such as dried peas, lentils and beans, some vegetables including broccoli and mushrooms, and spices are some of the best sources of chromium. If one insists on taking a supplement for "insurance" or "peace of mind," a separate chromium supplement is unnecessary. A multivitamin-mineral supplement containing chromium will do.

ENERGY BALANCE AND WEIGHT CONTROL

chapter 13

O f people you see on the street, one-fourth of the men and nearly half the women are struggling to control their weight. Still, despite all their efforts, the ranks of the obese in America and worldwide are growing. Recall from Chapter 1 that it is estimated that 1.1 billion people in the world are overweight. This problem is increasing not only in the United States but also in affluent peoples in Brazil, China, India, Russia, the United Kingdom, and Germany. This excess weight increases the likelihood of many health problems, such as coronary heart disease, cancer, hypertension and strokes, certain bone and joint disorders, and type 2 diabetes.[9, 23]

Currently, most weight-reduction efforts fizzle before bodies fall into a healthy weight range. Monotonous, ineffective, and confusing, typical fad diets even endanger some populations, such as children, teenagers, pregnant women, and people with various health disorders. Yet a more logical approach to weight loss is actually very straightforward: (1) Eat less; (2) increase physical activity; and (3) change problematic eating behaviors.[27]

Experts are calling for a national commitment to address the growing weight problem in the United States. They suspect that, without a national commitment to weight maintenance and effective new approaches to making the environment more favorable to maintaining healthy weight, the current trends will not be reversed.[13, 24] This chapter discusses these recommendations to help you understand obesity's effects, causes, and potential treatments.

■ KEY CHAPTER CONCEPTS

- Energy balance is energy intake minus energy output. Positive energy balance occurs when energy intake is greater than energy output.
- Total energy use by the body is accounted for by basal metabolism, the thermic effect of food, physical activity, and nonexercise activity thermogenesis. The first two factors typically account for about 70 to 80% of energy use.
- Energy use by the body can be measured directly from heat output or indirectly from oxygen uptake. Energy needs can be estimated using formulas based on various combinations of body weight, height, degree of physical activity, and age.
- A variety of related forces promote the desire to eat. The major determinants of food intake are most likely availability and related habits, as well as various social factors, rather than hunger per se.
- A person of healthy weight shows good health and performs daily activities without weight-related problems. A body mass index (weight [in kilograms] divided by height^2 [in meters]) of 18.5 to 25 is one measure of healthy weight, although weight in excess of this value may not necessarily indicate ill health. Overweight and overfat are not necessarily synonymous.
- Obesity can be defined as total body fat percentage over 25% in men and about 35% in women. A body mass index over 30 also generally represents obesity.
- Fat distribution partially determines health risks from obesity. Excess upper body fat storage distribution suggests higher risks of hypertension, cardiovascular disease, and type 2 diabetes than does excess fat distribution on the lower part of the body.
- Genetic factors influence the tendency to develop obesity. How a person is raised (or nurtured) is also an influence. Obesity can be viewed as nurture allowing nature to be expressed.
- When considering a treatment for obesity, remember these important points: (1) The emphasis should be on preventing obesity, because curing the disorder is very difficult; (2) the body resists weight loss; and (3) rapid weight loss and quick regain can be harmful to emotional health.
- A sound weight-loss plan recommends regular physical activity and meets the dieter's nutritional needs by emphasizing a wide variety of low-fat and nonfat food choices from the Food Guide Pyramid that total less calories than energy needs. Fruits, vegetables, and whole grain breads and cereals deserve special attention.
- Modifying problem eating behaviors is another important part of a weight-loss program.
- Above all, it is important to remember that a healthy, active lifestyle offers the best hope for weight control in the long term.

■ REFRESH YOUR MEMORY

As you begin your study of weight control in Chapter 13, you may want to review

- The concept of energy density and the use of the exchange system in Chapter 2
- The nervous and endocrine systems in Chapter 3
- The causes and consequences of ketosis in Chapter 4
- The fat content of various foods in Chapter 6
- The long-term risks of high protein diets in Chapter 7

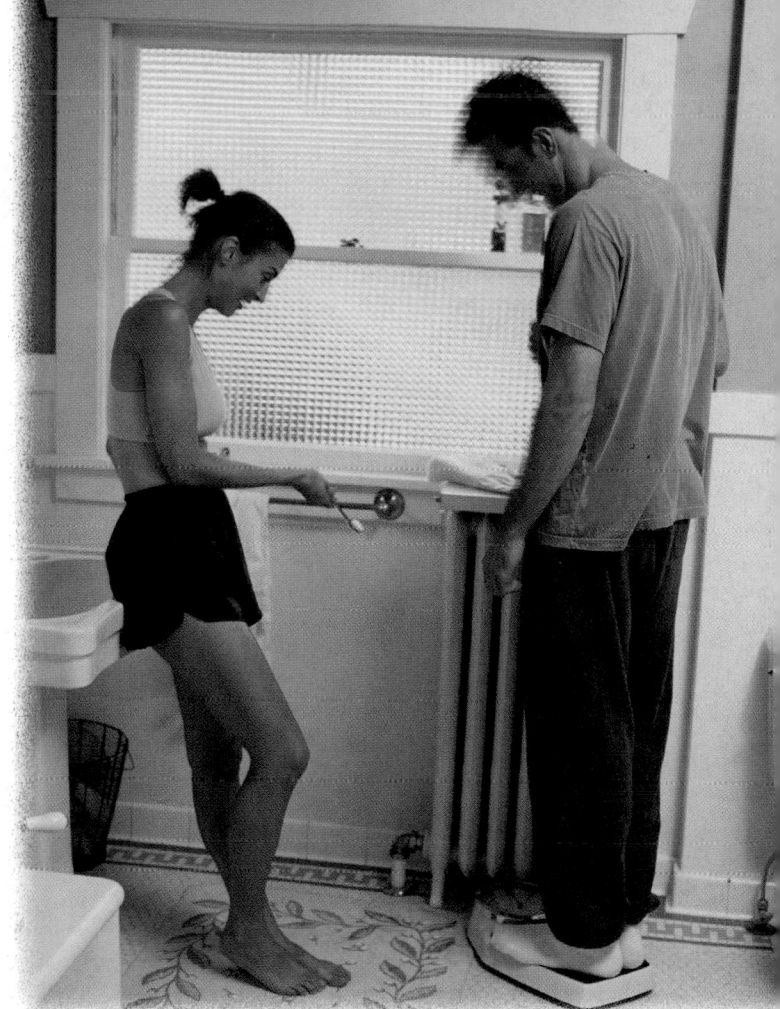

■ CASE SCENARIO

Crystal has a hectic schedule. She works during the day for a "temp" agency, primarily performing secretarial duties. At night, three times a week she attends class at the local community college in pursuit of computer certification. She has little time to think about what she eats—convenience rules. Unfortunately, over the past few years Crystal's weight has been climbing. Watching television a few nights ago, she saw an infomercial for a product that promises she can eat large portions of tasty foods but not gain weight. Famous celebrities support the claim that this product allows one to eat at will and not gain weight. She doesn't have a lot of spare money, but the claim that by taking this product you can eat whatever you want and never gain weight is tempting. What do you think she should do?

■ ENERGY BALANCE

This chapter on weight control starts with some good news and some bad news. The good news is that you are probably at a healthy body weight. An important life goal is to stay within the recommended range for healthy body weight. The bad news is that over 60% of all American adults are overweight (about 40% of these people are obese [25% of the total population]), and there is a good chance that any of us can join those ranks if we don't pay attention to the prevention of significant adult weight gain. Gaining more than 10 pounds or 2 inches in waist circumference should be a red flag that diet re-evaluation is in order. This preventive strategy is currently considered the most potent form of therapy for the problem of overweight in our society. Other strategies do exist; however, as you will see, they have not shown to be as successful as prevention.[13, 32]

Bathroom scales keep many of us emotionally off balance. We would all benefit by paying more attention to another scale—that of **energy balance.** This balance depends on energy input and energy output. These in turn influence energy stores, primarily, the amount of triglyceride in adipose tissue (Fig. 13-1). Energy balance can be thought of as an equation: energy consumed minus energy expended. You are in positive energy balance when energy consumed is greater than energy expended. The result of **positive energy balance** is the storage of the excess energy.

An example of when positive energy balance is necessary is during pregnancy because the surplus of energy supports the developing fetus. Infants and children also need to be in positive energy balance to grow. In adults, however, positive energy balance causes creeping weight gain.

Negative energy balance results from an energy deficit. Energy consumed is less than energy expended. Weight loss occurs when a person is in a state of negative energy balance. In adulthood, however, the weight that is lost consists of a combination of lean and adipose tissue.

As noted in the overview, the maintenance of energy balance—energy intake matching energy output over the long run—substantially contributes to health and well-being in adults by minimizing the risk of developing many common health problems. As well, adulthood is often a time of creeping weight gain, which eventually turns into obesity if not checked. However, increasing age is not the primary reason for this weight gain; it is caused primarily by the pattern of excess food intake and limited physical activity. Let's look in detail at the factors that affect the relationship between positive and negative energy balance.

■ Energy Intake

Energy needs are met by food intake, represented by the number of kcal eaten each day. Determining the appropriate amount and type of food to match energy needs over the long run is a challenge for many of us. Our ability to consume food and use it efficiently is an evolutionary survival mechanism. However, given modern North American food supplies, many of us are now too successful in obtaining food energy.[13] Given the wide availability of food in vending machines, drive-up windows, social gatherings, and fast-food (quick-service) restaurants—combined with the ubiquitous *super-sized* portions—it is no wonder that the average adult is 8 pounds heavier than just 10 years ago.[22] You might say "food hunts man" today, rather than man hunting food as in earlier times.

How much food energy is contained in a meal? A bomb calorimeter is used to determine the amount of energy in a food (Fig. 13-2). The process involves burning a portion of food inside a chamber of the calorimeter that is surrounded by water. As the food burns, it gives off heat, which raises the temperature of the water surrounding the chamber. The increase in water temperature measured after the food has burned indicates the amount of energy in the food. One kcal is the amount of energy required to increase the temperature of 1 kg (about 2.2 lb) of water 1° Celsius.

energy balance The state in which energy intake, in the form of food and/or alcohol, matches the energy expended, primarily through basal metabolism and physical activity.

positive energy balance The state in which energy intake is greater than energy expended, generally resulting in weight gain.

negative energy balance The state in which energy intake is less than energy expended, resulting in weight loss.

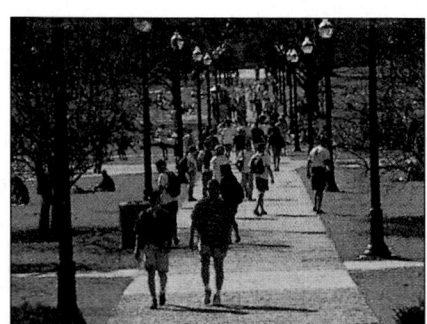

Student life is full of physical activity. This is not necessarily true for a person's later working life; hence, weight gain is a strong possibility.

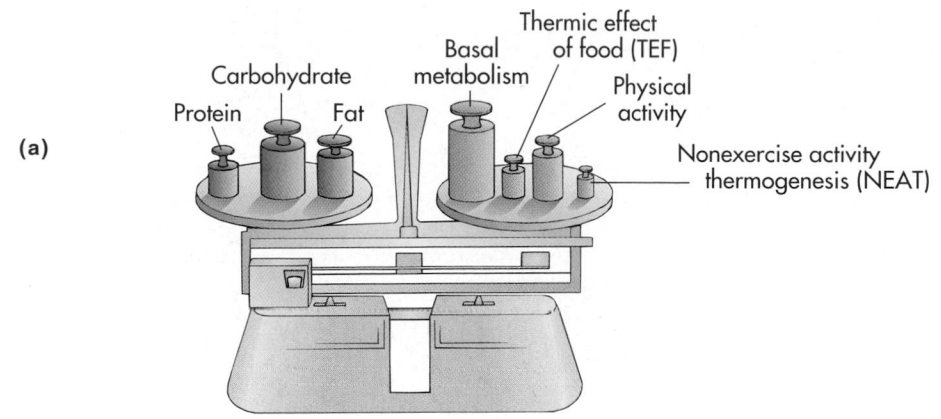

(a)

CRITICAL THINKING

A 26-year-old classmate of yours has been thinking about the process of aging. One of the things she fears most as she gets older is gaining weight. How would you explain energy balance to her?

(b)

Intake	Output	Weight change

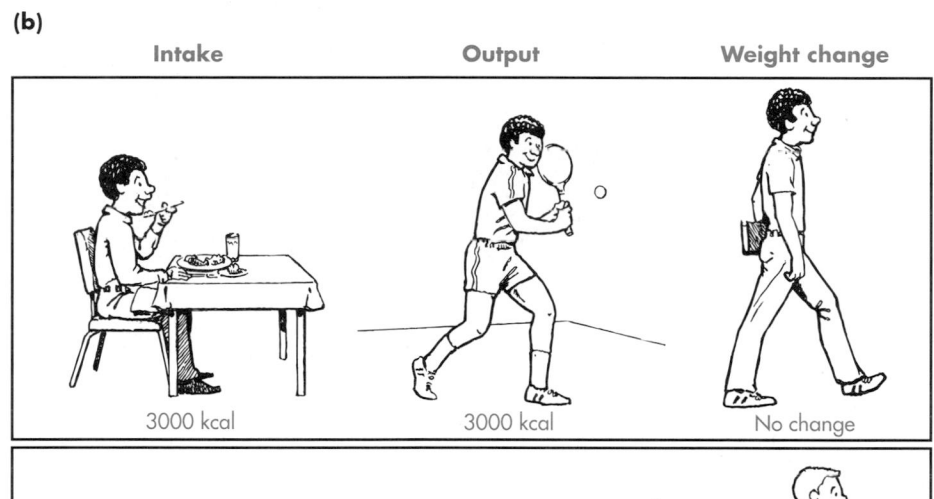

3000 kcal   3000 kcal   No change

Energy balance (equilibrium)

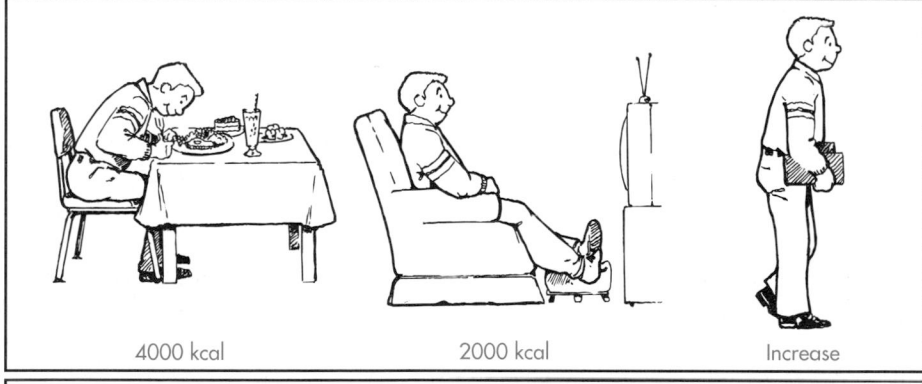

4000 kcal   2000 kcal   Increase

Positive energy balance

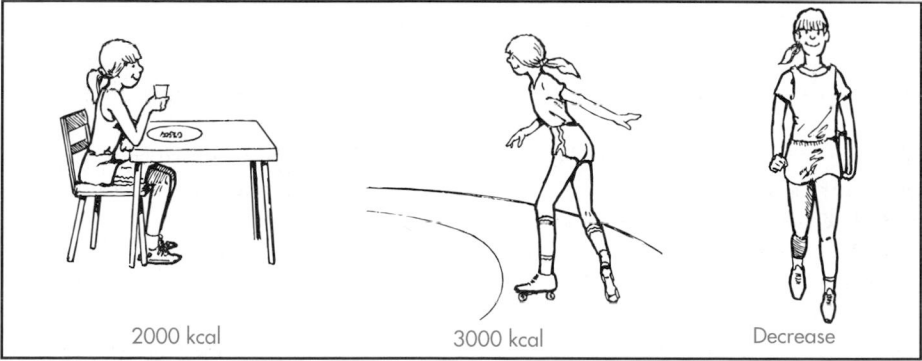

2000 kcal   3000 kcal   Decrease

Negative energy balance

▌FIGURE **13-1** A model for energy balance. (*a*) This model incorporates the major variables, discussed in the chapter, that influence energy balance. Note that alcohol is an additional source of energy for some of us. (*b*) Depiction of energy balance in practical terms.

Illustration by William Ober.

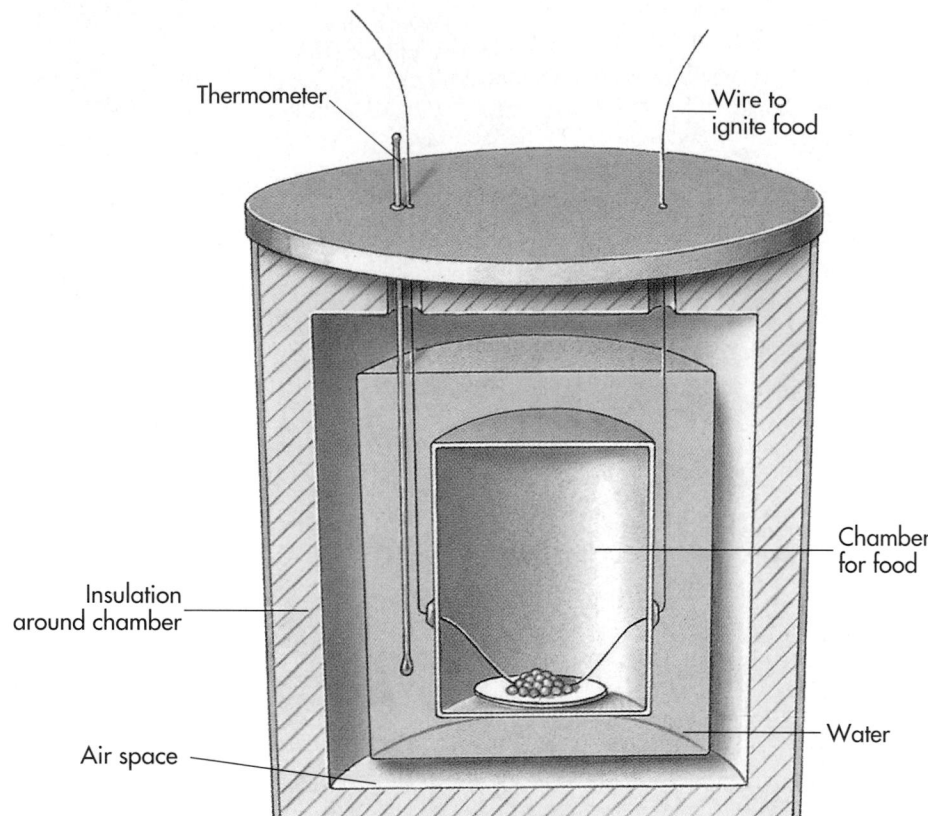

■ FIGURE 13-2 Cross section of a bomb calorimeter. To determine energy content, a dried portion of food is burned inside a chamber charged with oxygen and surrounded by water. As the food is burned, it gives off heat, which raises the temperature of the water surrounding the chamber. The amount of increase in water temperature indicates the number of kcal contained in the food. Recall that 1 kcal equals the amount of heat needed to raise the temperature of 1 kg of water 1°C.
Illustration by William Ober.

*T*oday, scientific journals often express energy intake and output in kjoules, rather than kcal (see Chapter 1).

The bomb calorimeter provides values for the amount of energy that can be derived from carbohydrate, fat, protein, and alcohol. Recall that carbohydrates yield about 4 kcal/g, proteins yield about 4 kcal/g, fats yield about 9/kcal/g, and alcohol yields 7 kcal/g. These energy figures have been adjusted for (1) digestibility and (2) substances in food, such as fibrous plant parts, that burn in the bomb calorimeter but are unusable by the human body for energy needs. The figures are then rounded to whole numbers.

In bomb calorimeter studies, fats produce close to 9 kcal/g. This value alone should warn us about the overconsumption of fat. However, most absorbed fats are not immediately burned in the body for energy needs. Instead, much fat goes directly into storage in adipose tissue. We have an essentially unlimited ability to do this.

In contrast, we have a limited ability to store carbohydrate as glycogen. As well, most carbohydrate is used at the time of consumption for energy needs or glycogen synthesis; generally little is converted to fat for storage in the body. This is not to say, however, that infinite amounts of carbohydrate can be consumed: Excessive amounts can lead to increased fat synthesis.

Protein is used for tissue synthesis, but adults generally eat more than enough protein for this. Beyond body needs, excess amounts of amino acids are generally metabolized for energy; only some are metabolized as fat.

Carbohydrate and protein intake also stimulate body use of these fuels. This is not true for fat. Finally, excess amounts of carbohydrate or protein are only inefficiently turned into fat, if this occurs at all.

Based on these observations, experts suggest that ideally fat intake should not exceed the amount of fat burned by the body. Active people can achieve this more easily than those who are sedentary can, since physical activity encourages burning of dietary fat. For a person who is sedentary and consumes a large amount of dietary fat, it is thought that any obesity that results actually represents an adaptation to this high-fat diet. This is because it is thought that only by reaching a certain point of body fatness will this sedentary person be able to balance the amount of fat burned by the body with fat intake: The greater fat mass present now allows for more release of body fat into circulation, so more fat is available for use. In other words, one needs enough fat mass to be able to burn the great amount of fat consumed.[26]

As noted in Chapters 2 and 6, it is also easier to overeat high-fat foods because they are energy dense and highly palatable. We can more easily eat a few extra cookies than a few extra apples, even though both may contain about the same amount of food energy. Laboratory animals become more obese when provided with high-fat foods than with their typical leaner fare. All these findings suggest that, to reduce or control body fatness, focus on controlling fat intake, substituting instead moderate amounts of foods rich in complex carbohydrates and dietary fiber.[19]

■ Energy Use

So far, some factors concerning energy intake have been discussed. Now let's look at the other side of the relationship—energy output.

The body uses energy for three general purposes: basal metabolism, physical activity, and the thermic effect of food. Fidgeting demonstrates another minor form of energy turned into heat production, and is part of what is called *nonexercise activity thermogenesis* (NEAT) (review Fig. 13-1).

Basal Metabolism

As covered in Chapter 12, basal metabolism represents the minimum energy expended in a fasting state (12 hours) to keep a resting, awake body alive in a warm, quiet environment. This requires about 60 to 70% of total energy use by the body. The processes involved include maintaining a heartbeat, respiration, temperature, and other functions. It does not include energy used for physical activity or food digestion. For an example of how basal metabolism contributes to energy needs, consider a 130-lb woman. Convert her weight, in pounds, into kilograms ($130 \div 2.2 = 59$ kg). Then, multiply 59 kg $\times$ 0.9 kcal/kg/hr $\times$ 24 hours = 1274 kcal needed for basal metabolism. Note that basal metabolism varies 25 to 30% among individuals.

The amount of energy used for basal metabolism depends primarily on **lean body mass.** That is, basal metabolism is generally higher in people with greater amounts of lean body mass than in those with large proportions of fat mass. The participating tissues—such as muscle, liver, brain, and kidney—show high metabolic activity at rest and have high energy needs. Other influences that determine basal metabolism include the following:

- The amount of body surface (the greater the area, the greater the heat loss)
- Gender (males average higher energy use because of greater lean body mass)
- Body temperature (fever increases basal metabolism)
- Thyroid hormones (increase basal metabolism)
- Aspects of nervous system activity, such as norepinephrine release (increases basal metabolism)
- Age (basal metabolism rate falls as we age through adulthood)
- Nutritional state (eating less slows basal metabolism rate in the short term)
- Pregnancy (increases basal metabolism)
- Caffeine and tobacco use (increase basal metabolism)

A low energy intake decreases the basal metabolism by about 10 to 20%, or about 150 to 300 kcal/day. This makes losing weight difficult. In addition, the effects of aging make weight maintenance hard. Basal metabolism declines about 2% each decade past age 30 as activity-metabolizing cells slowly and steadily decrease. However, because physical activity helps maintain lean body mass, remaining active as one ages helps maintain a high basal metabolism and, in turn, aids in weight control.[31]

Energy for Physical Activity

Physical activity increases energy expenditure above and beyond basal energy needs by as much as 25 to 40%. In choosing to be active or inactive, we determine much

While a person is resting, the percentage of total energy use by various organs is about as follows:

Liver	27%
Brain	19%
Skeletal muscle	18%
Kidney	10%
Heart	7%
Other	19%

lean body mass Body weight minus fat storage weight equals lean body mass. This includes organs such as the brain, muscles, and liver, as well as blood and other body fluids.

When planning a smoking cessation program, a plan to limit weight gain should also be implemented. Smoking cessation is linked to an increased risk of weight gain and obesity. Any form of regular physical activity can be extremely beneficial in an attempt to keep weight in check. Various risk factors associated with smoking, however, make it essential that this population obtain approval from a physician before beginning an intensive exercise regimen.

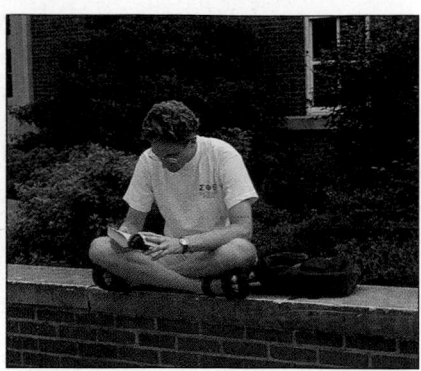

Studying leads to mental stress but puts little physical stress on the body. Hence, energy needs are only about 1.5 kcal/min.

thermic effect of food (TEF) The increase in metabolism occurring during the digestion, absorption, and metabolism of energy-yielding nutrients. This represents 5 to 10% of energy consumed.

*O*ther names for the thermic effect of food include *specific dynamic action* and *diet-induced thermogenesis.*

nonexercise activity thermogenesis (NEAT) Adaptive energy expended in heat production, such as fidgeting when one is subjected to overfeeding.

sympathetic nervous system Part of the nervous system that regulates involuntary vital functions, including the activity of the heart muscle, smooth muscle, and adrenal glands.

of our total energy expenditure for a day. Unlike basal metabolism, energy expenditure from physical activity varies widely among people.

Climbing stairs rather than riding the elevator, walking rather than driving to the store, and standing in a bus rather than sitting increase physical activity and, hence, energy use. People who fidget use more energy (an extra 100 to 800 kcal daily) than do those who readily relax.

The alarming rate of and recent increase in obesity in North America are caused in part by our inactivity. We eat little more than people did at the turn of the twentieth century, but we are less active. Jobs demand less physical activity, and leisure time is usually spent slouched before a television or computer.

Thermic Effect of Food (TEF)

In addition to basal metabolism and physical activity, the body uses energy to digest, absorb, and further process food nutrients. Energy used for these tasks accounts for the **thermic effect of food (TEF).** The energy cost of this thermic effect is analogous to a sales tax. It is like being taxed about 5 to 10% for the total energy you eat. The charge covers the cost of processing that energy. To supply the body with 100 kcal for basal metabolism and physical activity, you must eat between 105 and 110 kcal. The processes of digestion, absorption, and metabolism use the extra 5 to 10 kcal to modify the energy-yielding nutrients for use. Given a daily energy intake of 3000 kcal, the thermic effect of food uses 150 to 300 kcal ($3000 \times 0.05 = 150$; $3000 \times 0.1 = 300$). However, the total amount can vary somewhat among individuals.

The TEF value for a carbohydrate-rich or a protein-rich meal is higher than for a fat-rich meal. This is because it takes less energy to transfer absorbed fat into adipose stores than to convert glucose into glycogen or to metabolize excess amino acids into fat (see Chapter 4). In addition, large meals show higher values for TEF than the same amount of food eaten over many hours. Some possible mechanisms for this phenomenon include changes in central nervous system activity, greater production and release of hormones (such as insulin) and enzymes, and the rate of absorption and storage of macronutrients.

Nonexercise Activity Thermogenesis (NEAT)

Nonexercise activity thermogenesis represents the increase in nonvoluntary physical activity triggered by overeating. This activity includes fidgeting, maintenance of muscle tone, and maintenance of body posture when not lying down. The increase in food intake may lead to an increase in **sympathetic nervous system** activity, which in turn may increase fidgeting. One study has shown that some people resists weight gain from overfeeding by inducing NEAT, whereas others are not able to do so to as great an extent.[15]

Overall, a sedentary person uses 70 to 80% of energy for a combination of basal metabolism and the thermic effect of food. The remainder is used for physical activity and nonexercise activity thermogenesis.

CONCEPT CHECK

*E*nergy balance compares energy intake with energy output. Energy content of food is expressed in kcal and determined using a bomb calorimeter. This analysis yields the 4-9-4-7 estimates for carbohydrate, fat, protein, and alcohol.

The body uses this energy for four main purposes:

1. Basal metabolism represents the minimal amount of energy needed to maintain a body in a resting state. The rate of a person's basal metabolism depends greatly on the amount of lean body mass, the amount of body surface, and thyroid hormone concentrations in the bloodstream.
2. Physical activity expenditure represents energy use for total body cell metabolism above what is needed during rest (that is, basal metabolism).

3. The thermic effect of food represents the energy needed to digest, absorb, and process absorbed nutrients. This corresponds to 5 to 10% of energy used for basal metabolism and physical activity.

4. Nonexercise activity thermogenesis (NEAT) is heat production in response to over-feeding and other stimuli. Increased fidgeting is generally seen.

In a sedentary person, 70 to 80% of energy is used for basal metabolism and the thermic effect of food; the remainder is used for physical activity and nonexercise adaptive thermogenesis.

■ DETERMINATION OF ENERGY USE BY THE BODY

The amount of energy a body uses can be measured by both direct and indirect calorimetry or can be simply estimated based on height, weight, degree of physical activity, and age.

■ Direct and Indirect Calorimetry

Direct calorimetry measures the amount of body heat released by a person. The subject is put into an insulated chamber, often the size of a small bedroom, and body heat released raises the temperature of a layer of water surrounding the chamber. A kcal, as you recall, is related to the amount of heat available to raise the temperature of the water. By measuring the water temperature in the direct calorimeter before and after the body releases heat, scientists can determine the energy expended. This method resembles the bomb calorimeter method for measuring the energy content in food.

Direct calorimetry works because almost all the energy used by the body eventually leaves as heat. However, few studies use direct calorimetry, mostly because of its expense and complexity.

For **indirect calorimetry,** instead of measuring heat output, the most commonly used method measures the amount of oxygen a person uses (Fig. 13-3). A predictable relationship exists between the body's use of energy and oxygen. For example, when metabolizing a mixed diet of carbohydrate, fat, and protein—a typical blend of nutrients—the human body needs 1 liter of oxygen to metabolize about 4.85 kcal.

Instruments used to measure oxygen consumption for indirect calorimetry have great versatility. They can be mounted on carts and rolled up to a hospital bed or carried in backpacks while a person plays tennis or jogs. Tables showing energy demands of exercises rely on information gained from indirect calorimetry studies.

Another approach to indirect calorimetry uses **stable isotopes** of oxygen and hydrogen. In this method, a person consumes isotopically labeled water ($^2H_2^{18}O$). A technician measures the ^2H_2O and the $H_2^{18}O$ later that arises in body fluids, such as urine. Using the difference between the decline in the amount of ^2H_2O compared to $H_2^{18}O$ over a week or so and some mathematical formulas, total carbon dioxide (CO_2) output per day can be estimated. This method works because ^2H is only eliminated from the body via water production, while the ^{18}O is eliminated both as water and carbon dioxide. The difference between ^2H_2O production and $H_2^{18}O$ production predicts CO_2 production ($C^{18}O_2$). This ultimate estimate of CO_2 output is used to calculate energy expenditure, just as is done with oxygen use in indirect calorimetry. ^2H and ^{18}O are stable isotopes of hydrogen and oxygen (therefore, they are nonradioactive); special instruments can measure them in body fluids. This stable isotope method is quite accurate but also very expensive.

■ Estimates of Energy Needs

A method of estimating energy needs that is widely used by registered dietitians for hospitalized patients is the **Harris-Benedict equation.** This equation considers

Brown adipose tissue is a specialized form of adipose tissue found in small amounts in infants. The brown appearance results from its rich blood flow. Brown adipose tissue contributes to thermogenesis by uncoupling the use of energy-yielding nutrients and the production of ATP (it contains a protein called uncoupling protein [UPC-1]). In brown adipose tissue more of the energy released from metabolism is simply lost as heat compared to other types of cells. The role of brown adipose tissue in adults is unknown; it appears that adults have little brown adipose tissue. One interesting finding regarding brown adipose tissue is that hibernating animals contain much of it. This allows them to create the heat needed to withstand a long winter.

direct calorimetry A method of determining a body's energy use by measuring heat that emanates from the body, usually using an insulated chamber.

indirect calorimetry A method to measure the energy use by the body by measuring oxygen uptake. Formulas are then used to convert this gas exchange value into energy use.

stable isotope An isotope is a specific form of a chemical element. It differs from atoms of other forms (isotopes) of the same element in the number of neutrons in its nucleus. *Stable* means that the isotope is not radioactive, in contrast to some other types of isotopes.

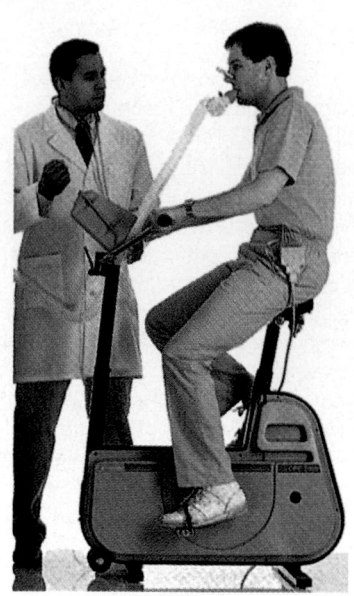

■ FIGURE 13-3 Indirect calorimetry. This method can be used to measure energy output during daily activities by monitoring oxygen uptake and carbon dioxide output.

weight, height, and age to provide an estimate of resting energy needs. (Resting energy needs are about 6% higher than basal metabolism because the conditions of measurement are not as strict, such as the need to be in a fasting state). Table 13-1 illustrates how to use the Harris-Benedict equation. The value for resting energy needs is then multiplied by predetermined factors to reflect a patient's degree of physical activity and illness, both of which raise energy needs above resting needs. The final value calculated gives total energy needs.

A rough estimate for energy needs uses a person's weight and degree of physical activity. Total energy needs for a sedentary person are set at 25 to 30 kcal/kg. The value may then decrease by 100 kcal for every 10 years of age over age 30. People performing moderate activity, such as routine walking, start with 35 kcal/kg; those regularly performing heavy activity, as required in some sports play, start at 40 kcal/kg. These values can then be adjusted for age, as mentioned previously. For example, a 68 kg (150-lb), 40-year-old woman performing moderate activity needs to eat about 2300 kcal ([68 kg × 35 kcal/kg] − 100) to meet total energy needs.

Rough guidelines for energy needs found in the Food Guide Pyramid publication are as follows:

• Sedentary women and some older adults	1600 kcal
• Children, teenage girls, active women, most men	2200 kcal
• Teenage boys, active men, very active women	2800 kcal
• Young children, pregnant and breastfeeding women	Check with a registered dietitian

These values then need to be fine-tuned based on personal characteristics and experiences, such as amount of physical activity performed.

A simple method of tracking your energy expenditure, and thus your energy needs, is to use the forms in Appendix E. Begin by taking an entire 24-hour period and listing all activities performed, including sleep. Record the number of minutes spent in each activity; the total should equal 1440 minutes (24 hours). Next record the energy cost for each activity in kcal/min following the directions in Appendix E; these values are based on your weight in kilograms (pounds ÷ 2.2). Multiply the energy cost by the minutes. This gives the energy expended for each activity. Total all the kcal values. This gives your estimated energy expenditure for the day.

CONCEPT CHECK

Energy use by the body can be measured by direct calorimetry as heat given off and by indirect calorimetry as oxygen used. Total energy needs can be estimated based on a person's characteristics: height, weight, age, and amount of physical activity. In addition, the Food Guide Pyramid publication provides rough guidelines for energy intake.

hunger The primarily physiological (internal) drive to find and eat food, mostly regulated by innate cues to eating.

appetite The primarily psychological (external) influences that encourage us to find and eat food, often in the absence of obvious hunger.

neuroendocrine Linked to the combined action of the endocrine glands and the nervous system. Examples include substances released from glands in response to nerve stimulation.

vagus nerves Nerves arising from the brain that branch off to other organs essential for control of speech, swallowing, and gastrointestinal function.

■ WHY AM I HUNGRY?

Two drives influence our desire to eat and thus take in food energy, **hunger** and **appetite.** These differ dramatically (Fig. 13-4). Hunger, our primarily physical drive to eat, is controlled by internal body mechanisms. Organs, such as the liver and brain, interact with hormones, hormonelike (**neuroendocrine**) factors, the nervous system, and other aspects of body physiology to influence feeding behavior (Table 13-2).[33] For example, as nutrients are absorbed, the liver and surrounding organs communicate with the brain through the two **vagus nerves.** This changes subsequent food choices by sending information about the rate of digestion and energy metabolism from the gastrointestinal tract and the liver to the brain.

TABLE 13-1   Calculating Energy Use

The following examples illustrate how to estimate energy expenditure. Nonexercise activity thermogenesis is not included because of limited knowledge regarding its contribution to daily energy output. Carlos weighs 154 lb (70 kg), is 5 feet 9 inches tall (175 cm), is 25 years old, and is involved in moderate muscular activity each day.

Basal Metabolism

Use the value 1 kcal/kg body weight/hour for *men*,

0.9 kcal/kg body weight/hour for *women*.

For Carlos:
1. Multiply his weight in kilograms by the appropriate value for men.

70 kg × 1 kcal/kg/hr = 70 kcal/hr

2. Multiply kcal used in an hour by hours in a day.

70 kcal/hr × 24 hr/day = 1680 kcal/day

Basal metabolism = 1680 kcal/day

Physical Activity

Select one of the following categories based on the amount of muscular activity performed in a day:
  Sedentary activity (mostly sitting): add 20 to 40% of basal metabolism
  Light activity (a clerk involved in a daily walking program): add 55 to 65% of basal metabolism
  Moderate activity (a teacher involved in daily vigorous exercise): add 70 to 75% of basal metabolism
  Heavy activity (a mail carrier who walks the route or an adult involved in a daily exercise program): add 80 to 100% or more of basal metabolism
If Carlos performs moderate activity,
  Take 70% of his basal metabolism.

1680 kcal/day × 0.70 = 1176 kcal/day.

Physical activity = 1176 kcal/day

Thermic Effect of Food

A quick way to approximate this value is to take 10% of the sum of the basal metabolism and physical activity kcal. For Carlos,
1. 1680 kcal/day + 1176 kcal/day = 2856 kcal/day.
2. 2856 kcal/day × 0.10 = 286 kcal/day.
   Thermic effect of food = 286 kcal/day

Total Energy Use

Now sum the energy contributions from each factor.
For Carlos,
  1680 kcal/day + 1176 kcal/day + 286 kcal/day = 3142 kcal/day
  Total energy use = 3142 kcal/day

Calculating Resting Energy Use Using Harris-Benedict Equation

We have estimated Carlos's total energy use. Let's calculate Carlos's resting energy expenditure using the appropriate Harris-Benedict equation and compare it with the basal metabolism we determined for him:

Harris-Benedict Equation

66.5 + 13.8 (weight in kg) + 5 (height in cm) − 6.8 (age in years)

Carlos weighs 70 kg, is 175 cm tall, and is 25 years old. Therefore, Carlos's resting energy expenditure is as follows:

66.5 + 13.8 (70 kg) + 5 (175 cm) − 6.8 (25) = 1738 kcal/day

Resting energy use = 1738 kcal/day

   Compare this with the estimate of basal metabolism of 1680 kcal/day we determined previously. The values are not very different. Note also that the Harris-Benedict equation for women is 655.1 + 9.6 (weight in kg) + 1.9 (height in cm) − 4.7 (age in years).

TABLE 13-2	Hormones, Neuroendocrine Substances, Medications, and Other Factors That Affect Feeding Behavior[20, 26, 28, 30, 33, 36]
Increase Food Intake	**Decrease Food Intake**
Neurotransmitters	
Norepinephrine	Serotonin
Growth hormone releasing hormone	Dopamine
Neuropeptides	
Opiods	Cholecystolcinin
Galanin	Enterostatin
Neuropeptide Y	Tumor necrosis factor
Agouti-related protein	Glucagon-like peptide (GLP-1)
Orexin	Corticotropin releasing hormone
Melanin-concentrating hormone	Melanocyte-stimulating hormone
	Melanocortin
Medications	
Corticosteroids	Sibutramine
Some tranquilizers	Leptin[†]
Progestins	Amphetamines
Some antidepressants	

[†]Some of these medications are also body hormones. Many of the neuropeptides are also found in the gastrointestinal tract (see Chapter 3).

[†]In conjunction with the hormone insulin when both are present in the brain.

Appetite, our primarily psychological drive to eat, is affected by external food choice mechanisms, such as seeing a tempting dessert. Fulfilling either or both drives by eating sufficient food normally brings a state of satiety, temporarily halting our desire to continue eating.

■ Hypothalamus: a Satiety Regulator

The **hypothalamus,** a portion of the brain, is the key integration site for the regulation of food intake. When stimulated, cells in the feeding centers of the hypothalamus signal us to eat. Then, as we eat, hunger decreases. Eventually, we stop eating as cells in the satiety centers of the hypothalamus are stimulated. The amount of blood glucose probably stimulates both groups of centers. When glucose drops, we eat. Various cues to eat come from other groups of cells in the vicinity of the hypothalamus, amino acids and fatty acids in the bloodstream, various hormones and other substances, and sympathetic nervous system activity. Overall, as sympathetic nervous system activity decreases, food intake increases. The opposite is also true. Thus, many internal signals both inhibit and encourage food intake.

Chemicals, surgery, and some cancers can destroy the feeding and satiety centers in the hypothalamus. Without satiety-center activity, laboratory animals (and humans) eat their way to obesity. Without feeding-center activity, animals eat little and eventually lose weight.

■ Satiety Regulation at Other Body Sites

As just mentioned, satiety is controlled by a network of mechanisms spread throughout the body. Satiety is maintained first by the sensory stimulation that food elicits, coupled with the knowledge that a meal was eaten. Second, the effects of nutrient digestion, absorption, and metabolism are felt. The satiety and feeding centers in the

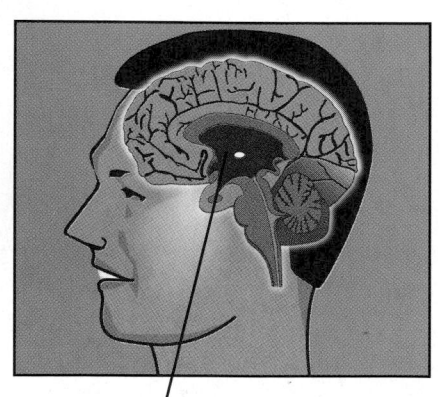

Hypothalamus

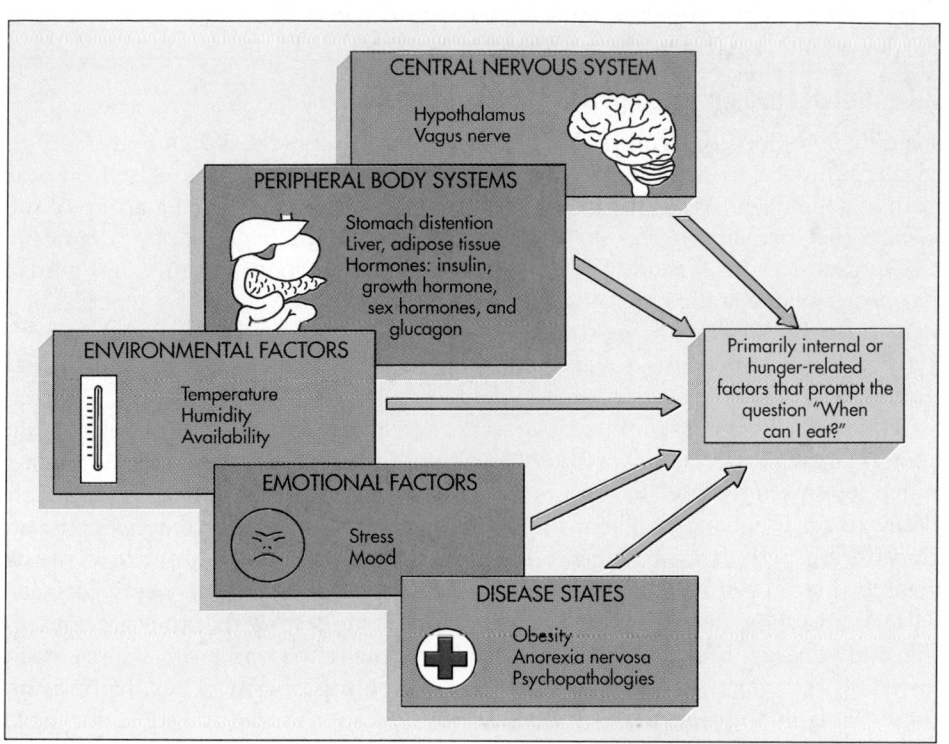

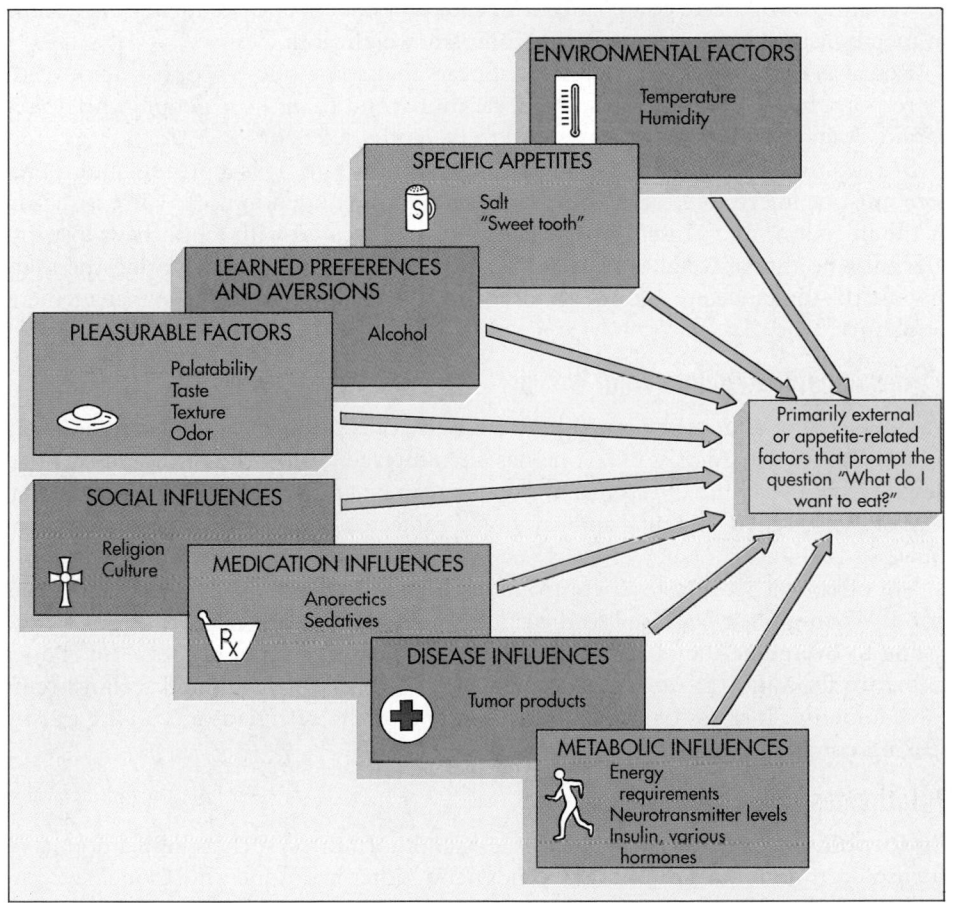

■ **FIGURE 13-4** A model incorporating many factors that influence satiety. Note that there is some overlap between influences on hunger and appetite. Overall, feeding is regulated by a group of complex and inter-related processes.

Illustration by William Ober.

hypothalamus communicate and interact with other decision points in the brain, small intestine, and liver.

Control of Feeding Through Body Composition

Feeding behavior also changes in response to body fat content. When body fat is surgically removed from animals, their food consumption increases. Based on work with genetic forms of obesity in animals, researchers have identified a group of substances that circulates in the blood and communicates the degree of body fatness to the central nervous system. The gene for one such substance in mice and humans has been isolated (called the ob gene). The product produced by the gene has been named **leptin.** Work with one strain of mice suggests that leptin partly decreases the activity of **neuropeptide Y** and other small proteins present in the brain (review Table 13-2). This then reduces food intake.[20, 28, 30]

Theoretically, when adipose tissues are increasing, leptin (and/or related substances) causes satiety. Conversely, when adipose tissue stores are decreasing, not as much leptin (and/or related substances) is released into the bloodstream, and the desire to eat is enhanced. The main function of leptin is probably energy conservation during periods of inadequate food supply.[28] Low leptin output leads to decreased thyroid gland activity and, thus, a fall in basal metabolism. Leptin-deficient animals also show decreased spontaneous activity, suggesting that they are conserving body energy. Experts suggest that leptin actually may be more important for lessening the effects of starvation than for preventing obesity. Thus, leptin is not there primarily to protect against obesity but, instead, to serve as a signal for inadequate energy intake. It may be in the future that leptin administration during times of weight loss will make compliance with the protocol easier by reducing the decline in metabolism and the hunger that accompany weight loss.[28]

Research on leptin is in progress. It appears that some obese people do not readily respond to the leptin signal and, so, eat more food than those people who do respond. A few children have been found to be leptin deficient.

Studies to date show that leptin administration is safe. It is a protein and therefore must be injected into the body; most problems with leptin use involve irritation at the injection site.[20] Interestingly, not all people treated with leptin have lost significant amounts of weight; some people have even gained weight during the therapy. At this time, we are a long way off from routine leptin use in the management of obesity.[11]

Does Appetite Regulate What We Eat?

Various feeding and satiety messages from body cells do not single-handedly determine what we eat. Almost everyone has encountered a mouthwatering dessert and devoured it, even on a full stomach. Appetite can be affected by a variety of external forces, such as environmental and psychological factors, as well as social customs (review Fig. 13-4).

We often eat because food confronts us. It smells good, tastes good, and looks good. We might eat because it is the right time of day, we are celebrating, or we are trying to overcome the blues. Appetite may not be a biological process, but it does influence food intake. After a meal, memories of pleasant tastes and feelings reinforce appetite. If stress or depression sends you to the refrigerator, you are mostly seeking comfort, not food energy.

Hormones That Affect Satiety

Endorphins, the body's natural painkillers, and hormones, such as high amounts of cortisol, can prod us to eat. On the other hand, other hormones, hormonelike compounds, and still other chemical factors in the body can contribute to the feeling of satiety. With eating, blood concentrations of some digestive hormones, such as cholecystokinin (CCK), increase. This increase, combined with **gastrointestinal distention,** helps shut off hunger.

leptin A hormone (167 amino acids) made by adipose tissue that influences long-term regulation of fat mass. Leptin also influences reproductive functions, as well as other physiological processes, such as insulin release.

neuropeptide Y A small protein (36 amino acids) that increases food intake and reduces energy expenditure when injected into the brains of experimental animals.

Social customs, peers, and authority figures can influence the desire to eat. Concern about appearance when on a date can influence the food choices made. A woman concerned about looking "petite" in company may choose a smaller portion of food than when alone. We are also likely to eat more at a meal when with a large group of people than when with a few people or alone, or when someone else is "picking up the check."

Certain parts of the nervous system also contribute to satiety, in part linked to the release of the neurotransmitter histamine. Increased production of **serotonin,** another brain neurotransmitter, has also been linked to intake of various nutrients, especially carbohydrate. High serotonin concentrations in the brain can be calming, induce sleepiness, and reduce food intake. Medications that prolong serotonin action are used to treat certain eating disorders for this reason (see Chapter 15).[7]

Following the influence of gastrointestinal distention, **nutrient receptors** in the small intestine are believed to take over in promoting satiety after a meal. This concept is supported by experiments in which an individual feels satiated when fats or carbohydrates are infused directly into his or her small intestine. This effect is not reported, however, when the same fats or carbohydrates are infused directly into the person's bloodstream.

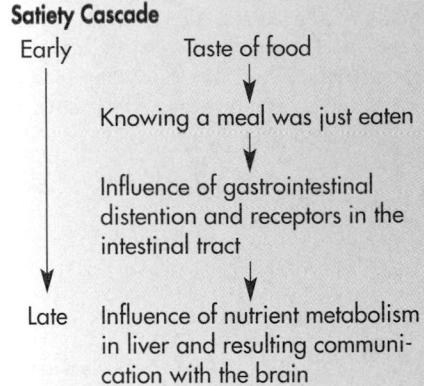

Satiety Cascade

Early — Taste of food
↓
Knowing a meal was just eaten
↓
Influence of gastrointestinal distention and receptors in the intestinal tract
↓
Late — Influence of nutrient metabolism in liver and resulting communication with the brain

■ Nutrients in the Blood That Affect Satiety

Accumulating evidence from both human and animal studies on the regulation of hunger suggests that an underlying hunger for food is never actually absent. After a meal, blood concentrations of glucose, fatty acids, amino acids, and other energy-yielding nutrients increase, the brain registers satiety, and hunger is temporarily relieved. Studies suggest that an apolipoprotein on the chylomicrons (apolipoprotein A-IV) also signals satiety to the brain as these appear in the blood after a meal.

Several hours after eating, when concentrations of nutrients in the blood begin to fall, the body must start using fuel from body stores; hunger then returns. This is because satiety is no longer registered by the metabolism of ingested energy-yielding compounds. In other words, feeding signals begin to dominate again.

Internal and external signals—driving hunger and appetite—generally operate simultaneously and combine into a momentary decision whether to reject or eat a food item. For example, visual and taste stimulation can cause something called *cephalic phase responses* by the body. Saliva flows and digestive hormones and insulin are released in response to seeing, smelling, and initially tasting food, such as a favorite hamburger. This readies the body for the meal. These internal forces are elicited by external cues, again showing the degree to which internal and external forces are intertwined.

■ Hunger and Appetite in Perspective

The next time you pick up a candy bar or ask for second helpings, remember the physiological influences on eating behavior. Body cells (brain, stomach, intestine, liver, and other organs), hormones (such as insulin and cortisol), neurological components (such as histamine and serotonin), and social customs all influence food intake. Where food is ample, appetite—not hunger—mostly triggers eating.[13] Keep track of what triggers your eating for a few days. Is it primarily hunger or appetite? Note as well that this system is not perfect; your body weight can increase (or decrease) over time if you are not careful to balance energy intake with energy output.

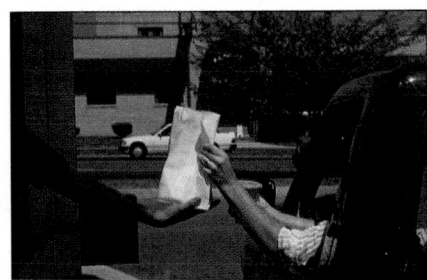

The easy availability of quick-service food in recent years has made weight control even harder for many people.

CONCEPT CHECK

*H*unger is the primarily physiological or internal desire to find and eat food. Appeasing it creates satiety—no further desire to eat exists. Satiety is influenced by hunger-related (internal) forces in the brain, gastrointestinal tract, adipose tissue, liver, and other organs. Various hormones and neuroendocrine compounds participate. Food intake is also affected by appetite-related (external) forces such as social custom, time of day, palatability, and presence of others. Americans probably respond more to external, appetite-related forces than to hunger-related ones in choosing when and what to eat.

■ ESTIMATION OF A HEALTHY WEIGHT

Numerous methods are used to set what body weight should be, typically called *healthy body weight*. Several tables exist, generally based on weight-for-height. These tables arise from studies of large population groups. When applied to a population, they provide good estimates of weight associated with health and longevity. These tables, however, do not necessarily refer directly to an individual's weight and health status.

Ideally, family history of weight-related disease and current health parameters should be considered when establishing a healthy weight for an individual, in addition to weight-for-height. Evidence of the following weight-related conditions is important:[34]

- Hypertension
- Elevated LDL
- Family history of obesity, cardiovascular disease, or certain forms of cancer (e.g., breast, colon)
- Pattern of fat distribution in the body
- Elevated blood glucose

On a more practical note, other questions can be pertinent: What is the least one has weighed as an adult for at least a year? What is the largest size clothing one would be happy with? What weight has one been able to maintain during previous diets without feeling constantly hungry? Overall, the individual, under a physician's guidance, should establish a "personal" healthy weight (or need for weight reduction) based on weight history, fat distribution patterns, family history of weight-related disease, and current health status. This assessment points out how well the person is tolerating any existing excess weight. Thus, current height/weight standards are only a rough guide. Furthermore, a healthy lifestyle may make a more important contribution to a person's health status than the number on the scale. Fit and overweight are, for the most part, not mutually exclusive. And neither is thin synonymous with healthy if the person is also not physically active. This topic is discussed at greater length later in the chapter with regard to the appropriateness of a recommendation for weight loss.

■ Using Body Mass Index (BMI) to Set Healthy Weight

For the past 50 years, weight-for-height tables issued by the Metropolitan Life Insurance Company have been the typical way healthy weight was established. These tables considered gender and frame size, predicting the weight range at a specific height that was associated with the greatest longevity. The latest table (issued in 1983) and methods for determining frame size are in Appendix G.

Currently in the medical and nutrition literature there is less use of the Metropolitan Life Insurance tables and greater use of **body mass index (BMI)** as a weight-for-height standard. Still, you may see either in current medical practice. This chapter will focus on body mass index. Research has shown it is the weight-for-height standard that is most closely related to body fat content.

Body mass index is calculated as

$$\frac{body\ weight\ (in\ kilograms)}{height^2\ (in\ meters)}$$

An alternate method for calculating BMI is

$$\frac{weight\ (pounds)\ \times\ 703.1}{height^2\ (inches)}$$

Table 13-3 lists BMI for various heights and weights. Health risks from excess weight begin when the body mass index exceeds 25. A healthy weight-for-height is

---

Healthy weight is currently the preferred term to use for weight recommendations. Older terms, such as *ideal weight* and *desirable weight,* are no longer used in the medical literature. However, you still may hear these terms in clinical practice.

body mass index (BMI) Weight (in kilograms) divided by height (in meters) squared; a value greater than 25 indicates a higher risk for obesity-related health disorders. As a rough estimate, 1 BMI unit equals 6-7 pounds.

BMI is not a standard for everyone. Adult BMI should not be applied to children, adolescents who are still growing, frail elderly people, pregnant and lactating women, and highly muscular individuals. Children and pregnant women have unique BMI standards (see Chapters 16 and 17).

TABLE 13-3	Body Weight in Pounds According to Height and Body Mass Index (BMI)

	BMI (kg/m²)													
	19	20	21	22	23	24	25	26	27	28	29	30	35	40
Height (Inches)	**Body Weight (Pounds)**													
58	91	96	100	105	110	115	119	124	129	134	138	143	167	191
59	94	99	104	109	114	119	124	128	133	138	143	148	173	198
60	97	102	107	112	118	123	128	133	138	143	148	153	179	204
61	100	106	111	116	122	127	132	137	143	148	153	158	185	211
62	104	109	115	120	126	131	136	142	147	153	158	164	191	218
63	107	113	118	124	130	135	141	146	152	158	163	169	197	225
64	110	116	122	128	134	140	145	151	157	163	169	174	204	232
65	114	120	126	132	138	144	150	156	162	168	174	180	210	240
66	118	124	130	136	142	148	155	161	167	173	179	186	216	247
67	121	127	134	140	146	153	159	166	172	178	185	191	223	255
68	125	131	138	144	151	158	164	171	177	184	190	197	230	262
69	128	135	142	149	155	162	169	176	182	189	196	203	236	270
70	132	139	146	153	160	167	174	181	188	195	202	207	243	278
71	136	143	150	157	165	172	179	186	193	200	208	215	250	286
72	140	147	154	162	169	177	184	191	199	206	213	221	258	294
73	144	151	159	166	174	182	189	197	204	212	219	227	265	302
74	148	155	163	171	179	186	194	202	210	218	225	233	272	311
75	152	160	168	176	184	192	200	208	216	224	232	240	279	319
76	156	164	172	180	189	197	205	213	221	230	238	246	287	328

Each entry gives the body weight in pounds for a person of a given height and BMI. Pounds have been rounded off. To use the table, find the appropriate height in the far left column. Move across the row to a weight. The number at the top of the column is the BMI for the height and weight.

a BMI 18.5 to 24.9. What is your BMI? How much would your weight need to change to yield a BMI of 25? 30? These are general cut-off values for the presence of overweight and obesity, respectively.

The concept of body mass index is convenient to use because the values apply to both men and women. However, any body weight-for-height standard is actually a crude measure because we are concerned about overfat, not simply overweight, individuals when setting guidelines for healthy weight. The husky athlete is a notable exception; he or she may be overweight but not overfat because the excess weight is from muscle mass, not fat mass. For this reason, any weight-for-height measurement should be used only as a screening test for obesity.

Still, overfat and overweight conditions generally appear together. The focus is on body weight-for-height standards in clinical settings mainly because these are easier to measure than total body fat.

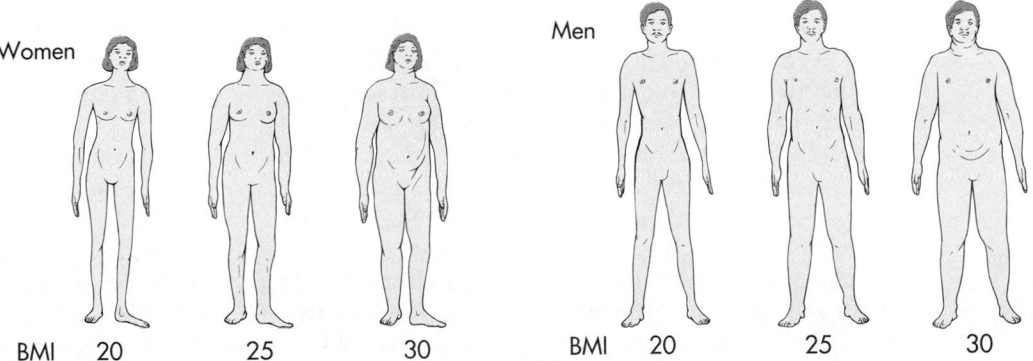

Women   BMI   20   25   30

Men   BMI   20   25   30

For your reference, these are estimates of body shapes at different BMI values.

Former Surgeon General Dr. C. Everett Koop is currently spearheading a campaign, called "Shape Up America," to convince overweight people to lose weight and increase physical activity. According to Dr. Koop, obesity is the number two killer in the United States. What many Americans don't understand, he explains, is how serious the problem of excess pounds is: Although many Americans are aware that smoking is responsible for more than 400,000 deaths per year, they are not aware that obesity is responsible for nearly as many—300,000—deaths annually in the United States. Before long, obesity will surpass cigarette smoking as a leading cause of death.

A shortcut method of estimating healthy body weight is the pounds per inch of height method. For women, allow 100 pounds for the first 5 feet, then add 5 pounds for every inch thereafter. To estimate a man's healthy body weight, allow 106 pounds for the first 5 feet and then add 6 pounds for each inch thereafter. Based on this system, a 6-foot-tall man should weight about 178 pounds ($106 + [12 \times 6]$).

■ Putting Healthy Weight into Perspective

One current school of thought is to let nature take its course with regard to body weight. According to this proposal, by trying to lose weight in order to fall within a specific (often unrealistic) height/weight range, people often regain their original weight plus more. In contrast, listening to the body for hunger cues, eating a healthy diet, and remaining physically active eventually helps one maintain an appropriate height/weight value. This concept will be further addressed in the upcoming discussion on treatment for obesity. It is a cornerstone of the current "size acceptance" movement.[18] The clearest idea regarding a healthy weight is that it is personal. Weight has to be considered in terms of health, not simply fashion.

CONCEPT CHECK

Healthy body weight is generally determined in a clinical setting using a body mass index or another weight-for-height standard. The presence of existing weight-related disease should be considered in determining healthy body weight. Total health and a healthy lifestyle, not simply fashion, should be the major considerations when determining healthy weight.

■ ENERGY IMBALANCE

If energy intake exceeds expenditure over time, obesity is likely to result. Often, health problems eventually follow (Table 13-4). In this context, medical experts recommend that an individual's cutoff value for obesity should not be based primarily on body weight but, rather, on the total amount of fat in the body, the location of body fat, and the presence or absence of weight-related medical problems.[8]

■ Estimating Body Fat Content and Diagnosing Obesity

Body fat can range from 2 to 70% of body weight. In this regard, men with over 24% body fat and women with over about 35% body fat are considered obese. Desirable amounts are about 8 to 24% body fat for men and 21 to 35% fat for women. Women need more body fat because some "sex-specific" fat is associated with reproductive functions. This fat is normal and factored into calculations.

Still other methods to estimate body fat include using instruments to measure air displacement by the body (plethysmography) and total-body electrical conductance when placed in an electromagnetic field (TOBEC).

underwater weighing A method of estimating total body fat by weighing the individual on a standard scale and then weighing him or her again submerged in water. The difference between the two weights is used to estimate total body fat.

bioelectrical impedance The method to estimate total body fat that uses a low-energy electrical current. The more fat storage a person has, the more impedance (resistance) to electrical flow will be exhibited.

Various methods are used to estimate body fat content. **Underwater weighing** (most accurate) works because fat tissue is less dense than lean tissue; because fat floats, the more fat tissue present, the less a person weighs when submerged. This procedure requires a trained technician and submersion (Fig. 13-5).

Although there are some limits to its accuracy, skinfold thickness is the method most widely used to estimate total body fat. Clinicians use calipers to measure the fat layer directly under the skin at multiple sites (Fig. 13-6).

Clinicians have begun measuring total body fat using **bioelectrical impedance.** This technique sends a painless, low-energy electrical current to and from the body via wires and electrode patches. Researchers surmise that fat resists electrical flow, so more fat proportionately means greater electrical resistance. Within a few min-

TABLE 13-4   Health Problems Associated with Excess Body Fat[9, 23]

Health Problem	Partially Attributable To
Surgical risk	Increased anesthesia needs and greater risk of wound infections
Pulmonary disease and sleep disorders	Excess weight over lungs and pharynx
Type 2 diabetes	Enlarged adipose cells, which poorly bind insulin and poorly respond to the message insulin sends to the cell
Hypertension and stroke	Increased miles of blood vessels found in the adipose tissue, increased blood volume, and increased resistance to blood flow
Cardiovascular disease	Increases in LDL and triglyceride values, low HDL, and decreased physical activity
Bone and joint disorders (including gout)	Excess pressure put on knee, ankle, and hip joints
Gallstones	Increased cholesterol content of bile
Skin disorders	Trapping of moisture and microbes in tissue folds
Various cancers	Estrogen production by adipose cells; animal studies suggest excess energy intake encourages tumor development
Shorter stature (in some forms of obesity)	Earlier onset of puberty
Pregnancy risks	More difficult delivery, increased number of birth defects, and increased needs for anesthesia
Reduced physical agility and increased risk of accidents and falls	Excess weight that impairs movement
Menstrual irregularities and infertility	Hormones produced by adipose cells, such as estrogen
Premature death	A variety of risk factors for disease, listed in this table

The greater the degree of obesity, the more likely and the more serious these health problems generally become. They are much more likely to appear in people who show an upper body fat distribution pattern and/or greater than twice healthy body weight.

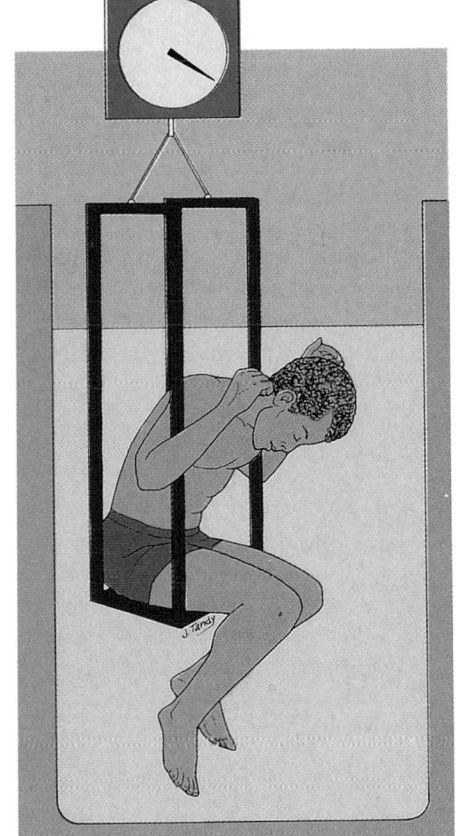

FIGURE 13-5 Underwater weighing. To get an accurate estimate of body fat, the subject exhales as much air as possible and then holds his or her breath and bends over at the waist. Once the subject is totally submerged, the underwater weight is recorded. For example, the loss of weight when submerged might yield a body density of 1.06 g/cm³. This would be put into the formula such as: % body fat = (495 ÷ body density) − 450. The subject is 17% body fat based on use of this formula.

utes, bioelectrical impedance analyzers convert body electrical resistance into an approximate estimate of total body fat, as long as body hydration status is normal (Fig. 13-7).

Another method for estimating total body fat exposes the biceps to infrared light, assessing the interactions with the fat and protein in arm muscle. After only 2 seconds, this flashlight-size device can give an estimate.

A further advance in determining body fat is use of dual x-ray photon absorptiometry (DEXA). This x-ray system allows the clinician to separate body weight into three components—fat, fat-free soft tissue, and bone mineral. The usual whole-body scan requires about 5 to 20 minutes and delivers a minimal radiation dose. Obesity, osteoporosis, and other aspects of nutritional health can be investigated using this method.

BMI offers an alternative way to define obesity (Fig. 13-8):

18.5	Underweight	Nutritional risk
18.5–24.9	Healthy	Acceptable range
25–29.9	Overweight	At risk for obesity and related health problems
30–39.9	Obese	Increased health risk
> 40	Severely obese	Major health risk

A planned treatment program should be implemented after BMI reaches 30.[4]

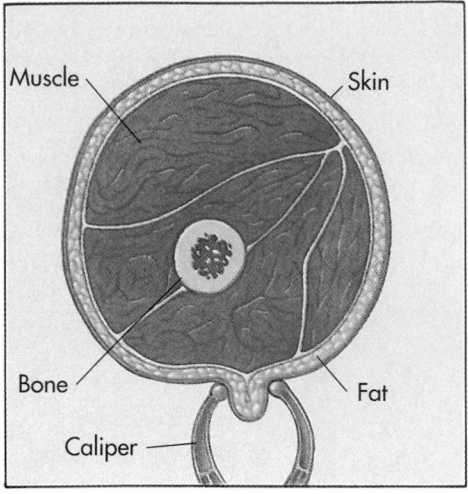

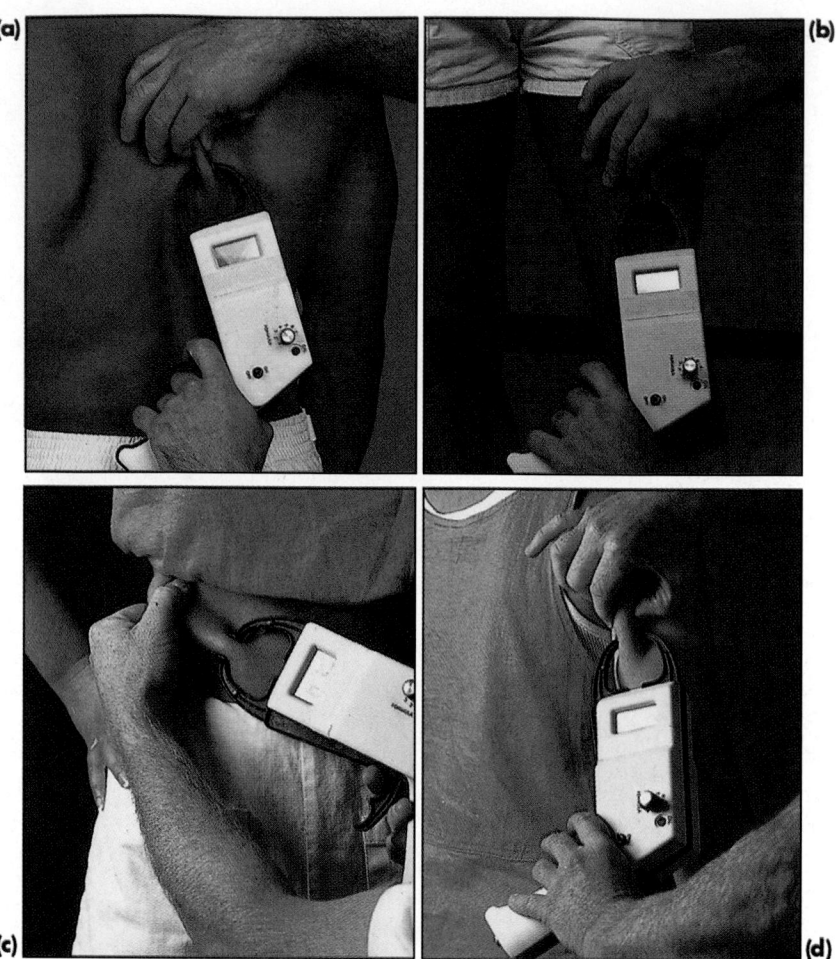

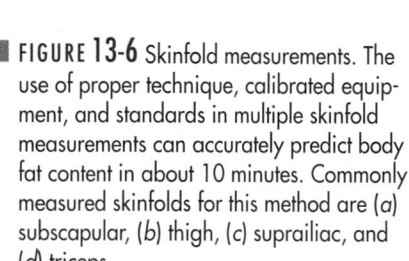

FIGURE 13-6 Skinfold measurements. The use of proper technique, calibrated equipment, and standards in multiple skinfold measurements can accurately predict body fat content in about 10 minutes. Commonly measured skinfolds for this method are (a) subscapular, (b) thigh, (c) suprailiac, and (d) triceps.

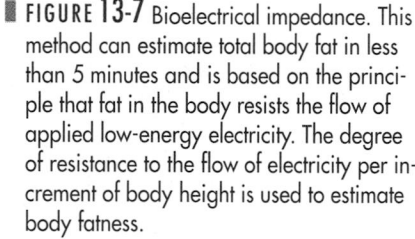

FIGURE 13-7 Bioelectrical impedance. This method can estimate total body fat in less than 5 minutes and is based on the principle that fat in the body resists the flow of applied low-energy electricity. The degree of resistance to the flow of electricity per increment of body height is used to estimate body fatness.

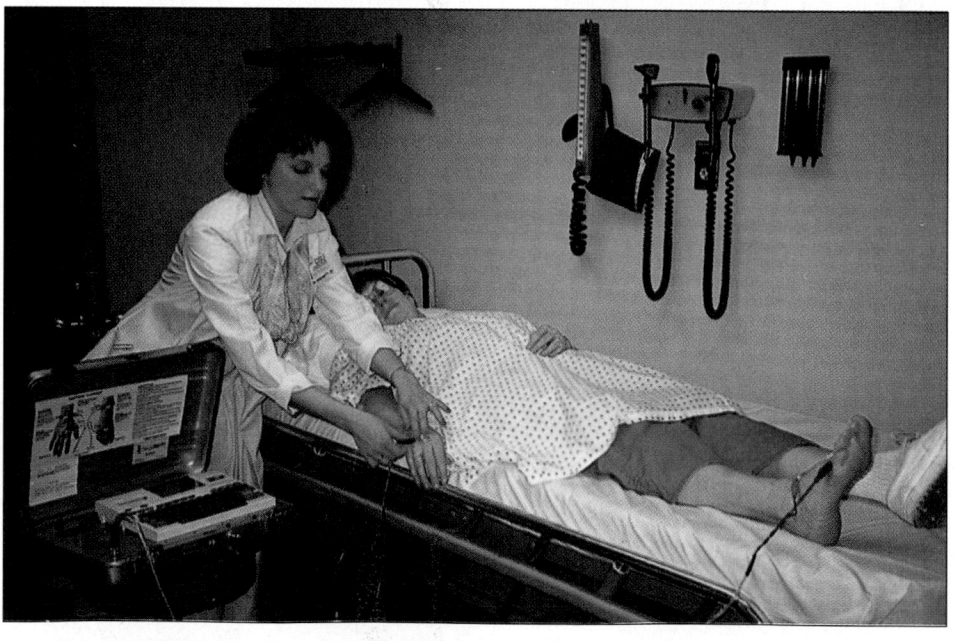

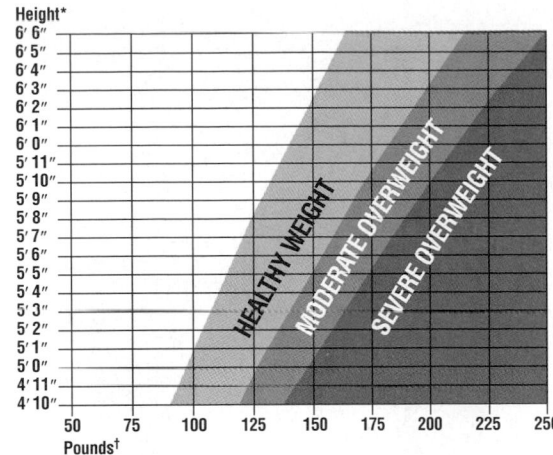

* Without shoes.
† Without clothes.The higher weights apply
  to people with more muscle and bone,
  such as many men.

■ **FIGURE 13-8** Height/weight table included as part of the latest Dietary Guidelines publication. The upper ends of the healthy weight ranges correspond to a body mass index of 25.

■ Using Body Fat Distribution to Establish Obesity

Where we store fat, as well as how much, can predict health risks. Some people store fat in upper body areas. Others hold fat lower on the body. Excess fat in either place generally spells trouble, but each storage space also has its unique risks. Fat deposited in the lower body often resists being shed. However, **upper-body (android) obesity** is related to more cardiovascular disease, hypertension, and type 2 diabetes. Whereas other fat cells empty fat directly into general circulation, the fat contents of abdominal fat cells go straight to the liver, by way of the portal vein, before being circulated to the muscles. This process interferes with the liver's ability to clear insulin and alters lipoprotein metabolism by the liver. Both changes spell trouble for the body.

High blood testosterone (a primarily male hormone) levels apparently encourage upper-body obesity, as does alcohol intake. This characteristic male pattern of fat storage appears in the "apple-on-a-stick" shape (large abdomen [pot belly] and small buttocks and thighs). This type of android-related risk is assessed by simply measuring the waist. A waist circumference more than 40 inches in men and more than 35 inches in women indicates such a shape (Fig. 13-9). If BMI is also ≥ 25, health risks are significantly increased.[8]

Estrogen and progesterone (primarily female hormones) encourage lower-body fat storage and **lower-body (gynecoid or gynoid) obesity**—the typical female pattern. The small abdomen and much larger buttocks and thighs give a pearlike appearance. After menopause, blood estrogen falls, encouraging upper-body fat distribution.

Overall, researchers suggest that women with lower-body fat distribution must be about 20 pounds more obese than men with a "pot belly" shape before they show the same health risks from an overfat state. Only a small percentage of women have upper-body obesity. Note also that the cutoff values are based on studies of Caucasians. More study of minorities is needed to verify use in those populations.

■ Using Age of Onset in the Evaluation of Obesity

Obesity can be classified as juvenile-onset or adult-onset. When obesity develops in infancy or childhood, numerous adipose cells develop, each with the ability to grow larger. (This is discussed further in Chapter 17, particularly in reference to weight control in childhood.) In adult obesity, fewer adipose cells are usually present, but these contain an excess amount of fat. Still, as obesity progresses in adulthood, adipose cells can increase in number again.

Juvenile-onset obesity presents a special concern because the greater number of adipose cells may increase the body's resistance to cutting down fat stores. Adipose

upper-body (android) obesity The type of obesity in which fat is stored primarily in the abdominal area; defined as a waist circumference > 40 inches (102 cm) in men and > 35 inches (89 cm) in women; closely associated with a high risk for cardiovascular disease, hypertension, and type 2 diabetes.

lower-body (gynecoid, gynoid) obesity The type of obesity in which fat storage is primarily located in the buttocks and thigh area.

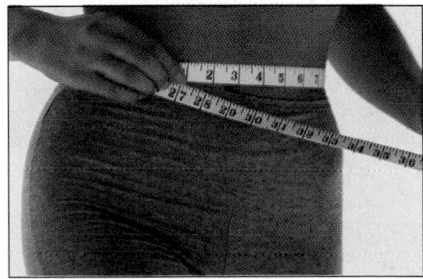

Waist circumference is an important measure of weight-related health risk.

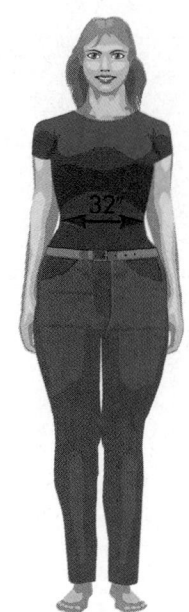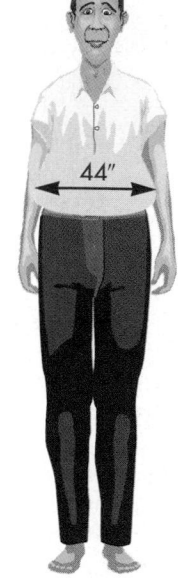

Lower-body obesity   Upper-body obesity

■ FIGURE 13-9 Body fat distribution, showing upper-body and lower-body obesity. The upper-body (android) form brings higher risks for ill health associated with obesity. The woman has a waist circumference of 32". The man has a waist circumference of 44". Thus, the man has upper-body obesity, but the woman does not, based on a cutoff of > 40 inches for men and > 35 inches for women.

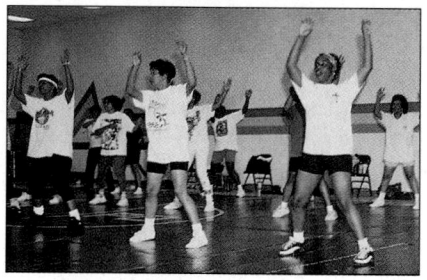

Even a moderate weight loss of 10 to 20 lb to a "healthier" weight can help improve blood glucose regulation and blood pressure.

cells have a long life span and apparently need to store some fat. If more adipose cells automatically require more fat storage, reducing total body fat becomes a tough task. Although the reasons are still puzzling, long-term obesity appears to make losing weight more difficult.

■ Putting Obesity into Perspective

Obesity is a very personal disorder. It can be measured in many ways, but statistics aside, each person has unique characteristics and problems. Treatment needs to account for current energy expenditure, weight range in adulthood, fasting blood glucose, family history of obesity, number of years the person has been obese, and extent of erroneous nutrition practices. Each person faces possible complications requiring individual treatment plans.[3]

On a positive note, however, only about a 10% weight loss is often needed for people to lower the risk for developing most weight-related diseases. Researchers are calling this a healthier weight. Although a person might not achieve a BMI of 25, he or she might still be healthier after a small weight loss.[4]

CONCEPT CHECK

besity is a state of excessive body fat storage. The risk of health problems related to obesity increases under the following conditions:
• A man's percentage of body fat exceeds 25%; a woman's exceeds about 35%.
• Body mass index (BMI) is over 25 (calculated as weight in kilograms divided by height squared in meters).
However, if a healthy lifestyle is being followed and no current health problems exist, these guidelines need to be re-evaluated.

Body fat storage can be estimated clinically using skinfold thickness or bioelectrical impedance. Fat storage distribution further specifies an obese state as either upper body or lower body. Obesity leads to an increased risk for cardiovascular disease, some types of cancer, hypertension, type 2 diabetes, certain bone and joint disorders, and some digestive disorders. The risks for some of these diseases are greater with upper-body fat storage.

■ WHY SOME PEOPLE ARE OBESE— NATURE VERSUS NURTURE

Both genetic traits and psychological factors can increase the risk for obesity. These diverse influences spark controversies concerning which factor yields the greater influence.

■ How Does Nature Contribute to Obesity?

Identical twins raised apart tend to show similar weight gain patterns, whether lean or obese (Fig. 13-10). It appears that nurture—what we learn about eating habits and nutrition, which varies between twins who are raised apart—has less to do with obesity than genes do. In fact, research using twins suggests that genetic background accounts for about 40% of weight differences between people. Twins even tend to accumulate fat in the same body sites. Our genes help determine rates of metabolism, fuel use, and differences in brain chemistry. All affect weight.[25]

We also inherit specific body types, such as pencil-thin or muscular. The specific body types—known as endomorph, mesomorph, and ectomorph—greatly determine human size and shape. Endomorphs, with their stocky builds, have short, stubby bones; short trunks; round heads; wide chest and hips; and very short fingers. Ectomorphs, such as Abraham Lincoln, are tall and slender with long, thin bones and narrow chests, hips, heads, and fingers. Mesomorphs exhibit a medium, muscular build.

Ectomorphs appear to have an inherently easier time maintaining healthy body weight. Basal metabolism increases as body surface increases. Tall people have more body surface (based on body weight comparisons) than short, stocky people. Therefore, taller people use more energy than do shorter ones, even when resting.

Some rats and mice have a genetic predisposition to obesity. They inherit a **thrifty metabolism,** one that uses energy frugally. This enables them to store fat more readily than the typical animal. Some people probably inherit a thrifty metabolism as well. Farmers once bred cows and hogs based on their ability to acquire fat. Today, because we know that eating too much animal fat can increase the risk for cardiovascular disease, farmers breed leaner animals.

A thrifty human metabolism requires less energy to get through the day. In earlier times, when food supplies were scarce, a thrifty metabolism helped protect people against starvation. With today's general abundance of food, people operating in this low gear require a high-energy output and wise food choices to prevent obesity.[13]

If you think your metabolism promotes weight gain, you may have inherited a thrifty metabolism. It is likely that this is true for many of us. As a consequence, a child with no obese parent has only a 10% chance of becoming obese. A child with one obese parent (common in U.S. society) has a 40% risk, and one with two obese parents has an 80% risk. It can be argued that these probabilities are related, in part, to the eating behaviors a child learns. **Fraternal twins** vary less in weight than do two unrelated people. This pattern supports the theory that environment, or nurture, affects obesity. Still, the close association of body weights between identical twins strongly supports a genetic linkage. This varied evidence shows how complicated it is to separate nature from nurture when searching for the causes of obesity.

■ Does the Body Have a Set Point for Weight?

The **set-point** theory of weight maintenance espouses the notion that weight is closely regulated by the body. It proposes that humans have a genetically predetermined body weight or body fat content, which the body attempts to defend. Some research suggests that the hypothalamus monitors the amount of body fat in humans and tries to keep that amount constant over time. This regulation of body fat content is referred to as a "set point." You have already seen in this chapter that the

identical twins Two offspring who develop from a single ovum and sperm and consequently have the same genetic makeup.

thrifty metabolism A metabolism that characteristically conserves more energy than normal, so that it increases the risk of weight gain and obesity.

fraternal twins Offspring that develop from two separate ova and sperm and therefore have separate genetic identities, although they develop simultaneously in the mother.

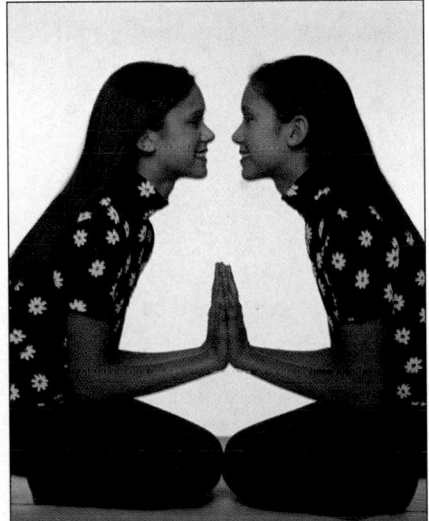

■ FIGURE 13-10 Nature or nurture: What causes these twins to have similar body weights?

hormone *leptin* forms one communication link between adipose cells and the brain that allows for some weight regulation.[20]

Analogies to the tight regulation of blood pressure and body temperature are used to support this concept of set point. You could view the set point as a coiled spring: The further you stray from your usual weight, the harder the force acts to pull you back to that weight.

In the major studies of humans cited to support the set-point theory, volunteers who lost weight through starvation later ate in a way to regain their original weight or a little more. In addition, studies in the 1960s using prisoners with no history of obesity found it was hard for some men to gain weight. This was supported by later studies in the 1990s (see the section on nonexercise adaptive thermogenesis). Also, after an illness is resolved, a person generally gains lost weight.

Sound physiological evidence also suggests that body weight tends to be regulated. If energy intake is reduced, the blood concentration of the thyroid hormones fall, and the metabolic rate slows. In addition, lower body weight decreases the energy cost of each future weight-bearing activity, and the total energy used by lean tissue falls because some of these tissues are also lost. Furthermore, the enzyme used by adipose and muscle cells to take up fat from the bloodstream (lipoprotein lipase) often increases its activity. Through these changes, the body resists further weight loss.

If a person overeats, in the short run the metabolic rate tends to increase because total body mass increases. This causes some resistance to further weight gain. People often recognize the body's resistance to weight loss when dieting but do not think much about the resistance to weight gain after eating a big holiday meal. However, in the long run, resistance to weight gain is much less than resistance to weight loss. When a person gains weight and stays at that weight for a while, the body tends to defend the new weight.

Arguments against the set-point theory cite the fact that, during pregnancy, women slowly increase body weight and fat. Also, an average person's weight does not remain constant throughout adulthood; it usually increases slowly, at least until old age. This means that a person must be able to shift his or her set point. It is also argued that, if an individual is placed in a different social, emotional, or physical environment, weight can become markedly higher or lower and is maintained. These arguments suggest that humans, rather than having a set point determined by genetics or number of adipose cells, actually settle into a particular stable weight based on an interaction between nature and nurture influences.

In the final analysis, we must bear much of the responsibility for weight maintenance ourselves since set point is weaker in preventing weight gain than in preventing weight loss.[26] The odds are against the likelihood that, even with a set point helping us, we can avoid creeping weight gain in adulthood without great attention to this tendency.

■ Does Nurture Have a Role?

Genetic factors determine some differences in energy metabolism and explain certain weight-gain variations among people. However, environmental factors, such as high-fat diets and inactivity, can literally shape us as well. Consider that our gene pool hasn't changed much in the past 50 years, but the ranks of obese people have grown.[22]

Family members often have similar eating habits and choose similar foods. Even husbands and wives—who have no genetic link—may behave similarly toward food and eventually assume similar degrees of leanness or chunkiness. Therefore, the family that bonds at the local quick-service restaurant can influence each other's eating habits and, ultimately, fatness.

Is poverty associated with obesity? Ironically, the answer is often yes. Americans of lower socioeconomic status, especially females, are more likely to be obese than those in upper socioeconomic groups. Are cultural expectations or socioeconomic stress the cause of this?

The importance of environment in the development of obesity is exhibited in the treatment of Prader-Willi syndrome. Children with this inherited disorder have an *extreme* appetite and become very obese if food availability is not carefully controlled. If such a child has become obese, however, further careful control of food availability (e.g., locking all kitchen cabinets and not allowing the child access to money) can lead to significant weight loss, often 100 pounds or more. This environmental therapy is effective, despite the fact that the children maintain their *extreme* appetite.

Adult obesity in women is often rooted in childhood obesity. In addition, relative inactivity, periods of stress and boredom, as well as excess weight gain in pregnancy, contribute to female obesity. (Chapter 16 notes that breastfeeding one's infant contributes to loss of some of this excess fat associated with pregnancy.) These patterns suggest both social and genetic links. Male obesity, however, is not strongly linked to childhood obesity and, instead, tends to appear after age 30. In part, marriage and a working life encourage a sedentary state for many men. This powerful and prevalent pattern suggests a primary role of nurture in obesity, with less genetic influence.

■ Nature and Nurture Together

Overall, both nature and nurture influence the tendency toward obesity (Table 13-5). Consider the possibility that obesity is nurture allowing nature to express itself, like an accident waiting to happen. Some people begin life with a slower metabolism. Put these people in an inactive environment, feed them high-calorie foods, and praise them for eating. Like any of us, they can be nurtured into gaining weight, which allows their natural tendency for obesity to blossom. The eventual location of fat storage is strongly influenced by genetics.[25]

If your parents are obese, you're likely to be at risk for obesity all your life. To avoid it will require eternal vigilance. Eat the right foods at the right times for the right reasons.[35] And, whatever the answer to the nature versus nurture question is, it is likely that all obese people or those at risk for obesity will face this lifelong struggle as well. Still, genes do not control this destiny. With increased physical activity and decreased food (especially fat) consumption, even those with a genetic tendency toward obesity can maintain a healthy or "healthier" body weight.[4]

Little relationship exists between how an infant was fed or how much weight was gained in the first year of life and the presence or absence of obesity in later childhood. The exception could be the infant who gains weight very rapidly in the first 6 weeks of life. Most overweight or obese infants become normal-weight schoolchildren. However, if a child has become obese by 5 years of age, immediate attention is necessary. Obesity in childhood is strongly related to obesity in adulthood.

CONCEPT CHECK

Genetic background plays a role in obesity, influencing body shape, sites of fat deposition, and rate of basal metabolism. The role of nurture is evident in families, who tend to have similar eating habits, activity patterns, and degrees of fatness. Men tend to develop obesity after age 30, and women tend to have both childhood and adult roots for obesity; this suggests an especially important influence of nurture in men. Because both factors have an impact, it makes sense to assume that nurture serves as a catalyst for expressing or denying a genetic tendency toward obesity.

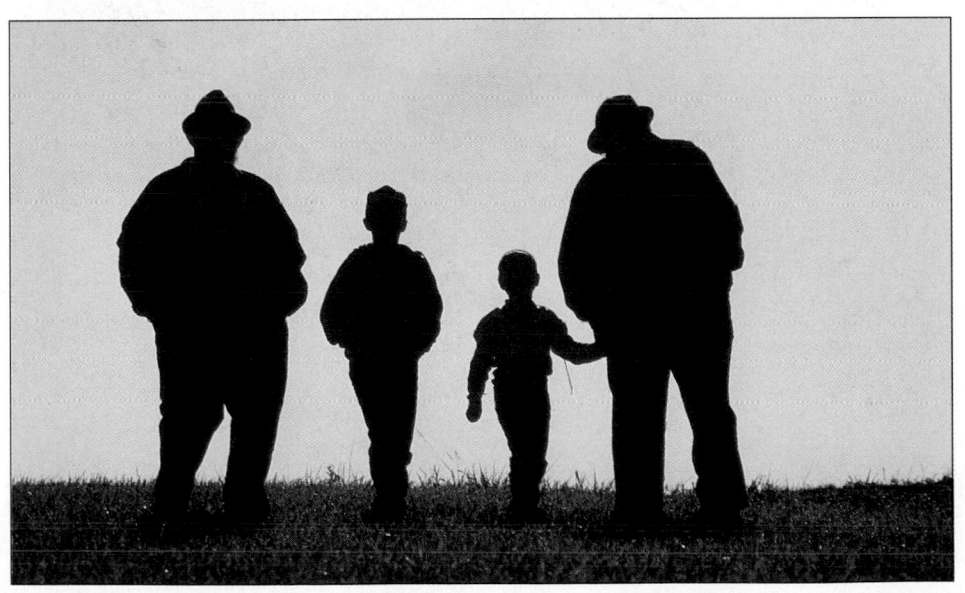

Does the difference in body fat between grandfathers and sons arise from nature, nurture, or both?

TABLE 13-5   What Encourages Excess Body Fat Stores and Obesity?

Factor	How Fat Storage Is Affected
Age	Excess body fat is more common in adults and middle-aged individuals.
Menopause	Increase in abdominal fat deposition is favored.
Gender	Females have more fat.
Insulin resistance	This often develops as obesity develops.
Positive energy balance	This is especially important if over a relatively long period.
Composition of diet	High fat intake, excess alcohol intake, and preference for sugary, fat-rich foods are likely to contribute to obesity.
Physical activity	Low or decreasing amount of physical activity ("couch potato") affects energy balance and body fat stores.
Resting metabolic rate	A low value with respect to lean body mass is linked to weight gain.
Sympathetic nervous system	Low activity favors weight gain.
Thermic effect of food	This is low for some obesity cases.
Use of fat for energy	There is limited fat release into the bloodstream.
Total fat mass	Leptin, produced by adipose tissue, affects food intake. Greater fat mass leads to greater leptin production.
Ratio of fat to lean tissue	A high ratio of fat mass to lean body mass is correlated with weight gain.
Fat uptake by adipose tissue	This is high in some obese individuals and remains high (perhaps even increases) with weight loss.
Blood cortisol value	Elevated values promote weight and fat gain.
Variety of social and behavioral factors	Obesity is associated with socioeconomic status; familial conditions; network of friends; busy lifestyles that discourage balanced meals; binge eating; easy availability of inexpensive, "supersized" high-fat food (such as in quick-service restaurants); pattern of leisure activities; television time; smoking cessation; excessive alcohol intake; and number of meals eaten away from home. These meals are often served in large portions and high in fat and energy content. Today, "food hunts man" to a great extent in Western societies.
Undetermined genetic characteristics	These affect energy balance, particularly via the energy expenditure components, the deposition of the energy surplus as fat or as lean tissue, and the relative proportion of fat and carbohydrate use by the body.
Race	In some ethnic groups, higher body weight may be more socially acceptable.
Certain medications	Food intake increases.
Childbearing	Women may not lose all weight gained in pregnancy, leading to creeping weight gain.
National region	Regional differences, such as high-fat diets and sedentary lifestyles in the Midwest and areas of the South, cause different rates of obesity in different places.

◼ TREATMENT OF OBESITY

Obesity should be considered similar to any chronic disease. Treatment requires long-term lifestyle changes, rather than simply taking medicine for 2 weeks, as for a sore throat, or following a quick fix promoted by a fad diet book.[27] We often, however, view a "diet" as something one goes on temporarily, only to resume prior (typically poor) habits once satisfactory results have been achieved. It is for this reason that so many people regain lost weight. In place of this, healthy, active living with dietary modifications one can live with should be the emphasis for both obese and thin people. Let's explore why obesity must be regarded and treated in this way.

◼ Some Basic Premises

As you begin to consider current treatment options for obesity, first focus on five important general principles concerning weight loss for adults. (Chapter 17 provides weight-loss strategies for children.)

Much of the Current Mania Surrounding Dieting Is Misdirected

People on diets often fall within a BMI of 18.5 to 25. Rather than worrying about weight loss, these individuals should be focusing on a healthy lifestyle that allows for weight maintenance. Incorporating necessary lifestyle changes and learning to accept one's particular body characteristics—such as an endomorphic shape—should be the overriding goal.

Actually, this dieting mania can be viewed as mostly a social problem, stemming from unrealistic weight expectations (especially for women) and lack of appreciation for the natural variety in body shape and weight. Not every woman can look like a Hollywood actress, nor can every man look like a Greek god, but all of us can strive for good health and, if physically possible, an active lifestyle.[4]

The Body Defends Itself Against Weight Change

As noted in the discussion on set point, the body makes numerous physiological adjustments during times of underfeeding or overfeeding that resist weight change. The compensation is most pronounced during times of underfeeding.

Weight Cycling Is a Common Phenomenon

Only about 5% of people who follow commercial diet programs actually lose weight and then remain close to that weight. Typically, one-third of the weight lost during dieting is regained within 1 year of the end of dietary restriction, and almost all weight lost is regained within 3 to 5 years. Some programs have slightly higher success rates than 5%, as do some people who simply lose weight on their own without enrolling in any supervised plan. Overall, however, the statistics are grim. Currently, only the surgical approaches to obesity treatment show much success in maintaining the weight loss in most people.[32]

Negative health consequences associated with this weight cycling are an increased risk for upper-body fat deposition, profound discouragement and erosion of self-esteem, and possibly a fall in blood HDL-cholesterol. Nevertheless, experts still encourage obese people to attempt weight loss, with a strong focus on maintaining that lower weight. Still, dieters need to be aware of the trap of today's crash diet, which too often leads to the next month's weight gain. Weight-loss programs that claim you can lose weight and keep it off without changing food intake or increasing physical activity are selling a fantasy. A weight-loss program should be considered successful only when the subjects involved in the process remain at or close to their lower weights.

Weight Gain in Adulthood Is All Too Common

In adulthood, weight gain is common, especially in those aged 25–44 years.[22] Particular care should be practiced in these decades, although childhood and the

The total costs attributable to weight-related disease approaches $100 billion annually.

Here are some practices that can stimulate metabolism while one is dieting:
- *Perform physical activity regularly throughout the day. Find opportunities for increasing activity, such as quick walks, stair climbing, or calisthenics (crunches, push-ups, etc.).*
- *Fidget when sitting and standing.*
- *Eat breakfast, so that food intake is spread throughout the day. Each time food is consumed, metabolism increases.*
- *Follow a carbohydrate-rich diet; much of this is further processed by the liver, which uses energy.*
- *Avoid "crash" dieting. Slow weight loss is a better idea because it leads to a smaller decline in metabolism during a diet.*

CRITICAL THINKING

Hal has been dieting to lose weight for 2½ months. However, like many dieters, he has reached a plateau. Although he continues to restrict his kcal intake, he's no longer losing weight. How would you explain to Hal the physical factors that fight weight loss?

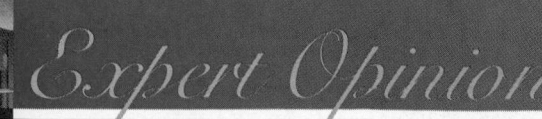

WHY IS WEIGHT MANAGEMENT SO DIFFICULT?

Sachiko T. St. Jeor, Ph.D., R.D.

Currently we are expecting a worldwide epidemic of obesity; 97 million or approximately 60% of adults in the United States are overweight (body mass index, or BMI, ≥ 85th percentile of 25.0 to 29.9 kg/m²) or obese (BMI in the ≥ 95th percentile or > 30.0 kg/m²). This is a sad commentary on the history of weight gain over the years. Although Americans are weight conscious, it appears that they are not successful in weight management overall.

Why is weight management so difficult? The first reason is that small weight gains overtime go unnoticed. According to the statistics of two nationally representative surveys, the National Health and Nutrition Examination Survey II, or NHANES II (1976–1980), and NHANES III (1988–1994), it appears that the average weight gain over 10 years is approximately 8 lbs (3.6 kg), or approximately 1 lb/year. We would rarely notice a 1-lb weight gain over a year but hopefully would notice a 10 to-20-lb weight gain over a 10- to 20-year period. In addition, many of us would rather not notice a small weight gain over time and certainly would

like to think that these small weight gains are temporary and will even out over time. Thus, new weight monitoring techniques may be of importance.

Second, little emphasis has been placed on weight maintenance or on the prevention of weight gain. This epidemic of obesity could have been partially halted if we did not gain so much weight and instead accept weight stability as our first goal. Since the conditions of overweight and obesity are associated with increased morbidity and mortality from at least five major diseases (hypertension, diabetes, dyslipidemia, cardiovascular disease, and stroke) as well as some types of cancers (endometrium, breast, prostate, and colon), the problem is of major significance. Our research group has defined weight maintenance as ± 5 lb between any two points in time. This reflects about a 3% change in body weight. However, there has been no standard definition broadly accepted for weight maintenance, and individual fluctuations vary widely.

Using this practical definition, only 20% of a group of both normal and overweight males and females of all ages

studied in my laboratory were weight maintainers over 4 years. Furthermore, more normal-weight individuals were weight maintainers (75%) than those who were overweight (25%). Older males, adults who experienced lower weight variability, and adults undergoing less dieting were also more successful at maintaining their weight. The weight maintainers tended to have better health profiles, were characterized by being more physically active, used more problem-solving and self-monitoring strategies, and had more "normalized" eating patterns, social support, and self-efficacy. These results point to the difficulty of implementing well-accepted strategies for weight management over the long term.

Third, we are a population with very unrealistic expectations. Weight maintenance is not a popular concept; instead, weight loss is always the goal. A fad diet is usually on the bestseller list, and losing large amounts of weight in short periods of time (10 lbs/10 days) is always attractive. Few individuals are really committed to putting in the long-term effort needed to lose weight gradually (1–3 lb/week) in a

adolescent years also deserve attention. Adults should generate a goal of not gaining greater than about 10 to 16 pounds more than their weight was on reaching age 21. People who gain weight rapidly should closely monitor food intake and activity patterns to discover the causes and then moderate the increases or reverse the trend in appropriate ways.[4]

Changes in Body Composition Deserve a Primary Focus in Weight Loss

Weight should be lost mostly from adipose stores, not from muscle and other lean tissues. Rapid weight loss at the start of a diet program often represents fluid lost as a result of decreased salt intake and loss of glycogen from the liver and muscle. Substantial muscle tissue may be lost as well, and this is mostly (about 73%) water. People are fooled when they weigh themselves after starting a fad diet. They lose weight, but very little of it represents fat loss. Any loss of lean tissue means a decrease in basal metabolism and thus a decrease in overall energy expenditure.

healthy manner, by making a conscious effort to decrease energy intake and increase physical activity daily. Furthermore, the amount of weight loss desired is always much higher than that which generally can be achieved and maintained in the longer term.

The fourth reason is that little emphasis is put on obesity prevention, and insurance reimbursement for weight-management counseling is very limited. Most individuals who seek professional counseling are those with medically related diseases. In contrast, the majority of the dieting population uses self-help methods (books, over-the-counter medications, supplements, clubs, etc.), which may work only temporarily. The most intelligent adults are also susceptible to diet fads, as they might be desperate to find quick and easy answers. Because the medical profession has put little emphasis on weight management, the burden of success and prevention lies on the individual and interested professionals. However, recent emphasis on obesity as a disease, its recognition as one of the leading health indicators in the Healthy People 2010 objectives, and emphasis on weight management in the major message of "aim for a healthy weight" in the 2000 Dietary Guidelines will certainly help put obesity

and weight management on the national agenda as higher priorities in the future.

The last reason is that healthy lifestyles are difficult to maintain in our busy and demanding lives. We need to be more physically active. Ways to more easily incorporate increased activity need facilitation and motivation. Simultaneously, since tasty foods and social occasions increase our food consumption, strategies to balance our energy intake and output need more emphasis. Health reasons for weight management are less immediate but should be stressed and somehow rewarded. Time is of the essence in all regards.

In summary, there are many reasons that weight management is difficult. However, a winning strategy is to take small steps in balancing energy intake with output. Small, additive changes, even in 100 kcal increments, will make a difference in the long run. On the intake side, 100 kcal is not much and can be as little as a bite of food in less than 1 minute. On the expenditure side, calories burned take more effort. For example, a mile walked in approximately 15–20 minutes is approximately 100 kcal. Still, the resulting 200-kcal deficit in one day and 1400 kcal deficit in 1 week equates to approximately 0.5 lb/week fat loss and could result in a

weight change of 26 lb/year. It takes time, education, awareness, motivation, and action for successful weight management. A good message is to start where you are and prevent weight gain—whether you currently are healthy-weight, overweight, or obese. Then, concentrate on small changes to implement additive weight losses over time. Initial targets of approximately 5 to 10% of weight loss in the first 6 months is reasonable. Prevention of weight gain or regain is more difficult (concentrate on weight maintenance at ± 5 lb or 3% of weight between any two points in time). Patience, realistic goals, and time without relapse will work. We can be successful at weight management if we place primary emphasis on weight maintenance, especially when weight loss is not possible.

Dr. St. Jeor is a professor and director of the Nutrition Education and Research Program at the University of Nevada School of Medicine, Reno. She is internationally known for her research focusing on efforts to improve weight control and overall health in adults.

Weight Loss in Perspective

All this shows the importance of preventing obesity, because curing the disorder is very difficult. Public-health and political strategies to address the obesity epidemic must begin with weight maintenance for the adult population and increased physical activity. There is a particular need to focus on children and adolescents, in which excess weight and sedentary lifestyle may form the basis for a lifetime of weight-related illness and increased mortality.[24]

Only the very motivated person should try to lose weight, and ideally this attempt should be preceded by a period of weight maintenance for about 6 months in order to begin the process of balancing energy intake with a degree of energy output that can be maintained.[2] Dr. Sach St. Jeor discusses this concept in greater detail in her Expert Opinion.

A typical fast-food hamburger in 1957 contained little more than 1 oz of cooked meat, compared with up to 6 oz in 1997. A theater serving of popcorn was 3 cups in 1957, compared with 16 cups (medium-size popcorn) in 1997.

For more information on weight control, obesity, and nutrition, visit the Weight-Control Information Network (WIN) at http://www.niddk.nih.gov/ NutritionDocs.html or call 800-WIN-8098. Other web sites include http://www.caloriecontrol.org, http://www.weight.com, http://www.obesity.org, and http://www.cyberdiet.com.

When you read brochures or research reports about specific diet plans, ask not only whether the people lost weight but also whether they maintained much of that weight loss. If this did not happen, then the entire dieting program was in vain.

■ Wishful Shrinking—Why Can't Quick Weight Loss Be Mostly Fat?

Rapid weight loss cannot consist mostly of fat loss because such a high energy deficit is needed to lose a large amount of adipose tissue. The body fat present in adipose tissue contains about 3500 kcal per pound. Fat storage, which includes body fat tissue plus supporting lean tissues, contains approximately 2700 kcal per pound. To lose 1 to 2 pounds of fat stores per week, energy intake must be decreased by approximately 500 to 1000 kcal/day, with the addition of participating in at least 30 minutes of physical activity on most days of the week. Behavioral strategies to reinforce lifestyle changes are also effective for weight loss and later weight maintenance.[27] Diets that promise 10 to 15 lb of weight loss per week can't ensure that the weight loss is from fat stores alone. Producing an energy deficit sufficient to lose that amount of fat storage simply isn't practical. Lean tissue, rather than fat, accounts for the major part of the weight lost.

■ What to Look for in a Sound Weight-Loss Diet

A dieter can try to devise a plan of action by seeking advice from health professionals or consulting current books. Either way, a sound weight-loss program should include three components: control of energy intake, especially fat intake; increased energy expenditure through physical activity; and acknowledgment that a lifelong change in habits is required, not simply a short-term weight-loss period. Focusing on just consuming less energy represents a difficult path to success. Adding regular physical activity and an appropriate psychological component contributes to success and later maintenance of the weight loss.

Specifically, any weight-loss plan should have the following characteristics:[8]

1. The plan should meet nutritional needs, except for energy. To do that, it should follow the Food Guide Pyramid, emphasizing a wide variety of low-fat and non-fat choices and adequate fluids (8 cups per day). Overall, this controlled eating should remain a satisfying and pleasurable experience.

2. Expect slow weight loss. This helps with later weight maintenance. A loss of 1 or so pounds of fat storage per week is desirable. Once about 10% of excess weight is lost, maintenance of that loss for about 6 months is recommended before more weight loss is attempted. That may seem like a disappointing prescription, but a more radical approach to weight loss is likely to produce a yo-yo episode. Recall that a person could view this as a "healthier" weight, because it will probably lead to health improvement. Then, careful evaluation should be made to determine whether further weight loss is needed, based on current health state.

3. The plan should allow adaptations to individual habits and tastes. The same plan does not work for everyone.

4. The plan should minimize hunger and fatigue. To do this, it should contain at least 1200 to 1500 kcal per day. Otherwise, consuming sufficient vitamins and minerals, especially enough iron for young women, is difficult. In reality, however, 1000 kcal per day is generally regarded as the minimum energy intake because many dieters perform so little physical activity and therefore need very restricted energy allowances. If the eating plan calls for an energy intake below 1200 to 1500 kcal per day, it should recommend the use of either fortified foods (breakfast cereals, for example) or a balanced vitamin and mineral supplement (see Chapter 9 for advice on supplement use).

5. The plan should contain common foods. There is no magical food that can speed weight loss. If a diet suggests that there is, whether ginseng, tofu, or garlic, advice should be sought elsewhere. Furthermore, if special foods were required, maintaining this practice indefinitely would be difficult.

6. The plan should fit into any social situation. The healthier lifestyle should allow attendance at parties, eating at restaurants, and participation in normal daily activities.

7. The plan should help change problem eating habits. It should promote reshaping food habits and lifestyle to make weight loss and then weight maintenance possible and, so, thwart weight regain. Eating at least three meals per day and avoiding binge eating are two important considerations. Maintenance should be a key concern of any plan—the plan must have a lifetime focus. For example, a 150-lb person should reduce energy intake, increase physical activity, and start eating like a 130-lb person to become a 130-lb person. Moreover, once the weight is lost, the person can't go back to the habits of his or her 150-lb self. The program should also focus on changing obesity-promoting beliefs and rallying healthy social support.

8. The plan should improve overall health. It should emphasize regular physical activity, proper rest, stress reduction, and other health changes in lifestyle. All too often, people know how to diet, but they don't know how to live. They find it easier to count calories and follow a plan than to deal with underlying issues that encourage eating, such as stress.

9. The plan should insist that the person see a physician before starting if any of the following are true:
   • He or she has existing health problems, such as heart disease or hypertension.
   • He or she plans to lose weight as quickly as possible.
   • He or she is over 40 years of age for men or 50 years of age for women and plans to perform substantially increased physical activity (according to the latest Dietary Guidelines publication).

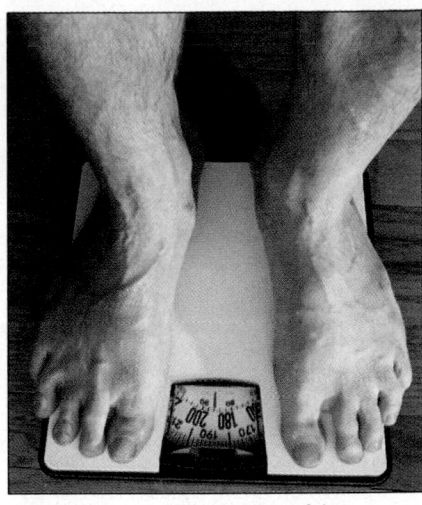

Slow, steady weight loss is one of the characteristics of a sound weight-loss plan.

CONCEPT CHECK

Obesity is a chronic disease that necessitates lifelong treatment. Key points to consider when attempting to treat obesity include the following: (1) The primary focus should be on a healthy lifestyle that can be maintained; (2) the body resists weight loss; (3) typical weight-loss attempts often are followed by weight regain; (4) emphasis should be placed on preventing obesity, since curing this disorder is very difficult; (5) weight should be lost from fat stores, not mostly from lean tissues. Appropriate weight-loss programs have the following characteristics in common: (1) They meet nutritional needs—this can be evaluated by checking for mostly low-fat and nonfat choices from the Food Guide Pyramid; (2) they can adjust to accommodate habits and tastes; (3) they emphasize readily obtainable foods; (4) they promote changing habits that lead to overeating; (5) they encourage regular physical activity; and (6) they help change obesity-promoting beliefs and rally healthy social support.

Weight-Control Objectives from _Healthy People 2010_

Increase by 40% the proportion of adults who are at a healthy weight (body mass index between 18.5 and 25).

Reduce by 50% the proportion of adults who are obese (body mass index of 30 or more).

Reduce by 50% the proportion of children and adolescents who are overweight or obese.

■ CONTROL OF ENERGY INTAKE— THE FIRST KEY TO WEIGHT LOSS

A goal of losing 1 to 2 lb of stored fat per week may require limiting energy intake to 1200 kcal per day for women and 1500 kcal for men, with less than 30% of energy intake coming from fat. Recall that adults currently consume about 33% of energy as fat. The calorie allowance could also be higher for very active people. Keep in mind that, in a very sedentary society, decreasing fat (and calories) is important because it is difficult to use much of either without ample physical activity.

Traditionally, dieters have counted calories. Many experts recommend counting mostly fat grams, assuming that control of energy intake follows. Chapter 6 contains a table to convert energy intake into an appropriate fat gram allowance. The new food labels simplify the task of counting fat grams. Note that not all food choices need to be low fat. Total fat intake for the day is the focus. This approach makes

Liquids are getting more attention, since liquid calories do not stimulate satiety mechanisms to the same extent as solid foods. The advice from experts is to use beverages that have few or no calories and limit calorie-containing beverages.

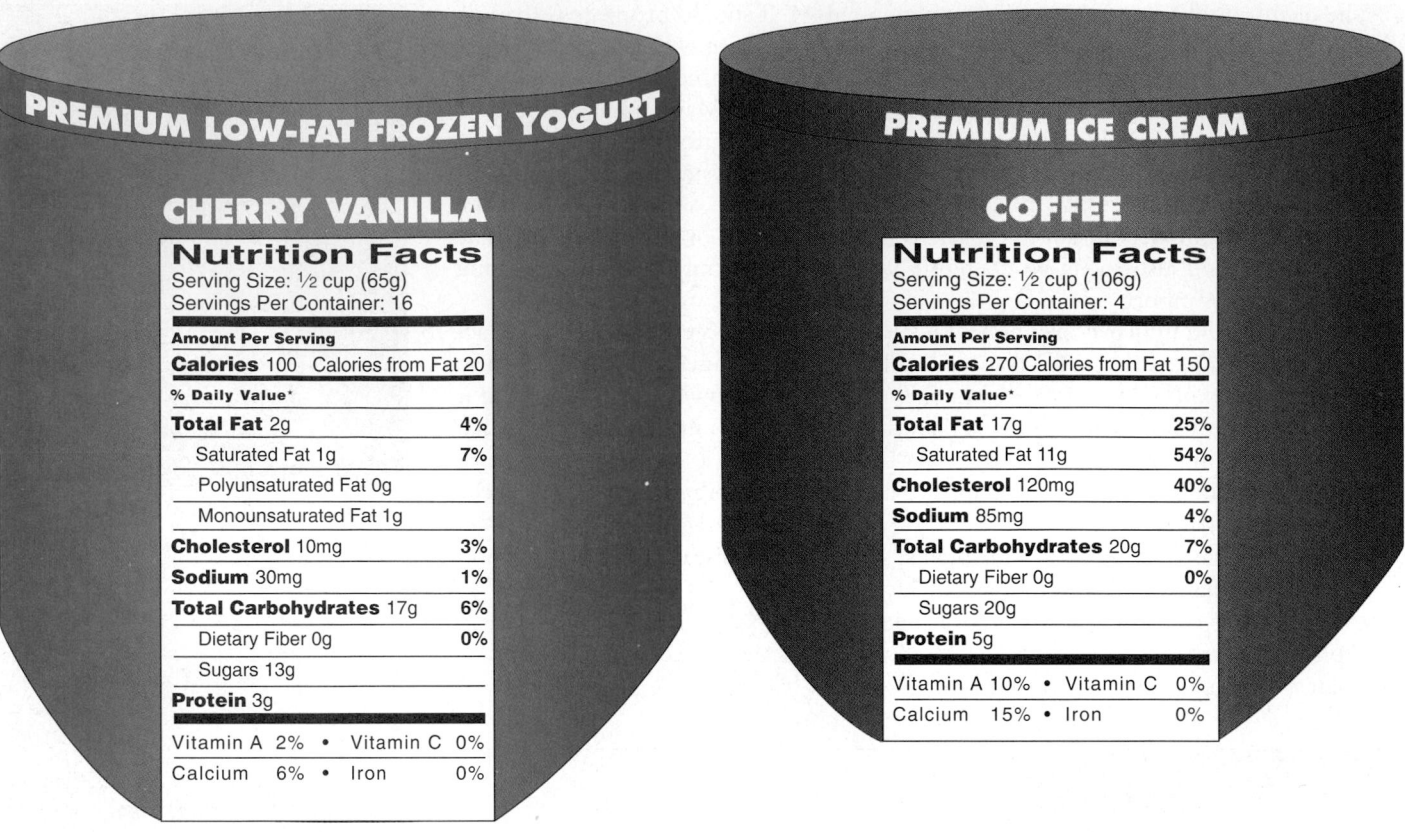

■ FIGURE 13-11 Reading labels helps you choose foods with less fat and energy. Which frozen dessert is the best choice for a person on a weight-loss diet? The % Daily Values are based on a 2000 kcal diet.

Compared with the late 1970s, the average American now eats about 160 calories more each day; that is especially a problem, since many of us engage in such little physical activity. Every food is fattening when you exceed your daily calorie needs.

sense because a lifelong restriction of energy intake is almost impossible, whereas a low-fat diet is easy to follow indefinitely if it allows the consumption of enough food—especially fruits, vegetables, and whole grains—to satisfy hunger. However, this method will work only if high-calorie fat-free foods—such as fat-free cakes and cookies—are not overeaten.

As discussed in Chapter 6, many of the fat-reduced products flooding the market substitute sugar for fat to maintain flavor. Consequently, they tend to be slightly lower in energy content. This makes it easy to gain weight, even on a low-fat diet, without careful portion control of fat-reduced foods. In addition, some experts think that certain fat-reduced foods, such as nonfat sour cream, merely remind dieters of what they are missing, driving them back to the high-fat food choice. In addition, some studies have shown that people eat more when told a food is fat reduced, even if it is not. This suggests it may be better to avoid high-fat foods and their fat-reduced counterparts, instead replacing them with a food choice naturally low in fat, such as nonfat yogurt for sour cream or a plain warm bagel for a doughnut. Fruits, vegetables, and whole grains also are recommended.[31]

In any case, dieters should consume at least 1000 kcal daily; fewer than that causes so much hunger that they will probably not be able to stick to the plan. A better idea is to first increase physical activity, allowing at least 1000 kcal (ideally, closer to 1500 kcal) to be eaten each day.

Two ways for a dieter to monitor energy intake at the start of a weight-loss program are reading labels and learning the exchange system. Label reading is important, because many foods are more energy dense than people suppose (Fig. 13-11). See the menu patterns listed in Table 2-10 in Chapter 2 for some possible exchange system approaches. Another method is to write down food intake for 24 hours and then calculate energy intake from the food table in Appendix A or your diet analysis software, adjusting future food choices as needed. Because people often underestimate portion size when recording food intake, measuring cups can help.

Whatever the method chosen, it is unreasonable to think that measuring food and keeping records will continue for a lifetime. These methods are suggested as a temporary practice for people who need to get a handle on their portion sizes. Once the eyes and stomach are trained to know what constitutes a specific portion size, it will be possible to then "eyeball" appropriate meals.

Decreasing fat in the diet from 40 to 30% does not result in much compensation. That is, people do not often feel the need to eat large volumes of food to make up for the missing fat. On the other hand, reducing dietary fat to 20% of calories frequently leaves people feeling hungry and leads to the overeating of fat-free foods, many of which are high in calories. It is only when the dietary fat is replaced by foods rich in complex carbohydrates and dietary fiber that this compensation can be minimized.[13]

Table 13-6 shows how to start reducing energy intake. As you should realize by now, it is best to consider healthy eating a lifestyle change, rather than simply a weight-loss plan.[27]

*S*pot-reducing using diet and physical activity is not possible. "Problem" local fat deposits can be reduced in size, however, using suction lipectomy. Lipectomy means surgical removal of fat. A pencil-thin tube is inserted into an incision in the skin, and the fat tissue, such as that in the buttocks and thigh area, is suctioned. This procedure carries some risks, such as infection; lasting depressions in the skin; and blood clots, which can lead to kidney failure and sometimes death. The procedure is designed to help a person lose about 4 lb per treatment. Cost is about $1600 per site; total costs range as high as $2600-$9000.

■ REGULAR PHYSICAL ACTIVITY—A SECOND KEY TO WEIGHT LOSS AND ESPECIALLY IMPORTANT FOR LATER WEIGHT MAINTENANCE

Regular physical activity is very important for everyone, especially those who are trying to lose weight or maintain a lower body weight. Fat use is enhanced. Therefore, it greatly complements a reduction in energy intake for weight loss but does not substitute for it.[1] Many of us rarely do more than sit, stand, and sleep. Obviously, much

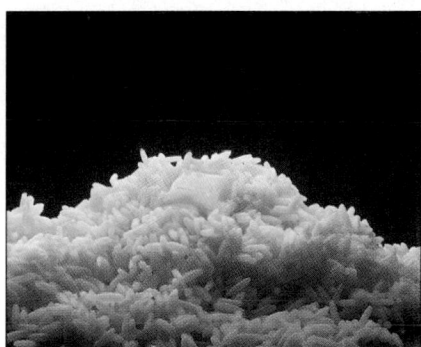

When controlling energy intake, it is especially important to watch the amount of added fats.

TABLE 13-6   Saving Kcal: Ideas to Help Get Started

Instead Of	Try	Number of kcal Saved
3 oz well-marbled meat (prime rib)	3 oz lean meat (eye of round)	140
½ chicken breast, batter-fried	½ chicken breast, broiled with lemon	175
½ cup beef stroganoff	3 oz lean roast beef	210
½ cup home-fried potatoes	1 medium baked potato	65
½ cup green bean-mushroom casserole	½ cup cooked green beans	50
½ cup potato salad	1 cup raw vegetable salad	140
½ cup pineapple chunks in heavy syrup	½ cup pineapple chunks canned in juice	25
2 tbsp bottled French dressing	2 tbsp low-calorie French dressing	150
⅙ 9-inch apple pie	1 baked apple	185
3 oatmeal-raisin cookies	1 oatmeal-raisin cookie	125
½ cup ice cream	½ cup ice milk	45
1 danish pastry	½ English muffin	150
1 cup sugar-coated corn flakes	1 cup plain corn flakes	60
1 cup whole milk	1 cup 1% low-fat milk	45
7-fluid-oz gin and tonic	6-fluid-oz wine cooler made with sparkling water	150
1-oz bag potato chips	1 cup plain popcorn	120
⅟₁₂ 8-inch white layer cake with chocolate frosting	⅟₁₂ angel food cake, 10-inch tube	185
Regular beer	Light beer	40

more energy is used during physical activity than at rest. In addition, expending only 200 to 300 extra kcal per day above and beyond normal daily activity, while controlling energy intake, can lead to about a half pound of fat loss per week, or about 25 pounds of fat loss per year. Furthermore, physical activity often boosts overall self-esteem.

Adding any of the activities in Table 13-7 to one's lifestyle leads to more energy expenditure. Duration and regular performance, rather than intensity, are the keys to success with this approach to weight loss. One should search for activities that can be continued over time. In this regard, walking vigorously 2 miles per day can be as

TABLE 13-7	Approximate Energy Costs of Various Activities, and those Projected for a 150-lb (68 kg) Person	
Activity	**Kcal per kg per Hour**	**Number of kcal per Hour**
Aerobics—heavy	8.0	544
Aerobics—light	3.0	204
Aerobics—medium	5.0	340
Backpacking	9.0	612
Basketball—vigorous	10.0	680
Bicycling (5.5 MPH)	3.0	204
Bowling	3.9	265
Calisthenics—heavy	8.0	544
Calisthenics—light	4.0	272
Canoeing (2.5 MPH)	3.3	224
Cleaning (female)	3.7	253
Cleaning (male)	3.5	236
Cooking	2.8	190
Cycling (13 MPH)	9.7	659
Dressing/showering	1.6	106
Driving	1.7	117
Eating (sitting)	1.4	93
Food shopping	3.6	245
Football—touch	7.0	476
Golf	3.6	244
Horseback trotting	5.1	346
Ice skating (10 MPH)	5.8	394
Jogging—medium	9.0	612
Jogging—slow	7.0	476
Lying—at ease	1.3	89
Racquetball—social	8.0	544
Roller-skating	5.1	346
Running or jogging (10 MPH)	13.2	897
Skiing (10 MPH)	8.8	598
Sleeping	1.2	80
Swimming (.25 MPH)	4.4	299
Tennis	6.1	414
Volleyball	5.1	346
Walking (2.5 MPH)	3.0	204
Walking (3.75 MPH)	4.4	299
Water skiing	7.0	476
Weight lifting—heavy	9.0	612
Weight lifting—light	4.0	272
Window cleaning	3.5	240
Writing (sitting)	1.7	118

The values in the table refer to total energy expenditure, including that needed to perform the physical activity, plus that needed for basal metabolism, the thermic effect of food, and nonexercise activity thermogenesis. Use your diet analysis software for your personal estimate.

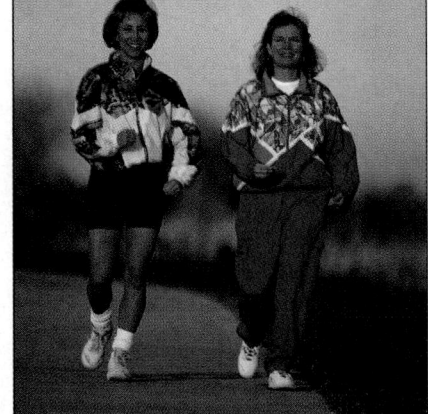

Physical activity complements any diet plan.

helpful as aerobic dancing or jogging if it is maintained. Moreover, walking is less likely to lead to injuries. Some resistance exercises (weight training) can also be added to increase lean body mass and, in turn, fat use (see Chapter 14). Exercise also helps maintain bone health during weight loss. Keep in mind that bone health suffers most in those involved in weight reduction programs that do not include an exercise component.

Opportunities in daily lives to expend energy have diminished: technology is systematically eliminating almost every reason to move our muscles.[13, 24] The easiest way to increase physical activity is to make it part of a daily routine. To start, one could consider walking every day and then incorporating some regular stair climbing. A simple trick is to park the car farther from school, work, and the shopping mall, so that one must walk farther.

■ BEHAVIOR MODIFICATION— A THIRD STRATEGY FOR WEIGHT LOSS

Controlling energy intake, so important to weight loss, also means modifying *problem* behaviors. Only the dieter can decide what behaviors keep the person from reaching for the wrong foods at the wrong times for the wrong reasons.[27]

What events start (or stop) eating? What factors influence food choices? Psychologists often use terms such as **chain-breaking, stimulus control, cognitive restructuring, contingency management,** and **self-monitoring** when discussing behavior modification (Table 13-8). This terminology helps place the problem in perspective and organize the intervention strategy into manageable steps.

Chain-breaking separates behaviors that tend to occur together—for example, snacking on chips while watching television. Although these activities do not have to occur together, they often do. Dieters may need to break the chain reaction (see the Take Action at the end of this chapter for more details).

Stimulus control puts us in charge of temptations. Options include pushing tempting food to the back of the refrigerator, removing fat-laden snacks from the kitchen counter, and avoiding the path by the vending machines. Provide a positive stimulus by keeping low-fat snacks ready to satisfy hunger/appetite. Note that alcohol and foods offer quick, easy stress relief. We need to plan healthful alternatives.

Cognitive restructuring changes our frame of mind. For example, after a hard day, respond with a walk or satisfying talk with a friend instead of a binge. Replace eating reactions to stress with healthful, relaxing alternatives.

Decreeing some food off limits sets up an internal struggle to resist the urge to eat that food. This hopeless battle can keep us feeling deprived. We lose the fight. Managing food choices with the principle of moderation is best. If a favorite food becomes troublesome, place it off limits only temporarily, until it can be enjoyed in moderation.

Contingency management prepares us for potential pitfalls and high-risk situations. We might rehearse in advance some appropriate responses to pressure—such as food being passed at a party.

Did you keep a record of what you ate and what catalysts urged you to pick up the fork or put it down as suggested in Take Action in Chapter 1? If so, you already know one key tool in modifying behavior—self-monitoring. A self-monitoring record can reveal patterns—such as unconscious overeating—that may explain problem eating habits. This record can encourage new habits to counteract unwanted behaviors. Obesity experts note that this is the key tool to use in any weight-loss program.

Overall, it's important to *address specific* problems, such as snacking, compulsive eating, and mealtime overeating. Behavior modification principles end up as critical components of weight reduction and maintenance. Without behavior modification, it is difficult to make lifelong lifestyle changes needed to meet weight-control goals.

chain-breaking Breaking the link between two or more behaviors that encourage overeating, such as snacking while watching television.

stimulus control Altering the environment to minimize the stimuli for eating—for example, removing foods from sight and storing them in kitchen cabinets.

cognitive restructuring Changing one's frame of mind regarding eating—for example, instead of using a difficult day as an excuse to overeat, substituting other pleasures for rewards, such as a relaxing walk with a friend.

contingency management Forming a plan of action to respond to a situation in which overeating is likely, such as when snacks are within arm's reach at a party.

self-monitoring Tracking foods eaten and conditions affecting eating; actions are usually recorded in a diary, along with location, time, and state of mind. This is a tool to help people understand more about their eating habits.

*R*eaching for fruit in a fruit bowl may prevent snacking on fat-laden foods. Although having the willpower to resist high-fat foods is desirable, a better alternative is to avoid the temptation.

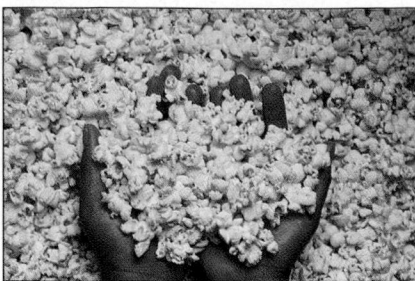

Popcorn is a wise snack choice when eaten in a reasonable quantity.

TABLE 13-8   Behavior Modification Principles for Weight Loss

Stimulus Control

Shopping
1. Shop for food after eating—buy nutritious foods.
2. Shop from a list; limit purchases of irresistible "problem" foods.
3. Avoid ready-to-eat foods.
4. Put off food shopping until absolutely necessary.

Plans
1. Plan to limit food intake as needed.
2. Substitute periods of physical activity for snacking.
3. Eat meals and snacks at scheduled times; don't skip meals.

Activities
1. Store food out of sight, preferably in the freezer, to discourage impulsive eating.
2. Eat all food in the same place.
3. Keep serving dishes off the table, especially dishes of sauces and gravies.
4. Use smaller dishes and utensils.

Holidays and Parties
1. Drink fewer alcoholic beverages.
2. Plan eating behavior before parties.
3. Eat a low-calorie snack before parties.
4. Practice polite ways to decline food.
5. Don't get discouraged by an occasional setback.

Eating Behavior
1. Put fork down between mouthfuls.
2. Chew thoroughly before taking the next bite.
3. Leave some food on the plate.
4. Pause in the middle of the meal.
5. Do nothing else while eating (for example, reading, watching television).

Reward
1. Plan specific rewards for specific behavior (behavioral contracts).
2. Solicit help from family and friends and suggest how they can help you. Encourage family and friends to provide this help in the form of praise and material rewards.
3. Use self-monitoring records as basis for rewards.

Self-Monitoring
1. Note the time and place of eating.
2. List the type and amount of food eaten.
3. Record who is present and how you feel.
4. Use the diet diary to identify problem areas.

Cognitive Restructuring
1. Avoid setting unreasonable goals.
2. Think about progress, not shortcomings.
3. Avoid imperatives such as *always* and *never*.
4. Counter negative thoughts with positive restatements.

■ Relapse Prevention Is Important

A dieter can tolerate an occasional lapse but needs to plan for lapses, encouraging not overreacting, but taking charge immediately. Change responses such as "I ate that cookie; I'm a failure" to "I ate that cookie, but I did well to stop after only one!" An occasional cookie is fine; a pound of cookies in an afternoon deserves reconsideration. When dieters lapse from their diet plan, newly learned food habits should steer them back toward the plan. This should enable dieters to avoid the lapse-relapse-collapse trap. Without a strong behavioral program for **relapse prevention** in place, a lapse frequently turns into a relapse. Once a pattern of poor food choices begins, dieters may feel that they have failed and stray further from the plan. As the relapse lengthens, the diet plan collapses, and dieters fall short of their weight-loss goal. Even with a good behavioral plan, one may fail at a diet. Losing weight is difficult. Overall, maintenance of weight loss is fostered by the "3 *M*s": motivation, movement, and monitoring.

■ Social Support Aids Behavioral Change

Healthy social support is helpful in weight control. Helping others understand how they can be supportive can make weight control easier. Family and friends can provide praise and encouragement. A weight-control professional can keep dieters accountable and help them learn from difficult situations. Long-term contact with a professional can be quite helpful for later weight maintenance.[27] Groups of individuals attempting to lose weight or maintain losses can provide empathetic support.

■ A RECAP

In the past, dieting emphasized the need for immediate results through unreasonable restrictions, willpower, and perfection. The emphasis today is on a well-balanced diet containing whole grains, fruits, and vegetables; regular physical activity; and behavior modification (Fig. 13-12). These components should be a part of an overall lifestyle change that is permanent.[14] No foods should be forbidden, and occasional overindulgence should be expected. Managing weight can be described as practicing healthy eating and maintaining a physically active lifestyle. In turn, this lifestyle can be continued for a lifetime and will result in improved health for the mind and the body.

Would-be dieters should choose and follow weight-control plans that are appropriate for them. They have a smorgasbord of options: lowered energy and fat intakes, behavior modification, increased physical activity, and group or individual counseling. Many tools are effective, but some are more useful than others, depending on the individual's lifestyle, personality, and motivation.

CONCEPT CHECK

*I*ncreasing physical activity in daily life should be part of any weight-loss plan. Daily activity, such as walking and stair climbing, is recommended. Behavior modification can improve conditions for losing weight. One behavioral area that requires change is habit chains that encourage overeating, such as snacking while watching television. Another tactic is to modify the environment to reduce temptation; for example, put foods into cupboards to keep them out of sight. In addition, rethinking attitudes about eating—for example, substituting pleasures other than food as a reward for coping with a stressful day—can be important for altering undesirable behavior. Advanced planning to prevent and deal with lapses is vital, as is rallying healthy social support. Finally, the careful observation and recording of eating habits can reveal subtle cues that lead to overeating. Overall, weight loss and maintenance are fostered by controlling energy intake, performing regular physical activity, and modifying problem behaviors.

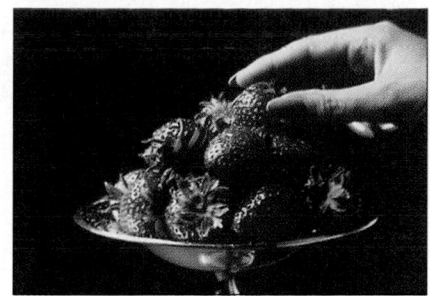

Fruit is a great low-cal snack—high nutrient density and low energy density.

relapse prevention A series of strategies used to help prevent and cope with weight-control lapses, such as recognizing high-risk situations and deciding beforehand on appropriate responses.

*T*he motivation to lose weight and keep it off generally comes with a proverbial "flip of the switch," in which the desire to lose weight finally becomes more important than the desire to overeat.

Control energy intake

Perform regular physical activity   **Control "problem" behaviors**

■ FIGURE 13-12 Weight-loss triad. The key to weight loss and maintenance can be thought of as a triangle in which the three corners consist of (1) controlling energy intake, (2) performing regular physical activity, and (3) controlling "problem" behaviors. The three corners of the triangle support each other in that without one corner the triangle becomes incomplete. In the same way, without one of the three keys to weight loss, weight loss and later maintenance become unlikely.

■ PROFESSIONAL HELP FOR WEIGHT LOSS

The first professional to see for advice about a weight-loss program is the family physician. Doctors are best equipped to assess overall health and the appropriateness of weight loss. The physician may then recommend a registered dietitian for a specific weight-loss plan and answers to diet-related questions. Registered dietitians are uniquely qualified to help design a weight-loss plan because they understand both food composition and the psychological importance of food. Exercise physiologists can provide advice about programs to increase physical activity.

Many communities have a variety of weight-loss organizations. These include self-help groups, such as Take Off Pounds Sensibly and Weight Watchers. Other programs, such as Jenny Craig and Physicians' Weight Loss Center, are less desirable for the average dieter. Often, the employees are not dietitians or other appropriately trained health professionals. These programs also tend to be expensive because of their requirements for intense counseling or mandatory diet foods and supplements. In addition, the Federal Trade Commission has charged these and other commercial diet-program companies with misleading consumers through unsubstantiated weight-loss claims and deceptive testimonials.

▌ Pharmacotherapy for Weight Loss

People who are candidates for pharmacotherapy for obesity include those with a BMI >30 or a BMI >27 with weight-related conditions, such as type 2 diabetes, cardiovascular disease, hypertension, or excess waist circumference; those with no contraindications to use of the medication; and those ready to undertake lifestyle change. Success with pharmacotherapy has been shown only in those who modify their behavior and energy intake and increase their physical activity. Pharmacotherapy alone has not been found to be successful. In addition, if a person has not lost at least 4.4 pounds (2 kg) after 4 weeks, it is not likely that the person will benefit from further use of the medication.[3]

With regard to the agents used, an **amphetamine**-like medication (phenteramine [Fastin or Ionamin]) is available. It prolongs the activity of epinephrine and norepinephrine in the brain. This therapy is effective for some people in the short run but has not yet been proved effective in the long run. Most state medical boards currently limit use to 12 weeks unless the person is participating in a medical study using the product. The drug should not be used in pregnant or nursing women or those under 18 years of age.

Sibutramine (Meridia) has been approved by FDA for weight loss. It enhances both norepinephrine and serotonin activity in the brain by reducing reuptake of these neurotransmitters by the secreting neurons. The neurotransmitters then remain active in the brain for a longer period of time, and so prolong a sense of reduced hunger. The most common side effects are constipation, dry mouth, insomnia, and a mild increase in blood pressure. Thus, sibutramine should be used with caution in people with a history of hypertension (or cardiovascular disease). Studies have shown that it is effective in helping some people who already eat healthy diets but just eat too much. The main effect is to moderately reduce appetite to allow people to eat less. Sibutramine is safe and effective only when combined with a comprehensive weight-control program and when supervised by a physician.[7]

Another medication approved by FDA for weight loss is orlistat (Xenical). This medication inhibits lipase action in the small intestine, reducing fat digestion and the subsequent absorption of dietary fat by one-third for about 2 hours when taken along with a meal containing fat. This malabsorbed fat simply is deposited in the feces. *Fat intake has to be controlled,* however, because large amounts of fat in the feces cause numerous side effects, such as gas, bloating, and oily discharge.[6] Interestingly, orlistat use can actually remind the person to follow a fat-controlled diet, as the symptoms resulting from consuming a high-fat meal quickly develop. Orlistat costs

amphetamine A group of medications that stimulate the central nervous system, among other effects. Abuse is linked to physical and psychological dependence.

*T*he only two medications approved by FDA for long-term use are sibutramine (Meridia) and orlistat (Xenical).

about $1.00 per pill, and a pill is taken with each meal. One way to reduce the cost of orlistat use is to eat a very-low-fat breakfast (e.g., breakfast cereal, juice, and skim milk) and use the medication to inhibit fat absorption at lunch and dinner.

Since the malabsorbed fat carries fat-soluble vitamins into the feces, the person taking orlistat must take a vitamin and mineral supplement at bedtime. In this way, any micronutrients not absorbed during the day can be replaced; fat malabsorption from the dinner meal will not greatly influence micronutrient absorption in the late evening.

Overall, in skilled hands, prescription medications can aid weight loss in some instances. However, they do not supplant the need for reducing energy and fat intake, modifying problem behavior, and increasing physical activity, both during and after therapy. And, more times than not, any weight loss during drug treatment can be attributed mostly to the individual's hard work.[7]

■ Treatment of Severe Obesity

Severe (morbid) obesity—weighing at least 100 pounds over healthy body weight (or twice one's healthy body weight)—requires professional treatment. Because of the serious health problems related to severe obesity, drastic measures may be necessary. Such treatments are recommended only when traditional diets fail. Drastic weight-loss procedures are not without side effects, both physical and psychological, making careful physician monitoring a necessity.

Very-Low-Calorie Diets

If more traditional diet changes have failed, treating severe obesity with a **very-low-calorie diet (VLCD)** is possible.[3] Optifast is one such commercial program. Some researchers believe that people with body weight greater than 30% above their healthy weight are also appropriate candidates. The diet allows a person to consume 400 to 800 kcal/day, often in liquid form. (These diets were known earlier as protein-sparing modified fasts.) Of this amount, about 30 to 120 g (120 to 480 kcal) is carbohydrate. The rest is high-quality protein, which supplies about 70 to 100 g per day (280 to 400 kcal). This low carbohydrate intake often causes ketosis, which may decrease hunger. However, the main reasons for weight loss are the minimal energy allowed and the absence of food choice. About 3 to 4 lb can be lost per week; men tend to lose at a faster rate than women. When physical activity and resistance training augment this diet, a greater loss of adipose tissue occurs. Careful physician monitoring is crucial throughout this very restrictive form of diet therapy during weight loss, refeeding, and later maintenance. Major health risks include heart problems and gallstones.

Weight regain remains a nagging problem with this type of therapy. If behavioral therapy and physical activity supplement a long-term support program, maintenance of the weight loss is more likely but still difficult. Any program under consideration should include a maintenance plan. Today, antiobesity medications also may be included in this phase of the program.

Gastroplasty

Gastroplasty, or stomach stapling, is the most common surgical procedure for treating severe obesity. The procedure works by reducing the stomach to about 30 ml (1 oz). Overeating of solid foods is consequently less likely, because rapid vomiting would result. The smaller stomach also promotes more rapid satiety. With the enforced food reduction, about 75% of people with severe obesity eventually lose 50% or more of excess body weight. The surgery's success at long-term loss maintenance often leads to dramatic health improvements, such as reduced blood pressure and elimination of type 2 diabetes. Risk of death from the surgery itself is about 1%.[32]

Gastroplasty has disadvantages. The surgery is costly and often not covered by medical insurance. In addition, follow-up surgery is often needed after weight loss

---

Chapter 9 discussed the risks of self-diagnosis and self-treatment of disease with megadose vitamin and mineral supplements. An even bigger danger exists using herbal substances to foster weight loss. Chapter 18 will discuss herbal remedies in detail. For now, know that, despite widespread advertising, ephedrine (also known as ma huang) and St. John's wort are neither effective nor safe treatments for weight loss. Ephedrine has been linked to numerous health problems and even deaths in recent years. St. John's wort should not be taken with any other antidepressants. Many experts advise staying away from any over-the-counter diet pills, and especially these herbal combinations.[29]

very-low-calorie diet (VLCD) Known also as *protein-sparing modified fast* (PSMF), this diet allows a person 400 to 800 kcal per day, often in liquid form. Of this, 120 to 480 kcal is carbohydrate, whereas the rest is mostly high-biological-value protein.

gastroplasty Surgery performed on the stomach to limit its volume to approximately 30 ml.

Gastroplasty Criteria
1. BMI should be > 40.
2. BMI between 36 and 40 is considered when there is a serious obesity-related health concern.
3. Obesity must be present for a minimum of 5 years, with several nonsurgical attempts to lose weight..
4. There should be no history of alcoholism or major psychiatric disorders.

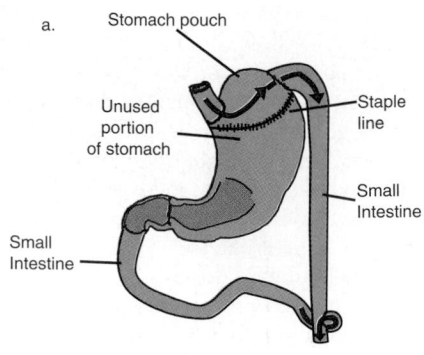

a.

Stomach pouch

Unused portion of stomach

Staple line

Small Intestine

Small Intestine

Roux-en-Y Gastroplasty

b.

Esophagus

Staple line

Stomach pouch

Banded outlet

Unused portion of stomach

Small intestine

Vertical Banded Gastroplasty

FIGURE 13-13 Two current forms of gastroplasty for treatment of severe obesity. The Roux-en-Y procedure (a) is the most effective method, but is more technically demanding for the surgeon than the Vertical-Banded Gastroplasty (b). In the latter the band prevents expansion of outlet for the stomach pouch.

underweight A body mass index below 18.5. The cutoff is less precise than for obesity because this condition has been less studied.

to correct stretched skin, which used to be filled with fat. Furthermore, months of difficult adjustments face the dieter who has chosen this drastic approach to weight loss. The elimination of simple carbohydrates (sugar) from the diet is necessary to avoid *dumping syndrome*. Dumping syndrome is characterized by severe diarrhea, which begins almost immediately following the ingestion of concentrated sugar, such as regular soft drinks, Jell-o, candy, cookies, and other high-sugar foods. Nutrient deficiencies are also possible if an appropriate diet and nutrient supplement plan is not followed.

Two gastroplasty approaches are common today (Fig. 13-13). For the Roux-en-Y gastroplasty procedure, the small intestine is cut at the jejunum. The distal portion of the jejunum is then relocated to the top portion of the stomach and sewed into place. A staple line is then created across the upper portion of the stomach, yielding a stomach pouch of about 30 ml. Food now traverses through the stomach pouch into this limb of small intestine, and eventually into the main flow of the small intestine. In the vertical-banded gastroplasty procedure, a verticle staple line is made to create a stomach pouch, again about 30 ml. The outlet for this pouch is surrounded by a band in order to control the diameter of the outlet. This eliminates the possibility that the outlet will eventually stretch and allow for greater food intake. Food travels through the stomach pouch into the main portion of the stomach.

Either surgery is not reversed, even after the desired weight loss is attained. Thus, however successful for weight loss, gastroplasty still requires major, lifelong lifestyle changes.

Concept Check

Severely obese people who have failed to lose weight with conservative weight-loss strategies may consider other options. Their doctors may recommend undergoing surgery to reduce the volume of the stomach to approximately 30 ml or following a very-low-calorie diet plan containing 400 to 800 kcal per day. Careful physician monitoring is crucial in both cases.

■ Treatment of Underweight

Underweight can be caused by a variety of factors, such as anorexia nervosa (see Chapter 15 for details), cancer, infectious disease, digestive tract disorders, and excessive physical activity. Genetic background may also lead to a higher resting metabolic rate, a slight body frame, or both. Significant underweight is also associated with increased death rates, especially when combined with cigarette smoking. Health problems associated with underweight include the loss of menstrual function, complications with pregnancy and surgery, and slow recovery after illness. We frequently hear about the risks of obesity, but seldom of underweight. In our culture, being underweight is much more socially acceptable than being obese.

Sometimes being underweight requires medical intervention. A physician should be consulted first to rule out hormonal imbalances, depression, cancer, infectious disease, digestive tract disorders, excessive physical activity, and other hidden disease, such as the eating disorders anorexia nervosa and bulimia nervosa (see Chapter 15 for a detailed discussion of eating disorders).

The causes of underweight are not altogether different from the causes of obesity. Internal and external satiety-signal irregularities, the rate of metabolism, hereditary tendencies, and psychological traits can all contribute to underweight.

In growing children, the demand for energy to support physical activity and growth can cause underweight. During growth spurts in adolescence, active children may not take the time to consume enough energy to support their energy needs. Moreover, gaining weight can be a formidable task for an underweight person. More than 500 extra kcal per day may be required to gain weight, even at a slow pace, in part because of the increased expenditure of energy in nonexercise activity thermogenesis. In contrast to the weight loser, the weight gainer may need to increase portion sizes.

When underweight requires a specific intervention, one approach for treating adults is to gradually increase their consumption of energy-dense foods (foods that provide a great deal of energy in a small volume), especially those high in vegetable fat. Italian cheeses, nuts, and granola can be good energy sources with low saturated-fat content. Dried fruit and bananas are energy-dense fruit choices. If eaten at the end of a meal, they don't cause early satiety. Underweight people should replace such foods as diet soft drinks with good energy sources, such as fruit juices.

Encouraging a regular meal and snack schedule aids in weight gain and maintenance. Sometimes people who are underweight have experienced stress at work or have been too busy to eat. Making regular meals a priority may not only help them attain an appropriate weight but also help with digestive disorders, such as constipation, which are sometimes associated with irregular eating times.

Excessively physically active people can reduce activity. If their weight remains low, they can add muscle mass through a resistance training (weight-lifting) program, but they must increase their energy intake to support that physical activity. Otherwise, weight gain will be hindered.

If these efforts fail to achieve the desired weight, they should at least prevent the health problems associated with being underweight. After achieving that, they may have to accept their lean frames.

*C*heck out the *Perspective in Nutrition* Online Learning Center http://www.mhhe.com/wardlaw for quizzes, flash cards, other activities, and web links designed to further help you learn about weight control.

■ SUMMARY

1. Energy balance is energy intake minus energy output. Negative energy balance occurs when energy output surpasses energy intake, resulting in weight loss. Positive energy balance occurs when energy intake is greater than energy output. The result is weight gain.

2. Groups of cells in the hypothalamus and other regions in the brain affect hunger, the primarily internal desire to find and eat food. These cells monitor nutrients and other substances in the blood and read low amounts as a signal to promote feeding.

3. A variety of external (appetite-related) forces affect satiety. Hunger cues combine with appetite cues, such as easy availability of food, to promote feeding.

4. In North America, the major determinants of food intake are probably appetite-driven forces because food is so readily available. The physiological influences affecting food consumption are often suppressed or ignored.

5. Basal metabolism, the thermic effect of food, physical activity, and nonexercise activity thermogenesis account for total energy use by the body. Basal metabolism, which represents the minimum energy expenditure needed to keep the resting, awake body alive, is primarily affected by lean body mass, surface area, and thyroid hormone concentrations. Physical activity represents energy use above that expended at rest. The thermic effect of food represents the increase in metabolism to facilitate the digesting, absorbing, and processing of nutrients recently consumed. Nonexercise activity thermogenesis is heat production caused by overfeeding and other stimuli. About 70 to 80% of energy use is accounted for by basal metabolism and the thermic effect of food in a primarily sedentary person.

6. Energy use by the body can be measured directly from heat output or indirectly from oxygen uptake, carbon dioxide output, or both. Energy use by the body can be estimated using formulas based on various combinations of body height and weight with degree of physical activity and age.

7. A person of healthy weight shows good health and performs daily activities without weight-related problems. A body mass index (weight [in kilograms] ÷ height^2 [in meters]) of 18.5 to 25 is one measure of healthy weight, although weight in excess of this value may not lead to ill health. This suggests that healthy weight is best determined in conjunction with a thorough health evaluation by a physician.

8. Obesity is usually defined as total body fat percentage over 25% in men and about 35% in women. A body mass index over 30 also represents obesity.

9. Fat distribution partially determines health risks from obesity. Upper-body fat-storage distribution (waist circumference > 40 inches in men and > 35 inches in women) suggests higher risks of hypertension, cardiovascular disease, and type 2 diabetes associated with obesity than does lower-body fat distribution.

10. Genetic factors influence the tendency toward obesity. Basal metabolism and body-fat distribution both have genetic links. How a person is raised (or nurtured) also influences the tendency toward obesity because family members often develop similar eating habits and activity patterns. Obesity can be viewed as nurture allowing nature to be expressed.

11. Those in search of a treatment for obesity should remember these five points: (1) A focus on healthy lifestyle rather than weight loss per se is more appropriate for many potential and current dieters; (2) the body resists weight loss; (3) the emphasis should be on preventing obesity because curing the disorder is very difficult; (4) weight loss should represent mostly a loss of fat storage and not primarily the loss of muscle and other lean tissues; and (5) rapid weight loss and quick regain can be especially harmful to emotional health.

12. A sound weight-loss program meets the dieter's nutritional needs by emphasizing a wide variety of low-fat and nonfat food choices from the Food Guide Pyramid; it adapts to the dieter's habits, consists of readily obtainable foods, strives to change poor eating habits, stresses regular physical activity, and stipulates the participation of a physician if weight is to be lost rapidly or if the person is over 40 (men) or 50 (women) years of age and plans to perform substantially greater physical activity than usual.

13. A pound of fat contains about 3500 kcal. A pound of adipose tissue—the fat itself plus lean support tissue—lost or gained represents approximately 2700 kcal. Thus, if energy output exceeds energy intake by about 500 kcal/day, a pound of fat storage can be lost per week. Decreasing the intake of high-fat foods is probably the best way to obtain this energy deficit, along with increasing physical activity.

14. Physical activity as part of a weight-loss program should be focused on duration rather than intensity. Ideally, vigorous activity should be part of each day.

15. Behavior modification is a vital part of a weight-loss program because the dieter may have many habits that encourage overeating and thus discourage weight maintenance. Specific behavior-modification techniques, such as stimulus control and self-monitoring, can be used to help change problem behavior.

16. Medications to blunt appetite, such as phenteramine [Fastin] and sibutramine (Meridia), can aid weight-reduction strategies. Orlistat (Xenical) reduces fat absorption in a meal when taken with the meal. Use is reserved for those who are obese or have or weight-related problems, and they must be administered under strict physician supervision.

17. The treatment of severe obesity may include surgery to reduce stomach volume to approximately 30 ml or very-low-calorie diets containing 400 to 800 kcal per day. Both these measures should be reserved for people who have failed at more conservative approaches to weight loss. They require close medical supervision.

18. Underweight can be caused by a variety of factors, such as excessive physical activity and genetic background. Sometimes being underweight requires medical intervention. A physician should be consulted first to rule out ongoing disease. The underweight person may need to increase portion sizes and learn to like energy-dense foods. In addition, encouraging a regular meal and snack schedule aids in weight gain and maintenance. A physically active person can reduce excessive activity and substitute some resistance exercise (weight training).

■ STUDY QUESTIONS

1. After re-examining the internal and external forces associated with hunger, satiety, and food intake, propose two hypotheses for the development of obesity.
2. Knowing the four contributors to human energy expenditure, propose two hypotheses for the development of obesity, based on the classes of energy expenditure.
3. Define a healthy weight in a way that makes the most sense to you.
4. Describe a practical method to define obesity in a clinical setting.
5. What are the two most convincing pieces of evidence that both genetic and environmental factors play significant roles in the development of obesity?
6. What three health problems do obese people typically face? Describe a possible reason that each problem arises.
7. When searching for a sound weight-loss program, what three key characteristics would you look for?
8. Why is the claim for quick, effortless weight loss by any method necessarily misleading?
9. Define the term *behavior modification*. Relate it to the terms *stimulus control, self-monitoring, chain-breaking, relapse prevention,* and *cognitive restructuring*. Give examples of each.
10. Why should the treatment of obesity be viewed as a lifelong commitment rather than just a short episode of weight loss?

■ ANNOTATED REFERENCES

1. Allara L: The return of the high-protein, low-carbohydrate diet: Weighing the risks. *Nutrition in Clinical Practice* 15:26, 2000.

   The weight problem in this country is not seen as due to one particular nutrient ingested—for example, too much carbohydrate or too little protein—but, instead, to an increase in total calorie intake without some compensation, such as increased physical activity.

2. Apovian CM: Medical management of obesity and the role of pharmacotherapy: An update. *Nutrition in Clinical Practice* 15:5, 2000.

   Medical treatment of obesity—diet modification, exercise therapy, and pharmacotherapy—can be combined and adapted to meet the needs of a specific person in order to yield weight loss and later weight maintenance. Assessment of the motivational level of the patient especially predicts success in weight loss and weight maintenance.

3. Atkinson RL: A 33-year-old woman with morbid obesity. *Journal of the American Medical Association* 283:3236, 2000.

   The history of an African-American woman who has struggled with weight control since her teenage years is presented. Dr. Atkinson reviews much of what is known about obesity treatment as he presents the options suggested to the patient, such as the use of diet control, exercise, behavior modification, pharmacotherapy, and possibly gastric bypass surgery.

4. Blackburn GL, He Y: The changing nature of obesity in the U.S.: How serious is the problem? *Nutrition & the M.D.* 25(6):25, 1999.

   Clinical and laboratory evidence shows that modest weight lose—as low as 5 to 10% of body weight—reduces or eliminates symptoms of weight-related diseases and metabolic risk factors, including elevated serum triglyceride levels, glucose intolerance, and hypertension.

5. Calle EE and others: Body mass index and mortality in a prospective cohort of U.S. adults. *The New England Journal of Medicine* 341:1097, 1999.

   Risk of death from all causes, cardiovascular disease, cancer, or other diseases increases throughout the range of moderate and severe overweight for both men and women in all age groups. In healthy people who have never smoked, ideal body mass index is 23.5 to 24.9 in men and 22.0 to 23.4 in women.

6. Davidson MH and others: Weight control and risk factor reduction in obese subjects treated for two years with orlistat. *Journal of the American Medical Association* 281:235, 1999.

   Two-year treatment with orlistat significantly promoted weight loss, lessened weight regain, and improved some weight-related risk factors. The majority of GI tract side effects occurred in people unable to maintain a moderate fat intake.

7. Dickerson LM, Carek PJ: Drug therapy for obesity. *American Family Physician* 61:2131, 2000.

   If drug therapy is recommended in the management of obesity, it should be used in combination with a structured diet and exercise program to achieve the greatest and longest-lasting results. The use of phenteramine (Ionamin), sibutramine (Meridia), and orlistat (Xenical) are reviewed, along with the potential use of fluoxetine (Prozac).

8. Expert panel on the identification, evaluation, and treatment of overweight in adults: clinical guidelines on the identification, evaluation, and treatment of overweight and obesity in adults: Executive summary. *American Journal of Clinical Nutrition* 68:899, 1998.

   Step-by-step plans are provided for the evaluation and treatment of weight and obesity. After successful weight loss, the likelihood of weight-loss maintenance is enhanced by a program consisting of dietary therapy, physical activity, and behavior therapy—this should be continued indefinitely.

9. Fine JT and others: A prospective study of weight change and health-related quality of life in women. *Journal of the American Medical Association* 282:2136, 1999.

   Current U.S. guidelines recommending that adult women avoid weight gain are supported. Weight maintenance and, in cases of overweight, weight loss are desirable and likely to be beneficial for physical function, vitality, and bodily pain.

10. Glanz K and others: Why Americans eat what they do: Taste, nutrition, cost, convenience, and weight control concerns as influences on food consumption. *Journal of the American Dietetic Association* 98:1118, 1998.

    Nutrition concerns are, unfortunately, less relevant to most people than taste and cost when it comes to food choice. One implication is that nutrition education programs should promote nutritious diets that are tasty and inexpensive.

11. Heymsfield SB and others: Recombinant leptin for weight loss in obese and lean adults. *Journal of the American Medical Association* 282:568, 1999.

    The administration of leptin via daily injections appears to induce weight loss in some obese subjects, even though they already have high circulating blood leptin concentrations. Additional research into the potential role of leptin and related hormones and the treatment of human obesity is needed before wide application of this therapy.

12. High-protein, low-carb diets: Are they right for you? *Mayo Clinic Health Letter*, p. 4, July 2000.

    Mayo Clinic physicians do not support the current craze for high-protein, low-carbohydrate diet, stating that ultimately most of the weight loss in high-protein diets is temporary. These diets are overly complicated and boring; eventually, the person goes off the diet and the weight comes back.

13. Hill JO, Peters JC: Environmental contributions to the obesity epidemic. *Science* 280:1371, 1998.

    The control of portion size, the consumption of a diet low in fat and energy density, and regular physical activity are behaviors that protect against obesity, but it is becoming difficult to adopt and maintain these behaviors in the current environment. Because obesity is difficult to treat, public health efforts need to be directed toward prevention.

14. Klem ML and others: A descriptive study of individuals successful at long-term maintenance of substantial weight loss. *American Journal of Clinical Nutrition* 66:239, 1997.

    Some individuals are highly successful at losing weight and keeping it off. For the most part, these individuals restrict intake of certain types or classes of foods, eat all types of foods but in limited quantity, count calories, limit percentage of daily energy intake from fat, and participate in regular physical activity.

15. Levine JA and others: Role of nonexercise activity thermogenesis in resistance to fat gain in humans. *Science* 283:212, 1999.

    The activation of nonexercise activity thermogenesis (NEAT) dissipates excess energy in part to preserve leanness during overfeeding. The failure to activate NEAT may result in ready weight gain. NEAT is the thermogenesis that accompanies physical activity other than which is voluntary exercise, such as fidgeting.

16. Liebman B: Diet vs. diet. *Nutrition Action Healthletter*, p. 9, May 2000.

    The false hopes of various high-protein, low-carbohydrate diets for weight loss are discussed. Also included are tips for staying lean, such as eating more fruits and vegetables, curbing energy density, shrinking serving size, and limiting (some) choices, such as sweets.

17. Lin BH and others: Popularity of dining out presents barriers to dietary improvements. *CNI Nutrition Week*, p. 4, December 10, 1999.

    Away-from-home foods generally contain more of the nutrients overconsumed and less of the nutrients underconsumed in the United States. The fat and saturated fat content of away-from-home foods has not declined as much as for home foods. As a result, the recent popularity of dining out represents a barrier to diet improvements.

18. Marcus J: Dietitians come in all sizes. *Today's Dietitian*, p. 26, October 1999.

    People who weigh more than current healthy BMI standards undergo unfair social hardship that erodes self-esteem. Some health professionals are calling for size acceptance—less emphasis on body size and more emphasis on healthy eating and personal fitness.

19. McBean LD: Insights into weight management. *Dairy Council Digest* 71(2):7, 2000.

    Many strategies are under study to reverse the obesity epidemic, including research into low-energy-density foods, emphasis on foods with low glycemic indexes, control of dietary variety for some food groups, and greater attention when eating out at restaurants.

20. McCamish M, Van Etten A: Leptin: A vital hormone and a potential therapy for obesity. *Nutrition & the M.D.* 25(2):1, 1999.

    Leptin is one of a dozen or more molecules involved in the regulation of energy metabolism in the body. Leptin administration has an acceptable safety profile; irritation at injection sites is the most common adverse problem reported.

21. McCrory MA and others: Dietary determinants of energy intake and weight regulation in healthy adults. *Journal of Nutrition* 130:276S, 2000.

    The increasing variety of high-energy-density foods available and the increasing proportion of household income spent on foods consumed away from home may help explain the rising U.S. national prevalence of obesity.

22. Mokdad AH and others: The spread of the obesity epidemic in the United States, 1991-1998. *Journal of the American Medical Association* 282:1519, 1999.

    The rapid increase in obesity throughout the United States is described. In 1990, obesity was primarily a problem in some midwestern and southeastern states. In 1998, obesity was common in all states except for those in the Rocky Mountain area and some in New England.

23. Must A and others: The disease burden associated with overweight and obesity. *Journal of the American Medical Association* 282:1523, 1999.

    Obesity increases the risk for type 2 diabetes, gallbladder disease, cardiovascular disease, hypertension, and osteoarthritis. The prevalence of weight-related diseases emphasizes the need for a concerted effort to prevent and treat obesity, rather than just its associated diseases.

24. Nestle M, Jacobson MF: Halting the obesity epidemic: The public health policy approach. *CNI Nutrition Week*, p. 4, March 31, 2000.

    Attention to changing the environment to promote physical activity; to decrease sedentary activities, such as television viewing; and to reduce advertisements for sugared snack foods and soft drinks are discussed as ways to aid the weight regulation of U.S. citizens. We must move beyond genetic, metabolic, and drug development studies to emphasize population-based interventions.

25. Perusse L, Bouchard C: Genotype-environment interaction in human obesity. *Nutrition Reviews* 57(5):S31, 1999.

    Genetic factors may play an important role in determining the response of body mass and body fat stores to alterations in energy balance. It is likely that genetic variation at several genes contributes to this difference in responses and to the susceptibility to obesity.

26. Peter JC and others: Control of energy balance in Stipanuk MH, *Physiological Aspects of Human Nutrition*, W.B. Saunders, Philadelphia, PA, 2000.

    Set point with respect to body weight is more effective in preventing weight loss than weight gain. Throughout adult life a person may settle at a variety of "set point" weights, rather than a single weight.

27. Poston WS, Foreyt JP: Successful management of the obese patient. *American Family Physician* 61:3615, 2000.

    Obesity is best thought of as a chronic disease requiring continuous care. Behavior modification provides an important part of the therapy.

28. Rosenbaum M, Leibel RL: Role of leptin in human physiology. *The New England Journal of Medicine* 341:913, 1999.

    During times of undernutrition, the fall in leptin production results in the preferential storage of ingested calories as fat, increased food intake, reduced metabolism (in rodents), and decreased fertility. Although leptin administration does not produce effortless weight loss, such treatment might have clinical value in making compliance with a low-calorie diet easier and in maintaining reduced body weight by lessening the fall in both metabolism and hunger that accompanies weight loss.

29. Schardt D: Fat burners. *Nutrition Action Healthletter*, p. 9, July/August 1999.

    There is no over-the-counter magic bullet that causes weight loss, including hydroxycitrate, chitosan, ephedrine, and pyruvate. The risks associated with the use of these products are reviewed.

30. Schwartz MW and others: Model for the regulation of energy balance and adiposity by the central nervous system. *American Journal of Clinical Nutrition* 69:584, 1999.

    Many hormones and neurotransmitters provide signals for food intake and weight regulation. Some compounds under study are neuropeptide Y, melanin-concentrating hormone, orexins, melanocortin, corticotropin-releasing hormone, and leptin.

31. Serdula MK and others: Prevalence of attempting weight loss and strategies for controlling weight. *Journal of the American Medical Association* 282:1353, 1999.

    Most persons trying to lose weight are not using the recommended combination of reducing calorie intake and increasing leisure-time physical activity (150 minutes or more per week). Of persons trying to lose weight, reduction in fat intake is a common strategy; however, reduction in fat intake is not effective unless calorie intake is also reduced.

32. Shikora SA: Surgical treatment for severe obesity: The state-of-the-art for the new millennium. *Nutrition in Clinical Practice* 15:13, 2000.

    For appropriately selected people, surgery can achieve the weight loss that is necessary to lessen or prevent the development of significant medical complications and improve quality of life. Until science finds the underlying biological derangements that cause obesity, surgery will continue to be the most cost-effective treatment option for serious cases.

33. Wilkinson DA: A weighty matter: Neuropeptides involved in appetite and energy homeostasis. *The Scientist*, p. 18, September 13, 1999.

    There is great interest in the brain chemicals that induce eating and then later satiety and their receptors. This is a very complex system, as is pointed out. A greater understanding of neuropeptide Y, melanin-concentrating hormone, melanocortin, corticotropin-releasing hormone, and leptin may ultimately provide important therapies for the treatment of obesity.

34. Willett WC and others: Guidelines for healthy weight. *The New England Journal of Medicine* 341:427, 1999.

    Body mass index is strongly linked to fat mass. Most excess body fat laid down in the adult years ends up in the abdominal area, leading to an increased waist circumference. The prevention of obesity must begin with an increased awareness that small weight gains should prompt people to modify diet and activity patterns to address the problem and should prompt them to seek professional counseling as necessary.

35. Williamson DF: The prevention of obesity. *The New England Journal of Medicine* 341:1140, 1999.

    The prevention of obesity needs to include more participants than just the health-care team, including food marketers and manufacturers, public and private purchasers of health care, large employers, transportation agencies or planners, and real estate developers. These efforts can reshape our environment to aid weight regulation, especially with regard to physical activity.

36. Yanovski JA, Yanovski SZ: Recent advances in basic obesity research. *Journal of the American Medical Association* 282:1504, 1999.

    A greater understanding of the behavioral and metabolic processes underlying body weight regulation provide great excitement for the future. It is likely that a greater understanding of brain neurotransmitters, in particular, will bring more targeted and effective treatments for obesity.

TAKE ACTION

I. A CLOSE LOOK AT YOUR WEIGHT STATUS

Determine the following two indices of your body status: body mass index and waist circumference.

Body Mass Index (BMI)

Record your weight in pounds: _____ lb
Divide your weight in pounds by 2.2 to determine your weight in kilograms (kg): _____ kg
Record your height in inches: _____ in
Divide your height in inches by 39.3 to determine your height in meters (m): _____ m
Calculate your BMI using the following formula:
BMI = weight (kg)/height(m)^2
BMI = _____ kg/ _____ m^2 = _____

Waist Circumference

Use a tape measure to measure the circumference of your waist (at the umbilicus with stomach muscles relaxed).
Circumference of waist (umbilicus) = _____ in

Interpretation

1. When BMI is greater than 25, health risks from obesity often begin. It is especially advisable to consider weight loss if your BMI exceeds 30. Does yours exceed 25?

    Yes _____   No _____

2. When a person has a BMI greater than 25 and a waist circumference of more than 40 inches in men or 35 inches in women, there is an increased risk of cardiovascular disease, hypertension, and type 2 diabetes. Does your circumference exceed the standard for your gender?

    Yes _____   No _____

3. Do you feel you need to pursue a program of weight loss?

    Yes _____   No _____

Application

From what you've learned in this chapter, what habits can you change in patterns of eating and physical activity to lose weight and help ensure maintenance of any loss?

_____

_____

_____

II. AN ACTION PLAN TO CHANGE WEIGHT STATUS

Now that you have assessed your current weight status, do you feel that you would like to make some changes? Following is a step-by-step guide to behavioral change. This process can be useful even for those who are satisfied with their current weight, as it can be applied to changing exercise habits, self-esteem, and a variety of other behaviors (Fig. 13-14).

Becoming Aware of the Problem

By calculating your current weight status, you have already become aware of the problem, if one exists. From here, it is important to find out more information about the cause of the problem and whether it is worth working toward a change.

1. Looking back at the food diary you completed in Chapter 1. What are some of the factors that most influence your eating habits? Do you eat due to stress, boredom, or depression? Is volume of food your problem, or do you eat mainly the wrong foods for you? Take some time to assess the root causes of your eating habits.

TAKE ACTION

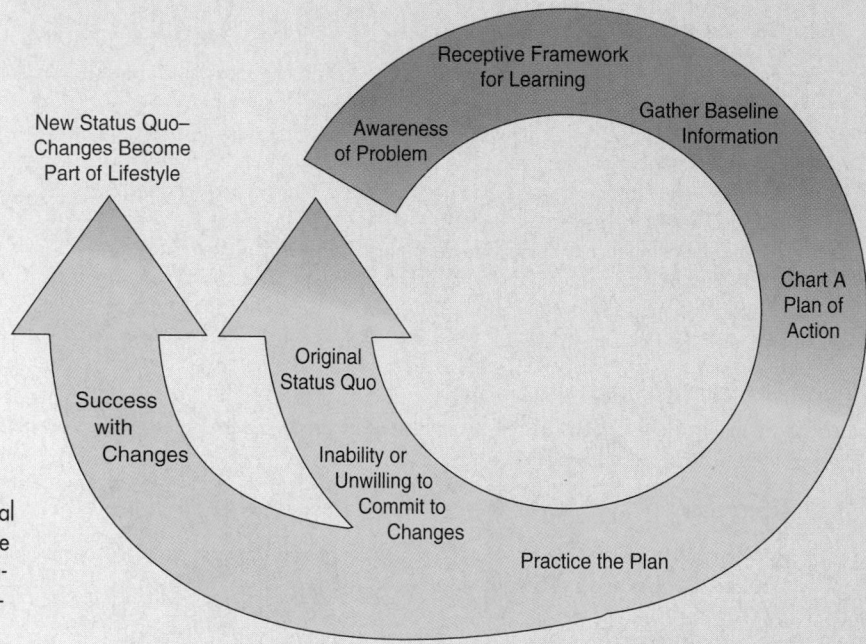

■ FIGURE 13-14 A model for behavioral change. It starts with awareness of the problem and ends with the incorporation of new behaviors intended to address the problem.

2. Once you have more information about your specific eating practices, you must decide if it is worth changing these practices. A benefits-and-costs analysis can be a useful tool in evaluating whether or not it is worth your effort to make life changes. Use the following example as a guide for listing benefits and costs pertinent to your own situation (Fig. 13-15).

Setting Goals

What can we accomplish, and how long will it take? Setting a realistic, achievable goal and allowing a reasonable amount of time to pursue it increase the likelihood of success.

1. Begin by determining the final outcome you would like to achieve. If you are trying to change your eating behaviors to be more healthy, list your reasons for doing so (e.g., overall health, weight loss, self-esteem).

   Overall goal:

   _____

   _____

   _____

   Reasons to pursue goal:

   _____

   _____

   _____

2. Now list several steps that will be necessary to achieve your goal. Keep in mind, however, that it is generally best to change only a few specific behaviors at first—walking briskly for 30 minutes five times a week, reducing fat intake, using more whole-grain products, and not eating after 7 P.M. Attempting small and perhaps easier dietary changes first reduces the scope of the problem and can increase the likelihood of success.

TAKE ACTION

BENEFITS AND COSTS ANALYSIS

1 Benefits of changing eating habits?

What do you expect to get, now or later, that you want? What do you get to avoid that would be unpleasant?

— *feel better physically and psychologically*
— *look better*
—
—
—
—

3 Costs involved in changing eating habits?

What do you have to do that you don't want to do? What do you have to stop doing that you would rather continue doing?

— *take time to plan meals and shop*
— *must give up some food volume*
—
—

2 Benefits of not changing eating habits?

What do you get to do that you enjoy doing? What do you avoid having to do?

— *no need for planning*
— *can eat without feeling guilty*
—
—
—
—

4 Costs of not changing eating habits?

What unpleasant or undesirable effects are you likely to experience now or in the future? What are you likely to lose?

— *creeping weight gain*
— *low self-esteem and poor health*
—
—
—

■ FIGURE **13-15** Benefits-and-costs analysis applied to increasing physical activity. This process helps put behavioral change into the context of total lifestyle.

Steps toward achieving goal:

1. _____
2. _____
3. _____

Note that, if you are having trouble deciphering the steps needed to achieve your goal, health professionals are an excellent resource for aid in planning.

Measuring Commitment

Now that you have collected information and know what is required to reach your goal, you must ask yourself, "Can I do this?" Commitment is an essential component in the success of behavioral change. Be honest with yourself. Permanent change is not quick or easy. Once you have decided that you have the commitment required to see this through, continue on to the following sections.

Making It Official With a Contract

Drawing up a behavioral contract often adds incentive to follow through with a plan. The contract could list goal behaviors and objectives, milestones for measuring progress, and regular rewards for meeting the terms of the contract. After finishing a contract, you should sign it in the presence of some friends. This encourages commitment.

Initially, plans should reward positive behaviors, and then they should focus on positive results. Positive behaviors, such as regular physical activity, eventually lead to positive outcomes, such as increased stamina.

Figure 13-16 is a sample contract for increasing physical activity. Keep in mind that this sample contract is only a suggestion; you can add your own ideas as well.

TAKE ACTION

Name *Alan Young*

Goal

I agree to *ride my exercise bike*
(specify behavior)

under the following circumstances *for 30 minutes, 4 times per week*
(specify where, when, how much, etc.)
in the evening

Substitute behavior and/or reinforcement schedule *I will reinforce myself if I've achieved my goal after a month with a weekend off campus with my roommate.*

Environmental planning

In order to help me do this, I am going to (1) arrange my physical and social environment by *buying a new jogging suit at the local sporting goods store*

and (2) control my internal environment (thoughts, images) by *coordinating riding the bike with the first T.V. watching I do in the evening*

Reinforcements

Reinforcements provided by me daily or weekly (if contract is kept):
I will buy myself a new piece of clothing for off campus trip

Reinforcements provided by others daily or weekly (if contract is kept):
at the end of a month if I've completed my goal my parents will buy me a fitness club membership for winter.

Social support

Behavior change is more likely to take place when other people support you. During the quarter/semester please meet with the other person at least three times to discuss your progress.

The name of my "significant helper" is: *Mr. and Mrs. Young*

This contract should include:

1. Baseline data (one week)
2. Well-defined goal
3. Simple method for charting progress (diary, counter, charts, etc.)
4. Reinforcements (immediate and long-term)
5. Evaluation method (summary of experiences, success, and/or new learnings about self).

■ FIGURE **13-16** A behavioral contract. Completing such a contract can help generate commitment to behavioral change. What would your contract look like?

TAKEACTION

Psyching Yourself Up

Once your contract is in place, you need to psych yourself up. Discouragement from peers and your own temptations to stray from your plan need to be anticipated. Psyching yourself up can enable you to progress toward your goals in spite of others' attitudes and opinions. Almost everyone benefits from some assertiveness training when it comes to changing behaviors. The following are a few suggestions. Can you think of any others?

- No one's feelings should be hurt if you say, "No, thank you," firmly and repeatedly when others try to dissuade you from a plan. Rather, ask them—and yourself—why they want you to eat their way. Your needs are as important as anyone else's.
- You don't have to eat a lot to accommodate anyone—your mother, business clients, or the chef. For example, at a party with friends, you may feel you have to eat a lot to participate, but you don't. Another trap is ordering a lot just because someone else is paying for the meal.
- Learn ways to handle put-downs—inadvertent or conscious. An effective response can be to communicate feelings honestly, without hostility. Tell criticizers that they have annoyed or offended you, that you are working to change your habits and would really like understanding and support from them.

Practicing the Plan

Once you've set up a plan, the next step is to implement it. Start with a trial of at least 6 to 8 weeks. Thinking of a lifetime commitment can be overwhelming. Aim for a total duration of 6 months of new activities before giving up. We may have to persuade ourselves more than once of the value of continuing the program. The following are some suggestions to help keep a plan on track:

- *Focus on reducing, but not necessarily extinguishing, undesirable behaviors.* For example, it's usually unrealistic to say, "I'll never eat a certain food again." It's better to say, "I won't eat that *problem* food as regularly as before."
- *Monitor progress.* Note your progress in a diary and reward yourself according to your contract. While conquering some habits and seeing improvement, you may find yourself quite encouraged, even enthusiastic, about your plan of action. That can give you the impetus to move ahead with the program.
- *Control environments.* In the early phases of behavioral change, try to avoid problem situations, such as parties, coffee breaks, and favorite restaurants. Once new habits are firmly established, you can probably more successfully resist the temptations in these environments.

Re-evaluating and Preventing Relapse

After practicing a program for several weeks to months, it is important to reassess the original plan. In addition, you may now be able to pinpoint other problem areas for which you need to plan appropriately.

1. Begin by taking a close and critical look at your original plan. Does it actually lead to the goals you set? Are there any new steps toward your goal that you feel capable of adding to your contract? Do you need new reinforcements? It may even be necessary to make a new contract. For permanent change, it is worth this time of reassessment.

2. In practicing your plan over the past weeks or months, you have likely experienced relapses. What triggered these relapses? To prevent a total retreat to your old habits, it is important to set up a plan for such relapses. You can do this by identifying high-risk situations, rehearsing a response, and remembering your goals.

You may have noticed a behavior chain in some of your relapses. That is, the relapse may stem from a series of interconnected habitual activities. The way to break the chain is to first identify the activities, pinpoint the weak links, break those links, and substitute other behaviors. In Figure 13-17 is a sample behavior chain and a substitute activities list. Consider compiling your own list based on your behavior chains.

Epilogue

If you have used the activities in this section, you are well on your way to permanent behavioral change. Recall that this exercise can be used for a variety of desired changes, including quitting smoking, increasing physical activity, and improving study habits. It is by no means an easy process, but the results can be well worth the effort. Overall, the keys to success are motivation (keeping the problem in the forefront of your mind), having a plan of action, securing the resources and skills needed for success, and looking for help from family, friends, or a group.

TAKE ACTION

ALTERNATIVE ACTIVITY SHEET

SUBSTITUTE ACTIVITIES

Pleasant activities
1. *Singing / washing hair*
2. *Reading comics / biking*
3. *Sewing / calling a friend*

Necessary activities
1. *Ironing*
2. *Vacuuming*
3. *Straightening apartment*

Situations when used
1. *Wanted ice cream – delayed with bath*
2. *Wanted wheat thins – cleaned up apt.*
3. *Wanted snack – went for walk*
4. *Wanted cookies – did dishes first*
5. *Saw leftovers – went for bike ride*
6. *Tempted by cookies – set timer*
7. *Wanted snack – read comics*

BEHAVIOR CHAIN

Identify the links in your eating response chain on the following diagram. Draw a line through the chain where it was interrupted. Add the link you substituted and the new chain of behavior this substitution started.

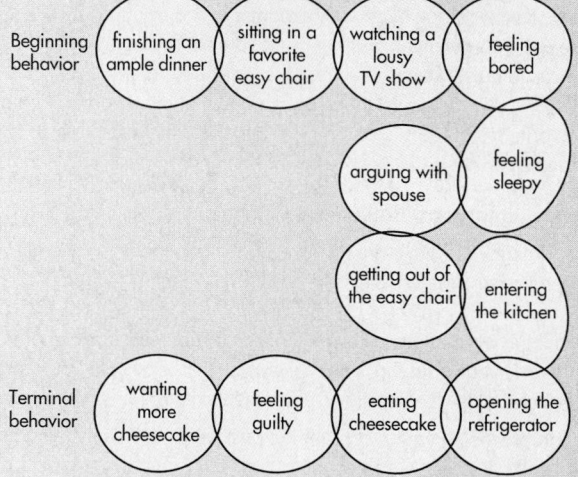

■ FIGURE 13-17 Identifying behavior chains. This is a good tool for understanding more about your habits and pinpointing ways to change unwanted habits. The earlier in the chain you substitute a nonfood link, the easier it is to intervene. Four types of behaviors can be substituted in an ongoing behavior chain.

1. Fun activities (taking a walk, reading a book)
2. Necessary activities (cleaning a room, balancing your checkbook)
3. Incompatible activities (taking a shower)
4. Urge-delaying activities (setting a kitchen timer for 20 minutes before allowing yourself to eat)

Using activities to interrupt behavior patterns that lead to inappropriate eating (or inactivity) can be a powerful means of changing eating habits.

FAD DIETS

Many overweight people try to help themselves by using the latest fad diet book. But, as you will see, most of these diets do not help, and some can actually harm those who follow them (Table 13-9).

You may wonder why fad diet books exist at all. Why doesn't the government put a stop to them? Many contain blatant misinformation. However, FDA concerns itself only when products are suspected of doing serious harm, as in the case of earlier forms of liquid protein diets. FDA is too busy and too underfunded to pursue every new fad diet plan. Ancient advice is still valid: "Let the buyer beware." Responsibility rests with the authors and publishers, who want to sell books and earn money and know there is little risk involved. Making outrageous claims sells more books than writing "eat less fat and walk more."

It is illegal in the United States to falsely represent worthless or dangerous cures and medical devices. Thus, U.S. citizens can use their rights under federal law to have FDA pursue a seller of a dangerous fad diet book in an attempt to have it removed from the market.

TABLE 13-9 Summary of Popular Diet Approaches to Weight Control

Approach and Examples*	Characteristics and Possible Negative Health Consequences
Moderate Calorie Restriction	
The Setpoint Diet	Usually 1000–1800 kcal per day, with moderate fat intake
Slim Chance in a Fat World	Reasonable balance of macronutrients
Weight Watcher's Diet	Encourage exercise
Mary Ellen's Help Yourself Diet Plan	May use behavioral approach
The Beyond Diet	Acceptable if vitamin and mineral supplement is used and permission of family physician is granted
Staying Thin	
The Callaway Diet	
Living Without Dieting	
Volumetrics	
Lose the Last 10 Pounds	
Dieting with the Duchess	
Dieting for Dummies	
The Wedding Dress Diet	
Dr. Shapiro's Picture Perfect Diet	
Macronutrient Restriction	
Low or Restricted Carbohydrate	
Dr. Atkins' Diet Revolution	Generally less than 100 g of carbohydrate per day
Calories Don't Count	Ketosis; reduced exercise capacity due to poor glycogen stores in the muscles; excessive animal fat intake
Miracle Diet for Fast Weight Loss	
Woman Doctor's Diet for Women	
The Doctor's Quick Weight Loss Diet	
The Complete Scarsdale Medical Diet	
Four Day Wonder Diet	
Endocrine Control Diet	
Enter the Zone	
Protein Power	
The Five-Day Miracle Diet	
Healthy for Life	
Carbohydrate Addicts Diet	
Sugar Busters	

*Diets may be listed in more than one category if multiple characteristics apply.

TABLE 13-9   continued

Approach and Examples	Characteristics and Possible Negative Health Consequences
Low Fat	
The Rice Diet Report	Less than 20% of energy from fat
The Macrobiotic Diet (some versions)	Limited (or elimination of) animal protein sources; also all fats, nuts, seeds
The Pritikin Diet	
Eat More, Weigh Less	Little satiety; flatulence; possibly poor mineral absorption from excess dietary fiber; limited food choices
The 35+ Diet	sometimes leads to deprivation
20/30 Fat and Fiber	
Fat to Muscle Diet	Not necessarily to be avoided, but certain aspects of many of the plans possibly unacceptable
T-Factor Diet	
Fit or Fat	
Two Day Diet	
Complete Hip and Thigh Diet	
The Maximum Metabolism Diet	
The Pasta Diet	
The McDougall Plan	
Ultrafit Diet	
Stop the Insanity	
G-Index Diet	
Outsmarting the Female Fat Cell	
Foods that Cause You to Lose Weight	
Lean Bodies	
Novelty Diets	
Dr. Abravenel's Body Type and Lifetime	Promotes certain nutrients, foods, or combinations of foods as having
Nutrition Plan (or his other books)	unique, magical, or previously undiscovered qualities
Dr. Berger's Immune Power Diet	Malnutrition; no change in habits leads to relapse; unrealistic food choices lead to possible bingeing
Fit for Life	
The Hilton Head Metabolism Diet	
The Beverly Hills Diet	
Dr. Debetz Champagne Diet	
Sun Sign Diet	
F-Plan Diet	
Fat Attack Plan	
Autohypnosis Diet	
The Ultrafit Diet	
The Princeton Diet	
The Diet Bible	
Eat to Succeed	
The Underburner's Diet	
Eat to Win	
Two Day Diet	
Paris Diet	
Cabbage-Soup Diet	
Eat Great, Lose Weight	
Eat Smart Think Smart	
Scentsational Weight Loss	
Eat Right 4 Your Type	
The Greenwich Diet	
3 Season Diet	
Metabolize	
God's Diet	
The Weigh Down Diet	

TABLE 13-9   concluded

Approach and Examples	Characteristics and Possible Negative Health Consequences
Very-Low-Calorie Diets (VLCDs)	
Optifast	
Cambridge Diet	Less than 800 kcal per day
HMR	Also known as protein-sparing modified fasts
Ultrafast	Must be under close physician scrutiny
Thin So Fast	Organ tissue loss—especially from the heart; low blood potassium leads to heart failure; expense; kidney stones; gout
Formula Diets	
Optifast	Can help people who find it easier not to eat whole foods while dieting to lose weight
Genesis	
Cambridge Diet	Based on formulated or packaged products
	Tend to be very-low-calorie diet regimens (see above); no change in habits, possibly leading to increased chance of relapse; expense; constipation
Slimfast	
Premeasured Diets	
Jenny Craig	Most food supplied in premeasured servings to take much of the decision making out of the process of eating
	Expense; may not allow for easy sound eating later

HOW TO RECOGNIZE A FAD DIET

Earlier in this chapter are listed the criteria for evaluating weight-loss programs with regard to their safety and effectiveness. In contrast, fad diets typically share some different common characteristics:

1. They promote quick weight loss. As mentioned before, this loss primarily results from glycogen, sodium, and lean muscle mass depletion. All lead to a loss of body water.

2. They limit food selections and dictate specific rituals, such as eating only fruit for breakfast or cabbage soup every day.

3. They use testimonials from famous people and tie the diet to well-known cities, such as Beverly Hills and New York.

4. They bill themselves as cure-alls. These diets claim to work for everyone, whatever the type of obesity or the person's specific strengths and weaknesses.

5. They often recommend expensive supplements.

6. No attempts are made to change eating habits permanently. Dieters follow the diet until the desired weight is reached and then revert to old eating habits—they are told to eat rice for a month, lose weight, and then return to old habits.

7. They are generally critical of and skeptical about the scientific community. They suggest that physicians and registered dietitians do not really want people to lose weight. They encourage people to look outside the medical establishment for correct advice.

Probably the cruelest characteristic of fad diets is that they essentially guarantee failure for the dieter. These diets are not designed for permanent weight loss. Habits are not changed, and the food selection is so limited that the person cannot follow the diet in the long run. Although dieters assume they have lost fat, they have actually lost mostly muscle and other lean tissue mass. As soon as they begin eating normally again, the lost tissue is replaced. In a matter of weeks, most of the lost weight is back. The dieter appears to have failed, when actually the diet has failed. This whole scenario can add more blame and guilt, challenging the self-worth of the dieter. If someone needs help losing weight, professional help is advised. It is unfortunate that current trends suggest people are spending more time and money on "quick fixes" rather than on such professional help.

TYPES OF FAD DIETS

▌ Low- or Restricted-Carbohydrate Approaches

This is the most common form of fad diet.[1] As discussed in Chapter 4, a very low-carbohydrate intake forces the liver to produce needed glucose. The source of carbons for this glucose is mostly tissue proteins. Thus, a low-carbohydrate diet results in protein tissue loss, as well as urinary loss of essential ions, such as potassium. Since protein tissue is mostly water, the dieter loses weight very rapidly. When a normal diet is resumed, the protein tissue is rebuilt and the weight is regained.

Low carbohydrate diets primarily work in the short run because they limit food intake.[16] Consider a visit to a fast-food restaurant. You plan to order a hamburger, French fries, and a soft drink and pay a bit more for the *supersize* option. This will yield about 1500 kcal. If you were on a low-carbohydrate plan, you can't have the French fries or the soft drink, as they contain too much carbohydrate. You can have the hamburger, but you will have to discard the bun. This leaves a lunch containing about 240 kcal. You will also soon tire of the limited food choices, and this will cause you to eat less.

In the short run, this low-carbohydrate gimmick can lead to weight loss. But this plan does not include the fruits, vegetables, and whole grains that nutrition experts point out are important components of a healthy diet. Thus, the low-carbohydrate diet is not intended for long-term use (no more than 4 to 6 weeks).[12] If one is just going to eat less, why not just eat less of the foods one likes?

Diet plans that use a low-carbohydrate approach are the Dr. Atkins' Diet Revolution, Dr. Stillman's Calories Don't Count Diet, the Scarsdale Diet, and the Four Day Wonder Diet. A more moderate approach is found in the various Zone diets (40% of energy intake as carbohydrate). When you see a new fad diet advertisement, look first to see how much carbohydrate it contains. If breads, cereals, fruits, and vegetables are extremely limited, you are probably looking at a low- or restricted-carbohydrate diet.

▌ Low-Fat Approaches

The very-low-fat diet turns out to be a very-high-carbohydrate diet. These diets contain approximately 5 to 10% of energy intake as fat. The most notable is the Pritikin Diet and the Dr. Dean Ornish diet plans. This approach is not harmful for healthy adults, but it is extremely difficult to follow. People get bored with this type of diet very quickly because they can't eat many of their favorite foods. Dieters eat primarily grains, fruits, and vegetables, which most people cannot do for very long. Eventually, the person wants some foods higher in fat or protein. Thus, the dieter suffers a lapse, then a relapse, and probably a collapse. These diets are just too different from the typical American diet for many adults to follow consistently.

▌ Novelty Diets

A variety of fad diets are built on gimmicks. Some novelty diets emphasize one food or food group and exclude almost all others. A rice diet was designed in the 1940s to lower blood pressure; now it has resurfaced as a weight-loss diet. The first phase consists of eating only rice and fruit until you can't stand them any longer. Another novelty diet is the egg diet, on which you eat all the eggs you want. On the Beverly Hills Diet, you eat mostly fruit.

The rationale behind these diets is that you can eat only eggs, fruit, or rice for just so long before becoming bored and, in theory, reducing your energy intake. However, chances are that you will abandon the diet entirely before losing much weight.

Since the 1960s, grapefruit has been touted for supposed unique ability to cause weight loss. No studies back up this claim. To add appeal to a grapefruit diet, proponents even suggest adding several "diet aids": lecithin to help release fat from the tissues, vitamin B-6 to act as a diuretic, vinegar to provide potassium, and kelp to stimulate the thyroid gland.

The most bizarre of the novelty diets proposes that "food gets stuck in your body." Fit for Life, the Beverly Hills Diet, and Eat Great, Lose Weight are examples. The supposition is that food gets stuck in the intestine, putrefies, and creates toxins, which invade the blood and cause disease. This is utter nonsense. Nevertheless, the same idea has been promoted in health-food books since the 1800s. Today, Fit for Life suggests that meat eaten with potatoes is not digested and that fresh fruit should be consumed only before noon. These recommendations are absurd. They are gimmicks that appear controversial but are really designed to sell books.

Finally, some commercial schemes are used to sell diet books. Books describing the allergy approach to dieting, for instance, suggest that diseases, including obesity, are due to food allergies. Supposedly, once your food allergies are found and treated, you will no longer have the disease. However, no research supports the claim. In addition, see the Sun Sign Diet if you believe in astrology, the Champagne Diet if you need a drink, the Cabbage Soup Diet if you want to eat it every day, or the Body Type and Lifetime Nutrition Diet if you have a "dominant" gland.

QUACKERY IS CHARACTERISTIC OF FAD DIETS

Fad diets fall under the category of quackery, people taking advantage of others. They usually involve a product or service that costs a considerable amount of money. Often, those offering the product or service don't realize that they are promoting quackery, because they were victims themselves. For example, they tried the product and by pure coincidence it worked for them, so they wish to sell it to all their friends and relatives.

Recent examples of dubious recommendations in the field of weight loss are herbal laxative teas and chromium picolinate. These laxative teas, many of which have oriental-type labels, contain senna, which induces diarrhea. However, this diarrhea does not sufficiently reduce the absorption of calories from the diet. FDA is concerned that these teas may also result in serious injury or death linked to the diarrhea and related intestinal damage that is inducted. To date, these teas are linked to deaths of four young women.

Chromium picolinate, a nutritional supplement, has been touted as an aid for reducing body fat, increasing lean body mass, suppressing hunger, and increasing metabolic rate. However, chromium picolinate has not been approved for weight loss by FDA, nor has the agency seen any convincing data on the claims being made (see Chapter 12).

Numerous other gimmicks for weight loss have come and gone and are likely to resurface. If in the future an important aid for weight loss is discovered, you can feel confident that major journals, such as the *Journal of the American Dietetic Association*, the *Journal of the American Medical Association*, or *The New England Journal of Medicine*, will report it. You don't need to rely on paperback books or newspaper advertisements for information about weight loss (Fig. 13-18).

Usually, quackery reduces only the bank account. Currently $6 billion dollars a year are spent on such false hope. However, it can lead to life-threatening results. The rule of thumb on seeing a new diet aid on the market is that, if it sounds too good to be true, it is.

■ CASE SCENARIO
Follow-Up

As you have probably surmised, Crystal will just be wasting her money if she buys the product seen in the infomercial. Unfortunately, regulation of the supplement industry currently is woefully lacking. In the future, if there is such a breakthrough in weight loss and weight control, authorities such as the Surgeon General's Office or the National Institutes of Health will make Americans aware of that fact. At this time, Crystal would be better off simply paying more attention to what she is eating and trying to find time for daily physical activity.

35 Pounds of Fat.

DR. EDISON'S OBESITY PILLS AND REDUCING TABLETS CURED MRS. MANNING.

No Other Remedies But Dr. Edison's Reduce Obesity— Take No Others.

SAMPLES FREE—USE COUPON.

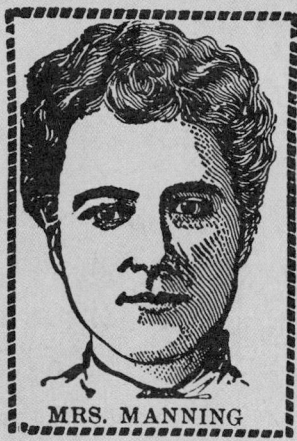

MRS. MANNING

Mary Hyde Manning, one of the best known of Troy's, New York, society women, grew too fleshy, and used Dr. Edison's Obesity Remedies. Read the letter telling of her reduction and restoration to health:—"In six weeks I was reduced 35 pounds, from 171 to 136, by Dr. Edison's Obesity Pills and Reducing Tablets. I recommend these remedies to all fat and sick men and women."

The following well-known men and women have been reduced by DR. EDISON'S OBESITY REMEDIES:

Mrs. H. Mershon, 156 South Jackson St., Lima, O., 148 lbs.
Mrs. Josephine McPherson, 7916 Wright St., Chicago, 42 lbs.
Rev. Edward R. Pierce, 410 Alma St., Chicago, 42 lbs.
C. C. Nichols, 145 Clark St., Aurora, Ill., 36 lbs.
Mrs. W. Davlin, Whitemore, O., 149 lbs.
W. H. Webster, 618 2d Ave., Troy, N. Y., 26 lbs.
J. M. McKinney, 4504 State St., Chicago, 30 lbs.
Mrs. J. M. McKinney, 4504 State St., Chicago, 33 lbs.
Mrs. A. Walker, 1104 Milton Place, Chicago, 20 lbs.

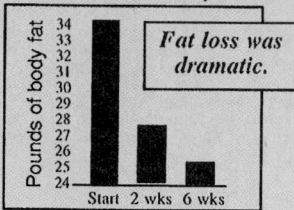

22% LESS BODY FAT IN SIX WEEKS

University studies have identified CHROMIUM PICOLINATE as a "trigger" for fat loss and lean muscle enhancement. 200 micrograms taken daily caused a 22% fat loss in only 6 weeks.

Fat loss was dramatic.

Men and women of every age are talking about the amazing benefits of this safe, essential nutrient:

**WEIGHT LOSS • FAT LOSS
MORE ENDURANCE AND STAMINA
MORE LEAN MUSCLE**

Our Product is made to the exact specifications of the capsules used in the studies cited above. Each bottle of 60 capsules is a 2-month supply.

SATISFACTION GUARANTEED
(Check or money order only. Canada: U.S. $ m.o.)

FIGURE 13-18 Outrageous weight-loss claims are not new. Even 100 years ago, people wanted to believe that fat can be lost without changing habits or without much effort, and many still do.

SPORTS NUTRITION

chapter *14*

*A*thletes invest a lot of time and effort in training. Because they are often seeking ways to modify their diets to improve their performances, athletes make easy targets for purveyors of nutrition misinformation. Still, most athletes don't want to miss out on any advantage, whether real or perceived, that might give them the winning edge.

Although good eating habits can't substitute for physical training and genetic endowment, proper diet choices are crucial to top-notch performance, contributing to endurance and helping speed the repair of injured tissues.[1]

In this chapter, you will also discover how physical fitness benefits the entire body; it is an essential ingredient in achieving maximal health.[16] Experts might disagree on how much carbohydrate, protein, and fat we should consume, but there is no argument over the health benefits of regular physical activity. It is even beneficial for overweight people who remain at that excess weight.[19]

Some people also are active simply because they enjoy it, whether they're swimming, playing basketball, walking briskly, or engaging in any of innumerable other activities. Let's now look further at nutrition as it relates to fitness.

■ KEY CHAPTER CONCEPTS

- Nutritional status affects one's ability to perform physical activity. Physical activity, in turn, affects nutrient use by the body.
- A minimum plan for physical activity includes a total of at least 30 minutes on most (and preferably all) days. A more intense program should begin with warm-up exercises to increase blood flow and warm the muscles, and then end with cooldown. Resistance training and stretching exercises on a regular basis provide even further health benefits.
- At rest, muscle cells use fat mainly for fuel, forming carbon dioxide (CO_2) and water (H_2O). For intense exercise of short duration, muscles use mostly phosphocreatine (PCr) for energy. During more sustained intense activity, such as sprinting, muscle glycogen breaks down into lactate.
- For endurance exercise, both fat and carbohydrate are used as fuels; carbohydrate is used increasingly as activity intensifies. Little protein is used to fuel muscles (10 to 15% of energy use at most).
- The body adapts to exercise by building muscles (hypertrophy) and by increasing both the maximum amount of work that can be done and the oxygen that can be utilized ($VO_{2\ max}$).
- Any athlete who regularly exercises vigorously for more than an hour per day should consume a diet that is moderate to high in carbohydrates, based primarily on whole grains, fruits, and vegetables. Most athletes can meet vitamin and mineral needs by the sheer volume of food consumed. Any use of supplements should be based on meeting known nutrient gaps in the diet.
- Athletes should consume enough fluid to minimize loss of body weight during sports activity and ultimately restore preexercise weight. Sports drinks aid fluid, electrolyte, and carbohydrate replacement. Their use especially should be considered when continuous activity is expected to last beyond 60 minutes.
- Rather than waiting for a magic bullet to enhance performance, athletes should concentrate their efforts on improving training routines and sport technique and consuming well-balanced diets. Adequate calorie, fluid, and carbohydrate intake are the primary diet-related ergogenic (work-producing) aids.

■ REFRESH YOUR MEMORY

As you begin your study of sports nutrition in Chapter 14, you may want to review

- The exchange system in Chapter 2
- The components of the cell and functions of various organelles in Chapter 3
- Metabolic pathways and the role of ATP in Chapter 4
- The concept of glycemic index in Chapter 5
- The various components of the macronutrient classes—carbohydrates, proteins, and lipids—in Chapters 5–7
- The food sources of calcium in Chapter 11 and iron in Chapter 12

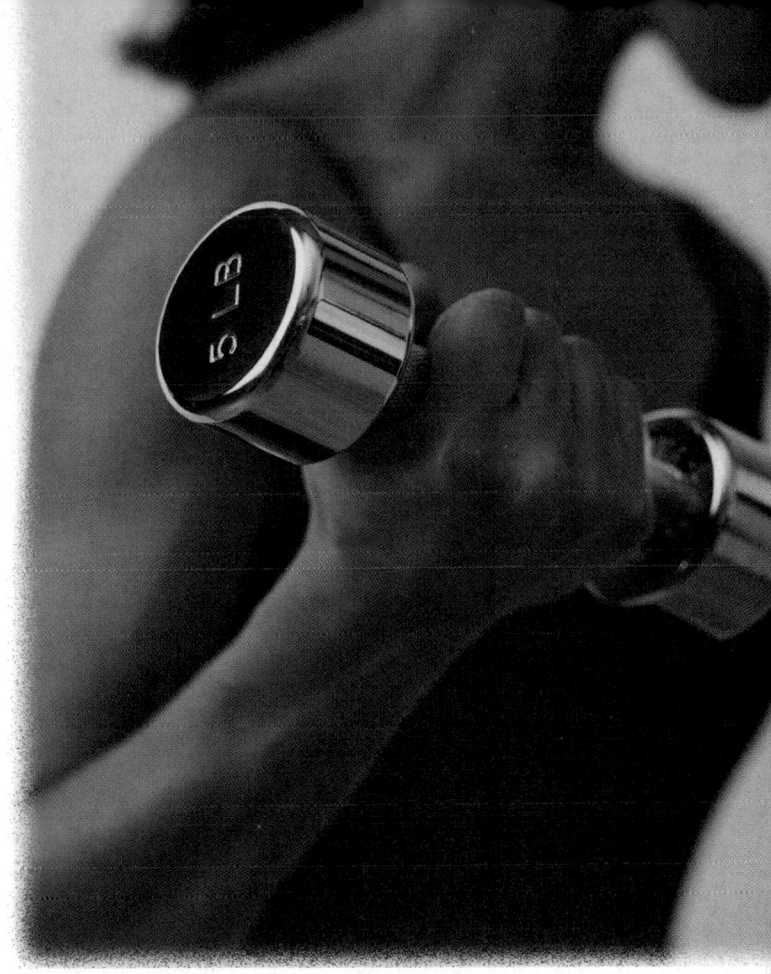

■ CASE SCENARIO

Marcella has become hooked on fitness in the past year and is training for a 10K run coming up in 3 weeks. She has read a lot about sports nutrition, and especially about the importance of eating a high-carbohydrate diet while in training. She also has been struggling to keep her weight in a range that she feels contributes to better speed and endurance. Consequently, she is also trying to eat as little fat as possible. Unfortunately, over the past week her workouts in the afternoon have not met her expectations. Her run times are slower, and she shows signs of fatigue after just 20 minutes into her training program.

Her breakfast yesterday was a large bagel, a small amount of cream cheese, and orange juice. For lunch, she had a small salad with fat-free dressing, a large plate of pasta with tomato marinara sauce and broccoli, and a diet soft drink. For dinner, she had a small broiled chicken breast, a cup of rice, some carrots, and iced tea. Later, she snacked on fat-free pretzels.

What advice would you provide Marcella regarding her training diet? Note current strengths and weaknesses. Is her diet likely contributing to her recent fatigue during workouts?

■ THE CLOSE RELATIONSHIP BETWEEN NUTRITION AND FITNESS

The ability to engage routinely in vigorous physical activity requires good health. The ability to perform also depends on a nutritious diet that supplies all the needed nutrients. Adequate carbohydrate intakes are especially important for enhancing the endurance of athletes and nonathletes who expend more than 2000 kcal daily.[7]

Once muscles have nutrients available to them, what determines the type of fuel muscles will use? Athletes do to an extent, depending on how physically fit they are and how hard they perform. This physical fitness—defined as the ability to do moderate to vigorous activity without undue fatigue—affects fat use by the body. The greater one's fitness, the more fat used to supply energy needed for activity, especially if the activity lasts for 20 minutes or more.[28]

Beyond affecting fuel use, the benefits of regular physical activity include improvement in several aspects of heart function, less injury, better sleep habits, and improvement in body composition (less body fat, more muscle mass). Physical activity also can reduce stress and positively affect blood pressure, blood cholesterol, and blood glucose regulation. In addition, it aids in weight control, both by transiently raising resting energy expenditure and by increasing overall energy expenditure.[12, 16] See Table 14-1 for a further look at the benefits of a physically active lifestyle.

For the most part, nutrition influences physical activity, and physical activity influences nutrient use and general health. Unfortunately, as noted in Chapter 13, many American adults lead sedentary lives. Only about 15% of adults practice moderate to vigorous physical activity on a regular basis, and about half of all adults quit their exercise program within 3 months of onset.[33] Does this discussion motivate you to assess your activity patterns and improve them as needed? Dr. Sheri A. Melton discusses how to plan your exercise program in her Expert Opinion.

Healthy People 2010 has set a number of specific objectives for the American public related to physical activity:

* Reduce by 50% the proportion of adults engaging in no leisure-time physical activity (currently 40% of adults)
* Double the proportion of adults engaging regularly, preferably daily, in moderate physical activity for at least 30 minutes per day (currently 15% of adults)
* Increase by 30% the proportion of adults engaging in vigorous physical activity that promotes the development and maintenance of cardiorespiratory fitness

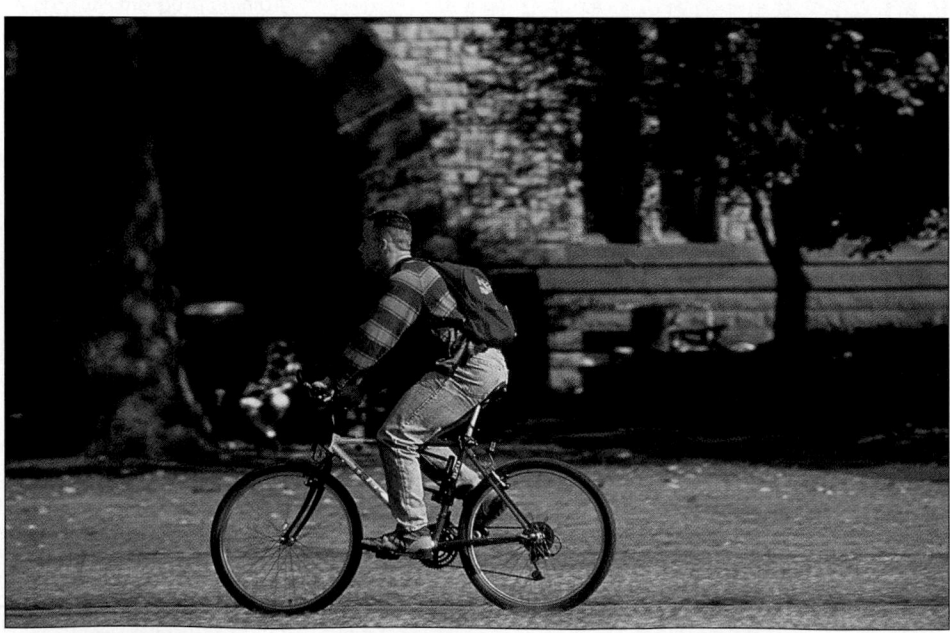

What is the best exercise? One you enjoy.

TABLE 14-1	**Exercise Is Medicine—the Benefits of Regular, Moderate Physical Activity**[13, 15, 22, 24, 27]
Cardiovascular health	Increases heart strength and overall cardiovascular function, which decreases chance of developing coronary heart disease and strokes
	Helps maintain healthy blood pressure
	Can increase HDL-cholesterol and lower LDL-cholesterol and triglycerides in the blood
	Aids in smoking-cessation programs
Obesity	Helps maintain lean tissue and promote loss of fat tissue
	Assists in better control of appetite and increases energy expenditure
	Helps prevent or reverse development of diseases associated with obesity, including type 2 diabetes, hypertension, and cardio-vascular disease, even if one can't attain a more healthy weight
Muscular health	Contributes to building and maintaining muscle mass and muscle tone
Diabetes	Increases glucose uptake by muscle tissue cells independent of insulin action
	Contributes to energy balance, which decreases risk of type 2 diabetes and related complications
Osteoporosis	Helps strengthen bones and contributes to joint health
Infections	Reduces susceptibility to respiratory and other infections by enhancing various functions of the immune system
Cancer	Reduces risk of colon cancer, and likely breast cancer
Gastrointestinal health	Improves peristaltic function and colonic mass movements
	Lessons risk for gallstones and related gallbladder disease
Fewer injuries (e.g., from falls)	Contributes to balance and agility, especially in older adulthood
Psychological health	Reduces depression, anxiety, and mental stress while enhancing a sense of well-being and self-image and improving sleep patterns

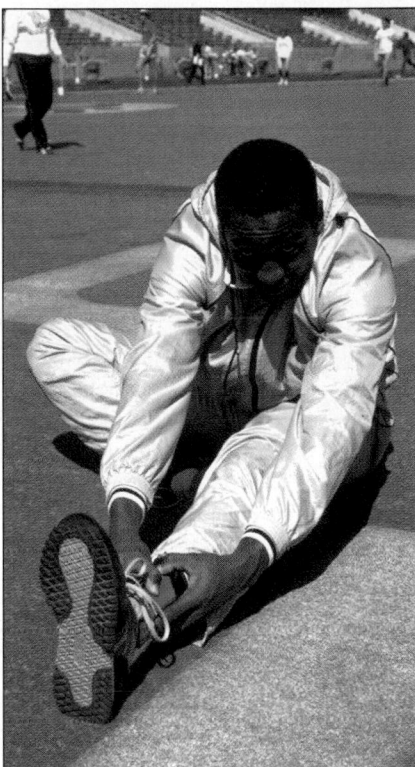

Stretching should be part of warm-up and cooldown activities.

3 or more days per week for 20 or more minutes per occasion (currently 23% of adults)

- Increase by 50% the proportion of adults who perform physical activities that enhance and maintain muscular strength and endurance (currently 19% of adults)

Experts recommend that, to help yourself stay with an exercise program,[3, 31]

- Start slowly
- Vary your workouts; make it fun
- Workout with friends and others
- Set specific attainable goals and monitor progress
- Set aside a specific time each day for exercise; build it into your routine, but make it convenient
- Reward yourself for being successful in keeping up with your goals
- Don't worry about occasional setbacks; focus on the long-term benefits to your health

CONCEPT CHECK

Regular physical activity is a vital part of a healthy lifestyle, ideally constituting a total of at least 30 minutes per day, including some aerobic and resistance activities. Physically active people show lower risks of coronary heart disease, hypertension and stroke, type 2 diabetes, obesity, and other common chronic diseases.

Expert Opinion

YOUR EXERCISE PRESCRIPTION

Sheri A. Melton, Ph.D.

The benefits of regular exercise, sometimes called "training effects," are well established. Most people can reap significant health benefits by participating in just a moderate amount of physical activity, even as little as 30 minutes on most (and preferably all) days in a week.

When developing a total exercise program, all components of fitness should be taken into consideration: cardiorespiratory (CR) endurance, muscular strength, muscular endurance, flexibility, and body composition (% body fat). However, the exercise prescription is usually developed specifically for the CR endurance component. CR endurance is defined as the ability of the heart, lungs, and circulatory system to supply oxygen to the working muscles during sustained physical activity. That is why this fitness component is also called aerobic capacity. Your exercise prescription should be tailor-made for you—depending on your current level of fitness, your activity preferences, and the goals you want to achieve.

A structured, formal exercise prescription has five distinct components: mode, frequency, intensity, duration, and progression. In order to gain a training effect and its accompanying cardiovascular benefits, the American College of Sports Medicine (ACSM) advises that each of these components meet certain criteria and thresholds.[2]

MODE

The mode of exercise is the type of exercise prescribed. It must be one that uses large muscle groups in a rhythmic fashion, such as running, walking, and cycling.

DURATION

Duration is the amount of time spent in an exercise session. It should last 20 to 30 minutes, not counting time for warm-up and cooldown. Ideally, this should be continuous (without stopping) exercise, but an individual may have to participate in intermittent exercise at the start (sessions lasting 10 minutes several times a day), eventually working up to one continuous session.

FREQUENCY

Frequency of exercise should be at least three times per week. Daily exercise reaps even more benefits.

INTENSITY

Intensity is the level of exertion that indicates the magnitude of energy expenditure required to sustain the activity. Health benefits are achieved with a moderate intensity of exercise. There are several methods of prescribing moderate-intensity exercise. One of the most popular, and simplest, methods is using a percentage of your age-predicted maximum heart rate. Subtract age from 220 (this is your age-predicted maximum heart rate); then multiply by 70% and 85%. The heart rate range that results is sometimes called the target zone. Beginner exercisers should stay close to the lower end of the range, so that a sufficient duration can be achieved.

Taking your pulse during the exercise session (count for 10 seconds and then multiply the result by 6) is recommended to ensure that you are in your target zone. Pulse meters are very popular, and they allow the exerciser immediate feedback without stopping to take the pulse. Another popular method for determining intensity is the Rating of Perceived Exertion scale (RPE). The original RPE scale is numbered 6 to 20; the revised rating scale is 0 to 10. Each number corresponds to a subjective feeling of exertion. For instance, in the revised scale, the number 0 is "nothing at all" (e.g., sitting at the table), and 10 is considered close to maximal effort, or very, very strong (e.g., sprinting at all out effort):

0	0.5	1	2
Nothing at all	Very, very weak	Very weak	Weak

3	4	5	6	7
Moderate	Somewhat strong		Strong	

8	9	10	*
Very strong		Very, very strong	Maximal

The goal is to aim for the number 4, "somewhat strong," which correspond to the original scale of 13, "somewhat hard." A good rule of thumb for knowing you are not exercising at a higher than moderate intensity is to try the talk test. The exerciser should be able to talk without getting breathless.

More exact methods for determining intensity may be used also, especially in the clinical setting. A maximum graded exercise test can be used to measure the true maximal physiological responses of heart rate, blood pressure, and oxygen consumption. The level attained is called functional capacity, and intensity is prescribed as a percentage of measured functional capacity.

PROGRESSION

The last component, progression, is how frequency, intensity, and duration of exercise are increased over a period of time. The first 3 to 6 weeks of your new exercise program is the initiation stage, which is the time it takes your body to adapt to the new behavior and routine. Generally, once the required duration is achieved, intensity is increased, so that work remains in the target zone. The next 5 or 6 months of training is the improvement stage, in which the intensity and possibly the duration of exercise are increased to a point of tapering off (and no appreciable gains are made in fitness). In this stage, intensity may be increased to the higher end of the target zone, depending on your goals. This plateau marks the beginning of your maintenance stage. Goals may be re-evaluated, but no changes need to be made to your exercise prescription in order to keep the gains that have already been accomplished.

A WORD OF CAUTION

Even though moderate exercise is considered safe for most individuals, it is recommended that all adults be screened prior to beginning an exercise program. Screening involves identifying risk factors that would compromise the safety of participation in exercise. It also identifies those who need to be medically evaluated prior to exercise. The ACSM uses the following risk factors in determining a person's risk: family history of heart disease, cigarette smoking, hypertension, high blood cholesterol, impaired fasting glucose (diabetes), obesity, and sedentary lifestyle. Younger individuals (males under 45 years old and females under 55 years) who are asymptomatic and have no more than one of these risk factors are considered at low risk. They may embark on a moderate or vigorous exercise program without a medical evaluation or an exercise test. Those at moderate risk are older individuals (males older than 44 and females older than 54) and anyone having at least two risk factors. (The current Dietary Guidelines use age 40 and 50 years, respectively, as cutoff points.) They may embark on a moderate exercise program without a medical evaluation or an exercise test prior to beginning a moderate exercise program, but both are recommended if embarking on a vigorous one.

A FINAL NOTE

Always start your exercise session with 5 to 10 minutes of a general warm-up, and a more specific warm-up for higher intensities. Be sure to round out your exercise program with daily stretching and some form of resistance (weight) training 2 to 3 days a week. Include a circuit of 8 to 10 exercises to condition major muscle groups of the upper body and lower body. Use an amount of weight that you can perform one (or more) set(s) of at least 8, but no more than 12, repetitions in proper form. If more than 12 repetitions are possible, increase the amount of weight. Finally, an appropriate cooldown is necessary (about 5 to 10 minutes). Following these basic guidelines for an individualized exercise prescription will help you safely optimize your efforts in achieving your health, fitness, and wellness goals and improve your overall quality of life.

Dr. Melton is an assistant professor in the Kinesiology Department, School of Health Sciences, at West Chester University in West Chester, Pennsylvania. She is certified as an exercise specialist by the American College of Sports Medicine. Her experience encompasses cardiac and orthopedic rehabilitation and personal training.

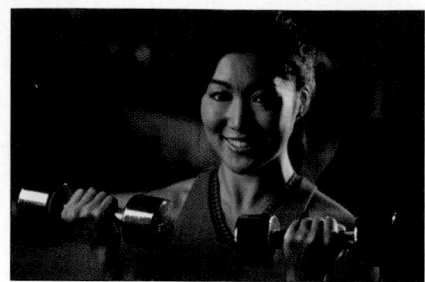

Resistance activities complement more aerobic activities and regular stretching exercises, rounding out a total fitness plan.[11, 25]

phosphocreatine (PCr) A high-energy compound that can be used to re-form ATP from ADP.

$\mathcal{S}$trength-training athletes have begun to use creatine supplements (see the Nutrition Perspective at the end of this chapter for details).

■ ENERGY SOURCES FOR MUSCLE USE

As you learned in Chapter 4, cells can't directly use the energy released from breaking down glucose or triglycerides. Rather, to utilize the chemical energy in foods, body cells must first convert the energy to a specific form, called adenosine triphosphate (ATP).

■ Adenosine Triphosphate (ATP)—Immediately Usable Energy

The partial breakdown of ATP by cells to yield ADP and Pi (the abbreviation for inorganic phosphate) releases usable energy for cell functions, including the muscle contractions required for locomotion. A resting muscle cell, however, contains just a small amount of ATP, enough to keep the muscle working maximally for about 2 to 4 seconds. To produce more ATP for muscle contraction over extended periods, the body uses **phosphocreatine (PCr),** a high-energy compound that is formed and stored in the muscle cells from the amino acid derivative creatine (glyine, arginine, and methionine participate in its synthesis). Dietary carbohydrates, fats, and proteins are also used as energy sources. The breakdown of all of these compounds releases enough energy to make more ATP (Table 14-2).

■ Phosphocreatine: The Initial Resupply of Muscle ATP

During periods of relaxation, muscles synthesize PCr from ATP and creatine and then store this in small amounts. As soon as ADP from the breakdown of ATP begins to accumulate in a contracting muscle, an enzyme is activated that transfers a high-energy Pi from PCr to ADP, thus reforming ATP (Fig. 14-1):

$$PCr + ADP \rightarrow Cr + ATP$$

If no other system for resupplying ATP were available, PCr could probably maintain maximal muscle contractions for about 10 seconds. However, since the energy released from the metabolism of glucose and fatty acids also begins to contribute ATP and thus spares some PCr use, this results in PCr functioning as the major source of energy for all events lasting up to about 1 minute (Table 14-2).

■ FIGURE 14-1 Quick energy for muscle use includes a supply of phosphocreatine (PCr). This can rapidly replenish ATP stores as activity begins. Phosphocreatine can be almost depleted in maximally contracting human forearm muscles in less than 60 seconds. It takes 4 minutes of rest to replenish half the PCr and 7 minutes to replenish 95% of the PCr. Similarly, it takes about 7 minutes of rest to replenish 95% of the PCr depleted with repeated knee extensions against resistance.
Illustration by William Ober.

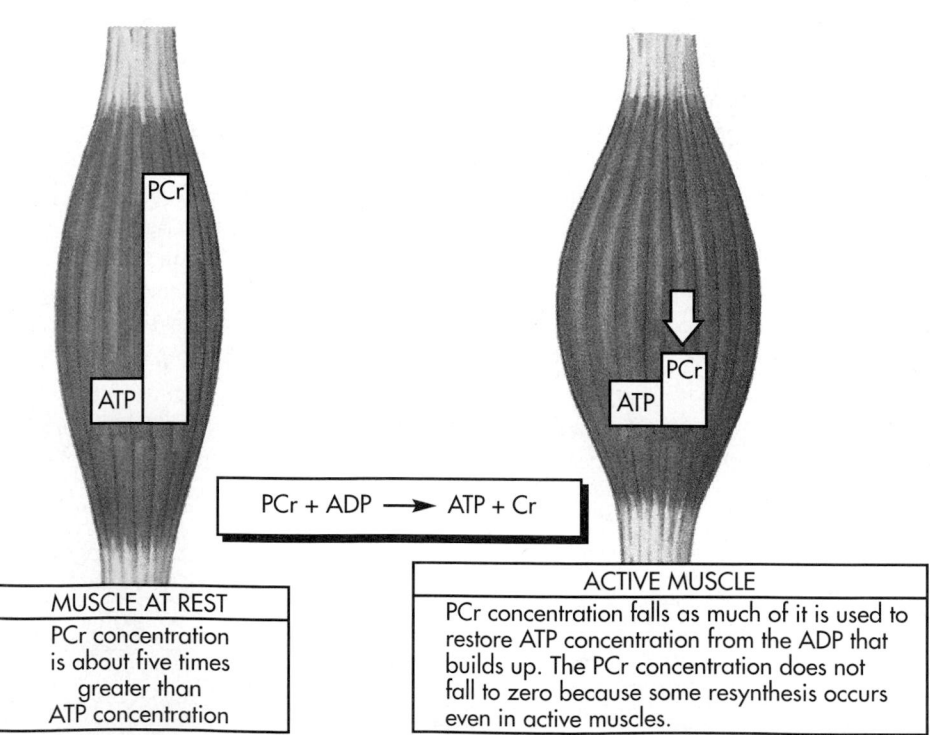

$$PCr + ADP \longrightarrow ATP + Cr$$

MUSCLE AT REST
PCr concentration is about five times greater than ATP concentration

ACTIVE MUSCLE
PCr concentration falls as much of it is used to restore ATP concentration from the ADP that builds up. The PCr concentration does not fall to zero because some resynthesis occurs even in active muscles.

The main advantage of PCr is that it can be activated instantly and can replenish ATP at rates fast enough to meet the energy demands of the fastest and most powerful sports events, including jumping, lifting, throwing, and sprinting actions. The disadvantage of PCr is that not enough is made and stored in the muscles to sustain a high rate of ATP resupply for more than a few minutes.

■ Glucose: Major Fuel for Short-Term, High-Intensity and Medium-Term Exercise

Recall from Chapter 4 that glucose breaks down during glycolysis, producing the three-carbon compound pyruvate. Glycolysis does not require oxygen and yields a small amount of ATP. If oxygen is present, the pyruvate is metabolized further, yielding additional ATP.

Anaerobic Pathway

When the oxygen supply in muscle is limited (**anaerobic** state) or when the physical activity is intense (e.g., running 400 meters or swimming 100 meters), pyruvate resulting from glycolysis accumulates in the muscle and is converted to **lactate.** Since the breakdown of 1 glucose to 2 pyruvates yields 2 ATP, glycolysis can resupply some ATP depleted in muscle activity. Carbohydrate is the only fuel that can be used for this process. The advantage of the anaerobic pathway is that, other than PCr breakdown, it is the fastest way to resupply ATP in muscle.

Glycolysis provides most of the energy for physical activity from about 30 seconds to 2 minutes after it has started. As you'll see shortly, fat utilization simply can't occur fast enough to meet the ATP demands of short-duration, high-intensity physical activity. If fat were the only available fuel, we would be unable to carry out physical activity more intense than a fast walk or jog.

The anaerobic pathway has three major disadvantages: (1) it can't sustain ATP production for long; (2) only about 5% of the energy available from glucose is released during glycolysis; and (3) the rapid accumulation of lactate greatly increases the acidity of muscle cells. Because high acidity inhibits the activity of key enzymes in glycolysis, anaerobic ATP production soon slows and fatigue sets in. We learn by trial-and-error a pace for these events that controls muscle lactate concentrations.

Most of the lactate that accumulates in active muscle cells is eventually released into the bloodstream. The liver picks up some of the lactate from the blood and

Recall from Chapter 4 that, when acids lose a hydrogen ion, as typically happens at the pH of the body, they are given the ending -ate. Thus, pyruvic acid is called pyruvate when in the context of body metabolism.

TABLE 14-2   Energy Sources Used by Resting and Working Muscle Cells

Source/System*	When in Use	Examples of an Exercise
ATP	At all times	All types
Phosphocreatine (PCr)	All exercise initially; extreme exercise thereafter	Shotput, jumping
Carbohydrate (anaerobic)	High-intensity exercise, especially lasting 30 seconds to 2 minutes	200-yard (20-meter) sprint
Carbohydrate (aerobic)	Exercise lasting 2 minutes to 4 to 5 hours; the higher the intensity (for example, running a 6-minute mile), the greater the use	Basketball, swimming, jogging
Fat (aerobic)	Exercise lasting more than a few minutes; greater amounts are used at lower exercise intensities	Long-distance running, long-distance cycling; much of the fuel used in a brisk walk is fat
Protein (aerobic)	Low quantity during all exercise; moderate quantity in endurance exercise, especially when carbohydrate fuel is lacking	Long-distance running

*At any given time, more than one system is operating.

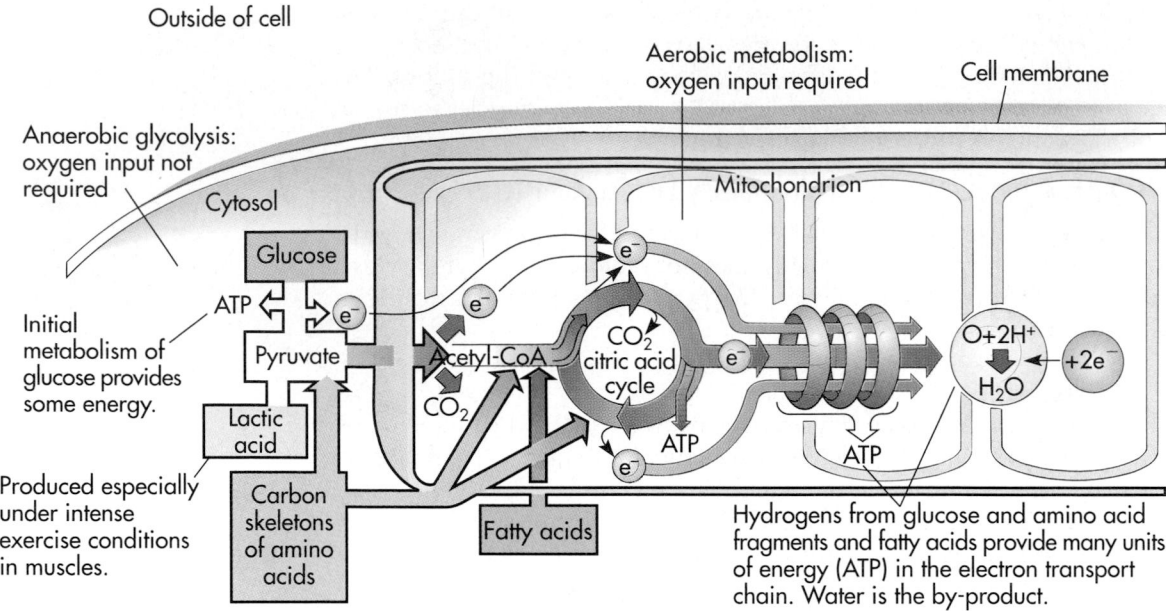

■ FIGURE 14-2 Metabolism of carbohydrate, fat, and protein supports ATP synthesis in a muscle cell. Carbohydrate metabolism occurs via both aerobic and anaerobic pathways, whereas fat and protein are metabolized for the most part via the aerobic pathway. Most of the ATP is produced as the hydrogen released from carbohydrate, fat, and protein metabolism combines with oxygen in the electron transport system to yield water. Recall from Chapters 10 through 12 that the B vitamins and many minerals are key participants in these metabolic pathways.

resynthesizes it into glucose, an energy-requiring process. This glucose then can re-enter the bloodstream, where it is available for cell uptake and breakdown. The heart can also use lactate directly for its energy needs, as can less active muscle cells situated near active ones.

Aerobic Pathway

If there is plenty of oxygen available in muscle (**aerobic** state) and the physical activity is of moderate to low intensity (e.g., jogging or distance swimming), the bulk of the pyruvate produced by glycolysis in the cytosol is shuttled to the mitochondria and further metabolized into carbon dioxide and water in a series of reactions. This requires oxygen. About 95% of the ATP produced from the complete metabolism of glucose is formed aerobically in mitochondria (Fig. 14-2).

Although the aerobic pathway supplies ATP more slowly than does the anaerobic pathway, it releases more energy. Furthermore, ATP production via the aerobic pathway can be sustained for hours. Accordingly, this pathway of glucose metabolism makes an important energy contribution to sports events lasting from about 2 minutes through 4 to 5 hours (Fig. 14-3).[10]

Glycogen Versus Blood Glucose as Muscle Fuel

Glycogen is the temporary storage form of glucose in the liver (about 100 g) and muscles (about 300 g in sedentary people). It is broken down to a form of glucose, which in turn can be metabolized by both the anaerobic and aerobic pathways. Glycogen is, in fact, the primary source of glucose for ATP production in muscle cells during fairly intense activities that last for less than about 2 hours. In such activities, the depletion of glycogen in the liver leads to a fall in blood glucose, whereas the depletion of glycogen in the muscles contributes to fatigue.

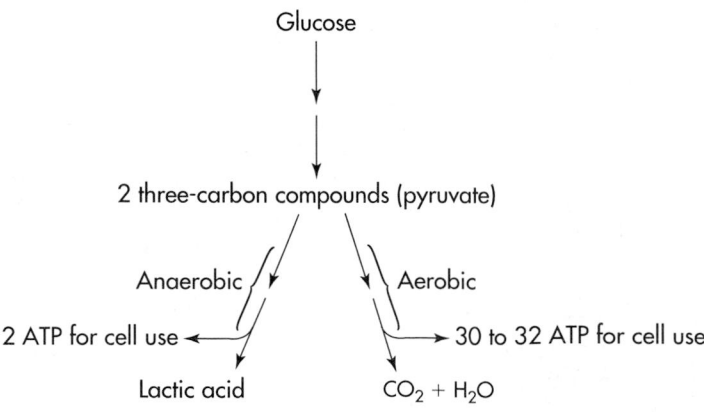

ATP yield for aerobic versus anaerobic glucose utilization.

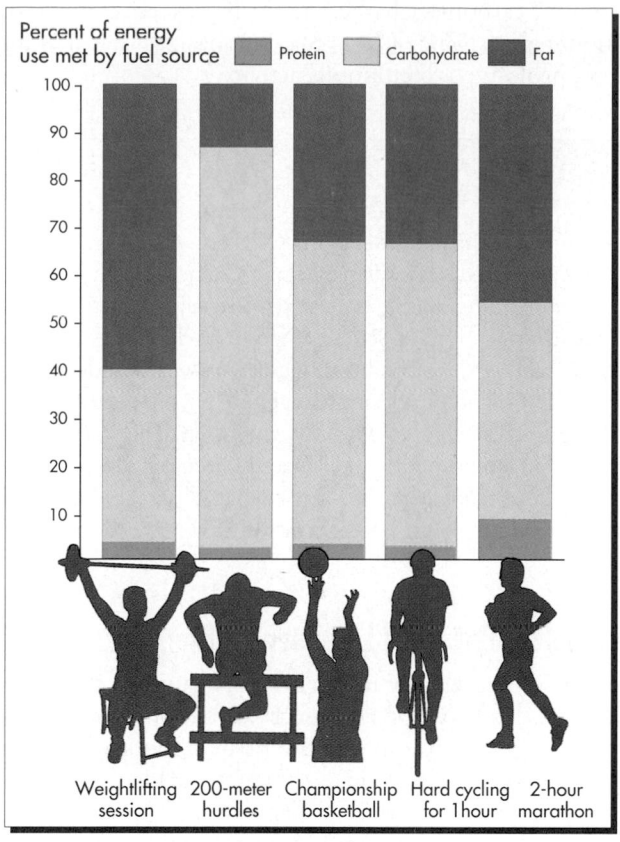

Percent of energy use met by fuel source — Protein, Carbohydrate, Fat

Weightlifting session | 200-meter hurdles | Championship basketball | Hard cycling for 1 hour | 2-hour marathon

FIGURE 14-3 Rough estimates of fuel use during various forms of physical activity.

Once these glycogen stores are exhausted, an athlete can continue working at only about 50% of maximal capacity. Athletes call this point of glycogen depletion "hitting the wall," as further exertion is hampered. Thus, when exertion meets or exceeds 70% of $VO_{2\ max}$ for more than an hour or so, athletes (e.g., long-distance runners or cyclists) should consider increasing the amount of carbohydrate stored in muscles. Diets high in carbohydrate can be used to build up muscle glycogen stores—up to double the typical amounts—in advance of competition, thereby forestalling fatigue and improving endurance.[1] A later section on carbohydrate needs discusses how to plan such a diet.

As exercise duration increases beyond about 20 to 30 minutes, the maintenance of blood glucose becomes an increasingly important consideration. This can spare the use of muscle glycogen, saving it in the muscle for sudden bursts of effort that may be required, such as a sprint to the finish in a marathon race. Linked to the importance of maintaining a normal concentration of glucose in the bloodstream during prolonged exercise, carbohydrate intake of about 30 to 60 g/hour during strenuous endurance exercise, such as cycling that lasts about 1 hour or more, can help maintain adequate blood glucose concentrations. This, in turn, results in delay of fatigue.[10] A later section on sports drinks discusses this in more detail. Such a high carbohydrate intake also helps one tolerate vigorous training on a daily basis.[1]

Without the maintenance of blood glucose in such endurance activities, there is a decline in mental function associated with low blood glucose (cyclists call this mental decline "bonking").

Carbohydrate intake is not as important for the muscles in shorter events (e.g., one-half hour or so) because the muscles do not take up much blood glucose during short-term exercise, relying instead primarily on glycogen stores for carbohydrate fuel. This is because the action of insulin to increase glucose uptake by muscles is blunted by other hormones, such as epinephrine and glucagon, that increase initially during exercise.[10]

VO_{2max} The maximum volume of oxygen that can be consumed per unit of time.

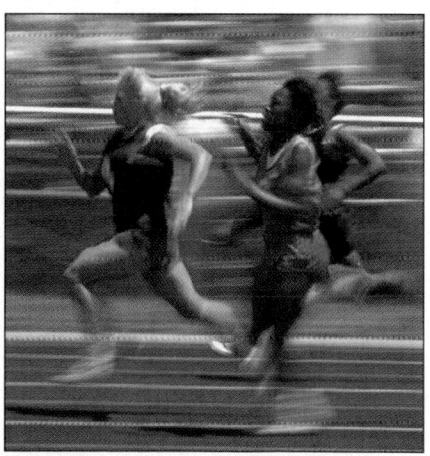

Bursts of muscle activity use a variety of energy sources, including PCr and ATP.

Overall, this use of carbohydrate feeding during exercise encompasses the advice of sports nutrition expert Nancy Clark. She emphasizes that it is important to fuel before and during prolonged, continuous activity.[7]

CONCEPT CHECK

ATP is the main form of energy that cells use. Carbohydrate metabolism to form ATP begins as glucose becomes available from the bloodstream or from glycogen breakdown. Carbohydrate feeding during exercise can also supply glucose. In a muscle cell, each glucose is broken down through a series of steps to yield either lactate or carbon dioxide (CO_2) plus water (H_2O). The breakdown of glucose to carbon dioxide and water is called the aerobic pathway because it requires oxygen. The conversion of glucose to lactate is called the anaerobic pathway because no oxygen is used. This latter process allows the cell to quickly reform ATP and supports the demand for energy during intense physical activity, as does phosphocreatine (PCr). The aerobic pathway takes longer to supply ATP but provides more energy in the end. This pathway is used more for endurance activities.

■ Fat: The Main Fuel for Prolonged Low-Intensity Exercise

The majority of the stored energy in the body is found in the fatty acids of stored triglycerides. Most of this resides in adipose tissue depots; some is stored in the muscle itself. When fat stores in various adipose tissue depots are broken down for energy, one triglyceride molecule first yields three fatty acids and one glycerol. The free fatty acids are then released into the bloodstream and travel to the muscles. Once fatty acids enter muscle cells, they combine with any of those released from intramuscular triglyceride storage. All these fatty acids then move into the mitochondria, using a shuttle system that uses carnitine. Then they are broken down into carbon dioxide and water, using in part the oxygen-requiring electron transport chain that yields much ATP. The rate at which muscles use fatty acids depends on a number of factors:

- *The more trained a muscle, the greater its ability to use fat as a fuel.* After a period of aerobic training, muscle cells contain more and larger mitochondria. These and other changes enable muscle cells to produce more ATP via oxygen-requiring pathways, including the pathway used to burn fat for fuel (Table 14-3).
- *The more fatty acids that are released from adipose tissue stores into the bloodstream, the more fat will be used by the muscles.* Some athletes have attempted to raise their blood concentrations of fatty acids by consuming caffeinated beverages. Because this practice actually can increase fatty-acid release from the adipose tissue, it can be helpful to some athletes (see the Nutrition Perspective at the end of this chapter).
- *As exercise becomes increasingly prolonged, fat use predominates,* especially when exercise remains at a low or moderate (aerobic) rate.[28] When energy is needed for long-duration exercise or physical labor, there is almost always plenty of fat that can be called on. In comparison, carbohydrate stores are quite limited.

The other advantage of fat over other sources of energy is that it provides more "bang for the buck." That is, for a given weight of fuel, fat supplies more than twice as much energy as carbohydrate. The aerobic breakdown of a 6-carbon glucose molecule yields 30 to 32 ATP (ratio of about 5 ATP to 1 carbon), whereas an 16-carbon fatty acid molecule produces 108 ATP (ratio of about 6.8 ATP to 1 carbon).

However, carbohydrate is more efficient than fat in one very important way: the amount of ATP produced per unit of oxygen consumed. It takes 6 O_2 molecules to produce 30 to 32 ATP molecules during the aerobic breakdown of a molecule of glucose (ratio of about 5 ATP to 1 O_2), whereas 23 O_2 molecules are needed to produce 108 ATP molecules from an 16-carbon fatty acid (ratio of about 4.5 ATP to 1 O_2). Thus, in situations when an athlete's maximal performance would be limited

The fatty acids can come from all over the body, not necessarily from depots near the active muscles. This is why spot reducing does not work. Exercise can tone the muscles underlying adipose tissue but does not preferentially use those stores. If this were not the case, we would all have lean cheeks and necks, because muscles in that vicinity are regularly used.

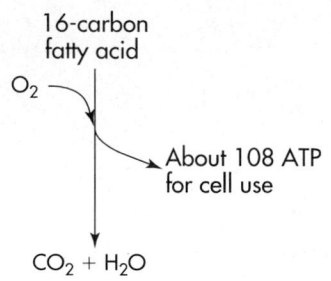

ATP yield from aerobic fatty acid utilization.

TABLE 14-3   Adaptations to Endurance Exercise in Skeletal Muscle

Changes	Advantage
Increased ability of muscle to store glycogen (high-carbohydrate diet increases this even further)	More glycogen fuel available for the final minutes of an event
Increased triglyceride storage in muscle	Conserves glycogen by allowing for increased fat use
Increased mitochondrial size and number	Conserves glycogen by allowing for increased fat use (even at high exercise outputs)
Increased myoglobin content	Increased oxygen delivery to muscles and increased ability to use fat for fuel

Overall, training allows an athlete to use fat for fuel more readily. This allows the athlete to conserve glycogen for when it is really needed—such as for a burst of speed at the end of a race.

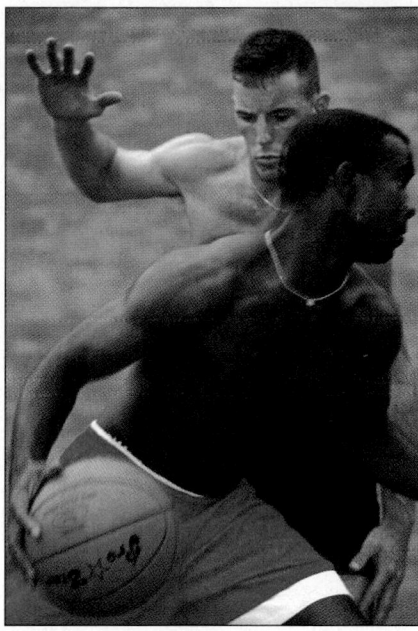

The energy to perform comes from carbohydrate, fat, and protein. The relative mix depends on the pace.

by the activity of oxygen-requiring pathways (as in competitive endurance exercise), it is necessary that muscle cells also use carbohydrate as long as the carbohydrate supply, especially muscle glycogen, lasts.[10]

During very lengthy activities, such as a triathlon, ultramarathon, manual labor in a foundry, or even work at a desk for 8 hours a day, fat supplies about 70 to 90% of the energy required. Overall, keep in mind that the only fuel we eat that can support intense (anaerobic) activity is carbohydrate; slow and steady (aerobic) activity uses all available energy sources: fat and carbohydrate, primarily.

■ Protein: A Minor Fuel Source, Primarily for Endurance Exercise

Although amino acids derived from protein are used to fuel muscles, their contribution is relatively small, compared with that of carbohydrate and fat. As a rough guide, only about 5% of the body's general energy needs, as well as the typical energy needs of exercising muscles, is supplied by the metabolism of amino acids.[1]

However, proteins can contribute significantly to energy needs in endurance exercise, perhaps as much as 10 to 15%, especially as glycogen stores in the muscle are exhausted. Most of the energy supplied from protein comes from metabolism of the branched-chain amino acids—leucine, isoleucine, and valine. Because a normal diet provides enough protein to supply this amount of fuel, protein supplements or amino acid supplements are not needed. Contrary to what many athletes believe, protein is used for fuel less in resistance types of exercise (e.g., weight lifting) than for endurance exercise (e.g., running) (review Fig. 14-3). The primary muscle fuels for weight lifting are phosphocreatine (PCr) and carbohydrate, with fat providing comparably less energy and little use of protein. Despite this fact, high-protein products such as Pro-Complex, Amino Fuel 2000, High Voltage Protein Drink, and Instant Egg Protein are marketed in nearly every health-food and fitness store, specifically for weight lifters and bodybuilders. Note also that consuming high-carbohydrate, moderate-protein foods immediately after a weight-training workout enhances the anabolic effect of the activity, most likely by increasing the concentrations of insulin and growth hormone release into the blood.[1]

CONCEPT CHECK

*F*at is a key aerobic fuel for muscle cells, especially at low to moderate exercise intensities. Training enhances the ability to use fat for fuel, in turn conserving glycogen stores. At rest, muscles burn primarily fat for energy needs. On the other hand, little protein is used to fuel muscles. It supplies roughly 5% of energy needs under most conditions, and perhaps 10 to 15% of energy needs during endurance exercise.

■ ADAPTATION OF MUSCLES AND BODY PHYSIOLOGY TO EXERCISE

hypertrophy An increase in tissue or organ size.

atrophy A wasting away of tissues or organs.

With training, muscle strength also becomes matched to the muscles' variable work demands. Muscles enlarge after being made to work repeatedly, a response called **hypertrophy.** Certain cells in the muscles gain bulk and improve their ability to work. Conversely, after several days without activity, muscles diminish in size and lose strength, a response called **atrophy.** Both hypertrophy and atrophy are forms of adaptation to the load applied. Thus, many marathon runners have well-developed leg muscles but little arm or chest muscle development.

Beyond the effects on individual muscles describe earlier, repeated aerobic exercise also produces beneficial changes in the heart and blood vessels that are responsible for delivering oxygen to the mitochondria of the muscle cells. Because the body needs more oxygen during exercise, it responds to training by producing more red blood cells and expanding total blood volume. Training also leads to an increase in the number of capillaries in muscle tissue; as a result, oxygen can be delivered more easily to muscles. Finally, training causes the heart, a muscle itself, to strengthen. Then each contraction empties the heart's chamber more efficiently, so more blood is pumped with each beat. As exercise increases the efficiency of the heart, its rate of beating at rest and during submaximal exercise decreases.

A*TP (energy) needs dictate the amount of oxygen used by cells. 1.5 or 2.5 ATP molecules are produced from each molecule of oxygen.

Oxygen consumption indicates how hard a person is exercising. The more physically fit a person is, the more work the muscles and body can do, and the more oxygen the person can consume. A treadmill test commonly is used to determine a person's $VO_{2\,max}$, based on the maximum amount of oxygen that can be consumed in a unit of time (ml/min). In this test, oxygen consumption is measured as the treadmill speed and/or grade is gradually increased until the subject becomes profoundly fatigued. The oxygen consumption measured right before total exhaustion is $VO_{2\,max}$.[12] Most people can improve their $VO_{2\,max}$ by 15% to 20% or more with exercise training.

Because of individual differences in $VO_{2\,max}$, it is generally best to express exercise intensity as a percentage of $VO_{2\,max}$. The percentage of $VO_{2\,max}$ required for exercise of various intensity is as follows:

- Low intensity (e.g., fast walk)—30 to 50% of $VO_{2\,max}$
- Moderate intensity (e.g., fast jog)—50 to 65% of $VO_{2\,max}$
- High intensity (e.g., 3-hour marathon pace)—70 to 80% of $VO_{2\,max}$
- Very high intensity (e.g., sprints)—85 to 150% of $VO_{2\,max}$

In very-high-intensity activities, the ATP equivalent to the "extra" 50% above 100% of $VO_{2\,max}$ is produced anaerobically from PCr and glycolysis.

Exercise output is sometimes expressed in units called METs. One MET is the expenditure of 1 kcal/kg/hr or, on average, 3.5 ml O_2/kg/min. This approximates resting energy expenditure. A brisk walk represents about 6–7 METs of energy expenditure. Exercise prescriptions given to people recovering from a heart attack are often given in MET units (see *ASCM Guidelines for Exercise Testing and Prescription* for details).[2]

CRITICAL THINKING

Marty started going to the gym about 8 weeks ago. At first, he noticed that he began huffing and puffing about 7 minutes into his aerobic workout. Now, however, he can work out for about 25 minutes without tiring. What is a possible explanation for his ability to work out longer?

Typical VO_{2max} Values	ml O_2/kg/min
Sedentary elderly person	15
Typical middle-aged adult	35–45
Elite athlete	65–75

■ POWER FOOD: DIETARY ADVICE FOR ATHLETES

Athletic training and genetic makeup are two very important determinants of athletic performance. A good diet won't substitute for either factor, but diet can further enhance and maximize an athlete's potential. More important, a poor diet can certainly harm performance.[1]

■ Energy Needs

Athletes need varying amounts of food energy, depending on each athlete's body size and current body composition and on the type of training or competition being considered. A small person may need only 1700 kcal daily to sustain normal daily activities without losing body weight; a large, muscular man may need 4000 kcal. These rough estimates can be viewed as starting points that need to be individualized by trial and error for each athlete.[1]

The energy required for sports training or competition has to be added to the basal energy needed just to carry on normal activities. Energy use averages 5 to 8 kcal/minute for moderate activity; again, this is just an estimate. For example, an hour of bowling requires little energy in addition to that required to sustain normal daily living. At the other extreme, a 12-hour endurance bicycle race over mountains can require an additional 4000 kcal/day. Therefore, some athletes may need as much as 7000 kcal or more daily just to maintain body weight while training, whereas others may need 1700 kcal or less. If an athlete experiences daily fatigue, the first consideration should be if he or she is consuming enough food.[14] Up to 6 meals per day may be needed, including one before each workout.

How can we know if an athlete is getting enough energy from food? Estimating daily intake from a food diary by the athlete is one way. Another step is to estimate the athlete's body fat percentage by measuring skinfold thicknesses, by using bioelectrical impedance, or by using the underwater weighing technique (see Chapter 13). Body fat should be in the desirable range—that is, 5 to 13% for most male athletes and 12% to 22% for most female athletes.[1] Then one goes on to monitor body weight changes on a daily or weekly basis. If body weight starts to fall, food energy should be increased; if weight rises and it is because of increases in body fat, the athlete should eat less.

If the body composition test shows that an athlete has too much body fat, the athlete should lower food intake by about 200 to 500 kcal/day, while maintaining a regular exercise program, until the desirable fat percentage is achieved. Reducing fat intake is the best nutrient-related approach. On the other hand, if an athlete needs to gain weight, increasing food intake by 500 to 700 kcal/day will eventually lead to the needed weight gain. A mix of carbohydrate, fat, and protein is advised, coupled with exercise to make sure this gain is mostly from lean tissue, and not mostly added fat stores.[1]

Wrestlers, boxers, judoists, jockeys, and oarsmen often try to lose weight, so that they can be certified to compete in a lower weight class. This helps them gain a mechanical advantage over an opponent of smaller stature. They usually lose this weight before stepping on the scale for weight certification. Athletes can lose up to 22 pounds (10 kg) of body water in 1 day by sitting in a sauna, exercising in a plastic sweat suit, or taking diuretic drugs, which speed water loss from the kidneys. Losing as little as 2 to 3% of body weight by dehydration can adversely affect endurance performance. A pattern of repeated weight loss or gain of more than 5% of body weight by dehydration carries some risk of kidney malfunction and heat-related illness. Death is also a possibility, as was seen in three collegiate wrestlers in late 1997.

To prevent such deaths in the future, the National Collegiate Athletic Association has begun requiring that a minimum safe weight be set by a physician or an athletic trainer for each wrestler at the start of the season. Several states also have adopted this practice. If athletes, such as wrestlers, wish to compete in a lower-body-weight class and have enough extra fat stores, they should begin a gradual, sustained reduction in food-energy intake long before the competitive season starts. In so doing, the athlete attains a healthier body composition (less fat) while avoiding the potentially harmful and certainly misery-creating effects of severe dehydration. Athletes who have no extra body fat should not attempt to compete at a lower-body-weight class. Coaches and trainers should be aware of the decreased performance and serious side effects of severe dehydration.[1]

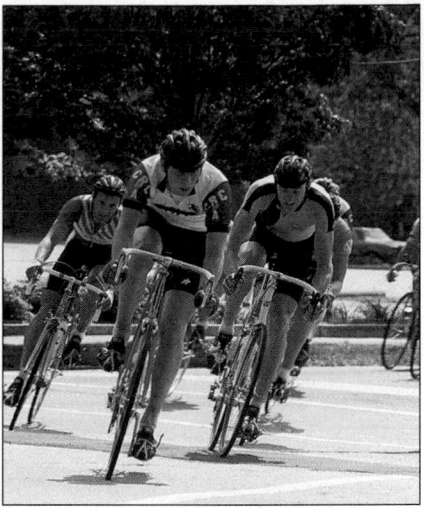

Athletes often expend much energy. Their resulting food intake should easily provide ample protein and other nutrients to support activity.

CRITICAL THINKING

Joe is a wrestler who qualified for the 125 pound weight classification in his annual high school competition. After a few matches, Joe began to feel dizzy and faint. He was disqualified because he was unable to continue the match. Later, the coach found out that Joe had spent 2 hours in the sauna before weighing in, which had made him dehydrated. What are the consequences of dehydration? What can you suggest as an alternative way to lose weight?

■ Carbohydrate Needs

Anyone who regularly exercises vigorously for more than 1 hour per day needs to consume a diet that includes moderate to high amounts of carbohydrates. The diet should include a variety of foods, such as recommended by the Food Guide Pyramid. Numerous servings of grains, starchy vegetables, and fruits provide enough carbohydrate to maintain adequate liver and muscle glycogen stores, especially for replacing glycogen losses from workouts on the previous day.[7] Relatively low-carbohydrate diets, such as *The Zone Diet*, are not recommended.[6]

Carbohydrate intake should be at least 5 g/kg body weight. People engaged in aerobic training and endurance athletes (duration >60 minutes per day) may need as much as 6 to 10 g/kg body weight. In other words, triathletes and marathoners should consider eating close to 500 to 600 g of carbohydrates daily, and even more if necessary, to (1) prevent chronic fatigue and (2) load the muscles and liver with glycogen. This is especially important when performing multiple training bouts in a day, such as swim practices, or heavy training on successive days, as in cross-country running.[1] Table 14-4 shows sample menus, based on the Food Guide Pyramid, for diets providing food energy ranging from 1500 to 5000 kcal/day. Table 14-5 lists

---

TABLE 14-4 Sample Daily Menus Based on the Food Guide Pyramid, That Provide Various Total Energy Intakes

1500 kcal Diet

Breakfast
Skim milk, 1 cup
Cheerios, ½ cup
Bagel, ½
Cherry jam, 2 tsp
Margarine, 1 tsp

Lunch
Chicken breast (roasted), 2 oz
Figs, 1
Skim milk ½ cup
Banana, 1

Snack
Oatmeal-raisin cookie, 1
Low-fat fruit yogurt, 1 cup

Dinner
Spaghetti w/meatballs, 1 cup
Romaine lettuce, 1 cup
Italian dressing, 2 tsp
Green beans, ½ cup
Cranberry juice, 1½ cups

18% protein (68 g)
64% carbohydrate (240 g)
19% fat (32 g)

2000 kcal Diet

Breakfast
Skim milk, 1 cup
Cheerios, 1 cup
Bagel, ½
Cherry jam, 1 tbsp
Margarine, 1 tsp

Lunch
Chicken breast (roasted), 2 oz
Wheat bread, 2 slices
Mayonnaise, 1 tsp
Raisins, ¼ cup
Cranberry juice, 1½ cups
Banana, 1

Snack
Oatmeal-raisin cookies, 3
Low-fat fruit yogurt, 1 cup

Dinner
Broiled beef sirloin, 3 oz
Romaine lettuce, 1 cup
Italian dressing, 2 tsp
Green beans, 1 cup
Skim milk, ½ cup

17% protein (85 g)
63% carbohydrate (315 g)
20% fat (44 g)

3000 kcal Diet

Breakfast
Skim milk, 1 cup
Cheerios, 2 cups
Bagel, 1
Cherry jam, 2 tsp
Margarine, 1 tsp
Oat bran muffins, 2

Lunch
Chicken breast (roasted), 2 oz
Wheat bread, 2 slices
Provolone cheese, 1 oz
Mayonnaise, 1 tsp
Raisins, ⅓ cup
Cranberry juice, 1½ cups
Low-fat fruit yogurt, 1 cup

Snack
Banana, 1
Oatmeal-raisin cookies, 3

Dinner
Broiled beef sirloin, 3 oz
Romaine lettuce, 1 cup
Garbanzo beans, 1 cup
Italian dressing, 2 tsp
Spinach pasta noodles, 1½ cups
Margarine, 1 tsp

Green beans, 1 cup
Skim milk, ½ cup

17% protein (128 g)
62% carbohydrate (465 g)
21% fat (70 g)

4000 kcal Diet

Breakfast
Orange, 1
Cheerios, 2 cups
Skim milk, 1 cup
Bran muffins, 2

Snack
Chopped dates, ¾ cup

Lunch
Romaine lettuce, 1 cup
Garbanzo beans, 1 cup
Grated carrots, ½ cup
French dressing, 2 tbsp
Macaroni and cheese, 3 cups
Apple juice, 1 cup

Snack
Wheat bread, 2 slices
Margarine, 1 tsp
Jam, 2 tbsp

Dinner
Skinless turkey breast, 2 oz
Mashed potatoes, 2 cups
Peas and onions, 1 cup
Banana, 1
Skim milk, 1 cup

Snack
Pasta, 1 cup cooked
Margarine, 2 tsp
Parmesan cheese, 2 tbsp
Cranberry juice, 1 cup

14% protein (140 g)
61% carbohydrate (610 g)
26% fat (116 g)

5000 kcal Diet

Breakfast
Cheerios, 2 cups
Bran muffins, 2
Orange, 1
2% milk, 1 cup

Snack
Low-fat yogurt, 1 cup
Chopped dates, 1 cup

Lunch
Apple juice, 1 cup
Chicken enchilada, 1
Romaine lettuce, 1 cup
Garbanzo beans, 1 cup
Shredded carrots, ¾ cup
Chopped celery, ½ cup
Seasoned croutons, 1 oz
French dressing, 2 tbsp
Wheat bread, 2 slices
Margarine, 1 tbsp

Snack
Banana, 1
Bagel, 1
Cream cheese, 1 tbsp

Dinner
2% milk, 1 cup
Beef sirloin, 5 oz
Mashed potatoes, 2 cups
Spinach pasta noodles, 1½ cups
Grated parmesan cheese, 2 tbsp
Green beans, 1 cup
Oatmeal-raisin cookies, 3

Snack
Cranberry juice, 2 cups
Air-popped popcorn, 4 cups
Raisins, ⅓ cup

14% protein (175 g)
63% carbohydrate (813 g)
24% fat (136 g)

the number of grams of carbohydrate in one exchange (serving) of the various groups in the Exchange System and some representative foods in each group. As shown in Chapter 2, the Exchange System is a very useful tool for planning all types of diets, including diets for athletes.

Note that one does not have to give up any specific food when planning a high-carbohydrate diet. The focus is to include more high-carbohydrate foods and moderation with concentrated fat sources. Sports nutritionists emphasize the difference between a high-carbohydrate meal and a high-carbohydrate/high-fat meal. Before endurance events, such as marathons or triathlons, some athletes seek to increase their carbohydrate reserves by eating potato chips, French fries, banana cream pie, and pastries. Although such foods contain carbohydrate, they also contain a lot of fat. Better high-carbohydrate food choices include pasta, rice, potatoes, bread, fruit and fruit juices, and many breakfast cereals (check the label for carbohydrate content). Sports drinks appropriate for carbohydrate loading, such as GatorLode and

TABLE 14-5 Grams of Carbohydrate per Exchange and Serving Size of Typical Foods

Starch list—15 g Carbohydrate per Serving

One Serving

½–¾ cup dry breakfast cereal*	1 small baked potato
½ cup cooked breakfast cereal	½ bagel
½ cup cooked grits	½ English muffin
⅓ cup cooked rice	1 slice bread
½ cup cooked pasta	¾ oz pretzels
¼ cup baked beans	6 saltine crackers
½ cup cooked corn	2 pancakes, 4 inches in diameter
½ cup cooked/dry beans	2 taco shells

Vegetable list—5 g Carbohydrate per Serving

One Serving
½ cup cooked vegetables
1 cup raw vegetables
½ cup vegetable juice
Examples: carrots, green beans, broccoli, cauliflower, onions, spinach, tomatoes, vegetable juice

Fruit List—15 g Carbohydrate per Serving

One serving:

½ cup canned fruit or berries	12 cherries or grapes
½ cup fruit juice	½ grapefruit
¼ cup dried fruit	1 nectarine
1 small apple	1 orange
4 apricots	1 peach
1 small banana	1¼ cups watermelon

Milk List—12 g Carbohydrate per Serving

One Serving
1 cup milk
¾ cup plain low-fat yogurt

Other Carbohydrates List—15 g Carbohydrate per Serving

One Serving

2-inch square typical slice of cake	
2 small cookies	½ cup ice cream
3 ginger snaps	½ cup sherbet

Modified from *Exchange Lists for Meal Planning* by the American Diabetes Association and American Dietetic Association, 1995, Chicago, American Dietetic Association.

*Note that the carbohydrate content of dry cereal varies widely. Check the labels of the ones you choose and adjust serving size accordingly. Most ready-to-eat breakfast cereals have the exchanges listed on the food label.

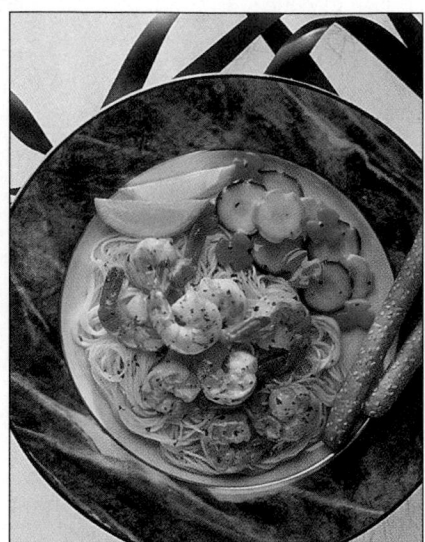

The athlete's plate should be covered two-thirds with grains and vegetables, and one-third with protein-rich sources.

Appropriate Activities for Carbohydrate Loading

Marathons
Long-distance swimming
Cross-country skiing
30-kilometer runs
Triathlons
Tournament-play basketball
Soccer
Cycling time trials
Long-distance canoe racing

Inappropriate Activities for Carbohydrate Loading

American football games
10-kilometer or shorter runs
Walking and hiking
Most swimming events
Single basketball games
Weight lifting
Most track and field events

UltraFuel, can also help. Consuming a moderate amount of dietary fiber during the final day of training is a good precaution to reduce the chances of bloating and intestinal gas during the next day's event.

As a general rule, athletes should obtain 60% or more of their total energy needs from carbohydrate, rather than the 50% typical of most American diets, especially if exercise duration is expected to exceed 2 hours and total caloric intake is about 3000 kcal/day or less. Diets containing 4000 to 5000 kcal/day can be as low as 50% carbohydrate, as these will still provide sufficient carbohydrate (500–600 g/day). Fat should provide 20 to 25% of total energy needs rather than the typical 33%. Protein then provides the rest of the total energy—about 15% of total needs.[1] This approach yields a training diet that is about two-thirds carbohydrate-rich foods and one-third protein-rich foods, with fat coming in as part of many of the food choices made.[7]

For athletes who compete in continuous intense aerobic events lasting more than 60 to 90 minutes (or in shorter events repeated over a 24-hour period), undertaking a **carbohydrate-loading** regimen is often advantageous to maximizing muscle glycogen fuel. (Note, however, that this duration applies to few athletes.) One possible regimen includes a gradual reduction, or "tapering," of exercise intensity and duration, coupled with a gradual increase in dietary carbohydrate as a percentage of energy intake. The procedure can begin 6 days before competition, with the athlete completing a hard workout lasting about 60 minutes. Workouts for the next 4 days then last about 40, 40, 20, and 20 minutes, respectively, with exercise intensities being progressively reduced each day. On the final day before the competition, the athlete rests.

The dietary carbohydrate on the first 3 days of this regimen (about 450 g per day) contributes 45 to 50% of energy intake. The carbohydrate contribution rises to 65 to 75% (about 600 g per day) for the last 3 days before competition. This carbohydrate-loading technique usually increases muscle glycogen stores by 50 to 85% over typical conditions (that is, when dietary carbohydrate constitutes about 50% of the total energy intake). A typical carbohydrate-loading schedule looks like this:

Days Before Competition	6	5	4	3	2	1
Exercise time (minutes)	60	40	40	20	20	Rest
Carbohydrate (grams)	450	450	450	600	600	600

Total energy intake should decrease as exercise time decreases

A potential disadvantage of carbohydrate loading is that some water is incorporated in the muscles with the extra glycogen. Although it aids in maintaining hydration, in some individuals this additional water weight and related muscle stiffness are sufficient to detract from their sports performance, making carbohydrate loading inappropriate. Athletes considering carbohydrate loading should try it during training (and well before an important competition) to experience its effects on performance. They can then determine whether it is worth the effort. Note also that carbohydrate feeding during exercise provides about the same advantage as carbohydrate loading. In fact, the trend is currently toward this second method coupled with a daily diet high in carbohydrate.[7]

Carbohydrate loading is safe for adolescents, but the activities for which this technique is useful, such as marathon runs, may not be. Adolescents should obtain the approval of their physician before participating in such a regimen.

■ Protein Needs

Looking at protein intake more specifically, typical recommendations for athletes range from 1.2 to 1.4 g of protein per kg of body weight, considerably higher than the RDA of 0.8 g/kg body weight (Table 14-6). Again, athletes engaged in endurance sports should aim for the higher value, as protein supplies a greater percentage of the energy used (up to 15%) in these sports than in other athletic endeavors. Overall, the vast majority of athletes can meet protein needs without having to exceed twice the RDA.[20] In addition, energy needs must be met or much of this protein will be diverted to fuel use.

For athletes beginning a weight-training program, some experts recommend up to 1.8 g of protein per kg of body weight.[20] That is up to approximately 2¼ times the RDA for protein. To date, the importance of such an excessive protein intake during the initial phases of weight training has not been supported by sufficient research. In addition, protein intakes above this amount simply result in an increase use of amino acids for energy needs; no further increase in muscle protein synthesis is seen. Note also that energy needs for weight lifting itself are not the reason for the high protein recommendation, as the fuel used in this activity is primarily fat and carbohydrate. The extra protein, theoretically, is required for the synthesis of new tissue brought on by the loading effect of weight training. Once the desired muscle mass is achieved, protein intake need not exceed twice the RDA.

Any athlete not specifically on a hypocaloric regimen can easily have a protein intake twice the RDA simply by eating a variety of foods (see Table 14-6). For example, a 123-lb (53-kg) woman can consume 82 g of her upper range of 85 g of protein (twice the RDA) by eating 4 oz of chicken (one chicken breast), 3 oz of beef (a small lean hamburger), and ½ cup of cooked beans and by drinking two glasses of milk during a single day. A 180-pound (77-kg) man needs to consume only 6 oz of chicken (a large chicken breast), ½ cup of cooked beans, a 6-oz can of tuna, and two glasses of milk a day to consume 122 g of his upper range of 123 g of protein (twice the RDA). And, for both athletes this does not even include the protein in the grains or vegetables they will also eat. In meeting their energy needs, many athletes consume even more protein. Thus, protein supplements are not needed despite marketing claims.[7]

Athletes who either feel they must significantly limit their energy intake or are vegetarians should specifically determine how much protein they eat. They should make sure to choose foods that provide overall at least 1.2 g of protein per kg of body weight. Skimping on protein is not a good idea.[1]

■ Vitamin and Mineral Needs

Vitamin and mineral needs are the same or slightly higher for athletes, compared with those of sedentary adults. Still, because athletes usually have such high food-energy intakes, they tend to consume plenty of vitamins and minerals.[1] An exception are athletes consuming hypocaloric diets (about 1200 kcal or less), such as seen with some female athletes participating in events in which maintaining a low body weight is crucial. They may not be meeting B-vitamin and other micronutrient needs. Vegetarian athletes are also a concern. In these cases, consuming fortified foods, such as breakfast cereals, or a balanced multivitamin and mineral supplement is recommended.[23] Athletes' needs for vitamin E and vitamin C may be somewhat greater because of the antioxidant protection these nutrients provide; this effect could be

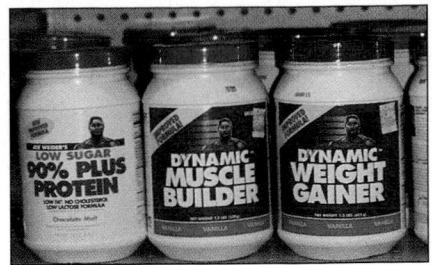

High-protein products, which are often marketed to athletes, are unnecessary. The same holds true for high protein bars, a current trend in marketing products to athletes.

*C*onsuming excessive amounts of protein is not without its drawbacks. As noted in Chapter 7, it increases calcium loss in the urine. It also leads to increased urine production, possibly compromising body hydration.

CRITICAL THINKING

Some athletes believe that their diets should consist of 25% of energy intake from protein because they are body building and working out. Your neighbor is a high school baseball player. He has been listening to many professional athletes talk about diet, and he plans to begin consuming 25% of his energy intake from protein. How would you explain to him that this is too much protein?

TABLE 14-6	Grams of Protein That Meet Recommendations for Individuals of Different Weights			
Pounds	Kilograms	RDA (0.8 g/kg)	1.5 × RDA (1.2 g/kg)	2 × RDA (1.6 g/kg)
110	50	40	60	80
130	60	48	72	96
155	70	56	84	112
175	80	64	96	128
200	90	72	108	144
220	100	80	120	160

Compare these quantities with protein intake from the diets listed in Table 14-5. Note that diets supplying enough total energy for athletes yield plenty of protein, even for those who make no special attempt to consume high-protein foods.

especially important in the face of high oxygen use by muscles. Still, the use of megadoses of vitamin E and vitamin C requires more study and is not currently an accepted part of the dietary guidance for athletes.[8] Experts first suggest following a diet containing foods rich in antioxidants, such as fruits, vegetables, whole grains, and vegetable oils. This diet is rich in vitamin C but still does not supply the amount of vitamin E currently used in studies of athletes (about 400 IU/day). Adding this amount of vitamin E to a diet is generally safe; it provides no benefit to exercise performance but may offer some protection from exercise-induced muscle damage, especially for athletes competing at high altitudes.[26] For other nutrients, if supplements are used, intakes below the Upper Level set for each is a safe guide.

Iron Deficiency Impairs Performance

Athletes, especially female and adolescent athletes (if they experience heavy monthly menstrual flows or follow a somewhat low-calorie diet), vegetarians, and distance runners in general, should pay special attention to their iron intake. They are at risk of what is called *sports anemia*. Much of the anemia results from hemodilution, in which the **plasma** volume expands to a greater extent than the red blood cells in response to training. (Note that hemodilutin is also common in pregnancy; see Chapter 16). Although an athlete has increased synthesis of red blood cells, this increase is diluted by an even larger plasma volume and, so, the red blood cell concentration falls. Iron deficiency may also be a cause. Iron status may be compromised by the loss of iron in sweat, urine, and gastrointestinal blood and by the increased use of iron required for the elevated production of red blood cells associated with physical fitness. A minor source of iron loss is foot-strike destruction of red blood cells in the blood passing through the feet; this results from the trauma created at the point of impact when a foot strikes the ground.

If iron status is low and not replenished, iron deficiency anemia and markedly impaired endurance performance can eventually result. Although true anemia (noted as a depressed blood hemoglobin concentration) is not that common among athletes, it is a good idea, especially for adult women athletes, to have their serum ferritin and/or related iron status indicators checked about once a year and to monitor dietary iron intake.[4] To see if iron deficiency is the cause of anemia in an athlete, iron supplements should be given for 1 month, and then the athlete should be retested to see if blood hemoglobin increases by at least 1 g/dl (see Chapter 12 for details on medicinal iron use). If so, the athlete was truly iron depleted, and the therapy was appropriate. A lesser or no response suggests that the problem may have been due merely to hemodilution.

Because iron deficiency can be caused by blood loss, it is important that physicians also investigate the cause of the deficiency. If caught early, some serious medical conditions can be treated or prevented. And, if blood iron is consistently low, the use of iron supplements by an athlete may be advisable. However, indiscriminate use of iron supplements is not advised because toxic effects are possible.

Some studies have suggested that iron deficiency without anemia may still have a negative effect on physical activity and performance. For this reason, athletes must be especially careful not to deplete iron stores.[1]

Calcium Intake Deserves Attention, Especially in Women

Athletes, especially women trying to lose weight by restricting their intake of dairy products, can have marginal or low dietary intakes of calcium. This practice compromises optimal bone health. Of still greater concern are women athletes who have stopped menstruating because their arduous exercise training interferes with the normal secretion of the reproductive hormones. Disturbing reports show that female athletes who do not menstruate regularly have far less dense spinal bones than both nonathletes and female athletes who menstruate regularly. This places them at increased risk for osteoporosis in later life, a risk that outweighs the benefit of weight-bearing exercise on bone density. This is discussed further in Chapter 15,

plasma The fluid, extracellular portion of the blood that results when blood is centrifuged but is not allowed to clot beforehand. This includes the blood serum plus all blood-clotting factors.

*A*t one time in his career, long-distance runner Alberto Salazar experienced problems sleeping and performed poorly because of low iron intake and related iron deficiency anemia.

with respect to the Female Athlete Triad, and in Chapter 11, where osteoporosis was reviewed in detail.

Research has clearly documented the importance of regular menstruation to maintain bone mineral density. Current studies imply that a woman runner who does not menstruate regularly may also have a higher risk for the development of a **stress fracture.** (Intakes below the Adequate Intake for calcium for one's age also increases the risk for stress fractures.) Female athletes whose menstrual cycles become irregular should consult a physician to ascertain the cause. Decreasing the amount of training or increasing energy intake and body weight often restores regular menstrual cycles. If irregular menstrual cycles persist, severe bone loss and osteoporosis can result. Extra calcium in the diet does not necessarily compensate for the effects of menstrual loss, but inadequate dietary calcium can make matters worse. Calcium intakes up to 1500 mg/day have been suggested, but the most effective measure is to have menstruation resume.

■ Fluid Needs

Water (fluid) needs for an average adult are about 1 ml/kcal expended. This is equivalent to about 8 cups of fluid per day. Athletes need this and generally even more water intake to maintain the body's ability to regulate internal temperature and to keep cool. Most energy released during metabolism appears immediately as heat. Furthermore, heat production in contracting muscles can rise 15 to 20 times above that of resting muscles. Unless this heat is quickly dissipated, heat exhaustion, heat cramps, and deadly heatstroke may ensue[9] (Fig. 14 4).

Heat exhaustion occurs when heat stress causes loss of body fluid and then depletion of blood volume. As environmental temperature rises above 95°F (35°C), virtually all body heat is lost through the evaporation of sweat from the skin. Sweat rates during prolonged exercise range from 3 to 8 cups (750 to 2000 ml) per hour. However, as the humidity rises, especially when it rises above 75%, evaporation slows and sweating becomes inefficient. The result is rapid fatigue, increased work for the heart, and difficulty with prolonged exertion. Clearly, for athletes, the combination of heat and humidity can be as dangerous for athletes as extreme cold.

Increased body temperature associated with dehydration is most evident when the amount of water loss exceeds 3% of body weight. This dehydration then leads to a fall in endurance, strength, and overall performance. Wearing football equipment in hot weather can lead to a loss of 2% of body weight in 30 minutes. Marathon runners have been shown to lose 6 to 10% of body weight during a race.

Common symptoms of heat exhaustion include profuse sweating, headache, dizziness, nausea, vomiting, muscle weakness, visual disturbances, and flushing of the skin. A person with heat exhaustion should be taken to a cool environment immediately, and excess clothing should be removed. The body should be sponged with tap water. Fluid replacement, as tolerated, then should suffice.

Heat cramps are a frequent complication of heat exhaustion, but they may appear alone, without other symptoms of dehydration. They usually occur in individuals exercising for several hours in a hot climate who have large sweat losses and have consumed a large volume of unsalted water. It is important not to confuse heat cramps with other forms of muscle cramps, such as those caused by gastrointestinal upset. Heat cramps occur in skeletal muscles, including those of the abdomen and the extremities. They consist of a contraction for 1 to 3 minutes at a time. The cramp moves down the muscle and is associated with excruciating pain. The best way to prevent heat cramps is to exercise moderately at first in the heat, with adequate salt intake, before engaging in long, strenuous exercise.

Heatstroke can occur when internal body temperature reaches 105°F or more. Related symptoms include nausea, confusion, irritability, poor coordination, seizures, and coma (in severe cases). Exertional heatstroke results from high blood flow to exercising muscles, which overloads the body's cooling capacity. Sweating generally ceases, and the body temperature may become dangerously high. If left

Hormone replacement therapy (e.g., estrogen replacement) has been suggested to increase bone density in women who exercise intensely and have irregular menstruation. More research is needed before this therapy can be widely used.

stress fracture A fracture that occurs from repeated jarring of a bone. Common sites include bones of the foot.

heat exhaustion The first stage of heat-related illness that occurs because of depletion of blood volume from fluid loss by the body. This increases body temperature and can lead to headache, dizziness, muscle weakness, and visual disturbances, among other effects.

heat cramps A frequent complication of heat exhaustion. They usually occur in people who have experienced large sweat losses from exercising for several hours in a hot climate and have consumed a large volume of unsalted water. The cramps occur in skeletal muscles and consist of contractions for 1 to 3 minutes at a time.

heatstroke Heatstroke can occur when internal body temperature reaches 105°F. Sweating generally ceases if left untreated, and blood circulation is greatly reduced. Nervous system damage may ensue, and death is likely. Often the skin of individuals who suffer heatstroke is hot and dry.

Heat index

Relative humidity (%) \ Air temperature (°F)	70°	75°	80°	85°	90°	95°	100°	105°	110°
100	72°	80°	91°	108°					
90	71°	79°	88°	102°	122°				
80	71°	78°	86°	97°	113°	136°			
70	70°	77°	85°	93°	106°	124°	144°		
60	70°	76°	82°	90°	100°	114°	132°	149°	
50	69°	75°	81°	88°	96°	107°	120°	135°	150°
40	68°	74°	79°	86°	93°	101°	110°	123°	137°
30	67°	73°	78°	84°	90°	96°	104°	113°	123°
20	66°	72°	77°	82°	87°	93°	99°	105°	112°
10	65°	70°	75°	80°	85°	90°	95°	100°	105°
0	64°	69°	73°	78°	83°	87°	91°	95°	99°

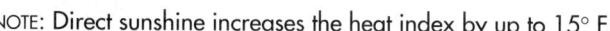

Heat index	Heat disorders possible with prolonged exposure and/or physical activity
80° to 89°	Fatigue
90° to 104°	Sunstroke, heat cramps, and heat exhaustion
105° to 129°	Sunstroke, heat cramps, or heat exhaustion likely and heatstroke possible
130° or higher	Heatstroke/sunstroke highly likely

■ FIGURE 14-4 Heat index chart, showing associated heat disorders.

NOTE: Direct sunshine increases the heat index by up to 15° F.

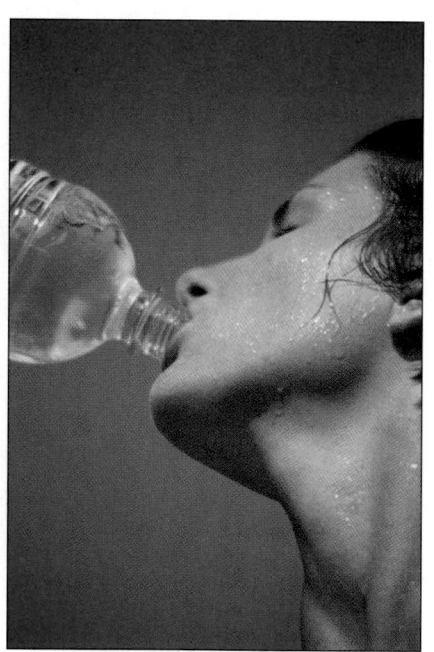

Fluid intake during physical activity is important.

untreated, circulatory collapse, central nervous system damage, and death are likely. Death rate is high, approximately 10%.

Many individuals who suffer heatstroke faint, and their skin becomes hot and dry. Ice packs or cold water is the usual recommended immediate treatment until medical help can be summoned. To decrease the risk of developing heatstroke, athletes should replace lost fluids, watch for rapid body-weight changes (2 to 3% or more of body weight), and avoid exercise under extremely hot, humid conditions.

Since dehydration during exercise leads to body-weight loss and sets the stage for heat exhaustion, heat cramps, and potentially fatal heatstroke, athletes must avoid becoming dehydrated. Fluid intake during exercise, when possible, should be adequate to minimize body-weight loss; this practice is a good idea even in the winter, when sweating can go unnoticed.[29]

The recommended goal is a loss of no more than 3% of body weight during exercise. Athletes should first calculate 2 to 3% of their body weight and then by trial and error determine how much fluid they must take in to avoid losing more than this amount of weight during exercise. This determination will be most accurate if an athlete is weighed before and after a typical workout. For every 1 lb (½ kg) lost, 2 cups (0.5 L) of water should be consumed during exercise or immediately afterward. However, most athletes find it very uncomfortable to replace more than 75 to 80% of this sweat loss during exercise.

Thirst is not a reliable indicator of an athlete's need to replace fluid during exercise. An athlete who drinks only when thirsty is likely to take 48 hours to replenish fluid loss. After several days of training, an athlete relying on thirst as an indicator can build up a large enough fluid debt to impair performance. The following fluid replacement approach can meet athletes' fluid needs in most cases:

- Freely drink beverages (e.g., water, diluted fruit juice, sports drinks) during the 24-hour period before an event, even if not particularly thirsty.
- Drink 1½ to 2½ cups of fluid (400 to 600 ml) 2 to 3 hours before exercise. This allows time for both adequate hydration and excretion of excess fluid.
- During events lasting more than 30 minutes, consume about ½ to 1½ cup (150 to 350 ml) of fluid every 15 to 20 minutes as possible beginning at the start of the exercise. Consuming more than 1 L per hour can cause discomfort. On hot days, cold drinks are preferable to help cool the body. Again, the athlete should not wait until he or she feels thirsty. In many cases, athletes especially children and teenagers, need to be reminded to do this.
- After exercise, about 2 cups of fluid should be consumed for every pound lost. If the weather is hot and/or humid, even more fluids may be required, about 3 cups for every pound lost. Weight should be restored before the next exercise period. Skipping fluids before or during events will almost certainly cause problems.[1, 9]

A question that often arises is whether to drink water or a sports-type carbohydrate-**electrolyte** drink (e.g., All Sport, Exceed Energy Drink, Gatorade, PowerAde, and Amino Force) during competition (Fig. 14-5). For sports that require less than 60 minutes of exertion or when total weight loss is less than 5 to 6 lb, the primary concern is replacing the water lost in sweat, because losses of carbohydrate stores and electrolytes (sodium, chloride, potassium, and other minerals) are not usually too great.[1] Although electrolytes are lost in sweat, the quantities lost in exercise of brief to moderate duration can be easily replaced later by consuming normal foods, such as orange juice, potatoes, and tomato juice. Keep in mind that sweat is about 99% water and only 1% electrolytes and other substances.

Beyond 60 minutes of exertion, electrolyte (e.g., sodium and chloride) and carbohydrate replacement becomes increasingly important, especially in hot weather. Use of a sports drink then provides water for hydration, electrolytes both to enhance water and glucose absorption from the intestine and to help maintain blood volume, as well as carbohydrate to provide energy.

Some experts prefer sports drinks over water for all athletes because sports drinks taste better than water. This may help the athlete drink more often—a clear advantage of this form of fluid replenishment. In addition, the carbohydrate in these drinks quickly replaces carbohydrate used during practice or competition, and the sodium present aids in glucose uptake in the small intestine. In addition, the sodium content stimulates thirst, so athletes drink more.

As mentioned before, optimum performance can be enhanced when carbohydrate is replaced throughout endurance exercise as opposed to replacement only near the end of exercise.[10] For this reason, it may be beneficial for endurance athletes to begin carbohydrate replacement using sports drinks or another convenient source early.

Overall, the decision to use a sports drink hinges primarily on the duration of the activity. As the projected duration of continuous activity approaches 60 minutes or longer, the advantages of the use of a sports drink over plain water begin to emerge. However, athletes should first experiment with the

wo Kansas high school football players and one in North Carolina died in the fall of 1998 from heat illness. Air temperatures were in the 90s to 100s°F during practice. Lack of attention to ongoing fluid replacement caused the deaths.

electrolytes Compounds that separate into ions in water and, in turn, are able to conduct an electrical current. These include sodium, chloride, and potassium.

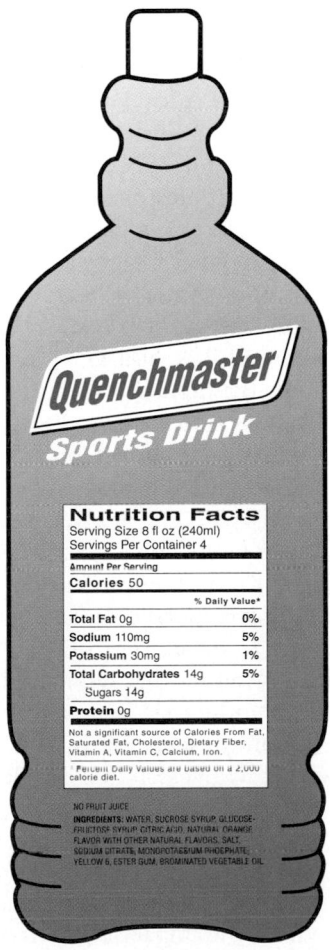

Nutrition Facts
Serving Size 8 fl oz (240ml)
Servings Per Container 4

FIGURE 14-5 Sports drinks for fluid and electrolyte replacement typically contain a form of simple carbohydrate plus sodium and potassium. The various sugars in this product total 14 g per 1 cup (240 ml) serving. In percentage terms based on weight, the sugar content is about 6% ([14 g sugar/serving ÷ 240 g/serving] × 100 = 5.8%). Sports drinks typically contain 6 to 8% sugar. This provides ample glucose and other monosaccharides to aid in fueling working muscles, and it is well tolerated. Drinks with a higher sugar content may cause stomach distress.

Rule of Thumb for Approximate Pre-event Carbohydrate Intake (g)[7]

Hours Before	g/kg Body Weight (70 kg person)
1	1 (70)
2	2 (140)
3	3 (210)
4	4 (280)

suggested protocol during practice, instead of trying it for the first time during competition.[1]

As an alternative to the use of sports drinks for providing a source of carbohydrate during prolonged physical activity, some athletes have begun to use carbohydrate gels (e.g., PowerGel) and so-called energy bars (e.g., PowerBar).[21] The amount to use can be calculated as follows. If one was to use 6 ounces of a sports drink every 15 minutes, this would provide 13 g of carbohydrate. One can use gels or energy bars in order to provide the same amount of carbohydrate (check the label for grams of carbohydrate per serving). Interestingly, one fig cookie also provides the 13 g carbohydrate dose (Gummy Bears work as well). Note that any use of these alternate carbohydrate sources must be accompanied by water consumption. In this way, the goal of fluid *and* carbohydrate replacement from the sports drink will be realized. Another thing to consider when using gels and energy bars is that they are relatively expensive.

It is also possible to drink too much water. Ultra-endurance athletes compete at relatively low exercise intensities for prolonged periods of time and therefore may not sweat as much as one might predict. Thus, water losses are not very high. In addition, some of these athletes have used one-half strength Coca-Cola as their fluid-replacement beverage, which is relatively low in sodium, and they drink this at every rest stop. This combination leads to hyperhydration, low blood sodium, and low blood chloride. Drinking less fluid and choosing a sports drink containing sodium chloride can help prevent this problem.[1]

■ Meals Before Endurance Events Should Emphasize Carbohydrate

A light meal supplying 300 to 1000 kcal should be eaten about 2 to 4 hours before an endurance event to top off muscle and liver glycogen stores, prevent hunger during the event, and provide extra fluid. The longer the period before an event, the larger the meal can be, as there will be more time available for digestion. A pre-event meal should consist primarily of carbohydrate, have little fat (<25% of energy intake) or dietary fiber, and include a moderate amount of protein (Table 14-7).[1] A pre-event meal eaten 1 to 2 hours before an event should be blended or liquid to promote rapid stomach emptying.

Good food choices for a pre-event meal include spaghetti, bagels, muffins, bread, bananas, apples, oranges, and breakfast cereals with low-fat or nonfat milk. Liquid meal-replacement formulas, such as Carnation Instant Breakfast, also can be used. Foods rich in dietary fiber should be eaten the previous day to help empty the colon before an event, but they should not be eaten the night before or in the morning before the event. Foods to avoid are those that are fatty or fried, such as sausage, bacon, sauces, and gravies. A meal high in carbohydrate is quickly digested, promotes maintenance of blood glucose, and avoids the need to dip right away into glycogen stores.

The selection of carbohydrates for the pre-event meal (and postevent meal) based on their glycemic index is becoming increasingly popular among athletes (see Chapter 5 for a review of glycemic index and a table of values for specific foods).[5] The rationale behind this practice is that the glycemic index of a carbohydrate is a major influence on the insulin response to that carbohydrate: high-glycemic-index carbohydrates generally cause high insulin responses, and low-glycemic-index carbohydrates result in lower insulin responses. You know, of course, that insulin is one of the hormones that regulates blood glucose.

An endurance athlete may wish to choose a low-glycemic-index food before an event in the attempt to achieve a moderate and sustained increase in blood glucose, which will lessen the insulin response (see Table 5-6). This decreased insulin response, in turn, may allow for greater access to the fatty acids from the adipose tissue as a fuel source, preserving glycogen stores for when they are needed late in the race.[1]

In such a pre-event situation, there have been a number of studies that have examined the impact of the feeding of low-glycemic-index foods and high-glycemic-

TABLE 14-7	Convenient Pre-event Meals

Breakfast

Cheerios, ¾ cup	450 kcal
2% milk, 1 cup	82% carbohydrate
Blueberry muffin, 1	(92 grams)
Orange juice, 4 oz	
Low-fat fruit yogurt, 1 cup	482 kcal
Plain bagel, ½	68% carbohydrate
Apple juice, 4 oz	(84 grams)
Peanut butter (for bagel), 1 tbsp	
Whole-wheat toast, 1 slice	491 kcal
Apple, 1 large	73% carbohydrate
2% milk, 1 cup	(94 grams)
Oatmeal, ½ cup	
2% milk, ½ cup	

Lunch or Dinner

Chili with beans, 8 oz	900 kcal
Baked potato with sour cream and chives	65% carbohydrate
Chocolate Frosty	(150 grams)
Spaghetti noodles, 2 cups	761 kcal
Spaghetti sauce, 1 cup	66% carbohydrate
2% milk, 1½ cups	(129 grams)
Green beans, 1 cup	
Orange, 1 large	829 kcal
2% milk, 1½ cups	70% carbohydrate
Chicken noodle soup, 1 cup	(160 grams)
Saltine crackers, 12	
Buttered beans, 1 cup	
Corn, 1 cup	
Angel food cake, 1 slice	

With regard to the timing of preactivity meals, the rule of thumb is to allow 4 hours for a big meal (about 1200 kcal), 3 hours for a moderate meal (about 800–900 kcal), 2 hours for a light meal (about 400–600 kcal), and an hour or less for a snack (about 300 kcal).

index foods 45 minutes to 1 hour prior to exercise. In general, these studies have shown a more favorable metabolic profile for endurance performance—lower blood insulin, higher blood free fatty acids, and more stable blood glucose—with low- versus high-glycemic-index pre-event meals. However, not all these studies have shown improved endurance exercise performance with low-glycemic-index foods.[1] Still, no detrimental effects have been observed, compared with higher-glycemic-index foods.

If an athlete feels a pre-event meal harms performance, eating a high-carbohydrate diet the day and night before can help meet the same goal. Overall, athletes should experiment with various pre-event carbohydrate feedings to see whether their performance is adversely or positively affected.

■ Carbohydrate Intake During Recovery from Prolonged Exercise

Carbohydrate-rich foods yielding about 1.5 g of carbohydrate per kg body weight should be consumed within 2 hours after extended (endurance) exercise, and the sooner the better, because this is when glycogen synthesis is greatest, as the muscles are very insulin-sensitive at this point.[1] This process should then be repeated over the next 2-hour interval. Athletes who are training hard can consume a simple sugar candy, sugared soft drink, fruit or fruit juice, or a sports-type carbohydrate

For more information on sports medicine, visit http://www.physsportsmed.com on the Web. This home page of *The Physician and Sportsmedicine* journal details current issues in sports medicine, including injury prevention, nutrition, and exercise. Also helpful are the web pages of the Gatorade Sports Science Institute (http://www.gssiweb.com), American College of Sports Medicine (http://www.acsm.org), Centers for Disease Control (http://www.cdc.gov/nccdphp/dnpa), and the American Council on Exercise (http://www.acefitness.org).

supplement right after training as they attempt to reload their muscles with glycogen. Later bread, mashed potatoes, and rice can contribute further carbohydrate. All these high-glycemic-index carbohydrates especially contribute to glycogen synthesis. Adding some rich protein sources is also recommended, with carbohydrate to protein in a 3:1 ratio. For a 154-lb (70-kg) athlete, this corresponds to about 70 g carbohydrate and 25 g protein in each 2-hour interval (see Table 14-8 for sample meals of this composition). In summary, the following are key factors for achieving the most rapid replenishment of muscle glycogen after exercise: (1) availability of adequate carbohydrate, (2) ingestion of carbohydrate as soon as possible after completion of exercise, (3) selection of high-glycemic-index carbohydrates, (4) combination of carbohydrate and protein foods, rather than either carbohydrate or protein alone.

Fluid and electrolyte (i.e., sodium and potassium) intake is also an essential component of an athlete's recovery diet. This helps replenish body fluids as quickly as possible. This is especially important if two workouts a day are followed and if the environment is hot and humid. If food and fluid intake is sufficient to restore weight loss, it generally will also supply enough electrolytes to meet needs during recovery from endurance activities.[1]

CASE SCENARIO
Follow-Up

Marcella is correct in following a high-carbohydrate diet. However, in her effort to minimize her fat intake, she is probably not consuming enough calories to support her training routine. Her diet is also low in protein. She has fallen into the bagel, pasta, and pretzel routine that sports nutritionists warn is not conducive to peak performance. Marcella would be smart to have a high-protein source at each meal. She could include milk with breakfast and possibly some low-fat yogurt or low-fat cheese at lunch. She should have a carbohydrate/protein snack before her workout, such as a half a sandwich and fruit and some water. The sandwich and fruit will help provide her with fuel to support her vigorous training. During her workouts, she could consume a sports drink to meet fluid needs and supply some carbohydrate, or she could consume water, along with a few fig cookies to provide the carbohydrate. In the evenings, she could substitute oil and vinegar dressing for the fat-free dressing on her salad and cheese and crackers for the pretzels to improve protein intake. Overall, it is important for Marcella to fuel her body before, during, and after workouts.

CONCEPT CHECK

All athletes would do well to plan a diet following the Food Guide Pyramid. High-carbohydrate foods should be emphasized, and these should dominate in pre-event meals. Protein intake above twice the RDA is not needed in most cases. If nutrient supplements are used, dosages generally should not exceed the Upper Level set for each nutrient. Fluid should be consumed as liberally as possible before, during, and after an event. Carbohydrate and electrolytes in the fluid are especially helpful when exercise duration is expected to exceed 60 minutes to help delay fatigue and maintain electrolyte balance.

TABLE 14-8 Sample Postexercise Meals for Rapid Muscle Glycogen Replacement

Option 1

1 regular bagel
2 tbsp peanut butter, smooth
8 fl oz skim milk
1 medium banana
562 kcal, 77 g carbohydrate, 23 g protein, 18 g fat

Option 2

1 packet, Carnation Instant Breakfast
8 oz skim milk
1 medium banana
1 tbsp peanut butter
Blend until smooth.
438 kcal, 70 g carbohydrate, 17 g protein, 10 g fat

Option 3

1.5 cans GatorPro (11 fl oz/can)
559 kcal, 89 g carbohydrate, 26 g protein, 11 g fat

SUMMARY

1. A gradual increase in regular physical activity is recommended for all healthy persons. A minimum plan includes at least a total of 30 minutes of physical activity per day. A more intense program should begin with warm-up exercises, to increase blood flow and warm the muscles, and end with cooldown exercises. Regular resistance activities and stretching add further benefits.

2. Human metabolic pathways extract chemical energy from food and transforms it into ATP, the compound that provides energy for body functions.

3. In glycolysis, glucose is broken down (oxidized) into pyruvate, a three-carbon compound, yielding some ATP. The pyruvate is metabolized further via the aerobic pathway to form carbon dioxide (CO_2) and water (H_2O) or via the anaerobic pathway to form lactate.

4. At rest, muscle cells mainly use fat for fuel. For intense exercise of short duration, muscles mostly use phosphocreatine (PCr) for energy. During more sustained intense activity, muscle glycogen breaks down to lactate. For endurance exercise, both fat and carbohydrate are used as fuels; carbohydrate is used increasingly as activity intensifies. Little protein is used to fuel muscles.

5. $VO_{2\ max}$ is a measure of the maximum volume of oxygen one can consume per unit of time. Oxygen consumption is measured by exercising the subject at an increasing pace and workload until fatigue occurs. The amount of oxygen consumed right before total exhaustion is $VO_{2\ max}$. The value of $VO_{2\ max}$ varies among individuals but usually improves with exercise training.

6. Anyone who exercises regularly should consume a diet that meets energy needs and is moderate to high in carbohydrates and fluid.

7. Athletes should consume enough fluid to both minimize loss of body weight and ultimately restore preexercise weight. Sports drinks aid fluid, electrolyte, and carbohydrate replacement. Their use especially should be considered when continuous activity lasts beyond 60 minutes.

8. High-glycemic-index carbohydrates should be consumed by an athlete within 2 hours after a workout to begin restoration of muscle glycogen stores. Some protein in the meal is also helpful. The use of low-glycemic-index carbohydrates in the pre-event meal may help some endurance athletes.

STUDY QUESTIONS

1. How does greater physical fitness contribute to greater aerobic metabolism? Explain the process.

2. The store of ATP in muscle is rapidly depleted once contraction begins. For physical activity to continue, ATP must be resupplied immediately. Describe how this occurs after initiation of physical activity and at various times thereafter.

3. What is the difference between anaerobic and aerobic exercise? At what point is the switch made from mostly anaerobic to mostly aerobic fuel metabolism? Explain how aerobic metabolism is enhanced by a regular exercise routine.

4. What is glycogen? How does the body obtain it? How much can be stored? How long does it last during exercise?

5. Are fat stores used as an energy source during exercise? If so, when?

6. What is the typical measure of physical fitness? Explain the physiological/biochemical bases for why this is an appropriate measure.

7. Physical activity can be classified into four types: low intensity; moderate intensity; prolonged high intensity (endurance); and brief maximal intensity (very high intensity). Compare and contrast the four types of exercise with respect to the percentage of $VO_{2\ max}$ used and the specific fuels used.

8. List five specific nutrients that athletes need and a nutrient-rich food source for each.

9. What advice would you give to your neighbor, who is planning to run a 50-kilometer (km) race, concerning fluid intake before and during the event?

10. One of your friends, who is a competitive athlete, asks your opinion about a nutritional supplement sold in a local sporting-goods store. She has read that such supplements, which contain vitamins, minerals, and amino acids, can help improve athletic performance. What would you tell her about the general effectiveness of such products?

*C*heck out the *Perspectives in Nutrition* Online Learning Center http://www.mhhe.com/wardlaw for quizzes, flash cards, other activities, and web links designed to further help you learn about sports nutrition.

■ ANNOTATED REFERENCES

1. American College of Sports Medicine and others: Nutrition and Athletic Performance, *Medicine & Science in Sports & Exercise* 32:2130, 2000.

   The athlete who wants to optimize exercise performance needs to follow good nutrition and hydration practices, use supplements and ergogenic aids carefully, minimize severe weight loss practices, and eat a variety of foods in adequate amounts.

2. American College of Sports Medicine: *ACSM's guidelines for exercise testing and prescription.* 6th ed. Philadelphia: Lippincott, Williams & Wilkins, 2000.

   Detailed protocols are listed for exercise testing and exercise prescriptions by the American College of Sports Medicine. This is a reference for all health professionals in the practice of sports nutrition.

3. Anderson RE: Exercise, an active lifestyle, and obesity. *The Physician and Sportsmedicine* 27 (10): 41, 1999.

   Traditional advice about vigorous exercise may need to be modified to increase rates of adoption and compliance. Recent evidence suggests that accumulating several short bouts of moderate to vigorous activity each day may improve adherence to an exercise program

4. Beard J, Tobin B: Iron status and exercise. *American Journal of Clinical Nutrition* 72 (Suppl): 594S, 2000.

   Athletes most likely to develop iron deficiency anemia are female athletes in general, distance runners, and vegetarian athletes. These groups are advised to pay particular attention to maintaining adequate amounts of iron in their diets. They also may want to consider using low-dose iron supplements under medical supervision.

5. Burke LM and others: Glycemic index—A new tool in sport nutrition? *International Journal of Sport Nutrition* 8: 401, 1998.

   With regard to using the glycemic index in planning diets for athletes, the clearest evidence is that moderate- to high-glycemic-index carbohydrates appear to enhance glycogen storage when consumed after exercise. There is insufficient evidence to indicate that a low-glycemic-index meal prior to exercise provides performance benefits.

6. Cheuvront SN: The zone diet and athletic performance. *Sports Medicine* 27: 213, 1999.

   Measurable improvements in endurance activities can be achieved by following a high-carbohydrate diet. This recommendation profoundly opposes that of The Zone Diet, which suggests that only 40% of calories come from carbohydrates. Thus, The Zone Diet is not recommended for improving performance in endurance athletes.

7. Clark N: *Nancy Clark's sports nutrition guidebook.* Champaign, IL: Human Kinetics, 1997.

   It is very important to meet daily energy needs during a training regimen. Otherwise, performance and endurance can suffer. The best advice is to fuel before, during, and after a training session. Other important advice is available in this comprehensive look at sports nutrition.

8. Clarkson PM, Thompson HS: Antioxidants: What role do they play in physical activity and health? *American Journal of Clinical Nutrition* 72(Suppl): 637S, 2000.

   There is general agreement that following a diet rich in antioxidants for all those who exercise regularly is beneficial. At present, data are insufficient to recommend antioxidant supplements for athletes or other persons who exercise regularly. With respect to vitamin E, such supplements do not appear to enhance exercise performance but may offer protection from exercise-induced muscle damage, although study results are equivocal.

9. Convertino VA and others: Exercise and fluid replacement: Position stand of the American College of Sports Medicine. *Medicine and Science in Sports and Exercise* 28(1): i, 1996.

   Athletes should drink about 500 ml of fluid about 2 hours before exercise. The addition of proper amounts of carbohydrate and/or electrolytes to a fluid replacement solution is recommended for exercise events of duration greater than 1 hour. Carbohydrate intake should be about 30–60 grams per hour, using a 4 to 8% carbohydrate solution that contains 0.5–0.7 g/liter of sodium.

10. Coyle E: Physical activity as a metabolic stressor. *American Journal of Clinical Nutrition* 72(Suppl): 512S, 2000.

    Blood glucose is a minor source of fuel during exercise lasting less than 30 minutes. As exercise duration increases to an hour or more, blood glucose becomes increasingly important, especially after 2 hours. Consuming carbohydrate during endurance exercise can help maintain blood glucose and reduce fatigue.

11. Get strong, get healthy. *Consumer Reports on Health*, p. 6, June 1999.

    Strength training can prevent or reverse muscle loss, making one far more mobile, active, and energetic than before. As well, it is never too late to start, and, the weaker one is, the more one stands to gain from strength training.

12. Getting active, staying active. Washington, DC: American Institute for Cancer Research, 1999.

    Exercise gets easier as one's body adapts. Before long, physical activity becomes a way of life—something one is eager to get back to after a break and something that is an enjoyable, comfortable part of the day.

13. Glass TA and others: Population based study of social and productive activities as predictors of survival among elderly Americans. *British Medical Journal* 319: 478, 1999.

    There is a strong survival advantage seen in people who remain active throughout life. This activity need not be strenuous and can include activity in traveling, gardening, and employment.

14. Horvath PJ: The effects of varying dietary fat on the nutrient intake in male and female runners. *Journal of the American College of Nutrition* 19: 42, 2000.

    Endurance runners may not be consuming enough calories on a low-fat diet. Increasing dietary fat will increase energy consumption. On a low-fat diet, essential fatty acids and some minerals (especially zinc) also may be too low.

15. Hu FB and others: Physical activity and risk of stroke in women. *Journal of the American Medical Association* 283: 2961, 2000.

    Moderate-intensity exercise, such as walking, is associated with a substantial reduction in risk of total and ischemic stroke in a dose-response manner.

16. JAMA Patient Page: The benefits of regular physical activity. *Journal of the American Medical Association* 283: 3030, 2000.

    Physical activity is one habit that should be unbreakable if one wants to maintain or improve health. It is not necessary to exercise all in one session—several 10- to 15-minute sessions can be just as effective.

17. Juhn MS: Oral creatine supplementation. *The Physician and Sportsmedicine* 27(5): 47, 1999.

    Creatine supplements appear to enhance performance in repeated, short bursts of stationary cycling and weight lifting, but the data on running, swimming, and single cycle sprints are not convincing of an ergogenic effect. Commonly reported side effects include muscle cramping, GI disturbances, kidney dysfunction, and possibly other organ damage.

18. King DS and others: The effect of oral androstenedione on serum testosterone and adaptations to resistance training in young men: A randomized controlled trial. *Journal of the American Medical Association* 281: 2020, 1999.

    Androstenedione does not enhance adaptations to resistance training and may result in potentially serious adverse health consequences in young men, such as a decrease in HDL-cholesterol.

19. Lee CO and others: Cardiorespiratory fitness, body composition, and all-cause and cardiovascular disease mortality in men. *American Journal of Clinical Nutrition* 69: 373, 1999.

   The health benefits of leanness are limited to fit men, and being fit may reduce the health hazards of obesity. Obese people should be encouraged to increase their cardiorespiratory fitness by engaging in regular, moderate-intensity physical activity; this provides benefits even when remaining overweight.

20. Lemon PWR: Beyond the Zone: Protein needs for active individuals, *Journal of the American College of Nutrition* 19:513S, 2000.

   Studies indicate that for physically active individuals daily protein intake needs could be as high as 1.6–1.8 g/kg (about twice the current recommendation). Despite these increased protein needs, assuming energy intake is sufficient to match the additional expenditures of training and competition (which can be excessive), special protein supplementation is unnecessary for most who consume a varied diet containing complete protein foods (meat, fish, eggs, and dairy products).

21. Ling N: Performance foods for active individuals: Sports drinks, energy bars and energy gels. *Today's Dietitian*, p. 26, March 2000.

   Sports drinks, energy bars, and energy gels are unnecessary for short workouts. If a preexercise meal or snack has been consumed, use need not begin until an hour into a workout. Bars and gels should be consumed with at least 8 ounces of water, but not with sports drinks. For high-intensity workouts, such as track running or swimming, an energy gel may be a better choice than an energy bar.

22. Manson, JE and others: A prospective study of walking as compared with vigorous exercise in the prevention of coronary heart disease in women. *New England Journal of Medicine* 341: 650, 1999.

   Brisk walking and other vigorous exercise are associated with a substantial reduction in heart attack risk in women. Enormous public health benefits would accrue from the adoption of regular, moderate-intensity exercise by those who are currently sedentary.

23. Manore MM: Effect of physical activity on thiamine, riboflavin, and vitamin B-6 requirements. *American Journal of Clinical Nutrition* 72(Suppl): 598S, 2000.

   Active individuals who restrict their energy intake or make poor dietary choices are at risk for poor B-vitamin status. However, the amount of these nutrients needed to cover losses or increased needs resulting from physical activity is small and can be met easily through wise food choices.

24. Marcus BH and others: The efficacy of exercise as an aide for smoking cessation in women. *Archives of Internal Medicine* 159: 1229, 1999.

   Relatively intense exercise appears to improve success in traditional smoking cessation programs. It also can decrease the weight gain expected from smoking cessation.

25. Roach M: Give yourself a lift. *Health*, p. 69, March 1999.

   Strength training is a growing trend among women. Six essential exercises are leg press, lateral pull-down, calf raise, seated chest press, crunch, and seated row.

26. Sarubin A: The Health Professionals Guide to Popular Dietary Supplements, The American Dietetic Association, Chicago Ill, 2000.

   The author provides a detailed look at individual dietary supplements, including those used by athletes. One example is creatine, which can increase strength/power during short bouts of exercise.

27. Shepard RJ, Shek PN: Exercise, immunity, and susceptibility to infection. *The Physician and Sportsmedicine* 27(6): 47, 1999.

   Regular, moderate-intensity exercise enhances immune function. Vigorous exercise may temporarily reduce resistance to viral infection. Persons who have such symptoms should avoid competition and heavy training until these remit.

28. Smith SR and others: Concurrent physical activity increases fat oxidation during a shift to a high fat diet. *American Journal of Clinical Nutrition* 72: 131, 2000.

   Physical activity increases fat oxidation. This may be especially important for people who consume a high-fat diet, in turn blunting the tendency for this type of diet to cause weight gain.

29. Sparling PB, Millard-Stafford M: Keeping sports participants safe in hot weather. *The Physician and Sportsmedicine* 27(7): 27, 1999.

   Sound strategies for sports participation in hot weather include heat acclimatization 10 to 14 days before competition. Prudent hydration includes drinking plenty of fluid 2 hours before exercise, 5 to 10 ounces of fluid every 10–15 minutes during exercise, and fluids containing sodium after exercise.

30. Steen SN, Coleman E: Selected ergogenic aids used by athletes. *Nutrition in Clinical Practice* 14: 287, 1999.

   Most athletes are not aware that the safety and efficacy of current ergonomic aids have not been established, and need not be, by FDA. Currently, ergogenic aids are typically marketed without any scientific claims, nor do they warn of possible adverse side effects.

31. Success stories: How the experts stay active. Consumer Reports on Health, p. 8, April 1999.

   Many experts find that they stick to their exercise best when they exercise early in the day. In essence, one can plan how the day will start, but not necessarily how the day is going to end. The workouts they enjoy doing most are the ones they are likely to keep doing.

32. Ten exercise myths. *Nutrition Action Health Letter*, p. 1, January/February 2000.

   Many people believe that you have to work at a very high intensity in order to get the benefits of exercise. In fact, moderate-intensity exercise lowers the risk of death just as much as high-intensity exercise does. Overall, regular exercise has numerous health benefits.

33. United States Department of Health and Human Services: *Physical activity and health: A report of the surgeon general.* Atlanta: U.S. Department of Health and Human Services, Centers for Disease Control and Prevention, National Center for Chronic Disease Prevention and Health Promotion, 1996.

   Moderate-intensity exercise of 30 minutes a day—broken into three 10-minute sessions, if necessary—provides substantial health benefits. Currently, many Americans follow a primarily sedentary lifestyle.

TAKE ACTION

I. IS YOUR DIET MEASURING UP TO THE NUMBERS?

In this chapter, several key nutrients were discussed in relation to exercise performance. The following guidelines were mentioned, not only for athletes but for everyone maintaining generally good fitness.

- Eat a moderate to high amount of carbohydrates generally (generally 60% or more of total energy intake).
- Athletes should eat a minimum of 1.2 grams of protein per kilogram of body weight.
- Consume the recommended standards of vitamins and minerals, making sure iron and calcium intakes are adequate (especially for women).
- Consume enough fluid, especially to maintain weight during prolonged exercise or in hot conditions.

Review the results of the dietary assessment you completed in Chapter 2. Remember that you analyzed a 1 day food intake. Now answer the following questions, whether or not you consider yourself an athlete.

1. What percentage of your energy intake came from carbohydrate? Was your carbohydrate intake 60% or more of your total energy intake?

   _____

2. Did you eat at least 0.8 gram of protein per kilogram of body weight? If you are an athlete, did you consume at least 1.2 grams per kilogram of body weight? Did intake exceed 1.8 grams per kilogram of body weight?

   _____

   _____

3. Did you consume your estimated needs of all vitamins and minerals, especially iron and calcium? Which ones were below the current nutrient standards?

   _____

   _____

4. For nutrients low in your diet, list one rich food source (see Chapters 9 through 12).

   _____

   _____

5. Did you consume sufficient fluid—about 8 cups for a good starting point?

   _____

   _____

6. What can you do to improve your dietary intake to aid general fitness and, if you are an athlete, to promote maximal performance in your chosen event(s)?

   _____

   _____

   _____

   _____

TAKE ACTION

II. EVALUATING PROTEIN INTAKE—A CASE STUDY

Marcus is a college student who has been lifting weights at the student recreation center. The trainer at the center recommended a protein drink to help Marcus build muscle mass. Evaluate Marcus's current food intake and determine whether a protein drink is needed to supplement Marcus's diet.

1. The following is a tally of yesterday's intake.

Breakfast	Frosted Mini-Wheats cereal, 2 oz
	1% milk, 1½ cups
	Orange juice, chilled, 6 oz
	Glazed yeast doughnut, 1
	Brewed coffee, 1 cup
Lunch	Double hamburger with condiments, 1
	French fries, 30
	Cola, 12 oz
	Medium apple, 1
Dinner	Frozen lasagna w/meat, 2 pieces
	1% milk, 1 cup
	Looseleaf lettuce, chopped, 1 cup
	Creamy Italian salad dressing, 2 tsp
	Medium tomato, ½
	Whole carrot, raw, 1
Evening snack	Vanilla ice milk, 1 cup
	Hot fudge chocolate topping, 2 tsp
	Soft chocolate chip cookies, 2

Evaluate Marcus's diet—is he meeting the minimum recommendations of the Food Guide Pyramid? _____

2. Marcus's weight has been stable at 70 kilograms (154 pounds). Determine his protein needs based on the RDA (0.8 grams per kilogram).

   a. Marcus's estimated protein RDA: _____

   b. What are the maximum recommendations for protein intake for strength-training athletes (see p. 579)? _____

   c. Apply the maximum recommendations to Marcus. _____
   _____

3. An analysis of the total kcal and protein content of Marcus's current diet is 3470 kcal, 125 grams of protein (14% of total calories supplied by protein). This diet is representative of the food choices and amounts of food that Marcus chooses on a regular basis.

   a. What is the difference between Marcus's estimated protein needs as an athlete (from Exercise 2) and the amount of protein that his current diet provides? _____

   b. Is his current protein intake inadequate, adequate, or excessive? _____

4. Marcus takes his trainer's advice and goes to the supermarket to purchase a protein drink to add to his diet. Four products are available; they contain the following label information.

	Amino Fuel	Joe Weider's Sugar-Free 90% Plus Protein	Joe Weider's Dynamic Muscle Builder	Victory Super Mega Mass 2000
Serving size	3 tbsp	3 tbsp	3 tbsp	¼ scoop
Kcal	104	110	103	104
Protein (grams)	15	24	10	5

TAKEACTION

The trainer recommends adding the supplement to Marcus's diet two times a day. Marcus chooses Joe Weider's Dynamic Muscle Builder.

a. How much protein would be added to Marcus's diet daily from two servings of the supplement alone (prior to mixing it with a beverage)?

b. Marcus mixes the powder with 8 ounces of milk at breakfast and dinner. How much protein total would Marcus now consume in 1 day? (Add the protein amount from the nutrition analysis to the value from the previous question.)

c. What is the difference between Marcus's estimated protein needs as an athlete and this total value?

5. What is your conclusion—does Marcus need the protein supplement?

Answers to Calculations

2a. Marcus's estimated protein RDA: 70 kilograms × 0.8 g/kg = 56 g

2b. Maximum recommendation for protein intake for athletes = 1.8g/kg

2c. Applied to Marcus: 1.8 × 70 = 126 g

3a. Difference between Marcus's estimated maximum protein needs if an athlete and the amount of protein provided by his current diet: 126 − 125 = 1 g protein

3b. Marcus's current diet is adequate

4a. Two servings of protein supplement alone = 20 g of protein

4b. Marcus's total protein consumption: 125 g + 20 g = 145 g protein

4c. Difference between Marcus's estimated maximum protein needs as an athlete and total value (from above): 145 g − 126 g = 19 g protein

EVALUATING ERGOGENIC AIDS TO ENHANCE ATHLETIC PERFORMANCE

Diet manipulation to improve athletic performance is not a recent innovation. As long as 30 years ago, American football players were encouraged on hot practice days to "toughen up" for competition by liberally consuming salt tablets before and during practice and by not drinking water. Now it is widely recognized that this practice can be fatal. Today's athletes are as likely as their predecessors to experiment with artichoke hearts, bee pollen, dried adrenal glands from cattle, seaweed, freeze-dried liver flakes, gelatin, and ginseng. These are just some of the ineffective substances used by athletes in hopes of gaining an ergogenic (work-producing) edge.

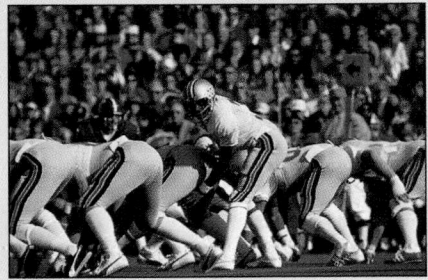

Attention to energy, carbohydrate, and fluid needs—along with overall nutrient needs—is the most important ergogenic aid.

Still, today's athletes can benefit from recent scientific evidence documenting the ergogenic properties of a few dietary substances. These ergogenic aids include sufficient water, lots of carbohydrates, and a balanced and varied diet consistent with the Food Guide Pyramid. Protein and amino acid supplements are not among those aids because athletes can easily meet protein needs from foods, as Table 14-4 demonstrated. Clearly, changing average athletes into champions is not possible simply by altering their diets. The use of nutrient supplements should be designed to meet a specific dietary shortcomings, such as an inadequate iron intake. These and other aids, which often have dubious benefits and may pose health risks, must be given close scrutiny before use. The risk-benefit ratio of any ergogenic aids especially needs to be examined.

As summarized in Table 14-9, no scientific evidence supports the effectiveness of many substances touted as performance-enhancing aids.[1, 30] Many are useless; some are dangerous. Athletes should be skeptical of any substance until its ergogenic effect is scientifically verified. FDA has a limited ability to regulate these dietary supplements (see the Nutrition Perspective in Chapter 18). As well, the manufacturing processes for dietary supplements are not as tightly regulated by FDA as they are for prescription drugs. Recent studies have called into question the quality control associated with the manufacturing of dietary supplements. For example, a study looked at 16 brands of dehydroepiandrosterone (DHEA) purchased from health-food stores. As noted in Table 14-9, DHEA is a supplement that is claimed to increase muscle mass, decrease body fat, and increase blood testosterone. The study showed that only 7 of the 16 brands had a DHEA content within 90 to 110% of the stated label claim; 3 products had essentially no DHEA at all.

These results add yet another worry for the athlete. Not only must the athlete determine whether there is evidence that a dietary supplement is safe and effective (FDA does not regulate dietary supplements) but now must also question if the dietary supplement contains what it is supposed to contain. To obtain information on independent laboratory tests on the quality of dietary supplements, the following web site is helpful: http://www.consumerlab.com. Even substances whose ergogenic effects have been supported by systematic scientific studies should be used with caution, as the testing conditions may not match those of the intended use.

Finally, rather than waiting for a magic bullet to enhance performance, athletes are advised to concentrate their efforts on improving their training routines and sport technique and consuming well-balanced diets, as described in this chapter. Adequate calories, fluid, and carbohydrate are the primary diet-related ergogenic aids.[1]

TABLE 14-9   An Evaluation of Ergogenic Aids Currently in the Limelight[1, 17, 18, 20, 26, 30]

Substance/Practice	Rationale	Reality
Useful in Some Circumstances		
Creatine	Increased phosphocreatine (PCr)	Use of 20 grams per day for 5 to 6 days and then a maintenance dose of 2 grams per day may improve performance in those who undertake repeated bursts of activity, such as in sprinting and weight lifting. Some of the muscle weight gain noted with use results from water retention. Little is known about the safety of long-term creatine use. Cost: $25–$65/month.
Bicarbonate	Counter lactic acid buildup	Partially effective in some circumstances, such as wrestling, but induces nausea and diarrhea. The dose used is 300 mg/kg, given 1–3 hours before exercise.
Caffeine	Increase use of fatty acids to fuel muscles, promote psychological effects	Drinking two to three 5-ounce cups of coffee (equivalent to 3–9 milligrams of caffeine per kilogram of body weight) about 1 hour before events lasting about 5 minutes or longer is useful for some athletes; benefits are less apparent in those who have ample stores of glycogen, are highly trained, or habitually consume caffeine; intake of more than about 600 milligrams (six to eight cups of coffee) elicits a urine concentration illegal under Olympic rules (12 micrograms per milliliter). A possible side-effect is reduced body hydration.
Possibly Useful, Still Under Study		
Beta-hydroxy-beta methylbutyric acid (HMB)	Decrease protein catabolism, causing a net growth-promoting effect	Research in livestock and humans suggests that supplementation with this may increase muscle mass. Still, safety and effectiveness of long-term HMB use in humans is unknown. Cost: $100/month
Glutamine	Enhance immune function, preserve lean body mass	Glutamine is the most abundant amino acid in plasma, and preservation of lean body mass levels fall in glycogen-depleted athletes. Overtrained athletes also have lower glutamine levels. Glutamine may be conditionally essential during metabolic stress and critical illness, and it is important for immunity. Some preliminary studies show decreased occurrence of upper respiratory tract infections in athletes with use. It also may promote muscle growth, but long-term studies are lacking.
Branched-chain amino acids (BCAA) (leucine, isoleucine, valine)	Important energy source, especially when carbohydrate stores are depleted. A high ratio of free tryptophan: BCAA in the brain increases serotonin in the brain, which depresses the central nervous system and causes fatigue	Supplementation of BCAA during exercise can increase BCAA in the blood when it has been lowered due to exercise, but there is no consistent evidence of improved performance. Carbohydrate feeding, by delaying use of BCAA as fuel, may negate the need for BCAA supplementation. Preliminary studies show that BCAA use increases muscle mass more than does carbohydrate supplementation alone in swimmers, but there are no studies regarding resistance training. Protein-rich foods are also rich in BCAA.
Useful in Some Circumstances, but Dangerous or Illegal		
Anabolic steroids	Increase muscle mass and strength	Although effective, are illegal in the United States; have numerous potential side effects, such as premature closure of growth plates in bones (thus possibly limiting the adult height of a teenage athlete), bloody cysts in the liver, increased risk of heart disease, high blood pressure, and reproductive dysfunction. Possible psychological consequences include increased aggressiveness, drug dependence (addiction), withdrawal symptoms (such as depression), sleep disturbances, and mood swings. Banned by the International Olympic Committee.
Growth hormone	Increase muscle mass	At critical ages may increase height; may also cause uncontrolled growth of the heart and other internal organs and even death; potentially dangerous; requires careful monitoring by a physician. Banned by the International Olympic Committee.

TABLE 14-9 continued

Substance/Practice	Rationale	Reality
Blood doping	Red blood cells harvested previously from the athlete and then injected into the bloodstream, or alternately the athlete may use the hormone erythropoietin (Epogen) to increase red blood cell number in order to try to enhance aerobic capacity	May offer aerobic benefit; very serious health consequences are possible, including thickening of the blood, which puts extra strain on the heart; is an illegal practice under Olympic guidelines.
Gamma hydroxybutyric acid (GHB)	Promoted as a steroid alternative for bodybuilding	FDA has never approved it for sale as a medical product; is illegal to produce or sell GHB in the United States. GHB-related symptoms includes vomiting, dizziness, tremors, and seizures. Many victims have required hospitalization, and some have died. Clandestine laboratories produced virtually all of the chemical accounting for GHB abuse. FDA is working with the U.S. Attorney's office to arrest, indict, and convict individuals responsible for the illegal operations.
Androstenedione	Increase muscle mass	Possibly converted to testosterone but does not increase muscle mass. Its use is banned by the NFL, NCAA, and International Olympic Committee. Side effects are acne, fits of rage, baldness, development of breasts in men, stunted growth, and sterility. Cost: $30/month.
Insulin	Promote muscle development and inhibit muscle breakdown	Use can lead to seizures, hypoglycemia, and resulting brain damage. The need for injection can lead to increased risk of hepatitis and other viral diseases. Overall, unsupervised use of this powerful hormone is fraught with danger to one's health.
Ephedrine	Increase stamina and exercise performance	No evidence that it enhances performance. Ephedrine (ephedra or ma huang in the herbal form) is currently under scrutiny by FDA due to more than 1000 reports of detrimental effects and at least 60 deaths. FDA is currently reviewing rules that would dictate amount of ephedrine allowed in each pill and taken within a 24-hour period, as well as a warning system on labels. Provisional advice is to consume no more than 25 milligrams per day for a total of 7 days, if at all. Ephedrine has caused heart attack, stroke, anxiety, seizure, and death.

Generally Not Effective

Substance/Practice	Rationale	Reality
Alcohol	Reduce fatigue, provide energy	Not a muscle fuel; actually impairs performance; abuse can lead to hypoglycemia and dehydration
Medium chain triglyceride (MCT oil)	Excellent fuel for muscles; transfers directly from GI tract into bloodstream	Can provide a source of energy for muscles but provides no advantage over carbohydrate intake alone, as is very expensive. Doses over 25–30 g at one time lead to nausea and diarrhea.
Phosphate loading	Improve oxygen delivery to muscles	Not effective
Inosine	Increase protein and ATP synthesis	Not effective
Coenzyme Q-10	Increase energy metabolism	Sufficient amount is produced by the body.
Carnitine	Shuttle fatty acids into mitochondria of cells	Body cells produce enough; therefore, use is ineffective.
Chromium	Enhance insulin function	No benefit in performance. American College of Sports Medicine states that supplementation is unnecessary. Generally, we consume enough chromium to meet needs.

TABLE 14-9   concluded

Substance/Practice	Rationale	Reality
Ornithine, arginine (human growth hormone releasers)	Used to increase human growth hormone output for muscle growth	Studies with unrealistically high doses of these amino acids (over 10 g/day) given intravenously have been shown to increase human growth hormone. However, recent studies with more reasonable doses (2–4 g/day) as commercial dietary supplements have shown no effects on human growth hormone. In addition, the increase in human growth hormone (even if the amino acids were effective) would be of questionable value and may even be harmful (see the section in this table on growth hormone).
Other amino acids	Increase bioavailability to promote protein synthesis and lessen the muscle loss that occurs during both strength and endurance exercise.	Of no value; dietary protein intake is sufficient to meet amino acid needs.
Deyhdroepiandrosterone (DHEA)	Increase production of testosterone and provide an anabolic steroid effect	Studies to date are inconclusive. Side effects are masculine traits in women, including hair loss and voice deepening. Men may develop irreversible breast development and prostate gland enlargement. Recently banned by International Olympic Committee. Use is not recommended. Cost: $14/month.
Albuterol	Train harder as to increase muscle strength and mass	No immediate ergogenic effect on either power or endurance
Pyruvate	Increase energy available to muscles	No benefit with use.
Vanadyl sulfate (vanadium)	Has insulin-like effects on carbohydrate and amino acid metabolism; used to promote muscle growth and decrease body fat	Doses of 0.5 mg/kg/day for 12 weeks did not alter body composition in weight trainers (normal diet contains 6–8 μg of vanadium/day, or about 0.1–0.3 mg/kg/day).
Hydroxycitrate (HCA) (*Garcinia cambogia*)	HCA is a competitive inhibitor of an enzyme involved in the synthesis of fat from carbohydrate; used as a fat-burner	Some poorly designed studies found body fat loss with HCA; however, the HCA was often given in combination with other herbs, vitamins, or minerals. A recent study with a more appropriate experimental design showed no impact of HCA (1500 mg/day), along with a 1200-kcal diet, on weight loss or body fat loss, compared to the diet alone.
Glycerol	Increase fluid retention in the body mass, enhancing body hydration	Limited research and small numbers of subjects used in studies provide conflicting evidence regarding the usefulness of glycerol in enhancing physical performance. Until more studies are completed, the claim that glycerol enhances sports performance is unsupported. Use of glycerol may produce headache and blurred vision, which could interfere with athletic performance.
Aspartates	May help reduce ammonia accumulation in muscles	Magnesium and/or potassium salts of aspartic acid have been used as potential aids to endurance performance. The small number of subjects used in current studies makes interpretation of the results difficult. To date, aspartate salts do not appear to reduce accumulation of ammonia in the blood. Until additional controlled trials with larger numbers of subjects are conducted, supplementation is not warranted. There appears to be no toxicity with the doses used in reported studies.
Ribose	Increase ATP synthesis	Although the monosaccharide ribose is part of the ATP molecule, no studies support the concept that increasing ribose intake increase ATP availability during physical activity.

EATING DISORDERS: ANOREXIA NERVOSA, BULIMIA NERVOSA, AND OTHER CONDITIONS

chapter 15

*M*any of us occasionally eat until we're stuffed and uncomfortable, such as at Thanksgiving dinner. Faced with savory and tempting foods, we find that we can't easily stop eating. Usually we forgive ourselves, vowing not to overeat the next time. Nevertheless, many of us have problems controlling our weight. Although creeping weight gain can eventually lead to medical problems, it is usually associated with simple overeating, coupled with too little physical activity.

Although obesity is the most common eating disorder in our society, the eating disorders explored in this chapter involve much more severe distortions of the eating process. The eating disorders discussed here are serious and can develop into life-threatening conditions if left untreated.[3] What's most alarming about these disorders—anorexia nervosa, bulimia nervosa, female athlete triad, binge-eating disorder, baryophobia and related disorders—is the increasing number of cases reported each year.[22]

Some people are more receptive and vulnerable to these disorders than other people are, for genetic, psychological, and physical reasons. And keep in mind that eating disorders are not restricted to any socioeconomic class or ethnicity. They can strike at any age in both females and males.[3] Let's examine the causes and treatments of these conditions in detail, because these eating disorders touch many of our lives.

KEY CHAPTER CONCEPTS

- Eating serves an extraordinary number of psychological, social, and cultural purposes.
- It is hard not to compare the media's ideal body images with our own, seemingly less than perfect bodies.
- Anorexia nervosa typically is seen in females, beginning around puberty. Warning signs include weight loss and abnormal eating habits, such as cooking a large meal and then only watching others eat it.
- Physical effects of anorexia nervosa are serious. Treatment requires professional—primarily, psychological—help. Slow weight gain is one of many desired outcomes.
- Bulimia nervosa is characterized by bingeing on a large amount of food at one sitting and then purging by vomiting, or misusing laxatives, diuretics, or enemas. Fasting and exercising excessively are other means to combat the caloric excess.
- Treatment of bulimia nervosa includes psychological as well as nutritional counseling. The latter focuses on establishing regular eating patterns.
- Binge-eating disorder includes grazing and food bingeing without purging. Treatment primarily addresses deeper emotional issues, as these are usually at the root of the disorder.
- Female athlete triad occurs when an athlete has disordered eating, amenorrhea, and osteoporosis. This problem is seen in appearance-related sports, such as gymnastics, ballet, and others.
- Baryophobia is diagnosed when caregivers have been found to underfeed children in order to prevent future disease, such as cardiovascular disease or obesity. Growth failure can result if not corrected.

REFRESH YOUR MEMORY

As you begin your study of eating disorders, such as anorexia nervosa and bulimia nervosa, in Chapter 15, you may want to review
- The role of genetic risk in disease susceptibility in Chapter 1
- Structure and function of female sexual organs in Chapter 3
- The effects and treatment of osteoporosis in Chapter 11
- The effects and treatment of iron deficiency anemia in Chapter 12
- Calculation of BMI in Chapter 13
- The effects of neurotransmitters on food intake in Chapter 13

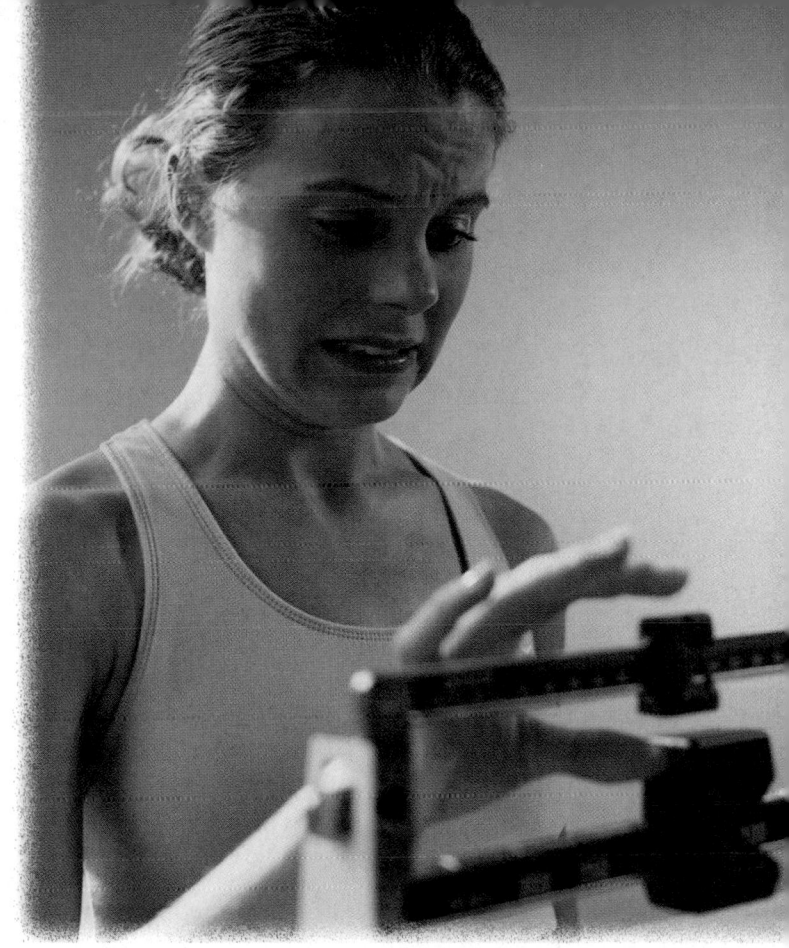

CASE SCENARIO

At age 13, Sarah suddenly became self-conscious about her weight when the neighborhood children teased her about being overweight. She began exercising to an aerobics video for an hour each day and found that she had success in losing weight; this was just the beginning of her obsession to be thin. Next, Sarah turned to eating less food to lose even more weight and began eliminating certain foods from her diet, such as candy and meat. She increased her water and vegetable intake and chewed sugarless gum to curb her appetite. Once she began dieting, it was impossible for her to stop. She really enjoyed having a high level of self-control over her body. She was literally obsessed with food and stared at others while they were eating a meal. She cooked large meals and then refused to eat all but a few bites. By the time Sarah was 19 years old and 5'6" tall, her weight had dropped from 150 lb to 85 lb in 20 months. Her family was concerned about her weight status, demanding that she go to a physician for an evaluation. Sarah was not happy about this idea but believed that her family would stop pestering her if she just went to the doctor's visit. Sarah did not think she had a problem; she truly thought she was still grotesquely overweight. She did notice, however, that she was intolerant of cold temperatures and had not menstruated in a year.

Does Sarah meet the qualifications to be diagnosed with an eating disorder? What types of therapy do you think the physician will suggest for Sarah? Where could she go for such therapy? What is the likelihood that she will fully recover from her condition?

■ FROM ORDERED TO DISORDERED EATING HABITS

Eating—a completely instinctive behavior for animals—serves an extraordinary number of psychological, social, and cultural purposes for humans. Eating practices may take on religious meanings; signify bonds among cultural, ethnic, and family groups; and be a means to express hostility and affection, prestige, and class values. Similarly, providing, preparing, and distributing food may be means of expressing love or hatred, or even power, in family relationships.

In our society, we are bombarded daily with images of the ideal body.[4] Dieting is promoted to achieve this ideal body—eternally young and acceptable to those around us. Television programs, billboard advertisements, magazine pictures, movies, and newspapers tell us that an ultra-slim body will bring happiness, love, and even success. This is despite the fact that much of society is becoming fatter. In response, some of us take this to the other extreme—the pathological pursuit of weight control or loss.[3]

Not comparing the media images with our own is hard. Not everyone can look like a fashion model. People who are overly susceptible to these messages, for genetic, psychological, and physical reasons, may be more likely than others to develop eating disorders.[22]

Given the multiple functions associated with normal eating and the media bombardment about ideal body image, it is not surprising that some people progress from typical responses to hunger and satiety cues, to obsessive weight loss, and then to a full-blown eating disorder, often associated with unusual and strange rituals.

■ Food: More Than Just a Source of Nutrients

From birth, we link food with personal and emotional experiences. As infants, we associate milk with security and warmth, so the bottle or breast becomes a source of comfort as well as food. Even when older, some people continue to derive comfort and great pleasure from food. This is both a biological and a psychological phenomenon. Food can be a symbol of comfort, but eating can also stimulate the release of certain neurotransmitters (e.g., serotonin) and *natural opioids* (including endorphins), which produce a sense of calm and euphoria in the human body.[22] Thus, in times of great stress some people turn to food for a druglike, calming effect.

Food is also used as a reward or a bribe. Haven't you heard or spoken something similar to the following comments?

You can have your dessert if you eat five more bites of your vegetables.

You can't play until you clean your plate.

I'll eat the broccoli if you let me watch TV.

If you love me, you'll eat what I fixed for dinner.

On the surface, using food as a reward or bribe seems harmless enough. Eventually, however, this practice encourages both caregivers and children to use food to achieve unstated goals. Food may then become much more than a source of nutrients. Regularly using food as a bargaining chip can contribute to abnormal eating patterns. Carried to the extreme, these patterns can lead to disordered eating behavior.

■ Overview of the Two Most Common Eating Disorders

The eating disorders **anorexia nervosa** and **bulimia nervosa** have been described since the time of the ancient Greeks. Both disorders are psychological problems expressed in part by food practices. Both erode medical, social, and psychological well-being. Currently, about 2 to 8% of young women have these disorders.[2, 3] This section provides a brief description of the characteristics and diagnoses of these two principal disorders. Detailed discussion of these and related disorders, including treatment, follows.

---

*P*arents may not consider a teenager mature enough to make decisions. If the teen disagrees and the situation is very tense, she may turn to purging or starving as a way to show her power: "You may try to control my life, but I can do anything I want with my body."

In the words of one young woman, "I couldn't get angry, because it would be like destroying someone else, like my mother. It felt like she would hate me forever, I got angry through anorexia nervosa. It was my last hope. It's my own body and this was my last-ditch effort."

Progression from Ordered to Disordered Eating

Attention to hunger and satiety signals; limitation of energy intake to restore weight to a healthful level

↓

Some disordered eating habits begin as weight loss is attempted, such as very restricted eating

↓

Clinically evident eating disorder recognized

---

anorexia nervosa An eating disorder involving a psychological loss or denial of appetite and self-starvation, related in part to a distorted body image and to various social pressures commonly associated with puberty.

bulimia nervosa An eating disorder in which large quantities of food are eaten at one time (binge eating) and then purged from the body by vomiting, or misuse of laxatives, diuretics, or enemas. Alternate means to counteract the caloric excess use are fasting and excessive exercise.

Anorexia nervosa is characterized by extreme weight loss, a distorted body image, and an irrational, almost morbid fear of obesity and weight gain. Anorexic patients irrationally believe they are fat, even though others constantly comment on their thin physique. Some anorexics realize they are thin but are habitually haunted by certain areas of their bodies that they believe to be fat (such as thighs, buttocks, and stomach) (Fig. 15-1). The discrepancy between actual and perceived body shape is an important gauge of the severity of the disease.[2]

The term *anorexia* implies a loss of appetite; however, denying one's appetite more accurately describes the behavior of people with anorexia nervosa. By rough estimate, approximately 1 in 100 girls between the ages of 12 and 18 years suffers from anorexia nervosa. This high number may be due to the tendency for these females to blame themselves for the weight gain seen at that age. It happens less commonly among adult women and African-American women. Men account for approximately 5 to 10% of the cases of anorexia nervosa, partly because the ideal image conveyed for men is big and muscular.[3]

Bulimia nervosa (*bulimia* means "great hunger") is characterized by episodes of binge eating followed by attempts to purge the excess energy taken up by the body by vomiting, or misuse of laxatives, diuretics, or enemas. Fasting and excessive exercise (**hypergymnasia**) also may be used to compensate for the caloric excess. People with this disorder may be difficult to identify because they keep their binge-purge behaviors secret, and their symptoms are not obvious. Between 5 and 17% of adolescent and college-age women suffer from bulimia nervosa. About 40% of the cases of binge eating occur in male athletes, especially those who participate in sports that require achieving lower weights to fit weight classes, such as boxers, wrestlers, and jockeys. Other activities that may foster eating disorders in men include swimming, dancing, and modeling.[3]

The *Diagnostic and Statistical Manual of Mental Disorders* lists specific criteria for diagnosing eating disorders (Table 15-1.).[2] People may exhibit some symptoms of an eating disorder but not enough to enable a medical worker to diagnose the disease. These people may fall under the category Eating Disorders Not Otherwise Specified (EDNOS). And, suggested in the diagnostic criteria, some people show characteristics of both anorexia nervosa and bulimia nervosa because the diseases overlap considerably (Fig. 15-2). About half of the women diagnosed as having anorexia nervosa eventually develop bulimic symptoms.[3] As shown in Table 15-1, bulimic characteristics are included as part of one type of anorexia nervosa, which blurs the distinction. Still, appreciating the differences between the disorders helps in understanding various approaches to prevention and treatment.

Table 15-2 lists some characteristics of people with anorexia nervosa and bulimia nervosa. Do you know someone who is at risk? If so, suggest that the person seek a professional evaluation because, the sooner treatment begins, the better.[3] However, do not try to diagnose eating disorders in your friends or family members. Only a professional can exclude other possible diseases and correctly evaluate the diagnostic criteria required to make a diagnosis of anorexia nervosa or bulimia nervosa. Once an eating disorder is diagnosed, immediate treatment is advisable. As a friend, the best you can do is to encourage an affected person to seek professional help. Note that such help is commonly available at student health centers and student guidance/counseling facilities on college campuses.

There are no simple causes of eating disorders, and there are no simple treatments. Stress may have an especially strong role in the development of eating disorders. An underlying commonality seems to be the lack of appropriate coping mechanisms as individuals begin to reach adolescence and young adulthood, coupled with dysfunctional family relationships.[3]

■ Is There a Genetic Connection to Eating Disorders?

A few research studies have investigated the possible link between genetic factors and the development of eating disorders.[6] These studies have involved a comparison

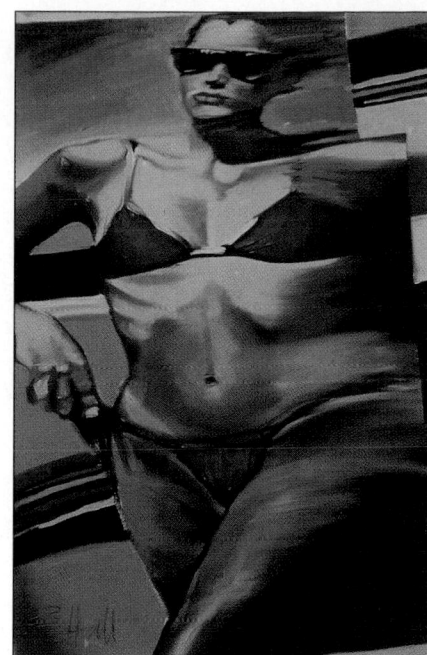

■ FIGURE 15-1 Self-image can be ever changing and deceiving. For people with eating disorders, the difference between the real and desired body images may be too difficult to accept.

hypergymnasia Exercising more than is required for good physical fitness or maximal performance in a sport; excessive exercise.

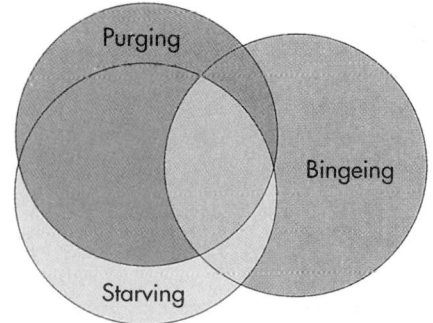

■ FIGURE 15-2 The overlap of eating disorders. A combination of binge eating, purging, and/or starving can be found in both anorexia nervosa and bulimia nervosa.

TABLE 15-1 Diagnostic Criteria for Anorexia Nervosa and Bulimia Nervosa[2]

Anorexia Nervosa

A. Refusal to maintain body weight at or above a minimally normal weight for age and height (e.g., weight loss leading to maintenance of body weight less than 85% of that expected; or failure to make expected weight gain during periods of growth, leading to body weight less than 85% of that expected)

B. Intense fear of gaining weight or becoming fat, even though underweight

C. Disturbance in the way in which one's body weight or shape is experienced, undue influence of body weight or shape on self-evaluation, or denial of the seriousness of the current low body weight

D. In postmenarcheal females, **amenorrhea**—i.e., the absence of at least three consecutive menstrual cycles. (A woman is considered to have amenorrhea if her periods occur only following hormone [e.g., estrogen] administration.)

Specify Type

Restricting type: During the current episode of anorexia nervosa, the person has not regularly engaged in binge-eating or purging behavior (such as self-induced vomiting and the misuse of laxatives, diuretics, or enemas).
Binge-eating/purging type: During the current episode of anorexia nervosa, the person has regularly engaged in binge-eating or purging behavior (such as self-induced vomiting and the misuse of laxatives, diuretics, or enemas).

Bulimia Nervosa

A. Recurrent episodes of binge eating. An episode of binge eating is characterized by both of the following:

1. Eating, in a discrete period of time (e.g., within any 2-hour period), an amount of food that is definitely larger than most people would eat during a similar period of time and under similar circumstances

2. A sense of lack of control over eating during the episode (e.g., a feeling that one cannot stop eating or control what or how much one is eating)

B. Recurrent inappropriate compensatory behavior to prevent weight gain, such as self-induced vomiting; misuse of laxatives, diuretics, enemas, or other medications; fasting; or excessive exercise

C. The binge eating and inappropriate compensatory behaviors both occur, on average, at least twice a week for 3 months.

D. Self-evaluation is unduly influenced by both body shape and weight.

E. The disturbance does not occur exclusively during episodes of anorexia nervosa.

Specify Type

Purging type: During the current episode of bulimia nervosa, the person has regularly engaged in self-induced vomiting or the misuse of laxatives, diuretics, or enemas.
Nonpurging type: During the current episode of bulimia nervosa, the person has used other inappropriate compensatory behaviors, such as fasting or excessive exercise, but has not regularly engaged in self-induced vomiting or the misuse of laxatives, diuretics, or enemas.

Eating Disorder Not Otherwise Specified (EDNOS)

This category is for disorders of eating that do not meet criteria for any specific eating disorder—for example:

1. For females, all of the criteria for anorexia nervosa are met except that the individual has regular menses.

2. All of the criteria for anorexia nervosa are met except that, despite significant weight loss, the individual's current weight is in the normal range.

3. All of the criteria for bulimia nervosa are met except that the binge eating and inappropriate compensatory mechanisms occur at a frequency of less than twice a week or for a duration of less than 3 months.

4. The regular use of inappropriate compensatory behavior by an individual of normal body weight after eating small amounts of food

5. Repeatedly chewing and spitting out, but not swallowing, large amounts of food

   Binge Eating Disorder (BED): Recurrent episodes of binge eating in the absence of the regular use of inappropriate compensatory behaviors characteristic of bulimia nervosa

Reprinted with permission from the *Diagnostic and Statistical Manual of Mental Disorders*, Fourth Edition. Copyright 1994 American Psychiatric Association.

This table will help you understand the characteristics of anorexia nervosa and bulimia nervosa. However, please do not attempt to diagnose these disorders in yourself or others. Instead, use this information to determine whether professional help is needed. Note also that for both anorexia nervosa and bulimia nervosa, all characteristics (A–D or A–E, respectively) must be present to make the diagnosis.

TABLE 15-2 Typical Characteristics of Anorexic and Bulimic Persons	
Anorexia Nervosa	**Bulimia Nervosa**
• Rigid dieting causing dramatic weight loss • False body perception—thinking "I'm too fat," even when emaciated; relentless pursuit of control • Rituals involving food, excessive exercise, and other aspects of life • Maintenance of rigid control in lifestyle; security found in control and order • Feeling of panic after a small weight gain; intense fear of gaining weight • Feelings of purity, power, and superiority through maintenance of strict discipline and self-denial • Preoccupation with food, its preparation, and observing another person eat • Helplessness in the presence of food • Lack of menses after what should be the age of puberty	• Secretive binge eating; never overeating in front of others • Eating when depressed or under stress • Bingeing followed by fasting, laxative abuse, self-induced vomiting, or excessive exercise • Shame, embarrassment, deceit, and depression; low-self-esteem and guilt (especially after a binge) • Fluctuating weight resulting from alternate bingeing and fasting (±10 lb or 5 kg) • Loss of control; fear of not being able to stop eating • Perfectionism, "people pleaser"; food as the only comfort/escape in an otherwise carefully controlled and regulated life • Erosion of teeth, swollen glands • Purchase of syrup of ipecac

Those who exhibit only one or a few of these characteristics may be at risk but probably do not have either disorder. They should, however, reflect on their eating habits and related concerns and take appropriate action.

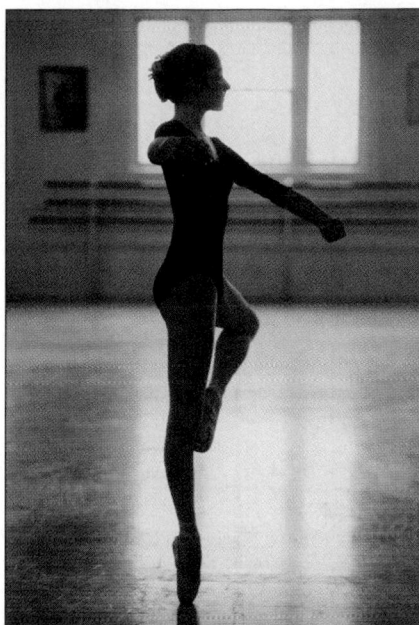

Eating disorders are commonly seen in people who must maintain low body weight, such as ballet dancers.

of identical twins with fraternal twins and the incidence of eating disorders. In general, these studies have shown that identical twins have a higher incidence of eating disorders among themselves than do fraternal twins. This indicates that genetics may have a strong role in development, since identical twins share the same DNA; however, these studies have not ruled out the impact of the environmental influences in eating disorder development. Identifying genes that cause eating disorders eventually could help in tailoring prevention efforts to those who are at risk, but affected individuals would still need the same interdisciplinary counseling that is part of therapy today.

The Nutrition Perspective at the end of this chapter adds further insight into this topic, as it reviews some sociological aspects of these disorders. This helps you further understand how the disorders develop and why some people are more susceptible than others. As is true for many health problems, both nature and nurture play a role.

A person with anorexia nervosa may use the disorder to gain attention from the family, sometimes in hopes of holding the family together.

■ ANOREXIA NERVOSA

Anorexia nervosa evolves from a dangerous mental state to an often life-threatening physical condition. People suffering from this disorder think they are fat and intensely fear obesity and weight gain. They lose much more weight than is healthful. Although food is entwined in this disease, it stems more from psychological conflict.

Depression is commonly found in conjunction with an eating disorder. In fact, a study done in the 1940s at the University of Minnesota found that depression and obsessional behaviors developed in the subjects during a 6-month period of restricted calorie intake. These abnormal behaviors did not reverse immediately after refeeding but, rather, took many weeks to return to normal. (see Chapter 20 for details).[11]

About 7% of people with anorexia die within 10 years of diagnosis—from suicide, heart ailments, and infections. About one quarter of those with anorexia nervosa recover within 6 years, whereas the rest simply exist with the disease or go on to

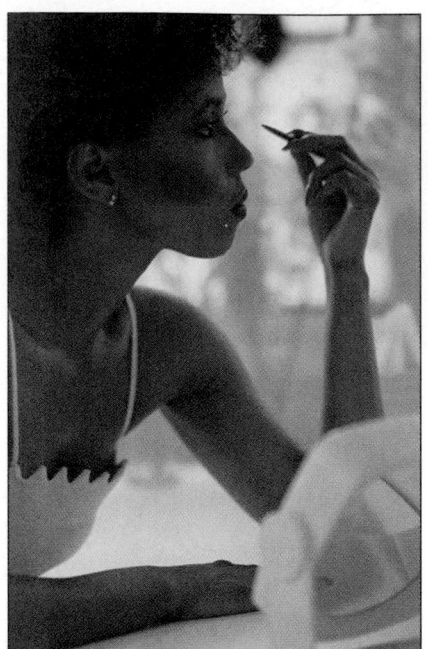

Concern over appearance begins early in life; a focus on healthful outlook with regard to body weight should also begin at this time.

*B*y severely restricting energy intake for long periods, adolescent girls and young adult women greatly compromise their nutritional status, impair their reproductive systems, and retard growth. The harm produced by milder, shorter periods of diet restriction is not clear. Evidence, however, suggests that even moderate diet restriction, if continued, contributes to the risks for various anemias, later pregnancy complications and low-birthweight infants, and permanently reduced bone density.

develop another form of eating disorder. The longer someone suffers from this eating disorder, the poorer the chances for complete recovery. A young patient with a brief episode and a cooperative family has a better outlook than those without these factors. Prompt and vigorous treatment with close follow-up improves the chances for success.[3]

Anorexia nervosa may begin as a simple attempt to lose weight. A comment from a well-meaning friend, relative, or coach suggesting that the person seems to be gaining weight or is too fat may be all that is needed. The stress of having to maintain a certain weight to look attractive or competent on a job can also lead to disordered eating. Physical changes associated with puberty, the stress of leaving childhood, or the loss of a friend may serve as another trigger for extreme dieting. Leaving home for boarding school or college or starting a job can reinforce the desire to appear more "socially acceptable." Still, looking "good" does not necessarily help people deal with anger, depression, low self-esteem, or past experiences with sexual abuse. If these issues are behind the disorder and are not resolved as weight is lost, the individual may intensify efforts to lose weight "to look even better," rather than work through unresolved psychological concerns.[3]

During adolescence, a period of turbulent sexual and social tensions, teenagers seek—and are often expected—to establish separate and independent lives. While declaring independence, they seek acceptance and support from peers and parents and react intensely to how they think others perceive them. At the same time, their bodies are changing, and much of the change is beyond their control. In response to the adolescent's or teenager's lack of control and coping mechanisms, dieting may start and then lead to a failure to gain appropriate weight for height. This may not be readily identified as a problem because the child has not actually lost any weight. Stunting (failure to grow in height) may also occur if inadequate calories are ingested during a period of growth.[21] If anorexia develops before puberty, sexual maturation and menstruation may be delayed.

Teens with chronic illnesses, such as diabetes or asthma, are at even greater risk for disordered eating. Any evidence of poor weight gain or excessive fitness among these individuals needs to be investigated as possible disordered eating.[17]

Extreme dieting is the most important predictor of an eating disorders.[14] (Adolescents expressing concern about their weight should be advised to focus on exercise, which does not appear to impart a risk for subsequent problems.)[18]

Once dieting begins, a person developing anorexia nervosa does not stop. The result is long periods of rigidly self-enforced semistarvation, practiced almost with a vengeance, in a relentless pursuit of control. Anorexia nervosa may eventually lead to bingeing on large amounts of food in a short time, then purging. Purging occurs primarily through vomiting, but laxatives, diuretics, and exercise are also used. Thus, a person with anorexia nervosa may exist in a state of semistarvation or may alternate periods of starvation with periods of bingeing and purging.[3]

■ Profile of the Typical Person with Anorexia Nervosa

A person with anorexia nervosa refuses to eat enough food to maintain an acceptable weight. This refusal is the hallmark of the disease, whether or not other practices, such as binge-purge cycles, appear. The most typical anorexic person is a white female from the middle or upper socioeconomic class. Perhaps her mother also has distorted views of desirable body shape and acceptable food habits. The girl is often described by parents and teachers as responsible, meticulous, and obedient.

She is competitive and often obsessive. Her parents set high standards for her. At home, she may not allow clutter in her bedroom. Physicians note that, after a physical examination, she may fold her examination gown very carefully and clean up the examination room before leaving. Even though such behavior may seem obvious, only a skilled professional can tell the difference between anorexia nervosa and other adolescent complaints, such as delayed puberty, fatigue, and depression.

A common thread underlying many—but not all—cases of anorexia nervosa is conflict within the family structure, typically manifested by an overbearing mother and an emotionally absent father. When family expectations are always too high—including those regarding body weight—resulting frustration leads to fighting. Overinvolvement, rigidity, overprotection, and denial are typical daily transactions of such families.[3]

Often, the eating disorder allows an anorexic person to exercise control over an otherwise powerless existence (Fig. 15-3). Losing weight may be the first independent success the person has had. People with anorexia evaluate their self-worth almost entirely in terms of self-control. Issues of control are central to the development of anorexia nervosa.[10, 22] Some sexually abused children develop anorexia nervosa, believing that, if they control their appetite for food, sexual relations, and human contact, they will feel in control and competent and will eliminate shameful feelings. Moreover, food restriction, which arrests development and shuts down sexual impulses, may be a strategy to prevent future victimization and guilt feelings in such cases. Often anorexic persons feel hopeless about human relationships and socially isolated because of their dysfunctional families. They substitute the world of food, eating, and weight for the world of human relationships.

■ Early Warning Signs

A person developing anorexia nervosa exhibits important warning signs. At first, dieting becomes the life focus. The person may think, "The only thing I am good at is dieting. I can't do anything else." This innocent beginning often leads to very abnormal self-perceptions and eating habits, such as cutting a pea in half before eating it. Other habits include hiding and storing food and or spreading food around a plate to make it look as if much has been eaten. An anorexic person may cook a large meal and watch others eat it while refusing to eat anything. Anorexics may also exercise compulsively to the point that it is obsessive and driven. It can interfere with life activities or occur at inappropriate times or settings—for example, doing squats while brushing teeth.[8]

As the disorder progresses, the range of foods may narrow and be rigidly divided into safe and unsafe ones, with the list of safe foods becoming progressively shorter. For people developing anorexia nervosa, these practices say, "I am in control." These people may be hungry, but they deny it, driven by the belief that good things will happen by just becoming thin enough. It becomes a question of willpower.[11]

Soon people with anorexia become irritable and hostile and begin to withdraw from family and friends. School performance generally crumbles. They refuse to eat out with family and friends, thinking, "I won't be able to have the foods I want to eat," or "I won't be able to throw up afterward."

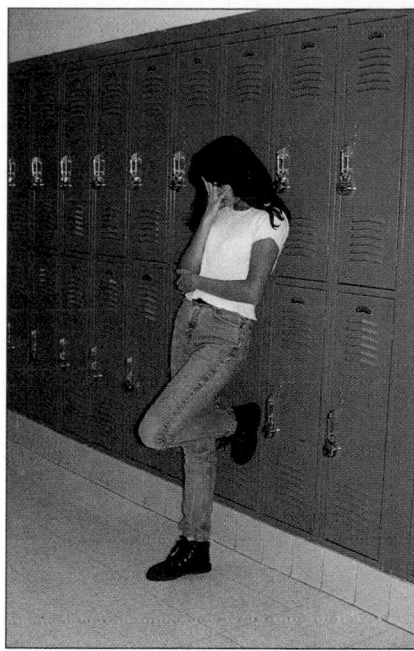

■ FIGURE 15-3 The stress of crossing from childhood into adulthood may trigger anorexia nervosa.

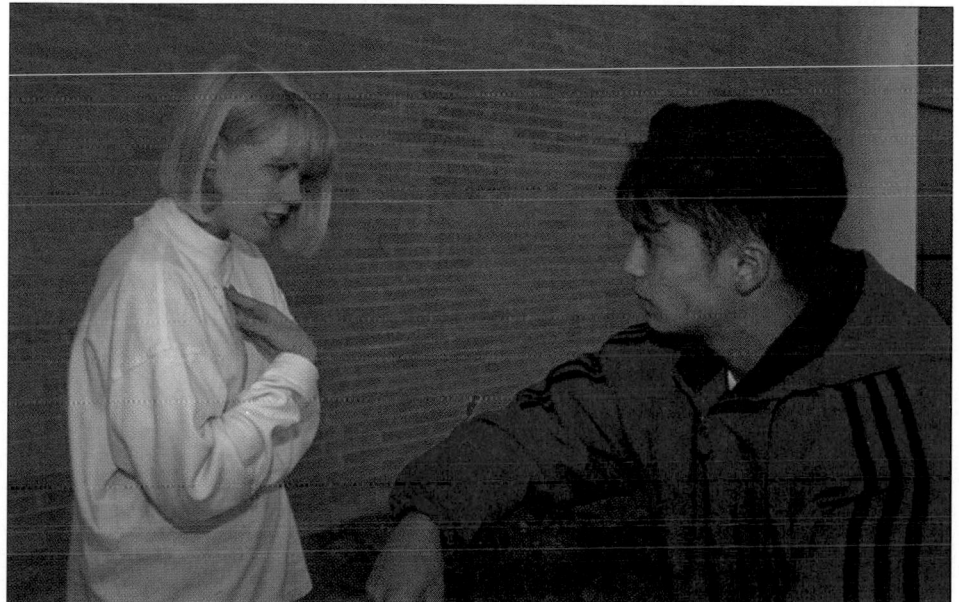

Stresses and changes are a common part of adolescence.

Anorexic persons see themselves as rational and others as irrational. They also tend to be excessively critical of themselves and others. Nothing is good enough. Because it cannot be perfect, life appears meaningless and hopeless. A sense of joylessness colors everything.

As stress increases in the person's life, sleep disturbances and depression are common. Many of the psychological and physical problems associated with anorexia nervosa arise from deficiencies of nutrients, such as thiamin and vitamin B-6, and semistarvation. For this reason, a multivitamin and mineral supplement is typically prescribed in therapy. For a female, the combination of problems—coupled with lower and lower body weight and fat stores—causes menstrual periods to cease. This may be the first sign of the disease that a parent notices and represents the hallmark of the disease.[3]

Ultimately, an anorexic person eats very little food; 300 to 600 kcal daily is not unusual. In place of food, the person may consume up to 20 cans of diet soft drinks and chew many pieces of sugarless gum each day.

■ Physical Effects of Anorexia Nervosa

Rooted in the emotional state of the victim, anorexia nervosa produces profound physical effects. The anorexic person often appears to be skin and bones. Body weight less than 85% of that expected is one clinical indicator of anorexia nervosa. This percentage can be calculated using the Metropolitan Life Insurance tables (see Appendix G), but it is important to note that body build and weight history should also be used when estimating an appropriate weight. BMI is a more reliable indicator of malnourishment; generally, a BMI of less than 17.5 indicates severe malnourishment (see Chapter 13 for more on BMI). For children less than 18 years old, growth charts should be used to assess weight status. (See Chapter 17).[3]

This state of semistarvation disturbs many body systems, as it forces the body to conserve as much energy as possible (Fig. 15-4). This attempt to conserve energy results in the most physical effects. Thus, many complications can be ended by returning to a healthy weight, provided the duration of the insult has not been too long. Following are predictable effects caused by hormonal responses to semistarvation:[3, 5]

- Lowered body temperature caused by loss of fat insulation.
- Slower metabolic rate caused by decreased synthesis of thyroid hormone
- Decreased heart rate as metabolism slows, leading to easy fatigue, fainting, and an overwhelming need for sleep. Other changes in heart function may also occur, including loss of heart tissue itself.
- Iron deficiency anemia from a deficient nutrient intake, which leads to further weakness
- Rough, dry, scaly, and cold skin from a deficient nutrient intake, iron-deficiency anemia, and estrogen deficiency. The skin may also show multiple bruises because of the loss of protection from the fat layer normally present under the skin.
- Low white blood cell count caused by a deficient nutrient intake. This condition increases the risk of infection, one cause of death in people with anorexia nervosa.
- Abnormal feeling of fullness or bloating, which can last for several hours after eating
- Loss of hair caused by a deficient nutrient intake
- Appearance of **lanugo,** downy hairs on the body that trap air, reducing heat loss and in turn replacing some insulation lost with the fat layer
- Constipation from semistarvation and laxative abuse
- Low blood potassium caused by a deficient nutrient intake, loss of potassium from vomiting, and use of some types of diuretics. This increases the risk of heart rhythm disturbances, another leading cause of death in anorexic people.
- Loss of menstrual periods because of low body weight, low body fat content, and the stress of the disease. Accompanying hormonal changes cause a loss of bone mass and increase the risk of osteoporosis later in life.
- Changes in neurotransmitter function in the brain and related depression

lanugo Downlike hair that appears after a person has lost much body fat through semistarvation. The hair stands erect and traps air, acting as insulation for the body to compensate for the relative lack of body fat, which usually functions as insulation.

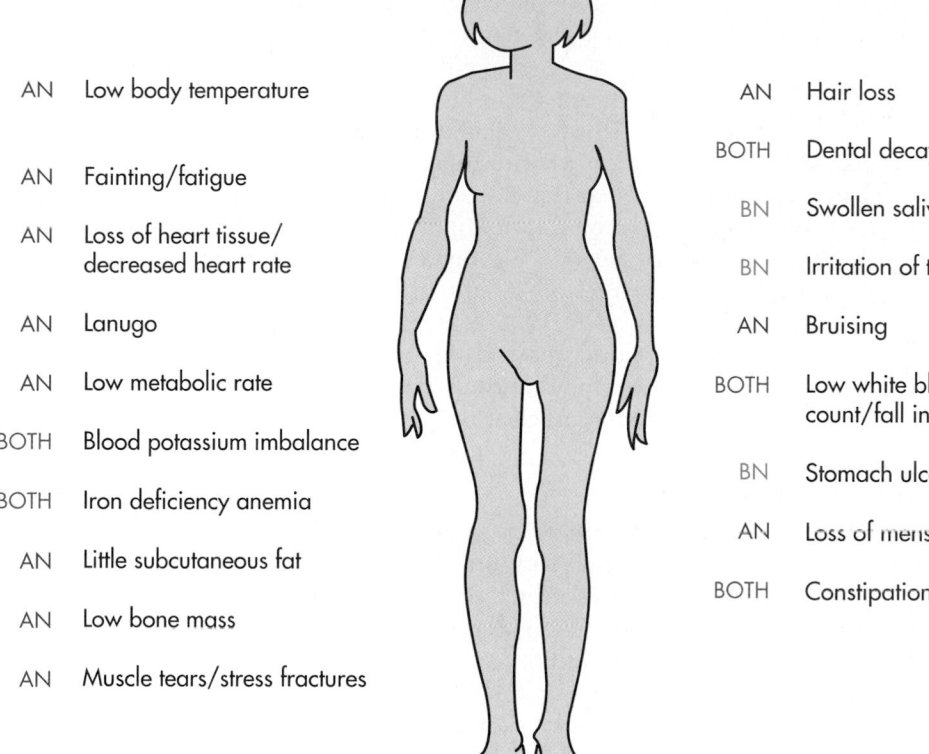

AN   Low body temperature

AN   Fainting/fatigue

AN   Loss of heart tissue/
      decreased heart rate

AN   Lanugo

AN   Low metabolic rate

BOTH Blood potassium imbalance

BOTH Iron deficiency anemia

AN   Little subcutaneous fat

AN   Low bone mass

AN   Muscle tears/stress fractures

AN   Hair loss

BOTH Dental decay

BN   Swollen salivary glands

BN   Irritation of the esophagus

AN   Bruising

BOTH Low white blood cell
      count/fall in immune function

BN   Stomach ulcers

AN   Loss of menstrual periods

BOTH Constipation

AN   = Associated primarily with anorexia nervosa

BN   = Associated primarily with bulimia nervosa

BOTH = Associated generally with both disorders

■ FIGURE 15-4 Signs and symptoms of eating disorders. A vast array of physical effects are associated with anorexia nervosa and bulimia nervosa. This figure contains many but is not an exhaustive list of all potential consequences. These physical effects can also serve as warning signs that a problem exists. Professional evaluation is then indicated.

- Eventual loss of teeth caused by acid erosion from frequent vomiting. Until vomiting ceases, one way to reduce this effect on teeth is to rinse the mouth with water right away and brushing teeth as soon as possible. Loss of teeth and bone mass can be lasting signs of the disease, even if the other physical and mental problems are resolved.
- Muscle tears and stress fractures in athletes because of decreased bone and muscle mass.

A person with this disorder is psychologically and physically ill and needs help.

CONCEPT CHECK

Anorexia nervosa is an eating disorder characterized by semistarvation. It is found primarily—but not exclusively—in adolescent girls, starting at or around puberty. People with anorexia dwindle essentially to skin and bones but often believe they are fat. Semistarvation produces hormonal and other changes, which lower body temperature, slow the heart rate, decrease immune response, stop menstrual periods, and contribute to hair, muscle, and bone loss. It is a very serious disease, which often produces lifelong consequences and may be fatal.

CRITICAL THINKING

Jennifer continues her pursuit of the perfect thin body into her late teens. She ignores the advice of her parents and the counselor. As a 19-year-old entering college, she is finally beginning to realize that her anorexic behavior might have serious consequences. She has been fluctuating 15 to 20% below her healthy body weight and has been amenorrheic for a few years. She would like to marry someday and have a family. What might some of the health consequences be for a person such as Jennifer with anorexia nervosa?

■ Treatment of Anorexia Nervosa

People with anorexia often sink into shells of isolation and fear. They deny that a problem exists. Frequently, their friends and family members meet with them to confront the problem in a loving way. This is called an *intervention*. They present evidence of the problem and encourage immediate treatment. Treatment then requires a multidisciplinary team of experienced physicians, registered dietitians, psychologists, and other health professionals working together.[3] An ideal setting is an eating disorders clinic in a medical center with inpatient facilities. Still, even in the most skilled hands and using the finest facilities, efforts may fail. This tells us that the prevention of anorexia nervosa is of utmost importance.[4]

Once a medical team has gained the cooperation of an anorexic patient, the team attempts to work together to restore a sense of balance, purpose, and future possibilities. As previously stated, anorexia nervosa is usually rooted in psychological conflict. However, a person who has been barely existing in a state of semistarvation cannot focus on much besides food. Dreams and even morbid thoughts about food will interfere with therapy until sufficient weight is regained.

Nutrition Therapy

Hospitalization is necessary once a person falls below 75% of expected weight, experiences acute medical problems, and/or exhibits severe psychological problems or suicidal risk.[5] Tube feeding and/or total parenteral nutrition support is used only if immediate renourishment is required, as this can cause the patient to distrust medical staff. The first goal of therapy is to gain the patient's cooperation and to increase oral food intake. Ideally, weight gain must be enough to raise the metabolic rate to normal and reverse as many physical signs of the disease as possible. Food intake is designed first to minimize or stop any further weight loss. Then the focus shifts to restoring appropriate food habits. After this, the expectation can be switched to slow weight gain. A range of 2 to 3 lb per week is appropriate.[3]

Energy needs begin at 1000 to 1600 kcal/day, increasing this in 100- to 200-kcal increments every few days as possible until an appropriate rate of weight gain is achieved. This appropriate weight is one in which normal menstruation is restored. A caloric distribution of about 50 to 55% carbohydrate, 15 to 20% protein, and 25 to 30% fat is appropriate. Multivitamin and mineral supplements are usually prescribed during refeeding to correct for nutrient deficiencies. To help prevent bone loss, clinicians prescribe approximately 1000 to 1500 mg/day of calcium and 400 to 800 IU of vitamin D. The use of typical osteoporosis medications in addition to supplementation are under investigation (see Chapter 11 for a list of these agents).

Patients need considerable reassurance during the refeeding process because of uncomfortable effects, such as bloating, increase in body heat, and increase in body fat. This is a frightening process because these changes can lead to feeling out of control. Monitoring for rapid changes in serum electrolytes and minerals, especially phosphorus and magnesium, is especially important during refeeding (see the discussion on phosphorus in Chapter 11).[3]

In addition to helping patients reach and maintain adequate nutritional status, the dietitian on the medical team also provides accurate nutrition information throughout treatment, promotes a healthy attitude toward food, and helps the patient learn to eat based on natural hunger and satiety. Therapy with many anorexic persons can be frustrating for a dietitian because many of those affected are knowledgeable regarding the calorie and fat gram content of most food products. The focus should be on helping these patients identify healthy and adequate food choices that promote weight gain to achieve and maintain a clinically estimated goal weight.[1] The medical team also should assure patients that they will not be abandoned after gaining weight.

Because excessive energy expenditure prevents weight gain, professionals must work with anorexic patients to help them moderate their activity. At many treatment centers, patients are placed on moderate bed rest in the early stages of treatment to help promote weight gain.

Experienced professional help is the key. An anorexic patient may be on the verge of suicide and near starvation. Today, suicide is the most common cause of death in people with anorexia nervosa. In addition, anorexic people are often very clever and resistant. They may try to hide weight loss by wearing many layers of clothes, putting coins in their pockets, and drinking numerous glasses of water.

Psychological and Related Therapy

Once the physical problems of anorexic patients are addressed, the treatment focus shifts to the underlying emotional problems that led to excessive dieting and other symptoms of the disorder. Dr. Laura Hill discusses various approaches in her Expert Opinion. To heal, these patients must reject the sense of accomplishment associated with an emaciated body. If therapists can discover reasons for the disorder, they can develop strategies for restoring normal weight and eating habits by resolving psychological conflicts. Education about the medical consequences of semistarvation is also helpful. A key aspect of psychological treatment is showing affected individuals how to regain control of some facets of their lives and cope with tough situations. As eating evolves into a normal routine, they then can turn to previously neglected activities.

Therapists may use **cognitive behavior therapy,** which involves helping the person confront and change irrational beliefs about body image, eating, relationships, and weight. Underlying issues that may be the cause for the disease, such as sexual abuse, must be identified and addressed by the therapist.[3]

Family therapy often is important in treating anorexia nervosa. It focuses on the role of the illness among family members, the reactions of individual family members, and ways in which their subconscious behavior might contribute to the abnormal eating patterns. Therapy includes all family members involved with the behavior problem. Frequently, a therapist finds family struggles at the heart of the problem. As the disorder resolves, patients must relate to family members in new ways to gain the attention previously tied to the disease. For example, the family may need to help the young person ease into adulthood and accept its responsibilities as well as its advantages.

Self-help groups for anorexic (and bulimic) people, as well as their families and friends, represent nonthreatening first steps into treatment. People can also attend to get a sense of whether they really do have an eating disorder.

Medications are generally not effective in treating the primary symptoms of anorexia nervosa. Fluoxetine (Prozac) may stabilize recovery in patients with anorexia who have attained 85% of their expected body weight.[5] Prozac works by increasing brain serotonin levels, which in turn regulates mood and feelings of satiety. A variety of other pharmacologic agents may have some role in treating mood changes, anxiety, or psychotic symptoms associated with anorexia nervosa but have limited value in patients unless weight gain is achieved. Food is the drug of choice for treating anorexic patients.

With professional help, many people with anorexia nervosa can lead normal lives. They then do not have to depend on unusual eating habits to cope with daily problems. Although they may not be totally cured, they do recover a sense of normality in their lives. No set answers or approaches exist, because each case is different. Establishing a strong

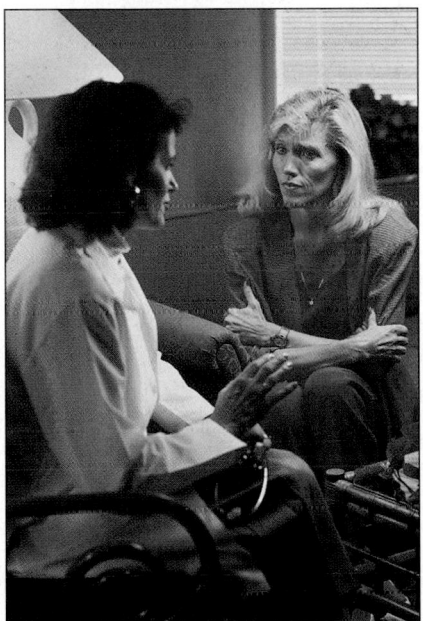

Anorexia nervosa is a potentially fatal disease that requires professional treatment.

A young woman in a self-help group for those with anorexia nervosa explained her feelings to the other group members: "I have lost a specialness that I thought it gave me. I was different from everyone else. Now I know that I'm somebody who's overcome it, which not everybody does."

cognitive behavior therapy Psychological therapy in which the person's assumptions about dieting, body weight, and related issues are challenged. New ways of thinking are explored and then practiced by the person. In this way, the person can learn new ways to control disordered eating behaviors and related life stress.

As noted in the Expert Opinion in this chapter, interpersonal therapy is another psychological approach used in anorexia nervosa. Rather than focusing on the patient's eating habits and assumptions about weight and shape, interpersonal therapy formulates the problem in terms of the interpersonal context, usually in one or more of four areas: grief, interpersonal problems (e.g., difficulty forming or maintaining close relationships), interpersonal disputes (e.g., unresolved conflict regarding the expectations of significant others in the person's life), or role transitions (e.g., fear of independence due to lack of self-confidence). Treatment focuses on assisting the patient to change in one or more of these areas.

relationship with either a therapist or another supportive person is an especially important key to recovery. Once anorexic patients feel understood and accepted by another person, they can begin to build a sense of self and exercise some autonomy. Then they can progress to substituting healthy relationships with others for a relationship with food, emphasizing alternative coping mechanisms.[3]

CASE SCENARIO
Follow-Up

Sarah does meet the DSM-IV qualifications to be diagnosed with anorexia nervosa because she refuses to maintain a healthy body weight for height, is at a weight below 85% of that expected, has a distorted view of her appearance, and has had amenorrhea for over 3 consecutive months.

Sarah would need to be hospitalized initially, due to her low BMI of 13.8. While in the hospital, her treatment would most likely consist of moderate bed rest to promote weight gain and an intake of 1000 to 1600 kcal initially, then increased by increments of about 100 to 200 kcal every few days until an acceptable rate of weight gain is achieved. The physician would likely prescribe a multivitamin and mineral supplement, along with 1200–1500 mg of calcium. A team of health professionals, most likely consisting of a physician, dietitian, and psychologist, would provide therapy. Sarah's cooperation would be the most important element for therapy to be successful. She needs to realize she has a problem and that she needs help, and she must be willing to accept the assistance these professionals are willing to offer. The team, especially the psychologist, may use cognitive behavior therapy to help Sarah improve her self-image.

Sarah's outlook for recovery is not good, unless she realizes she has a problem. Even if she is willing to accept the therapy and counseling, a relapse is likely to occur. Only about 50% of anorexia nervosa patients have been found to fully recover from the disease. Since Sarah's disordered eating habits have been in place for about 6 years, her problem is deep-rooted. The chances of recovery are greater if a vigorous treatment program is reinforced with close follow-up.

CONCEPT CHECK

To relieve the semistarved condition of most anorexic patients, the initial treatment focuses on moderately increased food intake and slow weight gain. Once this is accomplished psychotherapy can begin to uncover the causes of the disease and help patients develop the skills needed to return to a healthy life. Family therapy is an important tool in treatment, whereas medications have a limited role.

BULIMIA NERVOSA

Bulimia nervosa involves episodes of binge eating followed by various means to purge the food. This eating disorder was first described in 1979 and classified as a clinical psychiatric disorder in 1980. It is most common among young adults of college age, although some high school students are also at risk. Susceptible people often have genetic factors and lifestyle patterns that predispose them to becoming overweight, and many try frequent weight-reduction diets as teenagers. Like people with anorexia nervosa, those with bulimia nervosa are usually female and successful. Unlike anorexics, however, they are usually at or slightly above a normal weight. Females with bulimia nervosa are also more likely to be sexually active than those with anorexia nervosa.[3]

The person with bulimia nervosa may think of food constantly. In contrast to the anorexic person, who turns away from food when faced with problems, the bulimic person turns toward food in critical situations. Also, unlike those with anorexia nervosa, people with bulimia nervosa recognize their behavior as abnormal. These people often have very low self-esteem and are depressed. Approximately half of people with bulimia nervosa have major depression. Lingering effects of child abuse may be one reason for these feelings. Many bulimic persons report that they have been sexually abused.[3] The world sees their competence, while inside they feel out of control, ashamed, and frustrated.

Bulimic people tend to be impulsive, which may be expressed as stealing, drug and alcohol abuse, self-mutilation, or attempted suicide. Some experts have suggested that part of the problem may actually arise from an inability to control responses to impulse and desire.[15] Some studies have demonstrated that bulimic people tend to come from disengaged families, ones that are loosely organized. Roles for family members are not clearly defined. Too little protection is provided for family members, rules are very loose, and a great deal of conflict exists. Anorexic people tend to have families so actively engaged that roles may be too well defined.

■ Typical Behavior in Bulimia Nervosa

Many people with bulimic behavior are probably never diagnosed. The strict diagnostic criteria specify that, in order to be classified as having bulimia nervosa, a person must binge and purge at least twice a week for 3 months (review Table 15-1).[2] People with bulimia nervosa lead secret lives, hiding their abnormal eating habits. Moreover, it is impossible to recognize people with bulimia nervosa simply from their appearance. Because most diagnoses of bulimia nervosa are based on self-reports, current estimates of the number of cases are probably low. The disorder, especially in its milder forms, may be much more widespread than commonly thought.

Among sufferers of bulimia nervosa, bingeing often alternates with attempts to rigidly restrict food intake. Elaborate food rules are common, such as avoiding all sweets. Thus, eating just one cookie or donut may cause bulimic persons to feel they have broken a rule. Then the objectionable food must be eliminated. Usually, this leads to further overeating, partly because it is easier to regurgitate a large amount of food than a small amount. For intake to qualify as a binge, an atypically large amount of food must be consumed in a short time, and the person must exhibit a lack of control over this behavior.[2]

Binge-purge cycles may be practiced daily, weekly, or at longer intervals. A special time is often set aside. Most binge eating occurs at night, when other people are less likely to interrupt, and usually lasts from ½ to 2 hours. A binge can be triggered by a combination of hunger from recent dieting, stress, boredom, loneliness, and depression. It often follows a period of strict dieting and thus can be linked to intense hunger. The binge is not at all like normal eating; once begun, it seems to propel itself. The person not only loses control but generally doesn't even taste or enjoy the food that is eaten during a binge (Fig. 15-5).

Most commonly, bulimic people consume cakes, cookies, ice cream, and similar high-carbohydrate convenience foods during binges because these foods can be purged relatively easily and comfortably by vomiting. In a single binge, foods supplying up to 12,000 kcal or more may be eaten. Purging follows in hopes that no weight will be gained. However, even when vomiting follows the binge, 33 to 75% of the food energy taken in is still absorbed, which causes some weight gain. When laxatives or enemas are used, about 90% of the energy is absorbed, as these act in the large intestine, beyond the point of most nutrient adsorption. The common belief of bulimic persons that purging soon after bingeing will prevent excessive energy absorption and weight gain is clearly a misperception.

Early in the onset of bulimia nervosa, sufferers often induce vomiting by placing their fingers deep into the mouth. They may inadvertently bite down on these fingers. The resulting bite marks around the knuckles are a characteristic sign of this disorder. Once the disease is established, however, a person can often vomit simply by contracting the abdominal muscles. Vomiting may also occur spontaneously.[15]

Another way bulimic people attempt to compensate for a binge is by engaging in hypergymnasia—excessive exercise—to expend a large amount of energy. Some

*A*lice Machado, 1997's Miss Universe, reported being both anorexic and bulimic at the time she won the crown, stating, "Almost all of us are."

*F*requent binges can lead to enormous food bills for a bulimic person.

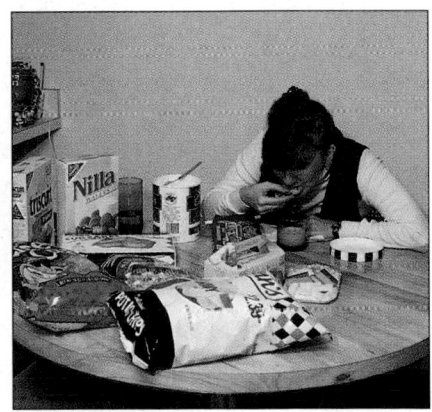

■ **FIGURE 15-5** The binge-purge cycle can lead to a sense of helplessness.

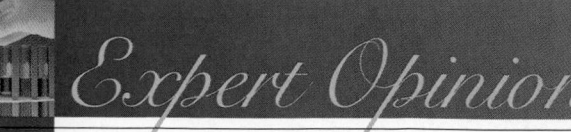

Expert Opinion

EATING DISORDERS

Laura Hill, Ph.D.

Eating disorders are serious health problems in the United States today. Approximately 5 million women will suffer at some time in their lives from eating disorders. There has been a consistent increase in the prevalence of eating disorders over the past 50 years in both the United States and Western Europe, especially among females within the age range of 15 to 24 years, as well as among identified subpopulations, such as some areas of athletics. Eating disorders consistently occur in 1 male for every 10 females.

Eating disorders are as old as history but relatively new to science. Hilde Bruch, a pioneer and leading authority on eating disorders, wrote that Socrates danced each morning so that he could remain slim. In the pre-Christian era, the Romans were as obsessed with fat as many in the United States are today. Women bound their breasts and starved themselves to look thin. Just as we design jacuzzis in our homes today, the Romans designed vomitoriums in their homes. The vomitoriums were used during the multiday feasts, when the Romans would binge over long periods of time and use the vomitoriums to make themselves vomit, only to continue to binge afterward.

CAUSES OF EATING DISORDERS

Cultures that demand slimness as an ideal for success, such as the United States and Western Europe, set the stage for a person to be vulnerable to eating disorders. In such cultures, the thinner one is, the more he or she is valued. In addition, psychological and biological factors play important roles in the development and maintenance of eating disorders. High achievement, perfectionism, and impulsivity are common psychological traits in persons with eating disorders. The newest genetic research shows that there may be a genetic predisposition for characteristics within a person, increasing vulnerability to develop an eating disorder. Common psychological disorders that coexist with eating disorders are depression, obsessive-compulsive disorder, and anxiety disorder. The family can also contribute to the development and maintenance of eating disorders, especially if depression or alcoholism runs in the family, or if acceptance and self-worth are evaluated through body shape. Hence, eating disorders are not caused by a single virus or biological abnormality. They are complicated and have factors that contribute to their development from the biological, psychological, social, and family areas. This is referred to as a biopsychosocial/familial problem.

WHAT TO LOOK FOR IN TREATMENT

A specialized team treatment approach is best. A general psychologist or family physician may not identify a patient with an eating disorder, due to the lack of experience or specialized training. To be most effective, eating disorders treatment should be comprehensive and multidimensional. This should include (1) specialized individual therapy that uses cognitive behavior therapeutic (CBT) or an interpersonal therapeutic (IPT) approach, (2) nutritional counseling by a person skilled in eating disorders treatment, (3) medication management as a supplement to individual therapy, and (4) family therapy if the person is still living with his or her family. Group therapy and support groups for eating disorders and some self-help books are also helpful for many who suffer with eating disorders.

In CBT individual therapy, the irrational thinking about body shape and dieting are confronted, along with the dysfunctional behaviors that are used to cope, such as binge eating or purging. Problem areas are addressed in the here and now. The person takes an active role in treatment. Research shows that CBT is more effective than medication management alone and other forms of individual therapy in the first 1 to 2 years. In CBT, the person learns to develop dietary regulation, problem-solving skills, and methods to prevent relapse. Interpersonal problems also need to be addressed through interpersonal therapy, which has proven to decrease eating disorders symptoms and to have better long-term effects.

The more severe the eating disorder, the more intense the treatment. If outpatient treatment is not sufficient, then other forms of treatment could be offered. Intensive outpatient treatment is usually 2 hours of group therapy a day, 3 to 5 days a week. If that is not enough, then day-hospital treatment could be offered, which is 6 to 12 hours a day, 5 to 7 days a week. The number of hours and days depends on the facility. Day-hospital is primarily offered in a group format, providing group therapy throughout the day, having planned meals in which all patients must participate, and offering family, nutritional, and medication management throughout the week. If the person still continues to demonstrate destructive eating disorder behaviors after returning home each night from treatment, then inpatient hospitalization is needed.

There are fewer and fewer inpatient eating disorders facilities in the United States. Many patients must travel out of state to receive both day or inpatient hospitalization for eating disorders. When an inpatient, the person is monitored to assure that the destructive eating disorder behaviors are not continuing during the 24-hour period. The patient learns to eat again. The nutritionist assigns him or her healthy portions of a wide variety of foods, and the patient is prevented from any form of purging. The patient may be in the day-hospital program and then monitored by professional staff after program hours to assure that the new healthier behaviors are practiced. Research shows that, when inpatient therapy is used to help persons with anorexia nervosa recover to normalized weight, the outcome is better because the intensive daily practice of healthier behaviors and the reframing of dysfunctional thinking around food and body shape allows the person to recover sooner and maintain a healthier body longer. Relapse is always a problem

with eating disorders; thus, outpatient treatment is needed after inpatient to help the person maintain newly developed healthier behaviors while he or she is reintegrating back into work or school.

OUTCOME

Do people get over eating disorders? Overall, there is a wide variety of outcomes. Some people have a full recovery and live normal lives, whereas other cases become chronic, and some even die. Long-term research shows that, after 10 years, 6.6% of patients with anorexia nervosa die, and 18% die after 30 years. Around one-fourth recover after 10 years. Up to half of those with anorexia may develop another form of an eating disorder, such as bulimia nervosa. Research shows that up to 3% of those with bulimia nervosa die, whereas around 50% fully recover. The course of recovery is unknown for binge-eating disorder. This is an area for further research.

If you or a friend experience many of the symptoms for an eating disorder listed in this chapter, then seek treatment. Eating disorders are one of the most difficult disorders to treat and overcome, but there is hope for better outcome if the treatment occurs early in the course of development. Otherwise, with each passing year the eating disorder becomes more deeply ingrained.

ILLUSTRATION

Assume you are a person with an eating disorder. This is similar to a person who is involved in an abusive relationship. The eating disorder is the abuser. The abuser may be charming and attractive and

someone with whom you want to be as much as possible. However, when alone with the abuser, the abuser begins to tell you how fat and incompetent you are. You begin to mistrust yourself and put in more and more effort to please the abuser living in your mind—dieting more, restricting more, and focusing on body shape to please the relentless voice of the abuser. The longer the abuser is allowed to reside in your mind, the more destroyed your self-esteem and life become. After a while, the eating disorder abuser controls all of your life, and there is rarely a moment in the day that you are not a slave to the abuser. Treatment helps you face the abusive eating disorder and leave it, knowing that it will stalk you and continually try to convince you that you cannot live well without it. The abuser tries to convince you that you are worthless without it. Treatment also works to help you realize that you are everything and more without an eating disorder abuser. With help and much support from friends and family, you may learn to live without an eating disorder.

You are the author of the end of your life story. What you do now to help yourself or a friend can make the difference for the rest of your life.

Dr. Laura Hill is a specialist in the field of eating disorders. She provides specialized treatment, consultations, and lectures nationally. She is the former director of the National Eating Disorders Organization and the author of numerous eating disorders publications. She is co-author of A 5 Day Lesson Plan on Eating Disorders.

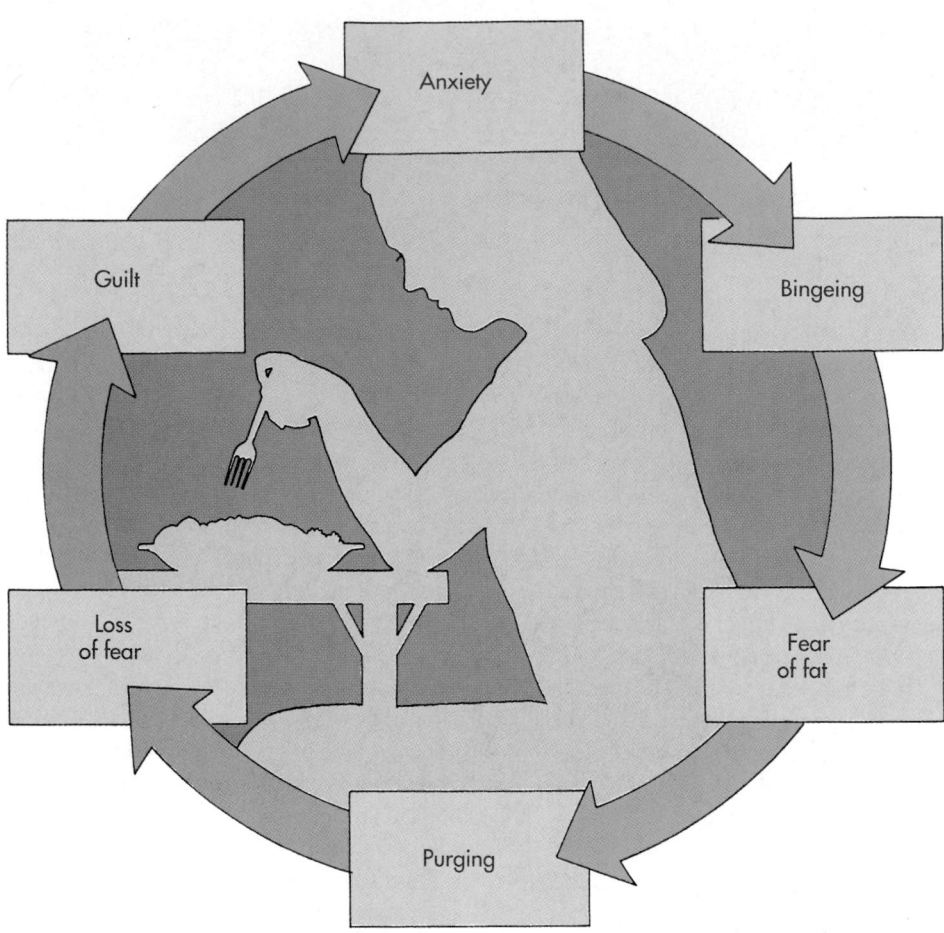

■ **FIGURE 15-6** Bulimia nervosa's vicious circle of obsession.

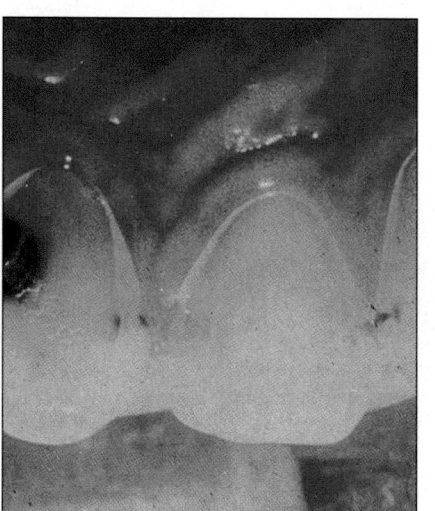

■ **FIGURE 15-7** Excessive tooth decay is common in bulimic patients.

bulimic people try to estimate the amount of energy eaten in a binge and then exercise to counteract this energy intake. This practice, referred to as "debting," represents an effort to control their weight.

People with bulimia nervosa are not proud of their behavior. After a binge, they usually feel guilty and depressed. Over time, they experience low self-esteem and feel hopeless about their situation (Fig. 15-6). Compulsive lying and drug abuse can further intensify these feelings. Bulimic people caught in the act of bingeing by a friend or family member may order the intruder to "get out" and "go away." Sufferers gradually distance themselves from others, spending more and more time preoccupied by and engaging in bingeing and purging.

■ Health Problems Stemming from Bulimia Nervosa

The vomiting that many bulimic sufferers induce is the most physically destructive method of purging. Indeed, the majority of health problems associated with bulimia nervosa arise from vomiting:[3, 19, 20]

- Repeated exposure of teeth to the acid in vomit causes demineralization, making the teeth painful and sensitive to heat, cold, and acids. Eventually, the teeth may severely decay, erode away from fillings, and finally fall out. Dental professionals are sometimes the first health professionals to notice signs of bulimia nervosa (Fig. 15-7). Until vomiting ceases, it is important to rinse the mouth with water after a vomiting episode, especially before brushing the teeth.
- Blood potassium can drop significantly with regular vomiting or the use of certain diuretics. This can disturb the heart's rhythm and even produce sudden death.
- Salivary glands may swell as a result of infection and irritation from persistent vomiting.

- Stomach ulcers and bleeding and tears in the esophagus develop in some cases.
- Constipation may result from frequent laxative use.
- Ipecac syrup, sometimes used to induce vomiting, is toxic to the heart, liver, and kidneys. It has caused accidental poisoning when taken repeatedly.

Overall, bulimia nervosa is a potentially debilitating disorder that can lead to death, usually from suicide, low blood potassium, or overwhelming infections.

■ Treatment of Bulimia Nervosa

Therapy for bulimia nervosa, as for anorexia nervosa, requires a team of experienced clinicians. These patients are less likely than those with anorexia to enter treatment in a state of semistarvation. However, if a bulimic patient has lost significant weight, this must be treated before psychological treatment begins. Although clinicians have yet to agree on the best therapy for bulimia nervosa, they generally agree that treatment should last at least 16 weeks. Hospitalization may be indicated in cases of extreme laxative abuse, regular vomiting, and substance abuse.[15]

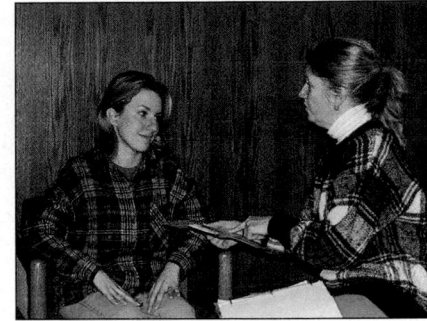

Bulimia nervosa affects many college students. Counselors are aware of this and are available to help.

The first goal of treatment for bulimia nervosa is to decrease the amount of food consumed in a binge session in order to decrease the risk of esophageal tears from related purging by vomiting. A decrease in the number of this type of purges will also decrease damage to the teeth.

The primary aim of psychotherapy is to improve patients' self-acceptance and help them to be less concerned about body weight. To correct the all-or-none thinking typical of bulimic persons—"If I eat one cookie, I'm a failure and might as well binge"—a patient may be asked to analyze the statement as a scientist would do when testing assumptions. In this way, patient and therapist together examine the validity of food and weight beliefs. The premise of this therapy is that, if abnormal attitudes and beliefs can be altered, normal eating will follow. In addition, the therapist guides the person in establishing food habits that will minimize bingeing: avoiding fasting, eating regular meals, and using alternative methods—other than eating—to cope with stressful situations.[15] Group therapy is often useful to foster strong social support. One goal of therapy is to help bulimic persons accept as normal some depression and self-doubt.

Although pharmacological agents should not be used as the sole treatment for bulimia nervosa, studies indicate that some medications may be beneficial in conjunction with other therapies. Fluoxetine (Prozac) is the only antidepressant that has been approved by FDA for use in the treatment of bulimia nervosa.[3] Physicians also may prescribe antidepressants (imipramine [Tofranil]) or mood stabilizers (lithium carbonate [Lithane]).

Nutritional counseling has two main goals: correcting misconceptions about food and re-establishing regular eating habits. Patients are given information about bulimia nervosa and its consequences. Avoiding binge foods and not constantly stepping on a scale may be recommended early in treatment. The primary goal, however, is to develop a normal eating pattern. To achieve this goal, some specialists encourage patients to develop daily meal plans and keep a food diary in which they record food intake, internal sensations of hunger, environmental factors that precipitate binges, and thoughts and feelings that accompany binge-purge cycles. Keeping a food diary not only is an accurate way to monitor food intake but also may help identify situations that seem to trigger binge episodes. With the help of a therapist, patients can develop alternative coping strategies.[3]

In general, the focus is not on stopping bingeing and purging per se but on developing regular eating habits. Once this is achieved, the binge-purge cycle should stop by itself. Patients are discouraged from following strict rules about healthy food choices, because this simply mimics the typical obsessive attitudes associated with bulimia nervosa. Rather, encouraging a mature perspective on nutrient intake—that is, regular consumption of moderate amounts of a variety of foods balanced among the food groups—helps patients overcome this disorder.

Setting time limits for the completion of meals and snacks is important for people with eating disorders. Many bulimic persons eat very quickly, reflecting their difficulties with satiety. Suggesting that the patient put his or her utensil down after each bite is a behavioral technique that a therapist might try with a recovering bulimic person. (Many anorexic persons eat in an excessively slow manner—for example, taking 1 hour to eat a muffin because it was cut into tiny, bite-size pieces.)

People with bulimia nervosa must recognize that it is a serious disorder that can have grave medical complications if not treated. Because relapse is likely, therapy should be long term. Note that those with bulimia nervosa need professional help because they can be very depressed and are at a high risk for suicide. About 50% of people with bulimia nervosa recover completely from the disorder. Others continue to struggle with it to varying degrees for the rest of their lives.[13, 22] This fact underscores the need for prevention because treatment is difficult.

■ EATING DISORDERS NOT OTHERWISE SPECIFIED (EDNOS)

EDNOS is a broad category of eating disorders in which the individuals have partial syndromes that do not meet the strict criteria for the other specific eating disorders. About 50% of people with eating disorders fall into this category, especially adolescents.[3] Examples of disordered eating in this category include (1) a woman who meets all the criteria for anorexia nervosa but continues to sustain menses; (2) an individual who meets all the criteria for anorexia nervosa but, despite a significant weight loss, the individual's current weight is in the normal range (this could be a person who was once obese); (3) a person who meets all the criteria for bulimia nervosa except that binge eating is less than two times a week; (4) a person who meets all the criteria for bulimia nervosa but does not binge (this person might eat normal amounts of food but purges regularly out of fear of weight or fat gain); and (5) a person who repeatedly chews and spits out food but does not swallow it.

Treatment as outlined for anorexia nervosa or bulimia nervosa should be sought in such cases, depending on the specific symptoms exhibited.

CONCEPT CHECK

Bulimia nervosa is characterized by episodes of binge eating followed by purging, usually by vomiting. Vomiting is very destructive to the body, often causing severe dental decay, stomach ulcers, irritation of the esophagus, and blood potassium imbalances. Treatment using nutrition counseling and psychotherapy attempts to restore normal eating habits, to help the person correct distorted beliefs about diet and lifestyle, and to find tools to cope with the stresses of life. Medications, such as fluoxetine (Prozac), can aid recovery when added to this regimen. Cases in which the symptoms and characteristics do not follow the strict guidelines for anorexia nervosa or bulimia nervosa typically fall under the category of Eating Disorders Not Otherwise Specified (EDNOS).

■ OTHER EXAMPLES OF DISORDERED EATING

In recent years, three other eating disorders—**female athlete triad, binge-eating disorder,** and **baryophobia**—have been recognized as requiring professional treatment. Although these disordered eating patterns share some characteristics with anorexia nervosa and bulimia nervosa, each has distinctive qualities.

■ Female Athlete Triad

Women participating in appearance-based and endurance sports are at risk of developing an eating disorder. A study of college-age female athletes found that 15% of

Female Athlete Triad A condition characterized by disordered eating, lack of menstrual periods, and osteoporosis.

binge-eating disorder An eating disorder characterized by recurrent binge eating and feelings of loss of control over eating. Binge episodes can be triggered by frustration, anger, depression, anxiety, permission to eat forbidden foods, and excessive hunger.

baryophobia A disorder of young children and young adults characterized by stunted growth. It results from parental underfeeding in an attempt to prevent the development of obesity and heart disease.

swimmers, 62% of gymnasts, and 32% of all varsity athletes exhibited disordered eating patterns. Estimates of eating disorders for college women not involved in competitive sports are much lower.

In addition to disordered eating, college women athletes tend to experience irregular menstruation more frequently than other college women. Disordered eating, particularly food restriction and stress, can precipitate this, causing women to have less dense and weaker bones than normal because of lower estrogen and higher cortisol concentrations in the blood. Some of these young women have bones equivalent to those of 50- to 60-year-olds, making them overly susceptible to fractures during both sports and general activities. Much of the bone loss is irreversible.[3]

The American College of Sports Medicine (ACSM) has named the syndrome female athlete triad because it consists of three parts, disordered eating, amenorrhea, and **osteoporosis.**[7] Not all athletes meet the criteria for eating disorders that are defined by the *Diagnostic and Statistical Manual of Mental Disorders* (review Table 15-1). Instead, they exhibit disordered eating tendencies and meet the other two criteria for female athlete triad. The ACSM has issued a call to teachers, coaches, health professionals, and parents to educate female athletes about the triad and its health consequences.

Many coaches/trainers and even some health professionals wrongly believe that amenorrhea is a normal consequence of a high level of physical activity. Amenorrhea has negative consequences on the body, such as fragile bones, because of decreased estrogen and increased cortisol concentrations in the blood. Correcting amenorrhea by increasing caloric intake should help normalize hormone levels and increase bone mineral density. During therapy, a physician may prescribe 1200–1500 mg of calcium and 400–800 IU of vitamin D per day to decrease bone mineral loss, as mentioned for anorexia nervosa.

Those exhibiting symptoms should seek treatment from a multidisciplinary team of health professionals. Involving the coach or trainer in therapy is usually a key factor in the success of the treatment plan. Suggestions for treatment are as follows:[12]

- Reduce preoccupation with food, weight, and body fat
- Gradually increase meals and snacks to an appropriate amount
- Achieve an appropriate weight for height
- Establish regular menstrual periods
- Decrease training time and/or intensity by 10 to 20%

The tragic case of Christy Henrich illustrates why anyone at risk for the female athlete triad should seek professional help. As a young teenager, Christy weighed 95 lb and was 4 feet 11 inches tall. She showed promise as a gymnast but was told that she was too fat to excel in gymnastics. Christy continued her training but often starved herself, some days consuming just an apple and frequently purging by vomiting. Her success in gymnastics continued, but at age 22 her weight had fallen to 52 pounds, and she died from the effects of long-term semistarvation.

■ Binge-Eating Disorder

In 1994, binge-eating disorder, commonly called *compulsive overeating*, was formally recognized by the American Psychiatric Association. The diagnostic criteria for this disorder are listed in Table 15-3. Generally, it can be defined as binge-eating episodes not accompanied by purging (as typifies bulimia nervosa) at least two times per week for at least 6 months. It thus falls under Eating Disorders Not Otherwise Specified. In the past, the catchall term *compulsive overeating* described a range of habitual excessive eating. Today, health-care professionals recognize this condition as complex and serious, as disturbing a problem as anorexia nervosa or bulimia nervosa.[2]

Approximately 30% of subjects in organized weight-control programs have binge-eating disorder, whereas among the general population only 2 to 5% have this disorder. However, many more people in the general population are likely to have less severe forms of the disorder that do not meet the formal criteria for diagnosis. The number of cases of binge-eating disorder is far greater than that of either anorexia

A female high school athlete recently admitted to a 3-year struggle with anorexia nervosa and bulimia nervosa. Even after her athletic performance declined and she suffered a related sports injury, which sidelined her for a year and required surgery, she continued to think that controlling both her weight and eating behaviors would make her the best—academically and physically. This example demonstrates several important points about eating disorders: certain groups of people are at greater risk for developing eating disorders; these people are often high achievers and are very careful about concealing their eating disorder; and eating disorders such as the female athlete triad, bulimia nervosa, and anorexia nervosa frequently overlap.

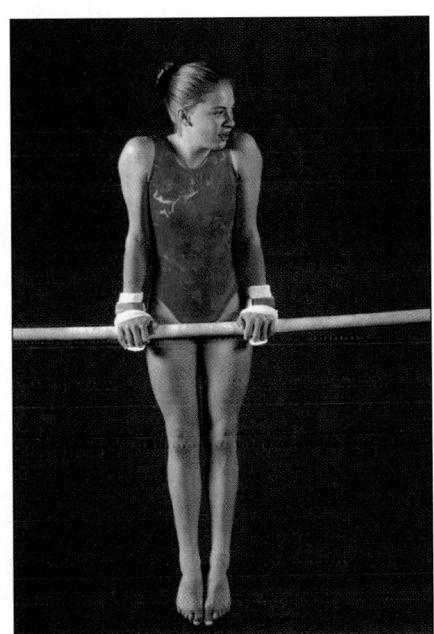

The female athlete triad occurs when the athlete has disordered eating, amenorrhea, and osteoporosis. This problem often is seen in appearance-related sports, such as gymnastics. Long-term health is at risk; thus, early treatment is most beneficial.

TABLE 15-3	Research Criteria for Binge-Eating Disorder

A. Recurrent episodes of binge eating, an episode being characterized by both of the following:
   (1) Eating, in a discrete period of time (e.g., within any 2-hour period), an amount of food that is definitely larger than most people would eat during a similar period of time in similar circumstances
   (2) A sense of lack of control during the episodes (e.g., a feeling that one can't stop eating or control what or how much one is eating)

B. During most binge episodes, at least three of the following occur:
   (1) Eating much more rapidly than usual
   (2) Eating until feeling uncomfortably full
   (3) Eating large amounts of food when not feeling physically hungry
   (4) Eating alone because of being embarrassed by how much one is eating
   (5) Feeling disgusted with oneself, depressed, or very guilty after overeating

C. Marked distress regarding binge eating

D. The binge eating occurs, on average, at least 2 days a week for 6 months.

E. The behavior does not occur only during the course of bulimia nervosa or anorexia nervosa.

Reprinted with permission from the *Diagnostic and Statistical Manual of Mental Disorders,* Fourth Edition. Copyright 1994 American Psychiatric Association.

nervosa or bulimia nervosa. This disorder is also more common among the severely obese and those with a long history of frequent restrictive dieting.

Development and Characteristics of Binge-Eating Disorder

Individuals with binge-eating disorder (about 40% of whom are males) often perceive themselves as hungry more often than normal. They usually started dieting at a young age, began bingeing during adolescence or in their early 20s, and did not succeed in commercial weight-control programs. Almost half of those with severe binge-eating disorder exhibit clinical depression.[5]

Typical binge eaters isolate themselves and eat large quantities of a favorite food. Stressful events and feelings of depression or anxiety can trigger this behavior. Giving themselves permission to eat a forbidden food can also precipitate a binge. Other triggers include loneliness, anxiety, self-pity, depression, anger, rage, alienation, and frustration. They sometimes binge on whatever is easy to eat in large amounts—noodles, rice, bread, leftovers. Characteristically, however, binge eaters consume foods that carry the social stigma of "junk" or "bad" foods—ice cream, cookies, sweets, potato chips, and similar snack foods.

In general, people engage in binge eating to induce a sense of well-being and perhaps even numbness, usually in an attempt to avoid feeling and dealing with emotional pain and anxiety. They eat without regard to biological need and often in a recurrent, ritualized fashion. Some people with this disorder eat food continually over an extended period, called *grazing;* others cycle episodes of bingeing with normal eating. For example, someone with a stressful or frustrating job might come home every night and graze until bedtime. Another person might eat normally most of the time but find comfort in consuming large quantities of food when an emotional setback occurs.

Although people with anorexia nervosa and bulimia nervosa exhibit persistent preoccupation with body shape, weight, and thinness, binge eaters do not necessarily share these concerns. Thus, neither purging nor prolonged food restriction is characteristic of binge-eating disorder. Some physicians classify binge-eating disorder as an addiction to food, involving psychological dependence. The person becomes attached to the behavior itself and has a drive to continue it, senses only limited control over it, and needs to persist at it despite negative consequences.

Food is used to reduce stress, produce feelings of power and well-being, avoid feelings of intimacy with others, and avoid life problems. Note that obesity and binge eating are not necessarily linked. Not all obese people are binge eaters, and, although obesity may result from trying to numb emotional pain with food, it is not necessarily an outcome.

Binge-eating disorder is most likely to develop in people who never learned to express and deal appropriately with their feelings. Rather than face their problems, they turn to food. They continue to do the things that perpetuate the experiences of frustration, anger, and pain. For example, people who regularly become frustrated because they don't assert themselves when necessary may eat to forget their frustration rather than learn to deal with this inhibition and practice assertiveness. The frustration will continue because they never attack the basic problem. Binge eating makes them feel they cannot control the behavior pattern and therefore cannot control their lives. Worse, the binge eating usually increases feelings of guilt, embarrassment, and shame.[2]

Often, people who practice binge eating have been shaped by families who do not address and express feelings in healthful ways. The parents nurture and comfort their children with food rather than engage in healthy exchanges of self-disclosure of feelings and potential solutions. Members of such families learn to eat in response to emotional needs and pain instead of hunger. Those who regularly practice binge eating may grow up nurturing others instead of themselves, avoiding their own feelings and taking little time for themselves. Not knowing how to satisfy their personal and emotional needs in more healthful ways, people in these families turn to food.

For some people, frequent dieting beginning in childhood or adolescence is a precursor to binge-eating disorder. During periods when little food is eaten, they get very hungry and obsessive about food. When allowed to eat more food, they feel driven to eat in a compulsive, uncontrolled way. The pattern of periods of strict dieting alternating with binge eating may continue over time.

Help for the Person with Binge-Eating Disorder

Those with binge-eating disorder must learn to eat in response to hunger—a biological signal—rather than in response to emotional needs or external factors (such as the time of day or the simple presence of food). Counselors often direct binge eaters to record their perceptions of physical hunger throughout the day and at the beginning and end of every meal. These people must learn to respond to a prescribed amount of fullness at each meal.[19] They should initially avoid weight loss diets because feelings of food deprivation can lead to more disruptive emotions and a greater sense of unmet needs. Diets are likely to encourage more intense problems, such as extreme hunger. Many people with binge eating disorder may experience difficulty in identifying personal emotional needs and expressing emotions. Because this problem is a common predisposing factor in binge eating, communication issues should be addressed during treatment. Binge eaters often must be helped to recognize their own buried emotions in anxiety-producing situations, and then encouraged to share them with their therapist or therapy group. Learning simple but appropriate phrases to say to oneself can help stop bingeing when the desire is strong.

Self-help groups, such as Overeaters Anonymous, aim to help recovery from binge-eating disorder. The treatment philosophy parallels that of Alcoholics Anonymous. Overeaters Anonymous attempts to create an environment of encouragement and accountability to overcome this eating disorder. Dietary advice typically ranges from avoiding restraint in eating to limiting binge foods. Some experts feel that learning to eat all foods—but in moderation—is an effective goal for binge eaters. This practice can prevent the feelings of desperation and deprivation that come from limiting particular foods. There is no set answer, but diet extremism is not needed. Antidepressants, such as fluoxetine (Prozac), and other types of medications have been found to help reduce binge eating in these individuals by

People with binge-eating disorder may come from families with alcoholism or may have suffered sexual abuse. Members of such dysfunctional families do not know how to deal effectively with emotions. They cope by turning to substances. Family members learn to cover up dysfunctional patterns for the alcoholic person and to nurture him or her at the expense of each other and their own needs.

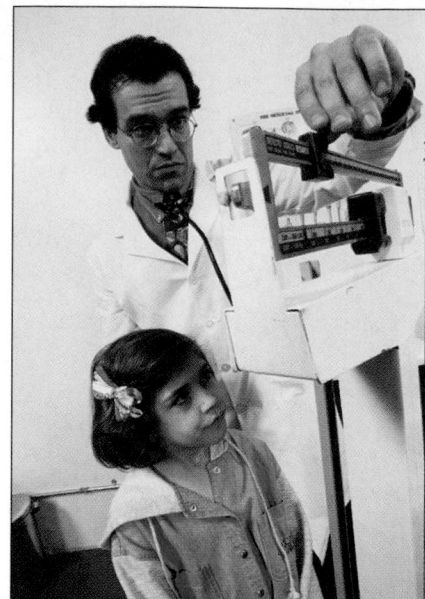

Gains in weight and height less than predicted for one's age can be a sign of baryophobia. If noted, this and other causes deserve further scrutiny.

CRITICAL THINKING

Tom, a high school teacher, is concerned about eating disorders. He wants to try to prevent young adults from falling into the discouraging traps of anorexia nervosa and bulimia nervosa. What are some of the topics and issues he should discuss with students in his health classes?

*N*ot only is treatment of eating disorders far more difficult than prevention, these disorders also have devastating effects on the entire family. For this reason, healthcare professionals and caregivers must emphasize the importance of an overall healthful diet and moderation, as opposed to restriction and perfection.

decreasing depression.[5] Overall, people who have this disorder are usually unsuccessful in controlling it on their own. Professional help is advised.

■ Baryophobia

Some children and young adults who grow more slowly and have a shorter stature than normal may suffer from baryophobia (literally, "the fear of becoming heavy"). Inadequate growth in children usually results from disease—commonly, a hormonal or other metabolic abnormality. In the absence of a recognized disease in such children, the possibility of baryophobia should be investigated.

This disorder occurs when children are given the same low-fat, high-carbohydrate diet that adults follow. Adults do this in an attempt to prevent children from developing obesity or cardiovascular disease later in life. Today's parents and caregivers, themselves frequently harassed by weight problems, may be determined that the children in their care will avoid such ordeals. Although these caregivers are well intended, such severely restricted diets are detrimental to children because they don't supply enough energy to sustain an adequate growth rate. In young adults, low-energy diets may be self-imposed to avoid a perceived risk of obesity.

Because this disorder results largely from lack of appropriate nutrition information leading to poor food choices, nutritional counseling to caregivers and young adults is the most effective response. They need to be informed about the nutrient requirements and normal weight-gain patterns for the relevant age group. This counseling will show caregivers that including some sweets and medium-fat foods in a child's diet is appropriate (see Chapter 17). The diet can still minimize saturated fat and cholesterol intake, a more important focus in a diet designed to reduce the risk of cardiovascular disease. Supplying adequate carbohydrate, protein, fat, and other nutrients is the key to promoting growth in both height and weight during childhood and the young-adult years, and it can be done in a healthful manner.

■ PREVENTION OF EATING DISORDERS

A key to developing and maintaining healthful eating behavior is to realize that some concern about diet, health, and weight is normal. It is also normal to experience variation in what we eat, how we feel, and even how much we weigh. For example, it is not abnormal to experience some minimal weight change (up to 2 to 3 lb) throughout the day and even more over the course of a week. A large weight fluctuation or ongoing weight gain or weight loss is a more likely to indicate that a problem is present. If you notice a large change in your diet, how you feel, or your body weight, it is a good idea to consult your personal physician. Treating physical and emotional problems early helps lead you to peace of mind and good health.

With a view to society as a whole, many people begin to form opinions about food, nutrition, health, weight, and body image prior or during puberty. Parents, friends, and professionals working with young adults should consider the following advice for preventing eating disorders:[3, 4, 12]

- Discourage restrictive dieting, meal skipping, and fasting.
- Provide information about normal changes that occur during puberty.
- Correct misconceptions about nutrition, healthy body weight, and approaches to weight loss.
- Carefully phrase weight-related recommendations and comments, and use them with caution.
- Don't overemphasize numbers on a scale. Instead, primarily promote healthful eating irrespective of body weight.
- Encourage normal expression of disruptive emotions.
- Encourage children to eat only when they're hungry.

- Teach the basics of proper nutrition and regular physical activity in school and at home.
- Provide adolescents with an appropriate but not unlimited degree of independence, choice, responsibility, and self-accountability for their actions.
- Increase self-acceptance and appreciation of the power and pleasure emerging from one's body.
- Enhance tolerance for diversity in weight, shape and ethnic food choices.
- Build respectful environments, supportive relationships.
- Encourage coaches to be sensitive to weight and body-image issues among athletes.
- Emphasize that thinness is not necessarily associated with better athletic performance.

Our society as a whole can benefit from a fresh focus on healthful food practices and a healthful outlook toward food and weight.

CONCEPT CHECK

The female athlete triad consists of disordered eating, amenorrhea, and osteoporosis, particularly those in appearance related and endurance sports. Parents, coaches, teachers, and health professionals need to initiate efforts to prevent and treat this problem. Grazing and food bingeing without purging are two behaviors characteristic of binge-eating disorder. Emotional disturbances are often at the root of this eating disorder. Treatment addresses deeper emotional issues and endorses avoiding food deprivation and restrictive diets, while restoring more normal eating behaviors. Baryophobia is a condition in which children are underfed by parents in an attempt to limit risk of future disease, such as obesity or cardiovascular disease. Growth failure—lack of expected weight and height gains—can result if nutrient intake is not increased to an appropriate amount.

Check out the *Perspectives in Nutrition* Online Learning Center http://www.mhhe.com/wardlaw for quizzes, flash cards, other activities, and web links designed to further help you learn about eating disorders.

■ BOOKS AND ORGANIZATIONS TO HELP YOU UNDERSTAND MORE ABOUT EATING DISORDERS

Along with the technical articles in the references, you can gain more insight into eating disorders from the following sources designed for the lay public:

Books

Barnhill J, Taylor N: *If you think you have an eating disorder.* New York: Dell, 1998.

Berg FM: *Women afraid to eat. Breaking free in today's weight obsessed world.* Hettinger, ND: Healthy Weight Network, 2000.

Cohen MA: *French toast for breakfast: Declaring peace with emotional eating.* Carlsbad, CA: Gruze, 1995.

Costin C: *The eating disorder sourcebook.* Chicago: RGA, 1996.

Gilbert SD, Commeford MC: *The unofficial guide to managing eating disorders.* Foster City, CA: IDG, 2000.

Gordon, RA: *Eating disorders: Anatomy of a social epidemic.* Malden, MA: Blackwell, 2000.

Hirshman JR, Munter CH: *When women stop hating their bodies.* New York: Ballantine, 1995.

Nash JD: *Binge no more: your guide to overcoming disordered eating.* Oakland, CA: New Harbinger, 1997.

Siegel M, Brisman J, Weinshel M: *Surviving an eating disorder. Strategies for families and friends.* New York: HarperCollins, 1998.

Organizations and Self-Help Groups

Academy for Eating Disorders, 6728 McClean Village Dr., McLean, VA 22101; 703-556-9222; http://www.acadeatdis.org

American Anorexia Bulimia Association, 165 West 46th St., #1108, New York, NY 10036; 212-575-6200; http://www.aabainc.org/home.html

Eating Disorders Awareness and Prevention (EDAP), 603 Stewart St., Suite 803, Seattle, WA 98101; 206-382-3587 or 8000 931-EDAP; http://www.edap.org

Harvard Eating Disorders Centers, 356 Boylston St., Boston, MA 02116 617-236-7766; http://www.hedc.org

The National Eating Disorders Organization, 6655 South Yale Ave., Tulsa, OK 74136; 918-481-4044; http://www.laureate.com

Summary

1. Anorexia nervosa is most common among high-achieving perfectionist girls from families marked by conflict, high expectations, rigidity, and denial. The disorder usually starts with dieting in early puberty and proceeds to the near-total refusal to eat. Early warning signs include intense concern about weight gain and dieting, as well as abnormal food habits, such as cooking food that they won't allow themselves to eat and classifying foods as safe and unsafe.

2. Anorexic persons become irritable, hostile, overly critical, and joyless; they tend to withdraw from family and friends. Eventually, anorexia nervosa can lead to numerous physical effects, including a profound decrease in body weight and body fat, a fall in body temperature and heart rate, iron deficiency anemia, a low white blood cell count, hair loss, constipation, low blood potassium, and the cessation of menstrual periods. Those with anorexia nervosa are physically very ill.

3. Treatment of anorexia nervosa includes increasing food intake to support slow weight gain. Psychological counseling attempts to help patients establish regular food habits and to find means of coping with the life stresses that led to the disorder. Hospitalization may be necessary, as well as use of certain medications.

4. Bulimia nervosa is characterized by bingeing on large amounts of food at one sitting and then purging by vomiting or misuse of laxatives, diuretics, or enemas. Alternately fasting and excessive exercise may be used. Both men and women are at risk. Vomiting as a means of purging is especially destructive to the body; it can cause severe tooth decay, stomach ulcers, irritation of the esophagus, low blood potassium, and other problems.

Bulimia nervosa poses a serious health problem and is associated with significant risk of suicide.

5. Treatment of bulimia nervosa includes psychological as well as nutritional counseling. During treatment, bulimic persons learn to accept themselves and to cope with problems in ways that do not involve food. Regular eating patterns are developed as these patients begin to plan meals in an informed, healthful manner. Certain medications can be a helpful addition to the regimen.

6. The female athlete triad consists of disordered eating, amenorrhea, and osteoporosis and is particularly common in appearance-related and endurance sports. If not corrected, this disorder eventually leads to decreased athletic performance and general health problems.

7. Binge-eating disorder, which is more widespread than either anorexia nervosa or bulimia nervosa, is most common among people with a history of frequent, unsuccessful dieting. Binge eaters typically either practice grazing (i.e., eating continually over extended periods) or bingeing without purging. Emotional disturbances are often at the root of this disordered form of eating. Treatment addresses deeper emotional issues, discourages food deprivation and restrictive diets, and helps restore normal eating behaviors. Certain medications may be a useful addition to this therapy.

8. Baryophobia is a condition in which children are underfed by caregivers in an attempt to limit the risk of future disease, such as obesity or cardiovascular disease. Growth failure—in weight and height gains—can result if nutrient intake is not increased to appropriate amounts.

Study Questions

1. What are the typical characteristics of a person with anorexia nervosa? What may influence a person to begin rigid, self-imposed dietary patterns?

2. List the detrimental physical and psychological side effects of bulimia nervosa. Describe important goals of the psychological and nutrition therapy used to treat bulimic patients.

3. What is the current thinking concerning medication use for anorexia nervosa and bulimia nervosa?

4. Explain the role of hypergymnasia in eating disorders. What is debting?

5. How might parents significantly contribute to the development of an eating disorder? Suggest an attitude that a parent or an adult friend of yours displayed that may not have been conductive to developing a normal relationship to food.

6. Based on your knowledge of good nutrition and sound dietary habits, answer the following questions:
   a. How can repeated bingeing and purging lead to significant nutrient deficiencies?
   b. How can significant nutrient deficiencies contribute to major health problems in later life?
   c. A friend asks you, the nutrition expert, if it is okay to "cleanse" the body by eating only grapefruit for a week. What is your response?

7. How, in your opinion, has society contributed to the development of various forms of disordered eating? Provide an example.

8. List the three symptoms that constitute the female athlete triad. What is the major health risk associated with amenorrhea in the female athlete?

9. How does binge-eating disorder differ from bulimia nervosa? Describe the factors that contribute to the development and treatment of binge-eating disorder.

10. Describe the common characteristics of a parent of a child with baryophobia.

ANNOTATED REFERENCES

1. ADA Reports: Position of the American Dietetic Association: Nutrition intervention in the treatment of anorexia nervosa, bulimia nervosa, and binge eating. *Journal of the American Dietetic Association* 94:902, 1994.

   The role of dietitians in nutritional assessment and treatment of eating disorders is fundamental to the overall therapy. The registered dietitian provides nutrition education or medical nutrition therapy and has the essential expertise to facilitate the highly individualized changes in food- and weight-related behaviors that are necessary for full recovery from an eating disorder.

2. American Psychiatric Association: *Diagnostic and statistical manual of mental disorders (DSM-IV)*. Washington, DC: American Psychiatric Association, 1994.

   This manual contains the criteria used in diagnosing an eating disorder. The specific criteria for anorexia nervosa, bulimia nervosa, and binge eating disorder are provided.

3. American Psychiatric Association: Practice guidelines for the treatment of patients with eating disorders (revision), *American Journal of Psychiatry* 157 (suppl): 4, 2000.

   People with eating disorders display a broad range of symptoms that occur along a continuum from between those of anorexia nervosa and those of bulimia nervosa. The care of these people requires a comprehensive array of approaches to provide the best chance of treatment success.

4. Anderson AE: Recognizing eating disorders, *Nutrition & the M.D.*, p. 1, August 1998.

   This article is from a physician's standpoint, concentrating on how to detect an eating disorder, as well as the role of a dietitian in treatment. The ultimate goal for health professionals should be to prevent eating disorders and to free adolescents from the burden of an unnecessary drive for thinness, in turn replacing this cultural insanity with healthy habits of eating and exercise.

5. Becker AE and others: Eating disorders. *The New England Journal of Medicine* 340:1092, 1999.

   This article reviews all facets of eating disorders, from detection to treatment, and is an excellent reference for more in-depth knowledge of eating disorders. All those with eating disorders should be evaluated and treated for medical complications of the disease at the same time psychotherapy and nutritional counseling are undertaken.

6. Chidley E: Eating disorders, nature or nurture. *Today's Dietitian*, p. 29, February 1999.

   Various studies that have shown correlations between genetics and eating disorder development. This new knowledge however is not going to change current therapy. We know that cognitive behavior therapy works for bulimia, and the fact that there are some genes that increase risk for developing the disease isn't going to change that practice.

7. Clairmont MA: The female athlete triad. *Today's Dietitian*, p. 47, September 1999.

   The author reviews the assessment and treatment of each of the three components of female athlete triad, as well as integrated treatment for the disorder as one entity. All too often amenorrhea is seen as a normal consequence of athletic training by athletes. Awareness and education efforts must be targeted to these individuals concerning the negative health consequences of this disorder.

8. Eating disorders and exercise: The connection. *Nutrition & the M.D.*, p. 5, July 1998.

   Excessive exercise is a predictor in the development of anorexia nervosa. Many people with anorexia nervosa misuse exercise. These individuals expend a tremendous amount of energy by staying in almost constant movement. The desire to exercise is so strong that it appears as if there is an addiction to exercise itself.

9. Faine M, Mobley C: Case problem: Balancing nutrition advice with dental care in patients with anorexia and bulimia. *Journal of the American Dietetic Association* 99(10):1291, 1999.

   Extensive loss of tooth enamel is common in people with bulimia nervosa. The authors provide a detailed description of therapy for a patient who presented with an eating disorder and dental health problems.

10. Fairburn CG and others: Risk factors for anorexia nervosa: Three integrated case-control comparisons. *Archives of General Psychiatry* 56:468, 1999.

    Perfectionism and negative self-evaluation are common personality traits associated with an eating disorder.

11. Halmi KA: A 24-year old with anorexia nervosa. *Journal of the American Medical Association* 279:1992, 1998.

    This article reviews an in-depth case study of a patient with anorexia nervosa; it broadens understanding of the psychological aspect of the disease. Also summarized the etiology, pathophysiology, clinical course, and treatment of anorexia nervosa.

12. Hobart JA, Smucker DR: The female athlete triad. *American Family Physician* 61(11):3357, 2000.

    This article discusses the importance of the physician in detecting female athlete triad during a preparticipation sports physical exam. The author provides helpful hints in obtaining important information from the patient during the exam. Many patients may benefit from a treatment plan that involves consultation with subspecialists. The involvement of a psychiatrist or psychologist and a dietitian who specialize in the management of the female athlete triad may facilitate prompt improvement.

13. Keel PK: Long-term outcome of bulimia nervosa. *Archives of General Psychiatry* 56:63, 1999.

Long-term follow-up of bulimia nervosa patients has shown that about 30% continue to engage in binge eating or purging behaviors. The predictors of poor long-term outcome were longer duration of symptoms at the time of clinical presentation and a history of substance abuse.

14. Krowchuk CP and others: Problem dieting behaviors among young adolescents. *Archives of Pediatric & Adolescent Medicine* 152:884, 1998.

There is a relationship between dieting behaviors in adolescents development of an eating disorder. Younger adolescents trying to lose weight typically engage in a variety of problem dieting and weight loss behaviors that can compromise health and may be associated with eating disorders.

15. McGilley BM, Pryor TL: Assessment and treatment of bulimia nervosa. *American Family Physician* 57: 2743, 1998.

This article discusses the clinical signs of bulimia nervosa and how to evaluate and treat patients with this eating disorder. The initial goal of cognitive—behavioral therapy is to restore control over dietary intake. Caloric restriction and dieting efforts that set patients up to binge should be avoided.

16. Morgan JF and others: The SCOFF questionnaire: Assessment of a new screening tool for eating disorders. *British Medical Journal* 319:1467, 1999.

British researchers have developed and tested a five-question screening tool for eating disorders, called the SCOFF questionnaire, in which each letter stands for a term in each question.

17. Neumark-Sztainer D and others: Disordered eating among adolescents with chronic illness and disability. *Archives of Pediatric & Adolescent Medicine* 152:871, 1998.

Adolescents with a physical disability or chronic illness, such as diabetes mellitus or asthma are at even greater risk for disordered eating than are those without a chronic illness.

18. Patton GC and others: Onset of adolescent eating disorders: Population based cohort study over 3 years. *British Medical Journal* 318:765, 1999.

Dieting was the most important predictor of an eating disorder in this study. Exercise did not pose a threat in eating disorder development, so it is suggested that adolescents be encouraged to exercise, rather than using dieting techniques, to maintain or improve weight status.

19. Ruud J, Calhoun A: Nondiet approach to binge disorder. *Today's Dietitian*, p. 30, March 2000.

This article includes two case studies that describe a nondiet approach to treating binge-eating disorder. This includes eating in response to hunger, normalizing feelings about food, and accepting one's size.

20. Steinberg L: Oral manifestations of eating disorders. *Nutrition & the M.D.*, 1997.

The oral manifestations of purging and typically obvious signs of eating disorders. Patients with purging behaviors need to follow the dental hygiene tips that are reviewed in this article, such as quickly rinsing one's mouth with water after vomiting.

21. Story M and others: Dieting status and its relationship to eating and physical activity behaviors in a representative sample of U.S. adolescents, *Journal of the American Dietetic Association* 98:1127. 1998.

Adolescents engaged in extreme weight control behaviors may be at risk for inadequate nutrient intake. In contrast, adolescents using more moderate approaches may be consuming a more healthful diet.

22. Walsh BT, Devlin MJ: Eating disorders: Progress and problems. *Science* 280:1387, 1998.

This article reviews the etiology of eating disorders with regard to biological, genetic, and cultural relationships. The authors also discuss the treatment approaches for each eating disorder. Although there is substantial variability among studies, overall the results suggest that a significant portion of the risk for developing an eating disorder is inherited.

TAKE ACTION

I. ASSESSING RISK OF DEVELOPING AN EATING DISORDER

British investigators have developed a five-question screening tool called the SCOFF Questionnaire for recognizing eating disorders:[16]

1. Do you make yourself Sick because you feel full?
2. Do you lose Control over how much you eat?
3. Have you lost more than One stone (about 13 lb) recently?
4. Do you believe yourself to be Fat when others say you are thin?
5. Does Food dominate your life?

Two or more positive responses suggest an eating disorder.

1. After completing this questionnaire, do you feel that you might have an eating disorder or the potential to develop one?

   _____

   _____

2. Do you think some of your friends might have an eating disorder?

   _____

   _____

3. What counseling and education resources exist in your area or on your campus to help with a potential eating disorder?

   _____

   _____

4. If a friend has an eating disorder, what do you think is the best way to assist him or her in getting help?

   _____

   _____

II. HELPING PREVENT EATING DISORDERS

You have been asked to speak to a junior high school class about eating disorders. What are four major points that you would make to help prevent disordered eating in this population?

1. _____
2. _____
3. _____
4. _____

Here are points you may consider:

1. Extreme thinness is oversold in the media. Extremely low weight (i.e., BMI of less than 19) is generally not healthy.
2. Self-induced vomiting is dangerous. Damage to the teeth, stomach, and esophagus often results.
3. Loss of menstrual periods (amenorrhea) is a sign of illness. It is important to see a physician about this. Bone deterioration is a common result.
4. The treatment of eating disorders in early phases aids success. These diseases are difficult to treat once firmly established.

EATING DISORDERS: A SOCIOLOGICAL PERSPECTIVE

One of the many criteria we use to evaluate ourselves is body image. We identify our bodies with our selves and judge them as we think others see us, knowing that our appearance affects their opinions of us.[4]

Early in life, we develop images of "acceptable" and "unacceptable" body types. Of all the attributes that constitute attractiveness, many people view body weight as the most important, partly because we can control our weight somewhat. Fatness is the most dreaded deviation from our cultural ideals of body image, the one most derided and shunned, even among schoolchildren.

Females in particular are likely to diet because they feel strongly about what is acceptable in both size and weight. In general, though, most dieting women aren't technically obese. Rather, they diet to correct some perceived flaw or because they simply feel they should weigh less than they do now. Their impulse "to please" fosters this desire to look socially acceptable.

A recent survey in the magazine *Redbook* found that, of more than 3000 respondents, only 3% of the women were happy with their bodies. In contrast, 42% wanted to lose more than 50 pounds, 22% wanted to lose 20 to 50 pounds, 19% wanted to lose 10 to 20 pounds, and 11% wanted to lose 5 to 10 pounds.

CHANGING TIMES

The cultural ideal of the "full-bodied" woman did not survive into the twentieth century in Western society, although it is still in fashion in many nonindustrialized countries, where a large body is a sign of wealth. Over the course of the twentieth century, the ideal female body form in the United States became progressively thinner. A thin waist with modest hips is now the overriding cultural "gold standard," at least as exemplified by models. Our passion for thinness may have its roots in the Victorian era, which specialized in denying "unpleasant" physical realities, such as appetite and sexual desire. Flappers of the 1920s cemented a trend for thinness (Fig. 15-8). Even as the ideal gradually moved toward a thinner, more angular body shape, the average weight among the general female population increased.

THINNESS AS AN INDICATOR OF COMPETENCE

Unfortunately, many Americans today view obesity as a failure of control, willpower, competence, and productivity. At stake are social acceptance and even access to scarce resources, such as good jobs and an attractive spouse. Whether we like it or not, in today's society our appearance says a lot about us, even though the way we were raised and our genetic background are beyond our control. Some people are simply much more likely to become obese than others. Implicit in our societal attitudes is the notion that those who can't control themselves enough to stay slim are unlikely to be good at supervising employees, organizing their work day, and shouldering heavy responsibilities. Clearly, fat is out. A prevailing myth is that thin people are more competent, energetic, and forceful than obese people.

MIXED MESSAGES AND SOCIAL TRENDS

Despite the pressure for thinness, our society is filled with mixed messages. Half the advertisements in women's magazines may describe diets or feature emaciated models; the other half displays tasty foods. Movie and television stars are almost always perfect physical specimens. Nevertheless, television advertisements encourage us to visit our local quick-service restaurant. There you can buy a hamburger, French fries, and large soft drink, totaling approximately

1200 kcal or more—about the amount of energy our daily basal metabolism uses—without even leaving the car.

In the past several decades, divorce, alcohol abuse in families, child abuse, school- and work-related stress, socioeconomic changes, and crowded urban conditions have all increased. These changes in our family and social environments encourage children, adolescents, and adults alike to find a release from the pressure. Many find relief in food, which sets the stage for the development of an eating disorder.

INTERNALIZING THE THINNESS IDEAL

Eating disorders are usually only a symptom of significant emotional trauma or psychological stress in a person's life. When psychiatrists are able to dig deeper, they find that eating disorders mask serious questions of self-worth, family struggles, and sometimes fears of puberty and the future.[3] The real illnesses are not the eating disorders—though they eventually contribute to poor health—but, rather, the way people feel about themselves. When people internalize the social value favoring thinness and can't meet that goal, their negative self-image is reinforced.

Researchers have linked this preference for a lean body type to the recent surge in eating disorders.[11] As the more full-figured woman (earth mother) was displaced by the ultrathin woman, the number of eating disorders increased, along with our society's preoccupation with obesity. The cultural pressures toward thinness seem to be stretching the physiological capabilities of many women (and men). For example, researchers surmise that the theoretical body fat content of the "Barbie doll" would not allow for menstruation. Given the natural variability in human basal metabolism and genetic makeup, as well as Americans' easy access to food and increasingly sedentary lifestyles, it is no surprise that some of us gain weight. People predisposed to eating disorders for either biological or emotional reasons may be nudged over the edge by these social changes.[3]

<table>
<tr>
<td>(a)</td>
<td>(b)</td>
<td>(c)</td>
<td>(d)</td>
</tr>
</table>

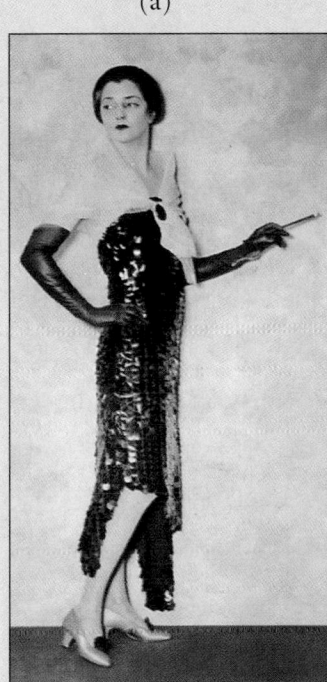 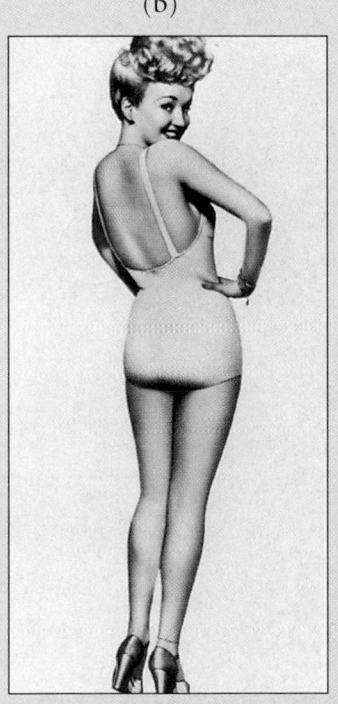 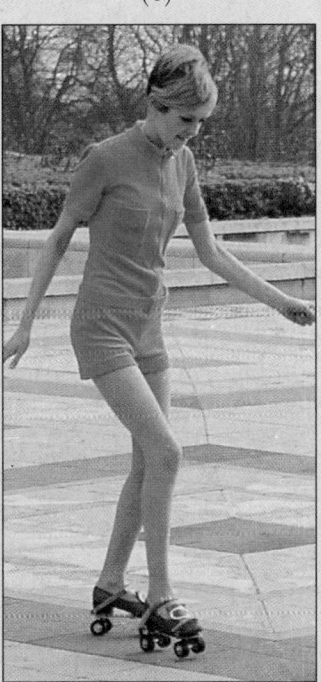 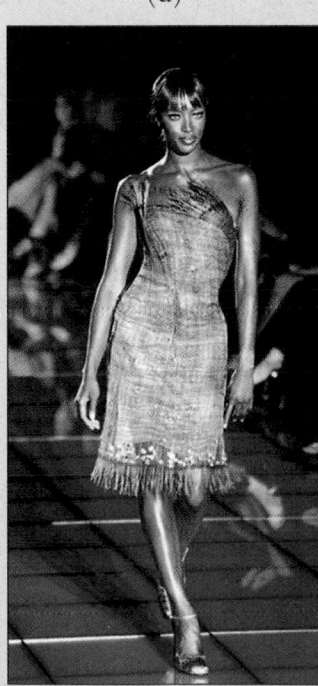

■ FIGURE 15-8 The changing views of desirable body weight. American society has imposed varying stereotypes for a desirable body weight, especially for women: (a) the svelte flapper of the 1920s; (b) the "thin but curvaceous" look of the 1940s; (c) ultrathin was in during the 1960s; (d) at the turn of the twenty-first century, women's fashion is trending toward the image of the muscularly fit, with little evidence of body fat.

Glimmers of Hope

Because eating disorders stem in part from certain cultural values, changing these values might reduce the pressures predisposing some people to various types of disordered eating behavior. Feminists, for example, assert that true liberation means being free to find one's natural weight. Women who combine careers and motherhood are saying that they have more important things to worry about; some fashion leaders are tolerating more curves; exercise programs are encouraging regular brisk walking, rather than mostly jogging and working out. Writers, therapists, and some registered dietitians are working to help women accept their bodies, as noted in the "size acceptance" approach discussed in Chapter 13.

What is the difference between people who can accept themselves—even with a few more pounds than the glamorous people have—and those who chronically diet and feel dissatisfied? Perhaps it is the willingness to recognize that satisfaction comes from within, not from the mirror or the approval of others. The challenge facing many Americans is achieving a healthy body weight without excessive dieting. This means adopting and maintaining sensible eating habits, a physically active lifestyle, and realistic and positive attitudes and emotions while practicing creative ways to handle stress.[4]

PREGNANCY AND BREASTFEEDING

chapter 16

Pregnancy can be a very special time for a couple. Along with the responsibility of shaping a child's health and personality comes the prospective exhilaration of watching the child develop and grow. These parents often feel an overriding desire to produce a healthy baby, which can pique new interest in nutrition and health information. The parents-to-be usually want to do everything possible to maximize their chances of having a robust, lively newborn.

Despite these possibilities, the infant mortality rate in the United States is higher than that of 24 other industrialized nations. In the United States, about 7.2 of every 1000 infants per year die before their first birthday,[13] and about 25 to 30% of pregnant women receive inadequate prenatal care in the early months of pregnancy.[22] Teenage mothers are at the highest risk.[7] These are alarming statistics for the country that has the highest per capita expenditure for health care in the world.

Producing a healthy baby is not just a matter of luck. True, some aspects of fetal and newborn health are beyond a parent's control. Still, conscious decisions about social, health, and nutritional factors significantly affect the baby's health and future.[31] What the parents do relates directly to the likelihood of having a healthy newborn. Then choosing to breastfeed the infant adds further benefit. Let's examine the practices that build toward having a healthy baby.

KEY CHAPTER CONCEPTS

- Pregnancy should be planned, as many hazardous health practices of the mother are modifiable, such as alcohol, drug, and certain medication use; smoking; and an inadequate diet.
- Adequate synthetic folate intake should be established at least 8 weeks before the time of conception to reduce the risk of neural tube defects.
- Certain diet and lifestyle habits throughout pregnancy, particularly in the first trimester, can cause birth defects, as well as harm to the mother. One example is alcohol use.
- Infants born preterm (before 37 weeks) or with low birth weight (less than 5.5 lb [2.5 kg]) usually have more medical problems than typical infants.
- An additional 300 kcal/day are usually needed to meet the energy needs of pregnancy in the second and third trimester. Gradual weight gain should reach a goal of approximately 25 to 35 lb throughout pregnancy.
- Protein, vitamin, and mineral needs increase during pregnancy and can often be met by increasing servings of dairy and lean meats and by consuming a ready-to-eat breakfast cereal on a regular basis.
- Iron and folate supplements may be prescribed during pregnancy, as it can be difficult to meet the needs for these nutrients from diet alone. A prenatal supplement generally is prescribed; this practice contributes to both needs.
- Almost all women are able to breastfeed. Advantages of breastfeeding over formula feeding include fewer intestinal, respiratory, and ear infections and fewer allergies and food intolerances for the infant. Breastfeeding is also less expensive and may be more convenient for the mother.

REFRESH YOUR MEMORY

As you begin your study of nutrition in pregnancy and breastfeeding in Chapter 16, you may want to review

- Reproductive and immune systems in Chapter 3
- The components of the macronutrient classes—carbohydrates, proteins, and lipids—in Chapters 5–7, especially omega-3 fatty aids
- Alcohol intake and fetal alcohol syndrome in Chapter 8
- The food sources of folate in Chapter 10, calcium in Chapter 11, and iron and zinc in Chapter 12
- The calculation of body mass index in Chapter 13.

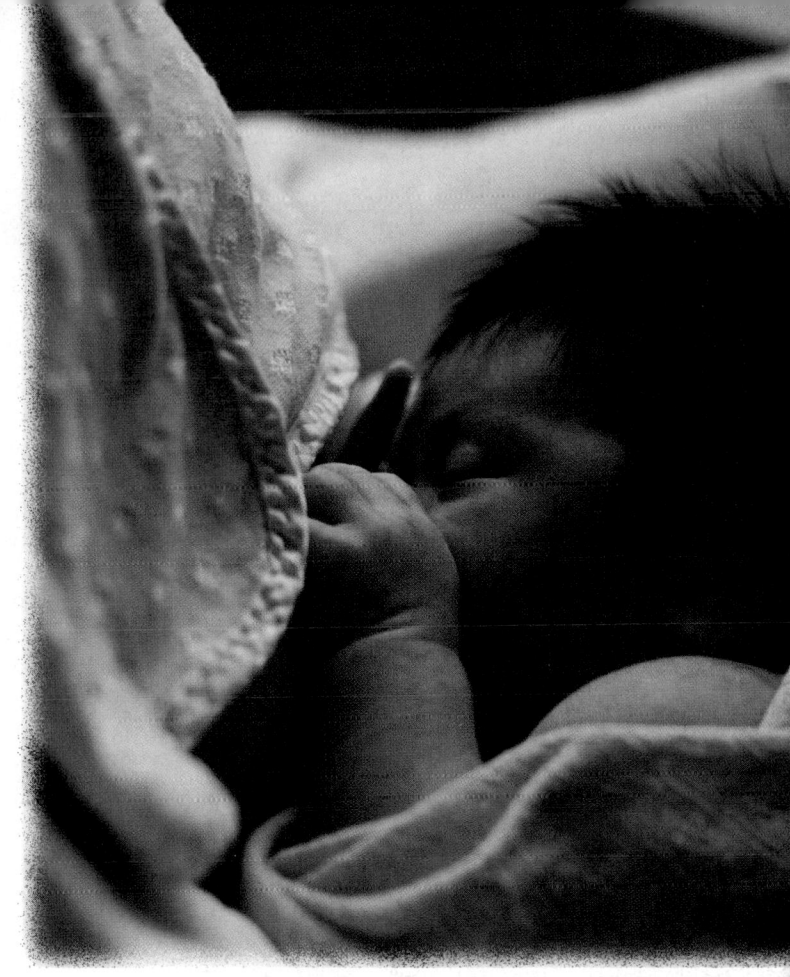

CASE SCENARIO

Tracey and her husband of 4 years have decided that they are ready to prepare for Tracey's first pregnancy. Tracey has been reading everything she can find on pregnancy because she knows that her prepregnancy health is important to the success of her pregnancy.

She just turned 25 and, so, is in the recommended childbearing age of 24 to 35 years. She knows to avoid alcohol, especially because she could become pregnant and not find that out right away. Alcohol is particularly toxic to the growing fetus in the first weeks of pregnancy. She is not a smoker, doesn't take any medications, and limits her coffee intake to 6 cups a day.

Based on her reading, she has decided to breastfeed her infant and has already checked out childbirth classes. She has modified her diet to include some extra protein, along with more fruits and vegetables. Recently, she started a running program 5 days a week, and she plans to continue running throughout her pregnancy. She has also started taking an over-the-counter vitamin and mineral supplement.

Tracey and her husband think that they have covered all the key areas of pre-pregnancy care. List a few positive attributes of her current practices you support. Can you identify some potential problems and what information they may have missed?

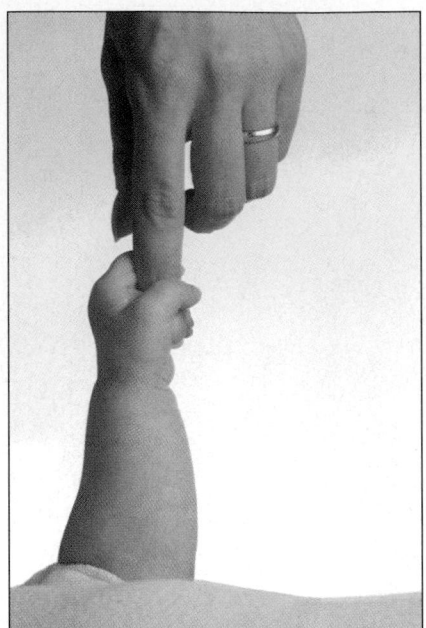

Attention to diet and lifestyle in pregnancy is worth the time and effort.

■ PLANNED PREGNANCY

Pregnancy deserves planning because many practices or conditions of the mother that can harm the developing fetus are modifiable, such as the following:[31]

- Alcohol consumption
- Use of certain medications, such as heavy use of aspirin
- Use of illegal drugs, such as cocaine
- Job-related hazards and stresses
- Smoking
- Inadequate diet, such as too little iron and too little synthetic folate intake
- Excess vitamin A intake and megadose use of other nutrient supplements
- Heavy caffeine use
- Lack of medical treatment with HIV-positive status or AIDS
- Poor control of ongoing diabetes or hypertension

Women need to pay attention to these risks in the months before conception. This precaution is necessary because women often do not suspect they are pregnant during the first few weeks after conception and may not seek medical attention until after the first 2 to 3 months.[22]

Still, even without fanfare, the child-to-be grows and develops daily. For that reason, the health and nutrition habits of a woman who is trying to become pregnant—or has the potential to become pregnant—are particularly important. Although some aspects of fetal and newborn health are beyond control, a woman's conscious decisions about social, health, and nutritional factors affect her infant's health and future. Much research suggests that an adequate vitamin and mineral intake at least 8 weeks before conception and during pregnancy can help prevent birth defects such as neural tube defects. This problem has been linked to folate deficiency (see Chapter 10). In addition, about 50% of pregnancies are unplanned. For these reasons, parents should be aware of the role nutrition plays in the development of a healthy infant both before and during pregnancy.[30]

■ PRENATAL GROWTH AND DEVELOPMENT

embryo In humans, the developing in utero offspring from about the beginning of the third week to the end of the eighth week after conception.

ovum The egg cell from which a fetus eventually develops if the egg is fertilized by a sperm cell.

placenta An organ that forms in pregnant women. Through this organ, oxygen and nutrients from the mother's blood are transferred to the fetus, and fetal wastes are removed. The placenta also releases hormones that maintain the pregnant state.

zygote The fertilized ovum; the cell resulting from the union of an egg cell (ovum) and sperm until it divides.

conceptus A generic term for any developmental stage derived from the fertilized ovum (zygote) until birth. The conceptus includes the extraembryonic membranes, as well as the embryo or fetus.

For 8 weeks after conception, a human **embryo** develops from an **ovum** into a **fetus.** For about another 32 weeks, the fetus continues to develop. When its body finally matures, the infant is born. Until birth, the mother nourishes it via a **placenta,** an organ that forms in her uterus to accommodate the growth and development of the fetus (Fig. 16-1).[32]

■ Early Growth—The First Trimester Is a Very Critical Time

The formation of the human organism begins when an egg and a sperm unite to form the **zygote** (Fig. 16-2). About 30 hours after the egg is fertilized, the zygote reproduces itself by dividing in half. The process of cell division then repeats many times. As the cluster of cells, commonly called the **conceptus,** drifts down the oviduct to the woman's uterus, several kinds of cells emerge. The entire genetic code is passed to every cell, but each cell uses only a segment of the code to produce proteins. If this were not the case, there would be no different organs or body parts. For example, all cells carry genes which dictate hair color and eye color, but only the cells of the hair follicles and irises respond to that specific information.

On about the fourth day after fertilization, the conceptus, now about 64 to 128 cells and hollow, arrives in the uterus. By the tenth day, the conceptus implants into the uterine lining. Two weeks after conception the cell number has increased further, and the conceptus is now termed an embryo. By day 35 of gestation, the heart is beating, and, although the embryo is only 8 mm (about 3/8 inch) long, the eyes and so-called limb buds, which ultimately form the arms and legs, are clearly visible.

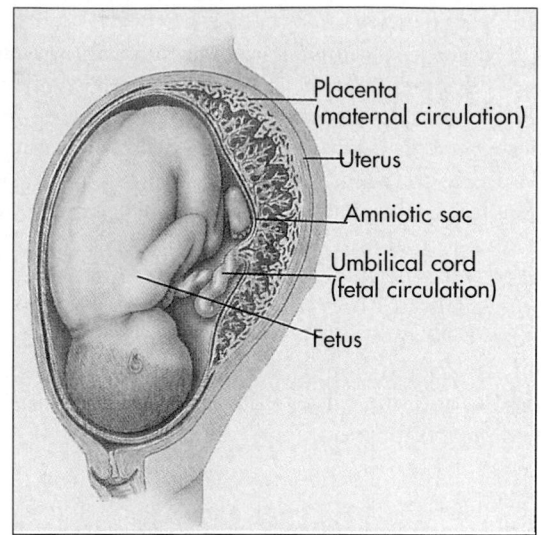

■ FIGURE 16-1 The fetus in relation to the placenta. The placenta is the organ through which nourishment flows to the fetus.
Illustration by William Ober.

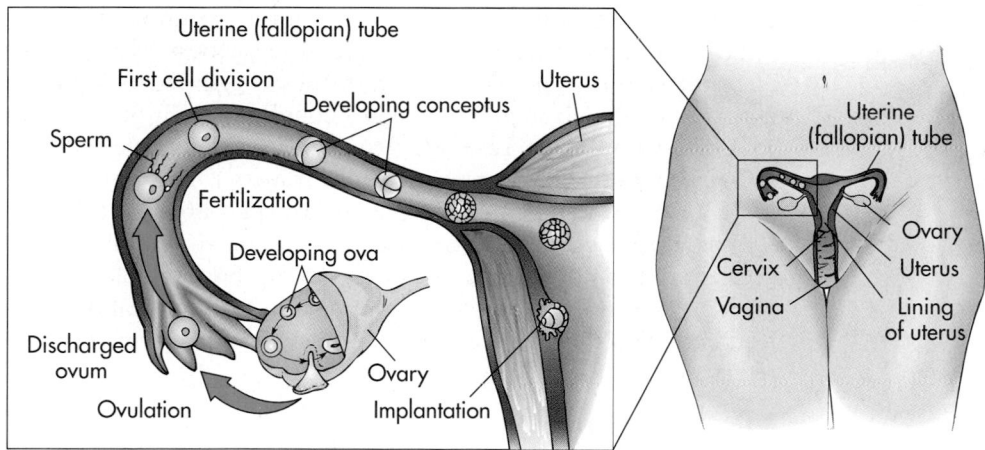

■ FIGURE 16-2 After ovulation, the discharged ovum first enters the abdominal cavity and then finds its way into the uterine (fallopian) tube, where conception, or fertilization, takes place. Sperm cells "swim" up the uterine tube toward the ovum. Fertilization most often occurs in the outer one-third of the oviduct. The ovum also takes an active role in the process of fertilization by attracting and "trapping" sperm with special receptor molecules on its surface. As soon as the head and neck of one spermatozoon enter the ovum (the tail drops off), complex mechanisms in the egg are activated to ensure that no more sperm enter. The 23 chromosomes from the sperm combine with the 23 chromosomes already in the ovum to make up the 46 chromosomes of the conceptus.

From about the end of the eighth week after conception to its birth about 32 weeks later, the developing offspring is known as a fetus.

For purposes of discussion, the duration of pregnancy—normally, 38 to 42 weeks—is commonly divided into three periods, called **trimesters.** Growth begins in the first trimester with a rapid increase in cell number (hyperplasia). This type of growth dominates embryonic and later fetal development. The newly formed cells then begin to grow larger (hypertrophy; see Chapter 13 to review these terms). Further growth and development then involve mostly hyperplasia with some hypertrophy. By the end of 13 weeks—the first trimester—most organs are formed and the fetus can move (Fig. 16-3).[32]

Nutritional deficiencies and other insults transmitted through the mother to the embryo or fetus—for example, injuries caused by medications and other drugs, high intakes of vitamin A, radiation, or trauma—can alter or arrest the current phase of development (review Fig. 16-3). The effects may last a lifetime. The most critical time for these problems to happen is during the first trimester. Most **spontaneous abortions**—premature terminations of pregnancy—occur at this time. Currently,

trimesters Three 13- to 14-week periods into which the normal pregnancy of 38 to 42 weeks is divided somewhat arbitrarily for purposes of discussion and analysis. Development of the embryo and fetus, however, is continuous throughout pregnancy, with no specific physiological markers demarcating the transition from one trimester to the next.

spontaneous abortion Any cessation of pregnancy and expulsion of the embryo or nonviable fetus as the result of natural causes, such as a genetic defect or developmental problem; also called miscarriage.

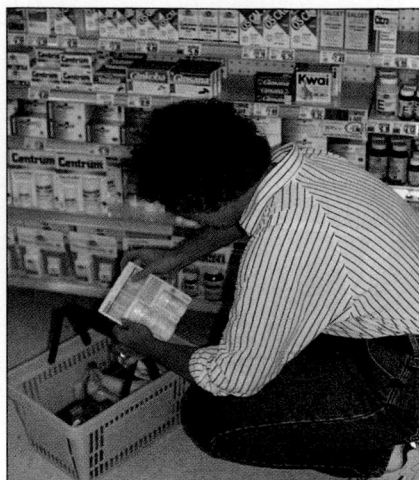

The time to begin thinking about prenatal nutrition is actually before becoming pregnant. This includes making sure that synthetic folate intake is adequate (400 µg/day) and that any supplemental use of vitamin A does not exceed 100% of the Daily Value (1000 RAE).

one-half or more of all pregnancies miscarry, often so early that a woman does not even realize she was pregnant. Early miscarriages usually result from a genetic defect or fatal error in fetal development.

A woman should avoid substances that may harm the developing fetus, especially during the first trimester.[31] This holds true for the time when a woman is trying to become pregnant. As previously mentioned, she is unlikely to be aware of her pregnancy for at least a few weeks. In addition, the fetus develops so rapidly during the first trimester that, if an essential nutrient is not available, the fetus may be affected even before evidence of the deficiency appears in the mother.

For this reason, the quality of one's nutritional intake is more important than quantity during the first trimester. In other words, women should consume the same amount of food, but the foods should be more nutrient dense. Although some women lose their appetite and feel nauseated during the first trimester, they should be careful to obtain adequate nutrition.

▪ Second Trimester

By the beginning of the second trimester, a fetus weighs about 1 oz. Arms, hands, fingers, legs, feet, and toes are fully formed. The fetus has ears and begins to form tooth sockets in its jawbone. Organs continue to grow and mature, and, with a stethoscope, physicians can detect the fetus's heartbeat. Most bones are distinctly evident through the body. Eventually, the fetus begins to look more like an infant. It may suck its thumb and kick strongly enough to be felt by the mother.[32]

As shown in Figure 16-3, the fetus can now still be affected by exposure to toxins, but not to the degree seen in the first trimester. During the second trimester, the mother's breast weight increases by approximately 30% due to the deposition of 2 to 4 lb of fat for lactation. Consequently, undernutrition in the second trimester has a greater effect on the mother than on the fetus. For example, if the mother does not meet her nutritional requirements during this time, her ability to successfully breast-feed her infant may be affected, as fat stored during pregnancy serves as an energy reserve for lactation.[32]

▪ Third Trimester

By the beginning of the third trimester, a fetus weighs about 2 to 3 lb. The third trimester is a crucial time for fetal growth. The fetus will double in length and will multiply its weight by five times. An infant that is born after about 26 weeks of

*A*lthough a mother's decisions, practices, and precautions during pregnancy contribute to the health of her fetus, she cannot guarantee her fetus good health because some genetic and environmental factors are beyond her control. Parents should not hold an unrealistic illusion of control.

▪ **FIGURE 16-3** Vulnerable periods of fetal development. The most serious damage to the fetus from exposure to toxins is likely to occur during the first 8 weeks after conception. The lighter bars indicate the time of greatest risk to the organ. As the chart shows, however, damage to vital parts of the body—including the eyes, brain, and genitals—can also occur during the last months of pregnancy.
Illustration by William Ober.

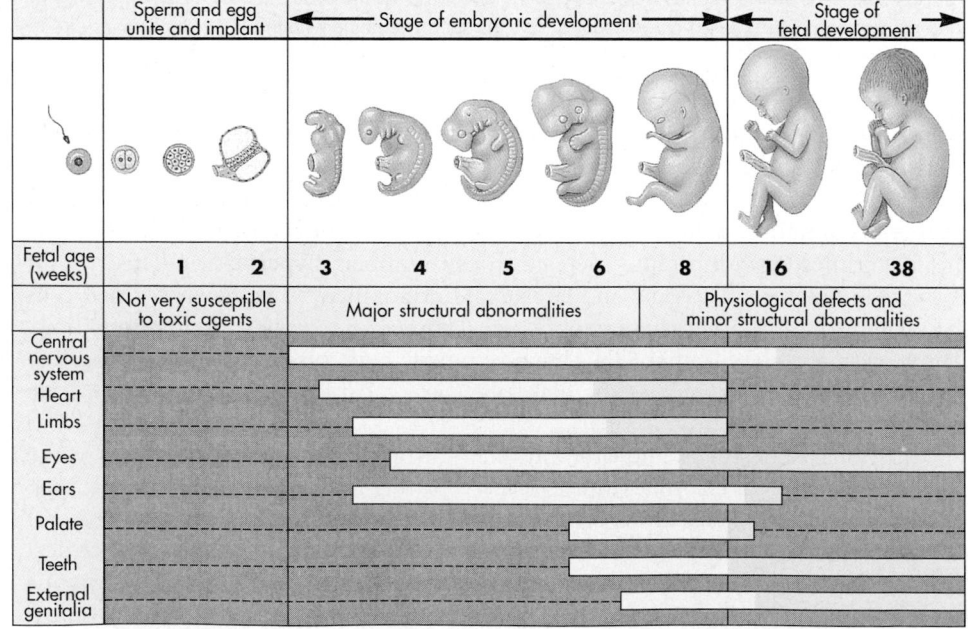

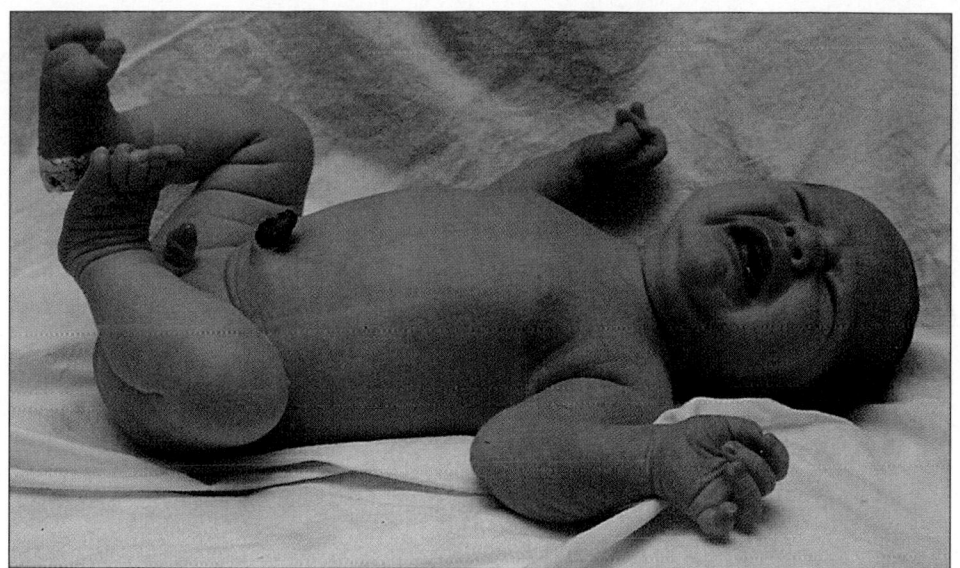

■ **FIGURE 16-4** A healthy 1-week-old baby. At birth, a baby usually weighs about 7.5 lb and is 20 in long.

gestation has a good chance of survival if it is cared for in a nursery for high-risk newborns. However, the infant will not contain the mineral (mainly iron and calcium) and fat stores normally accumulated during the last month of gestation. This and other medical problems, such as a poor ability to suck and swallow, complicate nutritional care for preterm infants. Note also that infants act as "parasites" with regard to iron, in that they deplete the stores of the mother. If the mother is not meeting her iron needs, she can be severely depleted after delivery.[32]

At 9 months, the fetus weighs about 7 to 9 lb (3 to 4 kg) and is about 20 inches (50 cm) long (Fig. 16-4). A soft spot in the forehead indicates where the skull bones (fontanels) are growing together. The bones finally close by the time the baby is about 12 to 18 months of age.

gestation The period of intrauterine development of offspring, from conception to birth; in humans, gestation lasts for about 40 weeks after the woman's previous menstrual period.

■ DEFINITION OF A SUCCESSFUL PREGNANCY

To define a successful pregnancy, one common criterion is the protection of the mother's physical and emotional health, so that she can return to her prepregnancy health status. As for the infant, two widely accepted criteria are (1) a gestation period longer than 37 weeks and (2) a birth weight greater than 5.5 pounds (2.5 kg). Sufficient lung development, which is likely to have occurred by 37 weeks' gestation, is critical to the survival of a newborn. The longer the gestation, the greater the ultimate birth weight and maturation and hence fewer medical problems are likely to occur.[32]

Low-birth-weight (LBW) infants are those weighing less than 5.5 lb (2.5 kg) at birth. Most commonly, LBW is associated with **preterm** birth. Full-term and preterm infants who weigh less than the expected weight for their duration of gestation, the result of insufficient growth, are described as **small for gestational age (SGA).** Thus, a full-term infant weighing less than 5.5 lb at birth is SGA but not preterm, whereas a preterm infant born at 30 weeks' gestation is probably LBW without SGA. Infants who are SGA are more likely than normal-weight infants to have medical complications, including problems with blood glucose control, temperature regulation, and growth and development in the early weeks after birth.

The newborn's quality of life must also be considered in rating the success of a pregnancy. Overall, prospective parents should strive toward producing a baby who is born healthy, on time, and with the mental, physical, and physiological capabilities to take advantage of whatever life offers, while also protecting the mother's health.

A goal of Healthy People 2010 is to reduce low birth weight and preterm births by one-third.

low-birth-weight (LBW) Referring to any infant weighing less than 2.5 kg (5.5 lb) at birth; most commonly results from preterm birth.

preterm An infant born before 37 weeks of gestation; also referred to as *premature*.

small for gestational age (SGA) Referring to infants who weigh less than the expected weight for their length of gestation. This corresponds to less than 2.5 kg (5.5 lb) in a full-term newborn. A preterm infant who is also SGA will most likely develop some medical complications.

*S*tudies from Britain suggest the low-birth-weight infants are likely to develop diabetes, hypertension and high blood cholesterol during later adult years. Reduced growth of the liver and other organs during gestation is one possible reason.[11]

Nutrition is one key to a successful pregnancy. Eating healthfully is vital during pregnancy to ensure the health of both the offspring and the mother. Fetal organs and body parts begin to develop very soon after conception. Again, the first trimester (13 weeks) is an especially critical period, when poor nutrition or drug use can result in birth defects.[22]

CONCEPT CHECK

*A*dequate nutrition, especially meeting folate needs from a synthetic source starting 8 weeks before pregnancy begins, is vital both before and during pregnancy to help ensure the optimal health of both the mother and her offspring. Organs and body parts in the offspring begin to develop very soon after conception. The first trimester is a critical period when inadequate nutrient intake or alcohol and drug use can result in birth defects.

Infants born after 37 weeks of gestation who weigh more than 5.5 lb (2.5 kg) have the fewest medical problems at birth. To reduce infant and maternal medical problems or death, those involved with the pregnancy should take the steps necessary to allow the mother to carry the baby in her uterus for the entire 9 months and contribute to adequate growth. Good nutrition and health practices aid in this goal.

*I*n the 1950s, physicians commonly recommended that women restrict weight gain to between 15 and 18 lb. At times, they also recommended severe energy and sodium restrictions to keep the baby small, in the hopes of easing labor and avoiding complications. Few of these practices were based on sound research, and we know now that many of these recommendations can actually harm the mother and fetus.

■ INCREASED NUTRIENT NEEDS TO SUPPORT PREGNANCY

The first comprehensive scientific report about nutrition and pregnancy was issued in 1970 by the National Academy of Sciences and was updated in 1990. Both documents emphasized an increase (not restrictions) in nutritional requirements during pregnancy and the importance of individually assessing and counseling mothers-to-be.

■ Increased Energy Needs

An average pregnancy requires approximately 300 extra kcal daily during the second and third trimesters. Energy needs during the first trimester are essentially the same as for the nonpregnant woman. An example of such a 300-kcal increase includes six whole-wheat crackers, 1 oz. cheese, and ½ cup of nonfat milk, or 1 cup of low-fat yogurt and an orange. Although she may "eat for two," the pregnant woman must not double her normal energy intake. She will want to seek the best-quality foods to ensure the best possible health for her child. Note that many vitamin and mineral needs are increased by 20 to 50% during pregnancy, whereas energy needs during the second and third trimesters represent only about a 15% increase, based on adding 300 kcal to an intake of 2000 kcal per day by nonpregnant women.[9]

Adequate energy intake is easy to achieve and can be assessed by appropriate weight gain throughout the pregnancy. However, to obtain the necessary vitamins and minerals without increasing her energy intake too much, a pregnant woman needs to seek nutrient-dense foods.

If a woman is active during pregnancy, she can add the extra energy she uses to the energy allowance for pregnancy. Her greater body weight requires more energy for activity. Women can continue most activities during pregnancy, except certain calisthenics, such as deep knee bends; scuba diving; downhill skiing; weight lifting; and contact sports (such as hockey). Walking, cycling, swimming, and light aerobics are generally advised, although it is not advised that normally inactive women begin an intense exercise program during pregnancy.[3] Because many women find that they are inactive during the later months, partly because of their increased size, an extra 300 kcal in their daily diet is usually enough.

Women with high-risk pregnancies may need to restrict their physical activity. To ensure optimal health for both herself and her infant, a pregnant woman should first consult her physician about physical activity and possible limitations.

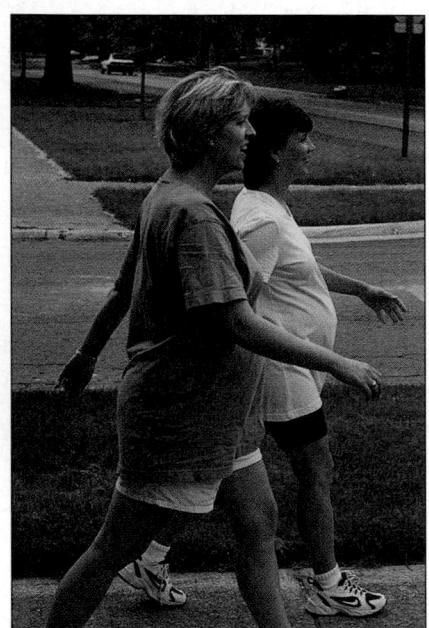

Walking, cycling, swimming, and light aerobics are all suitable exercises during pregnancy.

Adequate weight gain for a mother is one of the best predictors of pregnancy outcome. Her diet should allow for approximately 2 to 4 lb (0.9 to 1.8 kg) of weight gain during the first trimester and then a subsequent weight gain of 0.75 to 1 lb (0.3 to 0.5 kg) weekly during the second and third trimesters. Total weight gain goal normally averages about 25 to 35 lb (11.5 to 16 kg).[1] Adolescents and African-American women, who often have smaller babies, are strongly advised to aim for the greater amount. Women carrying twins should gain 35 to 45 lb.

For underweight women, the goal increases to 28 to 40 lb (12.5 to 18 kg). Body mass index (BMI) is currently the preferred means of establishing this weight status (Table 16-1). The goal decreases to 15 to 25 lb (7 to 11.5 kg) for obese women. Figure 16-5 shows why the typical recommendation begins at 25 lb.

A weight gain of between 25 and 35 lb has repeatedly been shown to yield optimal health for both mother and fetus if gestation lasts at least 38 weeks. The weight gain should yield a birth weight of 7.5 lb (3.5 kg). Although some extra weight gain during pregnancy is usually not harmful, it can set the stage for creeping obesity during the childbearing years if the mother does not return to about her prepregnancy weight. This is especially true if the woman intends to have more than one child.

Weight gain during pregnancy, especially in the teenage years, requires regular monitoring that approximately follows the pattern in Figure 16-5. Infant birth weights improve if the mother's weight gain meets the ranges previously mentioned.[18] Keeping weekly records of a pregnant woman's weight gain helps assess how much to adjust her food intake. Weight gain is a key issue in prenatal care and a concern of many mothers. Inadequate weight gain can cause many problems. If a woman deviates from the desirable pattern, she should be warned of this and counseled on how to make the appropriate adjustment.

For example, if a woman begins to gain too much weight during her pregnancy, she should not be encouraged to lose weight to get back on track. Even if a woman gains 35 lb in the first 7 months of pregnancy, she must still gain more during the last 2 months. She should simply slow the increase in weight to parallel the rise on the prenatal weight gain chart. In other words, the sources of the unnecessary food energy should be found and minimized. Alternately, if a woman has not gained the desired weight by a given point in pregnancy, she shouldn't be encouraged to gain the needed weight rapidly. Instead, she should slowly gain a little more weight than the typical pattern to meet the goal by the end of the pregnancy.

■ Increased Protein and Carbohydrate Needs

The RDA for protein increases by 10 to 15 g daily, depending on age. A glass of milk alone contains 8 g. Many nonpregnant women already eat the recommended 60 g of protein per day and therefore don't need to increase protein intake. However, all women should check to make sure they are actually eating enough protein.

The American College of Obstetrics and Gynecology suggests the following guidelines for physical activity during pregnancy:

1. Do not allow heart rate to exceed 140 beats per minute.
2. Avoid exercising in hot, humid weather.
3. Discontinue exercise that causes discomfort or overheating.
4. Drink plenty of liquids to avoid dehydration and overheating (>100°F).
5. After about the fourth month, don't exercise while lying on your back.
6. Avoid an abrupt decrease in exertion. In other words, don't just stop and stand around after a hard workout; rather, continue exercising but at a slow pace, gradually reducing pulse rate.

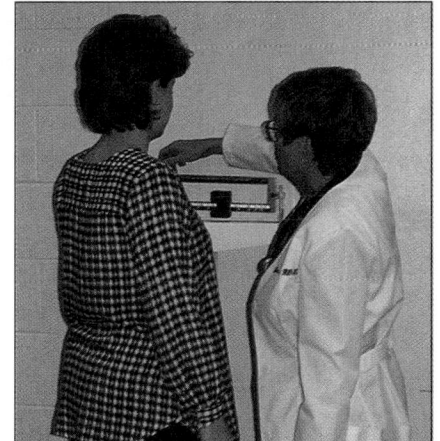

Weight gain is carefully monitored during pregnancy.

During pregnancy, women in the United States are more likely to gain excess weight and make poor food choices than to eat too little. Usually, the problem is how to limit weight gain. Excessive weight gain increases risk for complications during pregnancy and encourages excess fetal growth, which makes birth trauma more likely. Loose, accommodating maternity clothes and fluid retention can mask true weight gain during pregnancy.

TABLE 16-1	Recommended Weight Gain in Pregnancy Based on Prepregnancy Body Mass Index (BMI)	

| BMI Category | Total Weight Gain* | |
	(lb)	(kg)
Low (BMI < 19.8)	28–40	12.5–18
Normal (BMI 19.8 to 26)	25–35	11.5–16
High (BMI 26 to 29)	15–25	7–11.5
Obese (BMI > 29)	≤15	≤7

Reprinted with permission from *Nutrition During Pregnancy and Lactation*, Copyright 1992 by the National Academy of Sciences. Courtesy of the National Academy Press, Washington, DC.

*The listed values are for singleton pregnancies. For women of normal BMI who are carrying twins, the range is 35 to 45 pounds (16 to 20 kg). Adolescents within 2 years of menarche and African-American women should strive for gains at the upper end of the ranges; short women (<62 inches) should strive for gains at the lower end of the ranges.

Weight (lb)

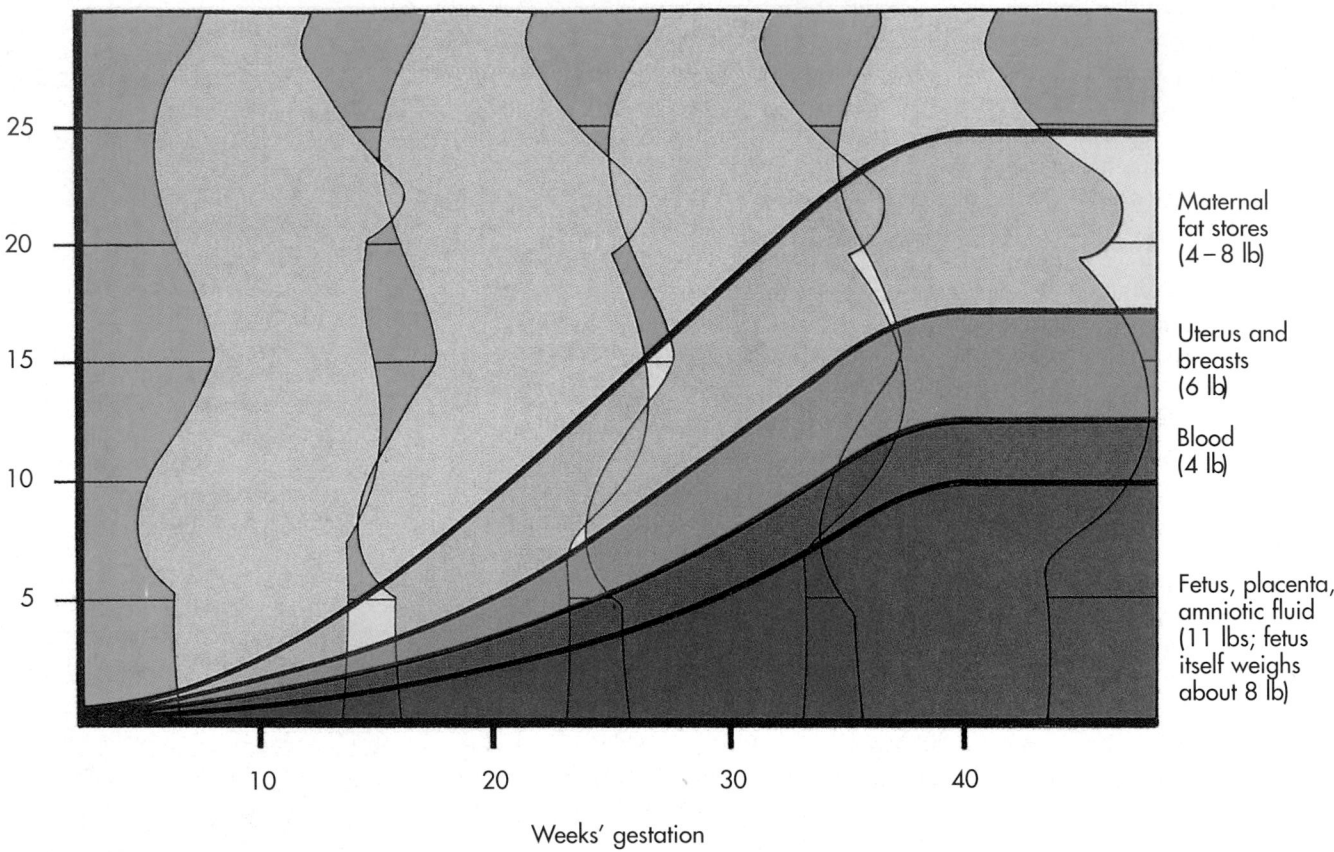

Maternal
fat stores
(4 – 8 lb)

Uterus and
breasts
(6 lb)

Blood
(4 lb)

Fetus, placenta,
amniotic fluid
(11 lbs; fetus
itself weighs
about 8 lb)

Weeks' gestation

■ **FIGURE 16-5** The components of weight gain in pregnancy. A weight gain of 25 to 35 lb is recommended for most women. Note that the various components total about 25 lb.

Healthy People 2010 has set a goal of increasing the number of pregnancies that begin with optimum folate status, to 80% from the current estimate of 21%, thus reducing the occurrence of neural tube defects.

Neural tube defects develop 28 days after conception, and may be reduced by 45% if all women of childbearing age were to meet the recommended 400 µg/day of synthetic folic acid. A recent survey found that 68% of women had heard of folate; 13% knew that folate helps prevent birth defects, but only 7% knew intake is important before they become pregnant.[30]

Carbohydrate needs are at least 100 g daily. This amount prevents ketosis, which can harm the fetus (see later section on the effects of nutrition and other factors on pregnancy outcome). Most women already consume almost twice this amount.

■ Increased Vitamin Needs

Vitamin needs generally increase by up to 30% for the B-vitamins, except vitamin B-6 (45%) and folate (50%).

The extra amount of vitamin B-6 and other B vitamins (except folate) needed in the diet is easily met via wise food choices, such as a serving of a typical breakfast cereal and some animal protein. Folate needs, however, often merit specific diet planning. Because the synthesis of DNA requires folate, this nutrient is especially crucial during pregnancy. Ultimately, both fetal and maternal growth depends on an ample supply of folate. Red blood cell formation, which requires folate, increases during pregnancy. Serious megaloblastic anemia can result if folate intake is inadequate. The RDA for folate increases during pregnancy to 600 µg per day. This is a critical goal in the nutritional care of a pregnant woman, whereas 400 µg per day is advocated for women who have the potential to become pregnant. In both cases, a synthetic form is emphasized. Folate deficiency at conception and thereafter has been associated with birth defects—specifically, neural tube defects, such as spina bifida. Still, about half of these birth defects arise from genetic and other reasons unrelated to folate intake.

Increasing synthetic folate intakes to meet 400 µg/day for a nonpregnant woman and 600 µg/day for a pregnant woman can be achieved through either dietary sources or supplemental folate, or a combination of both. Choosing a diet rich in synthetic folate, such as from breakfast cereals (look for 100% of the Daily Value) and enriched grains, can suffice. Otherwise, the use of a supplemental form is advised. The reason for this emphasis on synthetic folate is that it is the form that has been used in studies that have shown folate to be effective in reducing neural tube defects. Recall from Chapter 10 that the folate found in foods is often in the polyglutamate form, which is not as readily absorbed as is synthetic folate (which is in the monoglutamate form, also referred to as folic acid). This is not to say that the folate naturally found in foods is worthless. Experts are simply reluctant to say that food folate will suffice when all of the studies have used synthetic forms of folate.[9]

Women who have previously given birth to an infant with a neural tube defect should consult their physician about the need for folate supplementation; an intake of 4 mg per day is advocated but must be taken under a physician's supervision.

Meeting folate needs during pregnancy may be a problematic practice for women who have taken oral contraceptives for extended periods because this can inhibit folate absorption. A recent history of an inadequate diet or oral contraceptive use necessitates careful attention to folate intake during pregnancy. Ideally, the woman would begin a folate-rich diet (or take folate supplements) approximately 8 weeks before conception.[27]

■ Increased Mineral Needs

Mineral needs generally increase during pregnancy, especially the need for iodide and iron.

Pregnant women need extra iodide (total of 220 µg/day) for prevention of goiter. The extra iron (total of 27 mg/day) is needed to synthesize the greater amount of hemoglobin needed during pregnancy and to provide iron stores for the fetus. Typical iodide intakes suffice if the woman uses iodized salt. However, women often need an iron supplement, especially if they don't consume iron-fortified foods, such as highly-fortified breakfast cereals. Because iron supplements decrease appetite and can cause nausea and constipation, taking them between meals or just before going to bed is best. Milk, coffee, or tea should not be consumed with an iron supplement because these have substances that interfere with iron absorption. Eating foods rich in vitamin C along with nonheme iron–containing foods helps increase iron absorption. Pregnant women who are not anemic may wait until the second trimester, when pregnancy-related nausea generally lessens, to start iron supplementation.

Severe iron deficiency anemia in pregnancy, especially in the first half of pregnancy, may lead to preterm delivery, low birth weight, and increased risk for fetal death in the first weeks after birth.[20] As previously mentioned, infants are considered parasites when it comes to iron. This means that the fetus depletes the mother's iron stores during the third trimester. In other words, an inadequate iron intake may actually be more harmful to the mother than to the fetus.[32]

■ Is There an Instinctive Drive During Pregnancy to Consume More Nutrients?

Extra needs for folate, iron, and calcium are the most difficult for pregnant women to satisfy. These, then, should be the focus of diet planning for pregnant women. Before diet planning is discussed, however, one important misconception about pregnancy needs to be dispelled. You may have heard that mothers instinctively know what to eat and that their craving for pickles and ice cream is dictated by a natural desire to consume needed nutrients. These cravings are most common during the last two trimesters and could be related to hormonal changes in the mother, or just family traditions.

It remains an even greater mystery why some women crave nonfood items during pregnancy. The craving for and eating items such as starch, ice, chalk, burnt matchsticks, soap, plaster, and soil, especially noted during pregnancy, is called **pica**. This practice occurs more frequently among African-American women in the United States and essentially results from cultural influences and learned behaviors, rather than from a need for specific nutrients such as iron and zinc. It also poses some health risks. Eating soil raises the risk of infections from parasites or lead toxicity and can cause anemia, as well as life-threatening blockages of the intestinal tract. The consumption of laundry starch, wall plaster, moth balls, and toilet air fresheners are

The RDA for zinc during pregnancy is 11 mg/day, 35% higher than that for nonpregnant women. The protein foods in the diet of a healthy pregnant woman should supply this much zinc. Conditions such as cereal-based diets, high doses of supplemental iron, smoking, and alcohol abuse can reduce the amount of zinc available to the fetus. Women with these conditions may be given more zinc during pregnancy (approximately 25 mg/day, about two times the RDA).[17] This is the amount contained in a typical prenatal supplement.

pica The practice of eating nonfood items, such as dirt, laundry starch, or clay.

also dangerous because they contain toxic compounds. Eating ice can break teeth. Overall, although women may have a natural instinct to consume the right foods in pregnancy, humans are so far removed from living by instinct that relying on our desires is risky. Nutritional counseling can focus food choices more reliably.[32]

■ FOOD PLAN FOR PREGNANT WOMEN

One approach to a diet that supports a successful pregnancy is based on the Food Guide Pyramid. It includes at least the following:

- Two to three servings from the milk, yogurt, and cheese group (the range depends on the calcium content of other food choices)
- Three servings from the meat, poultry, fish, dry beans, eggs, and nuts group
- Three servings from the vegetable group
- Two servings from the fruit group
- Six servings from the bread, cereal, rice, and pasta group

Specifically, the servings from the milk, yogurt, and cheese group could include low-fat or nonfat versions of milk, yogurt, and cheese. These foods supply extra protein, calcium, riboflavin, and magnesium. Servings from the meat, poultry, fish, dry beans, eggs, and nuts group should include both animal and vegetable sources. Besides protein, the animal sources help provide the extra iron and zinc needed, and the vegetable sources help provide much of the extra magnesium needed during pregnancy.

The vegetable and fruit group servings provide a variety of vitamins and minerals. One serving from this combination should be a good vitamin C source, and one serving should be a green vegetable or other rich source of folate. Selections from the bread, cereal, and pasta group should focus on whole-grain and enriched foods. One serving of breakfast cereal significantly contributes to meeting many vitamin and mineral needs.

Table 16-2 illustrates one daily menu based on the basic diet plan shown. This daily menu supplies about 1800 kcal but still meets the extra nutrient needs associated with pregnancy. Women who need to consume more than this—and some do for various reasons—should add more servings from the fruit and vegetable groups and the bread, cereal, rice, and pasta group to the basic plan.

■ Use of Prenatal Vitamin and Mineral Supplements

Specially formulated supplements for pregnant women are prescribed routinely by most physicians. Some of these are dispensed by prescription because of their high folate content, which could pose problems for others, such as older people (see Chapter 10). This routine may exist because it is easier to prescribe supplements than to discuss diet changes. Also, some pregnant women are just not willing to change their diets to meet their increased nutrient needs, or they simply expect (or demand) this treatment. These prenatal supplements typically include the critical nutrients for pregnancy—that is, iron, and folate—and many others as well.

There is no evidence that potential supplements cause significant health problems in pregnancy, aside perhaps from the combined amounts of supplementary and dietary vitamin A. During pregnancy, supplemental preformed vitamin A should not exceed 3000 RAE/day (15,000 IU/day). Toxicity of vitamin A is linked with **teratogenesis** (see Chapter 9).[4] This occurs mainly during the first trimester. The primary instances when prenatal supplements may contribute to a successful pregnancy are with poor women, teenagers, those with a generally deficient diet, and women carrying multiple fetuses.

■ Pregnant Vegetarians

Women who practice either lactoovovegetarianism or lactovegetarianism generally do not face special difficulties in meeting their nutritional needs during pregnancy.

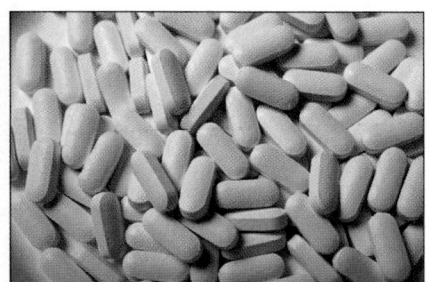

Pregnancy, in particular, is not a time to self-prescribe vitamin and mineral supplements.

teratogenic Tending to produce physical defects in a developing fetus.

TABLE 16-2 Sample 1800 kcal Daily Menu That Meets the Nutritional Needs of Most Pregnant and Breastfeeding Women	Vitamin D	Folate	Calcium	Iron	Zinc
Breakfast					
1½ cups Quaker Toasted Oatmeal Squares cereal	✓	✓		✓	✓
½ cup orange juice		✓			
¾ cup nonfat milk	✓		✓		
Snack					
2 tbsp peanut butter		✓		✓	✓
1 slice whole-wheat toast		✓		✓	✓
½ cup plain low-fat yogurt			✓		
½ cup strawberries					
Lunch					
1½ cups spinach salad with 1 tbsp oil and vinegar dressing		✓			
½ tomato					
1 slice whole-wheat toast		✓		✓	✓
1 oz provolone cheese			✓		
Snack					
4 whole-wheat crackers		✓		✓	✓
1 cup nonfat milk	✓		✓		
Dinner					
3 oz lean hamburger, broiled (with condiments)				✓	✓
½ cup baked beans		✓		✓	✓
1 hamburger bun		✓		✓	
½ sliced tomato					
¾ cup cooked broccoli		✓			
1 tsp soft margarine	✓				
Iced tea (milk if a teenager)					

This diet meets nutrient needs for pregnancy and lactation and supplies 24 mg of iron. The vitamin- and mineral-fortified breakfast cereal used in this example makes an important contribution to meeting nutrient needs, such as for synthetic folate (400 μg per cup). If more food energy is needed, 1 cup of nonfat milk, 1 slice of whole-wheat bread, and 5 baby carrots would increase intake to 2000 kcal.

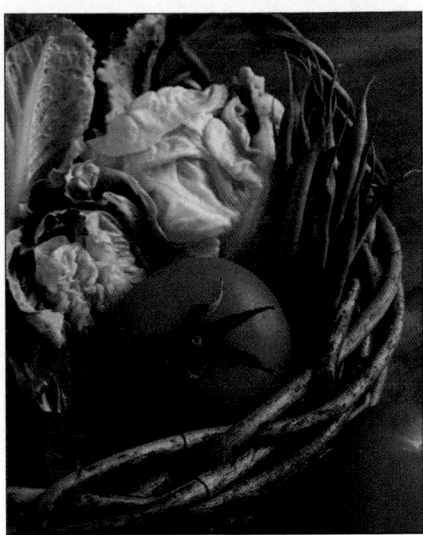

A salad each day provides many nutrients for the prenatal diet.

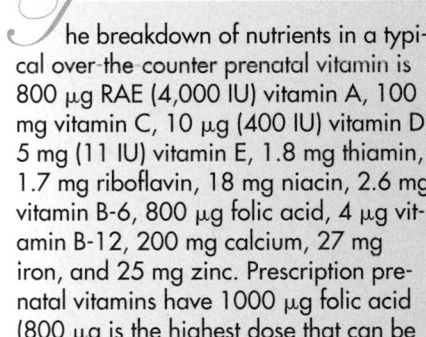

he breakdown of nutrients in a typical over-the-counter prenatal vitamin is 800 μg RAE (4,000 IU) vitamin A, 100 mg vitamin C, 10 μg (400 IU) vitamin D, 5 mg (11 IU) vitamin E, 1.8 mg thiamin, 1.7 mg riboflavin, 18 mg niacin, 2.6 mg vitamin B-6, 800 μg folic acid, 4 μg vitamin B-12, 200 mg calcium, 27 mg iron, and 25 mg zinc. Prescription prenatal vitamins have 1000 μg folic acid (800 μg is the highest dose that can be sold over the counter).

Like nonvegetarian women, they should be concerned primarily with meeting iron and folate needs.

On the other hand, when a total vegetarian (vegan) becomes pregnant, she must carefully plan a diet that includes sufficient protein, vitamin D (or sufficient sun exposure), vitamin B-6, iron, calcium, and zinc and must use a vitamin B-12 supplement. The basic vegan diet listed in Chapter 7 should be modified to include more grains, beans, nuts, and seeds to supply the necessary extra amounts of some of these nutrients. Because iron and calcium are poorly absorbed from most plant foods, iron and calcium supplements are probably necessary[26, 28]; however, to avoid competition for absorption, they should not be taken together. The amounts provided by typical prenatal supplements should suffice to meet iron needs but not calcium needs. The prenatal supplement also fulfills vitamin D needs if sufficient sun exposure does not take place.

CONCEPT CHECK

*E*nergy needs increase by an average of about 300 kcal per day during the second and third trimesters of pregnancy. Weight gain should be slow and steady up to a total of 25 to 35 lb for a woman of healthy weight. Protein, vitamin, and mineral needs all increase during pregnancy. Vitamin B-6, folate, iron, iodide, calcium, and zinc are nutrients of particular concern. A pregnant woman's diet should be varied and generally include more milk products than a prepregnancy diet. Prenatal supplemental vitamins and minerals are commonly prescribed but may not be necessary, depending on one's diet and current health status. Taking too many supplements—especially vitamin A—can be hazardous to the fetus.

■ EFFECT OF NUTRITION ON THE SUCCESS OF PREGNANCY

Is this attention to nutrition worth the effort? Yes; evidence shows that the effort is justified. Extra nutrients and energy are used for fetal growth, as well as the changes in the mother's body to accommodate the fetus. Her uterus and breasts grow, the placenta develops, her total blood volume increases, the heart and kidneys work harder, and stores of body fat increase.

Although it is difficult to specify what degree of poor nutrition will affect each pregnancy, a daily diet containing only 1000 kcal has been shown to greatly retard fetal growth and development. Increased maternal and infant death rates seen in famine-stricken areas of Africa supply further evidence (see Chapter 20).[32]

Genetic background can explain very little of the observed differences in birth weight in North America. Both environmental factors and nutritional factors are more important. The worse the nutritional condition of the mother at the beginning of pregnancy, the more valuable a good prenatal diet and/or use of prenatal supplements are in improving the course and outcome of her pregnancy.

During World War II, parts of Russia and much of Holland were blockaded. Food supplies were quickly exhausted. The resulting undernutrition greatly affected the birth weights of infants developing in the second or third trimester. Birth defects also occurred more commonly, and the number of new pregnancies fell. After the blockades were lifted, birth weights, subsequent infant health, and the numbers of new pregnancies quickly returned to prewar levels.

At the same time, researchers working in Boston noticed that a suficient protein intake is associated with a greater success of pregnancy. It appeared that the mother's diet—not only during pregnancy but also preceding conception—affects the health of both mother and infant. Studies in Toronto then showed that dietary supplements and nutritional counseling improve the health of the pregnant mother and produce a healthier baby. As health improved, complication rates also decreased. Researchers in Great Britain took this one step further. They showed that height and social class are better predictors of pregnancy outcome than dietary intake during pregnancy. Supporting this is a study of middle-class African-American women in Chicago. Even with nutritional supplements, their risk of having LBW infants still exceeded that of middle-class Whites, possibly reflecting the effects of poverty on previous generations. This finding suggests that long-term nutritional intake may be critical to pregnancy outcome.

Laboratory animal studies have supported the importance of diet during pregnancy. Food deprivation in pregnant laboratory animals led to smaller organ size in the offspring, affecting even the brain, which usually resists nutritional insults. In addition, placentas weighed less, and fewer healthy offspring survived the first weeks of life.

■ EFFECTS OF NUTRITIONAL AND OTHER FACTORS ON PREGNANCY OUTCOME

In the United States, about 8 of every 100,000 live births end in the mother's death. The infant mortality rate is even higher: for each 100,000 live births, about 720 infants die within the first year.[13] The infant death rate among African-Americans is more than double the rates among Whites and Hispanics in the United States. Based on the national statistics, the United States currently ranks 25th among industrialized nations in terms of maternal and infant death rates. Such grim and discomforting statistics can be attributed largely to the current number of teenage pregnancies in this country and to inadequate prenatal care, as well as marginal nutritional status among poor pregnant women.

■ Beyond the Nutrients

Many nutrition-related factors also affect the health of mother and fetus.[7, 12, 31, 33]

Low Socioeconomic Status

A constellation of characteristics that lead to poverty, inadequate health care, poor health practices, lack of education, and unmarried status is associated with problems in pregnancy. Currently, in the United States about 25% of all births are to unwed mothers, many of which are poor.

Closely Spaced Births

Siblings born in succession with less than a year between them are more likely to be born with low birth weights than are those further apart in age. In one study, the risks of low birth weight, preterm birth, or small size for gestational age was 30 to 40% higher for infants conceived less than 6 months apart compared to those conceived 18 to 23 months apart.[33] This danger is especially prevalent among African-American women.

Teenage Pregnancy

About half a million teenagers give birth in the United States each year, accounting for about 13% of all births. Teenage pregnancy poses special health problems for both the mother and child. Young women continue maturing into physical adulthood for 5 years after **menarche.** Because the average age for menarche is 13 years in the United States, a woman younger than 18 years is not as physically ready to be pregnant as she will be later.[7]

Pregnant teens frequently exhibit a variety of other risk factors that can complicate pregnancy and pose a risk to the fetus. For instance, teenagers are more likely than older women to be underweight at the beginning of pregnancy and to gain fewer than 16 lb during pregnancy. In addition, their bodies generally lack the maturity needed to safely carry a pregnancy. Sixteen percent of low-birth-weight infants are born to teenage mothers. This occurrence takes place, even with adequate prenatal care. Furthermore, the specific needs of pregnant teenagers vary according to their own growth patterns, body build, and physical activity habits. Thus, it is difficult to estimate their nutrient needs. Overall, mothers who are between 25 and 34 have the best pregnancy outcomes. Teenage pregnancy should be avoided.

Inadequate Prenatal Care

Inadequate, absent, or delayed prenatal care can allow maternal nutritional deficiencies to deprive a fetus of needed nutrients. Chronic diseases, such as hypertension or diabetes, increase the risk of fetal damage. Without prenatal care, a woman is three times more likely to give birth to an LBW baby—one who will be 40 times more likely to die during the first 4 weeks of life than a normal-birth-weight infant. (The ideal time to start prenatal care is before conception.) Still, about 20% of women in

The risks of low birth weight and preterm delivery increase modestly, but progressively, with maternal age. Given close monitoring, however, a woman older than 35 has an excellent chance of producing a healthy infant. Most women in this age group exhibit typical pregnancy-related problems, which usually are manageable if under close medical supervision.

menarche The onset of menstruation. Menarche usually occurs around age 13, 2 or 3 years after the first signs of puberty start to appear.

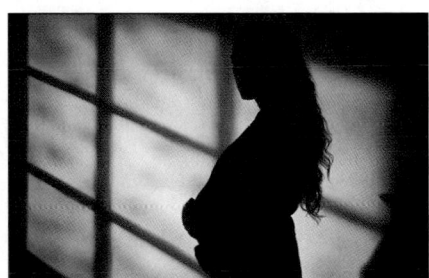

Pregnant teenagers need close monitoring throughout pregnancy. Ideally, teenage pregnancy should be avoided.

the United States receive no prenatal care in the first trimester—a critical time to change habits.[22]

Lifestyle Factors

Smoking, alcohol consumption, use of some medications, and illegal drug use in pregnancy all lead to harmful effects. The Nutrition Perspective at the end of this chapter reviews one effect of alcohol—fetal alcohol syndrome. Smoking is linked to preterm birth and low birth weight and appears to increase the risk of birth defects, sudden infant death, and childhood cancer. Problem drugs include aspirin (when used heavily), hormone ointments, nose drops, rectal suppositories, weight-control pills, and medications prescribed for previous illnesses.[31]

Of the illegal drugs, cocaine has the most devastating consequences for the developing fetuses. As cocaine use has become more common in recent years, the number of infants born to cocaine-using women has increased. Maternal use of cocaine during pregnancy has been linked to preterm birth, as well as to an undersized head and body and several other physical malformations in the newborn. Exposure of the fetus to cocaine appears to disrupt development of the brain and nervous system and may reduce interactive behaviors and responses to environmental stimuli in the infant.

Prenatal Ketosis

Ketosis is not desirable for the growing fetus. Ketone bodies are thought to be poorly used by the fetal brain, implying possible slowing of fetal brain development. Researchers oppose crash diets or fasting for more than 12 hours during pregnancy. A pregnant woman can develop significant ketosis after only 20 hours of fasting.[32] Eating about 100 g of carbohydrate every day prevents ketosis. Even nonpregnant women usually eat twice this amount.

Body Weight and Weight Gain

Obesity leads to an increased rate of hypertension and diabetes during pregnancy.[10] The need for surgery and other complications during delivery likewise increase. These pregnancies require intense monitoring and are linked to an increase in risk of birth defects in the infant, primarily because the fetus can grow very large.

Inadequate weight gain, especially among underweight women, often produces infants of low birth weight.[1] Undernourished women often have borderline vitamin and mineral intakes and need to build up body stores. They should try to reach healthy weight by the end of the first trimester. The recommendation for underweight women is to gain more weight (28 to 40 lb total) than a woman at healthy weight. Overweight women who try to avoid weight gain during pregnancy may rob both themselves and their fetuses of essential nutrients. Also, for efficient protein metabolism during pregnancy, enough carbohydrate and fat are needed to meet energy needs.

In the United States, about 7% of infants are born with low birth weight—that is, they weigh less than 5.5 lb (2.5 kg). Low-birth-weight infants are more susceptible to infections, illnesses, and disabilities and are more likely to die than normal-weight infants. Preterm birth, poor diet during pregnancy, some medical conditions in the mother, and the factors highlighted previously influence an infant's birth weight.[12] Reducing the number of LBW infants will help reduce infant deaths.

Caffeine Consumption

Research on the effects of caffeine consumption by pregnant women has produced some provocative findings. Caffeine decreases the absorption of iron and may reduce blood flow through the placenta, and studies have shown that the fetus is unable to detoxify caffeine. The risk of spontaneous abortion has been shown to increase in the first trimester and early in the second trimester with heavy caffeine consumption (>500 mg per day). About five cups of coffee per day contain this amount of caffeine (see Appendix H). In addition, as caffeine intake increases, so does the risk of delivering a low-birth-weight infant. Heavy caffeine use during pregnancy may also lead to caffeine withdrawal symptoms in the newborn. Finally, high caffeine intake often occurs in women who also smoke. In this case, it is the smoking that is the greater contributor to low birth weight.

Although more research is needed, it is advisable to limit caffeine intake. Drinking no more than two cups of coffee and no more than four cups of caffeinated soft drinks per day during pregnancy, or when pregnancy is possible, is advocated. Limiting intake from tea, over-the-counter medicines containing caffeine, and chocolate is also important. Some researchers advocate complete avoidance of caffeine during pregnancy in order to reduce the risk of miscarriage, birth defects, and underweight infants.[8]

Aspartame Use

Phenylalanine, a component of aspartame (Nutrasweet and Equal), causes concern for some pregnant women. High amounts of phenylalanine in maternal blood disrupt fetal brain development if the mother has a disease known as *phenylketonuria* (see Chapter 5). If the mother does not have this condition, however, it is unlikely that the baby will be affected by aspartame use. Some experts still recommend caution with regard to aspartame, but total abstinence is hardly warranted, based on current knowledge.[32]

Listeria Infection

Infection by the bacterium *Listeria monocytogenes* causes mild flulike symptoms, such as fever, headache, and vomiting, about 7 to 30 days after exposure. However, pregnant women, newborn infants, and people with depressed immune function may suffer more severe symptoms, including spontaneous abortion and serious blood infections. In these high-risk people, 25% of infections may be fatal.

Because unpasteurized milk, soft cheeses made from raw milk (brie, camembert, feta, and blue cheeses), and raw cabbage can be sources of listeria organisms, it is especially important that pregnant women and other people at high risk avoid these products. Experts advise consuming only pasteurized milk products and cooking meat, poultry, and seafood thoroughly to kill this and other foodborne organisms. It is unsafe in pregnancy to eat any raw meats or other raw animal products. Chapter 19 covers food-borne illness, such as listeria infections, in more detail.

■ Prenatal Care and Counseling

Education, an adequate diet, and early and consistent prenatal medical care maximize the chances of producing a healthy baby and avoiding the risks just covered, such as X-ray exposure, smoking, vitamin A supplements, medicines, illegal drugs, and alcohol use. If diabetes or hypertension is present or developing, it must be carefully controlled to minimize complications in the pregnancy.[31]

Again, women should receive these examinations and counseling strategies before becoming pregnant. Certainly, they should begin early in pregnancy. Many potential problems that develop associated with pregnancy can be diagnosed and quickly treated medically.

Food habits cannot be predicted from income, education, or lifestyle. Although some women already have good nutritional habits, most can benefit from nutritional advice. All should be reminded of habits that may harm the growing fetus, such as severe dieting or fasting. By focusing on appropriate prenatal care, good nutritional intake, and proper health habits, as well as using common sense, parents give their fetus—and, later, infant—the very best chance of thriving.

Several U.S. government programs exist to reduce infant mortality by providing high-quality health care and foods. These are designed to alleviate the effects of poverty and insufficient education. An example of such a program is the Special Supplemental Food Program for Women, Infants, and Children (WIC). This program offers health assessments and foods (or vouchers for foods) that supply high-quality protein, calcium, iron, and vitamins A and C to pregnant women, infants, and children (to age 5 years) from low-income populations.

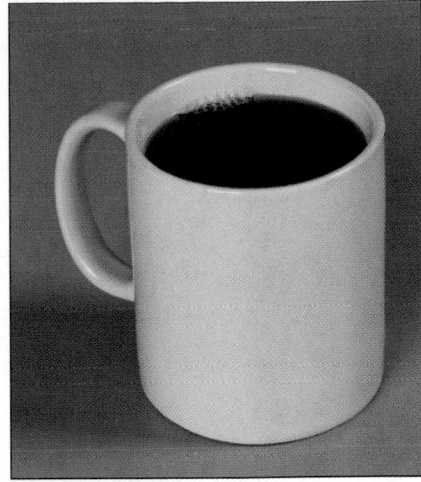

Coffee intake should be limited to two cups per day or so because the caffeine present can have deleterious effects on the fetus. In addition, caffeinated soft drinks and tea should also be limited.

Toxoplasmosis is another infection that causes birth defects. Pregnant women should limit exposure to the organism that causes toxoplasmosis by avoiding contact with cat feces (have someone else clean the cat's litter box), avoiding contact with kittens, bird feces, and garden soil, and by not eating raw or undercooked meat.

Women with acquired immune deficiency syndrome (AIDS) may pass the virus that causes this disease to the fetus during pregnancy or the birth process. About one in three infected newborns will develop AIDS symptoms and die within just a few years. Studies show that these odds of mother-infant transmission can be cut significantly if the woman begins taking the drug zidovudine (AZT) by the fourteenth week of pregnancy. Thus, screening pregnant women for AIDS and treating those with AIDS using AZT are currently advocated by some experts.

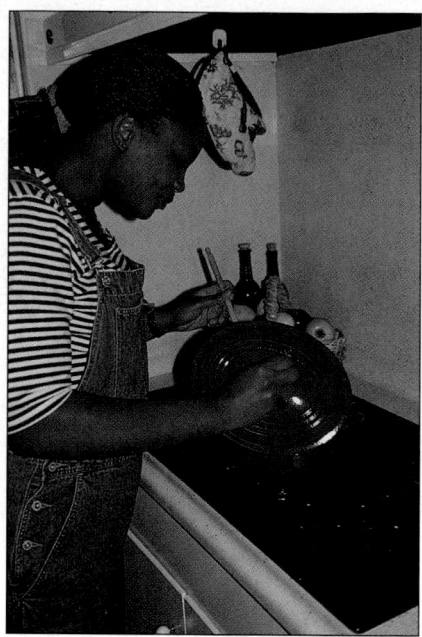

Attention to one's diet is especially important in pregnancy.

On the WIC program, participants' diets have improved markedly, as has the likelihood that women will have healthy babies. This program is credited with decreasing the cases of iron deficiency anemia and LBW infants within the population it serves. Studies have estimated that every dollar spent on the prenatal component of WIC saves about $3 in public health expenditures for the care of LBW babies.

The WIC program is available in all areas of the United States and has a staff trained to help women have healthy babies. More than 7 million women, infants, and young children are currently enrolled in the program. Many eligible pregnant women are not taking advantage of this program.

■ CASE SCENARIO
Follow-Up

From a dietary standpoint, Tracey is smart to take a close look at her protein intake because needs will increase slightly during pregnancy. More fruits and vegetables will provide some fiber to help prevent constipation, which is common in the later stages of pregnancy. These foods also supply folate, and her use of an over-the-counter vitamin and mineral supplement provides an ample amount of synthetic folate, the preferred form. Still, she should discuss this supplement use with her physician and would probably eventually benefit more from a prenatal supplement prescribed by her physician, as this will have more folate and iron than over-the-counter multivitamin and mineral supplements. Her diet may not have enough calcium, so she should pay as much attention to consuming some extra calcium as she does for protein. Avoiding alcohol is a smart move.

Many experts would say that she is consuming too much caffeine and would be wise to cut down to one to two cups of coffee per day, or possibly even eliminate coffee altogether. Her exercise routine is probably too vigorous if she hasn't already been practicing regular running. Tracey should not begin a new exercise routine upon becoming pregnant unless it is at a moderate pace, such as brisk walking or stationary biking.

A goal of *Healthy People 2010* is 100% abstinence from alcohol, cigarettes, and illicit drugs by pregnant women.

CONCEPT CHECK

*I*nfants born after 37 weeks of gestation and weighing more than 5.5 lb (2.5 kg) have the fewest medical problems at birth. Individual mothers and whole societies can attempt to reduce infant and maternal death and medical problems by limiting the factors that increase the risk of having a preterm or small-for-gestational-age infant. Such contributing factors, besides an inadequate diet in general, include low socioeconomic status; closely spaced births; obesity; inadequate or absent prenatal care; cigarette smoking; alcohol consumption; illegal drug use; teenage pregnancy; inadequate prenatal weight gain; heavy caffeine use; Listeria exposure; and prenatal ketosis. Adequate nutrition can reduce the risk of many medical problems in pregnancy.

■ PHYSIOLOGICAL CHANGES THAT CAN CAUSE DISCOMFORT IN PREGNANCY

During pregnancy, the fetus's needs for oxygen, nutrients, and excretion increase the burden on the mother's lungs, heart, and kidneys. Although a mother's digestive and metabolic systems work very efficiently, some discomfort accompanies the changes her body undergoes to accommodate the fetus.[32]

■ Heartburn, Constipation, and Hemorrhoids

Hormones produced by the placenta relax muscles in both the uterus and the intestinal tract. This often causes heartburn as stomach acid slips up into the esophagus (see Chapter 3). When this occurs, the woman should avoid lying down after eating, eat less fat so that foods pass more quickly from the stomach into the small intestine, and avoid spicy foods she can't tolerate. She should also consume liquids between meals to decrease stomach volume and pressure. Women with more severe cases may need antacids or related medications.

Constipation often results as the intestinal muscles relax during pregnancy. It is especially likely to develop late in pregnancy, as the fetus competes with the GI tract for space in the abdominal cavity. To offset these discomforts, a woman should perform regular exercise and consume more fluid, dietary fiber, and dried fruits, such as prunes (dried plums). These practices can help prevent constipation and a problem that frequently accompanies it, hemorrhoids. Straining during elimination can lead to hemorrhoids, which are already more likely to occur during pregnancy because of other body changes. A reevaluation of the need and dose of iron supplementation also should be considered, as this practice is linked to constipation.[32]

■ Edema

Placental hormones cause various body tissues to retain fluid during pregnancy. Blood volume also greatly expands during pregnancy. The extra fluid normally causes some swelling (edema). There is no reason to restrict salt severely or use diuretics to limit mild edema. However, the edema may limit physical activity late in pregnancy and occasionally require a woman to elevate her feet to control the symptoms. Overall, edema generally spells trouble only if hypertension and the appearance of protein in the urine accompany fluid retention (see later section on pregnancy-induced hypertension).

■ Morning Sickness

About 50% of pregnant women experience nausea during the early stages of pregnancy. This nausea may be related to the increased sense of smell induced by pregnancy-related hormones circulating in the bloodstream. Although commonly called "morning sickness," pregnancy-related nausea may occur at any time and persist all day. It is often the first signal to a woman that she is pregnant. To help control mild nausea, pregnant women can try the following: avoiding nauseating foods, such as fried or greasy foods; cooking with windows open to dissipate nauseating smells; eating soda crackers or dry cereal before getting out of bed; avoiding large fluid intakes early in the morning; and eating smaller, more frequent meals. Because the iron in prenatal supplements triggers nausea in some women, changing the type of supplement used or postponing use until the second trimester may provide relief in some cases. If a woman thinks her prenatal supplement is related to morning sickness, she should discuss switching to another supplement with her physician.

Overall, whether it is broccoli or soda crackers, if a food sounds good to a pregnant woman with morning sickness, she should eat it and eat when she can, while also striving to follow her prenatal diet. If she has a great deal of difficulty in following her diet, she should alert her physician to this and follow the advice given. Usually, nausea stops after the first trimester; however, in about 10 to 20% of cases, it can continue throughout the entire pregnancy. In cases of serious nausea the preceding practices offer little relief. When appetite is severely reduced or vomiting persists, medical guidance is warranted. Hospitalization may be needed if the mother exhibits significant dehydration or weight loss. This is called hyperemesis gravidarum. Sometimes total parenteral nutrition is needed in these cases to support the health of mother and fetus until the problem remits.[32]

■ Anemia

To supply fetal needs, the mother's blood volume expands to approximately 150% of normal. The amount of red blood cells expands only 20 to 30% above normal and occurs more gradually. This leaves proportionately fewer red blood cells in a

CRITICAL THINKING

Sandy, who is 4 months pregnant, has been having heartburn after meals, constipation, and difficult bowel movements. As a nutrition student, you understand the digestive system and the role of nutrition in health. What remedies might you suggest to Sandy to relieve her problems?

physiological anemia The normal increase in blood volume in pregnancy, that dilutes the concentration of red blood cells, resulting in anemia; also called *hemodilution*.

gestational diabetes A high blood glucose concentration that develops during pregnancy and returns to normal after birth; one cause is the placental production of hormones that antagonize the regulation of blood glucose by insulin.

pregnancy-induced hypertension A serious disorder that can include high blood pressure, kidney failure, convulsions, and even death of the mother and fetus. Although its exact cause is not known, good nutrition (especially adequate calcium intake) and prenatal care may prevent or limit its severity. Mild cases are known as *preeclampsia*; more severe cases are called *eclampsia* (formerly called toxemia).

pregnant woman's bloodstream. The lower ratio of red blood cells to total blood volume is a condition known as **physiological anemia.** It is a normal response to pregnancy, rather than the result of inadequate nutrient intake. If during pregnancy, however, iron stores and/or dietary iron intake are not sufficient to meet needs, any resulting iron deficiency anemia requires medical attention.[28]

■ Gestational Diabetes

Hormones synthesized by the placenta (human placental lactogen) antagonize the action of insulin. This antagonism can precipitate **gestational diabetes,** often beginning in weeks 20 to 28, particularly in women who have a family history of diabetes or who are obese. Nationwide, gestational diabetes develops in about 4% of pregnancies; however, it increases to 7% in the Caucasian population.[19] Today, pregnant women often are screened at 24 to 28 weeks for elevated blood glucose concentration 1 hour after consuming 50 g of glucose. If gestational diabetes is detected, a special diet distributing carbohydrate intake throughout the day and sometimes insulin injections are needed; regular physical activity is also helpful. Although gestational diabetes often disappears after the infant's birth, it is linked to the development of diabetes later in the mother's life, especially if she fails to maintain healthy body weight. Proper control of both gestational diabetes and diabetes present in the mother before pregnancy is extremely important. If not treated, the primary risks are that the fetus can grow quite large (fetal macrosomia). The fetus will produce too much insulin and this will cause increased fetal growth. The pregnancy may require a cesarean section due to the size of the fetus. Other concerns are the potential need for early delivery, increased risk of birth trauma and malformations, and hypoglycemia in the infant at birth.[32]

■ Pregnancy-Induced Hypertension

Pregnancy-induced hypertension is a high-risk disorder and occurs in about 7 to 8% of pregnancies.[6] In its mild forms, it is known as *preeclampsia* and, in severe forms, as *eclampsia*. Early symptoms include a rise in blood pressure, excess protein in the urine, edema, changes in blood clotting, and nervous system disorders. Very severe effects, including convulsions, can occur in the second and third trimesters. If not controlled, eclampsia eventually damages the liver and kidneys, and mother and fetus both may die. The population most at risk for this disorder is women over age 35 and those who have had multiple-birth pregnancies. A family history of pregnancy-induced hypertension in the mother or father, diabetes, African-American race, and a woman's first pregnancy also raise risk.

Pregnancy-induced hypertension resolves once the pregnancy ends, making delivery the most reliable treatment for the mother. However, since the problem often begins before the fetus is ready to be born, physicians in many cases must use treatments to prevent the worsening of the disorder. Bed rest and magnesium sulfate are possible treatment methods, although the effectiveness of these treatments varies and is often disappointing. Several other treatments such as various hypertension medications and low dose aspirin (60 mg/day) are under study, but no definite proof exists for success with any one approach.

CONCEPT CHECK

Heartburn, constipation, hemorrhoids, nausea and vomiting, edema, anemia, and gestational diabetes are possible discomforts and complications of pregnancy. Changes in food habits can often ease these problems. Pregnancy-induced hypertension, with high blood pressure and kidney failure, can lead to severe complications or even death of both the mother and fetus, if not treated.

■ BREASTFEEDING

Before the 1900s, if a mother didn't breastfeed (nurse) her infant, a substitute nursing mother (wet-nurse) was hired to do it. Formula feeding was fraught with complications, primarily because people did not know the importance of sterilizing formulas against bacteria. Nor did people know much about the nutritional needs of infants. During the early 1900s, the technology of formulas based on cow's milk and methods of feeding improved. From the 1920s and especially in the 1940s, when women worked in armament factories during World War II, more and more babies were fed formula. Throughout the 1950s and early 1960s, interest in breastfeeding further waned. In the 1970s, breastfeeding enjoyed a resurgence, which has since leveled off.

Healthy People 2010 has set a goal of 75% of women nursing their infants at time of hospital discharge, 50% breastfeeding for 6 months, and 25% still breastfeeding at 1 year. The American Dietetic Association and the American Academy of Pediatrics recommend breastfeeding exclusively for the first 4 to 6 months, with the continued combination of breastfeeding and infant foods until 1 year. The World Health Organization goes beyond that to recommend breastfeeding for at least 2 years, supplemented with other foods. Surveys show, however, that only about 55% of American mothers now nurse their infants in the hospital, and at 4 and 6 months only 33% and 20% are still breastfeeding their infants, respectively. Thus, many women are leaving the hospital breastfeeding, but there is a large dropoff, especially after 2 weeks.

Women who choose to breastfeed usually find it an enjoyable, special time in their lives and their relationship with their new infant. Bottle feeding with an infant formula is also safe for infants, as discussed in Chapter 17, but does not equal the benefits derived from human milk in all aspects.[32] If a woman doesn't nurse her child, breast weight returns to normal very soon after birth.

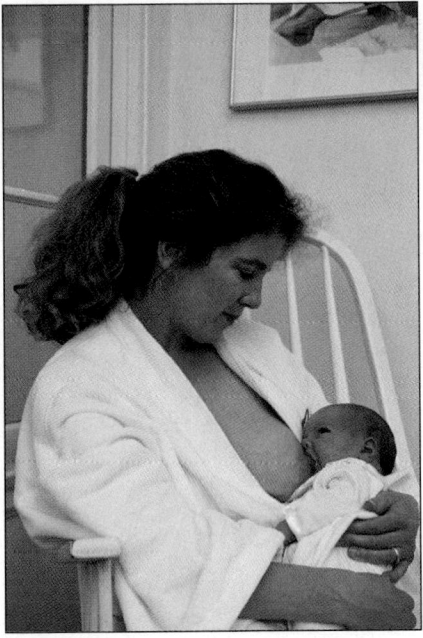

Breastfeeding fosters a closeness and bonding between the mother and the infant.

■ Ability to Breastfeed

In most cases, problems encountered in breastfeeding are due to a lack of appropriate information, because almost all women are physically capable of nursing their children (see later section on medical conditions precluding breastfeeding for exceptions). Anatomical problems in breasts, such as inverted nipples, can be corrected during pregnancy. Breast size is no indication of success in breastfeeding, and this generally increases during pregnancy. Most women notice a dramatic increase in the size and weight of their breasts by the third or fourth day of breastfeeding. If these changes don't occur, a woman needs to speak with her physician or a lactation consultant.[23]

Breastfed infants must be followed closely over the first days of life to ensure that the process is proceeding normally. Monitoring is especially important with a mother's first child, because the mother will be inexperienced with the process of breastfeeding. Nowadays, mothers and healthy infants are commonly discharged from the hospital 1 to 2 days after delivery, whereas 20 years ago they stayed in the hospital for 3 or 4 days or longer. One result of such rapid discharge is a decreased period of infant monitoring by health-care professionals. Incidents have been reported of infants developing dehydration and blood clots soon after hospital discharge when breastfeeding did not proceed smoothly. Careful monitoring in this first week by a physician or lacatation consultant is advised.[23]

First-time mothers who plan to breastfeed should learn as much as they can about the process early in their pregnancy. Interested women should learn the proper technique, what problems to expect, and how to respond to them. Overall, breastfeeding is a learned skill, and mothers need knowledge to nurse safely, especially with the first child.

Many of the benefits of breastfeeding can be found at http://www.4woman.gov./Breastfeeding/index.htm, sponsored by the US Surgeon General

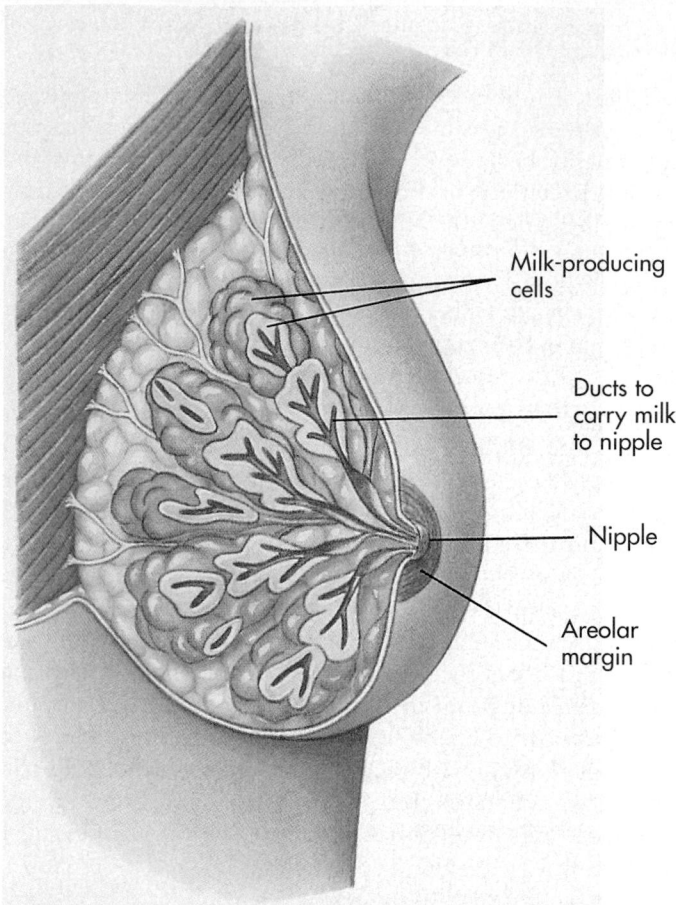

Milk-producing cells

Ducts to carry milk to nipple

Nipple

Areolar margin

FIGURE 16-6 The anatomy of the breast. Many types of cells form a coordinated network to produce and secrete human milk.
Illustration by William Ober.

lobules Saclike structures in the breast that store milk.

prolactin A hormone secreted by the mother that stimulates the synthesis of milk.

let-down reflex A reflex stimulated by infant suckling that causes the release (ejection) of milk from milk ducts in the mother's breasts.

oxytocin A hormone secreted by the posterior part of the pituitary gland. It causes contraction of the musclelike cells surrounding the ducts of the breasts, and the smooth muscle of the uterus.

■ Production of Human Milk

During pregnancy, cells in the breast form milk-producing **lobules** (Fig. 16-6). Hormones from the placenta stimulate these changes in the breast. After birth, the mother produces more **prolactin** hormone to maintain the changes in the breast and therefore the ability to produce milk. During pregnancy, breast weight increases by about 1 to 2 lb.[32]

The hormone prolactin also stimulates the synthesis of milk. Suckling stimulates prolactin release. Milk synthesis then occurs as an infant nurses. The more the infant suckles, the more milk is produced. Milk production closely parallels infant demand. Because of this fact, even twins can be nursed. Demand is the driving force for milk production.[32]

Most protein found in human milk is synthesized by breast tissue. Some proteins also enter the milk directly from the mother's bloodstream. These proteins include immune factors and enzymes (see the Expert Opinion by Dr. Lönnerdal). Fats in human milk come from the mother's diet, and some are synthesized by breast tissue. The sugar galactose is synthesized in the breast, whereas glucose enters from the mother's bloodstream. Together, these sugars form lactose, the main carbohydrate in human milk.

■ Let-Down Reflex

An important brain-breast connection—the **let-down reflex**—is necessary for breastfeeding.[32] The brain releases the hormone **oxytocin** to allow the breast tissues to let down (release) the milk from storage sites. It travels to the nipple area. A tingling sensation signals the let-down reflex shortly before milk flow begins. If the let-down reflex doesn't operate, little milk is available to the infant. The infant then gets frustrated, and this can frustrate the mother.

The let-down reflex is easily inhibited by nervous tension, a lack of confidence, and fatigue. Mothers should be especially aware of the link between tension and a weak let-down reflex. They need to find a relaxed environment where they can breastfeed.

After a few weeks, the let-down reflex becomes automatic. The mother's response can be triggered just by thinking about her infant or seeing or hearing another one. At first, however, the process can be a bit bewildering. Because she cannot measure the amount of milk the infant takes in, a mother may fear that she is not adequately nourishing the infant.

As a general rule, a well-nourished breastfed infant should (1) have six or more wet diapers per day after the second day of life, (2) show a normal weight gain, and (3) pass at least one or two stools per day that look like lumpy mustard. In addition, softening of the breast during the feeding helps indicate that enough milk is being consumed. Parents who sense their infant is not consuming enough milk should consult a physician immediately because dehydration can develop rapidly.[23]

It generally takes 2 to 3 weeks to fully establish the feeding routine: Infant and mother both feel comfortable, the milk supply meets infant demand, and initial nipple soreness disappears. Establishing the breastfeeding routine requires patience, but the rewards are great. The adjustments are easier if supplemental formula feedings are not introduced until breastfeeding is well established, after at least 3 to 4 weeks. Then a supplemental bottle or two of infant formula per day is fine.

Parents need not be concerned that breastfed infants grow a bit more slowly after about 3 months of age than formula-fed infants, based on increases in body weight. The infant's physician is the best judge of whether the rate of growth of the breastfed infant is satisfactory. Essentially, the difference is of no consequence, in part because some of it is related to increased fat deposition.[23]

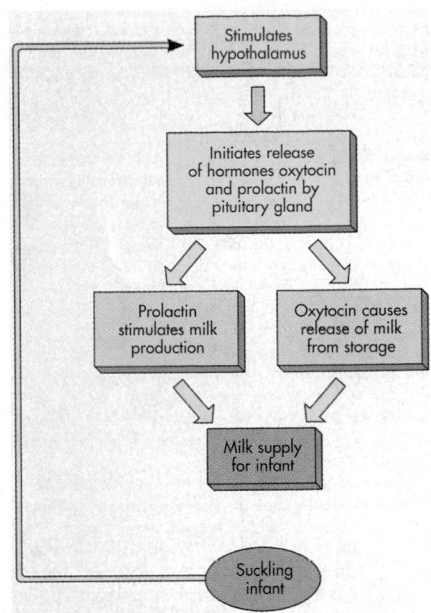

The let-down reflex—from suckling infant to human milk secretion from the breast.

▪ Nutritional Qualities of Human Milk

Human milk is very different in composition from cow's milk. Unless altered, cow's milk should not be used in infant feeding until the infant is 12 months old because cow's milk is too high in minerals and protein, does not contain enough carbohydrate to meet infant needs, and may trigger the development of diabetes in infants with a genetic predisposition to the disorder. In addition, the major protein in cow's milk, casein, is harder for an infant to digest than the major protein in human milk, lactalbumin. Finally, certain compounds in human milk presently under study show other possible benefits for the infant. These factors, such as the omega-3 fatty acids typically found in fish (see following discussion of mature milk), are not present in cow's milk or infant formulas.[16]

Colostrum

The first fluid made by the human breast is **colostrum.** This thick, yellowish fluid may leak from the breast during late pregnancy and is produced in earnest for a few days to a week after birth. Colostrum contains antibodies and immune-system cells, some of which pass unaltered through the immature GI tract of the infant into the bloodstream. These immune factors and cells protect the infant from some gastrointestinal diseases and other infectious disorders, compensating for the infant's own immature immune system during the first few months of life.[32]

Colostrum facilitates the passage of **meconium,** a stool produced during fetal life. One component of colostrum, the *Lactobacillus bifidus* factor, encourages the growth of *Lactobacillus bifidus* bacteria. These bacteria limit the growth of potentially toxic bacteria in the intestine. Overall, breastfeeding promotes the intestinal health of the breastfed infant in this way.

Mature Milk

Human milk composition gradually changes until several days after delivery, when it achieves the normal composition of mature milk. Human milk looks very different from cow's milk. (Table 17-1 in the next chapter provides a direct comparison.) Human milk is thin and almost watery in appearance and often has a slightly bluish tinge. Its nutritional qualities are quite impressive.

*D*isposable diapers can absorb so much urine that it is difficult to judge when they are wet. A strip of paper towel laid inside a disposable diaper makes a good wetness indicator. Or cloth diapers may be used for a day or two to assess whether nursing is supplying sufficient milk.

colostrum The first fluid secreted by the breast during late pregnancy and the first few days after birth. This thick fluid is rich in immune factors and protein.

meconium The first thick, mucuslike stool passed by the infant after birth.

Lactobacillus bifidus factor A protective factor secreted in the colostrum that encourages growth of beneficial bacteria in the newborn's intestines.

Expert Opinion

BREAST MILK PROVIDES MUCH MORE THAN NUTRIENTS TO THE NEWBORN

Bo Lönnerdal, Ph.D.

There is overwhelming support for breast milk being the optimum food for infant. Besides the fact that the mother-infant interaction during the process of breastfeeding provides many benefits for both the mother and her newborn, breast milk contains many unique components, which help the infant use nutrients, stimulate the immune system, protect against infection, and promote health and development.

Enzymes and binding proteins in breast milk help infants digest and absorb nutrients from the diet. A bile-salt stimulated lipase facilitates the complete digestion of triglycericdes and thus improves energy use. Specific nutrient-binding proteins—such as folate-binding protein, vitamin B-12–binding protein (haptocorrin), and lactoferrin, which binds iron—contribute to the efficient delivery of these micronutrients to the intestinal cells for further transport and metabolism in the body.

The immune system of a breastfed infant obtains a considerable boost from breast milk. Maternal immunity—that is, the mother's capacity to recognize harmful bacteria and viruses and develop antibodies against them—is transferred via the placenta but continues via breast milk, which contains high concentrations of a special form of immunoglobulin A (secretory IgA). This immunoglobulin can survive the conditions in the stomach and small intestine in an intact form. Live cells are also present in human milk, and some of these, so-called memory T-cells, are taken up by the infant and contribute to its immune competence. Additionally, breast milk contains biologically significant concentrations of cytokines (interleukins, interferon-gamma, tumor necrosis factor [TNF-alpha], etc.), signal substances that stimulate the immune system and help prevent allergy and inflammatory reactions. Several growth factors in human milk, such as epidermal growth factor (EGF), insulin-like growth factor (IGF), and transforming growth factor (TGF-beta) are believed to act both locally in the intestine by stimulating the growth and proliferation of cells and systemically by being absorbed and transported to vital organs via the bloodstream.

Other factors in breast milk that may affect the development of a breastfed infant include long-chain polyunsaturated fatty acids and nucleotides, the latter being the building blocks for DNA and RNA. Docosahexaenoic acid (DHA), which is incorporated specifically into certain regions of the brain; arachidonic acid, a precursor for prostaglandin and leukotriene synthyesis; and conjugated linoleic acid are fatty acids that are present in breast milk in low but biologically relevant concentrations, but not in infant formula. Research on the biological significance of these compounds is currently going on in preterm and term infants. Nucleotides are present at relatively high concentrations in breast milk, both in free and bound form. These nucleotides have been shown to stimulate the immune system in adult patients, and recent studies on infants suggest similar effects on their immune function.

There is a growing body of evidence showing that breastfed infants have fewer

Human milk's main protein forms a soft, light curd in the infant's stomach, easing digestion. Other human milk proteins bind iron, reducing the growth of iron-requiring bacteria. Many of these types of bacteria cause diarrhea. Still other proteins offer the important immune protection already noted.

The lipids in human breast milk are high in linoleic acid and cholesterol, which are needed for brain development. Breast milk also contains long-chain omega-3 fatty acids, such as docosahexaenoic acid (DHA). This unsaturated fatty acid is used for the synthesis of tissues in the brain and the rest of the central nervous system, and in the retina of the eye. Some evidence indicates that breastfed infants show greater visual acuity and better nervous system development than infants fed formulas, none of which currently contain DHA.[2] Breastfeeding for at least 6 months is advocated to obtain this benefit.

Researchers are currently determining the potential benefits of adding DHA to infant formulas. The long-term safety of this addition is under study. The World Health Organization (WHO) recommends adding DHA to infant formulas, whereas infections, such as upper respiratory and gastrointestinal infections, as well as otitis media (ear infection), and that, when they get ill, the duration of the illness is shorter than in formula-fed infants. Although part of this lower prevalence of infections may be a consequence of a more developed immune system, there are two more major lines of defense against infections in breastfed infants.

The gut microflora—that is, the microbial composition—of breastfed infants is different from that of formula-fed infants. Lactobacilli and bifidobacteria, which are beneficial to humans, dominate the gastrointestinal tracts of breastfed infants, whereas potentially harmful bacteria, such as *E. coli* and *Bacteroides*, are predominant in formula-fed infants. Breast milk contains several components, particularly oligosaccharides, which stimulate the growth of these beneficial bacteria. Lactobacilli and bifidobacteria in breastfed infants produce acids during their metabolism, which reduce the pH of the intestine and discourages the growth of many pathogenic bacteria (which prefer a higher pH).

Breast milk also contains so-called bioactive factors, which either inhibit the growth of harmful bacteria and viruses or directly kill them. These factors include the enzyme lysozyme, which degrades the cell walls of bacteria; lactoferrin, which can withhold iron from bacteria that require iron for growth; and lactoperioxidase, which can directly kill bacteria. The oligosaccharides, whether in free form or bound to milk proteins, can act as decoys and bind to harmful bacteria, thereby preventing them from attaching to the intestinal mucosa, which is a prerequisite for them to cause infection.

The nutritional quality of breast milk and the volume of milk produced by the mother are remarkably well maintained under various adverse conditions. Mal nourished women have generally been shown to produce adequate milk volumes and breast milk with normal contents of energy, protein, lipid, and carbohydrate. Concentrations of minerals, trace elements, and vitamins are usually normal, even if the mother is deficient in these nutrients, suggesting compensatory mechanisms in the mammary gland, although there are a few exceptions (e.g., vitamin A and selenium). Similarly, women with illnesses common in developing countries produce breast milk with normal composition in adequate volumes.

A recent dark shadow falling on the benefits of breast milk is the documented transmission of HIV by HIV-positive breastfeeding mothers. Although an immediate reaction to this finding was to recommend such women to abstain from nursing their infants, it also became obvious that this is virtually impossible in poor populations, where safe and adequate alternatives to breastfeeding are unavailable or economically unrealistic. The actual rate of transmission of HIV through breast milk is still unclear. Although HIV can be found in breast milk in both free and cell-bound form, human milk contains several bioactive factors that can inactivate viruses such as HIV, cytomegalovirus (CMV), and rotavirus. The extent to which these factors can inactivate HIV and/or limit its transmission is still unclear, as is the involvement of physical factors in the mother (such as sore nipples) or in the infant (integrity of the musocal lining, etc.). This represents a major health problem in several regions of the world and is in need of immediate action.

Dr. Lönnerdal is professor of nutrition and internal medicine, Department of Nutrition, University of California, Davis. He has spent his research career studying the nutritional and related benefits of human milk and is recognized internationally as an authority on the topic.

the American Academy of Pediatricians says that the data on DHA are still too sketchy, especially for full-term infants. DHA is predominantly a concern for preterm infants, as they are not receiving the normal amounts from the mother when in utero because of the shorter gestational period. Eventually, manufacturers may produce formulas for preterm and full-term infants with a fatty-acid composition equivalent to that of human milk, just as they have done for the protein and mineral content. Formulas with added DHA are in use in Europe. Providing this long-chain polyunsaturated fatty acid is also being considered for pregnant women. There is a concern that considerable amounts of DHA are lost through maternal (and lactation) processes.[16] However, until more research is completed, it is premature to make recommendations for consumption of this unsaturated fatty acid beyond fish consumption twice a week (or intake of 900 mg/day of omega-3 fatty acids from fish oil capsules; see Chapter 6).

Human milk changes in fat composition during each feeding. The consistency of milk released initially (about 60% of the volume) resembles that of skim milk. The next amount (about 35% of the total volume) has a greater fat proportion, similar to whole milk. Finally, the hindmilk (about 5% of the total) is essentially like cream and is usually released 10 to 20 minutes into the feeding. The overall energy content of human milk is about the same as that of infant formulas (67 kcal/100 ml). Babies need to nurse long enough (e.g., a total of 20 or more minutes) to get the energy in the rich hindmilk to be satisfied between feedings and to grow well.

Human milk also allows for adequate hydration of the infant, provided the baby is exclusively breastfed. A question commonly asked is whether the infant needs additional water, if stressed by hot weather, diarrhea, vomiting, or fever. Providing up to 4 ounces of water a day from a bottle to young breastfed infants is fine. Note, however, that greater amounts of supplemental water can lead to brain disorders, low blood sodium, and other problems. Thus, extra water may be given, but only with a physician's guidance.

Food Plan for Women Who Breastfeed

Nutrient needs for a breastfeeding mother change to some extent from those of the pregnant woman (see the inside cover of this book). Exceptions are decreases in folate and iron needs and an increase in the need for energy, vitamins A, E, and C, riboflavin, copper, chromium, iodide, magnanese, selenium, and zinc. The diet for breastfeeding women can be the same as that for pregnant women, except teenagers generally should have about four servings from the milk, yogurt, and cheese group (review Table 16-2). As in pregnancy, a serving of a fortified ready-to-eat breakfast cereal is advised (or use of a typical vitamin and mineral supplement) to meet extra nutrient needs. As mentioned for pregnant women, some researchers also recommend that women who are breastfeeding consume fish twice a week (or fish oil supplements) because the omega-3 fatty acids present in fish are thought to be important for brain development.[16]

A reasonable approach for a breastfeeding woman is to eat a balanced diet that supplies at least 1800 kcal per day, has a moderate fat content, and includes a variety of dairy products, fruits, vegetables, and grains. The woman should drink fluids every time the infant nurses, because drinking to quench thirst encourages ample milk production. If a woman restricts her energy intake too severely, the quantity of milk also decreases. This is not a time to crash diet. More than two alcoholic drinks a day also decreases milk output, as does smoking. Finally, the same fish precautions given to pregnant women apply to the breastfeeding mother.

Milk production requires approximately 800 kcal every day. The RDA for energy during lactation is an extra 500 kcal daily above prepregnancy recommendations. The difference between energy needs and intake—about 300 kcal—should contribute to gradual loss of the extra body fat accumulated during pregnancy, especially if breastfeeding is continued for 6 months or more and the woman performs some physical activity. This shows how practical the link is between pregnancy and breastfeeding. Weight loss of 1 to 4 lb per month in the nursing mother is appropriate. Milk output decreases at significantly greater rates of weight loss, as occur with severe dieting when energy intake is less than about 1500 kcal/day.[32]

Most substances the mother ingests are secreted into her milk. For this reason, she should limit intake of or avoid all alcohol and caffeine and check all medications with a pediatrician. Some mothers believe that some foods, such as garlic and chocolate, flavor the breast milk and upset the infant. If a woman notices a connection between a food she eats and the infant's later fussiness, she could consider avoiding that food. However, she might experiment again with it later, as infants become fussy for other reasons. Some researchers, on the other hand, feel that the passage of flavors from the mother's diet into her milk affords an opportunity for the infant to learn about the flavor of the foods of its family long before solids are introduced. These researchers suspect that bottle-fed infants are missing significant sensory experiences that until recent times in human history were common to all infants.

CONCEPT CHECK

Recognition of the importance of breastfeeding has contributed to its greater popularity during the past 20 years. Almost all women have the ability to breastfeed. The hormone prolactin stimulates breast tissue to synthesize milk. Some components of human milk come directly from the mother's bloodstream. Infant suckling triggers a let-down reflex, which releases the milk. The more an infant nurses, the more milk is synthesized. The nutrient composition of human milk is very different from that of cow's milk and changes as the infant matures. The first fluid produced, colostrum, is rich in immune factors. The diet for breastfeeding is generally similar to that for pregnancy, except for additional fluids, as well as four servings from the milk, yogurt, and cheese group for teenage mothers in general.

■ Pros and Cons of Breastfeeding

As noted already, the vast majority of women are capable of breastfeeding, and infants benefit from it. The many benefits are listed in Table 16-3 and the Expert Opinion. Nonetheless, a woman's decision to nurse depends on a variety of factors, some of which may make breastfeeding impractical or undesirable for a woman. Mothers who don't want to breastfeed their infants should not feel compelled to do so. Breastfeeding provides distinct advantages, but none so great that a woman who decides to bottle-feed should feel she is significantly penalizing her infant.

Advantages Of Breastfeeding

Human milk is tailored to meet infant nutrient needs for the first 4 to 6 months of life. The possible exceptions are the relative lack of fluoride, iron, and vitamin D. Infant supplements, used under the guidance of a pediatrician, can supply these and are often recommended. Some sun exposure also helps compensate for the gap in vitamin D nutriture, but will likely not be enough for dark-skinned (e.g., African-American) infants. Fluoride may be found in the household water supply. If it is not present in adequate amounts or the child is not receiving tap water, a fluoride supplement should be considered and a dentist consulted. Vitamin B-12 supplements are recommended for the breastfed infant whose mother is a complete vegetarian (vegan).

Fewer Infections. Breastfeeding reduces the general risk of infections to the infant. This is partially because of the antibodies in human milk that an infant can use. Breastfed infants also have fewer ear infections (otitis media) because they do not sleep with a bottle in the mouth. Experts strongly discourage allowing infants to sleep with a bottle in their mouths. When that happens, milk pools there, backs up through the throat, and eventually settles in the ears, creating a growth medium for bacteria. Infant ear infections are a common problem. By avoiding them, parents can decrease discomfort for the infant, avoid related trips to the doctor, and prevent possible hearing loss. Tooth decay from nighttime bottles is another likely consequence (see Chapter 17).

Frozen human milk should not be thawed in a microwave. The heat can destroy immune factors in the milk and create hot spots, which may scald the infant's tongue.

TABLE 16-3   Attributes of Breastfeeding

Infant

- Bacteriologically safe
- Always fresh and ready to go
- Provides antibodies while infant's immune system is still immature
- Contributes to maturation of gastrointestinal tract via *Lactobacillus bifidus* factor; decreases incidence of diarrhea and respiratory disease
- Reduces risk of food allergies and intolerances
- Establishes habit of eating in moderation, thus decreasing possibility of obesity later in life
- Contributes to proper development of jaws and teeth for better speech development
- Decreases ear infections
- Facilitates bonding with mother
- May enhance nervous system development

Mother

- Contributes to earlier recovery from pregnancy due to a quicker return of the uterus to the prepregnancy state
- Decreases the risk of ovarian and premenopausal breast cancer
- Lessens the economic strain of purchasing formula
- Facilitates bonding with infant

Fewer Allergies and Intolerances. Breastfeeding also reduces the chances of allergies, especially in allergy-prone infants (see the Nutrition Perspective in Chapter 17). The key time to attain this benefit from breastfeeding is during the first 4 to 6 months of an infant's life. Breastfeeding for even just the first few weeks is beneficial. A longer commitment than 4 to 6 months is better, but the first few months are most critical. Another benefit of breastfeeding is that infants are better able to tolerate human milk than formulas. Formulas must occasionally be switched several times until caregivers find the best one for the infant.

Convenience and Cost. Breastfeeding frees the mother from the time and expense involved in buying and preparing formula and washing bottles. Human milk is ready to go and sterile. This allows the mother to spend more time with her baby. On the other hand, if the child is bottle-fed, the mother may be free to do other things while others feed the baby.

Barriers to Breastfeeding

Widespread misinformation, return to jobs, and social reticence all serve as barriers to breastfeeding.

Misinformation. Probably the major barriers to breastfeeding are misinformation, such as one's breasts are too small, and lack of role models. One positive note has been the widespread increase in the availability of lactation consultants over the past several years. These consultants are a valuable source for new mothers in the adjustment to breastfeeding. If a woman is interested in breastfeeding, she should also talk to women who have done it successfully. Experienced mothers can be an enormous help to the first-time mother. The first-time mother should find a friend she can call on for advice. In almost every community, a group called La Leche League offers classes in breastfeeding and advises women who have problems with it (800-LALECHE or http://www.lalecheleague.org). Other resources are http://breastfeeding.com and http://breastfeeding.org.

Return to an Outside Job. Working outside the home can complicate plans to breastfeed. One possibility after a month or two of breastfeeding is for the mother to regularly express and save her own milk. She can express milk by breast pump or manually into a sterile plastic bottle or nursing bag (used in a disposable bottle system). Saving human milk requires careful sanitation and rapid chilling. It can be stored in the refrigerator for 1 day and be frozen for 1 month. There is a knack to learning how to express milk, but the freedom can be worth it, because it allows others to feed the infant the mother's milk. A schedule of expressing milk and using supplemental formula feedings is most successful if begun after 1 to 2 months of exclusive breastfeeding. After 1 month or so, the baby is well adapted to breastfeeding and probably feels enough emotional security and other benefits from nursing to drink both ways.

Some women can juggle both a job and breastfeeding, but others find it too cumbersome and decide to formula-feed. A compromise—balancing some breastfeedings, perhaps early morning and night, with formula-feedings during the day—is possible. However, too many supplemental formula feedings decrease milk production.

Social Reticence. Another barrier for some women is embarrassment about nursing a child in public. Historically our society has stressed modesty and has discouraged public displays of breasts—even for as good a cause as nourishing babies. Women who feel reticent should be reassured that, with appropriate clothing, they can nurse quite discreetly.

Medical Conditions Precluding Breastfeeding. Breastfeeding may be ruled out by certain medical conditions in either the infant or mother. For example, infants with the disease galactosemia can't break down galactose, the major sugar in breast milk. These infants do not grow well if nursed and often suffer from vomiting and diarrhea. If left untreated, the infants ultimately develop liver disease, cataracts, and mental retardation. A special infant formula free of galactose must be used. Breastfeeding may also be detrimental to infants with phenylketonuria; the high concentration of phenylalanine in breast milk may overwhelm the impaired ability of these infants to metabolize this amino acid, leading to production of toxic products.

Mothers who take certain medications, which pass into the milk and adversely affect the nursing infant, may be advised to avoid breastfeeding.[14, 15] In addition, a woman in the United States and other developed countries who has a serious chronic disease (such as tuberculosis, AIDS or HIV-positive status, or certain forms of hepatitis) or who is being treated with chemotherapy medications should not breastfeed.[24] Research remains unclear on whether or not hepatitis C is transmitted during breastfeeding; further research is needed. Note that this is a common infection, affecting about 4 million Americans (many of whom are undiagnosed).[25] A final group can include immature mothers and those with psychiatric problems.

■ Environmental Contaminants in Human Milk

Some women wonder whether breastfeeding is safe for their infant. There is some legitimate concern over the levels of various environmental contaminants in human milk. However, the benefits from human milk are very well established, and the risks from environmental contaminants are still largely theoretical. Thus, it is probably best to continue with what has been shown to work until sufficiently strong research data contradict it.

A few measures a woman could take to counteract some known contaminants are to (1) avoid freshwater fish from polluted waters, (2) carefully wash and peel fruits and vegetables, and (3) remove the fatty edges of meat, as this is where pesticides concentrate. In addition, a woman should not try to lose weight rapidly while nursing (more than ¾ to 1 lb per week), because contaminants stored in fat tissue might then enter her bloodstream and affect her milk. If a woman questions whether her milk is safe, especially if she has lived in an area known to have a high concentration of toxic wastes or environmental pollutants, she should consult her local health department.

■ Can a Preterm Infant Be Breastfed?

There is no clear-cut answer to whether a woman can breastfeed a preterm infant. In some cases, human milk is the most desirable form of nourishment, depending on weight and length of gestation. If so, it must usually be expressed from the breast and fed through a tube. This type of feeding demands great maternal dedication. Fortification of the milk with such nutrients as calcium, phosphorus, sodium, and protein is often necessary to match an infant's rapid growth. In other cases, special feeding problems may prevent the use of human milk or necessitate supplementing it with formula. Sometimes total parenteral nutrition support is the only option. Working as a team, the pediatrician, neonatal nurses, and registered dietitian must guide the parents in this decision.

CONCEPT CHECK

Human milk supplies most of an infant's nutritional needs for the first 6 months, although supplementation with vitamin D, iron, and fluoride may be needed. Breastfeeding is less expensive and often more convenient than formula feeding. Compared with formula-fed infants, breastfed infants have fewer intestinal, respiratory, and ear infections and are less susceptible to allergies and food intolerances. Despite the advantages of breastfeeding, misinformation, a return to work, and social reticence may dissuade a mother from breastfeeding. A combination of breastfeeding and formula feeding is possible when a mother is regularly away from the infant and is not able to express and store her milk for later use. Breastfeeding is not desirable if a mother has certain diseases or must take medication potentially harmful to the infant. The preterm infant, depending on its condition, may benefit from consuming human milk.

Breastfeeding mothers should get their physician's permission before embarking on a vigorous exercise program. Breastfeeding women must also take care to drink plenty of fluids before and after workouts and should avoid exercising when fatigued.[21]

Check out the *Perspectives in Nutrition* Online Learning Center http://www.mhhe.com/wardlaw for quizzes, flash cards, other activities, and web links designed to further help you learn about nutrition for pregnant and breastfeeding women

Summary

1. Adequate nutrition is vital during pregnancy to ensure the well-being of both the infant and mother. Poor maternal nutrition and use of some medications, especially during the first trimester, can cause birth defects. Growth retardation and altered development can also occur if these insults happen later in pregnancy.

2. Infants born preterm (before 37 weeks gestation) usually have more medical problems at and following birth than normal infants.

3. A woman typically needs an additional 300 kcal per day during the second and third trimesters of pregnancy to meet her energy needs. A better measure of meeting energy needs is adequate weight gain. This should occur slowly, reaching a total of 25 to 35 lb in a woman of healthy weight.

4. Protein, vitamin, and mineral needs increase during pregnancy. Extra servings from the milk, yogurt, and cheese group and the meat, poultry, fish, dry beans, eggs, and nuts group of the Food Guide Pyramid are recommended. Supplements of folate and iron, in particular, may be needed. Folate nutriture especially should be adequate at the time of conception. Any supplement use needs to be guided by a physician, as an excess intake of vitamin A and other nutrients during pregnancy can have harmful effects on the infant.

5. The factors that contribute to poor pregnancy outcome include inadequate health care in general and prenatal care in particular,
teenage pregnancy, closely spaced births, smoking, alcohol consumption, illegal drug use, insufficient carbohydrate intake (<100 g/day), obesity, heavy caffeine use, and various infections, such as *Listeria* and AIDS.

6. Pregnancy-induced hypertension, gestational diabetes, heartburn, constipation, nausea, vomiting, edema, and anemia are all possible discomforts and complications of pregnancy. Nutrition therapy can help minimize some of these problems.

7. Almost all women are able to nurse their infants. The nutrient composition of human milk is very different from that of unaltered cow's milk and is much more desirable. Colostrum, the first fluid produced by the human breast, is very rich in immune factors. Mature milk is rich in the protein lactalbumin and in lactose.

8. For the infant, the advantages of breastfeeding over formula feeding are numerous, including fewer intestinal, respiratory, and ear infections and fewer allergies and food intolerances. Moreover, breastfeeding is also less expensive and possibly more convenient for the mother than formula feeding. However, an infant can be adequately nourished with formula if the mother chooses not to breastfeed. Breastfeeding is not desirable if the mother has certain diseases or must take medication potentially harmful to the infant. Likewise, breastfeeding is not advised for infants with certain medical conditions, including some preterm infants.

Study Questions

1. What historical evidence established the importance of nutrition in pregnancy outcome?

2. Provide three key pieces of advice for parents seeking to maximize their chances of having a healthy infant. Why did you identify those specific factors?

3. Outline current weight-gain recommendations for pregnancy. What is the basis for these recommendations?

4. How is the Food Guide Pyramid adapted to meet the increased nutrient needs of pregnancy?

5. Why does teenage pregnancy receive so much attention these days? At what age do you think pregnancy is ideal? Why?

6. Give three reasons a woman should give serious consideration to breastfeeding her infant.

7. Describe the physiological mechanisms that stimulate milk production and release. How can knowing about these help mothers nurse successfully?

8. What guidelines can a woman use to determine whether her breastfed infant is receiving sufficient nourishment?

9. How should the basic food plan suitable for pregnancy be modified during breastfeeding?

10. Where can new mothers go for help in establishing successful breastfeeding?

■ ANNOTATED REFERENCES

1. Abrams B and others: Pregnancy weight gain: Still Controversial. *American Journal of Clinical Nutrition* 71(Suppl):1233S, 2000.

   There is a strong link between weight gain during pregnancy and fetal growth. Too little weight gain leads to reduced fetal growth, and excessive maternal weight gain is linked to large infants. Both conditions increase the infant's risk of health-related complications.

2. Anderson JW and others: Breast-feeding and cognitive development: A meta analysis. *American Journal of Clinical Nutrition* 70:525, 1999.

   Breastfeeding is associated with more rapid and better development of nervous system function. This may be because breast milk provides nutrients, such as very-long-chain fatty acids, that are needed for the development of the immature brain. Some increase in IQ is noted for breastfed compared with formula-fed infants; this is especially seen when comparing these forms of feeding in preterm infants.

3. Artal R, Sherman C: Exercise during pregnancy: Safe and beneficial for most. *The Physician and Sportsmedicine* 27:51, 1999.

   Regular, moderate exercise may ease pregnancy and subsequent labor. Moderate exercise does not significantly affect length of gestation or birth weight.

4. Azais-Braesco V, Pscal G: Vitmain A in pregnancy: Requirements and safety limits. *American Journal of Clinical Nutrition* 71(Suppl):1325S, 2000.

   During pregnancy, the daily use of vitamin A supplements should not exceed 10,000 IU. To avoid toxicity, estimated dietary vitamin A should be considered, along with supervision by a physician before supplement use is initiated.

5. Christensen D: Sobering work: Unraveling alcohol's effects on the developing brain. *Science News* 158:28, 2000.

   Studies report that 1 in 29 pregnant women drink the equivalent of a glass of wine a day. Total abstinence from alcohol is recommended during pregnancy.

6. Clairmont MA: Puzzling complications of pregnancy. *Today's Dietitian*, p. 32, December 1999.

   Pregnancy-induced hypertension has detrimental effects on the fetus, in part by reducing the blood flow to the uterus and placenta. It normally presents after the first 20 weeks of pregnancy, and it occurs in approximately 7% of pregnancies in the United States. Screening for its occurrence is important in midpregnancy.

7. Committee on Adolescents: Adolescent pregnancy—Current trends and issues: 1998. *Pediatrics* 103:516, 1999.

   The factors most associated with negative pregnancy results in teenagers are low prepregnancy weight and height, previous pregnancies, and poor pregnancy weight gain. Social factors associated with poor outcomes include poverty, unmarried status, limited education, drug use, and inadequate prenatal care.

8. Eskenazi B: Caffeine—Filtering the facts. *The New England Journal of Medicine* 341:1688, 1999.

   An estimated 75% of pregnant women consume caffeinated beverages. Caffeine and its metabolites cross from the mother to the fetus. Women who are pregnant (or breastfeeding) should limit their caffeine intake.

9. Food and Nutrition Board, Institute of Medicine: Dietary Reference Intakes for Thiamin, Riboflavin, Niacin, Vitamin B-6, Folate, Vitamin B-12, Pantothenic Acid, Biotin, and Choline, National Academy Press, Washington, DC, 1998.

   Adequate folate status is important at the time of conception in the mother in order to reduce the risk of producing a child with a neural tube defect. Meeting folate needs via a synthetic form is important for the mother-to-be because all studies that have shown a reduction in neural tube defects have used in this form of folate. Rich sources of food-borne folate is also advocated as part of a healthy diet for the pre-pregnant (and pregnant) woman.

10. Galtier-Dereure F and others: Obesity and pregnancy: Complications and cost. *American Journal of Clinical Nutrition* 71(Suppl):1242S, 2000.

    Maternal obesity and overweight increase the health risks for both mother and infant, such as gestational diabetes, hypertensive disorders, cesarean deliveries, and postoperative complications.

11. Godfrey KM, Barker DJP: Fetal nutrition and adult disease. *American Journal of Clinical Nutrition* 71(Suppl):1344S, 2000.

    Fetal undernutrition in middle and late pregnancy can lead to reduced fetal growth, especially in some organs, such as the liver and kidneys. This fetal undernutrition has been linked to disordered cholsterol metabolism and cardiovascular disease, insulin resistance, elevated blood pressure, and increased blood coagulation in adulthood.

12. Hickey CA: Sociocultural and behavioral influences on weight gain during pregnancy. *American Journal of Clinical Nutrition* 71(Suppl):1346S, 2000.

    During pregnancy, certain factors, such as socioeconomic status, age, education, and ethnicity, are associated with weight gain.

    Low prenatal weight gain may be more amenable to treatment if these factors are considered when planning the course of therapy.

13. Healthier mothers and babies—1900–1999. *Journal of the American Medical Association* 282:1807, 1999.

    The current infant mortality rate in the United States is 7.2 per 1000 live births, and the maternal mortality rate is 7.7 deaths per 100,000 live births. These statistics have declined substantially since 1900, indicating that the improved medical care given to pregnant women today has resulted in substantial gains in health for both mother and infant.

14. Ito S: Drug therapy for breast-feeding women. *The New England Journal of Medicine* 343:118, 2000.

    Certain medications and other hazards should be addressed with breastfeeding mothers. For example, maternal smoking is associated with decreased milk volume and early weaning from breastfeeding.

15. JAMA Patient Page: Feeding your newborn. *Journal of the American Medical Association* 283:1242, 2000.

    Women who should not breastfeed include those infected with HIV, hepatitis B, or untreated tuberculosis and those receiving cancer chemotherapy. Smoking, heavy drinking, and the use of drugs that can pass into breast milk should be avoided when breastfeeding.

16. Jensen CL and others: Effect of docosahexaenoic acid supplementation of lactating women on the fatty acid composition of breast milk lipids and maternal and infant plasma phospholipids. *American Journal of Clinical Nutrition* 71(Suppl):292S, 2000.

    Docosahexaenoic acid is found in breast milk, and it is an important component of the structural lipids of brain and retinal cell membranes. Despite the current interest in the supplementation of infant formulas with DHA, there are reasons for caution, such as the potential for reduced growth of the infant. Future studies are needed to establish the safety and efficacy of such use.

17. King JC: Determinants of maternal zinc status during pregnancy. *American Journal of Clinical Nutrition* 71(Suppl):1334S, 2000.

    Maternal zinc status can be reduced by alcohol abuse, high amounts of supplemental iron, and a cereal-based diet. Poor zinc status may limit fetal growth and cause serious birth defects. Supplemental zinc use may be prudent for women with any of these conditions during pregnancy.

18. King JC: Physiology of pregnancy and nutrient metabolism. *American Journal of Clinical Nutrition* 71(Suppl):1218S, 2000.

The energy needed for basal metabolism during pregnancy depends on maternal prepregnant nutritional status and on fetal size. When energy needs are not met, fetal growth may suffer. Efforts to achieve good maternal nutritional status preconception, as well as throughout gestation, best ensure a healthy outcome for fetal growth and development.

19. Kjos SL, Buchanan TA: Gestational diabetes mellitus. *The New England Journal of Medicine* 341:1750, 1999.

An increase from 4 to 7% of gestational diabetes has been seen in the U.S. Caucasian population in recent years. Women with gestational diabetes have a 17 to 63% risk of developing type 2 diabetes within 5 to 16 years after the pregnancy. The careful monitoring of blood pressure, weight gain, and urinary protein excretion is recommended, particularly during the second half of pregnancy.

20. Kurz KM, Galloway R: Improving iron status before childbearing. *Journal of Nutrition* 130:437S, 2000.

Iron status early in pregnancy (reflecting prepregnancy iron status) appears to have a stronger influence on birth outcomes than does status later in pregnancy. This supports the importance of improving iron status before childbearing. The prevalence of anemia and requirements for iron are particularly high in the third trimester of pregnancy, suggesting the need to provide iron supplementation throughout pregnancy.

21. Marcus MB: Don't rush the workout if you're a new mother. *U.S. News & World Report*, p. 57, May 15, 2000.

Breastfeeding mothers need to drink eight glasses or more of fluid a day, especially as they start back on an exercise program. Adequate fluid intake is needed to support the production of breast milk. If either the mother or the infant has dark yellow urine, or if the infant has fewer than six wet diapers a day, then fluid intakes need to be increased.

22. McGainty WJ and others: Maternal nutrition. In Shils ME and others (eds.): *Modern nutrition in health and disease.* 9th ed. Baltimore, MD. Williams & Wilkins, 1999.

Between 25 and 30% of all pregnant patients do not receive prenatal care prior to the second trimester. Ideally, improving diet and health habits should begin at least 8 weeks before conception. Thus, women should not wait until the first visit to their physician to begin improving their health habits as they anticipate becoming pregnant.

23. Moreland J, Coombs J: Promoting and supporting breast-feeding. *American Family Physician* 61:2093, 2000.

Breastfeeding should be discussed at the first and subsequent prenatal visits. Any history of early weaning or breastfeeding problems in previous pregnancies is predictive of future difficulties. Consultation by a lactation specialist may be helpful. A follow-up visit 2 to 4 days postdischarge for most breastfeeding newborns is recommended to make sure all is well.

24. Nduati R and others: Effect of breastfeeding and formula feeding on transmission of HIV-1: A randomized clinical trial. *Journal of the American Medical Association* 283:1167, 2000.

Transmission of human immunodeficiency virus type-1 (HIV-1) is known to occur through breastfeeding. Risks of transmission via breast milk are more so in early stages of infant life. Feeding of infant formula reduces the risk of contracting HIV, but many women throughout the world cannot afford formula for their infants. It is also unfortunate that, currently, many countries do not have the capacity to test for HIV status all women who want to breastfeed their infants.

25. Polywka S and others: Low risk of vertical transmission of hepatitis C virus by breast milk. *Clinical Infectious Disease* 29:1327, 1999.

It is estimated that 5% of infants born to mothers infected with hepatitis C will acquire the infection in utero. It is still uncertain whether the hepatitis C virus enters breast milk, but some studies have shown that this can happen.

26. Prentice A: Maternal calcium metabolism and bone mineral status. *American Journal of Clinical Nutrition* 71(Suppl):312S, 2000.

There is an increase in demand for calcium by the fetus, particularly in the third trimester. Additionally, calcium absorption and urinary exretion of calcium are both higher during pregnancy. Mothers with a customarily low calcium intake likely benefit from higher calcium intakes during pregnancy.

27. Scholl TO, Johnson WG: Folic acid: Influence on the outcome of pregnancy. *American Journal of Clinical Nutrition* 71(Suppl):1295S, 2000.

Poor dietary folate intake and low circulating concentrations of folate in pregnant women increase the risk of adverse birth outcomes. Supplementation studies likewise suggest that some women—most likely poor women—may benefit from receiving additional folate during, as well as before, pregnancy.

28. Scholl TO, Reilly T: Anemia, iron and pregnancy outcome. *Journal of Nutrition* 130:443S, 2000.

When maternal anemia is diagnosed before midpregnancy, it is associated with increased risk of preterm delivery. Maternal anemia detected during the later stages of pregnancy often reflects the expected (and necessary) expansion of maternal plasma volume. Thus, this anemia in the later stages of pregnancy is not associated with the same increased risk of preterm delivery.

29. Tolstoli LG, Josimovich JB: Gestational diabetes mellitus: Etiology and management. *Nutrition Today* 34:78, 1999.

The management of gestational diabetes mellitus includes diet therapy, regular exercise, and sometimes insulin therapy. The primary goal of this treatment is to achieve and maintain normal blood glucose concentration in the mother to improve the outcome of pregnancy for both the mother and the fetus. High blood glucose can adversely affect the well-being of both mother and fetus.

30. Vozenilek G: What they don't know could hurt them: Increasing public awareness of folic acid and neural tube defects. *Journal of the American Dietetic Association* 99:20, 1999.

Synthetic folate can be found in many fortified foods. However, it may be necessary for some women in their childbearing years to take a supplement to meet the standard of 400 µg of synthetic folate per day, if dietary choices do not suffice.

31. Williams R: Healthy pregnancy, healthy baby: Exercise, good food, and prenatal care are the keys. *FDA Consumer*, p. 18, March-April 1999.

Among the 2500 babies born with neural tube defects a year, an estimated 45% of these birth defects could be reduced if the recommended daily folate intake of 400 µg were met. In addition, women should receive early prenatal care; follow a well-balanced diet; exercise regularly (with a physician's permission); avoid alcohol, cigarettes, and illicit drugs; limit caffeine intake; and avoid X rays, hot tubs, and saunas.

32. Worthington-Robert BS, Williams SR: *Nutrition in pregnancy and lactation.* 6th ed. Boston: 1977. WCB McGraw-Hill.

This is a comprehensive textbook describing nutrient needs and desirable lifestyle habits for pregnant and lactating women. These recommendations are supported by numerous studies cited in the textbook.

33. Zhu BP and others: The effect of the interval between pregnancies on perinatal outcomes. *The New England Journal of Medicine* 340:589, 1999.

A pregnancy that occurs less than 6 months after previous delivery of an infant increases the risk for low birth weight, preterm birth, or small size for gestational age in the subsequent infant.

TAKEACTION

I. TARGETING NUTRIENTS NECESSARY FOR PREGNANT WOMEN

This chapter mentioned that pregnant women may have difficulty meeting their increased needs for folate, vitamin D, iron, calcium, and zinc. List five foods rich in each of these nutrients next to the appropriate heading below. Refer to Chapters 9 through 12 if necessary.

Nutrient	Foods	Nutrient	Foods
Folate		Calcium	
Vitamin D		Zinc	
Iron			

1. Foods rich in more than one of these nutrients would be especially valuable for pregnant women. Write on the line below any foods you listed that are good sources of more than one of these critical nutrients.

2. The need for folate, vitamin D, iron, calcium, and zinc increases considerably during pregnancy. For which of these nutrients can pregnant women usually obtain adequate intakes from dietary sources?

   Which of these nutrients are commonly taken in supplement form during pregnancy? Why might it be hard for pregnant women to meet their increased needs for these nutrients from food alone?

TAKE ACTION

II. PUTTING YOUR KNOWLEDGE ABOUT NUTRITION AND PREGNANCY TO WORK

A college friend tells you that she is newly pregnant. You are aware that this friend usually likes to eat the following foods for her meals:

Breakfast
Skips this meal, or gets a granola bar
Coffee

Lunch
Sweetened yogurt
Bagel with cream cheese
Occasional piece of fruit
Regular caffeinated soda

Snack
Chocolate candy bar

Dinner
Pizza, macaronic and cheese, or eggs with toast
Seldom eats a salad or vegetable
Regular caffeinated soda

Snacks
Pretzels or chips
Regular caffeinated soda

1. Using your software, or Appendix A, evaluate your friend's diet for protein, iron, folate, calcium, and zinc. How does her intake compare with the recommended amounts for pregnancy?

    _____

    _____

    _____

2. Now redesign her diet and make sure that her intake meets pregnancy needs for protein, folate, calcium, and zinc. (Hint: Fortified foods, such as breakfast cereal, are generally nutrient-rich foods, which can more easily help meet one's needs.) Increase the iron content as well, but it still may be below the RDA for pregnancy.

    _____

    _____

    _____

NUTRITION *Perspective*

FETAL ALCOHOL SYNDROME

Although much is known about diagnosing and treating some learning problems in children, many causes remain elusive. One particular question haunts many mothers: Did something happen while I was pregnant that created a learning disability in my child? This question leads directly to the topic of alcohol use during pregnancy, since alcohol is the most common damaging substance to which fetuses are exposed.

Conclusive evidence shows that large amounts of alcohol harm the fetus, especially when associated with binge drinking (for a woman, consumption of four or more alcoholic drinks at one sitting). Binge drinking is especially perilous during the first 12 weeks of pregnancy, as this is when critical early developmental events take place in the womb. Scientists don't know whether pregnant women must eliminate alcohol use entirely to avoid risk of damage to the fetus; however, until a safe level can be established, women are advised not to drink any alcohol during pregnancy or when there is a chance pregnancy might occur.[5]

When a pregnant woman drinks more alcohol than she can metabolize, the excess reaches the embryo (and, at later stages, the fetus), which has no means of detoxifying it. Women with chronic alcoholism produce children with a recognizable pattern of malformations called fetal alcohol syndrome (FAS). A diagnosis of FAS is based mainly on poor fetal and infant growth, physical deformities (especially of facial features), and mental retardation (Fig. 16-7). The infant is frequently irritable and may develop hyperactivity and a short attention span. Limited hand-eye coordination is common. Defects in vision, hearing, and mental processing often develop over time.

The range of abnormalities from alcohol exposure varies from the severe effects associated with FAS to reduced birth weight, behavioral effects, growth retardation, and hampered learning ability in infants born to women who report only social drinking. The latter condition, termed *fetal alcohol effects (FAE)*, is not marked by telltale facial abnormalities. For this reason, parents may not suspect the presence of subtle defects caused by alcohol, even when they exist. FAE can devastate learning potential.

Up to 30 per 10,000 infants exhibiting FAS are born each year; the incidence of FAS also has increased since the late 1970s. Many more infants are born annually with FAE. Today, 1 in 29 pregnant women reported drinking the equivalent of at least a glass of wine a day.[5] Alcohol use is, in fact, the leading cause of preventable birth defects and mental retardation in the United States and in the Western world as a whole.

Exactly how alcohol causes these defects is not known. One line of research suggests that alcohol or products produced by the metabolism of alcohol (acetaldehyde), cause faulty migration of cells in the brain during early stages of development or block the action of certain neurotransmitters in the brain. In addition, inadequate nutrient intake, reduced nutrient and

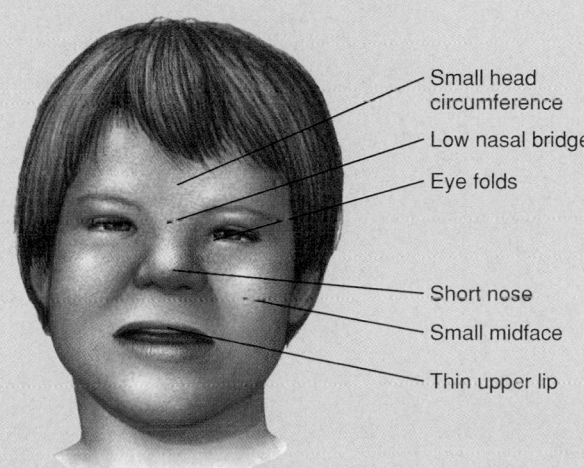

Small head circumference

Low nasal bridge

Eye folds

Short nose

Small midface

Thin upper lip

FIGURE 16-7 Fetal alcohol syndrome. Milder forms of alcohol-induced changes in the fetus and the infant are known as *fetal alcohol effects*. The facial features shown are typical of affected children. Additional abnormalities in the brain and other internal organs accompany fetal alcohol syndrome but are not immediately apparent from simply looking at the child.

oxygen transfer across the placenta, cigarette smoking commonly linked to alcohol intake, drug use, and possibly other factors contribute to the overall result. Furthermore, it is not known how much alcohol it takes to produce these adverse effects. Again, for this reason, many authorities—including the U.S. Surgeon General and the American Medical Association—believe it is best that mothers-to-be avoid alcohol altogether. In other words, there is no safe drinking.

Abstinence is especially important during the first trimester, when key growth and development occur. Alcohol reaches the fetal blood at the same concentration as the mother's blood within 15 minutes of her drinking. However, the effect on the fetus may be up to 10 times greater. For example, just one bout of binge drinking can arrest and alter cell division during critical phases of fetal development. The fetus then may develop an irreversible defect.

Physical damage to the embryo (and later the fetus) results more from first-trimester drinking because the basic structures of tissues and organs develop during this period. Emotional and learning problems stem more from third-trimester drinking because this is when critical further development of the brain occurs. And, throughout the pregnancy, alcohol interferes with growth. Overall, mothers who drink at least one to two drinks a day throughout pregnancy are much more likely to have growth-retarded infants, and mothers who drink only in late pregnancy are more likely to give birth to preterm infants.

Because alcohol has the capacity to adversely affect each stage of fetal development, the earlier in pregnancy that drinking ceases, the greater the potential for improved outcome. The best course is to consider alcohol an indulgence that must be eliminated from the time of conception until after pregnancy. Currently about half of all women are drinking at the time of conception (i.e., before learning they are pregnant). One step in the right direction is the mandated warnings about drinking during pregnancy that appear on all alcoholic beverage containers.

Pregnancy lasts only 9 months. In contrast, parents may spend a lifetime caring, often at great expense (estimated at $1.4 million in the United States), for their offspring needlessly handicapped by FAS or FAE. Keep in mind that fetal alcohol syndrome is a completely preventable disease.

Pregnant women should recognize that many cough syrups contain alcohol. Cases have been reported of infants with FAS born to mothers who consumed generous amounts of such cough syrups but no other alcoholic beverages.[32]

NUTRITION FROM INFANCY THROUGH ADOLESCENCE

chapter 17

A s humans grow through early years into adulthood, our needs for energy and nutrients change. Infants need more energy, protein, vitamins, and minerals per pound of body weight than do adults to support their tremendous growth and development. As growth tapers, children need and eat proportionately less.[34] The erratic eating behaviors of young children pose major challenges for parents and other caregivers. In turn, childhood becomes an important time to establish healthful habits, including those related to food choice and physical activity.[24]

The family wields a subtle but important influence over the child. Thus, education designed to change children's eating behaviors must be directed simultaneously at the main caregivers. They usually determine what foods are purchased and how they are prepared. To help children adopt a lifelong healthy dietary intake, parents and caregivers should provide a variety of foods at home, limit take-out food, and introduce new foods regularly.[1] Maintaining a healthful eating pattern should continue as children grow into teenagers. In exploring all these stages of life, this chapter looks at the key role nutrients play and how food choices should be tailored to meet those needs.

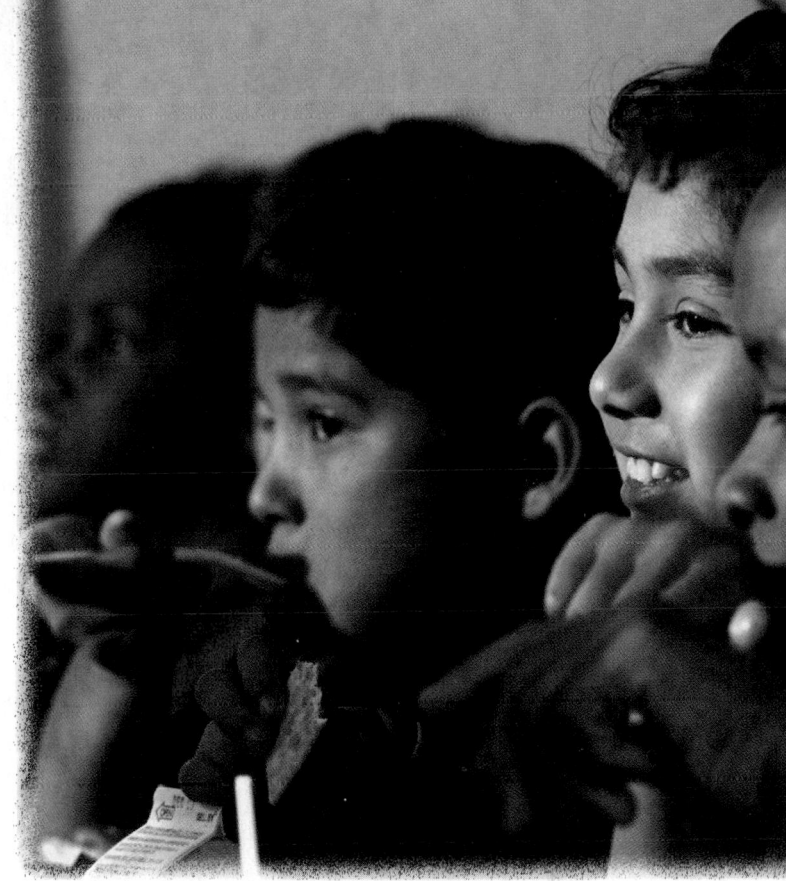

CASE SCENARIO

Damon is a 7-month-old who has been taken into a clinic for a routine checkup. On examination, he was found to be underweight and plotted on the growth chart at the 25th percentile for weight and the 50th percentile for height. His physician was concerned with his substandard weight gain, so she scheduled a follow-up appointment in 3 months. At the 3-month visit, Damon appeared sluggish. He was again plotted on the growth chart and was now at the 5th percentile for weight but still at the 50th percentile for height.

A registered dietitian interviewed Damon's 16-year-old mother to collect dietary intakes. The 24-hour diet recall consisted of two bottles of formula, three bottles of Kool-Ade, and a hot dog. However, the mother was still in school, and at night she often left Damon with the neighbor, so that she could go out for a few hours. Thus, she was not aware of all of what he ate, since much of her time was spent away from him.

What problems do you think are present in Damon's diet? What potential dangers await Damon if his health status continues along this current growth trend?

■ Nutrition and Child Health—An Introduction

Current trends in nutrition and overall health among children and adolescents in the United States have shown both positive and negative results. On a positive note, more children are receiving vaccinations than ever before, fewer teenagers are giving birth, and the poverty rate for children has fallen to a point equal to that of 1980. (Currently, 18% of children live in poverty.) In contrast to this good news, the number of children and teenagers with obesity and type 2 diabetes is rising, and physical activity in general is on the decline as more time is spent sitting in front of computer screens and television sets. Low calcium intakes are also receiving much attention, as soft drinks have replaced much of the milk that children and teenagers used to consume on a daily basis.[19] In this chapter, we will look at these trends, especially their effects on nutrition and overall health in this age group.

■ Infant Growth and Physiological Development

During infancy, a child's attitudes toward foods and the whole eating process begin to take shape. If parents and other caregivers practice good nutrition and are flexible, they can lead an infant into lifelong healthful food habits.[34] Such an infant has a good chance of starting life with the nutrients needed to support brain and body growth spurts and of developing a willingness to try new foods. However, these physical and psychological advantages alone don't guarantee that a child will thrive.

Children also need specific attention focused on them; they need to grow in a stimulating environment, and they need a sense of security. For example, children hospitalized for growth failure gain weight more quickly when loving care accompanies needed nutrients.

■ The Growing Infant

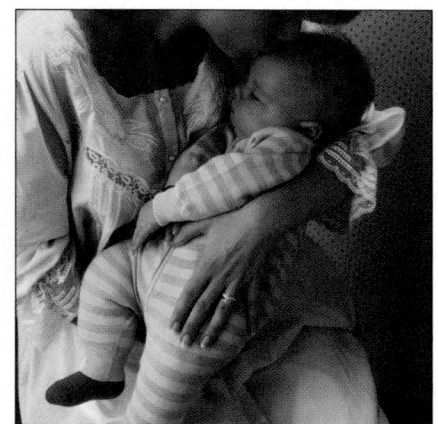

All babies seem to do is eat and sleep. There's a good reason for this. An infant's birth weight doubles in the first 4 to 6 months and triples within the first year. Such rapid growth requires a lot of both nourishment and sleep. Beyond the first year, growth is slower; it takes 5 more years to double the weight seen at 1 year. An infant also increases in length in the first year by 50% and then continues to gain height throughout, preschool and teen years. These gains are not necessarily continuous—spurts of growth alternate with plateaus. Height is essentially complete by age 19, although increases of several inches may occur in the early 20s (Fig. 17-1). Head size in proportion to total height shrinks from one-fourth to one-eighth during the climb from infancy to adulthood.[34]

The human body needs a lot more food to support growth and development than to merely maintain itself once growth ceases. When nutrients are missing at critical phases of growth and development, growth slows and may even stop. From observations of Egyptian mummies, we see that infants were about the same size in 300 B.C. as they are today. However, adult mummies are much smaller than adults today. Furthermore, the suits of armor in museum collections of the Middle Ages typically would not fit modern adults. The average height of American men in 1700 was approximately 5 feet, 8 inches, whereas today it is approximately 5 feet, 10 inches. This suggests that people of earlier times generally ate nutrient-poor diets, which did not support the growth we typically experience today.

In countries of the developing world today, about half the children are short and underweight for their ages. Poor nutrition—called *undernutrition*—is at the heart of the problem. This occurs to a lesser extent in the United States. The undernourished children are simply smaller versions of nutritionally fit children. In poorer countries, when breastfeeding ceases, children are often fed a high-carbohydrate,

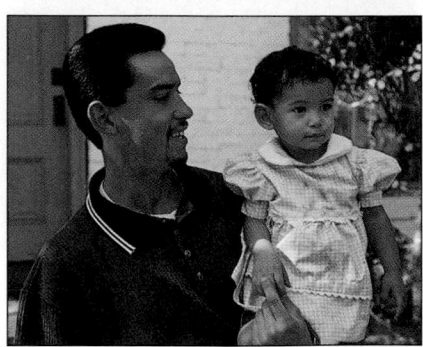

Children benefit from the love and attention of adults.

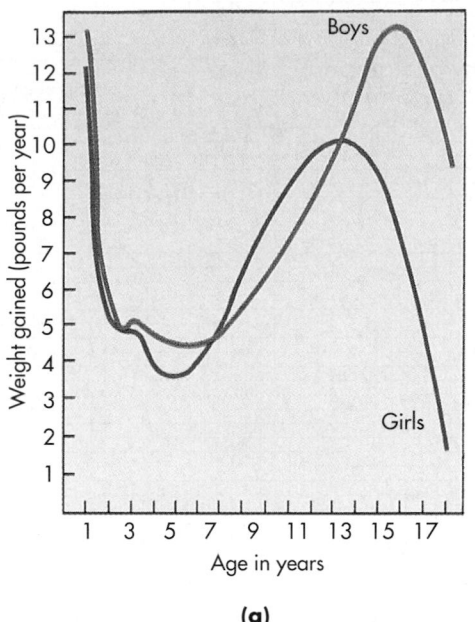

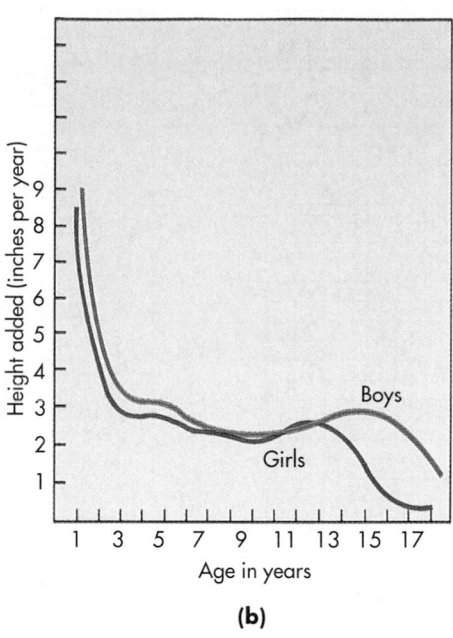

(a)

(b)

▌ FIGURE 17-1 Growth rates. (*a*) Average gains in weight for girls and boys. (*b*) Average additions to height for girls and boys. The higher the line in any one year, the greater the amount of annual gain compared with that in other years. Large gains in weight occur in both infancy and puberty, whereas the very high length gain in infancy is never reached again. If graphs such as these were plotted in smaller time segments, they would appear as zigzag lines, rather than smooth lines, reflecting short, periodic spurts in growth in the course of each year.

low-protein diet. This diet supports some growth but does not allow children to attain their full genetic potential. To grow, children must consume adequate amounts of energy, protein, iron, zinc, and other nutrients.

Infant development follows a pattern in which body water reduces from about 75% at birth to 60% at 1 year. The latter is also the proportion typical in adults. By age 1, an infant's body nitrogen content (and thus protein content) has increased from 2% of body weight at birth to 3%, indicating that the infant has synthesized much new lean tissue.[34]

▌ Effect of Undernutrition on Growth

As with the fetus in utero, the long-term effects of nutritional problems in infancy and childhood depend on the severity, timing, and duration of the nutritional insult to cell processes.

The single best indicator of a child's nutritional status is growth, particularly weight gain in the short run and length (height) in the long run.[34] Mild zinc deficiencies in American children have been linked to poor growth. Improving the diets of these children then leads to improved growth. Overall, eating a poor diet as an infant or a child hampers the cell division that occurs at that critical stage. Getting an adequate diet later usually won't compensate for lost growth, as the hormonal and other conditions needed for growth will not likely be present. In addition, growth ceases in girls and boys when the skeleton reaches its final size. Growth plates at the ends of the bones, called epiphyses, fuse at different ages, beginning around 14 years of age in girls and 15 years of age in boys. (see Chapter 3 for details). The final stages of this process end at about 19 years of age in girls and 20 years of age in boys. Furthermore, muscles can increase in diameter later in life but the growth is constrained by the length of the bone.

For these reasons, a 15-year-old Central American girl who is 4 feet, 8 inches tall cannot attain the adult height of a typical American girl simply by eating better. Girls experience their peak rate of growth before the onset of the menses. Once the time for growth ceases (in women, this is about 2 years after they start menstruating), a sufficient nutrient intake helps maintain health and weight but does not make up for all lost growth.

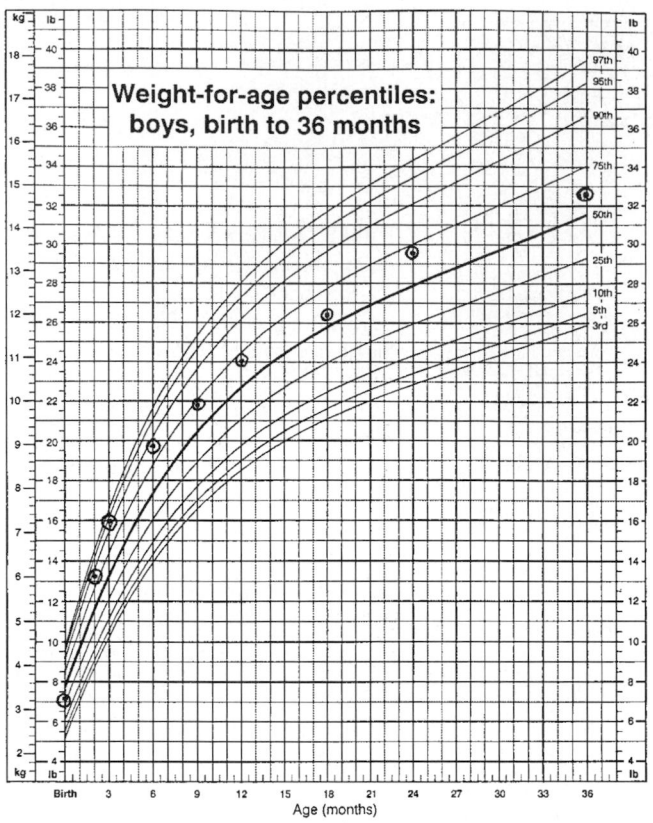

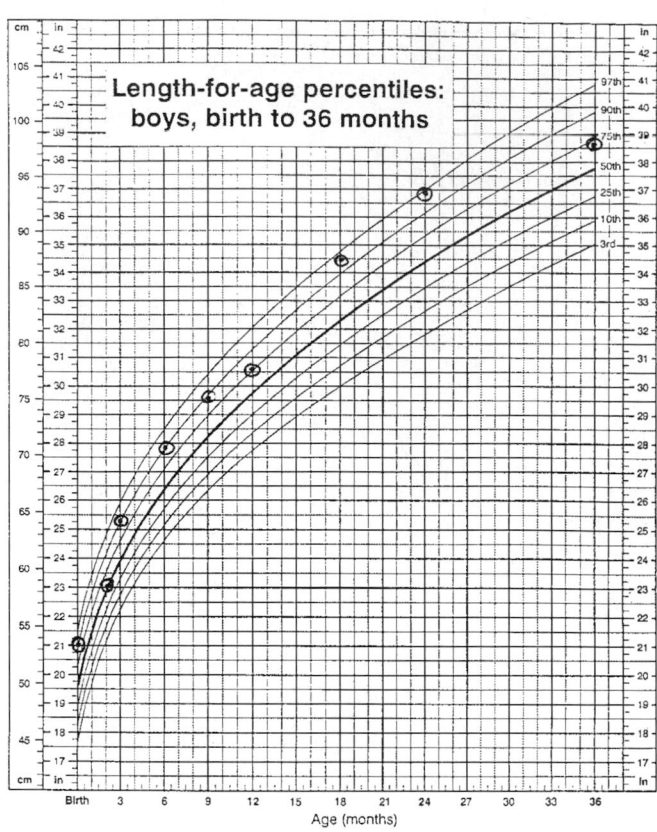

■ FIGURE 17-2 Growth charts used to assess length (height) in young boys. A certain weight and length (height) correspond to a percentile value, which is a ranking of the person among 100 peers. The growth pattern of Dr. Wardlaw's son is plotted to illustrate how this tool is used in clinical practice.

Children under 2 to 3 years of age are measured with knees unflexed and while lying on their backs, so the term length *is used rather than* height.

■ Assessment of Infant Growth and Development

Health professionals assess a child's increases in height and weight by comparing them with typical growth patterns recorded on charts. You can download the latest growth charts at http://www.cdc.gov/nchs/data/ad314.pdf. The typical charts contain 7 to 9 percentile divisions, which represent 90 to 96% of children (Fig. 17-2). A percentile represents the rank of the person among 100 peers matched for age and gender. If a young boy, for example, is at the 90th percentile height for age, he is shorter than 10 and taller than 89. A child at the 50th percentile is considered average. Fifty children will be taller than this child; 49 will be shorter. It is important to note that these charts were based primarily on observations of formula-fed infants. Breastfed infants may lag behind these typical patterns but eventually catch up in terms of height (see Chapter 16).

Individual growth charts are available for both males and females, for ages ranging from 0 to 36 months and 2 to 20 years. Height for age, weight for age, and weight for height can be plotted. Body mass index (BMI) is the weight for height standard used in the latter age range.[15] Infants and children should have their growth assessed during regular health checkups. It takes 1 to 3 years for an infant to establish his or her own genetic percentile. Once this figure is established, such as length (height) for age, the child's measurement should then track along that percentile. If the child's growth doesn't keep up with its length-for-age percentile, the physician needs to investigate whether a medical or nutritional problem is impeding the predicted growth. Inappropriate weight gain—too little or too much—should also be investigated.

Infants born preterm may catch up in growth in 2 to 3 years. This requires that the child jump up in the percentiles. If this occurs—especially in length for age—it is usually no cause for alarm. On the other hand, jumping percentiles in weight for height can be disturbing if the child approaches the 80th to 90th percentiles. A child at the 85th percentile or above for BMI is considered at risk for overweight. At or above the 95th percentile, the child is considered overweight. At the 95th percentile, the diagnosis of obesity can also be established if the physical exam of the child indicates he or she is truly overfat. This is generally the case at this percentile.[3]

■ Brain Growth

The brain grows faster in infancy than at any other time of life. To accommodate the growth, an infant's head must be very large in proportion to the rest of the body. The rapid growth stops at about 18 months of age. The rest of the body eventually grows to reach a typical proportion to head size. In early physical checkups, a health professional usually measures the head circumference as another means of assessing growth, especially brain growth. How nutritional status affects brain development and intelligence quotient (IQ) is difficult to measure because scientists haven't figured out how to separate the effects of nature from those of nurture. However, studies from Central America suggest that IQ after age 5 years relates more closely to the amount of schooling a child receives than to nutritional intake during childhood.

■ Adipose (Fat) Tissue Growth

Since 1970, researchers have speculated that overfeeding during infancy may increase adipose (fat) tissue cell numbers. Today, we know that adipose cells can also increase as adulthood obesity develops (see Chapter 13). Still, if energy intake is limited during infancy to keep down the number of adipose cells, the growth of other organ systems may also be severely retarded. Special concern revolves especially around proper brain and nervous system development. In addition, most obese infants become normal-weight preschoolers without excessive diet restrictions. For these reasons, it's unwise to restrict diet, and especially fat intake, before 2 years of age. About 40% of energy intake from fat is recommended until that age, but one study showed one can feed an infant 30 to 35% of energy as fat and still provide for normal growth and development.[26] Without adequate calories and essential nutrients, however, infants are unlikely to attain their potential adult height.

■ Failure to Thrive

Occasionally, an infant doesn't grow much in the first few months. Physical problems that may contribute to retarded growth range from poor oral cavity development, infections, and heart irregularities to constant diarrhea associated with intestinal problems. However, more than half the infants who fail to thrive have no apparent disease. Instead, the usual cause is poor infant-parent interaction. This stems from misinformation, lack of a parent role model, or apathy about the child's welfare. In general, the problems often arise from the parents' inexperience, rather than intentional negligence.

Infants not only need cuddling; they also respond to voices and eye contact, especially at feeding times. New parents need to appreciate the importance of these practices to their infant's well-being. Some parents also may be overcommitted to maintaining a lean child in the hope of preventing future obesity, as discussed in Chapter 15. The result, even though the intention was good, can be failure to thrive.

When **clinicians** encounter an infant who is failing to thrive from a nutritional standpoint, they must first determine whether formula-fed infants are consuming enough energy (see section on formula feeding of infants for details). For a breast-fed infant, the clinician needs to make sure that sufficient milk intake is possible (or taking place). The child should be nursing about six to eight times a day for about 20 minutes a session and have six to eight wet diapers each day.[34]

Children older than 2 years are less likely to experience failure to thrive because they can often get food for themselves. Younger children, for the most part, are limited to what caregivers provide.

clinician A person who works in the health-care field.

CONCEPT CHECK

Growth occurs rapidly during infancy: Birth weight doubles in about 4 to 6 months and triples within the first year. Lean tissue increases, and the percentage of body water falls during the first year. Undernutrition in childhood can irreversibly inhibit growth and maturation, so that an individual never attains his or her full genetic potential for height. Infant and child growth is assessed by tracking body weight, length (height), and head circumference over time. Body mass index (BMI) is used to assess weigh for height after 2 years of age. It is not desirable for infants to become obese, although no evidence strongly indicates that obese infants become obese adults. However, severe restriction of energy intake is not recommended for infants because it may slow the growth of organ systems. When infants do not grow properly, their failure to thrive may stem from physical disorders or inadequate care, including inappropriate feeding practices.

■ Infant Nutritional Needs

Infants' nutritional needs vary as they grow, and these differ from adult needs in both amount and proportion (Fig. 17-3). Initially, human milk or infant formula (generally using heat-treated cow's milk as a base) supplies needed nutrients. Solid foods are not needed until after 4 to 6 months. Even after solid foods are added, the basis of an infant's diet for the first year is still human milk or infant formula. Because of the critical importance of adequate nutrition in infancy and the difficulties

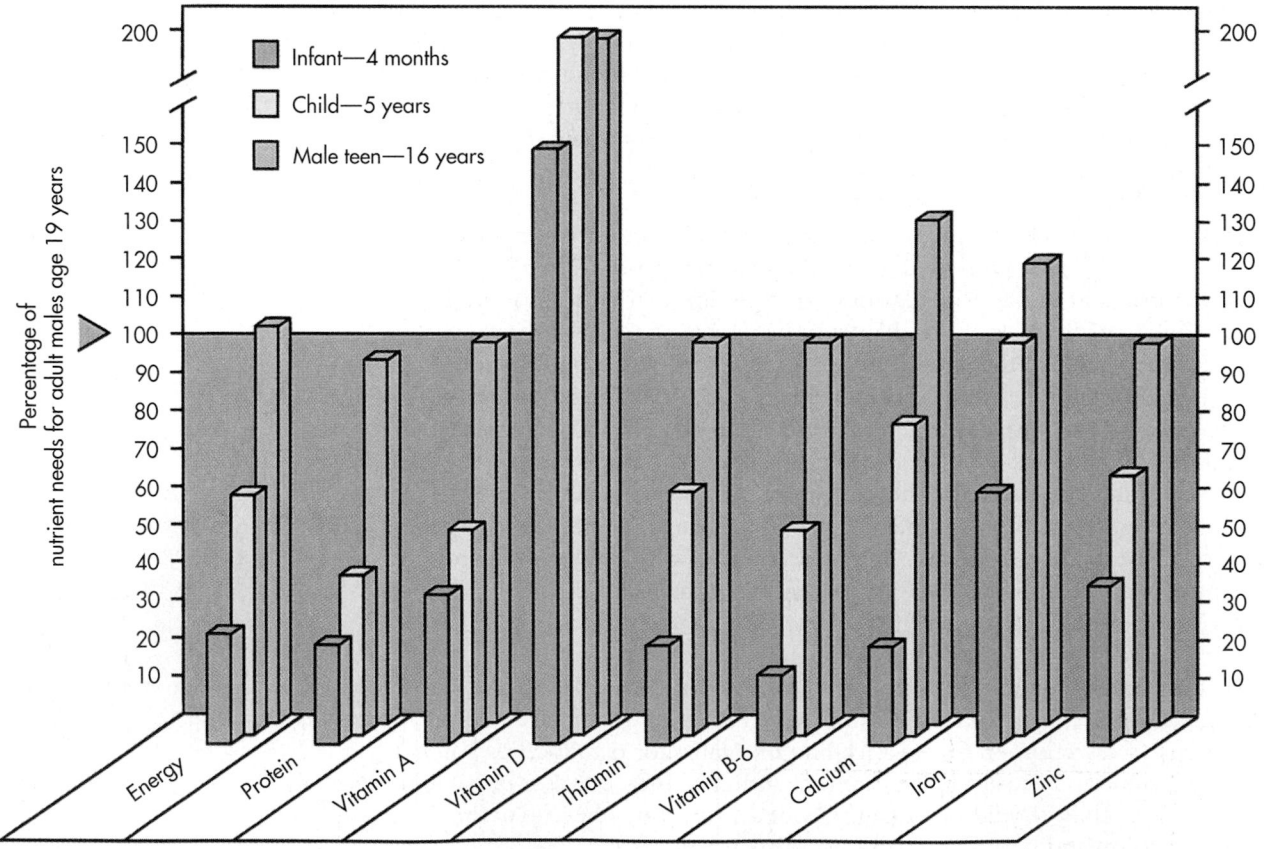

■ FIGURE 17-3 Nutrient needs for infants, children, and teenagers as percentages of those for adult males. Compared with adults, infants' relative energy needs are lower than are their needs for other nutrients, as illustrated by the different heights of the green bars. Thus, infants need to obtain relatively larger amounts of nutrients from a smaller intake of food than do adults. This is also true of young children (yellow bars), but to a lesser extent.

encountered in feeding some infants, more time is spent in this chapter on this developmental period than on the later periods of childhood.

Energy

Infants need about 45 to 50 kcal per pound of body weight daily (98–108 kcal/kg) to supply them with adequate energy. At 6 months of age, this amounts to about 700 kcal daily. Based on body weight, this amounts to two to four times more energy than adults need. Infants need an easy way to get this amount of energy. Either human milk or infant formula is ideal for the first few months. Both are high in fat and supply about 650 kcal per quart of fluid (about 700 kcal per liter; Table 17-1). Later, human milk or infant formula, supplemented by solid foods, can provide even more energy.[34]

The infant's high energy needs are primarily driven by its rapid growth and high metabolic rate. The high metabolic rate is caused in part by the ratio of the infant's body surface to its weight. More body surface allows more heat loss from the skin; the body must use extra energy to replace that heat.

Protein

Daily protein needs vary in infancy from 0.7 to 1 g of protein for each pound of body weight (1.6 to 2.2 g/kg). About half of total protein intake should come from essential (indispensable) amino acids. Both goals are satisfied by either human milk or infant formula. Total protein intake should not exceed 20% of energy needs.

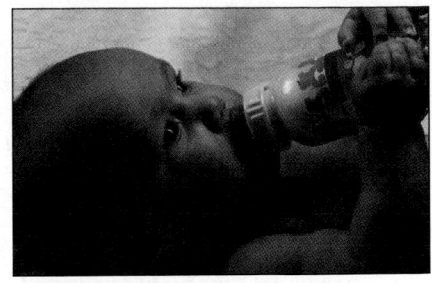

Infants who are formula-fed should remain on formula until 1 year of age. The formula should be iron fortified to reduce the risk of developing iron-deficiency anemia.

TABLE 17-1	Composition of Human and Cow's Milk and Infant Formulas per Liter (L)				
Milk or Formula	**Energy (kcal/L)**	**Protein (gram/L)**	**Fat (gram/L)**	**Carbohydrate (gram/L)**	**Minerals* (gram/L)**
Milk					
Human milk	750	11	45	70	2
Cow's milk, whole	670	36	36	49	7
Cow's milk, skim	360	36	1	51	7
Casein/Whey-Based Formulas					
Similac	680	14	36	71	3
Enfamil	670	15	37	69	3
Carnation	670	16	34	73	3
Soybean Protein-Based Formulas					
ProSobee	670	20	35	67	4
Isomil	680	16	36	68	4
Predigested Protein					
Nutramigen	670	19	26	89	1
Alimentum	680	18	37	68	1
Transition Formulas/Beverages†					
Similac Toddler's Best	670	25	33	75	3
Enfamil Next Step	670	17	33	74	3
Carnation Follow-Up	670	17	27	88	3

*Calcium, phosphorus, and other minerals.

†For use after 6 months of age or later (see label).

allergy A hypersensitive immune response that occurs when immune bodies produced by us react with a protein we sense as foreign (an antigen).

Excess nitrogen and minerals supplied by high-protein diets would exceed the ability of an infant's kidneys to excrete the resulting metabolic waste products.

In the United States, infant protein deficiency is unlikely, except in cases of mistaken feeding practices, such as when an infant's formula is excessively diluted with water. Protein deficiency may also be induced by elimination diets used to detect food **allergies** (hypersensitivities). As foods are eliminated from the diet, infants may not be offered enough protein to compensate for the high-protein sources no longer present (see the Nutrition Perspective at the end of this chapter).

Fat

As already mentioned, infants and children up to 2 years of age should get about 40% of their energy from fat. More than 50% from fat may lead to poor fat digestion. About half the energy supplied by both human milk and infant formula comes from fat. Essential fatty acids should make up at least 3% of total energy. Fats are an important part of the infant's diet because they are energy-dense and vital to the development of the nervous system. As a concentrated energy source, fat helps resolve the potential problem of the infant's high energy needs and small stomach capacity. Again, this is not an age to greatly restrict fat intake (Fig. 17-4).[19]

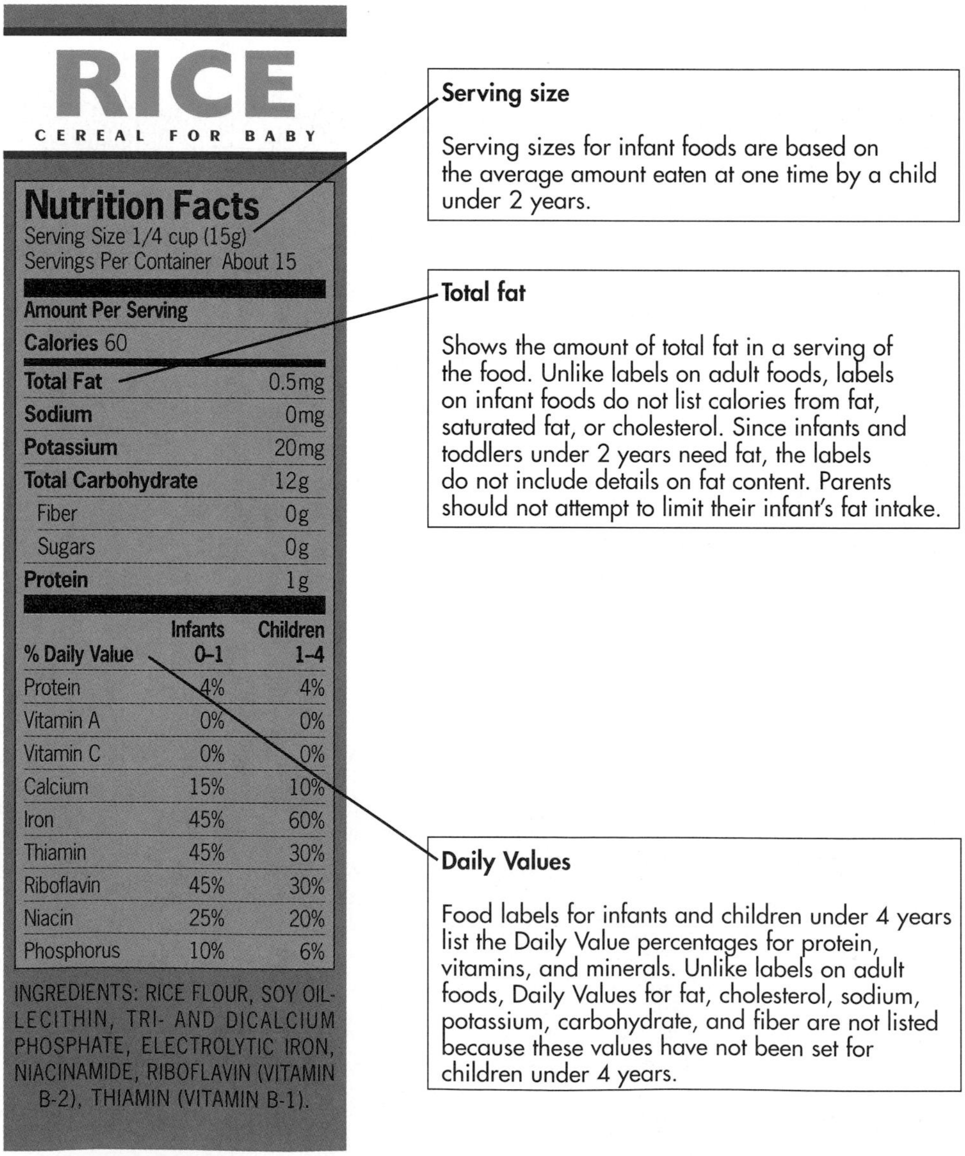

RICE
CEREAL FOR BABY

Nutrition Facts
Serving Size 1/4 cup (15g)
Servings Per Container About 15

Amount Per Serving

Calories 60

Total Fat	0.5mg
Sodium	0mg
Potassium	20mg
Total Carbohydrate	12g
Fiber	0g
Sugars	0g
Protein	1g

% Daily Value	Infants 0–1	Children 1–4
Protein	4%	4%
Vitamin A	0%	0%
Vitamin C	0%	0%
Calcium	15%	10%
Iron	45%	60%
Thiamin	45%	30%
Riboflavin	45%	30%
Niacin	25%	20%
Phosphorus	10%	6%

INGREDIENTS: RICE FLOUR, SOY OIL-LECITHIN, TRI- AND DICALCIUM PHOSPHATE, ELECTROLYTIC IRON, NIACINAMIDE, RIBOFLAVIN (VITAMIN B-2), THIAMIN (VITAMIN B-1).

Serving size

Serving sizes for infant foods are based on the average amount eaten at one time by a child under 2 years.

Total fat

Shows the amount of total fat in a serving of the food. Unlike labels on adult foods, labels on infant foods do not list calories from fat, saturated fat, or cholesterol. Since infants and toddlers under 2 years need fat, the labels do not include details on fat content. Parents should not attempt to limit their infant's fat intake.

Daily Values

Food labels for infants and children under 4 years list the Daily Value percentages for protein, vitamins, and minerals. Unlike labels on adult foods, Daily Values for fat, cholesterol, sodium, potassium, carbohydrate, and fiber are not listed because these values have not been set for children under 4 years.

FIGURE 17-4 The labels on infant foods, like those on adult foods, contain a Nutrition Facts panel. However, the information provided on infant food labels differs from that on adult food labels, especially with respect to saturated fat and cholesterol intake (review Fig. 2-4 in Chapter 2 for a comparison).

Vitamins of Special Interest

Vitamin K is routinely given by injection to all infants at birth. This dose lasts until the infant's intestinal bacteria are established and begin to synthesize vitamin K. Formula-fed infants receive the rest of the vitamins they need from the formula. Breast-fed infants, especially dark-skinned ones (e.g., African-Americans), likely require a vitamin D supplement if they are not exposed to much sunlight or if the mother has poor vitamin D status. (Sunlight exposure on human skin activates the synthesis of vitamin D; see Chapter 9) Breastfed infants whose mothers are total vegetarians (vegans) should receive a vitamin B-12 supplement. As well, infants who drink goat's milk need a dietary supplement of folate because this milk doesn't supply a sufficient amount of this essential nutrient. Goat's milk is also low in iron, vitamin C, and vitamin D, making it a poor choice for human infants.[34]

Minerals of Special Interest

The iron stores with which children are born are generally depleted by the time birth weight doubles, in 4 to 6 months. The American Academy of Pediatrics recommends that, to maintain a desirable iron status, formula-fed infants should be given an iron-fortified formula from birth. These experts also discourage the use of low-iron infant formulas, which are sometimes prescribed to treat infants with various gastrointestinal problems. Breastfed infants need solid foods to supply extra iron at about 6 months of age. The need for iron is a major consideration in deciding when to introduce solid foods. Some physicians recommend liquid iron supplements from birth or by 1 month of age for breastfed infants. Iron deficiency anemia can lead to poor cognitive development in infants.[17]

Infants need adequate amounts of zinc and iodide to support growth. Human milk and infant formula adequately supply these needs when they supply enough energy to meet needs. In addition, clinicians recommend fluoride supplements to aid tooth development for breastfed infants after 6 months of age. The same holds true for formula-fed infants if the water supply used in home formula preparation—either tap or bottled water—doesn't contain fluoride. Note that formula manufacturers use fluoride-free water in formula preparation. Parents should consult their dentist for advice on meeting the infant's need for fluoride.

Water

An infant needs about 2 oz of water and other fluids combined per pound of body weight (about 150 ml/kg.). Infants typically consume enough human milk or formula to supply this amount. In hot climates, however, supplemental water may be necessary. Furthermore, any conditions that lead to water loss—diarrhea, vomiting, fever, and too much sun—can call for supplemental water.

Infants are easily dehydrated, a condition that has serious effects if not remedied. Dehydration can result in rapidly decreasing kidney function, and the infant may then require hospitalization for rehydration. Special fluid-replacement formulas containing electrolytes such as sodium and potassium are available in supermarkets and pharmacies to treat dehydration. A physician should guide any use of these products.

Note that, in some stores, bottled water products marketed specifically for infants may be placed alongside infant formulas and electrolyte-replacement solutions. This placement may give parents and caregivers the mistaken impression that bottled water products are an appropriate feeding supplement or substitute for fluid replacement for infants; they are not and should not be used for such purposes. It is important to remember also that excessive fluid can also be harmful, especially to the brain.

Overall, it is best to limit supplemental fluids to about 4 oz (120 ml) per day, unless the physician thinks that a greater need exists because of disease or other conditions. In sum, extremes in fluid intake—either too little or too much—can lead to health problems.[34]

CRITICAL THINKING

Tatiana has been breastfeeding her baby exclusively since he was born 7 months ago. When she and her husband took the baby for his checkup, they were told that he was anemic. They were very surprised, since they thought that human milk contained all the nutrients the baby needed for the first year of life. How can you explain the baby's anemia?

■ Formula Feeding for Infants

Breastfeeding was covered in detail in Chapter 16. Let's now focus on formula feeding. You'll recall that a major advantage of breastfeeding is the provision of immune protection to the infant. Another advantage of breastfeeding is the supply of very-long-chain fatty acids (those typically found in fish such as docosahexaenoic acid [DHA]). DHA is found in high concentrations in the retina of the eye, and brain. Some research suggests that formula-fed infants are at a disadvantage, as DHA is not added at this time to commercial formulas. Currently, formula manufacturers are studying the safety and importance of doing so. Possible improvements in visual functions and cognitive development are two major effects being studied. Overall, in areas of the world where high standards for water purity and cleanliness are common, formula feeding is a safe alternative for infants but may not be as beneficial as breastfeeding.

Formula Composition

Infants cannot tolerate cow's milk as such because of its high protein and mineral content. Cow's milk reflects the greater growth needs of calves. Thus, cow's milk must be altered to be safe for infant feeding. It is important to note that goat's milk, sweetened condensed milk, and evaporated milk also are inappropriate substances for infants. Altered forms of cow's milk, known as infant formulas, were first available commercially in 1931. Since 1980, they have been required to conform to strict federal guidelines for nutrient composition and quality. Formulas generally contain lactose and/or sucrose for carbohydrate, heat-treated **casein** and **whey** proteins from cow's milk, and vegetable oils for fat (review Table 17-1). Soy protein–based formulas are available for infants who can't tolerate lactose or the types of proteins found in cow's milk. If the soybean-based formula is not tolerated, the next step is to try a predigested (hydrolyzed) protein formula, such as Nutramigen or Alimentum. A variety of other specialized formulas also are available for specific medical conditions.[34] In any case, it is important to use an iron-fortified formula.

Some transition formulas/beverages have been introduced for older infants and toddlers (review Table 17-1). Some of these products are intended for use after 6 months of age if the infant is consuming solid foods, whereas others are intended for use only by toddlers. These transition products are lower in fat than human milk or standard infant formulas; their iron content is higher than that of cow's milk, and their overall mineral content is generally more like that of human milk than cow's milk. According to the manufacturers, the advantages of these transition formulas/beverages over standard formulas for older infants and toddlers include reduced cost and better flavor. Parents should consult their physician with regard to the use of these products

Formula Preparation

In the 1950s, it was common to prepare a day's supply of bottles and then sterilize them in boiling water for about 30 minutes. Today, bottles are often prepared one at a time. Some infant formulas even come in ready-to-feed form. These are poured into a clean bottle and fed immediately. Room-temperature formula is acceptable for many infants. Otherwise, to warm a bottle of formula, a caregiver can run hot water over it or place it briefly in a pan of simmering water. Note that infant formulas

---

Soy-based formulas account for about 25% of the infant formula used in the United States. There is some concern over the use of soy milk in infant feeding because of the isoflavone content. Isoflavones may cause endocrine disruption, developmental delay in boys, and precocious puberty in girls.[8] Currently, the American Academy of Pediatrics states that soy formulas are safe but should be used only when typical breast-feeding or milk-based formulas are not appropriate: confirmed allergies to milk, lactose intolerance, galactosemia, or parents who insist on strict vegan diets.

casein A protein found in milk that forms curds when exposed to acid and is difficult for infants to digest.

whey Proteins, such as lactalbumin, that are found in great amounts in human milk and are easy to digest.

should not be heated in a microwave oven because hot spots may develop, which can burn the infant's mouth and esophagus.

Powdered and concentrated fluid formula preparations are more commonly used than ready-to-feed varieties. All utensils used in preparing formula from these preparations should be washed and thoroughly rinsed. Powdered or concentrated formulas are poured into a bottle, to which clean, cold water is added (following label directions) and then mixed. The formula is then warmed, if desired, and fed immediately to the infant. Hot water from the faucet should not be used to make formula, since it poses a risk for high lead content (see Chapter 19). Cold water poses much less risk.

Refrigerating diluted formula for 1 day is safe. However, formula left over from a feeding should be discarded because it will be contaminated by bacteria and enzymes in the infant's saliva. If well water is used, it should be boiled before making formula for at least the infant's first 3 months of life, and it should be analyzed for excessive concentration of naturally occurring nitrates, which can lead to a severe form of anemia. Note that, if nitrates are high in municipal water systems, consumers will be warned (such as in a local newspaper) not to use the water for making infant formula until the concentration falls to a safe amount. This problem with nitrates typically occurs in the summer, when these wash from fertilized farm fields into local rivers after heavy rains. Boiling tapwater is also advised by some groups, based on evidence that even municipal water may contain microbes that can harm the vulnerable, such as infants (see Chapter 11).

Feeding Technique

Because infants swallow a lot of air along with either formula or human milk, it's important to burp an infant after either 10 minutes of feeding or 1 to 2 oz (30 to 60 ml) from a bottle and again at the end of feeding. Spitting up a bit of milk is normal at this time. Once fed, infants should be placed on their backs. Infants should not be placed on their stomachs because this sleeping position has been linked to sudden infant death syndrome (SIDS).[6] The back to sleep campaign, started in 1994 in the United States, has reduced SIDS by 40%; however, plagiocephaly, otherwise known as flat-head syndrome, has increased as a result. Infant skulls are soft and can take on a different form. Flat-head syndrome can occur if an excessive amount of an infant's life is spent on his or her back, or against a highchair/car seat. In response to this concern The American Academy of Pediatrics has recommended periodic repositioning of an infant's head while asleep and allowing for time on his or her stomach while awake.

When the infant begins acting full, bottle-feeding should be stopped, even if some milk is left in the bottle. Common cues that signal that an infant has had enough include turning the head away, being inattentive, falling asleep, and becoming playful. Generally, the infant's appetite is a better guide than standardized recommendations concerning feeding amounts. Breastfeeding infants usually have had enough to eat after about 20 minutes. Although it's difficult to tell how much milk breastfed infants are getting, they also give signs when full. By carefully observing bottle-feeding or nursing infants and responding to their cues appropriately, caregivers not only can be assured that the infants' energy needs are being met but also can foster a climate of trust and responsiveness.

■ Development of Feeding Skills in Older Infants

By 6 to 7 months the infant has learned to grab and transfer objects from one hand to the other (Table 17-2). At about this time, teeth begin to appear, and the infant begins to handle finger foods with some dexterity. Dry toast, sliced in strips, offers hours of enjoyment.

By age 7 to 8 months, infants can push food around on a plate and play with a drinking cup, can hold a bottle, and, self-feed a cracker or piece of toast. In mastering these manipulations, infants develop self-confidence and self-esteem. It's important that parents be patient and support these early feeding attempts, even though they appear inefficient.

Not even all formula-like products are designed for infant use. A 5-month-old girl was admitted to a hospital in Arkansas with symptoms of heart failure, rickets, inflamed blood vessels, and possible nerve damage after being fed Soy Moo (a soy beverage sold in health stores) since 3 days of age. The symptoms suggest severe vitamin deficiencies. Parents should consult a physician when choosing an appropriate infant formula.

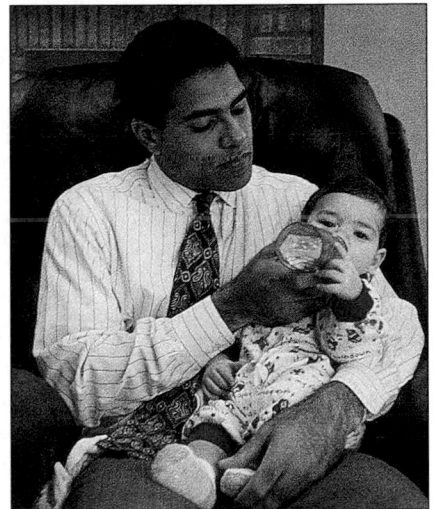

Careful attention during feeding allows the caregiver to pick up on the infant's signal as to when the feeding should cease.

TABLE 17-2   Typical Progression of Infant Eating Skills and Solid-Food Introduction*

Age	Feeding Skills	Oral Motor Skills	Types of Food	Suggested Activities
Birth–4 months		Rooting reflex Sucking reflex Swallowing reflex Extrusion reflex	Human milk Infant formula	Breastfeed or bottle-feed
5 months	Is able to grasp objects voluntarily Is learning to reach mouth with hands	Disappearance of extrusion reflex		Possibly introduce thinned cereal if baby not satisfied by breastfeeding or bottle-feeding
6 months	Sits with balance while using hands	Transfers food from front of tongue to back	Infant cereal Strained fruit Strained vegetables Egg yolk (if no family history of egg allergy)	Prepare cereal with formula or human milk to a semiliquid texture Use spoon Feed from a dish Advance to ⅓–½ cup cereal before adding fruits or vegetables
7 months	Has improved grasp Can transfer objects from hand to hand	Mashes food with lateral movements of jaw Learns side-to-side, or "rotary," chewing Tooth eruption	Infant cereal Strained to junior texture of fruits, vegetables, and meats	Thicken cereal to lumpier texture Sit in high chair with feet supported Introduce cup
8–10 months	Holds bottle without help Drinks from cup Decreases fluid intake and increases solids Coordinates hand-to-mouth movement		Juices (small amounts) Soft, mashed, or minced table foods	Begin finger foods, such as toast or crackers Avoid adding salt, sugar, or fats to food Present soft foods in chunks ready for finger-feeding
10–12 months	Feeds self Holds cup without help	Improved ability to bite and chew	Soft, chopped table foods Whole egg and whole milk (at 1 year of age)	Provide meals in pattern similar to rest of family Use cup at meals

Adapted with permission from *Handbook of Pediatric Nutrition*, Queen, p. 130. © 1993 Aspen Publishers, Inc.

*This time line is just an estimate, and individual infants may vary by several months from the ages given. A pediatrician should be consulted if caregivers are concerned about an infant's developmental progress. In general, there is no nutritional reason to begin introducing solid foods before 4 to 6 months of age.

At around 10 months of age, infants practice in earnest self-feeding finger foods and drinking from a cup. Feeding time is often very messy. Food is used as a means to explore the environment. By the first birthday, their bodies have developed sufficiently to accommodate crawling, probably walking, and self-feeding. Although attempts at feeding are still erratic, developing children take great pride in doing more things independently. As children drink from a cup more frequently, fewer bottle feedings and/or breastfeedings are necessary. The added mobility of walking should naturally lead to gradual weaning from the bottle or breast.

■ Introduction of Solid Foods at 4 to 6 Months of Age

The time to introduce solid foods into an infant's diet hinges on a few important factors:

1. *Nutritional need.* Iron stores are exhausted by about 6 months of age. Either solid foods or iron supplements are then needed to supply iron if the child is breastfed or fed a formula not supplemented with iron. Iron, however, is not the only nutrient missing from human milk and unfortified infant formulas. Vitamin D may also deserve attention, as previously mentioned. Still, before 4 to 6 months, it's unnecessary to add solid foods.

2. *Physiological capabilities.* Infants cannot readily digest starch before 3 months. As they age, their digestive capabilities increase. Kidney function likewise is quite limited until about 4 to 6 weeks of age. Until then, waste products from excessive amounts of dietary protein or minerals are difficult to excrete.

3. *Physical ability.* Three markers indicate that a child is ready for solid foods: (1) the disappearance of the extrusion reflex (thrusting the tongue forward and pushing food out of the mouth), (2) head and neck control, and (3) the ability to sit up with support. These usually occur around 4 to 6 months of age, but they vary with each infant.

4. *Allergy prevention.* An infant's intestinal tract can readily absorb whole proteins from birth until 4 to 5 months of age. Thus, early exposure to many types of proteins—particularly proteins in cow's milk and egg whites—may predispose a child to future allergies and other health problems because some types of these proteins may be absorbed intact. For this reason, it's best to minimize the number of different types of proteins in a child's diet, especially during the first 3 months.

With these considerations in mind—nutritional need, physiological and physical readiness, and allergy prevention—the American Academy of Pediatrics recommends that solid foods not be introduced until about 6 months of age and that infants receive no unaltered cow's milk before 1 year.

In general, a child starting solid foods should weigh at least 13 lb (6 kg) and should be drinking more than 32 oz (1 L) of formula daily or breastfeeding more than 8 to 10 times within 24 hours. This description generally applies to 6-month-old infants and to some 4-month-old infants.

Before 4 to 6 months, infants are not physically mature enough to consume much solid food. Attempts to push down solid foods have sometimes led to forcefeeding with a feeder (a giant syringe) or mixing infant cereal with milk and putting it in a bottle. Even if these are traditional alternatives in your family, there is no reason to carry on these practices. The inconvenience alone should make one consider whether all the effort is worth it. This practice is unnecessary nutritionally, tedious, and possibly dangerous for the infant because it increases the risk of allergies and choking or inhaling food when crying. Even so, many children are already eating solids before 4 months of age.[5] Only occasionally does a rapidly growing infant—one who consumes more than 32 oz (1 L) of formula daily—need solid foods at 4 months to meet high energy needs.

Solid Foods That Should Be Fed First

Before 6 months of age, the first solid foods should be iron-fortified cereals. A good idea is to offer foods after some breastfeeding or formula feeding, when the edge has been taken off the infant's hunger. This practice aids in early spoon-feeding. Rice cereal is the best cereal to begin with because it's least likely to cause allergies. After the age of 6 months, the first food is not such an important issue. Some pediatricians may recommend lean ground (strained) meats for more absorbable forms of iron. Although yogurt and cottage cheese are also well tolerated and their consistencies make them good candidates for early foods, they are not good sources of iron.

Start with teaspoon amounts of a single food item, such as rice cereal, and increase the serving size gradually. Once the new food has been fed for about a week without ill effects, another food can be added to the infant's diet. At first, this can be another type of cereal or perhaps a cooked and strained (blended) vegetable, meat, fruit, or egg yolk. It is best to add vegetables before fruits. If fruits are offered first, the infant will prefer the sweet taste and likely resist vegetables. Each feeding step builds on the last.

Waiting about 7 days between new foods is important because it can take that long for evidence of an allergy or intolerance to develop. Symptoms to look for are diarrhea, vomiting, a rash, or wheezing. If one or more of these symptoms appear, the suspected problem food should be avoided for several weeks and then reintroduced in a small quantity. If the problem continues, a physician should be consulted.

*P*arents may believe that the early addition of solid foods will help the infant sleep through the night. This achievement is a developmental milestone; the amount of food consumed by the infant is irrelevant.

Typical Solid Food Progression, Starting at 6 Months*

Week 1	Rice cereal
Week 2	Add strained carrots
Week 3	Add applesauce
Week 4	Add oat cereal
Week 5	Add cooked egg yolk
Week 6	Add strained chicken
Week 7	Add strained peas
Week 8	Add plums

*Extending the rice cereal step for a month or so is advised if solid food introduction begins at 4 months of age. Note also that, if at any point signs of allergy or intolerance develop, substitute another, similar food item.

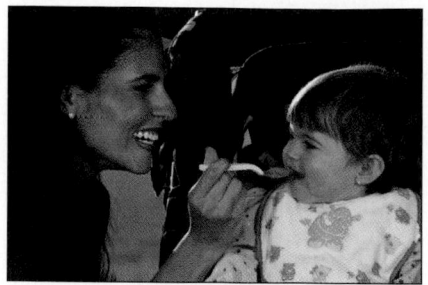

In the early stages of solid food introduction, these foods complement rather than replace human milk or infant formula in the diet.

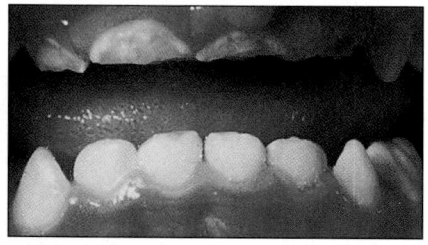

■ FIGURE 17-5 An extreme example of tooth decay caused by nursing-bottle syndrome. This child was probably put to bed with a bottle. The upper teeth have decayed almost all the way to the gum line.

It's important not to introduce mixed foods until each component of the mixed food has been given separately. Otherwise, if an allergy or intolerance develops, it will be difficult to identify the offending food. Note that many babies outgrow food sensitivities in childhood. Some foods that commonly cause an allergic response in infants are egg whites, chocolate, nuts, and cow's milk. It's best not to introduce these foods in infancy.[33]

A variety of strained foods is available for infant feeding. Investigate these and other foods intended for infants the next time you're in a supermarket. Single-food items are more desirable than mixed dinners and desserts, which are less nutrient-dense. Most brands have no added salt, but some fruit desserts contain a lot of added sugar.

As an alternative, plain foods from the table—vegetables, fruits, and meats (no seasoning added)—can be ground up in an inexpensive plastic baby food grinder/mill. Another option is to pureé a larger amount of food in a blender, freeze it in ice-cube portions, store in plastic bags, and defrost and warm as needed. Careful attention to cleanliness is necessary. Infant foods made at home should be ground before seasonings are added to please the rest of the family. The infant doesn't notice the difference if salt, sugar, or spices are omitted. It's best to introduce infants to a variety of foods, so that by the end of the first year the infant is consuming many foods—milk, meats, fruits, vegetables, and grains.

As early as possible, by about 8 months or so, juices and formulas should be offered in a cup. A heavy cup with a wide, flat bottom aids success. Drinking from a cup helps prevent nursing bottle syndrome (Fig. 17-5). As an infant plays with a bottle, the carbohydrate-rich fluid bathes the teeth, providing an ideal growth medium for bacteria. Bacteria on the teeth then make acids, which dissolve tooth enamel. Infants should never be put to bed with a bottle or placed in an infant seat with a bottle propped up. When children are allowed to do this, fluid (even milk) pools around the teeth, increasing the likelihood of dental caries. Again, infants need careful attention when being fed. Propping up a bottle does not constitute careful attention.

Getting a baby out of the bedtime-bottle habit is difficult. Determined caregivers can either wince through a few nights of their baby's crying or slowly wean the baby away from the bottle with either a pacifier or water (for a week or so).

In the first attempts to introduce solid foods, just getting the food into the infant's mouth proves to be a challenge. The caregiver must proceed slowly. Initially, table foods supplement—rather than replace—formula or human milk. These infants control the situation by signaling when they are hungry and when they have had enough to eat. Self-feeding skills require coordination and can develop only if the infant is allowed to practice and experiment. At 9 to 10 months, the infant's desire to explore, experience, and play with food can also hinder feeding. Presenting new foods for several consecutive days can aid in an infant's acceptance of that food.

Caregivers need to relax and take this phase of infant development in stride. Sloppy, friendly mealtimes actually make for good memories.

To ease efforts in feeding solid foods, consider the following tips:

- Use a baby-sized spoon; a small spoon with a long handle is best.
- Hold the infant comfortably on the lap, as for breastfeeding or bottle-feeding, but a little more upright to ease swallowing. When in this position, the infant expects food.
- Put a small dab of food on the spoon tip and gently place it on the infant's tongue.
- Convey a calm and casual approach to the infant, who needs time to get used to food.
- Expect the infant to take only two or three bites of the first meals. Anything more than that is real success.

By the end of the first year, finger-feeding becomes more efficient, drinking from a cup improves, and chewing is easier as more teeth erupt. Foods in the diet begin to resemble a balanced diet, such as a Food Guide Pyramid pattern (Table 17-3). Still, experimentation and unpredictability are to be expected.[34]

What Not to Feed an Infant

Following are several foods and practices to avoid when feeding an infant:

- *Honey and corn syrup.* These products may contain spores of *Clostridium botulinum.* The spores can eventually develop into bacteria in the stomach and lead to a foodborne illness known as *botulism.* This can be fatal in children under 1 year old (see Chapter 19).
- *Very salty and very sweet foods.* Infants don't need a lot of sugar or salt added to their foods. They enjoy bland foods much more than do adults.
- *Excessive infant formula or human milk.* After 6 to 8 months, solid foods should play a greater role in satisfying an infant's increasing appetite. The main reason to switch is that solid foods contain considerably more iron than do human milk, cow's milk, and low-iron formulas. About 24 to 32 oz (¾ to 1 L) of human milk or formula daily is ideal after 6 months, with food supplying the rest of the infant's energy needs.
- *Foods that tend to cause choking.* These foods include hot dogs (unless finely cut into sticks, not coin shapes), candy, whole nuts, grapes, coarsely cut meats, raw carrots, popcorn, and peanut butter. Caregivers should not allow younger children to gobble snack foods during playtime and should supervise all meals.
- *Cow's milk, especially low-fat or nonfat cow's milk.* Beyond 2 years, children can drink fat-reduced or 1% milk, because by then they are consuming enough solid foods to supply energy and fat needs. Before that age, the amount of fat-reduced, 1%, or nonfat milk needed for energy needs would supply too many minerals. That could overwhelm the kidneys' ability to excrete the excess. The lower fat intake might also harm nervous system development. The American Academy of Pediatrics strongly urges parents not to give children under age 2 fat-reduced, 1%, or nonfat milk.
- *Feeding excessive amounts of apple or pear juice.* The fructose and sorbitol contained in these juices can lead to diarrhea because they are slowly absorbed. Also, if fruit juice or related drink products are replacing formula or milk in the

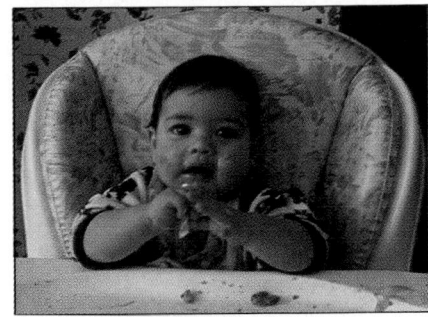

Early feeding attempts should be encouraged, even though they're messy.

*E*gg whites also should not be fed to children before 1 year of age to help prevent the development of allergies.

TABLE 17-3 Sample Daily Menu for a 1-Year-Old Child*	
Breakfast	**Snack**
1–2 tbsp applesauce	½ oz cheddar cheese
¼ cup Cheerios	4 wheat crackers
½ cup whole milk	½ cup whole milk
Snack	**Dinner**
½ hard-cooked egg	1 oz hamburger (crumbled)
½ slice wheat toast with ½ tsp margarine	1–2 tbsp mashed potatoes with ½ tsp margarine
½ cup orange juice	1–2 tbsp cooked carrots (cut in strips, not coins)
	½ cup whole milk
Lunch	**Snack**
1 oz roasted chicken, minced	½ banana
1–2 tbsp rice with ½ tsp margarine	2 oatmeal cookies (no raisins)
1–2 tbsp cooked peas	½ cup whole milk
½ cup whole milk	

Nutritional Analysis

Total energy (kcal)	1100
% energy from	
Carbohydrate	40%
Protein	19%
Fat	41%

A Summary of Infant Feeding Recommendations

Breastfed Infants
- Breastfeed for 6 months or longer, if possible. Then introduce infant formula if and when breastfeeding declines or ceases.
- Add iron-fortified cereal at about 6 months of age.
- Investigate the need for fluoride, iron, and vitamin D supplemental sources.
- Provide a variety of basic, soft foods after 6 months of age, advancing to a varied diet.

Formula-Fed Infants
- Use infant formula for the first year of life, preferably an iron-fortified type.
- Add iron-fortified cereal at about 6 months of age.
- Investigate the need for a fluoride supplement if the water supply is not fluoridated.
- Prove a variety of basic, soft foods after 6 months, advancing to a varied diet.

*This diet is just a start. A 1-year-old may need more or less food. In those cases, serving sizes should be adjusted. The milk can be fed by cup; some can be put into a bottle if the child has not been fully weaned from the bottle. The juice should be fed in a cup.

Damon's diet is inadequate for a 10 month old infant because it lacks enough of the nutritious foods his growing body needs to support weight gain. These foods include iron-fortified cereal, puréed infant foods, and appropriate table foods. Damon should stay on the infant formula until 1 year of age and should not be given sugary drinks, nor should these drinks be fed by bottle if used. Damon needs a more energy-dense diet containing a healthful variety of solid foods to provide him with enough calories and essential nutrients to grow and develop.

diet, the infant may not be receiving adequate amounts of calcium and other minerals that are essential for bone growth. In fact, studies have shown a link between excessive amounts of fruit juice and failure to thrive, gastrointestinal complications, obesity, short stature, and poor dental heath.[10] Thus, these substances should be used sparingly. Infants can usually safely consume 4 to 8 oz of juice in the course of a day, with no more than 2 to 4 oz at a time. Diluting juices with an equal part of water is a good idea, but it should be begun early, before the infant becomes accustomed to full-strength juices.

CONCEPT CHECK

Infant formulas generally contain lactose or sucrose, heat-treated proteins from cow's milk, and vegetable oil. Formulas may or may not be fortified with iron. Sanitation is very important in preparing and storing formula. Solid foods should not be added to an infant's diet until the child is both ready for and needs solid food, usually at about 4 to 6 months of age. The first solid food can be iron-fortified infant cereals, with very gradual additions of other foods—one at a time each week. Some foods to avoid giving infants in the first year are honey, cow's milk (particularly fat-reduced, 1%, or nonfat milk), very salty or sweet foods, foods that may cause the child to choke, and excessive amounts of fruit juice or related products (e.g., fruit drinks).

Dietary Guidelines for Infant Feeding

In response to various controversies surrounding infant feeding, The American Academy of Pediatrics has issued a number of statements concerning infant diets. The following guidelines are based on these statements:

- *Build to a variety of foods.* For the first months of life, human milk is all an infant needs. When the infant is ready, start adding new foods, one at a time. During the first year, the goal is to teach an infant to enjoy a variety of nutritious foods. A lifetime of healthy eating habits begins with this important first step.
- *Pay attention to your infant's appetite to avoid overfeeding or underfeeding.* Feed infants when they are hungry. Never force an infant to finish an unwanted serving of food. Watch for signs that indicate hunger or fullness.
- *Infants need fat.* Although fat is the cause of many adult health problems, it's an essential source of energy for growing infants. Fat also helps the nervous system develop.
- *Choose fruits, vegetables, and grains, but don't overdo high-fiber foods.* Although many adults benefit from higher-fiber diets, they are not good for infants. They are bulky, filling, and often low in energy. The natural amounts of fiber and nutrients in fruits, vegetables, and grains are appropriate as part of a healthy infant diet.
- *Infants need sugars in moderation.* Sugars are an additional source of energy for active, rapidly growing infants. Foods such as human milk, fruits, and juices are natural sources of sugars and other nutrients as well. Foods that contain artificial sweeteners should be avoided; they don't provide the energy growing infants need.
- *Infants need sodium in moderation.* Sodium is a necessary mineral found naturally in almost all foods. As part of a healthy diet, infants need sodium for their bodies to work properly.
- *Choose foods containing iron, zinc, and calcium.* Infants need good sources of iron, zinc, and calcium for optimum growth in the first 2 years. These minerals are important for healthy blood, proper growth, and strong bones.

In essence, there is no evidence that very restrictive diets during infancy have positive effects, whereas their hazards are well documented.

■ Health Problems Related to Infant Nutrition

Parents, other caregivers, and clinicians should be alert for a variety of potential health problems related to infant nutrition, so that corrective action can be taken quickly. In some cases, such problems stem from inappropriate feeding practices and inadequate nutrient intakes, including the following:

- Diet providing insufficient iron
- Absence from the diet of an entire food group of the Food Guide Pyramid (or other related Pyramid) as solid foods are introduced and become the main source of nutrients
- Drinking raw (unpasteurized) milk, which may be contaminated with bacteria or viruses
- Drinking goat's milk, which is low in folate, iron, vitamin C, and vitamin D; if used, it must be pasteurized and given in conjunction with a balanced vitamin and mineral supplement
- Failure to begin drinking from a cup by 1 year of age
- Continuing to feed from a bottle past 18 months of age
- Intake of supplemental vitamins or minerals above 100% of the appropriate RDA or other standard
- Drinking large amounts of fruit juice before 6 months of age, especially as a substitute for infant formula or human milk.

Now let's look more closely at four common infant health problems that cause concern for caregivers: colic, diarrhea, milk allergy, and iron deficiency anemia. Parents and other caregivers usually need to consult with a physician in dealing with these conditions. The web site of the American Academy of Pediatrics (http://www.aap.org) is another resourse.

Colic. The first time an otherwise healthy, well-fed infant has a lengthy, unexplained crying spell, most parents panic. Repeated crying episodes, lasting 3 or more hours that don't respond to typical remedies—such as feeding, holding, or changing diapers—are characteristic of infants who develop **colic.** Colic affects about 10 to 30% of all infants, so it is neither uncommon nor abnormal. Colicky infants typically cry during the late afternoon and early evening, and their nighttime sleeping is almost always disturbed by crying spells. In addition, these infants frequently pass gas rectally, clench their fists, draw up their legs, hold the body straight, and want to be held. The only good news is that colic usually goes away after a few months.

Colic generally occurs in the absence of any physical problem in the infant. It tends to be most common in "temperamental" infants—those who are more sensitive, more irritable, more intense, less adaptable, and less consolable than average for their age. In addition, a lack of harmonious interaction between parents and the infant may contribute to the problem. Some researchers have speculated that immature central nervous system mechanisms may cause colic.

Parents can do several things to help reduce excessive crying. For instance, many infants tend to become quiet and alert when held snugly to the shoulder. Parents should also check to see whether the infant is tired or bored or wants to suckle. Some infants can be calmed by rhythmic sounds or movement or with pacifiers.

Breastfeeding of colicky infants should continue. The breastfeeding mother's temporary decrease or cessation in consumption of dairy products, caffeine, chocolate, and vegetables such as broccoli and onions may help reduce colic in her infant. Formula-fed infants with severe colic are sometimes helped by changing from a standard formula to a soy-based or predigested protein formula (review Table 17-1). In addition, physicians may prescribe medication to calm colicky infants and reduce gas buildup.

Caring for an inconsolable, colicky infant is stressful and frustrating for parents. Most parents benefit from the counsel and support of other adults during this trying period, which may last for several months. Sharing with others who have been

colic Sharp abdominal pain that generally occurs in otherwise healthy infants and is associated with periodic inconsolable crying spells.

through similar experiences can help parents improve their tolerance of stress and ability to cope and can increase their confidence in their parenting abilities. Furthermore, to optimize their ability to be sensitive and responsive to their infant, parents need to be well rested and to set aside some time for themselves.

Diarrhea. Diarrhea in infants, characterized by numerous loose stools per day, results from various causes, including bacterial and viral infections. In the United States, about 500 infants die each year of simple dehydration resulting from diarrhea, and about 210,000 are hospitalized for this disorder. To prevent dehydration, infants with diarrhea should be given plenty of fluids, under the advice of a physician. Specialized electrolyte-replacement fluids, such as Pedialyte, may be recommended for very-short-term use.[34] These contain glucose, sodium, potassium, chloride, and water.

Once diarrhea subsides, a bottle-fed infant may be switched to a soy-based, lactose-free formula for a few days. This allows time for the intestine to produce sufficient lactase enzyme to digest the large amount of lactose typically found in formulas. A breastfed infant should continue at the breast for the duration of the diarrhea. If solid foods are consumed, the physician may also prescribe a BRAT (bananas, rice, applesauce, toast) diet for short-term use; this is not a nutritionally adequate diet for long-term use.

Milk Allergy. Cow's milk contains more than 40 proteins that can cause allergic reactions in infants. Although some of these proteins are inactivated by heating (scalding) milk, others are very heat stable. A true milk allergy develops in about 1 to 3% of formula-fed infants. Such infants may experience vomiting, diarrhea, blood in the stool, constipation, and other symptoms. If milk allergy is suspected, a formula-fed infant can be switched to a soy-based formula. In 20 to 50% of cases, however, the use of soy formula provides only temporary relief because the soy protein eventually triggers an allergic reaction in some infants. In such cases a predigested-protein formula is necessary (review Table 17-1). If the child is breastfeeding, the mother may experiment with eliminating cow's milk from her diet. Fortunately, such an allergy seldom lasts beyond 3 years of age.[33]

Iron Deficiency Anemia. Iron deficiency anemia typically occurs in older infants who consume few solid foods and whose diets are dominated by cow's milk, which contains little iron and causes intestinal bleeding in young infants. Iron stores are then quickly depleted by the daily need to synthesize new red blood cells. The best way to prevent iron deficiency anemia is to feed an iron-fortified formula beginning at birth, if formula is used; to start an infant on iron-fortified cereals and meats at about 6 months; and to limit formula to 16 to 25 oz (500 to 750 ml) daily at this age.[21] If anemia does develop, medicinal iron is used under a physician's guidance.

Feeding Preterm Infants

Preterm infants are fed either a specially designed formula or human milk. Total parenteral nutrition may also be required in the initial phase of hospitalization. As noted in Chapter 16, nutrients may be added to human milk to increase its protein, mineral, and energy content. Preterm infants must be fed immediately because their bodies store little fat or carbohydrate. The body composition of a full-term infant includes about 12% fat, whereas the composition of a very preterm infant can include as little as 2% fat.

CONCEPT CHECK

Colic is commonly associated with inconsolable crying. Switching to an infant formula made with soy or predigested proteins may reduce colic. It may also be helpful for breastfeeding mothers to decrease or avoid intake of dairy products, caffeine, chocolate, and certain vegetables, under a physician's guidance. Diarrhea requires additional fluids to prevent dehydration. Infants allergic to proteins in standard cow's milk formula can be switched to an infant formula containing soy protein or predigested protein. Introducing iron-containing solid foods at an appropriate time and avoiding the use of cow's milk during the first year can generally prevent iron deficiency anemia in infants.

■ PRESCHOOL CHILDREN

The rapid growth rate that characterizes infancy tapers off quickly during the subsequent few years. The average annual weight gain is only 4.5 to 6.6 lb (2 to 3 kg), and the average annual height gain is only 3 to 4 in (7.5 to 10 cm) between the ages of 2 and 5 (review Fig. 17-1). As a toddler's growth rate tapers off, eating behavior changes. For example, the decreased growth rate leads to a decreased appetite, compared with infants.[34]

Because of the reduced appetite of preschool children, planning a diet that meets their nutrient needs poses a challenge to caregivers. Choosing nutrient-dense foods is particularly important with children who eat relatively little. This is a good time to emphasize some whole grains, fruits, and vegetables without increasing fat and simple sugar intake. A whole-grain breakfast cereal with limited fat and sugar is an excellent choice. There is no need to decrease fat or simple sugar intake severely, but fatty and sweet food choices should not overwhelm more nutritious ones.[19]

The preschool years are the best time for a child to start a healthful pattern of living and eating, focusing on regular physical activity and nutritious foods (Fig. 17-6). Parents and other caregivers are role models: If they eat a variety of foods, the children will eat a variety of foods. One possible policy is the one-bite rule: Within reason, children should take at least one bite or taste of the foods presented to them. For snacks, parents should select several possibilities of acceptable choices and allow children to choose one; responsibility for food choice ideally should start early.

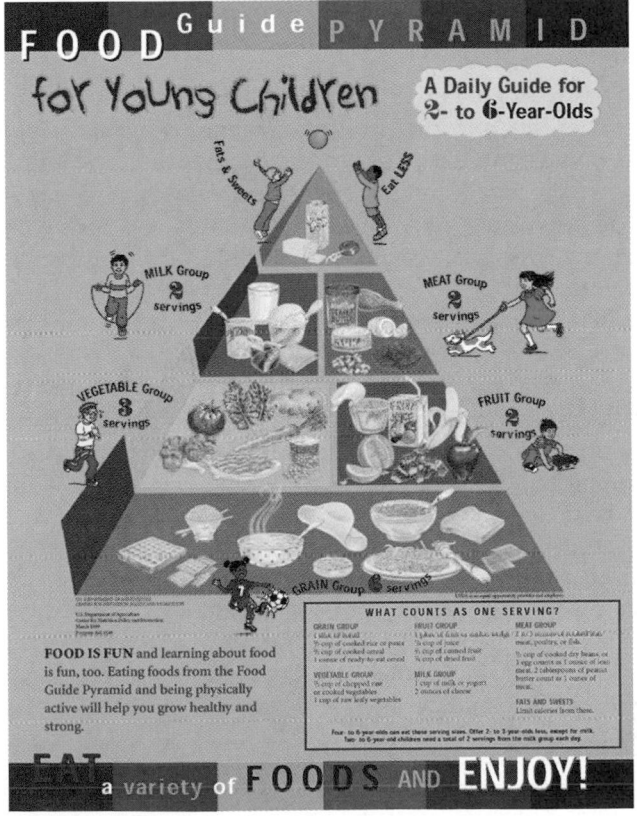

■ FIGURE **17-6** USDA has created a Food Guide Pyramid for children ages 2 through 6 years. The pyramid base recommends that young children consume six servings a day of grains such as bread, cereal, rice, and pasta; three servings of vegetables; and two servings each of fruit, milk, and meat. The pyramid is designed to be very child-friendly, showing foods children will recognize in appealing graphic format. It also emphasizes the importance of physical activity for good health by featuring many children playing actively around the pyramid to symbolize how eating and activity work hand-in-hand. The booklet accompanying this pyramid can be downloaded at http://www.usda.gov/cnpp.

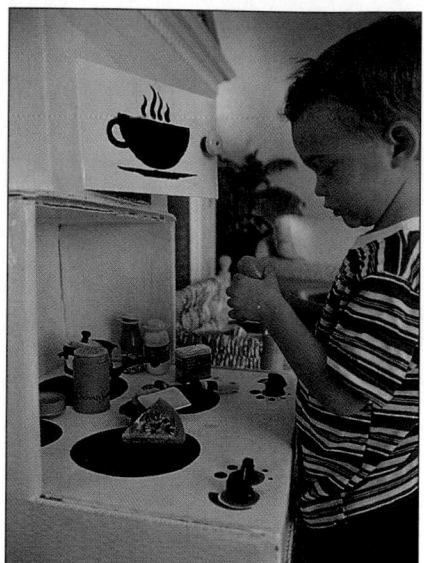

Interest in food starts early in life.

■ How to Help a Child Choose Nutritious Foods

One way adults can encourage young children to eat nutritious, well-balance meals is to serve new foods and repeat exposure to them. If a child observes adults and older children eating and enjoying a food, there's a good chance that, most of the time, he or she will eventually accept it. The dinner hour is a good time for children to experience new foods and to develop their own food preferences. Preschool children especially tend to be wary of new foods. One reason is that their taste buds are more sensitive than those of adults. In addition, they have a general distrust of unfamiliar foods. If adults can be patient and persevere, children will build good food habits. Above all, the dinner table should not become a battleground, and using one food as a bribe to eat another—for example, a piece of pie for peas—is strongly discouraged.

Perseverance with children is critical, because it takes effort and commitment to guide them into liking a variety of foods. Be ready for some surprises. Also, if left to their own devices, preschool children would find a few foods they like and eat them every day. However, by constantly being introduced to new foods, children at this age can expand their nutritional choices, develop an experimental approach, and learn to appreciate a variety of foods. It may take 10 to 15 exposures, but eventually children will accept most foods. A positive outlook by the caregivers helps a lot.

Children generally like certain foods—especially those with crisp textures and mild flavors—and familiar foods. Young children are especially sensitive to hot-temperature foods and tend to reject them.

Parents and other caregivers play a central role in teaching by example.[14] Children more readily learn good table manners alongside others who practice them. The harmony that comes from working at being polite creates a positive environment for learning good nutrition habits. Preschoolers eventually develop skill with spoons and forks and can even use dull knives (Table 17-4). However, it's still a good idea to serve some finger foods. A goal should be to make mealtime a happy, social time, sharing enjoyment of healthful foods. A regular family meal daily—whether breakfast, lunch, or dinner—is an appropriate setting for children to learn about healthful eating and to build good eating habits.

■ Childhood Feeding Problems

Tensions between parents, or between parents and children, often contribute to eating problems. Getting to the root of family problems and creating a more harmonious family atmosphere are important steps toward resolving many childhood feeding problems. In addition, many parents must be educated as to what to expect of a preschool child and what food-related goals to set (see Table 17-4). Let's consider some typical complaints and concerns of parents, the causes of the problems, and suggestions for correcting them.

"My Child Won't Eat as Much or as Regularly as He Did as an Infant"

This behavior is typical of preschoolers, because their growth rate slows after infancy; thus, they don't need as much food. Parents often need reminding that a 3-year-old can't be expected to eat as voraciously as an infant or to eat adult-size portions. Table 17-5 shows a general food plan, based on the Food Guide Pyramid, that is appropriate for preschool and school-age children. Until about 5 years of age, serving sizes in the vegetable group, fruit group, and meat, poultry, fish, dry beans, eggs, and nuts group can be estimated as about 1 tablespoon per year of life. The same restriction does not apply to cereals or milk. Normal-weight children have a built-in feeding mechanism, which adjusts hunger to regulate food intake at each stage of growth. If a child is developing and growing normally and the caregiver is providing a variety of healthful foods, all can be confident the child isn't starving. Caregivers should avoid nagging, forcing, and bribing.

Appetite also varies with activity level and general health. An initial symptom of a sick child is poor appetite. Picky eating is also just another indication of a child's

*T*wo-year-olds commonly prefer particular foods, but parents needn't worry about this. A child may switch from one specific food focus (often called a *jag*) to another with equal intensity. If the caregiver continues to offer choices, the child will soon begin to eat a wider variety of foods again, and the specific food focus will disappear as suddenly as it appeared.

TABLE 17-4 Observed Emotional Traits, Eating Behavior, and Food-Related Skills of Preschoolers

Age (years)	Emotional Traits	Eating Behavior	Food-Related Skills
1–2	• Fears new things • Sharing difficult • Requires constant supervision • Enjoys helping but can't be left alone • Curious • Often defiant • Eager for attention	• "Finicky" eater • Holds food in mouth without swallowing • May insist on eating the same food at meal after meal (called a food jag)	• Uses spoon with some skill (especially if hungry) • Can begin to tear, break, snap, and dip foods • Has good control of cup—lifts, drinks, sets it down, holds with one hand • Helps self-feed
3	• The "me too" age—wants to be included in everything • Responds well to options rather than demands • Sharing still difficult • Somewhat rigid about the "right" way to do things	• Eats most foods, except for certain vegetables • Dawdles over food when not hungry • Comments on how foods are served	• Uses spoon in semiadult fashion; may spear with fork • Medium hand muscle development • Feeds self independently, especially if hungry • Can pour milk and juice and serve individual portions from a serving dish if given instructions
4	• Shares well • Needs adult approval and attention—shows off • Understands; needs limits • Follows rules most of the time • Still rigid about the "right" way to do things	• Eating and talking get in the way—prefers to talk • Strong food likes and dislikes • Refuses to eat, to the point of tears	• Uses all eating utensils • Small-finger muscle development • Can wipe, wash, set table, and pour pre-measured ingredients • Can peel, spread, cut, roll mash foods; cracks eggs
5	• Helpful and cooperative with family chores and routines • Still somewhat rigid about the "right" way to do things • Very attached to parent, home, and family	• Likes familiar foods; prefers most vegetables raw • Latches on to food dislikes of family members and declares these as own	• Fine coordination in fingers and hands • Makes simple breakfast and lunch • Can measure, cut, grind, and grate

Modified from M. Sigman-Grant, "Feeding Preschoolers: Balancing Nutritional and Developmental Needs," *Nutrition Today*, July/August 1992, p. 13. Used with permission.

TABLE 17-5 Food Plan for Preschool and School-Age Children Based on the Food Guide Pyramid

Food Group	No. of Servings	Approximate Serving Size*			
		Age 1–2	Age 3–4	Age 5–6	Age 7–12
Milk, yogurt (cups), and cheese (oz)	3	½–¾ cup or 1 oz	¾ cup or 1½ oz	1 cup or 2 oz	1 cup or 2 oz
Meat, poultry, fish, dry beans, eggs, and nuts	2 or more	1 oz or 1–2 tbsp	1½ oz or 3–4 tbsp	1½ oz or ½ cup	2 oz or ½ cup
Vegetables	3 or more	1–2 tbsp	3–4 tbsp	½ cup	½ cup
Fruit	2 or more	1–2 tbsp or ½ cup juice	3–4 tbsp or ½ cup juice	½ cup or ½ cup juice	½ cup or ½ cup juice
Bread, cereal, rice, and pasta	6 or more	½ slice or ½ cup	1 slice or ½ cup	1 slice or ¾ cup	1 slice or ¾ cup

*Use as a starting point. Increase serving size as energy yields dictate, but maintain variety in the diet by making sure all food groups are still appropriately represented.
Adapted from Food and Nutrition Service, U.S. Department of Agriculture: *Meal pattern requirements and offer versus serve manual*, FNS-265, 1990.

striving toward independence and his or her strong desire to establish routines. Asserting himself or herself about food preferences is a relatively easy way for the child to do this, as this may worsen if parents are too restrictive.[12]

Parents should also be reminded that food likes and dislikes change rapidly in childhood and are influenced by food temperature, appearance, texture, and taste. Sometimes children object to having foods mixed, as in stews and casseroles, even if they normally like the ingredients separately.

In addition, parents should recognize that this is an important age for children to explore the world around them. Even good eaters are sometimes more interested in exploring than eating. There's room for occasional indulgences, a skipped meal or two, or once in a while "less than ideal" choices. It's eating and lifestyle habits over the course of a month and lifetime that matter. Children master their eating when adults provide opportunities to learn, give support for exploration, and limit inappropriate behavior.

"My Child Is Always Snacking, yet She Never Finishes Her Meal"

Children have small stomachs. Offering them six or so small meals succeeds better than limiting them to three meals each day. Sticking to three meals a day offers no special nutritional advantages; it's just a social custom. Snacking is fine, as long as good dental habits are practiced. When we eat isn't nearly as important as what we eat. If nutritious snacks are readily available, these are good to offer at midmorning or midafternoon when the child becomes hungry (Table 17-6). Fruits and vegetables (fresh, frozen, or juice) and whole-grain breads and crackers are good snack

TABLE 17-6   Ideas for Nutritious Snacks and Beverages

Snack	Serving Suggestion	Snack	Serving Suggestion	Snack	Serving Suggestion
Fresh raw vegetables	Serve with a dip of cottage cheese or yogurt blended with dried buttermilk dressing.	Ready-to-eat cereals	Use brands low in sugar and containing fiber; serve with raisins.	Parfait	Make with yogurt, fruit, and granola.
Celery	Spread with peanut butter and sprinkle on raisins, shredded carrots, or finely chopped nuts.	Pita bread	Place sliced meat, cheese, lettuce, and tomato in open pocket.	Gelatin	Add fruit or vegetable juice, vegetables, fruits, or cottage cheese
Bananas	Dip in sweetened yogurt or spread with peanut butter and roll in coconut, chopped nuts, or granola.	English muffins or pita bread	Top with spaghetti sauce, grated cheese, meats; broil or bake and cut in fourths.	Frozen fruit cubes	Freeze puréed applesauce or fruit juice into cubes.
Sliced apples or crackers	Serve with a dip of peanut butter, honey, nuts, raisins, and coconut.	Potato skins	Sprinkle with shredded cheese, broil, and top with yogurt and bacon bits.	Fruit fizz	Add club soda to juice instead of serving soft drinks.
Bagels	Spread with cream cheese or peanut butter and top with chopped bananas, crushed pineapple, or shredded carrots.	Canned chili with beans	Heat and top with onions, lettuce, and tomato; use as dip for Italian or French bread, biscuits, or cornbread.	Fruit shake	Blend milk with fresh fruit (bananas, berries, or a peach) and a dash of cinnamon or nutmeg.
Quick bread or muffins	Make with carrots, zucchini, pumpkin, bananas, nuts, dates, raisins, lemons, squash, or berries.	Kabobs	Make with any combination of fruit, vegetables, and sliced or cubed cooked meat (remove toothpicks before serving).	Yogurt frost	Combine fruit juice and yogurt; add fresh fruit, if desired.
Flour tortillas	Spread with refried beans or canned chili with beans, sprinkle with grated cheese and broil; top with chili sauce.	Popcorn	Serve plain or make 3 quarts and sprinkle with ¼ cup grated cheese and ½ tsp garlic or onion salt.	Hot chocolate	Make hot chocolate or cocoa with milk chocolate and a dash of cinnamon.
				Seeds	Choose shelled sunflower seeds.
				Fish	Put tuna salad on crackers.
				Canned soup	Serve a cup of vegetable or minestrone; nice on a cold winter day.

choices. Working parents should make sure their children are provided with nutritional snacks to tide them over until dinnertime.

When a child refuses to eat, it's best not to overreact. Doing so may give the child the idea that eating is a means of getting attention or manipulating a scene. Most children don't starve themselves to any point approaching physical harm. When children refuse to eat, have them sit at the table for a while; if they still aren't interested in eating, remove the food and wait until the next scheduled meal or snack.

"My Child Never Eats Vegetables"

Children generally eat enough fruit but not an adequate amount of vegetables. Everyone dislikes certain foods. Again, the one-bite policy can be encouraged, including for vegetable servings, and guidelines can be set to discourage fussing over unfamiliar foods. Children eventually learn that they can eat some of a food they don't particularly like without first gagging, choking, and yelling, "Oh, gross!" It takes time for a child to become enthusiastic about a new food; however, with continual exposure and a positive role model, chances are the child may even grow to like it.

Children cannot and should not be forced to eat. They need to develop independence and identities separate from their parents. In other words, children have to choose for themselves—a practice that should be encouraged. No one food is an essential part of a diet. Hunger is still the best means for getting a child to eat. It may be effective to feed children vegetables at the start of a meal, when they are hungriest. Offer new foods with familiar ones. A platter of raw or lightly cooked carrots, broccoli, green and red peppers, cabbage, and mushrooms eaten as a snack with friends can do a lot to remedy a vegetable problem. A 4- or 5-year-old child can safely eat raw vegetables without fear of choking. Recall that children often are more sensitive than adults to strong flavors and odors. Nutritious dips "sell" vegetables to many children. Vegetables may acquire more appeal when children help prepare them. And, as with any food, it is important to remember that children have likes and dislikes, too.

■ Do Children Need a Vitamin/Mineral Supplement?

Major scientific groups, such as the American Dietetic Association and the American Society for Clinical Nutrition, believe that vitamin and mineral supplements are unnecessary for healthy children; it's better to emphasize good foods. Fortified breakfast cereals are especially helpful in closing any gap between current vitamin and mineral intake and needs.[32] Two minerals of particular concern are iron and zinc. These may be lacking in children's diets because they consume such small portions of rich sources, such as animal protein foods. In addition, since the current Dietary Guidelines suggest that children over age 2 years follow a diet low in saturated fat and cholesterol, rich sources of iron and zinc may be lacking in their diets. To compensate, parents can search for a whole-grain breakfast cereal that the child likes that also has at least 50% of the Daily Value for iron and 25% of the Daily Value for zinc. (This will supply sufficient amounts of both nutrients since the Daily Values are based on the higher needs of adults.) If that's not possible, especially for a child who is ill or has a very erratic food preference pattern or appetite, the child may need a nutrient supplement not exceeding 100% of Daily Values on the label, especially if these conditions persist.[27] Diets for children who eat totally vegetarian fare should focus also on protein, vitamin B-12 and iron and zinc. Parents generally offer children conservative amounts of nutrient supplements, so toxicity is unlikely.

If current childhood feeding practices are to become more healthful, the focus should shift from high-fat food choices to lower-fat choices, as well as to the bottom half of the Food Guide or other pyramid shown in Chapter 2, including whole grains, fruits, and vegetables.[11, 16, 31] Caregivers can model this behavior by ordering from the salad bar more often and ordering French fries less often at quick-service restaurants. Children do not need to be severely restricted but, rather, should modify food habits with small changes.[19] Some easy diet changes to begin with are bagels

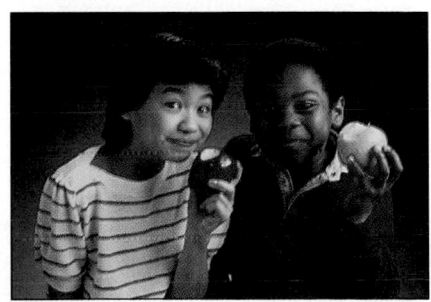

Childhood is an ideal time to begin to enjoy healthful foods.

Chapter 5 noted that it's unlikely that the use of sugar is the cause of hyperactivity or antisocial behavior in most children.

instead of doughnuts, nonfat frozen yogurt instead of ice cream, fat-reduced or 1% milk instead of whole milk, fruit instead of crackers and cheese for snacks, and air-popped popcorn instead of chips.

■ Nutritional Problems in Preschool Children

Three nutrition-related problems found in preschool children are iron deficiency anemia, constipation, and dental caries. Proper diet can help correct or relieve these conditions substantially.

Iron Deficiency Anemia

Childhood iron deficiency anemia is most likely to appear in children between the ages of 6 and 24 months. It can lead to decreases in both stamina and learning ability because the oxygen supply to cells decreases.[9] Another effect is lowered resistance to disease. Fortunately, childhood anemia is fairly uncommon in North America, probably because of children's use of iron-fortified breakfast cereals. Also deserving of credit in the United States is the Special Supplemental Food Program for Women, Infants, and Children (WIC), sponsored by the federal government. This program emphasizes the importance of iron-fortified formulas and cereals and distributes them—along with nutrition education—to low-income parents of infants and preschool children considered to be at nutritional risk.

The best way to prevent iron deficiency anemia in children is to regularly provide foods that are adequate sources of iron. Iron-fortified breakfast cereals and a few ounces of lean meat are convenient means of getting more iron into a child's diet. The high proportion of heme iron in many animal foods allows the iron to be more readily absorbed than is iron from plant foods. Consuming a vitamin C source along with the less readily absorbed iron in plants and supplements aids absorption.

Constipation

Constipation may be associated with another disease, and some young children experience constipation that is unrelated to any medical condition. When presented with a constipated child, a physician first has to rule out a medical cause, such as intestinal blockage. And, although the most common gastrointestinal symptom that reflects intolerance to cow's milk is diarrhea, chronic constipation may also result. This possibility should be investigated by the physician. Treatment for constipation generally consists of first evacuating the bowels, generally with an enema. The promotion of regular bowel habits then follows, with laxative use as directed by the physician. Several months to years of supportive intervention may be required for effective treatment.

Dietary interventions include eating more dietary fiber and drinking more fluids. Foods to emphasize for dietary fiber are fruits, vegetables, whole-grain breads and cereals, and beans. The current daily dietary fiber goal for children between ages 3 and 18 years is the child's age plus 5 g.[24] After age 18 years, typical adult recommendations are appropriate (see Chapter 5). Accompanying fluid recommendations are 5 cups per day for toddlers and up to 9 cups per day for older children.

Dental Caries

A proper diet goes a long way in reducing the risk for dental caries in young children. Earlier it was mentioned that infants are prone to nursing bottle syndrome, which can lead to excessive tooth decay. The following tips can help reduce dental problems in children:
- Begin oral hygiene when teeth start to appear.
- Seek early pediatric dental care.
- Drink fluoridated water.
- Use small amounts of fluoridated toothpaste twice daily.
- Snack in moderation.
- Have a dentist apply tooth sealants if needed.

• If toddlers or preschoolers are chewing gum, sugarless gum is the best choice, as this has been shown to reduce the incidence of dental caries.

Chapters 5 and 12 provide a fuller description of diet and dental health. If needed, these discussions will aid in putting this list of recommendations into perspective.

■ Modifications of Childhood Diets to Reduce Future Disease Risk

Earlier chapters covered the role of diet in development of cardiovascular disease and hypertension and the recommendations concerning diet to reduce the risk for these diseases. Parents sometimes wonder whether similar diet modifications are appropriate and beneficial during childhood.

Diets Designed to Limit Cardiovascular Disease for Children 2 Years of Age and Older

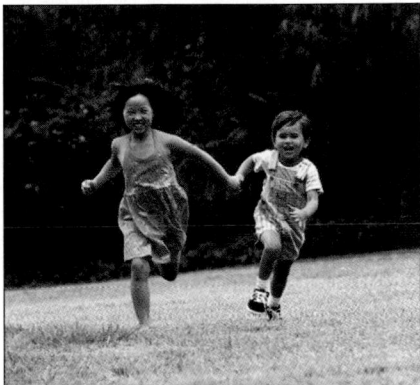

Children benefit from opportunities to be physically active. This contributes to cardiovascular health. The current goal is 60 minutes of such activity each day.

The development of atherosclerosis begins in childhood.[4] As a result, many experts recommend screening for blood cholesterol in children whose families have histories of early development of cardiovascular disease or high blood cholesterol and treating children found to have high blood cholesterol with appropriate diet and drug therapy, as discussed in Chapter 6. With regard to diet, children in the United States currently derive about 33% of their energy from fat, with about 13% of energy from saturated fat. Today, two schools of thought exist with regard to fat intake of children in preschool and later school years. The National Cholesterol Education Program and the Dietary Guidelines suggest that children 2 years and older consume no more than 30% of energy as fat, 10% of energy as saturated fat, and 300 mg of cholesterol.[30] (Note that this is the same recommendation given to adults.) The American Academy of Pediatrics recommends that children eat a similar diet and cautions against including less than 30% of energy as fat. However, other researchers have proposed that fat simply be gradually reduced from about 40% of energy intake in infancy to the 30% figure by either 5 years of age or the time a child's linear growth ceases (at about age 16 to 18 years). Note that, if diets contain about 30% of energy as fat and carefully planned (i.e., they follow the Food Guide Pyramid), normal childhood growth and development can be expected. Parents can choose which path to follow in conjunction with their child's physician. In general, it's unnecessary to discourage children from consuming nutrient-dense foods, such as milk and meat just because they contain some fat. The overriding message is moderation in fat intake.[35]

Salt–Restricted Diets

Scientific data neither confirm nor refute the notion that eating less salt (sodium) reduces the risk of future hypertension. Moderation in salt consumption does help build good health habits for the future—especially if the person later develops hypertension and needs to eat even less salt. If children become accustomed to less salt, they'll be less inclined to eat very salty foods as adults. This reduction in salt also contributes to better calcium retention in the body, as covered in Chapter 11. If a child with hypertension does not respond to diet and lifestyle therapy, typical antihypertensive medications may be used, but at lower doses.

■ Vegetarianism in Childhood

Vegetarian diets pose several risks for young children. These include the possibility of developing iron deficiency anemia, a deficiency of vitamin B-12, and rickets. During the first few years of life, children also may not consume enough energy when following a bulky vegetarian diet. But these known pitfalls are easily avoided by informed diet planning (see the Nutrition Perspective in Chapter 7). Diets for children who eat totally vegetarian fare should focus on protein, vitamin B-12, iron, and zinc content, with additional emphasis on vitamin D (or regular sun exposure) and calcium. Some of these dietary inadequacies can be compensated for by increasing oils, nuts, seeds, and fortified soy milk in the diet.

CONCEPT CHECK

The rapid growth rate of an infant's first year slows during the toddler and preschool years (ages 1 to 5). As a child's appetite decreases, adults need to serve nutrient-dense foods and allow the child to decide how much to eat. Sudden shifts in food preferences are to be expected. Snacking is fine if attention is given to the selection of healthful foods and good dental hygiene. Vitamin and mineral supplements are usually not needed—a plan following the Food Guide Pyramid that includes a serving of fortified breakfast cereal should meet nutrient needs. Children need plenty of iron-rich food to prevent iron deficiency anemia, as well as zinc for growth. Adequate dietary fiber and fluid help prevent constipation. Developing heart-healthy habits after the age of 2 years is advocated by some experts, but highly restrictive diets are not appropriate during childhood. Diets for children who eat totally vegetarian fare should focus on protein, vitamin D (or regular sun exposure), vitamin B-12, calcium, iron, and zinc content.

■ SCHOOL-AGE CHILDREN

In general, the nutritional concerns and goals applicable to school-age children are the same as those discussed in relation to preschoolers. The Food Guide Pyramid (or a related pyramid) continues to be a good basis for diet planning, with an emphasis on moderating fat intake and ensuring adequate iron, zinc, and calcium intake.[16, 18, 35] The only difference is that serving size increases as energy needs increase (review Table 17-5). Dr. Greg Miller discusses why greater attention to calcium intake in this age group is especially important. Now let's look at several other nutritional issues of particular concern during the school-age years.

■ Breakfast, Fat Intake, and Snacks

Once children enter school, their eating patterns become more scheduled, and the consumption of regular meals—especially breakfast—becomes an important focus. Fortified breakfast cereal is known to be the greatest source of iron, vitamin A, and folate for children ages 2 to 18.[32] Although there is controversy over the true benefit of breakfast for cognitive ability, children who eat breakfast likely meet their needs for vitamins and minerals compared to children not eating breakfast. To influence morning test performance, it currently appears that breakfast must be eaten within a few hours of a test; the rise in blood glucose is thought to change performance.[25]

Breakfast menus need not be limited to traditional fare. A little imagination can spark the interest of the most reluctant child. Instead of conventional breakfast foods, parents can offer leftovers from dinner—pizza, spaghetti, soups, yogurt topped with trail mix, chili with beans, or sandwiches, for starters.

Currently, the typical lunch served in school lunch programs contains 38% of total energy as fat. Based on current nutritional trends and changes in guidelines, the fat content of school lunches is expected to decrease to 30% of energy over the next few years.

There is general agreement that the diets of school-age children should include a variety of foods from each major group, not necessarily excluding any specific food because of its fat content.[19] Overemphasis on fat-reduced diets during childhood has been linked to an increase in eating disorders and encourages an inappropriate "good food," "bad food" attitude.

Steering children toward healthful foods, in school and at home, is likely to be more successful if children are exposed to nutrition education. Since children spend much of their younger years in school, it is a great place to learn about positive, healthy eating habits.[7] Such education can help children understand why eating a proper diet will make them feel more energetic, look better, and work more

In a recent survey, 17% of children aged 10 years old said they skip breakfast.

CRITICAL THINKING

Tim refuses to eat breakfast before school. He doesn't like cereal, toast, or any of the other usual breakfast foods. What can Tim's parents do to ensure that he eats nutritious foods before leaving for school?

efficiently. One survey of schoolchildren highlighted the need for nutrition education. On the day of the survey, 40% of the children ate no vegetables, except for potatoes or tomato sauce; 20% ate no fruits; and 75% snacked at least twice. Some 36% of the students ate at least four different types of snack foods. Another study showed that only 2% of about 3300 children 2 to 19 years old had met their recommended servings from all five Food Guide Pyramid groups. Clearly, the diets of many school-age students can stand general improvement, particularly with regard to fruit, vegetable, whole grain, and dairy choices.[16]

▪ Type 2 Diabetes

Type 2 diabetes is generally thought of as an adult condition. As reviewed in the Nutrition Perspective in Chapter 5, it frequently occurs in overweight people who are older than 40. However, recently physicians have noted an alarming increase in the frequency of the disease among children (and teenagers). This is primarily due to the rise in obesity in this age group, coupled with a decrease in physical activity.[3] Up to 85% of children with the disease are overweight at diagnosis. Experts are currently calling for the screening of fasting blood glucose in at-risk children every 2 years, starting at age 10 or the onset of puberty. Besides obesity and a sedentry lifestyle, risk factors include having a first- or second-degree relative with the disease, or belonging to an ethnic (non-Caucasian) population. Appropriate diet and lifestyle intervension should be implemented, along with the use of medications when necessary (see Chapter 5).

▪ Obesity

In the United States, about 25 to 30% of school-age children place above the 85th percentile for BMI and are considered at risk for or overweight, and the number of cases is currently increasing, especially in minority populations. Obesity is generally diagnosed when a child reaches the 95th percentile for BMI and a physical exam indicates the child is truly overfat. This usually is the case for child that reaches this degree of BMI.[3] In the short run, ridicule, embarrassment, and possibly depression are the main consequences of such obesity. In the long run, significant health problems associated with obesity, such as cardiovascular disease, type 2 diabetes, and hypertension, usually don't appear until adulthood. However, an increase in these health-related complications have been noted in children. Childhood obesity is a serious health threat, since about 40% of obese children (and about 80% of obese adolescents) become obese adults. Significant weight gain generally begins between ages 5 and 7, during puberty, or during the teenage years.[20]

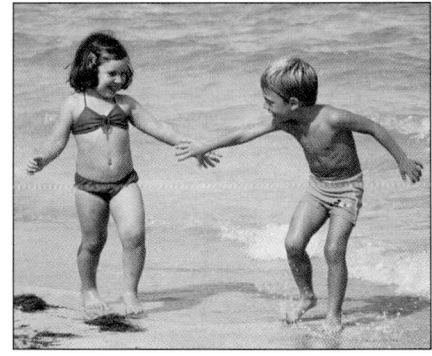

Many children start out life at an appropriate weight-for-height. A goal should be to retain that healthy proportion.

Current research points to many potential causes of childhood obesity. Recall the nature versus nurture discussion in Chapter 13. Some infants are born with lower metabolic rates; they use energy more efficiently and in turn can more easily save energy intake for fat storage. Thus, childhood obesity is linked to heredity. Obesity in children also has a correlation to sibling and maternal obesity. Studies also suggest, though, that this genetic link accounts for only one-third of individual differences in body weight.

Researchers believe that, although diet is still an important factor, inactivity is the key to the increase in childhood obesity.[13] The TV generation now glues itself to the tube for an average of 24 hours a week; many children spend another 10 hours or so playing computer and video games. And three out of every five children aged 12 to 17 have a TV in their bedroom.[29] The American Academy of Pediatrics recommends a limit of 14 hours of TV and computer time per week. In addition, excessive snacking, overreliance on quick-service restaurants, parental neglect, lack of safe areas to play, latchkey conditions, and high-fat/high-energy food choices most likely contribute to childhood obesity.

The initial approach in treating an obese child is to assess how much physical activity he or she engages in. If a child spends much free time in sedentary activities (such as watching television or playing video games), more physical activities should

Expert Opinion

CHILDREN: GOT CALCIUM?

Greg Miller, Ph.D., FACN

Calcium is an essential mineral nutrient responsible for a wide diversity of biological functions. These functions include structural support, cell adhesion, regulation of cell mitosis, blood clotting, nerve impulse transmission, muscle contraction, and glandular secretion. High calcium intake has been associated with reduced risk of osteoporosis, hypertension, premenstrual syndrome (PMS), lead poisoning, kidney stones, and colon cancer.

Adequate intake of dietary calcium is important for obtaining peak bone mass. This is particularly important during adolescence, when the rate of calcium accretion in bone is greatest. Teens achieve about 15% of adult height and 45% of adult skeletal mass during these prime bone-building years. Approximately 90 to 95% of bone acquisition is completed by 18 years of age, with a further 10 to 15% by about age 30–35 years. The age at which peak bone mass is attained depends on the bone site.

Government and health professional organizations have made recommendations for calcium intake. The Food and Nutrition Board of the National Academy of Sciences (NAS) has established Dietary Reference Intakes for calcium for Americans and Canadians. NAS has recommended daily intakes of 500 mg for children 1–3, 800 mg for children 4–8, 1300 mg for children 9–18, 1000 mg for adults 19–50, and 1200 mg for adults 50+ years of age.

The NAS calcium intake recommendations for children were based on a thorough review of data from epidemiological studies, randomized control trials, and balance studies. Results from epidemiological studies and randomized control trials indicated that calcium intakes greater than 1000 mg/day are needed by adolescents to avoid low bone mass. However, these data did not allow for an accurate quantitative assessment of calcium needs to maximize the bone health of adolescents. The calcium intake that produces maximal calcium retention in bone, as measured by balance studies, provided the strongest assessment for determining calcium requirements for adolescents. Research out of Dr. Connie Weaver's laboratory at Purdue University has indicated that a calcium intake of 1300 mg per day is the lowest intake that adolescent girls should consume if they are to achieve maximal calcium retention. This calcium requirement is in agreement with values using a factorial approach. This method sums calcium needs for bone accretion plus calcium losses (urine, feces, and sweat) while adjusting for degree of absorption.

Calcium deficiency is one of the chronic nutrition problems in the United States, and the lack of calcium begins in childhood. Approximately 30% of all children under age 5 fall short of recommendations, and more than half of children 6 to 11 fail to get the calcium they need. According to the 1988–1991 National Health and Nutrition Examination survey III (NHANES III) data, after age 11 the average female fails to meet recommendations for calcium intake. According to data from the United States Department of Agriculture's (USDA) Continuing Survey of Food Intakes by Individuals, two out of three Americans are not meeting calcium intake recommendations. USDA data indicate that roughly 9 out of 10 teen girls and 7 out of 10 teen boys are not meeting recommended intakes for calcium.

To achieve optimal calcium intakes, health professional organizations have recommended foods naturally containing calcium as the preferred source and that fortified foods and supplements be considered secondary sources. It has been demonstrated that diets low in calcium are low in many other essential nutrients, such as riboflavin, vitamin A, vitamin B-12, vitamin B-6, potassium, and magnesium. Thus, low calcium intake reflects a poor dietary pattern. Research findings have demonstrated that individuals who in-

be encouraged.[3] Both the federal government and health professionals recommend 60 minutes or more of moderate to intense physical activity per day for children and adolescents. An overall active lifestyle will help children not only to attain a healthy body weight but also to keep a similar body weight later in life. An increase in physical activity won't just happen; parents need to plan for it. Two good ideas are getting the family together for a brisk walk after dinner and finding an after-school sport the child enjoys.

Moderation in energy intake is important, especially the limitation of high-fat and high-energy foods, such as sugar-laden carbonated beverages and high-fat milk. The focus should be on more nutrient-dense foods and healthy snacks.[28]

crease their calcium intake through foods rich in this nutrient (e.g., dairy foods), rather than pills, increase their intake of many other nutrients as well, including protein, carbohydrate, magnesium, phosphorus, potassium, zinc, vitamin D, thiamin, and riboflavin.

Milk and other dairy foods are the major source of calcium in the United States, providing three-quarters of the calcium available in the U.S. food supply. In addition to being good sources of calcium, milk and other dairy foods are good sources of protein, vitamin A, vitamin B-6, vitamin D, riboflavin, potassium, magnesium, and phosphorus. USDA data from 1997 indicate that dairy foods contributed approximately 72% of the calcium, 32% of the phosphorus, 26% of the riboflavin, 22% of the vitamin B-12, 18% of the potassium, 19% of the protein, 16% of the magnesium, 16% of the zinc, 15% of the vitamin A, and 9% of the vitamin B-6 to the U.S. food supply. Research indicates that some of these nutrients may have health benefits that could be synergistic to calcium. As examples, vitamin D is important for good bone health; vitamins A and D may help reduce the risk of some forms of cancer; and potassium and magnesium may help reduce the risk of hypertension.

Inadequate intake of dairy foods is an important contributor to low calcium intake. USDA data indicate that the average consumption of dairy foods in the United States is about 1.5 servings, well below the recommended 3 servings for children, teenagers, and young adults. Boys 6–11 years of age consume about 2 servings a day, whereas those 12–19 have 2.5 servings. Girls 6–11 consume 1.8 servings per day, whereas those 12–19 have 1.5 servings. An analysis of USDA dietary intake data from 1965 to 1966 of individuals 11–18 years of age found that milk consumption decreased by 36%, whereas consumption of soft drinks and fruit drinks increased. Other studies have provided similar observations indicating that milk consumption may be displaced by other, less nutritious beverage choices, and loss of calcium intake is not being made up by the consumption of other dairy or calcium-rich foods.

Many young girls and women tend to avoid dairy products because of their concerns about fat and energy intake. However, recent studies have shown that adolescent girls and adults can consume at least 1400 mg of calcium per day, mainly through dairy foods, without negatively impacting weight gain, percentage body fat, or blood lipids while enhancing the nutritional quality of their diets. Newer data also indicate that women who consume adequate amounts of calcium with a moderate calorie intake can lose a significant amount of weight as body fat. The effect was strongest in women who obtained their calcium from dairy foods. Animal data indicate that the high calcium intake may be altering fat metabolism, such that fat is more readily used for energy and less likely to be stored as body fat.

Although calcium-fortified foods may be used to ensure adequate intake, this approach may fail to improve overall nutrient intake to the same extent as consuming foods that naturally contain calcium. Supplementation with calcium pills should be used only as a last alternative to increasing calcium intake. The use of calcium supplementation has many inherent limitations: a higher potential for calcium overconsumption, compared with calcium-containing foods; adverse interactions with other minerals; undesirable side effects (e.g., constipation, bloating); potential contamination with heavy metals; the need for a high degree of motivation to maintain intake; and a failure to correct poor dietary habits.

Health professionals need to promote dietary patterns that can be easily implemented to close the gap between the current calcium intakes of Americans and the recommended levels. Until calcium consumption reaches recommended levels, Americans can expect to experience a growing incidence of calcium deficiency–related chronic diseases.

Dr. Miller is vice president, nutrition research for the National Dairy Council. He has written and lectured extensively on the subject of diet and nutrition, especially with regard to calcium.

Resorting to a weight-loss diet is usually not necessary. As a start, it's best to emphasize changing habits. Children have an advantage over adults in dealing with obesity; their bodies can use stored energy for growth. Thus, if weight gain can be moderated, increases in height and resulting lean body tissue may reduce the percentage of body weight accounted for as stored fat, yielding a more healthful weight-to-height ratio. This is one reason it's desirable to treat obesity in childhood. Further growth can contribute to success.

If a child will still be obese after attaining ultimate adult height, a weight-loss regimen may be necessary. This is especially appropriate after the adolescent growth spurt. Weight loss should be gradual, perhaps ½ lb per week. If weight loss is

Unfortunately, fewer than half of all U.S. children engage in enough physical activity to benefit their health (60 minutes on most days). To get kids involved in exercise, new physical education classes have been introduced into schools. These classes provide lifelong fitness lessons, such as in rock climbing, in-line skating, and recreational jogging. These classes help promote activity because they take the focus away from teams and competition, which often discourage and embarrass kids who lack athletic talent.[13]

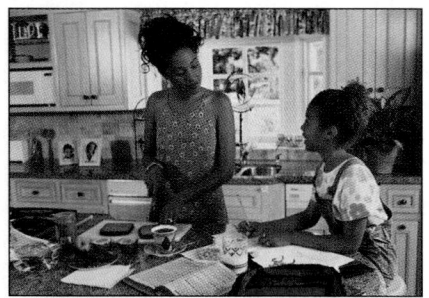

Nutrition education ideally begins in the home as parents and other caregivers provide a healthy, well-balanced diet.

A strictly vegetarian diet must be monitored for adequate energy, protein, iron, vitamin B-12, calcium, and vitamin D. This becomes particularly important in teenagers, as their diets are often already compromised.

necessary in younger children, the child should be watched closely to ensure that the rate of growth continues to be normal. The child's energy intake shouldn't be so low that gains in height diminish.[20]

Obese children often need to find a new way to relate to foods, especially snack foods. An important family rule could be that children are allowed to eat only while sitting at the dining table or in the kitchen. This could stop endless hours of snacking in front of the television and make all family members more conscious of when they are eating. It also might be helpful to put portions of snack foods on plates, rather than allow snacking to go on indefinitely, as often happens when children eat directly from a full box of crackers or cookies.

A child's self-esteem is extremely fragile. Obesity itself affects the child's psyche. Humiliation doesn't work; it only makes the child feel worse. Support, admiration, and encouragement of the child's efforts at weight control are more effective and should be emphasized.

Finally, it is important to understand that not all children are designed to look like society's ideal. In other words, some children simply weigh more than others. A healthful lifestyle with plenty of physical activity and nutritious foods remains the key concern.

CONCEPT CHECK

The school-age child is advised to follow the Food Guide Pyramid (or a related pyramid), moderating choices high in fat and simple sugars. Breakfast is an important meal to refuel the body for a new school day and to help ensure fulfilling nutrient needs for the day. Attention to regular physical activity and healthy diet should help prevent/treat childhood obesity and build a desirable lifestyle pattern for later life.

THE TEENAGE YEARS

Most girls begin a rapid growth spurt between the ages of 10 and 13, and most boys experience rapid growth between the ages of 12 and 15. Nearly every organ in the body grows during these periods. Most noticeable are increases in height and weight and the development of secondary sexual characteristics. Girls usually begin menstruating (reach menarche) during this growth spurt, and they grow very little beyond 2 years after menarche. Early-maturing girls may begin their growth spurt as early as age 7 to 8, whereas early-maturing boys may begin growing by age 9 to 10.

TABLE 17-7 Food Plan for Teenagers Based on the Food Guide Pyramid*

Food Category	Minimum Number of Daily Servings†
Milk, yogurt, and cheese (preferably low fat or nonfat)	3
Meat, poultry, fish, dry beans, eggs, and nuts	2–3
Vegetables	3–5
Fruit	2–4
Bread, cereal, rice, and pasta (preferably whole grain; otherwise, enriched or fortified)	6–11
Fats, oils, and sweets	Use sparingly.

*Here we define "teenager" as a person who has some gain in height in the past year and is at least 12 years old.
This food plan is applicable through age 18 years.
†Use same serving size as for adults (see Table 2-6 in Chapter 2).

During the growth spurt, girls gain about 10 in (25 cm) in height, and boys gain about 12 in (30 cm). Girls also tend to accumulate both lean and fat tissue, whereas boys tend to gain mostly lean tissue. This growth spurt provides about 50% of ultimate adult weight and about 15% of ultimate adult height (review Fig. 17-1).

As the growth spurt begins, teenagers begin to eat more. If teens choose nutritious food, they can take advantage of their increased hunger and easily satisfy their nutrient needs. As with older age groups, the Food Guide Pyramid can provide the basis for meeting these nutrient needs, with the major difference being three servings of milk and milk products (Table 17-7).

■ Nutritional Problems and Concerns of Teens

Anorexia nervosa and bulimia nervosa were covered in detail in Chapter 15. Other nutritional problems are more common during the teen years. A survey of high school students showed that only a little over 25% had eaten five servings of fruits and vegetables on the previous day. At the same time, the dietary fat content of teenagers is three to four percentage points higher than suggested amounts, and they are consuming approximately 25% more sodium than recommended. Another concern is that many teenage girls stop drinking milk, so they may not consume enough calcium to allow for maximal mineralization of bones through their early 20s.[18] Young women who don't consume enough calcium are likely to develop osteoporosis later, as discussed in Chapter 11.

The Adequate Intake for calcium for both males and females between ages 9 and 18 years is 1300 mg per day, compared with 800 mg per day for younger children. Unfortunately, most teenage girls do not consume the Adequate Intake for calcium. Three servings per day from the milk, yogurt, and cheese group are recommended for all teenagers and young adults.

A further concern is iron deficiency. Iron deficiency anemia sometimes appears in girls after they start menstruating (menarche) and in boys during their growth spurt. About 10% of teenagers have low iron stores or related anemia. Teens who strive to forge an identity by adopting dietary patterns unfamiliar to their families—vegetarianism, for example—may not know enough about the alternate diet pattern to keep from developing health problems, such as iron deficiency anemia. It's important that teenagers choose good food sources of iron, such as lean meats, whole grains, and enriched cereals. Teenage girls, particularly those with heavy menstrual flows, need to eat good sources of iron (or regularly consume an iron supplement). Iron deficiency anemia is a highly undesirable condition for a teen. It can produce increased fatigue and decreased ability to concentrate and learn. School and physical performance may suffer.

Acne is a common teen concern—about 80% of teens experience it. Although it's popularly believed that eating nuts, chocolate, and pizza can make acne worse, scientific studies have failed to show a strong link between any dietary factor and acne. It is important to note that many acne medications contain analogs of vitamin A. Although these treatments can be quite effective, the close supervision by a physician is crucial as these vitamin A analogs can be toxic. Vitamin A itself is no help in treating acne, and excess amounts of vitamin A or related analogs can cause birth defects. Thus, girls taking these vitamin A medications should not become pregnant.

■ A Closer Look at the Diets of Teenage Girls

Teenagers in general are apt to adopt fad diets, eat away from home or miss meals completely, and snack a lot. Teenage girls especially are very concerned with weight gain, appearance, and social acceptance. Government statistics reveal that female students are significantly more likely to report currently trying to lose weight (44%) than male students (15%). Moreover, 27% of female students who considered themselves the right weight report they were currently trying to lose weight. It is important to inform teenage girls that weight gain in the form of increased body fat is to be expected in the adolescent growth spurt.

Drinking soft drinks in place of milk causes many teenagers to have inadequate calcium intake. Because soft drinks are rich in phosphorus, this practice produces an imbalance in the intakes of calcium and phosphorus, a pattern that fails to promote optimal bone development, and it has been linked to increased bone fractures in this age group.

Free to Be Me is a Girl Scout badge program focusing on helping girls feel good about their bodies. It is designed to decrease unhealthy weight-control behaviors, but the benefits to date have been minimal. Peers and the media are stronger influences.

*A*lcoholism, a significant health problem that may have its roots in the teen years, is covered in detail in Chapter 8. Smoking—another habit that compromises health—also often begins in teen years and is currently increasing in this age group. Some of this is in an attempt to control body weight—not an advisable method.

*C*linicians who work with teenagers, including physicians, registered dietitians, and nurses, need to be prepared to discuss and deal with a variety of concerns: sports nutrition, eating disorders, use of steroids, and drug (and alcohol) abuse. Except for substance abuse, these topics usually are not a concern when working with older adult clients.

In an attempt to reach personal goals, teenage girls may eat dangerously little, select just a few items, and frequently skip meals altogether. If their limited food choices then consist of French fries, soft drinks, and pastries, little room is left for foods that are good nutrient sources. Another common practice among teenage girls is having a fat phobia, focusing primarily on foods that are fat-free. However, many teens may not realize that some fat is essential for body functions, thus emphasizing the need for some fat in the diet. This concept is discussed in Chapter 6. The diets of teenage girls often lack adequate sources of folate, calcium, zinc, and vitamins A and C.[23] The common use of diet pills and the increasing number of bulimia nervosa cases further add to these nutritional problems.

■ Helping Teens Eat More Nutritious Foods

Teenagers face a variety of challenges. They pursue their independence, experience identity crises, seek peer acceptance, and worry about physical appearance. All of these factors affect food choice. Advertisers take advantage of this by pushing a vast array of products—candy, gum, soft drinks, and snacks—at the teenage market. Potato chips and French fries make up more than one-third of the vegetable servings consumed by teens. Additionally, many schools offer French fries on a regular basis, and soft drink machines can be found in school hallways and cafeterias, in turn competing with the school lunch.

Teens often don't think about the long-term benefits of good health. They have a hard time relating today's actions to tomorrow's health outcomes. Many teenagers tend to think they can just change habits later; there's no hurry.

Still, healthful teen food habits don't have to include giving up favorite foods. Small portions of fatty foods can complement larger portions of nonfat and low-fat dairy products, lean meats, vegetable proteins, fruits, vegetables, and grain products. An example is a plain hamburger with a garden salad (minimize the amount of regular dressing or use a low-fat variety) and a small order of French fries or chili.

■ Overcoming the Teenage Mind-Set

One strategy for working with teenage boys is to stress the importance of nutrition and physical activity for physical development—especially muscular development—and for fitness, vigor, and health. With teenage girls, one approach is to help them understand how to choose nutrient-dense foods and activities that lead to better health while maintaining a healthy weight. For teenagers, it's more effective to focus on the benefits of healthful foods and regular physical activity they can reap right now than to talk about health hazards that may or may not happen later.[22]

■ Are Teenage Snacking Practices Harmful?

Teens often obtain one-fourth to one-third of all their energy and major nutrients from snacks. Unfortunately, studies have found just what you might expect—that teens snack mostly on potato and corn chips, cookies, candies, and ice cream. Key reasons for snacking include an opportunity to get out and socialize with friends, accessibility, hunger, and celebration of a special event. Teenagers can obtain many nutrients from snacking. Even quick-service restaurants offer some good food choices. By choosing wisely and eating in moderation, teens can eat at quick-service restaurants and still consume a very healthful diet. Snacks and quick-service restaurants themselves are not the problem; poor food choices are.

Poor dietary habits formed during teenage years often continue into adulthood, giving rise to an increased risk of chronic diseases, such as cardiovascular disease, osteoporosis, and some types of cancer. Getting this message across to teenagers is an important and challenging task for parents and health professionals.

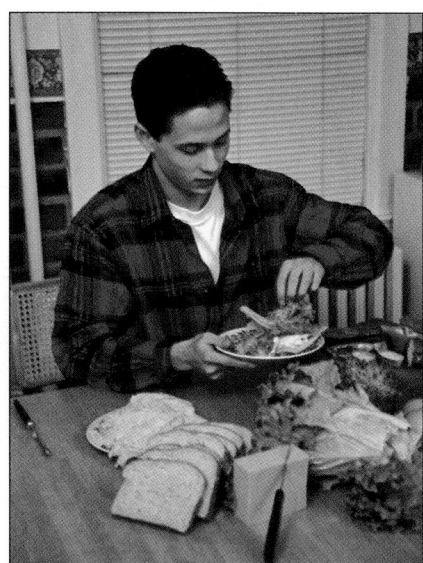

The teenage years are noted for snacking. With reasonable food choices, teenagers can have healthful diets.

CONCEPT CHECK

A second period of rapid growth occurs during the teen years. Girls generally start this growth spurt earlier than boys. The Food Guide Pyramid should guide meal planning. Common nutritional problems in these years arise from poor food choices and include inadequate calcium intake in girls, iron deficiency anemia, and sometimes excessive intake of total fat and saturated fat. Because changes occur so rapidly during these years, and in so many areas—psychological, social, and physical—it may be difficult to stress the importance of nutrition to teenagers. Moderation in fat intake is one goal to consider when choosing snacks.

*C*heck out the *Perspectives in Nutrition* Online Learning Center http://www.mhhe.com/wardlaw for quizzes, flash cards, other activities, and web links designed to further help you learn about issues surrounding nutrition from infancy through adolescence.

SUMMARY

1. Growth is very rapid during infancy; birth weight doubles in 4 to 6 months, and length increases by 50% in the first year. An adequate diet, especially in terms of energy, as well as the nutrients protein and zinc, is essential to support normal growth. Undernutrition can cause irreversible changes in growth and development. Growth in infants and children can be assessed by measuring body weight, height (or length), and head circumference over time. Growth charts have recently been revised to include a more valid measurement for determining children's growth, body mass index (BMI).

2. Nutrient needs in the first 6 months can be met by human milk or iron-fortified infant formula. Supplementary vitamin D and iron may be needed in the first 6 months for breastfed infants, and many infants may need supplemental fluoride after 6 months of age.

3. Infant formulas generally contain lactose or sucrose, heat-treated proteins from cow's milk, and vegetable oil. These formulas may or may not be fortified with iron. Sanitation is very important when preparing and storing formula.

4. Most infants don't need solid foods before about 4 to 6 months of age. Solid food should not be added to an infant's diet until the nutrients are needed, the GI tract can digest complex foods, the infant has the physical ability to control tongue thrusting, and the risk of developing food allergies has decreased.

5. The first solid food given should be iron-fortified infant cereals or ground meats. Other single foods can be added gradually, at the rate of about one each week. Some foods to avoid giving infants in the first year include honey, cow's milk (especially fat-reduced varieties), very salty or sweet foods, and foods that may cause choking.

6. Introducing iron-containing solid food at the appropriate time and not offering cow's milk until 1 year of age can generally prevent iron deficiency anemia in late infancy.

7. A slower growth rate in preschool years underlies the importance of children's eating nutrient-dense foods and reducing their food serving sizes. Choosing iron-rich foods, such as lean red meats, is important at this age. Portion sizes at meals of 1 tablespoon of each food for each year of life is a good rule of thumb for vegetables, fruits, and meats.

8. Preschoolers should be given some leeway in determining serving size and should be encouraged to try new foods. Highly restrictive diets designed to reduce the risk of cardiovascular disease or hypertension are not recommended for preschoolers or older children, unless prescribed by a physician.

9. Obese children and adolescents are more likely to become obese adults and, so, incur greater health risks. Parents can provide healthful food choices, and children should control portion sizes. When controlled early through diet and exercise interventions, a problem of obesity may correct itself as the child continues to grow in height.

10. During the adolescent growth spurt, both boys and girls have increased needs for iron and calcium. Inadequate calcium intake by teenage girls is a major concern because it can set the stage for the development of osteoporosis later in life. Teenagers generally should moderate their intake of high-fat foods—especially snacks and quick-service foods, which they often consume in abundance—and perform regular physical activity.

STUDY QUESTIONS

1. List two factors that limit "catch-up" growth in adulthood when a nutrient-deficient diet has been consumed throughout childhood.

2. Describe how you would assess whether an 8-month-old infant is consuming a healthful diet.

3. Outline three key factors that help determine when to introduce solid foods into an infant's diet.

4. A 3-month-old infant is taken to a clinic with failure to thrive. What are two possible explanations?

700   NUTRITION APPLICATIONS AND THE LIFE CYCLE   http://www.mhhe.com/wardlaw

5. List three reasons why preschoolers are noted for fussy eating. For each, describe an appropriate parent response.

6. What three factors are likely to contribute to obesity in a typical 10-year-old child?

7. Compare the guidelines for infant feeding summarized in the chapter with the Dietary Guidelines for children over 2 and adults discussed in Chapter 2. Which guidelines are similar? Do any contradict each other? If so, why?

8. Describe three pros and cons of snacking. What is the basic advice for healthful snacking from childhood through the teenage years?

9. Which two nutrients are of particular concern in planning diets for teenagers? Why does each deserve to be singled out?

10. List three nutrients of concern for a teenage vegetarian.

■ ANNOTATED REFERENCES

1. ADA Reports: Position of the American Dietetic Association: Dietary guidance for healthy children aged 2 to 11 years. *Journal of the American Dietetic Association* 99:93, 1999.

   Children older than 2 years of age should gradually adopt a diet by the age of 5 that reflects a lifelong healthy, nutrient-rich dietary pattern. The health status of U.S. children generally has improved over the past three decades; however, the number of children who are overweight has more than doubled.

2. Anderson RE and others: Relationship of physical activity and television watching with body weight and level of fatness among children. *Journal of the American Medical Association* 279:983, 1998.

   A relationship among television watching, physical activity, and body composition exists. Children with higher body mass index tend to watch more television than do their thinner peers. Next to sleeping, the greatest amount of leisure time for youngsters is spent watching television. It would be better for more of this time to be spent in physical activity.

3. Bellizzi MC, Dietz WH: Workshop on childhood obesity: Summary of the discussion. *American Journal of Clinical Nutrition* 70:173S, 1999.

   Early identification of childhood obesity is key in preventing obesity and health-related complications in later adulthood. Body mass index in children 2 years and older is favorable to other methods for assessing weight status.

4. Berenson GS and others: Association between multiple cardiovascular risk factors and atherosclerosis in children in young adults. *New England Journal of Medicine* 338:1650, 1998.

   As the number of cardiovascular risk factors increase in children, so does the severity of atherosclerosis. Interventions related to the risk factors, such as prevention of smoking, weight control, encouragement of physical exercise, and a prudent diet—if undertaken early in life, retard the development of atherosclerosis.

5. Bronner YL and others: Early introduction of solid foods among urban African-American participants in WIC. *Journal of the American Dietetic Association* 99:457, 1999.

   Current recommendations for infant feeding indicate that solid food should be withheld until 4 to 6 months of age. Unfortunately, by 7 to 10 days after birth, approximately a third of infants in this study were receiving some nonmilk liquids or solids, and by 8 weeks this increased to over three-quarters of infant. Early introduction of solid foods in this population was associated more with formula feeding than with breastfeeding.

6. Carroll JL: SIDS: Counseling parents to reduce the risk. *American Family Physician* 57:1566, 1998.

   The following guidelines exist to reduce the risk of sudden infant death syndrome: place sleeping babies on their backs, avoid exposure to cigarette smoke, breastfeed as opposed to bottle-feed, and provide a safe environment to sleep (no loose bedding).

7. Celebuski C, Farris E: Nutrition education in public elementary school classrooms, K–5. *CNI Nutrition Week*, p. 4, April 7, 2000.

   USDA encourages school meal programs to provide nutrition education to students. Most teachers reported that they taught nutrition lessons to their students, but generally not much class time was devoted to this topic.

8. Chidley E: Soy formula: Good or bad for babies. *Today's Dietitian* 26:28, 1999.

   Soy formula contains isoflavones. These may be linked to developmental delay in boys, precocious puberty in girls, and other hormonal problems. Thus, soy formulas should be used only when children have demonstrated intolerance to milk-based commercial formulas.

9. Cohen AR: Choosing the best strategy to prevent childhood iron deficiency. *Journal of the American Medical Association* 281:2247, 1999.

   Although there has been a decline in the prevalence of childhood iron deficiency in the United States, studies indicate that children who were diagnosed with the problem between the ages of 1 and 2 years were behind their peers in both mental and motor development. Targeted screening of iron status is important in younger children.

10. Dennison BA and others: Children's growth parameters vary by type of fruit juice consumed. *Journal of the American College of Nutrition* 18:346, 1999.

    Fruit juice consumption has increased over the past 40 years due to availability, convenience, and child's preference. Excessive fruit juice consumption by children—especially apple juice—has been linked with obesity, short stature, failure to thrive, and poor dental health. Parents should monitor the total amount of fruit juice consumed and make sure that use is not excessive.

11. Dennison BA and others: Fruit and vegetable intake in young children. *Journal of the American College of Nutrition* 17:371, 1998.

    Many preschool-age children meet the current recommendations for fruit intake but do not meet the recommended servings for vegetable intake. Low intake of vegetables is associated with inadequate intakes of vitamin A, vitamin C, and dietary fiber, in addition to high intakes of total fat and saturated fat. Serving vegetables several times a day and serving more than one type at a meal are ways to increase children's consumption of vegetables.

12. Fisher JO, Birth LL: Restricting access to palatable foods affects children's behavioral response, food selection, and intake. *American Journal of Clinical Nutrition* 69:1264, 1999.

    Greatly restricting fatty and sugary foods from children may appeal to parents; however, children often then crave and seek these forbidden foods more than they would if the foods were routinely available.

13. Ganley T, Sherman C: Exercise and children's health: A little counseling can pay lasting dividends. *The Physician and Sportsmedicine* 26(2):85, 2000.

    Despite the growing epidemic of childhood obesity and related health complications, nearly half of the children in the United States are not involved in regular activity sufficient for cardiovascular fitness. It is important for children—with the help of parents—to find activities that are interesting, enjoyable, and appropriate for their age and physical abilities. The goal of safe, enjoyable exercise is readily attainable by virtually all youngsters.

14. Gillman MW and others: Family dinner and diet quality among older children and adolescents. *Archives of Family Medicine* 9:235, 2000.

    Among children and adolescents, eating dinner with the family was associated with helpful dietary intake patterns, including the intake of more fruits and vegetables, fewer fried foods and soft drinks, less saturated and trans fatty acid intake, lower glycemic load, and more fiber and micronutrients from food. Generally, as children mature into adolescence, fewer meals are eaten with other family members.

15. Guo SS and others: The revised U.S. national growth charts. *Nutrition & the M.D.*, p. 1, July 1999.

The use of the latest growth charts, which use body mass index for children 2 years and older, helps identify overweight and obesity, as well as the potential risk for children to become overweight. The early indication of these problems can help parents and physicians in preventing worsening of the condition, and may help contribute to treatment.

16. Hampl JS and others: Intakes of vitamin C, vegetables, and fruits: Which school children are at risk? *Journal of the American College of Nutrition* 81:582, 1999.

A considerable number of children underconsume vitamin C and the recommended amount of vegetables and fruits. Overall, children with adequate vitamin C intakes had healthier diets. Health professionals should promote at least five daily servings of vegetables and fruits, with at least one serving rich in vitamin C.

17. Holst MC: Developmental and behavioral effects of iron deficiency anemia in infants. *Nutrition Today* 33(1):27, 1998.

Iron deficiency is probably the most common nutrition deficiency in childhood. Its effects can be long-lasting; there is evidence for direct central nervous system changes related to iron deficiency. This disease can be prevented, and it is important to do so if children are to attain their full development and behavioral potential.

18. McBean LD: Preventing osteoporosis: Starting in childhood. *Dairy Council Digest* 70:25, 1999.

Many factors influence calcium intake, including beverage and food choices, exercise, and meal skipping. An inadequate calcium intake during childhood has been linked to osteoporosis later in life. Currently, about 9 out of 10 teenage girls and 7 out of 10 teenage boys do not meet their daily calcium needs.

19. McBean LD, Miller GD: Enhancing the nutrition of America's youth. *Journal of the American College of Nutrition* 18:563, 1999.

Today, children's diets are out of balance with the Food Guide Pyramid recommendations. Dietary guidance should be conducive to consuming a variety of helpful foods in moderation, not food restrictions, and encouraging physical activity in children.

20. Moran R: Evaluation and treatment of childhood obesity. *American Family Physician* 59:861, 1999.

There are many causative factors attributed to the prevalence of childhood obesity. However, only a small percentage of factors can be associated with genetic or hormonal conditions. Treatment

should be initiated when the trend in increasing weight obviously surpasses the trend in increasing height, based on plotting children on growth charts.

21. Morey SS: CDC issues guidelines for prevention, detection and treatment of iron deficiency. *American Family Physician* 58:1475, 1998.

The Centers for Disease Control and Prevention recommends at least two servings of iron-fortified cereal a day, starting at age 4 to 6 months to prevent iron deficiency. To improve iron absorption, a daily serving of a food rich in vitamin C is recommended, starting at 6 months of age.

22. Neumark-Sztainer D and others: Factors influencing food choices of adolescents: Findings from focus-group discussions with adolescents. *Journal of the American Dietetic Association* 99:929, 1999.

Nutritional needs during adolescence are higher than at any other time in life due to the increased need for growth and development. Thus, adolescents should strive to make nutritious choices regarding their diet. One approach could be nutrition education to make it "cool" to eat healthfully.

23. Neumark-Sztainer D and others: Lessons learned about adolescent nutrition from the Minnesota Adolescent Health Survey. *Journal of the American Dietetic Association* 98:1449, 1998.

Adolescents typically have inadequate intakes of fruits, vegetables, and dairy products. Unhealthful weight-control practices and overweight status are also common. The challenge lies in the development of interventions that are effective in increasing motivation among youth and in decreasing barriers to eating a healthful diet and being physically active.

24. Picciano MF: How to grow a healthy child: A conference report. *Nutrition Today* 34(1):6, 1999.

Since children are not small adults, they require a separate list of dietary guidelines to meet their needs. For example, The American Health Foundation recommends that a child's dietary fiber intake equal his or her age plus 5 grams a day. Overall, caregivers should help children learn to enjoy a variety of nutritious foods and to appreciate the importance of regular physical activity.

25. Pollitt E: Breakfast and cognition: An integrative summary. *American Journal of Clinical Nutrition* 67:804S, 1998.

Skipping breakfast is linked with short-term metabolic and cognitive effects, along with reduced physical growth and cognitive development in adolescence. The effect is more pronounced in nutritionally at-risk children than in well-nourished children.

26. Rask-Nissila L and others: Neurological development of five-year-old children receiving a low saturated fat, low cholesterol diet since in-

fancy. *Journal of the American Medical Association* 284:993, 2000.

Diets containing 30 to 35% of daily energy as fat and low in saturated fat and cholesterol implemented at 7 months of age were shown to be a safe intervention. Neurological development was not affected by such a diet, and blood cholesterol was below that found in infants and children not following such an intervention.

27. Roberts SB, Heyman MB: Micronutrient shortfalls in young children's diets: Common, and owing to inadequate intakes both at home and at child care centers. *Nutrition Reviews* 58(1):27, 2000.

Although not currently supported by The American Academy of Pediatrics, the routine use of a multivitamin and mineral supplement may be needed to help young children in meeting their nutrient needs. This can be especially helpful for meeting iron and zinc needs, two nutrients that may be lacking in children's diets because they consume such small portions of rich sources, such as animal protein foods. In addition, since the current Dietary Guidelines for Americans suggest that children over age 2 years follow a diet low in saturated fat and cholesterol, rich sources of iron and zinc may be lacking in their diets. Fortified breakfast cereals are another potential source of these nutrients.

28. Robertson SM and others: Factors related to adiposity among children aged 3 to 7 years. *Journal of the American Dietetic Association* 99:938, 1999.

Most children who are overweight at ages 3 to 7 years follow high-fat diets. Targeting a heart-healthy diet at young ages increases the chance for a child to maintain an acceptable weight.

29. Robinson TN: Reducing children's television viewing to prevent obesity. *Journal of the American Medical Association* 282:1561, 1999.

Reducing television, videotape, and video game use may be a promising, population-based approach to preventing childhood obesity. Even a small shift downward in the population distribution of adiposity would be expected to have large effects on obesity-related morbidity and mortality.

30. Shamir R, Fisher EA: Dietary therapy for children with hypercholesterolemia. *American Family Physician* 61:675, 2000.

Recommendations by the National Cholesterol Education Program include low-fat dietary habits for children displaying high blood cholesterol (hypercholesterolemia). However, the total fat intake for these children (as well as adolescents) should not be less than 20% of total calories per day. In addition, if such a low-fat diet is used, a dietitian should be consulted to help manage this dietary intervention in order to make sure it remains otherwise adequate for normal growth and development.

31. Skinner JD and others: Longitudinal study of nutrient and food intakes of white preschool

TakeAction

I. GETTING YOUNG BILL TO EAT

Bill is 3 years old, and his mother is worried about his eating habits. He absolutely refuses to eat vegetables, meat, and dinner in general. Some days he eats very little food. He wants to eat snacks most of the time. His mother wants him to eat a sit-down lunch and dinner to make sure he gets all the nutrients he needs. Mealtime is a battle because Bill says he isn't hungry, but his mother wants him to eat everything served on his plate. He drinks five or six glasses of whole milk per day because that is the one food he likes.

When his mother prepares dinner, she makes plenty of vegetables, boiling them until they are soft, hoping this will appeal to Bill. Bill's dad waits to eat his vegetables last, regularly telling the family that he eats them only because he has to. He also regularly complains about how dinner has been prepared. Bill saves his vegetables until last and usually gags when his mother orders him to eat them. Bill has been known to sit at the dinner table for an hour until the war of wills ends. Bill's mother serves casseroles and stews regularly because these are her best dishes. Bill likes to eat breakfast cereal, fruit, and cheese and regularly requests these foods for snacks. However, his mother tries to deny his requests, so that he will have an appetite for dinner. Bill's mother comes to you and asks you what she should do to get Bill to eat.

Analysis

1. List four mistakes Bill's parents are making that contribute to Bill's poor eating habits.

2. List four strategies they might try to promote good eating habits in Bill.

children aged 24 to 60 months. *Journal of the American Dietetic Association* 99:1514, 1999.

Diets of preschool-age children often lack adequate sources of zinc, folate, vitamin E, and vitamin D. Foods most commonly consumed by preschoolers include fruit drinks, carbonated beverages, fat-reduced milk, and French fries. Parents should encourage their children to eat more vegetables, zinc- and folate-fortified breakfast cereals, lean red meats, seafood, vegetable oils, and fat-reduced milk.

32. Subar AF and others: Dietary sources of nutrients among U.S. children, 1989–1991. *Pediatrics* 102:913, 1998.

Fortified foods, such as breakfast cereals, are important contributors of many vitamins and minerals in the diets of children. Low-nutrient-dense foods are major contributors to energy, fat, and carbohydrate intake. These foods compromise the intake of more nutritious foods.

33. Taylor SL and others: Food allergies and avoidance diets. *Nutrition Today* 34(1):15, 1999.

Genetic background is a key contributing factor for allergy sufferers. Food allergies are frequently outgrown, sometimes within a few months. Allergies to certain foods, such as milk, eggs, and soybeans, are much more likely to be outgrown than are allergies to other foods, such as peanuts (an allergy that is almost never outgrown).

34. Trahms CM, Pipes PL: *Nutrition in Infancy and Childhood*, 6th edition, WCB/McGraw-Hill, Dubuque, IA 1997.

This text provides a comprehensive review of nutrition in infancy and childhood. The chapters' content is supported by numerous references, and is both easy to understand and quite informative.

35. Van Horn L: Primary prevention of cardiovascular disease starts in childhood. *Journal of the American Dietetic Association* 100:41, 2000.

Many of the problems in children's diets today are attributable to a lack of fruits, vegetables, and whole grains and to too many low-nutrient-dense foods, such as desserts, sweets, and snacks. These latter foods contribute excessive amounts of saturated fat, total fat, refined carbohydrate, and energy to the children's diets.

TAKE ACTION

II. EVALUATING A TEEN LUNCH

The following are two typical teen lunches and nutritional information for each:

Meal 1	Amount	Item
	2 pieces	Cheese pizza
	1 each	Milk chocolate candy bar
	20 fl oz	Cola

Meal 2	Amount	Item
	1	Hamburger with condiments
	30 each	French fries
	20 fl oz	Cola

	Meal 1	Meal 2	Nutrient Needs for Teens
kcal	990	1000	Males: 3000 Females: 2200
Protein	32	20	Males: 59 Females: 44
Vitamin C (mg)	5	18	45–75
Vitamin A (RAE)	300	10	Males: 900 Females: 700
Iron (mg)	3	4	Males: 11 Females: 15
Calcium (mg)	545	100	1300

1. Keeping in mind that meals should meet about one-third of nutrient needs, what are the shortcomings and excesses of these meals (i.e., given the nutritional information, compare these meals with one-third the RDA for calories, protein, vitamin C, vitamin A, and iron and the Adequate Intake for calcium?

   _____

   _____

   _____

2. How would you change these meals to improve balance and to meet the nutrient needs above? (Hint: use your software program or Appendix A.)

   _____

   _____

   _____

3. Reflect on your food choices as a teenager. Do you think your meal choices were balanced and varied? Why or why not? What could you have done to improve your nutritional habits at that time?

   _____

   _____

   _____

FOOD ALLERGIES AND INTOLERANCES

Adverse reactions to foods—indicated by sneezing, coughing, nausea, vomiting, diarrhea, hives, and other rashes—are broadly classed as food allergies (also called *hypersensitivities*) or **food intolerances.** Allergies involve responses of the immune system designed to eliminate foreign proteins, called **allergens.**[33] The symptoms experienced by susceptible people, such as rapid increase in heart rate and shortness of breath, are the result of this battle. In contrast, the symptoms of food intolerances do not result from a true allergic reaction. Rather, food intolerances are caused by an individual's inability to digest certain food components or by the direct effect of a food component or contaminant on the body. Let's examine each process, first allergies and then intolerances, so you can learn how to reduce the risk of becoming a victim of the food you eat.

food intolerance An adverse reaction to food that does not involve an allergic reaction.

allergen A foreign protein, or antigen, that induces excess production of certain immune system antibodies; subsequent exposure to the same protein leads to allergic symptoms. Whereas all allergens are antigens, not all antigens are allergens.

FOOD ALLERGIES: SYMPTOMS AND MECHANISM

Allergic reactions to foods are quite common and occur more frequently in females than males. Food allergies occur most frequently during infancy and young adulthood. Experts estimate that up to about 2% of adults and up to about 8% of children are allergic to certain foods. Three types of reactions may occur after the ingestion of problem foods by susceptible people:

- *Classic*—itching, reddening skin, asthma, swelling, choking, and a runny nose
- *GI tract*—nausea, vomiting, diarrhea, intestinal gas, bloating, pain, constipation, and indigestion
- *General*—headache, skin reactions, tension and fatigue, tremors, and psychological problems

Any reaction that is milder than these distinct allergic ones is referred to as a **food sensitivity.**

food sensitivity A mild reaction to a substance in a food, which might be expressed as light itching or redness of the skin.

Allergic reactions vary not only in the body system affected but also in their duration, ranging from seconds to a few days. A generalized, all-systems reaction is called anaphylactic shock. This severe allergic response results in low blood pressure and respiratory and GI tract distress. It can be fatal. A person who is extremely sensitive to a food may not be able to touch the food or even be in the same room where it is being cooked without responding to it. Although any food can trigger anaphylactic shock, the most common culprits are peanuts, tree nuts (walnuts, pecans, etc.), shellfish, milk, eggs, soybeans, wheat, and fish. For a small number of people, avoiding foods such as peanuts or shellfish is a matter of life and death.[33]

Almost all food allergies are caused by proteins in milk, eggs, corn, nuts (especially peanuts), seafood, soy products, and wheat. Other foods frequently identified with adverse reactions include meat and meat products, fruits, and cheese. These foods contain acidlike proteins, usually with a molecular weight between about 10,000 and 70,000, that stimulate the production of antibodies (specifically the immunoglobulin IgE) in susceptible people.

People with a history of serious allergic reactions should carry a self-administered form of epinephrine, such as EpiPen.

The American Academy of Allergy and Immunology has a 24-hour toll-free hot line (800-822-2762) to answer questions about food allergies and to help direct people to specialists who treat the problem. Free information on food allergies is available by writing to The Food Allergy Network, 4744 Holly Ave., Fairfax, VA 22030. The telephone number is 800-929-4040; the web site is http://www.foodallergy.org.

◼ Testing for a Food Allergy

The diagnosis of a food allergy can often be a difficult task (Table 17-8). It requires the advice of a skilled physician. The first step in determining whether a food allergy is present is to record in detail a history of symptoms, time from ingestion to onset of symptoms, most recent reaction, quantity and nature of food needed to produce a reaction, and food suspected of causing a reaction. A family history of allergic diseases can also help, as allergic reactions tend to run in families. A physical examination may reveal evidence of an allergy, such as skin diseases and asthma. Various diagnostic tests can rule out other conditions.

Perhaps the best laboratory test for determining which compounds a person is allergic to is the RAST test. This test estimates the blood concentration of antibodies that binds certain food-borne antigens. Skin tests can also be used; a drop of antigen is placed under the skin where it has been scratched or punctured. If a person is allergic to the test antigen, a red eruption will develop.

TABLE 17-8	Assessment Strategies for Food Allergies
History	Includes description of symptoms, time between food ingestion and onset of symptoms, duration of symptoms, most recent allergic episode, quantity of food required to produce reaction, suspected foods, and allergic diseases in other family members
Physical examination	Look for signs of an allergic reaction (rash, itching, intestinal bloating, etc.)
Skin test	Place a sample of the suspected allergen under the skin and watch for an inflamatory reaction.
RAST test	Determine presence of IgE antibodies in blood that bind to antigens tested
Elimination diet	Establish a diet lacking the suspected offending foods and stay on it for 1 to 2 weeks or until symptoms clear
Food challenge	Add back small amounts of excluded foods, one at a time, as long as anaphylactic shock is not a possible consequence

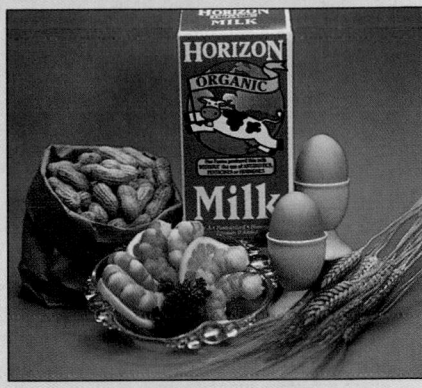

Eggs, wheat, milk, nuts, and seafood pose the greatest risk for food allergies in childhood.

The next step is to eliminate from the diet for 1 to 2 weeks all tested compounds that appear to cause allergic symptoms, plus all other foods suspected of causing an allergy based on the person's food history. The person generally starts out eating foods to which almost no one reacts, such as rice, vegetables, noncitrus fruits, and fresh meats and poultry. If symptoms are still present, the person can more severely restrict the diet or even use special formula diets that are hypoallergenic.

Once a diet is found that causes no symptoms, called an **elimination diet,** foods that are known not to trigger anaphylactic shock can be added back one at a time. Doses of ½ to 1 teaspoon (2.5 to 5 ml) are given at first. The amount is increased until the dose approximates usual intake. This should be done using a double-blind approach (see Chapter 1), especially when the reaction has a psychological component or when symptoms are vague or ill defined. Dried foods can be encapsulated and then given to the person. Any reintroduced food that causes significant symptoms to appear is identified as an allergen for the person.

elimination diet A restrictive diet that systematically tests foods that may cause an allergic response by first eliminating them for 1 to 2 weeks and then adding them back one at a time.

■ Treating Food Allergies

Once potential allergens are identified, the best treatment is to avoid them, especially for people with zero tolerance. Careful reading of food labels is essential for many allergic people and advisable for all.[33] A major challenge for the clinician treating a person with a food allergy is to make sure that what remains in the diet can still provide essential nutrients. The small food intake of children permits less leeway in removing the offending foods that may contain numerous nutrients. A registered dietitian can help guide the diet-planning process to ensure that what remains of the food choices still meets nutrient needs or to guide supplement use, if that is necessary.

If an allergy-prone woman is pregnant or breastfeeding, she should avoid offending foods—such as eggs and peanuts—because allergens can cross the placenta during pregnancy. Allergens are also secreted in her milk. She should work with her physician and registered dietitian to make sure she still consumes an adequate diet. In addition, when food allergies run in the family, women are advised to breastfeed their infants exclusively for 6 months. Human milk contains factors that play a role in the maturation of the small intestine. Formula-fed infants, especially those on formulas based on cow's milk, have a greater risk for developing allergies. Breastfeeding, thus, should continue for as long as possible, preferably to 1 year.

The **prognosis** for food allergies that first appear before 3 years of age is good. About 80% of young children with food allergies outgrow them before 3 years. Parents should be made aware of this and certainly not assume the allergy will be long-lived. Food allergies diagnosed after 3 years of age, however, are often more long-lived, but not always. In these cases, about 33% of people outgrow their food allergies within 3 years. For others, the condition may be prolonged; some food allergies can last a lifetime. Periodic reintroduction of offending foods

CRITICAL THINKING

Irene and Chris had a baby 11 months ago. At the last checkup, the doctor told them to start feeding the baby some new solid foods. After 5 days of eating a new food, the baby woke up with a runny nose and vomiting. The doctor told them to stop giving the baby that food. How can the doctor justify his recommendations?

prognosis A forecast of the course and end of a disease.

can be tried every 6 to 12 months or so to see whether the allergic reaction has decreased. If no symptoms appear, tolerance to the food has developed.

Food Intolerances

Food intolerances are adverse reactions to food that do not involve allergic mechanisms. Generally, larger amounts of an offending food are required to produce the symptoms of an intolerance than to trigger allergic symptoms. Common causes of food intolerances include

- Constituents of certain foods (e.g., red wine, tomatoes, pineapples) that have a druglike activity, causing physiological effects such as changes in blood pressure
- Certain synthetic compounds added to foods, such as sulfites, food-coloring agents, and monosodium glutamate (MSG)
- Food contaminants, including antibiotics and other chemicals used in the production of livestock and crops, as well as insect parts not removed during processing
- Toxic contaminants resulting from the ingestion of improperly handled and prepared foods containing *Clostridium botulinum*, *Salmonella* bacteria, or other food-borne microbes (see Chapter 19)
- Deficiencies in digestive enzymes, such as lactase (see Chapter 5)

Almost everyone is sensitive to one or more of these causes of food intolerance, many of which produce GI tract symptoms.

Sulfites, which are added to foods and beverages as antioxidants, cause flushing, spasms of the airways, and a loss of blood pressure in susceptible people. Wine, dehydrated potatoes, dried fruits, gravy, soup mixes, and restaurant salad greens commonly contain sulfites. A reaction to MSG may include an increase in blood pressure, numbness, sweating, vomiting, headache, and facial pressure. MSG is commonly found in Chinese food and many processed foods (e.g., soups). A reaction to tartrazine, a food-coloring additive, includes spasm of the airways, itching, and reddening skin. Tyramine, a derivative of the amino acid tyrosine, is commonly found in "aged" foods, such as cheeses and red wines. This natural food constituent can cause high blood pressure in people taking monoamine-oxidase inhibitor medications, which may be prescribed for mental depression.

The basic treatment for food intolerances is to avoid specific offending components. However, total elimination often is not required because people generally are not as sensitive to compounds causing food intolerances as they are to allergens. For instance, a slight amount of sulfites in a glass of wine may be tolerable, whereas a large amount from a chef's salad may cause a reaction.

NUTRITION DURING ADULTHOOD

chapter 18

Eating is one of our great pleasures. Guided by common sense and moderation, eating well is also a means to good health. Most of us want a long, productive life, free of illness, yet many people from early middle age onward suffer coronary heart disease, hypertension and strokes, type 2 diabetes, osteoporosis, and other chronic diseases. We can slow the development of, and in some cases even prevent, these diseases by pursuing a diet that works against them.[22] This action is most profitable if we begin early and continue throughout adulthood. We serve ourselves best—as individuals and as a nation—by striving to maintain vitality even in the later decades of life. This concept was first explored in Chapter 1 and is discussed again in this chapter, along with the special nutrition needs of older persons.

Keep in mind that present day-to-day health practices can significantly influence health during later life. Although genetics does play a role, as discussed in Chapter 1, many of the health problems that occur with age are not inevitable; they result from disease processes that influence physical health. Much can be learned from healthy older people whose attention to health and physical activity—along with a little luck—keeps them active and vibrant well beyond typical retirement years.[18] Successful aging is the goal. Age quickly or slowly—it is partly your choice.

CHAPTER OUTLINE

KEY CHAPTER CONCEPTS

- Delaying the symptoms of and disabilities from chronic disease for as many years of life as possible is a laudable life goal. Nutrient intake plays a part in this process.
- A basic plan for health promotion and disease prevention includes eating a proper diet that focuses on a variety of foods, performing regular physical activity, maintaining or improving body weight status, consuming an adequate amount of fluids, abstaining from smoking, getting adequate sleep, and moderating alcohol intake, if used.
- Although maximum life span hasn't changed, life expectancy has increased dramatically over the past century. Aging probably begins before birth. This aging likely results from automatic cellular changes and environmental influences, such as DNA damage, free-radical reactions, hormonal changes, alterations in immune function, elevated blood glucose, and excess energy intake.
- The nutritional problems of older people relate to the presence of chronic disease and the typical decreases in organ function that occur with age. These can include loss of teeth, a reduction in the senses of taste and smell, changes in gastrointestinal tract function, and deterioration in heart and bone health.
- Alzheimer's disease is a progressive brain disorder, which usually develops in older individuals and is identified by the inability to remember, reason, and understand what is going on. Risk factors include age, genetic variations, less education and occupational attainment, head trauma, and possibly loss of estrogen at menopause.
- Scientists are only now beginning to study specific nutrient requirements for older people. Diet plans should be based on the Food Guide Pyramid or another related plan, with consideration for present health problems, decreased physical abilities, the presence of drug-nutrient interactions, possible depression and alcoholism, and economic constraints.
- Nutrients such as protein, vitamin D, vitamin E, riboflavin, vitamin B-6, folate, vitamin B-12, zinc, and calcium, along with dietary fiber, often deserve special attention in diet planning in later life. Vitamin and mineral supplement use can help meet these needs if wise food choices don't suffice.
- Because of decreased mobility, minimal social contact, and an inability to prepare foods, many older people benefit from congregate meals, home-delivered food, and other related services in their area that support nutritional health.
- Currently, FDA has limited regulatory power over various dietary and herbal supplements marketed to adults and others. Some of these products yield health benefits when the directions on the label are followed. Knowing which of these products are helpful and which are potentially harmful is important to consumers. Generally, it is advisable to use only one product at a time, look closely for possible harmful side effects, and discuss any use with one's physician.

REFRESH YOUR MEMORY

As you begin your study of adult nutrition issues in Chapter 18, you may want to review
- The effect of genetics on health in Chapter 1
- The various body systems in Chapter 3
- The sources of dietary fiber in Chapter 5
- The dietary sources of vitamin D, the various B-vitamins, and calcium in Chapters 9, 10, and 11, respectively.
- The benefits of regular physical activity in Chapter 14

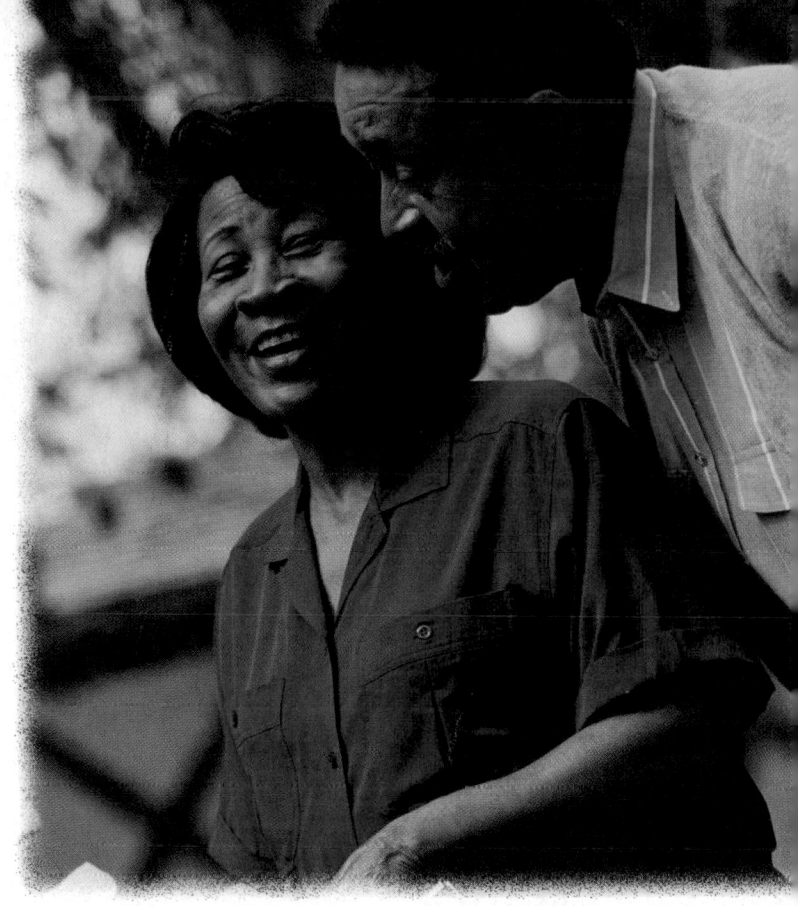

CASE SCENARIO

Francis is a 78-year-old woman who suffers from macular degeneration, osteoporosis, and arthritis. Since her husband died 1 year ago, she has moved from their family house to a small one bedroom apartment. Her eyesight is progressively getting worse, making it hard to go to the grocery store or even to cook for herself (for fear of burning herself). She is often lonely; her only son lives 1 hour away and works two jobs, but he visits her as often as he can. Francis has lost her appetite and, as a result, often skips meals throughout the week. She has resorted to eating mostly cold foods that are simple to prepare but at the same time is seriously limiting diet variety and palatability. She is slowly losing weight as a result of her dietary changes and loss of appetite.

Her typical diet usually consists of a breakfast that may include one slice of wheat toast with margarine, honey, and cinnamon and one cup of hot tea. If she has lunch, she normally has ½ can of peaches, ½ of a turkey and cheese sandwich, and ½ glass of water. For dinner, she might have ½ of a tuna fish sandwich made with mayonnaise and one cup of iced tea. Occasionally, she includes one or two cookies at bedtime.

What services do you think are available that could help Francis improve her diet and possibly increase her appetite? What other convenience foods could be included in her diet to make it more healthful and more varied?

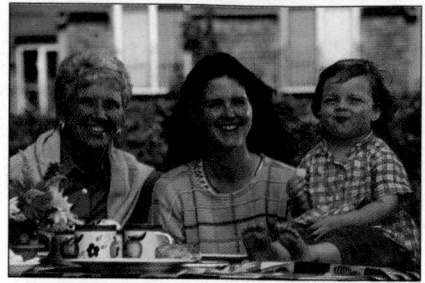

As we age, our nutrient needs change. For example, vitamin D needs are higher for older stages of adulthood than for younger stages or for childhood.

*K*eep in mind that extending life without delaying onset of chronic disease prolongs suffering in many cases. In addition, the greater number of disabled years is a great cost to all Americans. For these reasons, prolonging life without compressing the number of disabled years is called the "failure of success."

life expectancy The average length of life for a given group of people.

compression of morbidity The delay of the onset of disabilities caused by chronic disease.

*A*ppendix C reviews diet planning guidelines issued by the Canadian government for Canadians. In addition, Chapter 1 discussed *Healthy People 2010*, a U.S. federal agenda aimed at disease prevention and health promotion for Americans.

■ NUTRITION AND ADULTHOOD—AN INTRODUCTION

From a nutritional point of view, one's adult years are divided into four stages: 19 to 30, 31 to 50, 51 to 70, and beyond 70 years of age. The two intervals encompassing ages 19 to 50 can be seen as young adulthood; 51 to 70 then would be middle adulthood; and beyond 70 years of age would be older adulthood.

Nutritional needs change throughout these intervals. For example, calcium needs increase after age 50 for males and females. Vitamin B-12 needs also change after age 50, in that one should consume foods fortified with crystalline vitamin B-12 or take a supplement containing vitamin B-12.[28] Recall from Chapter 10 that this latter advice stems from the fact that about 10 to 30% of older people may malabsorb food-bound vitamin B-12 because of reduced acid production by the stomach. Vitamin D needs also change. Adults over age 70 need three times more vitamin D than they did when they were ages 19 to 50, and they need 50% more than they did during ages 51 to 70. In response to this increase in vitamin D needs for people over age 70, nutrition experts at Tufts University have suggested a modification of the Food Guide Pyramid to include a supplemental vitamin D source for this age group. Other such changes suggested by these experts for the Food Guide Pyramid will be mentioned in the section "Nutrient needs in middle and older adulthood."[24]

Attention to healthy nutrition and overall lifestyle habits is important at all ages. In this chapter, we will look particularly at adult nutrition issues. Applying the principles of the Dietary Guidelines will be the focus of advice for adults ages 19 to 50 years. Then we will look at additional recommendations for adults 51 and older, including appropriate vitamin and mineral supplement use for these individuals.

■ COMPRESSION OF MORBIDITY

Although most of us wish for long life, we do not like the thought of failing health in old age. And rightly so! Rather than suffer the ravages of heart disease, obesity, strokes, diabetes, osteoporosis, and other chronic diseases from age 40 or 60 years until death, we should strive to be as free of disease as possible and enjoy vitality throughout even our last decade. **Life expectancy** is at a record high of 77 years for the general population in the United States today, although the span of healthy life is only 65 years. Thus, an important focus here is not necessarily on living longer but on living healthier.

Striving to have the greatest number of healthy years and the fewest years of illness is often referred to as **compression of morbidity**.[32] In other words, a person tries to compress significant sickness related to aging into the last few years—or months—of life. An example of this concept is illustrated for coronary heart disease in Figure 18-1. Of the three lines shown, the line on the top depicts rapid deterioration in health; symptoms of this cardiovascular disease appear by about age 40, and death occurs at about age 60. In addition, between the ages of 40 and 60 years, symptoms of coronary heart disease, and therefore disability, are present.

A healthier lifestyle follows the middle line in Figure 18-1. Here, coronary heart disease is postponed so that the first symptoms are not apparent until age 60; severe symptoms occur at age 80, with death following a few years later. The line on the bottom is ideal. Disease progresses so slowly that symptoms do not appear during a person's lifetime; therefore, the disease process never hampers activities.

Body cells age no matter what health practices we follow. However, to a considerable extent, you can choose how quickly you age throughout your adult years. In light of the many studies showing the ability even to reverse atherosclerosis, we can say that the rate at which you age is partly your choice.

Although there is little doubt of the benefits of a healthy lifestyle, scientists have also found a strong genetic component to longevity, as well as to certain diseases

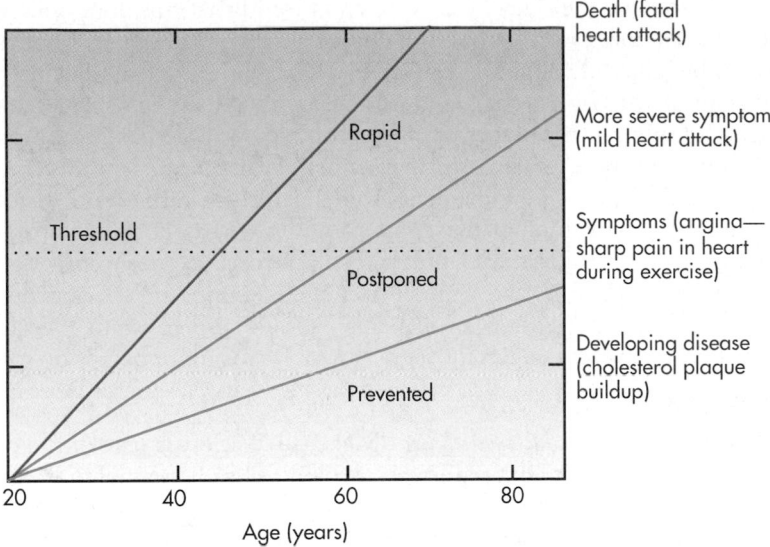

Death (fatal
heart attack)

Rapid

More severe symptoms
(mild heart attack)

Threshold

Symptoms (angina—
sharp pain in heart
during exercise)

Postponed

Developing disease
(cholesterol plaque
buildup)

Prevented

20   40   60   80
Age (years)

■ FIGURE 18-1 Compression of morbidity. The goal is to postpone illness until the final days of life. Coronary heart disease is used as an example. The line on the top shows rapid deterioration in health status, in which symptoms of this cardiovascular disease appear by about age 40 and death occurs at about age 60. In addition, between the ages of 40 and 60 years, symptoms of coronary heart disease—and therefore disability—are present. A healthier lifestyle follows the middle line pattern. Here, coronary heart disease is postponed, so that the first symptoms are not apparent until age 60; severe symptoms occur at age 80, with death following a few years later. The line on the bottom is the ideal: the disease progresses so slowly that symptoms do not appear during the lifetime; therefore, the disease process never hampers life's activities.

(see Chapter 1). Studies of families, and of twins in particular, provide support for a genetic contribution to human longevity.

Still, many adults in America today are doing what is within their control to achieve a healthy lifestyle, such as a healthful diet and a regimen of regular physical activity. Coupled with avoidance of tobacco products, limitation of or other adaptation to stress, adequate sleep, adequate fluid intake, and consultation with healthcare professionals on a regular basis, these actions contribute to a healthful, long life. Overall, the key to maximizing health throughout life is to establish harmony between one's physical, mental, psychological, and social states (see Part I in Take Action at the end of this chapter).[18]

■ DIET FOR THE ADULT YEARS

One diet approach that optimizes long-term nutritional health emphasizes low-fat and nonfat dairy products, some lean meats, plant proteins, a rich variety of fruits and vegetables, and generous amounts of whole-grain breads and cereals. The Food Guide Pyramid in Chapter 2 is one blueprint for this diet.

To further refine these food choices, recall also from Chapter 2 the latest Dietary Guidelines issued by the USDA/DHHS. The U.S. Surgeon General, the American Heart Association, the American Dietetic Association, the American Medical Association, the National Cancer Institute, the National Academy of Sciences, and the World Health Organization have added recommendations to the framework of the Dietary Guidelines. Following is a summary of the advice provided by the Dietary Guidelines, with additional comments from various health-related organizations.

Aim for Fitness

- *Aim for a healthy weight.* Use BMI to assess if you are at an acceptable weight for height. Measuring your waist circumference (just above your hip bones) is also a good way to determine your health risk (see Chapter 13 for more information on BMI and waist circumference). No matter what one's weight status is—acceptable, overweight, or underweight—the number one goal is to first maintain that weight. Then, if weight gain or loss is needed, set a reasonable weight goal that can be met by following the Dietary Guidelines for diet and exercise. Working closely with a registered dietitian can facilitate achieving that weight goal.
- *Be physically active each day.* Adults should strive to accumulate 30 minutes of moderate physical activity on most or all days of the week because this works in

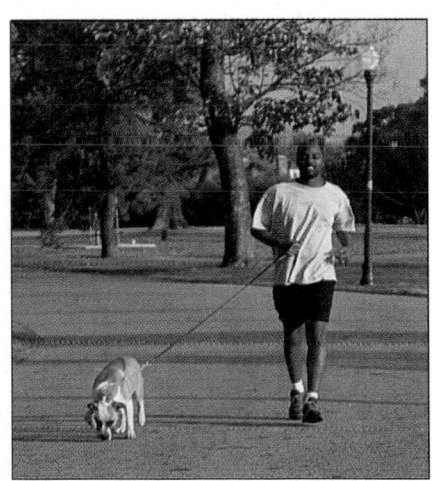

Many adults find that regular physical activity adds an important dimension to their lives.

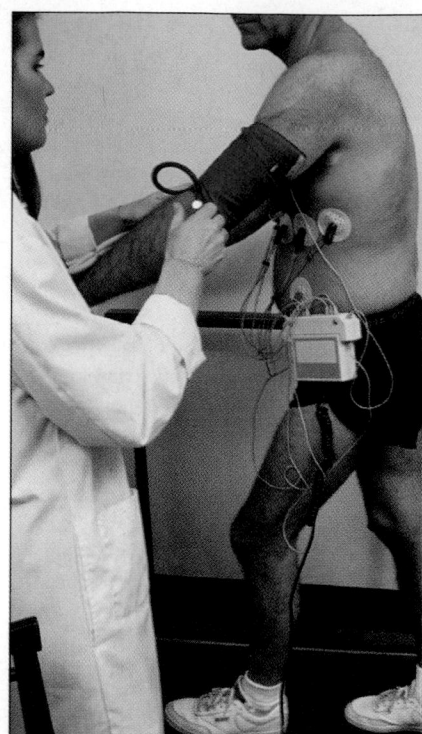

The Dietary Guidelines recommend that men over 40 and women over 50 years of age obtain physician approval before beginning a program of vigorous physical activity. This is especially important for people with evidence of cardiovascular disease, hypertension, or diabetes. The physician may suggest an exercise treadmill test be done to assess exercise tolerance.

many ways to keep the body healthy. Keep in mind that this does not have to come from 30 continuous minutes of a workout; the 30 minutes of physical activity can be tallied throughout the day. Daily activities such as walking up and down stairs at work, gardening, and washing a car can all be considered physical activity. Combining three types of physical activity—aerobic, strength training, and flexibility exercises—can assist in cardiovascular fitness, as well as building muscle strength and helping maintain bone health. It is important to consult a physician prior to beginning an exercise program when one has a chronic health problem, such as cardiovascular disease, osteoporosis, hypertension, diabetes, or obesity. Men over age 40 and women over age 50—especially if one has cardiovascular disease, hypertension, or diabetes—should also consult a physician before starting an exercise regimen (see Chapter 14 for more details on exercise).

Build a Healthy Base

- *Let the pyramid guide your food choices.* Make sure variety is part of the diet because no one food or food category can provide all the essential nutrients the body needs. Use the Food Guide Pyramid as a guide to choose healthy foods to include in the diet, and then select from the range of the recommended number of servings per day from each group. Also, use the Food Guide Pyramid serving size guide as a reference for what constitutes a serving (see Chapter 2 for more details on Food Guide Pyramid serving sizes). Vegetarian diets can be consistent with the Dietary Guidelines, but special care is needed to meet nutrient needs (see Chapter 7 for details). Some people need a vitamin-mineral supplement to meet specific nutrient needs. For example, women who could become pregnant are advised to consume foods fortified with folate or to take a supplement containing folate, in addition to consuming folate-rich foods. This practice reduces the risk of some serious birth defects. Older adults and people with little exposure to sunlight may need a supplemental source of vitamin D. Some people who seldom eat dairy products or other rich sources of calcium need a calcium supplement, and people who eat no animal foods need to take a supplement containing vitamin B-12. In addition, sometimes vitamins or minerals are prescribed for meeting nutrient needs for various medical purposes. For example, pregnant women may be advised to take an iron supplement. Still, supplements of some nutrients, such as vitamin A and selenium, can be harmful if taken in large amounts. Because foods contain many substances that promote health, one should use the Food Guide Pyramid as a starting point when planning a diet, rather than depending mostly on supplements to meet nutrient needs.[12]

- *Choose a variety of grains daily, especially whole grains.* Include six or more servings of a combination of bread, cereals, rice, and pasta, many of which are whole-grain varieties. These food choices should meet the goal of 20–35 g of dietary fiber per day. The current U.S. average for dietary fiber intake is closer to 15 g/day. Whole grains are rich in vitamins, minerals, and fiber. Fiber adds bulk to the diet, leading to an earlier feeling of satiety; in addition, it aids in proper elimination.

- *Choose a variety of fruits and vegetables daily.* Include at least five or more servings of vegetables and fruits daily. This recommendation enjoys the most overwhelming support of nutrition experts. Note that not many adults currently meet this goal, especially if potatoes are excluded from the vegetable category. Fruits and vegetables in combination with whole grains constitute a healthy diet because they are rich in the vitamins, minerals, and fiber that aid in preventing disease and maintaining health.

- *Keep food safe to eat.* Wash hands thoroughly prior to and during cooking, especially when handling raw meats and eggs, to prevent cross-contamination. To prevent further cross-contamination, separate raw, cooked, and ready-to-eat foods while shopping, for cooking, and storing food. Never thaw meats at room temperature; instead, thaw them in the refrigerator. To ensure you are cooking or reheating foods to a safe temperature, use a food thermometer. Keep cold foods cold and hot foods hot; do not leave cooked or refrigerated items at room temperature for more than 2 hours (see Chapter 19 for more details on food safety).

Choose Sensibly

- *Choose a diet that is low in saturated fat and cholesterol and moderate in total fat.* Be knowledgeable about the different kinds of fat—saturated, polyunsaturated, monounsaturated, trans fatty acids, and essential fatty acids. Saturated and trans fatty acids can raise blood cholesterol, whereas unsaturated fats generally have the opposite effect on blood cholesterol, and some of the essential fatty acids found in fatty fish offer additional protection against cardiovascular disease. Foods that are high in cholesterol (organ meats, egg yolks, and dairy fats) should be limited in the diet because they can also increase blood cholesterol in some people if consumed in abundant amounts (see Chapter 6 for more details on cardiovascular disease and the different types of fats).

- *Choose beverages and foods to moderate your intake of sugars.* Keep added sugars in the diet to a minimum by limiting soft drinks (nondiet types), fruit drinks, and fruitades, as well as sweets, candies, and cookies. Limiting these products is important because they supply excess calories, which can promote weight gain, and they take the place of nutrient-dense foods, such as fruits and vegetables. An excess amount of added sugars in the diet also promotes dental caries. Some authorities recommend that simple sugars supply no more than 10 to 15% of total energy intake. American adults currently consume about 16% of total energy intake as simple sugars (see Chapter 5 for more details on added sugars in the diet).

- *Choose and prepare foods with less salt.* Sodium and chloride found in salt are involved in regulating fluids in the body and blood pressure; limiting salt intake can reduce the risk of high blood pressure and more so in some people than others. Certain individuals (e.g., overweight people) are especially sensitive to salt causing a rise in blood pressure. Excess salt intake also increases the amount of calcium excreted in the urine. This can contribute to the development of osteoporosis if dietary calcium intake is inadequate.

   The recommended sodium intake is about 2.4 g/day (5g/day of salt); the average American consumes 4 to 7 g of sodium per day. To reduce sodium intake to the recommended 2.4 g/day would require a great change in food habits for many of us. It means not eating abundant amounts of processed (lunch) meats, salted snack foods, most canned and prepared soups, most types of cheese, and many tomato-based processed foods. Limiting the amount of salt used in cooking and avoiding adding it to food at the table also help reduce sodium intake.

- *If you drink alcoholic beverages, do so in moderation.* A moderate alcohol intake by men over age 45 and women over age 55 is associated with a decreased risk of cardiovascular disease and ischemic stroke. Younger adults enjoy few, if any, benefits of moderate alcohol consumption. Moderation of alcohol intake consists of two or fewer drinks of 12 oz of beer, 5 oz of wine, or 1 ½ oz of distilled spirits (80 proof) per day. Women, and all adults over age 65, are advised to drink no more than one drink per day. Women are more sensitive than men to alcohol-related cirrhosis of the liver. Remember that alcohol adds excess calories to the diet and is low in or devoid of essential nutrients (see Chapter 8 for more details on alcohol).

   Beyond these general recommendations, aim for the moderate use of salt-cured, smoked, and **nitrate**-cured foods because they are likely to increase the risk of certain forms of cancer (see Chapter 12). Obtain adequate fluoride to promote dental health and drink plenty of fluids. Finally, women of childbearing age need to eat iron-rich foods, primarily to avoid developing iron deficiency anemia.

   This group of guidelines provides a good general focus for diet planning. The practices recommended can accommodate many cultural dietary patterns (see the

nitrate A nitrogen-containing compound used to cure meats. Its use contributes a pink color to meats and confers some resistance to bacterial growth.

Nutrition Perspective in Chapter 2). They are broad enough to allow adults to include all the foods one enjoys in an eating plan—one just may have to eat some foods less frequently than others or in smaller portions, depending on health needs and preferences. Moderation, rather than elimination, should be the overriding consideration.[1]

■ Are Adults Following These Dietary Recommendations?

In general, American adults, both young and old, are trying to follow many of the diet recommendations listed. Since the mid-1950s, they have consumed less saturated fat as more people substitute nonfat and low-fat milk for cream and whole milk. They eat more cheese, however, which is usually a concentrated form of saturated fat. Since 1963, they have eaten less butter, fewer eggs, less animal fat, and more vegetable fats and oils and fish. These changes generally follow the recommendations to reduce the intake of saturated fat and cholesterol and, instead, to emphasize unsaturated fat. Today, animal breeders are raising much leaner cattle and hogs than in 1950, which helps. Our demand for chicken, a relatively lean source of animal protein, has skyrocketed.

Other aspects of the average U.S. diet are more mixed. The latest nutrition survey of eating habits shows that the major contributors of energy to the adult diet are white bread, beef, milk, doughnuts, cakes and cookies, soft drinks, chicken, cheese, salad dressing, mayonnaise, margarine, and sugars/syrups/jams. If the trend in diets were truly toward decreasing sugar and saturated fat, and increasing dietary fiber, many of these foods would not appear at the top of the list.

A list incorporating this book's suggestions for improvement would stress low-fat and nonfat milk, whole-wheat bread and whole-grain cereals, lean meat, salmon and tuna, peanuts and other nuts, kidney and pinto beans, oranges, carrots, and broccoli.

The overriding consideration should be quality and length of life and the impact dietary changes might have on them. Now is the time to design and begin to practice this plan. Adulthood is the key time to learn more about risk factors for chronic diseases and to do something about each one, where possible.[18]

■ A Note of Caution

Not all nutrition and health researchers agree with the blanket guidelines set by major health and science institutions, as noted in Chapter 2. Some scientists do not think that general recommendations for the public can be justified for sugar, salt (sodium), and cholesterol. Rather, they believe that these recommendations need to be individualized.

Although it can be argued that individualized dietary recommendations for such nutrients as sodium are best, that approach is generally too costly for the nation and therefore impractical. More global recommendations are appropriate if they benefit most people while not hampering the health of others. Not all people will benefit equally from following the general recommendations—for example, a reduction in salt intake—but no one is likely to be harmed. The dietary change may cause some inconvenience and necessitate the formation of new eating habits for some people. Nevertheless, we should all consider the general dietary recommendations, personalizing the advice when possible under the guidance of our health-care advisers.

CRITICAL THINKING

The "fountain of youth" remains a mystery. Many people believe a source exists that can stop the aging process, allowing youth to remain. However, Neil, a history student, asserts that the fountain of youth is not a place or a particular thing but, rather, a combination of diet and lifestyle. How can he justify this claim?

CONCEPT CHECK

Compression of morbidity, the delay of symptoms of and disabilities from chronic disease for as many years as possible, is a worthwhile goal. A basic plan to promote health and prevent disease includes eating a balanced, varied diet; performing regular physical activity; abstaining from smoking; limiting or abstaining from alcohol intake; and limiting or learning ways to deal with stress more effectively. More specific Dietary Guidelines direct people to eat a variety of foods; maintain healthy weight; choose a diet low in saturated fat, and cholesterol and moderate in total fat; choose a diet with plenty of vegetables, fruits, and grain products; use sugars only in moderation; use salt (sodium) only in moderation; and, if they drink alcoholic beverages, do so in moderation. Recommendations also include warnings against relying primarily on nutrient supplements to meet nutrient needs. Some scientists believe that these guidelines do not necessarily constitute an individual "prescription."

■ MIDDLE AND OLDER ADULTHOOD

How long do your family members generally live? Of those who died early in adulthood, can you pinpoint some causes? Do you plan to live longer than your parents did or will? How long will that be? Some basic statistics can help you predict this.

■ Life Span

Life span refers to the maximal number of years humans live. As far as we know, this hasn't changed in recorded time. The longest human life documented to date is 122 years. In contrast, the domestic dog has a life span of 20 years; a rat, 5 years.

life span The potential oldest age a person can reach.

■ Life Expectancy

Life expectancy is the time an average person born in a specific year, such as 2000, can expect to live. Currently, life expectancy in America is about 74 years for men and about 79 years for women, with a span of "healthy years" of about 64. Furthermore, if you survive to the age of 80, you can tack on another 7 to 9 years of life expectancy.

Worldwide, the highest average life expectancy is 82 years for women and 76 years for men in Japan. Researchers suggest that a diet based on rice, fish, vegetable protein sources, fruits, vegetables, and some meat contributes to this record longevity (see the Expert Opinion in Chapter 2).

Life expectancy hasn't always been this long; for primitive humans, it was about 20 to 35 years. It increased to 40 years in Medieval England and increased to 49 years by the turn of the twentieth century. During the last 80 years, life expectancy for nearly all people has increased, mainly because of changes in the principal causes of death.

In the early 1900s, infectious diseases were the first three causes of death. Vaccines and antibiotics have tremendously lowered death from disease. The decline in infant and childhood deaths, coupled with better diets and health care, has allowed more people to age first into maturity and then into older years. Now the principal causes of death in Western societies are related to cardiovascular diseases and cancer (Table 18-1).

Historically, the trend in the United States has been toward an ever older population. During Colonial times, half the population was over 16 years of age. By 1990, half were over 33. By 2050, half could be over 43, and approximately 20% of the entire U.S. population will be 65 years and older, twice as many as reach 65 today. This age—65 years—is arbitrarily listed as a dividing line for the beginning of later life because one can currently qualify for full Social Security benefits. The time at which old age occurs, however, varies for each person, according to health and independence.

Among the older population, the group constituting those aged 85+ years is the fastest growing segment. Between 1997 and 2050, the population aged 85+ years is expected to increase from 3.4 million to 19 million. This is the first time in history our society will need to deal with such a large population of older people. The associated expense will be enormous if a large percentage need special care because of ill health.[32]

This "graying" of America poses some problems. Today, although people older than age 65 account for 13% of the U.S. population, they account for more than

TABLE 18-1	Changes in Leading Causes of Death During the Twentieth Century in the United States

Chronic diseases, rather than infectious diseases, are now the major killers.

Rank	Cause of death	Percentage Mortality*
1900		
1	Pneumonia and influenza	12
2	Tuberculosis	11
3	Diarrhea and enteritis	8
4	Heart disease	8
5	Cerebrovascular disease (stroke)	6
6	Nephritis	5
7	Accidents	4
8	Cancer	4
9	Diphtheria	2
10	Meningitis	2
Today		
1	Heart disease	31
2	Cancer	23
3	Cerebrovascular disease (stroke)	7
4	Chronic obstructive pulmonary disease and allied conditions	5
5	Pneumonia and influenza	5
6	Accidents and adverse effects	4
	Motor vehicle accidents	(2)
	All other accidents and adverse effects	(2)
7	Diabetes	3
8	Suicide	1
9	Kidney disease	1
10	Liver disease	1

*Percentage of all deaths in that year.

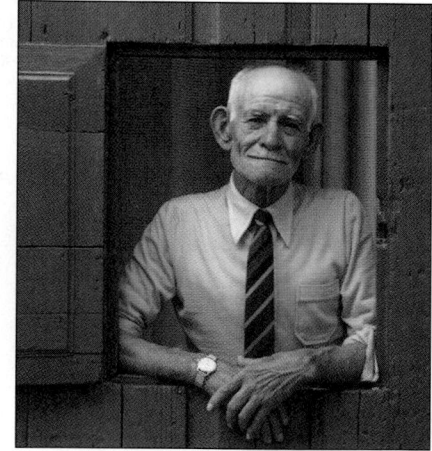

A diet based on vegetables, fruits, pasta, and olive oil as a source of fat—and with a small amount of alcohol in the form of red wine—provides southern Italians with many healthy years of life. Their active lifestyle is an additional contributing factor.

25% of all prescription medications used, 40% of acute care hospital stays, and 50% of the federal health budget. Hip fractures alone cost the nation about $10 billion per year. Of older persons, 85% have nutrition-related problems, such as heart problems, type 2 diabetes, hypertension, and osteoporosis.

Postponing these chronic diseases for as long as possible will help control health-care costs. The more independent, healthy years people live, the better life can be for them and the less they burden the health-care system, which will increasingly have to scramble to accommodate a growing elderly population. Keep in mind that aging is not a disease. Furthermore, diseases that commonly accompany old age—osteoporosis and atherosclerosis, for example—are not an inevitable part of aging. Many can be prevented or managed, for the most part.[17] Some people do die of old age, not as a direct result of disease.

▌Aging

One view of aging describes it as processes of slow cell death, beginning soon after fertilization. When we are young, aging is not apparent because the major metabolic activities are geared toward growth and maturation. We produce plenty of active cells to meet physiological needs. During late adolescence and adulthood, the body's major task is to maintain cells. Inevitably, though, cells age and die. Eventually, as more cells die, the body can't adjust to meet all physiological demands. Body functioning begins to decrease (Fig. 18-2). Still, organs usually retain enough **reserve capacity** that, for a long time, the body shows no outward disease. Although no symptoms appear, subclinical disease may develop, and, if the disease is allowed to progress unchecked, organ function and then body function eventually deteriorate noticeably.

The aging process is clearly illustrated by changes for many people in the function of the enzyme lactase. For some people, lactase activity in the small intestine slows during childhood. Generally, however, clear symptoms of the deficiency—gas and bloating after milk consumption—do not appear until adulthood. Although lactase output decreases in these cases, perhaps from birth, enough enzyme is present to digest the lactose consumed until adulthood.

Cells age probably because of automatic cellular changes and environmental influences. Even in the most supportive of environments, cell structure and function inevitably change. Eventually, cells lose their ability to regenerate the internal parts they need, and they die. This inevitable dying off of deteriorating cells is actually beneficial, as researchers have concluded it likely prevents diseases such as cancer.

Unfortunately, there are still consequences to this natural cell progression, because as more and more cells in an organ system die, organ function decreases. For example, **kidney nephrons** are continually lost as we age. In some people, this loss leads to eventual kidney failure, but most of us maintain sufficient kidney function throughout life. Again, in aging, there is first a reduction in reserve capacity. Only after that is exhausted does actual organ function noticeably decrease.

■ Hypotheses About the Causes of Aging

Although the causes of aging remain a mystery, many hypotheses have been promoted to explain it.

Errors Occur in Copying the Genetic Blueprint (DNA)

Some of the errors in copying DNA are spontaneous, and others arise from degradative processes that chemicals and radiation, and time alone, induce (recall the discussion of telomeres on DNA in Chapter 10). Once sufficient errors in DNA copying accumulate, a cell can no longer synthesize the major proteins needed to function, and it dies. Much attention is currently given to mitochondrial DNA. This DNA contains templates for synthesizing various compounds used in protein synthesis. Mitochondrial DNA undergoes a rapid mutation rate, due to exposure to toxins and free radicals. These mutations have been linked to diabetes, heart failure, and aging in general. The ability to combat this type of damage is primarily genetically determined. Gene variants that give rise to unusually efficient resistance to damage could contribute to life span by slowing the rate at which cells experience such lethal damage.

reserve capacity The extent to which an organ can preserve essentially normal function despite decreasing cell number or cell activity.

kidney nephrons The units of kidney cells that filter wastes from the bloodstream and deposits them into the urine.

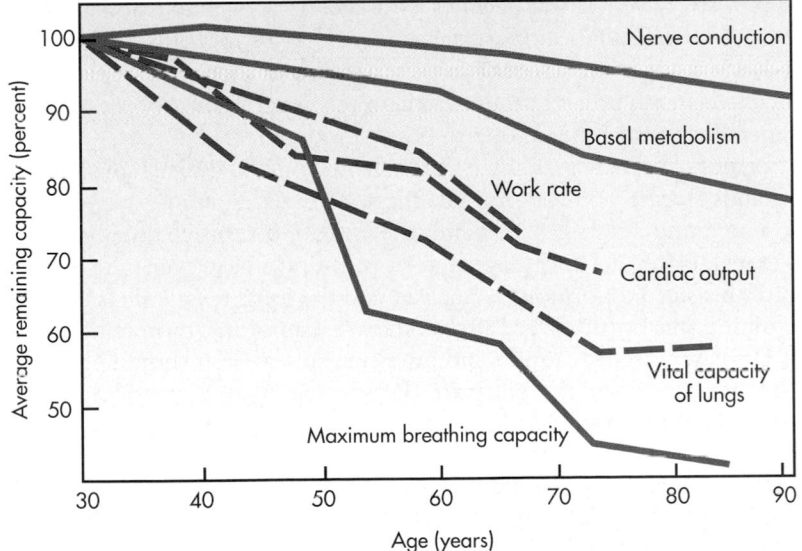

■ **FIGURE 18-2** The declines in physiological function seen with aging. The decline in many body functions is seen primarily in sedentary people.

lipofuscin A brown pigment characteristically found in aging cells. It is present in lysosomes and is the product of the breakdown of unsaturated fatty acids, and perhaps also membrane damage.

Connective Tissue Stiffens

Parallel collagen protein strands, found mostly in connective tissue, chemically bond and cross-link to each other. The bonding decreases flexibility in key body components, altering organ function. Skin wrinkles, and joints and arteries stiffen. The bonding may also restrict nutrients from entering cells.

Toxic Products Build Up

Breakdown products of lipids, called **lipofuscin**, may act as intracellular sludge, hampering normal metabolic processes by clogging cells.

Electron-Seeking Compounds Damage Cell Parts

Electron-seeking free radicals can break down cell membranes and proteins, such as in the eye. One way to prevent some damage from these compounds is to consume adequate amounts of vitamins E and C, selenium, and possibly carotenoids.[15] In contrast, it's not effective to consume cellular enzymes designed to break down the damaging compounds, such as superoxide dismutase. Ingested enzymes are themselves broken down during digestion before they can act in the body. Despite that, some health-food stores sell superoxide dismutase.

Hormone Function Changes

A fall in growth hormone concentration is also being investigated as a potentially treatable hormonal cause of aging. Growth hormone is secreted by the pituitary gland and stimulates protein synthesis in cells, such as muscle cells, as well as produces various other effects in the body. Growth hormone should only be used under physician supervision; it is routinely used in children who secrete abnormally low amounts.

Studies so far support the hypothesis that growth hormone–related loss of lean body mass in adults plays a role in aging. Research has shown that growth hormone injections increases lean body mass and skin thickness and decreases fat mass; however, this increase in lean body mass does not improve the strength or function of muscles. In addition, once treatment with growth hormone in adults is stopped, gains in lean body mass are lost. Growth hormone therapy also has significant adverse side effects, such as carpal tunnel syndrome, edema (swollen legs or ankles), hypertension, diabetes-like symptoms, and enlarged breasts in men and women.[5] These may limit its clinical usefulness in older people, and, since growth hormone signals muscle cells to replicate, many scientists fear that it may also trigger uncontrolled cell growth, leading to cancer. Researchers are currently concentrating on developing a synthetic hormone which would stimulate the release of growth hormone naturally and in doing so would avoid the negative side effects of supplementation.

Testosterone concentration declines with age. This decline is linked to a decline in muscle strength. Studies support the concept that a subgroup of older males who produce low amounts may benefit from testosterone therapy. Note that there are some side effects with use; treatment is still in the experimental phase and is not currently generally recommended, due to possible side effects.

The hormone known as dehydroepiandrosterone (DHEA), produced by the adrenal glands (located on top of the kidneys), circulates at an extremely high concentration in young adults but falls after the age of 30. This change has led to speculation that DHEA decline plays a role in aging. However, the physiological function of this steroid hormone is unclear, and the long-term effects of using products containing this hormone are also unknown. Until long-term studies ensure the safety of DHEA, extreme caution and physician supervision should accompany any use of this hormone (see the Nutrition Perspective at the end of this chapter for more information in DHEA).[4]

Melatonin, a hormone that regulates the cycle of sleeping and waking, is produced by the pineal gland (located in the center of the brain). The production of melatonin is highest at night and falls during the day. It was once thought that this hormone decreases with age, but new research has shown that melatonin production remains relatively constant during aging, with variations from person to person.

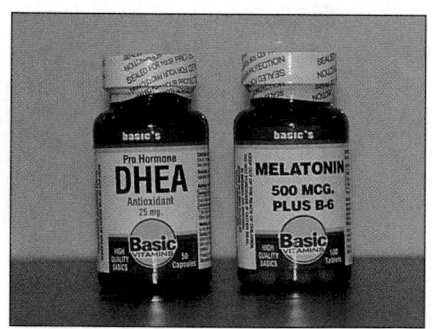

A variety of products are advocated to slow aging; however, little or no research supports their effectiveness.

With this knowledge, it is incorrect to think that melatonin is involved in the aging process and that supplementation is necessary (see the Nutrition Perspective at the end of this chapter for more information on melatonin).[21]

Immune System Loses Some Efficiency

The thymus gland (located in the upper part of the chest) is a major component of the immune system. During adolescence the thymus gland reaches its maximal size, and by age 50 it is barely visible. The immune system itself runs a somewhat parallel course. It is most efficient during childhood and young adulthood, but with advancing age it is less able to recognize and counteract foreign substances, such as viruses, that enter the body. As we age, then, the immune system's ability to detect and destroy developing cancer cells decreases, allowing them to multiply autonomously.

Nutrient deficiencies, particularly of protein, vitamin E, vitamin B-6, and zinc, hamper immune function, making matters worse for the aging body. Maintaining an adequate nutrient intake, especially in later life, is crucial for immune function.

Autoimmunity Develops

Autoimmune reactions occur when white blood cells and other immune bodies fail to distinguish between substances normally present in the body and invading foreign antigens. White blood cells and other immune bodies then begin to attack body tissues in addition to foreign antigens. Many diseases, including some forms of diabetes and arthritis, involve this autoimmune response.

Death Is Programmed into the Cell

Each human cell can divide only about 50 times. Once this number of divisions occurs, the cell automatically succumbs to death. This degradation occurs by design, probably as a way for the body to regulate cell number. Programmed cell death, called apoptosis, plays one of its most important roles in the maturation of cells used for immune function.

Some researchers believe the concept of programmed cell death to be the key to the aging process. Acceleration or deceleration of this natural process can lead to problems, such as cancer cell growth.

Glycosylation of Proteins Occurs

Blood glucose, especially when chronically elevated—as occurs in poorly controlled or undiagnosed diabetes—attaches to (glycates) various blood and body proteins. This decreases protein function and can encourage immune system attack on such altered proteins. Eventually, body health declines.

Excess Energy Intake Speeds Aging

For many years, scientists have known that underfed animals, such as spiders, mice, and rats, live longer. Scientists have not yet pinpointed the exact mechanism that allows for life extension in calorie-restricted animals, but they speculate that modified glucose use, decreased free radical damage, changes in gene function, slower cell turnover, and a variety of other factors contribute to longer life. Researchers are currently studying rhesus monkeys that are on a 30% lower energy intake than typical rhesus monkeys. Although the calorie-restricted monkeys have lower blood pressure, blood cholesterol and triglycerides, and higher HDL, it is too soon to analyze the full implications of this severe restriction. On the down side, the monkeys have the same appetite as typical monkeys, making them somewhat desperate for food; their bone density is reduced; and their reproductive ability is in question.[23]

Like the rhesus monkeys, humans housed in Biosphere II had to follow a limited diet because they overestimated their ability to grow their own food. They experienced declines in body weight, blood pressure, blood cholesterol, and blood glucose on the spartan 1800-kcal diets. These parameters remained at the low end of healthy values. It is unknown whether adults in general would voluntarily restrict themselves to this degree in order to obtain the same health benefits.

Hormones are not the only substances in the race for the fountain of youth. Coenzyme Q-10, an enzyme used in energy metabolism, is very popular in Japan and is sold in the United States. Early studies were promising in showing that the enzyme works as an antioxidant and may slow aging, but the studies were small and short term. More recent research casts doubt on the value of such supplementation. Additional research is needed to prove any benefits from use of Coenzyme Q-10.

As the number of possible cell divisions increases, so does life span. The Galapagos tortoise, whose cells divide about 140 times, has a life span of perhaps almost 200 years.

glycosylation The process by which glucose attaches to (glycates) other compounds, such as proteins.

Aging Results from an Interaction of Factors

Most likely, aging results from an interaction of events and changes. Even very healthy people have a shortened life expectancy if they are exposed to sufficient environmental stress, like radiation and certain chemical agents, such as industrial solvents. Because cell aging and diseases such as cancer are aggravated by environmental factors, it makes good sense to avoid such risks as excessive sunlight exposure and hazardous chemicals. Again, as has been stressed, we have some control over how quickly we age.

CONCEPT CHECK

Although life span has not changed, life expectancy has increased dramatically over the past century. In many societies, this means an increasing proportion of the population is, and will be, over 65 years of age. Avoiding continually rising health-care costs and maximizing satisfaction with life require postponing and minimizing chronic illness. Aging begins early in life and probably results from both automatic cellular changes and environmental influences. Some current hypotheses of aging suggest these possible causes: errors in DNA replication accumulate, connective tissue stiffens, lipid by-products build up, electron-seeking free radical compounds break down cell parts, hormonal and immune systems don't function well, and autoimmune responses and high blood glucose damage key body compounds. Researchers are also studying the possibility that excess energy intakes may be a factor in premature death. Diet can play a role in slowing some of these processes. The use of nutrient and related supplements, medical therapies, and energy restriction are in experimental phases.

■ EFFECTS OF AGING ON NUTRITIONAL HEALTH

Adults over age 50 vary more in health status among themselves than do persons in any other age group. This means that chronological age is not useful in predicting physical health status (physiological age). Among people aged 70 and over, some are totally independent, healthy people, whereas others are frail and require almost total care. To predict the nutritional problems of an older person, it is necessary to know the extent of physiological change caused by aging and whether the person shows early warning signs for long-term poor nutrition (Table 18-2).[1] As you examine how aging affects body systems and how these changes contribute to nutritional health, note the suggested ways to lessen health risks (Table 18-3).

TABLE 18-2   Selected Diseases Associated with Aging

Chronic Condition	Rate of Occurrence per 1000 People			
	All Americans	45–64 Years	65–74 Years	75+ Years
Arthritis	131	280	460	508
Hypertension	124	265	408	395
Hearing impairment	91	149	261	381
Heart condition	83	137	291	339
Visual impairment	35	46	72	136
Deformities or orthopedic impairment	121	175	191	198
Diabetes	26	55	98	92
Diverticula of intestines	8	15	36	45
Asthma	37	32	47	26

■ Decreased Appetite and Food Intake

Decreases in body weight are common in adults age 70 and older, who may not eat enough to meet energy needs.[27] This phenomenon is a problem for older people in particular because it increases the risk of nutrition-related illness, especially when the concentration of the blood protein albumin falls below about 4 g/dl.

Many causes of inadequate food intake in older people are possible. Researchers suggest that biological origins, such as changes in neuroendocrine factors that influence feeding, account for some of this decline (see Chapter 13 for a review of these factors). When older men are underfed in metabolic ward settings, they do not later increase food intake to compensate for reduced food consumption when given the opportunity. Changes in taste and smell may also be important. In addition, social aspects play a role in reduced food intake. Many older people live alone, a circumstance that is associated with less food consumption.

To maintain health, older adults need to address the issue of declining weight. Significant weight loss in older people, sometimes termed the "dwindles," increases risk of death. It may also indicate ongoing illness and reduced tolerance to medication or simple withdrawal from life itself. Even in apparently healthy older individuals, successful weight maintenance may require an increased conscious control over food intake, relative to younger individuals. Consuming energy-dense snacks, such as cheese, nuts, yogurt, oatmeal cookies, and bananas, between meals is one strategy. When assessing weight in older people, compare present weight with the previous year's weight.

*P*harmaceutical companies have begun to market liquid meal-replacement formulas to older adults. Previously, these products were primarily used in hospitals and nursing homes. These products are protein rich and have a fat content similar to 2% or whole milk, with added vitamins and minerals. It generally takes 4 cups (1 L) or more of the product to provide the Daily Values for vitamins and minerals, at an energy cost of about 1000 to 1500 kcal. Many of these products have an unusual taste because of the vitamins that have been added. Older adults can decide if the convenience, cost, and taste make this a wise diet choice.

TABLE 18-3   Typical Physiological Changes Experienced by Older Adults and Recommended Diet Lifestyle Responses[3,8,10,16,31]

Change	Response
Decrease in appetite and food intake	Monitor weight and strive to eat enough to maintain healthy weight
Decline in sense of taste and smell	Vary the diet and experiment with herbs and spices
Loss of teeth	Work with a dentist to maximize chewing ability; modify food consistency as necessary
Decreased sense of thirst	Consume about 8 cups of fluid each day, and watch for evidence of dehydration (e.g., minimal urine output or dark color)
Constipation	Consume 20 to 35 g of dietary fiber daily, choosing primarily fruits, vegetables, and whole grains; meet fluid needs
Decline in lactase production	Limit milk serving size at each use; consume yogurt or cheese; seek other calcium sources (see Chapter 11 for ideas)
Iron deficiency anemia	Include some lean meat in the diet; ask physician to monitor blood iron status
Decline in liver function	Consume alcohol in moderation, if at all
Decline in insulin function	Maintain healthy body weight and perform regular physical activity
Decline in kidney function	Modify protein and other nutrients in diet when advised by physician
Decline in immune function	Meet nutrient needs, especially protein, vitamin E, vitamin B-6, and zinc
Decline in lung function	Don't smoke tobacco products; perform regular physical activity
Decline in vision	Consume fruits, vegetables, and whole grains regularly to gain the benefit of carotenoids and vitamins C and E
Decrease in lean tissue	Meet nutrient needs and perform regular physical activity, including some resistance (strength-training) activity (see Chapter 14)
Decrease in cardiovascular function	Keep blood lipids and blood pressure within desirable range, using diet and medications when needed (see Chapters 6 and 11); stay physically active
Decrease in bone mass	Meet nutrient needs, especially calcium and vitamin D, and perform regular physical activity (see Chapter 11)

What is seen as the physiological changes associated with aging is the sum of natural processes and lifestyle practices. By adopting practices that minimize a decline in body function in the adult years, we invest in our future health.

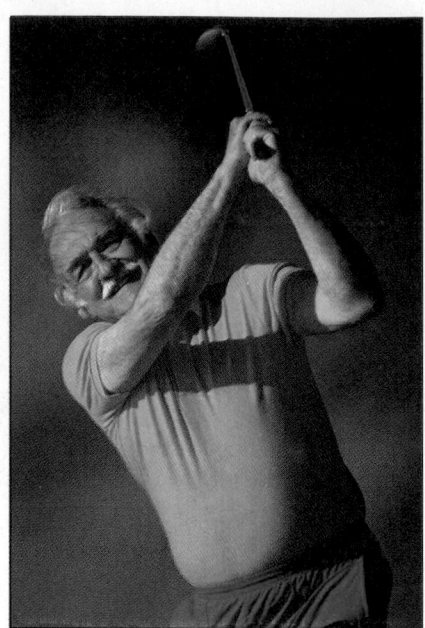

Age is no reason not to continue whatever physical activity is possible. This contributes to many aspects of health, including that of the GI tract.

ostomy A surgically created short circuit in intestinal flow where the end point usually opens from the abdominal cavity rather than the anus; for example, a colostomy.

Incontinence, the inability to control the muscle responsible for retaining urine, affects up to 20% of older adults living at home and about 75% of those in nursing homes. The embarrassment of having to wear diapers causes many to avoid fluids (resulting in dehydration and constipation) and to become socially isolated.

Changes in the Senses of Taste and Smell

Sensitivity to taste and smell often decreases with age, starting at about age 60. One reason is that the number of taste buds decline. Food may require stronger seasonings. Food companies are carving a niche in the marketplace by capitalizing on this change; by using a variety of flavor enhancers, they make foods tastier for older consumers. An inadequate diet, use of certain medications, and possibly a zinc deficiency can also contribute to a loss of taste, however. Therefore, a poor appetite should never be dismissed as a characteristic of old age. Many causes can be remedied by measures such as making sure to vary the diet.

■ Decline in Dental Health

About 30% or more older people in the United States have lost all their teeth. Attention to dental hygiene and dental care throughout life greatly lessens this risk. Periodontal (gum) disease commonly causes tooth loss. Replacement dentures enable some to chew normally, but many older adults—especially men—have denture problems. Solving individual dietary needs requires identifying foods that need to be modified in consistency. When people have problems chewing, nutrient-dense snacks can help. Sometimes just allowing extra time for chewing and swallowing encourages more eating.

■ Reduced Thirst Sensation

Older adults often partially lose their sense of thirst and in turn don't drink enough fluids. They are then more likely to become dehydrated, a condition that leads to confusion and sometimes hospitalization. In addition, 25% of fluid comes from food. If older adults are not eating enough food, they increase the risk of becoming dehydrated. It is important for older people to consume enough fluids, and, if necessary, they should be monitored to ensure they do so. About 8 cups of fluid daily is a good goal.[24] An approximate fluid recommendation is the same as for younger adults, 1 ml/kcal expended. This amount must be adjusted if diuretics are used or in certain other medical conditions, such as the presence of an **ostomy.** Some important signs of dehydration, other than confusion, include dry lips, sunken eyes, increased body temperature, decreased blood pressure, constipation, decreased urine output, and nausea.

■ Fall in Gastrointestinal Tract Function

The main intestinal problem for older people is constipation (see Chapter 3 for a review of this problem).[29] To keep the intestinal tract performing efficiently, older people generally need to consume more dietary fiber than they characteristically did in their youth. The goal is approximately 10 to 13 g/1000 kcal in the diet but generally no more than 35 g on a daily basis, unless a physician recommends otherwise. The regular consumption of nuts, fruits, vegetables, beans, and whole grains provides enough dietary fiber. Fiber medications are generally unnecessary but may be used if overall energy intake does not allow for enough dietary fiber intake. Older persons should also drink more fluid to move along masses that could form from high fiber intake. Physical activity likewise helps promote peristalsis. Because some medications can induce constipation, a physician should be consulted if constipation might be related to a medication. If mineral oil is taken as a laxative, it should always be used with caution—and not at mealtimes—because it binds fat-soluble vitamins and limits their absorption.

Lactase production frequently decreases with age. Chapter 5 listed several options for people with lactose intolerance.

The stomach slows its acid production as people age, as well as the synthesis of intrinsic factor. These changes can contribute to poor absorption of vitamin B-12 and eventually to pernicious anemia. Because of this, adults aged 51 years and older need to meet vitamin B-12 needs with crystalline sources, such as found in a fortified breakfast cereal or balanced multivitamin and mineral supplement.[28] Treatment of pernicious anemia, if it develops, includes regular injections of vitamin B-12, use of nasal preparations, or pharmacological oral doses.

Reduced stomach acid production may also hamper calcium and iron absorption. Other conditions that affect the body's iron status in particular occur with the regular use of aspirin, which frequently causes blood loss in the stomach, and the use of antacids, which may bind iron. Ulcers and hemorrhoids can also cause blood loss. Careful attention to iron status is necessary in these cases.

■ Changes in Liver, Gallbladder, and Pancreatic Function

With age, the liver functions less efficiently. When there is a history of significant alcohol consumption, fat buildup in the liver accounts for some decline. Alcohol abuse is a problem among a small but significant group of older individuals who may continue this pattern from earlier in life, or develop heavy drinking patterns and alcoholism later. Later development of this problem sometimes arises from the loneliness and social isolation of retirement or loss of a spouse. Alcohol-related sickness is high in older people, so the health consequences of this excess are considerable.[26] Also, older adults are more likely to take medications affected by alcohol intake. If cirrhosis then ultimately develops, the liver functions even less efficiently (see Chapter 8).

When its function significantly deteriorates, the liver cannot efficiently detoxify many substances. The possibility for vitamin A toxicity in turn increases. Older people should not take excessive amounts of vitamin A because toxic dosages can cause malaise, headache, bone pain, liver dysfunction, and a decrease in white blood cell count.

The gallbladder also functions less efficiently as we age. Gallstones may dam up the bile to be secreted through the gallbladder, causing it to pool and back up into the liver. Gallstones can also interfere with fat digestion by allowing less bile into the small intestine. Obesity is a prime risk factor for gallbladder disease. A low-fat diet or surgery to remove the organ may be necessary for treatment.

Although the digestive function of the pancreas may decline with age, the pancreas has a large reserve capacity. A sign of a failing pancreas is high blood glucose, which occurs under several conditions. Glucose may circulate in the bloodstream, instead of being taken up by cells, because the pancreas secretes less insulin or because cells resist insulin actions—especially adipose cells in obese people with upper-body fat storage. Another cause can be insufficient chromium intake. Where appropriate, improved nutrient intake, regular physical activity, and weight loss (when needed) can improve insulin action and blood glucose regulation.

■ Decline in Kidney Function

Over time, the kidneys filter wastes more slowly as they lose nephrons (filters). As noted in Chapter 7, kidneys deteriorate more often in people who have regularly eaten excessive protein and, in some cases, excess energy (as inferred from studies on laboratory animals). The deterioration significantly decreases the kidneys' ability to excrete the products of protein breakdown, such as urea. Although an increased protein intake of 1 g/kg of healthy body weight has been recommended for physically active older people, the recommendation does not apply to people whose decreased kidney function causes urea to accumulate in the bloodstream.

■ Reduced Immune Function

As previously mentioned, with age the immune system often operates less efficiently. Consuming adequate protein, the gamut of vitamins (especially vitamin E and vitamin B-6), and zinc helps maximize the health of the immune system. Recurrent sicknesses and poor wound healing are warning signs of a diet deficient especially in protein and zinc. Eating too little food in general or too few animal proteins is usually the reason. Older people often eliminate meat from their diet because it's too hard to chew. Balanced nutrient supplements can help bridge gaps in vitamin and mineral intake.[24] On the other hand, overnutrition appears to be equally harmful to the immune system. For example, obesity and excessive fat, iron, and zinc intake can suppress the immune system.

■ Reduced Lung Function

Lung efficiency declines somewhat with age and is especially pronounced in older people who have smoked and continue to smoke tobacco products. Breathing becomes shallower and faster and more difficult as the number of lung alveoli decreases. Smoking often leads to emphysema and lung cancer. The decrease in lung efficiency contributes to a general downward spiral in body function; breathing difficulties limit physical activity and endurance and frequently discourage eating. These changes eventually cancel other efforts to maintain overall health.

Besides not smoking, being physically active helps prevent lung problems. People need not lose their capacity to breathe deeply, as long as sufficient aerobic activity is part of their regular routine. Otherwise, merely walking can demand the exertion of a marathon pace. Coupled with poor muscle tone and decreased muscle mass, movement becomes continually more difficult. What is the answer? Stay physically active throughout life.

■ Reduced Hearing and Vision

Hearing and vision both decline in aging. Hearing impairment occurs mainly in members of industrial societies with urban traffic and aircraft noise and loud music. Older people may also avoid social contacts because they can't hear.

Degenerating eyesight, frequently caused by retinal degeneration, can affect a person's ability to physically get to a grocery store, locate the foods desired, read labels for nutritional content, and prepare the foods at home. Macular degeneration, one form of decreased eyesight, has been associated with cigarette smoking—yet another reason to avoid the habit.

On a positive note, the regular consumption of foods rich in carotenoids—in particular, dark green, leafy vegetables, such as kale, collard greens, spinach, swiss chard, mustard greens, and romaine lettuce—may decrease the risk of developing this retinal degeneration. These vegetables are rich in lutein and zeaxanthin, two carotenoids found in the portion of the eye subject to damage from age-related degeneration. Adequate zinc intake is also important.[15] Eventually, such vision changes may make people afraid to socialize, be active, or take care of important routines of daily life, such as shopping. Recall from Chapters 9 and 10 the possible role vitamins E and C play in reducing cataracts in the eye. This benefit serves as another reason adults should have a diet rich in fruits and vegetables.[8] Other causes of cataracts are smoking, certain medications, diabetes and ultraviolet light exposure.

■ Decrease in Lean Tissue

Some muscle cells shrink and others are lost as muscles age; some muscles lose their elasticity as they accumulate fat and collagen protein. Lifestyle greatly determines the rate of muscle mass deterioration. As you might predict, an active lifestyle tends to maintain muscle mass, whereas an inactive one encourages its loss.

The loss of muscle mass leads to a decrease in basal metabolism, muscle strength, and energy needs. Furthermore, less muscle mass leads to lower physical activity, which makes the prognosis for maintaining muscle mass even worse. Clearly, it is best to avoid this vicious cycle. Just when all seems lost, though, note that the benefits of exercise are quite striking, especially after the age of 50. Ideally, an active lifestyle should include some resistance activity (weight training) throughout life.

Physical activity increases muscle strength and mobility, improves mental outlook, eases daily tasks that require some strength, improves sleep and balance, slows bone loss, and increases joint movement, thus reducing injuries.[3,10,16] However, when older adults stop their strength-training program, gains in muscle strength are quickly lost. This illustrates the importance of regular physical activity throughout life.

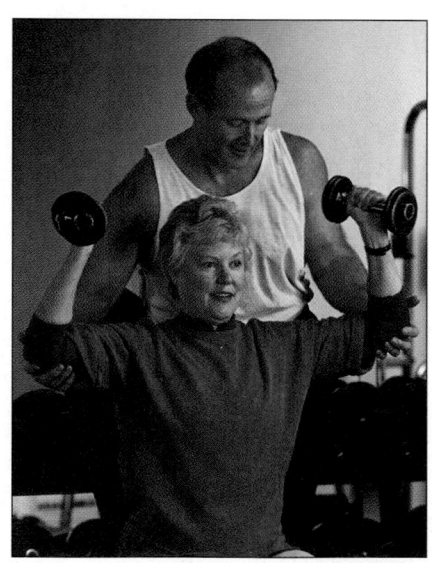

Older people benefit from both aerobic and strength-training exercises. Strength-training especially helps reverse some of the decline in daily function associated with the muscle loss typically seen in older adulthood.

After obtaining a physician's approval to get started, older people can seek out programs to begin strength and aerobic training at community recreation centers or the local YMCA or YWCA. Cardiac rehabilitation centers are another possibility. Most of these organizations have qualified trainers who can help set up a program. Dumbbells are inexpensive and thus ideal for performing strength training at home. Chapter 14 provides some general advice on this topic, including advice for warm-up, stretching, and cooldown activities.

Older adults also benefit from physical activity because it stimulates food intake by raising energy expenditure. By eating more, they increase their chances of consuming adequate amounts of nutrients. Overall, much of what we associate with aging in terms of physical health results from long-standing sedentary lifestyles.[3]

■ Increases in Fat Stores

As lean tissue decreases with age, the body often takes on more fat. Much of this results from overeating and minimal physical activity, although even athletic men gain some degree of midsection fat after the age of 50.

If obesity results, it can raise blood pressure and blood glucose and make walking and performing daily tasks more difficult. Although a small fat gain in adulthood may not compromise health, large gains are often problematic.

■ Reduced Cardiovascular Health

The heart often pumps blood less efficiently in older people, usually because of insufficient physical activity. Poor heart conditioning allows fatty and connective tissues to infiltrate the heart's muscular wall. However, this decline in **cardiac output** is not inevitable with aging and does not occur among older people who remain physically active. In fact, it is thought that the inactive lifestyles of nearly 60% of our country may contribute as much to the risk for cardiovascular disease as smoking a pack of cigarettes per day.

Heart attack and stroke, 2 of the 3 major causes of death in all adults, are caused primarily by atherosclerosis and hypertension. As we age, atherosclerotic plaque accumulates in the arteries, reducing their elasticity, constricting blood flow, and consequently elevating blood pressure.

You already know the main way to limit the buildup of atherosclerotic plaque: Keep LDL and the total cholesterol/HDL ratio in the desirable range (see Chapter 6). New evidence shows that a diet very low in fat can cause some plaques to decrease in size. Other studies use diet and medications to lower blood cholesterol, which in turn reduces the amount of plaque in the arteries supplying the heart. This suggests that a heart-healthy diet is more important during middle to late adulthood than researchers previously thought. Consuming sufficient vitamin B-6, folate, and vitamin B-12 is also important to avoid elevated blood homocysteine, an additional risk factor for cardiovascular disease.

Much controversy surrounds the treatment for elevated LDL-cholesterol in people over the age of 70. If these people adhere to extremely restrictive diets limited in fat and energy to the point that they can't keep up their weight, or if their diets lack variety, they may become undernourished. This may be a worse predicament for them than having high LDL-cholesterol. Therefore, treating elevated LDL-cholesterol in an older person who has other illnesses, such as chronic lung disease and **dementia** (which are likely to shorten life as well as hamper its quality) is probably inappropriate. However, if a healthy 70-year-old who is likely to live another 10 to 15 years has both elevated LDL-cholesterol and evidence of cardiovascular disease, an eating and exercise plan is probably in order to reduce the chance of heart attack. Overall, the pros and cons of different treatments to reduce cardiovascular disease need to be weighed carefully before they are advocated for an older adult.

Hypertension is heavily implicated in both stroke and heart attack in older adults. Blood pressure can be lowered in many people by restriction in salt intake. A limit of 2.4 g of sodium per day (5 g salt per day) helps many people with hypertension, but

*S*ince 1958, the number of Americans with diabetes has tripled, in part because the population is getting older and more obese. Currently, about 16 million Americans have diabetes, an increase of 5 million since 1983.

cardiac output The amount of blood pumped by the heart.

dementia General persistent loss or decrease in mental function.

that is a difficult diet to plan and follow. Alternatively, a mild sodium restriction (not to exceed 4 g of sodium daily) may be effective for salt-sensitive people but is not so helpful by itself for those who are not salt sensitive; it does, however, aid the action of certain diuretics used to treat hypertension. (The Nutrition Perspective in Chapter 11 reviews the effects of other nutrients such as calcium and potassium and lifestyle interventions on blood pressure.)

We can do much to prevent heart attack and stroke just by eating a balanced diet, walking briskly and otherwise performing regular physical activity, controlling blood pressure, not smoking, and maintaining healthy weight.[17] Regular physical activity and a diet rich in fruits and vegetables are also associated with fewer strokes as adults age, as is a moderate use of alcohol (e.g., ischemic strokes).

▪ Decline in Bone Health

Chapter 11 discussed the decline in bone density associated with aging. Recall that bone loss in women occurs primarily after menopause. Bone loss in men is slow and steady from middle age throughout later life. Estrogen replacement at menopause is one treatment to lessen bone loss in women, but other medication regimens are also effective (see the Expert Opinion in Chapter 11). For adults in general over age 50, increasing calcium intake to 1200 mg/day (200 mg/day greater than the young adult Adequate Intake) is recommended.

Other measures to prevent bone loss can be started earlier and continued throughout life. Maintaining adequate vitamin D nutriture (10–15 µg/day [5–10 µg/day greater than the young adult Adequate Intake]) is a first step. The 15 µg/day refers to adults > 70 years.

Many older people may suffer from hidden osteomalacia, a condition primarily caused by not enough sun exposure and therefore diminished vitamin D synthesis in the skin. When they can't get regular sun exposure—during the winter or when they are homebound—older people need a dietary (e.g., milk) or supplemental source of vitamin D.[24]

To these two measures, add not smoking and drinking alcohol moderately or not at all. In addition, underweight women are at especially high risk for developing osteoporosis. Performing weight-bearing activity, such as walking, can help sustain bone, in this case and in general.

Very severe osteoporosis limits the ability of older people to move about, shop, prepare food, and live normally. They eat less and as a result consume fewer nutrients.

Older people should also work with their physician to develop a plan for limiting falls. Falls may be caused by the side effects of medication, gait and balance disorders, impaired vision, and environmental hazards. Protective hip padding can reduce the risk of fracture in individuals who tend to fall.

▪ OTHER FACTORS THAT INFLUENCE NUTRIENT NEEDS IN AGING

*G*rapefruit juice can increase or decrease the potency of some prescription medications, such as certain blood pressure medications, tranquilizers, antihistamines, blood cholesterol-lowering medications (statins), and others, such as a class of drugs used to treat HIV/AIDS. For this reason, a physician or pharmacist should be consulted before grapefruit juice is ingested by those on prescription medication.

Medications and old age often go together. Medications can improve health and quality of life, but some of them also profoundly affect nutrient needs at all ages, including the later years (Table 18-4). Two-thirds of older adults take prescription drugs; one-quarter of the elderly population regularly take multiple prescription drugs, called polypharmacy. Many drugs affect appetite or the absorption of nutrients. Often, people must take medications for long periods. They should make sure to work with their physician and pharmacist to coordinate all medications taken. Pharmacists can advise when to take drugs—with or between meals—for maximum effectiveness.

Drug-related nutritional problems include (1) increased need for potassium when certain types of diuretics increase excretion from the body and (2) changes in ap-

TABLE 18-4	Potential Drug-Nutrient Interactions for Some Commonly Used Drugs		
Drugs	**Uses**	**Nutrients Affected**	**Potential Side Effects**
Antacids (Maalox)	Reduce stomach acidity	Calcium, vitamin B-12, and iron	Decreased absorption due to altered gastrointestinal pH
Anticoagulants (Coumadin)	Prevent blood clots	Vitamin K	Interfers with utilization
Aspirin	Anti-inflammatory; reduces pain	Iron	Anemia from blood loss
Cathartics (laxatives)	Induce bowel movement	Calcium and potassium	Poor absorption
Cholestyramine	Reduces blood cholesterol	Vitamins A, D, E, and K	Poor absorption
Cimetidine (Tagamet)	Treats ulcers	Vitamin B-12	Poor absorption
Colchicine	Treats gout	Vitamin B-12, carotenoids, and magnesium	Decreased absorption due to damaged intestinal mucosa
Corticosteroids (prednisone)	Anti-inflammatory	Zinc	Poor absorption
		Calcium	Poor utilization
Furosemide (Lasix)	Decreases blood pressure; potassium-wasting diuretic	Potassium and sodium	Increased loss
Hydrochlorothiazide	Decreases blood pressure; diuretic	Potassium and magnesium	Increased loss; decreased absorption
MAO inhibitors (Parnate)	Antidepressant	Tyramine (in aged foods)	High blood pressure caused by limited tyramine metabolism
Tricyclic antidepressants (Elavil)	Antidepressant	—	Weight gain from appetite stimulation

petite caused by antidepressant agents or certain antibiotics. Blood loss from the long-term use of aspirin or aspirin-like medications depletes iron reserves and can lead to anemia. People who must take one or more medications for more than just a few weeks should closely watch their diets, eat nutrient-dense foods, and possibly take nutrient supplements to counteract the effects of certain medications. A physician should supervise this last practice, because some supplements can interfere with the function of certain medications. For example, vitamin K can reduce the activity of oral anticoagulants (see Chapter 9).

■ Depression in Older Adults

Depression occurs in about 20% of nursing home residents. In contrast, it occurs in only 3% of older adults who reside outside of nursing homes. In the United States, about 16% of persons who are 65 years old or older experience depression, and this figure is projected to increase greatly by the year 2030. That—combined with isolation and loneliness as family and friends die, move away, or become less mobile—frequently contributes to apathetic eating and weight loss.[7] People living alone do not necessarily make poor food choices, but they often consume less energy, in part by skipping meals. Older men are especially prone to this habit. About one-third of all older people not in nursing homes live alone. Depression can be a downward spiral in which poor appetite produces weakness, which leads to even poorer appetite (Fig. 18-3). In older adults, the resulting poor nutritional state can produce further mental confusion and increased isolation and loneliness.

Many clinicians wrongly believe that depression is a typical consequence of old age, or they overlook its symptoms because they are similar to other characteristics of old age. If depression is left untreated, it is estimated that 15% of the cases may be fatal (suicide). Depression also may be a sign of an underlying illness, which is another reason that early detection is important in older adults. Depression is often treatable, but medication alone will not help those who are experiencing major life changes, such as the death of a spouse. Adequate social support also is essential.[7]

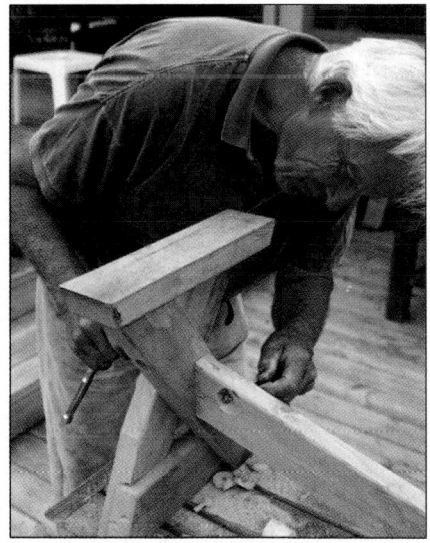

Aging is no reason to withdraw from life. Learning and practicing new skills throughout life contribute to overall health

Former president Jimmy Carter recommends that older adults stay connected to life to maximize health. This can include volunteering one's services and helping one's friends in their later years.

Social isolation; perhaps spouse has died

Loses interest in food; diet deteriorates

Poor diet leads to weakness; this increases a feeling of isolation and abandonment

Further isolation can then decrease desire for self–care

Health declines visibly; weakness remains

Self–care is seriously hampered

■ FIGURE 18-3 The decline of health often seen in older adults. This decline needs to be prevented whenever possible.

Ten Warning Signs of Alzheimer's Disease

1. Recent memory loss that affects job performance
2. Difficulty performing familiar tasks
3. Problems with language
4. Disorientation to time and place
5. Faulty or decreased judgment
6. Problems with abstract thinking
7. Tendency to misplace things
8. Changes in mood or behavior
9. Changes in personality
10. Loss of initiative

To find out more about Alzheimer's disease call the Alzheimer's Association at 800-272-3900, reach the association on the Internet at http://www.alz.org, or call the National Institute on Aging's Alzheimer's Disease Education and Referral center at 800-438-4380.

■ Alcoholism in Older Adults

Alcoholism is a problem in the older population, and about 17% of adults older than 60 are substance abusers. Many older people experience increased stressors, such as the loss of a spouse, loneliness, depression, or chronic diseases. Approximately two-thirds of these alcohol abusers turn to alcohol much earlier in life and simply continue the habit. About one-third begin the habit later in life, due to a variety of factors—more free time, social events centered around drinking, loneliness, or depression. Some of the symptoms of alcoholism in older persons include trembling hands, sleep problems, memory loss, and unsteady gait; these can be easily overlooked simply because they are similar to symptoms of old age.[26]

Older adults become intoxicated on a smaller amount of alcohol than when younger because they metabolize alcohol more slowly. And even small amounts of alcohol can react negatively with various medications that many older persons take routinely. In addition to having adverse effects on the liver, drinking large amounts of alcohol increases the risk of hemorrhagic stroke and may worsen hypertension in older adults. Since drinking large amounts of alcohol produces adverse effects, people over the age of 65 should limit alcohol consumption to no more than one drink per day. Recall from Chapter 8 that one drink per day is defined as 4–5 oz of wine, 12 oz of beer, or 1.5 oz shot of 80-proof liquor.

■ Alzheimer's Disease

In 1907, Dr. Alois Alzheimer documented several cases of what seemed to be early senility. Typical symptoms of the disease included personality changes, unreasonable fears, explosive outbursts, depression, wandering, and general forgetfulness. Today, the disease Dr. Alzheimer first described affects about 4 million people in the United States, including about 45% of all people over the age of 85 and 50% of all people in nursing homes. Age at diagnosis is generally about 75 years. It is estimated that Alzheimer's disease costs the nation $40 billion each year.

Old age is often accompanied by a general decline in mental function. What makes Alzheimer's disease different is that it can be diagnosed by the presence of specific protein (amyloid) deposits and tangled masses of nerves in areas of the brain that are linked to memory, motivation, emotions, voluntary muscle movement, and reasoning. However, this diagnosis can be done only at autopsy, so it is difficult to know precisely how many cases of dementia in old age are actually Alzheimer's disease. Clinical assessments can and should be made by an experienced physician. Because much is known about the typical course of the disease, clinical methods have become more reliable in differentiating between Alzheimer's disease and other causes of dementia.

Causes and Physical Effects

In general terms, Alzheimer's disease is best described as a progressive brain disorder marked by an inability to remember, reason, or understand what is going on. Age is the primary risk factor. Scientists propose causes, including altered cell development, altered brain proteins, and unidentified blood-borne agents. Research over the past few years suggests that a specific blood protein, called *apolipoprotein E-4*, increases the risk of developing Alzheimer's disease. It is thought that this compound interferes with the maintenance of nerve cells, whereas the E-2 or E-3 variant of this protein does not. If the E-4 gene is inherited from both parents, the risk of Alzheimer's disease is about nine times greater in the offspring than if neither gene is E-4. About 2 to 3% of Americans have two E-4 genes. Researchers note, however, that testing individuals for the presence of the E-4 variant is premature because this provides no guarantee that the person will or will not develop the disease. The presence of the E-4 variant is merely a risk factor. Still, there is some interest in developing medications that may compensate for the presence of E-4. Other risk factors under investigation include still more genetic variations, less educational and occupational attainment, physical inactivity, head trauma, aluminum in drinking water, atherosclerosis, and strokes, as well as loss of estrogen at menopause in women. Scientists are also studying the possibility that the regular use of ibuprofen and related drugs may reduce the risk of Alzheimer's disease by reducing related brain inflammation. Use of certain blood cholesterol-lowering medications (statins) may also reduce risk of Alzheimer's disease.

Prevention

The answer to preventing Alzheimer's disease is what scientists today are searching for because, once the disease progresses into its later stages, the damage done to the brain is probably irreversible. The most recent development is a vaccine that prevents amyloid accumulation in the brain. The vaccine was moderately effective in mice; with FDA approval, 24 people who have early signs of Alzheimer's have been treated with the vaccine. Scientists say it will take a few years before the results of its effectiveness are known.

In the meantime, scientists suggest exercising one's body as well as one's brain (e.g., read, do crossword puzzles, and be creative with daily tasks, such as taking another route to the store which is unfamiliar each day to prevent Alzheimer's disease. In addition, eating a diet rich in folate, vitamin B-6, and vitamin B-12 is suggested, due to the link between low levels of these vitamins and lower cognitive test results. If these vitamin intakes are low, then homocysteine in the blood is usually high, and this has been linked to the incidence of Alzheimer's disease.[25] Estrogen therapy and vitamin E and ginkgo biloba supplementation are being investigated further for use in prevention and treatment (see the Nutrition Perspective in this chapter). Current studies implicate mixed results, resulting in a need for further research.

Treatment

The environment of the person with Alzheimer's disease should be safe, with attention paid to risks such as wandering or forgetting about food cooking on a stove. Establishing routines is also helpful, along with regular physical activity and calming conversations. Nursing home placement can be delayed if the patient's family receives proper support and counseling on how to deal with the stress of caring for a patient with Alzheimer's disease.

Today, medical treatment of Alzheimer's disease is usually limited to the use of antidepressants and other drugs that target related symptoms of the disease. Two drugs are approved specifically for Alzheimer's disease. The first is tacrine (Cognex), a drug that may slow the brain's breakdown of a major neurotransmitter used in sending nerve messages. Side effects currently limit its usefulness to a subset of patients, and it does not cure the disease. The second drug, donepezil (Aricept), may maintain or improve cognitive function, behavioral function, and activities of daily living. Although donepezil works in the same way as tacrine, it is a breakthrough in that it leads to far fewer side effects, and fewer doses are required.

Nutritional Considerations

The main nutritional goal for people with this disease is a healthful diet that maintains body weight. Abnormal food behavior, such as gorging, is often seen early in the course of Alzheimer's disease. A craving for sweets may lead to a temporary weight gain, which can be managed by offering lower-energy snacks and meals. At the other extreme, many people refuse to eat. Frequent small meals and nutrient-dense snacks using favorite foods when possible may encourage more regular eating. People who are still leading reasonably independent lives may not be able to shop or to remember to eat meals. Congregate feeding programs and home-delivered meals may be helpful during the early stages of disease. Keep in mind that, by the time the disease has been diagnosed, some people have already developed nutritional problems.

As the disease progresses, people with Alzheimer's disease grow increasingly confused and distracted. At this stage, it is necessary for others to oversee food planning and mealtimes. Caretakers should also try to control distractions—such as television,

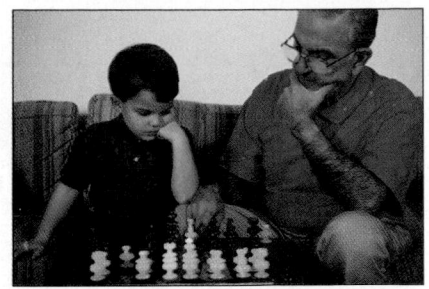

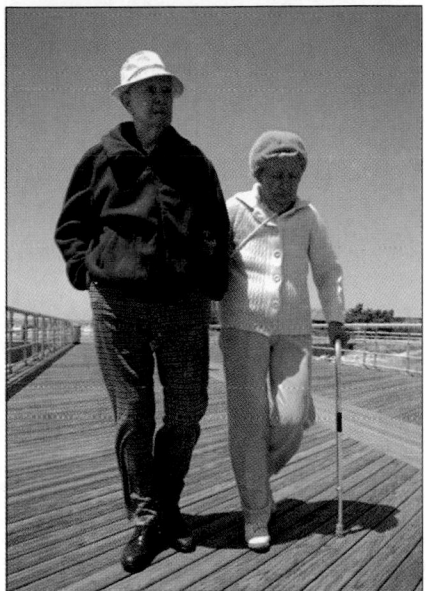

Exercising both the mind and body is important throughout life. The need for both is receiving great attention in the scientific literature.

radio, children, pets, and the telephone—that can disrupt a meal for someone with Alzheimer's disease.[2] Caretakers also should monitor food temperatures, because people with Alzheimer's disease may ignore discomfort and burn themselves. Tough or crunchy foods that may easily cause choking should be avoided. As people with Alzheimer's disease become less able to manage eating by themselves, feeding them becomes more of a challenge. They may hold food in the mouth, forget how to eat or swallow, spit out food, and play with and then refuse food. As you might surmise, caretakers bear much of the daily toll of this disease.

CONCEPT CHECK

Nutritional problems common to aging adults relate to both the process of chronic diseases and the normal decrease in organ function that occurs with time. All these organ systems and functions can decrease as we age: appetite; sense of taste, smell, thirst, hearing, and sight; digestion and absorption; liver, gallbladder, pancreatic, kidney, lung, and heart function; and the immune system. In addition, bone mass and muscle mass gradually decrease, the latter largely because of a deficient diet and inactivity. Appropriate dietary changes and regular physical activity can often help reduce the impact of these results of aging.

■ Nutrient Needs in Middle and Older Adulthood

The latest Dietary Reference Intakes for nutrients and energy include a category for both men and women who are 51 to 70 years of age and more than 70 years of age. Because the lifestyle of an active older person can differ considerably from that of a nursing home resident, establishing nutrient needs during these wide age ranges is problematic.

Do Nutrient Needs Change in Later Life?

Only during the past few years has much research focused on the question of whether nutrient needs change. Because DRIs apply only to healthy people, many older people—for example, those who have ulcers or are heavy aspirin users—are not covered by these standards. Indeed, it is particularly tricky to develop nutrient standards that are valid for most older people because so many are ill and/or regularly take medication.

Researchers have suggested that the current nutrient standards for healthy older people are probably too high for vitamin A; a bit too low in protein (for active people); and about right for the other vitamins. For most minerals, the nutrient standards are probably about right or a bit generous. The "about right" category reveals that we lack evidence to make a more definitive statement.

Still, a well-planned diet that follows the Food Guide Pyramid can meet all nutrient needs for older people within about 1600 to 1800 kcal, except for probably vitamin D, vitamin B-12, folate and calcium. It would take at least three servings from the milk, yogurt, and cheese group for calcium—a recommendation that most older people would find difficult to meet. Calcium-fortified foods can help when necessary (see Chapter 11 for details). Meeting the folate and vitamin B-12 standard also is aided by use of fortified foods, such as breakfast cereals.

The use of a balanced nutrient supplement is especially helpful for meeting vitamin D needs, but it should be low in or free of iron. Women after menopause have iron needs that are the same as men, as they no longer lose iron in menstruation. Recall from Chapter 12 that men should not take a supplement containing iron unless they have evidence of iron-deficiency anemia, as they consume enough iron and it can easily accumulate to toxic amounts in the body. This now applies to women, as they experience minimal iron loss in the postmenopausal state. Finally, if megadose vitamin E use is desired, this will require a separate supplement.

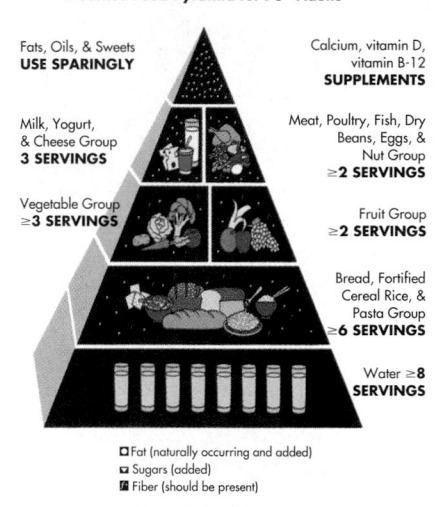

Tufts University's Modified Food Pyramid for 70+ Adults

Fats, Oils, & Sweets USE SPARINGLY

Calcium, vitamin D, vitamin B-12 SUPPLEMENTS

Milk, Yogurt, & Cheese Group 3 SERVINGS

Meat, Poultry, Fish, Dry Beans, Eggs, & Nut Group ≥2 SERVINGS

Vegetable Group ≥3 SERVINGS

Fruit Group ≥2 SERVINGS

Bread, Fortified Cereal Rice, & Pasta Group ≥6 SERVINGS

Water ≥8 SERVINGS

□ Fat (naturally occurring and added)
◨ Sugars (added)
▣ Fiber (should be present)

These symbols show fat, added sugars, and fiber in foods.

Nutrition experts at Tufts University recently suggested a modification of the Food Guide Pyramid to include vitamin D, vitamin B-12, and calcium supplements for adults over 70 years of age.[24] Other changes suggested were at least three servings from the milk, yogurt, and cheese group and at least eight servings of water (or other fluids). The use of a supplement to help meet vitamin D, vitamin B-12, and calcium needs is especially helpful for older people who require such a low energy intake that they are not able to consume enough food to supply these nutrients.

Planning a Diet for People in Their Later Years

To supply energy needs for males age 51 and older, the 1989 RDAs suggest 2300 kcal; for females, the recommendation is 1900 kcal. (These values are based on a 170-lb, 68-in tall man and a 143-lb, 63-in tall woman.) Studies show that older men eat closer to 1800 to 2100 kcal, whereas women eat about 1300 to 1600 kcal. Furthermore, surveys indicate that many older adults are consuming more fat than recommended and less calcium than is needed.

A good practice would be to decrease fat and sugar consumption to increase the diet's nutrient density and to make sure dietary fiber intake is adequate.[31] In addition, some protein should come from lean meats to help meet vitamin B-6 and zinc needs, two nutrients of additional concern.

Fluid needs are about 8 cups (about 2 L) per day. A high-fiber diet especially requires attention to fluid needs. Fiber intake should be slowly increased to about 35 g/day, with each serving of fiber accompanied by a glass of water (or other fluid).

Singles of all ages face logistical problems with food: Purchasing, preparing, storing, and using food with minimal waste are challenging. Economy packages of meats and vegetables are normally too large to be useful for a single person. Many singles live in small dwellings, some without kitchens and freezers. Creating a diet to accommodate a limited budget and facilities and a single appetite requires special considerations. Following are some practical suggestions for diet planning for singles:

- If one owns a freezer, cook large amounts, divide into portions, and freeze.
- Buy only what one can be used; small containers may be expensive, but letting food spoil is also costly.
- Ask the grocer to break open a family-sized package of wrapped meat or fresh vegetables and separate it into smaller units.
- Buy only several pieces of fruit—perhaps a ripe one, a medium-ripe one, and an unripe one—so that the fruit can be eaten over a period of several days.
- Keep a box of dry milk handy to add nutrients to recipes for baked foods and other foods for which this addition is acceptable.

Nutritional deficiencies and protein-energy undernutrition have been identified among some aging populations, particularly those in nursing homes or long-term care facilities and those who are hospitalized. These nutritional problems increase the risk for many diseases, including bed sores (pressure ulcers), and compromise recovery from illness and surgery. Friends, relatives, and health-care personnel should look for poor nutrient intake in all older people, including those who live in nursing home settings. About 40% of adults now age 65 will spend some time in a nursing home. Family members have a unique opportunity to make sure nutrient needs are met by looking for weight maintenance based on regular, healthful meal patterns. If problems arise in instituting a healthful diet, registered dietitians can offer professional and personalized advice.

Surveys show that the majority of older adults like most vegetables, despite misconceptions that they do not like broccoli (because it forms gas) or tomatoes (because they contain too much acid). By the time we reach adulthood, our eating habits reflect regional tastes, social class, ethnic group, and life experiences. There is no generic food list for older people. Dr. Nancy Wellman discusses this in detail in her Expert Opinion.

Overall, good nutrition benefits older adults in many ways. Meeting nutrient needs delays the onset of some diseases; improves the management of some existing diseases; hastens recovery from many illnesses; can increase mental, physical, and social well-being; and often decreases the need for and length of hospitalization.[22] A variety of strategies can promote healthful eating in later life (Table 18-5). These should focus on presenting nutritious, tasty foods in a pleasant environment.

Obtaining enough food may be difficult for some older persons, especially if they are unable to drive and relatives do not live close enough to help with cooking or shopping. Older persons tend to see asking for help as a symbolic loss of

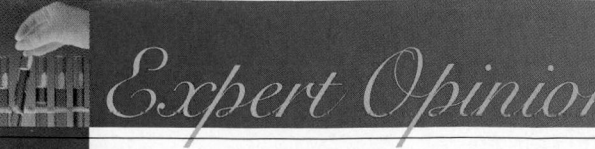

NUTRITION AND OLDER ADULTS—WHY SHOULD YOU CARE?

Nancy S. Wellman, Ph.D., RD, FADA

We all know people older than ourselves, yet whom we consider *old* depends a lot on our own age. Youngsters consider their *30-something* parents old. Almost everyone used to think anyone with gray hair or wrinkles or anyone who retired was old. Today, hair color, skin tone, or age 65 no longer defines *old*. In fact, many baby boomers and Xers have a goal to retire in their 40s or 50s—as soon as they can stockpile enough money for a comfortable lifestyle.

Before discounting older adults, just think how much more interesting you'll become as you add years and experiences to your own life. Although stereotypes about getting old abound, many just aren't true anymore.

How you age can be greatly influenced by your personal commitment to nutrition, fitness, health-risk reduction, and attitude. As a typical American, your goal is probably to stay young as long as possible. To make it happen, it's essential to eat healthfully, stay active, manage stress, and think positively. Certainly, genetics counts, too. Long-living family members are a definite plus; however, even longevity isn't enough. We want a good quality of life in our later years.

We are the most death-denying nation on earth, and most of us will refuse to grow old gracefully. Inevitably, some of us

will face similar health and nutrition problems if we live long enough. Let's look at some practical aspects of aging to determine why we should care about nutrition in older adults.

If it's too great a stretch to picture yourself in your 80s, in your 90s, or as a centenarian, think of some of the *oldest old* (those over 85) whom you know. They may be your great-grandparents, aunts, or neighbors, or they may be famous people. Many are living full, active, productive lives; others may not be as independent as they once were.

The following are some *likely* but not universal challenges as age and risk of malnutrition, frailty, and health problems increase. A lessened ability to taste, smell, chew, and digest food may interfere with getting all the nutrients we need. We might be too zealous in eliminating fat, salt, or sugar from our diets. If so, our food won't taste very good, and we may not bother to eat enough. The older we get, the tougher it is to keep weight up. In fact, losing a lot of weight without wanting to is a warning sign that shouldn't be ignored. You'll find few among the *oldest old* at the opposite end of the weight spectrum. The obese and overweight have already paid the price with a shorter life span.

Staying active pays off in greater and longer independence and a good quality

of life. If arthritis, osteoporosis, or other illnesses keep us from walking, we might not be able to grocery shop or cook—or even feed ourselves—all crucial to good nutritional status.

Our sense of thirst may diminish or we may intentionally drink less to avoid accidents or trips to the bathroom because of fear of falling or painful walking. Dehydration may make us more confused, cause us to be constipated, or place us at greater risk of heat illness and death.

Some medicines we take might drastically decrease our appetites. The more medicines taken, the greater risk of nutrition-related side effects. Medications can radically change the way food tastes and cause constipation, diarrhea, dry mouth, nausea, drowsiness, and weakness.

If we haven't taken care of our teeth or dentures or have mouth problems, we may be excluding harder-to-chew, higher-protein foods, such as meats, or higher-fiber foods, such as fruits and vegetables. Our diets might be quite monotonous if we are forced to skimp on food to pay for heat, medicine, or rent. Monotonous diets shortchange us on calories and nutrients. Having less—or choosing to spend less—than $3 to $4 a day on food makes it hard to eat healthfully, yet that is the daily situation for one in six older Americans.

If our memory isn't as sharp, we may forget if, what, and when we've eaten. Severe memory problems, whether labeled Alzheimer's, dementia, or senility may cause us to forget how to chew and swallow—even if a caregiver is helping us eat. If we live alone, we may not bother to fix a meal or to eat. The common tea and toast diet is not nutritious. Being with people daily improves our food intake and our morale. If we have recently lost a loved one, especially our spouse, it may be too painful to sit opposite the empty chair at the table. Among the one in four older adults who drinks too much alcohol, health problems usually worsen, and calories in alcohol are rarely replaced with nutritious foods.

Many of the challenges of nutrition and aging can be avoided. From a monetary perspective alone, the payoff is high. Reducing malnutrition in later years decreases costly health-care expenditures. Good nutritional status keeps us healthier and, should we become ill, we recover more quickly and have shorter hospital stays and fewer complications. Among the increasing numbers of frail, homebound older adults, 9 out of 10 are at considerable nutrition risk. Unless that risk is reduced, some will be admitted to hospitals again and again, others will be prematurely sent to nursing facilities, and others will die needlessly due to starvation or neglect.

Countries are rightfully measured by the care given their youngest and oldest.

We, as individuals—citizens, or relatives—must assume some responsibility for those born decades before us. It is easy and very personally rewarding to make a difference in the life of an older person. The following are some suggestions:

- Use service learning opportunities in courses to volunteer with older adults. College students have repeatedly had inspirational experiences interacting with older persons in adult day centers and in assisted living and nursing facilities, as well as in the delivery of meals to the homebound.
- Take your oldest relative or neighbor out to eat and ask his or her opinions on current or historical events, the most significant experiences in his or her life, his or her feelings about himself or herself, and his or her joys and needs today.
- Drop off a bag of easy to prepare groceries or ready to eat food to an older person. Help relatives set up a weekly system of fresh, frozen, or canned convenience meals labeled "morning," "afternoon," or "evening" plus the day of the week.
- Make a friendly phone call, even long distance, near mealtime. This may be just the needed reminder to eat for someone you care about.
- Arrange for transportation to meals at senior centers or for home delivery of meals.

- Provide a small, simple (inexpensive) microwave oven plus some supervised practice time as a gift. Give food gifts and generally discourage gifts of clothing and other nonedibles by other people.
- Encourage or arrange a visit to a dentist who specializes in the care of the older adults.
- If an older relative, friend, or neighbor is hospitalized, be that person's advocate. See that the person's weight is measured regularly, question what and how much is eaten, find out which staff member is responsible for monitoring nutritional status, be company at mealtimes, and, if needed, feed the person at a comfortable pace and with dignity. See that the person will receive meals when he or she goes home or that someone is available to help fix meals.

Think positively! It's never too early or too late to eat smarter, get more active, and be healthier, adding not only years to your life and life to your later years.

Dr. Wellman, a past president of the American Dietetic Association, is a professor of dietetics and nutrition at Florida International University. There she directs the National Policy and Resource Center on Nutrition and Aging. She chairs the Nutrition Screening Initiative, a nationwide campaign to reduce nutrition risk in older adults.

To learn about meal programs for senior citizens in your area, call the Administration on Aging's Elder Care Locator, 800-677-1116. For general information on programs for older persons, visit the following web sites: National Institute on Aging, http://www.nih.gov/nia/; American Geriatrics Society, http://www.americangeriatrics.org/; and Administration on Aging, http://www.aoa.dhhs.gov/.

TABLE 18-5   Guidelines for Healthful Eating in Later Years

- Eat regularly; small, frequent meals may be best. Use nutrient-dense foods as a basis for each menu.
- Find out which convenience foods and labor-saving devices can be of help.
- Try new foods, new seasonings, and new ways of preparing foods. Don't use just convenience foods and canned goods.
- Keep some easy-to-prepare foods on hand for times when you feel tired.
- Have a treat occasionally, perhaps an expensive cut of meat or a favorite fresh fruit.
- Eat in a well-lit or sunny area; serve meals attractively; use foods with different flavors, colors, shapes, textures, and smells.
- Arrange things so that food preparation and clean-up are easier.
- Eat with friends, relatives, or at a senior center when possible.
- Share cooking responsibilities with a neighbor.
- Use community resources for help in shopping and other daily care needs.
- Stay physically active.
- If possible, take a walk before eating to stimulate appetite.
- When necessary, chop, grind, or blend hard-to-chew foods. Softer, protein-rich foods can be substituted for meat when poor dental function limits normal food intake. Prepare soups, stews, cooked whole-grain cereals, and casseroles.
- If your feeding movements are limited, cut the food ahead of time, use utensils with deep sides or handles, and obtain more specialized utensils if needed.

independence. Pride, or fear of being victimized by those they hire, may stand in the way of much needed help. In these cases, friends can be a big help. Special transportation arrangements may also be available through a local transit company or taxi service.

Many eligible older people are missing meals and are poorly nourished simply because they don't know of available programs to help them. Irregular meal patterns and weight loss, often caused by difficulties in preparing food, are warning signs that undernutrition may be developing. An effort should be made to identify poorly nourished people and inform them of community services.

Determine:
- Disease
- Eating poorly
- Tooth loss or mouth pain
- Economic hardship
- Reduced social contact and interaction
- Multiple medications
- Involuntary weight loss or gain
- Need for assistance with self care
- Elder at an advanced age

■ Community Nutrition Services for Older People

Health-care advice and services for older people can come from clinics, private practitioners, hospitals, and health maintenance organizations. Home health-care agencies, adult day-care programs, adult overnight-care programs, and **hospice** units (for the terminally ill) can supply daily care.

The Nutrition Screening Initiative, a nutrition checklist for health-care workers, family members, and older persons, can be used as a tool to increase health and nutrition awareness and to plan related education of older persons (Fig. 18-4). The Nutrition Screening Initiative incorporates the acronym "DETERMINE" (see margin). Overall, professionals in the just-mentioned organizations should try to identify older people whose health needs require extra attention.

Nutrition programs for those age 60 and over offer congregate meal programs, which provide lunch at a central location, and home-delivered meals (often known as Meals-on-Wheels if sponsored by the local private or public agencies). About 2.3 million Americans are served each year. Currently about half of the meals use the home-delivered method.

The federal government sets specific standards for home-delivered meals and for those served in congregate feeding centers. The meals are designed to provide one-third of the nutrient needs. The social aspect often improves appetite and general outlook.

A Nutrition Test for Older Adults

Here's a nutrition check for anyone over age 65. Circle the number of points for each statement that applies. Then compute the total and check it against the nutritional score.

1. The person has a chronic illness or current condition that has changed the kind or amount of food eaten. (2 points)
2. The person eats fewer than two full meals per day. (3 points)
3. The person eats few fruits, vegetables, or milk products. (2 points)
4. The person drinks 3 or more servings of beer, liquor, or wine almost every day. (2 points)
5. The person has tooth or mouth problems that make eating difficult. (2 points)
6. The person does not have enough money for food. (4 points)
7. The person eats alone most of the time. (1 point)
8. The person takes three or more different prescription or over-the-counter drugs each day. (1 point)
9. The person has unintentionally lost or gained 10 pounds within the last 6 months. (2 points)
10. The person cannot always shop, cook, or feed himself or herself. (2 points)

Nutritional score:

0–2: Good. Recheck in 6 months.
3–5: Marginal. A local agency on aging has information about nutrition programs for the elderly. The National Association of Area Agencies on Aging can assist in finding help; call (800) 677-1116. Recheck in 6 months.
6 or more: High risk. A doctor should review this test and suggest how to improve nutritional health.

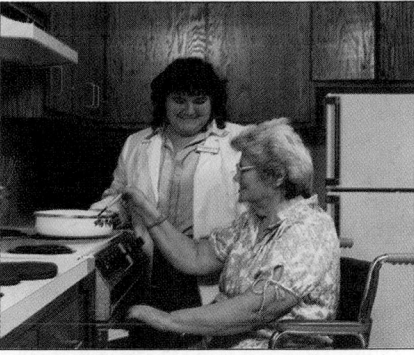

There are many resources in the community to help older adults maintain their health and independence.

■ FIGURE 18-4 A nutrition checklist for older adults.

Reprinted with permission by the Nutrition Screening Initiative, a project of the American Academy of Family Physicians, the American Dietetic Association and the National Council on Aging, Inc., and funded in part by a grant from Ross Products Division, Abbott Laboratories.

Still, congregate meal programs generally provide at most one meal a day and usually not every day of the week. The problem with home-delivered meals is that the one or two meals delivered may never be eaten, and, if not eaten on delivery and left at room temperature, they may become unsafe to eat later. Thus, these programs can help older adults but probably don't meet all their nutritional needs.

In addition to congregate and home-delivered meals, federal commodity distribution is available in some areas of the United States to low-income older people. Food stamps can benefit older people whose incomes are below the poverty level (see Chapter 20 for details on these programs). Food cooperatives and a variety of clubs and social organizations provide additional aid.

CONCEPT CHECK

*S*pecific nutrient requirements for older adults are only now being extensively studied. Diet plans should be modified for decreased physical abilities, the presence of drug-nutrient interactions, possible depression, and economic constraints. Particular attention should be paid to the opportunity for sun exposure and intake of the vitamins D, B-6, folate, and B-12, as well as the minerals calcium and zinc and dietary fiber. A nutrient-dense diet helps meet these needs. Carefully planned supplement use can also help, especially after age 70. In the United States, many nutrition services—such as congregate and home delivered meals—are available to help aging population obtain a healthful diet.

CASE SCENARIO

Follow-Up

Francis could contact a local government office that offers congregate meal programs at a central location. She could inquire about location and available transportation to the site. This would give her social contact with other older persons, which is probably an important element that is missing in her life. This could help alleviate her loneliness. She could also request Meals-on-Wheels (if available) to provide one hot meal a day. One hot meal a day that is prepared for her may be just what she needs to help stimulate her appetite. She could also have groceries delivered to her home if her budget could withstand the extra cost. Other convenience foods that could be included in her diet include milk, assorted nuts, peanut butter, breakfast cereals, canned chicken or deli meats, yogurt, sliced cheese, cottage cheese, calcium-fortified orange juice, canned or frozen fruits and vegetables, and some fresh fruits and vegetables that do not require preparation, such as prewashed lettuce and bananas. A further possibility is a liquid nutritional supplement, such as a can of Ensure, or a nutrition bar, such as an Ensure bar.

SUMMARY

1. Compression of morbidity means delaying symptoms of and disabilities from chronic disease for as many years of life as possible. Good nutritional habits, especially following the Food Guide Pyramid and the Dietary Guidelines for Americans, play a role in this process.

2. Although scientists disagree as to the best diet recommendations for the general public, most agree on some general principles, including those laid out by the Dietary Guidelines for Americans. Such authorities recommend that individuals eat a variety of foods; balance the food eaten with physical activity to maintain or improve weight; choose a diet with plenty of grain products, vegetables, and fruits; choose a diet low in saturated fat, and cholesterol; choose a diet moderate in sugars; choose a diet moderate in sodium (salt); and moderate or avoid alcoholic beverage intake. In addition, recommendations to reduce cancer risk emphasize moderation in the use of cured and smoked meats.

3. Although maximum life span hasn't changed, life expectancy has increased dramatically over the past century. For many societies, this means that an increasing proportion of the population is over 65 years of age. As health-care costs rise, the goal of delaying disease becomes even more important for all of us.

4. Aging begins before birth. Cell aging probably results from automatic cellular changes and environmental influences, such as DNA damage. Add to this list damage caused by electron-seeking free radical compounds, high blood glucose, hormonal changes, and alterations in the immune system as possible causes.

5. Nutritional problems of older adults are related to the presence of chronic diseases and to the normal decreases in organ function that occur with time. These include loss of teeth, lessened sensitivity to taste and smell, changes in gastrointestinal tract function, and deterioration in cardiovascular and bone health. Although disease affects nutritional state, the reverse is also true. Undernutrition adversely affects immune function, allowing for infection.

6. Alzheimer's disease is a progressive and irreversible brain disorder. Its causes are only beginning to be understood. It differs from other types of senile dementia in that the brain tissue accumulates abnormal protein plaques and tangled nerves (observable by autopsy). Nutritional health for people in advanced stages of disease is often complicated by special feeding problems.

7. Scientists are only now beginning extensive study of specific nutrient needs for older people. Diet plans should be based on a nutrient-dense approach and individualized for existing health problems, decreased physical abilities, presence of drug-nutrient interactions, possible depression, and economic constraints. Specific nutrients, such as protein, vitamin D, vitamin E, vitamin B-6, folate, vitamin B-12, zinc, and calcium, along with dietary fiber, often deserve special attention in diet planning.

Careful supplementation can help meet needs, especially for adults 70 years of age and older.

8. Health-care workers and family members should use available options for the procurement of food for the elderly, especially for those who are nutritionally compromised. Most communities have congregate or home-delivered meal systems, food stamps, and other provisions for those who qualify.

■ STUDY QUESTIONS

1. List four of the Dietary Guidelines and give an example of why each one may be difficult for the elderly to implement. What are some solutions to these barriers?
2. What is the difference between life span and life expectancy? As life expectancy increases, what consequence affects the entire population?
3. Name three hormones that decline with aging and the attributes of each.
4. Describe two hypotheses proposed to explain the causes of aging, and note evidence for each in your daily life experiences.
5. List four organ systems that can decline in function in later years, along with a diet/lifestyle response to help cope with the decline.
6. Defend the recommendation for regular physical activity during late adulthood, including some resistance activity (weight training).

7. How might the nutritional needs of older people differ from those of younger people? How are their needs similar? Be specific.
8. What three resources in a community are widely available to aid older adults in maintaining nutritional health?
9. Describe some early warning signs of Alzheimer's disease, and note some of the nutritional implications as this disease advances.
10. List four warning signs of undernutrition in older people that are part of the acronym DETERMINE. Briefly justify the inclusion of each.

■ ANNOTATED REFERENCES

1. ADA Reports: Position of the American Dietetic Association: Nutrition, aging, and the continuum of care. *Journal of the American Dietetic Association* 100:580, 2000.

   As the baby boomer population grows older, nutrition professionals need to focus more on developing successful interventions that will influence the proper nourishment of older adults, such as initiating nutrition screening of older adults and working with other health professionals to expand services to older persons. Multiple factors that influence nutritional status in older adults include medical problems, medications, housing, the availability of transportation, dental health, current diet modifications, and income.

2. Alzheimer's disease: Glimmers of hope: *Consumer Reports on Health,* p. 1, April 2000.

   Scientists are currently testing at least 50 new drugs in humans for the treatment of Alzheimer's disease. For people who have the disease, important precautions for caretakers are to monitor all medication used, arrange for the treatment of other health problems, reduce clutter and chaos, having calming conversations, and take walks together.

3. American College of Sports Medicine Position Stand: Exercise and physical activity for older adults. *The Physician and Sportsmedicine* 27(11):115, 1999.

   Participation in regular exercise is an effective intervention to reduce and/or prevent a number of functional declines associated with aging. Older people who have been shown to readily adapt and respond to endurance and strength-training activities. Together, these adaptations greatly improve the functional capacity of older men and women, thereby improving the quality of life for this population.

4. Anti-aging therapies. *Mayo Clinic Health Letter* 17(5):1, 1999.

   Despite tempting claims, there is no product proven to prevent or reverse aging. This includes DHEA and melatonin. Anyone considering a so-called anti-aging product should speak with a physician first. The physician can help one decide whether the potential benefits of a product outweigh any risks.

5. Are claims for growth hormone bulked up? *Harvard Health Letter* 24(6):1, 1999.

   Growth hormone supplementation in older adults is considered premature at this point in time because it is not clear how it will affect the body in the long run. Short-term supplementation has shown adverse side effects, such as glucose intolerance, high blood pressure, and swollen legs and ankles.

6. Barrett S, Herbert V: Alternative nutrition therapies. In Shils ME and others (eds.): *Modern nutrition in health and disease.* 9th ed. Baltimore MD: Williams & Wilkins, 1999.

   When someone feels better after using a product or procedure, it is natural to credit whatever was done. This can be misleading, however, because most ailments resolve spontaneously, and even those that persist can have symptoms that wax and wane. In addition, taking action for a problem often temporarily relieves symptoms via the placebo effect. People unaware of these facts often give undeserved credit to "alternative" methods of medical treatment.

7. Birrer RB: Depression and aging too often do mix. *Postgraduate Medicine* 104:143, 1998.

Depression is common among nursing home residents and should be diagnosed and treated as soon as possible. Treatment should include pharmacotherapy and psychotherapy.

8. Brown L and others: A prospective study of carotenoid intake and risk of cataract extraction in US men. *American Journal of Clinical Nutrition* 70:517, 1999.

   The carotenoids lutein and zeaxanthin may decrease the risk of cataracts. It is important for adults to consume vegetables and fruits high in carotenoids daily.

9. Can one substance treat both osteoarthritis and depression? *Tufts University Health & Nutrition Letter*, p. 3, November 1999.

   Research on the dietary supplement SAMe (S-adenosylmethionine) suggests that it may assist in rebuilding cartilage and affect brain levels of certain neurotransmitters, in turn decreasing depression symptoms.

10. Christmas C, Andersen RA: Exercise and older patients: Guidelines for the clinician. *Journal of the American Geriatric Society* 48:321, 2000.

    The goal for older persons is to exercise for 30 minutes with moderate intensity more days than not. Stretching and warm-up activities are particularly important in this age group. Including strength training on a regular basis further contributes to physical health.

11. Cupp MJ: Herbal remedies, adverse effects, and drug interactions. *Clinical Pharmacology* 59:1239, 1999.

    Because herbal products are not closely regulated, consumers and health practitioners need to be aware of the adverse effects that these products can produce alone or in conjunction with one another, or with prescription drugs.

12. JAMA Patient Page: Growing older in good health. *Journal of the American Medical Association* 283:560, 2000.

    The diets of older people should contain generous amounts of fruits, vegetables, whole grains, and fiber; small amounts of saturated fat and cholesterol; and only moderate amounts of sugar, and salt. Drinking about eight glasses of water and other fluids each day is beneficial. If one drinks alcohol, one should do so in moderation. Overall, one should make sure the foods eaten are full of the nutrients needed for a healthy body.

13. Kessler DA: Herbs and cancer. *The New England Journal of Medicine* 342:1742, 2000.

    Congress has shown little interest in protecting consumers from the hazards of dietary supplements. Recent examples of toxicity from herbs should persuade Congress to change the law to ensure the safety and efficacy of dietary supplements is established before marketing so more people are not harmed.

14. LeBars PL, Katz MM, Berman N and others: A placebo-controlled, double-blind, randomized trial of an extract of ginkgo biloba for dementia. *Journal of the American Medical Association* 278:1327, 1997.

    The extract of ginkgo biloba used in this trial was found to be safe and exhibited a modest positive effect on the dementia seen in the study participants.

15. Liebman B: Hocus-focus: Can diet protect your eyes? *Nutrition Action Healthletter*, p. 3, July/August 2000.

    Antioxidants such as vitamins C and E and two carotenoids (lutein and zeaxanthin) are strongly linked with cataract prevention. This protection comes from the ability to fight off free radicals produced from oxidative damage of light.

16. Live longer, feel younger. *Consumer Reports on Health*, p. 1, March 1999.

    It is never too late to improve physical or mental health, even if one is already ailing, by adopting healthy habits. Exercise is particularly useful, since it can ward off sickness, strengthen the body, sharpen the mind, and lift the spirits.

17. Living longer. *Mayo Clinic Health Letter* 17(1):1, 1999.

    Weight gain, hypertension, and chronic illness are not necessarily normal parts of aging. A person is, to a large extent, responsible for his or her own longevity. A person is never too old to start taking steps toward living longer and healthier, such as eating a balanced diet, exercising regularly, and investing time in relationships.

18. Malarkey WB: *Take control of your aging.* Wooster, OH: Wooster Book Co., 1999.

    Men and women who are healthy at ages 90 and 100 years typically have many characteristics in common, including daily exercise, excellent nutrition, ongoing learning, a spiritual dimension to their lives, lots of friends, and an excellent sense of humor. These habits are long-standing and are used to organize each day.

19. Mar C, Bent S: An evidence-based review of the 10 most commonly used herbs. *Western Journal of Medicine* 171:168, 1999.

    The most popular herbal supplements include echinacea, St. John's Wort, ginkgo biloba, garlic, saw palmetto, ginseng, and valerian. People should be advised to avoid using a wide variety of herbs at one time because herb-herb interactions are poorly understood. The starting dose for each herb should be the lowest in which desired effects occur. Long-term use of herbal products should be discouraged because long-term effects are unknown.

20. McAlindon TE and others: Glucosamine and chondroitin for treatment of osteoarthritis; a systemic quality assessment and meta-analysis. *Journal of the American Medical Association* 283:1483, 2000.

    Both glucosamine and chondroitin are building blocks of cartilage. When os-teoarthritis patients take them as supplements, they produce a moderate decrease in the pain associated with the disease.

21. Melatonin: Questions, facts, mysteries. *University of California, Berkeley Wellness Letter* 16(8):1, 2000.

    Melatonin in the blood remains at a constant concentration throughout life, so taking a supplement of melatonin is not necessary. Research on its purported benefits for the prevention of jet lag is weak.

22. Miller KE and others: The geriatric patient: A systematic approach to maintaining health. *American Family Physician* 61:1089, 2000.

    A nutritional health screening for older persons should consider whether an illness or a condition has made the person change that type or amount of food consumed. Other problems include eating fewer than two meals a day, consuming few fruits, vegetables, or milk products; consuming three or more alcoholic drinks a day; experiencing tooth loss; not having enough income to buy the food needed; eating alone most of the time; taking three or more different prescription drugs daily; losing or gaining 10 pounds in the past six months without particularly trying to do so; and not always being physically able to shop and feed oneself.

23. Mlot C: Running on one-third empty: Primates on a low-cal diet are in a metabolic slow lane, perhaps to longer life. *Science News* 151:162, 1997.

    Energy restriction has been shown to produce some positive and negative effects on rhesus monkeys. Whether a long-term energy restriction produces more positive or more negative benefits will need to be borne out by this and other research studies.

24. New Food Guide Pyramid specifically for people 70 and older. *Tufts University Health & Nutrition Letter*, p. 8, April 1999.

    Researchers at Tufts University have modified the Food Guide Pyramid to include at least eight servings of water, juice, or other source of fluid each day, as well as to consider increasing calcium, vitamin D, and vitamin B-12 intake via a supplemental source.

25. Nourhashemi F and others: Alzheimer disease: Protective factors. *American Journal of Clinical Nutrition* 71:643S, 2000.

    Many studies suggest that a dietary approach to protecting against Alzheimer's disease should include an abundant intake of the antioxidants found in vegetables and fruits, as well as a diet rich in folate, vitamin B-6, and vitamin B-12 (to counteract a rise in homocysteine in the blood).

26. Rigler S: Alcoholism in the elderly. *American Family Physician* 661:1710, 2000.

    Alcoholism goes unrecognized in many older adults because its symptoms are easily confused with symptoms of old age. It is, however,

TAKE ACTION

I. AM I AGING HEALTHFULLY?

Take Control of Your Aging by Dr. William B. Malarkey includes a plan that incorporates various diet and lifestyle factors that are associated with *successful* aging.[18] Indicate the degree to which you are following such a plan (or alternatively fill this out with a parent or another older relative in mind).

Physical: Do you eat a well-balanced diet, exercise on a regular basis, remain free of illness, abstain from smoking, not drink alcohol excessively, and experience refreshing sleep?

_____

_____

Intellectual: Are you analytical, do you read regularly, do you learn new things each day, do you engage your mental ability at work (or at school), and do you often reflect on your life?

_____

_____

Emotional: Are you at peace, do you like who you are, are you optimistic, and do you laugh and relax regularly?

_____

_____

Relational: Are you a good listener, do you feel supported by friends, do you attend social functions, do you talk with family members often, and do you feel close to coworkers (or fellow students)?

_____

_____

_____

Spiritual: Do you appreciate nature, give to or serve others, meditate or seek religious worship, and feel life has meaning?

_____

_____

_____

The more of these factors that you include in your life, the more well rounded is your plan for maintaining overall health. Any one of the five areas in which you are not achieving success should show you characteristics to work on in the future.

a real problem, which needs to be properly diagnosed and treated.

27. Roberts SB: Energy regulation and aging: Recent findings and their implications. *Nutrition Reviews* 58:91, 2000.

    Depression, social and environmental factors, prescription drugs, and underlying acute and chronic conditions can all negatively impact an elderly person's appetite. Health-care practitioners should manage the

problem by identifying such risk factors and implementing appropriate treatments.

28. Russell RM: The aging process as a modifier of metabolism. *American Journal of Clinical Nutrition* 72:529S, 2000.

    The aging gastrointestinal tract cannot adequately absorb various nutrients to meet the recommended amount because its function declines with age. In response, the latest DRI publication increased the recommendation

for vitamin D intake and recommended that individuals over age 50 obtain vitamin B-12 from fortified food products or vitamin supplements.

29. Schaeffer DC, Cheskin LJ: Constipation in the elderly. *American Family Physician* 58:907, 1998.

    Constipation is a common problem in the elderly population and could signify underlying gastrointestinal problems or an

TAKE ACTION

II. HELPING OLDER ADULTS EAT BETTER

During their lifetimes, most people usually eat meals with families or loved ones. As people reach their older ages, many of them are faced with living and eating alone. In a study of the diets of 4400 older Americans, one man in every five living alone and over age 55 ate poorly. One of four women between the ages of 55 and 64 years followed a low-quality diet. These poor diets can contribute to deteriorating mental and physical health. Consider the following example of the living situation of an older adult.

Neal, a 70-year-old man, lives alone in a home in a local suburban area. His wife died 1 year ago. He doesn't have many friends; his wife was his primary confidante. His neighbors across the street and next door are friendly, and Neal used to help them with yard projects in his spare time. Neal's health has been good, but he has had trouble with his teeth recently. His diet has been poor, and in the past 3 months his physical and mental vigor have deteriorated. He has been slowly lapsing into a depression and, so, keeps the shades drawn and rarely leaves his house. Neal keeps very little food in the house because his wife did most of the cooking and shopping and he just isn't that interested in food.

If you were one of Neal's relatives and learned of Neal's situation, what six things could you do or suggest to help improve his nutritional status and mental outlook? Look back into the chapter to get some ideas.

1. _____

2. _____

3. _____

4. _____

5. _____

6. _____

inadequate fluid, dietary fiber, or food intake. It is important to identify and treat constipation and its accompanying problems because patients who suffer from it often have a diminished outlook on their quality of life.

30. Schardt D: St. John's Worts and all. *Nutrition Action Healthletter*, pp. 6–8, September 2000.

    St. John's Wort is effective in treating mild depression in approximately half of the people who take it for at least 3 to 4 weeks. The herb's side effects are minimal.

31. Tucker KL: Nutritional consequences of dietary patterns of the elderly. *Nutrition & the M.D.*, 26(7):1, 2000.

    *Although a multivitamin and mineral supplement can help protect older persons' nutri-*tional status, there appears to be substantial benefit from healthy dietary patterns beyond that attained with supplements. A diet high in fruits, vegetables, low-fat dairy products, and whole grains can make important contributions to health maintenance and quality of life.

32. Vita A and others: Aging, health risks, and cumulative disability. *The New England Journal of Medicine* 338:1035, 1998.

    The compression of morbidity and the avoidance of disability should be goals for older adults. People with better health habits, such as not smoking, maintaining a healthy weight, and exercising regularly, live longer and avoid disability in the later years of life.

33. Wilt TJ and others: Saw palmetto extracts for treatment of benign prostatic hyperplasia: A systemic review. *Journal of the American Medical Association* 280:1604, 1998.

    The use of saw palmetto in the treatment of benign prostatic hyperplasia (BPH) indicates that it does improve urinary symptoms and flow measures. It also has fewer side effects than the medications available for treatment of this problem.

ALTERNATIVE MEDICAL PRACTICES

Consumer interest in complementary alternative medicine (CAM) (also called complementary care and integrative medicine) is growing; about 34% of people recently surveyed used alternative medical practices in the past year, and most of the associated expenses for these often expensive products and services ($5.1 billion per year) were paid out-of-pocket. The majority of the consumers did not discuss the practice with their primary care physician.

Given the phenomenal advances in medicine over the past decades, what brings people in such numbers and with such affinity to embrace alternative therapies? It may be that many people assume that natural substances are gentler forms of therapy, lacking the harsher side effects of some pharmacological medicines. People may also seek complementary medicine because standard medical treatments didn't work, standard medical treatments had too many adverse effects, they simply wanted to actively participate in treatment, or they wanted to combat poor doctor communication. The majority of alternative medicine consumers have illnesses for which conventional medicine cannot offer a cure, such as arthritis, terminal stages of AIDS, and stress-related conditions. These people will almost certainly benefit from the reassurance, hope, and relief that comes with being in a healing situation.[6]

In many instances, self-prescription or healing rituals involve the participants' optimism, commitment, attention, and high expectations for improvement. The mind is a powerful component of a treatment situation, which is proven in many trials as a placebo effect in which a person takes a "sugar pill" but believes that he or she is being treated with a real medication and subsequently feels and reacts better. It is likely that most alternative or natural treatments of the past probably have no intrinsic therapeutic value beyond the benefit of the placebo effect. And, besides the powerful placebo effect, there are many possible reasons that a folk remedy works, such as the natural ups and downs of symptoms, the remission of disease, the possibility that the remedy contains the effective dose of a pharmaceutical medicine or is adulterated with medicines not listed on the label, and the denial of symptoms or misrepresentation of effectiveness by people who believe the remedy is effective.[6]

In truth, little scientific evidence is available for physicians and health-care professionals to decipher the positive and negative aspects of natural therapies. Indeed, Western medicine is based on accurate scientific knowledge, which serves as a protective device to prevent harm. On the other hand, alternative therapies often involve **folk medicine** and weak scientific evidence (due to lack of large research trials). Still, health professionals should be aware of the scientific knowledge that does or does not exist on some alternative therapies, since clients will likely express interest in these therapies. Many clients wish clinicians would take the time to explain (in simple terms) the nature of the problem; to acknowledge nutritional influences on health, rather than just recommend drugs and surgery as the only approaches for treating illness; to answer questions intelligently about dietary supplements; to be sensitive to mind-body interactions; and to respect questions about alternative practices.

To date, few alternative therapies have been subjected to scientific scrutiny, and many of the practices are based on presumptions that are unconvincing at best, yet some of the therapies (e.g., acupuncture and chiropractic therapies) show promise in the treatment of certain conditions. The National Institutes of Health has created the following seven categories of alternative therapies:

1. Mind-body interventions: the use of the mind, such as hypnosis, meditation, biofeedback, and yoga, to enhance health. Integrative medicine teaches health-care providers to focus on the subtle yet complex interactions of mind, body, spirit, community, and environment. *Ayurveda* is a natural healing process from India, which includes eating healthful, fresh foods and taking medicinal herbs suited to one's particular mind-body type.
2. Bioelectrical magnetic therapies: the use of electrical currents or magnetic fields to promote healing, such as the use of electrical currents to help heal broken bones

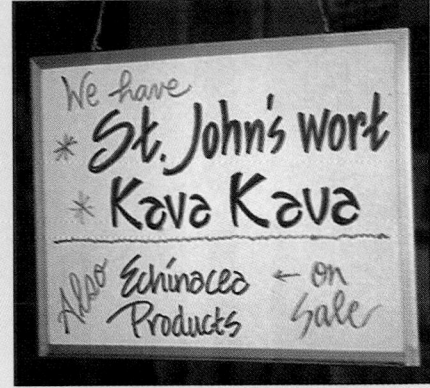

Some herbal products are active for treating specific medical problems. Follow label instructions carefully, if used. Note potential side effects listed, as well as who should not use the product.

folk medicine A medical treatment based on the beliefs, traditions, or customs of a particular society or ethnic/cultural group.

3. Alternative systems of medical practice: the use of medicine from another culture, such as Native American medicine and Chinese medicine (for example, acupuncture). Acupuncture likely works by stimulating sensory nerves leading to the spinal cord, eventually triggering the release of endorphins and corticosteroids (hormones that assist in pain management) into the brain and bloodstream. Acupuncture may be effective for treating people who experience nausea and vomiting following surgery or chemotherapy, nausea that accompanies pregnancy, pain experienced after certain dental procedures, and recovery from a drug addiction. Typically, a course of treatments end after 10 sessions if it is not showing benefit. FDA recently announced that acupuncture is no longer considered experimental. However, a qualified, certified practitioner must use sterile needles intended for single use and are made from nonreactive materials.

4. Manual healing methods: the use of the hands to promote healing, such as chiropractic or osteopathic manipulation or massage. FDA recognizes the effectiveness of chiropractic care for the treatment of acute low back pain.

5. Pharmacologic and biologic treatments: the use of various substances to treat specific medical problems. This includes **chelation** therapy.

6. Herbal medicine: the use of plants as medicines to treat or prevent disease. By definition, an herb is any plant or part of a plant that is used primarily for medicinal purposes. This includes **aromatherapy.** Dosage forms include capsules, tablets, extracts or tinctures, powders, dried herbs, teas, creams, and ointments. In March 1999, FDA established regulations that require the labels of such supplements to include name, quantity, dosage per day, and ingredient amounts.

7. Diet and nutrition: the use of foods, vitamins, and minerals to prevent illness and treat disease

The following are a few practical tips on using alternative medicine practices:

- We often tend to believe what we hear or what close acquaintances tell us. This well-meaning advice does not substitute for scientific verification of safety and effectiveness when it comes to health practices.
- The federal government provides little regulation regarding nutrient supplements or remedies. "Let the buyer beware" is prudent advice to follow when using these products. Knowledgeable, professional guidance is needed.
- Fraudulent claims for diet- and health-related remedies have always been a part of our culture. It is important to scrutinize carefully the credentials and motives of anyone providing medical or health advice. Phony credentials and bogus practitioners are widespread.
- If it sounds too good to be true, it probably is. The medical community gains nothing by holding back effective cures from the public, despite what the alternative practitioners may say.[6]

VITAMIN AND HERBAL SUPPLEMENTS ARE REGULATED LOOSELY BY FDA

Unless FDA has evidence that a supplement is inherently dangerous or marked with illegal claims, FDA will not regulate it closely. FDA is, in fact, prevented from doing so by the Proxmire Amendment to the 1938 Food, Drug, and Cosmetic Act, along with follow-up legislation—the Dietary Supplement Health and Education Act (DSHEA), which was passed in 1994. Currently, a product labeled as a dietary supplement can be marketed without FDA approval if there is a history of its use or other evidence that suggests it is reasonably safe (when used under the conditions recommended on the label). It is permissible for the labels on such products to claim a benefit related to a classic nutrient-deficiency disease, describe how a nutrient affects human body structure or function, and claim that general well-being results from consumption of the ingredient(s). These so called 'structure/function' claims are quite distinct from the health claims approved by FDA. The structure function claims are generally written in very vague terms, indicating only a general effect on the body, such as improvement in heart function or immune

chelation The use of medicinal compounds, such as ethylenediaminetetraacetic acid (EDTA), to bind metals and other constituents in the blood.

aromatherapy The use of the vapors of essential oils extracted from flowers, leaves, stalks, fruits, and roots for therapeutic purposes.

*A*nother concern regarding use of herbal and related supplements is the actual content of the active ingredient(s) in the product. Recently, many of these products have been tested by independent laboratories and found to contain either less than or more than the stated label content (see the web site http://consumerlabs.com for details).

function. Health claims are much more specific, such as the ability of the vitamin folate when consumed by pregnant women to reduce the risk of birth defects in their offspring. In addition, according to DSHEA, FDA must prove that a dietary supplement is unsafe before preventing its sale, rather than the manufacturer's having to prove its safety. In contrast, the safety of drugs must be demonstrated to FDA's satisfaction before they are marketed.

DIETARY SUPPLEMENT CLAIMS

Although structure/function claims do not have to be approved by FDA, they must have evidence that their marketing statements are truthful and not misleading. In addition, the labels of products bearing such claims must prominently display in boldface type the following disclaimer: **"This statement has not been evaluated by the Food and Drug Administration. This product is not intended to diagnose, treat, cure, or prevent any disease."** Despite this statement, consumers may mistakenly assume FDA has carefully evaluated the products.

Practice the following when evaluating dietary supplement claims:

1. Examine product labels carefully. A product is not likely to do something that is not specifically claimed on its label or package insert (legally part of the label). Be skeptical of any product promotion not clearly stated on the label, such as:

   - Testimonials about personal experience
   - Dramatic results (rarely true)
   - Lack of evidence from supporting studies made by other scientists
   - Statements that particular foods can cure specific diseases or that many harmful foods should be eliminated from the diet
   - Claims that only natural foods should be eaten because modern processing methods strip the nutritional value from foods
   - Warnings that stress greatly increases the need for nutrients

2. Examine the background and scientific credentials of the individual, organizations, or publication making the nutritional claim. Usually, a reputable author is one whose educational background or present affiliation is with a nationally recognized university or medical center that offers programs or courses in the field of nutrition, medicine, or another certified health profession.

3. Note the size and duration of any study cited in support of a nutrition claim. The larger it is and the longer it went on, the more dependable its findings. Check out the group studied; a study of men or women in Sweden may be less relevant than one of men or women of southern European, African, or Hispanic descent, because it involves more than one ethnicity. Keep in mind that "contributes to," "is linked to," or "is associated with" does not mean "causes." In addition, one study may not prove anything; many studies are needed to verify or strengthen the association or finding.

CRITICAL THINKING

Jamila went to her local pharmacy yesterday to look for a product to help her stay awake while studying. On the shelves she found a dietary supplement claiming to be a Chinese herbal remedy for sleepiness and fatigue. She thought that since a pharmacy carried the product, it should be safe, and work as indicated on the label.

Is she correct in these assumptions? Are there specific risks associated with taking such herbal remedies?

A CLOSER LOOK AT HERBAL THERAPY

Throughout history, healers have gone to the garden, forest, and sea to seek herbal remedies. Largely by trial and error, these healers have found the leaves and seeds of various herbs, roots, and barks to possess medicinal properties. As early as the second century B.C., the Egyptians use myrrh, cumin, peppermint, caraway, fennel, and clove oil for various ailments. In sixteenth-century Europe, physicians began experimenting with sarsaparilla, the dried root of the smilax plant, in an attempt to cure venereal disease. Later, the root was used to treat chronic rheumatism and skin disease. When late-nineteenth-century physicians abandoned a belief in its medicinal powers, sarsaparilla found new life as a syrup for soft drinks.

Some natural products may be harmless, others are potentially toxic, and still others may be effective for some problems but dangerous when taken in the wrong dose or by people with certain medical conditions (Table 18-6).[13] The National Cancer Institute is the world's leader in the search for medicinal compounds in plants. For example, the institute has tested extracts of

TABLE 18-6 Popular Herbal Remedies, Food Supplements, and Hormones[4,9,14,19,20,30,33]

Herbal Substance	Potential Effects	Side Effects	Who Should Avoid Them
Black cohosh	May reduce postmenopausal symptoms	Nausea, fall in blood pressure	Women taking estrogen, hypertension medications, or aspirin and related drugs
Echinacea	May stimulate the immune system and shorten the duration of flulike illnesses; studies show conflicting evidence	Nausea, skin irritation	Anyone with an autoimmune disease or who has allergic reactions to daisies
Feverfew	May reduce the pain and frequency of migraines	Abdominal pain, mouth sores, skin rash	Anyone allergic to ragweed or taking anti-inflammatory drugs, such as aspirin
Garlic	May have antibiotic properties	In large amounts, burning of the mouth, nausea, sweating, stomach irritation, lightheadedness, reduced blood clotting	Those taking anti-coagulant medications, such as warfarin, for cardiovascular disease
Ginger	May prevent motion sickness and nausea related to surgery	Gastrointestinal (GI) tract discomfort with high doses on an empty stomach	People with history of gallstones
Ginkgo biloba	Increases the circulation of blood in the body, especially to the brain and lower extremities; some studies have shown increased ability to think, reason, and remember in older persons	GI upset, headache, irritability, reduced blood clotting	Anyone taking anti-inflammatory or anti-coagulant medications, including vitamin E and aspirin; anyone who has had a stroke or is prone to them
Ginseng	May decrease weakness and fatigue and increase the body's resistance to stress; studies have not confirmed any benefit	Hypertension, asthma attacks, irregular heart beat, insomnia, headache, nervousness, GI upset, reduced blood clotting	Anyone taking anti-coagulant medications, such as warfarin; anyone with a chronic GI tract disease; anyone with diabetes
Kava kava	May alleviate mild anxiety and stress	GI complaints, headache, weakness, dizziness, pulmonary hypertension	Anyone taking antidepressants, anti-psychotics, barbiturates, and other sedatives, or those who use alcohol.
Ma huang (ephedra)	In combination with caffeine, stimulates the central nervous system and may increase metabolic rate (aiding in weight loss)	*Dangerous herb:* linked to over 60 deaths and 1200 reports of illness (hypertension, stroke, heart attack, seizure) in the United States	Generally, it is not regarded as safe for anyone to take more than 25 mg for longer than 7 days; people with cardiovascular disease should never take this herb
Milk thistle	May have a protective effect on the liver, which is thought to be due to its ability to prevent toxins from contaminating liver cell membranes	Loose stools	No specific persons are at risk
St. John's Wort	Mild antidepressant effect that may work by inhibiting monoamine oxidase (an enzyme in the brain that destroys "feel-good" hormones, such as serotonin, epinephrine, and dopamine); scientific research is promising	Nausea, fatigue, dry mouth, dizziness, photosensitivity; increases metabolism and removal of many prescription drugs from the body	People taking prescription drugs to control depression, HIV, epilepsy, cardiovascular disease, asthma, and drugs that suppress the immune system to keep the body from rejecting a transplanted organ
Saw palmetto	May reduce symptoms of enlarged prostate gland (otherwise known as BPH or benign prostatic hyperplasia), by increasing urinary flow and easing urination; studies show moderate evidence of effectiveness	Generally uncommon; when taken in large doses: headache, GI upset	Those taking medication to treat enlarged prostate or BPH, anyone with a chronic GI tract disease
Valerian	May alleviate restlessness and other sleeping disorders that stem from nervous conditions	Headache, morning grogginess, irregular heart beat, GI upset (also has a disagreeable odor)	Anyone taking central nervous system depressants, such as sedatives; anyone who drinks alcohol

TABLE 18-6   (concluded)

Related Substances	Potential Effects	Side Effects	Who Should Avoid Them
Chondroitin	Draws fluid to tissue and gives joints resistance and elasticity, which helps reduce the pain associated with osteoarthritis and improve mobility; research is encouraging for patients with osteoarthritis	None expected	Anyone taking an anticoagulant, such as vitamin E, warfarin, or aspirin
Glucosamine	Decreases joint inflammation and pain associated with osteoarthritis; research is encouraging for patients with osteoarthritis	GI discomfort, which may disappear after 2 weeks	May disrupt blood glucose regulation in people with diabetes
SAMe	S-adenosylmethionine is the active ingredient, may promote cartilage formation and decreases joint inflammation and pain associated with osteoarthritis; may also act as a mild antidepressant	Mild headaches, which last for short periods of time	Anyone with coronary heart disease, obsessive compulsive disorder, manic-depression, or addictive tendencies
Coenzyme Q-10	Fat-soluble vitamin-like substance with antioxidant properties; healthy individuals have normal body amounts, although some people with chronic conditions have lower amounts in the body	Mild gastrointestinal distress	No specific persons are at risk
Phytoestrogens: isoflavones from soy, lignans	May reduce postmenopausal symptoms and related bone loss	None expected	Women who are taking estrogen or who have breast cancer

Hormones	Potential Effects	Side Effects	Who Should Avoid Them
DHEA	Hormone that, when taken orally turns to estrogen and testosterone in the body; few, if any, benefits of supplementation are proven	Masculinization of women, acne, irritability, possible prostate or breast cancer	Women, due to possible irreversible masculinization qualities
Melatonin	Hormone that may help people fall asleep faster	Reduced ovulation in women, drowsiness, confusion, headache or morning grogginess	Anyone with cardiovascular disease, or anyone of childbearing age

Note that pregnant or breastfeeding women, children under 2 years old, anyone over the age of 65 years, and anyone with a chronic disease should never take supplements unless under the guidance of a physician.

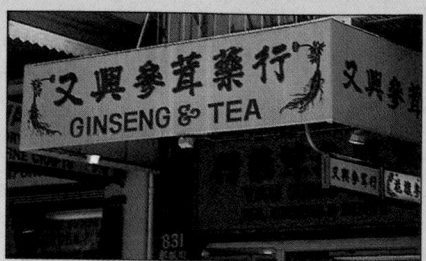

Herbal products are part of Chinese culture. The best advice for the use of herbal products is to stick to one herb at a time and to consult your physician first about any such use. Note especially that the use of herbal mixtures is very risky.

more than 30,000 plant species for activity against cancer. This work identified some anti-cancer compounds from flowering plants that have been approved for use in cancer patients. Other plant-derived compounds are currently being tested for safety and effectiveness in clinical trials but haven't yet been approved.

Traditional knowledge of the healing properties of plants provides leads for such scientists to explore. Any promising compounds they isolate are subjected to rigorous FDA-approved tests to determine safety, effectiveness, and side effects. This controlled testing provides a wealth of information far exceeding that available for herbal remedies.

The German government publishes a manual that is the most authoritative reference for the use of popular herbal products (Commission E Monographs). Unfortunately, little scientific data are available concerning the therapeutic value and safety of the 7000 or so herbs used in traditional medicine, which has been practiced and chronicled primarily by the Chinese. Proponents of Chinese herbal medicine suggest that its safety and efficacy have been well established during its 4000-year history. These individuals also point to the widespread use of herbal therapies in Europe. Still, numerous reports have documented significant health risks associated with the use of some herbal and alternative remedies, sometimes resulting in death. Studies especially implicate ephedra, germander, pokeroot, sassafras, mandrake, pennyroyal, comfrey, chaparral, yohimbe, lobelia, jin bu huan, products containing stephanie and magnolia, senna, hai gen fen, paraguay tea, kombucha tea, tung shueh (Chinese black balls), and willow bark.

There is also a distinct risk that a traditional herbal product may be mislabeled, adulterated with prescription drugs or contaminants, or subject to extreme variations in potency. Chinese combination herbs should always be avoided, due to the reported cases of adverse health effects and adulteration.

A recent concern also has been raised with regard to patients who abruptly end alternative medicines at the start of hospital treatments or simply deny that they are involved in alternative therapy. Interactions between alternative therapies and pharmaceutical drugs can be drastic and include complications such as delirium, clotting abnormalities, and rapid heart beat, resulting in the need for intensive care. If these patients had disclosed their treatments, many of the complications could have been prevented. The American Society of Anesthesiology recommends that, if time permits, patients stop taking herbal products 3 weeks before a scheduled surgery or otherwise take all original supplement containers to the hospital, so that the anesthesiologist can evaluate what was taken.

The following are questions that should be asked when evaluating a company's products. Still, what the label indicates as the active ingredient and the amount of the ingredient that a product claims to contain may or may not be valid, based on the recent analysis of many popular brands of herbal products.

- What forms of production control lab analysis are used to assure quality, quantity, and reproducibility of the ingredients in individual doses as labeled?
- Is the product labeled with Latin botanical names?
- Does the label have expiration dates and lot numbers, and if so what is the basis for the labeled expiration dates?
- Does the manufacturer offer a certificate of analysis for each product?
- Has the manufacturer been in business for at least 5 years and have national distribution of the product?

A rational approach to alternative therapy is to keep a diary of symptoms, follow only one therapy at a time, check with one's physician first before discontinuing a medication, and find out if the alternative practitioner has experience with the medical problem to be treated.[11] Interested consumers might also see if they can enter a study of the agent or procedure in question. In addition, FDA advises anyone who experiences adverse side effects from an herbal remedy to contact a physician. Physicians are encouraged to report such adverse effects to FDA's hot line for professionals. FDA also suggests contacting the state and local health departments and consumer protection agency.

Overall, herbal products should be used with great caution and only in consultation with a person's primary physician. Otherwise, potential side effects may go undiagnosed, or dangerous herb-medicine interactions may develop. Pregnant and nursing women, anyone with a chronic disease, and children under 2 years of age, especially, should not take herbal supplements unless their physicians consent to the practice and monitor them for potential complications.

Some herbalists claim that natural herbs cannot harm people. No evidence supports this claim. Indeed, if there's one thing experts agree on, it's this: An herb that has the ability to heal also has the ability, if misused, to harm. In addition, many conditions for which herbs are recommended (such as diabetes and arthritis) are not suitable for self-treatment. For a balanced, thoughtful discussion of herbal remedies, consult *The Honest Herbal* by Verro Taylor, an expert in the medicinal use of plants. Also, the following are helpful web sites:

Alternative Medicine Foundation

http://www.amfoundation.org/

The NCCAM Complementary and Alternative Medicine (CAM) Citation Index (CI)

http://nccam.nih.gov/nccam/resources/cam-ci/

American Botanical Council

http://www.herbalgram.org/

Complementary and Alternative Medicine Program at Stanford (CAMPS)

http://scrdp.stanford.edu/camps.html

Center for Complementary and Alternative Medicine Research in Asthma, located at the University of California, Davis

http://www.camra.ucdavis.edu/

National Council Against Health Fraud

http://www.ncahf.org

http://www.quackwatch.com

National Institutes of Health Office of Alternative Medicine

http://altmed.od.nih.gov/

PART SIX PUTTING NUTRITION KNOWLEDGE INTO PRACTICE

FOOD SAFETY *chapter* 19

At the turn of the twentieth century, conditions in Chicago's meat-packing industry were sickening. Moldy, spoiled meat was commonly doused with borax to cover up the smell, and glycerine was added to make it look fresh. By 1906, increasing public pressure forced the passage of the first Food and Drug Act in the United States. Federal inspection then safeguarded the public from worm-infested and diseased meat and generally improved food preparation standards.

Today, food safety warnings appear everywhere. Attention has turned to more contemporary food safety concerns, such as microbial and chemical contamination. On the one hand, we are told to eat more fruits, vegetables, fish, and poultry; on the other hand, we are warned that these foods may contain dangerous substances, so we still must ask, "How safe is our food?"

Scientists and health authorities agree that Americans enjoy a relatively safe food supply.[29] Over the past 90 or so years, tremendous progress has been made in food safety. Nonetheless, microbes and chemicals in foods still can pose a health risk.[7,14] This chapter focuses on these food-related hazards—how real they are and how you can minimize their effect on your life. Note that you bear much responsibility for this—government agencies and industry can do only so much.

- Bacteria and other microbes in food pose the greatest risk for food-borne illness. In the past, salt, sugar, smoke, fermentation, and drying were used to protect against food-borne illness. Today, careful cooking, pasteurization, and temperature control (keeping hot foods hot and cold foods cold) provide additional insurance.

- Cross-contamination, the transfer of microbes from one food to another, commonly causes food-borne illness, especially when bacteria on raw animal products contact foods that can support their growth. Because of the risk of cross-contamination, no perishable food should be kept at room temperature for more than 2 hours (depending on the environmental temperature), especially if the food may have come in contact with raw animal products.

- Treatment for food-borne illness usually requires drinking lots of fluids, avoiding contact with food while diarrhea is present, washing hands thoroughly, and getting bed rest. Botulism and hepatitis A are two types of food-borne illness that require prompt medical attention.

- Food additives are used primarily to extend shelf life of foods by preventing microbial growth and the destruction of food components by oxygen, metals, and other substances. In most cases, the Delaney Clause allows FDA to ban manufacturers from adding to foods any substance that causes cancer.

- Certain food additives, such as antioxidants, prevent oxygen and enzyme destruction of food products. Other preservatives prevent bacterial growth. Sequestrants bind metals and thus prevent spoilage of food from metal contamination. Emulsifiers suspend fat in water, improving the uniformity, smoothness, and body of foods such as ice cream.

- Toxic substances occur naturally in a variety of foods, such as green potatoes, raw fish, and some types of mushrooms. In many cases, cooking the foods limits their toxic effects.

- A variety of environmental contaminants can be found in foods. Because most of them are fat soluble, exposure can be minimized by trimming fat from meats and discarding fat that is rendered during the cooking of meats, fish, and poultry. In addition, it's helpful to wash fruits and vegetables thoroughly and discard the outer leaves of leafy vegetables. All these practices help reduce pesticide exposure.

REFRESH YOUR MEMORY

As you begin your study of food safety in Chapter 19, you may want to review

- Alternative sweeteners in Chapter 5
- Fat substitutes in Chapter 6
- The causes of cancer in Chapter 12

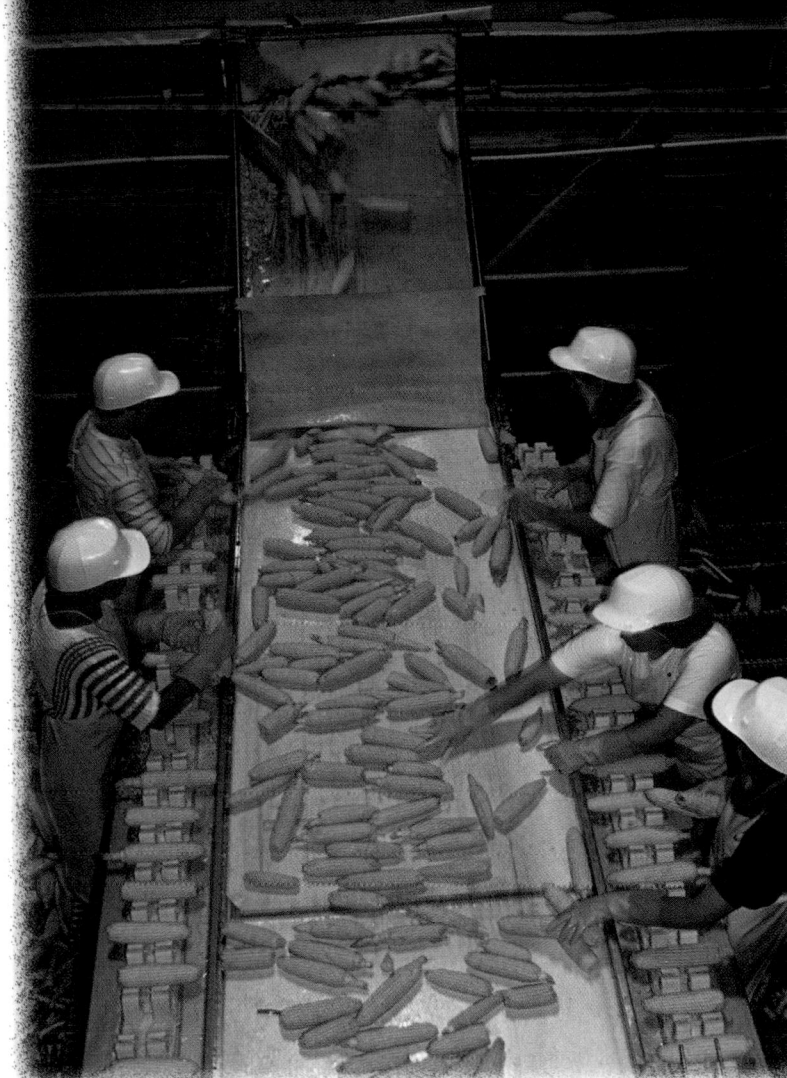

CASE SCENARIO

Aaron attended a gathering of his officemates on a warm July Saturday. The theme was international dining, and he and his wife were told to bring Argentine beef, a stewlike dish. They followed the recipe carefully, and it came out of the oven at 1 PM. The couple kept the dish warm by wrapping the pan in a towel. They traveled in their car to the party and set the dish out on the buffet table at 3 PM. Dinner was to be served at 4 PM. However, the guests were enjoying themselves so much lounging around the host's pool and drinking ginger beer (also on the menu) that no one began to eat until 6 PM. Aaron made sure he sampled the Argentine beef that he and his wife made, while his wife did not. He also had some salad, garlic bread, and a sweet dessert made with coconut.

The couple returned home at 11 PM and went to bed. About 2 AM Aaron knew something was wrong. He had severe abdominal pain and had to make a mad dash to the bathroom. For the next 3 hours he spent most of the time in the bathroom with severe diarrhea. By dawn, the diarrhea had subsided and he had started feeling better. After a few cups of tea and a light breakfast, he was feeling like himself by noon.

What type of food-borne illness did Aaron contract? What precautions for avoiding food-borne illness were ignored by Aaron and the rest of the people at the party? How could this scenario be rewritten, so that the party goers could substantially reduce their risk of food-borne illness?

pasteurizing The process of heating food products to kill pathogenic microorganisms.

bacteria Single-cell microorganisms; some produce poisonous substances, which cause illness in humans. They contain only one chromosome and lack many organelles found in human cells. Some can live without oxygen and survive by means of spore formation.

fungi Simple parasitic life forms, including molds, mildews, yeasts, and mushrooms. They live on dead or decaying organic matter. Fungi can grow as single cells, like yeast, or as a multicellular colony, as seen with molds.

food-borne illness Sickness caused by the ingestion of food containing toxic substances produced by microorganisms.

Food contamination presents a unique risk to older adults for a variety of reasons. Poor eyesight and reduced senses of smell and taste may make it harder to spot spoiled food or dirty utensils. Aging and their typically reduced food intake can lead to a weakened immune system. Older adults face further risks because their stomachs may not produce enough HCl, which destroys harmful bacteria, and because of poor blood circulation, which can prevent antibodies from reaching sites of infection.

toxins Poisonous compounds produced by an organism that can cause disease.

■ SETTING THE STAGE

During the early stages of urbanization in the United States, contaminated water and food—notably, milk—were responsible for many large outbreaks of typhoid fever, septic sore throat, scarlet fever, diphtheria, and other devastating human diseases. These experiences led to the development of processes for purifying water, treating sewage, and **pasteurizing** milk. Since that time, safe water and milk have become universally available, with only occasional problems from either.

The greatest health risk today from food is contamination from **bacteria** and, to a lesser extent, from various forms of **fungi** and viruses. These microbes can all cause **food-borne illness**.[2] For example, 1 child died and 50 others became ill from *Escherichia coli (E. coli)* bacteria, which was attributed to contaminated apple juice. In another case, 170 children became ill when served strawberries in their school lunch program that were contaminated by hepatitis A virus.

Even though microbial contamination is the cause of most incidents of food-borne illness, Americans seem more concerned about the health risks from chemicals in foods. Of consumers surveyed in a Gallup poll, about 75% said that pesticide contamination was a major concern to them. In the long run, this concern has some merit. On a day-to-day basis, however, food additives cause only about 4% of all cases of food-borne illness in the United States.

Since microbial contamination of food is by far the more important issue for our day-to-day health, it will be discussed first. This chapter will then cover the use and safety of food additives.

■ Effects of Food-Borne Illness

According to the Centers of Disease Control and Prevention, food-borne illness caused 76 million illnesses, 325,000 hospitalizations, and 5000 deaths in the United States in 1998. Some people can develop significant sickness from food-borne illness, including the following:[11]

- Infants and children
- Older adults
- Those with liver disease, diabetes, or HIV infection (and AIDS)
- Cancer patients
- Pregnant women
- People taking immunosuppressant agents

As you can see, food-borne illness has the greatest effect on the most vulnerable people in terms of health status. Some of these bouts of food-borne illness, coupled with the ongoing health conditions, are lengthy and lead to food allergies, seizures, blood poisoning (from **toxins** or microbes in the bloodstream), or other illnesses.

Because food-borne illness often results from the unsafe handling of food at home, we each bear some responsibility for preventing food-borne illness. Usually, you can't tell by taste, smell, or sight that a particular food contains harmful microbes, so you might not even be aware that food has caused your distress. In fact, your last case of diarrhea may have been caused by something you ate (Table 19-1).

■ Why Is Food-Borne Illness So Common?

The risk of contracting food-borne illness is high because—in addition to problems from consumers' mishandling of food—recent trends have added new causes.[2] First, there is greater consumer interest in eating foods of animal origin raw or undercooked. In addition, more people receive medication that suppresses their ability to combat food-borne infectious agents. Another factor is the continuing increase in the number of older adults in the population.

Furthermore, the food industry tries where possible to increase the shelf life of food products; however, a longer shelf life at room temperature allows more time for bacteria in foods to multiply. Some bacteria grow even at refrigeration temperatures.

TABLE 19-1   Some Examples of Cases of Food-Borne Illness

Bacteria

- A previously healthy 5-month-old girl suddenly died at home from contact with a pet iguana infected with *Salmonella*. Unpasteurized juice products were recalled after 57 cases of *Salmonella* illness were reported in California and Colorado. Eight people became ill from *Salmonella* after consuming tiramisu, a dessert that contains raw eggs.

- Six persons were reported ill from a *Shigella* infection after eating chopped, uncooked parsley that was served on chicken sandwiches and in coleslaw. A cruise ship had to return to port when more than 600 people developed shigellosis and one person died.

- The first documented food-borne illness caused by *Listeria* organisms in North America occurred in commercially prepared coleslaw. Later, incidents that involved 48 deaths were associated with soft Mexican-style cheeses. A listeriosis outbreak associated with undercooked hot dogs and cold cuts resulted in more than 82 illnesses and 17 deaths in 19 states.

- The first community outbreak in the United States of *E. coli* 0111:H8 sickened 58 teenagers at a cheerleading camp in Texas. Suspected sources of infection included the camp salad bar and a communal water barrel. One of the largest *E. coli* 0157:H7 outbreaks on record infected more than 1000 people in upstate New York at a county fair. The bacterium was found in infected well water. It killed a 79-year-old man and a 4-year-old girl, and it required 10 other children to undergo kidney dialysis. Six adults and a 2-year-old child were killed after an *E. coli* outbreak from contaminated drinking water in Canada. The bacteria entered the water supply from animal manure after flooding from a heavy storm. In northeastern Oklahoma, five children were infected with *E. coli* after consuming unpasteurized apple cider.

- A man in Arkansas developed botulism after eating stew that was cooked and then kept at room temperature for 3 days. He spent 49 days in the hospital—42 of them on mechanical ventilation.

- Since 1992, 17 people in Florida have died of *Vibrio vulnificus* infections after eating raw oysters.

- A teenage boy and his father experienced abdominal pain, vomiting, and diarrhea within 30 minutes of eating 4-day-old homemade pesto. The pesto had been reheated and left out a number of times during the 4-day period. It was apparently contaminated with *Bacillus cereus*. As a result the boy died of liver failure.

Viruses

- An estimated 6 million oysters from Louisiana were bathed with the *Norwalk virus* after ships with ill crewmembers dumped their sewage overboard. By the time the outbreak was recognized, an estimated 20,000 to 30,000 people had become ill. Another outbreak of the virus was attributed to an infected bakery worker, who stirred a vat full of buttercream frosting with his bare hand and arm. In Florida, 83 fraternity members caught the virus from the fraternity house ice machine. During the Gulf War, the Norwalk virus was one of the most common causes of gastroenteritis among U.S. troops.

Parasites

- A group attending a dinner banquet developed diarrhea after 3 to 9 days of eating green onions, which was the likely cause of the outbreak. Eight of 10 stool specimens obtained from the group with food-borne illness were positive for *Cryptosporidium*. Food workers at the restaurant reported they did not consistently wash green onions before using them to prepare food or serving them to patrons.

- Guatemalan raspberries have been associated with approximately 1000 cases of *Cyclospora* in the United States and Canada. Authorities speculate that contaminated water caused the outbreak. The United States has banned this source of the fruit until further precautions can be taken.

Risks from Seafood

- Four adults became ill with scrombroid fish poisoning after eating tuna-spinach salad at a restaurant in Pennsylvania.

- An outbreak of Ciguatera fish poisoning involved 17 crewmembers of a cargo ship that caught, cooked, and ate a barracuda in the Bahamas. All 17 men became ill with nausea, vomiting, abdominal cramps, and diarrhea within hours of eating the fish. Within 2 days, all of the men suffered from neurological symptoms, including muscle pain and weakness, dizziness, and numb or itchy feet, hands, and mouth.

- An outbreak of paralytic shellfish poisoning in Guatemala killed 26 people.

Partially cooked—and some fully cooked—products pose a particular risk because refrigerated storage may only slow, not prevent, bacterial growth.

The risk of illness from food-borne microbes increases as more of our foods are prepared in centralized kitchens outside the home. Supermarkets have become major food processors over the past decade and now offer a variety of prepared foods from specialty meat shops, salad bars, and bakeries. With the increasing number of two-income families, more people are looking for convenient, easy-to-prepare, nutritious foods. Supermarkets offer entrées that can be served immediately or reheated. The foods are usually prepared in central kitchens or processing plants and

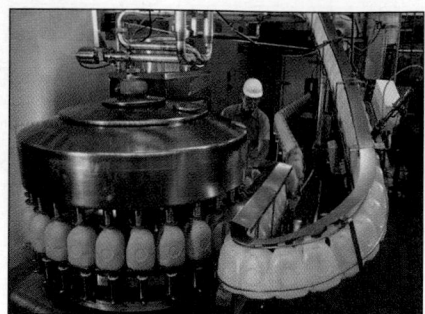

Food contaminated in a central plant can go on to produce illness in people in surrounding states or even across the nation. In the case of juices, it is important that these are pasteurized to reduce the risk of food-borne illness.

*W*hen traveling to developing countries, it is recommended that you "boil it, peel it, or don't eat it." Ironically, up to 70% of our fruits and vegetables during certain seasons comes from these countries. In other words, you do not have to travel to acquire traveler's diarrhea. In response, we should carefully inspect and wash produce, as we would in a foreign country.

A seafood hot line is also available through the American Seafood Institute. For free information on the purchase, preparation, and nutritional value of seafood products, call 1-800-328-3474 between 9 AM and 5 PM Eastern time on weekdays.

shipped to individual stores. If a food product is contaminated in the central kitchen or processing plant, patrons of stores over a wide area can suffer food-borne illness.

The centralization of food production by the food-processing industry also adds to the risk of food-borne illness. For example, a malfunction in an ice cream plant in 1994 resulted in 224,000 suspected cases of *Salmonella* bacterial infections, linked to the use of contaminated ice cream mix. In 1987, lettuce shredded in a Texas plant and then placed in large plastic bags was the cause of the largest *Shigella* bacterial outbreak ever reported in the United States. At least 347 people became ill. The nutrients released when the lettuce was shredded, coupled with the moist environment provided by the plastic bags, allowed growth and reproduction of the organism.

A survey showed that only 13% of restaurants implement the voluntary FDA Food Code for cooking temperatures for meat, eggs, fish and poultry. It is no surprise, then, that in 1993 at least 4 people died and 700 became ill in Washington and surrounding western states after eating at a chain of quick-service restaurants. The source of the problem was undercooked hamburger contaminated with the bacterium *E. coli 0157:H7*. Overall, the growth of large-scale food production and distribution technologies has introduced new and different food-borne risks.

Still another cause of increased food-borne illness in America is greater consumption of ready-to-eat foods imported from foreign countries. In the past, food imports were mostly raw products processed here under strict sanitation standards. Now, however, we import more processed foods—such as cheese from France and seafood from Asia—some of which are contaminated. Federal authorities are currently examining inspection procedures for these imports.

The use of antibiotics in animal feeds is increasing the severity of cases of food-borne illness. This use encourages bacteria to develop resistant strains, those that can grow even if exposed to typical antibiotic medicines.[12,33]

Finally, more cases of food-borne disease are reported now because scientists are more aware of the roles of various players in the process. In addition, physicians are more likely to suspect food-borne contaminants as a cause of illness. Every decade, the list of microorganisms suspected of causing food-borne illness lengthens (Table 19-2). Furthermore, we now know that food, besides serving as a good growth medium for some microorganisms, simply transmits many others as well. Seafood is receiving greater scrutiny and surveillance by FDA as a cause of food-borne illness. In addition, FDA is launching a $500,000 campaign to educate consumers about the risks of eating raw oysters. For more information about these risks, contact FDA's Seafood Hotline at 1-800-FDA-4010.

■ Food Preservation—Past, Present, and Future

For centuries, salt, sugar, smoke, fermentation, and drying have been used to preserve food. Ancient Romans used sulfites to disinfect wine containers and preserve wine. In the age of exploration, European adventurers traveling to the New World preserved their meat by salting it. Most preserving methods work on the principle of decreasing free water—that is, the amount of water not bound to other components in the food. Bacteria need abundant stores of water to grow; yeasts and molds can grow with less water, but some is still necessary. Adding sugar or salt decreases free water by binding to it. The process of drying drives off free water.

Decreasing the water content of some high-moisture foods, however, causes them to lose essential characteristics. To preserve such foods—cucumber pickles, sauerkraut, milk (yogurt), and wine—fermentation has been a traditional alternative. Selected bacteria are used to ferment or pickle foods. The fermenting bacteria make acids and alcohol, which minimize the growth of other microbes.

TABLE 19-2	Organisms That Cause Food-Borne Illness: Their Sources, Symptoms, and Prevention		
Organism	**Sources**	**Symptoms**	**Prevention Methods**
Bacteria			
Campylobacter jejuni	Found on poultry, beef, and lamb and can contaminate the meat and milk. Chief food sources are raw poultry and meat and unpasteurized milk.	Onset: 2–10 days after eating, or longer Diarrhea, abdominal cramping, fever, and sometimes bloody stools. Lasts 2–7 days.	• Thorough cooking of foods • Sanitary food-handling practices • Avoidance of unpasteurized milk
Salmonella	Found in raw meats, poultry, eggs, fish, unpasteurized milk, and products made with these items. Multiplies rapidly at room temperature. The bacteria themselves are toxic.	Onset: 8–48 hours after eating Nausea, fever, headache, abdominal cramps, diarrhea, and vomiting Can be fatal in infants, the elderly, and the sick.	• Sanitary food-handling practices • Thorough cooking of foods • Prompt and proper refrigeration of foods • Avoidance of cross-contamination
Shigella	Transmitted via fecal-oral route and somewhat in food and water.	Onset: 1–3 days. Abdominal cramps, diarrhea, fever, bloody stools	• Handwashing and sanitary food production
Escherichia coli (0157:H7 and other strains)	Undercooked beef, especially ground beef. Fruits, vegetables, and yogurt are also possibilities.	Onset: 2–4 days. Bloody diarrhea, abdominal cramps, kidney failure	• Thorough cooking, especially of beef • Avoidance of unpasteurized milk, untreated apple cider
Clostridium perfringens	Found throughout the environment. Generally found in meat and poultry dishes. Multiply rapidly in anaerobic conditions when foods are left for extended time at room temperature. The bacteria themselves are toxic.	Onset: 8–24 hours after eating (usually 12 hours) Abdominal pain and diarrhea Symptoms last a day or less, usually mild. Can be more serious in older or ill people.	• Sanitary handling of foods, especially meat and meat dishes, gravies, and leftovers • Thorough cooking and reheating of foods, especially leftovers • Prompt and proper refrigeration
Listeria monocytogenes	Found in soft cheeses made with unpasteurized milk and unpasteurized milk itself. Resists acid, heat, salt, and nitrate well.	Onset: 7–30 days. Fever, headache, vomiting, and sometimes more severe symptoms. May be fatal.	• Thorough cooking of foods • Sanitary food-handling practices • Avoidance of unpasteurized milk
Staphylococcus aureus	Found in nasal passages and in cuts on skin. Toxin is produced when food contaminated by bacteria is left for extended time at room temperature. Meats, poultry, egg products, tuna, potato salad, macaroni salads, and cream-filled pastries pose greatest risk.	Onset: 2–6 hours after eating Diarrhea, vomiting, nausea, and abdominal cramps Mimics flu Lasts 24–36 hours Rarely fatal	• Sanitary food-handling practices • Prompt and proper refrigeration of foods • Covering cuts on skin
Clostridium botulinum	Found throughout the environment. However, bacteria produce toxin only in a low-acid, anaerobic environment, such as in canned green beans, mushrooms, spinach, olives, and beef. Honey and corn syrup may carry spores.	Onset: 12–36 hours after eating Neurotoxic symptoms include double vision, inability to swallow, speech difficulty, and progressive paralysis of the respiratory system. OBTAIN MEDICAL HELP IMMEDIATELY. BOTULISM CAN BE FATAL.	• Use proper methods for canning low-acid foods • Avoidance of commercial cans of low-acid foods that have leaky seals or are bent, bulging, or broken • Discard if toxin is suspected (off odors are a sign)
Yersinia enterocolitica	Found throughout the environment; carried in food, water, and feces. They multiply rapidly at both room and refrigerator temperatures. Generally found in raw vegetables, meats, water, and unpasteurized milk.	Onset: 2–3 days Fever, headache, nausea, diarrhea, and general malaise Mimics flu and appendicitis May cause gastroenteritis in children.	• Thorough cooking • Sanitizing of cutting instruments and cutting boards before preparing foods to be eaten raw • Avoidance of unpasteurized milk and untreated water

continued

TABLE 19-2 concluded

Organism	Sources	Symptoms	Prevention Methods
Vibrio vulnificus and other vibrio species	Raw seafood, especially raw oysters.	Onset: 6–72 hours Diarrhea, fever, weakness, blood infection, death	• Thorough cooking of seafood
Vibrio cholerae	Human carriers, infected shellfish, contaminated water and food	Onset: 2–3 days Vomiting, severe watery diarrhea, which can lead to dehydration and cardiovascular collapse; death	• Handwashing after defecating
Viruses			
Hepatitis A virus	Fecal-oral route that contaminates food, beverages, or shellfish.	Onset: 30–60 day. Anorexia, diarrhea, fever, jaundice, and fatigue. May cause liver damage and death.	• Sanitary handling of foods • Use of pure drinking water • Adequate sewage disposal • Thorough cooking of foods
Norwalk, human rota-virus	Found in the human intestinal tract and feces. Contamination occurs: (1) when sewage is used to enrich garden/farm soil (2) by direct hand-to-food contact during the preparation of meals (3) when shellfish are harvested from waters contaminated by sewage.	Onset: 1–7 days Severe diarrhea, nausea, and vomiting. Respiratory symptoms. Usually lasts 4–5 days but may last for weeks.	• Sanitary handling of foods • Use of pure drinking water • Adequate sewage disposal • Adequate cooking of foods
Parasites			
Trichinella spiralis	Pork and wild game.	Onset: weeks to months Muscle weakness, fluid retention in face, fever, flulike symptoms	• Thorough cooking of pork and wild game
Anisakis	Raw fish.	Onset: 12 hours Stomach infection, severe stomach pain.	• Thorough cooking of fish
Tapeworms	Raw beef, pork, and fish.	May cause abdominal discomfort, diarrhea	• Thorough cooking of all animal products • Avoidance of raw fish dishes, such as sushi
Cyclospora cayetanensis	Carried to food via contaminated water; Guatemalan raspberries suspected in recent outbreaks.	Onset: 1 week Prolonged diarrhea, vomiting, muscle aches, fatigue	• Irradiation (not yet in practice)
Fungi			
A group of toxic compounds (mycotoxins) produced by molds, such as aflatoxin B-1	Found in foods that are relatively high in moisture. Chief food sources are beans and grains that have been stored in a moist place.	May cause liver and/or kidney disease	• Checking of foods for visible mold and discarding those that are contaminated • Proper storage of susceptible foods

Today, we can add pasteurization, sterilization, refrigeration, freezing, **irradiation,** canning, and chemical preservatives to the list of food preservation techniques. An additional method of food-preservation—**aseptic processing**—simultaneously sterilizes the food and package separately before the food enters the package. Liquid foods, such as fruit juices, are especially easy to process in this manner. With aseptic packaging, boxes of sterile milk and juices can remain on supermarket shelves, free of microbial growth, for many years.

Food irradiation is also a method used to treat food. It uses minimal doses of radiation in order to control pathogens such as *E. coli 0157:H7* and *Salmonella*. Even though FDA has permitted the irradiation of certain food products for more than a decade, the history of the technology goes back nearly a century, including scientific research, evaluation, and testing. The radiation used does not make the food radioactive. The rays essentially pass through the food, and no radioactive residues are left behind. However, the energy is strong enough to break chemical bonds, destroy cell walls and cell membranes, break down DNA, and link proteins together. Irradiation thereby controls the growth of insects, microorganisms, and parasites in foods.

FDA recently approved the use of irradiation for raw red meat to reduce the risk of *E. coli* and other infectious pathogens.[1] Other additions to the approved list are shell eggs and seeds. Prior to this, the only animal products so treated were pork and chicken. Irradiation also extends the shelf life of spices, dry vegetable seasonings, meats in general, and fresh fruits and vegetables. Due to recent *Listeria* outbreaks, manufacturers are petitioning the government for permission to irradiate processed meats, such as hot dogs.

Irradiated food, except for dried seasonings, must be labeled with the international symbol, the Radura, and a statement that the product has been treated by irradiation. Foods treated this way are safe in the opinion of FDA and many other health authorities. Although the demand for irradiated foods have yet to get off the ground in the United States, other countries, including Japan, France, Italy, and Mexico, all use food irradiation technology widely. Certain consumer groups continually try to block its use in the United States, claiming that irradiation diminishes the nutritional value of food and that it can lead to the formation of harmful compounds. Similar claims were once made about pasteurization. Many speculate that consumers will eventually accept the process, just as they did with pasteurization during the late nineteenth century.[16] Keep in mind also that, even when foods, especially meats, have been irradiated, it is still important to follow basic food-safety procedures, as later contamination in food preparation is possible.

■ FOOD-BORNE ILLNESS: WHEN UNDESIRABLE MICROBES ALTER FOODS

Most (about 75%) of the verifiable cases of food-borne illness are caused by specific toxin-producing bacteria and other microbes. These organisms cause health problems either directly by invading the intestinal wall and producing an infection via a toxin contained in the organism or indirectly by producing a toxin that is secreted into the food, which later harms us (called an *intoxication*). The main way to tell an infectious route from an intoxication is time: If symptoms appear in 4 hours or less, it is an intoxication.

Many types of bacteria cause food-borne illness, such as *Bacillus, Campylobacter, Clostridium, Escherichia, Listeria, Vibrio, Yersinia, Salmonella*, and *Staphylococcus*. Because each teaspoon of soil contains about 2 billion bacteria, we are constantly at risk for food-borne illness. Luckily, only a small number of all bacteria actually pose a threat. In addition, experts speculate that about 70% of cases of food-borne illness go undiagnosed because they result from viral causes, and there is no easy way to test for these pathogens. To learn more about the latest tools for investigating outbreaks of food-borne illness, see the Expert Opinion by Dr. Tammy Bannerman.

■ General Rules for Preventing Food-Borne Illness

You can greatly reduce the risk of food-borne illness by following some very important rules. It's a long list, because many risky habits need to be addressed.[6, 7, 14, 18]

irradiation A process in which radiation energy is applied to foods, creating compounds (free radicals) within the food that destroy cell membranes, break down DNA, link proteins together, limit enzyme activity, and alter a variety of other proteins and cell functions that can lead to food spoilage. This process does not make the food radioactive.

aseptic processing A method by which food and container are simultaneously sterilized; it allows manufacturers to produce boxes of milk that can be stored at room temperature.

This is the Radura, the international label denoting prior irradiation of the food product.

The World Health Organization's Golden Rules for Safe Food Preparation
1. Choose foods processed for safety.
2. Cook food thoroughly.
3. Eat cooked foods immediately.
4. Store cooked foods carefully.
5. Reheat cooked foods thoroughly.
6. Avoid contact between raw and cooked foods.
7. Wash hands repeatedly.
8. Keep all kitchen surfaces meticulously clean.
9. Protect foods from insects, rodents, and other animals.
10. Use pure water.

The USDA recently simplified these rules into four actions:
1. Clean. Wash hands and surfaces often.
2. Separate. Don't cross-contaminate.
3. Cook. Cook to proper temperatures.
4. Chill. Refrigerate promptly.

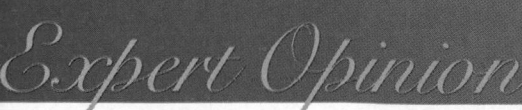

SURVEILLANCE OF EMERGING AND REEMERGING FOOD-BORNE PATHOGENS

Tammy L. Bannerman, Ph.D.

Every year, food-borne infections in the United States are known to cause millions of cases of illness and thousands of deaths. Substantial progress has been made in preventing various food-borne diseases; however, new food-borne pathogens continue to emerge. Factors that may contribute to their emergence include the ability of microorganisms to develop new pathogenic genes or resistance to standard therapeutic methods; changes in transmission pathways, which can allow a known pathogen to move into previously unexposed populations; an increase in the number of susceptible individuals; changes in food handling and processing due to consumer demands and trends; and the breakdown of public health standards.

EMERGING AND REEMERGING PATHOGENS

A food-borne pathogen may be a bacterium, a virus, or a parasite. The more common bacterial pathogens include *Bacillus cereus, Campylobacter, Clostridium botulinum,* enterohemorrhagic *Escherichia coli* (such as *E. coli 0157:H7, Listeria monocytogenes, Salmonella, Shigella, Staphylococcus aureus, Vibrio parahaemolyticus* and *Vibrio vulnificus,* and *Yersinia enterocolitica.* Emerging viral or parasitic pathogens include *Cyclospora, Cryptosporidium, Giardia,* hepatitis A, and the Norwalk family of viruses (small, round-structured viruses).

Many emerging pathogens share several characteristics. Most are food-borne zoonoses (acquired from vertebrate animals), which can rapidly spread globally. The animal reservoir appears to be healthy while harboring these pathogens; therefore, future research must focus on healthy animals and how they acquire and transmit emerging pathogens. Also, these pathogens are becoming increasingly resistant to antimicrobial agents, potentially due to the widespread use of antimicrobials in animals. *Salmonella enterica* serotype Typhimurium DT 104 (resistant to at least five antimicrobial agents) is such an example. Future control measures for emerging pathogens may include changing antimicrobial use in agriculture as well as in human populations.

Pathogens may contaminate food during preharvest or postharvest. Preharvest sources include the presence of the microbes in the soil, contaminated irrigation and surface runoff waters in the fields, and human handling. Postharvest sources include contaminated equipment, transport vehicles, improper food storage, and human handling. For example, an outbreak caused by *C. botulinum* was eventually traced to the improper storage of boxed foods. Contrary to popular belief, not all boxed foods are shelf-stable and

can be stored at ambient temperatures. Since the foods contaminated with the emerging pathogens usually look, smell, and taste normal, the food industry and consumers have limited warning signs. In addition, since the infective dose of these pathogens is generally low (particularly for the viruses and parasites), their ability to evolve and develop resistance to the traditional means of food preparation and storage is becoming more of a dilemma.

INVESTIGATION AND SURVEILLANCE OF FOOD-BORNE PATHOGENS

Investigation of a food-borne outbreak is a team effort, often involving sanitarians, epidemiologists, and laboratorians. When available, food samples that are suspected of being the vehicle for the pathogen and perhaps samples of other potentially hazardous foods are collected. These food items are then tested for the possible pathogen by considering (1) clinical signs, symptoms, and incubation periods in the victims; (2) types of foods; and (3) epidemiologic data. A vehicle can be epidemiologically suspect if food-specific attack rates are statistically high in persons who have eaten a specific food and low in persons who have not eaten the food. Further association can be made if a significant number of a specific pathogen that cause a syndrome similar to that seen

Purchasing Food

- When shopping, select frozen foods and perishable foods last, such as meat, poultry, or fish. Always have these products put in separate plastic bags, so that drippings don't contaminate other foods in the shopping cart. Then, don't let groceries sit in a warm car; this allows bacteria to grow. Get the perishable foods home and promptly refrigerate or freeze.
- Don't buy or use food from damaged containers that leak, bulge, or are severely dented or buy or use food from jars that are cracked or have loose or bulging

in victims are isolated from the food or if an enteric pathogen (such as *Salmonella*) are recovered from the food. However, to confirm the actual involvement of a food, the same pathogen or the same toxin as was found in specimens from the victims must be found in the epidemiologically implicated food.

Surveillance for food-borne pathogens in the United States has been conducted for many years. The surveillance has traditionally served three purposes: disease prevention and control, knowledge acquisition of disease causes, and administrative guidance for future food-processing and handling protocols. The Centers for Disease Control and Prevention (CDC) has expanded its national surveillance of food-borne pathogens by incorporating molecular DNA fingerprinting methods (or strain typing). Food-borne pathogens are being typed at state public health laboratories by a technique called pulsed-field gel electrophoresis. This technique has proven to be an invaluable tool for the investigation of food-borne outbreaks within and across states.

Another CDC surveillance strategy, known as FoodNet, is an active surveillance program. Since January 1996, five participating sites have been conducting this more intense surveillance of food-borne pathogens. FoodNet surveys the population, physicians, and laboratories to measure the proportion of diarrheal disease that is undiagnosed and unreported, so that the true disease incidence can be estimated. This surveillance is the platform on which more detailed investigations, including case-control studies of sporadic cases of common food-borne infections, are being conducted.

DETECTION/IDENTIFICATION OF FOOD-BORNE PATHOGENS

Traditional detection methods have been limited in terms of food safety because of the lack of timeliness, the limits of detection, and the poor separation of pathogenic from nonpathogenic isolates. Recent advances in diagnostic technology are starting to alter the ways in which food-borne pathogens are detected and identified. Molecular (DNA) methods may enable the food industry to overcome some of the previous obstacles.

Many commercial assay systems and kits that use miniaturized biochemical tests, new media formulations, automated instrumentation, DNA/RNA probes, antibody-dependent assays, and polymerase chain reaction (PCR) are currently being used or studied for their usefulness in the rapid detection of food-borne pathogens. PCR, a technique that amplifies a specific region of DNA, allows for the detection of pathogens present in low quantities. Detection of the pathogens can be accomplished in a number of hours, which could have taken days using traditional methods. A number of PCR-based assays have been developed, but they have been applied most often to clinical and environmental samples, rarely for the detection of food-borne pathogens. Much of the difficulty in implementing PCR for the analysis of food samples lies in the problems encountered from substances in the food that interfere with the procedure.

CONCLUSIONS

Each link in the production, preparation, and delivery of food can contribute a health hazard. Although new technologies that improve the safety of the food supply and early detection hold promise, changes in food processing, products, and practices will continue to allow for the emergence of food-borne pathogens. Actions must be taken to limit the possibility of the emergence of food-borne pathogens, such as a more prudent use of antimicrobial agents and increased research into the mechanisms involved in food-borne disease.

A rapid, coordinated response among state and federal agencies can help prevent widespread food-borne outbreaks. A continued vigilance and the ability to mobilize research capabilities must be integral parts of food safety programs if the impact of new food-borne microbial threats to human health is going to be minimized.

Dr. Bannerman is a molecular microbiologist at the Ohio Department of Health Laboratories. She is also a clinical assistant professor in the Medical Technology Division at The Ohio State University, Columbus.

---

lids. Don't taste or use food that has a foul odor or spurts liquid when the can is opened; the deadly *Clostridium botulinum* toxin may be present.

- Purchase only pasteurized milk and cheese (check the label). This is especially important for pregnant women because highly toxic bacteria and viruses that can harm the fetus thrive in unpasteurized milk.

- Purchase only the amount of produce needed for a week's time. The longer you keep fruits and vegetables, the more time is available for bacteria to grow.

A new website coordinating the federal efforts on food safety is http://www.foodsafety.gov.

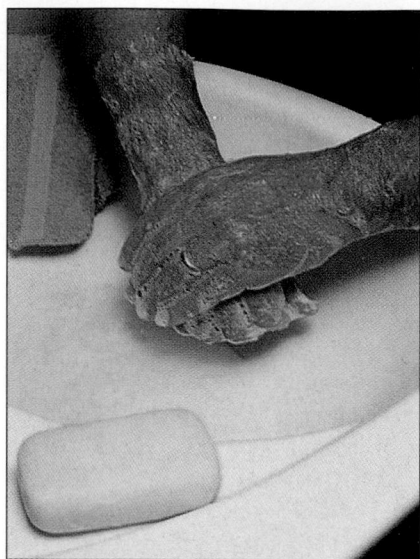

Washing hands thoroughly with hot water and soap should be the first step in food preparation. The 4 "F's" of food contamination are fingers, foods, feces, and flies. Handwashing especially combats the fecal and finger routes.

CRITICAL THINKING

Jon wants to buy a cutting board for his new kitchen. He's been looking at all of the possibilities: plexiglass, plastic, and wood. How would you advise him, so that he can minimize the risk of any foodborne illness from his food preparation?

*I*n one of the largest recalls of meat products in U.S. history, an Arkansas-based processing plant voluntarily recalled 25 million pounds of hamburger suspected of contamination with *E. coli 0157:H7.*

- When purchasing precut produce, avoid those that look slimy, brownish, or dry; these are signs of improper holding temperatures.

Preparing Food

- Thoroughly wash hands with hot, soapy water before and after handling food. This practice is especially important when handling raw meat, fish, poultry, and eggs, and after using the bathroom.
- Make sure counters, cutting boards, dishes, and other equipment are thoroughly cleaned and rinsed before use. Be especially careful to use hot, soapy water to wash surfaces and equipment that have come in contact with raw meat, fish, poultry, and eggs as soon as possible to remove *Salmonella* bacteria that may be present.
- If possible, cut foods to be eaten raw on a clean cutting board reserved for that purpose. Then clean this cutting board using hot, soapy water. If the same board must be used for both meat and other foods, cut any potentially contaminated items, such as meat, last. After cutting the meat, wash the cutting board thoroughly.

  USDA recommends cutting boards with unmarred surfaces made of easy-to-clean, nonporous materials, such as plastic, marble, or glass. If you prefer a wooden board, reserve it for a specific purpose; for example, set it aside for cutting raw meat and poultry. Then keep a separate wooden cutting board for chopping produce and slicing bread to prevent these products from picking up bacteria from raw meat. Note that many foods are served raw, so any bacteria clinging to them are not destroyed.

  Furthermore, USDA recommends that all cutting boards be replaced when they become streaked with hard-to-clean grooves or cuts, which may harbor bacteria. In addition, cutting boards should be sanitized once a week in a solution of 2 teaspoons of chlorine bleach per quart of water. Flood the board with the solution, let it sit a few minutes, and then rise thoroughly.
- When thawing foods, do so in the refrigerator for 1 to 3 days, under cold running water, or in a microwave oven. Also, cook foods immediately after thawing under cold water or in the microwave. Never let frozen foods thaw unrefrigerated all day or night. Also, marinate food in the refrigerator.
- Avoid coughing or sneezing over foods, even when you're healthy. Cover cuts on hands with a sterile bandage. This helps stop *Staphylococcus* from entering food.
- Carefully wash fresh fruit and vegetables under running water to remove dirt and bacteria clinging to the surface, using a vegetable brush if the skin is to be eaten. People have became ill from *Salmonella* that was introduced from melons used in making a fruit salad and from oranges used for freshly-squeezed orange juice. The bacteria were on the outside of the melons and oranges.
- Completely remove moldy portions of food, or don't eat the food. *When in doubt, throw the food out.* Mold growth is prevented by properly storing food at cold temperatures and using the food within a reasonable length of time.
- Use refrigerated ground meat and patties in 1 to 2 days and frozen meat and patties within 3 to 4 months.

Cooking Food

- Cook food thoroughly, especially beef, fish, and pork (160°F [71°C]), poultry (180°F [82°C]), and eggs (until the yolk and white are hard). Cooking is by far the most reliable way to destroy food-borne bacteria, such as toxic strains of *E. coli,* whereas freezing only halts growth. A good general precaution is to eat no raw animal products. USDA answers questions about the safe use of animal products (800-535-4555, 10 AM to 4 PM weekdays, Eastern time).

  Seafood also poses a risk of food-borne illness. Properly cooked fish should flake easily and be opaque or dull and firm. If it's translucent or shiny, it's not done. Raw fish dishes, such as sushi, can be safe for most people to eat if they are made with very fresh fish that has been commercially frozen and then thawed. The freezing is important to eliminate potential health risks from parasites. FDA recommends that the fish be frozen to an internal temperature of −10°F for 7 days. If you choose to eat uncooked fish, purchase the fish from reputable establishments that have high standards for quality and sanitation. People at high risk for food-borne illness would be wise to avoid raw fish products (Fig. 19-1).

- Cook stuffing separately from poultry (or wash poultry thoroughly, stuff immediately before cooking, and then transfer the stuffing to a clean bowl immediately after cooking). Make sure the stuffing reaches 165°F (74°C). Again, *Salmonella* is the major concern with poultry.
- Once a food is cooked, consume it right away, or cool it to 40°F (4°C) within 2 hours. If it is not to be eaten immediately, in hot weather (85°F and above) make sure this cooling is done within 1 hour. Do this by separating the food into as many shallow pans as needed to provide a large surface area. Be careful not to recontaminate cooked food by contact with raw meat or juices from hands, cutting boards, or dirty utensils or in other ways.
- Serve meat, poultry, and fish on a clean plate—never the same plate that was used to hold the raw product. For example, when grilling hamburgers, don't put cooked items on the same plate that was used to carry the raw product out to the grill.
- Cook food completely at a picnic site, with no partial cooking in advance.

Storing and Reheating Cooked Food

- Keep hot foods hot and cold foods cold. Hold food below 40°F (4°C) or above 140°F (60°C) (Fig. 19-2). Food-borne microbes thrive in more moderate temperatures (60° to 110°F [16° to 43°C]). Some microbes can even grow in the refrigerator. Again, don't leave cooked or refrigerated foods, such as meats and salads, at room temperature for more than 2 hours (or 1 hour in hot weather) because that gives microbes an opportunity to grow. Store dry food at 60°F to 70°F (16°C to 21°C).
- Reheat leftovers to 165°F (74°C); reheat gravy to a rolling boil to kill *Clostridium perfringens* bacteria, which may be present. Merely reheating to a good eating temperature isn't enough to kill sufficient bacteria.
- Store peeled or cut-up produce, such as melon balls, in the refrigerator.
- Make sure the refrigerator stays below 40°F (4°C). Either use a refrigerator thermometer or keep it as cold as possible without freezing milk and lettuce.

Microbes that cause food-borne illness commonly enter food through cross-contamination—from one source to another—and grow in temperatures favorable to them, as occurred at a large gathering where turkey franks were contaminated with bacteria. When the franks were later added to a salad, it too became contaminated, causing food-borne illness. Potential sources of cross-contamination are dirty kitchen towels and sponges. It's essential to practice sanitary food-handling procedures when preparing any food.

As one final precaution, watch for safe food-handling techniques when you eat out. Check that foods in a salad bar are iced; custard and pudding pies are chilled; hot foods served on a hot food bar are, in fact, hot; and vending machines are checked regularly, especially those containing sandwiches and milk. Send back any meat,

Current Safe Handling Instructions Issued by USDA for Labeling Meat and Poultry Products

This product was prepared from inspected and passed meat and/or poultry. Some food products may contain bacteria that could cause illness if the product is mishandled or cooked improperly. For your protection, follow these safe handling instructions.

Keep refrigerated or frozen.

Thaw in refrigerator or microwave.

Keep raw meat and poultry separate from other foods.

Wash working surfaces (including cutting boards), utensils, and hands after touching raw meat or poultry.

Cook thoroughly.

Keep hot foods hot. Refrigerate leftovers immediately or discard.

*T*o reduce the risk of bacteria surviving during microwave cooking,

- Cover food with glass or ceramic when possible to decrease evaporation and heat the surface.
- Stir and rotate food at least once or twice for even cooking. Then, allow microwaved food to stand, covered, after cooking is completed to help cook the exterior and equalize the temperature throughout.
- Use an oven temperature probe or a meat thermometer to check that food is done. Insert it at several spots.
- If thawing meat in the microwave, use the oven's defrost setting. Ice crystals in frozen foods are not heated well by the microwave oven and can create cold spots, which later cook more slowly.

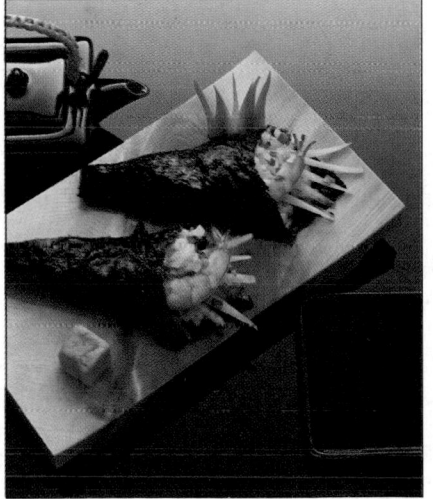

■ **FIGURE 19-1** Sushi, like all raw fish or meat dishes, is a high-risk food. For maximum protection from food-borne illness, you should cook animal foods thoroughly before eating. If you choose to eat uncooked fish, purchase fish from reputable establishments that have high standards for quality and sanitation. People at high risk for food-borne illness would be wise to avoid these products.

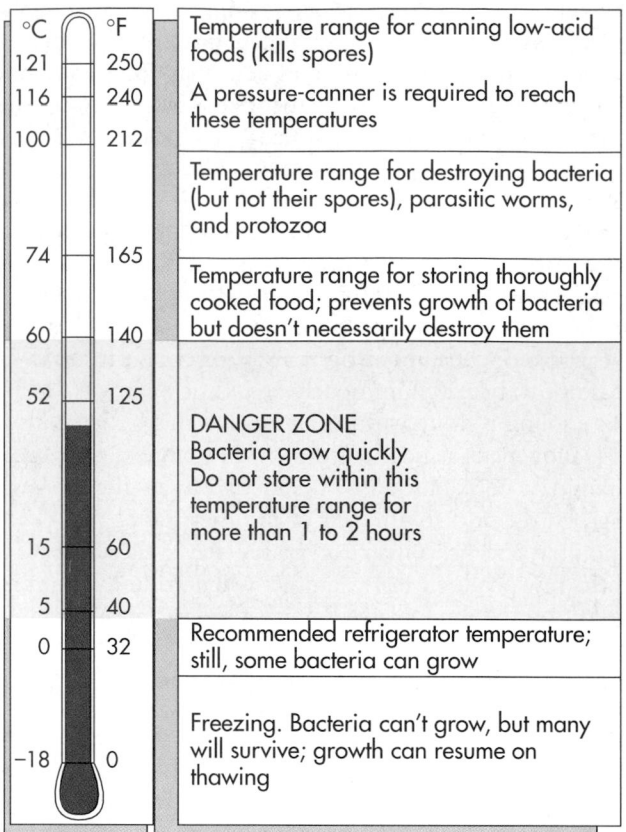

°C	°F	
121	250	Temperature range for canning low-acid foods (kills spores)
116	240	A pressure-canner is required to reach these temperatures
100	212	
		Temperature range for destroying bacteria (but not their spores), parasitic worms, and protozoa
74	165	
		Temperature range for storing thoroughly cooked food; prevents growth of bacteria but doesn't necessarily destroy them
60	140	
52	125	
		DANGER ZONE Bacteria grow quickly Do not store within this temperature range for more than 1 to 2 hours
15	60	
5	40	
0	32	Recommended refrigerator temperature; still, some bacteria can grow
		Freezing. Bacteria can't grow, but many will survive; growth can resume on thawing
−18	0	

▌ FIGURE 19-2 The effects of temperature on microbes that cause food-borne illness.
Adapted from Temperature guide to food safety: food and home notes, No. 25, Washington, DC, June 20, 1977, USDA.

*F*ightBAC! is a new program from USDA and FDA that emphasizes four messages designed to reduce food-borne illness:
  CLEAN: Wash hands and surfaces often.
  SEPARATE: Don't cross-contaminate.
  COOK: Cook food to proper temperatures.
  CHILL: Refrigerate promptly.
Check out: http://www.fightbac.org

poultry, seafood, or fish that does not appear thoroughly cooked. Food stored and served in dormitory cafeterias should also be properly handled.

CONCEPT CHECK

*B*acteria and the toxins they produce pose the greatest risk for food-borne illness. In the past, the addition to foods of sugar and salt, as well as smoking and drying, were used to prevent the growth of microorganisms. Today, we know that ensuring cleanliness, keeping hot foods hot and cold foods cold, and cooking foods thoroughly offer additional protection from food-borne illness. Commercial processes, such as pasteurization and irradiation, do the same. Treat all raw animal products, cooked food, and raw fruits and vegetables as potential sources of food-borne illness.

▌ A Closer Look at the Microbes That Cause Food-Borne Illness

As previously mentioned, bacteria pose the greatest risk for food-borne illness. Bacteria are extremely simple structures. They contain only one chromosome and lack mitochondria, endoplasmic reticulum, golgi body and lysosomes. Many bacteria are enclosed in a carbohydrate-like capsule, which protects them and aids their adherence to tissues. Some bacteria can survive harsh environmental conditions through **spore** formation. In the spore state, bacteria can remain stable for months or years.

Certain bacteria can thrive in almost freezing temperatures, whereas others thrive in very high temperatures. The optimum temperature for most disease-causing bacteria is about 98°F (body temperature; 37°C). Bacteria living in the presence of oxy-

spores Dormant reproductive cells capable of forming into adult organisms without the help of another cell. Various fungi and bacteria form spores.

gen are called *aerobes,* whereas those living in the absence of oxygen are called *anaerobes.* Those that prefer free oxygen but can live in its absence are called *facultative anaerobes.* Many bacteria produce toxins.

Finding the specific agent that has led to a food-borne illness requires some detective skills. Identifying the agent depends on knowing the food source, the incubation time for and types of symptoms, and the duration of the illness associated with an outbreak.[26] Let's look at the characteristics of the major contaminants individually. An informative web site on the topic is http://www.ama-assn.org/foodborne.

Campylobacter Jejuni (C. Jejuni)

In recent years, *Campylobacter* has jumped to the top of the list as the number one cause of all domestic food-borne illnesses, resulting in up to 4 million human infections a year in the United States.[17] The bacteria produce a toxin that destroys the mucosal surfaces of the small and large intestines.

Because *C. jejuni* is so difficult to detect in foods, an enormous number of cases of this food-borne illness probably go unreported in this country. Also, most infections are very sporadic and are not associated with a large outbreak, as are other food-borne infections, such as *E. coli* and *Salmonella.* In a study conducted by the U.S. Department of Agriculture's Poultry Microbiological Safety Research Unit, more than 90% of the poultry tested was positive for *Campylobacter.*

Symptoms of the illness are acute intestinal inflamation with fever, muscle pain, headache, and diarrhea. During the peak of the disease, 10 or more bowel movements per day are common, and stools are often bloody. Cases are associated with contaminated water, raw or inadequately cooked animal foods, including beef and unpasteurized milk. Poultry, especially chicken, is of most concern. Because this organism grows slowly, the onset of symptoms is delayed, occurring 2 to 10 days after ingesting the contaminated food; it may even take weeks. Older adults, children, and people with weakened immune systems are at particularly high risk.

Treatment uses antibiotic medication, with most people recovering in less than 1 week. Deaths are rare. However, a number of *Campylobacter* infections that are resistant to a class of antibiotics called fluoroquinolones have been on the rise. A recent study concluded that antibiotic use in the U.S. poultry industry is the main contributor to this antibiotic resistance. This creates a problem when physicians attempt to treat this food-borne illness, since those people found with the resistant infections are more likely to have severe infections and bloody diarrhea and to be hospitalized. Also, the bacterium is recognized as a major contributing factor to Guillain-Barre syndrome, which is the most common cause of acute paralysis in both children and adults.

Luckily, *Campylobacter* organisms are very sensitive to heat. This trait probably protects most people from infections. Prompt refrigeration, thorough cooking, avoidance of cross-contamination, thorough hand washing, and careful refrigeration of leftovers are important ways to prevent its growth.

Salmonella

There are 2000 strains of *Salmonella* bacteria, many of which cause food-borne illness.[19] *Salmonella* can be killed by normal cooking. Nonetheless, they are responsible for many cases of food borne illness, up to 1.4 million per year, many of which go unreported. Related deaths average 600 per year.

Commonly found in animal and human feces, these bacteria enter food via infected water, contaminated cutting boards, contaminated meat products, cracked eggs, and actual bits of feces in food. Ingesting the live bacteria causes the problem.[21, 23] Recent outbreaks of salmonellosis have been traced back to alfalfa sprouts.[11] It is thought that the seeds of these sprouts were contaminated by bird or rodent feces. According to FDA, children, older adults, and persons with weakened immune systems should not eat raw sprouts, such as alfalfa, clover, and radish. Feces

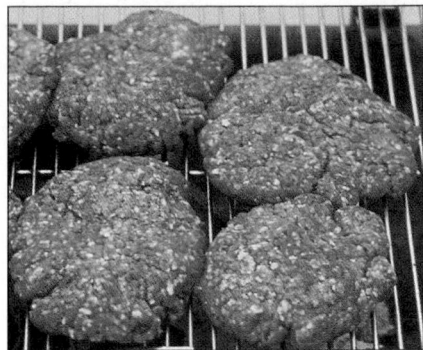

Cook hamburgers until they are brown throughout, the juices run clear, and the inside is hot.

A goal of *Healthy People 2010* is to reduce the number of cases of food-borne illness from *Campylobacter, E. coli, Listeria,* and *Salmonella* by 50%.

FDA warns us not to consume home-made ice cream, eggnog, and mayonnaise if made with unpasteurized, raw eggs because of the risk of *Salmonella* food-borne illness. Commercial forms of these products are safe because the egg products used have been pasteurized, which kills *Salmonella* bacteria. In addition, commercial mayonnaise contains enough acid to prevent bacterial growth.

Proposed Egg Safety Warning Label

Safe Handling Instructions: Eggs may contain harmful bacteria known to cause serious illness, especially in children, the elderly, and persons with weak immune systems. For your protection: Keep eggs refrigerated: cook eggs until yolks are firm: and cook foods containing eggs thoroughly.

from pet reptiles are also sources of *Salmonella* exposure.[28] Infants and young children are at high risk for salmonellosis from indrect or direct contact with reptiles.

Symptoms of *Salmonella* infections include nausea, fever, headache, abdominal cramps, diarrhea, and vomiting and can develop in 5 to 72 hours. Bed rest and fluids are the only effective treatment, and recovery usually occurs within 2 to 3 days. Deaths are rare. *Salmonella* attacks occur most frequently from consuming eggs, chicken, meat, meat products, custard made with infected eggs, raw milk, and inadequately refrigerated and reheated leftovers. Unpasteurized orange juice and milk may also be contaminated with *Salmonella*.[5] Raw chicken is often contaminated, and undercooked food—including eggs—poses a particular risk. FDA intends to add warning labels to egg cartons in an attempt to prevent up to 66,000 illnesses and 40 deaths per year from eggs contaminated with *Salmonella* inside the shell. The new warning label will inform people about potentially harmful bacteria, as well as instructions for safe handling to help prevent food-borne illness (see margin).

Most outbreaks of *Salmonella* infection can be traced to improper food handling. Picnics pose a special challenge, because food is frequently held for hours at a dangerously high temperature (between 40°F and 140°F or 4°C and 60°C). It takes only about 8 hours for *Salmonella* bacteria to multiply sufficiently to cause illness. Therefore, keep foods above 140°F (60°C) or below 40°F (4°C) to help prevent the growth of *Salmonella* bacteria.

Salmonella also poses a great risk for cross-contamination of foods. To avoid cross-contamination, keep produce, cooked foods, and ready-to-eat foods separate from uncooked meats and raw eggs. Thoroughly clean hands, cutting boards, counters, knives, and other utensils after handling uncooked foods, as well as in-between use.

Shigella sonnei (S. sonnei)

Food-borne illness caused by the *Shigella* bacterium is a common disease of youngsters in day-care centers, nurseries, and custodial institutions. The infection is transmitted by the fecal-oral route, primarily by way of the hands, as well as via food and water. The onset of symptoms usually occurs within 1 to 3 days of being infected. The symptoms include abdominal cramps, diarrhea, fever, and bloody stools. Some carriers of *Shigella* show no effect but represent a potential threat to all who are in their care. With as little as 10 organisms able to cause an infection, person-to-person transmission is easily accomplished where hygienic conditions are compromised.

Although reported infrequently, *Shigella* outbreaks have been associated with raw produce, including green onions, crisphead lettuce, and uncooked, raw parsley. Recent outbreaks have been traced back to raw, chopped parsley, which had been cut and stored at room temperature.[24] To avoid contamination from parsley, food handlers should store chopped parsley for short times, keeping it refrigerated, and chop smaller batches. Handwashing and sanitary food production offer the best protection against *Shigella* infections.

Escherichia coli (E. coli)

Escherichia coli (E. coli) is commonly found in the intestinal tract of humans and other animals. The bacteria first appeared in the late 1970s and now are found in entire herds of cattle. Since 1982, at least six strains—most notably, *E. coli 0157:H7*—have been shown to cause food-borne illness. Although there are hundreds of benign strains of the bacteria, 0157:H7 and 0111:H8 are especially virulent and cause severe illness. According to the Centers for Disease Control and Prevention, the *E. coli* bacterium, which is most commonly found in ground beef, kills about 60 people each year and causes illness in an estimated 73,000 more. It is quickly becoming a major threat for food-borne illness, with up to 4% of raw meat products in the United States possibly containing the bacteria.

Children and the elderly are most susceptible to the disease. The bacterium is transmitted primarily via contaminated ground beef and roast beef. In response, as previously mentioned, FDA has approved the irradiation of meat to reduce this risk. Although ground beef is the most common source of the *E. coli* bacteria, fruits, vegetables, and drinking water also can harbor the deadly pathogen.[9] Unpasteurized milk, untreated apple cider, salad greens grown in cow manure, cantaloupe, dry-cured salami (because it is not cooked during processing), and alfalfa sprouts have also been implicated in *E. coli* infections. In one case, fresh apple juice was contaminated with *E. coli* because the apples used to produce the juice had fallen to the ground and had come into contact with animal feces. New methods for apple juice production are being researched; pasteurization is becoming routine.

After an incubation period of 2 to 4 days, the disease normally lasts 4 to 10 days. The symptoms include severe abdominal cramps, bloody diarrhea, and hemolytic uremic syndrome, a condition that can lead to kidney failure. *E. coli* infection should be investigated in any case of bloody diarrhea.

Cooking meat until it is gray or brown in color and the juices run yellow to clear (no pink color left; see page 758) and then avoiding recontamination are important ways to prevent this type of food-borne illness. Cider that is not pasteurized or that does not contain preservatives can be heated to a slow simmer until steam rises from the pan before serving or refrigerating to reduce risk.

Clostridium perfringens (C. perfringens)

The bacterium *Clostridium perfringens* lives throughout the environment, especially in soil, the intestines of farm animals and humans, and sewage. It is called the "cafeteria germ," because most food-borne outbreaks caused by this organism are associated with the food service industry or with events where large quantities of food are prepared and served. The symptoms of an infection resemble those of *Salmonella* cases, but the victim usually doesn't vomit. The symptoms occur within 8 to 24 hours of consuming enough live bacteria. Again, bed rest and fluids are the only effective treatment, and recovery usually occurs within a day or so.

C. perfringens thrives in an oxygen-free environment. It forms heat-resistant spores, which become bacteria at temperatures between 70°F and 120°F (21°C and 49°C); and at the same time produces a toxin. The bacteria then can quickly multiply to disease-causing amounts. Foods stored in deep refrigerator pans are especially fertile media for the growth of these bacteria because the centers are isolated from air and they stay warm.

C. perfringens organisms are often found in cooked beef, turkey, gravy, dressing, stews, and casseroles. The best way to prevent their growth is to maintain proper holding temperatures and divide large leftover portions into smaller ones. Be especially careful to cook meats completely and cool them rapidly in small containers. Thoroughly reheat leftover meat to 165°F (74°C) before serving. Always bring leftover gravy to a rolling boil. Refrigerate cold cuts and sliced meats at 40°F or 4°C, and serve them cold.

Listeria monocytogenes (L. monocytogenes)

Listeria monocytogenes is widely distributed in the environment and often enters food from contamination with animal or human feces. It is a very hardy microbe, which resists heat, salt, and acidity much better than many other bacteria. This bacterium survives and even grows at refrigeration temperatures. Because pasteurization destroys *Listeria* organisms, reports of contaminated milk and cheese products suggest that contamination occurred following pasteurization, probably from the addition of unpasteurized milk. Listeriosis in the United States is estimated to kill 500 Americans a year and causes illness in 2000 more, which means that listeriosis kills 20% of the people it infects.[15]

Listeria infections cause fever, headache, and vomiting about 7 to 30 days after exposure. However, newborn infants, pregnant women, and people with depressed immune function may suffer severe symptoms, including meningitis, spontaneous abortion, serious blood infections, and death. It is especially important that pregnant

CRITICAL THINKING

Diana had a party at her house for her son's birthday. While cleaning up after the kids had gone home, she realized she had forgotten to put away the potato salad and coleslaw and decided to discard it. However, her husband, Tim, wanted her to just refrigerate it. "After all," he reasoned, "it was only left out for a couple of hours." Why was Diana right in wanting to throw away the leftover unrefrigerated food?

In a recent period of 6 months, more than 45 million pounds of hot dogs, luncheon meats, and other ready-to-eat meat products were recalled due to contamination with potentially deadly Listeria *bacteria.*

women and other people at high risk avoid products such as unpasteurized or expired milk, uncooked hot dogs, undercooked chicken, and Mexican soft cheeses (e.g., queso fresco), and other soft cheeses such as feta, brie, and blue-veined cheeses, all of which are suspected of being major sources of *Listeria* infection. USDA also warns pregnant women and other people at high risk to thoroughly cook all ready-to-eat meats, including hot dogs and cold cuts, until they are steaming.

Consuming only pasteurized milk products; cooking meat, poultry, and seafood thoroughly; keeping food refrigerated; and washing fresh produce thoroughly are ways to avoid *Listeria* infection.

Staphylococcus aureus (S. aureus)

The organism *Staphylococcus aureus (S. aureus)* produces toxins as it grows in food. Once ingested, the toxin causes nausea, vomiting, diarrhea, headache, and abdominal cramps. The symptoms usually develop within 2 to 6 hours of eating the contaminated food. People seldom die from the toxin, but they don't develop immunity against future attacks. And, as is true for almost all food-borne illnesses, continued unsafe food handling will result in repeated sickness. Bed rest and fluids are generally the only treatment needed. Recovery usually takes place within 2 to 3 days.

S. aureus bacteria live mainly in the nasal passages and skin sores. These microbes enter food when people sneeze and cough over food or handle food while they have open skin sores. Once present in significant numbers in a food, *S. aureus* can make enough toxin to cause human illness in about 4 hours if the food temperature stays near 100°F (38°C). The toxin is undetectable by flavor, odor, and appearance and can even withstand prolonged cooking.

Foods commonly associated with *S. aureus* intoxications are custard, ham, egg salad, cheese, seafood, cream-filled pastries, and milk. A frequent source is whipped cream left standing for hours at room temperature. Keeping these and other foods above 140°F (60°C) or below 40°F (4°C) prevents both the bacterium's growth and further toxin production. To limit the spread of this microbe, it's important to work with clean hands, working surfaces, and utensils; to direct coughs and sneezes away from food; and to cover skin cuts on hands and arms when handling food.

Clostridium botulinum (C. botulinum)

The *Clostridium botulinum* bacterium can cause botulism, a food-borne illness that can be fatal. This microbe comes from soil and may exist as a bacterium or spore in any food. As these bacteria multiply in food, they release a deadly toxin. The death rate for botulism receives much public attention; however, only a few cases are reported each year in the United States. At one time, botulism was a serious problem in the canning industry, but now adequate heating processing and intact containers have virtually eliminated this danger from North American manufactured canned foods.

The symptoms of botulism appear within 12 to 36 hours of ingesting contaminated food. The toxin blocks acetylcholine release at neuromuscular junctions, causing vomiting, abdominal pain, double vision, dizziness, and acute respiratory failure. The prompt administration of the botulism antitoxin can help prevent the progression of paralysis and reduce the duration of the illness. Sometimes treatment requires intensive care, including mechanical ventilation. The combination of the antitoxin and supportive care has reduced the incidence of mortality in the United States to less than 10%. If the person survives, recovery occurs within 10 days.[32]

C. botulinum grows only in the absence of air, so it thrives primarily in canned food, especially improperly home-canned, low-acid foods, such as string beans, corn, mushrooms, beets, and asparagus. Recently, other foods with oxygen-deprived centers—such as potato salad, sautéed onions, stew, and chopped garlic—have also caused botulism. FDA now requires that chopped garlic in oil be acidified to protect against *C. botulinum*. Consumers should look for a commercially prepared product that contains phosphoric or citric acid. Cured meats also pose a risk for botulism;

however, the nitrates and vitamin C used to preserve commercial products inhibit bacterial growth. Botulism has also occurred among Alaskan natives, as it is common practice to consume uncooked, fermented fish.

Home-canned foods are the most common sources of botulism. Although the canning process may kill all bacteria and the heat may drive out all oxygen, spores of *C. botulinum* can still survive if the heating is insufficient. When the can or jar cools, the spores germinate into bacteria, which produce the toxin. Even foods that were previously thought to be safe due to their acidity, such as tomatoes, require greater care, as new varieties tend to have a higher pH. To ensure the safety of home-canned foods, it is crucial to follow the canning directions exactly. To be safe, always check all cans carefully even those from commercial facilities. Look for holes, rust on the seams, and swollen sides or tops. Make sure the can sucks in air when opened to indicate the vacuum was maintained, and the liquid inside is clear, not milky or foul-smelling. If you see any signs of spoilage, return the can to the store or take it to the nearest public health department. Whatever you do, do not taste the food. One green bean can contain enough toxin to kill you. For questions on proper canning, call the Ball Consumer Hotline at 1-800-240-3340.

Botulism also may develop in vivo (inside the living body). Infants between 2 and 9 months of age are at the highest risk because of low stomach acid production. About 250 cases are reported each year. Fortunately, the death rate is low, 1 to 2%. Adults with low stomach acid production are also at risk. Bacteria spores germinate in the stomach and produce the exotoxin. For this reason, honey and corn syrup should not be given to young infants because these products can contain the spores of this bacterium.

Other Bacteria That Pose a Risk

Yersinia enterocolitica (Y. enterocolitica) has been linked to food-borne illnesses since 1976. Foods implicated include water, chocolate milk, reconstituted dry milk, wild animal meats, and tofu. Usually, the microbe enters the food after pasteurization. Symptoms of infection occur 24 to 36 hours after eating the contaminated food and include diarrhea, fever, headache, and severe abdominal pain that mimics appendicitis. (Unnecessary appendectomies have been performed after *Yersinia* infection.) The disease can last as long as 2 weeks, and even a year or longer in some cases. The disease may also trigger arthritis, inflammation of heart tissue, and blood infection. *Yersinia* organisms grow at cold temperatures, so refrigerated storage does not control its growth in food. Therefore, foods must be sterilized by sufficient cooking or pasteurization to destroy this microbe. Fortunately, the strains of *Yersinia* bacteria primarily associated with human illness are not common in food at this time.

Infection from *Vibrio vulnificus (V. vulnificus)*, a newly identified bacterium, has been linked to eating raw seafood, especially raw oysters. *V. vulnificus* causes a serious infection, which can be fatal in about 45 to 75% of cases, especially for people with liver disease and compromised immunity. Eating any raw or lightly (partially) cooked seafood, specifically that harvested from the Gulf Coast from April through October, poses a high risk. Symptoms include diarrhea, fever, weakness, blood infection, and other serious health problems. Prompt treatment is needed. Cooking destroys this organism.

Vibrio cholerae (V. cholerae) causes a severe form of GI tract infection. Sources of *V. cholerae* are food and water contaminated with fecal matter. Cholera is usually seen in developing countries with poor sanitation. Foreign travel and raw seafood, particularly raw shellfish, have accounted for all but a handful of the cholera cases in the United States during the past decade. The bacteria secrete a GI tract toxin. Handwashing after defecating is vital to reducing risk. The disease occurs 2 to 3 days after ingesting contaminated food or water. Symptoms include vomiting and severe watery diarrhea, which can lead to dehydration and cardiovascular collapse. The death rate can be as high as 60%. Treatment consists of replacing fluids and electrolytes.

A new tool in the battle against food-borne illness is HACCP, or Hazard Analysis and Critical Control Point. HACCP is a method of ensuring food safety. Rather than treating the cause after a food-borne illness outbreak has occurred, by applying the principles of HACCP, food handlers critically analyze how they approach food preparation and what conditions may exist that might allow pathogenic microorganisms to enter the food system. Once specific hazards and critical control points (where potential problems can occur) are identified, preventive measures can be used to reduce specific sources of contamination. Thus, the food handlers are using HACCP to stop a problem before it starts.

*R*ecovery from hepatitis A generally occurs of its own accord in 3 to 6 months. This food-borne illness constitutes the only exception to the rule of immunity, as it is the only one in which those infected with the virus are then immune for the rest of their lives.

Viruses

Viruses do not metabolize, grow, or move by themselves. Instead, they reproduce within a living host cell, and, thus, cannot grow in food once it is harvested or slaughtered. Viruses consist of a protein coat surrounding a nucleic acid core of either DNA or RNA. They have no cell wall. On entering a host cell, a virus takes over the cell's DNA replication processes and causes it to reproduce the virus's genetic material. Generally, the host cell dies in the process and bursts open, releasing new viruses into the surrounding medium. Many viruses cause disease in humans.

Because viruses cannot multiply in foods, they must enter in sufficient amounts through bits of feces that contaminate food. A well-known example is the hepatitis A virus, although this route accounts for only a small percentage of the total number of hepatitis A infections. This food-borne agent most often thrives because of unsanitary food handling by carriers of the virus in restaurants. People have also contracted hepatitis A infections from eating raw or undercooked shellfish—clams, oysters, and mussels—harvested from waters contaminated with raw or improperly treated sewage. The virus that causes hepatitis A can endure notable heat, cold, and drying. Cooking foods at 212°F (100°C) for more than 5 minutes inactivates the virus, as does irradiation.

Symptoms of the infection include intestinal problems, weakness, fatigue, jaundice, and sometimes even the development of serious liver disease, requiring hospitalization. Because the symptoms of hepatitis A infection do not usually occur until about 1 to 2 months after eating contaminated food, the source is difficult to identify. It is diagnosed by detection of hepatitis A antibodies. About 30,000 cases are reported annually.

Raw clams and oysters are particularly risky foods because they are filter feeders, a process that concentrates viruses and toxins present in the water as it is filtered for food. Consumption of these raw shellfish results in the consumption of live viruses and bacteria, too. It is important to buy oysters and clams only from the most reliable sources. By law, shellfish offered for sale must come from licensed beds, but often they do not, so be careful when you either purchase these foods or harvest them yourself. Check with the local health department if you question the safety of waters in an area.

Proper handwashing by food service personnel is especially important in restaurants, day-care centers, hospitals, and other institutions to lessen hepatitis outbreaks. The chlorination of drinking water is a reliable means of destroying the virus.

First noted in Norwalk, Ohio, in 1968, the Norwalk virus is a little known but leading cause of stomach and intestinal distress caused by a virus. Norwalk viral infections usually cause nausea, vomiting, diarrhea, weakness, abdominal pain, loss of appetite, headache, and fever. The virus is found in water and foods, and shellfish and salads are most often implicated. Cooking destroys the virus. Norwalk viruses are probably responsible for about 30 to 40% of all cases of viral intestinal infection in adults. The infection is typically found in nursing homes and hospitals, restaurants, and events with catered meals. Disease experts estimate that at least 180,000 Americans get sick from the Norwalk virus each year. The virus persists because it can survive chlorination and because a low amount of the virus can cause illness. The virus is of most concern for infants, young children, older adults, and people with chronic illnesses. Although there is no specific treatment, scientists are currently working on a vaccine.

Rotaviruses are another important cause of diarrhea, mainly in children, leading to about 55,000 hospitalizations per year. Symptoms appear in 1 to 7 days. Day-care centers are common sites for infections. Thorough, regular handwashing is a necessary practice at these sites, particularly after diaper changing.

Parasites

Parasites that enter the body through the intestinal tract include some single-celled protozoans, flukes, nematodes, roundworms, and tapeworms. In the United States, the parasite most apt to be in the food supply is *Trichinella spiralis.* This tiny organism may be present in raw and undercooked pork and pork products, such as sausage. Trichinosis is rare today, probably because people realize that pork must be cooked thoroughly to kill the nematode worm that causes it, and modern sanitary feeding practices have reduced *Trichinella* in hogs. About a hundred cases of trichinosis per year are reported in the United States.[27] However, other cases may be unreported. In addition to pork, bear meat and other raw meats are potential sources. It is seldom found in commercial meat.

Trichinosis begins with the consumption of meat containing the **larvae**. The larvae are released during digestion in the small intestine. Within 2 days, the larvae develop into adult nematodes. New larvae are then produced and move into the blood via the intestinal mucosa. The blood carries the larvae to muscle fibers, where they become resident.

In early stages, trichinosis is difficult to diagnose. The symptoms in mild cases develop over weeks to months and are usually thought to be flu. If enough larvae are present, muscle weakness, fever, and fluid retention in the face may eventually result. Thoroughly cooking meat, especially pork, destroys the larvae.

Anisakis is a roundworm parasite found in larval form in raw fish. They invade the stomach or intestinal tract, causing mild or serious effects, which are difficult to diagnose as *Anisakis*. A stomach infection is characterized by sudden onset of violent pain within 12 hours of eating raw fish. The larvae may penetrate the stomach lining. Serious stomach pain can continue until the larvae are surgically removed. The fresher the fish, the less likely this disease will occur because larvae move from the fish's stomach to the tissues only after the fish is dead. Thoroughly cooking fish or freezing it for at least 72 hours is a reliable method for eliminating the threat of *Anisakis* disease.

Cyclospora cayetanensis is a newly discovered parasite that infects the small intestine, producing diarrhea, vomiting, fatigue, and muscle aches. This parasite has been associated with two well-publicized outbreaks and several small outbreaks over the past 2 years. Guatemalan raspberries were associated with approximately 1000 cases of cyclosporiasis in the United States and Canada.[13] In response, the Guatemalan government agreed to implement a system for food safety after authorities speculated that contaminated water caused the outbreak (this is not known for certain). Following another outbreak, the United States banned the importation of this fruit from Guatemala until further precautions can be taken. Authorities are currently examining the use of irradiation, which would kill the *Cyclospora*, but this practice is not currently in use.

Problems with contaminated water in metropolitan Milwaukee were traced to a microscopic parasite few people had ever heard of before—*Cryptosporidium*. This parasite is found in many species of birds and animals, and in their feces. Consumption of food contaminated with the parasite can cause cryptosporidiosis, a rare but potentially serious disease. Outbreaks have occurred at public swimming pools and from unpasteurized apple cider. Fecal contamination was suspected in both cases. Symptoms include severe diarrhea, dehydration, nausea, fever, and abdominal cramps. Unknown as a human disease until 1976, cryptosporidiosis is now considered one of the foremost causes of diarrhea in the world, especially among children.

As with many other intestinal infections, people can contract the disease by ingesting food or water contaminated with fecal material. Safe food-handling practices and good personal hygiene, specifically handwashing, can lower infection rates. Pasteurization and common water treatment procedures render the parasite harmless. People with weakened immune systems (AIDS and cancer patients, for instance), infants, and older adults are particularly susceptible to these infections.

Other Risks from Seafood

Scombroidosis results from an acute allergic reaction to eating spoiled fish. Fish typically implicated are tuna, mackerel, and mahi-mahi.[31] An affected person develops facial flushing, a burning sensation in the month, a metallic taste, itching, intestinal upset, and headache within 10 to 60 minutes of consumption. The illness is caused

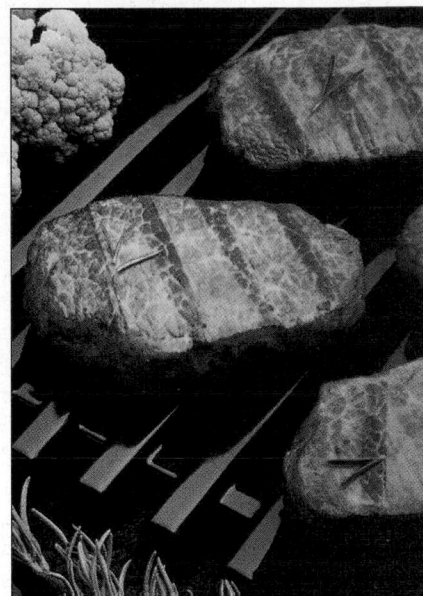

Grill pork to an internal temperature of 160°F (71°C) to eliminate the risk of trichinosis.

larva An early developmental stage in the life history of some organisms, such as parasites.

*M*ad cow disease is caused by an infectious protein, called a prion, and kills by creating voids in the brain tissue of cattle. The human condition, a variant of Creutzfeldt-Jakob disease, causes a form of dementia, which has killed about 100 people in Europe who apparently ate contaminated beef. Despite the recent evidence of mad cow disease in Europe, it is of little concern in the United States.[20] The U.S. government has taken steps to ban beef from Europe since the late 1980s; no case of the disease has been noted in humans in the United States. As a precaution, however, FDA has implemented a ban on the recycling of animal tissue from ruminant animals (e.g., cows, goats, sheep) for animal feed. These are suspected carriers of the prion that causes the fatal brain illness. In addition, the Red Cross will no longer accept blood donations from people who have recently resided in some European countries for six months or more.

by a toxin found in the flesh of the spoiled fish. Improperly refrigerated fish poses a special problem, and cooking does not destroy the toxin, so it is important to carefully refrigerate and use fresh fish soon after purchase.

Paralytic shellfish poisoning occurs when toxins produced by microscopic algae, called dinoflagellates, are consumed. These toxins are associated with the phenomenon known as a red tide, which is actually an explosive growth of the dinoflagellates in water. Symptoms, such as respiratory difficulty, appear within 4 hours. It is important that shellfish are harvested in clean waters, uncontaminated by sewage, industrial waste, and high amounts of toxic dinoflagellates.

Ciguatera fish poisoning is not a major cause of food-borne disease in general, but it is still the most common illness associated with fish consumption in the United States.[4] About 90% of cases occur in Hawaii and southern Florida. Ciguatera poisoning comes only from certain species of fish—notably grouper, snapper, amberjack, and barracuda—which live in warm waters near coral reefs. The toxin is produced by a type of dinoflagellate. These are eaten by small fish, which in turn are eaten by the larger fish that humans consume.

Researchers documented an outbreak of ciguatera fish poisoning in California, traced to frozen fillets shipped from Florida. Similar outbreaks have occurred in Vermont, Virginia, and Illinois, among other states. The symptoms tend to start in the GI tract within 6 hours after consumption of contaminated fish. Then, following a bout of diarrhea accompanied by abdominal pain, nausea, and perhaps vomiting, neurological problems begin, including tingling in the mouth, palms, and soles of the feet; aches throughout the body; and quite often the sensation that hot items are cold and cold items hot. This last symptom is considered the most definitive. Although recovery typically takes about a week, ciguatera fish poisoning has the potential for lingering neurological problems. The disease can last from several weeks to several months or longer. There is as yet no test for ciguatera toxicity. It can be diagnosed only by its symptoms.

There is no way to tell if fish is contaminated before it is eaten and no way to kill the ciguatera toxin; it is not destroyed by heating or freezing. Furthermore, medication cannot cure the illness. It can only relieve symptoms, and not in all cases.

Food safety experts advise staying away from potentially contaminated fish. The easiest way to exercise that caution is not to eat grouper, snapper, amberjack, moray eel, or barracuda from Caribbean waters. Small fish pose less risk. The larger the fish, the greater the chance that it has accumulated a lot of toxin because of its relatively long life.

Fungi

mycotoxins Toxic compounds produced by molds, such as aflatoxin B-1, found on moldy grains.

Fungi are mostly multicellular organisms. Those of concern in food safety do not infect people, but some mushrooms are intrinsically toxic, and molds growing on foods may produce toxins called **mycotoxins**. Fungi possess cell walls, a nucleus, and a nuclear membrane. They live on dead or decaying organic matter, living together with other organisms either in mutual advantage or as parasites. Fungi can grow as single cells, like yeasts, or as multicellular filamentous colonies, as with molds. They cannot synthesize their own food; rather, they digest their food outside their cell walls and absorb the simpler organic substances for use within the cell.

Most fungi are molds that consist of long, branched threads called *hyphae*. Hyphae form a tangled mass of filaments called *mycelium*. The mold often seen on bread is the mycelia of fungi.

Fungi require moisture to grow and can obtain water from the medium on which they live or from the atmosphere. When the atmosphere becomes dry, they can go into a resting state or form spores. They can live in a pH range of 2 to 9 and can grow in concentrated salt and sugar solutions. They thrive over a wide temperature range, even in the refrigerator. As spores, fungi can be scattered by the wind or carried by animals. When an air-borne spore lands on an appropriate target, such as a ripe peach, the spore germinates and begins to grow, producing the typical mold observed on spoiled fruit.

The best-known mycotoxins are the aflatoxins, substances believed to cause liver cancer. Aflatoxin B-1 causes cancer in animals; thus, human exposure is regulated by FDA. The foods most often contaminated with aflatoxins are tree nuts (e.g., walnuts and pecans), peanuts, corn, wheat, and oil seeds, such as cottonseed. FDA considers aflatoxins unavoidable contaminants on foods and therefore has set practical limits for aflatoxins in food and animal feed. Aflatoxins are also present in certain water supply sources, such as pond and ditch water. Some people in China use this type of water for cooking, and they experience a high incidence of liver cancer.

Cooking and freezing halt fungal growth but do not eliminate mycotoxins already produced. Thus, moldy food should not be eaten, or at least not without discarding the moldy portion and much of the surrounding area. Again, when in doubt, throw the food out. Mold growth is prevented by properly storing perishable foods at cold temperatures and using them within a reasonable length of time.

CONCEPT CHECK

Thoroughly cook all meat and poultry to reduce the risk of food-borne illness from *Campylobacter* and *Salmonella*. In addition, always separate raw meats and poultry products from cooked foods. To prevent food-borne intoxication from *Staphylococcus* organisms, cover cuts on hands and avoid sneezing on foods. To avoid intoxication from *Clostridium perfringens*, rapidly cool leftover foods and thoroughly reheat them. To avoid intoxication from *Clostridium botulinum,* carefully examine canned foods. Overall, don't allow cooked food to stand for more than 1 to 2 hours at room temperature. For other causes of food-borne illness, precautions already mentioned generally apply as well. In addition, thoroughly cook fish and other seafood; consume only pasteurized dairy products; wash all fruits and vegetables; and thoroughly wash your hands with soap and water before and after preparing food and after using the bathroom.

CASE SCENARIO
Follow-Up

Aaron likely contracted *Clostridium perfringens*, based on the fact that he had diarrhea but did not vomit, and the symptoms occurred about 8 hours after consuming the contaminated food. Spores of *Clostridium perfringens* are typically present in meat. Thorough cooking will kill any of the live bacteria present, but the product still may contain spores. These can later germinate if the product is kept in a warm setting for a few hours. The Argentine beef likely contained spores of *Clostridium perfringens*, and these germinated and produced a toxin as the product sat in the car and on the buffet table. Ideally, this product should have remained at room temperature for no longer than 1 hour, as the party took place in the summertime. Thus, soon after Aaron and his wife took it out of the oven, it should have been separated into a few smaller pans to speed cooling and then refrigerated. This is because they knew it was not going to be served within 1 hour. Before leaving, they could have recombined the dish into one clean pan. Once they arrived at the party, this again should have been refrigerated and then thoroughly reheated when it was time to eat. Overall, it is risky to leave perishable items such as meat, fish, poultry, eggs, and dairy products at room temperature for more than 1 to 2 hours.

FOOD ADDITIVES

By the time you see a food on the market shelf, it usually contains substances added to make it more palatable or to increase its nutrient content or shelf life. Manufacturers also add some substances to foods to make them easier to process. Other substances may have accidentally found their way into the foods you buy. All these extraneous substances are known as *additives,* and, although some may be beneficial,

When buying food products, especially perishables, check the product date for safety. Four types of dates are commonly used. The pack date is the day the product was manufactured. The pull or sell date indicates the last date the product should be sold. It allows some time for storing food at home before eating. Check the expiration date of foods stored at home, because that is the last date the food can safely be consumed. Last, baked goods may have a freshness date, indicating that the product may safely be eaten for a short time after the date but may not taste the same.

intentional food additives Additives knowingly (directly) incorporated into food products by manufacturers.

incidental food additives Additives that appear in food products indirectly, from environmental contamination of food ingredients or during the manufacturing process.

generally recognized as safe (GRAS) A list of food additives that in 1958 were considered safe for consumption. Manufacturers were allowed to continue to use these additives, without special clearance, when needed for food products. FDA bears responsibility for proving they are not safe but can remove unsafe products from the list.

*S*ome important definitions:

toxicology	The scientific study of harmful substances
safety	The relative certainty that a substance won't cause injury
hazard	The chance that injury will result from use of a substance
toxicity	The capacity of a substance to produce injury or illness at some dosage

others may be harmful for some people, such as sulfites. All purposefully added substances must be evaluated by FDA.

■ Why Are Food Additives Used?

Most additives are used to limit food spoilage. Food additives such as potassium sorbate are used to maintain the safety and acceptability of foods by retarding the growth of microbes implicated in food-borne illness.

Additives are also used to combat some enzymes that lead to undesirable changes in color and flavor in foods but don't cause anything as serious as food-borne illness. This second type of food spoilage occurs when enzymes in a food react to oxygen—for example, when apple and peach slices darken or turn rust color as they are exposed to air. Antioxidants are a type of preservative that retards the action of oxygen-requiring enzymes on food surfaces. These preservatives are not necessarily novel chemicals. They include vitamins E and C and a variety of sulfites.

Without the use of some food additives, it would be impossible to safely produce massive quantities of foods and distribute them nationwide or worldwide, as is now done. Despite consumer concerns about the safety of food additives, many have been extensively studied and proved safe when FDA guidelines for their use are followed.

■ Intentional Versus Incidental Food Additives

Food additives are classified into two types: **intentional food additives** (directly added to foods) and **incidental food additives** (indirectly added as contaminants). Both types of agents are regulated by FDA. Currently, more than 2800 substances are intentionally added to foods. As many as 10,000 other substances enter foods as contaminants. This includes substances that may reasonably be expected to enter food through surface contact with processing equipment or packaging materials.

■ The GRAS List

In 1958, all food additives used in the United States and considered safe at that time were put on a **generally recognized as safe (GRAS)** list. Congress established the GRAS list because it believed manufacturers did not need to prove the safety of substances that were already generally regarded as safe by knowledgeable scientists. Since that time, FDA has been responsible for proving that a substance does not belong on the GRAS list.

Since 1958, some substances on the list have been reviewed. A few, such as cyclamates, failed the review process and were removed from the list. The additive red dye #3 was banned because it is linked to cancer. Many chemicals on the GRAS list have not yet been rigorously tested, primarily because of expense. These chemicals have received a low priority for testing, mostly because they have long histories of use without evidence of toxicity or because their chemical forms do not suggest they are potential health hazards.

■ Are Synthetic Compounds Always Harmful?

Nothing about a natural product makes it inherently safer than a synthetic product. Many synthetic products are simply laboratory copies of chemicals that also occur in nature (see the discussion in Chapter 20 on biotechnology for some examples). Moreover, although human endeavors contribute some toxins to foods, such as synthetic pesticides and industrial chemicals, nature's poisons are often even more potent and prevalent. Some cancer researchers suggest that we ingest at least 10,000 times more (by weight) natural toxins produced by plants than we do synthetic pesticide residues. This comparison doesn't make synthetic chemicals any less toxic, but it does lend perspective.

Consider vitamin E, which is often added to food to prevent rancidity of fats. This chemical is safe when used within certain limits. However, high doses have been associated with health problem, such as interfering with vitamin K activity in the body (see Chapter 9). Thus, even well-known chemicals we are comfortable using can be toxic in some circumstances and at some concentrations.

■ Tests of Food Additives for Safety

Food additives are tested under FDA scrutiny for safety on at least two animal species, usually rats and mice. Scientists determine the highest dose of the additive that produces *no observable effects* in the animals. These doses are proportionately much higher than humans are ever exposed to. The maximum dosage is then divided by at least 100 to establish a margin of safety for human use. The rationale for reducing the **no-observable-effect level (NOEL)** by a 100-fold margin is that we assume humans are at least 10 times more sensitive to food additives than are laboratory animals and that any one person might be 10 times more sensitive than another. This very broad margin essentially ensures that the food additive in question will cause no harmful health effects in humans. In fact, many synthetic chemicals are probably less dangerous at these low doses than the natural compounds in apples or celery.

One important exception applies to the schema for testing intentional food additives: If an additive is shown to cause cancer, even though only in very high doses, no margin of safety is allowed. The food additive cannot be used, because it would violate the **Delaney Clause** in the 1958 Food Additive Amendments. This clause prohibits intentionally adding to foods a compound that was introduced after 1958 and causes cancer. Evidence for cancer could come from either laboratory animal or human studies. Very few exceptions to this clause are allowed; the few are discussed in the following section on curing and pickling agents.

Recently, the value of animal cancer tests has been questioned. Research suggests that, when rats are fed massive doses of chemicals, as they typically are in the tests, it may be the dose itself, rather than the chemical action, that causes cancer. The scientific community is currently debating which is the best method to test additives to evaluate cancer risk in humans. Nevertheless, until a better method is established, we are left with our current ban on the intentional addition of chemicals that cause cancer.

Incidental food additives are another matter altogether. FDA cannot simply ban various industrial chemicals, pesticide residues, and mold toxins from foods, even though some of these contaminants can cause cancer. These products are not purposely added to foods. FDA sets an acceptable level for these substances. Basically, an incidental substance found in a food cannot contribute to more than one cancer case during the lifetimes of 1 million people. If a higher risk exists, the amount of the compound in a food must be reduced until the guideline is met.

■ Approval for a New Food Additive

Today, before a new food additive can be added to foods, FDA must approve its use. Besides rigorously testing an additive to establish its safety margins, manufacturers must give FDA information that (1) identifies the new additive, (2) gives its chemical composition, (3) states how it is manufactured, and (4) specifies the laboratory methods used to measure its presence in the food supply at the amount of intended use.

Manufacturers must also offer proof that the additive will accomplish its intended purpose in a food, that it is safe, and that it is to be used in no higher amount than needed. Additives cannot be used to hide defective food ingredients, such as rancid oils; to deceive customers; or to replace good manufacturing practices. A manufacturer must establish that the ingredient is necessary for producing a specific food product.

■ Common Food Additives

A list of food additive categories appears in Table 19-3. Some serve the general function of preservatives: acidic or alkaline agents, antioxidants, antimicrobial agents,

no-observable-effects level (NOEL) The highest dose of an additive that produces no deleterious health effects in animals.

*N*ote that this 100-fold margin of safety is over 30 times that for vitamin A, when you compare the RDA with a potentially toxic dose for pregnant women.

*S*ugar, salt, corn syrup, and citric acid constitute 98% of all additives (by weight) used in food processing.

TABLE 19-3 Food Additive Categories

Anticaking agents	Flour treating agents	Processing aids: clarifying, clouding, catalyst, flocculants, filter aids, crystallization inhibitors
Antimicrobial agents	Formulation aids: carriers, binders, fillers, plasticizers	
Antioxidants		Propellants
Color and adjuncts	Fumigants	Sequestrants
Conditioners	Humectants	Solvents and vehicles
Curing and pickling agents	Leavening	Stabilizers and thickeners
Dough strengtheners	Lubricants and release agents	Surface active agents
Drying agents	Nonnutritive sweeteners	Surface-finishing agents
Emulsifiers	Nutritive sweeteners	Synergists
Enzymes	Oxidizing and reducing agents	Texturizers
Firming agents	pH controllers	
Flavor enhancers		
Flavoring agents		

sequestrants Compounds that bind free metal ions. By so doing, they reduce the ability of ions to cause rancidity in foods containing fat.

curing and pickling agents, and **sequestrants.** Let's look at some of the specific categories of additives to understand exactly why these are used and to learn more about the specific substances used.

Acidic or Alkaline Agents

Acids, such as calcium lactate, have many uses in foods. As flavor-enhancing agents, they impart a tart taste to soft drinks, sherbets, and cheese spreads. As preservatives, they inhibit microbial growth. As antioxidants, they prevent discoloration and rancidity. They also adjust acid and base balance. Adding acids during food processing reduces the later risk of botulism from eating naturally low-acid vegetables, such as beets.

Alkaline products, such as sodium hydroxide, can alter the texture and flavor of foods, including chocolate. In processing, alkaline products are sometimes used to produce a milder flavor by neutralizing the acids produced during fermentation.

Alternative Sweeteners

Currently, saccharin, sucralose, and acesulfame potassium (Sunette) are the only nonnutritive sweeteners used in foods. Because aspartame (Nutrasweet) yields some energy, it is considered a nutritive sweetener. (Cyclamates are available in Canada.) Recall from Chapter 5 that the moderate use of these alternative sweeteners are considered safe.

Anticaking Agents

By absorbing moisture, compounds such as calcium silicate, ammonium citrate, magnesium stearate, and silicon dioxide keep table salt, baking powder, powdered sugar, and other powdered food products free flowing. These chemicals prevent the caking and lumping that would make powdered or crystalline products hard to use.

Antimicrobial Agents

Sodium benzoate, sorbic acid, and calcium propionate are common preservatives. Sorbic acid is a potent inhibitor of molds and fungal growth. Calcium propionate, a natural part of some cheeses, inhibits mold growth.

Antioxidants

This type of food preservative helps delay food discoloration from oxygen exposure, such as occurs when potatoes are diced. It also helps keep fats from turning rancid. Two widely used antioxidants are BHA (butylated hydroxyanisole) and BHT (butylated hydroxytoluene). Alpha-tocopherol (vitamin E), which occurs naturally in nuts, whole grains, and oils, may be added to foods to keep them from becoming rancid. Ascorbic acid (vitamin C), which is another antioxidant, helps maintain the red color of luncheon meats and other cured foods, and it prevents the formation of cancer-promoting nitrosamines. (Vitamin C is also added to such foods as fruit drinks in order to increase the vitamin content; it is also used as a marketing tool for these products.)

Sulfites, a group of sulfur-based chemicals, are widely used as antioxidants in foods. Some people (1 in 100, according to FDA estimates) are extremely sensitive to sulfites added to foods and may have difficulty breathing, wheeze, and vomit, as well as develop hives, diarrhea, abdominal pain, cramps, and dizziness. As a result, FDA now limits the use of sulfites on raw fruits and vegetables—an action directed mainly at salad bars. FDA also requires manufacturers to declare the presence of sulfites on the labels of packaged foods containing at least 10 parts per million of sulfites. Labels on wine bottles often list a sulfite warning.

Colors

Color additives don't improve nutritional qualities, but they can make foods more visually appealing. Food colorings cannot be used to deceive consumers—for example, by covering blemishes, concealing any inferiority, or misleading people in any way. Although colorings are arguably unnecessary additives, manufacturers have satisfied FDA that color is "necessary" for the production of certain foods.

Controversy has surrounded the use of some food colors. Currently, the safety of using tartrazine (FD&C yellow No. 5) is disputed. It has caused allergic symptoms—such as hives, itching, and nasal discharge—in sensitive individuals, especially in people allergic to aspirin. Although few Americans are sensitive to tartrazine, FDA requires manufacturers to list FD&C yellow No. 5 on labels of food products containing it. Some red dyes have also raised alarms, and some have been banned. Currently, FDA requires manufacturers to list all forms of synthetic colors on the labels of foods that contain them. Pigments extracted from plant sources are exempted from specific description on food labels.

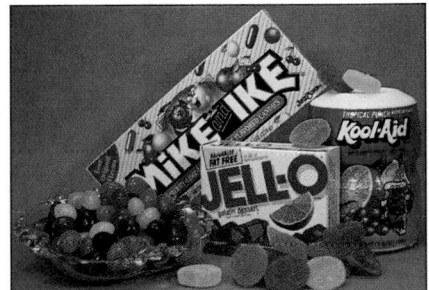

Color additives make some foods more desirable.

Curing and Pickling Agents

Nitrates and the related form, nitrites, are used as preservatives, especially to prevent the growth of *Clostridium botulinum*. Sodium and potassium nitrates and nitrites are used to preserve meats such as bacon, ham, salami, and hot dogs. Nitrates and nitrites have been used for centuries, in conjunction with salt, to preserve meat. An added effect of nitrates is their reaction with pigments in meat to form a bright pink color. This gives ham, hot dogs, and other cured meats their characteristic appearance.

Nitrate consumption from both cured foods and natural vegetables has been associated with the synthesis of nitrosamines in the stomach. Some nitrosamines are cancer-causing agents, particularly for the stomach and esophagus. The actual risk appears to be low, however, except for people who secrete little stomach acid (some older people, for example). A slightly increased risk for childhood leukemia and brain tumors is also suspected, but the data are inconclusive.

FDA surmises that consumers take for granted a margin of microbial safety gained from nitrite use in cured meats. People often serve these meats cold or at least underheated. Consequently, government agencies have chosen not to ban nitrate or nitrite use in foods but, rather, to change manufacturing practices to lower amounts of preformed nitrosamines and suggest moderation in the use of these food products. Since 1975, there has been an 80% decrease in the amount of nitrites in cured meats.

The addition of vitamin C (sodium ascorbate) to cured meats, such as bacon, is one way to reduce the amount of nitrosamines formed in foods. This is a common manufacturing practice. Other antioxidants, such as sodium erythrobate, also inhibit the synthesis of nitrosamines.

You might wonder why, if nitrates and nitrites form chemical substances that can cause cancer, they aren't banned by the Delaney Clause. In the United States, USDA regulates the use of chemicals in meats. The laws that govern USDA regulation of foods are separate from those that govern FDA regulation. Because of this, the Delaney Clause does not apply to USDA actions. Currently, USDA sees no clear threat to public safety from the regulated use of nitrates and nitrites in meats, so no action has been taken.

Emulsifiers

By distributing and suspending fat in water, emulsifiers improve the uniformity, smoothness, and body of foods such as baked goods, ice cream, and candies. In

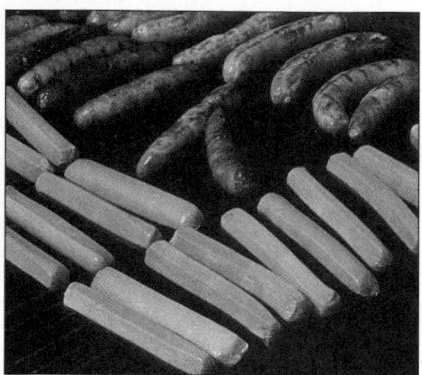

Cured meats derive their pink color from nitrates. The National Cancer Institute advises consuming these foods in moderation, as the nitrates/nitrites present some cancer risk.

*I*nfants are more sensitive to MSG than adults, in part because infants have not yet developed a complete blood-brain barrier. This means they cannot fully exclude such substances as MSG from the brain.

mayonnaise, for example, egg yolks act as emulsifiers in suspending the acids, such as vinegar or lemon juice in the oil. Lecithin, derived from soybeans, acts as an emulsifier in chocolate and margarine. Monoglycerides and diglycerides are used as emulsifiers in cake mixes.

Fat Replacements

Fat replacements—such as Paselli SA2, Dur-Low, Oatrim, Sta-Slim 143 Stellar, and Z-trim—are being produced for commercial use. These carbohydrate-based products are an addition to other fat replacement products—Simplesse and Olean—discussed in Chapter 6.

Flavors and Flavoring Agents

Both naturally occurring and artificial agents can impart more flavor to foods. These agents include extracts from spices and herbs, as well as synthetic agents. You've probably recognized flavors of some spices and of liquid derivatives of onion, garlic, cloves, and peppermint in foods. To meet the demand of industry, manufacturers have developed synthetic flavors that not only taste like natural flavors but also have the advantage of stability. Often artificial flavors, such as butter and banana flavors, have the same chemical composition as the natural flavor.

Flavor Enhancers

Flavor enhancers are substances, such as monosodium glutamate (MSG), that help bring out the natural flavors of foods. Note that the glutamate portion is simply a nonessential amino acid. A small percentage of people are sensitive to the glutamate in MSG and, after exposure, experience flushing, chest pain, facial pressure, dizziness, sweating, rapid heart rate, nausea, vomiting, high blood pressure, and headache. MSG is often used in preparation of Chinese food. The onset of symptoms occurs about 10 to 20 minutes after ingestion and may last from 2 to 3 hours. People who find themselves sensitive to MSG should avoid it. It may be present alone (look for the word *glutamate*), as well as in any isolated protein source (caseinate, texturized vegetable protein, etc.), yeast extract, bouillon, soup stock, and seasonings. Tomatoes, mushrooms, and parmesan cheese are also sources of free glutamate. Fortunately, most of us find that moderate use of MSG or glutamate in foods poses no significant risk to our health. FDA is currently contemplating label requirements for MSG.

Humectants

These chemicals—such as glycerol, propylene glycol, and sorbitol—are added to foods to help retain proper moisture, fresh flavor, and texture. They are often used in candies, shredded coconut, and marshmallows.

Leavening Agents

Air and steam can be used to create a light texture in breads and cakes; however, carbon dioxide bubbles are much more reliable for this purpose. Common leavening agents that produce carbon dioxide gas include yeast, baking powder, and baking soda. Baking soda must react with acids to generate carbon dioxide. Baking powder can be used in either acid or alkaline conditions.

Maturing and Bleaching Agents

Such compounds as bromates, peroxides, and ammonium chloride hasten the natural aging and whitening processes of milled flour. This shortens the time needed for flour to become usable in baking products. Without these agents, freshly milled flour lacks the qualities necessary to make a stable, elastic dough and requires several months of aging to be useful in baking.

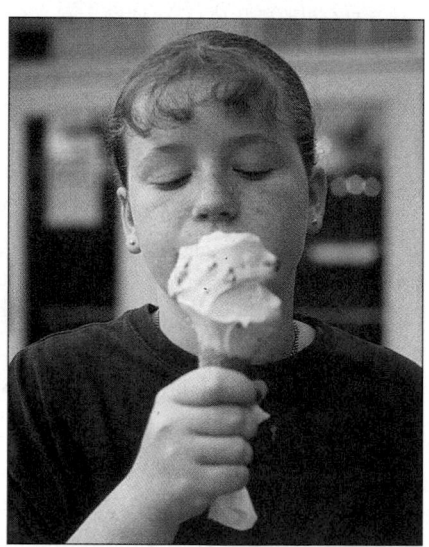

Emulsifiers improve the texture of foods such as ice cream, baked goods, and cookies.

Nutrient Supplements

Vitamin and mineral supplements are added to foods to improve their nutritional quality. Sometimes they replace nutrients lost in processing, as occurs when enriching flour. Vitamin A is added to margarine and some forms of milk. Vitamin D is added to some dairy products. Potassium iodide is added to salt and calcium and folate are added to some flours, fruit juices, and other products. Ready-to-eat breakfast cereals often contain a variety of added nutrients.

Stabilizers and Thickeners

Stabilizers and thickeners impart a smooth texture and uniform color and flavor to candies, ice creams and other frozen desserts, chocolate milk, and artificially sweetened beverages. Commonly used substances are pectins, vegetable gums (such as guar gum and carrageenan), gelatins, and agars. They work by absorbing water. Without stabilizers and thickeners, ice crystals form in ice cream and other frozen desserts, and particles of chocolate separate from chocolate milk. Stabilizers are also used to prevent the evaporation and deterioration of flavorings used in cakes, puddings, and gelatin mixes.

Sequestrants

Sequestrants include EDTA and citric acid. They bind many free chemical ions and, by doing so, help preserve food quality by reducing the ability of ions to cause rancidity in products containing fat.

Conclusion

In general, if you consume a variety of foods in moderation, the chances of food additives' jeopardizing your health are minimal. Pay attention to your body. If you suspect an intolerance or a sensitivity, consult your physician for further evaluation. Remember that, in the short run, you are more likely to suffer either from foodborne illness due to poor food-handling practices that allow bacteria to grow in food, or from the consumption of raw animal foods, than from consuming additives. Excess energy, saturated fat, salt, and other potential "problem" nutrients in our diets pose the greatest long-term risk.

CRITICAL THINKING

Recognizing that Joseph is taking a nutrition class, his roommate asks him, "What is more risky: the bacteria that can be present in food or the additives listed on the label of my favorite snack cake?" How should Joseph respond? On what information should he base his conclusions?

*I*f you are bewildered or concerned about all the additives creeping into your diet, you can easily avoid most of them by emphasizing unprocessed whole foods (Fig. 19-3). However, no evidence shows that this will necessarily make you healthier, nor can you avoid all additives, since some are used even on whole foods, such as with pesticides. It amounts to a personal decision. Do you have confidence that FDA and food manufacturers are adequately protecting your health and welfare, or do you want to take more personal control by minimizing your intake of compounds not naturally found in foods?

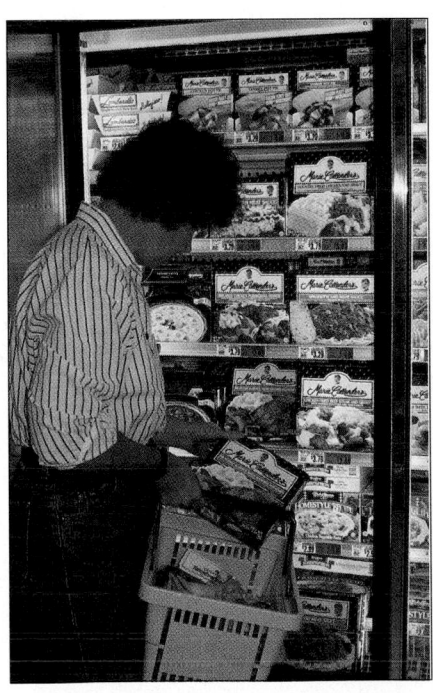

■ FIGURE 19-3 Depending on food choices, a diet can be either *(a)* essentially devoid of or *(b)* high in food additives.

CONCEPT CHECK

Food additives are used to reduce spoilage from microbial growth, oxygen, metals, and other compounds. Additives are also used to adjust pH, improve flavor and color, leaven, provide nutritional fortification, thicken, and emulsify food components. Additives are classified as intentional (direct), which are purposely added to foods, and incidental (indirect), which turn up in foods from environmental contamination or various manufacturing practices. The amount of an additive allowed in a food is limited to one-one-hundredth of the highest amount that has no observable effect when fed to animals. The Delaney Clause allows FDA to limit intentional addition of cancer-causing compounds to food under its jurisdiction. Also limited by law are the permissible amounts of carcinogens that incidentally enter foods.

■ SUBSTANCES THAT OCCUR NATURALLY IN FOODS AND CAN CAUSE ILLNESS

Foods contain a variety of naturally occurring substances that can cause illness. Here are some of the more important examples:

Safrole—found in sassafras, mace, and nutmeg; causes cancer

Solanine—found in potato shoots and green spots on potato skins; inhibits the action of neurotransmitters

Mushroom toxins—found in some species of mushrooms such as aminita; can cause stomach upset, dizziness, hallucinations, and other neurological symptoms. The more lethal varieties can cause liver and kidney failure, coma, and even death. FDA regulates commercially grown and harvested mushrooms. These are cultivated in concrete buildings or caves. However, there are no systematic controls on individual gatherers harvesting wild species, except in Michigan and Illinois.

Avidin—found in raw egg whites; binds the vitamin biotin in a way that prevents its absorption

Thiaminase—found in raw fish, clams, and mussels; destroys the vitamin thiamin

Tetrodotoxin—found in puffer fish; causes respiratory paralysis

Protease inhibitor—found in raw soybeans; inhibits digestive enzymes

Oxalic acid—found in spinach, strawberries, sesame seeds, and other foods; binds calcium and iron in the foods

Herbal teas—containing senna or comfrey; can cause diarrhea and liver damage

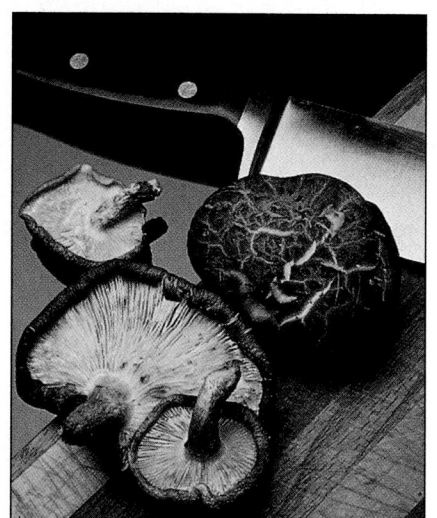

When hunting wild mushrooms, know what you are looking for. Many varieties contain deadly toxins.

People have coexisted for centuries with these naturally occurring substances and have learned to avoid some of them and limit intake in other cases. Today, they pose little health risk. Farmers know potatoes must be stored in the dark, so that solanine won't be synthesized. Furthermore, we've developed cooking and food-preparation methods to limit the potency of other substances, such as thiaminase. Spices are used in such small amounts that health risks don't result. Nevertheless, it's important to understand that some potentially harmful chemicals in foods occur naturally.

■ ENVIRONMENTAL CONTAMINANTS IN FOODS

A variety of environmental contaminants can be found in foods. Table 19-4 lists ways to limit pesticide residues in the diet. Aside from pesticide residues and products of fungal growth, though, other important contaminants deserve attention.

> **TABLE 19-4 What You Can Do to Reduce Dietary Exposure to Pesticides**
>
> FDA's sampling and testing show that pesticide residues in foods do not pose a health hazard. Nevertheless, if you want to reduce dietary exposure to pesticides, follow this advice from the Environmental Protection Agency:
>
> - Thoroughly rinse and scrub (with a brush if possible) fruits and vegetables. Peel them, if appropriate—although some nutrients will be peeled away.
> - Remove the outer leaves of leafy vegetables, such as lettuce and cabbage.
> - Trim fat from meat and poultry, remove skin (which contains most of the fat) from poultry and fish, and discard fats and oils in broths and pan drippings. Residues of some pesticides in feed concentrate in the animals' fat. Trim skin and fatty deposits from fish.
> - When fishing, throw back the big fish—the little ones have had less time to take up and concentrate pesticides and other harmful residues. In addition, pay attention to any warnings by local authorities (and the fishing license) about the high risk for contamination in specific waters or species of fish.

Adapted from Food and Drug Administration: Safety first: Protecting America's food supply. *FDA Consumer,* p. 26, November 1988.

■ Lead

Ingesting lead can cause anemia, kidney disease, and damage to the nervous system, which can interfere with nerve impulse conduction. Because lead has a high atomic weight, it is a heavy metal. Many heavy metals are toxic at low doses.

Lead toxicity is a particular problem for children because it is associated with IQ deficits, behavior disorders, slowed growth, impaired hearing, and possibly hypertension and kidney disease later in life. The precise mechanism by which lead affects the brain is not clear; however, because lead is chemically similar to calcium, it can disrupt brain mechanisms that depend on calcium. Despite the reduction of lead exposure in children over the past 20 years associated with the decline in leaded gasoline and lead solder used in homes and in the canning industry, approximately 1.7 million children have elevated blood lead.[22] Nearly 900,000 of all children affected are under the age of 6, which is when the brain and central nervous system are most vulnerable. Medical costs for a child with lead intoxication average $2500 per treatment, and most children require two or more treatments.

Exposed children who eat a high-fat diet low in calcium and low in iron absorb more lead than do those who eat a more healthful diet. For children with elevated lead levels, federal experts suggest nutritional and educational intervention, the location of the source of lead (and removal), and medical treatment.

Poor African-American children, who reside disproportionately in inner cities, are at increased risk for harmful lead exposure because of the lead-based paint present on the interiors and exteriors of older buildings. Of all U.S. children, 22% of African-American children who live in older homes are affected by lead. As this paint flakes off walls or is abraded from window trim as windows are opened and closed, lead paint chips enter the environment and may be ingested.[10, 30] Regular home cleaning can be a particularly effective way of removing contaminated household dust for those who, unfortunately, are unable to move to lead-free housing.

Approximately 90 to 95% of adult lead exposures occur in the work environment. Occupations that are linked to high blood lead levels in workers include radiator repair, battery manufacture and recycling, smelting, and construction or remodeling involving lead-based paint.

Other sources of lead include brass fittings on water pumps used in wells, imported wine from areas where leaded gasoline is still used (especially Eastern Europe), and lead caps on wine bottles in general. Wiping the neck of the bottle with a towel limits this type of exposure. An additional risk is posed by acidic products, such as fruit juice, sauerkraut, and pickled vegetables stored in galvanized, tin, or other metal containers (except stainless steel). Acid can dissolve the metal, and lead leaches into the food product. Foods packaged in ceramic jars from Mexico, some household candlewicks, and certain herbal remedies—such as Koo Soo pills, used to relieve menstrual cramping—have also been associated with lead poisoning. Because of this hazard, lead is no longer used on commercially produced dishes in the United States. However, there is no way to ensure the safety of homemade or imported pottery items, such as those from Mexico. Be sure not to use antiques or collectibles, including any made of leaded glass, for food or beverage storage.

Lead can leach from solder joints into copper pipes, so it is important to let tap water run a minute or so before drinking it or cooking with it, especially first thing in the morning or when the water has been off for a few hours. Use only cold water for drinking, cooking, and preparing infant formula. Lead in drinking water makes up about 20% of the average person's total lead exposure. Laboratories certified by Environmental Protection Agency (EPA) can test drinking water for lead content for about $20 to $50. Softening drinking water is also not advised, because soft water can leach lead from pipes.

Some signs of lead poisoning include tiredness, irritability, muscle and joint pain, headaches, stomach aches and cramps, changes in behavior, and changes in school performance. If you suspect that someone you know has lead poisoning, contact your physician or the local health department. For more information, visit www.hud.gov/lea, the web site for the U.S. Department of Housing and Urban Development Office of Lead Hazard Control, or call the National Lead Information Center and Clearinghouse at 1-800-424-LEAD.

■ Dioxin

Dioxin is a chemical that contains chlorine and benzene. It can be created by incinerating chlorine-based material, such as plastics, together with hydrocarbon-based material, such as paper. Dioxins are potent animal toxicants with the potential to produce adverse effects on reproduction and development, suppression of the immune system, and cancer.[8] Since dioxin causes cancer and other harmful effects in animals, even in small doses, it probably does so in humans as well. EPA characterizes most dioxins as likely human carcinogens. Besides trash-burning incinerators, other sources of dioxin are bottom-feeding fish from the Great Lakes—an area with a great deal of industrial activity and chemical production. Dioxin exposures also include small amounts from breathing air containing trace amounts of particles and in vapor form, from the inadvertent ingestion of soil containing dioxin, and from absorption through the skin contacting air, soil, or water containing small amounts.

For a typical person, dioxin exposure can also occur in the diet through the intake of animal fats. EPA presumes that most dioxin exposure that occurs through the diet is due to dioxin in the environment, which accumulates in the tissues of animals. This dioxin exposure from food is a problem primarily for people who frequently consume fish caught locally. People who eat commercial fish normally eat a variety, and even people who stick to one type of fish don't usually have a problem because fish in interstate commerce generally come from different waters, only a few of which may contain dioxin.

■ Mercury

FDA first limited mercury, another heavy metal, in foods in 1969, after 120 people in Japan became ill from eating fish contaminated with high amounts. Birth defects in the offspring of some of those people were also blamed on the mercury exposure. The fish most often contaminated was swordfish. Shark may also contain high amounts. Such large predatory fish that live for a long time can accumulate high amounts of mercury. Currently, these species are tested more frequently to ensure that the commercial supply is safe. FDA scientists responsible for seafood agree that these fish are safe for most people, provided they are eaten infrequently (no more than once a week). Since mercury is a neurotoxin, it slows fetal and child development and causes irreversible deficits in brain function. Therefore, pregnant women and women of childbearing age who may become pregnant are advised by FDA to limit their consumption of shark, swordfish, king mackeral, and tilefish. Note that other types of fish and seafood, especially smaller, younger varieties, generally contain little mercury.

■ Urethane in Some Alcoholic Beverages

Urethane forms during the fermentation of alcoholic beverages. If the fermented product is heated, as in the production of sherry and bourbon, urethane concentration increases. Although urethane causes cancer in laboratory animals, it's unclear whether it causes cancer in humans. FDA research on urethane in food products is now a high priority. A prudent choice might be to limit the consumption of products such as fruit brandies and sake because these show consistently high amounts of urethane.

■ Polychlorinated Biphenyls (PCBs)

PCBs were widely used for years in a variety of industrial products; however, because they are linked to liver tumors and reproductive problems in animals, they are no longer produced. FDA has banned their use in machinery associated with food and animal feed since 1977 and has established limits for PCBs in susceptible foods and in paper used for food-packaging material. The most significant food source of PCB residues is fish, primarily freshwater fish, such as coho and chinook salmon from the Great Lakes, and bottom-feeding freshwater species from waters in other industrial areas, such as the Hudson River Valley. Again, a key guideline for fish consumption is variety and moderation when local sources have the potential for contamination.

*G*enetic alteration of foods such as corn and soybeans has recently created concern, especially in Europe. FDA considers genetically-altered products safe if approval for human use has been granted (see Chapter 20 for details).

■ Protection from Environmental Toxins in Foods

Environmental toxins that cause disease can be present in foods. To reduce exposure, find out which foods pose a risk. In addition, emphasize variety and moderation in food selection. The presence of mercury in swordfish or shark may concern you, but it's normally not a health risk unless your diet is dominated by these fish. The small amount of mercury in most swordfish or shark isn't harmful if you're exposed to it infrequently. Table 19-4 offered some other practical tips for limiting pesticide exposure. These apply to reducing exposure to environmental contaminants as well.

CONCEPT CHECK

A general program to minimize exposure to environmental contaminants includes knowing which foods pose greater risks; consuming a wide variety of foods; thoroughly rinsing and scrubbing fruits and vegetables; removing the outer leaves of leafy vegetables; trimming fat from meat and poultry, including the skin; and discarding any fat that is rendered from meat or fish during cooking.

*C*heck out the *Perspectives in Nutrition* Online Learning Center http://www.mhhe.com/wardlaw for quizzes, flash cards, other activities, and web links designed to further help you learn about issues surrounding food safety.

■ SUMMARY

1. Bacteria and other microbes in food pose the greatest risk for food borne illness. In the past, salt, sugar, smoke, fermentation, and drying were used to protect against food-borne illness. Today, careful cooking, pasteurization, and keeping hot foods hot and cold foods cold provide additional insurance.

2. Major causes of food-borne illness are the bacteria *Campylobacter jejuni, Salmonella, Shigella, Staphylococcus aureus,* and *Clostridium perfringens.* In addition, such bacteria as *Clostridium botulinum, Listeria monocytogenes, Yersinia enterocolitica,* and *Escherichia coli* have been found to cause illness.

3. To protect against bacteria, cook susceptible foods thoroughly. In addition, cover cuts on the hands, do not sneeze or cough on foods, avoid contact between raw meat or poultry products and other food products, rapidly cool and thoroughly reheat leftovers, and use pasteurized dairy products.

4. Cross-contamination commonly causes food-borne illness. It occurs particularly when bacteria on raw animal products contact foods that can support bacterial growth. Because of the risk of cross-contamination, no perishable food should be kept at room temperature for more than 1 to 2 hours (depending on the environmental temperature), especially if it may have come in contact with raw animal products.

5. Treatment for food-borne illness usually requires drinking lots of fluids, avoiding touching food while diarrhea is present, washing hands thoroughly, and getting bed rest. Botulism, hepatitis A infections, and trichinosis are types of food-borne illness that require prompt medical attention.

6. Food additives are used primarily to extend shelf life by preventing microbial growth and the destruction of food components by oxygen, metals, and other substances. Food additives are classified as those intentionally added to foods and those that incidentally appear in foods. An intentional additive is limited to no more than one-one-hundredth of the greatest amount that causes no observed symptoms in animals. The Delaney Clause allows FDA to ban the use of any intentional food additive under its jurisdiction that causes cancer.

7. Antioxidants, such as BHA, BHT, vitamins E and C, and sulfites, prevent oxygen and enzyme destruction of food products. Emulsifiers suspend fat in water, improving the uniformity, smoothness, and body of foods such as ice cream. Common preservatives include sodium benzoate and sorbic acid, which prevent bacterial growth. Sequestrants bind metals and thus prevent spoilage of food from metal contamination.

8. Toxic substances occur naturally in a variety of foods, such as green potatoes, raw fish, mushrooms, raw soybeans, and raw egg whites. Cooking foods limits their toxic effects in some cases; others are best to avoid, such as toxic mushroom species and the green parts of potatoes.

9. A variety of environmental contaminants can be found in foods. Because most of them are fat soluble, trimming fat from meats and discarding fat that is rendered during the cooking of meats, fish, and poultry are good steps to minimize exposure. In addition, it's helpful to know which foods pose a special risk, to wash fruits and vegetables thoroughly, and to discard the outer leaves of leafy vegetables.

■ STUDY QUESTIONS

1. Identify three major classes of microorganisms that are responsible for food-borne illness.

2. Which kinds of foods are most likely to be involved in food-borne illness? Why are they targets for contamination?

3. What three trends in food purchasing and production have led to a greater number of cases of food-borne illness in recent years?

4. Why is thoroughly cooking food an important practice for reducing the risk of food-borne illness?

5. List four techniques other than thorough cooking that are important in preventing food-borne illness.

6. Define the term *food additive*, and give examples of four intentional food additives. What are their specific functions in foods? What is their relationship to the GRAS list?

7. Describe the federal process that governs the use of food additives, including the Delaney Clause.

8. Put into perspective the benefits and risks of using additives in food. Point out an easy way to reduce the consumption of food additives. Do you think this is worth the effort in terms of maintaining health? Why or why not?

9. Describe four recommendations for reducing the risk of toxicity from environmental contaminants.

10. Read the Nutrition Perspective before answering the following question. How do various federal agencies work together to maintain the safety of food?

■ ANNOTATED REFERENCES

1. ADA Reports: Position of the American Dietetic Association: Food irradiation. *Journal of the American Dietetic Association* 100:246, 2000.

It is the position of ADA that food irradiation enhances the safety and quality of the food supply and helps protect consumers from food-borne illness. ADA encourages qualified professionals to work together to educate consumers about this additional food safety tool.

2. Bender J and others: Food-borne disease in the 21st century: What challenges await us. *Postgraduate Medicine* 106(2):109, 1999.

The factors that contribute to an increasing incidence of food-borne disease include diet, the global distribution of foods, the expansion of commercial food services, and new methods of large-scale food production. Critical aspects to help reduce the risk for disease include improved surveillance, community education, the use of HACCP strategies, and ionizing radiation.

3. Carpy SA and others: Health risk of low dose-pesticide mixtures: A review of the 1985-1998 literature on combination toxicology and health risk assessment. *Journal of Toxicology and Environmental Health. Part B, Critical Reviews* 3:1, 2000.

Despite some exceptions, it has been demonstrated that interaction between various pesticide residues is not a common event at low levels of human exposure, such as those that may arise from food or drinking water. As a general rule, exposure to a mixture of pesticides at low doses of the individual constituents does not represent a potential source of concern to human health.

4. Centers for Disease Control and Prevention: Ciguatera fish poisoning—Texas, 1997. *Journal of the American Medical Association* 280:1394, 1998.

   An outbreak of Ciguatera fish poisoning involved 17 crewmembers of a cargo ship, which caught, cooked, and ate a barracuda in the Bahamas. Within hours of eating the fish, all 17 men became ill with nausea, vomiting, abdominal cramps, and diarrhea. Over the next 2 days, they suffered from muscle pain and weakness, dizziness, and numb or itchy feet, hands, and mouth.

5. Cook K and others: Outbreak of salmonella serotype Hartford infections associated with unpasteurized orange juice. *Journal of the American Medical Association* 280:1504, 1998.

   Unpasteurized orange juice caused an outbreak of salmonellosis in a large Florida theme park. Pasteurization (or other equally effective risk-management strategies) should be used in the production of all juices.

6. Corcoran L, Schardt D: Fighting food bugs. *Nutrition Action Healthletter*, p. 8, September 1998.

   Although lettuce, alfalfa sprouts, and unpasteurized apple juice are sources of E. coli 0157:H7 outbreaks, a person is most likely to acquire the illness from eating undercooked, contaminated ground beef. All of us should follow basic rules of cleaning, cooking, and chilling in order to protect ourselves from contracting food-borne illness.

7. Daniels R: Home food safety. *Food Technology* 52(2):54, 1998.

   Currently, 99% of households do not meet food safety standards. And, since proper preparation at home is the last chance people have to protect themselves, raising public awareness of home food safety is an important issue. For the general public, key efforts include avoiding cross-contamination, washing hands, cooking to appropriate temperature, and cooling of foods properly.

8. Dioxin more toxic than earlier estimates; spectrum of adverse effects found by EPA. *CNI Nutrition Week*, P. 4, June 30, 2000.

   Dioxins are potent animal toxicants with the potential to produce a broad spectrum of harmful effects in humans, including adverse effects on reproduction and development, suppression of the immune system, chloracne (a severe, acnelike condition), and cancer. EPA has characterized the most toxic dioxin, TCDD, as a human carcinogen. Other dioxins are classified as likely human carcinogens, based on the evidence of animal and human studies.

9. E. coli outbreak identified in Illinois: Cases in New York state top 1,000. *CNI Nutrition Week*, p. 1, September 17, 1999.

   Two deaths resulted from an E. coli outbreak in upstate New York during a county fair. The total number of people infected reached 1013, the largest number of confirmed and suspected cases to result from one outbreak in the United States. The source was identified as a private well which was contaminated by manure runoff from a nearby barn.

10. Farley D: Dangers of lead still linger. *FDA Consumer*, p. 16, January/February 1998.

    Although the percentage of potentially harmful blood lead concentrations has dropped dramatically in the past 20 years, lead is still a problem. Sources include lead paint in older housing, in the soil where leaded gasoline was once used, at some work sites, and occasionally in drinking water, ceramic ware, and a number of other products.

11. FDA advisory on consumption of raw sprouts. *American Family Physician* 60: 1573, 1999.

    According to FDA, children, older adults, and persons who have weakened immune systems are particularly at high risk of developing serious food-borne disease from raw sprouts. FDA is working closely with the sprout industry to establish preventive controls to protect consumers.

12. Food-borne antibiotic-resistant Campylobacter infections. *Nutrition Reviews* 57:224, 2000.

    In modern breeding of food animals, large amounts of antibiotics are used for a variety of reasons, including growth promotion. This has caused food-borne bacterial pathogens to become resistant to antibiotics and has caused an increase in morbidity and mortality among humans. Well-coordinated international programs are needed to assess the worldwide use of antibiotics in food animals.

13. Food safety fears prompt federal government to ban Guatemalan raspberries. *CNI Nutrition Week*, p. 1, December 12, 1997.

    A number of food-borne illness outbreaks have been associated with imported produce, including Cyclospora on raspberries, hepatitis A from strawberries, and E. coli on lettuce and alfalfa sprouts. FDA has taken action by banning imports of Guatemalan raspberries.

14. Food safety guide. *Nutrition Action Healthletter*, p. 3, October 1999.

    This article discusses the major causes of food-borne illnesses and precautions to take to prevent infections. Some ways to avoid contracting a food-borne illness are to marinate and defrost food in the refrigerator, not eat raw shellfish, discard cracked eggs, and wash fresh fruits and vegetables. These and other precautions should be taken in order to protect against harmful microbes.

15. FSIS unveils outline of proposed Listeria rule. *CNI Nutrition Week*, p. 6, May 26, 2000.

    USDA's Food and Safety and Inspection Service (FSIS) is discussing new strategies for preventing the Listeria monocytogenes contamination of ready-to-eat meat and poultry products. The new action plan will require processing plants to test finished products and the plant environment, to label food products concerning the risk of listeriosis, and to provide advice to high-risk populations—infants, older adults, pregnant women, and people with compromised immune systems.

16. Henkel J: Irradiation: A safe measure for safer food. *FDA Consumer*, p. 12, May/ June, 1998.

    Health experts say that irradiation can reduce E. coli 0157:H7 contamination and can help control the potentially harmful bacteria Salmonella and Campylobacter. The food industry needs to get more irradiated products into the marketplace; then the public can make up its mind with regard to acceptance.

17. Hingley A: Campylobacter. Low-profile bug is food poisoning leader. *FDA Consumer*, p. 14, September/October 1999.

    Although illnesses from Campylobacter are the most frequently diagnosed food-borne infections, it rarely makes the news. Most infections are sporadic and are not associated with an outbreak, but it causes up to 4 million human infections a year.

18. Hiser E: The top 10 food safety mistakes families make. *American Health*, p. 104, September 1999.

    More than 30 million Americans get sick every year from food-borne illnesses from the home and from restaurants. This article provides 10 of the most common fast fixes for food safety. Some ways to protect one's family include frequently washing hands, avoiding eating cookie dough, and asking for meat and seafood to be bagged separately at the checkout stand in the supermarket.

19. JAMA Patient Page: Protect against Salmonella. *Journal of the American Medical Association* 281:1866, 1999.

    Salmonella causes one of the most prevalent types of food-borne illnesses. New cases of isolated outbreaks have been reported, especially of strains that are resistant to certain antibiotics. Salmonella is usually transmitted through eating undercooked or raw eggs, poultry, and meat or unpasteurized dairy products.

20. Johnson R, Gibbs C: Creutzfeldt-Jakob disease and related transmissible spongiform encephalopathies. *New England Journal of Medicine* 339:1994, 1998.

    Creutzfeldt-Jakob disease is an obscure form of dementia, which occurs in humans from Europe and the United Kingdom. Studies have searched for risk factors. These point to dietary factors, such as beef and lamb. No human disease resembling new-variant

Creutzfeldt-Jakob disease has been found in North America, since the United States has banned the importation of European cattle and sheep.

21. Kurtzweil P: Safer eggs: Laying the groundwork. *FDA Consumer,* p. 10, September/October 1998.

    As many as 1 in 20,000 eggs, or about 2.7 million eggs annually in the United States, contains Salmonella bacteria. Contamination occurs as the egg develops in the oviduct—the canal through which the egg travels—of a Salmonella-infected chicken or from chicken waste matter coming into contact with an egg.

22. Matte T: Reducing blood lead levels: Benefits and strategies. *Journal of the American Medical Association* 281:2340, 1999.

    Despite dramatic reductions in population lead exposure over the past two decades, nearly 900,000 U.S. children younger than 6 years still have elevated blood lead levels. Progress toward the virtual eradication of childhood lead toxicity can be greatly accelerated by nutritional manipulation, such as increased dietary calcium intake, as well as by public and private efforts to increase testing for and the remediation of residential lead hazards.

23. Outbreaks of Salmonella serotype Enteritidis infection associated with eating raw or undercooked shell eggs—United States, 1996-1998. *Journal of the American Medical Association* 283:1132, 2000.

    Case-control studies of sporadic infections and outbreak investigations found that the increase in Salmonella serotype Enteritidis infections was associated with eating raw or undercooked shell eggs. In August 1997, 17 members of a Girl Scout troop and some of their parents became ill with salmonellosis after eating cheesecake that contained undercooked eggs.

24. Outbreaks of Shigella sonnei infection associated with eating fresh parsley—United States and Canada, July-August 1998. *Journal of the American Medical Association* 281:1785, 1999.

    Laboratory investigations have implicated parsley imported from a farm in Mexico as the source of recent Shigella sonnei outbreaks. On August 11, 1998, six people in Massachusetts reported illness after eating chicken sandwiches and coleslaw that was served with chopped, uncooked parsley.

25. Pesticide residues: Cause for concern? *Health News* p. 3, April 15, 1999.

    Since there's no firm evidence that eating produce with pesticide residues is unhealthy, consumers should not let the pesticide controversy scare them away from eating plenty of fruits and vegetables. Still, to be on the safe side, we should carefully rinse all fruits and vegetables under cold, running water before consumption.

26. Prescott LM and others: *Microbiology* 4th ed. WCB/McGraw-Hill Publishers, Boston, MA 1999.

    This text provides a detailed look at food and water-borne diseases. Much of this chapter was verified using this text.

27. Public health nutrition and food safety, 1900-1999. *Nutrition Reviews* 57:368, 1999.

    During the 1940s, studies of autopsied muscle samples showed that 16% of persons in the United States had trichinellosis. Since then, the rate of infection has declined markedly. From 1991 through 1996, only three deaths and an average of 38 cases per year were reported, showing the progress made in controlling this pathogen.

28. Reptile-associated salmonellosis—selected states, 1996-1998. *Journal of the American Medical Association* 282:2293, 1999.

    Salmonella infection can result in invasive illness, including sepsis and meningitis, particularly in infants. Despite educational efforts, some reptile owners remain unaware that reptiles place them and their children at risk for salmonellosis. A previously healthy 5-month-old girl suddenly died from salmonellosis due to indirect contact with a pet iguana.

29. *Residue monitoring 1999.* Washington, DC: Food and Drug Administration Pesticide Program, Food and Drug Administration, 1999.

    Based on FDA's Total Diet Study comprising 3500 different foods purchased from stores throughout the United States, only 0.8% of foods had pesticide residues exceeding EPA allowances. For imported products, 3.5% had pesticide residues exceeding EPA allowances. Otherwise, pesticide residues were either undetectable (about 60% of the time) or within allowable amounts for over 99% of domestic products and about 97% of imported products.

30. Rhoads G: The effect of dust lead control on blood lead in toddlers: A randomized trial. *Pediatrics* 103:551, 1999.

    Contaminated household dust is believed to be a major source of exposure for most children with elevated blood lead levels. Regular home cleaning, accompanied by parental education, is a safe and partially effective intervention, which should be recommended to those who are unable to move to lead-safe housing.

31. Scombroid fish poisoning—Pennsylvania , 1998. *Journal of the American Medical Association* 283:2927, 2000.

    Scombroid fish poisoning has been associated primarily with the consumption of tuna, mahi-mahi, and bluefish. The key to the prevention of scombroid fish poisoning is continuous icing or refrigeration at less than or equal to 32°F (0°C) of all potential scombrotoxin-producing fish from the time they are caught until they are cooked.

32. Villar R and others: Outbreak of type A botulism and development of a botulism surveillance and antitoxin release system in Argentina. *Journal of the American Medical Association* 281:1334, 1999.

    Botulism is a potentially fatal, neuroparalytic illness resulting from toxins produced by the bacterium Clostridium botulinum. Botulism antitoxin, the only specific therapy available to ameliorate illness, can help prevent the progression of paralysis, reduce the duration of illness, and decrease fatality rates.

33. When antibiotics stop working: Magic bullets under siege. *Nutrition Action Healthletter* 27(4):3, 2000.

    The more we use antibiotics—to treat humans and to promote growth in animals on factory farms—the more bacteria become resistant to those antibiotics. We need to minimize the unnecessary use of drugs—in both animals and people—to preserve the effectiveness of antibiotics as long as possible.

TAKEACTION

I. CAN YOU SPOT THE IMPROPER FOOD SAFETY PRACTICES?

In this chapter, you learned the following facts: (1) food-borne illness strikes up to 76 million Americans each year; (2) about 5000 deaths each year in the United States are caused by food-borne organisms.

Carefully preparing foods to prevent food-borne illness can minimize its occurrence for most of us. Read the following excerpt and find the food safety violations that could contribute to this risk.

A Local Health Department Instpector Gives the Following Account of His Visit to a Local Diner

As I walked through the kitchen of the Morningside Diner, I noticed that all food handlers washed their hands thoroughly with hot, soapy water before handling the food, especially after handling raw meat, fish, poultry, or eggs. Before preparing raw foods, they also thoroughly washed the cutting boards, dishes, and other equipment. As they used their cutting boards after cutting foods, they wiped them with a damp rag and used them again to cut more food.

When preparing fresh fruits and vegetables, they washed them but were careful to leave a little dirt on for fear of washing important nutrients from the outside. The cooks generally cooked meats to an internal temperature of 180°F (82°C). However, to preserve the flavor, pork was cooked to an internal temperature of 140°F (60°C). Some cooked foods to be served later were cooled to 40°F (4°C) within 2 hours, and foods such as beef stew were cooled in shallow pans.

The diner served canned foods, even when the cans were dented. When leftovers were reheated, they were raised to an internal temperature of 150°F (66°C) and served immediately. Food handlers took great care to remove moldy portions of food. The cooks prepared stuffing separately from the poultry. The temperature of the refrigerators was approximately 45°F (7°C).

1. List the violations of food safety practices that could contribute to food-borne illness.

    _____

    _____

    _____

2. If you were writing a report describing ways to correct these practices, what would you say?

    _____

    _____

    _____

TAKE ACTION

II. TAKE A CLOSER LOOK AT FOOD ADDITIVES

Evaluate a food label of a convenience food item either in the supermarket or one you have available.

1. Write out the list of ingredients.

   _____

   _____

   _____

   _____

2. Identify the ingredients that you think may be food additives.

   _____

   _____

   _____

   _____

3. Based on the information available in this chapter, what are the functions of these food additives?

   _____

   _____

   _____

   _____

4. How might this food product differ without these ingredients?

   _____

   _____

   _____

   _____

NUTRITION *Perspective*

PESTICIDES IN FOOD

Pesticides used in food production produce both beneficial and unwanted effects. Most health authorities believe that the benefits greatly outweigh the risks. Pesticides help ensure a safe and adequate food supply and help make foods available at reasonable cost. However, sentiment is growing nationwide that pesticides pose avoidable health risks. Consumers have come to assume that synthetic is dangerous and organic is safe. Some researchers believe that this sentiment is grounded in fear and fueled by unbalanced reports.[3] Other researchers say concern about pesticides is valid and overdue.

Most concern about pesticide residues in food appropriately focuses on chronic rather than acute toxicity because the amounts of residue present, if any, are extremely small. These low concentrations found in foods are not known to produce adverse effects in the short term, although harm has been caused by the high amounts that occasionally result from accidents or misuse. For humans, pesticides pose a danger mainly in their cumulative effects, so their threats to health are difficult to determine. However, growing evidence, including the problems of the contamination of underground water supplies and destruction of wildlife habitats, indicates that we would likely be better off as a nation if we could reduce our use of pesticides. Both the federal government and many farmers are working toward that end.

One of the problems with pesticides is that they create new pests because they destroy the spiders, wasps, and predatory beetles that naturally keep most plantfeeding insect populations in check. The brown plant hopper, which recently plagued Indonesian rice fields, was not a serious problem before heavy pesticide use began in the early 1970s. In the United States, such major pests as spider mites and the cotton bollworm were merely nuisances until pesticides decimated their predators.

WHAT IS A PESTICIDE?

Federal law defines a pesticide as any substance or mixture of substances intended to prevent, destroy, repel, or mitigate any pest. The built-in toxic properties of pesticides lead to the possibility that other, nontarget organisms, including humans, might also be harmed. The term *pesticide* tends to be used as a generic reference to many types of products, including insecticides, herbicides, fungicides, and rodenticides. A pesticide product may be chemical or bacterial, natural or synthetic. For agriculture, EPA allows about 10,000 pesticide uses, involving some 300 active ingredients. About 1.2 billion pounds of pesticides are used each year in the United States, much of which is applied to agricultural crops.

Once a pesticide is applied, it can turn up in a number of unintended and unwanted places. It may be carried in the air and dust by wind currents, remain in soil attached to soil particles, be taken up by organisms in the soil, decompose to other compounds, be taken up by plant roots, enter groundwater, or invade aquatic habitats. Each is a route to the food chain; some are more direct than others.

WHY USE PESTICIDES?

In the United States alone, pests destroy nearly $20 billion of food crops yearly, despite extensive pesticide use. The primary reason for using pesticides is economic—the use of agricultural chemicals increases production and lowers the cost of food, at least in the short run. Many farmers believe they would have a tough time staying in business without pesticides. Quick and direct, pesticides help protect farmers from ruinous losses caused by a sudden pest outbreak.

Consumer demands also have changed over the years. At one time, we wouldn't have thought twice about buying an apple with a worm hole; we simply took it home, cut out the wormy part, and ate the apple. Today, consumers find worm holes less acceptable, so farmers rely more and more on pesticides to produce cosmetically attractive fruits and vegetables. On the practical side, pesticides can protect against the rotting and decay of fresh fruits and vegetables. This is helpful because our food distribution system doesn't usually permit consumer purchase within hours of harvest. Also, food grown without pesticides can contain naturally occurring organisms that produce carcinogens at concentrations far above current standards for pesticide residues. For example, fungicides help prevent the carcinogen aflatoxin (caused by

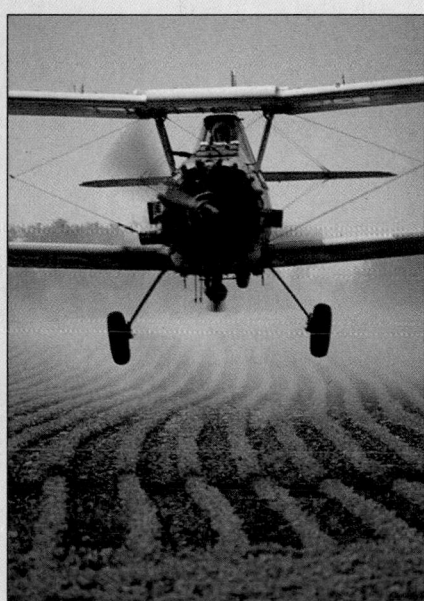

Pesticides use poses a risk-versus-benefit question. Each side has points that deserve to be considered.

growth of a fungus) from forming on some crops. Thus, although some pesticides may improve the appearance of food products, others help keep some foods fresher and safer to eat.

REGULATION OF PESTICIDES

The responsibility for ensuring that residues of pesticides in foods are below amounts that pose a danger to health is shared by FDA, EPA, and the Food Safety and Inspection Service of USDA (see Table 19-5 for the roles of various food protection agencies). FDA is responsible for enforcing pesticide tolerances in all foods except meat, poultry, and certain egg products, which are monitored by USDA. A newly proposed pesticide is exhaustively tested, perhaps over 10 years or more, before it is approved for use. EPA must decide both that the pesticide causes no unreasonable adverse effects on people and the environment and that benefits of use outweigh the risks of using it. However, there is concern about older chemicals registered before 1970, when less stringent testing conditions were permitted. EPA is now asking chemical companies to retest the old compounds using more rigorous tests. Unfortunately, inadequate funding at EPA has hampered the review of older pesticides. The slow pace of this retesting has angered the critics of pesticide use. When weighing whether to approve or cancel a pesticide, EPA considers how much more it would cost farmers to use an alternative pesticide or process and whether cancellation would decrease productivity. After determining the dollar cost to farmers, EPA then looks at costs to processors and consumers. Once a pesticide is approved for

TABLE 19-5   U.S. Agencies Responsible for Monitoring the Food Supply

Agency Name	Responsibilities	Methods	How to Contact
United States Department of Agriculture (USDA)	• Enforces wholesomeness and quality standards for grains and produce (while in the field), meat, poultry, milk, and eggs	• Inspection • Grading • "Safe Handling Label"	http://www.usda.gov/fsis or http://www.nal.usda.gov/fnic/foodborne/foodborn.htm or call 1-800-535-4555
Bureau of Alcohol Tobacco, and Fire Arms (ATF)	• Enforces laws on alcoholic beverages	• Inspection	http://www.atf.treas.gov/
Environmental Protection Agency (EPA)	• Regulates pesticides • Establishes water quality standards	• Approval required for all U.S. pesticides • Sets pesticide residue limits in food	http://www.epa.gov/
Food and Drug Administration (FDA)	• Ensures safety and wholesomeness of all foods in interstate commerce (except meat and poultry) • Regulates seafood • Controls product labels	• Inspection • Food sample studies • Sets standards for specific foods	http://www.fda.gov/ or call 1-800-FDA-4010
Centers for Disease Control and Prevention (CDC)	• Protects food safety	• Responds to emergencies concerning food-borne illness • Surveys and studies environmental health problems • Directs/enforces quarantines • National programs for prevention and control of food-borne and other diseases	http://www.cdc.gov/
The National Marine Fisheries Service or NOAA Fisheries	• Domestic and International conservation and management of living marine resources	• Voluntary seafood inspection program • Can use mark to show federal inspection	http://www.nmfs.noaa.gov/
State and local governments	• Milk safety • Monitors food industry within their borders	• Inspection of food-related establishments	Government pages of telephone book

use, it must follow the margin of safety provisions required of food additives (see the section on testing food additives for safety).

HOW SAFE ARE PESTICIDES?

Dangers from exposure to pesticides through food depend on how potent the chemical toxin is, how concentrated it is in the food, how much and how frequently it's eaten, and the consumer's resistance or susceptibility to the substance. Pesticide use is clearly associated with declining water quality. Accumulating information also links pesticide use to increased cancer rates in farm communities. For rural counties in the United States, the incidence of lymph, genital, brain, and digestive tract cancers increases with higher-than-average pesticide use. Respiratory cancer cases increase with greater insecticide use. In tests using laboratory animals, scientists have found that some of the chemicals present in pesticide residues cause birth defects, sterility, tumors, organ damage, and injury to the central nervous system. Some pesticides persist in the environment for years.

Still, some researchers argue that the cancer risk from minimal pesticide residues is hundreds of times less than the risk from eating such common foods as peanut butter, brown mustard, and basil. Plants manufacture their own toxic substances to defend themselves against insects, birds, and grazing animals (including humans). When plants are stressed or damaged, they produce even more of these toxins. Because of this, many foods contain naturally occurring chemicals considered toxic, and some are even carcinogenic. Other scientists argue that, if natural carcinogens are already in the food supply, then we should reduce the number of added carcinogens whenever possible. In other words, we should do what we can to decrease the problem.

THE RISKS OF PESTICIDES TO CHILDREN

Any discussions of pesticides and associated health risks must focus on children. They are not simply small adults in a biological sense. Children face a higher risk from pesticide exposure than do adults for several reasons:

1. Their exposure is greater; children eat more food in proportion to their body weight than do adults.

2. Children consume more foods that are potential sources of pesticide residues than do adults. For example, they eat more fruit.

3. Exposure at an early age carries a greater risk than does exposure later in life; residues can accumulate to toxic amounts over a longer period. Also, cancer has more time to develop.

4. Physiological susceptibility to the effects of carcinogens and neurotoxins in pesticides may be greater; the cells in children are dividing rapidly, and the enzyme systems that detoxify chemicals are not fully developed.

Until recent years, EPA did not consider these factors in risk calculations. However, the recent Food Quality Protection Act now requires EPA to look at age-related consumption data for the approval of new pesticides. Although children are at greater risk from pesticides, the magnitude of that risk and how best to calculate it are open to debate. Overall, experts stress the value of including fruits and vegetables in children's diets and caution parents not to change their children's diets to avoid certain foods. Carefully washing fruits and vegetables and consuming a wide variety are sufficient recommendations. Peeling fruits and vegetables is another option. A final general precaution is to keep children away from lawns, gardens, and flower beds that have recently been treated with pesticides and herbicides.

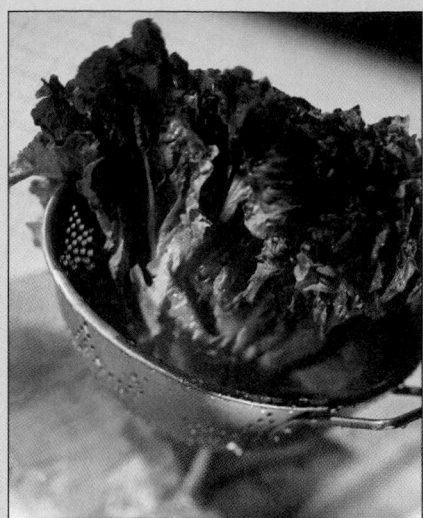

Rinsing fruits and vegetables under running water is advised to reduce pesticide exposure.

TESTS OF THE AMOUNTS OF PESTICIDES IN FOODS

FDA tests thousands of raw products each year for pesticide residues. (A pesticide is considered illegal in this case if it is not approved for use on the crop in question or if the amount used exceeds the allowed tolerance.) A 1999 FDA study showed no residues in about 60% of samples. Less than 1% of domestic and about 3% of import samples had residues that were over tolerance. The findings for 1999 continue to support previous FDA studies over the past 10 years that pesticide residues in foods are generally well below EPA tolerances, and they confirm the safety of the food supply relative to pesticide residues.[29]

Residues sometimes appear on the wrong crops or in excessive amounts because of contamination from nearby farms via wind or water. When a problem is identified, FDA takes steps to make sure it's corrected and that the tainted food in question never reaches the consumer. However, of 600 pesticides available on international markets, many are not even detected by any of FDA's multiresidue tests. This has raised concern by pesticide critics with regard to imported foods. Better tests, which detect single residues, are less frequently used because of cost.

PERSONAL ACTION

We often take risks in our own lives, but we prefer to have a choice in the matter after weighing the pros and cons. For instance, we can choose not to immunize a child, but we do so with the understanding that the child might get sick. We can also choose to risk cancer from smoking or to avoid that risk, or we can drive recklessly. In regard to pesticides in food, however, someone else is deciding what is acceptable and what is not. Our only choice is whether to buy or avoid pesticide-containing foods. In reality, it's almost impossible to avoid pesticides entirely, because even organic produce often contains traces of pesticides, probably as the result of cross-contamination from nearby farms.

Short-term studies of the effects of pesticides on laboratory animals cannot pinpoint long-term cancer risks precisely. It should be clearly understood, however, that the presence of minute traces of an environmental chemical in a food doesn't mean that any adverse effect will result from eating that food.

FDA and other scientific organizations believe that the hazards are comparatively low and in the short run are less than the hazards of food-borne illness created in our own kitchens. We can't avoid pesticide risks entirely, but we can limit exposure by following the advice given earlier in this chapter (review Table 9-4).[25]

We can also encourage farmers to use fewer pesticides to reduce exposure to our foods and water supplies, but we'll have to settle for produce that isn't perfect in appearance. Are you concerned enough about pesticides on food to change your shopping habits or take more political action?

*F*it is a product available to remove wax, dirt, pesticides, and other residues from fruits and vegetables. The ingredients include baking soda, citric acid, and water. Because some pesticide residues are not water soluble, Fit helps remove more water-resistant pesticide residue and wax than rinsing with water alone. There is currently no consensus on whether its use is important for the average consumer.

UNDERNUTRITION THROUGHOUT THE WORLD

chapter 20

The images are both vivid and heartrending. Emaciated children with enormous eyes and stomachs, too weak to cry, stare at us from news photos and television screens. Of the nearly 12 million children under 5 who die each year in developing countries, 55% of the deaths are attributable to undernutrition.[4, 31]

Today, nearly one in five people worldwide is chronically undernourished—too hungry to lead a productive, active life. Over the past 10 years, this problem has even worsened. Throughout the world the problems of poverty and undernutrition are widespread and growing.[5]

The majority (two-thirds) of undernourished people live in Asia. However, the largest increases in numbers of chronically hungry people currently occur in eastern Africa, particularly in Ethiopia, Sudan, Rwanda, Burundi, Kenya, Somalia, and Tanzania. Their eyes haunt us.[10]

This chapter examines the problem of undernutrition and the conditions that create it, as well as some possible solutions. If we are to eradicate undernutrition, we all have to understand the problem and assume responsibility for supplying some answers. It is important to recognize that many political leaders and citizens worldwide contribute directly and indirectly to the economic and social destruction that spawns hunger.[6]

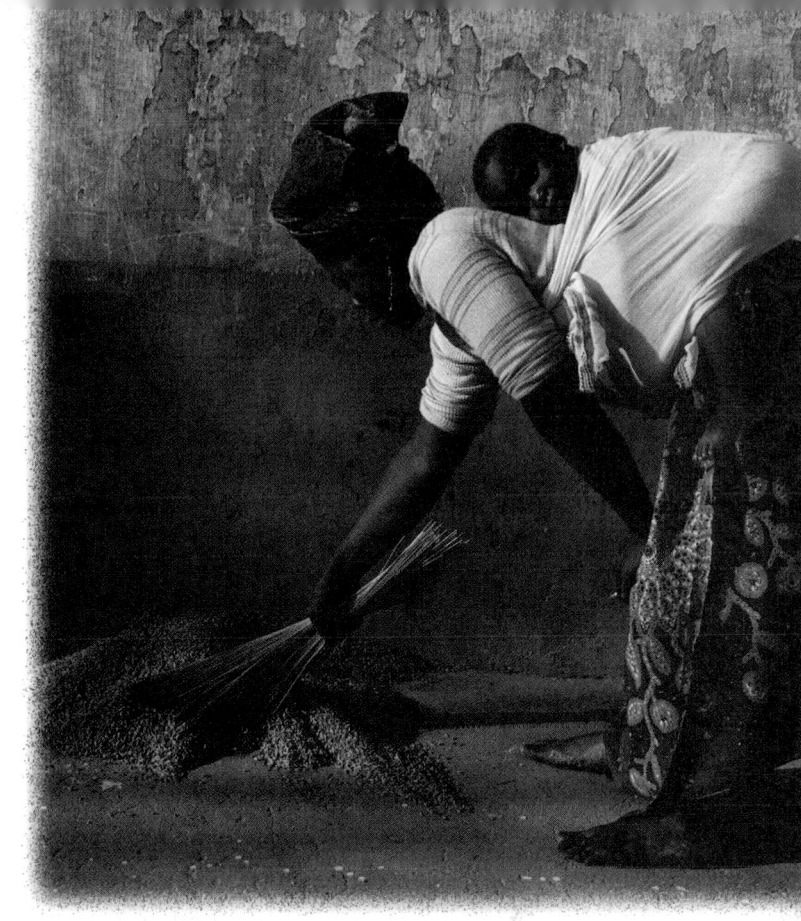

KEY CHAPTER CONCEPTS

- Poverty is common wherever people suffer from undernutrition.
- The greatest risk of undernutrition occurs during critical periods of growth, development, and old age. Low birth weight is a leading cause of infant deaths worldwide.
- Although famine has not existed in the United States since the 1930s, undernutrition is still a problem. In response, soup kitchens, the food stamp program, school lunch and breakfast programs, and the Special Supplemental Feeding Program for Women, Infants, and Children (WIC) have been created to help those in need.
- Reducing out-of-wedlock pregnancies and focusing more on the responsibilities of parents remain national priorities for the United States, because single parents and their children are likely to live in poverty.
- Multiple factors contribute to the problem of undernutrition in the developing world. Food resources may be inadequate. Farming methods often encourage erosion. Naturally occurring devastation from droughts, excessive rainfall, fire, crop infestation, and human causes—such as urbanization, war and civil unrest, debt, and poor sanitation—worsen the problem of undernutrition, as does AIDS.
- Direct food aid is only a short-term solution to undernutrition in developing countries. Sustainable subsistence-level farming and small-scale industrial development are ways to gain the resources to feed one's family.
- The world has both the food and technical expertise to end hunger. What is lacking is the political will to do so.

REFRESH YOUR MEMORY

As you begin your study of world hunger in Chapter 20, you may want to review
- Immune system function in Chapter 3
- The role of vitamin A and rich food sources in Chapter 9
- The roles of iron, zinc and iodide, and rich food sources in Chapter 12
- The advantage of breastfeeding to infants in Chapter 15
- Methods to monitor the adequacy of growth in Chapter 16

CASE SCENARIO

Jamal traveled during spring break with his church group to Guatemala. During their week-long stay, they were to help build shelters for people in the village in which a large fire had destroyed most of the housing a few weeks before. Jamal noticed that many of the children in the village are short, much shorter than the children in his neighborhood. Mothers in the village stated that their children often have diarrhea and are ill. Jamal also noticed that the children are not as lively as he would expect.

A nurse at the local health clinic pointed out that these children generally do not have enough to eat and that health problems are rampant. She hoped that the recent fire would spur the Guatemalan government to send supplies to the village, particularly food and medicines.

Should Jamal have been surprised by the high prevalence of disease and general listlessness of the children in the Guatemala village? What nutrients are likely to be deficient in the diets of these children, in turn contributing to their poor health status?

792 PUTTING NUTRITION KNOWLEDGE INTO PRACTICE   http://www.mhhe.com/wardlaw

■ WORLD HUNGER: A CONTINUING PLAGUE

In November 1974, the United Nations World Food Conference proclaimed its bold objective "that within a decade no child will go to bed hungry, that no family will fear for its next day's bread, and that no human being's future and capacities will be stunted by malnutrition." Today, this promise remains unfulfilled: Hunger remains a daily experience for one in seven people in the developing world (800 million) and one in nine households in the United States.[10, 12]

The famines that occurred in Ethiopia in the 1980s elicited widespread public support for immediate aid to the victims. Still, far from ending, hunger remains frequently in the news. The past 3 years of extended drought have once again left many people in Ethiopia without crops, livestock, and food. Civil wars and droughts in many parts of the world, have brought millions of people to the brink of starvation. About two-thirds of these people live in Africa. Relief aid has been arriving but often with too little, too late. The deadly combination of political corruption, administrative ineptness, war, and poor weather has also led to increasing hunger in Bangladesh, Afghanistan, Haiti, the Philippines, North Korea, and Cambodia.[10]

We must face the reality that the United Nations' members have yet to meet their pledge to elevate 3 billion people (half of the world's population) out of abject poverty. We also have to consider that 45% of the world's income currently goes to the 12% of the world's people who live in the rich industrial nations. Dr. Norman Meyers, an expert on world hunger, states that we have never had as rich a resource base to tackle the problem of worldwide undernutrition as we have today. Will we take advantage of this opportunity?

■ DEFINITION OF WORLD HUNGER

Let's begin our look at the problem of world hunger by first defining some key words.

Hunger is the physiological state that results when not enough food is eaten to meet energy needs. It also describes an uneasiness, a discomfort, a weakness, or a pain caused by lack of food. If hunger is not relieved, the resulting medical and social costs of **undernutrition** are high—preterm births and mental retardation, inadequate growth and development in childhood, poor school performance, decreased work output in adulthood, and chronic disease[30] (Table 20-1). Symptoms of chronic hunger are found not only among people in the developing world but also among many people living at or below the poverty level in America. Of any industrialized country, the United States has the largest number of children living in poverty (14 million under the age of 19). About one out of every six children in this country goes hungry or is at risk for inadequate food.[12]

Malnutrition is a condition of impaired development or function caused by either a long-term deficiency or an excess in energy and/or nutrient intake, the latter representing the state of overnutrition described in Chapter 4. When food supplies are low and the population is large, undernutrition is common, leading to nutritional deficiency diseases, such as goiter (from an iodide deficiency) and xerophthalmia (eye problems caused by poor vitamin A intake). However, when the food supply is ample or overabundant, incorrect food choices coupled with an excessive intake can lead to overnutrition-related chronic diseases, such as type 2 diabetes.

Undernutrition is the most common form of malnutrition among the poor in both developing and developed countries.[10] Currently, about half of the 4 million African children under 5 years of age who die annually are undernourished. Undernutrition is also the primary cause of specific nutrient deficiencies that can result in muscle wasting, xerophthalmia (blindness), scurvy, pellagra, beriberi, anemia, rickets, goiter, and a host of other problems (Table 20-2).

TABLE 20-1   The Realities of Undernutrition

- Nearly one in five people in the developing world is chronically undernourished—too hungry to lead a productive, active life. This includes one-third of the world's children.
- About 55,000 people die of hunger each day—two-thirds of them children.
- Three million newborns in the developing world die in the first week of life.
- Over half of all children who die each year in developing countries do so from causes that could be prevented at low cost.
- At least 350,000 children are permanently blinded each year simply from lack of vitamin A.
- Residents in developed countries spent more money on pet food, perfumes, and cosmetics than it would take to provide basic education, water and sanitation, health care, and nutrition for all those now deprived of it.
- About 20 million people worldwide have developed brain damage from maternal iodide deficiency; currently, 1.5 billion people are at risk for iodide deficiency.
- Women in poor countries average up to four times more births than women in the United States.
- Every day the world produces about 2400 kcal for each person, generally meeting average energy needs. A daily intake less than 2100 kcal would not likely sustain an older child or adult.
- Poor women in developing countries face a 50 to 200-fold increased risk of death in pregnancy, compared with women in the United States.
- In many developing countries, life expectancy of the population is one-half to two-thirds of that in the United States.
- Almost half of the world's people earn less than $200 a year—many use 80 to 90% of that income to obtain food. About $2000 to $3000 of income each year is needed for a person to reach the life expectancy seen in the United States.
- Of the 6 billion people on earth, more than 1 billion drink contaminated water. In India alone, 300,000 children die each year from drinking polluted water.
- About 3 billion people in the world live without proper sanitation, such as reliable toilet facilities.
- About 25% of children in the world have iron deficiency anemia.
- Developing countries have most of the 36 million AIDS cases worldwide.

The most critical micronutrients missing from diets worldwide are iron, vitamin A, and iodide. More than 1 billion people, mostly in the developing world, affected with iron deficiency, which impairs the cognitive development of children and likely is a permanent effect if the iron deficiency is prolonged in early infancy. It is estimated that 20 million people worldwide show brain damage from preventable maternal iodide deficiency. Although severe vitamin A deficiency, which causes blindness, is on the decline, up to 250 to 500 million preschool children are still affected by it. This vitamin deficiency also raises the risk for other diseases, such as measles.[4] The United Nations International Children's Fund reports that the lives of 1 to 3 million children could be saved annually in the developing world if vitamin A supplements were provided a few times a year. The annual cost per child would be about 6 cents.

Of the 6 billion people in the world, up to 2 billion may be affected by some form of micronutrient malnutrition.[24, 30] Death and disease from infections, particularly those causing acute and prolonged diarrhea or acute lower respiratory disease, increase dramatically when the infections are superimposed on a state of chronic undernutrition. Chronic undernutrition leaves many people in the developing world in a continual state of depressed immune function. Diarrhea alone is the number one killer of children in developing countries, responsible for over 2 million deaths of children under 5 years of age.

Protein-energy malnutrition (PEM) is a form of undernutrition caused by an extremely deficient intake of energy or protein generally accompanied by an illness.

TABLE 20-2   Effects of Nutrient-Deficiency Diseases That Commonly Accompany Undernutrition

Disease and Key Nutrient Involved	Typical Effects	Foods Rich in Deficient Nutrient	Where the Problem Currently Still Exists
Xerophthalmia Vitamin A	Blindness from chronic eye infections, retarded growth, dryness and keratinization of epithelial tissues	Liver, fortified milk, sweet potatoes, spinach, greens, carrots, cantaloupe, apricots	Asia, Africa
Rickets Vitamin D	Poorly calcified bones, bowed legs, other bone deformities	Fortified milk, fish oils, sun exposure	Asia and Africa where religious dress codes prevent women and children from receiving adequate sun exposure; elderly in developed nations
Beriberi Thiamin	Nerve degeneration, altered muscle coordination, cardiovascular problems	Sunflower seeds, pork, whole and enriched grains, dried beans	Areas of famine in Africa
Ariboflavinosis Riboflavin	Inflammation of tongue, mouth, face and oral cavity, nervous system disorders	Milk, mushrooms, spinach, liver, enriched grains	Areas of famine in Africa
Pellagra Niacin	Diarrhea, dermatitis, dementia	Mushrooms, bran, tuna, chicken, beef, peanuts, whole and enriched grains	Areas of famine in Africa
Scurvy Vitamin C	Delayed wound healing, internal bleeding, abnormal formation of bones and teeth	Citrus fruits, strawberries, broccoli	Areas of famine in Africa
Iron deficiency anemia Iron	Reduced work output, retarded growth, increased health risk in pregnancy	Meats, seafood, broccoli, peas, bran, whole-grain and enriched breads	Worldwide
Goiter Iodide	Enlarged thyroid gland in teenagers and adults, possible mental retardation, cretinism	Iodized salt, saltwater fish	South America, Eastern Europe, Africa

Often two or more nutrition-deficiency diseases are found in an undernourished person in the developing world. This separate discussion of nutrients just makes it easier to see the important role of each nutrient.

famine An extreme shortage of food, which leads to massive starvation in a population; often associated with crop failures, war, and political unrest.

The typically dramatic results of PEM—kwashiorkor and marasmus—were described in Chapter 7. This chapter focuses on the more subtle effects of a chronic lack of food.

Genetic background contributes to both forms of malnutrition. Nutrition expert Dr. Robert Olson states that not every child in Thailand who eats mainly rice develops protein-energy malnutrition; similarly, not every adult in New York City who consumes a high-fat, energy-rich diet experiences a heart attack. Genetic background influences the development of these diseases.

Famine is not the same thing as chronic hunger. Although both result from poverty and a lack of food, famine is the extreme form of chronic hunger. Periods of famine are characterized by large-scale loss of life, social disruption, and economic chaos that slows food production. As a result of these extreme events, the affected community experiences a downward spiral characterized by human distress; sales of land, livestock, and other important farm assets; migration; division and impoverishment of the poorest families; crime; and the weakening of customary moral codes, as seen in Sudan and Rwanda. In the midst of all this, undernutrition rates soar; infectious diseases, such as cholera, spread; and many people die.[10]

Special efforts are needed to eradicate the fundamental causes of famine. Causes vary by region and decade, but the most common underlying cause is crop failure. The most obvious causes of crop failure are bad weather, war, and civil strife, or all three. War, in fact, deserves a special focus; this will be specifically addressed in an upcoming section on war and political/civil unrest.

■ Critical Life Stages When Undernutrition Is Particularly Devastating

Prolonged undernutrition is detrimental to health at all stages of life but is particularly critical during some periods of growth and old age (Fig. 20-1).

Pregnancy

The period when undernutrition poses the greatest health risk is during pregnancy.[20] A pregnant woman needs extra nutrients to meet both her own needs and those of her developing fetus. Nourishing the fetus may deplete stores of maternal nutrients. Maternal iron deficiency anemia is one possible consequence (see Chapter 16).[10]

In Africa, women give birth, on average, to more than six live babies. Coupled with chronic undernutrition, these high birth rates create a 1 in 20 chance that a woman will die from pregnancy-related causes. In contrast, American women face a risk of 1 death in about 8000 births from pregnancy-related causes. No other social indicator, including literacy, life expectancy, and infant mortality, betrays a wider gap between the developing and industrialized worlds.

Fetal and Infant Stages

The fetus faces major health risks from undernutrition during gestation. To support growth and development of the brain and other body tissues, a growing fetus requires a rich supply of protein, vitamins, and minerals.[19] When these needs are not

More than 3 million people may have perished in the great famine of 1943 in Bengal, India. In 1974, another 1.5 million from that region starved in country of Bangladesh. China suffered an almost unbelievable famine from 1959 to 1961—estimates of mortality range from 16 million to 64 million.

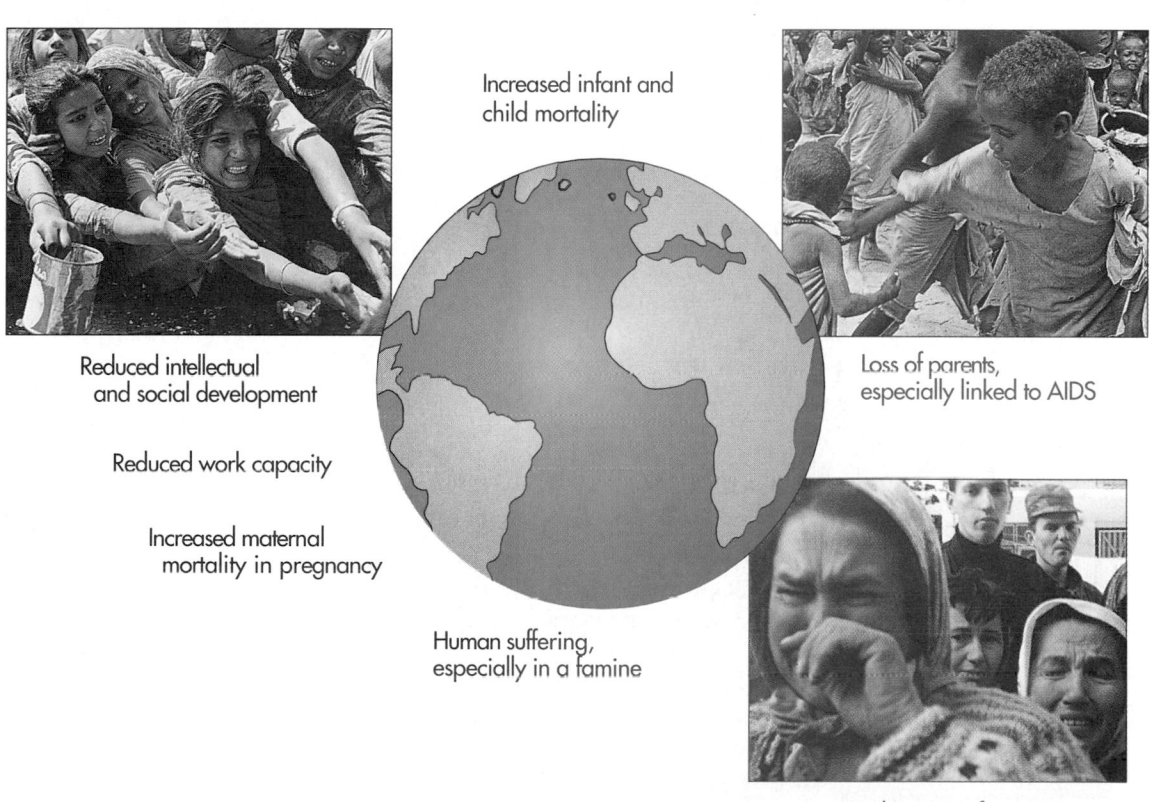

Increased infant and child mortality

Reduced intellectual and social development

Reduced work capacity

Increased maternal mortality in pregnancy

Human suffering, especially in a famine

Loss of parents, especially linked to AIDS

Exploitation of women in general

■ FIGURE 20-1 Undernutrition affects many aspects of human health and humanity in general.

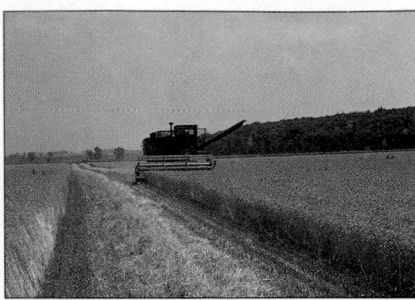

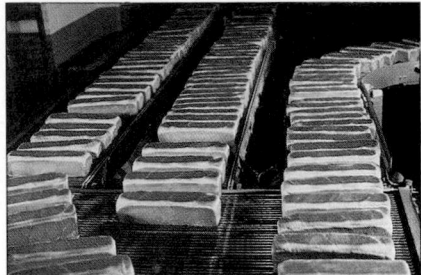

The bounty of food we enjoy in North America relies on its rich agricultural resources. Many developing countries do not have such resources.

*A*bout 40% of children in developing countries show evidence of growth failure.

CRITICAL THINKING

While studying early childhood development, Nakia was surprised to learn that some children in the United States are undernourished. What evidence might Nakia observe in children that would suggest undernourishment?

met, the infant is often born before 37 weeks of gestation, well before the 40 weeks of gestation that is considered ideal. The consequences of preterm birth include reduced lung function and a weakened immune system. These conditions not only compromise health but also increase the likelihood of premature death. Long-term problems in growth and development can result if the infant survives. In extreme cases, low-birth-weight babies (2500 g [about 5.5 lb] or less)—face 5 to 10 times the normal risk of dying before the age of 1 year, primarily because of reduced lung development. Chapter 17 pointed out that, when low birth weight is accompanied by other physical abnormalities, medical intervention can cost $200,000 or more. These costs can only be met in developed countries.

In the United States, low birth weight accounts for more than half of all infant deaths and for 75% of deaths of babies under 1 month of age. Currently, about 7.5% of infants born in the United States have low birth weights. Worldwide, more than 30 million infants are born with low birth weight.

Childhood

Early childhood, when growth is rapid, is another period when undernutrition is extremely risky. The central nervous system—including the brain—is particularly vulnerable because of rapid growth from conception through early childhood. After the preschool years, brain growth and development slow dramatically until maturity, when they cease. Nutritional deprivation, especially in early infancy, can lead to permanent brain impairment.[31] If more is not done, it is projected that ongoing undernutrition could leave more than 1 billion children with mental impairment by 2020.[14]

In general, poor children experience more nutritional deprivation and over-all illness and are more severely affected than other children. For example, iron deficiency anemia is much more common among poor children than children from less deprived families. This deficiency can lead to fatigue, reduced stamina, stunted growth, impaired motor development and learning problems. Undernutrition in childhood can also weaken resistance to infection, because immune function decreases when such nutrients as protein, vitamin A, and zinc are very low in a diet.[17, 24] Clearly, undernutrition and illness have a cyclical relationship. Not only does undernutrition cause illness, but illness worsens undernutrition, particularly by diarrhea and infectious diseases. For this reason, many children in developing countries are dying from the combination of malnutrition and infection. Conversely, when adequate nutrients are restored to children's diets, improvements in health can be obvious.

Later Years

Older adults are also at risk for undernutrition. They often require nutrient-dense foods, in amounts depending on their state of health and degree of physical activity. Because many of them have fixed incomes and incur significant medical costs, food often becomes a low-priority item. In addition, older adults are often unable to take care of all their own needs, are sometimes isolated, and may be depressed—all important factors that influence food intake (see Chapter 18).

■ General Effects of Semistarvation

In the initial stages, the results of undernutrition from semistarvation are often so mild that physical symptoms are absent and blood tests do not usually detect the slight metabolic changes. Even in the absence of clinical symptoms, however, undernourishment may affect reproductive capacity, resistance to and recovery from disease, physical activity and work output, and lead to lassitude and behavior problems.[10] Recall from Chapter 4 that, as tissues continue to be depleted of nutrients, blood tests eventually detect biochemical changes, such as a drop in blood hemoglobin concentration. Physical symptoms, such as body weakness, appear with further depletion. Finally, the full-blown symptoms of the predominating deficiency are recognizable, such as when edema accompanies a protein deficiency.

In general, when a few people in a population develop a severe deficiency, this represents only the tip of the iceberg. Typically, a much greater number have milder degrees of undernutrition. These deficiencies should not, therefore, be dismissed as trivial, especially in the developing world.[17] It is becoming clear that combined deficiencies of specific vitamins and the minerals iron and zinc can seriously reduce work performance, even when they don't cause obvious physical symptoms.

In the 1940s, a group of researchers led by Dr. Ansel Keys maintained 32 previously healthy men on a diet averaging about 1600 kcal daily for 6 months. During this time, the men lost an average of 24% of their body weight. After about 3 months, the participants complained of fatigue, muscle soreness, irritability, and hunger pains. They exhibited a lack of ambition and self-discipline and poor concentration. They were often moody and depressed. They became less able to laugh heartily, sneeze, and tolerate heat. Heart rate and muscle tone also decreased. When the men were permitted to eat normally again, the desire for more food and a feeling of fatigue continued, even after 12 weeks of rehabilitation. Full recovery required about 33 weeks.

The effects of undernutrition in poor countries are probably even greater than this research indicated because the participants in this study had adequate vitamin and mineral intakes. In addition, the inhabitants of poorer countries must contend with recurrent infections, poor sanitary conditions, extreme weather conditions, and regular exposure to extremely infectious diseases. They require greater amounts of certain nutrients—especially iron—to combat rampant parasite and other infections, which compounds the problem. Deficiencies in both iron and zinc can lead to reduced immune function and thereby increase the risk of disease caused by infections such as diarrhea, pneumonia, and dysentery.[24] This state of ill health, in turn, diminishes the ability of individuals, communities, and even whole countries to perform at peak levels of physical and mental capacity, creating a dearth in human resources.

A common consequence of undernutrition in the United States and worldwide is an increased rate of infant mortality. The U.S. infant mortality rate is currently higher than that of 24 other industrialized countries. Contributing to infant mortality here are teenage pregnancy and inadequate food intake. Young mothers frequently don't meet their nutrient needs, which increases their risk of delivering a low-birth-weight infant. These babies are much more likely to contract life-threatening infections.

CONCEPT CHECK

*H*unger is the uneasiness and pain that result when insufficient food is eaten to meet energy needs. Chronic hunger leads to undernutrition, which can cause growth failure in children and weakness in adults. Risk of infection increases, and nutrient-deficiency diseases result. The primary cause of undernutrition is poverty. The critical periods for undernutrition occur during pregnancy, infancy, childhood, and old age. Chronic undernutrition causes decreased work performance and motivation and compromises immune function. The adverse effects in pregnancy and infancy are quite dramatic, as evidenced by mortality rates much higher than those of healthy populations.

■ UNDERNUTRITION IN THE UNITED STATES

About 33 million Americans live at or near the poverty level, currently estimated at about $16,450 annually for a family of four (Table 20-3). These poor include about 20% of all children; children, in fact, comprise about 40% of the poor.[12]

Currently, 8% of Caucasians are poor, 24% of African-Americans are poor, 23% of Hispanics are poor. Many native Americans are also poor, as are a small proportion of Asian-Americans.

Poor Americans often face difficult choices: whether to buy groceries for the family or pay this month's rent; whether to have dental work done or pay the current utility bill; whether to replace clothes the children have outgrown or pay for

*H*unger reduces energy and strength; it diminishes concentration. Hunger reduces a child's ability to learn. Hunger hurts businesses when workers are more concerned about their next meal than the task at hand. Hunger among older adults makes chronic health conditions worse and can cause others. Hunger is patient, quiet, and persistent, and its effects can be life-long.

■ CASE SCENARIO
Follow-Up

Jamal should not be surprised that the children in the village were often sick and listless. Vitamin A, iron, iodide and zinc deficiencies contribute to poor growth and depressed immune function. One or more of these deficiencies are likely seen in many children in the village. The diets of these children may also be marginal in protein and calories, further contributing to poor growth and overall health. We know from many nutrition intervention studies that the provision of more calories, protein, vitamin A, iron, iodide, and zinc—along with other micronutrients—can reverse some of this disease pattern and improve health. Still, we know that many children throughout the world exist in a stunted and immune-depressed state associated with their chronically deficient diets.

Undernutrition in the United States is a much more subtle problem than in developing countries. To the untrained eye, undernourished children may just seem skinny, when, in fact, their growth is being stunted by insufficient nutrients. It is also possible that poverty-stricken children in this country are overweight. This is because quick-service restaurants provide cheap, accessible food, and, consequently, the poor often eat a diet high in fat and calories.

transportation to apply for a job. Food is one of the few flexible items in a poor person's budget. Rents are fixed, utility costs aren't negotiable, the price of medical care and prescription drugs can't be bargained down, and bus drivers won't accept less than the going rate to transport riders. A person can always eat less, however. The short-term consequences may be less dramatic than having the utilities shut off. The long-term cumulative effects, however, are disturbing.[12]

In sheer numbers, undernutrition in the United States is a troubling problem. Its existence is all the more disturbing because, although the threat of undernutrition for most Americans was virtually eliminated in the 1970s, it reemerged and spread rapidly in the 1980s. The fact that undernutrition and hunger remain today indicates that their roots are mainly political and socioeconomic, rather than technical. Clearly, American society is productive enough to generate the resources required to feed all its citizens. (In the developing world, far more factors complicate this problem.)

▪ Helping Hungry Americans: A Historical Perspective

Until the twentieth century, individuals and a wide variety of charitable, often church-related organizations provided most of the help to poor, undernourished people in the United States. Few early efforts distributed direct cash payments to poor people because these were thought to reduce recipients' motivation to improve their circumstances or change behavior, such as excessive drinking, that contributed to their poverty. Beginning in the early 1900s, the involvement of local, county, and state governments in providing assistance to the poor has steadily increased.

Depression Era to the Mid-1970s

The Great Depression of the 1930s marked a decisive change. Studies at the time documented both undernutrition and the existence of widespread pellagra (niacin deficiency) and rickets (vitamin D deficiency). In response, the federal government sponsored soup kitchens and other programs that distributed food commodities throughout the country. During World War II, a large percentage of the men

The presence of undernutrition in the United States raises a broad question for our society at large: Where can people in such situations turn when their own resources fail? The responsibility for helping those in need could lie with the federal, state, and local governments; religious groups; charitable organizations; and in many cases with the individuals themselves. All can be part of the solution.[17]

TABLE 20-3 The Realities of Poverty and Undernutrition in the United States

- About 7.5% of infants born in the United States are low birth weight. This accounts for more than half of all infant deaths and for 75% of deaths of babies under 1 month of age.
- The infant mortality rate in the United States is higher than that of 24 other industrialized countries. Teenage pregnancy contributes to infant mortality because young mothers frequently don't meet their nutrient needs.
- Single-parent families constitute about 25% of all families with children. The poverty rate (60%) for the approximately 14 million children in such families is five times higher than that for children in two-parent families.
- About 35 million Americans live at or near the poverty level. These poor include about 17% of all children; children, in fact, comprise 39% of the poor. Hunger frequently accompanies poverty.
- A family of four in the United States at the bottom 20% of households has an average income of $17,196. Contrast that to the average earnings of the top 20% of households: $79,375.
- In the United States, an estimated 12 million people, or 6.5% of all adults, have experienced homelessness sometime during their lives. An episode of homelessness nearly always lasts for at least 1 week and often for a month or more.
- The Food Stamp program for low-income people provides each household with $170 per month. About 1 American in 13 currently participates in this program.
- Second Harvest, the largest U.S. food bank, estimates that 26 million people, or more than 1 American in 10, rely on food depositories and soup kitchens to feed themselves and their families. Most of these people, the organization reports, are workers who have lost their jobs.
- Food thrown out in U.S. cafeterias, grocery stores, and restaurants could feed 49 million people per year.

rejected for physical reasons by the draft were found to have been undernourished 10 to 12 years earlier, during the Depression era. This practical demonstration of the long-term detrimental effects of childhood undernutrition led Congress to enact legislation setting up the school lunch program in 1946.

In the 1950s, it was assumed that all Americans had enough to eat. Nevertheless, occasional reports of undernutrition surfaced, mostly among the truly destitute: migrant workers, Native Americans, African-Americans in the South, unemployed minorities in general, and some older people.

After observing extensive hunger and poverty during his presidential campaign in the 1960s, John F. Kennedy revitalized the Food Stamp program, which actually had begun two decades earlier, and expanded commodity distribution programs. The Food Stamp program for low-income people allows recipients to use food stamps to purchase food and seeds—but not tobacco, cleaning items, alcoholic beverages, and nonedible products—at stores authorized to accept them. Each household currently receives about $170 per month, on average. Currently about 1 in 13 Americans participates in this program (Table 20-4).[16]

TABLE 20-4   Some Current Federally Subsidized Programs That Supply Food for Americans

Program	Eligibility	Description
Food Stamps	Low income; employment generally necessary	Coupons are given to purchase food at grocery stores; the amount is based on size of household and income.
Emergency Food System	Low income	Food stamps are issued on 24-hour notice for 1 month while eligibility for further use of the program can be investigated.
Commodity Supplemental Food Program	Certain low-income populations, such as pregnant women and young children	USDA surplus foods are distributed by county agencies.
Special Supplemental Feeding Program for Women, Infants, and Children (WIC)	Low-income pregnant/lactating women, infants, and children less than 5 years old at nutritional risk	Coupons are given to purchase milk, cheese, fruit juice, cereal, infant formula, and other specific food items at grocery stores.
School Lunch	Low income	Free or reduced-price lunch is distributed by the school; meal follows USDA pattern based on the Food Guide Pyramid; cost for the child depends on family income. In schools without a lunch program, special milk program may be available.
School Breakfast	Low income	Free or reduced-price breakfast is distributed by the school; meal follows USDA pattern; cost for the child depends on family income.
Child Care Food Program	Child enrolled in organized child-care program; income guidelines are the same as School Lunch program	Reimbursement is given for meals supplied to children at the site; meals must follow USDA guidelines based on the Food Guide Pyramid.
Congregate Meals for the Elderly	Age 60 or over (no income guidelines)	Free noon meal is furnished at a site; meal follows specific pattern based on one-third of nutrient needs.
Home-Delivered Meals	Age 60 or over, homebound	Noon meal is delivered at no cost or for a fee, depending on income, at least 5 days a week. Sometimes other meals for later consumption are delivered at the same time; private organizations that sponsor these programs often refer to them as "Meals on Wheels."
Summer Food Service Program	Low income	Free, nutritious meals and snacks are given to a group of children in a low-income area at a central site, such as a school or a community center during long school vacations.

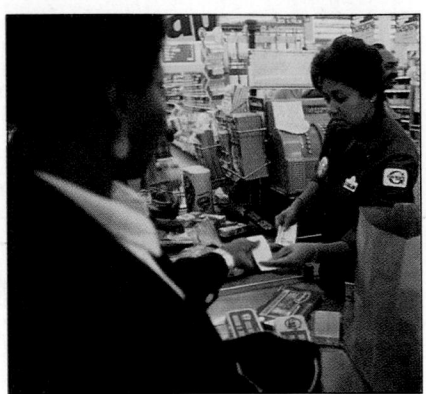

Food stamps are part of the social safety net in the United States.

Congress established the school breakfast program in 1965 as politicians were made aware of the number of children coming to school hungry. School lunch and breakfast programs still enable low-income students—6.4 million for breakfast and 27 million for lunch—to receive meals free or at reduced cost if certain income guidelines are met (under $26,500 annual income for a family of four). In the same year, Congress funded group noontime (called *congregate*) meals and home-delivered meals for all citizens over 60 years of age, regardless of income. Both remain active programs, serving about 1 million meals each day, but they still do not reach all who need help. In addition, in 1972 the Special Supplemental Feeding Program for Women, Infants, and Children (WIC) was authorized. This program provides food vouchers and nutrition education to low-income pregnant and lactating women and their young children. Today, it serves about 7 million people.[22]

Political and social awareness of hunger and undernutrition in the late 1960s was spurred on by the book *Hunger USA* and a resulting television documentary, *Hunger in America,* shown in May 1968. The film graphically demonstrated that hunger exists in all areas and ethnic groups in the United States. The response was dramatic. Between 1969 and 1971, some already large federal food programs were expanded and others were created. For example, the Food Stamp program served only 2 million people in 1968, but by 1971 it was serving 11 million. The School Lunch program, which served only 2 million poor children before 1970, was serving 8 million children by 1971. Soon after, the School Breakfast program, a pilot program for children living in impoverished areas, became nationally available. And, as just mentioned, in 1972 the Special Supplemental Feeding Program for Women, Infants, and Children (WIC) began.

A Reevaluation for Our Times

The first official recognition that widespread hunger had reappeared in the United States came from a conference of mayors in 1982. Why was there a sudden increase in hungry people in the United States? First, unemployment in the United States rose in early 1980. Second, the eligibility and funding for federal food assistance programs, such as the Food Stamp program and the School Lunch and Breakfast programs, were tightened and reduced, respectively. Overall, the safety net of the previous decade became more porous: hunger and related food insecurity has thus continued to be a problem in the United States.

USDA defines this food insecurity as not having enough food, enough money to buy food, or experiencing concern over having enough food. Food insecurity includes limiting or reducing food intake, cutting or skipping meals, or feeding children a less than nutritious diet, without resorting to unusual strategies to obtain food (e.g., stealing or scavenging). In contrast, food security means household members had access at all times to enough food for an active, healthy life.[12]

Privately funded programs have stepped in to take an important role in augmenting state and federal efforts to combat hunger and related food insecurity in the United States. There are currently more than 180 food banks, 23,000 food pantries, and 3300 soup kitchens helping to cope with this problem. A recent survey found that slightly more than two of every three people requesting such emergency food assistance were members of families—children and their parents. America's Second Harvest, the nation's largest domestic hunger-relief organization, has recently merged with Food Chain, a leader in food-rescue programs, to better serve the 36 million Americans who face hunger. Second Harvest estimates that more than 1 in 10 of all Americans rely on food depositories and soup kitchens to feed themselves and their families, and the number is on the rise. Nearly 40% of people asking for help lived in families with at least one working adult.

■ Socioeconomic Factors Related to Undernutrition

In the United States today, persistent hunger and food insecurity are largely associated with two interrelated conditions: poverty and homelessness. Thus, the economic, social, and political changes that lead to an increase in the number of poor or homeless people also tend to intensify the problem.[21]

Poverty

Although highly trained people are quite competitive in the increasingly global economy, there is a glut of unskilled manual labor available throughout the world. Many families have suffered economic hardship caused by massive layoffs in U.S. manufacturing industries, which began in the late 1980s and continue in the 1990s as the economy became more global. Furthermore, many jobs created in the 1980s were in the service sector, such as quick-service restaurants. When one or both parents have one of these low-paying jobs—even full-time—their families may still be at or below the poverty level. Note that parents in most poor families do work; nearly two in three contain at least one worker.

Another primary factor contributing to poverty has been the dramatic increase in the number of single-parent families in the United States, the result of high rates of divorce and out-of-wedlock births. Currently, single-parent families constitute about 25% of all families with children. The poverty rate (60%) for the approximately 19 million children in single-parent families is five times higher than the rate for those in two-parent families.

Some observers believe that many publicly funded assistance programs have actually provided an incentive for poor single women to have more children: The more children they have, the more welfare and other assistance benefits they receive. The new welfare reform laws reflect this thinking by requiring able-bodied Americans to get jobs, limiting future direct support to 3 years in a row and a total of 5 years in a lifetime. It is up to each state to determine how to implement this work requirement and establish exceptions, such as in the case of disability or other overwhelming hardships.[9]

Many politicians and political writers point out that we need greater wisdom in our approach to illegitimacy and single parenthood. Some suggestions have been to improve child care, to teach parenting skills, and to expand job opportunities. To a great extent, states are doing this as they help people end their dependence on welfare payments. Nationwide the number of people on welfare rolls has fallen 60% since 1992.

Homelessness

The economics of poverty and undernutrition have changed in one additional important way. Homelessness is much more evident now than in 1980. Families with children currently account for about 43% of the homeless. An estimated 12 million people, or 6.5% of all adults, in the United States have experienced homelessness sometime during their lives. Episodes of homelessness nearly always last for at least 1 week and often for a month or more. The estimated lifetime homelessness rate rises to about 15% of the adult population in the United States when it includes people who have moved into someone else's residence during periods when they had nowhere else to live.

Although many citizens of the United States in general are enjoying continuing prosperity, the economic status of many of the working poor has declined because affordable housing is harder and harder for them to find.[18] Due to the nation's rising prosperity, higher-income tenants have bid up the prices of the apartments in some cities beyond the abilities of the poorer tenants. The government considers housing costs, which include rent and utilities, to be affordable if they consume no more than 30% of a family's income. A recent federal report stated that 5.4 million low-income families pay more than half their incomes for housing or live in dilapidated units. These families, although not homeless, are likely to experience undernutrition without direct food assistance. Moreover, the continuing changes in the economic circumstances they face could force such poor families into actual homelessness, at least temporarily.[26]

The availability of cooking facilities affects nutrient intake among the poor. Without cooking facilities, people may buy expensive foods that require no preparation. These are typically processed snack foods, which provide food energy but are often lacking in nutrients.

Homeless children suffer higher rates of many medical problems than do other children, some of which include
- Upper respiratory tract infections
- Scabies and lice
- Tooth decay
- Ear and skin infections
- Diaper rash
- Conjunctivitis
- Developmental delays
- Visual problems
- Trauma-related injuries

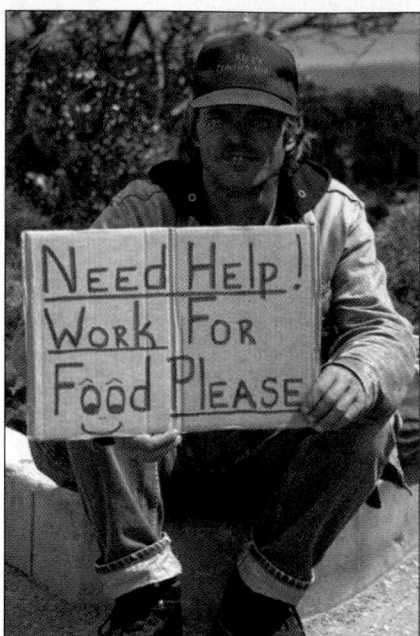

Major job layoffs in blue-collar industries have contributed to the twin problems of hunger and homelessness in the United States.

Other important causes of homelessness include the widespread release of mentally ill patients from mental institutions in the 1980s, unemployment, substance abuse, and personal crises. The abuse of alcohol and crack cocaine is another notable cause. Nationally, up to 85% of all homeless people in large cities abuse alcohol or drugs or have a mental illness. Most people with such problems are unable to find and hold employment; without support from family or friends, they and their dependents will probably become homeless.

■ Possible Solutions to Hunger in the United States

Few would argue the need to support physically and mentally handicapped Americans, as well as the multitude of poor children in this country. The debate begins when able-bodied adults are receiving public aid. Many of these people have extenuating circumstances or have dug such a deep hole for themselves financially that it is difficult to get out. It is also true that the United States has enough money and food to feed every citizen. The question is, can government programs provide a permanent solution to poverty?

Private emergency-food network systems are also important, as noted earlier, but are not sufficient to meet all food needs in the United States.[12] Furthermore, most of the donated items are limited in nutritional value. By necessity, processed and canned grocery items predominate, rather than protein-rich foods and perishable items, such as fresh produce and milk.

Still, a long-term solution to the problem of hunger in the United States can't be achieved by the government or private agencies alone. Change also requires a cultural shift emphasizing the responsibility of all citizens to provide as best they can for themselves, their families, and the less fortunate around them.[17] Many Americans consider an increase in individual responsibility as a critical goal for our society at this time. Government programs can't easily fix poverty and the resulting hunger that stem from irresponsible individual behavior. Government programs can, however, help reduce or prevent the poverty that results largely from lack of opportunity.[1]

Clearly, the victims of poverty don't deserve all the blame. Poorer Americans confront substantial difficulties: substandard education and training, poor communication skills, lack of reliable and safe child care, inability to relocate, little employment experience, and no economic reserves to fall back on during crises. Even with a strong desire for a better life, people may get discouraged and apathetic in the face of apparently insurmountable obstacles. Moreover, many poor Americans are unable to meet the demands of a modern, dynamic society—in particular, older adults, sick, and disabled people and young single mothers and their children. Regardless of how repugnant government assistance appears to some people, it will probably always be necessary to some extent.

Because long-term undernutrition—especially among children—has both individual and societal consequences, all Americans are affected by this problem, either directly or indirectly. The next few years are likely to bring further changes in both government and private assistance programs, demanding new initiatives from all Americans. As the welfare system is reformed and government programs are redesigned, it is likely that some will suffer. The hope is that these new approaches will lead to long-term progress and the eventual relief of poverty and hunger.

CONCEPT CHECK

Federal programs designed to reduce hunger and undernutrition began in the 1930s, during the Great Depression. In response to reports of widespread poverty and hunger during the early 1960s, Congress established several federal food assistance programs and substantially increased funding for already existing programs. Largely as a result of these federal programs, undernutrition had decreased substantially by the mid-1970s.

The improvement was short-lived, and the number of Americans experiencing poverty, homelessness, and undernutrition grew during the 1980s and 1990s linked to federal cutbacks in human services programs. The presence of these three interrelated problems is influenced by economic, cultural, and individual factors, as well as government policies. The serious questions about the long-term effectiveness of many government assistance programs are causing major changes in their future administration, funding mechanisms, and program design. All citizens can help reduce the problem of undernutrition.

∎ UNDERNUTRITION IN THE DEVELOPING WORLD

Undernutrition in the developing world is also tied to poverty, and any true solution must address this problem. However, these countries have a multitude of problems so complex and interrelated that they cannot be treated separately. Programs that have proved immensely helpful in the United States are only a starting point in this context. The following major obstacles challenge those seeking a solution:

- Extreme imbalances in the food/population ratio in different regions of a country
- War and political/civil unrest
- The rapid depletion of natural resources
- Cultural attitudes toward certain foods
- High external debt
- Poor **infrastructure,** especially poor housing, sanitation and storage facilities, education, communications, and transportation systems

Each problem deserves individual consideration. In this context, Figure 20-2 depicts key factors relating to a household's food intake.

infrastructure The basic framework of a system of organization. For a society, this includes roads, bridges, telephones, and other basic technologies.

∎ Food/Population Ratio

Whether the earth can produce enough food for all people has been a long-standing question. As early as 1798, English clergyman and political economist Thomas Malthus proposed a rather pessimistic view of our prospects. He said that, given the passion between the sexes (which he felt should be discouraged), the population would always increase faster than the food supply. Malthus felt that the growing population would therefore be subject to recurring checks imposed by widespread starvation, war, or natural catastrophe brought on by disease.

Malthus's proposals became the object of intense controversy in England and elsewhere, often meeting vigorous opposition. Eminent British scientists pointed out that scientific advances in agriculture would greatly increase food production. In fact, that has proved true. Nevertheless, the aptly named population explosion has undermined this progress. Overall population growth has not slowed significantly through natural checks, disease, or recent human interventions, such as birth control. In the year 1800, 1 billion people inhabited the earth. By the year 2000, this number has skyrocketed to more than 6 billion. By 2050, the United Nations estimates that the world population could reach almost 9 billion. (The recent spread of AIDS throughout the world has put into question these future population estimates [see the Nutrition Perspective]).

Currently, population growth exceeds economic growth in much of the world, and poverty is increasing. Because efforts to speed up economic development have failed, the only remaining way to improve the situation may be to slow down the growth of population, as Malthus recommended. If we want to ensure a decent life for a widening segment of humanity, the growth in the earth's population should slow.[6] According to the World Bank, the world's population increases by 1 billion people every 12 years, mostly in cities and in seacoast and river-basin areas, where the environment is most under stress. By 2050, the world will have more than 3 billion more people than today—2 billion of them in countries where the average

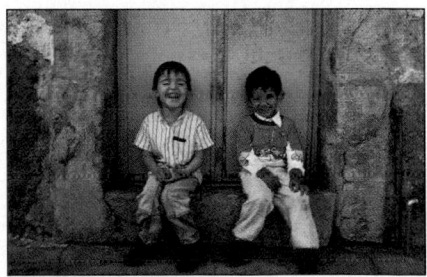

Minimal intakes of protein and zinc limit the growth of children worldwide.

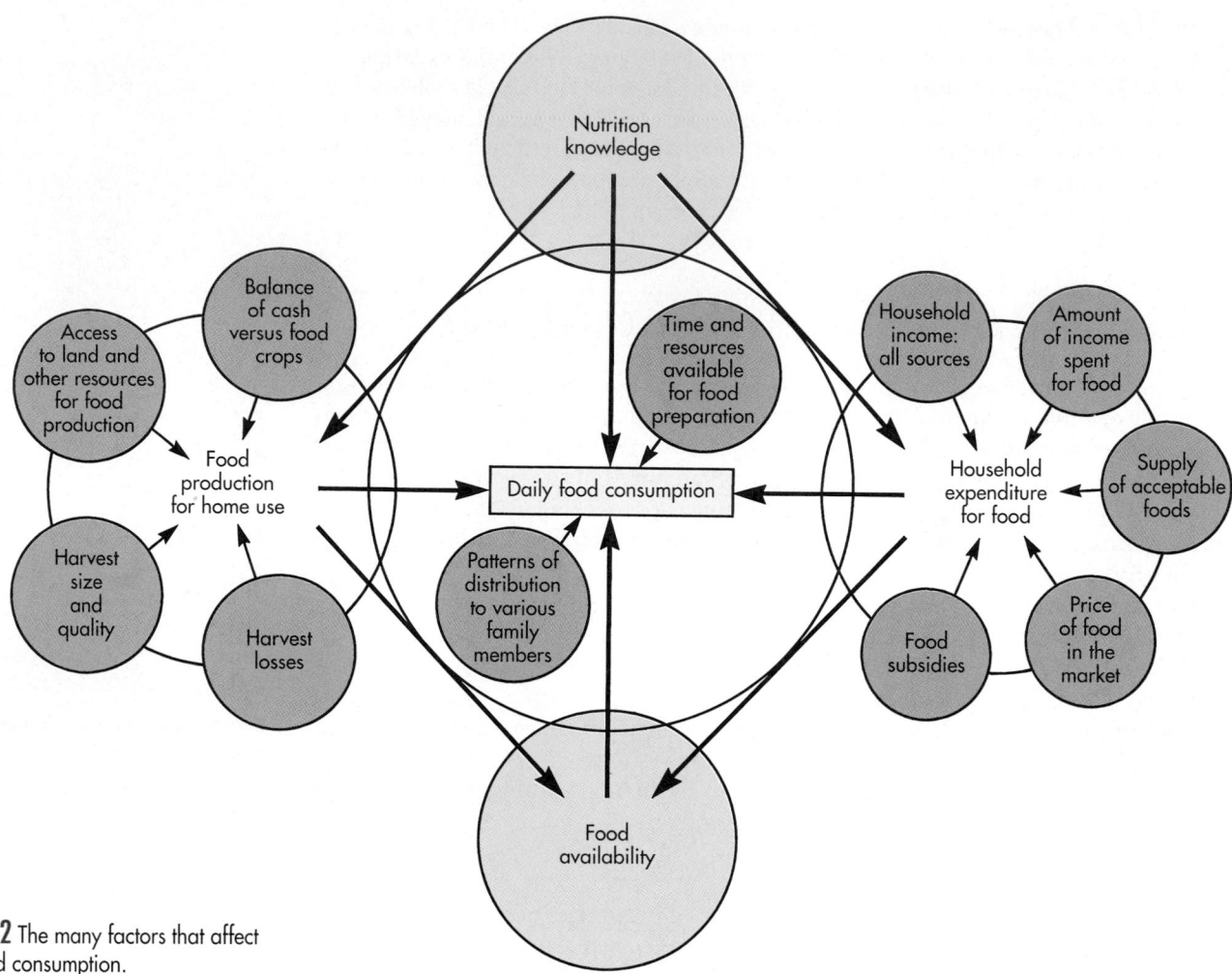

■ FIGURE 20-2 The many factors that affect household food consumption.

person earns less than $2 a day. Unless a catastrophe occurs, more than 9 of 10 infants in the next generation will be born in the poorest parts of the world.

Of the 6 billion people in the world, more than three-quarters live in countries in the developing world, and more than half live in Asia. A recent United Nations report on worldwide hunger revealed that 826 million people in the developing world are chronically undernourished, and almost two-thirds of the world's undernourished live in Asia and the Pacific. The world's food supplies also are not distributed equally among consumers. Gross disparities exist between developed and developing countries, among the rich and poor within countries, and even within families.[10]

Food supply and population trends within the developing world also vary greatly. Japan is facing a large decrease in its population over the next 50 years unless the birth rate increases from the average of 1.4 children per family to at least 2. On the other hand, the population in Africa will have more than doubled, constituting 19% of the world population. When the world's population hit 6 billion in 2000, it doubled the number of people on earth in less than 40 years.

Economists estimate that world food production will, in fact, continue to increase more rapidly than the world population in the near future, allowing the food/population ratio to increase through the year 2020. In the short run, then, the primary problem appears to be not food production but distribution and use, especially in poverty-stricken areas of the developing nations.

Eventually, though, food production will probably begin to lag behind population growth.[6] We are currently drifting in that direction. Most good farmland in the world is already in use, and because of poor farming practices or competing land-use demands, the number of farmable acres worldwide decreases annually. For many reasons, sustainable world food output—an amount that doesn't deplete the earth's resources—is now running well behind food consumption.[17] This discrepancy suggests that food production in less-developed countries will barely keep up with population growth and will soon lag behind.

Due to its exponential nature, reproduction is said to be the ultimate driving force behind consumption. Although efforts on the supply side of the food/population ratio are essential, many researchers still emphasize the need to reduce the demand side. They argue that the survival of our civilization depends on limiting reproduction.

For millions of years, maximizing reproduction has been a measure of biological success. Because disease and difficult living conditions often claimed young lives, couples produced many offspring in an attempt to ensure the longevity of the family. These conditions still exist in countries in the developing world, where children also provide the primary means of support to their parents in old age. More children also means more helpers to farm, hunt, and prepare food. In India, a rigid class structure, which leaves many people destitute, encourages large families. Traditionally, poorer people bear more children, contrary to what you might predict. Now, in an evolutionary blink of the eye—mere decades—poor people in developing nations are being asked to reverse their attitude toward having children. It is a difficult undertaking.

As one brake on population expansion, birth control programs have been effective in developed countries but relatively ineffective in developing countries—those that could really profit from them. Family planning and contraceptive use has increased to 60% of women today, up from 10% of women in 1969. If the United Nations, voluntary organizations, and governments had not started promoting family planning and contraceptive use, the population today may be as high as 7 or 8 billion. However, women (and men) in many countries are still lacking adequate access to contraceptives. There are women in Sri Lanka who want to control their fertility but are so poor that they have to buy oral contraceptive tablets 5 at a time, rather than in a monthly pack of 21.[23] Organizations such as Population Services International are trying to keep distribution costs low and make the products available to as many people as possible by subsidizing condoms and oral contraceptives to areas such as Bangladesh. Unless people are given the option of controlling their fertility, severe environmental and health problems loom in the near future throughout large parts of the world.[20]

Still, experience with family-planning programs in developing countries and historical changes in birth rates in many industrialized countries suggest an important conclusion: Only when people have enough to eat and are financially secure do they feel safe that having fewer children will still result in enough sons and/or daughters that survive in order to provide for care in older years. Increasing per capita income and improving education, especially for women in developing nations, are currently considered to be the most likely long-term solutions to excessive population growth.

In addition to economics, other obstacles to family-planning programs are ancient cultural, religious, and traditional beliefs. In sub-Saharan Africa, childlessness signifies the end of a line of descent, and women who don't have children are often perceived as evil. The Yoruba believe, for example, that a childless woman made a pact with evil spirits before her own birth to kill her children and, devoid of descendants, will return to join these evil spirits in some otherworldly sphere. These women fear being rendered functionally infertile by the death of all their children almost as much as they fear bearing none. Thus, female sterilization and even contraception have not been successful. Even women with four or five children fear, not unreasonably, that all their children may suddenly die. Also, Moslem religious practices typically promote a large, abundant family as a sign of prosperity and health.

By taking on the twin challenges of economic insecurity and population growth, the developing world can begin to escape the expensive trap of humanitarian intervention and crisis management for peoples in need.[17] Otherwise, it is likely that Malthus's gloomy prediction may soon become a fact.

In the 1960s, South Korean families averaged six children each. Through economic policies and family planning programs, this number has been decreased to two. Other countries, such as Indonesia and Thailand, prove that industrialization is not a prerequisite to population control but, rather, family-planning programs can lead to economic success.

Breastfeeding aids in family planning because it helps space births farther apart. If no supplemental nourishment is given, breastfeeding an infant decreases ovulation—and therefore, the likelihood of fertilization—for an average of about 6 months, although breastfeeding is not a completely reliable form of birth control. When childbirths are more widely spaced, mother and infant are healthier and fewer total births occur. Women who do not breastfeed generally begin to ovulate within a month or so after giving birth.

CONCEPT CHECK

*C*urrently, world food production is sufficient to meet the energy needs of the world's population. Despite adequate food resources, however, undernutrition exists because of poverty, politics, and unequal distribution. In addition, projected population growth may soon overwhelm food production. Most scientists and world leaders recommend limiting population growth, especially in developing countries where birth rates are high.

■ War and Political/Civil Unrest

The recent Millennium Summit of the United Nations pledged to "spare no effort to free our peoples from the scourge of war." Against that background stands the reality that worldwide military spending has doubled over the past 20 years. In the twentieth century, deadly weapons of war took an enormous toll on civilians living in poor, politically vulnerable, war-torn nations. Although Africa has been ravaged by economic decay and famines for years, military spending in Africa more than doubled in the 1970s and held firm through the 1990s. Currently, less than one-half of 1% of the world's yearly production of goods and services is devoted to economic development assistance, whereas approximately 6% goes to military expenditures.

Civil disruptions and wars are setting back the progress of the poor and contribute to massive undernutrition.[3] War-related famine affects at least 20 million people in southern and northeastern Africa. The border war between Ethiopia and neighboring Eritrea has had a tremendous impact on government resources. A World Bank official stated that the food shortage in Ethiopia is a problem that will persist until political changes are made. Currently, 12.4 million people in Ethiopia, Eritrea, Djibouti, Kenya, and Somalia are at risk for food shortages resulting in starvation. Other conflicts continue between Congo and the Republic of Congo, as well as in Angola, where millions have been left to starve. Most of these people are without shelter, clothing, food, and any means of obtaining them.[10] Worldwide this entire problem is projected to worsen over the next 15 years. Globally, civil strife currently involving 68 different conflicts puts 100 million people at risk for hunger.

Even when food is available, political divisions may impede distribution to the point that undernutrition will plague many people for years to come. Especially during emergencies, programs designed to help the poor have been undermined by poor administration, corruption, and political influence. During such political chaos, relief agencies are often caught between waring factions and those they are trying to help. This was the case in Zaire, where Rwandan refugee camps fell under the control of a militant group. The rebels controlled the food coming in the camps and would not allow relief agencies to do their work.

During the 1960s and 1970s, the problem of undernutrition in less-developed countries was perceived as a technical one: how to produce enough food for the growing world population. The problem is now seen as largely political: how to achieve cooperation among and within nations, so that gains in food production and infrastructure are not wiped out by war. Only a combination of approaches—finding technical solutions that may help with the problems of chronic hunger and poverty and solving political crises that push disadvantaged nations into a state of acute hunger and chaos—will help.[6]

■ Rapid Depletion of Natural Resources

As we quickly deplete the earth's resources, population control grows increasingly critical. The productive capacity of agriculture is approaching its limits in many areas worldwide. Environmentally unsustainable farming methods undermine food production, especially in parts of the developing world.[17]

The term **green revolution** describes a phenomenon that began in the 1960s when crop yields rose dramatically in some countries, such as the Philippines, India,

*T*he Nutrition Perspective at the end of this chapter discusses the impact of AIDS worldwide. Currently in the developing world, the impact of AIDS is analogous to that of ongoing war and civil strife, as it disrupts the lives of families, communities, and entire nations.

green revolution This refers to increases in crop yields that accompany the introduction of new agricultural technologies in less-developed countries, beginning in the 1960s. The key technologies were high-yielding, disease-resistant strains of rice, wheat, and corn; greater use of fertilizer and water; and improved cultivation practices.

and Mexico. The increased use of fertilizers, irrigation, and the development of superior crops through careful plant breeding made this rise possible. Many of the technologies associated with the green revolution have now achieved most of their potential. For example, rice yield has not increased significantly since the release of superior varieties in 1966.

Future gains in productivity may be much harder to accomplish because of the need to farm less productive soils. Until the introduction of another superior strain of rice or other grain, developing countries will not benefit greatly from recent, more modest breakthroughs in biotechnology (see the section on use of biotechnology). Actually, the green revolution was never intended to solve the world's food problems, according to Dr. Norman Borlaug, its chief architect. It was just a stop-gap measure until world leaders could control population growth.

Areas of the world that remain uncultivated or ungrazed are mostly unsuited to farming: rocky, steep, infertile, too dry, too wet, or inaccessible. Much of this land is nonetheless invaluable for the crucial **ecosystem** benefits it provides. This is particularly true for humid tropical areas, such as the Amazon basin rain forests, which significantly influence the earth's climate, most notably through oxygen production. Some nations, such as Brazil, can still expand onto arable land, but such countries are in the minority. Even then, this expansion in Brazil causes further rain forest devastation.

In Africa, an area of land twice the size of New Jersey is turned into unproductive desert each year because of soil erosion. The erosion results from overgrazing by livestock, destructive farming techniques, and burning of mature rain forests. Also, the cultivation of many **cash crops** in African countries damages the land, draining the soil of vital nutrients. Then, when the land has been used up, farmers move on to other areas, leaving behind desolate land vulnerable to soil erosion. In the short run, farmers can overplow and overpump water with impressive results, but in the long run they use up natural resources on which long-term productivity depends. Soil erosion is also a problem in the United States. Farmland equivalent in size to Ireland is currently lost in the United States to erosion every year. New farming techniques, such as "no till" planting, where plowing is kept to a minimum, are helping reverse this trend.

Nearly all irrigation water available worldwide is currently being used, and groundwater supplies are becoming depleted at rapid rates in many regions. The eventual water shortage this will create is projected to even increase war and civil unrest in arid areas of the world, such as Northern Africa and the Middle East. China, which has more than 20% of the world's irrigated land, as well is plagued with a growing scarcity of fresh water.

The prospects of obtaining substantially more food from the oceans are also poor. In recent years, the amount of fish caught worldwide has leveled off at about 80 million metric tons a year. Fish was once considered the poor person's protein. But, without actual farming of fish, this is unlikely to be true again.

Clearly, we can exploit the earth's resources only so far—world population probably can't continue to expand as it does today without the potential for serious famine and death. The Food and Agriculture Organization (FAO) of the United Nations works on this principle: "The fight to ensure that all people have enough nutritious food to eat is worthy of our greatest efforts, but it must be fought with the full recognition that it cannot be won unless agricultural, fishery, and forestry production returns to the earth as much as—or more than—it takes." This statement highlights the need for immediate action to protect the earth's already deteriorated environment from further destruction, if food production is to keep up with the expanding population.[17]

■ Cultural Attitudes Toward Certain Foods

Culture affects food use, just as it does family size. In India, for example, the Hindu reverence for cattle has worsened some already significant nutrition problems. These

ecosystem A community in nature that includes plants, animals, and their environment.

cash crop A crop grown specifically for export, so that goods from other countries can be purchased. Cultivation of cash crops diverts agricultural resources necessary to feed a country's own citizens. Examples of cash crops are coffee, tea, cocoa, and bananas.

In the United States, many people shun potential foods such as horse meat, insects, and algae.

sacred cows consume food rather than provide it; the wandering cows also damage vegetation that could otherwise feed humans. Although the cows provide milk, no attempt is made to improve milk production through selective breeding practices. In certain areas of India, a child may not be fed milk curds, because of a superstitious belief that they inhibit growth. Bananas may not be fed because they supposedly cause convulsions. These are obstacles, but not barriers, to good nutrition. Given adequate food resources, a healthful diet allowing for individual food taboos and prejudices is possible.

■ Inadequate Shelter and Sanitation

When people die from undernutrition in developing countries, other influences, such as inadequate shelter and sanitation, almost always contribute. Poor sanitation raises the risk of infection, as does undernutrition. Together these represent a lethal combination (Fig. 20-3). For example, the 1994 plague, which killed almost 5000 people and sparked the panicked exodus of another half a million in Surat, in northwest India, was linked mainly to unsanitary housing conditions.

Inadequate and deteriorating shelters threaten the lives of more than 500 million people today. Many of the 15 million annual deaths of children—half of them under 5 years old—in developing countries could be prevented by improving the standards of environmental hygiene. Urban populations of some developing countries are currently growing at an annual rate of 5 to 7%. Such a skewed population distribution will result in more poverty. The current urban explosion is the result of both high birth rates and continuing migration of people to the cities from the countryside. People go to the cities to find employment and resources the countryside can no longer provide. Worldwide, 38% of people lived in urban areas in 1975. The figure is now 50%, and is expected to reach 66% by 2025. Nine of the 10 largest cities 20 years from now will be in poor countries. Los Angeles, which is now the seventh largest city in the world, and New York, which is third, will drop far down the list.

In developing countries, the poor make up most of the urban population, and their needs for housing and community services often outstrip available governmental resources. Most of these urban poor live in overcrowded, self-made shelters, which lack a safe and adequate water supply and are only partially served by public utilities. The shantytowns and ghettos of the developing world are often worse than the rural areas the people left behind. Because the urban poor need cash to purchase food, they often subsist on diets that are even more meager than the homegrown rural fare. Making matters worse, haphazard shelters often lack facilities to protect food from spoilage or the ravages of insects and rodents. In some developing countries, food losses can amount to as much as 40% of the perishable foods.

The shift from rural to urban life takes its greatest toll on infants and children. Infants are often weaned early from the breast, partly because the mother must find employment and partly because she may be influenced by the images of sophisticated, formula-using women promoted in advertisements. Unfortunately, because infant formulas are relatively expensive, poor parents may overdilute the mixture or use too little to meet the baby's needs. Because the water supply may not be safe, the prepared formula is also likely to be contaminated with bacteria. Human milk, in contrast, is generally much more hygienic, readily available, and nutritious, and it provides infants with immunity to some ailments. Promoting breastfeeding when it is safe for a mother to breastfeed her baby is important (see the discussion of AIDS in the Nutrition Perspective for further details on when it is safe to breastfeed).[13]

Overall, the single most effective health advantage for people, wherever they live, is a safe and convenient water supply. Inadequate sanitation and the consumption of contaminated water cause 75% of all diseases and more than one-third of all deaths in developing countries. The World Health Organization (WHO) estimates that 1 billion people, about one-sixth of all people, have an unsafe and inadequate water supply. In addition, up to 90% of the diseases seen in developing countries may be attributed to contaminated water.

In Brazil, migrants displaced by multinational land developers have flooded from the north and northeast into Rio de Janeiro and São Paulo, attracted by the prospect of jobs. There they have built shantytowns next to apartment towers and affluent suburbs, but the jobs do not materialize, and urban poverty simply replaces rural impoverishment.

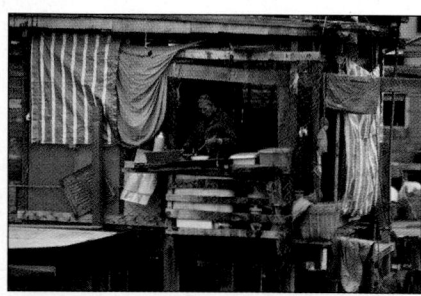

Inadequate sanitation facilities and the consumption of contaminated water cause 75% of all diseases, yet people in developing countries often lack access to a safe water supply.

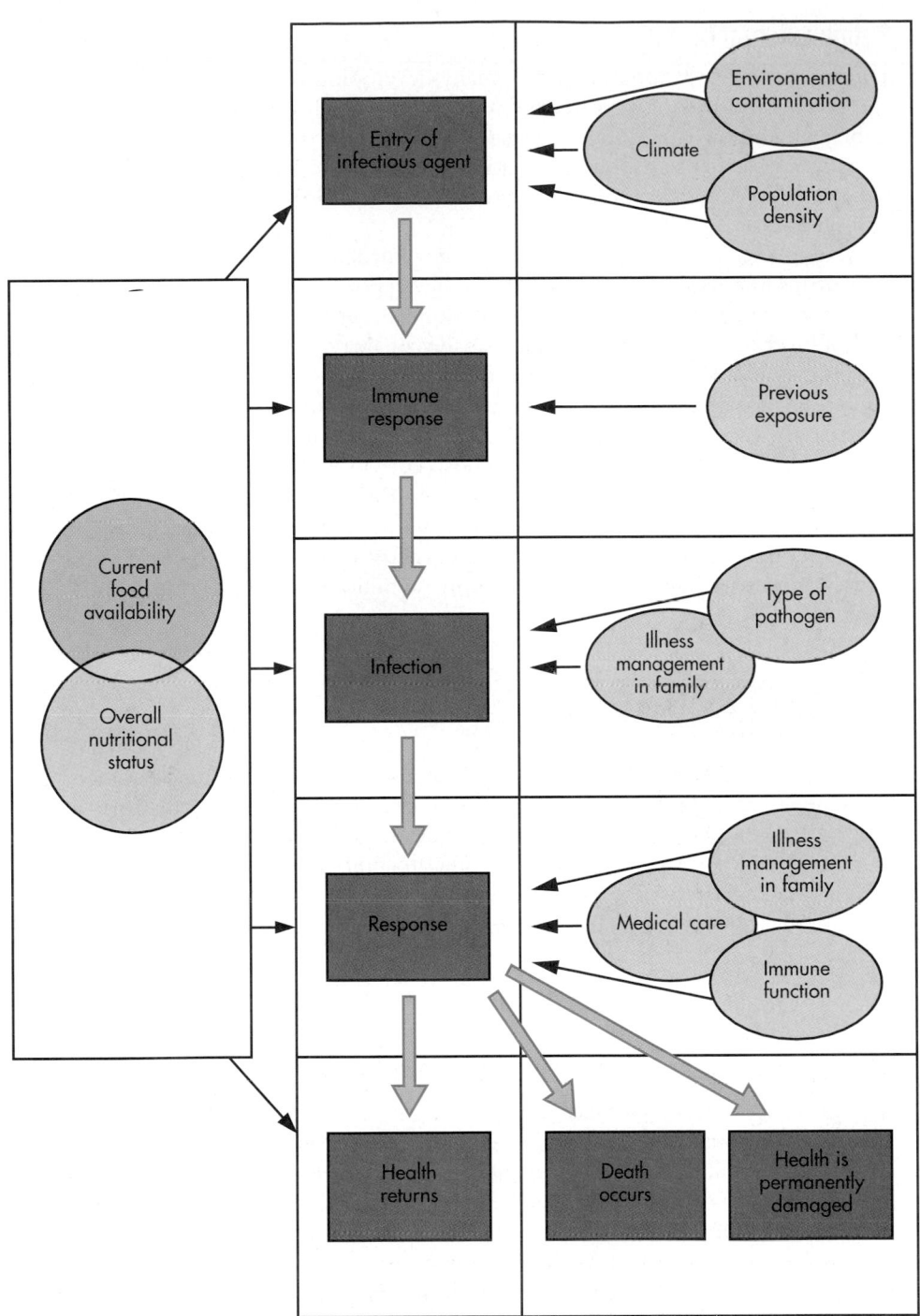

FIGURE 20-3 Nutritional status and overall food supply combine with a variety of environmental factors to influence the risk of infection and ultimate outcome.

Poor sanitation, another example of inadequate infrastructure in the developing world, creates another critical public health problem. Human feces, rotting garbage, and associated insect and rodent infestations are commonly seen in urban areas of the developing world. Potent sources of disease organisms, human urine and feces are two of the most dangerous substances people encounter in routine daily living. The inability to dispose of the massive numbers of dead people (and dead animls) resulting from civil wars causes additional sanitation problems. In some developing countries, diarrheal diseases account for as many as one-third of all deaths in children under 5 years of age. WHO estimates that, even with improvements in housing, 3 billion people in the world still lack proper sanitation facilities.

■ High External Debt

During the 1970s through to 1990, many developing countries became trapped in the cycle of borrowing repeatedly from foreign countries. Servicing these external debts, which now total about $2 trillion, has brought several countries to the verge of economic collapse. About $6 billion is owed to the United States. The external debt of Latin America represents 45% of the region's gross regional output of goods and services.

Many African nations also carry large debt burdens—currently, $350 billion. Recent drops in prices for raw commodities they export, higher prices for imported oil, and embezzlement of funds by high political officials are at the root of this problem. Although the African debts are much smaller in absolute terms than those of Brazil, Argentina, and Mexico, for example, the actual burden is greater when national incomes and export earnings are considered. Nearly half the money African nations earn from exports goes to paying off the continent's multibillion-dollar debt. As a result, African nations have had to impose cuts in domestic programs, which can cause widespread undernutrition in many of these poor nations, in part because these countries still need to import—and pay for—machinery, concrete, trucks, and consumer goods. To make up the difference between export income and import expenses, countries have been forced to borrow billions of dollars from international banks.

CONCEPT CHECK

War and civil strife, along with a decline in the world's natural resources, contribute to the difficulty of ending undernutrition in many developing countries. In addition, inadequate housing conditions, impure water, and inadequate sanitation worldwide increase the risk for infection and disease. Infection then combines with undernutrition to compromise further the health of impoverished people. Finally, many developing countries are burdened by extremely high external debts, which severely limit their ability to implement programs to reduce undernutrition.

■ Reduction of Undernutrition in the Developing World

As you have probably guessed, greatly reducing undernutrition in the developing world will be complicated and will take considerable time to accomplish. Today, it is a common practice for the more affluent nations to supply famine areas with direct food aid. However highly publicized and praised at the time, direct food aid is not a long-term solution. Although it reduces the number of deaths from famine, it can also reduce incentives for local production by driving down local prices. In addition, the affected countries may have little or no means of transporting the food to those who need it most. Furthermore, the donated foods may receive little cultural acceptance.

In the short run, there is no choice—aid must be given because people are starving. Still, improving the infrastructure for poor people, especially rural people, needs to be the long-term focus.[17] This long-term approach is necessary because the most significant factor affecting the undernutrition of people in impoverished areas of the world is their reliance on outside sources for basic needs. Their dependence makes them constantly vulnerable.[25]

One American program that has helped improve the infrastructure of developing nations is the Peace Corps, which provides education, distributes food and medical supplies, and builds structures for local use. The aim of the Peace Corps is to improve the infrastructure and education of developing countries and thereby help create independent, self-sustaining economies around the world.

Development Tailored to Local Conditions

Recall that, in the past 40 years, world food supplies have grown faster than the population. Thus, the increase in undernutrition during this period is caused by an increase in the number of people cut off from their share of this supply. Millions of farmers are losing access to resources they need to be self-reliant. In response, careful, small-scale regional development is one option. There is a growing realization that rural people who own no land will flock to the overcrowded cities unless economic opportunities can be created as part of a plan for sustainable development.[17]

For the most part, the solution lies in helping people meet their own needs and directing them to resources and employment opportunities, rather than simply giving them resources. Experience has shown that credit—along with training, food storage facilities, and marketing—allows rural people to participate in development to their benefit and that of their families and communities.[33]

Impoverished women are a special concern. In addition to working longer hours than men, they grow most of the food for family consumption and make up three-fourths of the labor force in the informal sector and an increasing proportion in the formal economy. Economic opportunities for women must be augmented.[20] Of the 1.3 billion people in the world living on less than $2 a day, 70% are women. Moreover, among the developing world's 900 million illiterate people, women outnumber men 2 to 1. Thus, an important means of propelling nations out of poverty is to end the cycle of female neglect. A United Nations Conference on Women in Beijing had one critical message: Providing women with education, entrepreneurship, and political power could pay off in numerous ways, ranging from slower population growth and higher incomes to healthier families.

Suitable technologies for processing, preserving, marketing, and distributing nutritious local staples also need to be encouraged, so that small farmers can flourish. Education on how to use these foods to create healthful diets, such as preparing vitamin A-rich vegetables, adds further benefit. Supplementing indigenous foods with nutrients that are in short supply, such as iron and iodide, also deserves consideration. One current program involves adding iron to sugar in various parts of the world. In addition, advances in water purification using ultraviolet light have the potential to cut energy expenditures by 20,000 times what is used now. This new method would result in a cost of 7 cents for a typical village's annual drinking water bill.

Promoting extensive landownership is a key part of the solution. Increasing the availability of food is one of the many advantages. If food resources are concentrated among a minority of people, as often happens with unequal landownership, food won't be equally distributed unless efficient transportation systems are in place. Inequitable distribution then proves a very difficult problem to resolve.

Raising the economic status of impoverished people by employing them is as important as expanding the food supply.[17] If an increase in food supply is achieved without an accompanying rise in employment, there may be no long term change in the number of undernourished people. Although food prices may fall with increased mechanization, use of fertilizers, and other modern technologies, these advances can also displace people from jobs.

A shipment of high-technology tractors, for example, might put local laborers out of work. From this perspective, it is of little consequence that jobs are technologically primitive by Western standards. As mentioned before, increasing both per capita income and education is necessary. That effort must include employment. Making full use of the human resources available in the developing world itself is more essential than ever.

Overemphasizing cash crops, such as coffee, tea, rubber, and cocoa—as some developing countries have done, especially in Latin America—is not likely to solve the nutritional problems of poor people. Cash crops are usually grown at the expense of food crops on the assumption that money earned from the cash crops will be used to purchase food for the families of the workers. However, this is not always the case.

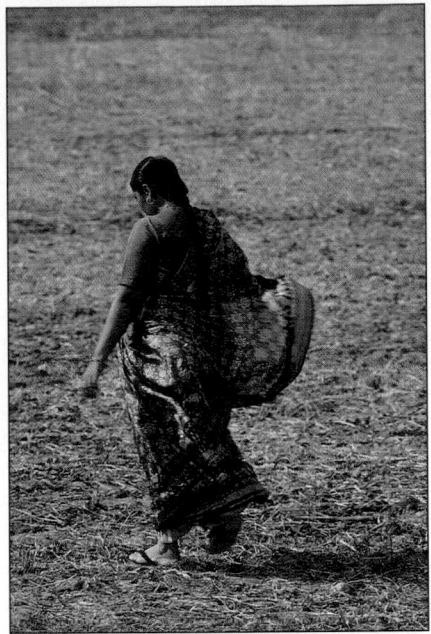

Women are receiving more attention as efforts to improve the health and welfare of the world's people evolve.

CRITICAL THINKING

Stan has read about various relief efforts to help undernourished people in developing countries, especially the emergency food aid programs for famine-ravaged areas. Many of these efforts appear to be only temporary, and he wonders what long-range approaches might help alleviate the problem of undernutrition. What suggestions would you give Stan about possible long-term solutions for undernutrition in developing countries?

Expert Opinion

GENETIC MODIFICATION OF FOODS

JOHN ALLRED, PH.D.

In the broadest sense, plants and domesticated animals have been genetically modified for thousands of years through the process of plant and animal breeding. To some, this type of genetic manipulation is "natural" in that cross-breeding can occur only between members of the same species. At the same time, these matings are not random, as might occur in nature but, rather, are planned to deliberately change the genetics of a species.

Developments in biotechnology have provided a more effective means of manipulating the gene pool of a particular species of plant. That is, in conventional breeding, each of the two parents that are crossed might contribute half of 40,000 genes in a corn plant. Some of the offspring will have the desirable characteristic that the scientist is trying to achieve but will also have many undesirable attributes. It takes successive generations of further cross-breeding, which may take years, in order to eliminate the undesirable characteristics while keeping the desirable ones. With biotechnology, a single gene for a desired trait can be incorporated into a plant without the introduction of undesirable ones. Although biotechnology can be much more efficient than conventional breeding, it still involves substantial developmental research to obtain the final product.

Another way that biotechnology differs significantly from conventional plant or animal breeding is that conventional breeding allows the mixing of the genetic pool only within species, whereas biochemical manipulation allows the transfer of genes between species. Such technology has long been used in human medicine. For example, in 1982, FDA approved the sale of human insulin produced by incorporating the gene for human insulin into the bacterium *Escherichia coli*. Insulin produced in this manner has been used in the intervening years without incident or controversy. Real controversy developed much more recently, when genes from bacteria were inserted into plants destined for human food. These plant products are herbicide-resistant soybeans and corn that produces a protein toxic to the European corn borer.

Is it dangerous for us to eat foods made from these soybean and corn varieties? FDA has concluded that it is not. Consider that the modified soybean and corn varieties differ from their conventional counterparts in two ways. First, they have additional genetic material, DNA; second, they make proteins that are not

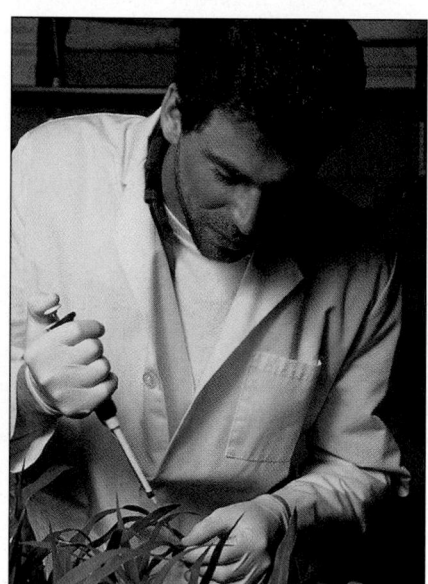

Traditional plant breeding and biotechnology have been used to produce improved plant varieties.

Food can be bought, but it may not be enough, and it is more expensive. In such a situation, poorer families are at greater risk than others, because the money earned from cash crops is often not enough to meet other basic family needs, let alone their food needs. As with poor families in the United States, buying quality foods often takes a secondary position, resulting in nutritional deprivation.

Use of Biotechnology

Current efforts in **biotechnology** may contribute to meeting the food needs of our current (and expanding) world population. Some visionaries even hope to one day produce a banana enhanced with vital oral vaccines, as well as fruits and vegetables that contain more beta-carotene and vitamins C and E. The beta-carotene will help counteract vitamin A deficiency, the leading cause of blindness in children in the developing world. A new form of rice called golden rice is being developed to do the same. Such improved nutrient content of foods eaten by indigenous people throughout the world is a major promise of biotechnology.

The type of biotechnology that can yield these results includes several methods that directly modify products. It differs from traditional methods of cross-breeding plants or animals because it directly changes some of the DNA of organisms to improve characteristics. The development of this new process, called **genetic engineering,** began in the 1970s as part of what is called **recombinant DNA technol-**

present in conventionally grown plants. Consuming the DNA is not a hazard. We do that all the time. Remember, it is the sequence of four chemical bases in DNA that constitutes the blueprint for making proteins. During the digestion of DNA by DNAase secreted by the pancreas, the deoxyribose/phosphate backbone is destroyed, so the base sequence, and therefore the blueprint, is destroyed. Fortunately, this scenario is true regardless of the source of DNA.

The protein made by the corn that is toxic to the European corn borer is not toxic to humans. In fact, we digest it as we would any other protein. The same is true of the extra protein made by the herbicide-resistant soybeans.

Critics of genetically modified foods have expressed concern that these types of hybrids could cause allergic reactions. However, more than 90% of food allergies are known to occur in response to specific proteins in eight foods, including peanuts, tree nuts, milk, eggs, soybeans, shell fish,

fish, and wheat. In general, allergies develop after prolonged exposure to large quantities of the allergen. In contrast, the quantity of new protein introduced in genetically modified soybeans and corn is extremely small. Thus, it is unlikely that the bacterial proteins introduced into a plant would be allergenic. Obviously, there would be potential danger if a gene for an allergenic protein, such as one from peanuts, were introduced into a nonallergenic food, such as corn. FDA is quite aware of this problem and has taken steps to monitor it.

In addition to showing that the food from a modified plant is neither allergenic nor toxic to humans, FDA also requires evidence that the nutrient content and other properties have not been changed. If the food is substantially equivalent to its conventional counterpart, FDA recognizes it as safe, and it therefore can be legally marketed. The guiding principle used by FDA is that the safety of a food will be de-

termined by the properties of the final product, not by the method of production.

Even if genetically modified foods are safe, is there a compelling reason for using them? Herbicide-resistant soybeans have the advantage that farmers can use a relatively nontoxic herbicide to make their fields weed-free. Corn that produces its own toxin to the European corn borer makes spraying with chemical pesticides less necessary. Both of these save money for farmers and are arguably good for the environment—but neither seems to have direct benefit for consumers. The expectations are, however, that future generations of modified products will have major benefits for both the quantity and quality of our food supply.

Dr. Allred is a professor in the Department of Food Science and Technology at The Ohio State University. He is well known for his research on biotin-related enzymes, as well as his contribution to the furthering of biochemical training of dietitians.

---

ogy. The field now features a wide range of cell and subcell techniques for the synthesis and placement of genetic material in organisms (Fig. 20-4). This allows access to a wider gene pool, and it permits the faster and more accurate production of new and more useful microbial, plant, and animal species. Traditional breeding has had inconsistent results, but this new use of biotechnology is precise. Scientists select the traits they want and introduce the gene that produces the desired trait into animals or plants (now called a genetically-modified organism [GMO]).

Currently about one-quarter of all corn and half of all soybeans produced in the United States has been genetically engineered in such a way to resist pests, in the case of corn, and to reduce pesticide use, in the case of soybeans. For example, corn is genetically altered by inserting a gene from the bacterium *Bacillus thurigiensis*, usually referred to as the Bt gene, into the corn DNA. The gene then allows the corn plant to make a protein that is lethal to certain caterpillars that destroy the plant. The Bt protein in the corn, which is present in the plant in very low concentrations, has no effect on humans, as it is digested along with the other proteins in corn. Dr. John Allred discusses this and other issues regarding genetically engineered foods in his Expert Opinion. Many experts agree with Dr. Allred that currently approved varieties of genetically engineered foods are safe to consume.[15, 29] (The controversy over use of StarLink corn in 2000 arose because this GMO corn variety was not approved for human consumption. It found its way, however, into some corn

biotechnology A collection of processes that involve the use of biological systems for altering and, ideally, improving the characteristics of plants, animals, and other forms of life.

genetic engineering The alteration of genetic material in plants and animals with the intent of improving growth, disease resistance, or other characteristics.

recombinant DNA A molecule composed of the DNA of two different species spliced together, such as a combination of bacterial and human DNA used to produce unique bacteria, which now can synthesize human proteins.

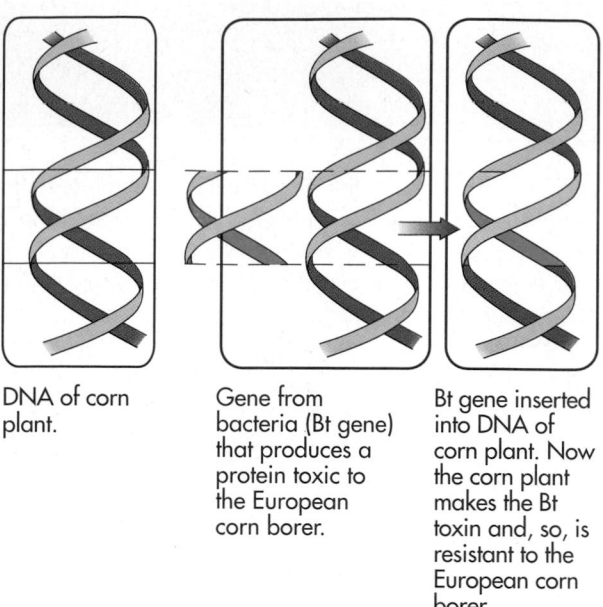

■ **FIGURE 20-4** Biotechnology involves various techniques for transferring foreign DNA into an organism. In this diagram, a sample of DNA is cleaved out of a larger DNA fragment and inserted into the DNA of a host cell. Thus, the host cell contains new genetic information, with the potential of providing the cell with new capabilities. For corn, this means resistance to the European corn borer. The corn plant is now referred to as a genetically-modified organism (GMO). In other applications, bacteria can be engineered to produce the human form of the hormone insulin and another hormone that increases milk production in cows.
Rollins Graphics

DNA of corn plant.

Gene from bacteria (Bt gene) that produces a protein toxic to the European corn borer.

Bt gene inserted into DNA of corn plant. Now the corn plant makes the Bt toxin and, so, is resistant to the European corn borer.

The European Economic Community is very skeptical regarding the use of genetic engineering in foods. This may be because these citizens feel they cannot rely on their governments to ensure food safety, given the problem with mad cow disease in Britain. In contrast, U.S. citizens show great confidence in FDA oversight of food safety. Activism is also much more prevalent in Europe than in the United States. Currently, it is illegal to import genetically engineered foods, such as products made from genetically engineered corn or soybeans, into Europe. (The same is true for Japan.) This is creating problems for U.S. food manufacturers; some have reduced their use of genetically engineered ingredients in order to make it easier to export the finished foods. This also has created a dilemma for U.S. farmers who wonder if they will have a market for their genetically-engineered grains.

CRITICAL THINKING

Bobbie is in a debate class and has been assigned to argue the biotechnologist's side of genetic engineering. Help her come up with a list of arguments in favor of biotechnology. What would the list look like if Bobbie were on the opposing side?

products, such as taco shells). The biggest debate in the United States surrounds the potential hazards to the environment from introducing genes from one species to another. There is also a question regarding the actual reduction in pesticide use that accompanies the cultivation of these products; it may not be as great as was originally predicted.

The extent to which genetically engineered applications will help *significantly* reduce undernutrition in the developing world remains to be seen.[28] Besides improved nutrient content, increased crop yields are another possibility. But, unless price cuts in foods accompany the increased production, landowners and suppliers of biotechnology will be the main ones to enjoy the benefits.

■ Some Concluding Thoughts

Clearly, the developing world will have to rely largely on its own resources to finance development. For decades, countries in Africa could count on the Cold War as an economic resource. The United States and the former Soviet Union opposed each other through African proxies, pouring in money to prop up pro-Western or pro-Communist governments. Now the big powers' priorities have turned inward.

Also detrimental is the economics of drug crops, such as cocaine, marijuana, and opium. Perceiving drugs as valuable cash crops, workers often believe that the large sums of money netted from these crops—which are often more easily grown than food crops—can meet family needs and increase the standard of living. An unfortunate reality is that many workers see little or no cash earnings and become victims of their trade. Cash from drug crops often lines the pockets of criminals and corrupt government officials and results in little incentive to initiate subsistence-level food crops that could provide employment and nourishment for many.

Today, the economic loss from undernutrition is staggering, and the amount of human pain and suffering is incalculable. With all the international relief efforts and assistance from governments and private organizations combined, we are still lacking when it comes to our battle against undernutrition.[10]

Currently, some experts are concerned about the "marginalization" of problems in the developing world, fearing rich nations might dismiss war, disease, and famine as a way of life for poorer nations. In a recent survey, Americans identified world famine as less of a concern than violence, drugs, and inflation. (Currently, U.S. food aid stands at $2.4 billion.) Ultimately, however, the depletion of world resources,

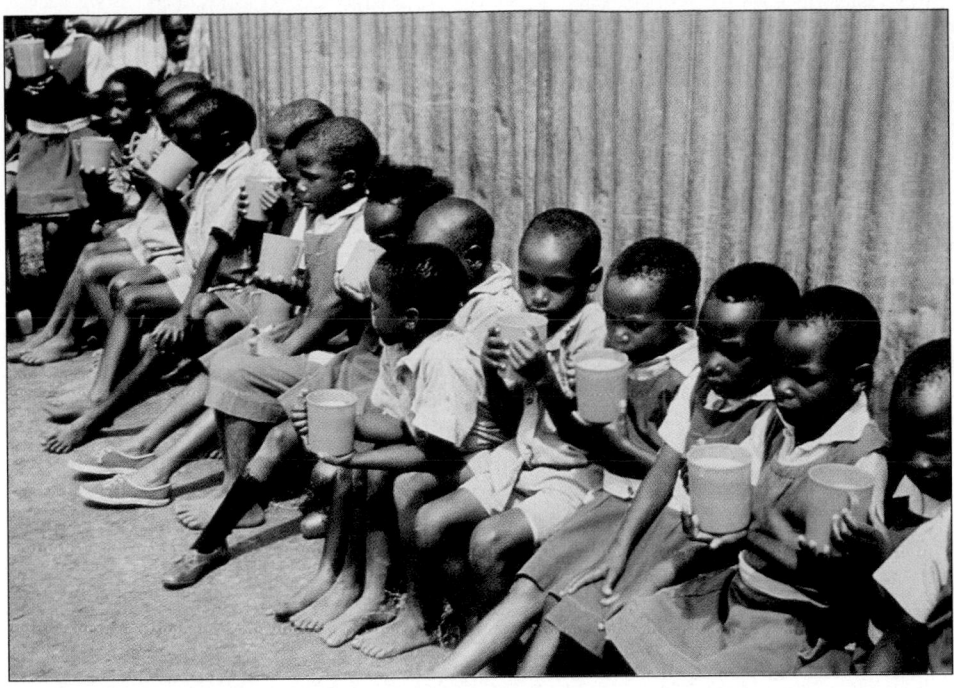

*W*ith regard to the world food supply, the current generation of young adults and the next will not likely have to face the absolute limits. Instead, they will have to make difficult choices if the outlook for future generations is to improve. The "live in the now" mentality has the potential to devastate a great part of humanity if it is not corrected.

There's no doubt that food aid is important in reducing death from famine, but it isn't a long-term solution.

the massive debt incurred by poorer countries, the threat of danger to more prosperous countries nearby, and the toll taken in human lives does affect the world economy and well-being.[5]

Leaders of rich and poor nations alike need to come to an agreement on the best possible means to serve all of the world's citizens. Perhaps if we rid ourselves of negative government policies worldwide, the task can become easier. Life is not necessarily fair, but the aim of civilization should be to make it fairer. The world has both the food and the technical expertise to end hunger. What is lacking is the political will to do so.[10, 17]

CONCEPT CHECK

*O*verall, one important solution to reducing undernutrition in the developing world lies in providing sufficient employment, so that people can purchase the food their families need or provide access to land and other food production resources. Development programs must be sensitive to regional conditions to ensure that the new technologies introduced don't intensify existing problems for the poorest people.

*C*heck out the *Perspectives in Nutrition* Online Learning Center http://www.mhhe.com/wardlaw for quizzes, flash cards, other activities, and web links designed to further help you learn about issues surrounding world hunger.

SUMMARY

1. Poverty is commonly linked to undernutrition. Malnutrition can occur when the food supply is either scarce or abundant. The resulting deficiency conditions and degenerative diseases are influenced by genetic makeup.
2. Undernutrition is the most common form of malnutrition in developing countries. It results from inadequate intake, absorption, or use of nutrients or food energy. Many deficiency conditions consequently appear, and infectious diseases thrive because the immune system cannot function properly.
3. The greatest risk of undernutrition occurs during critical periods of growth and development: gestation, infancy, and childhood. Low birth weight is a leading cause of infant deaths worldwide. Many developmental problems are caused by nutritional deprivation during critical periods of brain growth. People in their later years are also at greater risk.
4. Undernutrition diminishes both physical and mental capabilities. In poor countries, this is worsened by recurrent infections,

unsanitary conditions, extreme weather, inadequate shelter, and exposure to diseases.

5. In the United States, famine has been nonexistent since the 1930s, but undernutrition remains. Soup kitchens, food stamps, school lunch and breakfast programs, and the Special Supplemental Feeding Program for Women, Infants, and Children (WIC) have focused on improving the nutritional health of poor and at-risk people. When adequately funded, these programs have proved effective in reducing undernutrition. The need to reduce out-of-wedlock pregnancies remains a national priority because single parents and their children are likely to live in poverty.

6. Multiple factors contribute to the problem of undernutrition in the developing world. In densely populated countries, food resources, as well as the means for distributing food, may be inadequate. Farming methods often encourage erosion, which deprives the soil of valuable nutrients and thereby hampers future efforts to grow food. Limited water availability limits food production. Naturally occurring devastation from droughts, excessive rainfall, fire, crop infestation, and human causes—such as urbanization, war and civil unrest, debt, and poor sanitation—all contribute to the major problem of undernutrition.

7. Proposed solutions to world undernutrition must include consideration of the interaction of multiple factors, many of which are thoroughly embedded in cultural traditions. Family planning efforts, for example, may not succeed until life expectancy increases. Through education, efforts should be made to upgrade farming methods, improve crops through applications of biotechnology, encourage breastfeeding when it is safe to do so, and improve sanitation and hygiene. Direct food aid is only a short-term solution. In what may appear to be a step backward, many experts recommend sustainable subsistence-level farming, away from the specialization of cash crops, to increase the economic status of poor people. Small-scale industrial development is another way to create meaningful employment and purchasing power for vast numbers of the rural poor.

■ STUDY QUESTIONS

1. Describe the difference between malnutrition and undernutrition.

2. Describe in a short paragraph any evidence of undernutrition that you saw while you were growing up, such as on television. What are/were the likely roots of these problems?

3. What do you believe are the major factors contributing to undernutrition in wealthy nations, such as the United States? What are some solutions to this problem?

4. What three points would you make to a group of seventh-grade girls concerning the economic perils of teenage pregnancy and parenting?

5. Personal responsibility is a common theme in political circles. How does this relate to the problem of undernutrition in the United States? Does it apply to all causes of the problem?

6. Outline how war and civil unrest in developing countries have worsened problems of chronic hunger over the past few years.

7. How important is population control in addressing the problem of world hunger now and in the future? Support your answer with three main points.

8. Why is solving the problem of undernutrition a key factor in the development of the full potential of developing countries? What basic nutrients are keys to the health of these people?

9. Discuss how infrastructure could influence the causes and solutions of chronic hunger in a developing nation.

10. Name three nutrients that are often lacking in the diets of undernourished people. What effects can be expected with each deficiency?

■ ANNOTATED REFERENCES

1. ADA Reports: Position of the American Dietetic Association: Domestic food and nutrition security. *Journal of the American Dietetic Association* 98:337, 1998.

   Aggressive action is needed to bring an end to domestic hunger and to achieve food and nutrition security for all residents of the United States. Immediate and long-range interventions are needed, including adequate program funding of federal programs and assistance from private sources.

2. ADA Reports: Position of the American Dietetic Association and Dietitians of Canada: Nutrition intervention in the care of persons with human immunodeficiency virus infection. *Journal of the American Dietetic Association* 100:708, 2000.

   Malnutrition, various forms of tissue wasting, fat accumulation, and risk of additional chronic disease have become central issues in health-care plans for patients living with HIV. Efforts to optimize nutritional status, including nutrition therapy and nutrition-related education, should be components of the total health care provided to people infected with the HIV virus.

3. Brentlinger PE and others: Childhood malnutrition and postwar reconstruction in rural El Salvador. *Journal of the American Medical Association* 281:184, 1999.

   The 1992 peace settlement that ended the civil war in El Salvador included land redistribution and other provisions to improve socioeconomic status. Malnutrition persisted at high levels, especially in children, and was strongly associated with delay in the full cultivation of redistributed land and in the provision of water.

4. Brundtland GH: Nutrition and infection: Malnutrition and mortality in public health. *Nutrition Reviews* 58(II):S1, 2000.

   The combination of malnutrition and infectious disease is deadly. These conditions arise from poverty and keep people in poverty—not just for one generation, but for many generations. Many infections are preventable. For example, when vitamin A is introduced as part of measles management, the fatality rate can be reduced by greater than 50%.

5. Conway G: Agenda for a doubly green revolution. *Food Technology* 53(11):146, 1999.

   Three-quarters of a billion people—15% of the world's population—eat too little or too poorly. Poverty is the main cause of hunger in developing countries. Political stability in the world will erode further unless developing countries are helped to produce enough food, work, and shelter for their growing populations.

6. Daily G and others: Food production, population growth, and the environment. *Science* 281:1291, 1998.

   The nearly 1 billion people in poor countries who go to bed hungry each night do so because they are extremely poor. Further increases in world population are likely to create additional stresses in both local and global ecosystems.

7. Darnton-Hill I and others: Iron and folate fortification in the Americas to prevent and control micronutrient malnutrition: An analysis. *Nutrition Reviews* 57:25, 1999.

   Although micronutrient malnutrition is largely preventable, it is a serious threat to the health and productivity of more than 2 billion people worldwide. Interest in fortifying wheat flour and dry-milled maize flour, as done in the United States, is growing.

8. Ezzell C: Care for a dying continent. *Scientific American*, p. 96, May 2000.

   AIDS is destined to alter history in Africa—and, in fact, the world—to a degree not seen in humanity's past since the Black Death. It is estimated that between 20 and 25% of the population in Zimbabwe carries the virus, and an estimated 10 million children are destined to become orphaned on the continent of Africa due to the AIDS epidemic. The AIDS drugs available to many in the developed world—which cost upward of $14,000 per person per year—are unthinkable for the majority of people in Africa.

9. Fagoni C: Welfare reform: Implementation progress and information on former recipients. *CNI Nutrition Week*, p. 4, June 25, 1999.

   States have clearly made progress in restructuring their welfare programs to emphasize work and to reduce families' dependence on welfare. Several states have consistently shown that most families who have left welfare have at least some attachment to the workforce, but the percentage of families who initially left welfare then returned to the rolls is significant.

10. Food and Agriculture Organization: The state of food insecurity in the world: 2000, Food and Agriculture Organization of the United Nations, Rome Italy, 2000.

    Countries with the highest prevalence and greatest depth of hunger include 18 countries in Africa, as well as Afghanistan, Bangladesh, Haiti, the Democratic People's Republic of Korea, and Mongolia. These countries face difficult problems in feeding their people due to instability and conflict, poor governance, erratic weather, poverty, agricultural failure, population pressure, and fragile ecosystems.

11. Henkel J: Attacking AIDS with a "cocktail" therapy. *FDA Consumer*, p. 12, July/August 1999.

    The combined drug cocktail, including a protease inhibitor and two other drugs called reverse transcriptase inhibitors, has helped change AIDS from an automatic death sentence to what is now frequently called a chronic, but manageable, disease. This highly active antiretroviral therapy often drops viral load—a measure of new AIDS virus produced in the body—to undetectable levels. Patients need to adhere to their dosing schedule, so that there is not an emergence of HIV strains that are resistant to treatment.

12. Holben DH: Nuts & bolts of food security. *Today's Dietitian*, p. 14, May 2000.

    Food security, an essential, universal dimension of household and personal well-being, means that all people at all times have access to enough food for an active, healthy life. Currently in the United States, about 10% of families are food insecure and have to resort to emergency food supplies.

13. Hormann E: Breast-feeding and HIV: What choices does a mother really have? *Nutrition Today* 34:189, 1999.

    Because breastfeeding could be a route of HIV transmission from mother to infant, new guidelines on feeding the infants of HIV-positive mothers encourages replacement feeding, even in developing countries. However, when there is no access to nutritionally adequate human milk substitutes and infectious diseases and malnutrition are the primary causes of death during infancy, artificial feeding can substantially increase children's risk of illness and death. Many mothers have no choice, considering their circumstances.

14. Hurtado EK and others: Early childhood anemia and mild or moderate mental retardation. *American Journal of Clinical Nutrition* 69:115, 1999.

    Iron deficiency is directly associated with mild or moderate mental retardation. Since iron deficiency is most prevalent during the first 2 years of life, when the infant brain is still developing, adequate nutrition is essential during this time in order to prevent brain damage.

15. Institute of Food Technologists: Human food safety evaluation of rDNA biotechnology-derived foods. *Food Technology* 54(9): 53, 2000.

    Genetically modified foods are safe, based on scientific procedures used by FDA, despite the concern of some consumers. Recombinant DNA technology has great promise to increase world food production and improve the characteristics of plants in ways that will benefit farmers, consumers, and the environment.

16. Karp RJ: Head Start, nutrition, and problems of poverty in childhood. *Journal of the American College of Nutrition* 18:100, 1999.

    Federal food programs, such as food stamps, school lunches and breakfasts, and the Special Supplemental Feeding Program for Women, Infants, and Children (WIC), offer poor families food with a high nutrient density. These are one of the most effective ways of addressing poverty and the multiple, interrelated problems of poor families with children. Although some people believe that these programs create a welfare dependence, they actually benefit the children and the society by creating a healthy population able to learn, work, and earn.

17. Lappe FM and others: World hunger: Twelve myths, Grove Press, New York, NY, Second edition, 1998.

    Choices determine whether we are helping to end world hunger. Only as we make our choices conscious do we become less victims of the world handed to us, and more its creators. The more we consciously align our life choices with a vision of the world were working toward, the more powerful we become in solving this problem of world hunger.

18. McCoy F: In an age of plenty, a search for shelter: The crunch in affordable housing for the poor. *U.S. News & World Report*, p. 28, April 10, 2000.

    As the nation's economy soars to new heights, the gap between the supply and demand for affordable housing is growing ever wider. With the economy so strong, real-estate prices are rising at a rate faster than income is rising for those at the bottom, which leaves many people unable to find decent, affordable housing. To pay rent, people are skimping on food or medicine, or they are living in unfit housing.

19. Mendez MA, Adair L: Severity and timing of stunting in the first two years of life affect performance on cognitive tests in late childhood. *Journal of Nutrition* 129:1555, 1999.

    There is an urgent need to limit malnutrition during early childhood because it is associated with reduced cognitive development later in childhood and may have long-term implications. Ensuring that children with early stunting receive schooling comparable in quantity and quality with that received by nonstunted children may help improve their cognitive development.

20. Mora JO, Nestel PS: Improving prenatal nutrition in developing countries: Strategies, prospects, and challenges. *American Journal of Clinical Nutrition* 71(Suppl): 1353S, 2000.

The health and nutrition of females throughout their entire lives is affected by complex and highly interrelated factors. Prospects for improving prenatal nutrition are contingent on increasing one's education, delaying the age of marriage, reducing fertility rates, having smaller families, having greater health system coverage, and increasing women's participation in the labor force. Increasing women's access to health and nutrition services is especially important.

21. Nelson K and others: Hunger in an adult patient population. *Journal of the American Medical Association* 279:1211, 1998.

   Hunger and food insecurity are common among patients seeking care at an urban county hospital. In this case in Minneapolis, families with annual incomes of less than $10,000 did not receive food stamps, reflecting national data that half of the households living in poverty do not take advantage of food stamps. Recipients whose food stamps were reduced or nonexistent were more likely to report food insecurity and hunger.

22. Oliveira V, Gunderson C: WIC and the nutrient intake of children. *CNI Nutrition Week*, p. 4, May 12, 2000.

   Due to increased federal funding, the WIC program has expanded and has been able to serve more lower-priority children in recent years. The average intakes of iron, protein, and folate for the low-income, nutritionally at-risk children were significantly greater than those WIC income-eligible children. Overall, participation in the WIC program has shown a positive and significant effect on the nutrient intakes of children.

23. Potts M: The unmet need for family planning. *Scientific American*, p. 88, January 2000.

   Women and men in many countries still lack adequate funding and access to contraceptives. There are women in Sri Lanka who are eager to control their fertility but are so poor that they have to buy oral contraceptive tablets 5 at a time instead of in a packet of 21. Unless family planning options become more readily available, severe environmental and health problems loom in this century throughout large parts of the world.

24. Prasad AS: Zinc deficiency in humans: A neglected problem. *Journal of the American College of Nutrition* 17:542, 1998.

   Deficiency of zinc is very widespread throughout the world, and may even be as prevalent as iron deficiency anemia, affecting nearly 1 billion people. There are several adverse consequences related to zinc deficiency, including growth retardation, poor sexual development, delayed wound healing, and malabsorption syndromes.

25. Shapouri S, Rosen S: Food security assessment: Why countries are at risk. *CNI Nutrition Week*, p. 4, August 20, 1999.

   Uneven distribution of the world's resources means that the poor, low-resource countries are vulnerable to food insecurity. To improve food security, it is essential to promote policies that accelerate agricultural growth, particularly in sub-Saharan Africa. A few African countries have adopted high-yielding corn varieties and have significantly increased yields in the past two decades.

26. Starr P: The homeless and the public household. The *New England Journal of Medicine* 338:1761, 1998.

   Failure to deal with homelessness in the United States is creating added stress for supportive services, such as the police, prisons, and especially hospital care. Lack of housing, education, health insurance, and substance abuse prevention leads to added costs for these resource institutions, which are not equipped to deal with the homeless. If people with very low incomes are to afford homes, either their incomes must be higher or housing must be cheaper.

27. Stephenson J: Apocalypse now: HIV/ AIDS in Africa exceeds the experts' worst predictions. *Journal of the American Medical Association* 284:556, 2000.

   The HIV/AIDS epidemic is rampant in sub-Saharan Africa, taking a heavier toll on women than on men. With no preventive vaccine on the horizon and antiretroviral therapy currently being beyond economic reach for most Africans living with HIV, the best tool is prevention efforts, including education about the disease and the use of condoms and other means of reducing the risk of infection.

28. Tangley L: Engineering the harvest: Biotech could help fight hunger in the world's poorest nations—But will it? *U.S. News & World Report*, p. 46, March 13, 2000.

   The need to improve agriculture in the developing world is indisputable, and genetic engineering has the potential to help reduce hunger problems by allowing scientists to splice into crops genes that could boost yields and enhance the nutritional quality of food. However, the technology's potential hazards must not be ignored. Crops first should be tested for detrimental effects on human health and the environment.

29. Thompson L: Are bioengineered foods safe? *FDA Consumer*, p. 18, January/February 2000.

   There is no evidence that bioengineered foods pose any human health concerns or that they are in any way less safe than crops produced through traditional breeding. No matter how a new crop is created—using traditional methods or biotechnology tools—breeders must conduct field testing for several seasons to make sure the crops are safe for widespread use.

30. Underwood BE: Micronutrient malnutrition: Is it being eliminated? *Nutrition Today* 33:121, 1998.

   Micronutrient malnutrition has existed for centuries and remains as a global public health problem of concern. The focus of detecting consequences of iron deficiency has changed from anemia to the more subtle consequences, such as cognitive function and work performance. About 1 billion people are affected by iron deficiency anemia, and another 1 billion people are at risk of iron deficiency disorder. Micronutrient programs currently are being implemented in more countries than ever before, which gives reason for hope.

31. UNICEF: The state of the world's children 2001, United Nations Children Fund, New York, NY, 2001.

   Most brain development happens before a child reaches three years old. Long before many adults even realize what is happening, the brain cells of a new infant proliferate, synapses develop, and the patterns of a lifetime are established. In these early years, children develop their abilities to think and speak, learn and reason and lay the foundation for their values and social behavior as adults.

32. Wolfe PR: Practical approaches to HIV therapy: Recommendations for the year 2000. *Postgraduate Medicine* 107(4):127, 2000.

   In just the past 3 years, the outlook for patients with HIV infection has brightened remarkably. Although new pharmaceutical agents have increased the effectiveness of therapy, the potential toxic effects of these agents are a continuing problem for both patient and physician. Not only are patients concerned about suffering from side effects, but physicians are concerned about drug-resistant strains emerging in patients who are unable to take their medications on a regular basis.

33. Yunus M: The Grameen bank. *Scientific American*, p. 114, November 1999.

   The majority of poor people have few opportunities to escape from poverty. The Grameen Bank Center in Bangladesh allows women to start small businesses, such as raising chickens, by offering loans with no collateral. A Grameen loan empowers a woman by increasing her economic security and status within the family. Putting commercial funds to work is helping this society eradicate poverty.

TAKE ACTION

I. FIGHTING WORLD UNDERNUTRITION ON A PERSONAL LEVEL

If you want to do something about world and domestic undernutrition, the following activities are suggested. It is a noble act to try to make a difference, even if you make just one small step. As with any change in behavior, don't try to do too many things at once. Try one or two activities that represent your commitment to solving this problem.

1. Volunteer at a local soup kitchen or homeless shelter for a limited period of time (1 month, for example). What insights did you gain?

2. Coordinate the efforts of a campus organization to donate some money to a voluntary agency that does antihunger work, such as the following:

Bread for the World	Oxfam America	Save the Children Foundation
802 Rhode Island Ave., NE	115 Broadway	P.O. Box 970
Washington, DC 20018	Boston, MA 02116	Westport, CT 06881
Catholic Relief Services	CARE	Second Harvest
209 W. Fayette St.	660 First Ave.	116 Michigan Ave., Suite #4
Baltimore, MD 21201	New York, NY 10016	Chicago, IL 60603

3. Take a contribution for the ongoing offering of nonperishable foods at your church, or mosque, or synagoge, or one near you. If your church doesn't have this offering, start one.

4. Get on a food recovery program's mailing list and read its newsletters for information on upcoming fund-raisers and programs to become involved.

5. Participate in food drives organized by local grocery stores through contributing food or services. Food-drive organizers may need volunteers to transport the donations from the store to a food pantry.

6. Point, click, and fight hunger. Internet users can find information on hunger at several sites, including the following:
    *   Someone somewhere dies of hunger every 3.6 seconds. You can help stop the clock: go to http://www.thehungersite.com and click on Donate Free Food to send a meal to a needy someone. This site is affiliated with the UN World Food Program, which tracks the number of clicks and then sends a bill to one of its corporate or nonprofit sponsors.
    *   HungerWeb, at Brown University, offers information on hunger research, programs, mailing lists, education, and advocacy, as well as an overview of the Alan Shawn Feinstein World Hunger Program at Brown. This site contains web links to Internet sites run by the UN, U.S. AID, and the World Bank. http://www.netspace.org/hungerweb
    *   The Food and Agriculture Organization of the United Nations has worked to alleviate poverty and hunger by promoting agricultural development, improved nutrition, and the pursuit of food security. This web site will keep you up-to-date on recent issues and provides an extensive list of publications related to food security: http://www.fao.org
    *   America's Second Harvest, the largest domestic hunger-relief organization, shows you how to help online and has information about the latest updates. http://www.secondharvest.org
    *   Bread for the World is a nationwide Christian citizens' movement seeking justice for the world's hungry people by lobbying our nation's decision makers. http://www.bread.org
    *   CARE is one of the world's largest private international relief and development organizations, with the goal of saving lives, building opportunity, and bringing hope to people in need. http://www.care.org

II. JOINING THE BATTLE AGAINST UNDERNUTRITION

Imagine that you recently spent your summer vacation in a developing country and saw evidence of undernutrition and hunger. Then imagine that you are now asking a large corporation to support your efforts to ease hunger and suffering in this area. Develop a two-paragraph statement outlining why addressing hunger issues in this area is important. Address how you think a large corporation could assist you in your efforts.

THE IMPACT OF AIDS WORLDWIDE

The Black Plague left its grim mark on civilization by claiming the lives of approximately 25 million people in the fourteenth century. Today there are more than 36 million people around the world with **human immunodeficiency virus (HIV)** infection or **acquired immune deficiency syndrome (AIDS),** leading to an estimated 16.3 million deaths to date. This represents a current worldwide epidemic. Once infected with HIV, the person is said to be HIV-positive. If untreated, the viral disease progresses over the next few years, and the person develops clinical signs and symptoms, such as diarrhea, lung disease, weight loss, and a form of cancer called kaposis sarcoma.[11] The person is now said to have AIDS. In 1998, an estimated 5.8 million new HIV infections occurred worldwide—approximately 16,000 each day.

In the United States, it is estimated that 920,000 people are infected with HIV, of whom more than 200,000 are unaware of their infection. This means that as many as 1 of every 280 Americans may be infected. In more than 60 U.S. cities, AIDS is the number one killer of men ages 25 to 44. Minority populations account for more cases than Caucasians in the U.S., based on their percentage of the population. Stopping the spread of this disease is imperative for the United States, especially in minority communities.

In Africa, particularly sub-Saharan countries, the HIV virus is rampant throughout the entire population, with this region containing nearly 70% of the world's HIV-positive people.[27] In many villages, AIDS is creating orphans. In most areas of sub-Saharan Africa AIDS is reducing life expectancy by one-half. As noted in the chapter, world population projections for the next 50 years may have to be reduced to account for the impact of AIDS in Africa and in Asia.

Ten varieties of the HIV that infects humans (called clades) have been described; those found in Africa are more deadly than those found in the United States. The virus is a retrovirus. It takes the RNA it contains and converts that into DNA. The DNA is then used to direct the synthesis of the proteins by the infected cell that are needed to make new viral particles. T lymphocytes and macrophages of the immune system are prime targets of the virus; it is in these cells that the new viral particles are made. The resulting dramatic fall in immune function from HIV infection is the hallmark of the disease.

The virus is transferred between people via blood contact or body secretions, including sexual secretions. It has a very limited ability to exist outside the body. Experts have blamed sexual promiscuity in some African societies, as well as sexual practices that can make it easier for the virus to enter a woman's bloodstream, for the rapid spread of the disease in that area of the world.[8] Many people in Africa engage in unprotected sex because they can't afford condoms, or because the females cannot get their male partners to use them. Overall, 75 to 85% of all cases of HIV have been spread through sexual contact, homosexual as well as heterosexual. Intravenous drug use, via shared needles, accounts for a large number of the rest of the cases.

One drug used to treat HIV infection blocks the activity of the enzyme used by HIV to convert RNA to DNA, called reverse transcriptase. A common form of this drug is zidovudine (AZT). Other drugs used to treat HIV infection block specific enzymes in HIV that are needed to assemble the viral particle. These drugs are called protease inhibitors; a common form is Indinavir (Crixivan) (Fig. 20-5).[32] The latest therapies can significantly slow the progress of the disease, but this requires patients to take at least three different drugs and about 14 pills each day. This costs approximately $14,000 per year, not including any unforeseen hospital stays.[11] Making these drugs available to people in developing countries is a major roadblock to solving the AIDS crisis in those regions. Certain drug companies and governments are working to lower the cost of AIDS drugs to developing nations. Still, in many cases the cost will remain out of reach to many who need the drugs. It has been suggested that developed nations step in and cover most of the costs.

The main hope for addressing the problem of AIDS in the developing world is the creation and widespread use of a vaccine against the virus.[8] This would significantly reduce the spread to further individuals but would be of no help to those already infected with the virus. Aside from providing AIDS drugs used in the United States, there is currently no answer to the AIDS

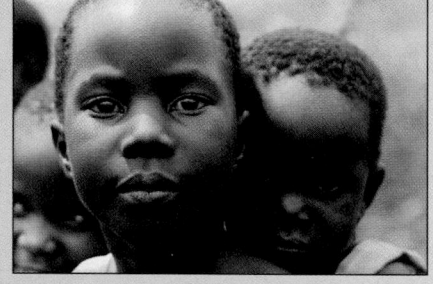

A particularly sad development of AIDS in Africa is the number of AIDS orphans, children whose parents have both died of AIDS.

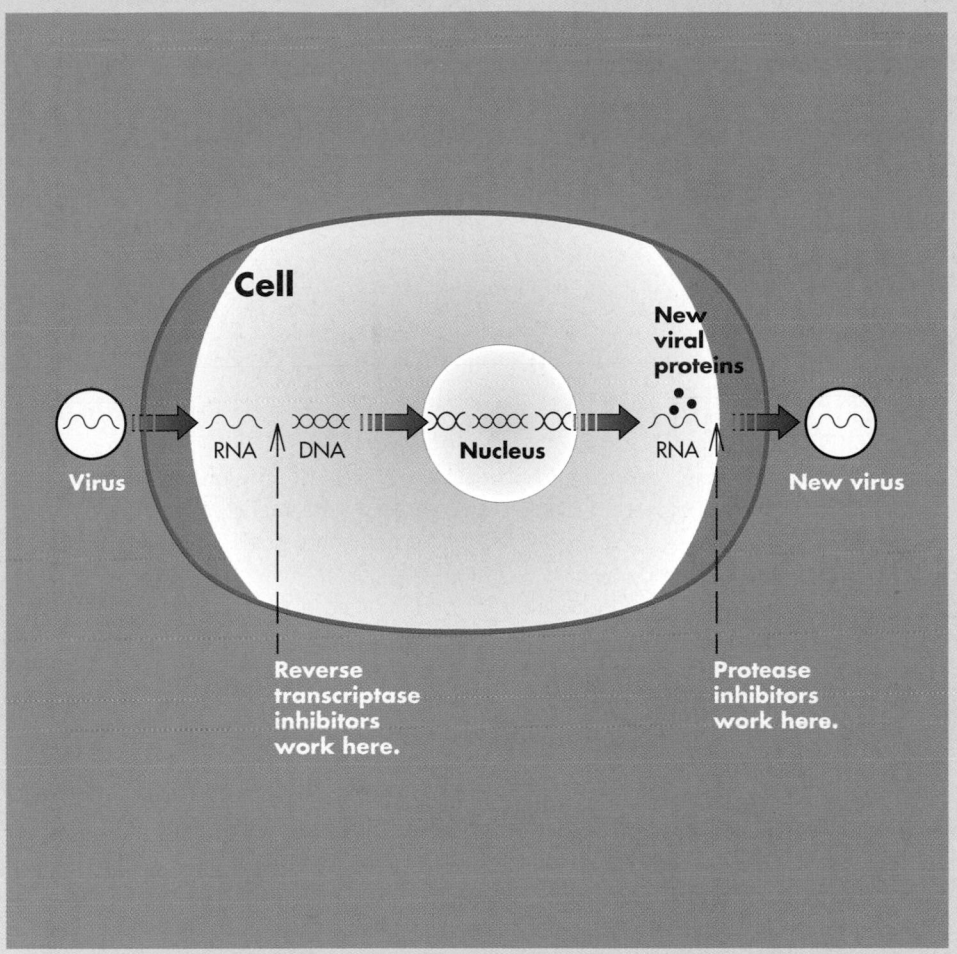

FIGURE 20-5 Medical Therapy for HIV. Normally, HIV enters the cell and uses the enzyme reverse transcriptase to convert its RNA to DNA. The DNA is then inserted into the cell's nucleus. Here, messenger RNA can be made from the DNA which carries the instructions from HIV. The RNA is then used in the cell cytoplasm to make the HIV proteins (see Chapter 7 for details on protein synthesis). These proteins are then assembled into new viral particles, and the particles are secreted from the cell. Reverse transcriptase inhibitors and protease inhibitors stop this entire process at two different points. This drug therapy can reduce the amount of virus in many cases to undetectable levels in a person infected with HIV. However, any lapse in therapy can allow the virus to mutate around the therapy, making further applications less effective. Recently, use of protease inhibitors has been declining due to side effects associated with long term use.

crisis in the developing world beyond safe sex, use of clean needles, and other behavior-linked approaches.[27]

The devastating effects of AIDS on our civilization have been very rapid when measured by earth's scale of time, and the true costs to societies—other than the cost of human lives—have yet to emerge. The very nature of the disease is likely to wreak significant human devastation here and worldwide, partly because its primary route of transmission is a basic human behavior—sexual activity.

An encouraging study done in rural Uganda suggests that people with minimal amounts of HIV in their blood show a low likelihood of spreading the virus to others during unprotected sex. This is a positive finding, since treatment reduces the viral load in infected patients, which in turn might help decrease the spread of this disease. On a more pessimistic note, highly drug-resistant strains of HIV are increasing, appearing in as many as 5% of newly infected patients in the United States. With their complicated drug regimens, many patients miss doses or quit taking their medicines for a period of time, which aid in the development of drug-resistant strains.

WHO IS AFFECTED?

The belief that AIDS is a novel disease affecting a limited population of homosexual males on the East and West Coasts of the United States is dangerously inaccurate. With the number of new cases per year among homosexual men dramatically decreasing, the number of new infections among heterosexuals, particularly among women, has accelerated dramatically. In fact, recent studies show that about 20% of people in some south Florida towns have HIV infections, with heterosexual contact being the main method of contracting the virus. Along with the increase in infection in women, there is an increased number of HIV-infected infants and children.

AIDS needs no passport. Heterosexually transmitted HIV flows freely in Thai sex brothels, along the truck routes of India, around Dominican Republic sugar-cane plantations, and in the copper mines of Zambia. It is likely that one-fourth of all adults in Zambia are infected with HIV. Heterosexual contact accounts for the majority of cases. A recent study warns us that 57 countries risk major HIV outbreaks. Reported HIV cases are increasing rapidly in Africa, Asia, and Russia, with an estimated 5.8 million men, women, and children becoming infected yearly worldwide.

NUTRITION AND AIDS

On a more individual scale, can eating a balanced diet prevent HIV or stave off AIDS? The answer is no. Consuming a balanced diet, however, helps lessen the impact of infections but does not cure the disease or make it less deadly, while poor nutritional status contributes to quicker onset of such symptoms as body wasting and fever. This ultimately leads to a quicker demise. Overall, AIDS patients should consider sufficient food an integral part of their treatment regimen.[2]

In addition, many AIDS patients experience diarrhea. Eating such foods as applesauce, potatoes without the skin, broth, hot cereal, rice, gelatin, bananas, and crackers may minimize the severity of the diarrhea. Patients should also stay hydrated with fluids such as fruit juice, sports drinks, water, and ice chips.

Breastfeeding becomes an issue for mothers who test HIV-positive. Research shows that babies have a 10% chance of getting the virus from their HIV-infected mothers' milk if they breastfeed for 2 years. Many experts recommend the avoidance of breastfeeding as an intervention to prevent the transmission of the virus from mother to child.[13] However, in many situations, nutritionally adequate breast-milk substitutes are not available, especially in an environment where infectious diseases and malnutrition are the primary causes of death during infancy. In these instances, feeding with infant formulas can increase a child's risk of illness and death. In the end, the choice is with the mother, based on current circumstances. Some African countries are now supplying infant formulas if an HIV positive mother chooses to use this option.

WHAT ARE THE COMBINED COSTS OF AIDS?

Although human life can't be tagged with a price, the cost of AIDS research and medical care for AIDS patients, the loss of labor force for industry, and the economic hardship experienced by families of victims can be quantified. A conservative estimate for the total lifetime cost of treating HIV-related illness in just one person is $154,000. Consider those dollars, and then think about the more than 36 million people around the world who are infected. In the United States in 1996, $6.7 billion, or about $20,000 per patient, was spent on HIV-related health care. This is money that could have been spent on goods and services to help maintain stable economies around the world.

The impact of AIDS is hitting poor countries worst because their economies are already small and their living standards low. Brazil, for example, would need to spend $600 million to adequately help its AIDS victims today. Such an economic burden would certainly mean rising budget deficits and expanding levels of debt, especially for a country that is still struggling with a foreign debt load of more than $100 billion. Other developing nations may well face a similar dilemma.[8]

Behind the mind-boggling statistics on AIDS are less obvious costs to businesses, families, schools and universities, and society in general. In India and Thailand, for example, a significant number of the adult male population will die of AIDS. Worker productivity will plummet because AIDS victims produce less and demand more, especially as they waste away in the latter stages of the disease. Business productivity drops even further when relatives take time away from work and school to care for family members afflicted with AIDS. Furthermore, AIDS demands a considerable amount of family income. Hard-pressed families, who have to devote much of their income to doctors and medicines, have little left for living expenses. Other family members must struggle to keep up with daily duties because they must care for orphans left behind in the disease's wake. The number of youngsters orphaned by AIDS could more than double in the next 3 years to reach 3.7 million worldwide.

INDIVIDUAL AND GOVERNMENT RESPONSE

Governments worldwide have come under fire for their slow response in fighting AIDS. Many governments of developing nations can't afford to supply AIDS counseling or treatment. More recently, governments are trying to take more responsibility in stopping the spread of AIDS. The U.S. government has formally designated the disease a threat to U.S. national security that could topple foreign governments, touch off ethnic wars, and undo decades of work in building free-market democracies abroad.

The world must act in concert to stop the spread of HIV. To do any less is to allow the problem of undernutrition to worsen throughout the world. The medical ramifications of caring for those already infected with HIV will be troubling enough, especially in the developing world. If the AIDS epidemic continues to spread at the current rate, however, the resulting social and economic burdens could spark crises that spread beyond national borders.[8]

For further information on HIV and AIDS, call the CDC national HIV/AIDS hot line at 1-800-458-5231. As well, visit the following web sites:

http://www.aegis.com

http://www.thebody.com

http://www.aids.org

Appendixes

Appendix A

FOOD COMPOSITION TABLE

Abbreviation Key:

Unit/Amt = Unit Amount

Wt (g) = Weight in grams

Energy (Kcal) = kilocalories

Prot (g) = Protein

Carb (g) = Carbohydrate

Fiber (g) = Dietary fiber

Fat (g) = Total fat

Mono (g) = Monounsaturated fat

Poly (g) = Polyunsaturated fat

Sat (g) = Saturated fat

Chol (mg) = Cholesterol

Cal (mg) = Calcium

Iron (mg) = Iron

Magn (mg) = Magnesium

Phos (mg) = Phosphorus

Pota (mg) = Potassium

Sodi (mg) = Sodium

Zinc (mg) = Zinc

Vit A (RE) = Vitamin A

Vit C (mg) = Vitamin C

Vit E (mg) = Vitamin E

Thia (mg) = Thiamin

Ribo (mg) = Riboflavin

Niac (mg) = Niacin

Vit B-6 (mg) = Vitamin B-6

Fol (μg) = Folate

Vit B-12 (μg) = Vitamin B-12

Wat (g) = Water

Code	Food Name	Unit/Amt	Wt (g)	Energy (Kcal)	Prot (g)	Carb (g)	Fiber (g)	Fat (g)	Mono (g)	Poly (g)
16104	Bacon, Vegetarian, Meatless	1 strip	5	15.5	0.5	0.3	0.1	1.5	0.4	0.8
18005	Bagel, Cinnamon-Raisin	1 mini bagel 2.5" dia	46	126.0	4.5	25.4	1.1	0.8	0.1	0.3
18003	Bagel, Egg	1 bagel 3.5" dia	64	177.9	6.8	33.9	1.5	1.3	0.3	0.4
18007	Bagel, Oatbran	1 bagel 3.5" dia	64	163.2	6.8	34.1	2.3	0.8	0.2	0.3
918008	Bagel, Oatbran, toasted, mini/small sizes	1 mini bagel 2.5" dia	46	126.0	5.3	26.4	1.7	0.6	0.0	0.0
18001	Bagel, Plain/Onion/Poppy/Sesame, enriched	1 bagel 3.5" dia	64	176.0	6.7	34.2	1.5	1.0	0.1	0.4
918801	Leavening Agent, Baking Powder	1 tsp	4	12.5	1.5	1.5	1.5	0.0	0.0	0.0
924037	Bean Burrito	8.0 oz	224	463.7	20.0	64.0	1.5	14.3	0.0	0.0
16115	Bean Flour, Soy, fullfat, raw	1 cup	85	370.6	29.4	29.9	8.2	17.6	3.9	9.9
16118	Bean Flour, Soy, lowfat	1 cup	88	327.4	40.9	33.4	9.0	5.9	1.3	3.3
16112	Bean Sauce, Fermented Soy Product, Miso	½ cup	138	284.3	16.3	38.6	7.5	8.4	1.9	4.7
16114	Bean Sauce, Fermented Soy Product, Tempeh	½ cup	83	165.2	15.7	14.1	0.0	6.4	1.4	3.6
16123	Bean Sauce, Soy & Wheat (Shoyu)	1 tbsp	15	8.0	0.8	1.3	0.1	0.0	0.0	0.0
16424	Bean Sauce, Soy & Wheat (Shoyu) low sodium	1 tbsp	15	8.0	0.8	1.3	0.1	0.0	0.0	0.0
16008	Beans, Baked w/franks, canned	1 cup	256	363.5	17.3	39.4	17.7	16.8	7.2	2.1
16011	Beans, Baked w/pork & tom sauce, canned	1 cup	227	222.5	11.7	44.0	10.9	2.3	1.0	0.3
16006	Beans, Baked, Plain or Vegetarian, canned	1 cup	254	236.2	12.2	52.1	12.7	1.1	0.1	0.5
16018	Beans, Black Turtle Soup, mature seeds, canned	1 cup	253	230.2	15.3	41.9	17.5	0.7	0.1	0.3
16054	Beans, Broadbeans (Fava) mature seeds, canned	½ cup	94	66.7	5.1	11.7	3.5	0.2	0.0	0.1
16026	Beans, Great Northern, mature seeds, canned	½ cup	131	149.3	9.7	27.5	6.4	0.5	0.0	0.2
16029	Beans, Kidney, mature seeds, canned	½ cup	128	103.7	6.7	19.0	4.5	0.4	0.0	0.2
16070	Beans, Lentils, mature seeds, boiled w/o salt	½ cup	99	114.8	8.9	19.9	7.8	0.4	0.1	0.2
16081	Beans, Mung, mature seeds, boiled w/o salt	½ cup	52	54.6	3.7	10.0	4.0	0.2	0.0	0.1
16039	Beans, Navy, mature seeds, canned	½ cup	91	102.8	6.9	18.6	4.6	0.4	0.0	0.2
16044	Beans, Pinto, mature seeds, canned	½ cup	113	97.2	5.5	17.2	5.2	0.9	0.2	0.3
16103	Beans, Refried, canned (includes USDA Commodity)	½ cup	126	118.4	6.9	19.6	6.7	1.6	0.7	0.2
16111	Beans, Soy, mature seeds, dry roasted	½ cup	144	648.0	57.0	47.1	11.7	31.1	6.9	17.6
16162	Beans, Soy, Tofu, Mori-Nu, silken, firm	¼ block	84	52.1	5.8	2.0	0.1	2.3	0.5	1.2
16164	Beans, Soy, Tofu, Mori-Nu, silken, lite firm	¼ block	84	31.1	5.3	0.9	0.0	0.7	0.1	0.4
16161	Beans, Soy, Tofu, Mori-Nu, silken, soft	¼ block	84	46.2	4.0	2.4	0.1	2.3	0.4	1.3
16132	Beans, Soy, Tofu, Nigari, Fuyu, salted & fermented	¼ block	84	97.4	6.8	4.3	0.0	6.7	1.5	3.8
913524	Beef Brisket, All Grades, lean (½"trim) braised	3.5 oz	100	241.0	29.4	0.0	0.0	12.8	0.0	0.0
913522	Beef Brisket, All Grades, lean&fat (½"trim) braised	3.5 oz	100	391.0	23.0	0.0	0.0	32.4	0.0	0.0
924324	Beef Burgundy, frz (Le Menu)	7.5 oz	213	315.2	25.1	12.3	0.0	18.5	0.0	0.0
924246	Beef Chop Suey	1 cup	250	300.0	26.0	12.5	1.3	17.0	0.0	0.0
924222	Beef Chow Mein/LaChoy	¾ cup	120	60.0	6.0	5.0	2.0	1.0	0.6	0.0
924022	Beef Goulash	7.5 oz	213	213.0	13.2	21.7	0.0	8.1	0.0	0.0
13326	Beef Liver, braised	3.5 oz	100	161.0	24.4	3.4	0.0	4.9	0.7	1.1
13327	Beef Liver, pan fried	4.0 oz	119	258.2	31.8	9.3	0.0	9.5	1.9	2.0
924002	Beef Pot Pie, frz (Banquet)	7.0 oz	198	485.1	19.8	36.8	1.7	28.3	12.2	7.0
924034	Beef Stroganoff, frz (Stouffers)	4.0 oz	142	200.2	15.6	5.8	0.0	12.8	0.0	0.0
913512	Beef, All Cuts, All Grades, lean (½"trim) ckd	3.5 oz	100	222.0	30.4	0.0	0.0	10.2	0.0	0.0
13012	Beef, All Cuts, All Grades, lean (¼"trim) ckd	3.5 oz	100	216.0	29.6	0.0	0.0	9.9	4.2	0.3
913504	Beef, All Cuts, All Grades, lean&fat (½"trim) ckd	3.5 oz	100	349.0	25.0	0.0	0.0	26.9	0.0	0.0
13004	Beef, All Cuts, All Grades, lean&fat (¼"trim) ckd	3.5 oz	100	305.0	25.9	0.0	0.0	21.5	9.2	0.8
13366	Beef, All Cuts, Select, lean (0"trim) ckd	3.5 oz	100	201.0	29.9	0.0	0.0	8.1	3.4	0.3
924108	Beef, Corned Beef Hash	3.5 oz	100	184.0	8.5	8.5	1.2	12.7	5.8	0.6
924325	Beef, Creamed Chipped	4.0 oz	113	174.0	9.3	8.0	0.0	11.6	4.6	0.6
13347	Beef, Cured Corned Beef Brisket, cooked	3.5 oz	100	251.0	18.2	0.5	0.0	19.0	9.2	0.7
13418	Beef, Eye of Round, All Grades, lean (0"trim) roasted	100	166.0	29.0	0.0	0.0	4.7	2.0	0.2	1.7
13300	Beef, Ground, extra lean, pan fried, medium	4.0 oz	119	303.5	29.7	0.0	0.0	19.5	8.6	0.7
13305	Beef, Ground, lean, broiled, medium	3.5 oz	100	272.0	24.7	0.0	0.0	18.5	8.1	0.7
13307	Beef, Ground, lean, pan fried, medium	3.5 oz	100	275.0	24.2	0.0	0.0	19.1	8.3	0.7
13312	Beef, Ground, regular, broiled, medium	3.5 oz	100	289.0	24.1	0.0	0.0	20.7	9.1	0.8
13314	Beef, Ground, regular, pan fried, medium	4.0 oz	119	364.1	28.5	0.0	0.0	26.8	11.8	1.0
13315	Beef, Ground, regular, pan fried, welldone	4.0 oz	119	340.3	32.1	0.0	0.0	22.5	9.9	0.8
14177	Beverage Mix, Chocolate Flavor, dry mix, prep w/milk	8.0 oz	224	190.4	7.4	26.0	1.1	7.4	2.2	0.3
14317	Beverage Mix, Chocolate Malt Milk Flavor Powder, no added nutrients	¾ oz (3 heaping tsp)	21	78.8	1.1	18.4	0.2	0.8	0.2	0.1
14316	Beverage Mix, Chocolate Malt Powder, fort, prep w/milk	8.0 oz	224	190.4	7.6	24.6	0.2	7.4	2.2	0.3
14318	Beverage Mix, Chocolate Malted Milk Powder, no added nutrients, prep w/milk	8.0 oz	224	192.6	7.6	25.3	0.2	7.6	2.2	0.3
14245	Beverage Mix, Eggnog, dry, prep w/milk	8.0 oz	224	215.0	6.7	32.0	0.7	6.9	2.0	0.3
14310	Beverage Mix, Natural Malt Powder, fortified, prep w/milk	8.0 oz	224	194.9	8.3	24.0	0.0	7.4	2.1	0.3
14351	Beverage Mix, Strawberry Flavor, dry, prep w/milk	8.0 oz	224	197.1	6.7	27.6	0.0	6.9	2.0	0.3
14006	Beverage, Alcoholic, Beer, Light	12.0 oz	360	100.8	0.7	4.7	0.0	0.0	0.0	0.0
14003	Beverage, Alcoholic, Beer, Regular	12.0 oz	360	147.6	1.1	13.3	0.7	0.0	0.0	0.0
914008	Beverage, Alcoholic, Bloody Mary, prep from recipe	5.0 oz	148	115.4	0.7	4.9	0.4	0.1	0.0	0.0
914870	Beverage, Alcoholic, Champagne	3.5 oz	103	72.1	0.2	2.6	0.0	0.0	0.0	0.0
14414	Beverage, Alcoholic, Coffee Liqueur 53 proof	1.5 oz	52	174.7	0.1	24.3	0.0	0.2	0.0	0.1
14009	Beverage, Alcoholic, Daiquiri, canned	6.8 oz	209	261.3	0.0	32.8	0.0	0.0	0.0	0.0

Sat (g)	Chol (mg)	Cal (mg)	Iron (mg)	Magn (mg)	Phos (mg)	Pota (mg)	Sodi (mg)	Zinc (mg)	Vit A (RE)	Vit C (mg)	Vit E (mg)	Thia (mg)	Ribo (mg)	Niac (mg)	Vit B-6 (mg)	Fol (µg)	Vit B-12 (µg)	Wat (g)
0.2	0.0	1.2	0.1	1.0	3.5	8.5	73.3	0.0	0.5	0.0	0.3	0.2	0.0	0.4	0.0	2.1	0.0	2.4
0.1	0.0	8.7	1.7	12.9	46.0	68.1	148.1	0.5	0.0	0.3	0.1	0.2	0.1	1.4	0.0	41.4	0.0	14.7
0.3	15.4	8.3	2.5	16.0	53.8	43.5	323.2	0.5	21.1	0.4	0.0	0.3	0.2	2.2	0.1	56.3	0.1	20.9
0.1	0.0	7.7	2.0	19.8	70.4	73.6	324.5	0.6	0.0	0.1	0.1	0.2	0.2	1.9	0.0	51.8	0.0	21.1
0.2	0.1	6.0	1.5	28.5	81.4	100.7	250.7	1.0	0.0	0.0	0.1	0.1	0.2	1.3	0.1	16.1	0.0	12.8
0.1	0.0	47.4	2.3	18.6	61.4	64.6	341.8	0.6	0.0	0.0	0.0	0.3	0.2	2.9	0.0	56.3	0.0	20.9
0.0	0.0	8.5	0.7	0.0	70.0	76.0	5.0	0.3	0.0	0.0	0.0	0.6	0.2	1.5	0.2	156.5	0.0	0.0
0.0	0.0	275.7	1.6	103.4	265.1	634.9	1387.7	0.0	0.0	0.0	0.0	0.0	0.0	0.0	0.0	0.0	0.0	0.0
2.5	0.0	175.1	5.4	364.7	419.9	2137.8	11.1	3.3	10.2	0.0	1.7	0.5	1.0	3.7	0.4	293.3	0.0	4.4
0.9	0.0	165.4	5.3	201.5	521.8	2261.6	15.8	1.0	3.5	0.0	0.2	0.3	0.3	1.9	0.5	360.8	0.0	2.4
1.2	0.0	91.1	3.8	58.0	211.1	226.3	5032.9	4.6	12.4	0.0	0.0	0.1	0.3	1.2	0.3	45.5	0.0	57.2
0.9	0.0	77.2	1.9	58.1	171.0	304.6	5.0	1.5	57.3	0.0	0.0	0.1	0.1	3.8	0.2	43.2	0.8	45.6
0.0	0.0	2.6	0.3	5.1	16.5	27.0	857.3	0.1	0.0	0.0	0.0	0.0	0.0	0.5	0.0	2.3	0.0	10.7
0.0	0.0	2.6	0.3	5.1	16.5	27.0	500.0	0.1	0.0	0.0	0.0	0.0	0.0	0.5	0.0	2.3	0.0	10.7
6.0	15.4	122.9	4.4	71.7	266.2	601.6	1100.8	4.8	38.4	5.9	1.2	0.1	0.1	2.3	0.1	76.8	0.0	177.5
0.9	15.9	127.1	7.4	79.5	265.6	681.0	998.8	13.3	27.2	7.0	1.2	0.1	0.1	1.1	0.2	51.1	0.0	165.0
0.3	0.0	127.0	0.7	81.3	264.2	751.8	1008.4	3.6	43.2	7.9	1.3	0.4	0.2	1.1	0.3	60.7	0.0	184.5
0.2	0.0	88.6	4.8	88.6	273.2	779.2	971.5	1.4	0.0	6.8	0.0	0.4	0.3	1.6	0.1	153.8	0.0	191.4
0.0	0.0	24.4	0.9	30.1	74.3	227.5	425.8	0.6	0.9	1.7	0.0	0.0	0.0	0.9	0.0	30.7	0.0	75.5
0.2	0.0	69.4	2.1	66.8	178.2	459.8	5.2	0.9	0.0	1.7	0.0	0.2	0.1	0.6	0.1	106.5	0.0	91.6
0.1	0.0	34.6	1.6	39.7	134.4	329.0	444.2	0.7	0.0	1.5	0.0	0.1	0.1	0.6	0.1	63.0	0.0	99.8
0.1	0.0	18.8	3.3	35.6	178.2	365.3	2.0	1.3	1.0	1.5	0.1	0.2	0.1	1.0	0.2	179.0	0.0	68.9
0.1	0.0	14.0	0.7	25.0	51.5	138.3	1.0	0.4	1.0	0.5	0.3	0.1	0.0	0.3	0.0	82.6	0.0	37.8
0.1	0.0	42.8	1.7	42.8	121.9	262.1	407.7	0.7	0.0	0.6	0.3	0.1	0.1	0.4	0.1	56.7	0.0	64.1
0.2	0.0	48.6	1.6	30.5	104.0	274.6	332.2	0.8	2.3	1.0	1.1	0.1	0.1	0.3	0.1	68.0	0.0	87.6
0.6	10.1	44.1	2.1	41.6	108.4	336.4	376.7	1.5	0.0	7.6	0.0	0.0	0.0	0.4	0.2	13.9	0.0	95.7
4.5	0.0	201.6	5.7	328.3	934.6	1964.2	2.9	6.9	2.9	6.6	0.0	0.6	1.1	1.5	0.3	294.6	0.0	1.2
0.3	0.0	26.9	0.9	22.7	75.6	163.0	30.2	0.5	0.0	0.0	0.2	0.1	0.0	0.2	0.0	0.0	0.0	73.4
0.1	0.0	30.2	0.6	8.4	68.0	52.9	71.4	0.3	0.0	0.0	0.1	0.0	0.0	0.1	0.0	0.0	0.0	76.8
0.3	0.0	26.0	0.7	24.4	52.1	151.2	4.2	0.4	0.0	0.0	0.2	0.1	0.0	0.3	0.0	0.0	0.0	74.8
1.0	0.0	38.6	1.7	43.7	61.3	63.0	2413.3	1.3	14.3	0.2	0.0	0.1	0.1	0.3	0.1	24.4	0.0	58.8
0.4	5.8	6.0	2.8	23.0	239.0	287.0	72.0	6.9	0.0	0.0	0.0	0.1	0.2	3.8	0.3	8.0	2.6	55.7
1.2	14.7	9.0	2.2	18.0	184.0	229.0	61.0	5.0	0.0	0.0	0.0	0.1	0.2	3.0	0.3	6.0	2.2	43.0
0.0	0.0	37.0	1.0	0.0	0.0	231.0	640.0	0.0	207.4	2.0	0.0	0.1	0.3	3.6	0.0	0.0	0.0	0.0
8.5	0.0	60.0	4.8	0.0	248.0	425.0	1053.0	0.0	120.0	33.0	0.0	0.3	0.4	5.0	0.0	0.0	0.0	188.5
0.4	16.0	80.0	1.4	0.0	0.0	150.0	890.0	0.0	150.0	2.0	0.0	0.1	0.1	1.2	0.0	0.0	0.0	0.0
0.0	0.0	49.0	1.7	0.0	0.0	357.0	753.0	0.0	144.4	1.0	0.0	0.0	0.2	1.7	0.0	0.0	0.0	167.2
1.9	389.0	7.0	6.8	20.0	404.0	235.0	70.0	6.1	10602.0	23.0	0.0	0.2	4.1	10.7	0.9	217.0	71.0	65.9
3.2	573.6	13.1	7.5	27.4	548.6	433.2	126.1	6.5	12767.5	27.4	0.8	0.2	4.9	17.2	1.7	261.8	133.0	66.3
7.4	39.6	27.3	3.6	0.0	140.5	314.9	561.9	3.0	795.8	5.7	0.0	0.3	0.3	4.5	0.2	27.3	0.0	0.0
0.0	56.0	33.9	1.4	0.0	0.0	270.2	795.5	0.0	8.5	0.0	0.0	0.1	0.3	2.6	0.0	0.0	0.0	105.1
0.4	4.5	9.0	3.2	27.0	245.0	352.0	65.0	7.1	0.0	0.0	0.0	0.1	0.3	4.2	0.4	9.0	2.7	57.8
3.8	86.0	9.0	3.0	26.0	233.0	360.0	67.0	6.9	0.0	0.0	0.1	0.1	0.2	4.1	0.4	8.0	2.6	59.3
1.0	12.0	10.0	2.6	21.0	193.0	287.0	59.0	5.5	0.0	0.0	0.0	0.1	0.2	3.5	0.3	7.0	2.4	46.9
8.5	88.0	10.0	2.6	22.0	203.0	313.0	62.0	5.9	0.0	0.0	0.2	0.1	0.2	3.6	0.3	7.0	2.4	51.4
3.1	86.0	8.0	3.0	26.0	231.0	354.0	66.0	6.8	0.0	0.0	0.0	0.1	0.2	4.0	0.4	8.0	2.6	60.1
4.9	155.3	34.1	5.2	0.0	172.9	517.6	672.9	5.2	0.0	9.4	0.0	0.1	0.5	5.3	0.5	17.6	0.0	0.0
6.3	29.5	118.5	0.9	0.0	158.2	173.0	809.0	0.0	81.2	0.5	0.0	0.1	0.2	0.7	0.0	0.0	0.0	81.4
6.3	98.0	8.0	1.9	12.0	125.0	145.0	1134.0	4.6	0.0	0.0	0.2	0.0	0.2	3.0	0.2	6.0	1.6	59.8
69.0	5.0	2.0	27.0	226.0	395.0	62.0		4.7	0.0	0.0	0.1	0.1	0.2	3.8	0.4	7.0	2.2	64.6
7.7	96.4	8.3	2.8	25.0	190.4	371.3	83.3	6.4	0.0	0.0	0.0	0.1	0.3	5.6	0.3	10.7	2.4	68.5
7.3	87.0	11.0	2.1	21.0	158.0	301.0	77.0	5.4	0.0	0.0	0.2	0.1	0.3	5.2	0.3	9.0	2.4	55.7
7.5	84.0	10.0	2.2	20.0	159.0	299.0	77.0	5.2	0.0	0.0	0.2	0.1	0.2	4.8	0.3	9.0	2.3	55.6
8.1	90.0	11.0	2.4	20.0	170.0	292.0	83.0	5.2	0.0	0.0	0.2	0.0	0.2	5.8	0.3	9.0	2.9	54.2
10.5	105.9	13.1	2.9	23.8	203.5	357.0	100.0	6.0	0.0	0.0	0.3	0.0	0.2	6.9	0.3	10.7	3.2	62.2
8.8	116.6	15.5	3.2	26.2	224.9	395.1	110.7	6.7	0.0	0.0	0.0	0.0	0.2	7.7	0.3	11.9	3.6	62.7
4.6	26.9	253.1	0.7	44.8	215.0	418.9	138.9	1.1	65.0	2.0	0.0	0.1	0.4	0.3	0.1	10.3	0.7	181.2
0.5	1.1	12.6	0.5	14.7	36.8	129.8	52.7	0.2	4.0	0.3	0.1	0.0	0.0	0.4	0.0	4.2	0.0	0.3
4.6	29.1	324.8	3.2	44.8	264.3	524.2	206.1	1.0	761.6	28.7	0.0	0.6	1.1	9.2	0.9	26.9	0.7	181.9
4.7	29.1	257.6	0.5	40.3	224.0	421.1	145.6	0.9	67.2	2.2	0.0	0.1	0.4	0.5	0.1	13.9	0.8	181.7
4.2	26.9	239.7	0.3	26.9	188.2	304.6	134.4	0.8	62.7	1.8	0.0	0.1	0.3	0.2	0.1	10.1	0.7	176.7
4.6	29.1	313.6	3.0	40.3	259.8	483.8	172.5	0.9	627.2	24.9	0.0	0.6	1.0	8.8	0.7	18.4	0.9	182.1
4.3	26.9	246.4	0.2	26.9	192.6	311.4	107.5	0.8	62.7	2.0	0.0	0.1	0.4	0.2	0.1	10.3	0.7	181.2
0.0	0.0	18.0	0.1	18.0	43.2	64.8	10.8	0.1	0.0	0.0	0.0	0.0	0.1	1.4	0.1	14.8	0.0	342.7
0.0	0.0	18.0	0.1	21.6	43.2	90.0	18.0	0.1	0.0	0.0	0.0	0.0	0.1	1.6	0.2	21.6	0.1	332.3
0.0	0.0	10.4	0.5	11.8	20.7	216.1	331.5	0.1	50.3	20.4	0.0	0.1	0.0	0.6	0.1	19.7	0.0	127.3
0.0	0.0	0.0	0.0	0.0	0.0	0.0	0.0	0.0	0.0	0.0	0.0	0.0	0.0	0.0	0.0	0.0	0.0	0.0
0.1	0.0	0.5	0.0	1.6	3.1	15.6	4.2	0.0	0.0	0.0	0.0	0.0	0.0	0.1	0.0	0.0	0.0	16.1
0.0	0.0	0.0	0.0	2.1	4.2	23.0	83.6	0.1	0.0	2.7	0.0	0.0	0.0	0.0	0.0	1.7	0.0	155.9

Code	Food Name	Unit/Amt	Wt (g)	Energy (Kcal)	Prot (g)	Carb (g)	Fiber (g)	Fat (g)	Mono (g)	Poly (g)
14037	Beverage, Alcoholic, Distilled Spirits (gin, rum, vodka or whisky) 80 proof	1.5 oz	42	97.0	0.0	0.0	0.0	0.0	0.0	0.0
914011	Beverage, Alcoholic, Gin and Tonic, prep from recipe	7.5 oz	225	171.0	0.0	15.8	0.0	0.0	0.0	0.0
914014	Beverage, Alcoholic, Martini, prep from recipe	2.5 oz	70	156.1	0.0	0.2	0.0	0.0	0.0	0.0
14015	Beverage, Alcoholic, Pina Colada, canned	6.8 oz	209	495.3	1.3	57.7	0.2	15.9	0.9	0.3
14027	Beverage, Alcoholic, Whiskey Sour, canned	6.8 oz	209	248.7	0.0	28.0	0.2	0.0	0.0	0.0
14084	Beverage, Alcoholic, Wine (all table)	3.5 oz	103	72.1	0.2	1.4	0.0	0.0	0.0	0.0
14115	Beverage, Alpine Spiced Cider, Instant Apple Flavor Drink Mix, h powder/Continenta	2 tsbp	8	31.6	0.0	7.9	0.0	0.0	0.0	0.0
14181	Beverage, Chocolate Syrup w/o added nutrients	2 tsbp	38	82.8	0.7	22.4	0.7	0.3	0.1	0.1
14186	Beverage, Chocolate Syrup, fortified, mixed w/milk	8.0 oz	224	168.0	7.2	20.2	0.2	7.2	2.1	0.3
14390	Beverage, Cocoa Mix w/aspartame, dry, low kcal, prep w/H$_2$O	8.0 oz	224	56.0	4.5	9.9	0.4	0.4	0.2	0.0
14194	Beverage, Cocoa Mix, dry, w/o added nutrients, prep w/H$_2$O	8.0 oz	224	112.0	3.4	24.4	2.7	1.3	0.4	0.0
14417	Beverage, Cocoa Mix, fortified, dry, prep w/H$_2$O	8.0 oz	224	127.7	2.0	25.8	0.9	3.1	1.1	0.1
14195	Beverage, Cocoa, Hot Cocoa Mix w/marshmallows/Carnation	2 tsbp	22	87.8	1.1	19.1	0.4	0.8	0.2	0.3
14418	Beverage, Coffee Mix w/sugar (Cappuccino) dry, prep w/H$_2$O	8.0 oz	224	71.7	0.4	12.5	0.0	2.5	0.1	0.0
14209	Beverage, Coffee, Brewed	6.0 oz	168	3.4	0.2	0.7	0.0	0.0	0.0	0.0
14219	Beverage, Coffee, Instant powder, decaffeinated, prep	1 rd tsp.	1.8	0.0	0.0	0.0	0.0	0.0	0.0	0.0
14215	Beverage, Coffee, Instant, prep	6.0 oz	168	3.4	0.2	0.7	0.0	0.0	0.0	0.0
14400	Beverage, Cola w/caffeine	12.0 oz	336	137.8	0.0	34.9	0.0	0.0	0.0	0.0
1057	Beverage, Eggnog	8.0 oz	254	341.9	9.7	34.4	0.0	19.0	5.7	0.9
914840	Beverage, Fruit Tea Punch	6.0 oz	168	107.5	0.0	27.0	0.0	0.0	0.0	0.0
14123	Beverage, Kiwi Strawberry Cocktail/Snapple	6.0 oz	168	80.0	0.2	19.8	0.0	0.0	0.0	0.0
14305	Beverage, Malt Beverage	6.0 oz	168	100.8	0.5	22.6	0.0	0.2	0.0	0.1
14137	Beverage, Nestea Ice Tea, Lemon Flavor	6.0 oz	168	61.7	0.0	14.3	0.0	0.5	0.0	0.0
914814	Beverage, Soft Drink, Chocolate Carbonated	12.0 oz	355	163.3	0.0	41.5	0.0	0.0	0.0	0.0
14121	Beverage, Soft Drink, Club Soda	12.0 oz	355	0.0	0.0	0.0	0.0	0.0	0.0	0.0
14166	Beverage, Soft Drink, Cola or Pepper-type, low kcal w/saccharin & caffeine	12.0 oz	355	0.0	0.0	0.4	0.0	0.0	0.0	0.0
14535	Beverage, Soft Drink, Cola, low kcal w/saccharin&aspartame, w/caffeine	12.0 oz	355	3.6	0.4	0.4	0.0	0.0	0.0	0.0
14416	Beverage, Soft Drink, Cola, w/aspartame, low kcal	12.0 oz	355	3.6	0.4	0.4	0.0	0.0	0.0	0.0
14130	Beverage, Soft Drink, Cream Soda	12.0 oz	355	181.1	0.0	47.2	0.0	0.0	0.0	0.0
914818	Beverage, Soft Drink, Diet Fruit Flavor	12.0 oz	355	3.6	0.0	0.0	0.0	0.0	0.0	0.0
914819	Beverage, Soft Drink, Diet Ginger Ale	12.0 oz	355	3.6	0.0	1.5	0.0	0.0	0.0	0.0
914820	Beverage, Soft Drink, Diet Lemon-Lime	12.0 oz	355	0.0	0.0	0.0	0.0	0.0	0.0	0.0
914887	Beverage, Soft Drink, Diet Root Beer	12.0 oz	355	0.0	0.0	0.4	0.0	0.0	0.0	0.0
14136	Beverage, Soft Drink, Ginger Ale	12.0 oz	355	120.7	0.0	30.9	0.0	0.0	0.0	0.0
14142	Beverage, Soft Drink, Grape	12.0 oz	355	152.7	0.0	39.8	0.0	0.0	0.0	0.0
14145	Beverage, Soft Drink, Lemon-Lime	12.0 oz	355	142.0	0.0	36.9	0.0	0.0	0.0	0.0
914888	Beverage, Soft Drink, Mineral H$_2$O	12.0 oz	355	0.0	0.0	0.0	0.0	0.0	0.0	0.0
14537	Beverage, Soft Drink, Not Cola or Pepper-type, w/saccharin, low kcal	12.0 oz	355	0.0	0.0	0.4	0.0	0.0	0.0	0.0
14150	Beverage, Soft Drink, Orange	12.0 oz	355	170.4	0.0	43.7	0.0	0.0	0.0	0.0
14153	Beverage, Soft Drink, Pepper type	12.0 oz	355	145.6	0.0	36.9	0.0	0.4	0.0	0.0
14157	Beverage, Soft Drink, Root Beer	12.0 oz	355	145.6	0.0	37.6	0.0	0.0	0.0	0.0
14376	Beverage, Tea Mix, Instant w/lemon flavor, w/saccharin, dry, prep	2 tsp	1.4	0.0	0.0	0.0	0.0	0.0	0.0	0.0
14369	Beverage, Tea Mix, Instant w/lemon, unsweetened, dry, prep	2 tsp	1.4	0.0	0.0	0.0	0.0	0.0	0.0	0.0
14367	Beverage, Tea Mix, Instant, unsweetened, dry, prep	2 tsp	1.4	0.0	0.0	0.0	0.0	0.0	0.0	0.0
14355	Beverage, Tea, Brewed	6.0 oz	240	2.4	0.0	0.7	0.0	0.0	0.0	0.0
14545	Beverage, Tea, Chamomile, Brewed	6.0 oz	240	2.4	0.0	0.5	0.0	0.0	0.0	0.0
914810	Beverage, Tea, Crystal Light	6.0 oz	240	2.4	0.1	0.4	0.0	0.0	0.0	0.0
14381	Beverage, Tea, Herbal (not chamomile) Brewed	6.0 oz	240	2.4	0.0	0.5	0.0	0.0	0.0	0.0
14549	Beverage, Tea, Instant, w/sugar, lemon-flavored, w/added Vit C, dry, prep	6.0 oz	240	81.6	0.2	20.4	0.0	0.0	0.0	0.0
914906	Beverage, Tea, sweetened, canned	12.0 oz	480	196.8	0.0	48.7	0.0	0.0	0.0	0.0
14133	Beverage, Tomato Cocktail/Bloody Mary mix, mild/Tabasco	6.0 oz	240	55.7	2.2	11.8	0.0	0.0	0.0	0.0
14429	Beverage, Water	1.0 fl oz	30	0.3	0.0	0.0	0.0	0.0	0.0	0.0
14155	Beverage, Water, Carbonated, Tonic (Quinine)	12.0 oz can or bottle	366	124.4	0.0	32.2	0.0	0.0	0.0	0.0
14384	Beverage, Water, Perrier	6.5 fl oz bottle	192	0.0	0.0	0.0	0.0	0.0	0.0	0.0
18615	Biscuit, Buttermilk Biscuit Mix, dry/Martha White	1 biscut	41	171.4	3.0	26.4	0.0	5.9	0.0	0.0
18017	Biscuit, Mixed Grain, refrig dough	1 biscuit (2.5" dia)	44	115.7	2.7	20.9	0.0	2.5	1.3	0.4
18633	Biscuit, Pillsbury Grands Buttermilk, refrigerated dough/Pillsbury	1 biscut	61	194.8	4.1	25.1	0.0	8.7	0.0	0.0
18009	Biscuit, Plain or Buttermilk, commercially baked	1 small (2.5" diam)	35	127.4	2.2	17.0	0.5	5.8	2.4	2.2
918011	Biscuit, Plain or Buttermilk, dry mix, prep	1 biscuit (3" dia)	57	191.0	4.2	27.6	1.0	6.9	0.0	0.0
18016	Biscuit, Plain or Buttermilk, homemade	1 medium biscuit (2.5" dia)	60	212.4	4.2	26.8	0.9	9.8	4.2	2.5
18013	Biscuit, Plain or Buttermilk, refrig dough, baked, reduced fat	1 biscuit (2.25" dia)	21	62.8	1.6	11.6	0.4	1.1	0.6	0.2
18015	Biscuit, Plain or Buttermilk, refrig dough, bkd	1 biscuit (2.5" dia)	27	93.4	1.8	12.8	0.4	4.0	2.2	0.5
20015	Bran, Corn, crude	1 tbsp	4.8	10.8	0.4	4.1	4.1	0.0	0.0	0.0
20034	Bran, Oat, ckd	1 tbsp	13.7	5.5	0.4	1.6	0.4	0.1	0.0	0.0
20060	Bran, Rice, crude	1 tbsp	7.4	23.4	1.0	3.7	1.6	1.5	0.6	0.6
20077	Bran, Wheat, crude	1 tbsp	3.5	7.6	0.5	2.3	1.5	0.1	0.0	0.1
18376	Bread Crumbs, dry, grated, seasoned	1 oz	28	102.8	4.0	19.7	1.2	0.7	0.3	0.2
18079	Bread Crumbs, Plain, grated, dry	¼ cup	27	106.7	3.4	19.6	0.6	1.5	0.6	0.3

Sat (g)	Chol (mg)	Cal (mg)	Iron (mg)	Magn (mg)	Phos (mg)	Pota (mg)	Sodi (mg)	Zinc (mg)	Vit A (RE)	Vit C (mg)	Vit E (mg)	Thia (mg)	Ribo (mg)	Niac (mg)	Vit B-6 (mg)	Fol (µg)	Vit B-12 (µg)	Wat (g)
0.0	0.0	0.0	0.0	0.0	1.7	0.8	0.4	0.0	0.0	0.0	0.0	0.0	0.0	0.0	0.0	0.0	0.0	28.0
0.0	0.0	4.5	0.0	2.3	2.3	11.3	9.0	0.2	0.0	0.9	0.0	0.0	0.0	0.0	0.0	1.1	0.0	193.1
0.0	0.0	1.4	0.1	1.4	2.1	12.6	2.1	0.0	0.0	0.0	0.0	0.0	0.0	0.0	0.0	0.1	0.0	47.3
13.7	0.0	2.1	0.1	12.5	75.2	173.5	148.4	0.4	4.2	3.1	0.0	0.0	0.0	0.2	0.0	12.5	0.0	114.7
0.0	0.0	0.0	0.0	2.1	12.5	23.0	92.0	0.1	2.1	3.3	0.0	0.0	0.0	0.0	0.0	0.0	0.0	160.7
0.0	0.0	8.2	0.4	10.3	14.4	91.7	8.2	0.1	0.0	0.0	0.0	0.0	0.0	0.1	0.0	1.1	0.0	91.6
0.0	0.0	0.0	0.0	0.0	0.0	0.0	0.1	0.0	0.0	29.0	0.0	0.0	0.0	0.0	0.0	0.0	0.0	0.0
0.2	0.0	5.3	0.8	24.7	49.0	85.1	36.5	0.3	1.1	0.1	0.0	0.0	0.0	0.1	0.0	1.5	0.0	14.1
4.4	29.1	248.6	2.3	26.9	194.9	392.0	125.4	0.8	273.3	2.0	0.0	0.1	0.5	5.6	0.1	10.3	0.7	187.7
0.3	2.2	105.3	0.9	38.1	156.8	472.6	201.6	0.6	0.0	0.0	0.0	0.0	0.2	0.2	0.1	2.7	0.3	207.0
0.7	2.2	105.3	0.4	26.9	96.3	219.5	161.3	0.5	0.0	0.4	0.0	0.0	0.2	0.2	0.0	0.0	0.4	193.5
1.9	0.0	112.0	1.9	24.6	118.7	434.6	221.8	0.3	161.3	6.5	0.0	0.2	0.2	2.1	0.0	0.0	0.4	190.8
0.3	1.3	32.3	0.2	12.8	45.5	111.5	75.5	0.2	0.0	0.0	0.0	0.0	0.1	0.1	0.0	0.9	0.1	0.4
2.1	0.0	9.0	0.2	11.2	31.4	138.9	121.0	0.1	0.0	0.0	0.0	0.0	0.0	0.4	0.0	0.0	0.0	207.4
0.0	0.0	3.4	0.1	8.4	1.7	90.7	3.4	0.0	0.0	0.0	0.0	0.0	0.0	0.4	0.0	0.2	0.0	166.8
0.0	0.0	0.1	0.0	0.1	0.1	0.6	0.1	0.0	0.0	0.0	0.0	0.0	0.0	0.0	0.0	0.0	0.0	1.8
0.0	0.0	5.0	0.1	6.7	5.0	60.5	5.0	0.1	0.0	0.0	0.0	0.0	0.0	0.5	0.0	0.0	0.0	166.3
0.0	0.0	10.1	0.1	3.4	40.3	3.4	13.4	0.0	0.0	0.0	0.0	0.0	0.0	0.0	0.0	0.0	0.0	300.4
11.3	149.1	330.2	0.5	47.0	277.9	419.6	138.2	1.2	203.2	3.8	0.6	0.1	0.5	0.3	0.1	2.3	1.1	188.9
0.0	0.0	0.0	0.0	0.0	0.0	0.0	9.1	0.0	0.0	0.0	0.0	0.0	0.0	0.0	0.0	0.0	0.0	
0.0	0.0	0.0	0.0	0.0	0.0	0.0	4.2	0.0	0.0	0.0	0.0	0.0	0.0	0.0	0.0	0.0	0.0	147.8
0.0	0.0	8.4	0.1	11.8	37.0	13.4	21.8	0.0	0.0	0.8	0.0	0.0	0.1	1.9	0.0	23.5	0.0	144.5
0.0	0.0	0.0	0.0	0.0	0.0	0.0	0.0	0.0	0.0	0.0	0.0	0.0	0.0	0.0	0.0	0.0	0.0	153.2
0.0	0.0	0.0	0.0	0.0	0.0	0.0	26.6	0.0	0.0	0.0	0.0	0.0	0.0	0.0	0.0	0.0	0.0	0.0
0.0	0.0	17.8	0.0	3.6	0.0	7.1	74.6	0.4	0.0	0.0	0.0	0.0	0.0	0.0	0.0	0.0	0.0	354.6
0.0	0.0	14.2	0.1	3.6	39.1	7.1	56.8	0.2	0.0	0.0	0.0	0.0	0.0	0.0	0.0	0.0	0.0	354.3
0.0	0.0	14.2	0.1	3.6	32.0	0.0	32.0	0.3	0.0	0.0	0.0	0.0	0.1	0.0	0.0	0.0	0.0	354.3
0.0	0.0	14.2	0.1	3.6	32.0	0.0	21.3	0.3	0.0	0.0	0.0	0.0	0.1	0.0	0.0	0.0	0.0	354.3
0.0	0.0	17.8	0.2	3.6	0.0	3.6	42.6	0.2	0.0	0.0	0.0	0.0	0.0	0.0	0.0	0.0	0.0	307.8
0.0	0.0	35.5	0.0	0.0	0.0	0.0	21.7	0.0	0.0	0.0	0.0	0.0	0.0	0.0	0.0	0.0	0.0	0.0
0.0	0.0	17.8	0.1	0.0	0.0	0.0	31.6	0.0	0.0	0.0	0.0	0.0	0.0	0.0	0.0	0.0	0.0	0.0
0.0	0.0	34.5	0.0	0.0	0.0	3.9	48.3	0.0	0.0	0.0	0.0	0.0	0.0	0.0	0.0	0.0	0.0	0.0
0.0	0.0	0.0	0.0	0.0	0.0	0.0	56.6	0.0	0.0	0.0	0.0	0.0	0.0	0.0	0.0	0.0	0.0	0.0
0.0	0.0	10.7	0.6	3.6	0.0	3.6	24.9	0.2	0.0	0.0	0.0	0.0	0.0	0.0	0.0	0.0	0.0	323.8
0.0	0.0	10.7	0.3	3.6	0.0	3.6	53.3	0.2	0.0	0.0	0.0	0.0	0.0	0.0	0.0	0.0	0.0	315.2
0.0	0.0	7.1	0.2	3.6	0.0	3.6	39.1	0.2	0.0	0.0	0.0	0.0	0.1	0.0	0.0	0.0	0.0	317.7
0.0	0.0	48.1	0.0	1.8	0.0	0.0	5.5	0.0	0.0	0.0	0.0	0.0	0.0	0.0	0.0	0.0	0.0	354.8
0.0	0.0	14.2	0.1	3.6	0.0	7.1	56.8	0.2	0.0	0.0	0.0	0.0	0.0	0.0	0.0	0.0	0.0	354.3
0.0	0.0	17.8	0.2	3.6	3.6	7.1	42.6	0.4	0.0	0.0	0.0	0.0	0.0	0.0	0.0	0.0	0.0	311.0
0.2	0.0	10.7	0.1	0.0	39.1	3.6	35.5	0.1	0.0	0.0	0.0	0.0	0.0	0.0	0.0	0.0	0.0	317.4
0.0	0.0	17.8	0.2	3.6	0.0	3.6	46.2	0.2	0.0	0.0	0.0	0.0	0.0	0.0	0.0	0.0	0.0	317.0
0.0	0.0	0.0	0.0	0.0	0.0	0.2	0.1	0.0	0.0	0.0	0.0	0.0	0.0	0.0	0.0	0.0	0.0	1.4
0.0	0.0	0.0	0.0	0.0	0.0	0.3	0.1	0.0	0.0	0.0	0.0	0.0	0.0	0.0	0.0	0.0	0.0	1.4
0.0	0.0	0.0	0.0	0.0	0.0	0.3	0.0	0.0	0.0	0.0	0.0	0.0	0.0	0.0	0.0	0.0	0.0	1.4
0.0	0.0	0.0	0.0	7.2	2.4	88.8	7.2	0.0	0.0	0.0	0.0	0.0	0.0	0.0	0.0	12.5	0.0	239.3
0.0	0.0	4.8	0.2	2.4	0.0	21.6	2.4	0.1	4.8	0.0	0.2	0.0	0.0	0.0	0.0	1.4	0.0	239.3
0.0	0.0	0.0	0.0	10.1	0.0	15.1	1.0	0.0	0.0	6.1	0.0	0.0	0.0	0.0	0.0	0.0	0.0	238.9
0.0	0.0	4.8	0.2	2.4	0.0	21.6	2.4	0.1	0.0	0.0	0.0	0.0	0.0	0.0	0.0	1.4	0.0	239.3
0.0	0.0	4.8	0.0	4.8	2.4	45.6	7.2	0.1	0.0	21.6	0.0	0.0	0.0	0.1	0.0	8.9	0.0	218.9
0.0	0.0	0.0	0.0	0.0	0.0	125.3	17.3	0.0	0.0	0.0	0.0	0.0	0.0	0.0	0.0	0.0	0.0	0.0
0.0	0.0	0.0	1.7	0.0	0.0	0.0	1164.0	0.0	0.0	0.0	0.0	0.0	0.0	0.0	0.0	0.0	0.0	221.5
0.0	0.0	0.6	0.0	0.3	0.0	0.0	0.9	0.0	0.0	0.0	0.0	0.0	0.0	0.0	0.0	0.0	0.0	30.0
0.0	0.0	3.7	0.0	0.0	0.0	0.0	14.6	0.4	0.0	0.0	0.0	0.0	0.0	0.0	0.0	0.0	0.0	333.4
0.0	0.0	26.9	0.0	0.0	0.0	0.5	1.9	0.0	0.0	0.0	0.0	0.0	0.0	0.0	0.0	0.0	0.0	191.8
1.1	0.0	60.7	0.0	0.0	0.0	0.0	504.3	0.0	0.0	0.0	0.0	0.0	0.0	0.0	0.0	0.0	0.0	3.6
0.6	0.0	7.5	1.2	13.2	103.8	200.6	294.8	0.3	0.0	0.0	0.0	0.2	0.1	1.5	0.0	36.5	0.0	16.6
2.4	0.0	0.0	1.5	0.0	0.0	0.0	605.1	0.0	0.0	0.0	0.0	0.0	0.0	0.0	0.0	0.0	0.0	21.2
0.9	0.4	17.2	1.2	6.0	150.5	78.4	368.2	0.2	0.4	0.0	1.0	0.1	0.1	1.2	0.0	20.7	0.0	9.3
2.5	2.4	105.5	1.2	14.3	267.9	107.2	544.4	0.3	14.8	0.2	0.0	0.2	0.2	1.7	0.0	3.4	0.1	16.5
2.6	1.8	141.0	1.7	10.8	98.4	72.6	348.0	0.3	13.8	0.1	0.8	0.2	0.2	1.8	0.0	36.6	0.0	17.3
0.3	0.0	4.0	0.6	3.6	97.7	38.9	304.7	0.1	0.0	0.0	0.1	0.1	0.0	0.7	0.0	14.5	0.0	5.8
1.0	0.0	5.4	0.7	3.8	104.0	42.4	324.5	0.1	0.0	0.0	0.5	0.1	0.1	0.8	0.0	11.6	0.0	7.5
0.0	0.0	2.0	0.1	3.1	3.5	2.1	0.3	0.1	0.3	0.0	0.1	0.0	0.0	0.1	0.0	0.2	0.0	0.2
0.0	0.0	1.4	0.1	5.5	16.3	12.6	0.1	0.1	0.0	0.0	0.0	0.0	0.0	0.0	0.0	0.8	0.0	11.5
0.3	0.0	4.2	1.4	57.8	124.1	109.9	0.4	0.4	0.0	0.0	0.4	0.2	0.0	2.5	0.3	4.7	0.0	0.5
0.0	0.0	2.6	0.4	21.4	35.5	41.4	0.1	0.3	0.0	0.0	0.1	0.0	0.0	0.5	0.0	2.8	0.0	0.3
0.2	0.3	27.7	0.9	10.6	37.2	75.6	742.0	0.3	0.8	0.1	0.0	0.0	0.0	0.8	0.0	30.5	0.0	1.6
0.3	0.0	61.3	1.7	12.4	39.7	59.7	232.7	0.3	0.0	0.0	0.2	0.2	0.1	1.8	0.0	29.4	0.0	1.7

Code	Food Name	Unit/Amt	Wt (g)	Energy (Kcal)	Prot (g)	Carb (g)	Fiber (g)	Fat (g)	Mono (g)	Poly (g)
18080	Bread sticks, plain	1 small stick (4.25″ long)	5	20.6	0.6	3.4	0.2	0.5	0.2	0.2
18085	Bread Stuffing, Corn, dry mix, prep	½ cup	100	179.0	2.9	21.9	2.9	8.8	3.9	2.7
18082	Bread Stuffing, Plain, dry mix, prep	½ cup	100	178.0	3.2	21.7	2.9	8.6	3.8	2.6
918083	Bread Stuffing, Plain, homemade	½ cup	100	168.0	3.8	22.2	0.0	7.2	0.0	0.0
918020	Bread, Banana, homemade w/vegetable shortening	½ cup	116	392.1	5.0	63.9	0.0	13.7	0.0	0.0
18021	Bread, Boston Brown, canned	1 slice	45	87.8	2.3	19.5	2.1	0.7	0.1	0.3
918023	Bread, Corn, dry mix, prep	1 piece	60	188.4	4.3	28.9	1.4	6.0	0.0	0.0
918026	Bread, Cracked Wheat, toasted	1 thin slice	18	50.9	1.7	9.7	1.1	0.8	0.0	0.0
18027	Bread, Egg	1 slice (5″ x 3″ x 0.5″)	40	114.8	3.8	19.1	0.9	2.4	0.9	0.4
18029	Bread, French/Vienna/Sourdough	1 medium slice (4.75 x 4 x 0.5″)	25	68.5	2.2	13.0	0.8	0.8	0.3	0.2
18604	Bread, Garlic, frozen/Campione	1 slice	50	181.2	4.3	22.2	2.4	8.4	0.0	0.0
18641	Bread, Hamburger Rolls/Wonder	1 roll	43	115.5	4.3	21.2	0.0	1.5	0.0	0.0
18033	Bread, Italian	1 medium slice	20	54.2	1.8	10.0	0.5	0.7	0.2	0.3
18035	Bread, Mixed Grain/7-Grain/Whole Grain	1 large slice	32	80.0	3.2	14.8	2.0	1.2	0.5	0.3
18037	Bread, Oatbran	1 slice	30	70.8	3.1	11.9	1.4	1.3	0.5	0.5
18049	Bread, Oatbran, reduced kcal	1.0 oz	28.35	57.0	2.3	11.7	3.4	0.9	0.2	0.5
18039	Bread, Oatmeal	1.0 oz	28.35	76.3	2.4	13.7	1.1	1.2	0.4	0.5
18041	Bread, Pita, White, enriched	1 small pita (4″ dia)	28	77.0	2.5	15.6	0.6	0.3	0.0	0.1
18042	Bread, Pita, Whole Wheat	1 small pita (4″ dia)	28	74.5	2.7	15.4	2.1	0.7	0.1	0.3
18044	Bread, Pumpernickel	1 thin slice	20	50.0	1.7	9.5	1.3	0.6	0.2	0.2
918046	Bread, Pumpkin, homemade	1 slice (3.75 x 3 x 0.5″)	60	198.6	2.4	30.7	0.0	7.7	0.0	0.0
18047	Bread, Raisin, enriched	1 slice	26	71.2	2.1	13.6	1.1	1.1	0.6	0.2
18059	Bread, Rice Bran	1 slice	27	65.6	2.4	11.7	1.3	1.2	0.4	0.5
18060	Bread, Rye	1 slice	32	82.9	2.7	15.5	1.9	1.1	0.4	0.3
18064	Bread, Wheat (includes wheat berry)	1 slice	25	65.0	2.3	11.8	1.1	1.0	0.4	0.2
18066	Bread, Wheat Bran	1 slice	36	89.3	3.2	17.2	1.4	1.2	0.6	0.2
18055	Bread, Wheat, reduced kcal	1 slice	23	45.5	2.1	10.0	2.8	0.5	0.1	0.2
18069	Bread, White, commercially prep, crumbs/cubes/slices	¼ cup of crumbs	12	32.0	1.0	5.9	0.3	0.4	0.2	0.1
18057	Bread, White, reduced kcal	1 slice	23	47.6	2.0	10.2	2.2	0.6	0.2	0.1
18075	Bread, Whole Wheat, commercially prep	1 slice	29	71.3	2.8	13.4	2.0	1.2	0.5	0.3
18022	Bread/Muffins, Corn, dry mix, enriched	¼ cup of crumbs	12	50.2	0.8	8.3	0.8	1.5	0.8	0.2
908918	Breakfast Bar, Chocolate Chip	1 bar	41	198.0	6.5	20.6	1.4	10.6	5.3	1.1
908919	Breakfast Bar, Chocolate Crunch	1 bar	38	183.2	6.8	18.6	1.2	9.8	4.3	1.6
908920	Breakfast Bar, Peanut Chocolate Chip	1 bar	40	196.0	7.0	19.4	1.4	10.6	5.4	2.2
908921	Breakfast Bar, Peanut Crunch	1 bar	38	188.9	7.1	17.9	1.0	10.4	5.3	2.3
1001	Butter, Regular (with salt)	1 pat (1″ sq, ⅓″ high)	5	35.9	0.0	0.0	0.0	4.1	1.2	0.2
1145	Butter, Unsalted	1 tbsp	14	100.4	0.1	0.0	0.0	11.4	3.3	0.4
1002	Butter, Whipped (with salt)	1 pat (1″ sq, ⅓″ high)	4	28.7	0.0	0.0	0.0	3.2	0.9	0.1
18086	Cake, Angelfood, commercially prep	1 piece (1/12 of 12 oz cake)	29	74.8	1.7	16.8	0.4	0.2	0.0	0.1
18088	Cake, Angelfood, dry mix, prep	1 piece (1/12 of 10″ dia)	50	128.5	3.1	29.4	0.1	0.2	0.0	0.1
918823	Cake, Apple Streusel Crumb	1 piece	52	240.2	2.0	33.0	0.3	11.0	5.0	3.0
918824	Cake, Banana	1/12 cake	75	249.8	3.0	36.0	0.3	11.0	0.0	0.0
18090	Cake, Boston Cream Pie, commercially prep	1 piece (⅙ of pie)	92	231.8	2.2	39.5	1.3	7.8	4.2	0.9
918093	Cake, Carrot, dry mix, prep, w/o icing	1 piece (1/12 of 9″ dia)	70	239.4	3.6	32.7	1.4	11.0	0.0	0.0
918828	Cake, Chocolate Fudge	⅙ cake	60	310.2	30.0	40.0	0.0	15.0	5.0	6.0
918858	Cake, Chocolate Suzy Q's/Hostess	2 cakes	128	480.0	4.0	74.0	0.5	20.0	0.0	0.0
18099	Cake, Chocolate, dry mix, regular	1 package (18.5 oz)	524	2242.7	30.9	382.5	12.6	81.7	33.1	26.4
918129	Cake, Chocolate, dry mix, special dietary	1 package (8 oz)	227	874.0	7.5	176.2	0.0	22.2	0.0	0.0
18101	Cake, Chocolate, homemade, w/o icing	1 piece (1/12 of 9″ dia)	95	340.1	5.0	50.7	1.5	14.3	5.7	2.6
918846	Cake, Cinnamon Streusel, frozen	⅛ cake	39	145.9	2.2	19.4	0.3	7.1	0.0	0.0
918851	Cake, Devil Square/LittleDeb	2 squares	62	295.1	1.9	32.9	0.5	17.3	11.3	1.3
918831	Cake, German Chocolate, frozen	⅛ cake	50	198.0	2.5	22.1	0.9	11.4	0.0	0.0
918115	Cake, Gingerbread, dry mix, prep	1.0 oz	28	86.5	1.1	14.2	0.3	2.9	0.0	0.0
918853	Cake, Ho Ho's/Hostess	2 cakes	56	240.2	2.0	34.0	0.5	12.0	0.0	0.0
918838	Cake, Pineapple Upside Down Mix	⅐ cake	68	250.2	2.0	39.0	0.7	10.0	5.0	0.0
18120	Cake, Pound, commercially prep w/butter	1 piece (1/10 of cake)	30	116.4	1.7	14.6	0.1	6.0	1.8	0.3
918855	Cake, Snoballs/Hostess	2 cakes	86	300.1	2.0	56.0	0.5	8.0	0.0	0.0
18133	Cake, Sponge, commercially prep	1 piece (1/12 of 16 oz cake)	38	109.8	2.1	23.2	0.2	1.0	0.4	0.2
918859	Cake, Twinkies/Hostess	2 cakes	86	319.9	2.0	52.0	0.5	10.0	0.0	0.0
918811	Cake, White w/chocolate icing, slice	1/16 cake	78	250.4	3.0	45.0	0.5	8.0	0.0	0.0
18137	Cake, White, dry mix, regular	1.0 oz	29	123.5	1.3	22.6	0.3	3.2	1.3	1.2
18140	Cake, Yellow w/chocolate icing, commercially prep	1 piece (⅛ of 18 oz cake)	64	242.6	2.4	35.5	1.2	11.1	6.1	1.4
18141	Cake, Yellow w/vanilla icing, commercially prep	1 piece (⅛ of 18 oz cake)	64	238.7	2.2	37.6	0.2	9.3	3.9	3.3
19159	Candy Bar, 3 Musketeers/M&M Mars	1 bar (.8 oz)	23	95.7	0.7	17.7	0.4	3.0	1.0	0.1
19065	Candy Bar, Almond Joy/Hershey	1.76 oz	50	233.5	2.1	29.2	2.4	13.4	3.3	0.8
19111	Candy Bar, Baby Ruth/Nestle	2.1 oz	60	288.6	4.5	39.1	1.7	12.7	3.9	2.0
19075	Candy Bar, Caramello/Hershey	1.6 oz	45	213.3	2.7	28.5	0.7	9.8	3.2	0.3
919944	Candy Bar, Chocolate Almond/Hershey	1.0 oz	28	157.1	3.2	13.9	0.4	9.8	2.8	1.3
19119	Candy Bar, Chunky	1.0 oz	28	138.6	2.5	16.0	1.3	8.2	0.1	1.2

Sat (g)	Chol (mg)	Cal (mg)	Iron (mg)	Magn (mg)	Phos (mg)	Pota (mg)	Sodi (mg)	Zinc (mg)	Vit A (RE)	Vit C (mg)	Vit E (mg)	Thia (mg)	Ribo (mg)	Niac (mg)	Vit B-6 (mg)	Fol (μg)	Vit B-12 (μg)	Wat (g)
0.1	0.0	1.1	0.2	1.6	6.1	6.2	32.9	0.0	0.0	0.0	0.1	0.0	0.0	0.3	0.0	6.1	0.0	0.3
1.8	0.0	26.0	0.9	13.0	34.0	62.0	455.0	0.2	85.0	0.8	1.4	0.1	0.1	1.2	0.0	97.0	0.0	64.9
1.7	0.0	32.0	1.1	12.0	42.0	74.0	543.0	0.3	81.0	0.0	1.4	0.1	0.1	1.5	0.0	101.0	0.0	64.8
2.1	3.2	64.0	1.6	15.0	49.0	131.0	461.0	0.3	69.0	1.7	0.0	0.2	0.1	1.6	0.1	17.0	0.0	65.2
3.4	5.8	20.9	1.6	16.2	65.0	152.0	229.7	0.4	27.8	2.0	0.0	0.2	0.2	1.7	0.2	12.8	0.1	32.2
0.1	0.5	31.5	0.9	28.4	50.4	143.1	284.0	0.2	5.0	0.0	0.3	0.0	0.1	0.5	0.0	5.0	0.0	21.2
0.7	3.1	43.8	1.1	12.0	225.6	76.8	466.8	0.4	26.4	0.1	0.0	0.1	0.2	1.2	0.1	6.6	0.1	19.1
0.1	0.4	8.5	0.5	10.3	29.9	34.6	105.3	0.2	0.0	0.0	0.1	0.1	0.0	0.6	0.1	5.4	0.0	5.4
0.6	20.4	37.2	1.2	7.6	42.4	46.0	196.8	0.3	9.2	0.0	0.2	0.2	0.2	1.9	0.0	42.0	0.0	13.9
0.2	0.0	18.8	0.6	6.8	26.3	28.3	152.3	0.2	0.0	0.0	0.1	0.1	0.1	1.2	0.0	23.8	0.0	8.6
1.4	0.0	0.0	0.5	0.0	0.0	0.0	275.0	0.0	0.0	0.0	0.0	0.0	0.0	0.0	0.0	0.0	0.0	14.3
0.4	0.0	74.8	1.0	0.0	0.0	0.0	256.3	0.0	0.0	0.0	0.0	0.0	0.0	0.0	0.0	0.0	0.0	15.0
0.2	0.0	15.6	0.6	5.4	20.6	22.0	116.8	0.2	0.0	0.0	0.1	0.1	0.1	0.9	0.0	19.0	0.0	7.1
0.3	0.0	29.1	1.1	17.0	56.3	65.3	155.8	0.4	0.0	0.0	0.1	0.2	0.1	1.4	0.1	25.6	0.0	12.1
0.2	0.0	19.5	0.9	10.5	42.3	44.1	122.1	0.3	0.0	0.0	0.2	0.1	0.1	1.4	0.0	24.3	0.0	13.2
0.1	0.0	16.2	0.9	15.6	39.4	28.9	99.5	0.3	0.0	0.0	0.1	0.1	0.1	1.1	0.0	18.7	0.0	13.0
0.2	0.0	18.7	0.8	10.5	35.7	40.3	169.8	0.3	0.6	0.0	0.2	0.1	0.1	0.9	0.0	17.6	0.0	10.4
0.0	0.0	24.1	0.7	7.3	27.2	33.6	150.1	0.2	0.0	0.0	0.2	0.0	0.1	1.3	0.0	26.6	0.0	9.0
0.1	0.0	4.2	0.9	19.3	50.4	47.6	149.0	0.4	0.0	0.0	0.3	0.1	0.0	0.8	0.1	14.0	0.0	8.6
0.1	0.0	13.6	0.6	10.8	35.6	41.6	134.2	0.3	0.0	0.0	0.1	0.1	0.1	0.6	0.0	16.0	0.0	7.6
4.1	1.9	10.8	1.0	7.8	31.8	55.2	187.8	0.2	334.2	0.6	0.0	0.1	0.1	0.8	0.0	6.6	0.0	18.5
0.3	0.0	17.2	0.8	6.8	28.3	59.0	101.4	0.2	0.0	0.0	0.1	0.1	0.1	0.9	0.0	22.6	0.0	8.7
0.2	0.0	18.6	1.0	21.6	48.1	58.1	118.8	0.4	0.0	0.0	0.2	0.2	0.1	1.8	0.1	17.6	0.0	11.1
0.2	0.0	23.4	0.9	12.8	40.0	53.1	211.2	0.4	0.3	0.1	0.1	0.1	0.1	1.2	0.0	27.5	0.0	11.9
0.2	0.0	26.3	0.8	11.5	37.5	50.3	132.5	0.3	0.0	0.0	0.1	0.1	0.1	1.0	0.0	19.3	0.0	9.3
0.3	0.0	26.6	1.1	29.2	66.6	81.7	175.0	0.5	0.0	0.0	0.2	0.1	0.1	1.6	0.1	24.8	0.0	13.6
0.1	0.0	18.4	0.7	9.0	23.5	28.1	117.5	0.3	0.0	0.0	0.0	0.1	0.1	0.9	0.0	16.3	0.0	9.9
0.1	0.1	13.0	0.4	2.9	11.3	14.3	64.6	0.1	0.0	0.0	0.0	0.1	0.0	0.5	0.0	11.4	0.0	4.4
0.1	0.0	21.6	0.7	5.3	27.8	17.5	104.2	0.3	0.2	0.1	0.0	0.1	0.1	0.8	0.0	21.9	0.1	9.9
0.3	0.0	20.9	1.0	24.9	66.4	73.1	152.8	0.6	0.0	0.0	0.2	0.1	0.1	1.1	0.1	14.5	0.0	10.9
0.4	0.2	6.8	0.3	2.9	58.7	13.6	133.3	0.1	1.4	0.0	0.2	0.1	0.0	0.4	0.0	12.6	0.0	0.9
4.2	0.0	20.0	4.5	60.0	60.0	98.0	177.0	3.0	350.0	28.0	0.0	0.3	0.0	5.0	0.4	100.0	0.6	1.9
3.9	0.0	20.0	4.5	60.0	60.0	127.0	151.0	3.0	350.0	28.0	0.0	0.3	0.0	5.0	0.4	100.0	0.6	1.7
3.0	0.0	20.0	4.5	60.0	60.0	110.0	167.0	3.0	350.0	28.0	0.0	0.3	0.0	5.0	0.4	100.0	0.6	1.4
2.8	0.0	20.0	4.5	60.0	60.0	107.0	177.0	3.0	350.0	28.0	0.0	0.3	0.0	5.0	0.4	100.0	0.6	1.5
2.5	10.9	1.2	0.0	0.1	1.2	1.3	41.3	0.0	37.7	0.0	0.1	0.0	0.0	0.0	0.0	0.2	0.0	0.8
7.1	30.6	3.3	0.0	0.3	3.2	3.6	1.5	0.0	105.6	0.0	0.2	0.0	0.0	0.0	0.0	0.4	0.0	2.5
2.0	8.8	0.9	0.0	0.1	0.9	1.0	33.1	0.0	30.2	0.0	0.1	0.0	0.0	0.0	0.0	0.1	0.0	0.6
0.0	0.0	40.6	0.2	3.5	9.3	27.0	217.2	0.0	0.0	0.0	0.0	0.0	0.1	0.3	0.0	10.2	0.0	9.6
0.0	0.0	42.0	0.1	4.0	116.0	67.5	254.5	0.1	0.0	0.0	0.0	0.0	0.1	0.1	0.0	15.0	0.0	16.5
3.0	45.0	11.0	0.8	0.0	31.0	50.0	190.0	0.0	13.0	15.0	0.0	0.1	0.1	0.9	0.0	0.0	0.0	0.0
0.0	0.0	0.0	0.0	0.0	0.0	80.0	290.0	0.0	0.0	0.0	0.0	0.0	0.0	0.0	0.0	0.0	0.0	0.0
2.2	34.0	21.2	0.3	5.5	45.1	35.9	132.5	0.1	21.2	0.2	1.0	0.4	0.2	0.2	0.0	13.8	0.1	41.8
5.0	3.4	77.0	0.9	4.9	122.5	84.0	249.2	0.2	172.9	1.7	0.0	0.1	0.1	0.8	0.1	8.4	0.8	21.6
4.0	35.0	0.0	0.0	0.0	0.0	80.0	300.0	0.0	0.0	0.0	0.0	0.0	0.0	0.0	0.0	0.0	0.0	0.0
0.0	32.0	42.0	1.6	0.0	0.0	0.0	600.0	0.0	0.0	0.0	0.0	0.0	0.1	1.0	0.0	5.0	0.0	0.0
17.1	0.0	786.0	23.6	246.3	1414.8	1729.2	4323.0	4.2	0.0	0.0	12.6	0.9	0.8	8.4	0.2	283.0	0.0	16.2
1.6	9.0	81.7	5.8	104.4	778.6	583.4	935.2	1.9	0.0	0.0	0.0	0.5	0.4	4.4	0.0	22.7	0.0	10.9
5.2	55.1	57.0	1.5	30.4	100.7	133.0	299.3	0.7	38.0	0.2	1.5	0.1	0.2	1.1	0.0	25.7	0.2	23.2
0.0	0.0	12.0	0.7	6.0	28.0	36.0	134.0	0.0	51.2	0.0	0.0	0.1	0.1	0.8	0.0	0.0	0.0	10.0
4.7	0.0	0.0	1.0	0.0	0.0	75.0	136.0	0.0	0.0	0.0	0.0	0.1	0.1	0.7	0.0	5.0	0.0	9.4
0.0	0.0	28.0	0.9	14.0	63.0	93.0	153.0	0.0	37.8	0.0	0.0	0.0	0.1	0.3	0.0	5.0	0.0	12.6
0.4	1.6	19.3	0.9	4.5	47.0	67.5	128.2	0.1	4.5	0.0	0.4	0.1	0.1	0.4	0.0	2.8	0.0	9.3
0.0	26.0	24.0	0.6	0.0	0.0	0.0	180.0	0.0	0.0	0.0	0.0	0.0	0.0	0.0	0.0	4.0	0.0	0.0
4.0	40.0	0.0	0.0	0.0	0.0	70.0	210.0	0.0	0.0	0.0	0.0	0.0	0.0	0.0	0.0	0.0	0.0	0.0
3.5	66.3	10.5	0.4	3.3	41.1	35.7	119.4	0.1	46.8	0.0	0.0	0.0	0.1	0.4	0.0	12.3	0.1	7.4
0.0	4.0	24.0	1.0	0.0	0.0	0.0	340.0	0.0	0.0	0.0	0.0	0.0	0.0	0.0	0.0	0.0	0.0	0.0
0.3	38.8	26.6	1.0	4.2	52.1	37.6	92.7	0.2	17.5	0.0	0.1	0.1	0.1	0.7	0.0	14.8	0.1	11.3
0.0	40.0	38.0	1.1	0.0	0.0	0.0	300.0	0.0	0.0	0.0	0.0	0.0	0.1	1.0	0.0	5.0	0.0	0.0
3.0	1.0	70.0	0.7	15.0	127.0	82.0	238.0	0.2	8.0	0.0	0.0	0.1	0.1	0.8	0.0	4.0	0.1	15.8
0.5	0.0	55.7	0.4	3.2	97.7	33.9	192.6	0.1	0.0	0.1	0.6	0.1	0.1	0.3	0.0	13.9	0.1	1.2
3.0	35.2	23.7	1.3	19.2	103.0	113.9	215.7	0.4	21.1	0.0	1.5	0.1	0.1	0.8	0.0	14.1	0.1	14.0
1.5	35.2	39.7	0.7	3.8	91.5	33.9	220.2	0.2	12.2	0.0	0.0	0.1	0.0	0.3	0.0	17.3	0.1	14.1
1.5	2.5	19.3	0.2	6.7	20.9	30.6	44.6	0.1	5.5	0.1	0.1	0.0	0.0	0.1	0.0	0.0	0.0	1.3
8.7	2.0	30.5	0.7	0.0	0.0	123.0	73.0	0.0	0.0	0.0	0.0	0.0	0.0	0.0	0.0	0.0	0.0	4.8
7.4	2.4	24.6	0.1	48.0	90.6	237.6	135.6	0.8	0.0	0.0	1.1	0.1	0.1	1.7	0.0	18.6	0.0	2.9
6.3	12.2	82.8	0.3	0.0	0.0	0.0	61.7	0.0	0.0	0.0	0.0	0.0	0.0	0.0	0.0	0.0	0.0	3.3
5.7	7.5	73.8	0.5	25.3	84.0	120.2	34.8	0.5	5.1	0.0	0.0	0.0	0.1	0.0	0.0	0.0	0.0	0.0
6.5	3.1	40.0	0.4	20.4	58.2	149.5	14.8	0.5	3.1	0.1	0.0	0.0	0.1	0.5	0.0	6.2	0.1	0.8

Code	Food Name	Unit/Amt	Wt (g)	Energy (Kcal)	Prot (g)	Carb (g)	Fiber (g)	Fat (g)	Mono (g)	Poly (g)
19130	Candy Bar, Golden Almond Chocolate Bar/Hershey	3.2 oz	91	522.3	11.2	41.6	4.4	34.7	16.1	3.5
19109	Candy Bar, Kit Kat Wafer/Hershey	1.62 oz	46	236.4	3.3	29.4	0.9	11.7	3.4	0.4
19115	Candy Bar, Mars Almond/M&M Mars	1.76 oz (69 pieces)	48	224.2	3.9	30.1	1.0	11.0	5.1	1.9
19135	Candy Bar, Mars Milky Way/M&M Mars	2.1 oz	60	253.8	2.7	43.0	1.0	9.7	3.6	0.4
19142	Candy Bar, Mounds/Hershey	1.55 oz	44	209.9	1.7	25.9	2.6	11.0	1.9	0.2
19143	Candy Bar, Mr. Goodbar/Hershey	1.75 oz	50	272.5	5.4	25.9	1.8	17.5	5.9	2.4
19136	Candy Bar, Skor Toffee Candy/Hershey	1.4 oz	40	222.4	1.8	23.1	0.6	13.6	4.4	0.6
19155	Candy Bar, Snickers/M&M Mars	2.16 oz	61	292.2	4.9	36.1	1.5	15.0	6.4	3.0
19164	Candy Bar, Special Dark Sweet Chocolate/Hershey	1.45 oz bar	41	226.3	2.0	24.8	2.1	13.3	4.6	0.4
919967	Candy Bar, Summit Bar	0.75 oz bar	22	100.1	1.0	11.0	0.4	6.0	0.0	0.0
19093	Candy Bar, Symphony Milk Chocolate/Hershey	1.4 oz	40	221.2	2.9	23.2	0.8	13.1	0.0	0.0
919951	Candy Bar, Tiger Milk Bar	2.0 oz	56	249.8	9.0	35.0	29.1	8.0	0.0	0.0
19160	Candy Bar, Twix Caramel Cookie/M&M Mars	2.0 oz	57	284.4	2.6	37.4	0.6	13.9	7.6	0.5
919912	Candy, Candy Corn	¼ cup	50	182.0	0.1	44.8	0.0	1.0	0.5	0.2
19074	Candy, Caramel	1 piece (0.75" cube)	10	38.2	0.5	7.7	0.1	0.8	0.1	0.0
19071	Candy, Carob	3.0 oz	87	469.8	7.1	49.0	3.3	27.3	0.4	0.3
919901	Candy, Chocolate Caramel Turtle	0.6 oz	17	81.9	1.1	9.9	0.0	4.7	1.9	0.8
19080	Candy, Chocolate Chips, semisweet	1 cup, large chips	182	871.8	7.6	114.8	10.7	54.6	18.1	1.8
919921	Candy, Chocolate Chips/Bakers	¼ cup	44	200.6	1.7	32.0	0.7	9.0	1.6	0.3
919956	Candy, Chocolate w/cream center	1.0 oz	28	122.9	1.1	19.9	0.4	4.8	2.8	0.6
919946	Candy, Chocolate, dietetic	1 bar	56	333.8	7.2	14.0	0.0	27.8	0.0	0.0
19014	Candy, Fruit Leather, roll	1 small roll	14	49.0	0.1	11.8	0.5	0.4	0.2	0.1
919970	Candy, Fruit Roll Snack	1 large roll	21	73.1	0.2	17.7	0.5	0.6	0.3	0.1
19100	Candy, Fudge, Chocolate, homemade	1 piece	17	64.8	0.3	13.5	0.1	1.4	0.4	0.1
19103	Candy, Fudge, Vanilla, homemade	1 piece	16	59.0	0.2	13.2	0.0	0.9	0.2	0.0
19105	Candy, Goobers Chocolate Covered Peanuts/Nestle	10 pieces	10	51.3	1.4	4.9	0.6	3.4	1.5	0.5
19106	Candy, Gumdrops/Gummy Bears/Fish/Worm/Dinosaur	1 small gumdrop (0.5" dia)	3	11.6	0.0	3.0	0.0	0.0	0.0	0.0
19117	Candy, Halvah, Plain	1 bar (8 oz)	227	1064.6	28.4	137.3	10.2	48.9	18.6	19.3
19107	Candy, Hard Candy	1 lollipop (0.75" diam)	6	23.6	0.0	5.9	0.0	0.0	0.0	0.0
19108	Candy, Jellybeans	10 small	11	40.4	0.0	10.2	0.0	0.1	0.0	0.0
19140	Candy, M&M's Peanut Chocolate	1 piece	2	10.3	0.2	1.2	0.1	0.5	0.2	0.1
19141	Candy, M&M's Plain Chocolate	1 piece	0.7	3.4	0.0	0.5	0.0	0.1	0.0	0.0
19148	Candy, Peanut Brittle, homemade	1.0 oz	28	126.8	2.1	19.4	0.6	5.3	2.4	1.3
19150	Candy, Peanut Butter Cups, Reese's/Hershey	1 miniature cup	7	37.9	0.7	3.8	0.2	2.2	0.9	0.4
19126	Candy, Peanuts, milk chocolate coated	10 pieces	40	207.6	5.2	19.8	1.9	13.4	5.2	1.7
919072	Candy, Pudding Pops, Chocolate, frozen	1 pop	47	71.9	1.9	11.9	0.2	2.2	0.0	0.0
919073	Candy, Pudding Pops, Vanilla, frozen	1 pop	47	74.7	1.9	12.6	0.0	2.1	0.0	0.0
19149	Candy, Raisinets/Nestle	10 pieces	10	41.2	0.5	7.1	0.5	1.6	0.6	0.2
19127	Candy, Raisins, milk chocolate coated	10 pieces	10	39.0	0.4	6.8	0.4	1.5	0.5	0.1
19152	Candy, Rolo Caramel, milk chocolate/Hershey	1.94 oz (8 pieces)	55	226.6	2.7	29.4	0.4	11.0	3.5	0.3
919923	Candy, Semisweet Chocolate Chips/Nestle	1.0 oz	28	148.1	1.0	17.8	1.0	7.9	2.2	0.7
919947	Candy, Semisweet Chocolate/Baker	1.0 oz	28	135.0	2.0	16.3	0.5	9.0	3.2	0.4
919948	Candy, Semisweet Chocolate/Hershey	1.0 oz	28	147.0	1.2	17.5	0.5	9.2	0.0	0.0
19370	Candy, Skittles, Original Bite Size Candy/M&M Mars	2.3 oz (59 pieces)	65	263.3	0.1	58.9	0.0	2.8	1.9	0.1
919958	Candy, Sno Caps	1 oz	28	131.9	1.5	20.6	0.2	5.6	2.0	0.5
19156	Candy, Starburst Fruit Chews/M&M Mars	2.07 oz	59	233.6	0.2	49.9	0.0	4.9	2.1	1.8
919966	Candy, Taffy	0.5 oz piece	15	56.0	0.0	13.7	0.0	0.4	0.1	0.0
19112	Candy, Twizzlers Strawberry/Hershey	1 package (2.5 oz)	71	237.1	2.4	55.0	1.0	1.1	0.0	0.0
19091	Candy, York Peppermint Patty	0.39 oz, 1 sm patty	11	43.2	0.2	8.8	0.2	0.8	0.3	0.0
8053	Cereal, 100% Bran (wheat bran & barley)	1 cup	66	177.5	8.3	48.1	19.5	3.3	0.6	1.9
908912	Cereal, 100% Natural/Quaker	¼ cup	28	127.1	3.3	18.0	2.0	5.5	0.9	0.6
8153	Cereal, 40% Bran Flakes/Ralston Purina	1.0 oz, @ ¾ cup	29	94.0	3.3	23.1	4.1	0.4	0.0	0.0
8001	Cereal, All-Bran/Kellogg	½ cup	30	79.2	3.7	22.8	9.7	0.9	0.2	0.5
8006	Cereal, Bran Chex (wheat & corn)	1 cup	49	156.3	5.0	39.1	7.9	1.4	0.3	0.7
8010	Cereal, Cap'n Crunch/Quaker	¾ cup	27	107.2	1.4	23.0	0.9	1.4	0.3	0.2
8013	Cereal, Cheerios/Gen Mills	1 cup	30	109.5	3.1	22.9	2.6	1.8	0.6	0.2
8014	Cereal, Cocoa Krispies/Kellogg	¾ cup	31	120.3	1.6	27.2	0.4	0.8	0.1	0.1
8017	Cereal, Cookie Crisp, Chocolate Chip & Vanilla	1 cup	30	120.0	1.5	26.3	0.4	1.1	0.2	0.2
8019	Cereal, Corn Chex	1 single serving box (.75 oz)	21.3	83.5	1.5	18.7	0.4	0.1	0.0	0.0
8022	Cereal, Corn Flakes, low sodium	1.0 oz	28.35	113.1	2.2	25.2	0.3	0.1	0.0	0.0
8020	Cereal, Corn Flakes/Kellogg	1 cup	28	102.2	1.8	24.2	0.8	0.2	0.0	0.1
8023	Cereal, Cracklin' Oat Bran/Kellogg	¾ cup	55	225.0	4.6	40.1	6.5	7.0	3.2	0.8
8101	Cereal, Cream of Rice, prep w/o salt	1 tbsp	15.2	7.9	0.1	1.7	0.0	0.0	0.0	0.0
8109	Cereal, Cream of Wheat, Plain, Mix 'n Eat, prep	1 packet, prep	142	102.2	2.7	21.4	0.4	0.3	0.0	0.2
8103	Cereal, Cream of Wheat, Regular, prep w/o salt	1 cup	251	133.0	3.8	27.6	1.8	0.5	0.1	0.3
8259	Cereal, Crispix/Kellogg	1 cup	29	108.5	2.1	25.0	0.6	0.3	0.1	0.1
8018	Cereal, Crunchy Bran/Quaker	¾ cup	27	89.9	1.9	22.7	4.8	0.9	0.2	0.3
8244	Cereal, Fiber One/Gen Mills	1 cup	60	123.0	5.6	48.0	28.5	1.7	0.3	0.1
8030	Cereal, Froot Loops/Kellogg	1 cup	30	117.3	1.5	26.5	0.6	0.9	0.2	0.3

Sat (g)	Chol (mg)	Cal (mg)	Iron (mg)	Magn (mg)	Phos (mg)	Pota (mg)	Sodi (mg)	Zinc (mg)	Vit A (RE)	Vit C (mg)	Vit E (mg)	Thia (mg)	Ribo (mg)	Niac (mg)	Vit B-6 (mg)	Fol (μg)	Vit B-12 (μg)	Wat (g)
14.9	13.7	203.8	1.6	0.0	0.0	0.0	61.0	0.0	0.0	0.0	0.0	0.0	0.0	0.0	0.0	0.0	0.0	1.9
7.5	2.8	75.9	0.4	17.9	109.5	133.9	34.5	0.6	22.1	0.3	0.4	0.1	0.2	1.2	0.1	65.3	0.1	0.8
3.5	8.2	80.6	0.5	34.6	112.3	156.0	81.6	0.5	24.0	0.3	2.2	0.0	0.1	0.5	0.0	9.1	0.2	2.2
4.7	8.4	78.0	0.5	20.4	86.4	144.6	144.0	0.4	19.2	0.6	0.4	0.0	0.1	0.2	0.0	6.0	0.2	3.8
8.9	0.9	6.6	0.9	24.6	40.0	108.7	65.6	0.4	0.4	0.2	0.3	0.0	0.0	0.1	0.0	1.3	0.0	4.8
7.5	4.0	54.0	0.7	43.0	124.0	223.5	74.5	0.9	18.5	0.2	1.4	0.1	0.1	1.7	0.0	19.5	0.2	0.4
8.7	20.4	52.0	0.2	0.0	0.0	0.0	110.4	0.0	0.0	0.0	0.0	0.0	0.0	0.0	0.0	0.0	0.0	1.0
5.5	7.9	57.3	0.5	43.9	135.4	197.6	162.3	1.4	23.8	0.4	0.9	0.1	0.1	2.6	0.1	24.4	0.1	3.3
8.3	0.4	11.1	1.0	45.5	61.5	122.6	2.9	0.6	1.6	0.0	0.2	0.0	0.0	0.2	0.0	0.8	0.0	0.4
0.0	0.0	0.0	0.0	0.0	0.0	0.0	0.0	0.0	0.0	0.0	0.0	0.0	0.0	0.0	0.0	0.0	0.0	0.0
0.0	8.8	86.0	0.5	0.0	0.0	0.0	36.8	0.0	0.0	0.0	0.0	0.0	0.0	0.0	0.0	0.0	0.0	0.2
0.0	0.0	0.0	6.3	0.0	0.0	0.0	0.0	0.0	0.0	0.0	0.0	0.0	0.5	0.7	0.6	0.0	0.0	0.0
5.1	2.9	51.3	0.5	18.2	68.4	115.1	110.0	0.4	14.3	0.2	0.7	0.1	0.1	0.7	0.0	13.7	0.1	2.4
0.3	0.0	7.0	0.6	0.0	3.0	2.0	106.0	0.0	0.0	0.0	0.0	0.0	0.0	0.0	0.0	0.0	0.0	3.8
0.7	0.7	13.8	0.0	1.7	11.4	21.4	24.5	0.0	0.8	0.1	0.0	0.0	0.0	0.0	0.0	0.5	0.0	0.9
25.2	2.6	263.6	1.1	31.3	109.6	550.7	93.1	3.1	7.0	0.4	1.4	0.1	0.2	0.9	0.1	24.4	0.9	1.3
1.8	4.0	27.0	0.2	0.0	0.0	52.0	16.0	0.0	6.0	0.0	0.0	0.0	0.0	0.1	0.0	0.0	0.0	0.0
32.3	0.0	58.2	5.7	209.3	240.2	664.3	20.0	2.9	3.6	0.0	2.2	0.1	0.2	0.8	0.1	5.5	0.0	1.3
7.1	0.0	66.5	0.9	35.8	82.9	227.2	26.6	0.5	0.8	0.0	0.0	0.0	0.1	0.1	0.0	2.0	0.1	0.4
1.4	0.0	36.0	0.2	0.0	31.0	50.0	52.0	0.0	0.0	0.0	0.0	0.0	0.0	0.0	0.0	0.0	0.0	2.1
0.0	0.0	0.0	0.0	0.0	0.0	0.0	0.0	0.0	0.0	0.0	0.0	0.0	0.0	0.0	0.0	0.0	0.0	0.0
0.1	0.0	4.5	0.1	2.8	4.3	41.2	8.5	0.0	1.7	0.9	0.0	0.0	0.0	0.0	0.0	1.1	0.0	1.5
0.1	0.0	7.0	0.2	4.0	7.0	62.0	13.0	0.0	2.0	1.0	0.0	0.0	0.0	0.0	0.1	0.0	0.0	2.3
0.9	2.4	7.1	0.1	4.3	9.9	17.5	10.5	0.1	7.8	0.0	0.0	0.0	0.0	0.0	0.0	0.3	0.0	1.6
0.5	2.6	6.2	0.0	0.8	5.1	8.0	10.7	0.0	8.0	0.0	0.0	0.0	0.0	0.0	0.0	0.2	0.0	1.7
1.2	0.9	12.7	0.1	11.9	29.6	50.2	4.1	0.2	0.0	0.0	0.0	0.0	0.0	0.5	0.0	0.8	0.0	0.2
0.0	0.0	0.1	0.0	0.0	0.0	0.2	1.3	0.0	0.0	0.0	0.0	0.0	0.0	0.0	0.0	0.0	0.0	0.0
9.4	0.0	74.9	10.3	494.9	1377.9	424.5	442.7	9.8	0.0	0.2	6.4	1.0	0.2	6.5	0.8	147.6	0.1	8.3
0.0	0.0	0.2	0.0	0.2	0.2	0.3	2.3	0.0	0.0	0.0	0.0	0.0	0.0	0.0	0.0	0.0	0.0	0.1
0.0	0.0	0.3	0.1	0.2	0.4	4.1	2.8	0.0	0.0	0.0	0.0	0.0	0.0	0.0	0.0	0.0	0.0	0.7
0.2	0.2	2.0	0.0	1.5	4.6	6.9	1.0	0.0	0.5	0.0	0.0	0.0	0.0	0.1	0.0	0.7	0.0	0.0
0.1	0.1	0.7	0.0	0.3	1.1	1.9	0.4	0.0	0.4	0.0	0.0	0.0	0.0	0.0	0.0	0.0	0.0	0.0
1.4	3.6	8.4	0.4	14.0	31.1	58.2	126.6	0.3	13.2	0.0	0.5	0.1	0.0	1.0	0.0	19.6	0.0	0.5
0.8	0.4	5.5	0.1	6.2	14.2	24.6	22.2	0.1	1.3	0.0	0.3	0.0	0.0	0.3	0.0	3.9	0.0	0.1
5.8	3.6	41.6	0.5	37.6	84.8	200.8	16.4	0.8	0.0	0.0	1.0	0.0	0.1	1.7	0.1	3.2	0.1	0.8
0.0	0.9	66.3	0.2	9.9	52.6	105.3	77.6	0.2	15.5	0.2	0.0	0.0	0.1	0.1	0.0	1.4	0.3	30.4
0.0	0.9	60.6	0.0	5.2	47.5	64.9	49.8	0.2	24.4	0.1	0.0	0.0	0.1	0.0	0.0	2.4	0.2	30.0
0.7	0.4	10.8	0.1	4.5	14.4	51.4	3.6	0.1	0.9	0.0	0.0	0.0	0.0	0.0	0.0	0.5	0.0	0.6
0.9	0.3	8.6	0.2	4.5	14.3	51.4	3.6	0.1	0.7	0.0	0.1	0.0	0.0	0.0	0.0	0.5	0.0	1.1
6.7	9.9	84.2	0.3	21.5	82.5	136.4	96.8	0.5	20.4	0.2	0.5	0.0	0.1	0.1	0.0	2.8	0.2	11.1
5.0	0.0	10.0	1.0	0.0	30.0	99.0	4.0	0.4	0.1	0.0	0.0	0.0	0.0	0.2	0.0	3.6	0.0	0.0
5.4	0.0	11.0	1.0	41.0	57.0	116.0	1.0	1.0	1.6	0.0	0.0	0.0	0.0	0.2	0.0	1.0	0.0	0.0
5.7	0.0	9.0	0.9	0.0	43.0	92.0	5.0	0.0	2.0	0.0	0.0	0.1	0.1	0.1	0.0	1.0	0.0	0.0
0.6	0.0	0.0	0.0	0.7	1.3	3.3	10.4	0.0	0.0	43.5	0.2	0.0	0.0	0.0	0.0	0.0	0.0	2.5
3.1	0.0	38.0	0.4	0.0	40.0	71.0	20.0	0.5	6.0	0.0	0.0	0.0	0.1	0.1	0.0	0.0	0.0	0.3
0.7	0.0	2.4	0.1	0.6	4.1	1.2	33.0	0.0	0.0	31.2	0.9	0.0	0.0	0.0	0.0	0.0	0.0	4.0
0.3	1.0	0.0	0.0	0.0	0.0	1.0	13.0	0.0	5.0	0.0	0.0	0.0	0.0	0.0	0.0	0.0	0.0	0.7
0.3	0.0	5.0	0.2	0.0	0.0	0.0	175.4	0.0	0.0	0.0	0.0	0.0	0.0	0.0	0.0	0.0	0.0	11.9
0.5	0.1	1.7	0.1	0.0	0.0	14.2	2.6	0.0	0.0	0.0	0.0	0.0	0.0	0.0	0.0	0.0	0.0	1.1
0.6	0.0	46.2	8.1	312.2	801.2	652.1	457.4	5.7	0.0	62.7	1.5	1.6	1.8	20.9	2.1	46.9	6.3	2.0
3.1	0.0	43.0	0.8	31.0	101.0	134.0	14.0	0.6	0.0	0.0	0.0	0.1	0.1	0.4	0.1	12.0	0.3	0.6
0.0	0.0	13.3	4.6	69.6	161.5	169.4	270.0	1.2	384.0	15.1	0.0	0.4	0.4	5.1	0.5	102.4	1.5	0.7
0.2	0.0	105.9	4.5	128.7	294.0	341.7	60.9	3.8	225.3	15.0	0.6	0.4	0.4	5.0	0.5	90.0	1.5	1.0
0.2	0.0	29.4	14.0	69.1	173.0	216.1	345.5	6.5	10.8	26.0	0.6	0.6	0.3	8.6	0.9	173.0	2.6	1.1
0.4	0.0	5.4	4.5	9.5	28.6	34.6	208.4	3.8	3.5	0.0	0.1	0.4	0.4	5.0	0.5	100.2	0.0	0.6
0.4	0.0	55.2	8.1	32.7	114.0	88.5	284.1	3.8	375.3	15.0	0.2	0.4	0.4	5.0	0.5	99.9	0.0	1.0
0.6	0.0	4.0	1.8	11.5	29.5	60.1	210.2	1.5	225.1	15.0	0.1	0.4	0.4	5.0	0.5	93.0	0.0	0.7
0.6	0.0	5.7	4.8	8.4	24.0	29.4	206.7	3.2	0.0	0.0	0.1	0.4	0.3	5.3	0.5	105.9	1.6	0.6
0.0	0.0	2.3	6.1	3.0	8.3	17.3	232.8	0.1	10.7	11.3	0.1	0.3	0.1	3.7	0.4	75.2	1.1	0.4
0.0	0.0	12.2	0.6	3.7	13.9	20.7	2.8	0.1	10.8	0.0	0.0	0.1	0.1	0.1	0.0	2.0	0.0	0.9
0.1	0.0	1.1	8.7	3.4	10.9	25.5	297.9	0.2	210.3	14.0	0.0	0.4	0.4	4.7	0.5	98.8	0.0	0.9
2.9	0.0	24.8	2.0	76.5	186.5	254.7	195.3	1.7	253.0	16.8	0.4	0.4	0.5	5.6	0.6	152.9	0.0	2.0
0.0	0.0	0.5	0.0	0.5	2.6	3.0	0.2	0.0	0.0	0.0	0.0	0.0	0.0	0.1	0.0	0.5	0.0	13.3
0.0	0.0	19.9	8.1	7.1	19.9	38.3	241.4	0.2	376.3	0.0	0.0	0.4	0.3	5.0	0.6	100.8	0.0	116.6
0.1	0.0	50.2	10.3	10.0	42.7	42.7	2.5	0.3	0.0	0.0	0.0	0.3	0.0	1.5	0.0	45.2	0.0	218.6
0.1	0.0	3.5	1.8	7.0	26.7	35.1	240.1	1.5	225.3	15.0	0.1	0.4	0.4	5.0	0.5	87.0	0.0	0.9
0.2	0.0	20.5	7.6	14.3	35.6	56.2	253.3	3.8	3.8	0.0	0.1	0.1	0.4	5.0	0.5	100.2	0.0	0.7
0.3	0.0	117.0	9.0	136.2	336.6	433.8	285.0	2.5	0.0	18.0	0.7	0.8	0.9	10.0	1.0	199.8	0.0	2.3
0.4	0.0	3.3	4.2	8.7	20.7	31.5	140.7	3.8	211.2	14.1	0.1	0.4	0.4	5.0	0.5	90.0	0.0	0.7

Code	Food Name	Unit/Amt	Wt (g)	Energy (Kcal)	Prot (g)	Carb (g)	Fiber (g)	Fat (g)	Mono (g)	Poly (g)
8319	Cereal, Frosted Mini-Wheats, bite size/Kellogg	1 cup, bite size	55	187.0	5.2	44.8	5.9	0.9	0.2	0.6
8035	Cereal, Golden Grahams/Gen Mills	¾ cup	30	115.5	1.6	25.7	0.9	1.1	0.3	0.2
8037	Cereal, Granola (oats & wheat germ) homemade	1.0 oz	29	135.4	4.3	15.4	3.0	7.1	2.3	3.1
908038	Cereal, Grape-Nuts	1-⅓ oz box	38	135.7	4.4	31.2	3.8	0.2	0.0	0.0
8040	Cereal, Heartland Natural, Plain (oats & wheat germ)	1 cup	115	499.1	11.6	78.5	7.0	17.7	4.8	7.1
8211	Cereal, Honey Graham Oh!s/Quaker	¾ cup	27	111.8	1.4	22.7	0.7	1.9	1.1	0.3
908046	Cereal, Honeycomb	1.0 oz	28	109.5	1.6	24.9	0.8	0.5	0.0	0.0
8242	Cereal, Just Right w/crunchy nuggets/Kellogg	1 cup	109	404.4	8.4	91.2	5.6	2.9	0.5	2.1
8048	Cereal, Kix/Gen Mills	1 cup	105	400.1	6.8	90.7	2.8	2.2	0.5	0.1
8049	Cereal, Life, Plain/Quaker	1 cup	110	416.9	10.8	86.6	7.0	4.4	1.4	1.9
8050	Cereal, Lucky Charms/Gen Mills	1 cup	115	445.1	8.3	96.5	4.6	4.2	1.5	0.6
8117	Cereal, Malt-O-Meal, plain & chocolate, prep w/o salt	1 cup	30	15.3	0.5	3.2	0.1	0.0	0.0	0.0
8277	Cereal, Nature Valley Low Fat Fruit Granola/Gen Mills	1 cup	22	84.9	1.8	17.5	1.4	1.2	0.6	0.2
8043	Cereal, Nut & Honey Crunch/Kellogg	¾ cup	27	109.4	2.0	22.6	0.4	1.2	0.6	0.4
8291	Cereal, Nutri-Grain Almond and Raisin/Kellogg	1-⅓ cup	30	110.1	2.4	23.3	2.4	1.7	0.8	0.9
8292	Cereal, Nutri-Grain Wheat/Kellogg	¾ cup	32	107.2	3.2	25.6	4.0	1.1	0.3	0.7
8202	Cereal, Oatmeal Crisp w/almonds/Gen Mills	1 cup	55	218.9	5.8	42.0	4.3	4.6	2.4	1.1
8190	Cereal, Oatmeal Crisp w/apples/Gen Mills	1 cup	55	205.2	4.3	46.2	4.5	1.8	0.6	0.2
8227	Cereal, Oatmeal, Instant w/fruit & cream, prep/Quaker	3.5 oz, @ 1 cup	100	118.0	2.5	23.1	1.9	2.2	0.7	0.5
8304	Cereal, Oatmeal, Quick 'N Hearty Regular Flavor, microwave/Quaker	1 packet	29	105.9	3.8	19.1	2.4	2.1	0.7	0.7
8127	Cereal, Oats, Instant w/bran & raisins, fortified, prep	1 packet prep	195	158.0	4.9	30.4	5.5	2.0	0.0	0.0
8123	Cereal, Oats, Instant, Plain, fortified, prep	1 cup, cooked	234	138.1	5.9	23.9	4.0	2.3	0.7	0.9
8180	Cereal, Oats, Regular/Quick/Instant, ckd w/salt	1 packet, prep	158	98.0	4.1	17.1	2.7	1.6	0.5	0.6
8058	Cereal, Product 19/Kellogg	¾ cup	175	640.5	15.6	145.6	5.8	2.3	0.9	1.2
8066	Cereal, Puffed Rice/Quaker	1 cup	30	114.9	2.1	26.3	0.4	0.3	0.1	0.1
908911	Cereal, Puffed Wheat/Quaker	1 cup	14	50.0	2.4	10.5	1.0	0.2	0.0	0.1
908061	Cereal, Raisin Bran, Post	1 single serving box (1.25 oz)	35	107.5	3.3	26.5	4.9	0.7	0.0	0.0
8261	Cereal, Raisin Nut Bran/Gen Mills	1 cup	55	209.0	5.2	41.5	5.1	4.4	1.9	0.5
8287	Cereal, Raisin Squares Mini-Wheats/Kellogg	¾ cup	55	187.0	4.4	42.9	5.2	1.5	0.1	0.5
8185	Cereal, Ralston, ckd w/salt	1 cup	253	134.1	5.6	28.3	6.1	0.8	0.0	0.0
8064	Cereal, Rice Chex	1 cup	33	130.4	1.7	29.4	0.6	0.1	0.0	0.0
8065	Cereal, Rice Krispies/Kellogg	⅝ oz box	18	67.9	1.1	15.6	0.2	0.2	0.1	0.1
8156	Cereal, Rice, Puffed, fortified	0.5 oz	14.2	57.1	0.9	12.8	0.2	0.1	0.0	0.0
8067	Cereal, Special K/Kellogg	0.63 oz box	18	66.6	3.7	13.0	0.6	0.2	0.0	0.1
8070	Cereal, Sugar Frosted Flakes/Ralston Purina	1 cup	38	148.6	2.0	34.2	0.8	0.5	0.1	0.1
8074	Cereal, Tasteeos	10 pieces	1	3.9	0.1	0.8	0.1	0.0	0.0	0.0
908075	Cereal, Team	1 cup	42	164.2	2.7	36.0	0.5	0.8	0.0	0.0
8077	Cereal, Total/Gen Mills	¾ cup	30	105.3	3.0	23.9	2.6	0.7	0.1	0.1
8082	Cereal, Wheat Chex	1 cup	46	168.8	4.6	37.8	4.1	1.2	0.1	0.5
8157	Cereal, Wheat, Puffed, fortified	1 cup	12	43.7	1.8	9.6	0.5	0.1	0.0	0.0
8148	Cereal, Wheat, Shredded, small biscuit	1 single serving box (.875 oz)	24.8	88.5	2.7	19.9	2.4	0.4	0.1	0.2
8089	Cereal, Wheaties/Gen Mills	1 cup	30	110.1	3.2	23.8	2.1	0.9	0.2	0.2
924035	Cheese Blintzes	8.0 oz	227	431.3	19.2	31.2	0.0	25.6	0.0	0.0
1163	Cheese Fondue	1.0 oz	28	64.1	4.0	1.1	0.0	3.8	1.0	0.1
1150	Cheese Spread, Pasteurized Process, American w/disodium phosphate	1.0 oz	28	81.3	4.6	2.4	0.0	5.9	1.7	0.2
1161	Cheese Substitute, Mozzarella	1.0 oz	28	69.4	3.2	6.6	0.0	3.4	1.7	0.5
1004	Cheese, Blue	1.0 oz	28	98.9	6.0	0.7	0.0	8.0	2.2	0.2
1005	Cheese, Brick	1.0 oz	28	103.9	6.5	0.8	0.0	8.3	2.4	0.2
1006	Cheese, Brie	1.0 oz	28	93.4	5.8	0.1	0.0	7.8	2.2	0.2
1007	Cheese, Camembert	1.0 oz	28	83.9	5.5	0.1	0.0	6.8	2.0	0.2
1008	Cheese, Caraway	1.0 oz	28	105.3	7.1	0.9	0.0	8.2	2.3	0.2
1009	Cheese, Cheddar	1.0 oz	28	112.7	7.0	0.4	0.0	9.3	2.6	0.3
1169	Cheese, Cheddar of Colby, low-sodium	1.0 oz	28	111.4	6.8	0.5	0.0	9.1	2.6	0.3
1168	Cheese, Cheddar or Colby, low fat	1.0 oz	28	48.4	6.8	0.5	0.0	2.0	0.6	0.1
1011	Cheese, Colby	1.0 oz	28	110.2	6.7	0.7	0.0	9.0	2.6	0.3
1012	Cheese, Cottage, Creamed, large or small curd	1.0 oz or 1 tbsp	28	28.9	3.5	0.8	0.0	1.3	0.4	0.0
1013	Cheese, Cottage, Creamed, w/fruit	1.0 oz or 1 tbsp	28	34.6	2.8	3.7	0.0	1.0	0.3	0.0
1016	Cheese, Cottage, Lowfat, 1% fat	1.0 oz or 1 tbsp	28	20.3	3.5	0.8	0.0	0.3	0.1	0.0
1015	Cheese, Cottage, Lowfat, 2% fat	1.0 oz or 1 tbsp	28	25.1	3.8	1.0	0.0	0.5	0.2	0.0
1014	Cheese, Cottage, Nonfat, Uncreamed, Dry, large or small curd	1.0 oz or 1 tbsp	28	23.7	4.8	0.5	0.0	0.1	0.0	0.0
1017	Cheese, Cream	1.0 oz or 1 tbsp	28	97.7	2.1	0.7	0.0	9.8	2.8	0.4
1186	Cheese, Cream, fat free	1.0 oz or 1 tbsp	28	26.9	4.0	1.6	0.0	0.4	0.1	0.0
1018	Cheese, Edam	1.0 oz	28	99.8	7.0	0.4	0.0	7.8	2.3	0.2
1019	Cheese, Feta	1.0 oz	28	73.8	4.0	1.1	0.0	6.0	1.3	0.2
1020	Cheese, Fontina	1.0 oz	28	108.9	7.2	0.4	0.0	8.7	2.4	0.5
1022	Cheese, Gouda	1.0 oz	28	99.8	7.0	0.6	0.0	7.7	2.2	0.2
1023	Cheese, Gruyere	1.0 oz	28	115.6	8.3	0.1	0.0	9.1	2.8	0.5
1165	Cheese, Mexican, Queso Anejo	1.0 oz	28	104.4	6.0	1.3	0.0	8.4	2.4	0.3
1025	Cheese, Monterey	1.0 oz	28	104.5	6.9	0.2	0.0	8.5	2.5	0.3

Sat (g)	Chol (mg)	Cal (mg)	Iron (mg)	Magn (mg)	Phos (mg)	Pota (mg)	Sodi (mg)	Zinc (mg)	Vit A (RE)	Vit C (mg)	Vit E (mg)	Thia (mg)	Ribo (mg)	Niac (mg)	Vit B-6 (mg)	Fol (μg)	Vit B-12 (μg)	Wat (g)
0.2	0.0	0.0	15.4	55.6	159.5	186.5	1.7	1.4	0.0	0.0	0.0	0.3	0.4	4.7	0.4	110.0	1.4	2.9
0.2	0.0	14.4	4.5	9.3	36.0	52.8	274.5	3.8	225.3	15.0	0.2	0.4	0.4	5.0	0.5	99.9	0.0	0.8
1.4	0.0	23.5	1.2	51.6	134.0	156.0	7.0	1.2	1.2	0.4	3.7	0.2	0.1	0.6	0.1	24.9	0.0	1.5
0.1	0.0	3.6	10.9	25.5	95.4	126.9	264.1	0.8	503.1	0.0	0.1	0.5	0.6	6.7	0.7	134.1	2.0	1.2
4.5	0.0	74.8	4.3	147.2	416.3	385.3	293.3	3.0	6.9	1.2	0.8	0.4	0.2	1.6	0.2	64.4	0.0	4.7
0.6	0.0	12.4	4.5	12.7	41.9	45.1	177.9	3.8	301.3	12.0	0.1	0.4	0.4	5.0	0.5	100.4	0.0	0.5
0.1	0.1	4.8	2.7	9.5	27.7	32.2	157.6	1.5	370.7	0.0	0.1	0.4	0.4	4.9	0.5	98.8	1.5	0.4
0.2	0.0	28.3	32.2	67.6	210.4	239.8	669.3	1.7	744.5	0.0	4.4	0.8	0.9	9.9	1.0	202.7	2.9	3.5
0.6	0.0	152.3	28.4	32.6	147.0	143.9	920.9	13.1	1313.6	52.5	0.3	1.3	1.5	17.5	1.8	349.7	0.0	2.1
0.8	0.0	335.5	30.8	106.7	466.4	271.7	599.5	13.8	4.4	0.0	0.6	1.4	1.6	18.3	1.8	367.4	0.0	4.4
0.8	0.0	124.2	17.3	74.8	289.8	207.0	778.6	14.4	863.7	57.5	0.5	1.4	1.6	19.2	1.9	383.0	0.0	2.7
0.0	0.0	0.6	1.2	0.6	3.0	3.9	0.3	0.0	0.0	0.0	0.0	0.1	0.0	0.7	0.0	0.6	0.0	26.3
0.1	0.0	15.8	0.6	7.5	72.2	64.7	82.1	0.3	0.0	0.0	0.3	0.0	0.0	0.4	0.0	2.9	0.0	1.0
0.2	0.0	2.7	2.2	2.4	17.8	29.4	181.7	0.2	110.7	7.4	0.1	0.2	0.2	2.5	0.2	54.0	0.0	0.7
0.1	0.0	91.5	0.8	6.9	102.3	107.1	106.5	2.0	0.0	0.0	3.0	0.2	0.2	2.7	0.3	60.0	0.8	1.9
0.1	0.0	10.2	1.1	25.9	115.5	116.8	235.5	4.0	0.0	16.0	5.8	0.4	0.4	5.3	0.5	96.0	1.6	1.2
0.6	0.0	35.8	4.5	57.2	144.1	184.8	250.3	3.8	0.0	9.0	3.1	0.4	0.4	5.0	0.5	99.6	0.0	1.3
0.4	0.0	23.1	4.5	45.1	121.6	159.5	281.6	3.8	0.0	9.0	0.4	0.4	0.4	5.0	0.5	99.6	0.0	1.3
0.5	0.0	94.0	3.5	25.0	92.0	85.0	150.0	0.6	277.0	0.1	0.1	0.3	0.3	3.7	0.4	74.0	0.0	71.2
0.4	0.0	107.9	8.5	38.6	136.3	110.2	152.5	0.9	315.2	0.0	0.0	0.3	0.4	4.2	0.4	84.1	0.0	2.8
0.4	0.0	173.6	7.6	56.6	206.7	236.0	247.7	1.3	479.7	0.0	0.0	0.6	0.6	8.1	0.8	156.0	0.0	156.0
0.4	0.0	215.3	8.3	56.2	175.5	131.0	376.7	1.1	599.0	0.0	0.3	0.7	0.4	7.2	1.0	198.9	0.0	200.1
0.3	0.0	12.6	1.1	37.9	120.1	88.5	252.8	0.8	3.2	0.0	0.2	0.0	0.2	0.0	0.2	6.3	0.0	134.8
0.2	0.0	15.8	105.0	71.8	192.5	236.3	1260.0	87.5	1314.3	350.0	129.5	8.8	10.0	116.7	11.7	2275.0	35.0	6.0
0.1	0.0	2.7	0.9	9.0	35.4	34.8	1.5	0.3	0.0	0.0	0.0	0.1	0.0	1.9	0.0	3.0	0.0	1.2
0.0	0.0	3.0	0.6	19.0	47.0	53.0	1.0	0.4	0.0	0.0	0.0	0.1	0.0	1.6	0.0	4.0	0.0	0.5
0.3	0.1	16.5	5.6	59.5	146.7	215.6	228.2	1.9	463.4	0.0	0.8	0.5	0.5	6.2	0.6	123.6	1.9	3.2
0.7	0.0	73.7	4.5	53.9	162.8	218.4	245.9	1.1	0.0	0.0	2.0	0.4	0.4	5.0	0.5	99.6	0.0	2.5
0.2	0.0	18.7	16.8	47.9	159.5	259.6	3.3	1.5	0.0	0.0	0.3	0.4	0.4	5.2	0.5	110.0	1.5	5.2
0.1	0.0	12.7	1.6	58.2	146.7	154.3	475.6	1.4	0.0	0.0	0.0	0.2	0.2	2.0	0.1	17.7	0.1	217.8
0.0	0.0	4.6	9.4	8.3	32.3	38.3	275.9	0.5	2.0	17.5	0.0	0.4	0.0	5.8	0.6	116.5	1.7	0.9
0.1	0.0	1.8	1.1	8.6	23.8	23.0	193.0	0.3	135.2	9.0	0.0	0.2	0.3	3.0	0.3	63.5	0.0	0.5
0.0	0.0	0.9	4.5	3.6	13.9	16.0	0.4	0.1	0.0	0.0	0.0	0.4	0.3	5.0	0.0	2.7	0.0	0.4
0.0	0.0	2.7	5.1	10.3	29.5	31.7	145.1	2.2	130.7	8.7	0.0	0.3	0.3	4.1	0.4	54.0	0.0	0.5
0.3	0.0	4.2	1.0	2.7	9.5	23.9	246.6	0.8	503.1	20.1	0.1	0.5	0.6	6.7	0.7	2.7	2.0	0.6
0.0	0.0	0.5	0.3	1.1	4.0	3.0	7.6	0.0	13.2	0.5	0.0	0.0	0.0	0.2	0.0	3.5	0.1	0.0
0.3	0.2	6.3	12.0	11.8	65.1	71.0	259.6	0.6	556.1	22.3	0.1	0.5	0.6	7.4	0.8	6.7	2.2	1.6
0.2	0.0	258.3	18.0	32.1	210.9	96.9	198.6	15.0	375.3	60.0	23.5	1.5	1.7	20.1	2.0	399.9	7.7	0.8
0.2	0.0	17.9	13.1	58.4	181.7	173.4	308.2	1.2	0.0	24.4	0.2	0.6	0.2	8.1	0.8	162.4	2.4	1.2
0.0	0.0	3.4	3.8	17.4	42.6	41.8	0.5	0.3	0.0	0.0	0.0	0.3	0.2	4.2	0.0	3.8	0.0	0.4
0.1	0.0	9.4	1.0	32.7	87.5	89.5	2.5	0.8	0.0	0.0	0.1	0.1	0.1	1.3	0.1	12.4	0.0	1.3
0.2	0.0	54.6	8.1	31.8	95.4	104.1	222.3	0.7	225.3	15.0	0.4	0.4	0.4	5.0	0.5	99.9	0.0	1.0
0.0	436.0	336.0	4.8	0.0	0.0	312.0	246.0	0.0	313.6	0.0	0.0	0.3	2.0	3.9	0.0	0.0	0.0	0.0
2.4	12.6	133.3	0.1	6.4	85.7	29.4	37.0	0.5	31.9	0.0	0.0	0.0	0.1	0.1	0.0	2.2	0.2	17.3
3.7	15.5	157.3	0.1	8.0	245.0	67.7	455.0	0.7	52.9	0.0	0.0	0.0	0.1	0.1	0.0	2.0	0.1	13.3
1.0	0.0	170.8	0.1	11.5	163.2	127.4	191.8	0.5	122.4	0.0	0.6	0.0	0.1	0.1	0.0	3.1	0.2	13.3
5.2	21.1	147.7	0.1	6.4	108.5	71.8	390.7	0.7	63.8	0.0	0.2	0.0	0.1	0.3	0.0	10.2	0.3	11.9
5.3	26.4	188.6	0.1	6.8	126.3	38.0	156.7	0.7	84.6	0.0	0.1	0.0	0.1	0.0	0.0	5.7	0.4	11.5
4.9	28.0	51.5	0.1	5.6	52.6	42.6	176.2	0.7	51.0	0.0	0.2	0.0	0.1	0.1	0.1	18.2	0.5	13.6
4.3	20.2	108.5	0.1	5.6	97.0	52.2	235.7	0.7	70.6	0.0	0.2	0.0	0.1	0.2	0.1	17.4	0.4	14.5
5.2	26.0	188.5	0.2	6.2	137.2	26.0	193.2	0.8	80.9	0.0	0.0	0.0	0.1	0.1	0.0	5.1	0.1	11.0
5.9	29.4	202.0	0.2	7.8	143.4	27.6	173.7	0.9	77.8	0.0	0.1	0.0	0.1	0.1	0.0	5.1	0.2	10.3
5.8	28.0	196.8	0.2	7.6	135.5	31.4	5.9	0.9	80.6	0.0	0.1	0.0	0.1	0.1	0.0	5.0	0.2	10.9
1.2	5.9	116.2	0.1	4.5	135.5	18.5	171.4	0.5	17.9	0.0	0.0	0.0	0.1	0.1	0.0	3.1	0.1	17.7
5.7	26.6	191.7	0.2	7.2	127.8	35.4	169.2	0.9	77.0	0.0	0.1	0.0	0.1	0.1	0.0	5.1	0.2	10.7
0.8	4.2	16.8	0.0	1.5	36.9	23.6	113.3	0.1	13.4	0.0	0.0	0.0	0.0	0.0	0.0	3.4	0.2	22.1
0.6	3.1	13.3	0.0	1.2	29.3	18.7	113.3	0.1	10.1	0.0	0.0	0.0	0.0	0.0	0.0	2.7	0.1	20.2
0.2	1.2	17.1	0.0	1.5	37.5	23.9	113.7	0.1	3.1	0.0	0.0	0.0	0.0	0.0	0.0	3.5	0.2	23.1
0.3	2.4	19.2	0.0	1.7	42.1	26.9	113.7	0.1	5.6	0.0	0.0	0.0	0.1	0.0	0.0	3.7	0.2	22.2
0.1	1.9	8.9	0.1	1.1	29.1	9.1	3.6	0.1	2.2	0.0	0.0	0.0	0.0	0.0	0.0	4.1	0.2	22.3
6.2	30.7	22.4	0.3	1.8	29.2	33.4	82.7	0.2	107.0	0.0	0.3	0.0	0.0	0.0	0.0	3.7	0.1	15.1
0.3	2.2	51.8	0.1	3.9	121.5	45.6	152.6	0.2	78.1	0.0	0.0	0.0	0.0	0.0	0.0	10.4	0.2	21.1
4.9	25.0	204.7	0.1	8.3	150.0	52.6	270.2	1.1	70.8	0.0	0.2	0.0	0.1	0.0	0.0	4.5	0.4	11.6
4.2	24.9	137.9	0.2	5.4	94.4	17.3	312.5	0.8	35.8	0.0	0.0	0.0	0.2	0.3	0.1	9.0	0.5	15.5
5.4	32.5	154.0	0.1	3.9	97.0	17.8	224.0	1.0	81.2	0.0	0.1	0.0	0.0	0.0	0.0	1.7	0.5	10.6
4.9	31.9	195.9	0.1	8.1	153.0	33.7	229.4	1.1	48.7	0.0	0.1	0.0	0.1	0.0	0.0	5.9	0.4	11.6
5.3	30.8	283.1	0.0	10.1	169.5	22.7	94.1	1.1	84.3	0.0	0.1	0.0	0.1	0.0	0.0	2.9	0.4	9.3
5.3	29.4	190.4	0.1	7.8	124.3	24.4	316.7	0.8	17.6	0.0	0.0	0.0	0.0	0.0	0.0	0.3	0.4	10.7
5.3	24.9	209.0	0.2	7.6	124.3	22.6	150.2	0.8	70.8	0.0	0.1	0.0	0.1	0.0	0.0	5.1	0.2	11.5

Code	Food Name	Unit/Amt	Wt (g)	Energy (Kcal)	Prot (g)	Carb (g)	Fiber (g)	Fat (g)	Mono (g)	Poly (g)
1028	Cheese, Mozzarella, Part Skim Milk	1.0 oz	28	71.2	6.8	0.8	0.0	4.5	1.3	0.1
1026	Cheese, Mozzarella, Whole Milk	1.0 oz	28	78.8	5.4	0.6	0.0	6.0	1.8	0.2
1030	Cheese, Muenster	1.0 oz	28	103.1	6.6	0.3	0.0	8.4	2.4	0.2
1031	Cheese, Neufchatel	1.0 oz or 1 tbsp	28	72.8	2.8	0.8	0.0	6.6	1.9	0.2
1032	Cheese, Parmesan, grated	1.0 oz	28	127.6	11.6	1.0	0.0	8.4	2.4	0.2
1033	Cheese, Parmesan, hard	1.0 oz	28	109.8	10.0	0.9	0.0	7.2	2.1	0.2
1146	Cheese, Parmesan, shredded	1.0 oz	28	116.2	10.6	1.0	0.0	7.7	2.4	0.2
1042	Cheese, Pasteurized Process, American with disodium phosphate	1 cup, shredded	113	424.3	25.0	1.8	0.0	35.3	10.1	1.1
1043	Cheese, Pasteurized Process, Pimiento	1 cup, shredded	113	424.2	25.0	2.0	0.0	35.3	10.1	1.1
1044	Cheese, Pasteurized Process, Swiss with disodium phosphate	1 cup, shredded	113	376.9	27.9	2.4	0.0	28.3	8.0	0.7
901903	Cheese, Process, Cheez Whiz	1.0 oz	28	77.0	4.6	1.8	0.0	5.7	2.3	0.1
901901	Cheese, Process, Velveeta	1 oz	28	84.0	5.2	2.2	0.0	6.1	2.0	0.2
1035	Cheese, Provolone	1 cup, diced	132	464.0	33.8	2.8	0.0	35.1	9.8	1.0
1037	Cheese, Ricotta, Part Skim Milk	1.0 oz or 1 tbsp	15.4	21.3	1.8	0.8	0.0	1.2	0.4	0.0
1036	Cheese, Ricotta, Whole Milk	1.0 oz or 1 tbsp	15.4	26.8	1.7	0.5	0.0	2.0	0.6	0.1
1038	Cheese, Romano	1.0 oz	28	108.3	8.9	1.0	0.0	7.5	2.2	0.2
1039	Cheese, Roquefort	1.0 oz	28	103.3	6.0	0.6	0.0	8.6	2.4	0.4
1040	Cheese, Swiss	1.0 oz	108	405.8	30.7	3.7	0.0	29.6	7.9	1.0
18147	Cheesecake, commercially prep	1 piece (½ of 9" dia)	128	410.9	7.0	32.6	0.5	28.8	11.1	2.1
918149	Cheesecake, homemade	1 piece (½ of 9" dia)	99	353.4	6.7	24.9	0.0	25.7	0.0	0.0
18148	Cheesecake, no bake mix, prep	1 piece (½ of 9" dia)	142	389.1	7.8	50.4	2.7	18.0	6.4	1.1
1045	Cheesefood, Cold Pack, American	1.0 oz	28	92.7	5.5	2.3	0.0	6.8	2.0	0.2
1149	Cheesefood, Pasteurized Process, American w/disodium phosphate	1.0 oz	28	91.9	5.5	2.0	0.0	6.9	2.0	0.2
1047	Cheesefood, Pasteurized Process, Swiss	1.0 oz	28	90.5	6.1	1.3	0.0	6.8	1.9	0.2
5028	Chicken Liver, simmered	3.5 oz	100	157.0	24.4	0.9	0.0	5.5	1.3	0.9
22703	Chicken & Dumplings, canned/Sweet Sue	1 package	681	619.7	42.9	64.7	7.5	21.1	8.4	4.6
924003	Chicken A la King frz (Le Menu 10. 5 oz meal)	1 package	299	574.1	32.9	14.6	0.1	41.5	16.4	7.6
924006	Chicken Chow Mein	10.0 oz	284	289.7	35.2	11.4	3.4	14.2	5.6	4.0
924005	Chicken Chow Mein, canned	¾ cup	200	76.0	5.6	14.4	1.6	0.8	0.1	0.6
924248	Chicken Chow Mein/Chun King	¾ cup	200	200.0	13.6	28.7	0.0	3.3	0.0	0.0
924068	Chicken Egg Roll/LaChoy	3 medium	37	89.9	3.0	12.0	0.0	3.0	1.1	1.3
924043	Chicken Kiev, frozen	1 breast w/ filling	280	604.8	22.3	41.4	0.0	39.0	0.0	0.0
924051	Chicken Parmigiana	11 .5 oz	356	548.2	38.4	39.3	0.0	26.3	0.0	0.0
22527	Chicken Pie, frozen/Stouffers	1 slice	232	468.6	19.0	29.9	2.6	30.4	10.1	8.6
924007	Chicken Pot Pie	7.0 oz	198	465.3	19.6	35.8	1.5	27.7	13.2	5.6
924171	Chicken Teriyaki/LaChoy	¾ cup	120	85.2	8.0	8.0	1.0	2.0	1.1	0.4
924242	Chicken w/vegetables&pasta	9.5 oz	269	121.1	10.8	13.7	0.0	2.4	0.0	0.0
924004	Chicken&Noodles	1 cup	240	364.8	22.0	26.0	0.1	18.0	7.1	3.9
924047	Chicken&Rice	7.0 oz pkg	200	364.0	22.0	26.0	1.0	18.0	7.0	4.0
5060	Chicken, Broiler or Fryer, Breast w/skin, roasted	3.5 oz	100	197.0	29.8	0.0	0.0	7.8	3.0	1.7
5061	Chicken, Broiler or Fryer, Breast w/skin, stewed	3.5 oz	100	184.0	27.4	0.0	0.0	7.4	2.9	1.6
5063	Chicken, Broiler or Fryer, Breast, no skin, fried	3.5 oz	100	187.0	33.4	0.5	0.0	4.7	1.7	1.1
5064	Chicken, Broiler or Fryer, Breast, no skin, roasted	3.5 oz	100	165.0	31.0	0.0	0.0	3.6	1.2	0.8
5065	Chicken, Broiler or Fryer, Breast, no skin, stewed	3.5 oz	100	151.0	29.0	0.0	0.0	3.0	1.0	0.7
5037	Chicken, Broiler or Fryer, Dark Meat w/skin, roasted	3.5 oz	100	253.0	26.0	0.0	0.0	15.8	6.2	3.5
5038	Chicken, Broiler or Fryer, Dark Meat w/skin, stewed	3.5 oz	100	233.0	23.5	0.0	0.0	14.7	5.8	3.2
5044	Chicken, Broiler or Fryer, Dark Meat, no skin, fried	4.0 oz	119	284.4	34.5	3.1	0.0	13.8	5.1	3.3
5045	Chicken, Broiler or Fryer, Dark Meat, no skin, roasted	3.5 oz	100	205.0	27.4	0.0	0.0	9.7	3.6	2.3
5046	Chicken, Broiler or Fryer, Dark Meat, no skin, stewed	3.5 oz	100	192.0	26.0	0.0	0.0	9.0	3.3	2.1
5078	Chicken, Broiler or Fryer, Leg w/skin, roasted	3.5 oz	100	232.0	26.0	0.0	0.0	13.5	5.2	3.0
5079	Chicken, Broiler or Fryer, Leg w/skin, stewed	3.5 oz	100	220.0	24.2	0.0	0.0	12.9	5.0	2.9
5081	Chicken, Broiler or Fryer, Leg, no skin, fried	4.0 oz	119	247.5	33.8	0.8	0.0	11.1	4.1	2.6
5082	Chicken, Broiler or Fryer, Leg, no skin, roasted	3.5 oz	100	191.0	27.0	0.0	0.0	8.4	3.1	2.0
5083	Chicken, Broiler or Fryer, Leg, no skin, stewed	3.5 oz	100	185.0	26.3	0.0	0.0	8.1	2.9	1.9
5032	Chicken, Broiler or Fryer, Light Meat w/skin, roasted	3.5 oz	100	222.0	29.0	0.0	0.0	10.9	4.3	2.3
5033	Chicken, Broiler or Fryer, Light Meat w/skin, stewed	3.5 oz	100	201.0	26.1	0.0	0.0	10.0	3.9	2.1
5040	Chicken, Broiler or Fryer, Light Meat, no skin, fried	4.0 oz	119	228.5	39.1	0.5	0.0	6.6	2.3	1.5
5041	Chicken, Broiler or Fryer, Light Meat, no skin, roasted	3.5 oz	100	173.0	30.9	0.0	0.0	4.5	1.5	1.0
5042	Chicken, Broiler or Fryer, Light Meat, no skin, stewed	3.5 oz	100	159.0	28.9	0.0	0.0	4.0	1.4	0.9
5009	Chicken, Broiler or Fryer, meat & skin, roasted	3.5 oz	100	239.0	27.3	0.0	0.0	13.6	5.3	3.0
5010	Chicken, Broiler or Fryer, meat & skin, stewed	3.5 oz	100	219.0	24.7	0.0	0.0	12.6	4.9	2.7
5094	Chicken, Broiler or Fryer, Thigh w/skin, roasted	3.5 oz	100	247.0	25.1	0.0	0.0	15.5	6.2	3.4
5095	Chicken, Broiler or Fryer, Thigh w/skin, stewed	3.5 oz	100	232.0	23.3	0.0	0.0	14.7	5.8	3.3
5097	Chicken, Broiler or Fryer, Thigh, no skin, fried	4.0 oz	119	259.4	33.5	1.4	0.0	12.3	4.5	2.9
5098	Chicken, Broiler or Fryer, Thigh, no skin, roasted	3.5 oz	100	209.0	25.9	0.0	0.0	10.9	4.2	2.5
5099	Chicken, Broiler or Fryer, Thigh, no skin, stewed	3.5 oz	100	195.0	25.0	0.0	0.0	9.8	3.7	2.2
5103	Chicken, Broiler or Fryer, Wing w/skin, roasted	3.5 oz	100	290.0	26.9	0.0	0.0	19.5	7.6	4.1
5104	Chicken, Broiler or Fryer, Wing w/skin, stewed	3.5 oz	100	249.0	22.8	0.0	0.0	16.8	6.6	3.6
5106	Chicken, Broiler or Fryer, Wing, no skin, fried	4.0 oz	119	251.1	35.9	0.0	0.0	10.9	3.7	2.5

Sat (g)	Chol (mg)	Cal (mg)	Iron (mg)	Magn (mg)	Phos (mg)	Pota (mg)	Sodi (mg)	Zinc (mg)	Vit A (RE)	Vit C (mg)	Vit E (mg)	Thia (mg)	Ribo (mg)	Niac (mg)	Vit B-6 (mg)	Fol (µg)	Vit B-12 (µg)	Wat (g)
2.8	16.2	180.8	0.1	6.5	129.6	23.4	130.5	0.8	49.6	0.0	0.1	0.0	0.1	0.0	0.0	2.5	0.2	15.1
3.7	22.0	144.8	0.1	5.2	103.8	18.8	104.5	0.6	67.5	0.0	0.1	0.0	0.1	0.0	0.0	2.0	0.2	15.2
5.4	26.8	200.8	0.1	7.7	131.0	37.6	175.8	0.8	88.5	0.0	0.1	0.0	0.1	0.0	0.0	3.4	0.4	11.7
4.1	21.3	21.1	0.1	2.1	38.2	31.9	111.8	0.1	84.0	0.0	0.0	0.0	0.1	0.0	0.0	3.2	0.1	17.4
5.3	22.0	385.2	0.3	14.2	226.0	30.0	521.2	0.9	48.4	0.0	0.2	0.0	0.1	0.1	0.0	2.2	0.4	4.9
4.6	19.0	331.4	0.2	12.2	194.4	25.8	448.4	0.8	41.7	0.0	0.2	0.0	0.1	0.1	0.0	1.9	0.3	8.2
4.9	20.2	350.8	0.2	14.2	205.8	27.2	474.9	0.9	48.4	0.0	0.0	0.0	0.1	0.1	0.0	2.2	0.4	7.0
22.3	106.7	695.5	0.4	25.1	841.7	183.1	1616.4	3.4	327.7	0.0	0.5	0.0	0.4	0.1	0.1	8.8	0.8	44.3
22.2	106.4	694.3	0.5	25.1	840.5	182.7	1613.1	3.4	363.9	2.5	0.5	0.0	0.4	0.1	0.1	8.8	0.8	44.2
18.1	95.8	872.2	0.7	32.9	860.5	243.5	1548.4	4.1	258.8	0.0	0.8	0.0	0.3	0.0	0.0	6.7	1.4	47.8
3.1	16.0	147.0	0.1	8.0	255.0	52.0	370.0	0.7	38.6	0.0	0.0	0.0	0.1	0.1	0.0	4.0	0.2	14.5
3.6	21.0	154.0	0.1	8.0	292.0	88.0	454.0	0.6	68.6	0.0	0.0	0.0	0.1	0.0	0.0	6.0	0.3	13.0
22.5	90.9	997.8	0.7	36.4	654.9	182.6	1155.7	4.3	348.5	0.0	0.5	0.0	0.4	0.2	0.1	13.7	1.9	54.1
0.8	4.7	41.9	0.1	2.3	28.1	19.3	19.2	0.2	17.4	0.0	0.0	0.0	0.0	0.0	0.0	2.0	0.0	11.5
1.3	7.8	31.9	0.1	1.7	24.3	16.1	13.0	0.2	20.6	0.0	0.1	0.0	0.0	0.0	0.0	1.9	0.1	11.0
4.8	29.1	297.9	0.2	11.5	212.8	24.2	336.0	0.7	39.5	0.0	0.2	0.0	0.1	0.0	0.0	1.9	0.3	8.7
5.4	25.2	185.3	0.2	8.3	109.8	25.4	506.5	0.6	83.7	0.0	0.0	0.0	0.2	0.2	0.0	13.7	0.2	11.0
19.2	99.0	1037.8	0.2	38.8	653.0	119.6	280.8	4.2	273.2	0.0	0.5	0.0	0.4	0.1	0.1	6.9	1.8	40.2
12.7	70.4	65.3	0.8	14.1	119.0	115.2	265.0	0.7	186.9	0.5	2.0	0.0	0.2	0.2	0.1	23.0	0.2	58.4
2.0	8.0	57.4	1.2	7.9	95.0	101.0	280.2	0.5	317.8	0.4	0.0	0.0	0.2	0.4	0.0	11.9	0.2	40.5
9.5	41.2	244.2	0.7	27.0	332.3	299.6	539.6	0.7	140.6	0.7	0.0	0.2	0.4	0.7	0.1	42.6	0.4	62.8
4.3	17.8	139.2	0.2	8.3	112.0	101.6	270.5	0.8	56.6	0.0	0.0	0.0	0.1	0.0	0.0	1.5	0.4	12.1
4.3	17.9	160.8	0.2	8.6	211.1	78.1	446.9	0.8	61.3	0.0	0.0	0.0	0.1	0.0	0.0	2.0	0.3	12.1
4.3	22.9	202.6	0.2	7.8	147.3	79.5	434.6	1.0	68.0	0.0	0.0	0.0	0.1	0.0	0.0	1.6	0.6	12.2
1.8	631.0	14.0	8.5	21.0	312.0	140.0	51.0	4.3	4913.0	15.8	1.4	0.2	1.7	4.5	0.6	770.0	19.4	68.3
5.1	102.2	0.0	7.3	0.0	0.0	0.0	2683.1	0.0	0.0	0.0	0.0	0.0	0.0	0.0	0.0	0.0	0.0	544.1
15.7	269.7	155.0	3.0	0.0	436.9	493.0	927.5	2.2	275.8	14.6	0.0	0.1	0.5	6.6	0.3	13.4	0.0	0.0
4.7	85.2	65.9	2.8	0.0	332.8	537.3	815.6	2.4	63.6	11.4	0.0	0.1	0.3	4.9	0.5	21.6	0.0	0.0
0.1	6.4	36.0	1.0	0.0	68.0	334.4	580.0	1.0	24.0	10.4	0.0	0.0	0.1	0.8	0.1	9.6	0.0	0.0
0.0	0.0	14.6	1.1	0.0	111.1	140.9	845.5	0.0	68.6	2.2	0.0	0.1	0.1	1.6	0.0	0.0	0.0	0.0
0.6	3.0	9.0	0.8	0.0	0.0	55.0	140.0	0.0	5.0	2.0	0.0	0.1	0.1	1.1	0.0	0.0	0.0	0.0
0.0	0.0	54.3	1.5	0.0	0.0	291.1	95.0	0.0	397.4	2.5	0.0	0.2	0.2	9.0	0.0	0.0	0.0	0.0
0.0	0.0	309.7	11.2	0.0	521.5	608.8	637.2	0.0	494.1	28.5	0.0	0.3	0.3	8.5	0.0	0.0	0.0	0.0
8.8	62.6	83.5	2.5	0.0	0.0	0.0	772.6	0.0	0.0	0.0	0.0	0.0	0.0	0.0	0.0	0.0	0.0	149.4
8.8	47.8	59.7	2.6	0.0	198.0	292.7	506.9	1.7	1232.4	4.3	0.0	0.3	0.3	4.2	0.4	24.8	0.0	0.0
0.5	20.0	20.0	1.1	0.0	0.0	230.0	850.0	0.0	200.0	12.0	0.0	0.0	0.1	2.0	0.0	0.0	0.0	0.0
0.0	0.0	50.0	1.3	0.0	0.0	195.0	965.0	0.0	493.4	5.0	0.0	0.1	0.1	2.9	0.0	0.0	0.0	0.0
5.1	103.0	26.0	2.2	0.0	247.0	149.0	600.0	2.1	86.0	0.0	0.0	0.1	0.2	4.3	0.2	9.0	0.0	0.0
5.0	103.0	26.0	2.4	0.0	247.0	211.0	600.0	2.1	26.0	1.0	0.0	0.1	0.2	4.3	0.2	9.0	0.0	0.0
2.2	84.0	14.0	1.1	27.0	214.0	245.0	71.0	1.0	27.0	0.0	0.3	0.1	0.1	12.7	0.6	4.0	0.3	62.4
2.1	75.0	13.0	0.9	22.0	156.0	178.0	62.0	1.0	24.0	0.0	0.3	0.0	0.1	7.8	0.3	3.0	0.2	66.2
1.3	91.0	16.0	1.1	31.0	246.0	276.0	79.0	1.1	7.0	0.0	0.4	0.1	0.1	14.8	0.6	4.0	0.4	60.2
1.0	85.0	15.0	1.0	29.0	228.0	256.0	74.0	1.0	6.0	0.0	0.3	0.1	0.1	13.7	0.6	4.0	0.3	65.3
0.9	77.0	13.0	0.9	24.0	165.0	187.0	63.0	1.0	6.0	0.0	0.3	0.0	0.1	8.5	0.3	3.0	0.2	68.3
4.4	91.0	15.0	1.4	22.0	168.0	220.0	87.0	2.5	58.0	0.0	0.0	0.1	0.2	6.4	0.3	7.0	0.3	58.6
4.1	82.0	14.0	1.3	18.0	133.0	166.0	70.0	2.3	54.0	0.0	0.0	0.1	0.2	4.5	0.2	6.0	0.2	63.0
3.7	114.2	21.4	1.8	29.8	222.5	301.1	115.4	3.5	28.6	0.0	0.0	0.1	0.3	8.4	0.4	10.7	0.4	66.3
2.7	93.0	15.0	1.3	23.0	179.0	240.0	93.0	2.8	22.0	0.0	0.3	0.1	0.2	6.5	0.4	8.0	0.3	63.1
2.5	88.0	14.0	1.4	20.0	143.0	181.0	74.0	2.7	21.0	0.0	0.3	0.1	0.2	4.7	0.2	7.0	0.2	65.8
3.7	92.0	12.0	1.3	23.0	174.0	225.0	87.0	2.6	39.0	0.0	0.3	0.1	0.2	6.2	0.3	7.0	0.3	60.9
3.6	84.0	11.0	1.4	20.0	139.0	176.0	73.0	2.4	36.0	0.0	0.3	0.1	0.2	4.6	0.2	6.0	0.2	64.0
3.0	117.8	15.5	1.7	29.8	229.7	302.3	114.2	3.5	23.8	0.0	0.0	0.1	0.3	8.0	0.5	10.7	0.4	72.1
2.3	94.0	12.0	1.3	24.0	183.0	242.0	91.0	2.9	19.0	0.0	0.3	0.1	0.2	6.3	0.4	8.0	0.3	64.7
2.2	89.0	11.0	1.4	21.0	149.0	190.0	78.0	2.8	18.0	0.0	0.3	0.1	0.2	4.8	0.2	8.0	0.2	66.4
3.1	84.0	15.0	1.1	25.0	200.0	227.0	75.0	1.2	32.0	0.0	0.0	0.1	0.1	11.1	0.5	3.0	0.3	60.5
2.8	74.0	13.0	1.0	20.0	146.0	167.0	63.0	1.1	28.0	0.0	0.3	0.0	0.1	6.9	0.3	3.0	0.2	65.1
1.8	107.1	19.0	1.4	34.5	274.9	313.0	96.4	1.5	10.7	0.0	0.0	0.1	0.1	15.9	0.7	4.8	0.4	71.6
1.3	85.0	15.0	1.1	27.0	216.0	247.0	77.0	1.2	9.0	0.0	0.3	0.1	0.1	12.4	0.6	4.0	0.3	64.8
1.1	77.0	13.0	0.9	22.0	159.0	180.0	65.0	1.2	8.0	0.0	0.3	0.0	0.1	7.8	0.3	3.0	0.2	68.0
3.8	88.0	15.0	1.3	23.0	182.0	223.0	82.0	1.9	47.0	0.0	0.3	0.1	0.2	8.5	0.4	5.0	0.3	59.5
3.5	78.0	13.0	1.2	19.0	139.0	166.0	67.0	1.8	42.0	0.0	0.3	0.0	0.1	5.6	0.2	5.0	0.2	63.9
4.3	93.0	12.0	1.3	22.0	174.0	222.0	84.0	2.4	48.0	0.0	0.3	0.1	0.2	6.4	0.3	7.0	0.3	59.4
4.1	84.0	11.0	1.4	19.0	139.0	170.0	71.0	2.3	44.0	0.0	0.3	0.1	0.2	4.9	0.2	6.0	0.2	63.1
3.3	121.4	15.5	1.7	30.9	236.8	308.2	113.1	3.3	25.0	0.0	0.0	0.1	0.3	8.5	0.5	10.7	0.4	70.6
3.0	95.0	12.0	1.3	24.0	183.0	238.0	88.0	2.6	20.0	0.0	0.3	0.1	0.2	6.5	0.4	8.0	0.3	62.9
2.7	90.0	11.0	1.4	21.0	149.0	183.0	75.0	2.6	19.0	0.0	0.3	0.1	0.2	5.2	0.2	7.0	0.2	65.6
5.5	84.0	15.0	1.3	19.0	151.0	184.0	82.0	1.8	47.0	0.0	0.3	0.1	0.2	6.6	0.4	3.0	0.3	55.0
4.7	70.0	12.0	1.1	16.0	121.0	139.0	67.0	1.6	40.0	0.0	0.3	0.0	0.1	4.6	0.2	3.0	0.2	62.2
3.0	100.0	17.9	1.4	25.0	195.2	247.5	108.3	2.5	21.4	0.0	0.0	0.1	0.2	8.6	0.7	4.8	0.4	71.2

Code	Food Name	Unit/Amt	Wt (g)	Energy (Kcal)	Prot (g)	Carb (g)	Fiber (g)	Fat (g)	Mono (g)	Poly (g)
5107	Chicken, Broiler or Fryer, Wing, no skin, roasted	3.5 oz	100	203.0	30.5	0.0	0.0	8.1	2.6	1.8
5108	Chicken, Broiler or Fryer, Wing, no skin, stewed	3.5 oz	100	181.0	27.2	0.0	0.0	7.2	2.3	1.6
22697	Chicken, Chicken Salad Ready To Serve Sandwich Salad/Libby Spreadable	1 package	227	329.2	11.1	22.9	0.0	21.3	6.7	8.1
5277	Chicken, meat only w/broth, canned	2.5 oz	71	117.2	15.5	0.0	0.0	5.6	2.2	1.2
51608	Chicken, Nugget, breaded/Pierre product #1879	3.5 oz	100	329.0	16.8	13.3	1.1	23.4	6.9	10.4
924008	Chili con Carne	¾ cup	120	159.6	8.9	14.6	2.8	7.5	3.4	0.5
22904	Chili con carne w/beans, canned entree	1 cup	255	293.3	23.2	28.1	9.4	9.4	2.5	1.7
924243	Chili w/beans	1 package	425	909.5	30.9	90.8	11.6	52.2	28.0	2.7
16059	Chili w/beans, canned	1 cup	220	246.4	12.6	26.2	9.7	12.1	5.1	0.8
924059	Chili w/beans, homemade	1 cup	247	328.5	18.5	30.1	1.5	15.1	0.0	0.0
924056	Chili w/o Beans, homemade	1 cup	236	472.0	24.3	13.7	0.5	34.9	18.6	2.1
22720	Chili, Vegetarian Chili w/beans, canned entree/Hormel	1 cup	247	205.0	11.9	38.0	9.9	0.7	0.1	0.4
18606	Chocolate Cake, Snack Cake, Chocolate Creme Filling-Ding Dongs/Hostess	1 cup	220	1015.5	6.8	130.2	4.6	51.9	0.0	0.0
918804	Chocolate, Baking, Choco-Bake/Nestle	1 serving	80	480.0	4.0	34.0	0.0	39.4	0.0	0.0
918805	Chocolate, Baking, Hershey	1 oz	28	185.1	4.0	6.7	0.7	15.8	4.8	1.0
19146	Chocolate, Baking, M&M's Milk Chocolate Mini Baking Bits	1 oz	28	139.4	1.3	18.8	0.8	6.5	2.1	0.2
19139	Chocolate, Baking, M&M's Semisweet Chocolate Mini Baking Bits	1 serving	14.2	73.6	0.6	9.4	1.0	3.7	1.2	0.1
19124	Chocolate, Baking, Mexican, squares	1 tbsp	14	59.6	0.5	10.8	0.5	2.2	0.7	0.2
918806	Chocolate, Baking, Unsweetened Liquid	1 tablet	20	95.8	2.4	6.9	0.0	9.6	1.9	2.1
918870	Cobbler, Peach	1 oz	28	44.8	0.3	7.1	0.3	1.8	0.0	0.0
14198	Cocoa Mix, No Sugar Added Hot Cocoa Mix/Carnation	⅓ cup	100	365.0	28.7	56.2	5.0	2.8	0.9	0.1
14197	Cocoa Mix, Rich Chocolate Hot Cocoa Mix/Carnation	1 envelope	15	60.0	0.7	13.0	0.4	0.6	0.2	0.1
1105	Cocoa, Hot, homemade w/whole milk	1 envelope	28	21.6	1.1	3.3	0.2	0.7	0.2	0.0
918844	Coffee Cake, Apple, frozen	1 fl oz	31.2	100.5	1.4	14.0	0.1	4.4	0.0	0.0
918845	Coffee Cake, Blueberry, frozen	⅛ cake	50	190.0	2.6	25.1	0.6	8.9	0.0	0.0
18103	Coffee Cake, Cheese	⅛ Ring	35	118.7	2.5	15.5	0.4	5.3	2.5	0.6
918109	Coffee Cake, Cinnamon Crumb, homemade	1.0 oz	28.4	113.6	1.8	14.3	0.0	5.7	0.0	0.0
18108	Coffee Cake, Cinnamon w/crumb topping, dry mix, prep	1.0 oz	28	89.0	1.5	14.8	0.3	2.7	1.1	0.9
18104	Coffee Cake, Cinnamon w/crumb topping, enriched, commercially prep	1.0 oz	29	121.2	2.0	13.5	0.6	6.8	3.8	0.9
18106	Coffee Cake, Fruit	1.0 oz	28.4	88.3	1.5	14.6	0.7	2.9	1.6	0.4
918847	Coffee Cake, Pecan, frozen	1.0 oz	29	110.8	1.7	13.8	0.3	6.2	0.0	0.0
918843	Coffee Cake/LittleDeb	⅙ cake	40	153.6	2.0	26.8	0.0	4.2	1.6	1.6
14210	Coffee, brewed, espresso, restaurant-prep	2.0 oz	57	5.1	0.0	0.9	0.0	0.1	0.0	0.1
902912	Condiment, A-1 Sauce	6 fl oz	177	118.6	0.0	29.5	0.0	0.0	0.0	0.0
902922	Condiment, Enchilada Sauce	¼ cup	60	21.0	0.0	2.8	0.0	0.0	0.0	0.0
2055	Condiment, Horseradish, prep	1 tbsp	15	7.2	0.2	1.7	0.5	0.1	0.0	0.1
902916	Condiment, Mustard, brown	1 tsp	5	5.0	0.3	0.3	0.1	0.3	0.0	0.0
902917	Condiment, Mustard, yellow	1 tsp	5	4.0	0.2	0.3	0.1	0.2	0.0	0.0
902925	Condiment, Picante Sauce	3 tbsp	57	16.0	0.0	4.0	0.0	0.0	0.0	0.0
902918	Condiment, Pickle, Sour Relish	1 tbsp	15	16.1	0.0	3.8	0.2	0.0	0.0	0.0
902926	Condiment, Salsa	3 tbsp	43	24.9	1.0	6.0	0.0	0.0	0.0	0.0
902927	Condiment, Taco Sauce, chunky	3 tbsp	43	24.9	1.0	6.0	0.0	0.0	0.0	0.0
902928	Condiment, Taco Sauce, hot/mild	3 tbsp	43	15.1	0.0	4.0	0.0	0.0	0.0	0.0
11935	Condiment, Vege, Tomato Catsup	1 tbsp	15	15.6	0.2	4.1	0.2	0.1	0.0	0.0
11949	Condiment, Vege, Tomato Catsup, low sodium	1 tbsp	15	15.6	0.2	4.1	0.2	0.1	0.0	0.0
902919	Condiment, Worcestershire Sauce	1 tbsp	15	11.0	0.3	2.7	0.0	0.0	0.0	0.0
18150	Cookie, Animal Crackers/Arrowroot/Tea Biscuits	1 cracker	2	8.9	0.1	1.5	0.0	0.3	0.2	0.0
918153	Cookie, Brownies, dry mix, prep	1 brownie (2″ square)	33	139.6	1.4	20.4	0.9	6.6	0.0	0.0
18197	Cookie, Brownies, dry mix, prep, special dietary	1 brownie (2″ square)	22	84.5	0.8	15.7	0.8	2.4	1.0	0.2
18154	Cookie, Brownies, homemade	1 brownie (2″ square)	24	111.8	1.5	12.0	0.0	7.0	2.6	2.3
18155	Cookie, Butter, enriched, commercially prep	1 cookie	5	23.4	0.3	3.4	0.0	0.9	0.3	0.0
918861	Cookie, Capri/PepFarm	1 cookie	16	81.9	0.8	9.7	0.1	4.6	0.0	0.0
18614	Cookie, Chewy Fudge Brownie Mix, dry/Martha White	1 serving	28	114.1	1.3	23.2	0.0	1.8	0.0	0.0
18198	Cookie, Chocolate Chip, commercially prep, special dietary	1 medium cookie (1.6″ dia)	7	31.5	0.3	5.1	0.1	1.2	0.5	0.4
918162	Cookie, Chocolate Chip, dry mix, prep	1 cookie (2″ dia)	16	79.4	0.9	10.3	0.2	4.1	0.0	0.0
18159	Cookie, Chocolate Chip, enriched, commercially prep	1 large Keebler RichnChip/ PecanChipDelux	14	67.3	0.8	9.4	0.4	3.2	1.6	0.3
18378	Cookie, Chocolate Chip, homemade w/butter	1 medium cookie (2.25″ dia)	16	78.1	0.9	9.3	0.0	4.5	1.3	0.7
18158	Cookie, Chocolate Chip, lower fat, commercially prep	1 cookie	10	45.3	0.6	7.3	0.4	1.5	0.6	0.5
918164	Cookie, Chocolate Chip, refrig dough, bkd	1.0 oz	28	137.8	1.4	19.1	0.5	6.3	0.0	0.0
18160	Cookie, Chocolate Chip, soft, commercially prep	1 cookie	15	68.7	0.5	8.9	0.5	3.6	2.0	0.5
918862	Cookie, Chocolate Chip/PepFarm	2 large	64	321.3	3.2	44.2	0.0	14.7	0.0	0.0
918895	Cookie, Chocolate Coated Graham/Lance	1.8 oz	50	249.0	3.5	32.7	0.0	13.5	7.5	0.6
918854	Cookie, Chocolate Marshmallow Pie/LittleDeb	1.4 oz	39	170.0	1.5	27.1	0.0	6.2	3.3	0.7
18169	Cookie, Coconut Macaroons, homemade	1 individual pkg (2 oz pkg w/2 3″-bars	57	230.3	2.1	41.2	1.0	7.2	0.3	0.1
18170	Cookie, Fig Bar	1 cookie	16	55.7	0.6	11.3	0.7	1.2	0.5	0.4
18171	Cookie, Fortune	1 cookie	8	30.2	0.3	6.7	0.1	0.2	0.1	0.0

Sat (g)	Chol (mg)	Cal (mg)	Iron (mg)	Magn (mg)	Phos (mg)	Pota (mg)	Sodi (mg)	Zinc (mg)	Vit A (RE)	Vit C (mg)	Vit E (mg)	Thia (mg)	Ribo (mg)	Niac (mg)	Vit B-6 (mg)	Fol (µg)	Vit B-12 (µg)	Wat (g)
2.3	85.0	16.0	1.2	21.0	166.0	210.0	92.0	2.1	18.0	0.0	0.3	0.0	0.1	7.3	0.6	4.0	0.3	62.8
2.0	74.0	13.0	1.1	18.0	134.0	153.0	73.0	2.0	16.0	0.0	0.3	0.0	0.1	5.2	0.3	3.0	0.2	67.0
4.4	59.0	0.0	0.0	0.0	0.0	0.0	1062.4	0.0	0.0	0.0	0.0	0.0	0.0	0.0	0.0	0.0	0.0	167.3
1.6	44.0	9.9	1.1	8.5	78.8	98.0	357.1	1.0	24.1	1.4	0.2	0.0	0.1	4.5	0.2	2.8	0.2	48.7
4.6	39.0	36.0	2.2	24.0	225.0	211.0	697.0	2.5	0.0	0.0	2.7	0.3	0.2	6.3	0.3	29.0	0.7	44.6
2.7	13.2	38.6	2.0	0.0	151.1	279.5	637.2	2.4	14.1	3.8	0.0	0.0	0.1	1.6	0.2	19.3	0.0	0.0
2.4	28.1	76.5	3.8	63.8	221.9	698.7	1185.8	2.8	107.1	1.0	0.3	0.2	0.2	2.4	0.2	66.3	0.7	189.3
18.9	125.6	183.5	12.4	0.0	388.3	2801.1	1931.8	3.9	566.0	77.3	0.0	0.8	0.6	8.5	0.5	48.3	0.0	0.0
5.2	37.4	103.4	7.5	99.0	338.8	803.0	1148.4	4.4	74.8	3.7	1.6	0.1	0.2	0.8	0.3	49.9	0.0	166.1
0.0	0.0	79.0	4.2	0.0	311.2	575.5	1311.6	0.0	29.6	0.0	0.0	0.1	0.2	3.2	0.0	0.0	0.0	178.8
14.2	101.5	89.7	3.3	0.0	358.7	2199.5	3138.8	11.8	70.8	4.7	0.0	0.0	0.3	5.2	0.6	0.0	0.0	157.9
0.1	0.0	96.3	3.5	81.5	0.0	802.8	778.1	1.7	0.0	1.2	0.0	0.0	0.0	0.0	0.0	0.0	0.0	192.5
30.6	30.1	0.0	5.1	0.0	0.0	0.0	547.8	0.0	0.0	0.0	0.0	0.0	0.0	0.0	0.0	0.0	0.0	28.2
0.0	0.0	0.0	0.0	0.0	0.0	817.1	8.6	0.0	0.0	0.0	0.0	0.0	0.0	0.0	0.0	0.0	0.0	0.0
10.0	0.0	20.0	2.0	84.0	123.0	224.0	3.0	1.1	1.2	0.0	0.0	0.0	0.1	0.3	0.0	3.0	0.0	0.0
4.0	4.2	32.5	0.3	12.9	46.5	82.0	19.0	0.3	12.6	0.2	0.3	0.0	0.1	0.1	0.0	1.4	0.1	0.7
2.2	0.4	4.8	0.4	15.1	17.3	47.7	0.4	0.2	1.0	0.0	0.1	0.0	0.0	0.1	0.0	4.0	0.0	0.2
1.2	0.0	4.8	0.3	13.3	19.9	55.6	0.4	0.2	0.3	0.0	0.1	0.0	0.0	0.3	0.0	0.3	0.0	0.2
5.1	0.0	10.7	0.8	53.6	68.6	236.4	2.1	0.7	2.4	0.0	0.0	0.0	0.1	0.4	0.0	0.0	0.0	0.2
0.8	0.0	2.0	0.1	0.0	4.5	24.6	44.2	0.0	26.8	7.3	0.0	0.0	0.0	0.3	0.0	0.0	0.0	0.0
1.4	19.0	823.0	2.6	180.0	900.0	1921.0	947.0	4.0	0.0	2.7	0.1	0.4	1.5	1.2	0.4	39.0	3.0	3.3
0.2	0.9	21.5	0.2	14.7	38.0	104.1	54.5	0.2	0.0	0.0	0.0	0.0	0.1	0.1	0.0	1.1	0.1	0.2
0.4	2.2	35.3	0.1	7.8	32.8	56.0	14.3	0.2	15.4	0.3	0.0	0.0	0.0	0.0	0.0	1.7	0.1	22.7
0.0	0.0	8.7	0.4	3.1	18.7	23.7	121.1	0.0	30.6	2.5	0.0	0.1	0.0	0.5	0.0	0.0	0.0	10.4
0.0	0.0	8.6	0.8	7.1	31.4	41.4	192.9	0.0	14.0	0.0	0.0	0.1	0.1	1.1	0.0	0.0	0.0	11.9
1.9	29.8	20.7	0.2	5.3	35.4	101.2	118.7	0.2	30.5	0.0	0.5	0.0	0.0	0.2	0.0	13.7	0.1	11.3
2.2	2.2	31.8	0.6	11.4	39.2	67.9	110.5	0.2	46.9	0.1	0.0	0.1	0.1	0.3	0.0	4.3	0.0	6.0
0.5	13.7	38.1	0.4	5.0	60.2	31.4	117.9	0.1	11.2	0.1	0.5	0.0	0.0	0.4	0.0	19.0	0.0	8.5
1.7	9.3	15.7	0.6	6.4	31.3	35.7	101.8	0.2	9.6	0.1	1.0	0.1	0.1	0.5	0.0	17.7	0.1	6.4
0.7	2.0	12.8	0.7	4.8	33.5	25.6	109.3	0.2	5.7	0.2	0.2	0.0	0.1	0.7	0.0	13.3	0.0	9.0
0.0	0.0	5.8	0.5	5.8	21.0	22.5	115.3	0.0	37.1	0.0	0.0	0.1	0.1	0.6	0.0	0.0	0.0	6.6
1.0	0.7	0.0	0.6	0.0	0.0	0.0	148.1	0.0	0.0	0.0	0.0	0.1	0.1	1.0	0.0	0.0	0.0	6.5
0.1	0.0	1.1	0.1	45.6	4.0	65.6	8.0	0.0	0.0	0.1	0.0	0.0	0.1	3.0	0.0	0.6	0.0	55.7
0.0	0.0	9.8	1.0	0.0	0.0	167.2	2625.5	0.0	0.0	0.0	0.0	0.0	0.0	0.0	0.0	0.0	0.0	0.0
0.0	0.0	9.8	0.6	0.0	0.0	9.8	209.3	0.0	99.1	7.0	0.0	0.0	0.0	0.4	0.0	0.0	0.0	0.0
0.0	0.0	8.4	0.1	4.1	4.7	36.9	47.1	0.1	0.0	3.7	0.0	0.0	0.0	0.1	0.0	8.6	0.0	12.8
0.0	0.0	6.0	0.1	0.0	7.0	7.0	65.0	0.0	0.0	0.0	0.0	0.0	0.0	0.0	0.0	0.0	0.0	3.9
0.0	0.0	4.0	0.1	0.0	4.0	7.0	63.0	0.0	0.0	0.0	0.0	0.0	0.0	0.0	0.0	0.0	0.0	4.0
0.0	0.0	12.0	0.2	0.0	0.0	130.0	650.0	0.0	45.0	10.0	0.0	0.0	0.1	0.5	0.0	0.0	0.0	0.0
0.0	0.0	4.3	0.2	0.0	3.2	0.0	75.0	0.0	4.7	0.0	0.0	0.0	0.0	0.1	0.0	0.0	0.0	0.0
0.0	0.0	35.0	0.2	0.0	0.0	130.0	350.0	0.0	94.0	17.0	0.0	0.0	0.3	0.7	0.0	0.0	0.0	0.0
0.0	0.0	20.0	0.7	0.0	0.0	100.0	310.0	0.0	87.0	16.0	0.0	0.0	0.2	0.7	0.0	0.0	0.0	0.0
0.0	0.0	25.0	0.2	0.0	0.0	130.0	310.0	0.0	46.0	7.0	0.0	0.0	0.0	0.5	0.0	0.0	0.0	0.0
0.0	0.0	2.9	0.1	3.3	5.9	72.2	177.9	0.0	15.3	2.3	0.2	0.0	0.0	0.2	0.0	2.3	0.0	10.0
0.0	0.0	2.9	0.1	3.3	5.9	72.2	3.0	0.0	15.3	2.3	0.2	0.0	0.0	0.2	0.0	2.3	0.0	10.0
0.0	0.0	15.0	0.9	0.0	0.0	120.0	234.0	0.0	10.2	27.0	0.0	0.0	0.0	0.1	0.0	2.0	0.0	0.2
0.1	0.0	0.9	0.1	0.4	2.3	2.0	7.9	0.0	0.0	0.0	0.0	0.0	0.0	0.1	0.6	1.7	0.0	0.1
2.8	2.0	6.3	0.6	10.9	25.7	60.7	83.2	0.2	4.3	0.0	0.0	0.0	0.0	0.5	0.0	2.6	0.0	4.3
1.1	0.0	2.6	0.3	1.3	11.4	69.1	20.7	0.0	0.0	0.0	0.4	0.0	0.0	0.2	0.0	7.5	0.0	2.9
1.8	17.5	13.7	0.4	12.7	31.7	42.2	82.3	0.2	47.8	0.1	0.0	0.0	0.0	0.2	0.0	7.0	0.0	3.0
0.6	5.9	1.5	0.1	0.6	5.1	5.6	17.6	0.0	8.4	0.0	0.0	0.0	0.0	0.2	0.0	2.0	0.0	0.2
0.0	0.0	6.0	0.0	0.0	16.0	36.0	39.0	0.0	0.0	0.0	0.0	0.0	0.0	0.2	0.0	0.0	0.0	0.0
0.4	0.0	0.0	1.1	0.0	0.0	0.0	138.3	0.0	0.0	0.0	0.0	0.0	0.0	0.0	0.0	0.0	0.0	1.2
0.3	0.0	3.2	0.2	1.5	7.6	13.9	0.8	0.0	0.0	0.0	0.2	0.0	0.0	0.2	0.0	3.2	0.0	0.4
0.4	2.1	7.5	0.3	5.8	15.2	34.1	46.9	0.1	3.0	0.0	0.0	0.0	0.0	0.3	0.0	1.3	0.0	0.6
1.0	0.0	3.5	0.4	4.3	15.1	18.9	44.1	0.1	0.0	0.0	0.4	0.0	0.0	0.4	0.0	5.9	0.0	0.6
2.3	11.2	6.1	0.4	8.8	16.0	35.4	54.6	0.2	23.5	0.0	0.0	0.0	0.0	0.2	0.0	5.3	0.0	0.9
0.4	0.0	1.9	0.3	2.8	8.4	12.3	37.7	0.1	0.0	0.0	0.0	0.0	0.0	0.3	0.0	7.0	0.0	0.4
0.6	3.2	7.8	0.7	7.6	21.3	56.0	65.0	0.2	4.8	0.0	0.0	0.0	0.1	0.6	0.0	2.0	0.0	0.6
1.1	0.0	2.3	0.4	5.3	7.5	14.0	48.9	0.1	0.0	0.0	0.0	0.0	0.0	0.2	0.0	5.9	0.0	1.7
0.0	0.0	15.0	0.8	0.0	0.0	141.0	182.0	0.0	0.0	0.0	0.0	0.0	0.0	0.3	0.0	0.0	0.0	1.3
5.4	0.0	120.0	0.1	0.0	0.0	50.0	79.0	0.0	0.0	0.0	0.0	0.1	0.1	0.6	0.0	0.0	0.0	1.0
2.2	0.0	0.0	0.7	0.0	0.0	0.0	77.0	0.0	0.0	0.0	0.0	0.1	0.0	0.0	0.0	0.0	0.0	3.9
6.4	0.0	4.0	0.4	12.0	24.5	88.9	140.8	0.4	0.0	0.0	0.2	0.0	0.1	0.1	0.1	2.3	0.0	6.0
0.2	0.0	10.2	0.5	4.3	9.9	33.1	56.0	0.1	0.6	0.0	0.2	0.0	0.3	0.4	0.0	4.3	0.0	2.6
0.1	0.2	1.0	0.1	0.6	2.8	3.3	21.9	0.0	0.1	0.0	0.0	0.0	0.0	0.1	0.0	4.4	0.0	0.6

Code	Food Name	Unit/Amt	Wt (g)	Energy (Kcal)	Prot (g)	Carb (g)	Fiber (g)	Fat (g)	Mono (g)	Poly (g)
918822	Cookie, Fudge Brownie/LittleDeb	1 brownie	57	236.0	2.7	38.6	0.0	8.0	4.5	1.5
18172	Cookie, Ginger Snaps	1 cookie	7	29.1	0.4	5.4	0.2	0.7	0.4	0.1
18609	Cookie, Golden Vanilla Wafers/Keebler	1 large (3.5" - 4" dia)	32	152.0	1.7	22.3	0.0	6.2	0.0	0.0
18174	Cookie, Graham Crackers, chocolate coated	1 cracker (2.5" square)	14	67.8	0.8	9.3	0.4	3.2	1.1	0.1
18173	Cookie, Graham Crackers, Plain/Honey/Cinnamon	1 large or 4 small rectangular piec	14	59.2	1.0	10.8	0.4	1.4	0.6	0.5
918812	Cookie, Iced Brownies w/nuts	1 ladyfinger	11	44.6	0.5	7.0	0.0	1.9	0.8	0.4
18423	Cookie, Ladyfinger/Egg Jumbo/Breakfast Treat/Anisette Sponge w/o lemon	1 ladyfinger	11	40.2	1.2	6.6	0.1	1.0	0.5	0.2
918863	Cookie, Lemon Nut/PepFarm	2 large	64	336.0	3.8	40.3	0.0	17.9	0.0	0.0
18612	Cookie, Little Debbie Nutty Bars, Chocolate Covered Wafers w/Peanut Butter	1 bar	57	312.4	4.6	31.5	0.0	18.7	0.0	0.0
18176	Cookie, Marshmallow, chocolate coated/Marshmallow Pie	1 marshmallow pie (3" dia x 0.75")	39	164.2	1.6	26.4	0.8	6.6	3.6	0.8
18177	Cookie, Molasses	1 large (3.5"-4" dia/ Archway Brand)	32	137.6	1.8	23.6	0.3	4.1	2.3	0.6
18178	Cookie, Oatmeal, commercially prep	1 cookie	18	81.0	1.1	12.4	0.5	3.3	1.8	0.5
18200	Cookie, Oatmeal, commercially prep, special dietary	1 small cookie (1.75" dia x 0.75")	13	58.4	0.6	9.1	0.4	2.3	1.0	0.9
918181	Cookie, Oatmeal, dry mix, prep	1 large cookie:3.5-4"dia Archway,Grandma	25	115.5	1.9	16.3	1.0	4.9	0.0	0.0
18377	Cookie, Oatmeal, homemade w/o raisins	1 medium cookie (1.6" dia)	7	31.3	0.5	4.6	0.0	1.3	0.5	0.4
918183	Cookie, Oatmeal, refrig dough, bkd	1 cookie (2.65" dia)	15	70.7	0.9	9.9	0.4	3.2	0.0	0.0
918809	Cookie, Oreos	3 cookies	28	100.0	2.0	16.0	0.6	4.0	0.0	0.0
918821	Cookie, Peanut Butter Brownie	1 brownie	25	120.0	3.0	16.0	0.2	5.0	3.0	1.0
18185	Cookie, Peanut Butter, commercially prep	1 cookie	15	71.6	1.4	8.8	0.3	3.5	1.9	0.6
18189	Cookie, Peanut Butter, homemade	1 cookie (3" dia)	20	95.0	1.8	11.8	0.0	4.8	2.2	1.4
918188	Cookie, Peanut Butter, refrig dough, bkd	1 cookie	12	60.4	1.1	6.9	0.1	3.3	0.0	0.0
18191	Cookie, Raisin, soft	1 cookie	15	60.2	0.6	10.2	0.2	2.0	1.1	0.3
18166	Cookie, Sandwich, Chocolate, cream filled	1.0 oz	10	47.2	0.5	7.0	0.3	2.1	0.9	0.7
18199	Cookie, Sandwich, Chocolate, cream filled, special dietary	1 cookie	10	46.1	0.5	6.8	0.4	2.2	0.9	0.8
18190	Cookie, Sandwich, Peanut Butter, regular	1 cookie	14	66.9	1.2	9.2	0.3	3.0	1.6	0.5
18201	Cookie, Sandwich, Peanut Butter, special dietary	1 cookie	10	53.5	1.0	5.1	0.0	3.4	1.5	1.2
18210	Cookie, Sandwich, Vanilla, cream filled	1 oval cookie (3-⅛ x 1.25 x ⅜")	15	72.5	0.7	10.8	0.2	3.0	1.3	1.1
918194	Cookie, Shortbread, homemade w/butter	1 medium cookie (1.5" dia)	11	60.1	0.7	6.2	0.0	3.7	0.0	0.0
18193	Cookie, Shortbread, Pecan, commercially prep	1 cookie (2" dia)	14	75.9	0.7	8.2	0.3	4.6	2.6	0.6
18192	Cookie, Shortbread, Plain, commercially prep	1 cookie (1.6" square)	8	40.2	0.5	5.2	0.1	1.9	1.1	0.3
18209	Cookie, Sugar Wafer, cream filled	1 large wafer (3.5 x 1 x 0.5")	9	46.0	0.4	6.3	0.1	2.2	0.9	0.8
18202	Cookie, Sugar Wafer, cream filled, special dietary	1 wafer	4	20.1	0.1	2.6	0.0	1.0	0.4	0.4
918207	Cookie, Sugar, homemade w/butter	1 cookie (3" diam)	14	65.9	0.8	8.4	0.0	3.3	0.0	0.0
18206	Cookie, Sugar, refrig dough, baked	1 cookie	12	58.1	0.6	7.9	0.1	2.8	1.6	0.3
18204	Cookie, Sugar/Vanilla, commercially prep	1 cookie	15	71.7	0.8	10.2	0.1	3.2	1.8	0.4
18213	Cookie, Vanilla Wafer	1 wafer	6	28.4	0.3	4.3	0.1	1.2	0.7	0.1
18212	Cookie, Vanilla Wafer, lower fat	1 large wafer	6	26.5	0.3	4.4	0.1	0.9	0.4	0.2
20018	Corn flour, degermed, unenriched, yellow	1 tbsp	7.9	29.6	0.4	6.5	0.2	0.1	0.0	0.1
924077	Corn Fritter	1 Fritter	35	132.0	2.7	13.9	1.0	7.5	0.0	0.0
13348	Corned Beef Brisket, canned	1 oz	28.35	70.9	7.7	0.0	0.0	4.2	1.7	0.2
20027	Cornstarch	1 tbsp	8	30.5	0.0	7.3	0.1	0.0	0.0	0.0
18214	Cracker, Cheese	1 cracker, (1" square)	1	5.0	0.1	0.6	0.0	0.3	0.1	0.0
18216	Cracker, Crispbread, Rye	1 crispbread, wafer or cracker	10	36.6	0.8	8.2	1.7	0.1	0.0	0.1
919977	Cracker, Goldfish/PepFarm	12 crackers	6	30.0	0.0	4.0	0.5	2.0	0.0	0.0
18218	Cracker, Matzo, Egg	1 matzo	28.35	110.8	3.5	22.3	0.8	0.6	0.2	0.1
18219	Cracker, Matzo, Whole Wheat	1 matzo	28.35	99.5	3.7	22.4	3.3	0.4	0.1	0.2
18220	Cracker, Melba Toast Rounds, Plain	1 melba round	3	11.7	0.4	2.3	0.2	0.1	0.0	0.0
18221	Cracker, Melba Toast, Rye or Pumpernickel	1 toast	5	19.5	0.6	3.9	0.4	0.2	0.0	0.1
18223	Cracker, Milk	1 cracker	11	50.1	0.8	7.7	0.2	1.7	1.0	0.2
18620	Cracker, Original Premium Saltine Crackers/Nabisco	1 serving	14	58.8	1.5	10.0	0.4	1.4	0.8	0.2
18621	Cracker, Ritz/Nabisco	1 serving	16	78.7	1.2	10.3	0.3	3.7	2.9	0.3
18224	Cracker, Rusk Toast	1 rusk	10	40.7	1.4	7.2	0.0	0.7	0.3	0.2
918808	Cracker, Rye Krisps	¼ large square	14	40.0	1.5	13.0	2.5	0.2	0.0	0.0
18425	Cracker, Saltine/Oyster/Soda/Soup, low salt	1 oyster cracker	1	4.3	0.1	0.7	0.0	0.1	0.1	0.0
18426	Cracker, Saltines/Oyster/Soda/Soup, unsalted	1 saltine	3	13.0	0.3	2.1	0.1	0.4	0.2	0.1
18230	Cracker, Sandwich, Cheese filled	1 sandwich cracker	7	33.4	0.7	4.3	0.1	1.5	0.8	0.2
18215	Cracker, Sandwich, Cheese w/peanut butter filling	1 sandwich cracker	7	33.7	0.9	4.0	0.2	1.6	0.8	0.3
18231	Cracker, Sandwich, Peanut Butter filled	1 sandwich cracker	7	34.2	0.8	4.1	0.2	1.7	0.9	0.3
18234	Cracker, Sandwich, Wheat w/peanut butter filling	1 sandwich cracker	7	34.7	0.9	3.8	0.3	1.9	0.8	0.6
18622	Cracker, Snackwell Zesty Cheese, Reduced Fat/Nabisco	1 serving	30	124.1	2.9	23.1	0.7	2.2	0.8	0.4
18229	Cracker, Standard Snack, regular	1 rectangular cracker	4	20.1	0.3	2.4	0.1	1.0	0.4	0.4
18624	Cracker, Wheat Thins, baked/Nabisco	1 serving	29	136.2	2.4	20.0	1.7	5.2	4.1	0.4
18235	Cracker, Whole Wheat	1 cracker	4	17.7	0.4	2.7	0.4	0.7	0.2	0.3

Sat (g)	Chol (mg)	Cal (mg)	Iron (mg)	Magn (mg)	Phos (mg)	Pota (mg)	Sodi (mg)	Zinc (mg)	Vit A (RE)	Vit C (mg)	Vit E (mg)	Thia (mg)	Ribo (mg)	Niac (mg)	Vit B-6 (mg)	Fol (µg)	Vit B-12 (µg)	Wat (g)
2.0	1.0	0.0	1.7	0.0	0.0	0.0	121.0	0.0	0.0	0.0	0.0	0.1	0.1	0.1	0.0	0.0	0.0	7.2
0.2	0.0	5.4	0.4	3.4	5.8	24.2	45.8	0.0	0.0	0.0	0.1	0.0	0.0	0.2	0.0	5.0	0.0	0.4
1.1	0.0	0.0	0.0	0.0	0.0	0.0	123.5	0.0	0.0	0.0	0.0	0.0	0.0	0.0	0.0	0.0	0.0	1.3
1.9	0.0	8.1	0.5	8.1	18.8	29.3	40.7	0.1	0.1	0.0	0.2	0.0	0.0	0.3	0.0	2.4	0.0	0.4
0.2	0.0	3.4	0.5	4.2	14.6	18.9	84.7	0.1	0.0	0.0	0.3	0.0	0.0	0.6	0.0	8.4	0.0	0.6
0.7	0.0	5.5	0.3	4.4	11.6	22.0	25.9	0.2	6.5	0.0	0.0	0.0	0.0	0.2	0.0	1.1	0.0	1.4
0.4	40.2	5.2	0.4	1.3	19.0	12.4	16.2	0.1	18.4	0.0	0.1	0.0	0.0	0.2	0.0	8.5	0.1	2.1
0.0	0.0	22.0	0.4	0.0	0.0	97.0	189.0	0.0	0.0	0.0	0.0	0.0	0.1	0.3	0.0	0.0	0.0	1.5
3.6	0.0	0.0	0.0	0.0	0.0	0.0	127.1	0.0	0.0	1.1	0.0	0.0	0.0	0.0	0.0	0.0	0.0	1.7
1.8	0.0	17.9	1.0	14.0	37.8	71.0	65.5	0.3	0.4	0.0	0.8	0.0	0.1	0.3	0.0	7.4	0.1	3.9
1.0	0.0	23.7	2.1	16.6	30.4	110.7	146.9	0.1	0.0	0.0	0.5	0.1	0.1	1.0	0.0	23.7	0.0	1.9
0.8	0.0	6.7	0.5	5.9	24.8	25.6	68.9	0.1	0.4	0.1	0.5	0.0	0.0	0.4	0.0	8.1	0.0	1.0
0.4	0.0	7.0	0.5	2.2	15.9	22.8	1.2	0.1	0.1	0.0	0.4	0.1	0.0	0.4	0.0	6.8	0.0	0.8
0.7	2.7	7.3	0.6	12.0	43.8	47.3	117.5	0.2	5.3	0.1	0.0	0.1	0.0	0.3	0.0	2.8	0.0	1.5
0.3	2.5	7.4	0.2	3.0	11.7	12.7	41.9	0.1	12.8	0.0	0.0	0.0	0.0	0.1	0.0	2.3	0.0	0.4
0.4	1.8	5.3	0.4	4.8	17.4	24.5	49.1	0.1	2.0	0.0	0.0	0.0	0.0	0.3	0.0	1.1	0.0	0.9
0.0	0.0	0.0	0.0	0.0	0.0	50.0	150.0	0.0	0.0	0.0	0.0	0.0	0.0	0.0	0.0	0.0	0.0	0.0
1.0	0.0	6.0	0.9	15.0	30.0	55.0	100.0	0.2	10.0	0.0	0.0	0.0	0.0	1.1	0.0	2.0	0.0	0.8
0.7	0.2	5.3	0.4	6.8	12.9	25.1	62.3	0.1	0.5	0.0	0.5	0.0	0.0	0.6	0.0	9.3	0.0	0.9
0.9	6.2	7.8	0.4	7.8	23.2	46.2	103.6	0.2	31.2	0.0	0.0	0.0	0.0	0.7	0.0	11.0	0.0	1.2
0.6	1.7	13.3	0.2	4.9	31.7	40.6	52.3	0.1	1.7	0.0	0.0	0.0	0.0	0.5	0.0	1.1	0.0	0.5
0.5	0.3	6.9	0.3	3.2	12.5	21.0	50.7	0.0	0.2	0.1	0.3	0.0	0.0	0.3	0.0	6.6	0.0	2.0
0.4	0.0	2.6	0.4	4.5	9.8	17.5	60.4	0.1	0.0	0.0	0.3	0.0	0.0	0.2	0.0	4.3	0.0	0.2
0.4	0.0	9.8	0.5	2.6	20.0	29.5	24.3	0.1	0.0	0.0	0.4	0.1	0.0	0.4	0.0	6.2	0.0	0.4
0.7	0.0	7.4	0.4	6.9	26.3	26.9	51.5	0.1	0.1	0.0	0.5	0.0	0.0	0.5	0.0	6.2	0.0	0.4
0.5	0.0	4.3	0.3	5.1	15.4	29.4	41.2	0.1	0.0	0.0	0.6	0.0	0.0	0.5	0.0	5.4	0.0	0.4
0.4	0.0	4.1	0.3	2.1	11.3	13.7	52.4	0.1	0.0	0.0	0.5	0.0	0.0	0.4	0.0	8.9	0.0	0.3
0.2	1.0	2.0	0.3	1.4	7.6	7.6	51.2	0.0	33.6	0.0	0.0	0.0	0.0	0.3	0.0	1.2	0.0	0.3
1.1	4.6	4.2	0.3	2.5	11.9	10.2	39.3	0.1	0.1	0.0	0.0	0.0	0.0	0.3	0.0	8.8	0.0	0.5
0.5	1.6	2.8	0.2	1.4	8.6	8.0	36.4	0.0	1.0	0.0	0.3	0.0	0.0	0.3	0.0	4.7	0.0	0.3
0.3	0.0	1.6	0.2	1.0	5.0	5.3	13.2	0.0	0.0	0.0	0.4	0.0	0.0	0.2	0.0	3.9	0.0	0.1
0.2	0.0	2.1	0.1	0.2	1.4	2.4	0.4	0.0	0.0	0.0	0.0	0.0	0.0	0.1	0.0	1.7	0.0	0.2
0.2	0.9	9.9	0.3	1.7	12.6	10.2	64.3	0.1	31.2	0.0	0.0	0.0	0.0	0.3	0.0	1.7	0.0	1.2
0.7	3.8	10.8	0.2	1.0	22.4	19.6	56.2	0.0	1.3	0.0	0.4	0.0	0.0	0.3	0.0	6.4	0.0	0.6
0.8	7.7	3.2	0.3	1.8	12.0	9.5	53.6	0.1	4.1	0.0	0.4	0.0	0.0	0.4	0.0	6.8	0.0	0.7
0.3	0.0	1.5	0.1	0.7	3.8	6.4	18.4	0.0	0.0	0.0	0.0	0.0	0.0	0.2	0.0	2.6	0.0	0.3
0.2	3.1	2.9	0.1	0.8	6.2	5.8	18.7	0.0	0.5	0.0	0.1	0.0	0.0	0.2	0.0	3.0	0.0	0.3
0.0	0.0	0.2	0.1	1.4	4.7	7.1	0.1	0.0	0.4	0.0	0.0	0.0	0.0	0.2	0.0	3.8	0.0	0.8
2.0	0.0	22.0	0.6	0.0	54.0	47.0	167.0	0.0	28.0	1.0	0.0	0.1	0.1	0.6	0.0	0.0	0.0	10.2
1.8	24.4	3.4	0.6	4.0	31.5	38.6	285.2	1.0	0.0	0.0	0.0	0.0	0.0	0.7	0.0	2.6	0.5	16.4
0.0	0.0	0.2	0.0	0.2	1.0	0.2	0.7	0.0	0.0	0.0	0.0	0.0	0.0	0.0	0.0	0.0	0.0	0.7
0.1	0.1	1.5	0.0	0.4	2.2	1.5	10.0	0.0	0.3	0.0	0.0	0.0	0.0	0.0	0.0	0.8	0.0	0.0
0.0	0.0	3.1	0.2	7.8	26.9	31.9	26.4	0.2	0.0	0.0	0.0	0.1	0.0	0.1	0.0	4.7	0.0	0.6
0.0	0.0	4.0	0.2	0.0	6.0	12.0	50.0	0.0	0.2	0.0	0.0	0.0	0.0	0.2	0.0	0.0	0.0	0.0
0.2	23.5	11.3	0.8	6.8	42.0	42.5	6.0	0.2	3.7	0.0	0.0	0.2	0.2	1.4	0.0	33.2	0.1	1.8
0.1	0.0	6.5	1.3	38.0	86.5	89.6	0.6	0.7	0.0	0.0	0.4	0.1	0.1	1.5	0.0	13.6	0.0	1.4
0.0	0.0	2.8	0.1	1.8	5.9	6.1	24.9	0.1	0.0	0.0	0.0	0.0	0.0	0.1	0.0	3.7	0.0	0.2
0.0	0.0	3.9	0.2	2.0	9.2	9.7	45.0	0.1	0.0	0.0	0.0	0.0	0.0	0.2	0.0	4.3	0.0	0.2
0.3	1.2	18.9	0.4	2.4	33.3	12.5	65.1	0.1	0.8	0.0	0.3	0.1	0.0	0.5	0.0	9.0	0.0	0.5
0.3	0.0	27.0	0.7	2.9	13.9	13.9	177.8	0.0	0.0	0.0	0.0	0.0	0.1	0.6	0.0	11.8	0.0	0.5
0.6	0.0	23.5	0.6	3.2	48.0	14.9	124.2	0.2	0.0	0.0	0.0	0.0	0.0	0.6	0.0	9.6	0.0	0.5
0.1	7.8	2.7	0.3	3.6	15.3	24.5	25.3	0.1	1.2	0.0	0.0	0.0	0.0	0.5	0.0	8.7	0.0	0.6
0.0	0.0	12.0	0.4	34.0	93.0	63.0	112.0	0.8	0.0	0.0	0.0	0.0	0.1	0.3	0.1	7.0	0.0	0.0
0.0	0.0	1.2	0.1	0.3	1.1	7.2	6.4	0.0	0.0	0.0	0.0	0.0	0.0	0.1	0.0	1.2	0.0	0.0
0.1	0.0	3.6	0.2	0.8	3.2	3.8	23.0	0.0	0.0	0.0	0.0	0.0	0.0	0.2	0.0	3.7	0.0	0.1
0.4	0.1	18.0	0.2	2.5	28.4	30.0	98.1	0.0	1.3	0.0	0.0	0.0	0.0	0.3	0.0	5.9	0.0	0.3
0.4	0.4	5.5	0.2	4.1	22.7	17.2	69.4	0.1	2.4	0.0	0.3	0.0	0.0	0.5	0.1	6.2	0.0	0.3
0.4	0.0	6.8	0.2	3.7	16.9	15.6	65.9	0.1	0.0	0.0	0.3	0.0	0.0	0.4	0.0	5.9	0.0	0.2
0.3	0.0	11.9	0.2	2.7	24.3	20.8	56.5	0.1	0.0	0.0	0.0	0.0	0.0	0.4	0.0	4.9	0.0	0.3
0.5	1.5	40.5	1.0	9.6	98.4	47.7	275.1	0.5	0.0	0.1	0.0	0.1	0.1	1.3	0.1	17.4	0.0	0.8
0.2	0.0	4.8	0.1	1.1	9.1	5.3	33.9	0.0	0.0	0.0	0.2	0.0	0.0	0.2	0.0	3.1	0.0	0.1
0.9	0.0	25.8	1.0	15.1	60.3	56.3	167.6	0.0	0.0	0.0	0.0	0.1	0.1	1.2	0.0	12.2	0.0	0.7
0.1	0.0	2.0	0.1	4.0	11.8	11.9	26.4	0.1	0.0	0.0	0.0	0.0	0.0	0.2	0.0	1.6	0.0	0.1

Code	Food Name	Unit/Amt	Wt (g)	Energy (Kcal)	Prot (g)	Carb (g)	Fiber (g)	Fat (g)	Mono (g)	Poly (g)
18429	Cracker, Whole Wheat, low sodium	1 cracker	4	17.7	0.4	2.7	0.4	0.7	0.2	0.3
18434	Crackers, Cheese, Cheez-its/Goldfish, low sodium	1 gold fish	0.6	3.0	0.1	0.3	0.0	0.2	0.1	0.0
18457	Crackers, Saltines, fat-free, low-sodium	3 saltines	15	59.0	1.6	12.3	0.4	0.2	0.0	0.1
1067	Cream Substitute, Nondairy, liquid w/hydrogenated vege oil and soy protein	1 tbsp	15	20.3	0.2	1.7	0.0	1.5	1.1	0.0
1069	Cream Substitute, Nondairy, powder	1 tsp	2	10.9	0.1	1.1	0.0	0.7	0.0	0.0
1058	Cream, Filled Cream, Nonbutterfat Sour Dressing, cultured	1 cup	235	417.5	7.6	11.0	0.0	38.9	4.6	1.1
1049	Cream, Half and Half	1 tbsp	15	19.6	0.4	0.6	0.0	1.7	0.5	0.1
1053	Cream, Heavy Whipping	1 tbsp	15	51.7	0.3	0.4	0.0	5.6	1.6	0.2
1052	Cream, Light Whipping	1 tbsp	15	43.9	0.3	0.4	0.0	4.6	1.4	0.1
1056	Cream, Sour, cultured	1 tbsp	12	25.7	0.4	0.5	0.0	2.5	0.7	0.1
1074	Cream, Sour, Imitation, cultured	1.0 oz	29	60.5	0.7	1.9	0.0	5.7	0.2	0.0
1055	Cream, Sour, Reduced Fat (Half and Half) cultured	2 tbsp	30	40.4	0.9	1.3	0.0	3.6	1.0	0.1
1054	Cream, Whipped Cream Topping, Pressurized	1 tbsp	3	7.7	0.1	0.4	0.0	0.7	0.2	0.0
18242	Croutons, Plain	1 cup	30	122.1	3.6	22.1	1.5	2.0	0.9	0.4
18243	Croutons, Seasoned	4 cubes	1	4.7	0.1	0.6	0.1	0.2	0.1	0.0
919168	Custard, Egg, baked, homemade	½ cup	141	148.1	7.2	15.1	0.0	6.6	0.0	0.0
19205	Custard, Egg, dry mix prep w/reduced fat (2%) milk	1 cup	266	297.9	11.2	47.1	0.0	7.4	2.4	0.5
919186	Dessert, Apple Crisp, homemade	½ cup	141	229.8	2.5	45.5	2.4	5.1	0.0	0.0
919094	Dessert, Flan (Caramel Custard) homemade	½ cup	153	220.3	6.9	34.9	0.0	6.3	0.0	0.0
902923	Dip, Jalapeno Bean	1 oz	28	33.0	1.5	2.9	0.3	1.1	0.0	0.0
18251	Donut, Cake, Chocolate w/sugar or glaze	1 small doughnut (3" dia)	42	175.1	1.9	24.1	0.9	8.4	4.7	1.0
18249	Donut, Cake, Plain w/chocolate icing	1 small doughnut (2" dia)	28	132.7	1.4	13.4	0.6	8.7	4.9	1.1
18250	Donut, Cake, Plain w/sugar or glaze	1 oz	28.35	120.8	1.5	14.4	0.4	6.5	3.6	0.8
918865	Donut, Cake/Hostess	1 doughnut	28	110.0	1.0	12.0	0.5	7.0	0.0	0.0
918866	Donut, Chocolate/Hostess	1 doughnut	28	129.9	1.0	14.0	0.5	8.0	0.0	0.0
918867	Donut, Cinnamon/Hostess	1 doughnut	28	110.0	1.0	15.0	0.5	6.0	0.0	0.0
18253	Donut, French Cruller, glazed	1 cruller (3" dia)	41	168.9	1.3	24.4	0.5	7.5	4.3	0.9
918868	Donut, Powdered Sugar/Hostess	1 mini donut	28	110.0	1.0	15.0	0.5	5.0	0.0	0.0
18254	Donut, Yeast Leavened, cream filled	1 doughnut (3.5 x 2.5" oval)	85	306.9	5.4	25.5	0.7	20.8	10.3	2.6
18256	Donut, Yeast Leavened, jelly	1 doughnut (3.5 x 2.5" oval)	85	289.0	5.0	33.2	0.7	15.9	8.7	2.0
18255	Donut/Honey Bun, Yeast Leavened, glazed	1 extra large (~ 5" dia)	122	491.7	7.8	54.0	1.5	27.8	15.7	3.5
5140	Duck, Domestic, Meat & Skin, roasted	½ duck	382	1287.3	72.5	0.0	0.0	108.3	49.3	13.9
5142	Duck, Domestic, Meat, no skin, roasted	½ duck	221	444.2	51.9	0.0	0.0	24.8	8.2	3.2
924066	Egg Foo Young/LaChoy	2 patties	120	159.6	8.0	19.0	1.0	7.0	0.8	4.0
924181	Egg Souffle w/cheese	1 cup	95	207.1	9.4	5.9	0.0	16.2	0.0	0.0
924182	Egg Souffle w/spinach, frozen/Stouffer	4.0 oz	113	141.3	6.7	9.4	0.0	8.6	0.0	0.0
901910	Egg Substitute, Country Morning	½ cup	121	173.0	14.6	1.3	0.0	12.1	0.0	0.0
1142	Egg Substitute, frozen	¼ cup	60	95.9	6.8	1.9	0.0	6.7	1.5	3.7
1143	Egg Substitute, liquid	1 tbsp	15.7	13.2	1.9	0.1	0.0	0.5	0.1	0.3
901912	Egg Substitute, Scramblend	½ cup	121	142.8	12.1	3.0	0.0	9.1	0.0	0.0
924272	Egg&Cheese Bagel, frozen/Swanson	3.6 oz	102	256.0	12.7	29.0	0.0	9.9	0.0	0.0
924323	Egg, Omelet w/bacon&onion	6.5 oz	186	364.6	17.4	12.7	0.1	27.1	0.0	0.0
924322	Egg, Omelet w/cheese	4.0 oz	113	313.0	15.5	1.3	0.0	27.1	0.0	0.0
924012	Egg, Quiche Lorraine	1 slice	176	600.2	13.0	29.0	1.0	48.0	17.8	4.1
1128	Egg, Whole, fried	1 large	46	91.5	6.2	0.6	0.0	6.9	2.7	1.3
1129	Egg, Whole, hard-cooked	1 large egg	50	77.5	6.3	0.6	0.0	5.3	2.0	0.7
1130	Egg, Whole, omelet	1 tbsp	15.2	23.1	1.6	0.2	0.0	1.7	0.7	0.3
1131	Egg, Whole, poached	large egg	50	74.5	6.2	0.6	0.0	5.0	1.9	0.7
1123	Egg, Whole, raw	1 large	50	74.5	6.2	0.6	0.0	5.0	1.9	0.7
1132	Egg, Whole, scrambled	1 large egg	61	101.3	6.8	1.3	0.0	7.4	2.9	1.3
1125	Egg, Yolk, raw, fresh	1 large egg yolk	16.6	59.4	2.8	0.3	0.0	5.1	1.9	0.7
18260	English Muffin, Mixed Grain/Granola	1 muffin	66	155.1	6.0	30.6	1.8	1.2	0.5	0.4
18258	English Muffin, Plain/Sourdough, enriched	1 muffin	57	134.0	4.4	26.2	1.5	1.0	0.2	0.5
18262	English Muffin, Raisin-Cinn/Apple Cinnamon	1 muffin	57	138.5	4.3	27.8	1.7	1.5	0.3	0.8
18264	English Muffin, Wheat	1 muffin	57	127.1	5.0	25.5	2.6	1.1	0.2	0.5
18266	English Muffin, Whole Wheat	1 muffin	66	134.0	5.8	26.7	4.4	1.4	5.1	0.7
921897	Fast Food, Apple Pie/MCD	1 pie	83	259.8	2.2	30.0	0.5	14.8	9.1	0.9
921915	Fast Food, Bean Burrito/TB	1 burrito	206	447.0	15.0	63.0	9.6	14.0	8.0	2.0
921916	Fast Food, Beef Burrito/TB	1 burrito	206	492.3	25.0	48.0	2.2	21.0	11.0	2.0
921805	Fast Food, Biscuit/MCD	1 biscuit	75	260.3	4.6	31.9	0.5	12.7	8.6	0.6
921919	Fast Food, Burrito Supreme/TB	1 burrito	255	502.4	20.0	55.0	5.8	22.0	11.0	2.0
21069	Fast Food, Burrito w/apples or cherries	1 small burrito	74	230.9	2.5	35.0	0.0	9.5	3.4	1.1
21060	Fast Food, Burrito w/beans	2 burritos	217	447.0	14.1	71.4	0.0	13.5	4.7	1.2
21061	Fast Food, Burrito w/beans & cheese	2 burritos	186	377.6	15.1	55.0	0.0	11.7	2.5	1.8
21063	Fast Food, Burrito w/beans & meat	2 burritos	231	508.2	22.5	66.0	0.0	17.8	7.0	1.2
21064	Fast Food, Burrito w/beans, cheese & beef	2 burritos	203	330.9	14.6	39.7	0.0	13.3	4.5	1.0
21066	Fast Food, Burrito w/beef	2 burritos	220	523.6	26.6	58.5	0.0	20.8	7.4	0.9
21068	Fast Food, Burrito w/beef, cheese & chili peppers	2 burritos	304	632.3	40.9	63.7	0.0	24.8	9.9	2.2
921813	Fast Food, Chicken Center Breast, extra crispy/KFC	1 piece	135	341.6	33.0	11.7	0.5	19.7	12.5	2.1

Sat (g)	Chol (mg)	Cal (mg)	Iron (mg)	Magn (mg)	Phos (mg)	Pota (mg)	Sodi (mg)	Zinc (mg)	Vit A (RE)	Vit C (mg)	Vit E (mg)	Thia (mg)	Ribo (mg)	Niac (mg)	Vit B-6 (mg)	Fol (μg)	Vit B-12 (μg)	Wat (g)
0.1	0.0	2.0	0.1	4.0	11.8	11.9	9.9	0.1	0.0	0.0	0.0	0.0	0.0	0.2	0.0	1.6	0.0	0.1
0.1	0.1	0.9	0.0	0.2	1.3	0.6	2.7	0.0	0.2	0.0	0.0	0.0	0.0	0.0	0.0	0.5	0.0	0.0
0.0	0.0	3.3	1.2	3.9	17.0	17.3	95.4	0.1	0.0	0.0	0.0	0.1	0.1	0.9	0.0	18.6	0.0	0.5
0.3	0.0	1.4	0.0	0.0	9.6	28.6	11.9	0.0	1.4	0.0	0.2	0.0	0.0	0.0	0.0	0.0	0.0	11.6
0.7	0.0	0.4	0.0	0.1	8.4	16.2	3.6	0.0	0.4	0.0	0.0	0.0	0.0	0.0	0.0	0.0	0.0	0.0
31.2	12.7	265.8	0.1	23.3	204.7	379.5	113.3	0.9	4.7	2.2	0.3	0.1	0.4	0.2	0.0	27.7	0.8	175.8
1.1	5.5	15.7	0.0	1.5	14.3	19.4	6.1	0.1	16.1	0.1	0.0	0.0	0.0	0.0	0.0	0.4	0.0	12.1
3.5	20.6	9.7	0.0	1.1	9.4	11.3	5.6	0.0	63.2	0.1	0.1	0.0	0.0	0.0	0.0	0.6	0.0	8.7
2.9	16.7	10.4	0.0	1.1	9.2	14.5	5.1	0.0	44.3	0.1	0.1	0.0	0.0	0.0	0.0	0.6	0.0	9.5
1.6	5.3	14.0	0.0	1.3	10.2	17.3	6.4	0.0	23.4	0.1	0.1	0.0	0.0	0.0	0.0	1.3	0.0	8.5
5.2	0.0	0.7	0.1	1.9	12.9	46.5	29.6	0.3	0.0	0.0	0.0	0.0	0.0	0.0	0.0	0.0	0.0	20.6
2.2	11.6	31.3	0.0	3.0	28.4	38.7	12.2	0.2	33.6	0.3	0.1	0.0	0.0	0.0	0.0	3.2	0.1	24.0
0.4	2.3	3.0	0.0	0.3	2.7	4.4	3.9	0.0	6.2	0.0	0.0	0.0	0.0	0.0	0.0	0.1	0.0	1.8
0.5	0.0	22.8	1.2	9.3	34.5	37.2	209.4	0.3	0.0	0.0	0.0	0.2	0.1	1.6	0.0	39.6	0.0	1.7
0.1	0.1	1.0	0.0	0.4	1.4	1.8	12.4	0.0	0.1	0.0	0.0	0.0	0.0	0.0	0.0	0.9	0.0	0.0
0.5	2.1	157.9	0.4	19.7	159.3	215.7	108.6	0.7	84.6	0.7	0.0	0.0	0.3	0.1	0.1	14.1	0.4	111.0
3.8	149.0	393.7	0.7	53.2	351.1	574.6	399.0	1.4	149.0	2.1	0.0	0.1	0.6	0.3	0.2	21.3	1.2	197.6
1.5	2.2	39.5	1.1	9.9	35.3	136.8	256.6	0.2	43.7	3.2	0.0	0.1	0.1	1.1	0.1	7.1	0.0	86.7
0.5	2.1	131.6	0.5	16.8	145.4	185.1	85.7	0.7	87.2	0.8	0.0	0.0	0.3	0.1	0.1	13.8	0.4	103.9
0.0	1.0	7.0	0.4	0.0	23.0	77.0	163.0	0.1	8.4	0.0	0.0	0.0	0.0	1.1	0.0	0.0	0.0	0.0
2.2	23.9	89.5	1.0	14.3	68.0	44.5	142.8	0.2	4.6	0.0	1.1	0.0	0.0	0.2	0.0	16.0	0.0	6.8
2.3	17.1	9.8	0.7	11.2	56.6	54.9	120.1	0.2	3.1	0.1	1.2	0.0	0.0	0.4	0.0	8.1	0.1	4.0
1.7	9.1	17.0	0.3	4.8	33.2	28.9	114.0	0.1	0.9	0.0	0.0	0.1	0.1	0.4	0.0	13.0	0.1	5.6
0.0	7.0	12.0	0.4	0.0	0.0	0.0	135.0	0.0	0.0	0.0	0.0	0.1	0.0	0.5	0.0	0.0	0.0	0.0
0.0	4.0	10.0	0.4	0.0	0.0	0.0	150.0	0.0	0.0	0.0	0.0	0.0	0.0	0.3	0.0	0.0	0.0	0.0
0.0	6.0	10.0	0.3	0.0	0.0	0.0	140.0	0.0	0.0	0.0	0.0	0.0	0.0	0.4	0.0	0.0	0.0	0.0
1.9	4.5	10.7	1.0	4.9	50.4	32.0	141.5	0.1	1.2	0.0	1.0	0.1	0.1	0.9	0.0	14.4	0.0	7.3
0.0	6.0	9.0	0.3	0.0	0.0	0.0	140.0	0.0	0.0	0.0	0.0	0.0	0.0	0.4	0.0	0.0	0.0	0.0
4.6	20.4	21.3	1.6	17.0	64.6	68.0	262.7	0.7	16.2	0.0	2.3	0.3	0.1	1.9	0.1	54.4	0.1	32.5
4.1	22.1	21.3	1.5	17.0	72.3	67.2	249.1	0.6	13.6	0.0	2.1	0.3	0.1	1.8	0.1	52.7	0.2	30.3
7.1	7.3	52.5	2.5	26.8	113.5	131.8	417.2	0.9	4.9	0.1	3.7	0.4	0.3	3.5	0.1	52.5	0.1	31.0
36.9	320.9	42.0	10.3	61.1	595.9	779.3	225.4	7.1	240.7	0.0	2.7	0.7	1.0	18.4	0.7	22.9	1.1	198.0
9.2	196.7	26.5	6.0	44.2	448.6	556.9	143.7	5.7	50.8	0.0	1.5	0.6	1.0	11.3	0.6	22.1	0.9	141.9
2.2	275.0	60.0	1.8	0.0	0.0	270.0	1250.0	0.0	50.0	0.0	0.0	1.2	0.1	0.0	0.0	0.0	0.0	0.0
8.2	184.0	191.0	1.0	0.0	185.0	115.0	346.0	1.2	152.0	0.0	0.0	0.1	0.2	0.2	0.0	0.0	0.0	61.8
0.0	88.0	107.0	1.5	0.0	0.0	249.0	599.0	0.0	316.4	4.0	0.0	0.1	0.3	0.5	0.0	0.0	0.0	85.9
0.0	594.0	52.0	2.1	0.0	197.0	133.0	180.0	0.0	227.6	0.0	0.0	0.1	0.5	0.0	0.0	0.0	0.0	0.0
1.2	1.2	43.7	1.2	9.0	43.0	128.0	119.6	0.6	81.0	0.3	1.3	0.1	0.2	0.1	0.1	9.8	0.2	43.9
0.1	0.2	8.3	0.3	1.4	19.0	51.8	27.8	0.2	33.9	0.0	0.1	0.0	0.0	0.0	0.0	2.3	0.0	13.0
0.0	466.0	77.0	1.7	0.0	190.0	150.0	173.0	0.0	214.2	0.0	0.0	0.1	0.4	0.0	0.0	0.0	0.0	0.0
0.0	0.0	137.0	2.1	0.0	0.0	102.0	621.0	0.0	55.8	0.0	0.0	0.2	0.4	1.6	0.0	0.0	0.0	0.0
0.0	365.0	267.0	2.2	0.0	621.0	160.0	1148.0	0.0	141.8	2.0	0.0	0.2	0.5	1.2	0.0	0.0	0.0	0.0
0.0	328.0	245.0	1.6	0.0	0.0	128.0	398.0	0.0	0.0	0.0	0.0	0.1	0.0	0.0	0.0	0.0	0.0	0.0
23.2	285.0	211.0	1.0	0.0	276.0	283.0	653.0	2.0	328.0	0.0	0.0	0.1	0.3	0.0	0.1	17.0	0.0	0.0
1.9	211.1	25.3	0.7	5.1	89.2	60.7	162.4	0.5	114.1	0.0	0.8	0.0	0.2	0.0	0.1	17.5	0.4	31.5
1.6	212.0	25.0	0.6	5.0	86.0	63.0	62.0	0.5	84.0	0.0	0.5	0.0	0.3	0.0	0.1	22.0	0.6	37.3
0.5	53.2	6.4	0.2	1.4	22.5	15.4	41.0	0.1	28.4	0.0	0.2	0.0	0.1	0.0	0.0	4.4	0.1	11.5
1.5	211.5	24.5	0.7	5.0	88.5	60.0	140.0	0.6	95.0	0.0	0.5	0.0	0.2	0.0	0.1	17.5	0.4	37.5
1.6	212.5	24.5	0.7	5.0	89.0	60.5	63.0	0.6	95.5	0.0	0.5	0.0	0.3	0.0	0.1	23.5	0.5	37.7
2.2	214.7	43.3	0.7	7.3	103.7	84.2	170.8	0.6	119.0	0.1	0.8	0.0	0.3	0.0	0.1	18.3	0.5	44.6
1.6	212.6	22.7	0.6	1.5	81.0	15.6	7.1	0.5	96.9	0.0	0.5	0.0	0.1	0.0	0.1	24.2	0.5	8.1
0.2	0.0	129.4	2.0	27.1	53.5	103.0	274.6	0.9	0.0	0.0	0.2	0.3	0.2	2.4	0.0	52.8	0.0	26.5
0.1	0.0	99.2	1.4	12.0	75.8	74.7	264.5	0.4	0.0	0.0	0.1	0.3	0.2	2.2	0.0	46.2	0.0	24.0
0.2	0.0	83.8	1.4	8.6	39.3	118.6	254.8	0.6	0.0	0.0	0.2	0.2	0.2	2.0	0.0	46.2	0.0	22.0
0.2	0.0	101.5	1.6	21.1	61.0	106.0	217.7	0.6	0.0	0.0	0.3	0.2	0.2	1.9	0.0	31.4	0.0	24.1
8.8	0.0	174.9	1.6	46.9	186.1	138.6	420.4	1.1	0.0		0.5	0.2	0.1	2.3	0.1	27.7	0.0	30.2
4.8	6.0	11.0	0.7	0.0	6.0	39.0	240.0	0.2	0.0	11.0	0.0	0.1	0.0	0.3	0.0	5.0	0.0	0.0
4.0	9.0	144.0	2.6	0.0	253.0	495.0	1148.0	2.4	156.0	2.4	0.0	0.8	0.5	3.3	1.2	66.0	0.0	0.0
8.0	57.0	113.0	2.4	0.0	247.0	380.0	1311.0	4.4	22.0	2.2	0.0	0.3	0.5	3.7	0.2	30.0	0.0	0.0
3.4	1.0	75.0	1.3	0.0	299.0	108.0	730.0	0.3	0.0	0.0	0.0	0.2	0.1	1.7	0.0	9.0	0.0	0.0
8.0	33.0	163.0	2.5	0.0	261.0	501.0	1181.0	3.5	212.8	10.4	0.0	0.5	0.5	3.6	0.6	46.0	0.5	26.4
4.6	3.7	15.5	1.1	7.4	14.8	104.3	211.6	0.4	37.0	0.7	0.0	0.2	0.2	1.9	0.1	24.4	0.1	26.4
6.9	4.3	112.8	4.5	86.8	97.7	653.2	985.2	1.5	32.6	2.0	0.0	0.6	0.6	4.1	0.3	86.8	1.1	114.0
6.8	27.9	213.9	2.3	80.0	180.4	496.6	1166.2	1.6	238.1	1.7	0.0	0.2	0.7	3.6	0.2	74.4	0.9	100.3
8.3	48.5	106.3	4.9	83.2	140.9	656.0	1335.2	3.8	64.7	1.8	0.0	0.5	0.8	5.4	0.4	115.5	1.7	119.9
7.1	123.8	129.9	3.7	50.8	140.1	410.1	990.6	2.4	150.2	5.1	0.0	0.3	0.7	3.9	0.2	75.1	1.1	131.8
10.5	63.8	83.6	6.1	81.4	173.8	739.2	1491.6	4.7	28.6	1.1	0.0	0.2	0.9	6.4	0.3	129.8	2.0	109.1
10.4	170.2	221.9	7.8	69.9	316.2	665.8	2091.5	7.9	112.5	3.6	0.0	0.6	1.2	8.3	0.4	139.8	2.1	167.8
4.8	114.0	33.0	0.9	0.0	205.0	270.0	790.0	0.7	12.0	0.0	0.0	0.1	0.1	13.1	0.3	8.0	0.5	0.0

Code	Food Name	Unit/Amt	Wt (g)	Energy (Kcal)	Prot (g)	Carb (g)	Fiber (g)	Fat (g)	Mono (g)	Poly (g)
921867	Fast Food, Chicken Center Breast, original recipe/KFC	1 piece	115	282.9	27.5	8.8	0.1	15.3	9.0	2.0
921812	Fast Food, Chicken Drumstick, extra crispy/KFC	1 piece	69	204.2	13.6	6.1	0.5	13.9	8.0	1.7
921866	Fast Food, Chicken Drumstick, original recipe/KFC	1 piece	57	145.9	13.1	4.2	0.1	8.5	5.0	1.3
921946	Fast Food, Chicken McNuggets/MCD	1 serving	113	290.4	19.0	16.5	0.5	16.3	10.4	1.8
921884	Fast Food, Chicken Peg Legs/Long John	5 pieces	125	350.0	22.0	26.0	0.5	28.0	0.0	0.0
921876	Fast Food, Chicken Planks/Long John	4 pieces	166	456.5	27.0	35.0	1.0	23.0	0.0	0.0
921963	Fast Food, Chicken Strips/JB	4 pieces	125	348.8	29.0	28.0	0.0	14.0	5.9	0.7
921800	Fast Food, Chicken Tenders/BK	6 pieces	90	235.8	16.0	14.0	0.0	13.0	5.0	3.0
921815	Fast Food, Chicken Thigh, extra crispy/KFC	1 piece	119	405.8	20.0	14.4	0.5	29.9	18.0	4.2
921869	Fast Food, Chicken Thigh, original recipe/KFC	1 piece	104	294.3	17.9	11.1	0.1	19.7	9.0	3.1
921816	Fast Food, Chicken Wing, extra crispy/KFC	1 piece	65	254.2	12.4	9.3	0.5	18.6	11.0	2.5
921870	Fast Food, Chicken Wing, original recipe/KFC	1 piece	55	178.2	12.2	6.0	0.2	11.7	6.5	1.8
921807	Fast Food, Chicken, Hot Wings/KFC	6 pieces	119	376.0	22.4	17.3	0.5	24.1	14.0	4.1
21042	Fast Food, Chili con Carne	8 fl oz cup	253	255.5	24.6	21.9	0.0	8.3	3.4	0.5
921927	Fast Food, Chili/Wendy	1 serving	255	219.3	21.0	23.0	6.0	7.0	2.0	2.6
21070	Fast Food, Chimichanga w/beef	1 chimichanga	174	424.6	19.6	42.8	0.0	19.7	8.1	1.1
21071	Fast Food, Chimichanga w/beef & cheese	1 chimichanga	183	442.9	20.1	39.3	0.0	23.4	9.4	0.7
921951	Fast Food, Chocolate Chip Cookies/MCD	1 box	56	329.8	4.2	41.9	1.0	15.6	10.2	0.4
21043	Fast Food, Clams (shellfish) breaded, fried	1 tbsp	9.6	37.6	1.1	3.2	0.0	2.2	1.0	0.6
921896	Fast Food, Cookies, McDonaldland	1 box	56	290.1	4.2	47.1	1.0	9.2	6.8	0.5
21128	Fast Food, Corn on the Cob w/butter	1 ear	146	154.8	4.5	31.9	0.0	3.4	1.0	0.6
921044	Fast Food, Crab (shellfish) baked	1 crab	109	160.2	28.5	4.2	0.0	2.3	0.0	0.0
921045	Fast Food, Crab (shellfish) soft shell, fried	1 crab	125	333.8	11.0	31.2	0.0	17.9	0.0	0.0
21046	Fast Food, Crab Cake (shellfish)	1 cake	60	159.6	11.3	5.1	0.2	10.4	4.3	3.1
21015	Fast Food, Danish Pastry, Cheese	1 pastry	91	353.1	5.8	28.7	0.0	24.6	15.6	2.4
21016	Fast Food, Danish Pastry, Cinnamon	1 pastry	88	349.4	4.8	46.9	0.0	16.7	10.6	1.6
21017	Fast Food, Danish Pastry, Fruit	1 pastry	94	334.6	4.8	45.1	0.0	15.9	10.1	1.6
21074	Fast Food, Enchilada w/cheese	1 enchilada	163	319.5	9.6	28.5	0.0	18.8	6.3	0.8
21075	Fast Food, Enchilada w/cheese & beef	1 enchilada	192	322.6	11.9	30.5	0.0	17.6	6.1	1.4
21076	Fast Food, Enchirito w/cheese, beef & beans	1 enchirito	193	343.5	17.9	33.8	0.0	16.1	6.5	0.3
921933	Fast Food, Fish Tenders/BK	1 serving	99	267.3	12.0	18.0	0.0	16.0	7.0	4.0
921879	Fast Food, Fish, 2 pieces/Long John	2 pieces	136	651.4	30.0	53.0	1.0	36.0	0.0	0.0
921986	Fast Food, French Fries, large/Hardee	1 large	113	360.5	4.0	48.0	1.8	17.0	8.0	6.0
921984	Fast Food, French Fries, regular/Hardee	1 regular	71	230.0	3.0	30.0	1.2	11.0	5.0	4.0
921837	Fast Food, French Fries, small/DQ	1 small	71	200.2	2.0	25.0	1.0	10.0	3.0	1.0
21024	Fast Food, French Toast Sticks	5 sticks	141	513.2	8.3	57.9	2.7	29.0	12.6	9.9
21077	Fast Food, Frijoles (beans) w/cheese	8.0 oz	167	225.5	11.4	28.7	0.0	7.8	2.6	0.7
921834	Fast Food, Frozen Dessert, Freeze/DQ	1 serving, 14.0 oz	397	500.2	9.0	89.0	0.0	12.0	0.0	0.0
921835	Fast Food, Frozen Dessert, Mr Misty Freeze/DQ	1 serving, 15.0 oz	411	501.4	9.0	91.0	0.0	12.0	0.0	0.0
921841	Fast Food, Frozen Dessert, Mr Misty Kiss/DQ	1 serving 3.0 oz	89	70.3	0.0	17.0	0.0	0.0	0.0	0.0
921842	Fast Food, Frozen Dessert/DQ	1 serving 4.0 oz	113	179.7	5.0	27.0	0.0	6.0	0.0	0.0
921802	Fast Food, Ham & Cheese Sandwich	1 sandwich	230	471.5	24.0	44.0	0.5	23.0	8.0	4.0
21202	Fast Food, Hamburger, large, one meat patty w/condiments	1 sandwich	171.5	425.3	23.0	36.7	2.1	20.9	9.3	1.6
921895	Fast Food, Hot Cakes w/butter & syrup/MCD	1 serving	176	410.1	8.2	74.4	1.0	9.3	3.1	2.5
21119	Fast Food, Hot Dog w/chili, plain	1 hot dog	114	296.4	13.5	31.3	0.0	13.4	6.6	1.2
21120	Fast Food, Hot Dog w/corn flour coating, Corn Dog	1 hot dog	175	460.3	16.8	55.8	0.0	18.9	9.1	3.5
21118	Fast Food, Hot Dog, plain	1 hot dog	98	242.1	10.4	18.0	0.0	14.5	6.9	1.7
21129	Fast Food, Hush Puppies	5 hush puppies	78	256.6	4.9	34.9	0.0	11.6	7.8	0.4
921850	Fast Food, Ice Cream Cone, dipped, regular/DQ	1 regular	156	340.1	6.0	42.0	0.0	16.0	0.0	0.0
921849	Fast Food, Ice Cream Cone, dipped, small/DQ	1 small	78	190.3	3.0	25.0	0.0	9.0	0.0	0.0
921847	Fast Food, Ice Cream Cone, regular/DQ	1 regular	142	240.0	6.0	38.0	0.0	7.0	2.0	1.0
921846	Fast Food, Ice Cream Cone, small/DQ	1 small	71	139.9	3.0	22.0	0.0	4.0	1.0	1.0
921852	Fast Food, Ice Cream Parfait/DQ	1 serving	284	428.8	8.0	76.0	0.5	8.0	0.0	0.0
921853	Fast Food, Ice Cream Sandwich/DQ	1 sandwich	60	139.8	3.0	24.0	0.5	4.0	0.0	0.0
921859	Fast Food, Ice Cream Sundae, regular/DQ	1 regular	177	309.8	5.0	56.0	0.5	8.0	0.0	0.0
921858	Fast Food, Ice Cream Sundae, small/DQ	1 small	106	189.7	3.0	33.0	0.5	4.0	0.0	0.0
921823	Fast Food, Ice Cream, Banana Split/DQ	1 split	383	540.0	9.0	103.0	1.0	11.0	0.0	0.0
921824	Fast Food, Ice Cream, Buster Bar/DQ	1 bar	140	460.6	10.0	41.0	0.5	29.0	0.0	0.0
921829	Fast Food, Ice Cream, Dilly Bar/DQ	1 bar	85	210.0	3.0	21.0	0.5	13.0	0.0	0.0
921832	Fast Food, Ice Cream, Float/DQ	1 serving	397	408.9	5.0	82.0	0.0	7.0	0.0	0.0
921839	Fast Food, Ice Cream, Malt, regular/DQ	1 regular	418	760.8	14.0	134.0	0.5	18.0	0.0	0.0
921838	Fast Food, Ice Cream, Malt, small/DQ	1 small	291	520.9	10.0	91.0	0.5	13.0	0.0	0.0
21028	Fast Food, Ice Milk Cone, soft, vanilla	1 cone	103	163.8	3.9	24.1	0.1	6.1	1.8	0.4
14346	Fast Food, Milk Beverage, Chocolate Shake/MCD	1 fl oz	20.8	26.4	0.7	4.3	0.2	0.8	0.2	0.0
14428	Fast Food, Milk Beverage, Strawberry Shake	10 fl oz	283	319.8	9.6	53.5	1.1	7.9	0.0	0.0
14347	Fast Food, Shake, Vanilla/MCD	1 fl oz	20.8	23.1	0.7	3.7	0.1	0.6	0.2	0.0
21078	Fast Food, Nachos w/cheese	6-8 nachos	113	345.8	9.1	36.3	0.0	19.0	8.0	2.2
21079	Fast Food, Nachos w/cheese & jalapeno peppers	6-8 nachos	204	607.9	16.8	60.1	0.0	34.1	14.4	4.0
21080	Fast Food, Nachos w/cheese, beans, ground beef & peppers	6-8 nachos	255	568.7	19.8	55.8	0.0	30.7	11.0	5.7

Sat (g)	Chol (mg)	Cal (mg)	Iron (mg)	Magn (mg)	Phos (mg)	Pota (mg)	Sodi (mg)	Zinc (mg)	Vit A (RE)	Vit C (mg)	Vit E (mg)	Thia (mg)	Ribo (mg)	Niac (mg)	Vit B-6 (mg)	Fol (μg)	Vit B-12 (μg)	Wat (g)
3.8	93.0	36.0	1.0	0.0	205.0	267.0	672.0	0.7	12.0	0.0	0.0	0.1	0.2	11.5	0.3	8.0	0.4	0.0
3.4	71.0	13.0	0.7	0.0	100.0	147.0	324.0	1.3	8.0	0.0	0.0	0.1	0.1	3.7	0.2	6.0	0.4	0.0
2.2	67.0	21.0	1.1	0.0	95.0	125.0	275.0	1.3	6.0	1.0	0.0	0.1	0.1	3.2	0.1	4.0	0.4	0.0
4.1	65.0	13.0	1.0	0.0	283.0	302.0	520.0	0.9	0.0	0.0	0.0	0.1	0.1	9.0	0.4	11.0	0.0	0.0
0.0	0.0	0.0	0.0	0.0	0.0	0.0	0.0	0.0	0.0	0.0	0.0	0.0	0.0	0.0	0.0	0.0	0.0	0.0
0.0	0.0	0.0	0.0	0.0	0.0	0.0	0.0	0.0	0.0	0.0	0.0	0.0	0.0	0.0	0.0	0.0	0.0	0.0
6.8	68.0	0.0	0.0	0.0	0.0	0.0	748.0	0.0	0.0	0.0	0.0	0.0	0.0	0.0	0.0	0.0	0.0	0.0
3.0	46.0	18.0	0.7	24.0	236.0	200.0	541.0	0.6	19.0	0.0	0.0	0.1	0.1	7.3	0.3	10.0	0.0	0.0
7.7	129.0	49.0	1.2	0.0	170.0	217.0	688.0	1.7	26.2	0.0	0.0	0.1	0.2	6.5	0.2	9.0	1.0	0.0
5.3	123.0	65.0	1.3	0.0	170.0	220.0	619.0	1.7	20.8	0.0	0.0	0.1	0.3	5.5	0.2	9.0	1.0	0.0
4.4	67.0	18.0	0.6	0.0	77.0	90.0	422.0	0.6	6.0	0.0	0.0	0.0	0.1	3.3	0.1	5.0	0.3	0.0
3.0	64.0	48.0	1.2	0.0	75.0	85.0	372.0	0.6	11.2	0.0	0.0	0.0	0.1	3.7	0.1	4.0	0.3	0.0
5.3	148.0	0.0	0.0	0.0	0.0	0.0	677.0	0.0	0.0	0.0	0.0	0.0	0.0	0.0	0.0	0.0	0.0	0.0
3.4	134.1	68.3	5.2	45.5	197.3	690.7	1006.9	3.6	167.0	1.5	0.0	0.1	1.1	2.5	0.3	45.5	1.1	194.1
2.4	45.0	64.0	4.5	0.0	320.0	497.0	750.0	3.8	237.6	6.0	0.0	0.2	0.2	3.0	0.3	40.0	0.0	0.0
8.5	8.7	62.6	4.5	62.6	123.5	586.4	910.0	5.0	15.7	4.7	0.0	0.5	0.6	5.8	0.3	83.5	1.5	88.2
11.2	51.2	237.9	3.8	60.4	186.7	203.1	957.1	3.4	126.3	2.7	0.0	0.4	0.9	4.7	0.2	91.5	1.3	96.4
5.0	4.0	24.0	2.2	0.0	108.0	170.0	280.0	0.5	0.0	0.0	0.0	0.2	0.2	2.5	0.0	6.0	0.1	0.0
0.6	7.3	1.7	0.3	2.6	19.9	22.2	69.6	0.1	3.1	0.0	0.0	0.0	0.2	0.0	0.0	3.6	0.1	2.8
1.9	10.0	9.0	2.1	0.0	74.0	52.0	300.0	0.3	0.0	0.0	0.0	0.2	0.2	2.5	0.0	6.0	0.0	0.0
1.6	5.8	4.4	0.9	40.9	108.0	359.2	29.2	0.9	96.4	6.9	0.0	0.2	0.1	2.2	0.3	43.8	0.0	105.2
0.8	0.6	415.3	1.4	81.8	336.8	597.3	549.4	7.0	22.9	2.6	0.0	0.3	0.2	4.5	0.5	20.7	15.8	71.6
4.9	7.7	55.0	1.8	25.0	131.3	162.5	1117.5	1.1	3.8	0.8	0.0	0.1	0.1	1.8	0.2	20.0	4.5	62.3
2.2	82.2	202.2	1.1	25.2	226.8	162.0	491.4	2.1	82.2	0.2	0.0	0.1	0.1	1.2	0.1	24.6	4.4	32.0
5.1	20.0	70.1	1.8	15.5	80.1	116.5	319.4	0.6	42.8	2.6	0.0	0.3	0.2	2.5	0.1	54.6	0.2	30.8
3.5	27.3	37.0	1.8	14.1	73.9	95.9	326.5	0.5	5.3	2.6	0.0	0.3	0.2	2.2	0.1	54.6	0.2	18.4
3.3	18.8	21.6	1.4	14.1	68.6	110.0	332.8	0.5	24.4	1.6	0.0	0.3	0.2	1.8	0.1	31.0	0.2	27.3
10.6	44.0	324.4	1.3	50.5	133.7	239.6	784.0	2.5	185.8	1.0	0.0	0.1	0.4	1.9	0.4	65.2	0.7	103.1
9.0	40.3	228.5	3.1	82.6	167.0	574.1	1319.0	2.7	142.1	1.3	0.0	0.1	0.4	2.5	0.3	67.2	1.0	128.4
7.9	50.2	218.1	2.4	71.4	223.9	559.7	1250.6	2.8	133.2	4.6	0.0	0.2	0.7	3.0	0.2	59.8	1.6	121.0
3.0	28.0	0.0	0.0	0.0	0.0	0.0	870.0	0.0	0.0	0.0	0.0	0.0	0.0	0.0	0.0	0.0	0.0	0.0
0.0	27.0	0.0	0.0	0.0	0.0	0.0	1543.0	0.0	0.0	0.0	0.0	0.0	0.0	0.0	0.0	0.0	0.0	0.0
3.0	0.0	19.0	1.0	0.0	86.0	560.0	135.0	0.1	0.0	16.0	0.0	0.1	0.0	0.6	0.0	0.0	0.0	0.0
2.0	0.0	12.0	1.0	0.0	62.0	350.0	85.0	0.1	0.0	10.0	0.0	0.1	0.0	1.0	0.0	0.0	0.0	0.0
4.0	10.0	0.0	0.3	16.0	60.0	450.0	115.0	0.0	0.0	9.0	0.0	0.1	0.0	0.8	0.2	15.0	0.0	0.0
4.7	74.7	77.6	3.0	26.8	122.7	126.9	499.1	0.9	12.7	0.0	4.0	0.2	0.3	3.0	0.3	81.8	0.1	42.2
4.1	36.7	188.7	2.2	85.2	175.4	604.5	881.8	1.7	70.1	1.5	0.0	0.1	0.3	1.5	0.2	111.9	0.7	115.4
0.0	30.0	300.0	1.8	0.0	350.0	0.0	180.0	0.0	80.0	0.0	0.0	0.2	0.5	0.0	0.0	0.0	0.9	0.0
0.0	30.0	300.0	1.4	0.0	200.0	0.0	140.0	0.0	80.0	0.0	0.0	0.1	0.5	0.0	0.0	0.0	0.6	0.0
0.0	0.0	0.0	0.0	0.0	0.0	0.0	10.0	0.0	0.0	0.0	0.0	0.0	0.0	0.0	0.0	0.0	0.0	0.0
0.0	20.0	150.0	0.0	0.0	100.0	0.0	0.0	0.0	20.0	0.0	0.0	0.1	0.2	0.0	0.0	0.0	0.6	0.0
10.0	70.0	195.0	3.2	42.0	384.0	419.0	1534.0	2.4	170.0	7.0	0.0	0.9	0.4	6.0	0.3	25.0	0.0	0.0
7.9	70.3	133.8	4.1	34.3	212.7	394.5	728.9	4.8	0.0	2.6	0.0	0.3	0.3	6.5	0.2	61.7	2.6	88.8
3.7	21.0	114.0	2.1	0.0	501.0	187.0	640.0	0.7	34.6	0.0	0.0	0.3	0.3	2.8	0.1	9.0	0.2	0.0
4.9	51.3	19.4	3.3	10.3	191.5	166.4	479.9	0.8	5.7	2.7	0.0	0.2	0.4	3.7	0.0	73.0	0.3	54.5
5.2	78.8	101.5	6.2	17.5	166.3	262.5	973.0	1.3	36.8	0.0	0.0	0.3	0.7	4.2	0.1	103.3	0.4	81.7
5.1	44.1	23.5	2.3	12.7	97.0	143.1	670.3	2.0	0.0	0.1	0.0	0.2	0.3	3.6	0.0	48.0	0.5	52.9
2.7	134.9	68.6	1.4	16.4	190.3	188.0	964.9	0.4	26.5	0.0	0.0	0.0	0.0	2.0	0.1	13.3	0.2	25.2
0.0	20.0	150.0	0.7	0.0	200.0	220.0	100.0	0.7	40.0	0.0	0.0	0.1	0.3	0.0	0.1	3.0	0.6	0.0
0.0	10.0	100.0	0.4	0.0	100.0	134.0	55.0	0.5	40.0	0.0	0.0	0.1	0.3	0.0	0.0	2.0	0.4	0.0
4.0	15.0	150.0	0.7	0.0	200.0	220.0	80.0	0.7	40.0	0.0	0.0	0.1	0.3	0.0	0.1	3.0	0.6	0.0
2.0	10.0	100.0	0.4	0.0	100.0	135.0	45.0	0.5	20.0	0.0	0.0	0.0	0.2	0.0	0.0	2.0	0.4	0.0
0.0	30.0	250.0	1.4	0.0	300.0	0.0	140.0	0.0	80.0	0.0	0.0	0.1	0.4	0.4	0.0	0.0	0.9	0.0
0.0	5.0	60.0	0.0	0.0	60.0	0.0	40.0	0.0	20.0	0.0	0.0	0.0	0.1	0.4	0.0	0.0	0.1	0.0
0.0	20.0	200.0	1.1	0.0	200.0	290.0	120.0	0.9	40.0	0.0	0.0	0.1	0.3	0.3	0.1	4.0	0.6	0.0
0.0	10.0	100.0	0.4	0.0	150.0	145.0	75.0	0.5	20.0	0.0	0.0	0.0	0.2	0.2	0.0	2.0	0.4	0.0
0.0	30.0	250.0	1.8	0.0	350.0	670.0	150.0	2.1	150.0	15.0	0.0	0.1	0.5	0.4	0.8	9.0	0.9	0.0
0.0	10.0	100.0	1.1	0.0	250.0	0.0	175.0	0.0	20.0	0.0	0.0	0.1	0.2	2.0	0.0	0.0	0.4	0.0
0.0	10.0	100.0	0.4	0.0	100.0	0.0	50.0	0.0	20.0	0.0	0.0	0.0	0.2	0.0	0.0	0.0	0.4	0.0
0.0	20.0	200.0	1.1	0.0	200.0	0.0	85.0	0.0	40.0	0.0	0.0	0.1	0.3	0.0	0.0	0.0	0.6	0.0
0.0	50.0	450.0	4.5	0.0	600.0	690.0	260.0	0.1	150.0	0.0	0.0	0.3	0.8	0.8	0.2	4.0	2.1	0.0
0.0	35.0	350.0	2.7	0.0	400.0	480.0	180.0	0.1	100.0	0.0	0.0	0.2	0.6	0.4	0.1	3.0	1.2	0.0
3.5	27.8	153.5	0.2	15.5	139.1	168.9	91.7	0.6	51.5	1.1	0.4	0.1	0.3	0.3	0.1	12.4	0.2	67.4
0.5	2.7	23.5	0.1	3.5	21.2	41.6	20.2	0.1	4.8	0.1	0.0	0.0	0.1	0.0	0.0	0.7	0.1	14.9
4.9	31.1	319.8	0.3	36.8	283.0	515.1	234.9	1.0	82.1	2.3	0.0	0.1	0.6	0.5	0.1	8.5	0.9	209.7
0.4	2.3	25.4	0.0	2.5	21.2	36.2	17.1	0.1	6.7	0.2	0.0	0.0	0.0	0.0	0.0	0.7	0.1	15.5
7.8	18.1	272.3	1.3	55.4	275.7	171.8	815.9	1.8	91.5	1.2	0.0	0.2	0.4	1.5	0.2	10.2	0.8	45.7
14.0	83.6	620.2	2.4	108.1	393.7	293.8	1736.0	2.9	471.2	1.0	0.0	0.1	0.5	2.8	0.4	18.4	1.0	87.1
12.5	20.4	385.1	2.8	96.9	387.6	451.4	1800.3	3.6	469.2	4.8	0.0	0.2	0.7	3.3	0.4	38.3	1.0	142.7

Code	Food Name	Unit/Amt	Wt (g)	Energy (Kcal)	Prot (g)	Carb (g)	Fiber (g)	Fat (g)	Mono (g)	Poly (g)
21081	Fast Food, Nachos w/cinnamon & sugar	6-8 nachos	109	591.9	7.2	63.4	0.0	36.0	11.8	4.1
21130	Fast Food, Onion Rings, breaded, fried	8-9 onion rings	83	275.6	3.7	31.3	0.0	15.5	6.7	0.7
21048	Fast Food, Oysters (shellfish) battered/breaded, fried	6 oysters	139	368.4	12.5	39.9	0.0	17.9	6.9	4.6
21025	Fast Food, Pancakes w/butter & syrup	3 cakes	232	519.7	8.3	90.9	0.0	14.0	5.3	2.0
21049	Fast Food, Pizza w/cheese	1 slice (⅛ 12"-pizza)	63	140.5	7.7	20.5	0.0	3.2	1.0	0.5
21050	Fast Food, Pizza w/cheese, meat & veges	1 slice (⅛ 12"-pizza)	79	184.1	13.0	21.3	0.0	5.4	2.5	0.9
21051	Fast Food, Pizza w/pepperoni	1 slice (⅛ 12"-pizza)	71	181.1	10.1	19.9	0.0	7.0	3.1	1.2
921911	Fast Food, Pizza, Cheese Pan/PH	2 slices	205	492.0	30.0	57.0	5.0	18.0	0.0	0.0
921906	Fast Food, Pizza, Cheese, thin/PH	2 slices	148	398.1	28.0	37.0	4.0	17.0	0.0	0.0
921912	Fast Food, Pizza, Pepperoni Pan/PH	2 slices	211	540.2	29.0	62.0	5.0	22.0	0.0	0.0
921905	Fast Food, Pizza, Pepperoni, personal/PH	1 pizza	256	675.8	37.0	76.0	8.0	29.0	0.0	0.0
921907	Fast Food, Pizza, Pepperoni, thin/PH	2 slices	146	413.2	26.0	36.0	4.0	20.0	0.0	0.0
921913	Fast Food, Pizza, Super Supreme Pan/PH	2 slices	257	562.8	33.0	53.0	6.0	26.0	0.0	0.0
921908	Fast Food, Pizza, Super Supreme, thin/PH	2 slices	203	462.8	29.0	44.0	5.0	21.0	0.0	0.0
921914	Fast Food, Pizza, Supreme Pan/PH	2 slices	255	589.1	32.0	53.0	7.0	30.0	0.0	0.0
921910	Fast Food, Pizza, Supreme Personal/PH	1 pizza	264	646.8	33.0	76.0	9.0	28.0	0.0	0.0
921909	Fast Food, Pizza, Supreme, thin/PH	2 slices	200	460.0	28.0	41.0	5.0	22.0	0.0	0.0
21132	Fast Food, Potato, baked, topped w/cheese & bacon	1 potato	299	451.5	18.4	44.4	0.0	25.9	9.7	4.8
21133	Fast Food, Potato, baked, topped w/cheese & broccoli	1 potato	339	403.4	13.7	46.6	0.0	21.4	7.7	4.2
21134	Fast Food, Potato, baked, topped w/cheese & chili	1 potato	395	481.9	23.2	55.9	0.0	21.8	6.8	0.9
21131	Fast Food, Potato, baked, topped w/cheese sauce	1 potato	296	473.6	14.6	46.5	0.0	28.7	10.7	6.0
21135	Fast Food, Potato, baked, topped w/sour cream & chives	1 potato	302	392.6	6.7	50.0	0.0	22.3	7.9	3.3
21139	Fast Food, Potato, mashed	1 tbsp	15	12.5	0.3	2.4	0.0	0.2	0.1	0.0
21026	Fast Food, Potatoes, Hash Brown	1 tbsp	9	18.9	0.2	2.0	0.0	1.2	0.5	0.1
21122	Fast Food, Roast Beef Sandwich w/cheese	1 sandwich	176	473.4	32.2	45.4	0.0	18.0	3.7	3.5
21121	Fast Food, Roast Beef Sandwich, plain	1 sandwich	139	346.1	21.5	33.4	0.0	13.8	6.8	1.7
4021	Fast Food, Salad Dressing, Italian, w/salt, diet (2kcal/tsp)	1 tbsp	15	15.8	0.0	0.7	0.0	1.5	0.3	0.9
4025	Fast Food, Salad Dressing, Mayonnaise, Soybean Oil, w/salt	1 cup	220	1577.0	2.4	5.9	0.0	174.7	49.9	90.9
921983	Fast Food, Salad, Chef/Hardee	1 salad	294	241.1	22.0	5.0	0.0	15.0	5.0	1.0
921864	Fast Food, Salad, Chunky Chicken/BK	1 salad	258	141.9	20.0	8.0	0.0	4.0	1.0	1.0
21127	Fast Food, Salad, Cole Slaw	1 tbsp	8.3	12.3	0.1	1.1	0.0	0.9	0.2	0.5
921871	Fast Food, Salad, Cole Slaw/KFC	1 serving	91	119.2	1.5	13.2	1.0	6.6	2.0	3.4
921803	Fast Food, Salad, Garden/BK	1 salad	223	95.9	6.0	8.0	0.0	5.0	1.0	0.0
21140	Fast Food, Salad, Potato	1 tbsp	17.8	20.3	0.3	2.4	0.0	1.1	0.3	0.5
21083	Fast Food, Salad, Taco	1 tbsp	8.1	11.4	0.5	1.0	0.0	0.6	0.2	0.1
21084	Fast Food, Salad, Taco w/chili con carne	1 tbsp	10.9	12.1	0.7	1.1	0.0	0.5	0.2	0.1
921974	Fast Food, Sandwich, Beef & Cheddar/Arby	1 sandwich	168	490.6	24.0	51.0	0.5	21.0	11.0	5.0
921981	Fast Food, Sandwich, Big Deluxe Hamburger/Hardee	1 burger	216	499.0	27.0	32.0	0.5	30.0	12.0	5.0
921971	Fast Food, Sandwich, Big Roast Beef/Hardee	1 sandwich	134	300.2	18.0	32.0	0.5	12.0	5.0	2.0
921989	Fast Food, Sandwich, Big Twin/Hardee	1 sandwich	173	449.8	23.0	34.0	0.0	25.0	9.0	5.0
21002	Fast Food, Sandwich, Biscuit w/egg	1 biscuit	136	315.5	11.1	24.2	0.0	20.2	8.2	4.2
21003	Fast Food, Sandwich, Biscuit w/egg & bacon	1 biscuit	150	457.5	17.0	28.6	0.8	31.1	13.4	7.5
21004	Fast Food, Sandwich, Biscuit w/egg & ham	1 biscuit	192	441.6	20.4	30.3	0.8	27.0	11.0	7.7
21005	Fast Food, Sandwich, Biscuit w/egg & sausage	1 biscuit	180	581.4	19.2	41.1	0.9	38.7	16.4	4.4
21006	Fast Food, Sandwich, Biscuit w/egg & steak	1 biscuit	148	410.0	17.9	21.3	0.0	28.4	11.7	5.8
21007	Fast Food, Sandwich, Biscuit w/egg, cheese & bacon	1 biscuit	144	476.6	16.3	33.4	0.0	31.4	14.2	3.5
21093	Fast Food, Sandwich, Cheeseburger (2 patty) condiments & veges	1 burger	166	416.7	21.2	35.2	0.0	21.1	7.8	2.7
21092	Fast Food, Sandwich, Cheeseburger (2 patty) plain	1 burger	155	457.3	27.7	22.1	0.0	28.5	11.0	1.9
921969	Fast Food, Sandwich, Cheeseburger, ¼ pound/Hardee	1 burger	182	500.5	29.0	34.0	0.4	29.0	12.0	2.0
921952	Fast Food, Sandwich, Cheeseburger, Big Classic/Wendy	1 burger	295	640.2	30.0	46.0	2.0	38.0	14.0	4.0
921926	Fast Food, Sandwich, Cheeseburger, junior/Wendy	1 burger	123	300.1	17.0	31.0	0.0	13.0	0.0	0.0
21100	Fast Food, Sandwich, Cheeseburger, large (2 patty) w/condiments & vege	1 burger	258	704.3	38.0	39.7	0.0	43.7	17.4	4.7
21096	Fast Food, Sandwich, Cheeseburger, large, one meat patty, plain	1 burger	185	608.7	30.1	47.4	0.0	33.0	12.7	2.4
21089	Fast Food, Sandwich, Cheeseburger, one meat patty, plain	1 burger	102	319.3	14.8	31.8	0.0	15.1	5.8	1.5
21090	Fast Food, Sandwich, Cheeseburger, one meat patty, w/condiments	1 burger	113	294.9	16.0	26.5	0.0	14.1	5.3	1.1
21102	Fast Food, Sandwich, Chicken Filet, plain	1 sandwich	182	515.1	24.1	38.7	0.0	29.4	10.4	8.4
921934	Fast Food, Sandwich, Chicken/BK	1 sandwich	229	684.7	26.0	56.0	0.5	40.0	11.0	20.0
921979	Fast Food, Sandwich, Club/Arby	1 sandwich	252	559.4	30.0	43.0	1.0	30.0	0.0	0.0
921809	Fast Food, Sandwich, Colonel's Chicken/KFC	1 sandwich	166	481.4	20.8	38.6	1.0	27.3	12.6	8.0
921801	Fast Food, Sandwich, Croissandwich/BK	1 sandwich	144	345.6	19.0	19.0	0.5	21.0	11.0	2.0
21011	Fast Food, Sandwich, Croissant w/egg & cheese	1 croissant	127	368.3	12.8	24.3	0.0	24.7	7.5	1.4
21012	Fast Food, Sandwich, Croissant w/egg, cheese & bacon	1 croissant	129	412.8	16.2	23.6	0.0	28.4	9.2	1.8
21013	Fast Food, Sandwich, Croissant w/egg, cheese & ham	1 croissant	152	474.2	18.9	24.2	0.0	33.6	11.4	2.4
21020	Fast Food, Sandwich, English Muffin w/cheese & sausage	1 muffin	115	393.3	15.3	29.2	1.5	24.3	10.1	2.7
21021	Fast Food, Sandwich, English Muffin w/egg, cheese & Canadian bacon	1 sandwich	137	289.1	16.7	26.7	1.5	12.6	4.7	1.6
21047	Fast Food, Sandwich, Fish Filet, battered/breaded, fried	1 fillet	91	211.1	13.3	15.4	0.5	11.2	2.3	5.7
21105	Fast Food, Sandwich, Fish w/tartar sauce	1 sandwich	158	431.3	16.9	41.0	0.0	22.8	7.7	8.2
21106	Fast Food, Sandwich, Fish w/tartar sauce & cheese	1 sandwich	183	523.4	20.6	47.6	0.0	28.6	8.9	9.4
921977	Fast Food, Sandwich, Ham & Cheese/Arby	1 sandwich	154	352.7	26.0	33.0	0.5	13.0	6.0	3.0

Sat (g)	Chol (mg)	Cal (mg)	Iron (mg)	Magn (mg)	Phos (mg)	Pota (mg)	Sodi (mg)	Zinc (mg)	Vit A (RE)	Vit C (mg)	Vit E (mg)	Thia (mg)	Ribo (mg)	Niac (mg)	Vit B-6 (mg)	Fol (μg)	Vit B-12 (μg)	Wat (g)
18.2	39.2	85.0	2.9	19.6	32.7	78.5	439.3	0.6	10.9	8.0	0.0	0.2	0.4	3.9	0.2	7.6	1.7	1.1
7.0	14.1	73.0	0.8	15.8	86.3	129.5	429.9	0.3	0.8	0.6	0.3	0.1	0.1	0.9	0.1	54.8	0.1	30.8
4.6	108.4	27.8	4.5	23.6	196.0	182.1	676.9	15.6	108.4	4.2	0.0	0.3	0.3	4.4	0.0	30.6	1.0	66.7
5.9	58.0	127.6	2.6	48.7	475.6	250.6	1104.3	1.0	69.6	3.5	1.4	0.4	0.6	3.4	0.1	30.2	0.2	115.4
1.5	9.5	116.6	0.6	15.8	112.8	109.6	335.8	0.8	73.7	1.3	0.0	0.2	0.2	2.5	0.0	34.7	0.3	30.1
1.5	20.5	101.1	1.5	18.2	131.1	178.5	382.4	1.1	101.1	1.6	0.0	0.2	0.2	2.0	0.1	32.4	0.4	37.7
2.2	14.2	64.6	0.9	8.5	75.3	152.7	267.0	0.5	54.7	1.6	0.0	0.1	0.2	3.0	0.1	36.9	0.2	33.0
9.0	34.0	500.0	5.4	0.0	0.0	320.0	940.0	0.0	200.0	0.0	0.0	0.7	0.7	7.0	0.0	0.0	0.0	0.0
10.4	33.0	450.0	4.5	0.0	0.0	261.0	867.0	0.0	150.0	0.0	0.0	0.3	0.5	5.0	0.0	0.0	0.0	0.0
9.2	42.0	400.0	5.4	0.0	0.0	405.0	1127.0	0.0	250.0	4.0	0.0	0.7	0.7	8.0	0.0	0.0	0.0	0.0
12.5	53.0	0.0	0.0	0.0	0.0	408.0	1335.0	0.0	0.0	0.0	0.0	0.0	0.0	0.0	0.0	0.0	0.0	0.0
10.6	46.0	300.0	4.5	0.0	0.0	287.0	986.0	0.0	200.0	4.0	0.0	0.3	0.5	6.0	0.0	0.0	0.0	0.0
12.0	55.0	400.0	7.2	0.0	0.0	532.0	1447.0	0.0	150.0	1.0	0.0	0.9	0.8	9.0	0.0	0.0	0.0	0.0
10.3	56.0	350.0	6.3	0.0	0.0	463.0	1336.0	0.0	200.0	1.0	0.0	0.4	0.7	7.0	0.0	0.0	0.0	0.0
13.8	48.0	400.0	7.2	0.0	0.0	580.0	1363.0	0.0	200.0	9.0	0.0	0.7	0.8	9.0	0.0	0.0	0.0	0.0
11.2	49.0	0.0	0.0	0.0	0.0	487.0	1313.0	0.0	0.0	0.0	0.0	0.0	0.0	0.0	0.0	0.0	0.0	0.0
11.0	42.0	350.0	7.2	0.0	0.0	544.0	1328.0	0.0	250.0	2.0	0.0	0.4	0.7	7.0	0.0	0.0	0.0	0.0
10.1	29.9	308.0	3.1	68.8	346.8	1178.1	971.8	2.2	173.4	28.7	0.0	0.3	0.2	4.0	0.7	29.9	0.3	194.4
8.5	20.3	335.6	3.3	78.0	345.8	1440.8	484.8	2.0	278.0	48.5	0.0	0.3	0.3	3.6	0.8	61.0	0.3	237.4
13.0	31.6	410.8	6.1	110.6	497.7	1572.1	699.2	3.8	173.8	31.6	0.0	0.3	0.4	4.2	0.9	47.4	0.2	276.8
10.6	17.8	310.8	3.0	65.1	319.7	1166.2	381.8	1.9	227.9	26.0	0.0	0.2	0.2	3.3	0.7	26.6	0.2	194.6
10.0	24.2	105.7	3.1	69.5	184.2	1383.2	181.2	0.9	277.8	33.8	0.0	0.3	0.2	3.7	0.8	33.2	0.2	209.7
0.1	0.3	3.2	0.1	2.7	8.3	44.1	34.1	0.0	1.5	0.1	0.0	0.0	0.0	0.2	0.0	1.2	0.0	11.9
0.5	1.2	0.9	0.1	2.0	8.6	33.4	36.3	0.0	0.4	0.7	0.0	0.0	0.0	0.1	0.0	1.0	0.0	5.4
9.0	77.4	183.0	5.1	40.5	401.3	345.0	1633.3	5.4	45.8	0.0	0.0	0.4	0.5	5.9	0.3	63.4	2.1	76.6
3.6	51.4	54.2	4.2	30.6	239.1	315.5	792.3	3.4	20.9	2.1	0.0	0.4	0.3	5.9	0.3	57.0	1.2	67.6
0.2	0.9	0.3	0.0	0.0	0.8	2.3	118.1	0.0	0.0	0.0	0.2	0.0	0.0	0.0	0.0	0.0	0.0	12.3
26.0	129.8	39.6	1.1	2.2	61.6	74.8	1250.5	0.4	184.8	0.0	25.9	0.0	0.0	0.0	1.3	16.9	0.6	33.7
9.0	115.0	279.0	2.0	0.0	0.0	590.0	930.0	0.0	0.0	0.0	0.0	0.0	0.0	0.0	0.0	0.0	0.0	0.0
1.0	49.0	0.0	0.0	0.0	0.0	0.0	443.0	0.0	0.0	0.0	0.0	0.0	0.0	0.0	0.0	0.0	0.0	0.1
0.1	0.4	2.8	0.1	0.7	3.0	14.9	22.4	0.0	4.2	0.7	0.0	0.0	0.0	0.0	0.0	3.2	0.0	6.1
1.0	5.0	33.0	0.2	0.0	20.0	115.0	197.0	0.1	62.0	22.0	0.0	0.0	0.2	0.1	0.1	10.0	0.0	0.0
3.0	15.0	0.0	0.0	0.0	0.0	0.0	125.0	0.0	0.0	0.0	0.0	0.0	0.0	0.0	0.0	0.0	0.0	0.0
0.2	10.7	2.5	0.1	1.4	10.0	48.1	58.4	0.0	3.0	0.2	0.0	0.0	0.0	0.0	0.0	4.5	0.0	14.0
0.3	1.8	7.9	0.1	2.1	5.8	17.0	31.2	0.1	3.2	0.1	0.0	0.0	0.0	0.1	0.0	3.4	0.0	5.9
0.3	0.2	10.2	0.1	2.2	6.4	16.4	37.0	0.1	8.9	0.1	0.0	0.0	0.0	0.1	0.0	3.8	0.0	8.4
5.0	51.0	80.0	5.4	0.0	0.0	355.0	1520.0	0.0	14.2	3.0	0.0	0.1	0.3	5.0	0.0	0.0	0.0	0.0
12.0	70.0	185.0	5.0	0.0	0.0	390.0	760.0	0.0	0.0	0.0	0.0	0.0	0.0	0.0	0.0	0.0	0.0	0.0
5.0	45.0	106.0	5.0	0.0	0.0	320.0	880.0	0.0	129.6	8.0	0.0	1.0	0.2	5.2	0.0	0.0	0.0	0.0
11.0	55.0	180.0	4.0	0.0	0.0	280.0	580.0	0.0	0.0	0.0	0.0	0.0	0.0	0.0	0.0	0.0	0.0	0.0
6.2	232.6	153.7	3.1	20.4	185.0	160.5	654.2	1.1	178.2	0.0	0.0	0.3	0.3	0.7	0.1	61.2	0.7	69.5
8.0	352.5	189.0	3.7	24.0	238.5	250.5	999.0	1.6	52.5	2.7	2.1	0.1	0.2	2.4	0.1	60.0	1.0	70.0
5.9	299.5	220.8	4.6	30.7	316.8	318.7	1382.4	2.2	240.0	0.0	2.2	0.7	0.6	2.0	0.3	65.3	1.2	104.9
15.0	302.4	154.8	4.0	25.2	489.6	320.4	1141.2	2.2	163.8	0.0	2.8	0.5	0.5	3.6	0.2	64.8	1.4	77.2
8.6	272.3	137.6	5.3	25.2	225.0	306.4	888.0	2.8	190.9	0.1	0.0	0.4	0.5	3.1	0.2	56.2	1.4	77.7
11.4	260.6	164.2	2.5	20.2	459.4	230.4	1260.0	1.5	165.6	1.6	0.0	0.3	0.4	2.3	0.1	53.3	1.1	59.3
8.7	59.8	171.0	3.4	29.9	242.4	335.3	1050.8	3.5	64.7	1.7	0.0	0.3	0.3	8.1	0.2	61.4	1.9	85.0
13.0	110.1	232.5	3.4	32.6	373.6	308.5	635.5	5.0	79.1	0.0	1.2	0.2	0.4	6.0	0.2	68.2	2.3	65.7
14.0	70.0	248.0	5.0	0.0	355.0	350.0	1060.0	3.6	101.6	33.0	0.0	0.3	0.6	14.0	0.3	0.0	0.7	0.0
14.0	100.0	180.0	5.4	0.0	489.0	590.0	1370.0	9.0	87.8	2.3	0.0	0.5	0.7	11.4	0.5	31.0	0.0	0.0
0.0	45.0	0.0	0.0	0.0	0.0	220.0	745.0	0.0	0.0	0.0	0.0	0.0	0.0	0.0	0.0	0.0	0.0	0.0
17.7	141.9	239.9	5.9	51.6	394.7	596.0	1148.1	6.7	54.2	1.0	0.0	0.4	0.5	7.2	0.4	74.8	3.4	131.8
14.8	96.2	90.7	5.5	38.9	421.8	643.8	1589.2	5.6	148.0	0.0	0.0	0.5	0.6	11.2	0.3	74.0	2.5	71.5
6.5	50.0	140.8	2.4	21.4	195.8	164.2	499.8	2.4	36.7	0.0	0.0	0.4	0.4	3.7	0.1	54.1	1.0	38.0
6.3	37.3	110.7	2.4	20.3	176.3	222.6	615.9	2.1	93.8	1.9	0.5	0.2	0.2	3.7	0.1	54.2	0.9	53.9
8.5	60.1	60.1	4.7	34.6	233.0	353.1	957.3	1.9	30.9	8.9	0.0	0.3	0.2	6.8	0.2	100.1	0.4	86.1
8.0	82.0	79.0	3.3	54.0	274.0	375.0	1417.0	1.1	25.2	0.0	0.0	0.5	0.3	9.6	0.4	18.0	0.0	0.0
0.0	100.0	200.0	3.6	0.0	0.0	0.0	1610.0	0.0	0.0	0.0	0.0	0.7	0.4	7.0	0.0	0.0	0.0	0.0
5.7	47.0	46.0	1.3	0.0	0.0	0.0	1060.0	0.0	0.0	0.0	0.0	0.4	0.3	11.1	0.0	0.0	0.0	0.0
7.0	241.0	136.0	2.2	24.0	317.0	256.0	962.0	1.9	85.2	0.0	0.0	0.5	0.3	3.2	0.0	0.0	0.0	0.0
14.1	215.9	243.8	2.2	21.6	348.0	174.0	551.2	1.8	255.3	0.1	0.0	0.2	0.4	1.5	0.1	47.0	0.8	57.7
15.4	215.4	150.9	2.2	23.2	276.1	201.2	888.8	1.9	120.0	2.2	0.0	0.3	0.3	2.2	0.1	45.2	0.9	56.7
17.5	212.8	144.4	2.1	25.8	335.9	272.1	1080.7	2.2	117.0	11.4	0.0	0.5	0.3	3.2	0.2	45.6	1.0	77.7
9.9	58.7	167.9	2.3	24.2	186.3	215.1	1036.2	1.7	86.3	1.3	0.5	0.7	0.3	4.1	0.1	66.7	0.7	43.4
4.7	234.3	150.7	2.4	23.3	269.9	198.7	728.8	1.6	156.2	1.8	0.9	0.5	0.4	3.3	0.1	43.8	0.7	77.8
2.6	30.9	16.4	1.9	21.8	155.6	291.2	484.1	0.4	10.9	0.0	0.0	0.1	0.1	1.9	0.1	15.5	1.0	48.7
5.2	55.3	83.7	2.6	33.2	211.7	339.7	614.6	1.0	30.0	2.8	0.9	0.3	0.2	3.4	0.1	85.3	1.1	74.8
8.1	67.7	184.8	3.5	36.6	311.1	353.2	938.8	1.2	97.0	2.7	1.8	0.5	0.4	4.2	0.1	91.5	1.1	82.7
4.0	50.0	200.0	1.8	0.0	405.0	312.0	1655.0	2.4	40.0	24.0	0.0	1.0	0.5	6.0	0.3	26.0	0.0	0.0

Code	Food Name	Unit/Amt	Wt (g)	Energy (Kcal)	Prot (g)	Carb (g)	Fiber (g)	Fat (g)	Mono (g)	Poly (g)
21110	Fast Food, Sandwich, Hamburger (2 patty) plain	1 burger	176	543.8	29.9	42.9	0.0	27.9	12.1	2.3
21111	Fast Food, Sandwich, Hamburger (2 patty) w/condiments	1 burger	215	576.2	31.8	38.7	0.0	32.5	14.1	2.8
921929	Fast Food, Sandwich, Hamburger, Big Classic/Wendy	1 burger	277	570.6	27.0	46.0	1.0	33.0	13.0	8.0
921887	Fast Food, Sandwich, Hamburger, Big Mac/MCD	1 burger	215	559.0	25.2	42.5	1.0	32.5	20.9	1.5
921931	Fast Food, Sandwich, Hamburger, junior/Wendy	1 burger	111	259.7	14.0	30.0	0.0	9.0	0.0	0.0
21107	Fast Food, Sandwich, Hamburger, plain	1 burger	90	274.5	12.3	30.5	0.0	11.8	5.5	0.9
921930	Fast Food, Sandwich, Hamburger, single/Wendy	1 burger	126	340.2	24.0	38.0	1.0	17.0	9.0	1.0
921894	Fast Food, Sandwich, Hamburger/MCD	1 burger	102	260.1	12.2	30.6	0.5	9.5	5.1	0.8
921825	Fast Food, Sandwich, Hot Dog w/cheese/DQ	1 hot dog	113	330.0	15.0	21.0	0.5	21.0	8.0	2.0
921827	Fast Food, Sandwich, Hot Dog w/chili/DQ	1 hot dog	128	320.0	13.0	23.0	0.5	20.0	8.0	2.0
921844	Fast Food, Sandwich, Hot Dog/DQ	1 hot dog	99	280.2	11.0	21.0	0.5	16.0	7.0	2.0
921976	Fast Food, Sandwich, Jr Roast Beef/Arby	1 sandwich	74	218.3	12.0	22.0	0.5	8.0	3.0	2.0
921973	Fast Food, Sandwich, Roast Beef/Arby	1 sandwich	140	350.0	22.0	32.0	0.5	15.0	5.0	2.0
921972	Fast Food, Sandwich, Roast Beef/Hardee	1 sandwich	114	259.9	15.0	31.0	0.5	10.0	4.0	2.0
921806	Fast Food, Sandwich, Sausage McMuffin/MCD	1 sandwich	117	369.7	16.5	27.3	0.5	21.9	11.7	2.4
921978	Fast Food, Sandwich, Turkey Deluxe/Arby	1 sandwich	236	375.2	24.0	32.0	0.5	17.0	5.0	8.0
921890	Fast Food, Scrambled Eggs/MCD	1 serving	100	140.0	12.4	1.2	0.0	9.8	5.0	1.4
921988	Fast Food, Shake, Chocolate/Hardee	1 shake	341	460.4	11.0	85.0	0.0	8.0	2.0	0.0
921932	Fast Food, Shake, Frosty/Wendy	1 shake	243	401.0	8.0	59.0	0.0	14.0	3.0	2.0
921903	Fast Food, Shake, Strawberry/MCD	1 shake	239	320.3	10.7	67.0	0.0	1.3	0.6	0.1
921821	Fast Food, Shake, Vanilla/BK	1 shake	284	335.1	9.0	51.0	0.0	10.0	3.0	0.0
921904	Nutrient/Protein Supplement, Liquid Nutrition, Boost, vanilla	8 oz.	260	239.2	10.1	41.1	0.0	4.1	0.0	0.0
21059	Fast Food, Shrimp (shellfish) breaded, fried	6-8 shrimp	164	454.3	18.9	40.0	0.0	24.9	17.4	0.6
21123	Fast Food, Steak Sandwich	1 sandwich	204	459.0	30.3	52.0	0.0	14.1	5.3	3.3
21124	Fast Food, Submarine Sandwich, cold cuts	1 sub	228	456.0	21.8	51.0	0.0	18.6	8.2	2.3
21125	Fast Food, Submarine Sandwich, roast beef	1 sub	216	410.4	28.6	44.3	0.0	13.0	1.8	2.6
21126	Fast Food, Submarine Sandwich, tuna salad	1 sub	256	583.7	29.7	55.4	0.0	28.0	13.4	7.3
21082	Fast Food, Taco	1 small taco	171	369.4	20.7	26.7	0.0	20.6	6.6	1.0
921958	Fast Food, Taco/JB	1 taco	81	191.2	8.0	16.0	1.2	11.0	4.4	1.0
21085	Fast Food, Tostada w/beans & cheese	1 tostada	144	223.2	9.6	26.5	0.0	9.9	3.1	0.7
21086	Fast Food, Tostada w/beans, beef & cheese	1 tostada	225	333.0	16.1	29.7	0.0	16.9	3.5	0.6
4002	Fat, Animal, Lard, Pork	1 cup	205	1849.1	0.0	0.0	0.0	205.0	92.5	23.0
924073	Fish Cakes, fried	4.0 oz	120	206.4	17.6	11.2	0.0	9.6	0.0	0.0
924074	Fish Cakes, frozen	4.0 oz	119	253.5	11.6	27.3	0.0	10.8	0.0	0.0
15187	Fish, Bass, Freshwater, cooked w/dry heat	3.5 oz	100	146.0	24.2	0.0	0.0	4.7	1.8	1.4
15188	Fish, Bass, Striped, cooked w/dry heat	1 fillet	124	153.8	28.2	0.0	0.0	3.7	1.0	1.2
15189	Fish, Bluefish, cooked w/dry heat	1 fillet	117	186.0	30.1	0.0	0.0	6.4	2.7	1.6
15009	Fish, Carp, baked or broiled (dry heat)	1 fillet	170	275.4	38.9	0.0	0.0	12.2	5.1	3.1
15235	Fish, Catfish, Channel, Farmed, cooked w/dry heat	1 fillet	143	217.4	26.8	0.0	0.0	11.5	5.9	2.0
15233	Fish, Catfish, Channel, Wild, cooked w/dry heat	1 fillet	143	150.2	26.4	0.0	0.0	4.1	1.6	0.9
15012	Fish, Caviar, black/red, granular	1.0 oz	29	73.1	7.1	1.2	0.0	5.2	1.3	2.1
15016	Fish, Cod, Atlantic, baked/broiled (dry heat)	1 fillet	180	189.0	41.1	0.0	0.0	1.5	0.2	0.5
15018	Fish, Cod, Atlantic, dried & salted	1 piece (5.5" x 1.5" x 0.5")	80	232.0	50.3	0.0	0.0	1.9	0.3	0.6
15192	Fish, Cod, Pacific, cooked w/dry heat	3.0 oz	85	89.3	19.5	0.0	0.0	0.7	0.1	0.3
15027	Fish, Fish Sticks, frozen & reheated	1 piece (4" x 2" x 0.5")	57	155.0	8.9	13.5	0.0	7.0	2.9	1.8
15032	Fish, Grouper, baked or broiled (dry heat)	3.0 oz	85	100.3	21.1	0.0	0.0	1.1	0.2	0.3
15034	Fish, Haddock, baked or broiled (dry heat)	3.0 oz	85	95.2	20.6	0.0	0.0	0.8	0.1	0.3
15035	Fish, Haddock, smoked	1 cubic inch, boneless	17	19.7	4.3	0.0	0.0	0.2	0.0	0.1
15037	Fish, Halibut, Atlantic & Pacific, baked or broiled (dry heat)	3.0 oz	85	119.0	22.7	0.0	0.0	2.5	0.8	0.8
15196	Fish, Halibut, Greenland, cooked w/dry heat	3.0 oz	85	203.2	15.7	0.0	0.0	15.1	9.1	1.5
15040	Fish, Herring, Atlantic, baked or broiled (dry heat)	3.5 oz	100	203.0	23.0	0.0	0.0	11.6	4.8	2.7
15042	Fish, Herring, Atlantic, kippered	1.5 oz (1 piece 4⅜" x 1 ¾ " x ¼ ")	44	95.5	10.8	0.0	0.0	5.4	2.2	1.3
15041	Fish, Herring, Atlantic, pickled	0.5 oz (1 piece ¾ " x ⅞" x ½ ")	15	39.3	2.1	1.4	0.0	2.7	1.8	0.3
15121	Fish, Light Tuna, canned in H₂O, drained	3.5 oz	100	116.0	25.5	0.0	0.0	0.8	0.2	0.3
15183	Fish, Light Tuna, canned in oil w/o salt, drained	3.5 oz	100	198.0	29.1	0.0	0.0	8.2	2.9	2.9
15119	Fish, Light Tuna, canned in oil, drained	3.0 oz, 1 sm can	85	168.3	24.8	0.0	0.0	7.0	2.5	2.5
15047	Fish, Mackerel, Atlantic, baked or broiled (dry heat)	3.5 oz	100	262.0	23.9	0.0	0.0	17.8	7.0	4.3
15200	Fish, Mackerel, King, cooked w/dry heat	3.5 oz	100	134.0	26.0	0.0	0.0	2.6	1.0	0.6
15058	Fish, Ocean Perch, Atlantic, baked or broiled (dry heat)	3.5 oz	100	121.0	23.9	0.0	0.0	2.1	0.8	0.5
15061	Fish, Perch, baked or broiled (dry heat)	3.5 oz	100	117.0	24.9	0.0	0.0	1.2	0.2	0.5
15063	Fish, Pike, Northern, baked or broiled (dry heat)	3.5 oz	100	113.0	24.7	0.0	0.0	0.9	0.2	0.3
15204	Fish, Pike, Walleye, cooked w/dry heat	3.5 oz	100	119.0	24.5	0.0	0.0	1.6	0.4	0.6
15205	Fish, Pollock, Atlantic, cooked w/dry heat	3.5 oz	100	118.0	24.9	0.0	0.0	1.3	0.1	0.6
15067	Fish, Pollock, Walleye, baked or broiled	3.5 oz	100	113.0	23.5	0.0	0.0	1.1	0.2	0.5
15069	Fish, Pompano, Florida, baked or broiled (dry heat)	3.5 oz	100	211.0	23.7	0.0	0.0	12.1	3.3	1.5
915902	Fish, Roe, canned	1.0 oz	28	33.0	6.0	0.1	0.0	0.8	0.0	0.0
15232	Fish, Roughy, Orange, cooked w/dry heat	3.5 oz	100	89.0	18.9	0.0	0.0	0.9	0.6	0.0
15237	Fish, Salmon, Atlantic, Farmed, cooked w/dry heat	3.5 oz	100	206.0	22.1	0.0	0.0	12.4	4.4	4.4
15209	Fish, Salmon, Atlantic, Wild, cooked w/dryheat	3.5 oz	100	182.0	25.4	0.0	0.0	8.1	2.7	3.3

Sat (g)	Chol (mg)	Cal (mg)	Iron (mg)	Magn (mg)	Phos (mg)	Pota (mg)	Sodi (mg)	Zinc (mg)	Vit A (RE)	Vit C (mg)	Vit E (mg)	Thia (mg)	Ribo (mg)	Niac (mg)	Vit B-6 (mg)	Fol (µg)	Vit B-12 (µg)	Wat (g)
10.4	98.6	86.2	4.6	37.0	234.1	362.6	554.4	5.7	0.0	0.0	1.3	0.3	0.4	8.3	0.3	77.4	2.9	72.3
12.0	103.2	92.5	5.5	45.2	283.8	526.8	741.8	5.8	4.3	1.1	0.0	0.3	0.4	6.7	0.4	83.9	3.3	108.6
7.0	85.0	48.0	6.3	0.0	339.0	590.0	1075.0	8.4	25.6	0.0	0.0	0.2	0.4	9.0	0.5	29.0	0.0	0.0
10.1	103.0	256.0	4.0	0.0	314.0	249.0	950.0	4.7	70.4	2.0	0.0	0.5	0.4	6.8	0.3	21.0	1.8	0.0
0.0	34.0	0.0	0.0	0.0	0.0	220.0	545.0	0.0	0.0	0.0	0.0	0.0	0.0	0.0	0.0	0.0	0.0	0.0
4.1	35.1	63.0	2.4	18.9	102.6	144.9	387.0	2.0	0.0	0.0	0.5	0.3	0.3	3.7	0.1	53.1	0.9	33.8
7.0	65.0	32.0	4.5	0.0	118.0	275.0	475.0	2.0	18.8	0.0	0.0	0.2	0.2	5.0	0.1	0.5	0.0	0.0
3.6	37.0	122.0	2.3	0.0	126.0	142.0	500.0	2.1	30.4	2.0	0.0	0.3	0.2	3.8	0.1	17.0	0.8	0.0
8.0	55.0	150.0	1.4	0.0	200.0	140.0	990.0	1.9	20.0	0.0	0.0	0.1	0.2	3.0	0.1	25.0	1.2	0.0
8.0	55.0	80.0	1.8	0.0	150.0	175.0	985.0	1.8	30.0	0.0	0.0	0.1	0.3	4.0	0.2	30.0	1.2	0.0
6.0	45.0	80.0	1.4	21.0	80.0	130.0	830.0	1.4	0.0	0.0	0.0	0.1	0.1	3.0	0.1	20.0	0.9	0.0
3.0	20.0	40.0	1.8	0.0	60.0	197.0	345.0	1.2	0.0	0.0	0.0	0.2	0.3	4.0	0.1	7.0	0.0	0.0
7.0	39.0	80.0	3.6	0.0	0.0	422.0	590.0	0.0	17.0	1.0	0.0	0.2	0.4	7.6	0.2	14.0	0.0	0.0
4.0	34.0	105.0	4.0	0.0	0.0	260.0	730.0	0.0	108.4	3.0	0.0	0.9	0.2	3.7	0.0	0.0	0.0	0.0
7.8	64.0	235.0	2.3	0.0	353.0	231.0	820.0	1.3	48.0	0.0	0.0	0.6	0.3	4.8	0.1	12.0	0.0	0.0
4.0	39.0	80.0	2.7	0.0	250.0	346.0	850.0	2.2	60.0	4.8	0.0	0.2	0.4	12.0	0.5	20.0	0.0	0.0
3.3	399.0	57.0	2.1	0.0	264.0	135.0	290.0	1.7	103.6	0.0	0.0	0.1	0.3	0.1	0.2	65.0	0.9	0.0
5.0	45.0	480.0	1.0	0.0	429.0	520.0	340.0	1.6	58.4	0.0	0.0	0.2	0.8	0.4	0.1	0.0	1.1	0.0
5.0	50.0	45.0	0.9	0.0	238.0	585.0	220.0	0.9	71.0	0.0	0.0	0.2	0.6	0.5	0.1	17.0	0.0	0.0
0.6	10.0	327.0	0.1	0.0	289.0	487.0	170.0	1.0	61.2	0.0	0.0	0.1	0.5	0.3	0.1	11.0	1.6	0.0
6.0	33.0	295.0	0.0	32.0	284.0	508.0	213.0	1.0	0.0	0.0	0.0	0.1	0.6	0.0	0.0	0.0	0.0	0.0
0.5	4.9	299.0	3.6	100.0	249.6	400.4	130.0	4.4	249.6	59.8	29.9	0.4	0.4	5.0	0.7	140.4	2.1	199.9
5.4	200.1	83.6	3.0	39.4	344.4	183.7	1446.5	1.2	36.1	0.0	0.0	0.2	0.9	0.0	0.1	36.1	0.1	78.4
3.8	73.4	91.8	5.2	49.0	297.8	524.3	797.6	4.5	44.9	5.5	0.0	0.4	0.4	7.3	0.4	89.8	1.6	104.2
6.8	36.5	189.2	2.5	68.4	287.3	394.4	1650.7	2.6	79.8	12.3	0.0	1.0	0.8	5.5	0.1	86.6	1.1	131.8
7.1	73.4	41.0	2.8	67.0	192.2	330.5	844.6	4.4	49.7	5.6	0.0	0.4	0.4	6.0	0.3	71.3	1.8	127.4
5.3	48.6	74.2	2.6	79.4	220.2	335.4	1292.8	1.9	41.0	3.6	0.0	0.5	0.3	11.3	0.2	102.4	1.6	139.0
11.4	56.4	220.6	2.4	70.1	203.5	473.7	802.0	3.9	147.1	2.2	0.0	0.2	0.4	3.2	0.2	68.4	1.0	99.9
5.2	21.0	100.0	1.1	0.0	146.0	257.0	406.0	1.2	80.0	2.8	0.0	0.1	0.2	1.0	0.1	0.0	0.5	0.0
5.4	30.2	210.2	1.9	59.0	116.6	403.2	542.9	1.9	85.0	1.3	0.0	0.1	0.3	1.3	0.2	43.2	0.7	95.4
11.5	74.3	189.0	2.5	67.5	173.3	490.5	870.8	3.2	173.3	4.1	0.0	0.1	0.5	2.9	0.2	85.5	1.1	158.5
80.4	194.8	0.1	0.0	0.0	0.0	0.0	0.0	0.2	0.0	0.0	2.5	0.0	0.0	0.0	0.0	0.0	0.0	0.0
0.0	0.0	56.0	0.9	0.0	266.0	0.0	0.0	12.8	0.0	0.0	0.0	0.0	0.0	0.0	0.0	0.0	0.0	79.2
0.0	0.0	79.0	1.6	0.0	0.0	242.2	824.6	0.0	0.0	0.0	0.0	0.2	0.3	1.6	0.0	0.0	0.0	0.0
1.0	87.0	103.0	1.9	38.0	256.0	456.0	90.0	0.8	35.0	2.1	0.0	0.1	0.1	1.5	0.1	17.0	2.3	68.8
0.8	127.7	23.6	1.3	63.2	315.0	406.7	109.1	0.6	38.4	0.0	0.0	0.1	0.0	3.2	0.4	12.4	5.5	91.0
1.4	88.9	10.5	0.7	49.1	340.5	558.1	90.1	1.2	161.5	0.0	0.0	0.1	0.1	8.5	0.5	2.3	7.3	73.3
2.4	142.8	88.4	2.7	64.6	902.7	725.9	107.1	3.2	15.3	2.7	0.0	0.2	0.1	3.6	0.4	29.4	2.5	118.4
2.6	91.5	12.9	1.2	37.2	350.4	459.0	114.4	1.5	21.5	1.1	0.0	0.6	0.1	3.6	0.2	10.0	4.0	102.4
1.1	103.0	15.7	0.5	40.0	434.7	599.2	71.5	0.9	21.5	1.1	0.0	0.3	0.1	3.4	0.2	14.3	4.1	111.1
1.2	170.5	79.8	3.4	87.0	103.2	52.5	435.0	0.3	162.4	0.0	2.0	0.1	0.2	0.0	0.1	14.5	5.8	13.8
0.3	99.0	25.2	0.9	75.6	248.4	439.2	140.4	1.0	25.2	1.8	0.5	0.2	0.1	4.5	0.5	14.6	1.9	136.7
0.4	121.6	128.0	2.0	106.4	760.0	1166.4	5621.6	1.3	33.6	2.8	0.5	0.2	0.2	6.0	0.7	19.8	8.0	12.9
0.1	40.0	7.7	0.3	26.4	189.6	439.5	77.4	0.4	8.5	2.6	0.0	0.0	0.0	2.1	0.4	6.8	0.9	64.6
1.8	63.8	11.4	0.4	14.3	103.2	148.8	331.7	0.4	17.7	0.0	0.8	0.1	0.1	1.2	0.0	10.4	1.0	26.4
0.3	40.0	17.9	1.0	31.5	121.6	403.8	45.1	0.4	42.5	0.0	0.0	0.1	0.0	0.3	0.3	8.7	0.6	62.4
0.1	62.9	35.7	1.1	42.5	204.9	339.2	74.0	0.4	16.2	0.0	0.0	0.0	0.0	3.9	0.3	11.3	1.2	63.1
0.0	13.1	8.3	0.2	9.2	42.7	70.6	129.7	0.1	3.7	0.0	0.1	0.0	0.0	0.9	0.1	2.6	0.3	12.2
0.4	34.9	51.0	0.9	91.0	242.3	489.6	58.7	0.5	45.9	0.0	0.9	0.1	0.1	6.1	0.3	11.7	1.2	60.9
2.6	50.2	3.4	0.7	28.1	178.5	292.4	87.6	0.4	15.3	0.0	0.0	0.1	0.1	1.6	0.2	0.9	0.8	52.6
2.6	77.0	74.0	1.4	41.0	303.0	419.0	115.0	1.3	31.0	0.7	1.3	0.1	0.3	4.1	0.3	11.5	13.1	64.2
1.2	36.1	37.0	0.7	20.2	143.0	196.7	403.9	0.6	17.2	0.4	0.4	0.1	0.1	1.9	0.2	6.0	8.2	26.3
0.4	2.0	11.6	0.2	1.2	13.4	10.4	130.5	0.1	38.7	0.0	0.2	0.0	0.0	0.5	0.0	0.4	0.6	8.3
0.2	30.0	11.0	1.5	27.0	163.0	237.0	338.0	0.8	17.0	0.0	0.5	0.0	0.1	13.3	0.4	4.0	3.0	74.5
1.5	18.0	13.0	1.4	31.0	311.0	207.0	50.0	0.9	23.0	0.0	0.0	0.0	0.1	12.4	0.1	5.3	2.2	59.8
1.3	15.3	11.1	1.2	26.4	264.4	176.0	300.9	0.8	19.6	0.0	1.0	0.0	0.1	10.5	0.1	4.5	1.9	50.9
4.2	75.0	15.0	1.6	97.0	278.0	401.0	83.0	0.9	54.0	0.4	0.0	0.2	0.4	6.9	0.5	1.5	19.0	53.3
0.5	68.0	40.0	2.3	41.0	318.0	558.0	203.0	0.7	252.0	1.6	0.0	0.1	0.6	10.5	0.5	9.0	18.0	69.0
0.3	54.0	137.0	1.2	39.0	277.0	350.0	96.0	0.6	14.0	0.8	0.0	0.1	0.1	2.4	0.3	10.4	1.2	72.7
0.2	115.0	102.0	1.2	38.0	257.0	344.0	79.0	1.4	10.0	0.0	0.0	0.1	0.1	1.9	0.1	5.8	2.2	73.3
0.2	50.0	73.0	0.7	40.0	282.0	331.0	49.0	0.9	24.0	3.8	0.0	0.1	0.1	2.8	0.1	17.3	2.3	73.0
0.3	110.0	141.0	1.7	38.0	269.0	499.0	65.0	0.8	24.0	0.0	0.0	0.3	0.2	2.8	0.1	17.0	2.3	73.5
0.2	91.0	77.0	0.6	86.0	283.0	456.0	110.0	0.6	12.0	0.0	0.0	0.1	0.2	4.0	0.3	3.0	3.7	72.0
0.2	96.0	6.0	0.3	73.0	482.0	387.0	116.0	0.6	23.0	0.0	0.2	0.1	0.1	1.7	0.1	3.6	4.2	74.1
4.5	64.0	43.0	0.7	31.0	341.0	636.0	76.0	0.7	36.0	0.0	0.0	0.7	0.2	3.8	0.2	17.3	1.2	63.0
0.0	0.0	4.2	0.3	0.0	96.9	0.0	0.0	0.0	0.0	0.0	0.0	0.0	0.0	0.0	0.0	0.0	0.0	20.3
0.0	26.0	38.0	0.2	38.0	256.0	385.0	81.0	1.0	24.0	0.0	0.0	0.1	0.2	3.7	0.3	8.0	2.3	69.1
2.5	63.0	15.0	0.3	30.0	252.0	384.0	61.0	0.4	15.0	3.7	0.0	0.3	0.1	8.0	0.6	34.0	2.8	64.8
1.3	71.0	15.0	1.0	37.0	256.0	628.0	56.0	0.8	13.0	0.0	0.0	0.3	0.5	10.1	0.9	29.0	3.1	59.6

Code	Food Name	Unit/Amt	Wt (g)	Energy (Kcal)	Prot (g)	Carb (g)	Fiber (g)	Fat (g)	Mono (g)	Poly (g)
15210	Fish, Salmon, Chinook, cooked w/dry heat	3.5 oz	100	231.0	25.7	0.0	0.0	13.4	5.7	2.7
15077	Fish, Salmon, Chinook, smoked	3.5 oz	100	117.0	18.3	0.0	0.0	4.3	2.0	1.0
15179	Fish, Salmon, Chinook, smoked, lox, regular	1.0 oz	28	32.8	5.1	0.0	0.0	1.2	0.6	0.3
15239	Fish, Salmon, Coho, Farmed, cooked w/dry heat	3.5 oz	100	178.0	24.3	0.0	0.0	8.2	3.6	2.0
15247	Fish, Salmon, Coho, Wild, cooked w/dry heat	3.5 oz	100	139.0	23.5	0.0	0.0	4.3	1.6	1.3
15082	Fish, Salmon, Coho, Wild, cooked w/moist heat	3.5 oz	100	184.0	27.4	0.0	0.0	7.5	2.7	2.5
15084	Fish, Salmon, Pink, canned, solids & liquid	3.5 oz	100	139.0	19.8	0.0	0.0	6.1	1.8	2.0
15212	Fish, Salmon, Pink, cooked w/dry heat	3.5 oz	100	149.0	25.6	0.0	0.0	4.4	1.2	1.7
15088	Fish, Sardine, Atlantic, w/bone, canned in oil, drained	1 small fish (2.66 x 0.5" x 0.25")	12	25.0	3.0	0.0	0.0	1.4	0.5	0.6
15089	Fish, Sardine, Pacific, w/bone, canned in tom sauce, drained	1 sardine	38	67.6	6.2	0.0	0.0	4.6	2.1	0.9
15092	Fish, Sea Bass, baked or broiled (dry heat)	3.5 oz	100	124.0	23.6	0.0	0.0	2.6	0.5	1.0
15214	Fish, Sea Trout, cooked w/dry heat	3.5 oz	100	133.0	21.5	0.0	0.0	4.6	1.1	0.9
15215	Fish, Shad, American, cooked w/dry heat	3.5 oz	100	252.0	21.7	0.0	0.0	17.7	0.0	0.0
15096	Fish, Shark, battered, fried	4.0 oz	120	273.6	22.3	7.7	0.0	16.6	7.1	4.4
15102	Fish, Snapper, baked or broiled (dry heat)	3.5 oz	100	128.0	26.3	0.0	0.0	1.7	0.3	0.6
15218	Fish, Sunfish/Pumpkin Seed, cooked w/dry heat	3.5 oz	100	114.0	24.9	0.0	0.0	0.9	0.2	0.3
15109	Fish, Surimi	3.0 oz	85	84.2	12.9	5.8	0.0	0.8	0.1	0.4
15111	Fish, Swordfish, baked or broiled (dry heat)	3.5 oz	100	155.0	25.4	0.0	0.0	5.1	2.0	1.2
15219	Fish, Trout, cooked w/dry heat	3.5 oz	100	190.0	26.6	0.0	0.0	8.5	4.2	1.9
15241	Fish, Trout, Rainbow, Farmed, cooked w/dry heat	3.5 oz	100	169.0	24.3	0.0	0.0	7.2	2.1	2.3
15116	Fish, Trout, Rainbow, Wild, cooked w/dry heat	3.5 oz	100	150.0	22.9	0.0	0.0	5.8	1.7	1.8
924207	Fish, Tuna Noodle Casserole	6.0 oz	170	193.8	11.4	15.8	1.0	9.4	0.0	0.0
924208	Fish, Tuna Pot Pie, frozen/Banquet	7.0 oz	198	540.5	17.0	44.0	0.0	33.0	0.0	0.0
15128	Fish, Tuna Salad	3.0 oz	85	159.0	13.6	8.0	0.0	7.9	2.5	3.5
15118	Fish, Tuna, Bluefin, baked or broiled (dry heat)	3.0 oz	85	156.4	25.4	0.0	0.0	5.3	1.7	1.6
915905	Fish, Tuna, canned, low sodium	2.0 oz	58	70.2	15.0	0.0	0.0	1.0	0.0	0.8
15221	Fish, Tuna, Yellowfin, fresh, cooked w/dry heat	3.5 oz	100	139.0	30.0	0.0	0.0	1.2	0.2	0.4
15222	Fish, Turbot, European, cooked w/dry heat	3.5 oz	100	122.0	20.6	0.0	0.0	3.8	0.0	0.0
15126	Fish, White Tuna, canned in H20, drained	3.0 oz	85	108.8	20.1	0.0	0.0	2.5	0.7	0.9
15124	Fish, White Tuna, canned in oil, drained	3.0 oz	85	158.1	22.6	0.0	0.0	6.9	2.1	2.9
15223	Fish, Whitefish, cooked w/dry heat	3.0 oz	85	146.2	20.8	0.0	0.0	6.4	2.2	2.3
15133	Fish, Whiting, baked or broiled (dry heat)	1 fillet	72	83.5	16.9	0.0	0.0	1.2	0.3	0.4
15225	Fish, Yellowtail, cooked w/dry heat	3.5 oz	85	159.0	25.2	0.0	0.0	5.7	0.0	0.0
2050	Flavoring, Vanilla Extract	1 tsp	4.2	12.1	0.0	0.5	0.0	0.0	0.0	0.0
20003	Flour, Arrowroot	1 tbsp	8	28.6	0.0	7.1	0.3	0.0	0.0	0.0
20130	Flour, Barley Flour or Meal	1 tbsp	9.25	31.9	1.0	6.9	0.9	0.1	0.0	0.1
20131	Flour, Barley Malt Flour	1 tbsp	10.1	36.5	1.0	7.9	0.7	0.2	0.0	0.1
920904	Flour, Bisquick Mix	½ cup	57	240.0	4.0	37.0	0.0	8.0	5.0	1.0
20090	Flour, Brown Rice	1 cup	158	573.5	11.4	120.8	7.3	4.4	1.6	1.6
20011	Flour, Buckwheat, Whole Groat	1 cup	120	402.0	15.1	84.7	12.0	3.7	1.1	1.1
20017	Flour, Corn, Masa, enriched	1 cup	114	416.1	10.6	86.9	10.9	4.3	1.1	2.0
20316	Flour, Corn, White, Whole Grain	1 cup	117	422.4	8.1	89.9	11.2	4.5	1.2	2.1
20016	Flour, Corn, Yellow, Whole Grain	1 cup	117	422.4	8.1	89.9	15.7	4.5	1.2	2.1
924291	Flour, Potato	½ cup	90	315.9	7.2	71.9	0.0	0.7	0.0	0.3
20061	Flour, Rice, White	1 cup	163	596.6	9.7	130.6	3.9	2.3	0.7	0.6
920906	Flour, Rye&Wheat	1 cup	128	457.0	14.1	96.5	0.0	1.7	0.0	0.0
20063	Flour, Rye, Dark	1 cup	128	414.7	18.0	88.0	28.9	3.4	0.4	1.5
20065	Flour, Rye, Light	1 cup	128	469.8	10.7	102.7	18.7	1.7	0.2	0.7
20064	Flour, Rye, Medium	1 cup	128	453.1	12.0	99.2	18.7	2.3	0.3	1.0
20070	Flour, Triticale, Whole Grain	1 cup	128	432.6	16.9	93.6	18.7	2.3	0.2	1.0
20081	Flour, Wheat, White, All Purpose, bleached, enriched	1 cup	125	455.0	12.9	95.4	3.4	1.2	0.1	0.5
20082	Flour, Wheat, White, All Purpose, Selfrise, enriched	1 cup	125	442.5	12.4	92.8	3.4	1.2	0.1	0.5
20083	Flour, Wheat, White, Bread, enriched	1 cup	125	451.3	15.0	90.7	3.0	2.1	0.2	0.9
20084	Flour, Wheat, White, Cake, enriched	1 cup	125	452.5	10.3	97.5	2.1	1.1	0.1	0.5
20086	Flour, Wheat, White, Tortilla Mix, enriched	1 cup	125	506.3	12.1	83.9	0.0	13.3	5.7	1.9
20080	Flour, Whole Wheat, whole grain	1 cup	125	423.8	17.1	90.7	15.3	2.3	0.3	1.0
18268	French Toast, frozen	1 piece	59	125.7	4.4	18.9	0.7	3.6	1.2	0.7
18269	French Toast, homemade w/reduced fat (2%) milk	1 slice	65	148.9	5.0	16.3	0.0	7.0	2.9	1.7
918381	French Toast, homemade w/whole milk	1 slice	65	150.8	5.0	16.2	0.0	7.3	0.0	0.0
924287	Frozen Meal, Beef Chop Suey	12.0 oz	340	282.2	13.6	38.8	0.0	8.2	0.0	0.0
924062	Frozen Meal, Beef Chop Suey/Banquet	8.0 oz	227	104.4	9.8	9.8	0.0	3.0	0.0	0.0
924255	Frozen Meal, Beef Enchilada/Banquet	7.0 oz	198	269.3	10.0	28.0	0.0	13.0	0.0	0.0
22402	Frozen Meal, Beef Macaroni/Healthy Choice	1 serving	240	211.2	14.1	33.5	4.6	2.2	1.2	0.3
924026	Frozen Meal, Beef Oriental/LeMenuLite	10.0 oz	284	221.5	18.8	24.5	0.0	5.4	3.0	0.9
924080	Frozen Meal, Beef Pepper Steak, diet/Armour	11.25 oz	319	220.1	17.0	29.0	0.0	4.0	0.0	0.0
22578	Frozen Meal, Beef Pot Roast w/whipped potatoes/ Stoffer Lean Cuisine Homestyle	1 package	255	206.6	17.3	22.4	3.6	5.4	2.3	0.8
22616	Frozen Meal, Beef Sirloin Salisbury Steak w/red skinned pots & vege/ Budget Gourm	1 package	311	261.2	18.3	33.9	7.2	5.9	1.8	0.9

Sat (g)	Chol (mg)	Cal (mg)	Iron (mg)	Magn (mg)	Phos (mg)	Pota (mg)	Sodi (mg)	Zinc (mg)	Vit A (RE)	Vit C (mg)	Vit E (mg)	Thia (mg)	Ribo (mg)	Niac (mg)	Vit B-6 (mg)	Fol (µg)	Vit B-12 (µg)	Wat (g)
3.2	85.0	28.0	0.9	122.0	371.0	505.0	60.0	0.6	149.0	4.1	0.0	0.0	0.2	10.0	0.5	35.0	2.9	65.6
0.9	23.0	11.0	0.9	18.0	164.0	175.0	784.0	0.3	26.0	0.0	1.4	0.0	0.1	4.7	0.3	1.9	3.3	72.0
0.3	6.4	3.1	0.2	5.0	45.9	49.0	560.0	0.1	7.3	0.0	0.0	0.0	0.1	1.3	0.1	0.5	0.9	20.2
1.9	63.0	12.0	0.4	34.0	332.0	460.0	52.0	0.5	59.0	1.5	0.0	0.1	0.1	7.4	0.6	14.0	3.2	67.0
1.1	55.0	45.0	0.6	33.0	322.0	434.0	58.0	0.6	39.0	1.4	0.8	0.1	0.1	8.0	0.6	13.0	5.0	71.5
1.6	57.0	46.0	0.7	35.0	298.0	455.0	53.0	0.5	32.0	1.0	0.0	0.1	0.2	7.8	0.6	9.0	4.5	65.4
1.5	55.0	213.0	0.8	34.0	329.0	326.0	554.0	0.9	17.0	0.0	1.4	0.0	0.2	6.5	0.3	15.4	4.4	68.8
0.7	67.0	17.0	1.0	33.0	295.0	414.0	86.0	0.7	41.0	0.0	0.0	0.2	0.1	8.5	0.2	5.0	3.5	69.7
0.2	17.0	45.8	0.4	4.7	58.8	47.6	60.6	0.2	8.0	0.0	0.0	0.0	0.0	0.6	0.0	1.4	1.1	7.2
1.2	23.2	91.2	0.9	12.9	139.1	129.6	157.3	0.5	26.6	0.4	1.4	0.0	0.1	1.6	0.0	9.2	3.4	26.0
0.7	53.0	13.0	0.4	53.0	248.0	328.0	87.0	0.5	64.0	0.0	0.0	0.1	0.2	1.9	0.5	5.8	0.3	72.1
1.3	106.0	22.0	0.4	40.0	321.0	437.0	74.0	0.6	35.0	0.0	0.0	0.1	0.2	2.9	0.5	6.0	3.5	71.9
0.0	96.0	60.0	1.2	38.0	349.0	492.0	65.0	0.5	36.0	0.0	0.0	0.2	0.3	10.8	0.5	17.0	0.1	59.2
3.8	70.8	60.0	1.3	51.6	232.8	186.0	146.4	0.6	64.8	0.0	0.0	0.1	0.1	3.3	0.4	18.0	1.5	72.1
0.4	47.0	40.0	0.2	37.0	201.0	522.0	57.0	0.4	35.0	1.6	0.0	0.1	0.0	0.3	0.5	5.8	3.5	70.4
0.2	86.0	103.0	1.5	38.0	231.0	449.0	103.0	2.0	17.0	1.0	0.0	0.1	0.1	1.5	0.1	17.0	2.3	73.7
0.2	25.5	7.7	0.2	36.6	239.7	95.2	121.6	0.3	17.0	0.0	0.0	0.0	0.0	0.2	0.0	1.4	1.4	64.9
1.4	50.0	6.0	1.0	34.0	337.0	369.0	115.0	1.5	41.0	1.1	0.0	0.0	0.1	11.8	0.4	2.3	2.0	68.8
1.5	74.0	55.0	1.9	28.0	314.0	463.0	67.0	0.9	19.0	0.5	0.0	0.4	0.4	5.8	0.2	15.0	7.5	63.4
2.1	68.0	86.0	0.3	32.0	266.0	441.0	42.0	0.5	86.0	3.3	0.0	0.2	0.1	8.8	0.4	24.0	5.0	67.5
1.6	69.0	86.0	0.4	31.0	269.0	448.0	56.0	0.5	15.0	2.0	0.0	0.2	0.1	5.8	0.3	19.0	6.3	70.5
0.0	27.0	102.0	1.0	0.0	0.0	238.0	731.0	0.0	13.6	0.0	0.0	0.1	0.3	3.4	0.0	0.0	0.0	130.9
0.0	30.0	146.0	2.0	0.0	228.0	280.0	810.0	0.0	116.0	2.0	0.0	0.4	0.4	6.3	0.0	0.0	0.0	
1.3	11.1	14.5	0.9	16.2	151.3	151.3	341.7	0.5	23.0	1.9	0.0	0.0	0.1	5.7	0.1	6.8	1.0	53.7
1.4	41.7	8.5	1.1	54.4	277.1	274.6	42.5	0.7	642.6	0.0	0.0	0.2	0.3	9.0	0.4	1.9	9.2	50.2
0.2	20.0	3.0	0.7	54.0	83.0	85.0	120.0	0.3	0.0	0.0	0.0	0.0	0.0	7.5	0.2	2.0	0.8	0.0
0.3	58.0	21.0	0.9	64.0	245.0	569.0	47.0	0.7	20.0	1.0	0.0	0.5	0.1	11.9	1.0	2.0	0.6	62.8
0.0	62.0	23.0	0.5	65.0	165.0	305.0	192.0	0.3	12.0	1.7	0.0	0.1	0.1	2.7	0.2	9.0	2.5	70.5
0.7	35.7	11.9	0.8	28.1	184.5	201.5	320.5	0.4	5.1	0.0	1.4	0.0	0.0	4.9	0.2	1.7	1.0	62.2
1.4	26.4	3.4	0.6	28.9	227.0	283.1	336.6	0.4	20.4	0.0	0.0	0.0	0.1	9.9	0.4	3.9	1.9	54.4
1.0	65.5	28.1	0.4	35.7	294.1	345.1	55.3	1.1	33.2	0.0	0.0	0.1	0.1	3.3	0.3	14.5	0.8	55.3
0.3	60.5	44.6	0.3	19.4	205.2	312.5	95.0	0.4	24.5	0.0	0.2	0.0	0.0	1.2	0.1	10.8	1.9	53.8
0.0	60.4	24.7	0.5	32.3	170.9	457.3	42.5	0.6	26.4	2.5	0.0	0.1	0.2	7.4	0.2	3.4	1.1	57.2
0.0	0.0	0.5	0.0	0.5	0.3	6.2	0.4	0.0	0.0	0.0	0.0	0.0	0.0	0.0	0.0	0.0	0.0	2.2
0.0	0.0	3.2	0.0	0.2	0.4	0.9	0.2	0.0	0.0	0.0	0.0	0.0	0.0	0.0	0.0	0.6	0.0	0.9
0.0	0.0	3.0	0.2	8.9	27.4	28.6	0.4	0.2	0.0	0.0	0.0	0.0	0.0	0.6	0.0	0.7	0.0	1.1
0.0	0.0	3.7	0.5	9.8	30.6	22.6	1.1	0.2	0.2	0.1	0.0	0.0	0.0	0.6	0.1	3.8	0.0	0.8
2.0	0.0	0.0	0.0	0.0	0.0	0.0	80.0	0.0	700.0	0.0	0.0	0.0	0.0	0.0	0.0	0.0	0.0	0.0
0.9	0.0	17.4	3.1	177.0	532.5	456.6	12.6	3.9	0.0	0.0	1.1	0.7	0.1	10.0	1.2	25.3	0.0	18.9
0.8	0.0	49.2	4.9	301.2	404.4	692.4	13.2	3.7	0.0	0.0	1.2	0.5	0.2	7.4	0.7	64.8	0.0	13.4
0.6	0.0	160.7	8.2	125.4	254.2	339.7	5.7	2.0	0.0	0.0	0.3	1.6	0.9	11.2	0.4	213.2	0.0	10.3
0.6	0.0	8.2	2.8	108.8	318.2	368.6	5.9	2.0	0.0	0.0	0.3	0.3	0.1	2.2	0.4	29.3	0.0	12.8
0.6	0.0	8.2	2.8	108.8	318.2	368.6	5.9	2.0	55.0	0.0	0.3	0.3	0.1	2.2	0.4	29.3	0.0	12.8
0.2	0.0	30.0	15.5	0.0	160.0	1429.0	31.0	0.0	0.0	17.0	0.0	0.4	0.1	3.1	0.0	0.0	0.0	6.8
0.6	0.0	16.3	0.6	57.1	159.7	123.9	0.0	1.3	0.0	0.0	0.0	0.2	0.2	4.2	0.7	6.5	0.0	19.4
0.0	0.0	27.4	4.6	0.0	224.0	190.9	2.3	0.0	0.0	0.0	0.0	0.6	0.3	5.0	0.0	0.0	0.0	14.7
0.4	0.0	71.7	8.3	317.4	809.0	934.4	1.3	7.2	0.0	0.0	3.3	0.4	0.3	5.5	0.6	76.8	0.0	14.2
0.2	0.0	26.9	2.3	89.6	248.3	298.2	2.6	2.2	0.0	0.0	0.7	0.4	0.1	1.0	0.3	28.2	0.0	11.2
0.3	0.0	30.7	2.7	96.0	265.0	435.2	3.8	2.5	0.0	0.0	1.7	0.4	0.1	2.2	0.3	24.3	0.0	12.6
0.4	0.0	44.8	3.3	195.8	410.9	596.5	2.6	3.4	0.0	0.0	2.4	0.5	0.2	3.7	0.5	94.7	0.0	12.8
0.2	0.0	18.8	5.8	27.5	135.0	133.8	2.5	0.9	0.0	0.0	0.1	1.0	0.6	7.4	0.1	192.5	0.0	14.9
0.2	0.0	422.5	5.8	23.8	743.8	155.0	1587.5	0.8	0.0	0.0	0.1	0.8	0.5	7.3	0.1	192.5	0.0	13.2
0.3	0.0	18.8	5.5	31.3	121.3	125.0	2.5	1.1	0.0	0.0	0.1	1.0	0.6	9.4	0.0	192.5	0.0	16.7
0.2	0.0	17.5	9.2	20.0	106.3	131.3	2.5	0.8	0.0	0.0	0.1	1.1	0.5	8.5	0.0	192.5	0.0	15.6
5.1	0.0	256.3	8.8	26.3	262.5	125.0	846.3	0.8	0.0	0.0	0.0	0.9	0.6	7.3	0.1	170.0	0.0	12.8
0.4	0.0	42.5	4.9	172.5	432.5	506.3	6.3	3.7	0.0	0.0	1.5	0.6	0.3	8.0	0.4	55.0	0.0	12.8
0.9	48.4	63.1	1.3	10.0	82.0	79.1	292.1	0.5	31.9	0.2	0.4	0.2	0.2	1.6	0.3	30.7	1.0	31.0
1.8	75.4	65.0	1.1	11.1	76.1	87.1	311.4	0.4	85.8	0.2	0.0	0.1	0.2	1.1	0.0	28.0	0.2	35.6
1.7	3.0	64.4	1.1	11.1	76.1	86.5	310.7	0.4	80.6	0.2	0.0	0.1	0.2	1.1	0.0	15.0	0.2	35.4
0.0	0.0	44.0	2.4	0.0	116.0	173.0	1802.0	0.0	68.0	4.0	0.0	0.1	0.1	3.0	0.0	0.0	0.0	0.0
1.5	0.0	32.0	2.1	0.0	68.0	136.0	1334.0	0.0	32.2	2.0	0.0	0.0	0.1	1.1	0.0	0.0	0.0	0.0
0.0	0.0	52.0	1.0	0.0	207.0	92.0	1477.0	0.0	35.8	0.0	0.0	0.2	0.1	1.9	0.0	0.0	0.0	0.0
0.7	14.4	45.6	2.7	36.0	134.4	364.8	444.0	1.2	50.4	58.1	1.5	0.3	0.2	3.1	0.2	105.6	0.1	187.7
1.5	39.0	39.0	3.4	0.0	0.0	362.0	560.0	0.0	289.8	9.0	0.0	0.1	0.5	3.4	0.0	0.0	0.0	0.0
0.0	35.0	50.0	2.0	0.0	139.0	320.0	970.0	0.0	105.4	15.0	0.0	0.2	0.3	1.6	0.0	0.0	0.0	0.0
1.3	38.3	0.0	0.0	0.0	0.0	0.0	494.7	0.0	0.0	0.0	0.0	0.0	0.0	0.0	0.0	0.0	0.0	206.8
2.0	43.5	0.0	3.0	0.0	0.0	0.0	494.5	0.0	0.0	51.0	0.0	0.0	0.0	0.0	0.0	0.0	0.0	249.7

Code	Food Name	Unit/Amt	Wt (g)	Energy (Kcal)	Prot (g)	Carb (g)	Fiber (g)	Fat (g)	Mono (g)	Poly (g)
924032	Frozen Meal, Beef Stew/Stouffer	5.0 oz	142	129.2	9.7	7.2	0.0	6.8	0.0	0.0
924229	Frozen Meal, Beef Stroganoff, diet/Armour	11.25 oz	319	248.8	18.0	33.0	0.0	6.0	0.0	0.0
924230	Frozen Meal, Beef Stroganoff/LeMenu	10.0 oz	284	383.4	26.5	23.8	0.0	20.3	0.0	0.0
924137	Frozen Meal, Beef Szechuan/LeanCuisine	9.2 oz	262	280.3	20.0	25.0	0.0	11.0	6.0	2.0
924231	Frozen Meal, Beef Teriyaki	9.0 oz	255	270.3	20.0	36.0	0.0	5.0	0.0	0.0
924025	Frozen Meal, Beef w/gravy/Banquet	4.0 oz	113	99.4	8.0	5.0	0.0	5.0	0.0	0.0
924268	Frozen Meal, Belgian Waffles&Berries/Swanson	3.5 oz	99	201.0	3.2	30.8	0.0	7.1	0.0	0.0
22679	Frozen Meal, Breakfast Burrito, Ham & Cheese Flavor	1 package	99	211.9	9.6	27.8	1.4	6.9	2.1	1.8
924031	Frozen Meal, Cannelloni/LeanCuisine	9.6 oz	273	270.3	19.0	25.0	0.0	10.0	5.0	1.0
924232	Frozen Meal, Cheese Cannelloni/Stouffer	5.5 oz	156	171.6	10.1	13.7	0.0	8.7	0.0	0.0
924292	Frozen Meal, Cheese Enchilada/Banquet	12.0 oz	340	550.8	22.0	71.0	0.0	19.0	0.0	0.0
924122	Frozen Meal, Cheese Lasagna/DiningLite	9.0 oz	225	261.0	14.0	36.0	0.0	6.0	0.0	0.0
924233	Frozen Meal, Cheese Tomato Cannelloni/LeanCuisine	9.1 oz	258	270.9	22.0	24.0	0.0	10.0	4.0	1.0
22577	Frozen Meal, Chicken & Vegetables w/vermicelli/Stouffer Lean Cuisine	1 package	297	252.5	18.7	32.1	5.0	5.6	2.1	1.4
22581	Frozen Meal, Chicken a l'Orange in Sauce w/broccoli & rice/ Stouffer's Lean Cuisi	1 package	255	267.8	24.5	38.5	0.0	1.8	0.5	0.4
924040	Frozen Meal, Chicken ala King&Rice/Swanson	9.0 oz	255	275.4	14.4	32.1	1.0	9.9	0.0	0.0
22610	Frozen Meal, Chicken Alfredo w/fettucini & vege/Stouffer's Lunch Express	1 package	272	372.6	19.0	32.6	3.8	18.5	6.3	2.4
924048	Frozen Meal, Chicken Cacciatore/LeanCuisine	10.9 oz	308	280.3	23.0	25.0	0.0	10.0	7.0	2.0
924234	Frozen Meal, Chicken Cannelloni, diet/LeMenu	10.3 oz	291	261.9	14.9	39.2	0.0	5.0	1.6	1.8
924254	Frozen Meal, Chicken Chow Mein/LeanCuisine	11.3 oz	319	248.8	14.0	36.0	0.0	5.0	3.0	1.0
22588	Frozen Meal, Chicken Enchilada Suprema w/green chili sauce, rice, corn&apple ras	1 package	320	297.6	13.0	46.0	4.2	6.7	2.6	1.0
924257	Frozen Meal, Chicken Enchilada/LeMenuLite	8.25 oz	234	269.1	19.1	33.2	0.0	6.6	2.7	1.9
924084	Frozen Meal, Chicken Fettucini/Armour	11.0 oz	312	259.0	17.0	28.0	0.0	9.0	0.0	0.0
924326	Frozen Meal, Chicken Fried Steak/Worthington	6.2 oz	176	580.8	28.0	25.0	1.0	41.0	0.0	0.0
924244	Frozen Meal, Chicken Parmesan/LeanCuisine	10.0 oz	283	249.0	25.0	19.0	0.0	8.0	4.0	2.0
924240	Frozen Meal, Chicken Piccata	11.0 oz	312	343.2	21.0	22.9	0.0	18.5	0.0	0.0
22906	Frozen Meal, Chicken Pot Pie, frozen entree	1 serving	217	483.9	13.0	42.7	1.7	29.1	12.5	4.5
22587	Frozen Meal, Chicken Teriyaki w/rice, mixed vege w/butter sauce& apple cherry com	1 package	312	268.3	17.1	37.1	2.8	5.6	2.2	0.5
924283	Frozen Meal, Chicken&Noodle/Armour	11.0 oz	312	230.9	19.0	23.0	0.0	7.0	0.0	0.0
924091	Frozen Meal, Chicken, Sweet&Sour Dinner/LeMenu	10.5 oz	298	381.4	18.8	41.0	0.0	15.7	0.0	0.0
924289	Frozen Meal, Corned Beef Hash	10.0 oz	284	372.0	19.9	42.6	0.0	13.3	0.0	0.0
924180	Frozen Meal, Egg Souffle w/broccoli&cheese/Stouffer	4.0 oz	113	151.4	8.4	7.7	0.0	9.6	0.0	0.0
22614	Frozen Meal, Escalloped Chicken & Noodles/Stouffer's	1 package	283	365.1	17.0	3.7	0.0	31.4	7.7	13.6
924294	Frozen Meal, Filet of Sole/LeMenu	10.0 oz	284	355.0	17.9	43.5	3.7	12.1	0.0	0.0
924216	Frozen Meal, Fried Chicken/Banquet	10.0 oz	284	400.4	15.0	45.0	0.0	22.0	0.0	0.0
924046	Frozen Meal, Glazed Chicken/LeanCuisine	8.5 oz	241	269.9	26.0	23.0	0.0	8.0	3.0	4.0
924261	Frozen Meal, Green Pepper Steak/Stouffer	3.0 oz	85	85.9	7.7	3.8	0.0	4.4	0.0	0.0
22673	Frozen Meal, Italian Sausage Lasagna/Budget Gourmet	1 package	298	455.9	20.6	39.9	3.0	23.8	9.8	2.0
924296	Frozen Meal, Lasagna	13.0 oz	369	391.1	19.0	54.0	0.0	14.0	0.0	0.0
22570	Frozen Meal, Lasagna w/meat & sauce/Stouffer	1 package	595	767.6	51.8	73.2	8.9	29.8	9.6	1.5
924117	Frozen Meal, Lasagna/LeanCuisine	10.3 oz	291	279.4	27.0	24.0	0.0	8.0	5.0	0.0
924267	Frozen Meal, Linguini w/clam sauce/LeanCuisine	9.6 oz	272	261.1	16.0	32.0	0.0	7.0	4.0	2.0
22576	Frozen Meal, Macaroni & Beef in Tomato Sauce/Stouffer Lean Cuisine	1 package	283	249.0	13.9	36.5	3.4	5.4	2.1	0.7
22680	Frozen Meal, Macaroni & Beef in Tomato Sauce/WW	1 package	269	282.5	15.6	44.7	6.7	4.6	1.8	0.6
924092	Frozen Meal, Macaroni&Cheese Dinner/Banquet	10.0 oz	284	420.3	14.0	46.0	0.0	20.0	0.0	0.0
924280	Frozen Meal, Manicotti w/tomato sauce/LeMenu	11.7 oz	333	392.9	20.0	44.3	0.0	15.2	0.0	0.0
22675	Frozen Meal, Meat Loaf w/tomato sauce, mashed pot & carrots in seasoned sauce/B	1 package	453	611.6	29.1	33.6	6.3	40.0	17.3	7.2
924114	Frozen Meal, Meatballs Italian Style/Stouffer	13.0 oz	369	483.4	24.5	60.4	0.2	15.9	0.0	0.0
924093	Frozen Meal, Meatloaf/LeMenu	10.0 oz	284	301.0	17.8	27.3	0.0	13.3	0.0	0.0
924302	Frozen Meal, Mexican Combo Dinner/Banquet	12.0 oz	340	520.2	20.0	72.0	0.0	17.0	0.0	0.0
924305	Frozen Meal, Noodles&Chicken/Banquet	10.0 oz	284	349.3	10.0	42.0	0.0	15.0	0.0	0.0
22571	Frozen Meal, Original Fried Chicken Meal w/mashed pots & corn in seasoned sauce/	1 package	228	469.7	21.5	35.1	2.1	27.0	15.4	2.4
924238	Frozen Meal, Pasta Primavera/Campbell	10.0 oz	284	14.2	22.2	39.9	0.0	0.0	0.0	0.0
924177	Frozen Meal, Pasta, Cheese Tortellini/Stouffer	4.5 oz	128	267.5	15.4	26.9	0.0	10.9	0.0	0.0
924308	Frozen Meal, Pasta, Ravioli Dinner/Swanson	16.0 oz	468	486.7	16.1	68.3	0.0	16.8	0.0	0.0
924193	Frozen Meal, Pasta, Spaghetti w/meat sauce/Banquet	8.0 oz	227	270.1	14.0	35.0	1.0	8.0	0.0	0.0
924191	Frozen Meal, Pasta, Spaghetti w/meat sauce/LeMenuLite	9.5 oz	269	285.1	12.6	44.6	0.0	6.1	3.6	1.3
924311	Frozen Meal, Pasta, Spaghetti&Meatballs/Swanson	12.5 oz	354	375.2	13.5	46.0	0.0	15.1	0.0	0.0
22569	Frozen Meal, Pepper, Stuffed w/Beef in Tomato Sauce/Stouffer	1 package	439	377.5	15.8	41.7	10.5	16.2	7.5	1.1
924090	Frozen Meal, Pork Ham/LeMenu	10.0 oz	284	286.8	18.3	31.0	0.0	10.1	0.0	0.0
22609	Frozen Meal, Rice & Chicken Stir-Fry w/vegetables/ Stouffer's Lean Cuisine Lunch	1 package	255	270.3	11.7	39.5	5.9	7.4	3.5	2.0
924156	Frozen Meal, Rigatoni Pasta/Stouffer	6.0 oz	170	180.2	11.7	17.0	0.0	7.1	0.0	0.0

Sat (g)	Chol (mg)	Cal (mg)	Iron (mg)	Magn (mg)	Phos (mg)	Pota (mg)	Sodi (mg)	Zinc (mg)	Vit A (RE)	Vit C (mg)	Vit E (mg)	Thia (mg)	Ribo (mg)	Niac (mg)	Vit B-6 (mg)	Fol (μg)	Vit B-12 (μg)	Wat (g)
0.0	28.0	14.0	1.3	0.0	0.0	213.0	540.0	0.0	213.0	3.0	0.0	0.1	0.1	1.4	0.0	0.0	0.0	116.4
0.0	55.0	56.0	2.0	0.0	196.0	320.0	510.0	0.0	580.8	43.0	0.0	0.3	0.2	1.6	0.0	0.0	0.0	0.0
0.0	0.0	107.0	4.3	0.0	0.0	469.0	867.0	0.0	220.6	1.0	0.0	0.1	0.3	5.1	0.0	0.0	0.0	0.0
3.0	95.0	40.0	1.8	0.0	0.0	320.0	720.0	0.0	250.0	12.0	0.0	0.1	0.3	4.0	0.0	0.0	0.0	0.0
0.0	45.0	29.0	2.0	0.0	152.0	370.0	850.0	0.0	146.4	2.0	0.0	0.2	0.2	3.4	0.0	0.0	0.0	0.0
0.0	40.0	10.0	2.0	0.0	0.0	81.0	426.0	0.0	5.8	0.0	0.0	0.0	0.1	1.2	0.0	0.0	0.0	0.0
0.0	0.0	45.0	1.1	0.0	0.0	165.0	235.0	0.0	3.8	3.0	0.0	0.1	0.1	0.7	0.0	0.0	0.0	0.0
2.0	192.1	0.0	3.2	0.0	0.0	0.0	404.9	0.0	0.0	0.0	0.0	0.0	0.0	0.0	0.0	0.0	0.0	53.3
4.0	45.0	200.0	1.4	0.0	0.0	400.0	940.0	0.0	400.0	0.0	0.0	0.2	0.3	2.0	0.0	0.0	0.0	0.0
0.0	20.0	218.0	0.6	0.0	0.0	218.0	608.0	0.0	156.0	17.0	0.0	0.1	0.2	0.9	0.0	0.0	0.0	121.7
0.0	0.0	281.0	3.0	0.0	388.0	420.0	2170.0	0.0	142.2	7.0	0.0	0.4	0.3	2.4	0.0	0.0	0.0	0.0
0.0	0.0	307.0	2.0	0.0	0.0	770.0	800.0	0.0	397.6	7.0	0.0	0.2	0.3	1.9	0.0	0.0	0.0	0.0
5.0	30.0	300.0	0.7	0.0	0.0	330.0	900.0	0.0	150.0	6.0	0.0	0.1	0.3	1.2	0.0	0.0	0.0	0.0
1.0	23.8	104.0	1.3	0.0	0.0	0.0	582.1	0.0	0.0	14.6	0.0	0.0	0.0	0.0	0.0	0.0	0.0	237.9
0.4	45.9	0.0	0.0	0.0	0.0	0.0	359.6	0.0	0.0	18.1	0.0	0.0	0.0	0.0	0.0	0.0	0.0	188.4
0.0	0.0	64.0	0.9	0.0	0.0	217.0	859.0	0.0	116.6	2.0	0.0	0.1	0.3	5.0	0.0	0.0	0.0	0.0
7.0	57.1	146.9	0.0	0.0	0.0	0.0	587.5	0.0	0.0	24.2	0.0	0.0	0.0	0.0	0.0	0.0	0.0	199.1
1.0	45.0	40.0	1.8	0.0	0.0	440.0	950.0	0.0	100.0	12.0	0.0	0.1	0.2	5.0	0.0	0.0	0.0	0.0
1.6	38.0	93.0	3.1	0.0	0.0	368.0	621.0	0.0	350.6	9.0	0.0	0.6	0.4	3.2	0.0	0.0	0.0	0.0
1.0	30.0	40.0	1.1	0.0	0.0	270.0	1030.0	0.0	20.0	15.0	0.0	0.1	0.2	4.0	0.0	0.0	0.0	0.0
3.1	38.4	134.4	0.8	0.0	236.8	384.0	563.2	0.0	0.0	18.2	0.0	0.0	0.0	0.0	0.0	0.0	0.0	251.5
2.0	33.0	215.0	1.8	0.0	0.0	624.0	537.0	0.0	68.8	11.0	0.0	0.1	0.4	3.2	0.0	0.0	0.0	0.0
0.0	50.0	146.0	2.0	0.0	300.0	400.0	660.0	0.0	329.8	61.0	0.0	0.2	0.2	3.8	0.0	0.0	0.0	0.0
0.0	95.0	20.0	4.1	0.0	198.0	390.0	1040.0	0.0	9.4	0.0	0.0	0.2	0.2	4.9	0.0	0.0	0.0	0.0
2.0	70.0	150.0	1.4	0.0	0.0	750.0	850.0	0.0	100.0	6.0	0.0	0.2	0.3	7.0	0.0	0.0	0.0	0.0
0.0	0.0	96.0	2.9	0.0	0.0	135.0	1148.0	0.0	178.6	6.0	0.0	0.2	0.1	8.0	0.0	0.0	0.0	0.0
9.7	41.2	32.6	2.1	23.9	119.4	256.1	857.2	1.0	342.9	1.5	3.8	0.3	0.4	4.1	0.2	52.1	0.2	130.0
3.0	43.7	37.4	1.1	0.0	224.6	424.3	602.2	0.0	0.0	12.2	0.0	0.0	0.0	0.0	0.0	0.0	0.0	249.6
0.0	50.0	87.0	2.0	0.0	213.0	540.0	660.0	0.0	895.6	57.0	0.0	0.2	0.2	4.7	0.0	0.0	0.0	0.0
0.0	0.0	80.0	2.1	0.0	0.0	400.0	1020.0	0.0	329.6	5.0	0.0	0.1	0.2	5.5	0.0	0.0	0.0	0.0
0.0	0.0	65.0	4.0	0.0	148.0	318.0	1752.0	0.0	70.4	13.0	0.0	0.2	0.1	3.1	0.0	0.0	0.0	0.0
0.0	141.0	130.0	0.9	0.0	0.0	158.0	509.0	0.0	65.6	9.0	0.0	0.1	0.3	0.5	0.0	0.0	0.0	84.8
6.6	76.4	116.0	1.1	0.0	0.0	0.0	1211.2	0.0	0.0	0.0	0.0	0.0	0.0	0.0	0.0	0.0	0.0	202.9
0.0	0.0	105.0	2.0	0.0	0.0	341.0	956.0	0.0	415.8	2.0	0.0	0.2	0.3	2.4	0.0	0.0	0.0	0.0
0.0	0.0	46.0	1.0	0.0	0.0	480.0	1100.0	0.0	112.8	8.0	0.0	0.1	0.1	4.9	0.0	0.0	0.0	0.0
1.0	60.0	20.0	0.7	0.0	0.0	390.0	710.0	0.0	20.0	2.0	0.0	0.1	0.1	8.0	0.0	0.0	0.0	0.0
0.0	19.0	14.0	0.9	0.0	0.0	170.0	527.0	0.0	27.2	7.0	0.0	0.0	0.1	1.5	0.0	0.0	0.0	67.2
8.2	47.7	315.9	2.7	0.0	0.0	0.0	902.9	0.0	0.0	0.0	0.0	0.0	0.0	0.0	0.0	0.0	0.0	209.5
0.0	0.0	0.0	0.0	0.0	0.0	0.0	825.0	0.0	0.0	0.0	0.0	0.0	0.0	0.0	0.0	0.0	0.0	0.0
13.0	113.1	636.7	0.0	0.0	0.0	0.0	2034.9	0.0	0.0	0.0	0.0	0.0	0.0	0.0	0.0	0.0	0.0	431.4
3.0	70.0	250.0	1.4	0.0	0.0	540.0	1000.0	0.0	400.0	5.0	0.0	0.9	0.4	4.0	0.0	0.0	0.0	0.0
1.0	30.0	20.0	1.8	0.0	0.0	100.0	800.0	0.0	0.0	0.0	0.0	0.1	0.1	1.2	0.0	0.0	0.0	0.0
1.6	22.6	0.0	2.2	0.0	0.0	0.0	563.2	0.0	0.0	157.3	0.0	0.0	0.0	0.0	0.0	0.0	0.0	224.7
1.6	13.5	0.0	5.7	0.0	0.0	0.0	492.3	0.0	0.0	27.4	0.0	0.0	0.0	0.0	0.0	0.0	0.0	201.5
0.0	30.0	272.0	3.0	0.0	0.0	340.0	450.0	0.0	1517.6	7.0	0.0	0.3	0.4	2.4	0.0	0.0	0.0	0.0
0.0	0.0	493.0	3.1	0.0	0.0	4.0	871.0	0.0	22.0	17.0	0.0	0.3	0.4	4.0	0.0	0.0	0.0	0.0
15.5	113.3	77.0	3.9	0.0	0.0	0.0	1943.4	0.0	0.0	7.7	0.0	0.0	0.0	0.0	0.0	0.0	0.0	343.4
0.0	0.0	148.0	5.7	0.0	0.0	645.0	935.0	0.0	335.8	16.0	0.0	0.3	0.4	4.9	0.0	0.0	0.0	0.0
0.0	0.0	97.0	4.0	0.0	0.0	626.0	860.0	0.0	934.4	5.0	0.0	0.2	0.3	4.3	0.0	0.0	0.0	0.0
0.0	0.0	194.0	3.0	0.0	418.0	420.0	1980.0	0.0	107.8	7.0	0.0	0.4	0.2	2.7	0.0	0.0	0.0	0.0
0.0	45.0	29.0	2.0	0.0	0.0	250.0	460.0	0.0	1378.0	2.0	0.0	0.2	0.2	3.8	0.0	0.0	0.0	0.0
9.3	88.9	38.8	1.4	0.0	0.0	0.0	1500.2	0.0	0.0	1.4	0.0	0.0	0.0	0.0	0.0	0.0	0.0	140.8
0.0	0.0	265.0	2.4	0.0	0.0	80.0	882.0	0.0	204.4	2.0	0.0	0.1	0.3	2.1	0.0	0.0	0.0	0.0
0.0	77.0	243.0	1.0	0.0	0.0	95.0	326.0	0.0	7.6	1.0	0.0	0.1	0.2	1.2	0.0	0.0	0.0	73.0
0.0	0.0	162.0	4.4	0.0	0.0	275.0	975.0	0.0	196.6	25.0	0.0	0.3	0.3	4.2	0.0	0.0	0.0	0.0
0.0	0.0	29.0	3.0	0.0	188.0	421.0	1250.0	0.0	179.6	14.0	0.0	0.1	0.1	3.2	0.0	0.0	0.0	0.0
1.2	14.0	45.0	3.9	0.0	0.0	494.0	406.0	0.0	146.4	32.0	0.0	0.2	0.3	3.0	0.0	0.0	0.0	0.0
0.0	0.0	113.0	3.1	0.0	177.0	411.0	1097.0	2.4	242.4	14.0	0.0	0.2	0.2	3.4	0.2	0.0	0.5	0.0
5.4	43.9	0.0	0.0	0.0	0.0	0.0	1154.6	0.0	0.0	173.0	0.0	0.0	0.0	0.0	0.0	0.0	0.0	360.9
0.0	0.0	67.0	2.2	0.0	0.0	426.0	1486.0	0.0	1479.4	31.0	0.0	0.6	0.3	4.5	0.0	0.0	0.0	0.0
0.9	25.5	0.0	0.0	0.0	0.0	0.0	632.4	0.0	0.0	23.7	0.0	0.0	0.0	0.0	0.0	0.0	0.0	193.8
0.0	22.0	170.0	1.7	0.0	0.0	357.0	510.0	0.0	85.0	9.0	0.0	0.1	0.2	2.2	0.0	0.0	0.0	130.9

Code	Food Name	Unit/Amt	Wt (g)	Energy (Kcal)	Prot (g)	Carb (g)	Fiber (g)	Fat (g)	Mono (g)	Poly (g)
22712	Frozen Meal, Roasted Chicken w/garlic sauce, pasta & vegetable medley/Tyson	1 package	255	214.2	16.9	21.5	3.6	6.7	2.3	2.1
22583	Frozen Meal, Salisbury Steak in gravy & macaroni & cheese/ Stouffer Homestyle	1 package	272	386.2	22.6	26.4	0.0	21.2	7.9	1.8
924157	Frozen Meal, Salisbury Steak/Banquet	5.0 oz	142	190.3	9.0	8.0	0.5	14.0	0.0	0.0
924204	Frozen Meal, Sliced Beef/Swanson	15.2 oz	432	453.6	37.8	50.0	0.0	11.3	0.0	0.0
22580	Frozen Meal, Spaghetti w/meat sauce/Stouffer's Lean Cuisine	1 package	326	313.0	14.3	50.5	5.5	5.9	2.3	1.3
924260	Frozen Meal, Stuffed Shells/LeMenuLite	10.0 oz	284	269.8	17.3	33.5	0.0	7.3	2.8	1.2
22573	Frozen Meal, Swedish Meatballs w/pasta/Stouffer's Lean Cuisine	1 package	258	276.1	21.7	31.2	2.6	7.2	2.3	1.0
924101	Frozen Meal, Swiss Steak/Swanson	10.0 oz	284	346.5	26.2	37.0	0.0	10.5	0.0	0.0
22683	Frozen Meal, Teriyaki Chicken Breast w/Oriental veges/ Budget Gourmet Light & Hea	1 package	311	317.2	18.7	52.2	4.0	3.7	0.9	1.6
924176	Frozen Meal, Turkey w/gravy	5.0 oz	142	95.1	8.4	6.6	0.1	3.7	1.4	0.7
924215	Frozen Meal, Turkey w/gravy/Banquet	5.0 pz	142	99.4	7.0	5.0	0.1	6.0	0.0	0.0
924175	Frozen Meal, Turkey&Dressing/Armour	11.5 oz	326	319.5	19.0	34.0	0.0	12.0	0.0	0.0
924103	Frozen Meal, Turkey/Banquet	10.5 oz	298	390.4	18.0	35.0	0.0	20.0	0.0	0.0
924304	Frozen Meal, Veal Marsala/LeMenuLite	10.0 oz	284	249.9	25.3	25.4	0.0	5.2	3.2	1.0
924314	Frozen Meal, Veal Parmigiana Dinner/Armour	11.25 oz	319	398.8	18.0	34.0	0.0	22.0	0.0	0.0
924061	Frozen Meal, Vegetable Chow Mein/LeanCuisine	¾ cup	128	34.6	2.0	6.0	2.0	0.0	0.0	0.0
924115	Frozen Meal, Vegetable Lasagna/LeMenuLite	10.5 oz	298	253.3	12.4	34.0	0.0	7.4	3.2	1.5
924121	Frozen Meal, Vegetarian Lasagna	7.8 oz	221	316.0	20.0	30.0	2.0	14.0	5.0	1.5
924301	Frozen Meal, Ziti w/meat sauce/Swanson	17.6 oz	489	557.5	28.4	58.4	2.0	23.5	0.0	0.0
914896	Fruit Beverage Mix, Fruit Punch Drink, dry, prep	8 fl oz	262	96.9	0.0	24.8	0.0	23.6	0.0	0.0
914847	Fruit Beverage Mix, Grape/Crystal Light	8 fl oz	238	2.4	0.1	0.3	0.0	0.0	0.0	0.0
914844	Fruit Beverage Mix, Kool-Aid	8 fl oz	240	98.4	0.0	25.1	0.0	0.0	0.0	0.0
14127	Fruit Beverage Mix, Kool-Aid, sugar free w/aspartame & Vit C, dry mix, cherry fl	⅛ envelope	1.2	3.5	0.1	1.0	0.0	0.0	0.0	0.0
14290	Fruit Beverage Mix, Lemonade w/aspartame, low kcal, dry, prep	1 fl oz	29.6	0.6	0.0	0.1	0.0	0.0	0.0	0.0
14288	Fruit Beverage Mix, Lemonade, dry, prep w/H₂O	1 cup H₂O & 2 tbsp mix	264	103.0	0.0	26.9	0.0	0.0	0.0	0.0
914845	Fruit Beverage Mix, Lemonade/CountryTime	8 fl oz	240	81.6	0.0	20.5	0.0	0.0	0.0	0.0
14408	Fruit Beverage Mix, Orange Flavor Drink, dry, prep w/H₂O	1 fl oz	31	14.3	0.0	3.7	0.0	0.0	0.0	0.0
914807	Fruit Beverage Mix, w/sugar/Kool-Aid	8 fl oz	240	81.6	0.0	21.0	0.0	0.0	0.0	0.0
914897	Fruit Beverage, Cherry Juice Drink	6 fl oz	182	96.5	0.2	23.6	0.0	0.1	0.0	0.1
14263	Fruit Beverage, Citrus Drink, frozen concentrate, prep w/H₂O	1 cup (8 fl oz)	245	112.7	0.7	28.2	0.0	0.0	0.0	0.0
14238	Fruit Beverage, Cranberry-Apple Drink, bottled	1 cup (8 fl oz)	245	164.2	0.2	41.9	0.2	0.0	0.0	0.0
14242	Fruit Beverage, Cranberry Cocktail, bottled	12 fl oz can	435	248.0	0.0	62.6	0.4	0.4	0.1	0.2
14431	Fruit Beverage, Cranberry Juice Cocktail, frozen concentrate, prep w/H₂O	1 cup (8 fl oz)	262	144.1	0.0	36.7	0.3	0.0	0.0	0.0
14267	Fruit Beverage, Fruit Punch, canned	1 cup	247	116.1	0.0	29.4	0.2	0.0	0.0	0.0
14269	Fruit Beverage, Fruit Punch, frozen concentrate, prep w/H₂O	1 cup	247	113.6	0.0	28.9	0.2	0.0	0.0	0.0
14282	Fruit Beverage, Grape Juice Drink, canned	6 fl oz glass	188	94.0	0.2	24.3	0.2	0.0	0.0	0.0
914848	Fruit Beverage, Grapefruit Juice Cocktail	6 fl oz	180	79.2	0.0	20.0	0.1	0.0	0.0	0.0
914842	Fruit Beverage, Hawaiian Punch	8 fl oz	247	121.0	0.0	29.0	0.0	0.0	0.0	0.0
14406	Fruit Beverage, Juice Drink, frozen concentrate, prep	1 fl oz	31	15.5	0.0	3.8	0.0	0.1	0.0	0.0
914898	Fruit Beverage, Lemonade, canned	6 fl oz	184	64.4	0.0	16.5	0.0	0.0	0.0	0.0
14543	Fruit Beverage, Lemonade, Pink, frozen conc, prep w/H₂O	6 fl oz	186	74.4	0.2	19.5	0.0	0.0	0.0	0.0
14293	Fruit Beverage, Lemonade, White, frozen, prep w/H₂O	6 fl oz	186	74.4	0.2	19.5	0.2	0.0	0.0	0.0
14303	Fruit Beverage, Limeade, frozen concentrate, prep w/H₂O	6 fl oz	186	76.3	0.0	20.5	0.2	0.0	0.0	0.0
914843	Fruit Beverage, low kcal/Hawaiian Punch	8 fl oz	247	34.6	0.1	8.0	0.0	0.0	0.0	0.0
14323	Fruit Beverage, Orange Drink, canned	6 fl oz	186	94.9	0.0	24.0	0.2	0.0	0.0	0.0
914900	Fruit Beverage, Orange-Pineapple Juice Drink	6 fl oz	180	93.6	0.6	23.0	1.0	0.0	0.0	0.0
14334	Fruit Beverage, Pineapple & Grapefruit Juice Drink, canned	6 fl oz	186	87.4	0.4	21.6	0.2	0.2	0.0	0.1
14341	Fruit Beverage, Pineapple & Orange Juice Drink, canned	6 fl oz	186	93.0	2.4	21.9	0.2	0.0	0.0	0.0
914808	Fruit Beverage, Sugar Free/Kool-Aid	8 fl oz	240	2.4	0.1	0.3	0.0	0.0	0.0	0.0
914903	Fruit Beverage, Wild Berry Juice Drink	6 fl oz	185	90.7	0.0	23.0	0.0	0.0	0.0	0.0
9101	Fruit Cocktail (peach,pineapple,pear,grape&cherry)canned in ex-heavy syrup	½ cup	130	114.4	0.5	29.8	1.4	0.1	0.0	0.0
9098	Fruit Cocktail (peach,pineapple,pear,grape&cherry)canned in extralite syrup	½ cup	122	54.9	0.5	14.2	1.3	0.1	0.0	0.0
914839	Fruit Juice, Apple Juice Works/Campbells	6 fl oz	180	97.2	0.3	23.7	0.0	0.1	0.0	0.0
9400	Fruit Juice, Apple, canned or bottled, unsweetened w/added Vit C	6 fl oz	180	84.6	0.1	21.0	0.2	0.2	0.0	0.1
9411	Fruit Juice, Apple, frozen concentrate, unsweetened w/added Vit C, prep	6 fl oz container	211	99.2	0.3	24.3	0.2	0.2	0.0	0.1
9403	Fruit Juice, Apricot Nectar, canned, w/added Vit C	6 fl oz container	211	118.2	0.8	30.4	1.3	0.2	0.1	0.0
914910	Fruit Juice, Cranberry Apple Juice	6 fl oz container	211	192.0	1.1	48.8	1.1	10.2	0.0	0.0
914907	Fruit Juice, Cranberry Apple Juice, low kcal	6 fl oz container	211	35.9	0.2	8.4	0.0	0.2	0.0	0.2
9137	Fruit Juice, Grape, frozen concentrate, sweetened w/added Vit C, prep	6 fl oz container	216	110.2	0.4	27.5	0.2	0.2	0.0	0.0
9124	Fruit Juice, Grapefruit, canned, sweetened	6 fl oz container	216	99.4	1.3	24.0	0.2	0.2	0.0	0.0
9123	Fruit Juice, Grapefruit, canned, unsweetened	6 fl oz container	216	82.1	1.1	19.4	0.2	0.2	0.0	0.0
9126	Fruit Juice, Grapefruit, frozen concentrate, unsweetened, prep	1 fl oz	30.9	12.7	0.2	3.0	0.0	0.0	0.0	0.0
9404	Fruit Juice, Grapefruit, Pink or Red, fresh	1 cup	247	96.3	1.2	22.7	0.0	0.2	0.0	0.1
9128	Fruit Juice, Grapefruit, white, fresh	juice from 1 fruit	196	76.4	1.0	18.0	0.2	0.2	0.0	0.0
9153	Fruit Juice, Lemon, canned or bottled	1 tbsp	15.2	3.2	0.1	1.0	0.1	0.0	0.0	0.0

Sat (g)	Chol (mg)	Cal (mg)	Iron (mg)	Magn (mg)	Phos (mg)	Pota (mg)	Sodi (mg)	Zinc (mg)	Vit A (RE)	Vit C (mg)	Vit E (mg)	Thia (mg)	Ribo (mg)	Niac (mg)	Vit B-6 (mg)	Fol (μg)	Vit B-12 (μg)	Wat (g)
1.3	28.1	0.0	1.6	0.0	0.0	0.0	466.7	0.0	0.0	0.0	0.0	0.0	0.0	0.0	0.0	0.0	0.0	207.5
8.0	62.6	195.8	2.3	0.0	0.0	0.0	1014.6	0.0	0.0	0.0	0.0	0.0	0.0	0.0	0.0	0.0	0.0	198.0
0.0	35.0	49.0	1.9	0.0	0.0	180.0	766.0	0.0	5.8	0.0	0.0	0.1	0.1	1.1	0.2	0.0	1.2	0.0
0.0	0.0	43.0	5.9	0.0	0.0	772.0	1003.0	0.0	105.2	7.0	0.0	0.2	0.4	7.7	0.0	0.0	0.0	0.0
1.4	13.0	0.0	2.1	0.0	0.0	0.0	609.6	0.0	0.0	34.9	0.0	0.0	0.0	0.0	0.0	0.0	0.0	252.3
3.3	20.0	241.0	2.7	0.0	0.0	315.0	686.0	0.0	268.2	34.0	0.0	0.1	0.1	2.0	0.0	0.0	0.0	0.0
2.4	46.4	0.0	2.1	0.0	0.0	0.0	562.4	0.0	0.0	0.0	0.0	0.0	0.0	0.0	0.0	0.0	0.0	195.6
0.0	0.0	49.0	4.4	0.0	0.0	483.0	701.0	0.0	112.6	11.0	0.0	0.2	0.2	4.6	0.0	0.0	0.0	0.0
0.6	24.9	0.0	0.0	0.0	0.0	0.0	674.9	0.0	0.0	44.5	0.0	0.0	0.0	0.0	0.0	0.0	0.0	233.9
1.2	45.0	20.0	1.3	12.0	114.0	0.0	786.0	1.0	11.8	0.0	0.0	0.0	0.2	2.6	0.1	0.0	0.0	120.8
0.0	45.0	19.0	0.7	0.0	0.0	83.0	586.0	0.0	1.6	0.0	0.0	0.0	0.1	1.7	0.0	0.0	0.0	0.0
0.0	50.0	95.0	2.0	0.0	206.0	520.0	1280.0	0.0	601.2	8.0	0.0	0.3	0.2	5.5	0.0	0.0	0.0	0.0
0.0	40.0	49.0	1.0	0.0	228.0	500.0	1110.0	0.0	109.2	6.0	0.0	0.1	0.2	5.8	0.0	0.0	0.0	0.0
1.0	112.0	33.0	1.8	0.0	0.0	492.0	728.0	0.0	243.2	3.0	0.0	0.2	0.5	7.4	0.0	0.0	0.0	0.0
0.0	55.0	164.0	3.0	0.0	169.0	520.0	1320.0	0.0	220.4	27.0	0.0	0.3	0.3	3.6	0.0	0.0	0.0	0.0
0.0	0.0	80.0	0.7	0.0	0.0	175.0	780.0	0.0	200.0	15.0	0.0	0.0	0.0	0.4	0.0	0.0	0.0	0.0
2.7	24.0	174.0	2.8	0.0	0.0	531.0	462.0	0.0	367.6	44.0	0.0	0.2	0.4	2.8	0.0	0.0	0.0	0.0
7.0	30.0	457.0	2.4	0.0	345.0	424.0	760.0	2.0	33.6	7.0	0.0	0.2	0.3	2.0	0.2	14.0	0.0	0.0
0.0	0.0	255.0	7.5	0.0	0.0	1027.0	1689.0	0.0	476.2	38.0	0.0	0.4	0.4	6.6	0.0	0.0	0.0	0.0
0.0	0.0	41.0	0.1	3.0	52.0	2.0	38.0	0.1	0.0	31.0	0.0	0.0	0.0	0.0	0.0	0.0	0.0	236.8
0.0	0.0	0.0	0.0	14.0	0.0	0.0	0.0	0.0	0.0	6.0	0.0	0.0	0.0	0.0	0.0	0.0	0.0	236.8
0.0	0.0	15.0	0.0	0.0	7.0	1.0	14.0	0.0	0.0	6.0	0.0	0.0	0.0	0.0	0.0	0.0	0.0	0.0
0.0	0.0	0.0	0.0	0.0	0.0	0.0	5.1	0.0	0.0	6.7	0.0	0.0	0.0	0.0	0.0	0.0	0.0	0.0
0.0	0.0	6.2	0.0	0.3	3.0	0.0	0.9	0.0	0.0	0.7	0.0	0.0	0.0	0.0	0.0	0.0	0.0	29.4
0.0	0.0	71.3	0.2	2.6	34.3	34.3	13.2	0.1	0.0	8.4	0.0	0.0	0.0	0.0	0.0	3.4	0.0	236.8
0.0	0.0	1.0	0.0	16.0	0.0	12.0	21.0	0.0	0.0	6.0	0.0	0.0	0.0	0.0	0.0	0.0	0.0	220.0
0.0	0.0	7.8	0.0	0.3	4.7	6.2	1.6	0.0	68.8	15.1	0.0	0.0	0.0	0.0	0.0	17.9	0.0	27.3
0.0	0.0	26.0	0.0	0.0	11.0	1.0	19.0	0.0	0.0	6.0	0.0	0.0	0.0	0.0	0.0	0.0	0.0	0.0
0.0	0.0	20.0	0.9	0.0	0.0	118.0	18.0	0.0	0.0	7.0	0.0	0.0	0.0	0.4	0.0	0.0	0.0	0.0
0.0	0.0	22.1	2.7	14.7	24.5	274.4	7.4	0.1	9.8	66.4	0.0	0.0	0.0	0.4	0.1	4.9	0.0	215.1
0.0	0.0	17.2	0.1	4.9	7.4	66.2	4.9	0.1	0.0	78.4	0.0	0.0	0.0	0.1	0.1	0.5	0.0	202.9
0.0	0.0	13.1	0.7	8.7	8.7	78.3	8.7	0.3	0.0	154.0	0.0	0.0	0.0	0.2	0.1	0.9	0.0	371.9
0.0	0.0	13.1	0.2	5.2	2.6	36.7	7.9	0.1	2.6	25.9	0.0	0.0	0.0	0.0	0.0	0.0	0.0	225.1
0.0	0.0	19.8	0.5	4.9	2.5	61.8	54.3	0.3	2.5	73.1	0.0	0.1	0.1	0.1	0.0	3.2	0.0	217.4
0.0	0.0	9.9	0.2	4.9	2.5	32.1	9.9	0.1	2.5	108.4	0.0	0.0	0.0	0.1	0.0	2.2	0.0	217.9
0.0	0.0	5.6	0.2	7.5	7.5	65.8	1.9	0.1	0.0	30.1	0.0	0.0	0.0	0.2	0.0	1.5	0.0	163.6
0.0	0.0	14.0	0.2	8.0	16.0	125.0	15.0	0.1	0.0	100.0	0.0	0.0	0.0	0.0	0.0	0.0	0.0	0.0
0.0	0.0	4.0	0.4	0.0	3.0	40.0	23.0	0.0	2.6	80.0	0.0	0.0	0.0	0.0	0.0	0.0	0.0	0.0
0.0	0.0	2.2	0.1	1.2	0.0	23.9	1.6	0.1	0.3	1.7	0.0	0.0	0.0	0.0	0.0	0.0	0.0	27.1
0.0	0.0	0.0	0.0	0.0	0.0	5.5	33.0	0.0	0.0	22.0	0.0	0.0	0.0	0.0	0.0	0.0	0.0	0.0
0.0	0.0	5.6	0.3	3.7	3.7	27.9	5.6	0.1	0.0	7.3	0.0	0.0	0.0	0.0	0.0	4.1	0.0	166.1
0.0	0.0	5.6	0.3	3.7	3.7	27.9	5.6	0.1	3.7	7.3	0.0	0.0	0.0	0.0	0.0	4.1	0.0	166.1
0.0	0.0	5.6	0.1	1.9	1.9	24.2	3.7	0.0	0.0	5.0	0.0	0.0	0.0	0.0	0.0	1.9	0.0	165.4
0.0	0.0	0.0	0.0	0.0	0.0	0.0	0.0	0.0	0.0	0.0	0.0	0.0	0.0	0.0	0.0	0.0	0.0	0.0
0.0	0.0	11.2	0.5	3.7	1.9	33.5	29.8	0.2	3.7	63.4	0.0	0.0	0.0	0.1	0.0	4.1	0.0	161.6
0.0	0.0	0.0	0.0	0.0	0.0	64.0	1.0	0.0	115.2	60.0	0.0	0.0	0.0	0.0	0.0	0.0	0.0	157.3
0.0	0.0	13.0	0.6	11.2	11.2	113.5	26.0	0.1	7.4	85.6	0.0	0.1	0.0	0.5	0.1	19.5	0.0	163.5
0.0	0.0	9.3	0.5	11.2	7.4	85.6	5.6	0.1	98.6	41.9	0.0	0.1	0.0	0.4	0.1	20.3	0.0	161.6
0.0	0.0	24.0	0.0	0.0	17.0	9.0	13.0	0.0	0.0	6.0	0.0	0.0	0.0	0.0	0.0	0.0	0.0	0.0
0.0	0.0	2.0	0.4	0.0	2.0	26.0	19.0	0.0	2.8	60.0	0.0	0.0	0.0	0.0	0.0	0.0	0.0	0.0
0.0	0.0	7.8	0.4	6.5	14.3	111.8	7.8	0.1	26.0	2.5	0.0	0.0	0.0	0.5	0.1	3.4	0.0	99.4
0.0	0.0	9.8	0.4	7.3	14.6	126.9	4.9	0.1	28.1	3.7	0.0	0.0	0.0	0.6	0.1	3.3	0.0	107.0
0.0	0.0	19.0	0.9	0.0	0.0	125.0	30.0	0.0	0.0	5.0	0.0	0.0	0.0	0.3	0.0	0.0	0.0	0.0
0.0	0.0	12.6	0.7	5.4	12.6	214.2	5.4	0.1	0.0	74.9	0.0	0.0	0.0	0.0	0.1	0.2	0.0	158.3
0.0	0.0	12.7	0.5	10.6	14.8	265.9	14.8	0.1	0.0	52.8	0.0	0.0	0.0	0.1	0.1	0.6	0.0	185.5
0.0	0.0	14.8	0.8	10.6	19.0	240.5	6.3	0.2	278.5	114.8	0.0	0.0	0.0	0.5	0.0	2.7	0.0	179.1
0.0	0.0	20.4	0.2	0.0	7.9	77.1	5.7	0.1	0.2	90.8	0.0	0.0	0.1	0.2	0.1	1.1	0.0	0.0
0.0	0.0	19.3	0.1	0.0	2.3	90.8	9.1	0.0	0.0	68.1	0.0	0.0	0.0	0.0	0.0	0.0	0.0	0.0
0.1	0.0	8.6	0.2	8.6	8.6	45.4	4.3	0.1	2.2	51.6	0.1	0.0	0.1	0.3	0.1	2.8	0.0	187.7
0.0	0.0	17.3	0.8	21.6	23.8	349.9	4.3	0.1	0.0	58.1	0.1	0.1	0.0	0.7	0.0	22.5	0.0	188.7
0.0	0.0	15.1	0.4	21.6	23.8	330.5	2.2	0.2	2.2	63.1	0.1	0.1	0.0	0.5	0.0	22.5	0.0	194.6
0.0	0.0	2.5	0.0	3.4	4.3	42.0	0.3	0.0	0.3	10.4	0.0	0.0	0.0	0.1	0.0	1.1	0.0	27.6
0.0	0.0	22.2	0.5	29.6	37.1	400.1	2.5	0.1	108.7	93.9	0.0	0.1	0.0	0.5	0.1	25.2	0.0	222.3
0.0	0.0	17.6	0.4	23.5	29.4	317.5	2.0	0.1	2.0	74.5	0.1	0.1	0.0	0.4	0.0	20.0	0.0	176.4
0.0	0.0	1.7	0.0	1.2	1.4	15.5	3.2	0.0	0.3	3.8	0.0	0.0	0.0	0.0	0.0	1.5	0.0	14.1

Code	Food Name	Unit/Amt	Wt (g)	Energy (Kcal)	Prot (g)	Carb (g)	Fiber (g)	Fat (g)	Mono (g)	Poly (g)
9152	Fruit Juice, Lemon, fresh	1 tbsp	15	3.8	0.1	1.3	0.1	0.0	0.0	0.0
9161	Fruit Juice, Lime, canned or bottled unsweetened	1 tbsp	15	3.2	0.0	1.0	0.1	0.0	0.0	0.0
9160	Fruit Juice, Lime, fresh	1 tbsp	15	4.1	0.1	1.4	0.1	0.0	0.0	0.0
9207	Fruit Juice, Orange, canned, unsweetened	1 fl oz	31.1	13.1	0.2	3.1	0.1	0.0	0.0	0.0
9206	Fruit Juice, Orange, fresh	juice from 1 fruit (2.6" diam)	86	38.7	0.6	8.9	0.2	0.2	0.0	0.0
9215	Fruit Juice, Orange, frozen concentrate, unsweetened, prep	1 fl oz	31.1	14.0	0.2	3.4	0.1	0.0	0.0	0.0
914889	Fruit Juice, Orange-Grapefruit Juice	1 cup	245	110.3	1.6	25.5	0.1	0.1	0.0	0.0
9229	Fruit Juice, Papaya Nectar, canned	6 fl oz	213	121.4	0.4	30.9	1.3	0.3	0.1	0.1
9232	Fruit Juice, Passion Fruit, Purple, fresh	6 fl oz	218	111.2	0.9	29.6	0.4	0.1	0.0	0.1
9407	Fruit Juice, Peach Nectar, canned, w/added Vit C	6 fl oz	213	115.0	0.6	29.6	1.3	0.0	0.0	0.0
9408	Fruit Juice, Pear Nectar, canned, w/added Vit C	6 fl oz	213	127.8	0.2	33.6	1.3	0.0	0.0	0.0
9409	Fruit Juice, Pineapple, canned, unsweetened w/added Vit C	6 fl oz	213	119.3	0.7	29.4	0.4	0.2	0.0	0.1
9294	Fruit Juice, Prune, canned	6 fl oz	213	151.2	1.3	37.2	2.1	0.1	0.0	0.0
9223	Fruit Juice, Tangerine, canned, sweetened	6 fl oz	213	106.5	1.1	25.6	0.4	0.4	0.0	0.1
9105	Fruit Salad (peach,pineapple,pear,apricot&cherry)canned in heavy syrup	½ cup	127	92.7	0.4	24.3	1.3	0.1	0.0	0.0
9103	Fruit Salad (peach,pineapple,pear,apricot&cherry)canned in juice	½ cup	124	62.0	0.6	16.2	1.2	0.0	0.0	0.0
9104	Fruit Salad (peach,pineapple,pear,apricot&cherry)canned in lite syrup	½ cup	126	73.1	0.4	19.1	1.3	0.1	0.0	0.0
9003	Fruit, Apple w/skin, raw	1 medium (2.75" dia) (3/lb)	138	81.4	0.3	21.0	3.7	0.5	0.0	0.1
9009	Fruit, Apple, dehydrated, sulfured	1 cup	60	207.6	0.8	56.1	7.4	0.3	0.0	0.1
9014	Fruit, Apple, frozen, unsweetened	1 cup slices	173	83.0	0.5	21.3	3.3	0.6	0.0	0.2
9004	Fruit, Apple, peeled, raw, medium	1 fruit (2.75" dia) (3/lb)	128	73.0	0.2	19.0	2.4	0.4	0.0	0.1
9007	Fruit, Apple, slices, sweetened, canned, drained	½ cup slices	102	68.3	0.2	17.0	1.7	0.5	0.0	0.1
9402	Fruit, Applesauce, canned, sweetened w/added Vit C	½ cup	127	96.5	0.2	25.3	1.5	0.2	0.0	0.1
9401	Fruit, Applesauce, canned, unsweetened w/added Vit C	½ cup	122	52.5	0.2	13.8	1.5	0.1	0.0	0.0
9024	Fruit, Apricot w/skin, canned in juice	½ cup of halves	123	59.0	0.8	15.2	2.0	0.0	0.0	0.0
9026	Fruit, Apricot w/skin, canned in lite syrup	½ cup of halves	123	77.5	0.7	20.3	2.0	0.1	0.0	0.0
9032	Fruit, Apricot, dried, sulfured	½ cup of halves	3.5	8.3	0.1	2.2	0.3	0.0	0.0	0.0
9035	Fruit, Apricot, frozen, sweetened	1 tbsp cup	121	118.6	0.8	30.4	2.7	0.1	0.1	0.0
9023	Fruit, Apricot, peeled, canned in H₂O	4 halves & 2 tbsp liquid	90	19.8	0.6	4.9	1.0	0.0	0.0	0.0
9028	Fruit, Apricot, peeled, canned in heavy syrup	4 halves & 2 tbsp liquid	90	74.7	0.5	19.3	1.4	0.1	0.0	0.0
9021	Fruit, Apricot, raw	1 apricot	35	16.8	0.5	3.9	0.8	0.1	0.1	0.0
9037	Fruit, Avocado, All Varieties, peeled, raw	1 fruit w/o pit	115	185.2	2.3	8.5	5.8	17.6	11.0	2.2
9041	Fruit, Banana, dried or powder	1 tbsp	50	173.0	1.9	44.1	3.8	0.9	0.1	0.2
9046	Fruit, Blackberries, canned in heavy syrup	½ cup	122	112.2	1.6	28.2	4.1	0.2	0.0	0.1
9048	Fruit, Blackberries, frozen, unsweetened	1 cup	255	163.2	3.0	40.0	12.8	1.1	0.1	0.6
9042	Fruit, Blackberries, raw	1 cup	144	74.9	1.0	18.4	7.6	0.6	0.1	0.3
9052	Fruit, Blueberries, canned in heavy syrup	½ cup	129	113.5	0.8	28.5	1.9	0.4	0.1	0.4
9054	Fruit, Blueberries, frozen, unsweetened	½ cup	142	72.4	0.6	17.3	3.8	0.9	0.1	0.4
9050	Fruit, Blueberries, raw	1 cup	145	81.2	1.0	20.5	3.9	0.6	0.1	0.2
9056	Fruit, Boysenberries, canned in heavy syrup	½ cup	142	125.0	1.4	31.7	3.7	0.2	0.0	0.1
9057	Fruit, Boysenberries, frozen, unsweetened	½ cup	142	71.0	1.6	17.3	5.5	0.4	0.0	0.2
9059	Fruit, Breadfruit, peeled, raw	¼ small fruit w/o seeds	96	98.9	1.0	26.0	4.7	0.2	0.0	0.1
9060	Fruit, Carambola (Starfruit) raw	1 small (3" long)	70	23.1	0.4	5.5	1.9	0.2	0.0	0.1
9061	Fruit, Carissa (Natal-plum) peeled, raw	1 fruit w/o seeds	20	12.4	0.1	2.7	0.0	0.3	0.0	0.0
9062	Fruit, Cherimoya, peeled, raw	1 fruit w/o seeds	547	514.2	7.1	131.3	13.1	2.2	Mono	Poly
9065	Fruit, Cherries, Sour, Red, canned in lite syrup	½ cup	126	94.5	0.9	24.3	1.0	0.1	0.0	0.0
9068	Fruit, Cherries, Sour, Red, frozen, unsweetened	½ cup	125	57.5	1.2	13.8	2.0	0.6	0.2	0.2
9063	Fruit, Cherries, Sour, Red, raw	1 cup w/pits	103	51.5	1.0	12.5	1.6	0.3	0.1	0.1
9064	Fruit, Cherries, Sour/Tart, Red, canned in H₂O	½ cup	122	43.9	0.9	10.9	1.3	0.1	0.0	0.0
9072	Fruit, Cherries, Sweet, canned in juice	½ cup w/o pits	125	67.5	1.1	17.3	1.9	0.0	0.0	0.0
9073	Fruit, Cherries, Sweet, canned in lite syrup	½ cup w/o pits	126	84.4	0.8	21.8	1.9	0.2	0.1	0.1
9076	Fruit, Cherries, Sweet, frozen, sweetened	10 oz package	142	126.4	1.6	31.8	3.0	0.2	0.1	0.1
9070	Fruit, Cherries, Sweet, raw	1 cup w/pits, edible part	117	84.2	1.4	19.4	2.7	1.1	0.3	0.3
9078	Fruit, Cranberries, raw	1 cup whole	95	46.6	0.4	12.0	4.0	0.2	0.0	0.1
9082	Fruit, Cranberry-Orange Relish, canned	½ cup	138	245.6	0.4	63.8	0.0	0.1	0.0	0.0
9081	Fruit, Cranberry Sauce, canned, sweetened	1 slice (0.5" thick, ~8 slices/can)	57	86.1	0.1	22.2	0.6	0.1	0.0	0.0
9083	Fruit, Currant, European, Black, raw	1 cup	112	70.6	1.6	17.2	0.0	0.5	0.1	0.2
9084	Fruit, Currant, Red or White, raw	1 cup	112	62.7	1.6	15.5	4.8	0.2	0.0	0.1
9087	Fruit, Dates, Domestic, Natural, dried	1 date	8.3	22.8	0.2	6.1	0.6	0.0	0.0	0.0
9091	Fruit, Figs, canned in lite syrup	1 fig w/liquid	28	19.3	0.1	5.0	0.5	0.0	0.0	0.0
9094	Fruit, Figs, Dried, raw	1 fig	19	48.5	0.6	12.4	2.3	0.2	0.0	0.1
9095	Fruit, Figs, Dried, stewed	½ cup	130	140.4	1.7	35.8	6.6	0.6	0.1	0.3
9089	Fruit, Figs, raw	1 small (1.5" dia)	40	29.6	0.3	7.7	1.3	0.1	0.0	0.1
9107	Fruit, Gooseberries, raw	½ cup	75	33.0	0.7	7.6	3.2	0.4	0.0	0.2
9120	Fruit, Grapefruit, canned in juice	½ cup	125	46.3	0.9	11.5	0.5	0.1	0.0	0.0
9121	Fruit, Grapefruit, canned in lite syrup	½ cup	158	94.8	0.9	24.4	0.6	0.2	0.0	0.0
9111	Fruit, Grapefruit, Red, White or Pink, peeled, raw	1.2 cup sections w/ juice	135	43.2	0.9	10.9	1.5	0.1	0.0	0.0
9131	Fruit, Grapes, American type (slip skin) raw	1 cup	92	61.6	0.6	15.8	0.9	0.3	0.0	0.1
9139	Fruit, Guava, Common, raw	½ cup	85	43.4	0.7	10.1	4.6	0.5	0.0	0.2

Sat (g)	Chol (mg)	Cal (mg)	Iron (mg)	Magn (mg)	Phos (mg)	Pota (mg)	Sodi (mg)	Zinc (mg)	Vit A (RE)	Vit C (mg)	Vit E (mg)	Thia (mg)	Ribo (mg)	Niac (mg)	Vit B-6 (mg)	Fol (µg)	Vit B-12 (µg)	Wat (g)
0.0	0.0	1.1	0.0	0.9	0.9	18.6	0.2	0.0	0.3	6.9	0.0	0.0	0.0	0.0	0.0	1.9	0.0	13.6
0.0	0.0	1.8	0.0	1.1	1.5	11.3	2.4	0.0	0.3	1.0	0.0	0.0	0.0	0.0	0.0	1.2	0.0	13.9
0.0	0.0	1.4	0.0	0.9	1.1	16.4	0.2	0.0	0.2	4.4	0.0	0.0	0.0	0.0	0.0	1.2	0.0	13.5
0.0	0.0	2.5	0.1	3.4	4.4	54.4	0.6	0.0	5.6	10.7	0.0	0.0	0.0	0.1	0.0	5.6	0.0	27.7
0.0	0.0	9.5	0.2	9.5	14.6	172.0	0.9	0.0	17.2	43.0	0.1	0.1	0.0	0.3	0.0	26.1	0.0	75.9
0.0	0.0	2.8	0.0	3.1	5.0	59.1	0.3	0.0	2.5	12.1	0.1	0.0	0.0	0.1	0.0	13.6	0.0	27.4
0.0	0.0	24.0	0.3	25.0	41.0	459.0	1.0	0.2	56.2	107.0	0.0	0.2	0.0	0.7	0.1	7.0	0.0	217.3
0.1	0.0	21.3	0.7	6.4	0.0	66.0	10.7	0.3	23.4	6.4	0.0	0.0	0.0	0.3	0.0	4.5	0.0	181.1
0.0	0.0	8.7	0.5	37.1	28.3	606.0	13.1	0.1	157.0	65.0	0.1	0.0	0.3	3.2	0.1	15.3	0.0	186.7
0.0	0.0	10.7	0.4	8.5	12.8	85.2	14.9	0.2	55.4	57.1	0.0	0.0	0.0	0.6	0.0	3.0	0.0	182.4
0.0	0.0	10.7	0.6	6.4	6.4	27.7	8.5	0.1	0.0	57.5	0.0	0.0	0.0	0.3	0.0	2.6	0.0	178.9
0.0	0.0	36.2	0.6	27.7	17.0	285.4	2.1	0.2	0.0	51.1	0.0	0.1	0.0	0.5	0.2	49.2	0.0	182.2
0.0	0.0	25.6	2.5	29.8	53.3	587.9	8.5	0.4	0.0	8.7	0.0	0.1	0.1	1.7	0.5	0.9	0.0	173.0
0.0	0.0	38.3	0.4	17.0	29.8	379.1	2.1	0.1	89.5	46.9	0.2	0.1	0.0	0.2	0.1	9.8	0.0	185.3
0.0	0.0	7.6	0.4	6.4	11.4	101.6	7.6	0.1	63.5	3.0	0.6	0.0	0.0	0.4	0.0	3.2	0.0	101.9
0.0	0.0	13.6	0.3	9.9	17.4	143.8	6.2	0.2	74.4	4.1	0.0	0.0	0.0	0.4	0.0	3.2	0.0	106.8
0.0	0.0	8.8	0.4	6.3	11.3	103.3	7.6	0.1	54.2	3.2	0.0	0.0	0.0	0.5	0.0	3.3	0.0	106.1
0.1	0.0	9.7	0.2	6.9	9.7	158.7	0.0	0.1	6.9	7.9	0.4	0.0	0.0	0.1	0.1	3.9	0.0	115.8
0.1	0.0	11.4	1.2	13.2	33.0	384.0	74.4	0.2	4.8	1.3	2.1	0.0	0.1	0.4	0.2	0.6	0.0	1.8
0.1	0.0	6.9	0.3	5.2	13.8	133.2	5.2	0.1	5.2	0.2	0.0	0.0	0.0	0.1	0.1	1.2	0.0	150.3
0.1	0.0	5.1	0.1	3.8	9.0	144.6	0.0	0.1	5.1	5.1	0.1	0.0	0.0	0.1	0.1	0.5	0.0	108.1
0.1	0.0	4.1	0.2	2.0	5.1	69.4	3.1	0.0	5.1	0.4	0.0	0.0	0.0	0.1	0.0	0.3	0.0	84.0
0.0	0.0	5.1	0.4	3.8	8.9	77.5	35.6	0.1	1.3	2.2	0.0	0.0	0.0	0.2	0.0	0.8	0.0	101.1
0.0	0.0	3.7	0.1	3.7	8.5	91.5	7.4	0.0	3.7	25.9	0.0	0.0	0.0	0.2	0.0	0.7	0.0	107.8
0.0	0.0	14.8	0.4	12.3	24.6	203.0	4.9	0.1	207.9	6.0	1.1	0.0	0.0	0.4	0.1	2.1	0.0	106.5
0.0	0.0	13.5	0.5	9.8	16.0	169.7	4.9	0.1	162.4	3.3	1.1	0.0	0.0	0.4	0.1	2.1	0.0	101.5
0.0	0.0	1.6	0.2	1.6	4.1	48.2	0.4	0.0	25.3	0.1	0.1	0.0	0.0	0.1	0.0	0.4	0.0	1.1
0.0	0.0	12.1	1.1	10.9	23.0	277.1	4.8	0.1	203.3	10.9	1.1	0.0	0.0	1.0	0.1	2.1	0.0	88.7
0.0	0.0	7.2	0.5	8.1	14.4	138.6	9.9	0.1	162.9	1.6	0.0	0.0	0.0	0.4	0.0	1.5	0.0	84.1
0.0	0.0	8.1	0.4	7.2	11.7	120.6	9.9	0.1	111.6	2.5	0.0	0.0	0.0	0.4	0.0	1.5	0.0	69.9
0.0	0.0	4.9	0.2	2.8	6.7	103.6	0.4	0.1	91.4	3.5	0.3	0.0	0.0	0.2	0.0	3.0	0.0	30.2
2.8	0.0	12.7	1.2	44.9	47.2	688.9	11.5	0.5	70.2	9.1	1.5	0.1	0.1	2.2	0.3	71.2	0.0	85.4
0.3	0.0	11.0	0.6	54.0	37.0	745.5	1.5	0.3	15.5	3.5	0.0	0.1	0.1	1.4	0.2	7.0	0.0	1.5
0.0	0.0	25.6	0.8	20.7	17.1	120.8	3.7	0.2	26.8	3.4	0.9	0.0	0.0	0.4	0.0	32.3	0.0	91.6
0.0	0.0	74.0	2.0	56.1	76.5	357.0	2.6	0.6	28.1	7.9	1.8	0.1	0.1	3.1	0.2	86.7	0.0	209.6
0.0	0.0	46.1	0.8	28.8	30.2	282.2	0.0	0.4	23.0	30.2	1.0	0.0	0.1	0.6	0.1	49.0	0.0	123.3
0.0	0.0	6.5	0.4	5.2	12.9	51.6	3.9	0.1	7.7	1.4	1.3	0.0	0.1	0.1	0.0	2.1	0.0	99.0
0.1	0.0	11.4	0.3	7.1	15.6	76.7	1.4	0.1	11.4	3.6	1.4	0.0	0.1	0.7	0.1	9.5	0.0	123.0
0.0	0.0	8.7	0.2	7.3	14.5	129.1	8.7	0.2	14.5	18.9	1.5	0.1	0.1	0.5	0.1	9.3	0.0	122.7
0.0	0.0	25.6	0.6	15.6	14.2	127.8	4.3	0.3	5.7	8.8	1.0	0.0	0.0	0.3	0.1	48.8	0.0	108.3
0.0	0.0	38.3	1.2	22.7	38.3	197.4	1.4	0.3	9.9	4.4	0.6	0.1	0.1	1.1	0.1	89.9	0.0	122.0
0.0	0.0	16.3	0.5	24.0	28.8	470.4	1.9	0.1	3.8	27.8	1.1	0.1	0.0	0.9	0.1	13.4	0.0	67.8
0.0	0.0	2.8	0.2	6.3	11.2	114.1	1.4	0.1	34.3	14.8	0.3	0.0	0.0	0.3	0.1	9.8	0.0	63.6
0.0	0.0	2.2	0.3	3.2	1.4	52.0	0.6	0.0	0.8	7.6	0.0	0.0	0.0	0.0	0.0	0.0	0.0	16.8
0.0	0.0	125.8	2.7	0.0	218.8	0.0	0.0	0.0	5.5	49.2	0.0	0.5	0.6	7.1	0.0	0.0	0.0	402.0
0.0	0.0	12.6	1.7	7.6	12.6	119.7	8.8	0.1	92.0	2.5	0.0	0.0	0.0	0.2	0.1	9.7	0.0	100.3
0.1	0.0	16.3	0.7	11.3	20.0	155.0	1.3	0.1	108.8	2.1	0.2	0.1	0.0	0.2	0.1	5.6	0.0	109.0
0.1	0.0	16.5	0.3	9.3	15.5	178.2	3.1	0.1	131.8	10.3	0.1	0.0	0.0	0.4	0.0	7.7	0.0	88.7
0.0	0.0	13.4	1.7	7.3	12.2	119.6	8.5	0.1	91.5	2.6	0.2	0.0	0.1	0.2	0.1	9.8	0.0	109.7
0.0	0.0	17.5	0.7	15.0	27.5	163.8	3.8	0.1	16.3	3.1	0.1	0.0	0.0	0.5	0.0	5.3	0.0	106.2
0.0	0.0	11.3	0.5	11.3	22.7	186.5	3.8	0.1	20.2	4.7	0.2	0.0	0.1	0.5	0.0	5.3	0.0	102.8
0.0	0.0	17.0	0.5	14.2	22.7	282.6	1.4	0.1	27.0	1.4	0.2	0.0	0.1	0.3	0.1	6.0	0.0	107.3
0.3	0.0	17.6	0.5	12.9	22.2	262.1	0.0	0.1	24.6	8.2	0.2	0.1	0.1	0.5	0.0	4.9	0.0	94.5
0.0	0.0	6.7	0.2	4.8	8.6	67.5	1.0	0.1	4.8	12.8	0.0	0.0	0.0	0.1	0.1	1.6	0.0	82.2
0.0	0.0	15.2	0.3	5.5	11.0	52.4	44.2	0.0	9.7	24.8	0.0	0.0	0.0	0.1	0.0	0.0	0.0	73.4
0.0	0.0	2.3	0.1	1.7	3.4	14.8	16.5	0.0	1.1	1.1	0.1	0.0	0.0	0.1	0.0	0.6	0.0	34.6
0.0	0.0	61.6	1.7	26.9	66.1	360.6	2.2	0.3	25.8	202.7	0.1	0.1	0.1	0.3	0.1	0.0	0.0	91.8
0.0	0.0	37.0	1.1	14.6	49.3	308.0	1.1	0.3	13.4	45.9	0.1	0.0	0.1	0.1	0.1	9.0	0.0	94.0
0.0	0.0	2.7	0.1	2.9	3.3	54.1	0.2	0.0	0.4	0.0	0.0	0.0	0.0	0.2	0.0	1.0	0.0	1.9
0.0	0.0	7.6	0.1	2.8	2.8	28.6	0.3	0.0	1.1	0.3	0.2	0.0	0.0	0.1	0.0	0.6	0.0	22.8
0.0	0.0	27.4	0.4	11.2	12.9	135.3	2.1	0.1	2.5	0.2	0.0	0.0	0.0	0.1	0.0	1.4	0.0	5.4
0.1	0.0	79.3	1.2	32.5	37.7	391.8	6.5	0.3	20.8	5.7	0.0	0.0	0.1	0.8	0.2	1.3	0.0	90.7
0.0	0.0	14.0	0.1	6.8	5.6	92.8	0.4	0.1	5.6	0.8	0.4	0.0	0.0	0.2	0.0	2.4	0.0	31.6
0.0	0.0	18.8	0.2	7.5	20.3	148.5	0.8	0.1	21.8	20.8	0.3	0.0	0.0	0.2	0.1	4.5	0.0	65.9
0.0	0.0	18.8	0.3	13.8	15.0	211.3	8.8	0.1	0.0	42.4	0.3	0.0	0.0	0.3	0.0	11.0	0.0	112.1
0.0	0.0	22.1	0.6	15.8	15.8	203.8	3.2	0.1	0.0	33.7	0.4	0.1	0.0	0.4	0.0	13.4	0.0	132.1
0.0	0.0	16.2	0.1	10.8	10.8	187.7	0.0	0.1	16.2	46.4	0.3	0.0	0.0	0.3	0.1	13.8	0.0	122.7
0.1	0.0	12.9	0.3	4.6	9.2	175.7	1.8	0.0	9.2	3.7	0.3	0.1	0.0	0.3	0.0	3.6	0.0	74.8
0.1	0.0	17.0	0.3	8.5	21.3	241.4	2.6	0.2	67.2	156.0	1.0	0.0	0.0	1.0	0.1	11.9	0.0	73.2

Code	Food Name	Unit/Amt	Wt (g)	Energy (Kcal)	Prot (g)	Carb (g)	Fiber (g)	Fat (g)	Mono (g)	Poly (g)
9148	Fruit, Kiwifruit (Chinese Gooseberry) peeled, raw	1 medium fruit	76	46.4	0.8	11.3	2.6	0.3	0.0	0.2
9149	Fruit, Kumquat, raw	1 fruit	19	12.0	0.2	3.1	1.3	0.0	0.0	0.0
9150	Fruit, Lemon, peeled, raw	1 medium fruit (2.1″ dia)	58	16.8	0.6	5.4	1.6	0.2	0.0	0.1
9165	Fruit, Lychee (Litchi) shelled, dried	1 fruit	2.5	6.9	0.1	1.8	0.1	0.0	0.0	0.0
9176	Fruit, Mango, peeled, raw	1 fruit w/o seed	207	134.6	1.1	35.2	3.7	0.6	0.2	0.1
9185	Fruit, Melon Balls (cantaloupe & honeydew) frozen	1 cup thawed	173	57.1	1.5	13.7	1.2	0.4	0.0	0.2
9183	Fruit, Melon, Casaba, peeled, raw	1 cup cubes	170	44.2	1.5	10.5	1.4	0.2	0.0	0.1
9184	Fruit, Melon, Honeydew, peeled, wedges, raw	10 honeydew balls	138	48.3	0.6	12.7	0.8	0.1	0.0	0.1
9188	Fruit, Mixed (prune, apricot & pear) dried	3.5 w/o pits	100	243.0	2.5	64.1	7.8	0.5	0.2	0.1
9187	Fruit, Mixed, (peach, pear & pineapple) canned in heavy syrup	1 tbsp	15.9	11.4	0.1	3.0	0.2	0.0	0.0	0.0
9191	Fruit, Nectarine, raw	1 fruit w/o pit (2.5″ diam)	136	66.6	1.3	16.0	2.2	0.6	0.2	0.3
9193	Fruit, Olives, Ripe, pitted, canned	1 tsp	2.8	3.2	0.0	0.2	0.1	0.3	0.2	0.0
9216	Fruit, Orange Peel, raw	1 tsp	2	1.9	0.0	0.5	0.2	0.0	0.0	0.0
9200	Fruit, Orange, All Varieties, peeled, raw	1 cup sections w/o membrane	180	84.6	1.7	21.2	4.3	0.2	0.0	0.0
9226	Fruit, Papayas, peeled, cubed/mashed, raw	1 cup cubes	140	54.6	0.9	13.7	2.5	0.2	0.1	0.0
9231	Fruit, Passion Fruit/Granadilla, Purple, peeled, raw	1 fruit	18	17.5	0.4	4.2	1.9	0.1	0.0	0.1
9241	Fruit, Peach, canned in heavy syrup	1 half w/liquid	98	72.5	0.4	19.5	1.3	0.1	0.0	0.0
9238	Fruit, Peach, canned in juice	1 half w/liquid	98	43.1	0.6	11.3	1.3	0.0	0.0	0.0
9240	Fruit, Peach, canned in lite syrup	1 half w/liquid	98	52.9	0.4	14.3	1.3	0.0	0.0	0.0
9246	Fruit, Peach, dried, sulfured	1 half	13	31.1	0.5	8.0	1.1	0.1	0.0	0.0
9250	Fruit, Peach, frozen, sweetened	10 slices	155	145.7	1.0	37.2	2.8	0.2	0.1	0.1
9236	Fruit, Peach, peeled, raw	1 large (2.75″ dia) (2.5/lb)	157	67.5	1.1	17.4	3.1	0.1	0.1	0.1
9254	Fruit, Pear, canned in juice	½ cup halves	124	62.0	0.4	16.0	2.0	0.1	0.0	0.0
9256	Fruit, Pear, canned in lite syrup	½ cup halves	126	71.8	0.2	19.1	2.0	0.0	0.0	0.0
9259	Fruit, Pear, dried, sulfured	10 halves	175	458.5	3.3	122.0	13.1	1.1	0.2	0.3
9252	Fruit, Pear, raw	1 large pear (2/lb)	209	123.3	0.8	31.6	5.0	0.8	0.2	0.2
9265	Fruit, Persimmon, Native, raw	1 fruit w/o seeds	25	31.8	0.2	8.4	0.0	0.1	0.0	0.0
9268	Fruit, Pineapple, canned in juice	½ cup crushed, sliced of chunks	125	75.0	0.5	19.6	1.0	0.1	0.0	0.0
9269	Fruit, Pineapple, canned in lite syrup	½ cup crushed, sliced of chunks	126	65.5	0.5	16.9	1.0	0.2	0.0	0.1
9272	Fruit, Pineapple, frozen, chunks, sweetened	½ cup of chunks, frz sweetened	123	104.6	0.5	27.3	1.4	0.1	0.0	0.0
9266	Fruit, Pineapple, peeled, raw	1 fruit	472	231.3	1.8	58.5	5.7	2.0	0.2	0.7
9276	Fruit, Pitanga (Surinam Cherry) peeled, raw	1 fruit w/o seeds	7	2.3	0.1	0.5	0.0	0.0	0.0	0.0
9277	Fruit, Plantain, peeled, raw	1 medium fruit	179	218.4	2.3	57.1	4.1	0.7	0.1	0.1
9282	Fruit, Plum, Purple, canned in juice	½ cup w/o pits	126	73.1	0.6	19.1	1.3	0.0	0.0	0.0
9283	Fruit, Plum, Purple, canned in lite syrup	½ cup w/o pits	126	79.4	0.5	20.5	1.3	0.1	0.1	0.0
9279	Fruit, Plum, raw	1 fruit (2.1″ diam) w/o pit	66	36.3	0.5	8.6	1.0	0.4	0.3	0.1
9286	Fruit, Pomegranates, peeled, raw	1 fruit: 3.35″ dia	154	104.7	1.5	26.4	0.9	0.5	0.1	0.1
9287	Fruit, Prickly Pear, peeled, raw	1 fruit	103	42.2	0.8	9.9	3.7	0.5	0.1	0.2
9292	Fruit, Prune, dried, stewed w/o added sugar	1 tbsp w/o pits	15.5	16.6	0.2	4.4	1.0	0.0	0.0	0.0
9290	Fruit, Prunes, dehydrated, stewed	½ cup	140	158.2	1.7	41.6	0.0	0.3	0.2	0.1
9291	Fruit, Prunes, dried	1 prune	8.4	20.1	0.2	5.3	0.6	0.0	0.0	0.0
9295	Fruit, Pummelo, peeled, raw	1 fruit w/o seeds & membrane	609	231.4	4.6	58.6	6.1	0.2	0.0	0.0
9296	Fruit, Quinces, peeled, raw	1 fruit w/o seeds	92	52.4	0.4	14.1	1.7	0.1	0.0	0.0
9297	Fruit, Raisins, Golden, seedless	½ cup packed	83	250.7	2.8	66.0	3.3	0.4	0.0	0.1
9298	Fruit, Raisins, seedless	½ cup packed	83	249.0	2.7	65.7	3.3	0.4	0.0	0.1
9302	Fruit, Raspberries, raw	10 raspberries	19	9.3	0.2	2.2	1.3	0.1	0.0	0.1
9304	Fruit, Raspberries, Red, canned in heavy syrup	½ cup	128	116.5	1.1	29.9	4.2	0.2	0.0	0.1
9306	Fruit, Raspberries, Red, frozen, sweetened	10 oz package	284	292.5	2.0	74.3	12.5	0.5	0.0	0.3
9310	Fruit, Rhubarb, frozen, cooked w/sugar	½ cup	120	139.2	0.5	37.4	2.4	0.1	0.0	0.0
9307	Fruit, Rhubarb, raw	½ cup diced	61	12.8	0.5	2.8	1.1	0.1	0.0	0.1
9317	Fruit, Strawberries, canned in heavy syrup	½ cup	77	70.8	0.4	18.1	1.3	0.2	0.0	0.1
9320	Fruit, Strawberries, frozen, sliced, sweetened	1 cup thawed	255	244.8	1.4	66.1	4.8	0.3	0.0	0.2
9318	Fruit, Strawberries, unsweetened, frozen	1 cup	149	52.2	0.6	13.6	3.1	0.2	0.0	0.1
9322	Fruit, Tamarind, raw	1 fruit w/o pods & seeds:3x1″	2	4.8	0.1	1.3	0.1	0.0	0.0	0.0
9326	Fruit, Watermelon, balls, raw	1 cup balls	154	49.3	1.0	11.1	0.8	0.7	0.2	0.2
5308	Game, Cornish Game Hen w/skin, roasted	½ bird	129	335.4	28.7	0.0	0.0	23.5	10.3	4.6
5310	Game, Cornish Game Hens, no skin, roasted	½ bird	110	147.4	25.6	0.0	0.0	4.3	1.4	1.0
17167	Game, Elk, roasted	3.0 oz	85	124.1	25.7	0.0	0.0	1.6	0.4	0.3
17179	Game, Rabbit, Domestic, Composite, roasted	3.0 oz	85	167.5	24.7	0.0	0.0	6.8	1.8	1.3
17161	Game, Venison/Deer, roasted	3.0 oz	85	134.3	25.7	0.0	0.0	2.7	0.7	0.5
5150	Goose Liver Pate/Pate de Fois Gras, Smoked, canned	2 tsbp	28	129.4	3.2	1.3	0.0	12.3	7.2	0.2
5148	Goose, Domestic, meat & skin, roasted	3.5 oz	100	305.0	25.2	0.0	0.0	21.9	10.3	2.5
20001	Goose, Domestic, meat only, no skin, roasted	3.5 oz	100	238.0	29.0	0.0	0.0	12.7	4.3	1.5
20005	Grain, Barley	1 tbsp	11.5	40.7	1.4	8.5	2.0	0.3	0.0	0.1
20008	Grain, Barley, Pearled, ckd	1 tbsp	9.8	12.1	0.2	2.8	0.4	0.0	0.0	0.0
20009	Grain, Buckwheat Groats, roasted, ckd	1 tbsp	10.5	9.7	0.4	2.1	0.3	0.1	0.0	0.0
20012	Grain, Bulgar, ckd	1 tbsp	8.4	7.0	0.3	1.6	0.4	0.0	0.0	0.0
20014	Grain, Corn, White	1 tbsp	10.4	38.0	1.0	7.7	0.0	0.5	0.1	0.2
20029	Grain, Corn, Yellow	1 tbsp	10.4	38.0	1.0	7.7	0.0	0.5	0.1	0.2

Sat (g)	Chol (mg)	Cal (mg)	Iron (mg)	Magn (mg)	Phos (mg)	Pota (mg)	Sodi (mg)	Zinc (mg)	Vit A (RE)	Vit C (mg)	Vit E (mg)	Thia (mg)	Ribo (mg)	Niac (mg)	Vit B-6 (mg)	Fol (µg)	Vit B-12 (µg)	Wat (g)
0.0	0.0	19.8	0.3	22.8	30.4	252.3	3.8	0.1	13.7	74.5	0.9	0.0	0.0	0.4	0.1	28.9	0.0	63.1
0.0	0.0	8.4	0.1	2.5	3.6	37.1	1.1	0.0	5.7	7.1	0.0	0.0	0.0	0.1	0.0	3.0	0.0	15.5
0.0	0.0	15.1	0.3	4.6	9.3	80.0	1.2	0.0	1.7	30.7	0.1	0.0	0.0	0.1	0.0	6.1	0.0	51.6
0.0	0.0	0.8	0.0	1.1	4.5	27.8	0.1	0.0	0.0	4.6	0.0	0.0	0.0	0.1	0.0	0.3	0.0	0.6
0.1	0.0	20.7	0.3	18.6	22.8	322.9	4.1	0.1	805.2	57.3	2.3	0.1	0.1	1.2	0.3	29.0	0.0	169.1
0.1	0.0	17.3	0.5	24.2	20.8	484.4	53.6	0.3	306.2	10.7	0.3	0.3	0.0	1.1	0.2	44.5	0.0	156.1
0.0	0.0	8.5	0.7	13.6	11.9	357.0	20.4	0.3	5.1	27.2	0.3	0.1	0.0	0.7	0.2	28.9	0.0	156.4
0.0	0.0	8.3	0.1	9.7	13.8	374.0	13.8	0.1	5.5	34.2	0.2	0.1	0.0	0.8	0.1	8.3	0.0	123.7
0.0	0.0	38.0	2.7	39.0	77.0	796.0	18.0	0.5	244.0	3.8	0.0	0.0	0.2	1.9	0.2	3.9	0.0	31.2
0.0	0.0	0.2	0.1	0.8	1.6	13.4	0.6	0.0	3.0	11.0	0.0	0.0	0.0	0.1	0.0	0.5	0.0	12.8
0.1	0.0	6.8	0.2	10.9	21.8	288.3	0.0	0.1	100.6	7.3	1.2	0.0	0.1	1.3	0.0	5.0	0.0	117.3
0.0	0.0	2.5	0.1	0.1	0.1	0.2	24.4	0.0	1.1	0.0	0.1	0.0	0.0	0.0	0.0	0.0	0.0	2.2
0.0	0.0	3.2	0.0	0.4	0.4	4.2	0.1	0.0	0.8	2.7	0.0	0.0	0.0	0.0	0.0	0.6	0.0	1.5
0.0	0.0	72.0	0.2	18.0	25.2	325.8	0.0	0.1	37.8	95.8	0.4	0.2	0.1	0.5	0.1	54.5	0.0	156.2
0.1	0.0	33.6	0.1	14.0	7.0	359.8	4.2	0.1	39.2	86.5	1.6	0.0	0.0	0.5	0.0	53.2	0.0	124.4
0.0	0.0	2.2	0.3	5.2	12.2	62.6	5.0	0.0	12.6	5.4	0.2	0.0	0.0	0.3	0.0	2.5	0.0	13.1
0.0	0.0	2.9	0.3	4.9	10.8	90.2	5.9	0.1	32.3	2.7	0.9	0.0	0.0	0.6	0.0	3.1	0.0	77.7
0.0	0.0	5.9	0.3	6.9	16.7	125.4	3.9	0.1	37.2	3.5	1.5	0.0	0.0	0.6	0.0	3.3	0.0	85.7
0.0	0.0	2.9	0.4	4.9	10.8	95.1	4.9	0.1	34.3	2.4	0.9	0.0	0.0	0.6	0.0	3.2	0.0	83.0
0.0	0.0	3.6	0.5	5.5	15.5	129.5	0.9	0.1	28.1	0.6	0.0	0.0	0.0	0.6	0.0	0.0	0.0	4.1
0.0	0.0	4.7	0.6	7.8	17.1	201.5	9.3	0.1	43.4	146.0	1.4	0.0	0.1	1.0	0.0	5.0	0.0	115.8
0.0	0.0	7.9	0.2	11.0	18.8	309.3	0.0	0.2	84.8	10.4	1.1	0.0	0.1	1.6	0.0	5.3	0.0	137.6
0.0	0.0	11.2	0.4	8.7	14.9	119.0	5.0	0.1	1.2	2.0	0.6	0.0	0.0	0.2	0.0	1.5	0.0	107.2
0.0	0.0	6.3	0.4	5.0	8.8	83.2	6.3	0.1	0.0	0.9	0.6	0.0	0.0	0.2	0.0	1.5	0.0	106.4
0.1	0.0	59.5	3.7	57.8	103.3	932.8	10.5	0.7	0.0	12.3	0.0	0.0	0.3	2.4	0.1	0.0	0.0	46.7
0.0	0.0	23.0	0.5	12.5	23.0	261.3	0.0	0.3	4.2	8.4	1.0	0.0	0.1	0.2	0.0	15.3	0.0	175.2
0.0	0.0	6.8	0.6	0.0	6.5	77.5	0.3	0.0	0.0	16.5	0.0	0.0	0.0	0.0	0.0	0.0	0.0	16.1
0.0	0.0	17.5	0.4	17.5	7.5	152.5	1.3	0.1	5.0	11.9	0.1	0.1	0.0	0.4	0.1	6.0	0.0	104.4
0.0	0.0	17.6	0.5	20.2	8.8	132.3	1.3	0.2	1.3	9.5	0.1	0.1	0.0	0.4	0.1	5.9	0.0	108.0
0.0	0.0	11.1	0.5	12.3	4.9	123.0	2.5	0.1	3.7	9.8	0.1	0.1	0.0	0.4	0.1	13.0	0.0	94.8
0.2	0.0	33.0	1.7	66.1	33.0	533.4	4.7	0.4	9.4	72.7	0.5	0.4	0.2	2.0	0.4	50.0	0.0	408.3
0.0	0.0	0.6	0.0	0.8	0.8	7.2	0.2	0.0	10.5	1.8	0.0	0.0	0.0	0.0	0.0	0.0	0.0	6.4
0.3	0.0	5.4	1.1	66.2	60.9	893.2	7.2	0.3	202.3	32.9	0.5	0.1	0.1	1.2	0.5	39.4	0.0	116.9
0.0	0.0	12.6	0.4	10.1	18.9	194.0	1.3	0.1	127.3	3.5	0.9	0.0	0.1	0.6	0.0	3.3	0.0	105.9
0.0	0.0	11.3	1.1	6.3	16.4	117.2	25.2	0.1	32.8	0.5	0.9	0.0	0.0	0.4	0.0	3.3	0.0	104.4
0.0	0.0	2.6	0.1	4.6	6.6	113.5	0.0	0.1	21.1	6.3	0.4	0.0	0.1	0.3	0.1	1.5	0.0	56.2
0.1	0.0	4.6	0.5	4.6	12.3	398.9	4.6	0.2	0.0	9.4	0.8	0.0	0.0	0.5	0.2	9.2	0.0	124.7
0.1	0.0	57.7	0.3	87.6	24.7	226.6	5.2	0.1	5.2	14.4	0.0	0.0	0.1	0.5	0.1	6.2	0.0	90.2
0.0	0.0	3.6	0.2	3.1	5.4	51.8	0.3	0.0	4.8	0.4	0.0	0.0	0.0	0.1	0.0	0.0	0.0	10.8
0.0	0.0	33.6	1.6	29.4	51.8	494.2	2.8	0.4	72.8	0.0	0.0	0.1	0.3	1.4	0.3	0.3	0.0	95.2
0.0	0.0	4.3	0.2	3.8	6.6	62.6	0.3	0.0	16.7	0.3	0.1	0.0	0.0	0.2	0.0	0.3	0.0	2.7
0.0	0.0	24.4	0.7	36.5	103.5	1315.4	6.1	0.5	0.0	371.5	0.0	0.2	0.2	1.3	0.2	0.0	0.0	542.6
0.0	0.0	10.1	0.6	7.4	15.6	181.2	3.7	0.0	3.7	13.8	0.5	0.0	0.0	0.2	0.0	2.8	0.0	77.1
0.1	0.0	44.0	1.5	29.1	95.5	619.2	10.0	0.3	3.3	2.7	0.6	0.0	0.2	0.9	0.3	2.7	0.0	12.4
0.1	0.0	40.7	1.7	27.4	80.5	623.3	10.0	0.2	0.8	2.7	0.6	0.1	0.1	0.7	0.2	2.7	0.0	12.8
0.0	0.0	4.2	0.1	3.4	2.3	28.9	0.0	0.1	2.5	4.8	0.1	0.0	0.0	0.2	0.0	4.9	0.0	16.4
0.0	0.0	14.1	0.5	15.4	11.5	120.3	3.8	0.2	3.8	11.1	0.6	0.0	0.0	0.6	0.1	13.4	0.0	96.4
0.0	0.0	42.6	1.8	36.9	48.3	323.8	2.8	0.5	17.0	46.9	1.3	0.1	0.1	0.7	0.1	73.8	0.0	206.6
0.0	0.0	174.0	0.3	14.4	9.6	115.2	1.2	0.1	8.4	4.0	0.2	0.0	0.0	0.2	0.0	6.4	0.0	81.3
0.0	0.0	52.5	0.1	7.3	8.5	175.7	2.4	0.1	6.1	4.9	0.1	0.0	0.0	0.2	0.0	4.3	0.0	57.1
0.0	0.0	10.0	0.4	6.2	9.2	66.2	3.1	0.1	2.3	24.4	0.1	0.0	0.0	0.0	0.0	21.6	0.0	58.0
0.0	0.0	28.1	1.5	17.9	33.2	249.9	7.7	0.2	5.1	105.6	0.4	0.0	0.1	1.0	0.1	38.0	0.0	186.6
0.0	0.0	23.8	1.1	16.4	19.4	220.5	3.0	0.2	6.0	61.4	0.4	0.0	0.1	0.7	0.0	25.0	0.0	134.1
0.0	0.0	1.5	0.1	1.8	2.3	12.6	0.6	0.0	0.1	0.1	0.0	0.0	0.0	0.0	0.0	0.3	0.0	0.6
0.1	0.0	12.3	0.3	16.9	13.9	178.6	3.1	0.1	57.0	14.8	0.2	0.1	0.0	0.3	0.2	3.4	0.0	140.9
6.5	169.0	16.8	1.2	23.2	188.3	316.1	82.6	1.9	41.3	0.6	0.3	0.1	0.3	7.6	0.4	2.6	0.4	75.7
1.1	116.6	14.3	0.8	20.9	163.9	275.0	69.3	1.7	22.0	0.7	0.3	0.1	0.2	6.9	0.4	2.2	0.3	79.1
0.6	62.1	4.3	3.1	20.4	153.0	278.8	51.9	2.7	0.0	0.0	0.0	0.0	0.0	0.0	0.0	0.0	0.0	56.3
2.0	69.7	16.2	1.9	17.9	223.6	325.6	40.0	1.9	0.0	0.0	0.0	0.1	0.2	7.2	0.4	9.4	7.1	51.5
1.1	95.2	6.0	3.8	20.4	192.1	284.8	45.9	2.3	0.0	0.0	0.0	0.2	0.5	5.7	0.0	0.0	0.0	55.4
4.0	42.0	19.6	1.5	3.6	56.0	38.6	195.2	0.3	280.0	0.6	0.0	0.0	0.1	0.7	0.0	16.8	2.6	10.4
6.9	91.0	13.0	2.8	22.0	270.0	329.0	70.0	2.6	21.0	0.0	1.7	0.1	0.3	4.2	0.4	2.0	0.4	52.0
4.6	96.0	14.0	2.9	25.0	309.0	388.0	76.0	3.2	12.0	0.0	0.0	0.1	0.4	4.1	0.5	12.0	0.5	57.2
0.1	0.0	3.8	0.4	15.3	30.4	52.0	1.4	0.3	0.2	0.0	0.1	0.1	0.0	0.5	0.0	2.2	0.0	1.1
0.0	0.0	1.1	0.1	2.2	5.3	9.1	0.3	0.1	0.1	0.0	0.0	0.0	0.0	0.2	0.0	1.6	0.0	6.7
0.0	0.0	0.7	0.1	5.4	7.4	9.2	0.4	0.1	0.0	0.0	0.0	0.0	0.0	0.1	0.0	1.5	0.0	7.9
0.0	0.0	0.8	0.1	2.7	3.4	5.7	0.4	0.0	0.0	0.0	0.0	0.0	0.0	0.1	0.0	1.5	0.0	6.5
0.1	0.0	0.7	0.3	13.2	21.8	29.8	3.6	0.2	0.0	0.0	0.0	0.0	0.0	0.4	0.1	2.0	0.0	1.1
0.1	0.0	0.7	0.3	13.2	21.8	29.8	3.6	0.2	4.9	0.0	0.1	0.0	0.0	0.4	0.1	2.0	0.0	1.1

Code	Food Name	Unit/Amt	Wt (g)	Energy (Kcal)	Prot (g)	Carb (g)	Fiber (g)	Fat (g)	Mono (g)	Poly (g)
20030	Grain, Couscous, dry	1 tbsp	10.8	40.6	1.4	8.4	0.5	0.1	0.0	0.0
20330	Grain, Hominy, Yellow	1 cup	242	128.3	2.7	27.9	1.6	0.6	0.0	0.0
20031	Grain, Millet, ckd	1 tbsp	10.9	13.0	0.4	2.6	0.1	0.1	0.0	0.1
20035	Grain, Oats	1 tbsp	9.8	38.1	1.7	6.5	1.0	0.7	0.2	0.2
20036	Grain, Rice, Brown, Long grain, ckd	1 tbsp	12.2	13.5	0.3	2.8	0.2	0.1	0.0	0.0
20040	Grain, Rice, Brown, Medium grain, ckd	1 tbsp	12.2	13.7	0.3	2.9	0.2	0.1	0.0	0.0
20054	Grain, Rice, White, Glutinous, ckd	1 tbsp, cooked	10.9	10.6	0.2	2.3	0.1	0.0	0.0	0.0
20047	Grain, Rice, White, Long grain, enriched, ckd w/salt	1 tbsp	9.9	12.9	0.3	2.8	0.0	0.0	0.0	0.0
20048	Grain, Rice, White, Long grain, Precooked/Instant, enriched, ckd	1 tbsp	10.3	10.1	0.2	2.2	0.1	0.0	0.0	0.0
20044	Grain, Rice, White, Long grain, Regular, enriched, ckd	1 tbsp	9.9	12.9	0.3	2.8	0.0	0.0	0.0	0.0
20444	Grain, Rice, White, Long Grain, Regular, unenriched, ckd w/o salt	1 tbsp	9.8	12.7	0.3	2.8	0.0	0.0	0.0	0.0
20051	Grain, Rice, White, Long Grain, unenriched, ckd w/salt	1 tbsp	9.9	12.9	0.3	2.8	0.0	0.0	0.0	0.0
20050	Grain, Rice, White, Medium grain, ckd	1 tbsp	11.6	15.1	0.3	3.3	0.0	0.0	0.0	0.0
20450	Grain, Rice, White, Medium grain, unenriched, ckd	1 tbsp	11.6	15.1	0.3	3.3	0.0	0.0	0.0	0.0
20056	Grain, Rice, White, w/pasta, ckd	1 tbsp	12.6	15.4	0.3	2.7	0.3	0.4	0.1	0.1
20066	Grain, Rye	1 tbsp	10.6	35.5	1.6	7.4	1.5	0.3	0.0	0.1
20466	Grain, Semolina, enriched	1 tbsp	10.4	37.4	1.3	7.6	0.4	0.1	0.0	0.0
20068	Grain, Sorghum	1 tbsp	12	40.7	1.4	9.0	0.0	0.4	0.1	0.2
20069	Grain, Tapioca, Pearl, dry	1 tbsp	9.5	34.0	0.0	8.4	0.1	0.0	0.0	0.0
20076	Grain, Wheat Germ, crude	1 tbsp	9.6	34.6	2.2	5.0	1.3	0.9	0.1	0.6
20071	Grain, Wheat, Durum	1 tbsp	12	40.7	1.6	8.5	0.0	0.3	0.0	0.1
6115	Gravy, Au Jus, canned	1 cup	238.4	38.1	2.9	6.0	0.0	0.5	0.2	0.0
6116	Gravy, Au Jus, dry, made w/H_2O	1 cup (8 fl oz)	246	32.0	1.2	4.0	0.0	1.3	0.5	0.0
6561	Gravy, Beef, canned	1 cup	233	123.5	8.7	11.2	0.9	5.5	2.2	0.2
6118	Gravy, Brown Gravy, dry mix/Nestle Trio	1 tbsp	6	24.4	0.6	3.5	0.2	0.9	0.2	0.5
6119	Gravy, Brown, dry, made w/H_2O	1 cup (8 fl oz)	258	74.8	2.4	13.0	0.0	1.7	0.7	0.1
6120	Gravy, Chicken, canned	1 cup	238	188.0	4.6	12.9	1.0	13.6	6.1	3.6
6572	Gravy, Chicken, dry, made w/H_2O	1 cup (8 fl oz)	260	83.2	2.6	14.4	0.0	1.9	0.9	0.4
6746	Gravy, dry, made w/H_2O	¼ cup	66	21.8	0.8	3.6	0.0	0.5	0.2	0.1
6579	Gravy, Hearty Beef Gravy, glass jar/PepFarm	1 package	340	146.2	10.2	21.1	0.0	2.4	0.9	0.2
6122	Gravy, Mushroom, canned	¼ cup	60	30.0	0.8	3.3	0.2	1.6	0.7	0.6
6124	Gravy, Onion, dry, made w/H_2O	¼ cup	60	18.0	0.5	3.7	0.0	0.2	0.0	0.0
6563	Gravy, Pork, dry, made w/H_2O	¼ cup	60	18.0	0.4	3.1	0.2	0.4	0.2	0.0
6126	Gravy, Turkey, canned	1 tbsp	15	7.7	0.4	0.8	0.1	0.3	0.1	0.1
5151	Gravy, Turkey, dry, made w/H_2O	1 tbsp	15	5.0	0.2	0.9	0.1	0.1	0.0	0.0
22700	Hamburger Helper	1 serving	144	341.3	20.3	30.0	0.0	15.7	0.0	0.0
2023	Herb, Ginger Root, peeled, sliced, raw	5 slices (1"diam x 0.12"thick)	11	7.6	0.2	1.7	0.2	0.1	0.0	0.0
17170	Hopping John (rice&blackeyed peas)	⅓ cup	100	118.0	5.0	17.8	0.5	3.6	0.0	0.0
901932	Ice Cream Bar, Vanilla	1 bar	67	162.1	2.1	14.5	0.0	10.6	0.0	0.0
18272	Ice Cream Cone, Cake or Wafer	1 cone	4	16.7	0.3	3.2	0.1	0.3	0.1	0.1
901920	Ice Cream Cone, Sugar, Rolled	1 cone	10	40.2	0.8	8.4	0.2	0.4	0.1	0.1
19270	Ice Cream Sandwich	1 bar	62	166.8	3.1	26.1	0.1	6.2	0.0	0.3
901917	Ice Cream, Chocolate	1 individual container (3.5 fl oz)	58	125.3	2.2	16.4	0.7	6.4	1.9	0.2
901918	Ice Cream, Creamsicle	1 bar	67	103.2	1.2	17.6	0.0	3.1	0.0	0.0
19264	Ice Cream, Drumstick	1 stick	67	186.3	2.6	21.5	0.2	9.9	0.0	0.0
19090	Ice Cream, Eskimo Pie Vanilla Ice Cream Bar w/dark chocolate coating	1 bar	50	165.7	2.1	12.3	0.0	12.1	0.0	0.0
901919	Ice Cream, French Vanilla custard, soft serve	1 cup (8 fl oz)	172	369.8	7.1	38.2	0.0	22.4	6.0	0.8
19262	Ice Cream, Fudgsicle	1 bar	73	91.3	3.8	18.6	0.0	0.2	0.0	0.0
901922	Ice Cream, Klondike Vanilla Ice Cream Bar w/chocolate coating	1 bar (5 fl oz)	148	488.5	6.2	35.7	0.0	35.7	0.0	0.0
901923	Ice Cream, Light, Chocolate (ice milk)	2/3 cup	90	136.8	4.3	20.2	0.0	4.6	1.5	0.2
19088	Ice Cream, Light, Strawberry (ice milk)	2/3 cup	90	133.2	4.3	22.1	0.1	3.1	0.9	0.1
19096	Ice Cream, Light, Vanilla	1 cup (8 fl oz)	132	183.5	5.0	30.0	0.0	5.7	1.6	0.2
19260	Ice Cream, Light, Vanilla, soft serve	1 cup (8 fl oz)	176	221.8	8.6	38.4	0.0	4.6	1.3	0.2
19271	Ice Cream, Light, w/aspartame, no sugar, vanilla	1 tbsp	8.1	12.3	0.4	1.5	0.0	0.5	0.1	0.0
19095	Ice Cream, Strawberry	1 individual container (3.5 fl oz)	58	111.4	1.9	16.0	0.2	4.9	0.0	0.0
19089	Ice Cream, Vanilla	1 individual container (3.5 fl oz)	58	116.6	2.0	13.7	0.0	6.4	1.8	0.2
17003	Lamb, Domestic, Choice, Composite, lean (¼" trim) ckd	3.0 oz	85	175.1	24.0	0.0	0.0	8.1	3.5	0.5
17001	Lamb, Domestic, Choice, Composite, lean (¼" trim) raw	3.5 oz	100	134.0	20.3	0.0	0.0	5.3	2.1	0.5
17226	Lamb, Domestic, Choice, Composite, lean&fat (⅛" trim) cooked	3.5 oz	100	271.0	25.5	0.0	0.0	18.0	7.6	1.3
18370	Leavening Agent, Baking Powder, Double Acting, Na Al sulfate	1 tsp	4.6	2.4	0.0	1.3	0.0	0.0	0.0	0.0
18373	Leavening Agent, Baking Soda	1 tbsp	13.8	0.0	0.0	0.0	0.0	0.0	0.0	0.0
18375	Leavening Agent, Cream of Tartar	1 tsp	3	7.7	0.0	1.8	0.0	0.0	0.0	0.0
18374	Leavening Agent, Yeast, Baker's, Active	1 package (0.25 oz)	7	20.7	2.7	2.7	1.5	0.3	0.2	0.0
7001	Lobster (shellfish) Egg Roll/LaChoy	1 medium	13	26.4	0.7	4.2	0.0	0.7	0.1	0.4
7274	Lunch Meat, Barbecue Loaf (Pork & Beef)	1.0 oz, 1 slice	28	48.4	4.4	1.8	0.0	2.5	1.2	0.2
7042	Lunch Meat, Beef Pastrami, cooked, smoked, chopped, pressed/Carl Buddig	2.5 oz, 1 pkg	71	100.1	13.9	0.7	0.0	4.6	0.0	0.2
7043	Lunch Meat, Beef, smoked, sliced/Carl Buddig	2.5 oz, 1 pkg	71	98.7	13.7	0.4	0.0	4.6	0.0	0.2
7008	Lunch Meat, Beef, thin slices	1.0 oz, 6 paper-thin slices	28	49.6	7.9	1.6	0.0	1.1	0.5	0.1
7202	Lunch Meat, Bologna (Beef & Pork)	1.0 oz, 1 slice	28	88.5	3.3	0.8	0.0	7.9	3.7	0.7

Sat (g)	Chol (mg)	Cal (mg)	Iron (mg)	Magn (mg)	Phos (mg)	Pota (mg)	Sodi (mg)	Zinc (mg)	Vit A (RE)	Vit C (mg)	Vit E (mg)	Thia (mg)	Ribo (mg)	Niac (mg)	Vit B-6 (mg)	Fol (μg)	Vit B-12 (μg)	Wat (g)
0.0	0.0	2.6	0.1	4.8	18.4	17.9	1.1	0.1	0.0	0.0	0.0	0.0	0.0	0.4	0.0	2.2	0.0	0.9
0.0	0.0	9.0	2.3	0.0	0.0	33.0	701.0	0.0	55.4	0.0	0.0	0.0	0.1	0.1	0.0	0.0	0.0	211.0
0.0	0.0	0.3	0.1	4.8	10.9	6.8	0.2	0.1	0.0	0.0	0.0	0.0	0.0	0.1	0.0	2.1	0.0	7.8
0.1	0.0	5.3	0.5	17.3	51.3	42.0	0.2	0.4	0.0	0.0	0.1	0.1	0.0	0.1	0.0	5.5	0.0	0.8
0.0	0.0	1.2	0.1	5.2	10.1	5.2	0.6	0.1	0.0	0.0	0.1	0.0	0.0	0.2	0.0	0.5	0.0	8.9
0.0	0.0	1.2	0.1	5.4	9.4	9.6	0.1	0.1	0.0	0.0	0.0	0.0	0.0	0.2	0.0	0.5	0.0	8.9
0.0	0.0	0.2	0.0	0.5	0.9	1.1	0.5	0.0	0.0	0.0	0.0	0.0	0.0	0.0	0.0	0.1	0.0	8.4
0.0	0.0	1.0	0.1	1.2	4.3	3.5	37.8	0.0	0.0	0.0	0.0	0.0	0.0	0.1	0.0	5.7	0.0	6.8
0.0	0.0	0.8	0.1	0.5	1.4	0.4	0.3	0.0	0.0	0.0	0.0	0.0	0.0	0.1	0.0	4.2	0.0	7.9
0.0	0.0	1.0	0.1	1.2	4.3	3.5	0.1	0.0	0.0	0.0	0.0	0.0	0.0	0.1	0.0	5.7	0.0	6.8
0.0	0.0	1.0	0.0	1.2	4.2	3.4	0.1	0.0	0.0	0.0	0.0	0.0	0.0	0.0	0.0	0.3	0.0	6.7
0.0	0.0	1.0	0.0	1.2	4.3	3.5	37.8	0.0	0.0	0.0	0.0	0.0	0.0	0.0	0.0	0.3	0.0	6.8
0.0	0.0	0.3	0.2	1.5	4.3	3.4	0.0	0.0	0.0	0.0	0.0	0.0	0.0	0.2	0.0	6.7	0.0	8.0
0.0	0.0	0.3	0.0	1.5	4.3	3.4	0.0	0.0	0.0	0.0	0.0	0.0	0.0	0.2	0.0	0.2	0.0	8.0
0.1	0.1	1.0	0.1	1.5	4.7	5.3	71.6	0.0	0.0	0.0	0.0	0.0	0.0	0.2	0.0	5.5	0.0	9.0
0.0	0.0	3.5	0.3	12.8	39.6	28.0	0.6	0.4	0.0	0.0	0.2	0.0	0.0	0.5	0.0	6.4	0.0	1.2
0.0	0.0	1.8	0.5	4.9	14.1	19.3	0.1	0.1	0.0	0.0	0.0	0.1	0.1	0.6	0.0	16.0	0.0	1.3
0.1	0.0	3.4	0.5	0.0	34.4	42.0	0.7	0.0	0.0	0.0	0.0	0.0	0.0	0.4	0.0	0.0	0.0	1.1
0.0	0.0	1.9	0.2	0.1	0.7	1.0	0.1	0.0	0.0	0.0	0.0	0.0	0.0	0.0	0.0	0.4	0.0	1.0
0.2	0.0	3.7	0.6	22.9	80.8	85.6	1.2	1.2	0.0	0.0	0.0	0.2	0.0	0.7	0.1	27.0	0.0	1.1
0.1	0.0	4.1	0.4	17.3	61.0	51.7	0.2	0.5	0.0	0.0	0.0	0.1	0.0	0.8	0.1	5.2	0.0	1.3
0.2	0.0	9.5	1.4	4.8	71.5	193.1	119.2	2.4	0.0	2.4	0.0	0.0	0.1	2.1	0.0	4.8	0.2	225.3
0.6	2.5	22.1	0.0	7.4	0.0	0.0	964.3	0.1	0.0	0.0	0.0	0.0	0.0	0.0	0.0	0.0	0.2	236.5
2.7	7.0	14.0	1.6	4.7	69.9	188.7	1304.8	2.3	0.0	0.0	0.1	0.1	0.1	1.5	0.0	4.7	0.2	203.8
0.3	0.0	2.2	0.1	0.5	7.3	0.8	261.8	0.0	0.0	0.0	0.0	0.0	0.0	0.0	0.0	1.6	0.0	0.3
0.8	2.6	67.1	0.2	10.3	43.9	56.8	1075.9	0.3	0.0	0.0	0.0	0.0	0.1	0.8	0.0	0.0	0.0	237.0
3.4	4.8	47.6	1.1	4.8	69.0	259.4	1373.3	1.9	264.2	0.0	0.4	0.0	0.1	1.1	0.0	4.8	0.2	203.1
0.5	2.6	39.0	0.3	10.4	46.8	62.4	1133.6	0.3	0.0	2.6	0.0	0.1	0.1	0.8	0.0	2.6	0.2	237.7
0.2	0.0	9.2	0.1	2.6	12.5	16.5	359.0	0.1	0.0	0.5	0.0	0.0	0.0	0.2	0.0	0.9	0.0	60.0
0.8	17.0	0.0	0.0	0.0	0.0	0.0	2145.4	0.0	0.0	0.0	0.0	0.0	0.0	0.0	0.0	0.0	0.0	300.6
0.2	0.0	4.2	0.4	1.2	9.0	63.6	342.0	0.4	0.0	0.0	0.0	0.0	0.0	0.4	0.0	7.2	0.0	53.4
0.1	0.0	16.8	0.0	0.6	0.0	0.0	232.8	0.1	0.0	0.0	0.0	0.0	0.0	0.0	0.0	0.0	0.0	54.7
0.2	0.6	7.2	0.1	2.4	10.2	13.2	287.4	0.1	0.0	0.4	0.0	0.0	0.0	0.2	0.0	0.7	0.0	55.2
0.1	0.3	0.6	0.1	0.3	4.4	16.4	86.6	0.1	0.0	0.0	0.0	0.0	0.0	0.2	0.0	0.3	0.0	13.3
0.0	0.2	2.9	0.0	0.6	2.9	3.8	86.0	0.0	0.0	0.1	0.0	0.0	0.0	0.1	0.0	0.2	0.0	13.6
0.0	0.0	0.0	0.0	0.0	0.0	436.0	1043.0	0.0	0.0	0.0	0.0	0.0	0.0	0.0	0.0	0.0	0.0	78.0
0.0	0.0	2.0	0.1	4.7	3.0	45.7	1.4	0.0	0.0	0.6	0.0	0.0	0.0	0.1	0.0	1.2	0.0	9.0
0.0	0.0	22.0	1.0	0.0	81.0	112.0	447.0	0.0	4.2	2.0	0.0	0.5	0.0	0.3	0.0	0.0	0.0	0.0
0.0	0.0	70.0	0.0	8.0	52.0	107.0	28.0	0.0	41.8	0.0	0.0	0.0	0.1	0.1	0.0	0.0	0.0	0.0
0.0	0.0	1.0	0.1	1.0	3.9	4.5	5.7	0.0	0.0	0.0	0.1	0.0	0.0	0.2	0.0	4.1	0.0	0.2
0.1	0.0	4.4	0.4	3.1	10.3	14.5	32.0	0.1	0.0	0.0	0.0	0.1	0.0	0.5	0.0	8.3	0.0	0.3
3.7	0.0	73.0	0.1	8.0	72.0	102.0	92.0	0.0	38.6	0.0	0.0	0.0	0.1	0.5	0.0	0.0	0.0	0.0
3.9	19.7	63.2	0.5	16.8	62.1	144.4	44.1	0.3	69.0	0.4	0.2	0.0	0.1	0.1	0.0	9.3	0.2	32.3
0.0	0.0	46.0	0.0	5.0	37.0	82.0	27.0	0.0	25.0	0.0	0.0	0.1	0.3	0.0	0.0	0.0	0.0	0.0
0.0	0.0	67.0	0.1	7.0	59.0	99.0	57.0	0.0	37.0	0.0	0.0	0.0	0.1	0.5	0.0	0.0	0.0	0.0
7.3	14.2	59.5	0.0	0.0	0.0	0.0	34.2	0.0	0.0	0.0	0.0	0.0	0.0	0.0	0.0	0.0	0.0	23.2
12.9	156.5	225.3	0.4	20.6	199.5	304.4	104.9	0.9	264.9	1.4	0.6	0.1	0.3	0.2	0.1	15.5	0.9	102.9
0.2	0.0	129.0	0.1	14.0	99.0	173.0	55.0	0.0	0.0	0.0	0.0	0.2	0.7	0.0	0.0	0.0	0.0	0.0
19.4	39.8	211.6	0.0	0.0	0.0	0.0	107.9	0.0	0.0	0.0	0.0	0.0	0.0	0.0	0.0	0.0	0.0	69.1
2.9	13.0	140.0	0.1	12.0	111.0	175.0	61.0	0.8	38.0	1.0	0.0	0.0	0.2	0.1	0.1	5.0	1.4	
2.1	13.0	161.0	0.3	12.0	121.0	412.0	64.0	0.9	25.8	0.0	0.0	0.1	0.2	0.1	0.1	5.0	1.4	0.0
3.5	18.5	183.5	0.1	19.8	143.9	278.5	112.2	0.6	62.0	1.1	0.0	0.1	0.3	0.1	0.1	7.9	0.9	90.0
2.9	21.1	276.3	0.1	24.6	213.0	389.0	123.2	0.9	51.0	1.6	0.0	0.1	0.3	0.2	0.1	10.6	0.9	122.5
0.3	1.3	15.9	0.0	0.0	0.0	0.0	7.2	0.0	0.0	0.0	0.0	0.0	0.0	0.0	0.0	0.0	0.0	5.6
3.0	16.8	69.6	0.1	8.1	58.0	109.0	34.8	0.2	45.2	4.5	0.0	0.0	0.1	0.1	0.0	7.0	0.2	34.8
3.9	25.5	74.2	0.1	8.1	60.9	115.4	46.4	0.4	67.9	0.3	0.0	0.1	0.1	0.1	0.0	2.9	0.2	35.4
2.9	78.2	12.8	1.7	22.1	178.5	292.4	64.6	4.5	0.0	0.0	0.2	0.1	0.2	5.4	0.1	19.6	2.2	52.7
1.9	65.0	10.0	1.8	26.0	189.0	280.0	66.0	4.1	0.0	0.0	0.2	0.1	0.2	6.0	0.2	23.0	2.6	73.4
7.5	96.0	16.0	1.9	24.0	193.0	318.0	72.0	4.7	0.0	0.0	0.2	0.1	0.3	6.6	0.1	19.0	2.6	55.8
0.0	0.0	270.3	0.5	1.2	100.8	0.9	487.6	0.0	0.0	0.0	0.0	0.0	0.0	0.0	0.0	0.0	0.0	0.2
0.0	0.0	0.0	0.0	0.0	0.0	0.0	3775.7	0.0	0.0	0.0	0.0	0.0	0.0	0.0	0.0	0.0	0.0	0.0
0.0	0.0	0.2	0.1	0.1	0.2	495.0	1.6	0.0	0.0	0.0	0.0	0.0	0.0	0.0	0.0	0.0	0.0	0.1
0.0	0.0	4.5	1.2	6.9	90.3	140.0	3.5	0.4	0.0	0.0	0.0	0.2	0.4	2.8	0.1	163.8	0.0	0.5
0.1	0.0	3.9	0.2	0.0	0.0	24.6	52.7	0.0	1.8	1.1	0.0	0.0	0.0	0.3	0.0	0.0	0.0	0.0
0.9	10.4	15.4	0.3	4.8	37.0	92.1	373.5	0.7	2.0	0.0	0.0	0.1	0.1	0.6	0.1	2.5	0.5	18.1
2.1	46.2	12.1	1.7	0.0	0.0	259.2	749.8	0.0	0.0	0.0	0.0	0.1	0.2	2.9	0.0	0.0	0.0	49.6
1.8	47.6	9.9	1.6	0.0	0.0	238.6	1016.0	0.0	0.0	0.0	0.0	0.1	0.2	2.7	0.0	0.0	0.0	49.3
0.5	11.5	3.1	0.8	5.3	47.0	120.1	402.9	1.1	0.0	0.0	0.1	0.0	0.1	1.5	0.1	3.1	0.7	16.3
3.0	15.4	3.4	0.4	3.1	25.5	50.4	285.3	0.5	0.0	0.0	0.1	0.0	0.0	0.7	0.1	1.4	0.4	15.2

Code	Food Name	Unit/Amt	Wt (g)	Energy (Kcal)	Prot (g)	Carb (g)	Fiber (g)	Fat (g)	Mono (g)	Poly (g)
7007	Lunch Meat, Bologna (Beef light)/Oscar Mayer	1.0 oz, 2 slices	28	55.4	3.3	1.7	0.0	4.0	2.0	0.1
7201	Lunch Meat, Bologna (Beef)	1.0 oz, 1 slice	28	87.4	3.4	0.2	0.0	8.0	3.9	0.3
7010	Lunch Meat, Bologna (Chicken, Pork & Beef)/Oscar Mayer	1.0 oz, 1 slice	28	89.0	3.1	0.7	0.0	8.2	4.1	1.1
7011	Lunch Meat, Bologna (Pork)	1.0 oz, 1 slice	28	69.2	4.3	0.2	0.0	5.6	2.7	0.6
7206	Lunch Meat, Bologna (Turkey)	1.0 oz, 1 slice	28	55.7	3.8	0.3	0.0	4.3	1.3	1.2
7039	Lunch Meat, Bologna, fat free/Oscar Mayer	1.0 oz, 1 slice	28	22.1	3.5	1.7	0.0	0.2	0.1	0.0
7249	Lunch Meat, Braunschweiger Liver Sausage, sliced/Oscar Mayer	1.0 oz, 1 slice	28	94.1	3.9	0.6	0.1	8.5	4.3	1.0
7209	Lunch Meat, Chicken Breast Classic Baked/Grill, carving board/Louis Rich	1.0 oz, 1 slice	28	27.4	5.5	1.0	0.0	0.1	0.0	0.0
7250	Lunch Meat, Chicken Breast, honey glazed/Oscar Mayer	1.0 oz, 1 slice	28	30.5	5.5	1.2	0.0	0.4	0.2	0.1
7210	Lunch Meat, Chicken Breast, oven roasted deluxe/Louis Rich	1.0 oz, 1 slice	28	28.3	5.1	0.7	0.0	0.6	0.2	0.1
7053	Lunch Meat, Chicken Breast, oven roasted, fat free/Oscar Mayer	1.0 oz, 1 slice	28	23.8	5.1	0.5	0.0	0.2	0.0	0.0
7018	Lunch Meat, Chicken Roll, light meat	2.0 oz, 2 slices	57	90.6	11.1	1.4	0.0	4.2	1.7	0.9
7271	Lunch Meat, Chicken Spread, canned	1.5 oz.	43	82.6	6.6	2.3	0.0	5.0	2.1	1.1
7251	Lunch Meat, Chicken, light and dark meat, sliced, smoked/Carl Buddig	2.5 oz, 1 pkg	71	117.2	12.7	0.5	0.0	7.2	0.0	1.5
7021	Lunch Meat, Corned Beef, cooked, chopped, pressed/Carl Buddig	2.5 oz, 1 pkg	71	100.8	13.7	0.7	0.0	4.8	0.0	0.2
7252	Lunch Meat, Dutch Brand (Old Fashion) Loaf (Pork & Beef)	1.0 oz, 1 slice	28	67.2	3.8	1.6	0.0	5.0	2.3	0.5
7253	Lunch Meat, Franks (Turkey & Chicken Cheese)/Louis Rich	1.6 oz, 1 frank	45	90.5	5.7	2.3	0.0	6.5	2.8	1.3
7054	Lunch Meat, Franks (Turkey & Chicken)/Louis Rich	1.6 oz, 1 frank	45	84.6	5.0	2.4	0.0	6.1	2.5	1.4
7033	Lunch Meat, Ham & Cheese Loaf or Roll	1.0 oz, 1 slice	28	72.5	4.7	0.4	0.0	5.7	2.6	0.6
7211	Lunch Meat, Ham & Cheese Spread	3 tbsp	43	105.4	7.0	1.0	0.0	8.0	3.0	0.6
7031	Lunch Meat, Ham and Cheese Loaf/Oscar Mayer	1.0 oz, 1 slice	28	64.4	3.9	1.0	0.0	5.0	2.3	0.5
7212	Lunch Meat, Ham Salad Spread	1.0 oz, 1tbsp	28	60.5	2.4	3.0	0.0	4.3	2.0	0.8
7030	Lunch Meat, Ham, honey, water added/Oscar Mayer	1 slice	21	23.3	3.5	0.7	0.0	0.7	0.4	0.1
7028	Lunch Meat, Ham, minced	1 slice	21	55.2	3.4	0.4	0.0	4.3	2.0	0.5
7029	Lunch Meat, Ham, slices, extra lean (5% fat)	1 slice : 6.25 x 4 x 0.06"	28.35	37.1	5.5	0.3	0.0	1.4	0.7	0.1
7217	Lunch Meat, Ham, slices, regular (11% fat)	1 slice : 6.25 x 4 x 0.06"	28.35	51.6	5.0	0.9	0.0	3.0	1.4	0.3
7216	Lunch Meat, Ham, smoked, sliced/Carl Buddig	2.5 oz, 1 pkg	71	115.7	13.1	0.8	0.0	6.6	0.0	0.8
7214	Lunch Meat, Ham, water added, baked, 96% fat free/Oscar Mayer	2.25 oz	63	64.9	10.4	0.6	0.0	2.3	0.7	0.8
7035	Lunch Meat, Head Cheese/Oscar Mayer	1.0 oz, 1 slice	28	51.8	4.4	0.0	0.0	3.8	1.9	0.4
7219	Lunch Meat, Honey Loaf (Pork & Beef)	2 slices: 4 x 4 x 0.09"	57	73.0	9.0	3.0	0.0	2.5	1.1	0.3
7220	Lunch Meat, Jellied, Beef	1 slice (4 x 4 x 0.9" thick)	29	32.2	5.5	0.0	0.0	1.0	0.4	0.0
7055	Lunch Meat, Liver Cheese (Pork)	1.0 oz slice	28	85.1	4.3	0.6	0.0	7.2	3.4	1.0
7041	Lunch Meat, Liver Pate, canned	1.0 oz, 2 tsbp	28	89.3	4.0	0.4	0.0	7.8	3.5	0.9
7221	Lunch Meat, Liver Sausage (Liverwurst)	1 slice: 2.5"diam x 0.25"thick	18	58.7	2.5	0.4	0.0	5.1	2.4	0.5
7060	Lunch Meat, Luncheon Loaf, spiced/Oscar Mayer	1.0 oz, 1 slice	28	65.5	3.8	2.0	0.0	4.7	2.1	0.8
7223	Lunch Meat, Old Fashioned Loaf/Oscar Mayer	1.0 oz, 1 slice	28	64.7	3.7	2.2	0.0	4.6	2.2	0.7
7051	Lunch Meat, Olive Loaf (Chicken, Pork & Turkey)/Oscar Mayer	1.0 oz, 1 slice	28	73.6	2.8	1.9	0.0	6.1	3.1	0.7
13355	Lunch Meat, Olive Loaf (Pork)	1.0 oz, 1 slice	28	65.8	3.3	2.6	0.0	4.6	2.2	0.5
7052	Lunch Meat, Pastrami (Beef)	1.0 oz, 1 slice	28	97.7	4.8	0.9	0.0	8.2	4.1	0.3
7056	Lunch Meat, Pastrami (Turkey)	1.0 oz, 1 slice	28	39.5	5.1	0.5	0.0	1.7	0.6	0.4
7058	Lunch Meat, Peppered Loaf (Pork & Beef)	1.0 oz, 1 slice	28	41.4	4.8	1.3	0.0	1.8	0.8	0.1
7224	Lunch Meat, Pickle & Pimiento Loaf	1.0 oz, 1 slice	28	73.4	3.2	1.7	0.0	5.9	2.7	0.7
7045	Lunch Meat, Pork Sausage Links, cooked/Oscar Mayer	1 link	24	82.3	3.9	0.2	0.0	7.3	3.6	0.9
7067	Lunch Meat, Pork, canned	0.75 oz, 1 slice	21	70.1	2.6	0.4	0.0	6.4	3.0	0.7
7227	Lunch Meat, Salami Beef Cotto/Oscar Mayer	0.75 oz, 1 slice	21	43.3	3.0	0.4	0.0	3.3	1.5	0.2
7230	Lunch Meat, Salami Cotto (Beef, Pork & Chicken)/Oscar Mayer	0.75 oz, 1 slice	21	51.5	2.8	0.5	0.0	4.3	2.1	0.4
7073	Lunch Meat, Salami, hard/Oscar Mayer	0.33 oz, 1 slice	9	35.8	2.5	0.3	0.0	2.8	1.4	0.3
7231	Lunch Meat, Sandwich Spread (Pork & Beef)	1.0 oz, 2 tbsp	28	65.8	2.1	3.3	0.1	4.9	2.1	0.7
7232	Lunch Meat, Sandwich Spread (Pork, Chicken & Beef)/Oscar Mayer	1.0 oz, 2 tbsp	28	66.4	1.8	4.3	0.1	4.6	2.0	0.7
7233	Lunch Meat, Smokie Links Sausage/Oscar Mayer	1.5 oz, 1 link	43	129.9	5.3	0.7	0.0	11.7	5.7	1.2
7236	Lunch Meat, Smokies Sausage Little (Pork & Turkey)/Oscar Mayer	0.33 oz, 1 sm link	9	27.1	1.1	0.2	0.0	2.4	1.2	0.3
7237	Lunch Meat, Smokies Sausage Little Cheese (Pork & Turkey)/Oscar Mayer	0.33 oz, 1 sm link	9	28.4	1.2	0.2	0.0	2.5	1.2	0.3
7254	Lunch Meat, Summer Sausage Thuringer Cervalat/Oscar Mayer	1.0 oz, 1 slice	28	85.1	4.2	0.3	0.0	7.5	3.4	0.6
7255	Lunch Meat, Turkey Bacon/Louis Rich	0.5 oz, 1 slice	14	34.2	2.2	0.3	0.0	2.7	1.1	0.7
7256	Lunch Meat, Turkey Bologna/Louis Rich	1.0 oz, 1 slice	28	51.5	3.2	1.3	0.0	3.7	1.5	1.0
7259	Lunch Meat, Turkey Breast Meat	1.5 oz, 2 slices	42	46.2	9.5	0.0	0.0	0.7	0.2	0.1
7260	Lunch Meat, Turkey Breast, oven roasted, fat free/Louis Rich	1.0 oz, 1 slice	28	23.5	4.2	1.3	0.0	0.2	0.1	0.0
7239	Lunch Meat, Turkey Breast, smoked, carving board/Louis Rich	2, 1.0 oz slices	45	42.3	8.9	0.7	0.0	0.5	0.1	0.1
7080	Lunch Meat, Turkey Ham, 10% water added/Louis Rich	1.0 oz slice	28	31.6	5.1	0.3	0.0	1.1	0.3	0.2
7265	Lunch Meat, Turkey Ham, cured	2 slices	57	73.0	10.8	0.2	0.0	2.9	0.7	0.9
7081	Lunch Meat, Turkey Roll, light & dark meat	2.0 oz slice	56	83.4	10.2	1.2	0.0	3.9	1.3	1.0
7267	Lunch Meat, Turkey Roll, light meat	2.0 oz slice	56	82.3	10.5	0.3	0.0	4.0	1.4	1.0
7266	Lunch Meat, Turkey Salami Cotto/Louis Rich	1.0 oz, 1 slice	28	41.7	4.2	0.3	0.0	2.7	1.1	0.7
5300	Lunch Meat, Turkey Smoked Sausage/Louis Rich	2 oz, slice	56	89.6	8.1	2.2	0.0	5.4	2.0	1.5
7273	Lunch Meat, Turkey, honey roasted, fat free/Louis Rich	2.0 oz slice	56	57.1	10.8	2.5	0.0	0.4	0.1	0.1
7243	Lunch Meat, Wieners (Beef Franks) bun length/Oscar Mayer	1 frank	57	183.5	6.4	1.6	0.0	16.9	8.3	0.5
7241	Lunch Meat, Wieners (Beef Franks) light/Oscar Mayer	1 frank	57	110.0	6.1	2.3	0.0	8.5	4.3	0.6
7246	Lunch Meat, Wieners (Cheese Hot Dogs w/turkey)/Oscar Mayer	1 frank	45	143.1	5.4	1.3	0.0	12.9	5.9	1.7
7247	Lunch Meat, Wieners (Hot Dogs) fat free/Oscar Mayer	1 frank	50	36.5	6.3	2.2	0.0	0.3	0.1	0.1

Sat (g)	Chol (mg)	Cal (mg)	Iron (mg)	Magn (mg)	Phos (mg)	Pota (mg)	Sodi (mg)	Zinc (mg)	Vit A (RE)	Vit C (mg)	Vit E (mg)	Thia (mg)	Ribo (mg)	Niac (mg)	Vit B-6 (mg)	Fol (µg)	Vit B-12 (µg)	Wat (g)
1.6	12.6	3.6	0.3	3.9	49.8	43.7	313.9	0.5	0.0	0.0	0.0	0.0	0.0	0.0	0.0	0.0	0.0	18.2
3.4	16.2	3.4	0.5	3.4	24.6	44.0	274.7	0.6	0.0	0.0	0.1	0.0	0.0	0.7	0.0	1.4	0.4	15.5
2.9	28.8	19.3	0.5	5.9	55.7	43.1	289.2	0.4	0.0	0.0	0.0	0.0	0.0	0.0	0.0	0.0	0.0	15.0
1.9	16.5	3.1	0.2	3.9	38.9	78.7	331.5	0.6	0.0	0.0	0.1	0.1	0.0	1.1	0.1	1.4	0.3	17.0
1.4	27.7	23.5	0.4	3.9	36.7	55.7	245.8	0.5	0.0	0.0	0.1	0.0	0.0	1.0	0.1	2.0	0.1	18.2
0.1	7.0	4.2	0.3	6.2	43.1	43.7	273.6	0.3	0.0	0.0	0.0	0.0	0.0	0.0	0.0	0.0	0.0	21.8
3.1	49.0	2.5	2.7	3.9	55.7	56.6	324.0	1.0	0.0	2.5	0.0	0.1	0.4	2.6	0.1	13.2	5.3	14.1
0.0	14.6	2.2	0.4	9.0	79.0	81.5	319.8	0.2	0.0	0.0	0.0	0.0	0.0	0.0	0.0	0.0	0.0	20.4
0.1	15.1	2.8	0.3	10.1	80.9	92.1	388.1	0.2	0.0	0.0	0.0	0.0	0.0	0.0	0.0	0.0	0.0	19.7
0.2	13.7	2.0	0.3	6.7	74.5	74.2	332.6	0.2	0.0	0.0	0.0	0.0	0.0	0.0	0.0	0.0	0.0	20.6
0.0	12.3	3.4	0.4	10.1	71.7	88.5	347.8	0.2	0.0	0.0	0.0	0.0	0.0	0.0	0.0	0.0	0.0	21.2
1.2	28.5	24.5	0.6	10.8	89.5	130.0	332.9	0.4	13.7	0.0	0.2	0.0	0.1	3.0	0.1	1.1	0.1	39.1
1.5	22.4	53.8	1.0	5.2	38.3	45.6	166.0	0.5	10.8	0.0	0.0	0.0	0.0	1.2	0.1	1.3	0.1	28.5
1.8	37.6	88.0	1.1	0.0	0.0	181.8	677.3	0.0	0.0	0.0	0.0	0.0	0.2	4.8	0.0	0.0	0.0	48.4
2.0	46.2	12.1	1.7	0.0	0.0	249.9	952.8	0.0	0.0	0.0	0.0	0.0	0.1	0.2	3.0	0.0	0.0	49.1
1.8	13.2	23.5	0.3	5.9	45.4	105.3	350.0	0.5	0.0	0.0	0.1	0.1	0.1	0.7	0.1	0.6	0.4	16.6
2.3	42.3	109.4	0.9	9.9	91.8	71.1	481.5	0.8	0.0	0.0	0.0	0.0	0.0	0.0	0.0	0.0	0.0	28.8
1.7	41.4	59.0	1.0	10.4	66.2	72.0	511.2	0.8	0.0	0.0	0.0	0.0	0.0	0.0	0.0	0.0	0.0	30.1
2.1	16.0	16.2	0.3	4.5	70.8	82.3	376.0	0.6	6.4	0.0	0.1	0.2	0.1	1.0	0.1	0.8	0.2	16.2
3.7	26.2	93.3	0.3	7.7	212.9	69.7	514.7	1.0	39.1	0.0	0.0	0.1	0.1	0.9	0.1	1.3	0.3	25.4
1.8	18.5	18.8	0.2	5.3	75.6	74.2	350.8	0.5	0.0	0.0	0.2	0.1	1.0	0.1	0.8	0.2	17.0
1.4	10.4	2.2	0.2	2.8	33.6	42.0	255.4	0.3	0.0	0.0	0.5	0.1	0.0	0.6	0.0	0.3	0.2	17.5
0.2	9.5	2.1	0.3	6.5	54.4	59.0	262.1	0.4	0.0	0.0	0.0	0.0	0.0	0.0	0.0	0.0	0.0	15.3
1.5	14.7	2.1	0.2	3.4	33.0	65.3	261.5	0.4	0.0	0.0	0.0	0.1	0.0	0.9	0.1	0.2	0.2	12.0
0.5	13.3	2.0	0.2	4.8	61.8	99.2	405.1	0.5	0.0	0.0	0.0	0.1	0.3	1.4	0.1	1.1	0.2	20.0
1.0	16.2	2.0	0.3	5.4	70.0	94.1	373.4	0.6	0.0	0.0	0.1	0.2	0.1	1.5	0.1	0.9	0.12	18.3
2.2	39.1	11.4	1.4	0.0	0.0	241.4	980.5	0.0	0.0	0.0	0.0	0.5	0.2	3.7	0.0	0.0	0.0	47.6
0.5	30.2	6.3	0.8	19.5	146.8	168.8	764.8	1.1	0.0	0.0	0.0	0.0	0.0	0.0	0.0	0.0	0.0	47.1
1.2	25.5	5.9	0.5	3.1	17.6	8.1	300.4	0.3	0.0	0.0	0.0	0.0	0.0	0.3	0.0	0.3	0.3	18.9
0.8	19.4	9.7	0.8	9.7	81.5	195.5	752.4	1.4	0.0	0.0	0.1	0.3	0.1	1.8	0.2	4.6	0.6	40.2
0.4	9.9	2.9	1.0	5.2	40.3	116.6	383.4	1.0	0.0	0.0	0.0	0.0	0.1	1.4	0.1	2.0	1.5	21.6
2.5	48.7	2.2	3.0	3.4	58.0	63.3	343.0	1.0	1470.6	0.8	0.0	0.1	0.6	3.3	0.1	29.1	6.9	15.0
2.7	71.4	19.6	1.5	3.6	56.0	38.6	195.2	0.8	279.7	0.6	0.0	0.0	0.2	0.9	0.0	16.8	0.9	15.1
1.9	28.4	4.7	1.2	2.2	41.4	30.6	154.8	0.4	1494.0	0.0	0.0	0.0	0.2	0.8	0.0	5.4	2.4	9.4
1.5	18.8	30.5	0.4	6.7	54.6	75.6	343.3	0.5	0.0	0.0	0.0	0.0	0.0	0.0	0.0	0.0	0.0	16.4
1.6	17.1	31.6	0.4	6.4	58.2	82.3	331.5	0.5	0.0	0.0	0.0	0.0	0.0	0.0	0.0	0.0	0.0	16.5
2.0	19.9	31.1	0.5	7.6	37.0	52.1	369.0	0.3	0.0	0.0	0.0	0.0	0.0	0.0	0.0	0.0	0.0	16.1
1.6	10.6	30.5	0.2	5.3	35.6	83.2	415.5	0.4	5.6	0.0	0.1	0.1	0.1	0.5	0.1	0.6	0.4	16.3
2.9	26.0	2.5	0.5	5.0	42.0	63.8	343.6	1.2	0.0	0.0	0.1	0.0	0.0	1.4	0.1	2.0	0.5	13.1
0.5	15.1	2.5	0.5	3.9	56.0	72.8	292.6	0.6	0.0	0.0	0.1	0.0	0.1	1.0	0.1	1.4	0.1	19.8
0.6	12.9	15.1	0.3	5.6	47.6	110.3	426.4	0.9	0.0	0.0	0.1	0.1	0.1	0.9	0.1	0.6	0.5	18.9
2.2	10.4	26.6	0.3	5.0	39.2	95.2	388.9	0.4	2.0	0.0	0.1	0.1	0.1	0.6	0.1	1.4	0.3	16.0
2.6	18.5	3.8	0.4	4.3	37.9	57.1	200.6	0.6	0.0	0.0	0.0	0.0	0.0	0.0	0.0	0.0	0.0	11.9
2.3	13.0	1.3	0.2	2.1	17.2	45.2	270.7	0.3	0.0	0.2	0.1	0.1	0.0	0.7	0.0	1.3	0.2	10.8
1.4	17.4	1.5	0.6	3.6	47.0	43.5	274.9	0.4	0.0	0.0	0.0	0.0	0.0	0.0	0.0	0.0	0.0	13.5
1.8	16.8	15.8	0.6	6.1	51.9	45.6	230.0	0.4	0.0	0.0	0.0	0.0	0.0	0.0	0.0	0.0	0.0	12.7
1.0	8.6	1.1	0.2	1.9	16.2	32.0	169.4	0.3	0.0	0.0	0.0	0.1	0.0	0.5	0.0	0.3	0.2	3.0
1.7	10.6	3.4	0.2	2.2	16.5	30.8	283.6	0.3	2.5	0.0	0.5	0.0	0.0	0.5	0.0	0.6	0.3	16.9
1.6	12.6	7.6	0.2	3.4	19.3	33.0	229.9	0.2	0.0	0.0	0.0	0.0	0.0	0.0	0.0	0.0	0.0	16.6
4.0	27.1	4.3	0.5	7.3	103.2	77.4	433.0	0.9	0.0	0.0	0.0	0.0	0.0	0.0	0.0	0.0	0.0	23.9
0.8	5.8	1.0	0.1	1.5	19.1	15.6	92.0	0.2	0.0	0.0	0.0	0.0	0.0	0.0	0.0	0.0	0.0	5.0
1.0	6.0	6.0	0.1	1.9	22.3	13.7	93.2	0.2	0.0	0.0	0.0	0.0	0.0	0.0	0.0	0.0	0.0	4.8
3.0	23.5	2.5	0.6	4.2	36.4	63.8	400.4	0.6	0.0	0.0	0.0	0.1	0.1	1.2	0.1	1.4	1.1	14.9
0.7	12.5	5.6	0.2	2.7	27.9	29.1	184.2	0.4	0.0	0.0	0.0	0.0	0.0	0.0	0.0	0.0	0.0	8.3
1.1	19.0	34.7	0.5	6.2	54.9	42.6	269.9	0.5	0.0	0.0	0.0	0.0	0.0	0.0	0.0	0.0	0.0	19.0
0.2	17.2	2.9	0.2	8.4	96.2	116.8	601.0	0.5	0.0	0.0	0.0	0.0	0.0	3.5	0.2	1.7	0.8	30.2
0.1	9.0	3.1	0.3	7.6	65.0	57.4	333.8	0.2	0.0	0.0	0.0	0.0	0.0	0.0	0.0	0.0	0.0	21.4
0.1	19.4	6.8	0.7	14.0	143.1	140.4	540.5	0.4	0.0	0.0	0.0	0.0	0.0	0.0	0.0	0.0	0.0	33.4
0.3	18.8	1.4	0.4	6.2	82.3	81.2	315.6	0.7	0.0	0.0	0.0	0.0	0.0	0.0	0.0	0.0	0.0	20.5
1.0	31.9	5.7	1.6	9.1	108.9	185.3	567.7	1.7	0.0	0.0	0.4	0.0	0.1	2.0	0.1	3.4	0.1	40.7
1.1	30.8	17.9	0.8	10.1	94.1	151.2	328.2	1.1	0.0	0.0	0.2	0.1	0.2	2.7	0.2	2.8	0.1	39.3
1.1	24.1	22.4	0.7	9.0	102.5	140.6	273.8	0.9	0.0	0.0	0.1	0.0	0.1	3.9	0.2	2.2	0.1	40.1
0.8	21.6	8.7	0.5	5.9	76.2	61.6	285.0	0.7	0.0	0.0	0.0	0.0	0.0	0.0	0.0	0.0	0.0	20.0
1.5	35.8	14.6	0.8	11.8	114.2	112.6	515.2	1.2	0.0	0.0	0.0	0.0	0.0	0.0	0.0	0.0	0.0	38.7
0.1	22.4	8.4	0.6	15.7	154.6	146.7	660.8	0.6	0.0	0.0	0.0	0.0	0.0	0.0	0.0	0.0	0.0	40.3
7.1	32.5	7.4	0.9	8.6	59.9	90.1	575.7	1.3	0.0	0.0	0.0	0.0	0.0	0.0	0.0	0.0	0.0	30.6
3.6	27.9	12.0	0.9	10.3	93.5	228.6	615.0	1.2	0.0	0.0	0.0	0.0	0.0	0.0	0.0	0.0	0.0	38.1
4.5	33.3	73.8	0.7	11.3	96.8	59.0	514.4	0.8	0.0	0.0	0.0	0.0	0.0	0.0	0.0	0.0	0.0	23.8
0.1	14.5	7.5	0.5	10.5	81.0	235.5	487.0	0.6	0.0	0.0	0.0	0.0	0.0	0.0	0.0	0.0	0.0	39.4

Code	Food Name	Unit/Amt	Wt (g)	Energy (Kcal)	Prot (g)	Carb (g)	Fiber (g)	Fat (g)	Mono (g)	Poly (g)
7248	Lunch Meat, Wieners (Pork & Turkey)/Oscar Mayer	1 frank	45	144.9	5.0	1.3	0.0	13.3	6.2	1.9
924132	Macaroni&Beef/FrancoAm	7.5 oz	213	191.7	9.0	30.1	0.0	3.8	0.0	0.0
924274	Macaroni&Cheese Mix/Kraft	¾ cup	147	254.3	10.8	36.3	1.0	7.5	2.0	0.6
924275	Macaroni&Cheese, frozen	6.0 oz	170	195.5	11.0	21.8	1.0	7.1	0.0	0.0
924276	Macaroni&Cheese/FrancoAm	7.5 oz	213	166.1	6.5	23.1	1.0	5.4	0.0	0.0
20099	Macaroni, enriched, ckd	1 cup elbow shaped	140	197.4	6.7	39.7	1.8	0.9	0.1	0.4
20499	Macaroni, unenriched, ckd	1 cup	115	162.2	5.5	32.6	1.5	0.8	0.1	0.3
20105	Macaroni, Vegetable, enriched, ckd	1 cup elbow shaped	140	179.2	6.3	37.3	6.0	0.2	0.1	0.1
20107	Macaroni, Whole Wheat, ckd	1 cup	134	166.2	7.1	35.6	3.8	0.3	0.1	0.3
4585	Margarine (about 40% fat) Imitation	1 cup elbow shaped	140	483.3	0.7	0.6	0.0	54.3	22.0	19.3
4132	Margarine, blend: 60% corn oil & 40% butter	1 cup spiral shaped	105	753.9	0.9	0.7	0.0	84.7	34.4	16.7
4522	Margarine, Hard w/salt	1 tbsp	15	107.8	0.1	0.1	0.0	12.1	5.4	3.8
4067	Margarine, Hard, Corn, Corn-Hydrogenated	1 tbsp	15	107.8	0.1	0.1	0.0	12.1	5.8	3.6
4068	Margarine, Hard, Corn, Soybean-Hydrogenated & Cottonseed-Hydrogenated w/salt	1 tbsp	15	107.8	0.1	0.1	0.0	12.1	5.5	3.8
4071	Margarine, Hard, Corn, Soybean-Hydrogenated & Cottonseed-Hydrogenated, no salt	1 tbsp	15	107.1	0.1	0.1	0.0	12.0	5.5	3.8
4091	Margarine, Hard, Corn-Hydrogenated	1 tbsp	15	107.8	0.1	0.1	0.0	12.1	6.9	2.7
4131	Margarine, Hard, Lard-Hydrogenated	1 tbsp	15	110.0	0.1	0.1	0.0	12.1	5.7	1.1
4089	Margarine, Hard, no salt	1 tbsp	15	107.1	0.1	0.1	0.0	12.0	5.5	3.8
4079	Margarine, Hard, Safflower, Soybean-Hydrogenated	1 tbsp	15	107.8	0.1	0.1	0.0	12.1	4.8	4.7
4081	Margarine, Hard, Soybean, Soybean-Hydrogenated	1 tbsp	15	107.8	0.1	0.1	0.0	12.1	5.6	3.9
4076	Margarine, Hard, Soybean-Hydrogenated	1 tbsp	15	107.8	0.1	0.1	0.0	12.1	5.9	3.1
4082	Margarine, Hard, Soybean-Hydrogenated & Palm-Hydrogenated	1 tbsp	15	107.8	0.1	0.1	0.0	12.1	4.8	4.5
4521	Margarine, Hard, Soybean-Hydrogenated, Cottonseed	1 tbsp	15	107.8	0.1	0.1	0.0	12.1	6.1	3.0
4109	Margarine, Imitation (about 40% fat) Corn, Corn-Hydrogenated	1 tbsp	15	51.8	0.1	0.1	0.0	5.8	2.2	2.4
4112	Margarine, Imitation (about 40% fat) Soybean-Hydrogenated	1 tbsp	15	51.8	0.1	0.1	0.0	5.8	2.5	2.1
4130	Margarine, Liquid, Soybean-Hydrogenated, Soybean, Cottonseed	1 tbsp	15	108.2	0.3	0.0	0.0	12.1	4.2	5.4
4092	Margarine, Soft w/salt	1 tbsp	15	107.5	0.1	0.1	0.0	12.1	4.3	5.2
4129	Margarine, Soft, Corn, Corn-Hydrogenated	1 tbsp	15	107.5	0.1	0.1	0.0	12.1	4.7	4.7
4101	Margarine, Soft, no salt	1 tbsp	15	107.5	0.1	0.1	0.0	12.0	5.6	3.9
4094	Margarine, Soft, Safflower, Safflower-Hydrogenated	1 tbsp	15	107.5	0.1	0.1	0.0	12.1	3.5	6.7
4093	Margarine&Soft, Soybean, Soybean-Hydrogenated w/salt	1 tbsp	15	107.5	0.1	0.1	0.0	12.1	5.5	4.0
4103	Margarine, Soft, Soybean, Soybean-Hydrogenated, no salt	1 tbsp	15	107.5	0.1	0.1	0.0	12.0	5.5	4.0
4099	Margarine, Soft, Soybean, Soybean & Cottonseed-Hydrogenated	1 tbsp	15	107.5	0.1	0.1	0.0	12.1	4.6	4.5
4095	Margarine, Soft, Soybean-Hydrogenated & Safflower	1 tbsp	15	107.5	0.1	0.1	0.0	12.1	4.7	5.3
4523	Margarine, Soft, Soybean-Hydrogenated, Cottonseed	1 tbsp	15	107.5	0.1	0.1	0.0	12.1	4.7	4.4
4525	Margarine, Soft, Soybean-Hydrogenated, Palm-Hydrogenated & Palm	1 tbsp	15	107.5	0.1	0.1	0.0	12.1	3.8	5.2
4527	Margarine-Like Spread (about 60% fat) tub	1 tbsp	15	80.9	0.1	0.0	0.0	9.1	4.7	2.1
920900	Mayonnaise Dressing, low kcal	2 tbsp	30	42.9	0.0	4.3	0.0	4.3	1.3	2.1
20324	Meal, Corn, enriched, ckd	1 cup	170	85.0	2.1	18.4	2.1	0.2	0.1	0.1
20322	Meal, Corn, White w/wheat flour, Selfrise, enriched, bolted	1 cup	170	591.6	14.3	124.8	10.7	4.8	1.3	2.2
20325	Meal, Corn, White, Selfrise, enriched, bolted	1 cup	122	407.5	10.1	85.7	8.2	4.1	1.1	1.9
20024	Meal, Corn, White, Whole Grain	1 cup	122	441.6	9.9	93.8	8.9	4.4	1.2	2.0
20025	Meal, Corn, Yellow, Degermed, enriched	1 cup	138	505.1	11.7	107.2	10.2	2.3	0.6	1.0
20020	Meal, Corn, Yellow, Degermed, unenriched	1 cup	138	505.1	11.7	107.2	10.2	2.3	0.6	1.0
18236	Meal, Corn, Yellow, Whole Grain	1 cup	122	441.6	9.9	93.8	8.9	4.4	1.2	2.0
16106	Meal, Crackermeal	1 tbsp	1.2	4.6	0.1	1.0	0.0	0.0	0.0	0.0
902934	Meat Extender, Vegetarian, Meatless	1 cup	88	275.4	33.5	33.7	15.4	2.6	0.6	1.5
902935	Meat Tenderizer	1 tsp	5	2.0	0.0	0.0	0.0	0.0	0.0	0.0
924327	Meat&Shrimp (shellfish) Egg Roll/LaChoy	3 medium	37	79.9	3.0	11.0	0.0	3.0	1.2	1.2
14422	Meatloaf	3.5 oz	98	159.7	17.0	4.6	0.2	7.6	0.0	0.0
14423	Milk Beverage Mix, Chocolate Dairy Drink w/aspartame, low kcal, dry	½ cup H₂O, 3 icecubes, ¾ oz pkt	204	607.9	51.0	102.4	3.3	5.3	1.0	0.1
901916	Milk Beverage Mix, Dairy Drink w/aspartame, low kcal, dry, prep w/H₂O	½ cup	74	22.9	1.9	3.8	0.1	0.2	0.0	0.0
901900	Milk Dessert, frozen, Vanilla/Simple Pleasures	½ cup	89	115.7	5.9	21.1	0.0	0.7	0.1	0.0
19220	Milk Dessert, frozen, Vanilla/Simple Pleasures Lite	½ cup	74	71.8	4.6	15.0	1.0	0.4	0.1	0.1
19221	Milk Dessert, Rennin, Chocolate, dry mix prep w/reduced fat (2%) milk	½ cup	137	111.0	4.4	18.5	0.7	2.9	0.8	0.1
19225	Milk Dessert, Rennin, Chocolate, dry mix prep w/whole milk	½ cup	137	126.0	4.4	18.2	0.7	4.5	1.3	0.2
19223	Milk Dessert, Rennin, Vanilla, dry mix prep w/reduced fat (2%) milk	½ cup	137	104.1	4.2	16.9	0.0	2.5	0.7	0.1
919224	Milk Dessert, Rennin, Vanilla, dry mix prep w/whole milk	½ cup	137	119.2	4.1	16.7	0.0	4.2	1.2	0.2
901905	Milk Dessert, Rennin, Vanilla, homemade	½ cup	137	112.3	4.0	15.3	0.0	4.1	0.0	0.0
1110	Milk Drink, Vanilla Cream	12 fl oz	360	194.4	0.0	48.0	0.0	0.0	0.0	0.0
1111	Milk Shake, Thick, Chocolate	1 container (10.6 oz net wt)	300	355.8	9.2	63.5	0.9	8.1	2.3	0.3
1094	Milk Shake, Thick, Vanilla	1 container (11 oz net wt)	313	350.0	12.1	55.6	0.0	9.5	2.7	0.4
1088	Milk, Buttermilk, Dry	1 tbsp	6.5	25.1	2.2	3.2	0.0	0.4	0.1	0.0
1059	Milk, Buttermilk, Lowfat, Cultured	1 cup	245	99.0	8.1	11.7	0.0	2.2	0.6	0.1
1082	Milk, Human, Mature Breast	1 fl oz	30.8	21.4	0.3	2.1	0.0	1.3	0.5	0.2
1083	Milk, Lowfat, 1% fat w/added vitamin A	1 cup	244	102.1	8.0	11.7	0.0	2.6	0.7	0.1
1104	Milk, Lowfat, 1% fat w/NFDM & Vit A added	1 cup	245	104.4	8.5	12.2	0.0	2.4	0.7	0.1

Sat (g)	Chol (mg)	Cal (mg)	Iron (mg)	Magn (mg)	Phos (mg)	Pota (mg)	Sodi (mg)	Zinc (mg)	Vit A (RE)	Vit C (mg)	Vit E (mg)	Thia (mg)	Ribo (mg)	Niac (mg)	Vit B-6 (mg)	Fol (µg)	Vit B-12 (µg)	Wat (g)
4.3	32.4	27.0	0.5	7.7	61.7	72.9	434.7	0.8	0.0	0.0	0.0	0.0	0.0	0.0	0.0	0.0	0.0	24.0
0.0	0.0	43.0	2.2	0.0	113.0	333.0	792.0	0.0	192.6	7.0	0.0	0.2	0.2	3.2	0.0	0.0	0.0	0.0
4.2	18.0	123.0	1.9	29.0	345.0	94.0	652.0	1.3	77.6	0.0	0.0	0.3	0.2	1.7	0.0	12.0	0.2	90.3
0.0	17.0	269.0	0.7		197.0	73.0	358.0	4.0	17.6	4.0	0.0	0.2	0.2	0.9	0.0	0.0	0.0	0.0
0.0	0.0	95.0	1.5	0.0	117.0	114.0	934.0	1.4	173.4	0.0	0.0	0.2	0.2	2.1	0.0	0.0	0.0	0.0
0.1	0.0	9.8	2.0	25.2	75.6	43.4	1.4	0.7	0.0	0.0	0.0	0.3	0.1	2.3	0.0	98.0	0.0	92.4
0.1	0.0	8.1	0.6	20.7	62.1	35.7	1.2	0.6	0.0	0.0	0.0	0.0	0.0	0.5	0.0	8.1	0.0	75.9
0.0	0.0	15.4	0.7	26.6	70.0	43.4	8.4	0.6	7.0	0.0	0.1	0.2	0.1	1.5	0.0	91.0	0.0	95.7
0.1	0.0	20.1	1.4	40.2	119.3	59.0	4.0	1.1	0.0	0.0	0.1	0.1	0.1	0.9	0.1	6.7	0.0	90.0
10.8	0.0	24.9	0.0	2.2	19.2	35.4	1343.4	0.0	1118.6	0.1	3.3	0.0	0.0	0.0	0.0	1.0	0.1	81.3
29.9	92.4	29.4	0.1	2.1	24.2	37.8	941.9	0.0	839.0	0.1	8.0	0.0	0.0	0.0	0.0	2.1	0.1	16.6
2.4	0.0	4.5	0.0	0.4	3.4	6.4	141.5	0.0	119.9	0.0	1.9	0.0	0.0	0.0	0.0	0.2	0.0	2.4
2.1	0.0	4.5	0.0	0.4	3.4	6.4	141.5	0.0	119.9	0.0	2.2	0.0	0.0	0.0	0.0	0.2	0.0	2.4
2.3	0.0	4.5	0.0	0.4	3.4	6.4	141.5	0.0	119.9	0.0	0.0	0.0	0.0	0.0	0.0	0.2	0.0	2.4
2.3	0.0	2.6	0.0	0.2	2.0	3.7	0.3	0.0	119.9	0.0	1.7	0.0	0.0	0.0	0.0	0.1	0.0	2.8
2.0	0.0	4.5	0.0	0.4	3.4	6.4	141.5	0.0	119.9	0.0	0.0	0.0	0.0	0.0	0.0	0.2	0.0	2.4
4.7	7.7	0.0	0.0	0.0	0.0	6.4	141.5	0.0	0.0	0.0	0.0	0.0	0.0	0.0	0.0	0.0	0.0	2.4
2.3	0.0	2.6	0.0	0.2	2.0	3.7	0.3	0.0	119.9	0.0	1.9	0.0	0.0	0.0	0.0	0.1	0.0	2.8
2.1	0.0	4.5	0.0	0.4	3.4	6.4	141.5	0.0	119.9	0.0	0.0	0.0	0.0	0.0	0.0	0.2	0.0	2.4
2.0	0.0	4.5	0.0	0.4	3.4	6.4	141.5	0.0	119.9	0.0	0.0	0.0	0.0	0.0	0.0	0.2	0.0	2.4
2.5	0.0	4.5	0.0	0.4	3.4	6.4	141.5	0.0	119.9	0.0	1.6	0.0	0.0	0.0	0.0	0.0	0.0	2.4
2.3	0.0	4.5	0.0	0.4	3.4	6.4	141.5	0.0	119.9	0.0	0.0	0.0	0.0	0.0	0.0	0.0	0.0	2.4
2.4	0.0	4.5	0.0	0.4	3.4	6.4	141.5	0.0	119.9	0.0	0.0	0.0	0.0	0.0	0.0	0.2	0.0	2.4
1.0	0.0	2.7	0.0	0.2	2.1	3.8	143.9	0.0	119.9	0.0	0.0	0.0	0.0	0.0	0.0	0.1	0.0	8.7
1.0	0.0	2.7	0.0	0.2	2.1	3.8	143.9	0.0	119.9	0.0	0.0	0.0	0.0	0.0	0.0	0.1	0.0	8.7
2.0	0.0	9.9	0.0	0.9	7.6	14.1	117.1	0.0	119.9	0.1	0.8	0.0	0.0	0.0	0.0	0.4	0.0	2.4
2.1	0.0	4.0	0.0	0.3	3.0	5.7	161.8	0.0	119.9	0.0	1.8	0.0	0.0	0.0	0.0	0.2	0.0	2.4
2.1	0.0	4.0	0.0	0.3	3.0	5.7	161.8	0.0	119.9	0.0	0.0	0.0	0.0	0.0	0.0	0.2	0.0	2.4
2.1	0.0	4.0	0.0	0.3	3.0	5.7	4.1	0.0	119.9	0.0	1.3	0.0	0.0	0.0	0.0	0.2	0.0	2.7
1.4	0.0	4.0	0.0	0.3	3.0	5.7	161.8	0.0	119.9	0.0	0.0	0.0	0.0	0.0	0.0	0.2	0.0	2.4
2.0	0.0	4.0	0.0	0.3	3.0	5.7	161.8	0.0	119.9	0.0	0.0	0.0	0.0	0.0	0.0	0.2	0.0	2.4
2.0	0.0	4.0	0.0	0.3	3.0	5.7	4.1	0.0	119.9	0.0	0.0	0.0	0.0	0.0	0.0	0.2	0.0	2.7
2.4	0.0	4.0	0.0	0.3	3.0	5.7	161.8	0.0	119.9	0.0	0.0	0.0	0.0	0.0	0.0	0.2	0.0	2.4
1.6	0.0	4.0	0.0	0.3	3.0	5.7	161.8	0.0	119.9	0.0	0.0	0.0	0.0	0.0	0.0	0.2	0.0	2.4
2.5	0.0	4.0	0.0	0.3	3.0	5.7	161.8	0.0	119.9	0.0	0.0	0.0	0.0	0.0	0.0	0.2	0.0	2.4
2.6	0.0	4.0	0.0	0.3	3.0	5.7	161.8	0.0	119.9	0.0	0.0	0.0	0.0	0.0	0.0	0.2	0.0	2.4
1.9	0.0	3.1	0.0	0.3	2.4	4.5	149.1	0.0	119.9	0.0	1.4	0.0	0.0	0.0	0.0	0.1	0.0	5.6
0.9	4.3	6.4	0.0	0.0	8.6	2.1	40.7	0.0	17.1	0.0	0.0	0.0	0.0	0.0	0.0	0.0	0.0	0.0
0.0	0.0	1.4	1.0	70.8	24.1	26.9	0.0	0.2	19.8	0.0	0.0	0.1	0.1	0.9	0.0	4.3	0.0	0.0
0.7	0.0	508.3	8.4	91.8	1106.7	351.9	2242.3	2.4	0.0	0.0	0.0	1.2	0.7	8.8	0.7	312.8	0.0	17.6
0.6	0.0	440.4	7.0	104.9	980.9	311.1	1521.3	2.4	0.0	0.0	0.0	0.8	0.5	6.5	0.7	228.1	0.0	15.4
0.6	0.0	7.3	4.2	154.9	294.0	350.1	42.7	2.2	0.0	0.0	0.4	0.5	0.2	4.4	0.4	31.0	0.0	12.5
0.3	0.0	6.9	5.7	55.2	115.9	223.6	4.1	1.0	56.6	0.0	0.5	1.0	0.6	6.9	0.4	258.1	0.0	16.0
0.3	0.0	6.9	1.5	55.2	115.9	223.6	4.1	1.0	56.6	0.0	0.5	0.2	0.1	1.4	0.4	66.2	0.0	16.0
0.6	0.0	7.3	4.2	154.9	294.0	350.1	42.7	2.2	57.3	0.0	0.8	0.5	0.2	4.4	0.4	31.0	0.0	12.5
0.0	0.0	0.3	0.1	0.3	1.2	1.4	0.3	0.0	0.0	0.0	0.0	0.0	0.0	0.1	0.0	1.4	0.0	0.1
0.4	0.0	179.5	10.6	190.1	562.3	1673.8	8.8	1.9	2.6	0.0	0.0	0.6	0.8	19.4	1.2	174.2	5.3	6.6
0.0	0.0	11.0	0.1	2.0	0.0	2.0	1695.0	0.0	1.0	0.0	0.0	0.0	0.0	0.0	0.0	0.0	0.0	0.0
0.6	4.0	9.0	0.8	0.0	0.0	65.0	115.0	0.0	2.0	3.0	0.0	0.1	0.1	1.0	0.0	0.0	0.0	0.0
0.0	92.0	38.0	2.3	0.0	162.0	374.0	653.0	0.0	35.8	2.0	0.0	0.1	0.2	8.0	0.0	0.0	0.0	0.0
3.8	16.3	1795.2	15.7	428.4	1740.1	4569.6	1591.2	7.3	701.8	2.4	0.2	0.2	4.0	2.6	0.2	85.7	4.9	26.1
0.1	0.7	69.6	0.6	17.0	65.9	173.9	62.2	0.3	26.6	0.1	0.0	0.0	0.2	0.1	0.0	3.3	0.2	67.2
0.2	12.0	162.0	0.1	12.0	122.0	114.0	50.0	0.7	103.6	0.0	0.0	0.0	0.2	0.1	0.0	0.0	0.0	61.0
0.2	9.0	128.0	0.6	13.0	105.0	201.0	68.0	0.4	69.2	0.0	0.0	0.1	0.2	0.1	0.1	0.0	0.9	0.7
1.7	9.6	172.6	0.4	27.4	134.3	249.3	71.2	0.7	60.3	1.2	0.0	0.0	0.2	0.1	0.1	6.9	0.5	110.1
2.8	16.4	169.9	0.4	27.4	132.9	245.2	69.9	0.7	32.9	1.1	0.0	0.0	0.2	0.1	0.1	6.9	0.4	108.6
1.5	9.6	165.8	0.1	17.8	130.2	194.5	63.0	0.5	71.2	1.2	0.0	0.0	0.2	0.1	0.1	6.9	0.5	112.5
2.6	17.8	163.0	0.1	16.4	127.4	191.8	63.0	0.5	34.3	1.2	0.0	0.0	0.2	0.1	0.1	6.9	0.5	111.0
0.2	1.2	150.7	0.1	16.4	115.1	185.0	95.9	0.5	37.0	1.1	0.0	0.0	0.2	0.1	0.1	5.5	0.4	112.6
0.0	0.0	0.0	0.0	0.0	0.0	0.0	28.0	0.0	0.0	0.0	0.0	0.0	0.0	0.0	0.0	0.0	0.0	0.0
5.0	31.5	396.0	0.9	48.0	378.0	672.0	333.0	1.4	63.0	0.0	0.3	0.1	0.7	0.4	0.1	14.7	0.9	216.6
5.9	36.9	457.3	0.3	36.8	360.6	571.9	298.6	1.2	87.6	0.0	0.3	0.1	0.6	0.5	0.1	20.7	1.6	233.0
0.2	4.5	77.0	0.0	7.1	60.6	103.5	33.6	0.3	3.5	0.4	0.0	0.0	0.1	0.1	0.0	3.1	0.2	0.2
1.3	8.6	285.2	0.1	26.8	218.5	370.7	257.0	1.0	19.6	2.4	0.1	0.1	0.4	0.1	0.1	12.3	0.5	220.8
0.6	4.3	9.9	0.0	1.0	4.2	15.8	5.2	0.1	19.7	1.5	0.3	0.0	0.0	0.1	0.0	1.6	0.0	27.0
1.6	9.8	300.1	0.1	33.7	234.7	380.9	123.2	1.0	144.0	2.4	0.1	0.1	0.4	0.2	0.1	12.4	0.9	219.8
1.5	9.8	312.9	0.1	35.2	244.8	397.1	128.4	1.0	144.6	2.5	0.1	0.1	0.4	0.2	0.1	13.0	0.9	220.0

Code	Food Name	Unit/Amt	Wt (g)	Energy (Kcal)	Prot (g)	Carb (g)	Fiber (g)	Fat (g)	Mono (g)	Poly (g)
1084	Milk, Lowfat, 1% fat, Chocolate	1 cup	250	157.6	8.1	26.1	1.3	2.5	0.8	0.1
1154	Milk, Lowfat, 1% fat, protein fortified, Vit A added	1 cup	246	119.1	9.7	13.6	0.0	2.9	0.8	0.1
1093	Milk, Nonfat, Dry w/addedVit A	¼ cup	30	108.7	10.8	15.6	0.0	0.2	0.1	0.0
1092	Milk, Nonfat, Dry, Calcium Reduced	1.0 oz	28.35	100.3	10.1	14.7	0.0	0.1	0.0	0.0
1155	Milk, Nonfat, Dry, Instant w/added Vit A	1 cup	68	243.6	23.9	35.5	0.0	0.5	0.1	0.0
1091	Milk, Nonfat, Dry, Instant w/o Vit A added	1 cup	68	243.4	23.9	35.5	0.0	0.5	0.1	0.0
1097	Milk, Nonfat, Dry, Regular w/o Vit A added	1 tbsp	7.5	27.2	2.7	3.9	0.0	0.1	0.0	0.0
1085	Milk, Nonfat, Skim, Evaporated, canned	1 tbsp	16	12.5	1.2	1.8	0.0	0.0	0.0	0.0
1086	Milk, Nonfat/Fat Free, Skim w/added Vit A	1 cup	245	85.5	8.4	11.9	0.0	0.4	0.1	0.0
1151	Milk, Nonfat/Fat Free, Skim w/NFDM & Vit A added	1 cup	245	90.3	8.7	12.3	0.0	0.6	0.2	0.0
1087	Milk, Nonfat/Fat Free, Skim w/o added Vit A	1 cup	245	85.8	8.4	11.9	0.0	0.4	0.1	0.0
1079	Milk, Nonfat/Fat Free, Skim, protein fortified, Vit A added	1 cup	246	99.9	9.7	13.7	0.0	0.6	0.2	0.0
1080	Milk, Reduced Fat, 2% fat w/added vitamin A	1 cup	244	121.2	8.1	11.7	0.0	4.7	1.4	0.2
1152	Milk, Reduced Fat, 2% fat w/NFDM & Vit A added	1 cup	245	124.9	8.5	12.2	0.0	4.7	1.4	0.2
1103	Milk, Reduced Fat, 2% fat w/NFDM, w/o added Vit A	1 cup	245	136.0	9.7	13.5	0.0	4.9	0.2	0.0
1081	Milk, Reduced Fat, 2% fat, Chocolate	1.0 fl oz	31.2	22.3	1.0	3.2	0.2	0.6	0.2	0.0
16120	Milk, Reduced Fat, 2% fat, protein fortified, Vit A added	1 cup	246	136.6	9.7	13.5	0.0	4.9	1.4	0.2
1075	Milk, Soy, fluid	1 cup	240	79.2	6.6	4.3	3.1	4.6	0.8	2.0
1076	Milk, Substitute w/hydrogenated vege oils	1 cup	244	150.0	4.3	15.0	0.0	8.3	4.9	1.2
1095	Milk, Substitute w/lauric acid oil	1 cup	244	150.0	4.3	15.0	0.0	8.3	0.4	0.0
1077	Milk, Sweetened Condensed, canned	1.0 fl oz	38.2	122.5	3.0	20.8	0.0	3.3	0.9	0.1
1078	Milk, Whole, 3.25% fat	1 tbsp	15.2	9.3	0.5	0.7	0.0	0.5	0.1	0.0
1102	Milk, Whole, 3.7% fat	1 cup	244	156.6	8.0	11.3	0.0	8.9	2.6	0.3
1090	Milk, Whole, Chocolate	8.0 fl oz	266	221.7	8.4	27.5	2.1	9.0	2.6	0.3
1153	Milk, Whole, Dry	1 tbsp	8	39.7	2.1	3.1	0.0	2.1	0.6	0.1
1096	Milk, Whole, Evaporated, canned, w/added Vit A	1 fl oz	31.5	42.3	2.1	3.2	0.0	2.4	0.7	0.1
1106	Milk, Whole, Evaporated, canned, w/o Vit A added	1 tbsp	15.75	21.2	1.1	1.6	0.0	1.2	0.4	0.0
1108	Milk, Whole, Goat	1 fl oz	30.5	21.0	1.1	1.4	0.0	1.3	0.3	0.0
1089	Milk, Whole, Indian Buffalo	8.0 fl oz	244	235.8	9.2	12.6	0.0	16.8	4.4	0.4
1109	Milk, Whole, low sodium	1 cup	244	148.6	7.6	10.9	0.0	8.4	2.4	0.3
924033	Milk, Whole, Sheep	1 cup	244	263.1	14.6	13.1	0.0	17.1	4.2	0.8
18613	Muffin, Almond Poppyseed Mix, dry/Krusteaz	1 piece	2	8.4	0.1	1.5	0.0	0.2	0.0	0.0
18274	Muffin, Blueberry Mix/Martha White	1 small muffin	40	161.6	2.0	30.4	0.0	3.5	0.0	0.0
18275	Muffin, Blueberry, commercially prep	1 serving	40	110.8	2.2	19.2	1.0	2.6	0.8	1.0
18278	Muffin, Blueberry, dry mix, prep	1 muffin (2.25" dia x 1.75")	50	149.5	2.6	24.4	0.6	4.4	0.0	0.0
918391	Muffin, Blueberry, homemade w/reduced fat (2%) milk	1 muffin	57	162.5	3.7	23.2	0.0	6.2	1.5	3.1
18279	Muffin, Blueberry, homemade w/whole milk	1 muffin (2.75" dia x 2")	57	165.3	3.7	23.1	0.0	6.4	0.0	0.0
918280	Muffin, Corn, commercially prep	1 muffin (2.5" dia x 2.25")	57	173.9	3.4	29.0	1.9	4.8	1.2	1.8
918393	Muffin, Corn, homemade w/reduced fat (2%) milk	1 muffin (2.75" dia x 2")	57	180.1	4.0	25.2	0.0	7.0	1.7	3.5
18605	Muffin, Corn, homemade w/whole milk	1 muffin (2.75" dia x 2")	57	183.0	4.0	25.2	0.0	7.4	0.0	0.0
18273	Muffin, Oatbran	1 muffin (2.5" dia x 2.25")	57	153.9	4.0	27.5	2.6	4.2	1.0	2.4
918389	Muffin, Plain, homemade w/reduced fat (2%) milk	1 muffin	57	168.7	3.9	23.6	1.5	6.5	1.6	3.3
18639	Muffin, Plain, homemade w/whole milk	1 muffin (2.75" dia x 2")	57	171.6	3.9	23.6	1.5	6.8	0.0	0.0
18284	Muffin, Thomas' English Muffins, plain/Best Foods	1.0 oz	29	66.9	2.5	13.2	0.0	0.4	0.5	0.9
918287	Muffin, Wheat Bran, dry mix, prep	1 muffin (2.25" dia x 1.75")	50	138.0	3.3	23.3	2.1	4.6	0.0	0.0
918394	Muffin, Wheat Bran, homemade w/reduced fat (2%) milk	1 muffin (2.75" dia x 2")	57	161.3	4.0	23.9	0.0	7.0	0.0	0.0
18601	Muffin, Wheat Bran, homemade w/whole milk	1 muffin (2.75" dia x 2")	57	164.2	4.0	23.8	0.0	7.3	0.0	0.0
20134	Muffin, Wild Blueberry, dry mix/General Mills-Betty Crocker	1 serving	40	128.4	2.1	26.0	0.0	1.8	0.0	0.0
22702	Noodle Weenee/VanCamp	1 cup	220	244.2	9.3	32.9	0.0	8.5	0.0	0.0
16082	Noodles, Alfredo Egg Noodles in a Creamy Sauce, dry mix/Lipton	1 cup	93	388.6	14.4	58.0	0.0	11.0	3.6	1.2
20113	Noodles, Beans, Mung, Long Rice or Cellophane, dry	1 tbsp	8.8	30.9	0.0	7.6	0.0	0.0	0.0	0.0
20110	Noodles, Chinese, Chow Mein	1 tbsp	2.8	14.8	0.2	1.6	0.1	0.9	0.2	0.5
20310	Noodles, Egg, enriched, ckd w/salt	1 tbsp	10	13.3	0.5	2.5	0.1	0.1	0.0	0.0
20111	Noodles, Egg, Spinach, enriched, ckd	1 cup	160	211.2	8.1	38.8	3.7	2.5	0.8	0.6
20510	Noodles, Egg, unenriched, ckd w/o salt	1 cup	160	212.8	7.6	39.7	1.8	2.4	0.7	0.7
20409	Noodles, Egg, unenriched, ckd w/salt	1 cup	160	212.8	7.6	39.7	0.0	2.4	0.7	0.7
20114	Noodles, Japanese, Soba, ckd	1 cup	114	112.9	5.8	24.4	0.0	0.1	0.0	0.0
20116	Noodles, Japanese, Somen, ckd	1 cup	176	230.6	7.0	48.5	0.0	0.3	0.0	0.1
20133	Noodles, Ramen	1 cup	227	231.5	6.2	34.1	4.1	8.4	4.3	2.9
12195	Nut Butter, Almond Butter w/honey & cinnamon, w/salt	1 cup	250	1505.0	39.6	67.4	9.3	130.5	84.7	27.4
12088	Nut Butter, Almond Butter, Plain, w/salt	1 cup	250	1582.5	37.7	53.1	9.3	147.8	95.9	31.0
12060	Nut Butter, Cashew Butter, Plain, w/salt	1 tbsp	16	93.9	2.8	4.4	0.3	7.9	4.7	1.3
12168	Nut Flour, Acorn, full-fat	3.5 oz	100	501.0	7.5	54.7	0.0	30.2	19.1	5.8
12697	Nut Flour, Pecan	3.5 oz	100	329.0	31.9	50.7	0.0	1.4	0.7	0.3
12197	Nut Meal, Almond, partly defatted, w/salt	3.5 oz	100	408.0	39.5	28.9	0.0	18.3	11.9	3.8
16420	Nut Paste, Almond Paste	1 cup firmly packed	227	1039.7	20.4	108.5	10.9	63.0	40.9	13.2
16421	Nutrient/Protein Supplement, Soy Protein Conc prep w/acid wash	3.5 oz	100	332.0	58.1	31.2	5.5	0.5	0.1	0.2
16122	Nutrient/Protein Supplement, Soy Protein Conc, prep w/R-OH extraction	3.5 oz	100	332.0	58.1	31.2	5.5	0.5	0.1	0.2
16422	Nutrient/Protein Supplement, Soy Protein Isolate	3.5 oz	100	338.0	80.7	7.4	5.6	3.4	0.6	1.6

Sat (g)	Chol (mg)	Cal (mg)	Iron (mg)	Magn (mg)	Phos (mg)	Pota (mg)	Sodi (mg)	Zinc (mg)	Vit A (RE)	Vit C (mg)	Vit E (mg)	Thia (mg)	Ribo (mg)	Niac (mg)	Vit B-6 (mg)	Fol (μg)	Vit B-12 (μg)	Wat (g)
1.5	7.3	286.8	0.6	33.3	256.5	425.5	151.8	1.0	147.5	2.3	0.1	0.1	0.4	0.3	0.1	12.0	0.9	211.3
1.8	9.8	349.3	0.1	39.3	273.3	443.5	143.4	1.1	145.1	2.8	0.0	0.1	0.5	0.2	0.1	14.5	1.0	218.3
0.1	5.9	377.1	0.1	33.0	290.5	538.2	160.6	1.2	198.0	2.0	0.0	0.1	0.5	0.3	0.1	15.0	1.2	0.9
0.0	0.6	79.4	0.1	17.0	286.6	192.8	646.4	1.1	0.6	1.9	0.0	0.0	0.5	0.2	0.1	14.0	1.1	1.4
0.3	12.4	836.9	0.2	79.6	669.6	1159.7	373.1	3.0	482.8	3.8	0.0	0.3	1.2	0.6	0.2	33.9	2.7	2.7
0.3	12.2	837.1	0.2	79.6	669.8	1159.4	373.3	3.0	3.4	3.8	0.0	0.3	1.2	0.6	0.2	34.0	2.7	2.7
0.0	1.5	94.3	0.0	8.3	72.6	134.6	40.1	0.3	0.6	0.5	0.0	0.0	0.1	0.1	0.0	3.8	0.3	0.2
0.0	0.6	46.3	0.0	4.3	31.2	53.0	18.4	0.1	18.7	0.2	0.0	0.0	0.0	0.0	0.0	1.4	0.0	12.7
0.3	4.4	302.3	0.1	27.8	247.2	405.7	126.2	1.0	149.5	2.4	0.1	0.1	0.3	0.2	0.1	12.7	0.9	222.5
0.4	4.9	316.3	0.1	35.5	254.8	418.2	129.9	1.0	149.5	2.5	0.1	0.1	0.4	0.2	0.1	13.2	0.9	221.4
0.3	4.9	301.4	0.1	27.0	247.5	406.7	127.4	1.0	2.5	2.4	0.1	0.1	0.3	0.2	0.1	12.3	0.9	222.5
0.4	4.9	351.8	0.1	39.5	275.3	446.5	144.4	1.1	150.1	2.8	0.0	0.1	0.5	0.2	0.1	14.8	1.1	219.8
2.9	18.3	296.7	0.1	33.4	232.0	376.7	121.8	1.0	139.1	2.3	0.2	0.1	0.4	0.2	0.1	12.4	0.9	217.7
2.9	18.4	312.9	0.1	35.2	244.8	397.1	128.4	1.0	139.7	2.5	0.2	0.1	0.4	0.2	0.1	13.0	0.9	217.7
3.0	18.9	350.6	0.1	35.5	274.4	445.2	144.1	1.0	149.5	2.7	0.0	0.1	0.5	0.2	0.1	13.2	0.9	214.9
0.4	2.1	35.4	0.1	4.1	31.7	52.7	18.8	0.1	17.8	0.3	0.0	0.0	0.1	0.0	0.0	1.5	0.1	26.1
3.0	18.9	352.0	0.1	39.6	275.5	447.0	144.6	1.1	140.2	2.8	0.0	0.1	0.5	0.2	0.1	14.8	1.1	215.8
0.5	0.0	9.6	1.4	45.6	117.6	338.4	28.8	0.6	7.2	0.0	0.0	0.4	0.2	0.4	0.1	3.6	0.0	223.8
1.9	0.5	79.3	1.0	15.6	181.0	278.9	191.1	2.9	0.0	0.0	2.6	0.0	0.2	0.0	0.0	0.0	0.0	215.2
7.4	0.5	79.3	1.0	15.6	181.0	278.9	191.1	2.9	0.0	0.0	0.0	0.0	0.2	0.0	0.0	0.0	0.0	215.2
2.1	12.9	108.3	0.1	9.8	96.8	141.9	48.5	0.4	30.9	1.0	0.1	0.0	0.2	0.1	0.0	4.3	0.2	10.4
0.3	2.1	18.1	0.0	2.0	14.2	23.0	7.4	0.1	4.7	0.1	0.0	0.0	0.0	0.0	0.0	0.8	0.1	13.4
5.6	34.9	290.4	0.1	32.7	227.2	368.4	119.1	0.9	83.0	3.6	0.2	0.1	0.4	0.2	0.1	12.2	0.9	214.0
5.6	32.5	298.2	0.6	34.7	267.3	444.0	158.5	1.1	77.1	2.4	0.2	0.1	0.4	0.3	0.1	12.5	0.9	218.9
1.3	7.8	73.0	0.0	6.8	62.0	106.4	29.7	0.3	22.4	0.7	0.1	0.0	0.1	0.1	0.0	3.0	0.3	0.2
1.4	9.3	82.2	0.1	7.6	63.8	95.5	33.3	0.2	17.0	0.6	0.0	0.0	0.1	0.1	0.0	2.5	0.1	23.3
0.7	4.6	41.1	0.0	3.8	31.9	47.7	16.7	0.1	8.5	0.3	0.0	0.0	0.0	0.0	0.0	1.2	0.1	11.7
0.8	3.5	40.7	0.0	4.3	33.8	62.3	15.2	0.1	17.1	0.4	0.0	0.0	0.1	0.0	0.0	0.2	0.0	26.5
11.2	46.4	412.4	0.3	75.9	286.5	433.6	127.4	0.5	129.3	5.5	0.0	0.1	0.3	0.2	0.1	13.7	0.9	203.5
5.3	33.2	246.0	0.1	12.2	208.6	616.8	6.1	0.9	78.1	2.3	0.2	0.0	0.3	0.1	0.1	12.2	0.9	215.2
11.2	65.9	471.9	0.2	44.8	385.5	333.1	107.6	1.3	102.5	10.2	0.0	0.2	0.9	1.0	0.1	17.1	1.7	196.9
0.1	0.0	0.0	0.0	0.0	0.0	0.0	12.1	0.0	0.0	0.0	0.0	0.0	0.0	0.0	0.0	0.0	0.0	0.1
0.8	0.0	0.0	0.0	0.0	0.0	0.0	343.2	0.0	0.0	0.0	0.0	0.0	0.0	0.0	0.0	0.0	0.0	2.7
0.6	12.0	22.8	0.6	6.4	78.8	49.2	178.8	0.2	3.6	0.4	0.4	0.1	0.0	0.4	0.0	18.0	0.2	15.3
1.5	1.8	12.5	0.6	5.5	94.5	39.0	218.5	0.2	11.0	0.5	0.0	0.1	0.2	1.1	0.0	5.5	0.0	17.8
1.2	21.1	107.7	1.3	9.1	82.7	70.1	251.4	0.3	22.2	0.9	0.0	0.2	0.2	1.3	0.0	27.4	0.1	22.5
3.1	1.6	107.2	1.3	9.1	82.1	69.5	250.8	0.3	16.0	0.9	0.0	0.2	0.2	1.3	0.0	6.8	0.1	22.2
0.8	14.8	42.2	1.6	18.2	161.9	39.3	297.0	0.3	20.5	0.0	1.0	0.2	0.2	1.2	0.0	35.3	0.1	18.6
1.3	23.9	147.6	1.5	13.1	100.9	82.7	333.5	0.3	29.1	0.2	0.0	0.2	0.2	1.4	0.1	35.3	0.1	18.8
3.5	1.8	147.1	1.5	13.1	100.3	82.1	333.5	0.3	22.8	0.2	0.0	0.2	0.2	1.4	0.1	9.7	0.1	18.5
0.6	0.0	35.9	2.4	89.5	214.3	289.0	224.0	1.0	0.0	0.0	0.7	0.1	0.1	0.2	0.1	29.6	0.0	20.0
1.2	22.2	114.0	1.4	9.7	87.2	69.0	266.2	0.3	22.8	0.2	0.0	0.2	0.2	1.3	0.0	29.1	0.1	21.5
3.3	1.7	113.4	1.4	9.1	86.6	68.4	266.2	0.3	16.5	0.2	0.0	0.2	0.2	1.3	0.0	6.8	0.1	21.2
0.4	0.0	38.9	0.9	0.0	0.0	0.0	107.0	0.0	0.0	0.0	0.5	0.0	0.0	0.0	0.0	42.1	0.1	12.4
0.7	2.3	16.0	1.3	28.5	167.0	73.5	233.5	0.6	15.5	0.0	0.0	0.1	0.1	1.4	0.1	8.0	0.1	17.7
3.6	1.7	106.6	2.4	44.5	162.5	181.3	335.2	1.6	142.5	4.4	0.0	0.2	0.3	2.3	0.2	29.6	0.1	20.2
3.6	1.8	106.6	2.4	44.5	162.5	180.7	335.2	1.6	136.2	4.4	0.0	0.2	0.3	2.3	0.2	29.6	0.1	19.9
0.4	0.0	0.0	0.0	0.0	0.0	0.0	186.0	0.0	0.0	0.0	0.0	0.0	0.0	0.0	0.0	0.0	0.0	9.5
0.0	0.0	47.0	6.0	0.0	0.0	289.0	1245.0	0.0	134.4	0.0	0.0	0.1	0.2	2.1	0.0	0.0	0.0	187.2
4.3	104.2	118.1	2.8	0.0	0.0	0.0	1646.1	0.0	0.0	0.0	0.0	0.0	0.0	0.0	0.0	0.0	0.0	4.6
0.0	0.0	2.2	0.2	0.3	2.8	0.9	0.9	0.0	0.0	0.0	0.0	0.0	0.0	0.0	0.0	0.2	0.0	1.2
0.1	0.2	0.6	0.1	1.5	4.5	3.4	12.3	0.0	0.3	0.0	0.0	0.0	0.0	0.2	0.0	2.5	0.0	0.0
0.0	3.3	1.2	0.2	1.9	6.9	2.8	0.7	0.1	0.6	0.0	0.0	0.0	0.0	0.1	0.0	6.4	0.0	6.9
0.6	52.8	30.4	1.7	38.4	91.2	59.2	19.2	1.0	22.4	0.0	0.1	0.4	0.0	2.4	0.2	102.4	0.2	109.6
0.5	52.8	19.2	1.0	30.4	110.4	44.8	11.2	1.0	9.6	0.0	0.1	0.0	0.0	0.6	0.1	11.2	0.1	109.9
0.5	52.8	19.2	1.0	30.4	110.4	44.8	264.0	1.0	9.6	0.0	0.0	0.0	0.0	0.6	0.1	11.2	0.1	109.9
0.0	0.0	4.6	0.5	10.3	28.5	39.9	68.4	0.1	0.0	0.0	0.0	0.1	0.0	0.6	0.0	8.0	0.0	83.2
0.0	0.0	14.1	0.9	3.5	47.5	51.0	283.4	0.4	0.0	0.0	0.0	0.0	0.1	0.2	0.0	3.5	0.0	119.5
1.1	0.0	7.2	2.1	0.0	0.0	41.3	892.5	0.0	0.0	0.0	0.0	0.2	0.2	2.4	0.0	0.0	0.0	0.0
12.4	0.0	667.5	9.2	750.0	1295.0	1875.0	425.0	7.5	0.0	1.8	0.0	0.3	1.5	7.1	0.2	161.3	0.0	5.0
14.0	0.0	675.0	9.3	757.5	1307.5	1895.0	1125.0	7.6	0.0	1.8	50.7	0.3	1.5	7.2	0.2	163.0	0.0	2.5
1.6	0.0	6.9	0.8	41.3	73.1	87.4	98.2	0.8	0.0	0.0	0.0	0.2	0.0	0.3	0.0	10.9	0.0	0.5
3.9	0.0	43.0	1.2	110.0	103.0	712.0	0.0	0.6	5.0	0.0	0.0	0.1	0.2	2.4	0.7	113.5	0.0	6.0
0.1	0.0	32.0	2.0	120.0	274.0	334.0	1.0	5.1	12.0	1.8	0.0	0.8	0.1	0.8	0.2	36.7	0.0	10.7
1.7	0.0	424.0	8.5	288.0	914.0	1400.0	746.0	2.8	0.0	0.6	0.0	0.3	1.7	6.3	0.1	57.0	0.0	7.2
6.0	0.0	390.4	3.6	295.1	585.7	712.8	20.4	3.4	0.0	0.2	46.0	0.2	0.9	3.2	0.1	165.7	0.0	32.0
0.1	0.0	363.0	10.8	140.0	839.0	450.0	900.0	4.4	0.0	0.0	0.0	0.3	0.1	0.7	0.1	340.0	0.0	5.8
0.1	0.0	363.0	10.8	315.0	839.0	2202.0	3.0	4.4	0.0	0.0	0.0	0.3	0.1	0.7	0.1	340.0	0.0	5.8
0.4	0.0	178.0	14.5	39.0	776.0	81.0	1005.0	4.0	0.0	0.0	0.0	0.2	0.1	1.4	0.1	176.1	0.0	5.0

Code	Food Name	Unit/Amt	Wt (g)	Energy (Kcal)	Prot (g)	Carb (g)	Fiber (g)	Fat (g)	Mono (g)	Poly (g)
16423	Nutrient/Protein Supplement, Soy Protein Isolate, potassium type	3.5 oz	100	326.0	80.7	10.2	5.6	0.5	0.6	1.6
925044	Nutrient/Protein Supplement, Soy Protein Isolate, potassium type	3.5 oz	100	321.0	88.3	2.6	2.0	0.5	0.1	0.3
925074	Nutrient/Vitamin Supplement, 1-A-Day Essential	1 tablet	1	0.0	0.0	0.0	0.0	0.0	0.0	0.0
925042	Nutrient/Vitamin Supplement, 1-A-Day Maximum	1 tablet	1	0.0	0.0	0.0	0.0	0.0	0.0	0.0
925058	Nutrient/Vitamin Supplement, 1-A-Day plus Extra C	1 tablet	1	0.0	0.0	0.0	0.0	0.0	0.0	0.0
925033	Nutrient/Vitamin Supplement, Allbee C-800	1 tablet	1	0.0	0.0	0.0	0.0	0.0	0.0	0.0
925040	Nutrient/Vitamin Supplement, Bugs Bunny	1 tablet	1	0.0	0.0	0.0	0.0	0.0	0.0	0.0
925050	Nutrient/Vitamin Supplement, Bugs Bunny Extra C	1 tablet	1	0.0	0.0	0.0	0.0	0.0	0.0	0.0
925091	Nutrient/Vitamin Supplement, Bugs Bunny plus Iron	1 tablet	1	0.0	0.0	0.0	0.0	0.0	0.0	0.0
925045	Nutrient/Vitamin Supplement, Centrum Jr.	1 tablet	1	0.0	0.0	0.0	0.0	0.0	0.0	0.0
925088	Nutrient/Vitamin Supplement, Chew Vits	1 tablet	1	0.0	0.0	0.0	0.0	0.0	0.0	0.0
925046	Nutrient/Vitamin Supplement, Engran-HP	1 tablet	1	0.0	0.0	0.0	0.0	0.0	0.0	0.0
925098	Nutrient/Vitamin Supplement, FemIron	1 tablet	1	0.0	0.0	0.0	0.0	0.0	0.0	0.0
925034	Nutrient/Vitamin Supplement, Fero-Grad-500	1 tablet	1	0.0	0.0	0.0	0.0	0.0	0.0	0.0
925073	Nutrient/Vitamin Supplement, Flintstones	1 tablet	1	0.0	0.0	0.0	0.0	0.0	0.0	0.0
925041	Nutrient/Vitamin Supplement, Flintstones Complete	1 tablet	1	0.0	0.0	0.0	0.0	0.0	0.0	0.0
925023	Nutrient/Vitamin Supplement, Flintstones plus Iron	1 tablet	1	0.0	0.0	0.0	0.0	0.0	0.0	0.0
925024	Nutrient/Vitamin Supplement, Geritol Complete	1 tablet	1	0.0	0.0	0.0	0.0	0.0	0.0	0.0
925097	Nutrient/Vitamin Supplement, Geritol Tonic	15 ml	1	0.0	0.0	0.0	0.0	0.0	0.0	0.0
925093	Nutrient/Vitamin Supplement, Iron & Vitamin C	1 tablet	1	0.0	0.0	0.0	0.0	0.0	0.0	0.0
925055	Nutrient/Vitamin Supplement, Lifestage, Children	1 tablet	1	0.0	0.0	0.0	0.0	0.0	0.0	0.0
925059	Nutrient/Vitamin Supplement, Lifestage, Men	1 tablet	1	0.0	0.0	0.0	0.0	0.0	0.0	0.0
925025	Nutrient/Vitamin Supplement, Lifestage, Teen	1 tablet	1	0.0	0.0	0.0	0.0	0.0	0.0	0.0
925049	Nutrient/Vitamin Supplement, Lifestage, Women	1 tablet	1	0.0	0.0	0.0	0.0	0.0	0.0	0.0
925096	Nutrient/Vitamin Supplement, Minute Man plus Iron	1 tablet	1	0.0	0.0	0.0	0.0	0.0	0.0	0.0
925054	Nutrient/Vitamin Supplement, Mol-Iron with C	1 tablet	1	0.0	0.0	0.0	0.0	0.0	0.0	0.0
925089	Nutrient/Vitamin Supplement, Myadec	1 tablet	1	0.0	0.0	0.0	0.0	0.0	0.0	0.0
925035	Nutrient/Vitamin Supplement, Natalins	1 tablet	1	0.0	0.0	0.0	0.0	0.0	0.0	0.0
925052	Nutrient/Vitamin Supplement, Neovadrin child	1 tablet	1	0.0	0.0	0.0	0.0	0.0	0.0	0.0
925087	Nutrient/Vitamin Supplement, Neovadrin with Iron	1 tablet	1	0.0	0.0	0.0	0.0	0.0	0.0	0.0
925086	Nutrient/Vitamin Supplement, Os-Cal Forte	1 tablet	1	0.0	0.0	0.0	0.0	0.0	0.0	0.0
925047	Nutrient/Vitamin Supplement, Os-Cal Plus	1 tablet	1	0.0	0.0	0.0	0.0	0.0	0.0	0.0
925061	Nutrient/Vitamin Supplement, Pac-man plus Iron	1 tablet	1	0.0	0.0	0.0	0.0	0.0	0.0	0.0
925084	Nutrient/Vitamin Supplement, Poly-Vi-Flor	0.5 mg tab	1	0.0	0.0	0.0	0.0	0.0	0.0	0.0
925085	Nutrient/Vitamin Supplement, Poly-Vi-Flor 0.25mg drops	1 ml	1	0.0	0.0	0.0	0.0	0.0	0.0	0.0
925076	Nutrient/Vitamin Supplement, Poly-Vi-Flor 0.5 mg drops	1 ml	1	0.0	0.0	0.0	0.0	0.0	0.0	0.0
925077	Nutrient/Vitamin Supplement, Poly-Vi-Flor tablets	1 mg tab	1	0.0	0.0	0.0	0.0	0.0	0.0	0.0
925081	Nutrient/Vitamin Supplement, Poly-Vi-Flor w/iron	1 mg tab	1	0.0	0.0	0.0	0.0	0.0	0.0	0.0
925063	Nutrient/Vitamin Supplement, Poly-Vi-Sol w/iron & zinc	1 tablet	1	0.0	0.0	0.0	0.0	0.0	0.0	0.0
925095	Nutrient/Vitamin Supplement, Stresstab 600 Adv Formula	1 tablet	1	0.0	0.0	0.0	0.0	0.0	0.0	0.0
925094	Nutrient/Vitamin Supplement, Stresstabs 600 w/iron	1 tablet	1	0.0	0.0	0.0	0.0	0.0	0.0	0.0
925092	Nutrient/Vitamin Supplement, Stresstabs 600 w/zinc	1 tablet	1	0.0	0.0	0.0	0.0	0.0	0.0	0.0
925030	Nutrient/Vitamin Supplement, Theragran-M	1 tablet	1	0.0	0.0	0.0	0.0	0.0	0.0	0.0
925100	Nutrient/Vitamin Supplement, Theragran	1 tablet	1	0.0	0.0	0.0	0.0	0.0	0.0	0.0
925082	Nutrient/Vitamin Supplement, Theragran Stress Formula	1 tablet	1	0.0	0.0	0.0	0.0	0.0	0.0	0.0
925065	Nutrient/Vitamin Supplement, Tri-Vi-Flor	1 tablet	1	0.0	0.0	0.0	0.0	0.0	0.0	0.0
925031	Nutrient/Vitamin Supplement, Tri-Vi-Sol w/iron drops	1 dose	1	0.0	0.0	0.0	0.0	0.0	0.0	0.0
925032	Nutrient/Vitamin Supplement, Unicap	1 tablet	1	0.0	0.0	0.0	0.0	0.0	0.0	0.0
925057	Nutrient/Vitamin Supplement, Unicap Jr	1 tablet	1	0.0	0.0	0.0	0.0	0.0	0.0	0.0
925048	Nutrient/Vitamin Supplement, Unicap M	1 tablet	1	0.0	0.0	0.0	0.0	0.0	0.0	0.0
925070	Nutrient/Vitamin Supplement, Unicap plus Iron	1 tablet	1	0.0	0.0	0.0	0.0	0.0	0.0	0.0
925056	Nutrient/Vitamin Supplement, Unicap Senior	1 tablet	1	0.0	0.0	0.0	0.0	0.0	0.0	0.0
925039	Nutrient/Vitamin Supplement, Unicap T	1 tablet	1	0.0	0.0	0.0	0.0	0.0	0.0	0.0
925043	Nutrient/Vitamin Supplement, Z-Bec	1 tablet	1	0.0	0.0	0.0	0.0	0.0	0.0	0.0
12059	Nutrient/Vitamin Supplement, Zymacap	1 capsule	1	0.0	0.0	0.0	0.0	0.0	0.0	0.0
12072	Nuts, Acorns, raw	1.0 oz	28	108.4	1.7	11.4	0.0	6.7	4.2	1.3
12061	Nuts, Almonds, dried, blanched	1 tbsp	9.1	53.3	1.9	1.7	0.6	4.8	3.1	1.0
12066	Nuts, Almonds, oil roast, blanched w/salt	1 whole kernel	1	6.1	0.2	0.2	0.1	0.6	0.4	0.1
12563	Nuts, Almonds, toasted, unblanched	1.0 oz	28	164.9	5.7	6.4	3.1	14.2	9.2	3.0
12565	Nuts, Almonds, unblanched, dry roasted w/salt	1 kernel	1	5.9	0.2	0.2	0.1	0.5	0.3	0.1
12078	Nuts, Beechnuts, dried	1.0 oz	28	161.3	1.7	9.4	0.0	14.0	6.1	5.6
12084	Nuts, Brazilnuts, dried, unblanched	1.0 oz, 6-8 kernals	28	183.7	4.0	3.6	1.5	18.5	6.4	6.8
12585	Nuts, Butternuts, dried	1 cup	120	734.4	29.9	14.5	5.6	68.4	12.5	51.3
12085	Nuts, Cashews, dry roasted w/salt	1 nut	2	11.5	0.3	0.7	0.1	0.9	0.5	0.2
912903	Nuts, Cashews, dry roasted, w/o salt	1 cup, halves and whole	137	786.4	21.0	44.8	4.1	63.5	37.4	10.7
12586	Nuts, Cashews, honey roasted	1.0 oz	28	150.1	4.0	7.0	2.0	13.0	7.0	3.0
12086	Nuts, Cashews, oil roasted w/salt	1 nut	2	11.5	0.3	0.6	0.1	1.0	0.6	0.2
12095	Nuts, Cashews, oil roasted, w/o salt	1.0 oz, 18 kernals	28	161.3	4.5	8.0	1.1	13.5	8.0	2.3
12203	Nuts, Chestnuts, European, roasted	1 kernel	8	19.6	0.3	4.2	0.4	0.2	0.1	0.1

Sat (g)	Chol (mg)	Cal (mg)	Iron (mg)	Magn (mg)	Phos (mg)	Pota (mg)	Sodi (mg)	Zinc (mg)	Vit A (RE)	Vit C (mg)	Vit E (mg)	Thia (mg)	Ribo (mg)	Niac (mg)	Vit B-6 (mg)	Fol (µg)	Vit B-12 (µg)	Wat (g)
0.4	0.0	178.0	14.5	39.0	776.0	1590.0	50.0	4.0	0.0	0.0	0.0	0.2	0.1	1.4	0.1	176.1	0.0	5.0
0.1	0.0	178.0	14.5	39.0	776.0	1590.0	50.0	4.0	0.0	0.0	0.0	0.2	0.1	1.4	0.1	176.1	0.0	5.0
0.0	0.0	0.0	0.0	0.0	0.0	0.0	0.0	0.0	1000.0	60.0	0.0	1.5	1.7	20.0	2.0	0.4	6.0	0.0
0.0	0.0	0.0	18.0	0.0	0.0	0.0	0.0	15.0	1000.0	60.0	0.0	1.5	1.7	20.0	2.0	0.4	6.0	0.0
0.0	0.0	0.0	0.0	0.0	0.0	0.0	0.0	0.0	1000.0	300.0	0.0	1.5	1.7	20.0	2.0	0.4	6.0	0.0
0.0	0.0	0.0	0.0	0.0	0.0	0.0	0.0	0.0	0.0	800.0	0.0	15.0	17.0	100.0	25.0	0.0	12.0	0.0
0.0	0.0	0.0	0.0	0.0	0.0	0.0	0.0	0.0	500.0	60.0	0.0	1.0	1.2	13.5	1.0	0.3	4.5	0.0
0.0	0.0	0.0	0.0	0.0	0.0	0.0	0.0	0.0	500.0	250.0	0.0	1.0	1.2	13.5	1.0	0.3	4.5	0.0
0.0	0.0	0.0	15.0	0.0	0.0	0.0	0.0	0.0	500.0	60.0	0.0	1.0	1.2	13.5	1.0	0.3	4.5	0.0
0.0	0.0	0.0	18.0	0.0	0.0	0.0	0.0	0.0	1000.0	300.0	0.0	1.5	1.7	20.0	2.0	0.4	6.0	0.0
0.0	0.0	0.0	0.0	0.0	0.0	0.0	0.0	0.0	500.0	60.0	0.0	1.0	1.2	13.5	1.0	0.3	4.5	0.0
0.0	0.0	325.0	9.0	0.0	0.0	0.0	0.0	0.0	800.0	30.0	0.0	0.9	1.0	10.0	1.3	0.4	4.0	0.0
0.0	0.0	0.0	20.0	0.0	0.0	0.0	0.0	0.0	1000.0	60.0	0.0	1.5	1.7	20.0	2.0	0.4	6.0	0.0
0.0	0.0	0.0	105.0	0.0	0.0	0.0	0.0	0.0	0.0	500.0	0.0	0.0	0.0	0.0	0.0	0.0	0.0	0.0
0.0	0.0	0.0	0.0	0.0	0.0	0.0	0.0	0.0	500.0	60.0	0.0	1.0	1.2	13.5	1.0	0.3	4.5	0.0
0.0	0.0	0.0	18.0	0.0	0.0	0.0	0.0	15.0	1000.0	60.0	0.0	1.5	1.7	20.0	2.0	0.4	6.0	0.0
0.0	0.0	0.0	15.0	0.0	0.0	0.0	0.0	0.0	500.0	60.0	0.0	1.0	1.2	13.5	1.0	0.3	4.5	0.0
0.0	0.0	0.0	50.0	0.0	0.0	0.0	0.0	0.0	1000.0	60.0	0.0	1.5	1.7	20.0	2.0	0.4	6.0	0.0
0.0	0.0	0.0	50.0	0.0	0.0	0.0	0.0	0.0	0.0	0.0	0.0	2.5	2.5	50.0	0.5	0.0	0.8	0.0
0.0	0.0	0.0	50.0	0.0	0.0	0.0	0.0	0.0	0.0	25.0	0.0	0.0	0.0	0.0	0.0	0.0	0.0	0.0
0.0	0.0	0.0	4.5	0.0	0.0	0.0	0.0	0.0	500.0	30.0	0.0	0.8	0.9	10.0	1.0	0.2	3.0	0.0
0.0	0.0	0.0	18.0	0.0	0.0	0.0	0.0	22.5	2000.0	500.0	0.0	20.0	10.0	100.0	10.0	0.4	25.0	0.0
0.0	0.0	0.0	18.0	0.0	0.0	0.0	0.0	0.0	1000.0	100.0	0.0	15.0	10.0	50.0	7.5	0.4	12.5	0.0
0.0	0.0	0.0	27.0	0.0	0.0	0.0	0.0	0.0	1000.0	100.0	0.0	3.0	3.4	40.0	4.0	0.4	12.0	0.0
0.0	0.0	0.0	18.0	0.0	0.0	0.0	0.0	0.0	1000.0	60.0	0.0	1.5	1.7	20.0	2.0	0.4	6.0	0.0
0.0	0.0	0.0	39.0	0.0	0.0	0.0	0.0	0.0	0.0	75.0	0.0	0.0	0.0	0.0	0.0	0.0	0.0	0.0
0.0	0.0	0.0	20.0	0.0	0.0	0.0	0.0	20.0	2000.0	250.0	0.0	10.0	10.0	100.0	5.0	0.4	6.0	0.0
0.0	0.0	200.0	45.0	0.0	0.0	0.0	0.0	0.0	1600.0	90.0	0.0	1.7	2.0	20.0	4.0	0.8	8.0	0.0
0.0	0.0	0.0	0.0	0.0	0.0	0.0	0.0	0.0	500.0	60.0	0.0	1.0	1.2	13.5	1.0	0.3	4.5	0.0
0.0	0.0	0.0	15.0	0.0	0.0	0.0	0.0	0.0	500.0	60.0	0.0	1.0	1.2	13.5	1.0	0.3	4.5	0.0
0.0	0.0	250.0	5.0	0.0	0.0	0.0	0.0	0.5	333.6	50.0	0.0	1.7	1.7	15.0	2.0	0.0	1.6	0.0
0.0	0.0	250.0	16.6	0.0	0.0	0.0	0.0	0.8	333.2	33.0	0.0	0.5	0.7	3.3	0.5	0.0	0.0	0.0
0.0	0.0	0.0	18.0	0.0	0.0	0.0	0.0	0.0	1000.0	60.0	0.0	1.5	1.7	20.0	2.0	0.4	6.0	0.0
0.0	0.0	0.0	0.0	0.0	0.0	0.0	0.0	10.0	500.0	60.0	0.0	1.0	1.2	13.5	1.0	0.3	4.5	0.0
0.0	0.0	0.0	0.0	0.0	0.0	0.0	0.0	0.0	300.0	35.0	0.0	0.5	0.6	8.0	0.4	0.0	2.0	0.0
0.0	0.0	0.0	0.0	0.0	0.0	0.0	0.0	0.0	300.0	35.0	0.0	0.5	0.6	8.0	0.4	0.0	2.0	0.0
0.0	0.0	0.0	0.0	0.0	0.0	0.0	0.0	0.0	500.0	60.0	0.0	1.0	1.2	13.5	1.0	0.3	4.5	0.0
0.0	0.0	0.0	12.0	0.0	0.0	0.0	0.0	10.0	500.0	60.0	0.0	1.0	1.2	13.5	1.0	0.3	4.5	0.0
0.0	0.0	0.0	12.0	0.0	0.0	0.0	0.0	0.0	500.0	60.0	0.0	1.1	1.2	13.5	1.1	0.3	4.5	0.0
0.0	0.0	0.0	0.0	0.0	0.0	0.0	0.0	0.0	0.0	600.0	0.0	15.0	15.0	100.0	5.0	0.4	12.0	0.0
0.0	0.0	0.0	27.0	0.0	0.0	0.0	0.0	0.0	0.0	600.0	0.0	15.0	15.0	100.0	5.0	0.4	12.0	0.0
0.0	0.0	0.0	0.0	0.0	0.0	0.0	0.0	23.9	0.0	600.0	0.0	20.0	10.0	100.0	5.0	0.4	12.0	0.0
0.0	0.0	40.0	27.0	0.0	0.0	0.0	0.0	15.0	1100.0	120.0	0.0	3.0	3.4	30.0	3.0	0.4	9.0	0.0
0.0	0.0	0.0	0.0	0.0	0.0	0.0	0.0	0.0	1100.0	120.0	0.0	3.0	3.4	30.0	3.0	0.4	9.0	0.0
0.0	0.0	0.0	27.0	0.0	0.0	0.0	0.0	0.0	0.0	600.0	0.0	15.0	15.0	100.0	5.0	0.4	12.0	0.0
0.0	0.0	0.0	0.0	0.0	0.0	0.0	0.0	0.0	500.0	60.0	0.0	0.0	0.0	0.0	0.0	0.0	0.0	0.0
0.0	0.0	0.0	10.0	0.0	0.0	0.0	0.0	0.0	300.0	35.0	0.0	0.0	0.0	0.0	0.0	0.0	0.0	0.0
0.0	0.0	0.0	0.0	0.0	0.0	0.0	0.0	0.0	1000.0	60.0	0.0	1.5	1.7	20.0	2.0	0.4	6.0	0.0
0.0	0.0	0.0	0.0	0.0	0.0	0.0	0.0	0.0	1000.0	60.0	0.0	1.5	1.7	20.0	2.0	0.4	6.0	0.0
0.0	0.0	0.0	18.0	0.0	0.0	0.0	0.0	15.0	1000.0	600.0	0.0	15.0	10.0	100.0	5.0	0.4	12.0	0.0
0.0	0.0	0.0	18.0	0.0	0.0	0.0	0.0	0.0	1000.0	60.0	0.0	1.5	1.7	20.0	2.0	0.4	6.0	0.0
0.0	0.0	0.0	10.0	0.0	0.0	0.0	0.0	15.0	1000.0	60.0	0.0	1.2	1.7	14.0	2.0	0.4	6.0	0.0
0.0	0.0	0.0	18.0	0.0	0.0	0.0	0.0	15.0	1000.0	500.0	0.0	10.0	10.0	100.0	6.0	0.4	18.0	0.0
0.0	0.0	0.0	0.0	0.0	0.0	0.0	0.0	22.5	0.0	600.0	0.0	15.0	10.2	100.0	10.0	25.0	6.0	0.0
0.0	0.0	0.0	0.0	0.0	0.0	0.0	0.0	0.0	1000.0	90.0	0.0	2.3	2.6	30.0	3.0	0.4	9.0	0.0
0.9	0.0	11.5	0.2	17.4	22.1	150.9	0.0	0.1	1.1	0.0	0.0	0.0	0.0	0.5	0.1	24.4	0.0	7.8
0.5	0.0	22.5	0.3	26.0	48.4	68.3	0.9	0.3	0.0	0.1	1.8	0.0	0.1	0.3	0.0	3.5	0.0	0.5
0.1	0.0	1.9	0.1	2.9	5.8	6.9	7.8	0.0	0.0	0.0	0.1	0.0	0.0	0.0	0.0	0.6	0.0	0.0
1.3	0.0	79.2	1.4	85.4	154.0	216.4	3.1	1.4	0.0	0.2	4.5	0.0	0.2	0.8	0.0	17.9	0.0	0.7
0.0	0.0	2.8	0.0	3.0	5.5	7.7	7.8	0.0	0.0	0.0	0.1	0.0	0.0	0.0	0.0	0.6	0.0	0.0
1.6	0.0	0.3	0.7	0.0	0.0	284.8	10.6	0.1	0.0	4.3	0.0	0.1	0.1	0.2	0.2	31.6	0.0	1.8
4.5	0.0	49.3	1.0	63.0	168.0	168.0	0.6	1.3	0.0	0.2	2.1	0.3	0.0	0.5	0.1	1.1	0.0	0.9
1.6	0.0	63.6	4.8	284.4	535.2	505.2	1.2	3.8	14.4	3.8	4.2	0.5	0.2	1.3	0.7	79.4	0.0	4.0
0.2	0.0	0.9	0.1	5.2	9.8	11.3	12.8	0.1	0.0	0.0	0.0	0.0	0.0	0.0	0.0	1.4	0.0	0.0
12.5	0.0	61.7	8.2	356.2	671.3	774.1	21.9	7.7	0.0	0.0	0.8	0.3	0.3	1.9	0.4	94.8	0.0	2.3
3.0	0.0	12.0	1.2	0.0	120.0	135.0	90.0	1.4	0.0	0.0	0.0	0.1	0.1	0.4	0.1	20.0	0.0	0.0
0.2	0.0	0.8	0.1	5.1	8.5	10.6	12.5	0.1	0.0	0.0	0.0	0.0	0.0	0.0	0.0	1.4	0.0	0.1
2.7	0.0	11.5	1.1	71.4	119.3	148.4	4.8	1.3	0.0	0.0	0.4	0.1	0.0	0.5	0.1	19.0	0.0	1.1
0.0	0.0	2.3	0.1	2.6	8.6	47.4	0.2	0.0	0.2	2.1	0.1	0.0	0.0	0.1	0.0	5.6	0.0	3.2

Code	Food Name	Unit/Amt	Wt (g)	Energy (Kcal)	Prot (g)	Carb (g)	Fiber (g)	Fat (g)	Mono (g)	Poly (g)
12118	Nuts, Coconut Meat, raw	1 cup shredded or grated	80	283.2	2.7	12.2	7.2	26.8	1.1	0.3
12176	Nuts, Coconut Milk, canned (liquid expressed from grated meat&water)	1 tbsp	15	29.6	0.3	0.4	0.0	3.2	0.1	0.0
12177	Nuts, Coconut Water (liquid from coconuts)	1 tbsp	15	2.9	0.1	0.6	0.2	0.0	0.0	0.0
12114	Nuts, Coconut, Creamed, dried, creamed	1.0 oz	28	191.5	1.5	6.0	0.0	19.3	0.8	0.2
12109	Nuts, Coconut, dried, toasted	1.0 oz	28	165.8	1.5	12.4	0.0	13.2	0.6	0.1
12108	Nuts, Coconut, Sweetened, shredded, dried	7 oz pkg	199	997.0	5.7	94.9	9.0	70.6	3.0	0.8
12121	Nuts, Coconut, Unsweetened, dried	1.0 oz	28	184.8	1.9	6.8	4.6	18.1	0.8	0.2
12120	Nuts, Filberts/Hazelnuts, dried, blanched	1.0 oz	28	188.2	3.6	4.5	1.8	18.8	14.8	1.8
12633	Nuts, Macadamia, dried	1 kernel	2	14.0	0.2	0.3	0.2	1.5	1.2	0.0
12138	Nuts, Mixed (no peanuts) oil roasted w/salt	1.0 oz	28	172.2	4.3	6.2	1.5	15.7	9.3	3.2
12135	Nuts, Mixed w/o peanuts, oil roasted, w/o salt	1.0 oz	28	172.2	4.3	6.2	1.5	15.7	9.3	3.2
12635	Nuts, Mixed w/peanuts, dry roast, w/o salt	1.0 oz	28	166.3	4.8	7.1	2.5	14.4	8.8	3.0
12137	Nuts, Mixed w/peanuts, dry roasted w/salt	1.0 oz	28	166.3	4.8	7.1	2.5	14.4	8.8	3.0
12637	Nuts, Mixed w/peanuts, oil roast, w/o salt	1 tbsp	8.9	54.9	1.5	1.9	0.9	5.0	2.8	1.2
12142	Nuts, Mixed w/peanuts, oil roasted w/salt	1 nut	1	6.2	0.2	0.2	0.1	0.6	0.3	0.1
12143	Nuts, Pecans, dried	2 halves	3	20.0	0.2	0.5	0.2	2.0	1.3	0.5
12643	Nuts, Pecans, dry roasted w/o salt	1.0 oz	28	184.5	2.2	6.3	2.6	18.1	11.3	4.5
12144	Nuts, Pecans, dry roasted w/salt	1.0 oz	28	184.5	2.2	6.3	2.6	18.1	11.3	4.5
12644	Nuts, Pecans, oil roasted w/o salt	2 halves	4	27.4	0.3	0.6	0.3	2.8	1.8	0.7
12145	Nuts, Pecans, oil roasted w/salt	2 halves	4	27.4	0.3	0.6	0.3	2.8	1.8	0.7
12149	Nuts, Pine Nut, Pignolias, dried	1 cup	136	769.8	32.6	19.3	6.1	69.0	25.9	29.0
12152	Nuts, Pistachios, dried	2 kernels	1	5.8	0.2	0.2	0.1	0.5	0.3	0.1
12652	Nuts, Pistachios, dry roasted w/o salt	1.0 oz	28	169.7	4.2	7.7	3.0	14.8	10.0	2.2
12154	Nuts, Pistachios, dry roasted w/salt	1.0 oz	28	169.7	4.2	7.7	3.0	14.8	10.0	2.2
12155	Nuts, Walnut, Black, dried	1 tbsp	7.8	47.3	1.9	0.9	0.4	4.4	1.0	2.9
4590	Oil, Fish, Cod Liver	1 cup	218	1966.4	0.0	0.0	0.0	218.0	101.8	49.1
4501	Oil, Vegetable, Canola	1 tbsp	13.6	120.2	0.0	0.0	0.0	13.6	8.0	4.0
4047	Oil, Vegetable, Cocoa Butter	1 tbsp	13.6	120.2	0.0	0.0	0.0	13.6	4.5	0.4
904902	Oil, Vegetable, Coconut	1 tbsp	13.6	117.2	0.0	0.0	0.0	13.6	0.8	0.2
4541	Oil, Vegetable, Crisco	1 tbsp	13.6	120.5	0.0	0.0	0.0	13.6	4.8	7.1
4532	Oil, Vegetable, Grapeseed	1 tbsp	13.6	120.2	0.0	0.0	0.0	13.6	2.2	9.5
4055	Oil, Vegetable, Oat	1 tbsp	13.6	120.2	0.0	0.0	0.0	13.6	4.8	5.6
4513	Oil, Vegetable, Palm	1 tbsp	13.6	120.2	0.0	0.0	0.0	13.6	5.0	1.3
4514	Oil, Vegetable, Palm Kernel	1 tbsp	13.6	117.2	0.0	0.0	0.0	13.6	1.6	0.2
4037	Oil, Vegetable, Poppyseed	1 tbsp	13.6	120.2	0.0	0.0	0.0	13.6	2.7	8.5
4536	Oil, Vegetable, Rice Bran	1 tbsp	13.6	120.2	0.0	0.0	0.0	13.6	5.3	4.8
4060	Oil, Vegetable, Soybean Lecithin	1 tbsp	13.6	103.8	0.0	0.0	0.0	13.6	1.5	6.2
4506	Oil, Vegetable, Sunflower, linoleic <60%	1 tbsp	13.6	120.2	0.0	0.0	0.0	13.6	6.2	5.5
4584	Oil, Vegetable, Sunflower, linoleic >60%	1 tbsp	13.6	120.2	0.0	0.0	0.0	13.6	2.7	8.9
4545	Oil, Vegetable, Sunflower, oleic >70%	1 tbsp	13.6	120.2	0.0	0.0	0.0	13.6	11.4	0.5
4516	Oil, Vegetable, Sunflower-Hydrogenated, linoleic	1 tbsp	13.6	120.2	0.0	0.0	0.0	13.6	6.3	5.0
4528	Oil, Vegetable, Ucuhuba Butter	1 tbsp	13.6	120.2	0.0	0.0	0.0	13.6	0.9	0.4
4502	Oil, Vegetable/Salad/Cooking, Corn	1 tbsp	13.6	120.2	0.0	0.0	0.0	13.6	3.3	8.0
4053	Oil, Vegetable/Salad/Cooking, Cottonseed	1 tbsp	13.6	120.2	0.0	0.0	0.0	13.6	2.4	7.1
4042	Oil, Vegetable/Salad/Cooking, Olive	1 tbsp	13.5	119.3	0.0	0.0	0.0	13.5	9.9	1.1
4510	Oil, Vegetable/Salad/Cooking, Peanut	1 tbsp	13.5	119.3	0.0	0.0	0.0	13.5	6.2	4.3
4511	Oil, Vegetable/Salad/Cooking, Safflower, linoleic >70%	1 tbsp	13.6	120.2	0.0	0.0	0.0	13.6	1.6	10.1
4058	Oil, Vegetable/Salad/Cooking, Safflower, oleic >70%	1 tbsp	13.6	120.2	0.0	0.0	0.0	13.6	10.2	1.9
4044	Oil, Vegetable/Salad/Cooking, Sesame	1 tbsp	13.6	120.2	0.0	0.0	0.0	13.6	5.4	5.7
4034	Oil, Vegetable/Salad/Cooking, Soybean	1 tbsp	13.6	120.2	0.0	0.0	0.0	13.6	3.2	7.9
4543	Oil, Vegetable/Salad/Cooking, Soybean, hydrogenated	1 tbsp	13.6	120.2	0.0	0.0	0.0	13.6	5.8	5.1
18294	Pancake/Waffle, Buttermilk, Eggo/Kellogg	1 serving (2 waffles)	78	181.7	4.7	29.7	0.9	5.2	2.3	1.7
18295	Pancakes, Blueberry, homemade	1 pancake (4" dia)	38	84.4	2.3	11.0	0.0	3.5	0.9	1.6
18611	Pancakes, Buckwheat, incomplete dry mix, prep	1 pancake (4" dia)	30	62.4	2.4	8.5	0.7	2.3	0.0	0.0
918298	Pancakes, Buttermilk, homemade	1 pancake (4" dia)	38	86.3	2.6	10.9	0.0	3.5	0.9	1.7
18297	Pancakes, dry mix, prep, special dietary	1 pancake (4" dia)	38	75.6	1.9	16.0	0.0	0.3	0.0	0.0
918292	Pancakes, Plain, homemade	1.0 oz	28	63.6	1.8	7.9	0.0	2.7	0.7	1.2
18289	Pancakes, Plain, incomplete dry mix, prep	1 pancake (4" dia)	38	82.8	3.0	11.0	0.7	2.9	0.0	0.0
18288	Pancakes, Plain/Buttermilk, complete dry mix, prep	1 pancake (4" dia)	38	73.7	2.0	13.9	0.5	1.0	0.0	0.0
18291	Pancakes, Plain/Buttermilk, frozen	1 pancake (4" dia)	36	82.4	1.9	15.7	0.6	1.2	0.4	0.3
20097	Pancakes, Whole Wheat, incomplete dry mix, prep	1 pancake (4" dia)	38	79.0	3.2	11.2	1.1	2.5	0.0	0.0
22907	Pasta w/egg, homemade, ckd	2.0 oz, ckd	57	74.1	3.1	13.4	0.0	1.0	0.3	0.3
20098	Pasta w/meatballs in tomato sauce, canned entree	1 can	425	437.8	18.4	52.2	11.5	17.3	7.1	1.0
22522	Pasta w/o egg, homemade, ckd	2.0 oz	57	70.7	2.5	14.3	0.0	0.6	0.1	0.3
22515	Pasta w/sliced franks in tomato sauce, canned entree	1 can	418	434.7	15.5	49.7	3.8	19.2	7.9	2.5
924169	Pasta, Beef Ravioli w/meat sauce, canned	1 can, 7.8 oz serving	213	268.4	9.8	34.8	0.0	10.1	0.0	0.0
924206	Pasta, Beefaroni, Macaroni w/beef in tomato sauce, canned entree/ Chef Boyardee	1 package	212	184.4	8.2	31.1	3.0	2.9	1.3	0.3
20092	Pasta, Cheese Ravioli/Contadina	4.5 oz	128	369.9	18.0	39.0	0.0	15.0	5.0	0.0

Sat (g)	Chol (mg)	Cal (mg)	Iron (mg)	Magn (mg)	Phos (mg)	Pota (mg)	Sodi (mg)	Zinc (mg)	Vit A (RE)	Vit C (mg)	Vit E (mg)	Thia (mg)	Ribo (mg)	Niac (mg)	Vit B-6 (mg)	Fol (µg)	Vit B-12 (µg)	Wat (g)
23.8	0.0	11.2	1.9	25.6	90.4	284.8	16.0	0.9	0.0	2.6	0.6	0.1	0.0	0.4	0.0	21.1	0.0	37.6
2.8	0.0	2.7	0.5	6.9	14.4	33.0	2.0	0.1	0.0	0.2	0.0	0.0	0.0	0.1	0.0	2.0	0.0	10.9
0.0	0.0	3.6	0.0	3.8	3.0	37.5	15.8	0.0	0.0	0.4	0.0	0.0	0.0	0.0	0.0	0.4	0.0	14.2
17.2	0.0	7.3	0.9	25.8	58.5	154.3	10.4	0.6	0.0	0.4	0.0	0.0	0.0	0.2	0.1	2.5	0.0	0.5
11.7	0.0	7.6	0.9	25.8	59.1	155.1	10.4	0.6	0.0	0.4	0.0	0.0	0.0	0.2	0.1	2.6	0.0	0.3
62.6	0.0	29.9	3.8	99.5	212.9	670.6	521.4	3.6	0.0	1.4	2.7	0.1	0.0	0.9	0.5	16.1	0.0	25.0
16.0	0.0	7.3	0.9	25.2	57.7	152.0	10.4	0.6	0.0	0.4	0.4	0.0	0.0	0.2	0.1	2.5	0.0	0.8
1.4	0.0	54.6	0.9	82.9	90.4	129.4	0.8	0.7	2.0	0.3	7.2	0.1	0.0	0.3	0.2	20.9	0.0	0.5
0.2	0.0	1.4	0.0	2.3	2.7	7.4	0.1	0.0	0.0	0.0	0.0	0.0	0.0	0.0	0.0	0.3	0.0	0.1
2.5	0.0	29.7	0.7	70.3	125.7	152.3	196.0	1.3	0.6	0.1	1.7	0.1	0.1	0.5	0.1	15.8	0.0	0.9
2.5	0.0	29.7	0.7	70.3	125.7	152.3	3.1	1.3	0.6	0.1	1.7	0.1	0.1	0.5	0.1	15.8	0.0	0.9
1.9	0.0	19.6	1.0	63.0	121.8	167.2	3.4	1.1	0.3	0.1	1.7	0.1	0.1	1.3	0.1	14.1	0.0	0.5
1.9	0.0	19.6	1.0	63.0	121.8	167.2	187.3	1.1	0.3	0.1	1.7	0.1	0.1	1.3	0.1	14.1	0.0	0.5
0.8	0.0	9.6	0.3	20.9	41.3	51.7	1.0	0.5	0.2	0.0	0.5	0.0	0.0	0.5	0.0	7.4	0.0	0.2
0.1	0.0	1.1	0.0	2.4	4.6	5.8	6.5	0.1	0.0	0.0	0.1	0.0	0.0	0.1	0.0	0.8	0.0	0.0
0.2	0.0	1.1	0.1	3.8	8.7	11.8	0.0	0.2	0.4	0.1	0.1	0.0	0.0	0.0	0.0	1.2	0.0	0.1
1.4	0.0	9.8	0.6	37.2	85.1	103.6	0.3	1.6	3.6	0.6	0.9	0.1	0.0	0.3	0.1	11.4	0.0	0.3
1.4	0.0	9.8	0.6	37.2	85.1	103.6	218.4	1.6	3.6	0.6	0.0	0.1	0.0	0.3	0.1	11.4	0.0	0.3
0.2	0.0	1.4	0.1	5.2	11.8	14.4	0.0	0.2	0.5	0.1	0.0	0.0	0.0	0.0	0.0	1.6	0.0	0.2
0.2	0.0	1.4	0.1	5.2	11.8	14.4	30.2	0.2	0.5	0.1	0.0	0.0	0.0	0.0	0.0	1.6	0.0	0.2
10.6	0.0	35.4	12.5	316.9	690.9	814.6	5.4	5.8	4.1	2.6	4.8	1.1	0.3	4.9	0.1	77.9	0.0	9.1
0.1	0.0	1.4	0.1	1.6	5.0	10.9	0.1	0.0	0.2	0.1	0.1	0.0	0.0	0.0	0.0	0.6	0.0	0.0
1.9	0.0	19.6	0.9	36.4	133.3	271.6	1.7	0.4	6.7	2.0	1.5	0.1	0.1	0.4	0.1	16.5	0.0	0.6
1.9	0.0	19.6	0.9	36.4	133.3	271.6	218.4	0.4	6.7	2.0	1.8	0.1	0.1	0.4	0.1	16.5	0.0	0.6
0.3	0.0	4.5	0.2	15.8	36.2	40.9	0.1	0.3	2.3	0.2	0.2	0.0	0.0	0.1	0.0	5.1	0.0	0.3
49.3	1242.6	0.0	0.0	0.0	0.0	0.0	0.0	0.0	65406.5	0.0	0.0	0.0	0.0	0.0	0.0	0.0	0.0	0.0
1.0	0.0	0.0	0.0	0.0	0.0	0.0	0.0	0.0	0.0	0.0	2.8	0.0	0.0	0.0	0.0	0.0	0.0	0.0
8.1	0.0	0.0	0.0	0.0	0.0	0.0	0.0	0.0	0.0	0.0	0.0	0.0	0.0	0.0	0.0	0.0	0.0	0.0
11.8	0.0	0.0	0.0	0.0	0.0	0.0	0.0	0.0	0.0	0.0	0.0	0.0	0.0	0.0	0.0	0.0	0.0	0.0
1.7	0.0	0.0	0.0	0.0	0.0	0.0	0.0	0.0	0.0	0.0	0.0	0.0	0.0	0.0	0.0	0.0	0.0	0.0
1.3	0.0	0.0	0.0	0.0	0.0	0.0	0.0	0.0	0.0	0.0	0.0	0.0	0.0	0.0	0.0	0.0	0.0	0.0
2.7	0.0	0.0	0.0	0.0	0.0	0.0	0.0	0.0	0.0	0.0	2.0	0.0	0.0	0.0	0.0	0.0	0.0	0.0
6.7	0.0	0.0	0.0	0.0	0.0	0.0	0.0	0.0	0.0	0.0	3.0	0.0	0.0	0.0	0.0	0.0	0.0	0.0
11.1	0.0	0.0	0.0	0.0	0.0	0.0	0.0	0.0	0.0	0.0	0.5	0.0	0.0	0.0	0.0	0.0	0.0	0.0
1.8	0.0	0.0	0.0	0.0	0.0	0.0	0.0	0.0	0.0	0.0	0.0	0.0	0.0	0.0	0.0	0.0	0.0	0.0
2.7	0.0	0.0	0.0	0.0	0.0	0.0	0.0	0.0	0.0	0.0	0.0	0.0	0.0	0.0	0.0	0.0	0.0	0.0
2.0	0.0	0.0	0.0	0.0	0.0	0.0	0.0	0.0	0.0	0.0	0.7	0.0	0.0	0.0	0.0	0.0	0.0	0.0
1.4	0.0	0.0	0.0	0.0	0.0	0.0	0.0	0.0	0.0	0.0	0.0	0.0	0.0	0.0	0.0	0.0	0.0	0.0
1.4	0.0	0.0	0.0	0.0	0.0	0.0	0.0	0.0	0.0	0.0	6.9	0.0	0.0	0.0	0.0	0.0	0.0	0.0
1.3	0.0	0.0	0.0	0.0	0.0	0.0	0.0	0.0	0.0	0.0	0.0	0.0	0.0	0.0	0.0	0.0	0.0	0.0
1.8	0.0	0.0	0.0	0.0	0.0	0.0	0.0	0.0	0.0	0.0	6.9	0.0	0.0	0.0	0.0	0.0	0.0	0.0
11.6	0.0	0.0	0.0	0.0	0.0	0.0	0.0	0.0	0.0	0.0	0.0	0.0	0.0	0.0	0.0	0.0	0.0	0.0
1.7	0.0	0.0	0.0	0.0	0.0	0.0	0.0	0.0	0.0	0.0	2.9	0.0	0.0	0.0	0.0	0.0	0.0	0.0
3.5	0.0	0.0	0.0	0.0	0.0	0.0	0.0	0.0	0.0	0.0	5.2	0.0	0.0	0.0	0.0	0.0	0.0	0.0
1.8	0.0	0.0	0.1	0.0	0.2	0.0	0.0	0.0	0.0	0.0	1.7	0.0	0.0	0.0	0.0	0.0	0.0	0.0
2.3	0.0	0.0	0.0	0.0	0.0	0.0	0.0	0.0	0.0	0.0	1.7	0.0	0.0	0.0	0.0	0.0	0.0	0.0
1.2	0.0	0.0	0.0	0.0	0.0	0.0	0.0	0.0	0.0	0.0	5.9	0.0	0.0	0.0	0.0	0.0	0.0	0.0
0.8	0.0	0.0	0.0	0.0	0.0	0.0	0.0	0.0	0.0	0.0	4.7	0.0	0.0	0.0	0.0	0.0	0.0	0.0
1.9	0.0	0.0	0.0	0.0	0.0	0.0	0.0	0.0	0.0	0.0	0.6	0.0	0.0	0.0	0.0	0.0	0.0	0.0
2.0	0.0	0.0	0.0	0.0	0.0	0.0	0.0	0.0	0.0	0.0	2.5	0.0	0.0	0.0	0.0	0.0	0.0	0.0
2.0	0.0	0.0	0.0	0.0	0.0	0.0	0.0	0.0	0.0	0.0	2.5	0.0	0.0	0.0	0.0	0.0	0.0	0.0
1.1	8.6	27.3	2.4	14.0	266.0	80.3	413.4	0.5	0.0	1.1	0.0	0.2	0.2	2.7	0.3	40.6	0.8	36.8
0.8	21.3	78.3	0.7	6.1	57.4	52.4	156.6	0.2	19.4	0.8	0.0	0.1	0.1	0.6	0.0	13.7	0.1	20.2
0.8	0.6	76.8	0.6	16.8	122.1	69.9	159.9	0.4	20.1	0.2	0.0	0.1	0.1	0.4	0.0	5.1	0.1	16.1
0.7	22.0	59.7	0.6	5.7	52.8	55.1	198.4	0.2	11.4	0.2	0.0	0.1	0.1	0.6	0.0	14.4	0.1	20.0
0.1	0.1	22.0	0.7	10.3	129.2	146.7	99.6	0.3	3.8	0.0	0.0	0.1	0.0	0.6	0.0	1.9	0.0	18.6
0.6	16.5	61.3	0.5	4.5	44.5	37.0	122.9	0.2	15.1	0.1	0.0	0.1	0.1	0.4	0.0	10.6	0.1	14.8
1.1	0.8	81.7	0.5	8.4	118.9	75.6	191.9	0.3	27.4	0.2	0.0	0.1	0.1	0.5	0.0	4.2	0.1	20.1
0.3	0.3	47.9	0.6	7.6	126.9	66.5	238.6	0.1	3.4	0.1	0.0	0.1	0.1	0.7	0.0	3.4	0.1	20.1
0.3	3.2	22.3	1.3	5.0	133.9	26.3	183.2	0.2	10.4	0.1	0.1	0.1	0.2	1.4	0.0	18.0	0.1	16.3
0.9	0.7	95.0	1.2	17.5	141.7	106.0	217.4	0.4	24.3	0.2	0.0	0.1	0.2	0.9	0.0	8.0	0.1	20.1
0.2	23.4	5.7	0.7	8.0	29.6	12.0	47.3	0.3	9.7	0.0	0.0	0.1	0.1	0.7	0.0	24.5	0.1	39.2
6.8	34.0	46.8	4.0	59.5	195.5	701.3	1776.5	3.1	157.3	12.8	2.1	0.3	0.3	5.6	0.3	89.3	1.0	330.8
0.1	0.0	3.4	0.6	8.0	22.8	10.8	42.2	0.2	0.0	0.0	0.0	0.1	0.1	0.8	0.0	24.5	0.0	39.3
6.1	37.6	0.0	3.8	0.0	0.0	0.0	2014.8	0.0	0.0	0.0	0.0	0.0	0.0	0.0	0.0	0.0	0.0	326.9
0.0	0.0	51.0	2.2	0.0	0.0	371.0	814.0	0.0	196.0	7.0	0.0	0.2	0.2	3.3	0.0	0.0	0.0	0.0
1.2	17.0	17.0	1.5	0.0	0.0	0.0	799.2	0.0	0.0	0.4	0.0	0.0	0.0	0.0	0.0	0.0	0.0	167.0
10.0	110.0	340.0	1.4	34.0	320.0	120.0	540.0	1.1	103.0	0.0	0.0	0.2	0.3	1.2	0.1	13.0	0.5	0.0

Code	Food Name	Unit/Amt	Wt (g)	Energy (Kcal)	Prot (g)	Carb (g)	Fiber (g)	Fat (g)	Mono (g)	Poly (g)
20094	Pasta, Fettucini Alfredo	2.0 oz dry, @ 1 cup cooked	29	30.7	1.3	46.0	0.0	0.9	0.0	0.0
20093	Pasta, Fresh-refrigerated, Plain, ckd	2.0 oz dry, @ 1 cup cooked	57	74.7	2.9	14.2	0.0	0.6	0.1	0.2
20095	Pasta, Fresh-refrigerated, Spinach, ckd	2.0 oz	57	74.1	2.9	14.3	0.0	0.5	0.2	0.1
924170	Pasta, Mini beef Ravioli in tomato & meat sauce, canned entree/Chef Boyardee	1 package	425	403.8	14.8	68.5	5.5	8.0	3.4	0.3
924270	Pasta, Ravioli, frozen	1.0 oz	28	59.9	2.0	7.0	0.0	2.0	0.0	0.0
924014	Pasta, Spaghetti w/meat sauce	1 cup	248	332.3	18.6	38.7	0.0	11.7	0.0	0.0
924126	Pasta, Spaghetti w/tomato sauce&cheese	1 cup	250	260.0	9.0	37.0	2.0	9.0	3.6	1.2
924189	Pasta, Spaghetti&Meatballs	1 cup	248	329.8	19.0	39.0	1.0	12.0	4.4	2.2
20121	Pasta, Spaghetti, canned	1 cup	250	190.0	6.0	39.0	2.0	2.0	0.4	0.5
20321	Pasta, Spaghetti, enriched, ckd w/o salt	1 cup	140	197.4	6.7	39.7	2.4	0.9	0.1	0.4
20120	Pasta, Spaghetti, enriched, ckd w/salt	1 cup	140	197.4	6.7	39.7	2.4	0.9	0.1	0.4
20126	Pasta, Spaghetti, Spinach, ckd	1 cup	140	182.0	6.4	36.6	0.0	0.9	0.1	0.4
20521	Pasta, Spaghetti, unenriched, ckd w/o salt	1 cup	140	197.4	6.7	39.7	2.4	0.9	0.1	0.4
20420	Pasta, Spaghetti, unenriched, ckd w/salt	1 cup	140	197.4	6.7	39.7	0.0	0.9	0.1	0.4
20124	Pasta, Spaghetti, Whole Wheat, ckd	1 cup	140	173.6	7.5	37.2	6.3	0.8	0.1	0.3
924172	Pasta, Spaghettios&Franks/FrancoAm	8.0 oz	227	227.0	8.3	28.3	1.1	9.1	0.0	0.0
924194	Pasta, Spaghettios&Meatballs/FrancoAm	8.0 oz	227	222.5	9.9	27.3	0.9	8.2	0.0	0.0
22520	Pasta, Spinach Tortellini/Contadina	8.0 oz	227	656.0	31.9	97.5	0.0	14.2	5.3	1.8
18640	Pasta, Whole Wheat Macaroni and Cheese Dinner, dry mix/Hodgson Mill	8.0 oz	227	852.4	32.0	157.1	17.3	10.7	0.0	0.0
18635	Pastry, Chocolate Eclairs, frozen/WW	1 eclair, frozen	59	140.5	2.4	23.5	0.9	4.1	0.0	0.0
18238	Pastry, Cinnamon Rolls w/icing, refrigerated dough/Pillsbury	1 serving	44	150.2	2.4	23.9	0.0	5.0	0.0	0.0
18237	Pastry, Cream Puff/Eclair Shell, homemade w/custard	1 miniature cream puff	23	59.3	1.5	5.3	0.1	3.6	1.5	1.0
18240	Pastry, Cream Puff/Eclair Shell, homemade	1 cream puff shell	66	238.9	5.9	15.0	0.5	17.1	7.3	4.9
18241	Pastry, Croissant, Butter	1 mini croissant	29	117.7	2.4	13.3	0.8	6.1	1.6	0.3
918816	Pastry, Croissant, Cheese	1 small croissant	42	173.9	3.9	19.7	1.1	8.8	2.7	1.0
18244	Pastry, Danish, Cheese	1 pastry	71	265.5	5.7	26.4	0.7	15.5	8.0	1.8
18431	Pastry, Danish, Fruit (Apple/Cinn/Raisin/Lemon/Raspberry/Strawberry)enrich	1 large (7″ dia)	142	526.8	7.7	67.9	2.7	26.3	14.2	3.4
18435	Pastry, Danish, Nut (Almond/Raisin Nut/Cinnamon Nut)	1 piece (⅛ of 15 oz ring)	53	227.9	3.8	24.2	1.1	13.4	7.3	2.3
18338	Pastry, Eclair/Cream Puff, homemade, custard filled w/chocolate icing	1 eclair (5″ x 2″ x 1.75″)	100	262.0	6.4	24.2	0.6	15.7	6.5	3.9
18337	Pastry, Phyllo Dough	1.0 oz	28	83.7	2.0	14.7	0.5	1.7	0.9	0.3
18354	Pastry, Puff, frozen, baked	1 shell	40	223.2	3.0	18.3	0.6	15.4	3.5	8.9
18368	Pastry, Strudel, Apple	1 piece	71	194.5	2.3	29.2	1.6	8.0	2.3	3.8
16398	Peanut Butter, chunky w/salt	2 tbsp	32	188.5	7.7	6.9	2.1	16.0	7.5	4.5
16099	Peanut Butter, smooth w/salt	2 tbsp	32	189.8	8.1	6.2	1.9	16.3	7.8	4.4
16100	Peanut Flour, defatted	1 cup	60	196.2	31.3	20.8	9.5	0.3	0.1	0.1
912902	Peanut Flour, low fat	1 cup	60	256.8	20.3	18.8	9.5	13.1	6.5	4.2
16090	Peanuts, All Types, dry roasted w/o salt	1 peanut	1	5.9	0.2	0.2	0.1	0.5	0.2	0.2
16389	Peanuts, All Types, dry roasted w/salt	1.0 oz	28	163.8	6.6	6.0	2.2	13.9	6.9	4.4
16089	Peanuts, All Types, oil roasted w/o salt	1 nut	1	5.8	0.3	0.2	0.1	0.5	0.2	0.2
16087	Peanuts, All Types, oil roasted w/salt	1 peanut	0.9	5.2	0.2	0.2	0.1	0.4	0.2	0.1
912901	Peanuts, All Types, raw	1.0 oz	28	158.8	7.2	4.5	2.4	13.8	6.8	4.4
16392	Peanuts, honey roasted	1.0 oz	28	150.1	7.0	4.0	3.0	13.0	7.0	4.0
16394	Peanuts, Spanish, raw	¼ cup (@ 1 handful)	37	210.9	9.7	5.9	3.5	18.4	8.3	6.4
16158	Peas, Chickpea/Garbanzo, Falafel, homemade	1 (2.25″ diam) patty	17	56.6	2.3	5.4	0.0	3.0	1.7	0.7
16357	Peas, Chickpea/Garbanzo, Hummus, commercial	½ cup	125	207.5	9.9	17.9	7.5	12.0	0.0	0.0
16056	Peas, Chickpea/Garbanzo/Bengal gram, mature seeds, canned	½ cup	120	142.8	5.9	27.1	5.3	1.4	0.3	0.6
16063	Peas, Cowpea, Catjang, mature seeds, raw	½ cup	65	223.0	15.5	38.8	7.0	1.3	0.1	0.6
16363	Peas, Cowpea, Common (blackeyed,crowder,southern) mature seed, boiled w/o salt	½ cup	66	76.6	5.1	13.7	4.3	0.3	0.0	0.1
16101	Peas, Pigeon (red gram) mature seeds, boiled w/salt	½ cup	84	101.6	5.7	19.5	5.6	0.3	0.0	0.2
16086	Peas, Split, mature seed, boiled w/salt	½ cup	93	109.7	7.8	19.6	7.7	0.4	0.1	0.2
18398	Pie Crust, Chocolate Cookie	⅛ crust	20	96.0	1.2	13.4	0.0	4.2	3.4	0.2
18618	Pie Crust, Chocolate Wafer, baked	1 piece (⅛ of 9″ dia)	27	139.3	1.4	15.0	0.0	8.6	0.0	0.0
18332	Pie Crust, Cookie Type Nilla Wafer, ready to use/Nabisco	1.0 oz	28	143.7	1.0	17.7	0.3	7.6	5.2	0.4
18335	Pie Crust, dry mix, prep, baked	1 piece (⅛ of 9″ dia)	20	100.2	1.3	10.1	0.4	6.1	0.0	0.0
18334	Pie Crust, frozen, baked	1 piece (⅛ of 9″ dia)	16	82.2	0.7	7.9	0.2	5.2	2.5	0.6
18336	Pie Crust, Graham Cracker/Cookie Type, baked	1 piece (⅛ of 9″ dia)	30	148.2	1.3	19.6	0.5	7.5	3.4	2.1
18402	Pie Crust, homemade, baked	1 piece (⅛ of 9″ dia)	23	121.2	1.5	10.9	0.4	8.0	3.5	2.1
19312	Pie Crust, Vanilla Wafer, baked	1 piece (⅛ of 9″ dia)	22	119.0	0.8	11.3	0.4	8.1	0.0	0.0
19314	Pie Filling, Apple, canned	⅛ can	74	74.7	0.1	19.4	0.7	0.1	0.0	0.0
918888	Pie Filling, Cherry, canned	⅛ can	74	85.1	0.4	21.7	0.4	0.1	0.0	0.0
18628	Pie, Apple Snack Pie/Hostess	1 pie	128	390.4	5.0	45.0	0.0	20.0	0.0	0.0
18443	Pie, Apple Turnover, frozen, ready to bake/PepFarm	1 serving	89	284.1	3.7	31.2	1.6	16.0	0.0	0.0
18302	Pie, Apple, frozen/Banquet	1 serving	112	292.3	2.9	41.4	1.0	13.2	6.1	1.4
918871	Pie, Apple, homemade	1 oz	28.35	75.1	0.7	10.5	0.0	3.5	1.5	0.9
18304	Pie, Banana Cream, frozen	⅙ pie	66	180.2	2.0	21.0	2.0	10.0	0.0	0.0
18303	Pie, Banana Cream, homemade	1 piece (⅛ of 9″ dia)	144	387.4	6.3	47.4	1.0	19.6	8.2	4.7
918872	Pie, Banana Cream, no bake mix	1 piece (⅛ of 9″ dia)	92	230.9	3.1	29.1	0.6	11.9	4.2	0.7
918873	Pie, Banana Custard	⅛ pie	114	251.9	5.1	35.0	1.0	10.6	0.0	0.0

Sat (g)	Chol (mg)	Cal (mg)	Iron (mg)	Magn (mg)	Phos (mg)	Pota (mg)	Sodi (mg)	Zinc (mg)	Vit A (RE)	Vit C (mg)	Vit E (mg)	Thia (mg)	Ribo (mg)	Niac (mg)	Vit B-6 (mg)	Fol (μg)	Vit B-12 (μg)	Wat (g)
0.0	5.7	13.2	0.3	0.0	18.9	8.9	47.3	0.0	0.0	0.0	0.0	0.0	0.0	0.2	0.0	0.0	0.0	0.0
0.1	18.8	3.4	0.6	10.3	35.9	13.7	3.4	0.3	3.4	0.0	0.0	0.1	0.1	0.6	0.0	36.5	0.1	39.1
0.1	18.8	10.3	0.6	13.7	32.5	21.1	3.4	0.4	8.0	0.0	0.0	0.1	0.1	0.6	0.1	36.5	0.1	39.1
3.0	29.8	38.3	4.1	0.0	0.0	0.0	2018.8	0.0	0.0	0.0	0.4	0.0	0.0	0.0	0.0	0.0	0.0	327.5
0.0	0.0	12.0	0.7	0.0	34.0	40.0	80.0	0.0	0.0	0.0	0.0	0.1	0.1	0.8	0.0	0.0	0.0	0.0
3.3	0.0	124.0	3.7	0.0	236.0	665.0	1009.0	0.0	318.0	22.0	0.0	0.3	0.3	4.0	0.0	0.0	0.0	173.8
3.0	8.0	80.0	2.3	0.0	135.0	408.0	955.0	1.3	216.0	13.0	0.0	0.3	0.2	2.3	0.2	8.0	0.0	0.0
3.9	89.0	124.0	3.7	0.0	236.0	665.0	1009.0	2.5	318.0	22.0	0.0	0.3	0.3	4.0	0.2	10.0	0.0	0.0
0.4	3.0	40.0	2.8	0.0	88.0	303.0	955.0	1.1	186.0	10.0	0.0	0.4	0.3	4.5	0.1	6.0	0.0	0.0
0.1	0.0	9.8	2.0	25.2	75.6	43.4	1.4	0.7	0.0	0.0	0.1	0.3	0.1	2.3	0.0	98.0	0.0	92.4
0.1	0.0	9.8	2.0	25.2	75.6	43.4	140.0	0.7	0.0	0.0	0.0	0.3	0.1	2.3	0.0	98.0	0.0	92.4
0.1	0.0	42.0	1.5	86.8	151.2	81.2	19.6	1.5	21.0	0.0	0.0	0.1	0.1	2.1	0.1	16.8	0.0	95.4
0.1	0.0	9.8	0.7	25.2	75.6	43.4	1.4	0.7	0.0	0.0	0.1	0.0	0.0	0.6	0.0	9.8	0.0	92.4
0.1	0.0	9.8	0.7	25.2	75.6	43.4	140.0	0.7	0.0	0.0	0.0	0.0	0.0	0.6	0.0	9.8	0.0	92.4
0.1	0.0	21.0	1.5	42.0	124.6	61.6	4.2	1.1	0.0	0.0	0.1	0.2	0.1	1.0	0.1	7.0	0.0	94.0
0.0	0.0	34.8	2.4	0.0	118.4	325.8	1074.2	1.7	111.0	4.3	0.0	0.2	0.2	3.5	0.1	0.0	0.5	0.0
0.0	0.0	32.0	2.4	0.0	137.7	342.7	1024.8	2.2	112.8	4.4	0.0	0.2	0.2	3.3	0.1	0.0	0.8	0.0
7.1	115.3	540.9	6.4	16.0	532.0	478.8	1064.1	0.6	94.0	0.0	0.0	1.3	1.0	11.4	0.0	12.4	0.3	0.0
3.1	17.9	258.8	5.9	0.0	0.0	0.0	1387.0	0.0	0.0	0.0	0.0	0.0	0.0	0.0	0.0	0.0	0.0	19.3
0.7	30.1	0.0	0.0	0.0	0.0	0.0	185.9	0.0	0.0	0.0	0.0	0.0	0.0	0.0	0.0	0.0	0.0	28.3
1.2	0.0	0.0	0.0	0.0	0.0	0.0	334.4	0.0	0.0	0.0	0.0	0.0	0.0	0.0	0.0	0.0	0.0	11.7
0.8	30.8	15.2	0.3	2.8	25.1	26.5	78.4	0.1	45.8	0.1	0.5	0.0	0.1	0.2	0.0	6.4	0.1	12.3
3.7	129.4	23.8	1.3	7.9	78.5	64.0	367.6	0.5	203.3	0.0	2.5	0.1	0.2	1.0	0.0	31.7	0.3	26.7
3.4	19.4	10.7	0.6	4.6	30.5	34.2	215.8	0.2	53.9	0.1	0.1	0.1	0.1	0.6	0.0	18.0	0.0	6.7
4.5	23.9	22.3	0.9	10.1	54.6	55.4	233.1	0.4	82.7	0.1	0.4	0.2	0.1	0.9	0.0	31.1	0.1	8.8
4.8	11.4	24.9	1.1	10.7	76.7	69.6	319.5	0.5	32.0	0.1	1.8	0.1	0.2	1.4	0.0	42.6	0.1	22.3
6.9	161.9	65.3	2.5	21.3	126.4	117.9	502.7	0.8	31.2	5.5	3.5	0.4	0.3	2.8	0.1	46.9	0.1	38.5
3.1	24.4	49.8	1.0	17.0	58.3	50.4	192.4	0.5	7.4	0.9	1.9	0.1	0.1	1.2	0.1	44.0	0.1	10.8
4.1	127.0	63.0	1.2	15.0	107.0	117.0	337.0	0.6	191.0	0.3	2.1	0.1	0.3	0.8	0.1	28.0	0.3	52.4
0.4	0.0	3.1	0.9	4.2	21.0	20.7	135.2	0.1	0.0	0.0	0.3	0.2	0.1	1.1	0.0	20.7	0.0	9.1
2.2	0.0	4.0	1.0	6.4	24.0	24.8	101.2	0.2	0.0	0.0	1.0	0.1	0.1	1.5	0.0	18.8	0.0	3.0
1.5	4.3	10.7	0.3	6.4	23.4	105.8	191.0	0.1	6.4	1.2	2.2	0.0	0.0	0.2	0.0	9.9	0.2	30.9
3.1	0.0	13.1	0.6	50.9	101.4	239.0	155.5	0.9	0.0	0.0	0.0	0.0	0.0	4.4	0.1	29.4	0.0	0.4
3.3	0.0	12.2	0.6	50.9	118.1	214.1	149.4	0.9	0.0	0.0	3.2	0.0	0.0	4.3	0.1	23.7	0.0	0.4
0.0	0.0	84.0	1.3	222.0	456.0	774.0	108.0	3.1	0.0	0.0	0.0	0.4	0.3	16.2	0.3	148.9	0.0	4.7
1.8	0.0	78.0	2.8	28.8	304.8	814.8	0.6	3.6	0.0	0.0	0.0	0.3	0.1	6.9	0.2	80.0	0.0	4.7
0.1	0.0	0.5	0.0	1.8	3.6	6.6	0.1	0.0	0.0	0.0	0.1	0.0	0.0	0.1	0.0	1.5	0.0	0.0
1.9	0.0	15.1	0.6	49.3	100.2	184.2	227.6	0.9	0.0	0.0	2.1	0.1	0.0	3.8	0.1	40.7	0.0	0.4
0.1	0.0	0.9	0.0	1.9	5.2	6.8	0.1	0.1	0.0	0.0	0.1	0.0	0.0	0.1	0.0	1.3	0.0	0.0
0.1	0.0	0.8	0.0	1.7	4.7	6.1	3.9	0.1	0.0	0.0	0.1	0.0	0.0	0.1	0.0	1.1	0.0	0.0
1.9	0.0	25.8	1.3	47.0	105.3	197.4	5.0	0.9	0.0	0.0	2.6	0.2	0.0	3.4	0.1	67.1	0.0	1.8
2.0	0.0	15.0	0.6	0.0	100.0	160.0	110.0	0.9	0.0	0.0	0.0	0.1	0.0	3.8	0.1	41.0	0.0	2.4
2.8	0.0	39.2	1.4	69.6	143.6	275.3	8.1	0.8	0.0	0.0	0.0	0.2	0.0	5.9	0.1	88.8	0.0	2.4
0.4	0.0	9.2	0.6	13.9	32.6	99.5	50.0	0.3	0.2	0.3	0.0	0.0	0.0	0.2	0.0	15.8	0.0	5.9
0.0	0.0	47.5	3.1	88.8	220.0	285.0	473.8	2.3	3.8	0.0	0.0	0.2	0.1	0.7	0.3	103.8	0.0	83.2
0.1	0.0	38.4	1.6	34.8	108.0	206.4	358.8	1.3	2.4	4.6	0.0	0.0	0.0	0.2	0.6	80.2	0.0	83.6
0.4	0.0	55.3	6.5	216.5	284.7	893.8	37.7	4.0	2.0	1.0	0.0	0.4	0.1	1.8	0.2	415.4	0.0	7.2
0.1	0.0	15.8	1.7	35.0	103.0	183.5	2.6	0.9	1.3	0.3	0.2	0.1	0.0	0.3	0.1	137.2	0.0	46.2
0.1	0.0	36.1	0.9	38.6	100.0	322.6	202.4	0.8	0.0	0.0	0.0	0.1	0.0	0.7	0.0	93.1	0.0	57.6
0.1	0.0	13.0	1.2	33.5	92.1	336.7	221.3	0.9	0.9	0.4	0.0	0.2	0.1	0.8	0.0	60.4	0.0	64.6
0.6	0.0	5.0	0.6	0.0	0.0	62.0	107.0	0.0	0.0	0.0	0.0	0.1	0.2	0.6	0.0	0.0	0.0	0.9
2.1	4.1	8.4	0.8	11.1	28.9	46.2	185.2	0.2	60.2	0.0	0.0	0.0	0.1	0.6	0.0	0.0	0.0	1.5
1.4	2.8	11.5	0.5	2.2	23.2	19.3	62.7	0.1	0.0	0.0	0.0	0.0	0.1	0.7	0.0	8.4	0.0	0.9
0.8	3.5	12.0	0.4	3.0	16.8	12.4	145.8	0.1	0.0	0.0	0.0	0.0	0.1	0.5	0.0	2.4	0.0	2.1
1.7	0.0	3.4	0.4	2.9	9.4	17.6	103.5	0.1	0.0	0.0	0.8	0.0	0.1	0.4	0.0	6.2	0.0	1.8
1.6	0.0	6.3	0.7	5.4	19.5	26.4	171.3	0.1	60.6	0.0	1.2	0.0	0.1	0.6	0.0	7.2	0.0	1.3
2.0	0.0	2.3	0.7	3.2	15.4	15.4	124.7	0.1	0.0	0.0	0.0	0.1	0.1	0.8	0.0	15.4	0.0	2.3
2.4	3.5	9.5	0.4	2.4	17.4	17.8	115.7	0.1	64.0	0.0	0.0	0.0	0.1	0.5	0.0	1.5	0.0	1.5
0.0	0.0	3.0	0.2	1.5	5.2	33.3	32.6	0.0	0.7	0.8	0.0	0.0	0.0	0.0	0.0	0.0	0.0	54.3
0.0	0.0	8.1	0.2	5.2	11.1	77.7	6.7	0.0	15.5	2.7	0.0	0.0	0.0	0.1	0.0	3.0	0.0	51.6
0.0	18.0	26.0	1.4	0.0	0.0	0.0	540.0	0.0	0.0	1.0	0.0	0.1	0.1	1.6	0.0	0.0	0.0	0.0
4.0	0.0	0.0	1.2	0.0	0.0	0.0	176.2	0.0	0.0	0.0	0.0	0.0	0.0	0.0	0.0	0.0	0.0	37.3
5.7	8.7	10.1	0.3	0.0	0.0	0.0	360.6	0.0	0.0	0.0	0.0	0.0	0.0	0.0	0.0	0.0	0.0	54.3
0.9	0.0	2.0	0.3	2.0	7.9	22.4	59.8	0.1	3.4	0.5	0.0	0.0	0.0	0.3	0.0	6.8	0.0	13.4
0.0	0.0	32.0	1.0	0.0	100.0	120.0	150.0	0.0	1.4	1.0	0.0	0.2	0.1	2.0	0.3	15.0	0.0	0.0
5.4	73.4	108.0	1.5	23.0	132.5	237.6	345.6	0.7	100.8	2.3	2.1	0.2	0.3	1.5	0.2	38.9	0.4	69.0
6.4	26.7	67.2	0.4	11.0	153.6	104.0	266.8	0.3	92.0	0.5	0.0	0.1	0.1	0.7	0.0	19.3	0.2	46.8
3.4	0.0	75.0	0.6	0.0	93.0	231.0	221.0	1.0	58.0	1.0	0.0	0.1	0.2	0.3	0.0	0.0	0.0	60.2

Code	Food Name	Unit/Amt	Wt (g)	Energy (Kcal)	Prot (g)	Carb (g)	Fiber (g)	Fat (g)	Mono (g)	Poly (g)
918889	Pie, Blackberry	⅛ pie	118	286.7	3.1	40.6	5.0	13.0	0.0	0.0
18305	Pie, Blueberry Snack Pie/Hostess	1 pie	128	390.4	3.0	49.0	0.0	20.0	0.0	0.0
18306	Pie, Blueberry, commercially prep	1 piece (⅛ of 9″ dia)	125	290.0	2.3	43.6	1.3	12.5	5.3	4.4
918307	Pie, Blueberry, homemade	1 piece (⅛ of 9″ dia)	147	360.2	4.0	49.2	0.0	17.5	7.5	4.5
918890	Pie, Butterscotch Pudding, homemade	1 piece (⅛ of 9″ dia)	127	354.3	6.0	42.3	0.0	18.2	0.0	0.0
18308	Pie, Cherry Snack Pie/Hostess	1 pie	128	390.4	5.0	55.0	0.0	20.0	0.0	0.0
18444	Pie, Cherry, commercially prep	1 piece (⅛ of 9″ dia)	125	325.0	2.5	49.8	1.0	13.8	7.3	2.6
18309	Pie, Cherry, fried	1.0 oz	28	88.5	0.8	11.9	0.7	4.5	2.1	1.5
918874	Pie, Cherry, homemade	1.0 oz	29	78.3	0.8	11.2	0.0	3.5	1.5	0.9
18310	Pie, Chocolate Cream, frozen/Banquet	⅙ pie	66	190.1	2.0	24.0	1.0	10.0	0.0	0.0
918311	Pie, Chocolate Creme, commercially prep	1 piece (⅙ of 8″ pie)	113	343.5	2.9	38.0	2.3	21.9	12.6	2.7
18312	Pie, Chocolate Creme, homemade	1 piece (⅛ of 9″ dia)	142	400.4	6.8	44.3	0.0	22.9	0.0	0.0
918875	Pie, Chocolate Mousse, no bake mix	1 piece (⅛ of 9″ dia)	95	247.0	3.3	28.1	0.0	14.6	4.8	0.8
18313	Pie, Coconut Cream, frozen	1 piece (⅙ of 8″ pie)	100	288.0	3.0	33.3	0.0	16.7	0.0	0.0
918315	Pie, Coconut Creme, commercially prep	1 piece (⅛ of 7″ pie)	48	143.0	1.0	17.9	0.6	8.0	3.5	0.7
18314	Pie, Coconut Creme, homemade	1 piece (⅛ of 9″ dia)	133	396.3	6.4	45.5	0.0	21.3	0.0	0.0
918318	Pie, Egg Custard, commercially prep	1 piece (⅙ of 8″ pie)	105	220.5	5.8	21.8	1.7	12.2	5.0	3.9
18319	Pie, Egg Custard, homemade	1 piece (⅛ of 9″ dia)	127	261.6	6.5	34.0	0.0	11.3	0.0	0.0
918876	Pie, Fruit Pie, fried	1 fried pie (5 x 3.75″)	128	404.5	3.8	54.5	3.3	20.6	9.5	6.9
918877	Pie, Lemon Chiffon	1 piece (⅙ of 8″ pie)	81	254.3	5.7	35.5	1.0	10.2	0.0	0.0
18320	Pie, Lemon Cream, frozen/Banquet	1 piece (⅙ of 8″ pie)	66	170.3	2.0	23.0	1.0	9.0	0.0	0.0
18321	Pie, Lemon Meringue, commercially prep	1 piece (⅙ of 8″ pie)	113	302.8	1.7	53.3	1.4	9.8	3.0	4.1
18445	Pie, Lemon Meringue, homemade	1 piece (⅛ of 9″ dia)	127	362.0	4.8	49.7	0.0	16.4	7.1	4.2
18322	Pie, Lemon, fried	1 fried pie (5 x 3.75″)	128	404.5	3.8	54.5	3.3	20.6	9.5	6.9
918878	Pie, Mince, homemade	1 piece (⅛ of 9″ dia)	165	476.9	4.3	79.2	4.3	17.8	7.7	4.7
18323	Pie, Mincemeat, frozen/Banquet	1 piece (⅙ of 8″ pie)	94	260.4	3.0	38.0	0.0	11.0	0.0	0.0
918891	Pie, Peach	1.0 oz	28.5	63.6	0.5	9.4	0.2	2.9	1.2	1.1
918892	Pie, Peach Snack Pie/Hostess	1 pie	128	399.4	4.0	53.0	0.0	20.0	0.0	0.0
18324	Pie, Pecan Snack Pie/LittleDeb	1 pie	52	201.8	1.8	33.1	1.0	6.9	4.0	1.2
18325	Pie, Pecan, commercially prep	1 piece (⅙ of 8″ pie)	113	452.0	4.5	64.6	4.0	20.9	12.1	3.6
918879	Pie, Pecan, homemade	1 piece (⅛ of 9″ dia)	122	502.6	6.0	63.7	0.0	27.1	13.6	7.0
918880	Pie, Pineapple	1 piece (⅛ of 9″ dia)	118	298.5	2.6	45.0	0.6	12.6	0.0	0.0
918881	Pie, Pineapple Chiffon	1 piece (⅛ of 9″ dia)	81	233.3	5.3	31.7	0.3	9.8	0.0	0.0
18326	Pie, Pineapple Custard	1 piece (⅛ of 9″ dia)	114	250.8	4.6	36.6	0.5	9.9	0.0	0.0
18327	Pie, Pumpkin, commercially prep	1 piece (⅙ of 8″ pie)	180	378.0	7.0	49.1	4.9	17.1	7.3	5.7
918882	Pie, Pumpkin, homemade	1 piece (⅛ of 9″ dia)	114	232.6	5.1	30.1	0.0	10.6	4.2	2.1
918883	Pie, Raisin	1 piece (⅛ of 9″ dia)	118	318.6	3.1	50.7	0.8	12.6	0.0	0.0
918885	Pie, Rhubarb	1 piece (⅛ of 9″ dia)	118	298.5	3.0	45.1	2.0	12.6	0.0	0.0
18328	Pie, Strawberry	1 piece (⅛ of 9″ dia)	93	184.1	1.8	28.7	1.8	7.3	0.0	0.0
22531	Pie, Vanilla Creme, homemade	1 piece (⅛ of 9″ dia)	93	258.5	4.5	30.3	0.6	13.4	5.6	3.2
22533	Pizza Rolls Pizza Snacks, Hamburger, frozen/Totinos	1 serving (⅓ pkg)	85	231.2	9.4	26.4	0.0	9.8	0.0	0.0
22532	Pizza Rolls Pizza Snacks, Pepperoni, frozen/Totinos	1 serving	141	384.9	14.4	39.5	2.3	18.9	9.2	2.2
924142	Pizza Rolls Pizza Snacks, Sausage, frozen/Totinos	1 serving	141	351.1	14.1	40.2	2.8	14.9	7.2	2.2
924146	Pizza, Cheese Meat Vegetable	⅛ of alarge pizza	79	184.1	13.0	21.3	0.0	5.4	2.5	0.9
924141	Pizza, Cheese, frozen/Celeste	¼ of a medium pizza	126	317.5	14.2	27.8	2.2	16.6	3.0	1.0
22545	Pizza, Cheese, homemade	1 slice	65	152.8	7.8	18.4	1.0	5.4	0.0	0.0
924262	Pizza, Combination, Sausage & Pepperoni, frozen/Jeno's Crisp'n Tasty	1 package	198	491.0	16.8	51.7	2.8	24.2	11.9	3.1
22548	Pizza, Combo, frozen/Totino	⅙ pizza	91	234.8	11.3	20.0	0.0	12.2	0.0	0.0
22554	Pizza, Deep Dish Sausage, frozen/Tony's D'Primo	1 package	569	1576.1	50.1	163.9	0.0	80.2	29.3	17.0
22542	Pizza, Deluxe French Bread w/Sausage, Pepperoni & Mushroom, frozen/Stouffer	1 package	350	857.5	32.2	88.9	7.0	41.3	17.4	5.0
924148	Pizza, Deluxe w/Sausage, Green & Red Pepper & Mushrooms, frozen/Celeste	1 package	666	1538.5	66.6	132.5	0.0	82.6	30.4	9.7
924133	Pizza, Deluxe, frozen/Celeste	¼ pizza	158	377.6	15.5	29.3	3.1	22.1	7.0	2.0
22553	Pizza, French Bread Pizza/Pillsbury	5.7 oz	161	389.6	18.5	43.0	0.0	15.8	0.0	0.0
924149	Pizza, French Bread w/sausage & pepperoni, frozen/Stouffers	1 package	354	895.6	35.4	87.1	5.0	45.0	18.5	5.6
924264	Pizza, Ground Beef/Totino	3.5 oz	100	240.0	10.5	24.4	0.0	11.0	0.0	0.0
22560	Pizza, Mexican, frozen/Totino	½ pizza	145	381.4	13.1	35.5	0.0	20.3	0.0	0.0
22555	Pizza, Original Pepperoni, frozen, 12″/Tombstone	1 serving	113	311.9	14.5	28.3	0.0	15.7	5.3	2.0
22557	Pizza, Original Pepperoni, frozen, 9″/Tombstone	1 serving	152	413.4	17.8	38.6	0.0	20.8	7.1	2.4
22559	Pizza, Original Sausage & Mushroom, frozen/Tombstone	1 serving	132	306.2	14.4	31.2	0.0	13.7	4.4	2.1
22566	Pizza, Original Sausage & Pepperoni, frozen/Tombstone	1 serving	125	327.5	14.4	30.6	2.1	16.4	5.6	2.3
22562	Pizza, Pepperoni	⅛ pizza	71	181.1	10.1	19.9	0.0	7.0	3.1	1.2
22903	Pizza, Pepperoni w/Italian Pastry Crust, frozen/Tony's	1 seving	140	411.6	15.1	36.8	0.0	22.7	9.2	2.6
924151	Pizza, Pepperoni, frozen	1 seving	138	378.1	15.3	34.2	2.2	20.0	8.0	2.3
22546	Pizza, Pepperoni, frozen/Jack's Original	1 serving	122	323.3	15.0	29.5	0.0	16.1	5.2	2.1
22551	Pizza, Pepperoni/Pillsbury	½ pizza	120	302.4	13.4	29.0	2.0	14.4	0.0	0.0
22563	Pizza, Premium Deep Dish Singles, Pepperoni, frozen/Red Baron	1 serving	168	480.5	16.0	47.9	0.0	25.0	10.8	2.8
22543	Pizza, Sausage & pepperoni, frozen	1 serving	146	385.4	15.8	36.2	2.3	19.7	7.8	2.6
924158	Pizza, Sausage & Pepperoni, frozen/Jack's Great Combination	1 serving	137	348.0	17.4	30.1	0.0	17.5	6.1	2.3
924155	Pizza, Sausage Mushroom, frozen/Celentano	8.5 oz	241	592.9	23.9	51.3	4.5	32.3	10.0	3.0

Sat (g)	Chol (mg)	Cal (mg)	Iron (mg)	Magn (mg)	Phos (mg)	Pota (mg)	Sodi (mg)	Zinc (mg)	Vit A (RE)	Vit C (mg)	Vit E (mg)	Thia (mg)	Ribo (mg)	Niac (mg)	Vit B-6 (mg)	Fol (μg)	Vit B-12 (μg)	Wat (g)
3.2	0.0	22.0	0.6	0.0	31.0	118.0	316.0	0.0	22.0	5.0	0.0	0.0	0.0	0.4	0.0	0.0	0.0	60.2
0.0	18.0	28.0	1.5	0.0	0.0	0.0	450.0	0.0	0.0	2.0	0.0	0.2	0.1	1.8	0.0	0.0	0.0	0.0
2.1	0.0	10.0	0.4	6.3	28.8	62.5	406.3	0.2	42.5	3.4	2.5	0.0	0.0	0.4	0.0	27.5	0.0	65.6
4.3	0.0	10.3	1.8	11.8	44.1	73.5	272.0	0.3	5.9	1.0	0.0	0.2	0.2	1.8	0.0	33.8	0.0	75.3
4.3	7.6	128.3	1.6	21.6	134.6	221.0	335.3	0.7	106.7	0.6	0.0	0.2	0.3	1.3	0.1	14.0	0.4	58.8
0.0	18.0	29.0	1.4	0.0	0.0	0.0	530.0	0.0	0.0	2.0	0.0	0.2	0.1	1.6	0.0	0.0	0.0	0.0
3.2	0.0	15.0	0.6	10.0	36.3	101.3	307.5	0.2	67.5	1.1	1.9	0.0	0.0	0.3	0.1	27.5	0.0	57.8
0.7	0.0	6.2	0.3	2.8	12.0	18.2	104.7	0.1	4.8	0.4	0.0	0.0	0.0	0.4	0.0	5.0	0.0	10.5
0.9	0.0	2.9	0.5	2.6	8.7	22.3	55.4	0.1	13.9	0.3	0.0	0.0	0.0	0.4	0.0	7.8	0.0	13.3
0.0	0.0	38.0	1.0	0.0	0.0	86.0	110.0	0.0	1.4	0.0	0.0	0.0	0.1	0.2	0.0	0.0	0.0	0.0
5.6	5.7	40.7	1.2	23.7	76.8	143.5	153.7	0.3	0.0	0.0	3.1	0.0	0.1	0.8	0.0	14.7	0.0	49.2
4.8	9.4	115.0	1.8	36.9	156.2	208.7	347.9	0.9	103.7	0.7	0.0	0.2	0.3	1.5	0.1	14.2	0.4	66.2
7.8	33.3	73.2	1.0	30.4	219.5	270.8	437.0	0.6	96.0	0.5	0.0	0.0	0.1	0.6	0.0	24.7	0.2	47.2
0.0	0.0	45.5	1.5	0.0	0.0	116.7	181.8	0.0	0.3	0.0	0.0	0.0	0.1	0.3	0.0	0.0	0.0	0.0
3.3	0.0	13.9	0.4	9.6	40.8	31.2	122.4	0.2	0.0	0.0	0.9	0.0	0.0	0.1	0.0	3.4	0.1	20.7
4.5	8.0	113.1	1.5	21.3	139.7	183.5	356.4	0.8	105.1	0.7	0.0	0.2	0.3	1.3	0.1	14.6	0.4	58.1
2.5	34.7	84.0	0.6	11.6	117.6	111.3	252.0	0.5	70.4	0.6	2.0	0.0	0.2	0.3	0.1	21.0	0.5	63.9
2.4	4.6	106.7	1.0	16.5	124.5	158.8	256.5	0.6	81.3	0.5	0.0	0.1	0.3	0.8	0.1	12.7	0.3	73.9
3.1	0.0	28.2	1.6	12.8	55.0	83.2	478.7	0.3	3.8	1.7	3.8	0.2	0.1	1.8	0.0	23.0	0.1	48.1
2.7	0.0	19.0	0.7	0.0	67.0	66.0	211.0	0.0	28.0	2.0	0.0	0.0	0.1	0.2	0.0	0.0	0.0	28.8
0.0	0.0	30.0	1.0	0.0	0.0	70.0	120.0	0.0	0.4	2.0	0.0	0.0	0.0	0.2	0.0	0.0	0.0	0.0
2.0	50.9	63.3	0.7	17.0	118.7	100.6	165.0	0.6	58.8	3.6	2.5	0.1	0.2	0.7	0.0	14.7	0.2	47.1
4.0	67.3	15.2	1.3	7.6	53.3	82.6	307.3	0.4	55.9	4.2	0.0	0.1	0.2	1.2	0.0	31.8	0.2	55.0
3.1	0.0	28.2	1.6	12.8	55.0	83.2	478.7	0.3	3.8	1.7	0.0	0.2	0.1	1.8	0.0	23.0	0.1	48.1
4.4	0.0	36.3	2.5	23.1	69.3	335.0	419.1	0.4	3.3	9.7	3.1	0.2	0.2	2.0	0.1	38.0	0.0	61.7
0.0	0.0	19.0	1.0	0.0	45.0	110.0	370.0	0.0	0.4	1.0	0.0	0.0	0.0	0.3	0.0	0.0	0.0	0.0
0.4	0.0	2.3	0.1	1.7	6.3	35.6	77.0	0.0	6.3	0.3	0.6	0.0	0.0	0.1	0.0	6.8	0.0	15.5
0.0	18.0	37.0	2.0	0.0	0.0	0.0	445.0	0.0	0.0	1.0	0.0	0.2	0.2	2.3	0.0	0.0	0.0	0.0
1.6	1.0	8.0	0.6	0.0	50.0	50.0	184.0	0.5	0.0	0.0	0.0	0.1	0.1	0.5	0.0	5.0	0.0	9.8
4.0	36.2	19.2	1.2	20.3	87.0	83.6	479.1	0.6	53.1	1.2	2.1	0.1	0.1	0.3	0.0	30.5	0.1	21.8
4.9	106.1	39.0	1.8	31.7	114.7	162.3	319.6	1.2	108.6	0.2	0.0	0.2	0.2	1.0	0.1	31.7	0.2	23.8
3.1	0.0	15.0	0.6	0.0	25.0	85.0	320.0	0.0	4.0	1.0	0.0	0.0	0.0	0.5	0.0	0.0	0.0	56.6
2.6	0.0	19.0	0.7	0.0	62.0	79.0	207.0	0.0	56.0	1.0	0.0	0.1	0.3	0.0	0.0	0.0	0.0	33.3
3.0	0.0	27.0	0.5	0.0	74.0	111.0	212.0	0.0	42.0	1.0	0.0	0.1	0.1	0.5	0.0	0.0	0.0	61.9
3.2	36.0	108.0	1.4	27.0	127.8	277.2	507.6	0.8	669.6	1.8	3.1	0.1	0.3	0.3	0.1	36.0	0.5	104.6
3.6	47.9	107.2	1.4	21.7	111.7	212.0	256.5	0.5	891.5	1.9	0.0	0.1	0.2	0.9	0.1	23.9	0.1	66.7
3.1	0.0	21.0	1.1	0.0	47.0	227.0	336.0	0.0	2.0	1.0	0.0	0.0	0.4	0.0	0.0	0.0	0.0	50.2
3.1	0.0	76.0	0.8	0.0	31.0	188.0	319.0	0.0	12.0	4.0	0.0	0.0	0.4	0.0	0.0	0.0	0.0	55.9
1.8	0.0	15.0	0.7	0.0	23.0	112.0	180.0	0.0	8.0	23.0	0.0	0.0	0.4	0.0	0.0	0.0	0.0	54.3
3.7	57.7	83.7	0.9	12.1	96.7	117.2	241.8	0.5	79.1	0.5	1.3	0.1	0.2	0.9	0.0	24.2	0.3	43.7
0.0	0.0	0.0	0.0	0.0	0.0	0.0	417.4	0.0	0.0	0.0	0.0	0.0	0.0	0.0	0.0	0.0	0.0	37.7
5.0	31.0	102.9	0.0	0.0	0.0	0.0	865.7	0.0	0.0	0.0	0.0	0.0	0.0	0.0	0.0	0.0	0.0	65.3
3.5	24.0	101.5	0.0	0.0	0.0	0.0	631.7	0.0	0.0	0.0	0.0	0.0	0.0	0.0	0.0	0.0	0.0	69.2
1.5	21.0	101.0	1.5	18.0	131.0	178.0	382.0	1.1	101.0	2.0	0.0	0.2	0.2	2.0	0.1	27.0	0.4	37.7
7.0	20.0	204.0	1.0	30.0	266.0	268.0	770.0	3.0	155.8	0.0	0.0	0.1	0.4	1.1	0.1	14.0	1.0	62.1
2.1	0.0	144.0	0.7	0.0	127.0	85.0	456.0	3.0	82.0	5.0	0.0	0.0	0.1	0.7	0.2	100.0	2.0	31.4
5.7	25.7	166.3	0.0	0.0	0.0	0.0	1239.5	0.0	0.0	0.0	0.0	0.0	0.0	0.0	0.0	0.0	0.0	101.0
0.0	0.0	177.0	1.5	0.0	196.0	177.0	539.0	0.0	65.8	3.0	0.0	0.3	0.2	2.0	0.0	0.0	0.0	46.4
23.2	62.6	574.7	11.7	0.0	0.0	0.0	3351.4	0.0	0.0	0.0	0.0	0.0	0.0	0.0	0.0	0.0	0.0	261.7
12.7	66.5	462.0	5.4	0.0	0.0	0.0	1680.0	0.0	0.0	59.9	0.0	0.0	0.0	0.0	0.0	0.0	0.0	181.0
32.4	146.5	1118.9	0.0	0.0	0.0	0.0	3050.3	0.0	0.0	0.0	0.0	0.0	0.0	0.0	0.0	0.0	0.0	369.6
7.0	20.0	267.0	1.9	38.0	357.0	352.0	903.0	3.0	190.0	0.0	0.0	0.2	0.5	2.7	0.2	57.0	2.0	86.3
0.0	0.0	309.0	2.2	0.0	250.0	274.0	708.0	0.0	33.4	1.0	0.0	0.4	0.2	2.7	0.0	0.0	0.0	79.5
14.3	74.3	308.0	6.0	0.0	0.0	0.0	1720.4	0.0	0.0	0.0	0.0	0.0	0.0	0.0	0.0	0.0	0.0	179.5
0.0	0.0	134.0	1.7	0.0	190.0	178.0	712.0	0.0	53.2	3.0	0.0	0.1	0.2	2.4	0.0	0.0	0.0	51.2
0.0	0.0	213.0	3.3	0.0	296.0	270.0	973.0	0.0	84.2	10.0	0.0	0.4	0.3	3.3	0.0	0.0	0.0	64.2
6.0	31.6	202.3	0.0	0.0	0.0	0.0	551.4	0.0	0.0	0.0	0.0	0.0	0.0	0.0	0.0	0.0	0.0	52.1
7.8	41.0	272.1	0.0	0.0	0.0	0.0	869.4	0.0	0.0	0.0	0.0	0.0	0.0	0.0	0.0	0.0	0.0	71.0
5.1	26.4	200.6	0.0	0.0	0.0	0.0	718.1	0.0	0.0	0.0	0.0	0.0	0.0	0.0	0.0	0.0	0.0	69.7
6.1	31.3	178.8	0.0	0.0	0.0	0.0	790.0	0.0	0.0	0.0	0.0	0.0	0.0	0.0	0.0	0.0	0.0	60.8
2.2	14.0	65.0	0.9	8.0	75.0	153.0	267.0	0.5	54.0	2.0	0.0	0.1	0.2	3.1	0.0	53.0	0.2	33.0
7.7	32.2	218.4	2.8	0.0	0.0	0.0	845.6	0.0	0.0	0.0	0.0	0.0	0.0	0.0	0.0	0.0	0.0	61.7
6.7	31.7	0.0	2.5	23.5	209.8	209.8	830.8	1.7	62.1	1.7	1.6	0.4	0.3	3.4	0.1	51.1	0.1	65.1
6.2	40.3	220.8	0.0	0.0	0.0	0.0	612.4	0.0	0.0	0.0	0.0	0.0	0.0	0.0	0.0	0.0	0.0	58.4
0.0	0.0	194.0	1.6	0.0	184.0	205.0	790.0	4.0	87.8	9.0	0.0	0.2	0.2	2.3	0.0	0.0	0.0	60.2
8.2	28.6	152.9	3.5	0.0	0.0	0.0	888.7	0.0	0.0	0.0	0.0	0.0	0.0	0.0	0.0	0.0	0.0	75.6
6.3	30.7	191.3	2.8	26.3	207.3	255.5	854.1	1.6	62.8	3.2	1.4	0.4	0.3	3.6	0.1	51.1	0.4	71.0
6.6	43.8	224.7	0.0	0.0	0.0	0.0	708.3	0.0	0.0	0.0	0.0	0.0	0.0	0.0	0.0	0.0	0.0	68.8
11.0	20.0	362.0	2.4	60.0	504.0	459.0	1179.0	5.0	240.0	0.0	0.0	0.3	0.9	3.9	0.3	82.0	2.0	127.7

Code	Food Name	Unit/Amt	Wt (g)	Energy (Kcal)	Prot (g)	Carb (g)	Fiber (g)	Fat (g)	Mono (g)	Poly (g)
924153	Pizza, Sausage, frozen/LeanCuisine	6 oz	170	329.8	21.0	40.0	0.0	10.0	6.0	1.0
924139	Pizza, Sausage, homemade	1 slice	67	156.8	5.2	19.8	1.0	6.2	0.0	0.0
924140	Pizza, Sicilian Cheese, frozen	¼ pizza	140	329.0	15.4	42.5	1.5	10.6	0.0	0.0
924145	Pizza, Sicilian Deluxe	¼ pizza	182	425.9	18.6	43.8	1.5	19.5	0.0	0.0
22550	Pizza, Sicilian Sausage	¼ pizza	168	399.8	18.2	44.5	1.2	16.5	0.0	0.0
22598	Pizza, Supreme Italian Pastry Crust w/sausage, pepperoni, mushroom, green&red pe	1 serving	155	399.9	15.8	39.1	0.0	20.0	7.9	2.8
22564	Pizza, Supreme, Sausage, Mushrooms, Pepperoni, frozen/Red Baron	1 serving	136	344.1	13.6	31.8	0.0	18.1	7.2	2.5
924263	Pizza, Taco/Mexican Sausage & Tangy Taco Sauce on a Corn Crust, frozen/Tony's	1 serving	154	437.4	14.3	42.8	0.0	23.3	8.9	3.5
18339	Pizza, Vegetable, frozen/Totino	½ pizza	152	304.0	10.6	36.0	0.0	13.4	0.0	0.0
18447	Popover, dry mix, prep	1 popover	33	66.7	2.6	10.4	0.0	1.5	0.0	0.0
918395	Popover, homemade w/reduced fat (2%) milk	1 popover	40	87.6	3.5	11.2	0.4	3.0	0.0	0.0
10131	Pork Back Rib, Fresh, lean&fat, roasted	3.5 oz	100	370.0	24.3	0.0	0.0	29.6	13.5	2.3
10130	Pork Bacon, Canadian, Cured, grilled	3.5 oz	100	185.0	24.2	1.4	0.0	8.4	4.0	0.8
10123	Pork Bacon, Cured, broiled, pan-fried, or roasted	3.5 oz	100	576.0	30.5	0.6	0.0	49.2	23.7	5.8
10041	Pork Centerloin/Chop, Fresh, lean&fat w/bone, broiled	3.5 oz	100	240.0	28.7	0.0	0.0	13.1	5.9	1.0
10039	Pork Centerloin/Roast, Fresh, lean w/bone, roasted	3.5 oz	100	199.0	27.6	0.0	0.0	9.0	4.0	0.7
10098	Pork Centerloin/Roast, Fresh, lean&fat w/bone, roasted	3.5 oz	100	234.0	26.3	0.0	0.0	13.5	5.9	1.2
10093	Pork Chow Mein, canned/LaChoy	¾ cup	120	45.6	5.0	4.0	2.0	1.0	0.5	0.2
10137	Pork Ham, Cured, boneless, extra lean (4% fat) canned, roasted	3.5 oz	100	136.0	21.2	0.5	0.0	4.9	2.5	0.4
10140	Pork Ham, Cured, boneless, regular fat (11% fat) roasted	3.5 oz	100	178.0	22.6	0.0	0.0	9.0	4.4	1.4
10151	Pork Ham, Smoked	3.5 oz	100	122.0	18.9	0.0	0.0	4.7	2.6	0.4
10032	Pork Loin, Blade/Chops, Fresh, lean&fat w/bone, broiled	3.5 oz	100	320.0	22.5	0.0	0.0	24.9	10.7	2.3
10048	Pork Loin, Blade/Roasts, Fresh, lean&fat w/bone, roasted	3.5 oz	100	323.0	23.7	0.0	0.0	24.6	10.6	2.2
10045	Pork Loin, Center Rib Chop, Fresh, lean w/bone, broiled	3.5 oz	100	219.0	30.8	0.0	0.0	9.7	4.5	0.6
10200	Pork Loin, Center Rib Chop, Fresh, lean&fat, boneless, pan-fried	4.0 oz	119	266.6	32.9	0.0	0.0	14.0	6.3	1.8
10203	Pork Loin, Center Rib Roast, Fresh, lean&fat, boneless, roasted	3.5 oz	100	252.0	27.0	0.0	0.0	15.2	6.7	1.3
10215	Pork Sirloin Chop, Fresh, lean&fat, boneless, broiled	3.5 oz	100	208.0	30.5	0.0	0.0	8.6	3.8	0.7
10213	Pork Sirloin Chop, Fresh, lean, boneless, broiled	3.5 oz	100	193.0	31.1	0.0	0.0	6.7	2.9	0.5
10056	Pork Sirloin Roast, Fresh, lean&fat, boneless, roasted	3.5 oz	100	207.0	28.5	0.0	0.0	9.4	4.1	0.9
10053	Pork Sirloin, Chop, Fresh, lean w/bone, broiled	3.5 oz	100	213.0	28.5	0.0	0.0	10.1	4.5	0.9
10059	Pork Sirloin, Fresh, lean, boneless, roasted	3.5 oz	100	198.0	28.9	0.0	0.0	8.3	3.6	0.7
10218	Pork Tenderloin, Fresh, lean&fat, broiled	3.5 oz	100	201.0	29.9	0.0	0.0	8.1	3.3	0.7
10223	Pork Tenderloin, Fresh, lean&fat, roasted	3.5 oz	100	173.0	27.8	0.0	0.0	6.1	2.5	0.5
51612	Pork, Bacon Bits	¼ oz	7	21.0	2.6	0.2	0.0	1.1	0.6	0.2
10219	Pork, Ground, Fresh, ckd	3.5 oz	100	297.0	25.7	0.0	0.0	20.8	9.3	1.9
10088	Pork, Spareribs, Fresh, lean&fat, braised	3.5 oz	100	397.0	29.1	0.0	0.0	30.3	13.5	2.7
924165	Pork, Sweet&Sour, canned/LaChoy	¾ cup	128	249.6	6.0	48.0	3.0	4.0	2.4	0.2
19318	Pudding Pop, Chocolate/Vanilla swirl	1 pop	47	78.0	1.9	13.0	0.0	1.9	0.1	0.0
919167	Pudding, Banana, RTE	1.0 oz	28.35	36.0	0.7	6.0	0.0	1.0	0.4	0.4
901924	Pudding, Bread Pudding, homemade	½ cup	126	211.7	6.6	31.0	1.3	7.4	0.0	0.0
901927	Pudding, Chocolate, RTE	4.0 oz (1 snack-sized can)	113	150.3	3.1	25.8	1.1	4.5	1.9	1.6
19191	Pudding, Chocolate, sugar free	½ cup	133	91.8	4.5	13.0	0.0	2.7	1.0	0.1
901928	Pudding, Flan (Caramel Custard) dry mix prep w/whole milk	1 cup	266	300.6	8.0	50.8	0.3	8.2	2.3	0.3
19330	Pudding, Indian	⅔ cup	158	161.2	5.4	22.6	0.0	5.6	0.0	0.0
919182	Pudding, Lemon, RTE	1 oz	28.35	35.4	0.0	7.1	0.0	0.9	0.4	0.3
901929	Pudding, Mousse, Chocolate, homemade	½ cup	202	446.4	8.7	33.1	1.2	32.9	0.0	0.0
19194	Pudding, Pistachio	½ cup	147	170.5	4.2	28.2	0.0	4.8	1.9	0.3
19198	Pudding, Rice, RTE	1 oz	28.35	46.2	0.6	6.2	0.0	2.1	0.9	0.8
919210	Pudding, Tapioca, RTE	1 can (5 oz)	142	169.0	2.8	27.5	0.1	5.3	2.2	1.9
901930	Pudding, Vanilla, RTE	1 cup (8 oz)	226	293.8	5.2	49.5	0.2	8.1	3.5	3.0
14342	Pudding, Vanilla, sugar free	½ cup	131	82.5	4.2	11.0	0.0	2.4	0.8	0.1
924152	Rice Beverage, Rice Dream, canned/Imagine Foods	1 cup	245	120.1	0.4	24.8	0.0	2.0	1.3	0.3
924042	Rice, Chicken Fried Rice/Chun King	8 fl oz	227	261.1	14.0	41.0	0.0	4.0	0.0	0.0
924197	Rice, Pork Fried Rice/Chun King	8 fl oz	227	270.1	10.0	44.0	0.0	6.0	0.0	0.0
918814	Rice, Spanish	1 cup	245	213.2	4.4	40.7	1.6	4.2	0.0	0.0
918815	Roll, Brown & Serve	1 roll	28	80.1	2.0	13.0	0.5	2.0	0.0	0.0
18344	Roll, Buttermilk	1 roll	28	80.1	2.0	13.0	0.5	2.0	0.0	0.0
918343	Roll, Dinner, Egg	1 roll, (2.5" dia)	35	107.5	3.3	18.2	1.3	2.2	1.0	0.4
18396	Roll, Dinner, Oat Bran	1 roll	33	77.9	3.1	13.3	1.4	1.5	0.5	0.5
18347	Roll, Dinner, Rye	1 large (3.5" - 4" dia)	43	123.0	4.4	22.8	2.1	1.5	0.5	0.3
18342	Roll, Dinner, Wheat	1 roll (3 oz)	85	232.1	7.3	39.1	3.2	5.4	2.6	0.9
18351	Roll, French	1 roll	38	105.3	3.3	19.1	1.2	1.6	0.7	0.3
18350	Roll, Hamburger/HotDog, Mixed Grain	1 roll	43	113.1	4.1	19.2	1.6	2.6	0.8	0.4
18352	Roll, Hamburger/HotDog, Plain	1 roll	43	123.0	3.7	21.6	1.2	2.2	0.4	1.1
18353	Roll, Hamburger/HotDog, Whole Wheat	1 frankfurter roll	43	114.4	3.7	22.0	3.2	2.5	0.5	0.9
918817	Roll, Hard/Kaiser	1 roll (3.5" dia)	57	167.0	5.6	30.0	1.3	2.5	0.6	1.0
4023	Salad Dressing, 1000 Island, regular, w/salt	2.0 tsbp	30	113.2	0.3	4.6	0.0	10.7	2.5	5.9

Sat (g)	Chol (mg)	Cal (mg)	Iron (mg)	Magn (mg)	Phos (mg)	Pota (mg)	Sodi (mg)	Zinc (mg)	Vit A (RE)	Vit C (mg)	Vit E (mg)	Thia (mg)	Ribo (mg)	Niac (mg)	Vit B-6 (mg)	Fol (µg)	Vit B-12 (µg)	Wat (g)
3.0	30.0	300.0	3.6	0.0	0.0	390.0	1040.0	0.0	60.0	6.0	0.0	0.5	0.4	5.0	0.0	0.0	0.0	0.0
1.8	0.0	11.0	0.8	0.0	62.0	113.0	488.0	3.0	76.0	6.0	0.0	0.1	0.1	1.0	0.2	100.0	2.0	33.9
0.0	0.0	269.0	2.1	0.0	0.0	0.0	0.0	0.0	123.6	6.0	0.0	0.4	0.3	2.0	0.0	0.0	0.0	69.2
0.0	0.0	267.0	2.0	0.0	375.0	400.0	1000.0	4.0	200.0	6.0	0.0	0.3	0.7	3.0	0.2	65.0	2.5	96.8
0.0	0.0	267.0	1.6	0.0	300.0	300.0	1000.0	3.0	213.2	2.0	0.0	0.3	0.5	2.1	0.2	90.0	1.0	85.6
6.9	27.9	212.4	2.9	0.0	0.0	0.0	771.9	0.0	0.0	0.0	0.0	0.0	0.0	0.0	0.0	0.0	0.0	76.6
6.1	23.1	223.0	2.3	0.0	0.0	0.0	738.5	0.0	0.0	0.0	0.0	0.0	0.0	0.0	0.0	0.0	0.0	69.2
7.7	27.7	187.9	2.5	0.0	0.0	0.0	756.1	0.0	0.0	0.0	0.0	0.0	0.0	0.0	0.0	0.0	0.0	70.4
0.0	0.0	210.0	2.6	0.0	284.0	205.0	909.0	0.0	104.6	13.0	0.0	0.3	0.3	2.9	0.0	0.0	0.0	88.5
0.2	0.6	9.2	0.6	4.6	29.7	25.1	143.2	0.2	16.5	0.0	0.0	0.1	0.1	0.4	0.0	5.6	0.1	18.0
1.0	0.9	37.6	0.8	7.2	56.4	65.2	82.0	0.3	34.0	0.2	0.4	0.1	0.1	0.7	0.0	7.2	0.1	21.8
11.0	118.0	45.0	1.4	21.0	195.0	315.0	101.0	3.4	3.0	0.3	0.0	0.4	0.2	3.6	0.3	3.0	0.6	45.4
2.8	58.0	10.0	0.8	21.0	296.0	390.0	1546.0	1.7	0.0	0.0	0.3	0.8	0.2	6.9	0.5	4.0	0.8	61.7
17.4	85.0	12.0	1.6	24.0	336.0	486.0	1596.0	3.3	0.0	0.0	0.5	0.7	0.3	7.3	0.3	5.0	1.8	12.9
4.8	82.0	33.0	0.8	25.0	232.0	358.0	58.0	2.3	3.0	0.4	0.0	1.1	0.3	5.2	0.4	6.0	0.7	57.6
3.3	79.0	25.0	1.0	22.0	219.0	362.0	66.0	2.1	2.0	1.0	0.0	0.9	0.3	5.5	0.4	4.0	0.6	63.0
5.1	80.0	27.0	1.0	20.0	215.0	352.0	63.0	2.0	2.0	0.9	0.0	0.9	0.3	5.2	0.4	4.0	0.6	59.8
0.3	50.0	80.0	0.7	0.0	0.0	280.0	820.0	0.0	150.0	10.0	0.0	0.0	0.0	0.4	0.0	0.0	0.0	0.0
1.6	30.0	6.0	0.9	21.0	209.0	348.0	1135.0	2.2	0.0	0.0	0.3	1.0	0.2	4.9	0.5	5.0	0.7	69.5
3.1	59.0	8.0	1.3	22.0	281.0	409.0	1500.0	2.5	0.0	0.0	0.3	0.7	0.3	6.2	0.3	3.0	0.7	64.5
1.5	38.8	6.1	1.0	17.3	228.6	371.4	1280.6	2.0	0.0	27.6	0.0	0.9	0.2	5.4	0.5	6.1	0.8	75.0
9.3	86.0	29.0	0.9	22.0	212.0	344.0	70.0	3.4	2.0	0.7	0.0	0.7	0.3	4.1	0.4	4.0	0.8	51.8
9.2	93.0	34.0	1.1	20.0	210.0	326.0	30.0	3.3	3.0	0.2	0.0	0.5	0.3	4.2	0.4	4.0	0.7	51.1
3.5	81.0	31.0	0.8	28.0	245.0	420.0	65.0	2.4	2.0	0.3	0.3	1.1	0.3	6.2	0.5	3.0	0.8	57.0
5.1	83.3	6.0	0.9	32.1	282.0	540.3	61.9	2.5	2.4	0.4	0.3	0.9	0.4	6.1	0.5	9.5	0.7	72.4
5.4	81.0	6.0	0.9	22.0	214.0	346.0	48.0	2.6	3.0	0.4	0.0	0.6	0.3	5.0	0.4	8.0	0.6	57.3
2.9	91.0	18.0	1.2	27.0	243.0	372.0	56.0	2.6	2.0	0.4	0.3	1.0	0.4	4.7	0.5	6.0	0.8	60.1
2.2	92.0	18.0	1.2	27.0	246.0	377.0	56.0	2.7	2.0	0.4	0.3	1.0	0.4	4.8	0.5	6.0	0.8	61.4
3.4	86.0	16.0	1.2	26.0	252.0	402.0	56.0	2.5	2.0	1.0	0.3	0.9	0.4	5.1	0.5	5.0	0.8	60.5
3.6	85.0	13.0	1.1	31.0	257.0	401.0	72.0	2.7	2.0	1.0	0.3	1.0	0.4	4.8	0.5	5.0	0.8	60.5
3.0	86.0	17.0	1.2	27.0	254.0	405.0	56.0	2.5	2.0	1.0	0.3	0.9	0.4	5.1	0.5	5.0	0.8	61.3
2.9	94.0	5.0	1.4	35.0	290.0	444.0	64.0	2.9	2.0	1.0	0.0	1.0	0.4	5.1	0.5	6.0	1.0	61.1
2.1	79.0	6.0	1.5	27.0	257.0	433.0	55.0	2.6	2.0	0.4	0.3	0.9	0.4	4.7	0.4	6.0	0.6	65.4
0.3	6.0	1.0	0.1	2.0	40.0	38.0	181.0	0.3	0.0	1.0	0.0	0.0	0.0	0.7	0.0	1.0	0.2	2.6
7.7	94.0	22.0	1.3	24.0	226.0	362.0	73.0	3.2	2.0	0.7	0.3	0.7	0.2	4.2	0.4	6.0	0.5	52.8
11.1	121.0	47.0	1.9	24.0	261.0	320.0	93.0	4.6	3.0	0.0	0.3	0.4	0.4	5.5	0.4	4.0	1.1	40.4
1.4	18.0	20.0	1.4	0.0	0.0	215.0	1540.0	0.0	125.0	4.0	0.0	0.1	0.1	1.2	0.0	0.0	0.0	0.0
1.8	1.0	71.0	0.2	7.0	51.0	70.0	66.0	0.1	13.4	0.0	0.0	0.0	0.1	0.1	0.0	2.0	0.1	30.4
0.2	0.0	24.1	0.0	2.3	19.6	31.2	55.6	0.1	8.5	0.1	0.0	0.0	0.0	0.0	0.0	0.6	0.1	20.4
1.2	2.7	143.6	1.4	23.9	137.3	282.2	291.1	0.7	81.9	1.0	0.0	0.1	0.3	0.8	0.1	16.4	0.3	79.3
0.8	3.4	101.7	0.6	23.7	90.4	203.4	145.8	0.5	12.4	2.0	0.1	0.0	0.2	0.4	0.0	3.4	0.0	78.3
1.6	9.0	152.0	0.3	25.0	289.0	256.0	381.0	0.6	50.2	1.0	0.0	0.1	0.2	0.1	0.1	6.0	0.4	1.6
5.1	31.9	300.6	0.2	31.9	228.8	383.0	130.3	0.9	69.2	1.9	0.0	0.1	0.4	0.2	0.1	10.6	0.7	197.4
0.0	0.0	221.0	1.4	0.0	151.0	0.0	0.0	0.0	79.0	0.0	0.0	0.1	0.3	0.4	0.0	0.0	0.0	0.0
0.1	0.0	0.6	0.0	0.3	1.4	0.3	39.7	0.0	0.0	0.0	0.0	0.0	0.0	0.0	0.0	0.0	0.0	20.3
1.7	10.3	202.0	1.3	44.4	258.6	296.9	86.9	1.4	323.2	1.2	0.0	0.1	0.4	0.3	0.1	32.3	0.9	125.4
2.6	17.0	149.0	0.1	19.0	307.0	194.0	408.0	0.5	30.8	1.0	0.0	0.1	0.2	0.1	0.1	7.0	0.4	107.8
0.3	0.3	14.7	0.1	2.3	19.3	17.0	24.1	0.1	9.9	0.1	0.4	0.0	0.0	0.0	0.0	0.9	0.1	19.2
0.9	1.4	119.3	0.3	11.4	112.2	137.7	225.8	0.4	0.0	1.0	0.1	0.0	0.1	0.4	0.0	4.3	0.3	105.4
1.3	15.8	198.9	0.3	18.1	153.7	255.4	305.1	0.6	13.6	0.0	0.3	0.0	0.3	0.6	0.0	0.0	0.2	160.9
1.5	9.0	152.0	0.1	18.0	117.0	189.0	199.0	0.3	30.0	1.0	0.0	0.0	0.2	0.1	0.0	6.0	0.6	100.6
0.2	0.0	19.6	0.2	9.8	34.3	68.6	85.8	0.2	0.0	1.2	1.8	0.1	0.0	1.9	0.0	90.7	0.0	217.5
0.0	0.0	38.0	2.0	0.0	128.0	190.0	1460.0	0.0	136.0	7.0	0.0	0.7	0.2	1.5	0.0	0.0	0.0	0.0
0.0	0.0	26.0	1.0	0.0	129.0	180.0	1210.0	0.0	170.0	4.0	0.0	0.3	0.2	1.5	0.0	0.0	0.0	0.0
0.0	0.0	34.0	1.5	0.0	96.0	566.0	774.0	0.0	324.0	37.0	0.0	0.1	0.1	1.7	0.0	0.0	0.0	192.3
0.0	5.0	14.0	0.6	0.0	25.0	28.0	140.0	0.0	0.0	1.0	0.0	0.1	0.1	0.6	0.0	0.0	0.0	0.0
0.0	5.0	0.0	0.0	0.0	0.0	0.0	140.0	0.0	0.0	0.0	0.0	0.0	0.0	0.0	0.0	0.0	0.0	0.0
0.6	17.5	20.7	1.2	8.8	35.4	36.4	190.8	0.4	2.8	0.0	0.3	0.2	0.2	1.2	0.0	36.8	0.1	10.6
0.2	0.0	28.1	1.4	10.9	38.0	39.9	136.3	0.3	0.0	0.0	0.2	0.1	0.1	1.6	0.0	31.4	0.0	14.5
0.3	0.0	12.9	1.2	23.2	68.4	77.4	383.6	0.4	0.4	0.0	0.2	0.2	0.1	1.7	0.0	37.0	0.0	12.9
1.3	0.0	149.6	3.0	30.6	88.4	97.8	289.0	0.8	0.0	0.0	0.8	0.4	0.2	3.5	0.1	43.4	0.0	31.5
0.4	0.0	34.6	1.0	7.6	31.9	43.3	231.4	0.3	0.0	0.0	0.2	0.2	0.1	1.7	0.0	36.1	0.0	13.2
0.4	0.0	40.9	1.7	18.9	52.5	68.8	196.9	0.5	0.0	0.0	0.2	0.2	0.1	1.9	0.0	40.9	0.0	16.3
0.5	0.0	59.8	1.4	8.6	37.8	60.6	240.8	0.3	0.0	0.0	0.7	0.2	0.1	1.7	0.0	40.9	0.0	14.6
0.4	0.0	45.6	1.0	36.6	96.3	117.0	205.5	0.9	0.0	0.0	0.6	0.1	0.1	1.6	0.1	13.3	0.0	14.2
0.3	0.0	54.2	1.9	15.4	57.0	61.6	310.1	0.5	0.0	0.0	0.2	0.3	0.2	2.4	0.0	54.2	0.0	17.7
1.8	7.8	3.3	0.2	0.6	5.1	33.9	210.0	0.0	28.8	0.0	0.3	0.0	0.0	0.0	0.0	1.9	0.1	13.8

Code	Food Name	Unit/Amt	Wt (g)	Energy (Kcal)	Prot (g)	Carb (g)	Fiber (g)	Fat (g)	Mono (g)	Poly (g)
902921	Salad Dressing, 1000 Island, w/salt, low kcal (10kcal/tsp)	2.0 tsbp	30	47.6	0.2	4.9	0.4	3.2	0.7	1.9
4539	Salad Dressing, Blue Cheese, low kcal	2.0 tsbp	30	80.1	0.6	3.0	0.0	7.4	1.8	3.8
4140	Salad Dressing, Blue/Roquefort Cheese, regular w/salt	2.0 tsbp	30	151.2	1.4	2.2	0.0	15.7	3.7	8.3
4120	Salad Dressing, French, low fat, w/salt, diet (5kcal/tsp)	2.0 tsbp	30	40.3	0.1	6.5	0.0	1.7	0.4	1.0
4141	Salad Dressing, French, regular w/salt	2.0 tsbp	30	128.9	0.2	5.3	0.0	12.3	2.4	6.5
4114	Salad Dressing, Italian, no salt, diet (2kcal/tsp)	2.0 tsbp	30	31.6	0.0	1.5	0.0	2.9	0.6	1.8
4143	Salad Dressing, Italian, regular w/salt	2.0 tsbp	30	140.2	0.2	3.1	0.0	14.5	3.4	8.4
4145	Salad Dressing, Mayonnaise, Safflower & Soybean Oil, w/salt	2.0 tsbp	30	215.0	0.3	0.8	0.0	23.8	3.9	16.5
18625	Salad Dressing, Mayonnaise-type, regular, w/salt	2.0 tsbp	30	116.9	0.3	7.2	0.0	10.0	2.7	5.4
4022	Salad Dressing, Russian w/salt	2.0 tsbp	30	148.2	0.5	3.1	0.0	15.2	3.5	8.8
4030	Salad Dressing, Russian, w/salt, low kcal	2.0 tsbp	30	42.4	0.2	8.3	0.1	1.2	0.3	0.7
4016	Salad Dressing, Sandwich Spread w/chopped pickle, regular	2.0 tsbp	30	116.7	0.3	6.7	0.1	10.2	2.2	6.0
902932	Salad Dressing, Sesame Seed	2.0 tsbp	30	132.9	0.9	2.6	0.3	13.6	3.6	7.5
902933	Salad Dressing, Sweet & Sour	2.0 tsbp	30	57.9	0.4	13.8	0.2	0.6	0.0	0.0
4135	Salad Dressing, Vinaigrette	2.0 tsbp	30	99.9	0.0	8.0	0.0	7.6	3.2	2.8
902910	Salad Dressing, Vinegar & Oil, homemade	2.0 tsbp	30	134.6	0.0	0.8	0.0	15.0	4.4	7.2
902909	Salt Substitute, lite/Morton	1 tsp	6	0.0	0.0	0.0	0.0	0.0	0.0	0.0
22539	Salt Substitute/Morton	1 tsp	6	0.0	0.0	0.1	0.0	0.0	0.0	0.0
2047	Salt, Table (Sodium Chloride)	1 tsp	6	0.0	0.0	0.0	0.0	0.0	0.0	0.0
22535	Sandwich, Hot Pockets, Beef & Cheddar Stuffed, frozen	1 package	142	403.3	16.3	39.2	0.0	20.2	6.7	1.2
22537	Sandwich, Hot Pockets, Croissant Pocket w/chicken, broccoli, & cheddar, frozen	1 package	256	601.6	22.8	77.8	2.8	22.0	8.8	3.3
22002	Sandwich, Lean Pockets, Glazed Chicken Supreme Stuffed, frozen	1 package	255	464.1	19.6	68.1	0.0	12.5	4.9	1.9
22540	Sandwich, Pizza Burger	1 burger	92	243.8	18.2	2.3	0.5	18.0	0.0	0.0
6931	Sandwich, Sausage Biscuits, breakfast sandwich, frozen/Jimmy Dean	1 package	96	384.6	9.5	23.1	1.4	28.2	0.0	0.0
6932	Sauce, Pasta, Spaghetti/Marinara, RTE	½ cup	125	71.3	1.8	10.3	2.0	2.6	1.1	0.9
906961	Sauce, 100% Natural Spaghetti Sauce, Traditional, jar/Prego	½ cup	125	130.9	2.1	20.0	3.9	4.9	0.0	0.0
6721	Sauce, Alfredo	1 tbsp	16	42.6	1.6	0.4	0.0	3.8	0.0	0.0
6921	Sauce, Barbecue, RTE	1 tbsp	18	13.5	0.3	2.3	0.2	0.3	0.1	0.1
6140	Sauce, Bearnaise, dry, made w/milk & butter	1 cup (8 fl oz)	250	687.5	8.2	17.2	0.0	67.0	19.6	3.0
906978	Sauce, Cheddar Cheese Sauce/LaVictoria	1 tbsp	16.29	26.2	0.3	1.5	0.0	2.1	1.0	0.5
6713	Sauce, Cheese	2.0 oz	56	59.9	2.3	3.5	0.0	4.1	0.0	0.0
6139	Sauce, Chili	1 tbsp	15	17.0	0.2	3.8	0.0	0.0	0.0	0.0
6923	Sauce, Chunky Chili Dip, Salsa, canned/LaVictoria	1 tbsp	15	4.7	0.1	1.0	0.1	0.0	0.0	0.0
6135	Sauce, Con Queso Sauce, RTE/Nestle Que Bueno	1 cup	252	335.2	15.4	14.3	0.0	24.1	6.8	3.0
6903	Sauce, Coney Island Style Hot Dog Sauce, RTE/Nestle Chef-Mate	¼ cup	62	75.6	2.2	5.6	1.4	4.9	1.5	2.1
6104	Sauce, Creole Sauce, RTE/Nestle Chef-Mate	¼ cup	62	24.8	0.9	3.7	0.8	0.7	0.2	0.3
6901	Sauce, Curry, dry, made w/milk	¼ cup	68	67.3	2.7	6.4	0.0	3.7	1.3	0.7
6152	Sauce, Deluxe Marinara Sauce, RTE/Contadina	¼ cup	64	37.1	0.8	4.4	0.8	1.8	0.9	0.5
6153	Sauce, Deluxe Pizza Sauce, RTE/Contadina	¼ cup	63	34.0	1.4	5.5	1.3	0.7	0.3	0.1
6179	Sauce, Enchilada Sauce/LaVictoria	1 tbsp	15.08	5.0	0.0	0.7	0.1	0.2	0.0	0.0
6273	Sauce, Green Chile Salsa, mild/LaVictoria	1 tbsp	15.23	3.8	0.2	0.7	0.1	0.0	0.0	0.0
6259	Sauce, Green Taco Sauce, medium/LaVictoria	1 tbsp	15.09	4.5	0.1	0.9	0.1	0.1	0.0	0.0
906965	Sauce, Hoisin, RTE	1 tbsp	16	35.2	0.5	7.1	0.4	0.5	0.2	0.3
6155	Sauce, Hollandaise	¼ cup	50	264.0	3.1	6.7	0.0	25.6	8.8	1.1
6181	Sauce, Hot Dog Chili Sauce, RTE/Nestle Chef-Mate	2.25 oz , ¼ cup	63	69.3	2.7	9.2	1.7	2.4	1.0	0.2
6922	Sauce, Italian Sauce, RTE/Nestle Chef-Mate	2.25 oz , ¼ cup	63	61.7	1.1	11.6	0.9	1.2	0.8	0.2
6905	Sauce, Jalapeno Cheese Sauce, RTE/Nestle Que Bueno	1 package	3005	3876.5	95.9	369.6	0.0	224.2	81.3	35.8
906970	Sauce, Lemon Sauce, RTE/Nestle Chef-Mate	1 package	2126	2848.8	4.7	678.6	0.0	12.5	3.6	6.0
906960	Sauce, Marinara/Contadina	7.5 oz	213	100.1	4.0	12.0	0.0	4.0	0.0	0.0
906966	Sauce, Medium White	1 cup	250	395.0	10.0	24.0	0.5	30.0	11.9	7.2
6136	Sauce, Mole Poblano, dry mix	1 tbsp	16.5	94.2	1.2	6.9	1.7	6.9	0.0	0.0
6714	Sauce, Mushroom, dry, made w/milk	1 cup (8 fl oz)	267	227.0	11.3	23.8	0.0	10.3	3.3	1.1
6910	Sauce, Nacho Cheese Sauce, mild, RTE/Nestle Que Bueno	1 cup	252	476.3	18.1	10.1	2.0	40.5	12.4	8.5
6168	Sauce, Oyster, RTE	1 tbsp	4	2.0	0.1	0.4	0.0	0.0	0.0	0.0
6169	Sauce, Pepper or Hot, RTE	¼ tsp	1.2	0.1	0.0	0.0	0.0	0.0	0.0	0.0
924173	Sauce, Pepperoni Pizza/Contadina	¼ cup	60	40.2	1.0	5.0	0.0	2.2	1.1	0.7
6157	Sauce, Pesto	1 oz	28	155.1	2.8	3.0	0.7	14.6	0.0	0.0
906968	Sauce, Picante Sauce, RTE/Que Bueno Nestle	1 serving	30	10.2	0.4	2.0	0.0	0.1	0.0	0.0
6151	Sauce, Pizza/Contadina	¼ cup	60	30.0	1.0	5.0	0.0	1.0	0.0	0.0
6153	Sauce, Plum, RTE	1 tbsp	19	35.0	0.2	8.1	0.1	0.2	0.0	0.1
6274	Sauce, Red Clam (Shellfish)	4 oz	112	80.6	3.6	9.3	1.0	3.2	0.0	0.0
6907	Sauce, Salsa, RTE	1 packet	8.9	2.5	0.1	0.6	0.1	0.0	0.0	0.0
906969	Sauce, Sofrito, homemade	1 tbsp	14.9	35.3	1.9	0.8	0.3	2.7	0.0	0.0
6148	Sauce, Sour Cream	¼ cup	52	123.8	2.8	1.9	0.0	11.9	4.6	1.2
906134	Sauce, Sour Cream, dry, made w/milk	1 cup (8 fl oz)	314	508.7	19.1	45.3	3.5	30.2	9.9	2.8
924192	Sauce, Soy Sauce, RTE	1 tbsp	18	9.5	0.9	1.5	0.0	0.0	0.0	0.0
924195	Sauce, Spaghetti Sauce w/meat	4 oz	113	70.1	2.0	12.0	2.0	2.0	0.8	0.9
6904	Sauce, Spaghetti Sauce w/mushrooms	4 oz	113	107.4	1.6	14.5	0.6	4.7	0.0	0.0
924162	Sauce, Spaghetti w/mushrooms, dry	2 tsp	10	30.4	1.0	4.9	0.0	0.9	0.3	0.0

Sat (g)	Chol (mg)	Cal (mg)	Iron (mg)	Magn (mg)	Phos (mg)	Pota (mg)	Sodi (mg)	Zinc (mg)	Vit A (RE)	Vit C (mg)	Vit E (mg)	Thia (mg)	Ribo (mg)	Niac (mg)	Vit B-6 (mg)	Fol (µg)	Vit B-12 (µg)	Wat (g)
0.5	4.5	3.3	0.2	0.2	5.1	33.9	300.0	0.0	28.8	0.0	0.4	0.0	0.0	0.0	0.0	1.7	0.1	20.8
1.6	2.0	0.0	0.0	0.0	0.0	0.0	394.0	0.0	0.0	0.0	0.0	0.0	0.0	0.0	0.0	0.0	0.0	20.8
3.0	5.1	24.3	0.1	0.0	22.2	11.1	328.2	0.1	19.8	0.6	2.8	0.0	0.0	0.0	0.0	2.4	0.1	9.7
0.2	3.3	3.3	0.1	0.0	4.2	23.7	236.1	0.1	39.0	0.6	0.4	0.0	0.0	0.0	0.0	0.0	0.0	20.8
2.9	0.0	3.3	0.1	0.0	4.2	23.7	411.0	0.0	39.0	0.0	2.5	0.0	0.0	0.0	0.0	1.3	0.0	11.4
0.4	1.8	0.6	0.1	0.0	1.5	4.5	9.0	0.0	0.0	0.0	0.0	0.0	0.0	0.0	0.0	0.0	0.0	25.1
2.1	0.0	3.0	0.1	0.2	1.5	4.5	236.1	0.0	7.2	0.0	3.1	0.0	0.0	0.0	0.0	1.5	0.0	11.5
2.6	17.7	5.4	0.2	0.3	8.4	10.2	170.5	0.0	25.2	0.0	0.0	0.0	0.0	0.2	0.0	2.3	0.1	4.6
1.5	7.8	4.2	0.1	0.6	7.8	2.7	213.2	0.1	25.2	0.0	1.2	0.0	0.0	0.0	0.0	1.9	0.1	12.0
2.2	5.4	5.7	0.2	0.5	11.1	47.1	260.4	0.1	62.1	1.8	3.1	0.0	0.0	0.2	0.0	3.1	0.1	10.4
0.2	1.8	5.7	0.2	0.1	11.1	47.1	260.4	0.0	4.8	1.8	0.2	0.0	0.0	0.0	0.0	1.0	0.0	19.5
1.5	22.8	4.2	0.1	0.6	7.8	10.5	300.0	0.2	25.2	0.0	2.1	0.0	0.0	0.0	0.0	1.8	0.1	12.2
1.9	0.0	5.7	0.2	0.0	11.1	47.1	300.0	0.0	62.1	0.0	0.0	0.0	0.0	0.0	0.0	0.0	0.0	11.8
0.0	0.0	2.0	0.0	0.0	2.0	28.0	136.0	0.0	0.0	0.0	0.0	0.0	0.0	0.0	0.0	0.0	0.0	0.0
1.2	0.0	0.0	0.0	0.0	0.0	0.0	432.0	0.0	0.0	0.0	0.0	0.0	0.0	0.0	0.0	0.0	0.0	0.0
2.7	0.0	0.0	0.0	0.0	0.0	2.3	0.2	0.0	0.0	0.0	2.6	0.0	0.0	0.0	0.0	0.0	0.0	14.2
0.0	0.0	0.0	0.0	4.0	0.0	1500.0	1100.0	0.0	0.0	0.0	0.0	0.0	0.0	0.0	0.0	0.0	0.0	0.0
0.0	0.0	30.0	0.0	0.0	28.0	2800.0	0.0	0.0	0.0	0.0	0.0	0.0	0.0	0.0	0.0	0.0	0.0	0.0
0.0	0.0	1.4	0.0	0.1	0.0	0.5	2325.5	0.0	0.0	0.0	0.0	0.0	0.0	0.0	0.0	0.0	0.0	0.0
8.8	52.5	336.5	2.9	0.0	0.0	0.0	906.0	0.0	0.0	0.0	0.0	0.0	0.0	0.0	0.0	0.0	0.0	62.5
6.7	74.2	0.0	7.6	0.0	0.0	0.0	1303.0	0.0	0.0	12.5	0.0	0.0	0.0	0.0	0.0	0.0	0.0	128.0
3.8	45.9	242.3	0.0	0.0	0.0	0.0	1119.5	0.0	0.0	0.0	0.0	0.0	0.0	0.0	0.0	0.0	0.0	150.2
0.0	62.0	109.0	2.3	16.0	205.0	263.0	615.0	3.3	72.6	4.0	0.0	0.1	0.2	6.5	0.0	0.0	0.0	51.0
8.6	31.4	75.5	1.6	0.0	0.0	0.0	881.3	0.0	0.0	0.0	0.0	0.0	0.0	0.0	0.0	0.0	0.0	32.2
0.4	0.0	27.5	0.9	21.3	40.0	368.8	515.0	0.2	47.5	10.0	1.6	0.1	0.1	1.3	0.1	12.5	0.0	108.6
1.1	0.0	0.0	0.0	0.0	0.0	0.0	537.5	0.0	0.0	13.0	0.0	0.0	0.0	0.0	0.0	0.0	0.0	96.0
0.0	0.0	28.9	0.2	0.0	0.0	4.6	104.4	0.0	4.2	0.1	0.0	0.0	0.0	0.0	0.0	0.0	0.0	0.0
0.0	0.0	3.4	0.2	3.2	3.6	31.3	146.7	0.0	15.7	1.3	0.2	0.0	0.2	0.0	0.0	0.7	0.0	14.6
41.0	185.0	225.0	0.3	25.0	182.5	292.5	1240.0	0.8	742.5	1.8	0.0	0.1	0.3	0.3	0.1	10.0	0.5	153.1
0.6	0.5	15.0	0.1	0.0	0.0	0.0	158.2	0.0	0.0	0.0	0.0	0.0	0.0	0.0	0.0	0.0	0.0	11.9
0.0	0.0	63.0	0.2	0.0	0.0	23.0	288.0	3.5	32.2	0.0	0.0	0.0	0.0	0.1	0.0	0.0	0.0	0.0
0.0	0.0	3.0	0.1	0.0	8.0	56.0	191.0	0.0	42.0	2.0	0.0	0.0	0.0	0.2	0.0	9.0	0.0	0.0
0.0	0.0	2.1	0.0	0.0	0.0	0.0	74.0	0.0	0.0	1.6	0.0	0.0	0.0	0.0	0.0	0.0	0.0	13.6
11.7	63.0	471.2	0.0	15.1	206.6	65.5	2220.1	1.3	148.7	0.0	1.3	0.0	0.2	0.2	0.0	7.6	0.2	190.8
0.9	1.9	19.8	1.1	11.8	29.1	197.8	383.2	0.3	63.2	0.1	1.1	0.0	0.0	0.8	0.1	8.1	0.0	47.9
0.1	0.0	34.7	0.3	8.7	17.4	187.2	339.1	0.1	23.6	0.0	0.6	0.0	0.0	0.5	0.1	8.7	0.0	55.3
1.5	8.8	121.0	0.3	11.6	70.0	123.8	318.9	0.3	10.2	0.7	0.0	0.0	0.1	0.1	0.0	4.1	0.3	53.9
0.3	0.0	12.2	0.4	7.7	16.6	132.5	240.0	0.1	22.4	4.5	0.0	0.0	0.0	0.4	0.1	5.8	0.0	56.1
0.3	1.9	34.0	0.6	13.2	31.5	223.0	116.6	0.2	42.2	7.1	1.6	0.0	0.0	0.9	0.0	6.3	0.0	54.6
0.0	0.0	1.8	0.0	0.0	0.0	0.0	99.2	0.0	0.0	0.7	0.0	0.0	0.0	0.0	0.0	0.0	0.0	13.9
0.0	0.0	2.3	0.1	0.0	0.0	0.0	87.4	0.0	0.0	2.0	0.0	0.0	0.0	0.0	0.0	0.0	0.0	14.0
0.0	0.0	1.2	0.0	0.0	0.0	0.0	95.7	0.0	0.0	0.7	0.0	0.0	0.0	0.0	0.0	0.0	0.0	13.7
0.1	0.5	5.1	0.2	3.8	6.1	19.0	258.4	0.1	0.2	0.1	0.0	0.0	0.0	0.2	0.0	3.7	0.0	7.1
15.7	71.0	23.0	0.9	0.0	78.0	0.0	425.0	0.0	205.4	0.0	0.0	0.0	0.0	0.0	0.0	0.0	0.0	58.5
1.0	4.4	19.5	1.0	12.6	39.7	149.3	398.8	0.5	42.2	0.1	0.3	0.0	0.0	0.7	0.1	22.1	0.1	47.2
0.2	0.0	34.7	0.4	20.2	43.5	383.0	308.7	0.3	24.6	4.2	1.2	0.1	0.0	1.1	0.2	16.4	0.0	47.8
86.2	300.5	2554.3	5.7	180.3	2464.1	781.3	27255.4	16.2	811.4	24.0	15.7	0.1	2.0	2.0	0.4	90.2	2.7	2230.3
1.5	0.0	85.0	8.1	42.5	85.0	425.2	170.1	0.9	0.0	182.8	0.9	0.1	0.1	0.7	0.2	21.3	0.0	1427.6
0.0	0.0	73.0	2.6	0.0	0.0	810.0	700.0	0.0	413.2	20.0	0.0	0.2	0.4	2.2	0.0	0.0	0.0	0.0
9.1	32.0	292.0	0.9	0.0	238.0	381.0	888.0	0.5	238.0	2.0	0.0	0.2	0.4	0.8	0.1	12.0	0.0	0.0
0.0	0.0	49.8	0.9	21.0	41.9	99.3	192.1	0.4	0.0	0.0	0.0	0.0	0.1	0.4	0.1	12.2	0.0	0.7
5.4	34.7	293.7	0.5	37.4	165.5	494.0	1535.3	1.3	93.5	1.9	0.0	0.2	0.8	4.8	0.2	40.1	0.8	215.7
16.9	80.6	471.2	0.8	25.2	420.8	80.6	1968.1	2.6	126.0	0.3	1.0	0.0	0.3	0.1	0.0	12.6	0.4	177.5
0.0	0.0	1.3	0.0	0.2	0.9	2.2	109.3	0.0	0.3	0.0	0.0	0.0	0.0	0.1	0.0	0.6	0.0	3.2
0.0	0.0	0.1	0.0	0.1	0.1	1.7	31.7	0.0	0.4	0.9	0.0	0.0	0.0	0.0	0.0	0.1	0.0	1.1
0.4	0.0	13.0	0.7	8.0	16.0	260.0	390.0	0.0	131.8	13.0	0.0	0.0	0.0	0.1	0.0	0.0	0.0	48.2
0.0	0.0	98.0	0.3	0.0	0.0	27.0	244.0	0.0	98.8	0.0	0.0	0.0	0.1	0.2	0.0	0.0	0.0	0.0
0.0	0.0	12.6	0.2	4.5	8.4	80.4	252.0	0.1	8.4	0.6	0.4	0.0	0.0	0.3	0.0	3.0	0.0	26.8
0.0	0.0	13.0	0.7	8.0	14.0	220.0	330.0	0.0	133.8	14.0	0.0	0.0	0.0	0.6	0.0	0.0	0.0	50.0
0.0	0.0	2.3	0.3	2.3	4.2	49.2	102.2	0.0	0.8	0.1	0.0	0.0	0.0	0.2	0.0	1.1	0.0	10.2
0.0	0.0	32.0	1.2	0.0	0.0	274.0	556.0	0.0	128.2	9.0	0.0	0.1	0.1	0.9	0.0	0.0	0.0	0.0
0.0	0.0	2.7	0.1	1.2	2.3	19.0	38.6	0.0	5.3	1.2	0.1	0.0	0.0	0.1	0.0	1.4	0.0	8.1
0.0	0.0	3.0	0.1	3.7	20.7	59.7	170.6	0.2	0.0	3.0	0.0	0.0	0.0	0.4	0.1	6.4	0.0	8.9
6.1	1966.0	23.0	0.3	3.0	75.0	13.0	7.0	0.5	82.0	0.0	0.0	0.0	0.1	0.0	0.0	23.0	0.6	11.9
16.1	91.1	546.4	0.6	44.0	310.9	731.6	1004.8	1.4	144.4	2.5	0.0	0.1	0.7	0.6	0.1	15.7	0.9	215.5
0.0	0.0	3.1	0.4	6.1	19.8	32.4	1028.7	0.1	0.0	0.0	0.0	0.0	0.0	0.6	0.0	2.8	0.0	12.8
0.3	2.0	18.0	1.8	0.0	51.0	650.0	570.0	0.0	156.0	18.0	0.0	0.1	0.1	1.8	0.0	0.0	0.0	0.0
0.0	0.0	21.0	1.1	0.0	30.0	428.0	499.0	0.0	129.8	12.0	0.0	0.1	0.1	1.3	0.0	0.0	0.0	0.0
0.6	2.8	39.9	0.2	3.6	28.6	41.1	942.0	0.2	4.9	0.2	0.0	0.0	0.0	0.0	0.0	2.8	0.0	0.3

Code	Food Name	Unit/Amt	Wt (g)	Energy (Kcal)	Prot (g)	Carb (g)	Fiber (g)	Fat (g)	Mono (g)	Poly (g)
6107	Sauce, Spaghetti&Meat/FrancoAm	7.5 oz	212	212.0	8.5	26.2	1.0	8.1	0.0	0.0
906972	Sauce, Steak	1 tbsp	15	18.0	0.0	2.5	0.1	0.0	0.0	0.0
6109	Sauce, Steak & Mushrooms	1 fl oz	30	9.0	0.3	1.9	0.2	0.1	0.1	0.0
6716	Sauce, Stroganoff, dry, made w/H$_2$O	1 cup (8 fl oz)	296	272.3	11.7	33.9	0.0	10.7	3.0	0.4
6110	Sauce, Sweet & Sour	¼ cup	59	54.9	0.2	13.6	0.0	0.0	0.0	0.0
906975	Sauce, Szechuan, RTE/Nestle Chef-Mate	1 tbsp	16	20.8	0.2	2.9	0.0	0.9	0.3	0.4
906974	Sauce, Tabasco	1 tsp	5	0.8	0.1	0.1	0.0	0.0	0.0	0.0
6111	Sauce, Tartar	1 tbsp	14	70.0	0.2	0.1	0.1	8.1	2.4	4.5
6129	Sauce, Teriyaki, RTE	1 tbsp	18	15.1	1.1	2.9	0.0	0.0	0.0	0.0
906977	Sauce, Thick White	¼ cup	66	130.7	2.6	7.3	0.3	10.3	3.8	1.3
924111	Sauce, Thin White	¼ cup	61	73.8	2.4	4.6	0.1	5.2	1.9	0.7
6113	Sauce, White Clam (Shellfish)	4.0 oz	112	121.0	4.5	4.2	0.5	9.6	0.0	0.0
7006	Sausage, Blood	1slice: 5 x 4.6 x 0.06"	25	94.5	3.7	0.3	0.0	8.6	4.0	0.9
7014	Sausage, Bratwurst (Pork) ckd	1 link (4/12 oz)	85	255.9	12.0	1.8	0.0	22.0	10.4	2.3
7022	Sausage, Frankfurter (weiner) (Beef & Pork)	1 frank:0.85"diam x 5"long-8/lb	57	182.4	6.4	1.5	0.0	16.6	7.8	1.6
7024	Sausage, Frankfurter (weiner) (Beef)	1 frank:0.75"diam x 5"long-10/lb	45	141.8	5.4	0.8	0.0	12.8	6.1	0.6
7025	Sausage, Frankfurter (weiner) (Chicken)	1 frank	45	115.7	5.8	3.1	0.0	8.8	3.8	1.8
7016	Sausage, Frankfurter (weiner) (Turkey)	1 frank	45	101.7	6.4	0.7	0.0	8.0	2.5	2.3
7089	Sausage, Italian (Pork & Beef)	1 slice: 4"diam x 0.12"thick	23	59.8	3.5	0.4	0.0	4.8	2.3	0.5
7038	Sausage, Kielbasa (Kolbassy) (Pork, Beef & NFD Milk)	1slice: 6 x 3.75 x 0.06"	26	80.6	3.4	0.6	0.0	7.1	3.4	0.8
7091	Sausage, Mortadella (Beef & Pork)	1 slice (15/8 oz)	15	46.7	2.5	0.5	0.0	3.8	1.7	0.5
7059	Sausage, Pepperoni (Pork & Beef)	1 sausage @ 9.0 oz.	251	1247.5	52.6	7.1	0.0	110.4	53.0	11.0
7064	Sausage, Pork, bulk/links/patties, frozen, raw/USDA Commodity	3.5 oz	100	231.0	15.0	0.0	0.0	18.6	8.1	2.2
7068	Sausage, Salami (Cotto) (Beef & Pork) ckd	1 slice: 4"diam x 0.12"thick (10/8 oz)	23	57.5	3.2	0.5	0.0	4.6	2.1	0.5
7072	Sausage, Salami, (Turkey) ckd	2 slices	57	111.7	9.3	0.3	0.0	7.9	2.6	2.0
7074	Sausage, Smoked Link (Pork & Beef)	2.4 oz	68	228.5	9.1	1.0	0.0	20.6	9.6	2.2
7077	Sausage, Smoked Link (Pork)	2.4 oz	68	264.5	15.1	1.4	0.0	21.6	10.0	2.6
7076	Sausage, Smoked Link (Pork, Beef & NFD Milk)	2.4 oz	68	212.8	9.0	1.3	0.0	18.8	8.6	2.1
7083	Sausage, Vegetarian, Meatless	2.4 oz	68	174.1	12.6	6.7	1.9	12.3	3.1	6.3
924160	Sausage, Vienna, canned (Beef & Pork)	1 sm sausage	16	44.6	1.6	0.3	0.0	4.0	2.0	0.3
12037	Seeds, Sunflower Kernels, dried	1 cup w/hulls (edible part)	46	262.2	10.5	8.6	4.8	22.8	4.4	15.1
12537	Seeds, Sunflower Kernels, dry roast w/o salt	1.0 oz	28.35	165.0	5.5	6.8	3.1	14.1	2.7	9.3
12538	Seeds, Sunflower Kernels, oil roast w/o salt	1.0 oz	28.35	174.4	6.1	4.2	1.9	16.3	3.1	10.8
15155	Shellfish, Abalone, fried	3.0 oz	85	160.7	16.7	9.4	0.0	5.8	2.3	1.4
15158	Shellfish, Clams, boiled/steamed (moist heat)	3.0 oz	85	125.8	21.7	4.4	0.0	1.7	0.1	0.5
15162	Shellfish, Clams, breaded & fried	3.0 oz	85	171.7	12.1	8.8	0.0	9.5	3.9	2.4
15160	Shellfish, Clams, canned with liquid	3.0 oz	85	1.7	0.3	0.1	0.0	0.0	0.0	0.0
15157	Shellfish, Clams, canned, drained	3.0 oz	85	125.8	21.7	4.4	0.0	1.7	0.1	0.5
15138	Shellfish, Crab, Alaskan King, boiled/steamed	3.0 oz	85	82.5	16.4	0.0	0.0	1.3	0.2	0.5
15136	Shellfish, Crab, Alaskan King, imitation surimi	3.0 oz	85	86.7	10.2	8.7	0.0	1.1	0.2	0.6
15139	Shellfish, Crab, Blue, Crab Cakes	1 cake	60	93.0	12.1	0.3	0.0	4.5	1.7	1.4
15143	Shellfish, Crab, Dungeness, cooked w/moist heat	3.0 oz	85	93.5	19.0	0.8	0.0	1.1	0.2	0.3
15147	Shellfish, Lobster, Northern, boiled/steamed (moist heat)	3.0 oz	85	83.3	17.4	1.1	0.0	0.5	0.1	0.1
15154	Shellfish, Lobster, Spiny, cooked w/moist heat	3.0 oz	85	121.6	22.4	2.7	0.0	1.6	0.3	0.6
15164	Shellfish, Mussel, Blue, boiled/steamed	3.0 oz	85	146.2	20.2	6.3	0.0	3.8	0.9	1.0
15246	Shellfish, Oyster, Eastern, breaded & fried	3.0 oz	85	167.5	7.5	9.9	0.0	10.7	4.0	2.8
15245	Shellfish, Oyster, Eastern, Farmed, cooked w/dry heat	6 medium oysters	59	46.6	4.1	4.3	0.0	1.3	0.1	0.4
15244	Shellfish, Oyster, Eastern, Farmed, raw	6 medium oysters	84	49.6	4.4	4.6	0.0	1.3	0.1	0.5
15174	Shellfish, Scallops, breaded, fried	2 large scallops	31	66.7	5.6	3.1	0.0	3.4	1.4	0.9
15172	Shellfish, Scallops, imitation surimi	3.0 oz	85	84.2	10.9	9.0	0.0	0.3	0.1	0.2
924252	Shellfish, Shrimp Chow Mein, frozen	1 cup	227	72.6	5.9	10.9	0.0	0.7	0.0	0.0
15151	Shellfish, Shrimp Egg Roll/LaChoy	3 medium	37	75.1	2.0	12.0	0.0	2.4	0.5	1.5
15150	Shellfish, Shrimp, boiled/steamed (moist heat)	1 large shrimp	6	5.9	1.3	0.0	0.0	0.1	0.0	0.0
15152	Shellfish, Shrimp, breaded & fried	1 large shrimp	7	16.9	1.5	0.8	0.0	0.9	0.3	0.4
15153	Shellfish, Shrimp, canned	1 cup	128	153.6	29.5	1.3	0.0	2.5	0.4	1.0
15149	Shellfish, Shrimp, Imitation Surimi	3.0 oz	85	85.9	10.5	7.8	0.0	1.2	0.2	0.6
4550	Sherbet, Orange	1 sherbert bar	66	91.1	0.7	20.1	0.0	1.3	0.3	0.1
4546	Shortening, Animal & Vegetable Fat, Lard & Vege Oil	1 cup	205	1845.0	0.0	0.0	0.0	205.0	91.0	22.3
4556	Shortening, Vegetable Fat, Crisco	1 tbsp	12	106.0	0.0	0.0	0.0	12.0	5.3	3.6
19002	Snack, Banana Chips	1.0 oz	28.35	147.1	0.7	16.6	2.2	9.5	0.6	0.2
919972	Snack, Beef Jerky	1.0 oz	28.35	116.2	9.4	3.1	0.5	7.3	3.2	0.3
18501	Snack, Bugles	1.0 oz	28	150.1	2.0	18.0	0.0	8.0	0.0	0.0
19419	Snack, Chex Party Mix	1.0 oz (⅔ cup)	28	119.0	3.1	18.2	1.6	4.8	0.0	0.0
19800	Snack, Corn Cakes	1 cake	9	34.8	0.7	7.5	0.2	0.2	0.1	0.1
919973	Snack, Corn Chips, BBQ flavor	1.0 oz	28.35	148.3	2.0	15.9	1.5	9.3	2.7	4.6
19003	Snack, Corn Chips, light/Fritos	1.0 oz	28	155.1	1.9	15.9	0.8	9.7	0.0	0.0
19803	Snack, Corn Chips, Plain	1.0 oz	28.35	152.8	1.9	16.1	1.4	9.5	2.7	4.7
19401	Snack, Corn Cones, Plain	1.0 oz	28.35	144.6	1.6	17.8	0.3	7.6	0.5	0.2

Sat (g)	Chol (mg)	Cal (mg)	Iron (mg)	Magn (mg)	Phos (mg)	Pota (mg)	Sodi (mg)	Zinc (mg)	Vit A (RE)	Vit C (mg)	Vit E (mg)	Thia (mg)	Ribo (mg)	Niac (mg)	Vit B-6 (mg)	Fol (µg)	Vit B-12 (µg)	Wat (g)
0.0	0.0	28.0	2.2	0.0	138.0	391.0	1101.0	0.0	185.6	5.0	0.0	0.2	0.2	3.5	0.0	0.0	0.0	0.0
0.0	0.0	6.0	0.4	0.0	1.0	64.0	149.0	0.0	10.2	11.0	0.0	0.0	0.1	0.0	0.0	0.0	0.0	0.0
0.0	0.0	2.0	0.2	0.0	5.0	10.0	157.0	0.0	0.8	2.0	0.0	0.0	0.1	0.0	0.0	0.0	0.0	0.0
6.8	38.5	521.0	1.3	38.5	301.9	671.9	1829.3	1.1	127.3	1.5	0.0	0.9	0.8	0.8	0.1	8.9	0.6	231.4
0.0	0.0	8.0	0.3	0.0	0.0	12.0	146.0	0.0	0.0	0.0	0.0	0.0	0.0	0.0	0.0	0.0	0.0	44.7
0.1	0.0	1.8	0.1	1.6	5.9	12.8	218.1	0.0	9.9	0.3	0.1	0.0	0.0	0.1	0.0	0.6	0.1	11.3
0.0	0.0	0.0	0.0	0.0	0.0	3.0	22.0	0.0	0.0	0.0	0.0	0.0	0.0	0.0	0.0	0.0	0.0	0.0
1.2	5.0	2.0	0.0	0.0	4.0	1.0	190.0	0.0	30.0	0.0	0.0	0.0	0.0	0.0	0.0	0.0	0.0	5.2
0.0	0.0	4.5	0.3	11.0	27.7	40.5	689.9	0.0	0.0	0.0	0.0	0.0	0.2	0.0	0.0	3.6	0.0	12.2
5.2	24.0	71.0	0.2	0.0	0.0	0.0	263.0	0.0	75.2	0.0	0.0	0.0	0.1	0.2	0.0	0.0	0.0	44.8
2.6	18.0	73.0	0.1	0.0	59.0	89.0	214.0	0.3	42.6	0.0		0.0	0.1	0.1	0.0	0.0	0.0	48.0
0.0	0.0	28.0	1.3	0.0	0.0	139.0	639.0	0.0	22.4	2.0	0.0	0.0	0.4	0.0	0.0	0.0	0.0	0.0
3.3	30.0	1.5	1.6	2.0	5.5	9.5	170.0	0.3	0.0	0.0	0.1	0.0	0.0	0.3	0.0	1.3	0.3	11.8
7.9	51.0	37.4	1.1	12.8	126.7	180.2	473.5	2.0	0.0	0.9	0.2	0.4	0.2	2.7	0.2	1.7	0.8	47.7
6.1	28.5	6.3	0.7	5.7	49.0	95.2	638.4	1.0	0.0	0.0	0.1	0.1	0.1	1.5	0.1	2.3	0.7	30.7
5.4	27.5	9.0	0.6	1.4	39.2	74.7	461.7	1.0	0.0	0.0	0.1	0.0	0.0	1.1	0.1	1.8	0.7	24.6
2.5	45.5	42.8	0.9	4.5	48.2	37.8	616.5	0.5	17.1	0.0	0.1	0.0	0.1	1.4	0.1	1.8	0.1	25.9
2.7	48.2	47.7	0.8	6.3	60.3	80.6	641.7	1.4	0.0	0.0	0.3	0.0	0.1	1.9	0.1	3.6	0.1	28.3
1.8	14.7	3.0	0.3	3.2	28.1	56.4	271.9	0.6	0.0	0.0	0.0	0.0	0.0	0.8	0.0	0.7	0.5	13.5
2.6	17.4	11.4	0.4	4.2	38.5	70.5	279.8	0.5	0.0	0.0	0.1	0.1	0.1	0.7	0.0	1.3	0.4	14.0
1.4	8.4	2.7	0.2	1.7	14.6	24.5	186.9	0.3	0.0	0.0	0.0	0.0	0.0	0.4	0.0	0.5	0.2	7.8
40.5	198.3	25.1	3.5	40.2	298.7	871.0	5120.4	6.3	0.0	0.0	0.6	0.8	0.6	12.4	0.6	10.0	6.3	67.9
5.0	73.0	9.0	1.0	17.0	162.0	231.0	507.0	2.4	8.0	0.0	0.6	0.7	0.2	2.6	0.2	3.0	0.8	64.9
1.9	15.0	3.0	0.6	3.5	26.5	45.5	245.0	0.5	0.0	0.0	0.1	0.1	0.1	0.8	0.0	0.5	0.8	13.9
2.3	46.7	11.4	0.9	8.6	60.4	139.1	572.3	1.0	0.0	0.0	0.3	0.0	0.1	2.0	0.1	2.3	0.1	37.5
7.2	48.3	6.8	1.0	8.2	72.8	128.5	642.6	1.4	0.0	0.0	0.1	0.2	0.1	2.2	0.1	1.4	1.0	35.5
7.7	46.2	20.4	0.8	12.9	110.2	228.5	1020.0	1.9	0.0	1.4	0.2	0.5	0.2	3.1	0.2	3.4	1.1	26.7
6.6	44.2	27.9	1.0	10.9	93.2	194.5	797.6	1.3	0.0	0.0	0.0	0.1	0.1	1.9	0.1	1.4	1.1	36.7
2.0	0.0	42.8	2.5	24.5	153.0	157.1	603.8	1.0	43.5	0.0	1.4	1.6	0.3	7.6	0.6	17.7	0.0	34.3
1.5	8.3	1.6	0.1	1.1	7.8	16.2	152.5	0.3	0.0	0.0	0.0	0.0	0.0	0.3	0.0	0.6	0.2	9.6
2.4	0.0	53.4	3.1	162.8	324.3	316.9	1.4	2.3	2.3	0.6	23.1	1.1	0.1	2.1	0.4	104.6	0.0	2.5
1.5	0.0	19.8	1.1	36.6	327.4	241.0	0.9	1.5	0.0	0.4	14.3	0.0	0.1	2.0	0.2	67.3	0.0	0.3
1.7	0.0	15.9	1.9	36.0	322.9	136.9	0.9	1.5	1.4	0.4	14.3	0.1	0.1	1.2	0.2	66.3	0.0	0.7
1.4	79.9	31.5	3.2	47.6	184.5	241.4	502.4	0.8	1.7	1.5	0.0	0.2	0.1	1.6	0.1	11.9	0.6	51.1
0.2	57.0	78.2	23.8	15.3	287.3	533.8	95.2	2.3	145.4	18.8	0.0	0.1	0.4	2.9	0.1	24.5	84.1	54.1
2.3	51.9	53.6	11.8	11.9	159.8	277.1	309.4	1.2	76.5	8.5	0.0	0.1	0.2	1.8	0.1	30.6	34.2	52.3
0.0	2.6	11.1	0.3	9.4	96.9	126.7	182.8	0.1	7.7	0.9	0.9	0.0	0.0	0.2	0.0	1.7	4.3	83.0
0.2	57.0	78.2	23.8	15.3	287.3	533.8	95.2	2.3	145.4	18.8	0.9	0.1	0.4	2.9	0.1	24.5	84.1	54.1
0.1	45.1	50.2	0.6	53.6	238.0	222.7	911.2	6.5	7.7	6.5	0.0	0.0	0.0	1.1	0.2	43.4	9.8	65.9
0.2	17.0	11.1	0.3	36.6	239.7	76.5	714.9	0.3	17.0	0.0	0.1	0.0	0.0	0.2	0.0	1.4	1.4	62.6
0.9	90.0	63.0	0.6	19.8	127.8	194.4	198.0	2.5	48.6	1.7	0.0	0.1	0.0	1.7	0.1	31.8	3.6	42.6
0.1	64.6	50.2	0.4	49.3	148.8	346.8	321.3	4.6	26.4	3.1	0.0	0.0	0.2	3.1	0.1	35.7	8.8	62.3
0.1	61.2	51.9	0.3	29.8	157.3	299.2	323.0	2.5	22.1	0.0	0.9	0.0	0.1	0.9	0.1	9.4	2.6	64.6
0.3	76.5	53.6	1.2	43.4	194.7	176.8	193.0	6.2	5.1	1.8	0.0	0.0	0.0	4.2	0.1	0.9	3.4	56.7
0.7	47.6	28.1	5.7	31.5	242.3	227.8	313.7	2.3	77.4	11.6	0.0	0.3	0.4	2.6	0.1	64.3	20.4	52.0
2.7	68.9	52.7	5.9	49.3	135.2	207.4	354.5	74.1	76.5	3.2	0.0	0.1	0.2	1.4	0.1	26.4	13.3	55.0
0.4	22.4	33.0	4.6	19.5	67.9	89.7	96.2	26.6	11.2	3.5	0.0	0.1	0.0	1.1	0.0	14.2	14.3	48.4
0.4	21.0	37.0	4.9	27.7	78.1	104.2	149.5	31.9	6.7	3.9	0.0	0.1	0.1	1.1	0.1	15.1	13.6	72.4
0.8	18.9	13.0	0.3	18.3	73.2	103.2	143.8	0.3	6.8	0.7	0.0	0.0	0.0	0.5	0.0	11.5	0.4	18.1
0.1	18.7	6.8	0.3	36.6	239.7	87.6	675.8	0.3	17.0	0.0	0.0	0.0	0.0	0.3	0.0	1.4	1.4	62.7
0.0	0.0	0.0	0.0	0.0	0.0	0.0	985.0	0.0	0.0	0.0	0.0	0.0	0.0	0.0	0.0	0.0	0.0	0.0
0.4	4.0	11.0	0.8	0.0	0.0	65.0	120.0	0.0	5.0	4.0	0.0	0.1	0.1	0.8	0.0	0.0	0.0	0.0
0.0	11.7	2.3	0.2	2.0	8.2	10.9	13.4	0.1	4.0	0.1	0.0	0.0	0.0	0.2	0.0	0.2	0.1	4.6
0.1	12.4	4.7	0.1	2.8	15.3	15.8	24.1	0.1	3.9	0.1	0.0	0.0	0.0	0.2	0.0	0.6	0.1	3.7
0.5	221.4	75.5	3.5	52.5	298.2	268.8	216.3	1.6	23.0	2.9	1.2	0.0	0.0	3.5	0.1	2.3	1.4	92.9
0.2	30.6	16.2	0.5	36.6	239.7	75.7	599.3	0.3	17.0	0.0	0.0	0.0	0.0	0.1	0.0	1.4	1.4	63.7
0.8	4.0	35.6	0.1	5.3	26.4	63.4	30.4	0.3	9.2	2.0	0.1	0.0	0.1	0.0	0.0	3.3	0.1	43.6
82.6	114.8	0.0	0.0	0.0	0.0	0.0	0.0	0.0	0.0	0.0	2.5	0.0	0.0	0.0	0.0	0.0	0.0	0.0
3.1	0.0	0.0	0.0	0.0	0.0	0.0	0.0	0.0	0.0	0.0	0.0	0.0	0.0	0.0	0.0	0.0	0.0	0.0
8.2	0.0	5.1	0.4	21.5	15.9	152.0	1.7	0.2	2.3	1.8	1.5	0.0	0.0	0.2	0.0	4.0	0.0	1.2
3.1	13.6	5.7	1.5	14.5	115.4	169.2	627.4	2.3	0.0	0.0	0.1	0.0	0.0	0.5	0.1	38.0	0.3	6.6
0.0	0.0	2.0	0.2	0.0	13.0	20.0	290.0	0.0	0.0	0.0	0.0	0.0	0.0	0.3	0.0	0.0	0.0	0.0
1.5	0.0	9.8	6.9	17.6	52.4	75.3	284.8	0.6	3.9	13.3	0.0	0.4	0.1	4.7	0.4	0.0	3.5	1.0
0.0	0.0	1.7	0.1	10.3	14.1	14.1	43.9	0.2	2.2	0.0	0.0	0.0	0.0	0.5	0.0	1.7	0.0	0.4
1.3	0.0	37.1	0.4	21.8	58.7	66.9	216.3	0.3	17.3	0.5	0.0	0.0	0.1	0.5	0.1	11.1	0.0	0.3
0.0	0.0	25.0	0.3	21.0	52.0	48.0	194.0	0.3	7.4	0.0	0.0	0.0	0.0	0.0	0.0	0.0	0.0	0.2
1.3	0.0	36.0	0.4	21.5	52.4	40.3	178.6	0.4	2.6	0.0	0.4	0.0	0.1	0.3	0.1	5.7	0.0	0.3
6.4	0.0	0.9	0.7	3.1	12.5	23.0	289.7	0.1	9.1	0.0	0.0	0.1	0.1	0.4	0.0	0.9	0.0	0.6

Code	Food Name	Unit/Amt	Wt (g)	Energy (Kcal)	Prot (g)	Carb (g)	Fiber (g)	Fat (g)	Mono (g)	Poly (g)
19402	Snack, Corn Nuts, BBQ flavor	1.0 oz	28.35	123.6	2.6	20.3	2.4	4.1	2.1	0.9
19008	Snack, Corn Nuts, Plain	1.0 oz	28.35	124.5	2.4	20.8	2.0	4.0	2.1	0.9
19016	Snack, Doo Dads Party Mix, Original flavor	1 tbsp	3.5	16.0	0.4	2.3	0.2	0.6	0.0	0.0
19015	Snack, Granola Bar, Hard, peanut butter	28.35	28.35	136.9	2.8	17.7	0.8	6.7	2.0	3.4
19017	Snack, Granola Bar, Hard, Plain	1.0 oz bar	28.35	133.5	2.9	18.3	1.5	5.6	1.2	3.4
19405	Snack, Granola Bar, Hard, w/chocolate chips	1.0 oz	28.35	124.2	2.1	20.4	1.2	4.6	0.7	0.4
19024	Snack, Granola Bar, Soft, chocolate chip, graham & marshmallow	1.0 oz bar	28.35	121.1	1.7	20.1	1.1	4.4	0.8	0.7
19406	Snack, Granola Bar, Soft, Chocolate Chip, milk chocolate cover	1.0 oz bar	28.35	132.1	1.6	18.1	1.0	7.1	2.2	0.5
19027	Snack, Granola Bar, Soft, Peanut Butter	1.0 oz bar	28.35	120.8	3.0	18.3	1.2	4.5	1.9	1.2
19022	Snack, Granola Bar, Soft, Plain	1.0 oz bar	28.35	125.6	2.1	19.1	1.3	4.9	1.1	1.5
19404	Snack, Granola Bar, Soft, Raisin	1.0 oz bar	28.35	127.0	2.2	18.8	1.2	5.0	0.8	0.9
19440	Snack, Granola Bar, Soft, w/chocolate chips	1.0 oz bar	28.35	119.1	2.1	19.6	1.4	4.7	1.0	0.6
19439	Snack, Kudos Whole Grain Bars, chocolate chip/M&M Mars	4.0 oz bar	100	437.0	5.8	67.7	3.6	16.4	5.2	0.9
19407	Snack, Low Fat Granola Bar, Crunchy Almond/Brown Sugar/Kellogg's	4.0 oz bar	100	390.0	8.0	78.0	6.2	7.4	1.8	4.5
19441	Snack, Meat-Based Sticks, smoked	1.0 oz	28.35	155.9	6.1	1.5	0.0	14.1	5.8	1.3
19031	Snack, Nutri-Grain Cereal Bars, fruit/Kellogg's	4.0 oz bar	100	368.0	4.4	72.9	2.1	7.5	5.0	0.9
19034	Snack, Popcorn Cakes	1 cake	10	38.4	1.0	8.0	0.3	0.3	0.1	0.1
19806	Snack, Popcorn, air-popped	1 tbsp	0.5	1.9	0.1	0.4	0.1	0.0	0.0	0.0
19039	Snack, Popcorn, caramel coated w/peanuts	1.0 oz (⅔ cup)	28.35	113.4	1.8	22.9	1.1	2.2	0.8	0.9
19040	Snack, Popcorn, caramel coated, no peanuts	1.0 oz	28.35	122.2	1.1	22.4	1.5	3.6	0.8	1.3
19807	Snack, Popcorn, Cheese flavor	1 tbsp	0.7	3.7	0.1	0.4	0.1	0.2	0.1	0.1
19035	Snack, Popcorn, oil-popped, white corn	1.0 oz	28.35	141.8	2.6	16.2	2.8	8.0	2.3	3.8
19408	Snack, Popcorn, prep in microwave	3 cups	40	210.0	3.0	20.4	1.0	13.2	8.3	3.2
19412	Snack, Pork Skins, Plain	1.0 oz	28.35	154.5	17.4	0.0	0.0	8.9	4.2	1.0
19042	Snack, Potato Chips w/o salt	1.0 oz	28.35	157.9	2.1	14.5	1.0	10.6	2.0	5.7
919975	Snack, Potato Chips, BBQ flavor	1.0 oz	28.35	139.2	2.2	15.0	1.2	9.2	1.9	4.6
19809	Snack, Potato Chips, light	1.0 oz	28.35	133.5	2.0	19.0	1.7	5.9	1.4	3.1
19411	Snack, Potato Chips, Plain, no salt	1.0 oz	28.35	152.0	2.0	15.0	1.4	9.8	2.8	3.5
19043	Snack, Potato Chips, Plain, salted	1.0 oz	28.35	152.0	2.0	15.0	1.3	9.8	2.8	3.5
919985	Snack, Potato Chips, sour cream & onion	1.0 oz	28.35	150.5	2.3	14.6	1.5	9.6	1.7	4.9
19047	Snack, Pretzel, Hard, Plain, no salt	1.0 oz	28.35	108.0	2.6	22.5	0.8	1.0	0.4	0.3
19813	Snack, Pretzel, Hard, Plain, salted	1.0 oz	28.35	108.0	2.6	22.5	0.9	1.0	0.4	0.3
19050	Snack, Pretzels, Hard, chocolate coated	1.0 oz	28.35	129.8	2.1	20.1	0.0	4.7	1.5	0.6
919978	Snack, Pretzels, Hard, whole wheat	1.0 oz, (2 sm pretzels)	28	101.4	3.1	22.7	2.2	0.7	0.3	0.2
19052	Snack, Rice Cake	1 cake	5	21.0	0.5	4.6	0.4	0.0	0.0	0.0
19818	Snack, Rice Cake, brown rice & multigrain	1 cake	9	34.8	0.8	7.2	0.3	0.3	0.1	0.1
19816	Snack, Rice Cake, brown rice, Plain	1 cake	9	34.8	0.7	7.3	0.4	0.3	0.1	0.1
19524	Snack, Sesame Stick, wheat based, no salt	1.0 oz	28.35	153.4	3.1	13.2	0.0	10.4	3.1	4.9
19857	Snack, Taro Chips	1.0 oz	28.35	141.2	0.7	19.3	2.0	7.1	1.3	3.7
19424	Snack, Tortilla Chips, Nacho flavor	1.0 oz	28.35	141.2	2.2	17.7	1.5	7.3	4.3	1.0
19056	Snack, Tortilla Chips, Nacho, light	1.0 oz	28.35	126.2	2.5	20.3	1.4	4.3	2.5	0.6
19058	Snack, Tortilla Chips, Plain	1.0 oz	28.35	142.0	2.0	17.8	1.8	7.4	4.4	1.0
19063	Snack, Tortilla Chips, Ranch flavor	1.0 oz	28.35	138.9	2.2	18.3	1.1	6.7	4.0	0.9
19059	Snack, Tortilla Chips, Taco flavor	1.0 oz	28.35	136.1	2.2	17.9	1.5	6.9	4.1	1.0
19062	Snack, Trail Mix, regular	1.0 oz	28.35	131.0	3.9	12.7	0.0	8.3	3.6	2.7
6201	Soup, Asparagus, canned, made w/H$_2$O	1 cup (8 fl oz)	244	85.4	2.3	10.7	0.5	4.1	1.0	1.9
6009	Soup, Beans w/ham, chunky, RTE, canned	1 cup (8 fl oz)	243	230.9	12.6	27.1	11.2	8.5	3.8	0.9
6748	Soup, Beef Noodle, condensed, canned	1 cup (8 fl oz)	251	168.2	9.7	18.0	1.5	6.2	2.5	1.0
6008	Soup, Beef Broth or Bouillon, dry, made w/H$_2$O	1 packet (6 fl oz)	183	14.6	1.0	1.4	0.0	0.5	0.2	0.0
6147	Soup, Beef Mushroom, canned, made w/H$_2$O	1 cup (8 fl oz)	244	73.2	5.8	6.3	0.2	3.0	1.2	0.1
6743	Soup, Beef Vegetable, canned, RTE/Progresso Healthy Classics	1 cup	250	160.0	10.5	25.6	6.0	1.6	0.6	0.2
6722	Soup, Beef, chunky, RTE, canned	1 cup	240	170.4	11.7	19.6	1.4	5.1	2.1	0.2
6724	Soup, Beefy Mushroom, dry mix/Lipton Recipe Secrets	1 serving	11	32.8	0.9	6.6	0.1	0.4	0.0	0.0
6402	Soup, Beefy Onion, dry mix/Lipton Recipe Secrets	1 serving	8	25.1	0.5	4.7	0.4	0.6	0.0	0.0
6002	Soup, Black Bean, canned, made w/H$_2$O	1 cup (8 fl oz)	247	116.1	5.6	19.8	4.4	1.5	0.5	0.5
906161	Soup, Broccoli & Cheese, dry mix/Lipton Soup Secrets	1 serving	16	66.9	1.8	8.9	0.7	2.9	0.0	0.0
6411	Soup, Cauliflower, dry, made w/H$_2$O	1 cup (8 fl oz)	256.1	69.1	2.9	10.7	0.0	1.7	0.7	0.6
6011	Soup, Cheese, canned, made w/milk	1 cup (8 fl oz)	251	230.9	9.5	16.2	1.0	14.6	4.1	0.5
6413	Soup, Chicken Broth or Bouillon, dry, made w/H$_2$O	1 cup (8 fl oz)	244	22.0	1.3	1.4	0.0	1.1	0.4	0.4
6017	Soup, Chicken Gumbo, canned, made w/H$_2$O	1 cup (8 fl oz)	244	56.1	2.6	8.4	2.0	1.4	0.7	0.3
6549	Soup, Chicken Mushroom Chowder, chunky, RTE		0.0	0.0	0.0	0.0	0.0	0.0	0.0	0.0
6727	Soup, Chicken Noodle, chunky, canned, RTE	1 cup (8 fl oz)	240	175.2	12.7	17.0	3.8	6.0	2.7	1.5
6022	Soup, Chicken Rice, canned, made w/H$_2$O	1 cup (8 fl oz)	241	60.3	3.5	7.2	0.7	1.9	0.9	0.4
6025	Soup, Chicken Vegetable, chunky, RTE, canned	1 cup (8 fl oz)	240	165.6	12.3	18.9	0.0	4.8	2.2	1.0
6012	Soup, Chicken w/dumplings, canned, made w/H$_2$O	1 cup (8 fl oz)	241	96.4	5.6	6.0	0.5	5.5	2.5	1.3
6034	Soup, Consomme w/gelatin, dry, made w/H$_2$O	1 cup (8 fl oz)	250	17.5	2.2	2.1	0.0	0.0	0.0	0.0
6001	Soup, Crab, RTE, canned	1 cup (8 fl oz)	244	75.6	5.5	10.3	0.7	1.5	0.7	0.4
6410	Soup, Cream of Broccoli, canned, RTE/Progresso Healthy Classics	1 cup (8 fl oz)	356	128.2	3.5	19.4	3.6	4.1	1.3	0.8
6210	Soup, Cream of Celery, canned, made w/H$_2$O	1 cup (8 fl oz)	244	90.3	1.7	8.8	0.7	5.6	1.3	2.5

Sat (g)	Chol (mg)	Cal (mg)	Iron (mg)	Magn (mg)	Phos (mg)	Pota (mg)	Sodi (mg)	Zinc (mg)	Vit A (RE)	Vit C (mg)	Vit E (mg)	Thia (mg)	Ribo (mg)	Niac (mg)	Vit B-6 (mg)	Fol (µg)	Vit B-12 (µg)	Wat (g)
0.7	0.0	4.8	0.5	30.9	80.2	81.1	276.7	0.5	9.6	0.1	0.0	0.1	0.0	0.4	0.1	0.0	0.0	0.5
0.7	0.0	2.6	0.5	32.0	78.0	78.8	155.6	0.5	0.0	0.0	0.3	0.0	0.0	0.5	0.1	0.0	0.0	0.4
0.1	0.0	2.6	0.1	2.1	10.4	9.7	44.5	0.1	1.5	0.0	0.0	0.0	0.0	0.2	0.0	1.4	0.0	0.1
0.9	0.0	11.6	0.7	15.6	39.4	82.5	80.2	0.4	0.6	0.1	0.0	0.1	0.0	0.6	0.0	5.1	0.0	0.7
0.7	0.0	17.3	0.8	27.5	78.5	95.3	83.3	0.6	4.3	0.3	0.0	0.1	0.0	0.4	0.0	6.5	0.0	1.1
3.2	0.0	21.8	0.9	20.4	57.8	71.2	97.5	0.5	1.1	0.0	0.0	0.1	0.0	0.2	0.0	3.7	0.0	0.7
2.6	0.3	25.2	0.7	20.1	57.3	78.0	89.6	0.4	1.4	0.0	0.0	0.0	0.0	0.3	0.0	6.0	0.0	1.7
4.0	1.4	29.2	0.7	18.7	56.4	88.7	56.7	0.4	2.0	0.0	0.0	0.0	0.1	0.2	0.0	7.4	0.2	1.0
1.0	0.3	25.8	0.6	24.4	70.9	82.5	116.0	0.5	0.6	0.0	0.0	0.1	0.0	0.9	0.0	9.1	0.1	2.1
2.1	0.3	29.8	0.7	21.0	65.2	92.1	78.8	0.4	0.0	0.0	0.0	0.1	0.0	0.1	0.0	6.8	0.1	1.8
2.7	0.3	28.6	0.7	20.4	62.4	102.6	79.9	0.4	0.0	0.0	0.0	0.1	0.0	0.3	0.0	6.0	0.1	1.8
2.9	0.3	26.4	0.7	22.1	65.2	96.4	77.1	0.4	1.4	0.0	0.0	0.1	0.0	0.3	0.0	6.2	0.0	1.5
9.5	136.0	783.0	9.2	70.0	207.0	279.0	280.0	1.4	1253.0	46.6	10.8	0.2	0.2	1.5	0.1	13.0	0.1	4.9
1.1	0.0	35.0	8.6	87.0	248.0	249.0	291.0	2.2	713.0	0.0	0.0	0.7	0.8	9.5	1.0	0.0	0.0	5.0
5.9	37.7	19.3	1.0	6.0	51.0	72.9	419.6	0.7	47.9	1.9	0.0	0.0	0.1	1.3	0.1	0.0	0.3	5.4
1.5	0.0	41.0	4.9	27.0	103.0	197.0	297.0	4.1	614.0	0.0	0.0	1.0	1.1	13.5	1.4	108.0	0.0	14.5
0.0	0.0	0.9	0.2	15.9	27.7	32.7	28.8	0.4	0.7	0.0	0.0	0.0	0.0	0.6	0.0	1.8	0.0	0.5
0.0	0.0	0.1	0.0	0.7	1.5	1.5	0.0	0.0	0.1	0.0	0.0	0.0	0.0	0.0	0.0	0.1	0.0	0.0
0.3	0.0	18.7	1.1	22.7	36.0	100.6	83.6	0.4	1.7	0.0	0.4	0.0	0.0	0.6	0.1	4.5	0.0	0.9
1.0	1.4	12.2	0.5	9.9	23.5	30.9	58.4	0.2	2.8	0.0	0.3	0.0	0.0	0.6	0.0	0.6	0.0	0.8
0.0	0.1	0.8	0.0	0.6	2.5	1.8	6.2	0.0	0.3	0.0	0.0	0.0	0.0	0.0	0.0	0.1	0.0	0.0
1.4	0.0	2.8	0.8	30.6	70.9	63.8	250.6	0.7	0.6	0.1	0.0	0.0	0.0	0.4	0.1	4.8	0.0	0.8
1.7	0.0	8.0	0.7	0.0	73.0	96.0	415.0	0.0	10.8	3.0	0.0	0.1	0.3	0.7	0.0	0.0	0.0	0.0
3.2	26.9	8.5	0.2	3.1	24.1	36.0	521.1	0.2	11.1	0.1	0.2	0.0	0.1	0.4	0.0	0.0	0.2	0.5
2.9	0.0	6.1	0.4	19.2	50.6	384.8	4.1	0.2	1.6	12.1	0.0	0.1	0.0	1.1	0.2	13.2	0.2	0.5
2.3	0.0	14.2	0.5	21.3	52.7	357.5	212.6	0.3	6.2	9.6	1.4	0.1	0.1	1.3	0.2	23.5	0.0	0.5
1.2	0.0	6.0	0.4	25.2	54.7	494.4	139.5	0.0	0.0	7.3	0.8	0.1	0.1	2.0	0.2	7.7	0.0	0.3
3.1	0.0	6.8	0.5	19.0	46.8	361.5	2.3	0.3	0.0	8.8	1.4	0.0	0.1	1.1	0.2	12.8	0.0	0.5
3.1	0.0	6.8	0.5	19.0	46.8	361.5	168.4	0.3	0.0	8.8	1.4	0.0	0.1	1.1	0.2	12.8	0.0	0.5
2.5	2.0	20.4	0.5	21.0	49.9	377.3	177.2	0.3	6.0	10.6	0.0	0.1	0.1	1.1	0.2	17.6	0.3	0.5
0.2	0.0	10.2	1.2	9.9	32.0	41.4	81.9	0.2	0.0	0.0	0.1	0.1	0.2	1.5	0.0	23.5	0.0	0.9
0.2	0.0	10.2	1.2	9.9	32.0	41.4	486.2	0.2	0.0	0.0	0.1	0.1	0.2	1.5	0.0	48.5	0.0	0.9
2.2	0.0	21.0	0.6	11.6	41.1	63.8	161.3	0.3	0.6	0.1	0.0	0.0	0.1	0.2	0.0	2.6	0.0	0.7
0.2	0.0	7.8	0.8	8.4	35.0	120.4	56.8	0.2	0.0	0.3	0.0	0.1	0.1	1.8	0.1	15.1	0.0	1.1
0.0	0.0	0.0	0.1	0.0	0.0	25.0	16.0	0.0	2.8	0.0	0.0	0.0	0.0	0.6	0.0	0.0	0.0	0.0
0.1	0.0	1.9	0.2	12.3	33.3	26.5	22.7	0.2	0.0	0.0	0.0	0.0	0.0	0.6	0.0	1.8	0.0	0.6
0.1	0.0	1.0	0.1	11.8	32.4	26.1	29.3	0.3	0.5	0.0	0.1	0.0	0.0	0.7	0.0	1.9	0.0	0.5
1.8	0.0	48.2	0.2	12.8	39.1	50.2	8.2	0.3	2.6	0.0	0.0	0.0	0.0	0.4	0.0	6.2	0.0	0.6
1.8	0.0	17.0	0.3	23.8	37.1	214.0	97.0	0.1	0.0	1.4	1.4	0.0	0.0	0.1	0.1	5.7	0.0	0.6
1.4	0.9	41.7	0.4	23.2	69.2	61.2	200.7	0.3	11.6	0.5	0.0	0.0	0.1	0.4	0.1	4.0	0.0	0.5
0.8	0.9	45.1	0.5	27.5	90.2	77.1	284.4	0.0	11.9	0.1	0.0	0.1	0.1	0.1	0.1	7.4	0.0	0.4
1.4	0.0	43.7	0.4	24.9	58.1	55.8	149.7	0.4	5.7	0.0	0.4	0.0	0.1	0.4	0.1	2.8	0.0	0.5
1.3	0.3	40.0	0.4	25.2	67.8	69.2	173.5	0.4	7.7	0.3	0.0	0.0	0.1	0.4	0.1	4.8	0.0	0.5
1.3	1.4	43.9	0.6	24.9	67.8	61.5	223.1	0.4	25.8	0.3	0.0	0.1	0.1	0.6	0.1	6.0	0.0	0.5
1.6	0.0	22.1	0.9	44.8	97.8	194.2	64.9	0.9	0.6	0.4	0.0	0.1	0.1	1.3	0.1	20.1	0.0	2.6
1.0	4.9	29.3	0.8	4.9	39.0	173.2	980.9	0.9	43.9	2.7	0.7	0.1	0.1	0.8	0.0	22.0	0.0	224.0
3.3	21.9	77.8	3.2	46.2	143.4	425.3	972.0	1.1	396.1	4.4	0.0	0.1	0.1	1.7	0.1	29.2	0.1	191.1
2.3	10.0	30.1	2.2	12.6	92.9	198.3	1905.1	3.1	125.5	0.8	0.0	0.1	0.1	2.1	0.1	37.7	0.4	211.9
0.3	0.0	7.3	0.0	5.5	18.3	27.5	1021.1	0.1	0.0	0.0	0.0	0.0	0.0	0.0	0.0	0.0	0.0	177.0
1.5	7.3	4.9	0.9	9.8	34.2	153.7	941.8	1.5	0.0	4.6	0.0	0.0	0.1	1.0	0.0	9.8	0.0	225.9
0.6	15.0	15.0	1.9	32.5	102.5	627.5	420.0	1.3	215.0	4.8	0.5	0.1	0.1	2.9	0.3	25.0	0.3	212.5
2.5	14.4	31.2	2.3	4.8	120.0	336.0	866.4	2.6	261.6	7.0	0.2	0.2	0.2	2.7	0.1	13.4	0.6	200.0
0.1	0.2	10.8	0.1	0.0	0.0	0.0	645.2	0.0	0.0	0.2	0.0	0.0	0.0	0.1	0.0	0.0	0.0	0.4
0.1	0.0	11.2	0.1	0.0	0.0	0.0	606.6	0.0	0.0	0.7	0.0	0.0	0.0	0.1	0.0	0.0	0.0	0.3
0.4	0.0	44.5	2.1	42.0	106.2	274.2	1198.0	1.4	49.4	0.7	0.1	0.1	0.1	0.5	0.1	24.7	0.0	215.6
0.8	2.9	46.4	0.2	0.0	0.0	0.0	545.3	0.0	0.0	3.0	0.0	0.0	0.0	0.1	0.0	3.7	0.0	0.6
0.3	0.0	10.2	0.5	2.6	51.2	105.0	842.6	0.3	0.0	2.6	0.0	0.1	0.0	0.5	0.0	2.6	0.2	238.0
9.1	41.7	288.7	0.8	20.1	251.0	341.4	1019.1	0.7	148.1	1.3	0.3	0.1	0.3	0.5	0.1	10.0	0.4	206.9
0.3	0.0	14.6	0.1	4.9	12.2	24.4	1483.5	0.0	12.2	0.0	0.0	0.0	0.0	0.2	0.0	2.4	0.0	236.2
0.3	4.9	24.4	0.9	4.9	24.4	75.6	954.0	0.4	14.6	4.9	0.0	0.0	0.0	0.7	0.1	4.9	0.0	229.0
0.0	0.0	0.0	0.0	0.0	0.0	0.0	0.0	0.0	0.0	0.0	0.0	0.0	0.0	0.0	0.0	0.0	0.0	
1.4	19.2	24.0	1.4	9.6	72.0	108.0	849.6	1.0	122.4	0.0	0.8	0.1	0.2	4.3	0.0	38.4	0.3	201.6
0.5	7.2	16.9	0.7	0.0	21.7	101.2	814.6	0.3	65.1	0.2	0.1	0.0	0.0	1.1	0.0	1.0	0.1	226.1
1.4	16.8	26.4	1.5	9.6	105.6	367.2	1068.0	2.2	600.0	5.5	0.0	0.0	0.2	3.3	0.1	12.0	0.2	200.3
1.3	33.7	14.5	0.6	4.8	60.3	115.7	860.4	0.4	53.0	0.0	0.1	0.0	0.1	1.8	0.0	2.4	0.2	221.2
0.0	0.0	7.5	0.1	7.5	40.0	57.5	3312.5	0.0	0.0	0.0	0.0	0.0	0.0	0.6	0.0	4.0	0.1	237.4
0.4	9.8	65.9	1.2	14.6	87.8	327.0	1234.6	1.5	51.2	0.0	0.0	0.0	0.1	1.3	0.1	14.6	0.2	223.3
1.0	7.1	60.5	1.8	21.4	57.0	235.0	843.7	0.4	46.3	8.5	0.6	0.0	0.1	0.5	0.1	42.7	0.0	327.5
1.4	14.6	39.0	0.6	7.3	36.6	122.0	949.2	0.2	31.7	0.2	0.9	0.0	0.1	0.3	0.1	2.4	0.2	225.1

Code	Food Name	Unit/Amt	Wt (g)	Energy (Kcal)	Prot (g)	Carb (g)	Fiber (g)	Fat (g)	Mono (g)	Poly (g)
6216	Soup, Cream of Chicken, canned, made w/H2O	1 cup (8 fl oz)	240	115.2	3.4	9.1	0.2	7.2	3.2	1.5
6243	Soup, Cream of Mushroom, canned, made w/H2O	1 cup (8 fl oz)	244	129.3	2.3	9.3	0.5	9.0	1.7	4.2
6246	Soup, Cream of Onion, canned, made w/H2O	1 cup (8 fl oz)	244	107.4	2.8	12.7	1.0	5.3	2.1	1.5
6253	Soup, Cream of Potato, canned, made w/H2O	1 cup (8 fl oz)	244	73.2	1.8	11.5	0.5	2.4	0.6	0.4
6256	Soup, Cream of Shrimp, canned, made w/H2O	1 cup (8 fl oz)	244	90.3	2.8	8.2	0.2	5.2	1.5	0.2
6582	Soup, Cream of Vegetable, dry, made w/H2O	1 cup (8 fl oz)	260	106.6	1.9	12.3	0.5	5.7	2.5	1.5
6035	Soup, Cup Noodles, Ramen, chicken flavor, dry/Nissin	1 individual container	64	296.2	5.6	36.8	0.0	14.1	0.0	0.0
6283	Soup, Gazpacho, RTE, canned	1 cup (8 fl oz)	244	46.4	7.1	4.4	0.5	0.2	0.0	0.1
6249	Soup, Green Pea, canned, made w/H2O	1 cup (8 fl oz)	250	165.0	8.6	26.5	2.8	2.9	1.0	0.4
6287	Soup, Hearty Chicken Noodle, dry mix/Lipton Cup-a-Soup	1 envelope	16	61.4	2.6	10.2	0.3	1.2	0.0	0.0
6204	Soup, Lentil Ham, RTE, canned	1 cup (8 fl oz)	248	138.9	9.3	20.2	0.0	2.8	1.3	0.3
6027	Soup, Manhattan Clam Chowder, canned, made w/H2O	1 cup (8 fl oz)	244	78.1	2.2	12.2	1.5	2.2	0.4	1.3
6039	Soup, Minestrone, canned, RTE/Progresso Healthy Classics	1 cup (8 fl oz)	241	122.9	4.8	20.3	1.2	2.5	0.9	1.0
6430	Soup, Nacho Cheese	1 cup (8 fl oz)	251	105.4	3.8	6.40	0.0	7.2	0.0	0.0
6230	Soup, New England Clam Chowder, canned, made w/H2O	1 cup (8 fl oz)	244	95.2	4.8	12.4	1.5	2.9	1.2	1.1
6302	Soup, Noodle w/real Chicken Broth, dry mix/Lipton Soup Secrets	1 tbsp	16	62.1	2.1	9.2	0.3	1.9	0.0	0.0
6045	Soup, Onion, canned, made w/H2O	1 cup (8 fl oz)	241	57.8	3.8	8.2	1.0	1.7	0.7	0.7
6730	Soup, Split Pea w/ham, canned, made w/H2O	1 cup (8 fl oz)	253	189.8	10.3	28.0	2.3	4.4	1.8	0.6
6192	Soup, Split Pea w/ham, chunky, RTE, canned	1 cup (8 fl oz)	240	184.8	11.1	26.8	4.1	4.0	1.6	0.6
6099	Soup, Tomato Rice, made w/H2O	1 cup (8 fl oz)	247	118.6	2.1	21.9	1.5	2.7	0.6	1.4
6559	Soup, Tomato Vegetable, dry, made w/H2O	1 cup (8 fl oz)	253	55.7	2.0	10.2	0.5	0.9	0.3	0.1
6359	Soup, Tomato, canned, made w/H2O	1 cup (8 fl oz)	244	85.4	2.0	16.6	0.5	1.9	0.4	1.0
6159	Soup, Tomato, canned, made w/milk	1 cup (8 fl oz)	248	161.2	6.1	22.3	2.7	6.0	1.6	1.1
6065	Soup, Turkey Noodle, canned, made w/H2O	1 cup (8 fl oz)	251	70.3	4.0	8.9	0.8	2.1	0.8	0.5
6066	Soup, Turkey Vegetable, canned, made w/H2O	1 cup (8 fl oz)	240	72.0	3.1	8.6	0.5	3.0	1.3	0.7
6471	Soup, Turkey, chunky, RTE, canned	1 cup (8 fl oz)	236	134.5	10.2	14.1	0.0	4.4	1.8	1.1
6301	Soup, Vegetable, chunky, RTE, canned	1 cup (8 fl oz)	240	122.4	3.5	19.0	1.2	3.7	1.6	1.4
6068	Soup, Vegetarian Vegetable, canned, made w/H2O	1 cup (8 fl oz)	241	72.3	2.1	12.0	0.5	1.9	0.8	0.7
22693	Stew, Beef Stew, canned entree	1 cup	232	218.1	11.5	15.7	3.5	12.5	5.5	0.5
924055	Stew, Beef&Vegetable	1 cup	245	220.5	16.0	15.0	2.0	11.0	4.5	0.5
906162	Stew, Chicken Vegetable/Bounty	7.5 oz	213	166.1	10.5	15.1	0.0	7.0	0.0	0.0
924190	Stew, Ratatouille, homemade	½ cup	107	132.7	1.2	5.9	0.0	12.3	9.0	1.1
19337	Stuffing, Brownberry Sage and Onion Stuffing Mix, dry mix/Best Foods	½ cup	67	255.3	8.9	47.2	3.6	3.4	0.0	0.0
919908	Sugar Substitute, Aspartame/Nutrasweet/Equal	1 tsp	3.5	12.3	0.1	3.00	0.0	0.0	0.0	0.0
924174	Sugar Substitute, Equal	1 package	1	4.0	0.0	1.0	0.0	0.0	0.0	0.0
18356	Sweet Roll, Cheese	1 oz	28.4	102.2	2.0	12.4	0.3	5.2	2.6	0.6
18357	Sweet Roll, Cinnamon-Raisin, commercially prep	1 large	83	308.8	5.1	42.2	2.0	13.6	4.0	6.2
919959	Sweet, All-Fruit Strawberry Spread/Polaner	1 tbsp	18	41.5	0.1	10.3	0.0	0.0	0.0	0.0
919904	Sweet, Baking Chocolate/Bakers	1 oz	28	141.1	3.1	9.0	0.5	14.6	5.5	0.4
919916	Sweet, Chewing Gum	1 stick	3	10.2	0.0	2.9	0.0	0.0	0.0	0.0
919902	Sweet, Chewing Gum, Sugarless	1 piece	3	8.0	0.0	2.0	0.0	0.0	0.0	0.0
19166	Sweet, Cocoa, dry powder, unsweetened	1 tbsp	5.4	12.4	1.1	2.9	1.8	0.7	0.2	0.0
19240	Sweet, Frosting, Chocolate creamy, RTE, no added phosphorus & Vit A	1/12 package	38	150.9	0.4	24.0	0.2	6.7	3.4	0.8
19375	Sweet, Frosting, Cream Cheese flavor, RTE	1/12 package	38	156.9	0.0	25.3	0.0	6.6	3.4	0.9
19714	Sweet, Frosting, Glaze, homemade	1/12 recipe	27	96.9	0.2	19.8	0.0	2.1	0.9	0.6
919377	Sweet, Frosting, Sour Cream flavor, RTE	1/12 package	38	156.6	0.0	25.7	0.0	6.5	3.4	0.9
19715	Sweet, Frosting, Vanilla, Creamy, RTE	1/12 package	38	159.2	0.0	26.4	0.0	6.4	3.3	0.9
19712	Sweet, Frosting, White, fluffy, dry mix prep w/H2O	1/12 package	26	63.4	0.4	16.3	0.0	0.0	0.0	0.0
19172	Sweet, Fruit Butter, Apple	1 tbsp	17	29.4	0.1	7.3	0.3	0.0	0.0	0.0
19703	Sweet, Gelatin, dry mix, low kcal w/aspartame, prep w/H2O	1 cup	234	16.4	2.6	1.6	0.0	0.0	0.0	0.0
19296	Sweet, Gelatin, dry, prep w/H2O	1 cup	270	159.3	3.2	37.8	0.0	0.0	0.0	0.0
19283	Sweet, Honey, strained/extracted	1 tbsp	21	63.8	0.1	17.3	0.0	0.0	0.0	0.0
19717	Sweet, Ice Popsicle	1 double stick	128	92.2	0.0	24.2	0.0	0.0	0.0	0.0
19280	Sweet, Ices/Sorbet, pineapple-coconut	1 tbsp	12.4	14.0	0.0	3.0	0.1	0.3	0.0	0.0
918860	Sweet, Ices/Sorbet/Water, fruit, low kcal w/aspartame	1 bar	51	12.2	0.3	3.2	0.0	0.1	0.0	0.0
919905	Sweet, Italian Ice, restaurant-prep	1.0 fl oz	29	15.4	0.0	3.9	0.0	0.0	0.0	0.0
19297	Sweet, Jam, low kcal	1 tbsp	6	18.0	0.0	5.1	0.5	0.0	0.0	0.0
19719	Sweet, Jams & Preserves	1 tbsp	20	48.4	0.1	12.9	0.2	0.0	0.0	0.0
919907	Sweet, Jellies	1 tbsp	19	51.5	0.1	13.5	0.2	0.0	0.0	0.0
919906	Sweet, Jelly, low kcal	1.0 oz	28	4.2	0.0	1.0	0.5	0.0	0.0	0.0
19303	Sweet, Maraschino Cherry	1.0 oz	28	96.0	0.1	24.6	0.3	0.1	0.0	0.1
19304	Sweet, Marmalade, orange	1 tbsp	20	49.2	0.1	13.3	0.2	0.0	0.0	0.0
19305	Sweet, Molasses	1 tbsp	20	53.2	0.0	13.8	0.0	0.0	0.0	0.0
19251	Sweet, Pectin, unsweetened, dry mix	¼ package	12	39.0	0.0	10.8	1.0	0.0	0.0	0.0
19334	Sweet, Solo Poppy Seed Filling/Sokol	1 tbsp	18	59.7	0.9	10.5	0.0	1.6	0.2	1.0
19335	Sweet, Sugar, brown	1 tsp, packed	4.6	17.3	0.0	4.5	0.0	0.0	0.0	0.0
19340	Sweet, Sugar, granulated, white	1 tsp	4.2	16.3	0.0	4.2	0.0	0.0	0.0	0.0
19336	Sweet, Sugar, Maple	1 piece (1 oz/1.75 x 1.25 x 0.5")	28	99.1	0.0	25.5	0.0	0.1	0.0	0.0
19113	Sweet, Sugar, powdered/confectioner's, white	1 tsp	2.5	9.7	0.0	2.5	0.0	0.0	0.0	0.0

Sat (g)	Chol (mg)	Cal (mg)	Iron (mg)	Magn (mg)	Phos (mg)	Pota (mg)	Sodi (mg)	Zinc (mg)	Vit A (RE)	Vit C (mg)	Vit E (mg)	Thia (mg)	Ribo (mg)	Niac (mg)	Vit B-6 (mg)	Fol (μg)	Vit B-12 (μg)	Wat (g)
2.0	9.6	33.6	0.6	2.4	36.0	86.4	969.6	0.6	55.2	0.2	0.2	0.0	0.1	0.8	0.0	1.7	0.1	217.5
2.4	2.4	46.4	0.5	4.9	48.8	100.0	880.8	0.6	0.0	1.0	1.2	0.0	0.1	0.7	0.0	4.9	0.0	220.4
1.5	14.6	34.2	0.6	4.9	36.6	119.6	927.2	0.1	29.3	1.2	0.0	0.1	0.1	0.5	0.0	6.8	0.0	220.8
1.2	4.9	19.5	0.5	2.4	46.4	136.6	1000.4	0.6	29.3	0.0	0.0	0.0	0.0	0.5	0.0	2.9	0.0	225.7
3.2	17.1	17.1	0.5	9.8	31.7	58.6	976.0	0.8	14.6	0.0	0.8	0.0	0.0	0.4	0.0	3.7	0.6	225.0
1.4	0.0	31.2	0.5	10.4	54.6	96.2	1170.0	0.3	2.6	3.9	1.2	1.2	0.1	0.5	0.0	7.8	0.1	237.1
6.3	0.0	0.0	2.2	0.0	0.0	0.0	1433.6	0.0	0.0	0.0	0.0	0.0	0.0	0.0	0.0	0.0	0.0	3.8
0.0	0.0	24.4	1.0	7.3	36.6	224.5	739.3	0.2	261.1	7.1	0.5	0.0	0.0	0.9	0.1	9.8	0.0	228.8
1.4	0.0	27.5	2.0	40.0	125.0	190.0	917.5	1.7	20.0	1.8	0.1	0.1	0.1	1.2	0.1	1.8	0.0	208.7
0.4	14.2	5.9	0.5	0.0	0.0	0.0	591.4	0.0	0.0	0.1	0.0	0.1	0.1	1.3	0.0	17.0	0.0	0.6
1.1	7.4	42.2	2.7	22.3	183.5	357.1	1319.4	0.7	34.7	4.2	0.0	0.2	0.1	1.4	0.2	49.6	0.3	212.7
0.4	2.4	26.8	1.6	12.2	41.5	187.9	578.3	1.0	97.6	3.9	0.7	0.0	0.0	0.8	0.1	9.8	4.1	224.2
0.4	0.0	38.6	1.7	31.3	86.8	306.1	470.0	0.7	135.0	0.7	0.7	0.1	0.1	1.0	0.1	60.3	0.0	208.9
0.0	0.0	78.0	0.6	0.0	0.0	56.0	754.0	0.0	270.8	5.0	0.0	0.0	0.1	0.3	0.0	0.0	0.0	0.0
0.4	4.9	43.9	1.5	7.3	53.7	146.4	915.0	0.8	0.0	2.0	0.1	0.0	0.0	1.0	0.1	3.7	8.0	220.9
0.6	14.4	3.4	0.5	0.0	0.0	0.0	723.8	0.0	0.0	0.1	0.0	0.2	0.1	1.0	0.0	19.8	0.0	0.6
0.3	0.0	26.5	0.7	2.4	12.1	67.5	1053.2	0.6	0.0	1.2	0.3	0.0	0.0	0.6	0.0	15.2	0.0	224.3
1.8	7.6	22.8	2.3	48.1	212.5	399.7	1006.9	1.3	45.5	1.5	0.0	0.1	0.1	1.5	0.1	2.5	0.3	206.9
1.6	7.2	33.6	2.1	38.4	177.6	304.8	964.8	3.1	487.2	7.0	0.1	0.1	0.1	2.5	0.2	4.6	0.2	194.3
0.5	2.5	22.2	0.8	4.9	34.6	331.0	815.1	0.5	76.6	14.8	0.8	0.1	0.0	1.1	0.1	13.6	0.0	217.6
0.4	0.0	7.6	0.6	20.2	30.4	103.7	1146.1	0.2	20.2	6.1	0.8	0.1	0.0	0.8	0.1	10.1	0.0	236.6
0.4	0.0	12.2	1.8	7.3	34.2	263.5	695.4	0.2	68.3	66.4	2.5	0.1	0.1	1.4	0.1	14.6	0.0	220.5
2.9	17.4	158.7	1.8	22.3	148.8	448.9	744.0	0.3	109.1	67.7	2.6	0.1	0.2	1.5	0.2	20.8	0.4	209.8
0.6	5.0	12.6	1.0	5.0	50.2	77.8	838.3	0.6	30.1	0.3	0.1	0.1	0.1	1.4	0.0	20.1	0.2	233.4
0.9	2.4	16.8	0.8	4.8	40.8	175.2	902.4	0.6	242.4	0.0	0.1	0.0	0.0	1.0	0.0	4.8	0.2	222.9
1.2	9.4	49.6	1.9	23.6	103.8	361.1	922.8	2.1	715.1	6.4	0.0	0.0	0.1	3.6	0.3	11.1	2.1	203.8
0.6	0.0	55.2	1.6	7.2	72.0	396.0	1010.4	3.1	588.0	6.0	0.6	0.1	0.1	1.2	0.2	16.6	0.0	210.2
0.3	0.0	21.7	1.1	7.2	33.7	209.7	821.8	0.5	301.3	1.4	0.8	0.1	0.0	0.9	0.1	10.6	0.0	222.5
5.2	37.1	27.8	1.6	32.5	127.6	403.7	946.6	1.9	494.2	10.2	0.2	0.2	0.1	2.9	0.3	25.5	0.9	189.1
4.4	71.0	29.0	2.9	0.0	184.0	613.0	292.0	5.3	1138.0	17.0	0.0	0.1	0.2	4.7	0.3	37.0	0.0	0.0
0.0	0.0	29.0	1.2	0.0	109.0	315.0	1055.0	0.0	1463.4	5.0	0.0	0.0	0.1	3.4	0.0	0.0	0.0	0.0
1.7	0.0	27.8	0.6	16.1	31.0	242.9	164.8	0.2	40.7	20.7	0.0	0.1	0.0	0.6	0.1	17.1	0.0	86.6
0.6	0.0	0.0	2.6	0.0	0.0	0.0	1125.6	0.0	0.0	0.0	0.0	0.0	0.0	0.0	0.0	0.0	0.0	4.2
0.0	0.0	0.0	0.0	0.0	0.0	0.1	0.1	0.0	0.0	0.0	0.0	0.0	0.0	0.0	0.0	0.0	0.0	0.4
0.0	0.0	0.0	0.0	0.0	0.0	0.0	0.0	0.0	0.0	0.0	0.0	0.0	0.0	0.0	0.0	0.0	0.0	0.0
1.7	21.6	33.5	0.2	5.4	27.8	38.9	101.4	0.2	21.9	0.1	0.0	0.0	0.0	0.2	0.0	12.2	0.1	8.3
2.6	54.8	59.8	1.3	14.1	63.1	92.1	317.9	0.5	53.1	1.7	3.6	0.3	0.2	2.0	0.1	43.2	0.1	20.6
0.0	0.0	0.0	0.0	0.0	0.0	0.0	3.6	0.0	0.0	0.0	0.0	0.0	0.0	0.0	0.0	0.0	0.0	7.5
8.7	0.0	23.0	2.0	86.0	113.0	245.0	1.0	1.0	3.4	0.0	0.0	0.0	0.1	0.4	0.0	3.0	0.0	0.4
0.0	0.0	0.0	0.0	0.0	0.0	0.1	0.2	0.0	0.0	0.0	0.0	0.0	0.0	0.0	0.0	0.0	0.0	0.1
0.0	0.0	5.0	0.0	0.0	0.0	0.0	0.0	0.0	0.0	0.0	0.0	0.0	0.0	0.0	0.0	0.0	0.0	0.0
0.4	0.0	6.9	0.7	26.9	39.6	82.3	1.1	0.4	0.1	0.0	0.0	0.0	0.0	0.1	0.0	1.7	0.0	0.2
2.1	0.0	3.0	0.5	8.0	22.4	74.5	69.5	0.1	0.0	0.0	0.0	0.0	0.0	0.0	0.0	0.0	0.0	6.5
1.9	0.0	1.1	0.1	0.8	1.1	13.3	90.1	0.0	44.1	0.0	0.0	0.0	0.0	0.0	0.0	0.0	0.0	5.7
0.5	0.5	5.9	0.0	0.8	4.9	8.1	25.4	0.0	21.9	0.1	0.2	0.0	0.0	0.0	0.0	0.3	0.0	4.8
1.9	0.0	0.8	0.0	0.8	1.5	73.7	77.5	0.0	46.4	0.0	0.0	0.0	0.0	0.3	0.0	0.4	0.0	5.4
1.9	0.0	1.1	0.0	0.4	14.8	14.1	34.2	0.0	85.9	0.0	1.8	0.0	0.0	0.0	0.0	0.0	0.0	5.0
0.0	0.0	1.0	0.0	0.5	1.3	20.0	40.6	0.0	0.0	0.0	0.0	0.0	0.0	0.2	0.0	0.5	0.0	9.2
0.0	0.0	2.4	0.1	0.9	1.7	15.5	15.5	0.7	2.0	0.1	0.0	0.0	0.0	0.0	0.0	0.2	0.0	9.6
0.0	0.0	4.7	0.0	2.3	63.2	0.0	112.3	0.1	0.0	0.0	0.0	0.0	0.0	0.0	0.0	0.0	0.0	229.3
0.0	0.0	5.4	0.1	2.7	59.4	2.7	113.4	0.1	0.0	0.0	0.0	0.0	0.0	0.0	0.0	0.0	0.0	228.4
0.0	0.0	1.3	0.1	0.4	0.8	10.9	0.8	0.0	0.0	0.1	0.0	0.0	0.0	0.0	0.0	0.4	0.0	3.6
0.0	0.0	0.0	0.0	1.3	0.0	5.1	15.4	0.0	0.0	0.0	0.0	0.0	0.0	0.0	0.0	0.0	0.0	102.4
0.3	0.0	0.0	0.4	0.6	1.1	2.1	4.3	0.0	0.0	1.6	0.0	0.0	0.0	0.0	0.0	0.1	0.0	9.1
0.0	0.0	1.0	0.1	1.0	0.0	13.3	2.6	0.0	0.0	0.0	0.0	0.0	0.0	0.0	0.0	0.0	0.0	47.5
0.0	0.0	0.3	0.0	0.0	0.0	1.7	1.2	0.0	0.0	0.1	0.0	0.0	0.0	0.2	0.0	1.5	0.0	25.1
0.0	0.0	1.0	0.0	0.0	8.0	9.0	7.0	0.0	0.0	0.0	0.0	0.0	0.0	0.0	0.0	1.0	0.0	3.8
0.0	0.0	4.0	0.1	0.8	2.2	15.4	8.0	0.0	0.2	1.8	0.0	0.0	0.0	0.0	0.0	6.6	0.0	6.9
0.0	0.0	1.5	0.0	1.1	1.0	12.2	6.8	0.0	0.4	0.2	0.0	0.0	0.0	0.0	0.0	0.2	0.0	5.4
0.0	0.0	1.0	0.0	0.0	8.0	20.0	4.0	0.0	0.0	0.0	0.0	0.0	0.0	0.0	0.0	5.0	0.0	0.0
0.0	0.0	0.0	0.0	0.0	0.0	0.0	0.0	0.0	0.0	0.0	0.0	0.0	0.0	0.0	0.0	0.0	0.0	3.4
0.0	0.0	7.6	0.0	0.4	1.2	7.4	11.2	0.0	1.0	1.0	0.0	0.0	0.0	0.0	0.0	7.2	0.0	6.6
0.0	0.0	41.0	0.9	48.4	6.2	292.8	7.4	0.1	0.0	0.0	0.0	0.0	0.2	0.1	0.0	0.0	0.0	5.2
0.0	0.0	0.8	0.3	0.1	0.2	0.8	24.0	0.0	0.0	0.0	0.0	0.0	0.0	0.0	0.0	0.1	0.0	1.0
0.2	0.0	58.0	0.0	0.0	0.0	0.0	13.3	0.0	0.0	0.0	0.0	0.0	0.0	0.0	0.0	0.0	0.0	4.8
0.0	0.0	3.9	0.1	1.3	1.0	15.9	1.8	0.0	0.0	0.0	0.0	0.0	0.0	0.0	0.0	0.0	0.0	0.1
0.0	0.0	0.0	0.0	0.0	0.1	0.1	0.1	0.0	0.0	0.0	0.0	0.0	0.0	0.0	0.0	0.0	0.0	0.0
0.0	0.0	25.2	0.5	5.3	0.8	76.7	3.1	1.7	0.6	0.0	0.0	0.0	0.0	0.0	0.0	0.0	0.0	2.2
0.0	0.0	0.0	0.0	0.0	0.1	0.1	0.0	0.0	0.0	0.0	0.0	0.0	0.0	0.0	0.0	0.0	0.0	0.0

Code	Food Name	Unit/Amt	Wt (g)	Energy (Kcal)	Prot (g)	Carb (g)	Fiber (g)	Fat (g)	Mono (g)	Poly (g)
19349	Sweet, Syrup, Chocolate, fudge-type	1 tbsp	17	59.5	0.8	10.7	0.5	1.5	0.7	0.0
19351	Sweet, Syrup, Corn, dark	1 tbsp	20	56.4	0.0	15.3	0.0	0.0	0.0	0.0
19362	Sweet, Syrup, Corn, light	1 tbsp	20	56.4	0.0	15.3	0.0	0.0	0.0	0.0
19129	Sweet, Syrup, Maple	1 tbsp	20	52.4	0.0	13.4	0.0	0.0	0.0	0.0
19360	Sweet, Syrup, pancake	1 tbsp	20	57.4	0.0	15.1	0.0	0.0	0.0	0.0
19355	Sweet, Syrup, pancake, reduced-kcal	¼ cup	60	98.4	0.0	26.6	0.0	0.0	0.0	0.0
19365	Sweet, Topping, Butterscotch or Caramel	tbsp	20.5	51.7	0.3	13.5	0.2	0.0	0.0	0.0
19367	Sweet, Topping, Marshmallow Cream	1.0 oz	28	90.2	0.2	22.1	0.0	0.1	0.0	0.0
19137	Sweet, Topping, Pineapple	2 tbsp	42	106.3	0.0	27.9	0.4	0.0	0.0	0.0
919984	Sweet, Topping, strawberry	1 tbsp	21	53.3	0.0	13.9	0.2	0.0	0.0	0.0
924200	Syrups, Chocolate, Genuine Chocolate Flavor,lite/Hershey	1 tbsp	17.5	25.0	0.3	5.8	0.4	0.1	0.0	0.0
924201	Taco	6.0 oz	171	369.4	20.7	26.7	2.0	20.6	6.6	1.0
18386	Toaster Muffin, Blueberry	1 toaster muffin	33	103.3	1.5	17.6	0.6	3.1	0.7	1.8
918387	Toaster Muffin, Corn	1 toaster muffin	33	114.2	1.7	19.1	0.5	3.7	0.9	2.1
18493	Toaster Pastry, Pop Tart, Brown Sugar Cinnamon/Kellogg	1 pastry	50	219.0	2.7	32.2	0.8	9.2	3.6	4.6
18480	Toaster Pastry, Pop Tart, Cherry, low fat/Kellogg	1 pastry	52	191.9	2.3	39.8	0.6	2.9	1.6	0.7
18477	Toaster Pastry, Pop Tart, Frosted Apple Cinnamon, low fat/Kellogg	1 pastry	52	191.4	2.2	40.0	0.6	2.9	1.5	0.8
18479	Toaster Pastry, Pop Tart, Frosted Brown Sugar Cinnamon, low fat/Kellogg	1 pastry	50	188.0	2.4	39.2	0.6	2.8	1.5	0.7
18481	Toaster Pastry, Pop Tart, Frosted Brown Sugar Cinnamon/Kellogg	1 pastry	50	211.0	2.5	34.2	0.7	7.4	3.9	2.4
18489	Toaster Pastry, Pop Tart, Frosted Strawberry, low fat/Kellogg	1 pastry	52	190.8	2.1	40.3	0.6	3.0	1.4	1.0
18490	Toaster Pastry, Pop Tart, Frosted Strawberry/Kellogg	1 pastry	52	202.8	2.3	37.6	0.5	5.0	2.9	0.7
11693	Toaster Pastry/Pop Tart, Fruit (Apple/Blueberry/Cherry/Strawberry)	1 Pop Tart	52	204.4	2.4	37.0	1.1	5.3	2.2	2.0
18363	Tomato, crushed, canned	½ cup	50	16.0	0.8	3.6	1.0	0.1	0.0	0.1
18449	Tortilla, Corn, ready-to-cook	1 medium tortilla (6" dia)	26	57.7	1.5	12.1	1.4	0.7	0.2	0.3
18616	Tortilla, Flour, ready-to-cook	1 12" diameter	75	243.8	6.5	41.7	2.5	5.3	2.8	0.8
18360	Tortilla, Flour, w/o added calcium, ready to cook	1 8" diameter	50	162.5	4.4	27.8	1.7	3.6	1.9	0.5
18448	Tortilla, Taco Shell, baked	1 large (6.5" dia)	21	98.3	1.5	13.1	1.6	4.7	1.9	1.8
5600	Tuna Helper	1 serving	184	301.8	14.4	29.4	0.0	14.0	0.0	0.0
924187	Turkey Patty, breaded, fried	1 patty	94	266.0	13.2	14.8	0.5	16.9	7.0	4.4
5296	Turkey Pot Pie, frozen/Swanson	7.0 oz	198	380.2	10.9	36.1	0.0	21.4	0.0	0.0
5295	Turkey Roast, Light & Dark Meat, no bone, frozen, seasoned, ckd	3.5 oz	100	155.0	21.3	3.1	0.0	5.8	1.2	1.7
5189	Turkey w/gravy, frozen	1 pkg (5.0 oz)	142	95.1	8.3	6.5	0.0	3.7	1.4	0.7
5293	Turkey, Breaded Turkey Nuggets w/USDA commodity meat, cooked/ Pierre product #193	3.5 oz	100	347.0	18.2	10.2	0.3	25.8	7.5	11.3
924210	Turkey, Breast w/skin, roasted	3.5 oz	100	189.0	28.7	0.0	0.0	7.4	2.5	1.8
5187	Turkey, Dark Meat w/skin, roasted	3.5 oz	100	221.0	27.5	0.0	0.0	11.5	3.7	3.1
51619	Turkey, Dark Meat, no skin, roasted	3.5 oz	100	187.0	28.6	0.0	0.0	7.2	1.6	2.2
5211	Turkey, Fryer/Roaster, Dark Meat w/skin, roasted	3.5 oz	100	182.0	27.7	0.0	0.0	7.1	2.3	1.9
5221	Turkey, Fryer/Roaster, Dark Meat, no skin, roasted	3.5 oz	100	162.0	28.8	0.0	0.0	4.3	1.0	1.3
5209	Turkey, Fryer/Roaster, Light Meat w/skin, roasted	3.5 oz	100	164.0	28.8	0.0	0.0	4.6	1.7	1.1
5201	Turkey, Fryer/Roaster, Light Meat, no skin, roasted	3.5 oz	100	140.0	30.2	0.0	0.0	1.2	0.2	0.3
51617	Turkey, Fryer/Roaster, Wing, no skin, roasted	3.5 oz	100	163.0	30.9	0.0	0.0	3.4	0.6	0.9
5305	Turkey, Ground, cooked	3.5 oz	100	235.0	27.4	0.0	0.0	13.2	4.9	3.2
5285	Turkey, Leg w/skin, roasted	3.5 oz	100	208.0	27.9	0.0	0.0	9.8	2.9	2.7
5181	Turkey, Light & Dark Meat, diced, seasoned	3.5 oz	100	138.0	18.7	1.0	0.0	6.0	2.0	1.5
5185	Turkey, Light Meat w/skin, roasted	3.5 oz	100	197.0	28.6	0.0	0.0	8.3	2.8	2.0
5165	Turkey, Light Meat, no skin, roasted	3.5 oz	100	157.0	29.9	0.0	0.0	3.2	0.6	0.9
5294	Turkey, Smoked	3.5 oz	100	118.0	19.6	0.7	0.0	3.9	1.4	1.1
5245	Turkey, Wing w/skin, roasted	3.5 oz	100	229.0	27.4	0.0	0.0	12.4	4.7	2.9
17089	Veal, Breast, Whole, boneless, lean, braised	3.5 oz	100	218.0	30.3	0.0	0.0	9.8	4.5	0.8
17138	Veal, Sirloin, lean&fat, roasted	6.0 oz	170	343.4	42.7	0.0	0.0	17.8	6.9	1.2
11886	Vege Juice, Carrot, canned	6.0 oz	184	73.6	1.7	17.1	1.5	0.3	0.0	0.1
11001	Vege Juice, Tomato, canned w/o salt	6.0 oz	184	31.3	1.4	7.8	1.5	0.1	0.0	0.1
11004	Vege, Alfalfa Seeds, sprouted, raw	1 cup	33	9.6	1.3	1.2	0.8	0.2	0.0	0.1
11009	Vege, Artichokes (Globe or French) boiled, drained, no salt	1 medium	300	150.0	10.4	33.5	16.2	0.5	0.0	0.2
11705	Vege, Arugula/Roquette, raw	1 cup	20	5.0	0.5	0.7	0.3	0.1	0.0	0.1
11015	Vege, Asparagus, boiled, drained	½ cup	90	21.6	2.3	3.8	1.4	0.3	0.0	0.1
11707	Vege, Asparagus, canned, drained	½ cup	90	17.1	1.9	2.2	1.4	0.6	0.0	0.3
11011	Vege, Asparagus, frozen, boiled, drained, no salt	4 spears	60	16.8	1.8	2.9	1.0	0.3	0.0	0.1
11028	Vege, Bamboo Shoots, canned, drained	½ cup	60	7.2	0.9	1.2	0.6	0.1	0.0	0.1
11045	Vege, Bean Sprouts, Mung, mature seeds, sprouted, stir fried	½ cup	30	3.6	0.4	0.6	0.2	0.0	0.0	0.0
11046	Vege, Bean Sprouts, Navy, mature seeds, sprouted, raw	1 cup	120	93.6	8.5	18.0	0.0	1.0	0.1	0.6
11052	Vege, Beans, Snap, Green, raw	1 cup	125	35.0	1.9	8.1	3.8	0.2	0.0	0.1
11722	Vege, Beans, Snap, Yellow, raw	1 cup	135	37.8	2.0	8.7	4.1	0.2	0.0	0.1
11081	Vege, Beets, boiled, drained	½ cup	85	37.4	1.4	8.5	1.7	0.2	0.0	0.1
11090	Vege, Broccoli florets, raw	1 cup	88	63.4	4.9	10.3	3.7	0.5	0.0	0.3
22600	Vege, Broccoli in Cheese Flavored Sauce, frozen/GreenGiant	½ cup	142	39.8	4.2	7.4	0.0	0.5	0.0	0.2
11095	Vege, Broccoli Spears, frozen, boiled, drained, no salt	½ cup	78	21.8	2.4	4.2	2.3	0.1	0.0	0.0
11093	Vege, Broccoli, chopped, frozen, boiled, drained, no salt	½ cup	84	23.5	2.6	4.5	2.5	0.1	0.0	0.0

Sat (g)	Chol (mg)	Cal (mg)	Iron (mg)	Magn (mg)	Phos (mg)	Pota (mg)	Sodi (mg)	Zinc (mg)	Vit A (RE)	Vit C (mg)	Vit E (mg)	Thia (mg)	Ribo (mg)	Niac (mg)	Vit B-6 (mg)	Fol (μg)	Vit B-12 (μg)	Wat (g)
0.7	0.3	13.8	0.2	8.7	23.0	61.5	58.8	0.1	0.7	0.0	0.5	0.0	0.0	0.1	0.0	0.7	0.0	3.7
0.0	0.0	3.6	0.1	1.6	2.2	8.8	31.0	0.0	0.0	0.0	0.0	0.0	0.0	0.0	0.0	0.0	0.0	4.6
0.0	0.0	0.6	0.0	0.4	0.4	0.8	24.2	0.0	0.0	0.0	0.0	0.0	0.0	0.0	0.0	0.0	0.0	4.6
0.0	0.0	13.4	0.2	2.8	0.4	40.8	1.8	0.8	0.0	0.0	0.0	0.0	0.0	0.0	0.0	0.0	0.0	6.4
0.0	0.0	0.2	0.0	0.4	1.8	0.4	16.6	0.0	0.0	0.0	0.0	0.0	0.0	0.0	0.0	0.0	0.0	4.8
0.0	0.0	0.6	0.0	0.0	25.8	1.8	120.0	0.0	0.0	0.0	0.0	0.0	0.0	0.0	0.0	0.0	0.0	32.9
0.0	0.2	10.9	0.0	1.4	9.6	17.2	71.5	0.0	5.5	0.1	0.0	0.0	0.0	0.0	0.0	0.4	0.0	6.6
0.0	0.0	0.8	0.1	0.6	2.2	1.4	13.7	0.0	0.0	0.0	0.0	0.0	0.0	0.0	0.0	0.3	0.0	5.5
0.0	0.0	9.2	0.2	0.8	3.4	133.1	26.5	0.2	0.8	24.6	0.0	0.0	0.0	0.0	0.0	1.3	0.0	13.9
0.0	0.0	5.0	0.2	0.8	2.7	15.3	4.4	0.1	0.4	5.2	0.0	0.0	0.0	0.1	0.0	0.0	0.0	6.9
0.0	0.0	1.9	0.0	2.6	4.0	13.5	24.0	0.0	0.0	0.0	0.0	0.0	0.0	0.0	0.0	0.2	0.0	11.3
11.4	57.0	221.0	2.4	71.0	203.0	473.0	802.0	3.9	147.0	2.0	0.0	0.2	0.1	3.2	0.2	23.0	1.0	99.9
0.5	2.0	4.3	0.2	4.0	19.5	27.4	157.7	0.1	22.1	0.0	0.6	0.1	0.1	0.7	0.0	18.2	0.0	10.2
0.6	4.3	6.3	0.5	4.6	49.8	30.4	141.9	0.1	6.6	0.0	0.0	0.1	0.1	0.8	0.0	18.8	0.0	7.8
1.0	0.0	15.5	1.8	8.0	31.5	67.5	214.0	0.6	0.0	0.0	0.0	0.2	0.2	2.0	0.2	40.0	0.0	5.3
0.6	0.0	5.7	1.8	4.7	22.4	29.6	221.5	0.2	0.0	0.0	0.0	0.2	0.2	2.0	0.2	52.0	0.0	6.5
0.6	0.0	5.7	1.8	4.7	21.3	28.1	205.9	0.2	0.0	0.0	0.0	0.2	0.2	2.0	0.2	52.0	0.0	6.5
0.6	0.0	7.0	1.8	5.0	22.5	30.5	209.5	0.2	0.0	0.0	0.0	0.2	0.2	2.0	0.2	50.0	0.0	5.3
1.1	0.0	14.5	1.8	7.5	46.5	55.5	184.5	1.2	0.0	0.0	0.0	0.2	0.2	2.0	0.2	40.0	0.0	5.3
0.6	0.0	5.2	1.8	4.2	20.3	25.5	201.2	0.2	0.0	0.0	0.0	0.2	0.2	2.0	0.2	52.0	0.0	6.5
1.4	0.0	11.4	1.8	5.2	26.5	44.2	169.0	0.2	0.0	0.0	0.0	0.2	0.2	2.0	0.2	52.0	0.0	6.5
0.8	0.0	13.5	1.8	9.4	57.7	58.2	217.9	0.3	1.6	0.3	1.2	0.2	0.2	2.0	0.2	33.8	0.0	6.4
0.0	0.0	17.0	0.7	10.0	16.0	146.5	66.0	0.1	35.0	4.6	0.3	0.0	0.0	0.6	0.1	6.5	0.0	44.7
0.1	0.0	45.5	0.4	16.9	81.6	40.0	41.9	0.2	0.0	0.0	0.0	0.0	0.0	0.4	0.1	29.6	0.0	11.5
1.3	0.0	93.8	2.5	19.5	93.0	98.3	358.5	0.5	0.0	0.0	0.7	0.4	0.2	2.7	0.0	92.3	0.0	20.1
0.9	0.0	19.5	1.7	13.0	62.0	65.5	239.0	0.4	0.0	0.0	0.5	0.3	0.1	1.8	0.0	61.5	0.0	13.4
0.7	0.0	33.6	0.5	22.1	52.1	37.6	77.1	0.3	0.0	0.0	0.8	0.0	0.0	0.3	0.1	22.1	0.0	1.3
0.0	0.0	0.0	0.0	0.0	0.0	239.0	916.0	0.0	0.0	0.0	0.0	0.0	0.0	0.0	0.0	0.0	0.0	126.2
4.4	58.3	13.2	2.1	14.1	253.8	258.5	752.0	1.4	10.3	0.0	2.2	0.1	0.2	2.2	0.2	26.3	0.2	46.7
0.0	0.0	29.0	2.4	0.0	0.0	138.0	719.0	0.0	393.4	2.0	0.0	0.3	0.2	3.1	0.0	0.0	0.0	0.0
1.9	53.0	5.0	1.6	22.0	244.0	298.0	680.0	2.5	0.0	0.0	0.4	0.0	0.2	6.3	0.3	5.0	1.5	67.8
1.2	25.6	19.9	1.3	11.4	115.0	86.6	786.7	1.0	18.5	0.0	0.0	0.0	0.2	2.6	0.1	5.7	0.3	120.8
5.1	57.0	28.0	1.9	15.0	205.0	178.0	567.0	1.9	0.0	0.0	2.8	0.2	0.2	4.3	0.2	22.0	0.2	44.2
2.1	74.0	21.0	1.4	27.0	210.0	288.0	63.0	2.0	0.0	0.0	0.0	0.1	0.1	6.4	0.5	6.0	0.4	63.2
3.5	89.0	33.0	2.3	23.0	196.0	274.0	76.0	4.2	0.0	0.0	0.6	0.1	0.2	3.5	0.3	9.0	0.4	60.2
2.4	85.0	32.0	2.3	24.0	204.0	290.0	79.0	4.5	0.0	0.0	0.6	0.1	0.2	3.6	0.4	9.0	0.4	63.1
2.1	117.0	27.0	2.3	23.0	190.0	237.0	76.0	3.8	0.0	0.0	0.0	0.0	0.2	3.4	0.3	9.0	0.4	64.8
1.5	112.0	26.0	2.4	24.0	196.0	246.0	79.0	4.1	0.0	0.0	0.0	0.1	0.2	3.5	0.4	10.0	0.4	66.4
1.3	95.0	18.0	1.6	26.0	205.0	262.0	57.0	2.1	0.0	0.0	0.0	0.0	0.1	6.3	0.5	6.0	0.4	66.5
0.4	86.0	15.0	1.6	28.0	216.0	277.0	56.0	2.1	0.0	0.0	0.0	0.0	0.1	6.9	0.6	6.0	0.4	68.6
1.1	102.0	26.0	1.8	22.0	174.0	204.0	78.0	3.8	0.0	0.0	0.1	0.0	0.2	4.1	0.6	7.0	0.4	65.6
3.4	102.0	25.0	1.9	24.0	196.0	270.0	107.0	2.9	0.0	0.0	0.3	0.1	0.2	4.8	0.4	7.0	0.4	59.4
3.1	85.0	32.0	2.3	23.0	199.0	280.0	77.0	4.3	0.0	0.0	0.6	0.1	0.2	3.6	0.4	9.0	0.4	61.2
1.8	55.0	1.0	1.8	17.0	240.0	310.0	850.0	2.0	0.0	0.0	0.0	0.0	0.1	4.8	0.3	5.0	0.2	71.7
2.3	76.0	21.0	1.4	26.0	208.0	285.0	63.0	2.0	0.0	0.0	0.1	0.1	0.1	6.3	0.5	6.0	0.4	62.8
1.0	69.0	19.0	1.4	28.0	219.0	305.0	64.0	2.0	0.0	0.0	0.1	0.1	0.1	6.8	0.5	6.0	0.4	66.3
1.4	42.9	7.1	0.5	92.9	260.7	271.4	996.4	1.9	0.0	0.0	0.0	0.0	0.1	3.6	0.4	0.0	0.7	256.8
3.4	81.0	24.0	1.5	25.0	197.0	266.0	61.0	2.1	0.0	0.0	0.2	0.1	0.1	5.7	0.4	6.0	0.3	59.5
3.7	116.0	9.0	0.8	22.0	208.0	289.0	68.0	4.2	0.0	0.0	0.4	0.1	0.3	9.0	0.3	15.0	1.5	59.7
7.7	173.4	22.1	1.6	44.2	379.1	596.7	141.1	5.7	0.0	0.0	0.7	0.1	0.6	15.1	0.5	25.5	2.4	106.5
0.0	0.0	44.2	0.8	25.8	77.3	537.3	53.4	0.3	2014.8	15.6	0.0	0.2	0.1	0.7	0.4	7.0	0.0	163.5
0.0	0.0	16.6	1.1	20.2	35.0	404.8	18.4	0.3	103.0	33.7	1.7	0.1	0.1	1.2	0.2	36.6	0.0	172.8
0.0	0.0	10.6	0.3	8.9	23.1	26.1	2.0	0.3	5.3	2.7	0.0	0.0	0.0	0.2	0.0	11.9	0.0	30.1
0.1	0.0	135.0	3.9	180.0	258.0	1062.0	285.0	1.5	54.0	30.0	0.6	0.2	0.2	3.0	0.3	153.0	0.0	251.9
0.0	0.0	32.0	0.3	9.4	10.4	73.8	5.4	0.1	47.4	3.0	0.1	0.0	0.0	0.1	0.0	19.4	0.0	18.3
0.1	0.0	18.0	0.7	9.0	48.6	144.0	9.9	0.4	48.6	9.7	0.3	0.1	0.1	1.0	0.1	131.4	0.0	83.0
0.1	0.0	14.4	1.6	9.0	38.7	154.8	258.3	0.4	47.7	16.6	0.4	0.1	0.1	0.9	0.1	86.0	0.0	84.6
0.1	0.0	13.8	0.4	7.8	33.0	130.8	2.4	0.3	49.2	14.6	0.8	0.0	0.1	0.6	0.0	80.8	0.0	54.7
0.0	0.0	7.2	0.1	1.8	12.0	319.8	2.4	0.3	0.0	0.0	0.0	0.0	0.0	0.2	0.1	1.4	0.0	57.6
0.0	0.0	4.2	0.1	2.7	9.6	8.1	42.0	0.1	0.6	0.1	0.0	0.0	0.0	0.1	0.0	2.9	0.0	28.8
0.1	0.0	19.2	2.5	133.2	123.6	380.4	16.8	1.2	0.0	20.8	0.0	0.5	0.3	1.5	0.2	127.6	0.0	91.2
0.1	0.0	61.3	1.1	30.0	38.8	157.5	11.3	0.6	50.0	5.1	0.2	0.0	0.1	0.5	0.1	28.8	0.0	114.3
0.1	0.0	66.2	1.2	32.4	41.9	170.1	12.2	0.6	14.9	5.5	0.2	0.0	0.1	0.5	0.1	31.1	0.0	123.4
0.0	0.0	13.6	0.7	19.6	32.3	259.3	242.3	0.3	3.4	3.1	0.0	0.0	0.0	0.3	0.1	68.0	0.0	74.0
0.1	0.0	19.4	1.7	33.4	83.6	220.0	44.0	0.5	30.8	29.0	0.0	0.1	0.1	1.3	0.0	84.7	0.0	71.3
0.1	0.0	68.2	1.2	35.5	93.7	461.5	38.3	0.6	426.0	132.3	2.4	0.1	0.2	0.9	0.2	100.8	0.0	128.8
0.0	0.0	39.8	0.5	15.6	42.9	140.4	202.8	0.2	147.4	31.3	1.3	0.0	0.1	0.4	0.1	23.4	0.0	70.8
0.0	0.0	42.8	0.5	16.8	46.2	151.2	218.4	0.3	158.8	33.7	1.4	0.0	0.1	0.4	0.1	47.4	0.0	76.2

Code	Food Name	Unit/Amt	Wt (g)	Energy (Kcal)	Prot (g)	Carb (g)	Fiber (g)	Fat (g)	Mono (g)	Poly (g)
11099	Vege, Brussels Sprouts, boiled, drained, no salt	½ cup, 4 sprouts	78	32.0	2.0	6.8	2.0	0.4	0.0	0.2
11110	Vege, Cabbage, boiled, drained, no salt	½ cup	60	13.2	0.6	2.7	1.7	0.3	0.0	0.1
11749	Vege, Cabbage, Common (Danish/Domestic/Pointed) Fresh Harvest, raw	1 cup	70	15.4	0.7	3.1	1.6	0.3	0.0	0.1
11970	Vege, Cabbage, Napa, cooked	½ cup	35	8.4	0.4	1.9	0.8	0.1	0.0	0.0
11960	Vege, Carrots, Baby, raw	1 cup, or 6 baby carrots	140	28.0	1.0	6.8	2.2	0.1	0.0	0.1
11128	Vege, Carrots, canned, drained	½ cup	73	32.9	0.8	7.7	2.4	0.1	0.0	0.1
11131	Vege, Carrots, frozen, boiled, drained, no salt	½ cup	73	26.3	0.9	6.0	2.6	0.1	0.0	0.0
11136	Vege, Cauliflower, boiled, drained, no salt	½ cup	62	14.3	1.1	2.5	1.7	0.3	0.0	0.1
11138	Vege, Cauliflower, frozen, boiled, drained, no salt	½ cup	62	11.8	1.0	2.3	1.7	0.1	0.0	0.1
11967	Vege, Cauliflower, green, cooked, no salt	½ cup	90	28.8	2.7	5.7	3.0	0.3	0.0	0.1
11965	Vege, Cauliflower, Green, head, raw	1 cup	100	32.0	3.0	6.3	3.3	0.3	0.0	0.1
11142	Vege, Celeriac, boiled, drained, no salt	½ cup	100	27.0	1.0	5.9	0.0	0.2	0.0	0.0
11143	Vege, Celery, raw	½ cup or 2 stalks	80	14.4	0.7	3.2	1.3	0.1	0.0	0.1
11148	Vege, Chard, Swiss, boiled, drained, no salt	½ cup	88	17.6	1.7	3.6	1.8	0.1	0.0	0.0
11162	Vege, Collards, boiled, drained, no salt	½ cup	74	19.2	1.6	3.6	2.1	0.3	0.0	0.1
11656	Vege, Corn Pudding, homemade	1 cup	250	232.5	7.8	55.8	7.0	1.9	0.5	0.9
11190	Vege, Corn Salad, raw	⅔ cup (#6 scoop)	167	182.0	7.3	21.3	0.0	8.9	2.9	1.1
11774	Vege, Corn, Yellow, kernels, frozen, boiled w/salt, drained	½ cup	82	52.5	1.6	12.6	1.4	0.4	0.1	0.2
11771	Vege, Corn, Yellow, Sweet, canned, solids & liquid, no added salt	½ cup	123	88.6	2.1	22.3	1.5	0.5	0.2	0.2
11174	Vege, Corn, Yellow, Sweet, cream style, regular pack, canned	½ cup	105	83.0	2.5	20.4	2.1	0.5	0.2	0.2
11179	Vege, Corn, Yellow, Sweet, kernels, frozen, boiled, drained, no salt	½ cup	84	73.9	2.5	17.5	2.0	0.6	0.2	0.3
11172	Vege, Corn, Yellow, Sweet, whole kernel, canned, drained	½ cup	84	67.2	2.3	16.4	2.0	0.4	0.1	0.2
11192	Vege, Cowpeas (Blackeyes), immature seeds, boiled, drained, no salt	½ cup	84	81.5	2.7	17.1	4.2	0.3	0.0	0.1
11205	Vege, Cucumber, raw	1 cup	40	4.8	0.2	1.0	0.3	0.1	0.0	0.0
11210	Vege, Eggplant (Brinjal) boiled, drained, no salt	½ cup, 1" cubes	99	27.7	0.8	6.6	2.5	0.2	0.0	0.1
11213	Vege, Endive (Escarole) raw	1 tbsp, 1" pieces	5.1	1.3	0.1	0.3	0.1	0.0	0.0	0.0
11957	Vege, Fennel Bulb, raw	1 cup	100	150.0	4.6	31.7	0.0	1.8	0.0	0.0
11950	Vege, Fungi, Mushroom, Enoki, raw	1 cup	28	79.5	2.6	20.4	19.6	0.2	0.0	0.0
11987	Vege, Fungi, Mushroom, Oyster, raw	1 medium: 3.35" long	3	1.0	0.1	0.2	0.1	0.0	0.0	0.0
11269	Vege, Fungi, Mushroom, Shiitake, ckd, no salt	½ cup, 4 mushrooms	72	39.6	1.1	10.3	1.5	0.2	0.0	0.0
11261	Vege, Fungi, Mushrooms, boiled, drained, no salt	1 mushroom	12	3.2	0.3	0.6	0.3	0.1	0.0	0.0
11260	Vege, Fungi, Mushrooms, slices, raw	10 slices	40	9.6	0.7	2.0	1.0	0.1	0.0	0.0
924135	Vege, Green Pepper, Stuffed, homemade	1 pepper	185	172.1	10.4	32.0	20.4	3.9	0.1	2.0
11961	Vege, Hearts of Palm, canned	½ cup	72	122.4	9.4	12.1	0.4	4.0	0.0	0.0
11971	Vege, Herb, Cilantro, raw	1 tbsp, chopped	8.1	2.3	0.2	0.4	0.2	0.1	0.0	0.0
11234	Vege, Kale, boiled, drained, no salt	½ cup	65	18.2	1.2	3.7	1.3	0.3	0.0	0.1
11242	Vege, Kohlrabi, boiled, drained, no salt	½ cup	85	24.7	1.5	5.7	0.9	0.1	0.0	0.0
11245	Vege, Lambsquarters, boiled, drained, no salt	1 tbsp, chopped	11.3	3.6	0.4	0.6	0.2	0.1	0.0	0.0
11246	Vege, Leeks (bulb & lower leaf-portion) raw	1 leek	124	38.4	1.0	9.4	1.2	0.2	0.0	0.1
11972	Vege, Lemon Grass (citronella), raw	1 leek	124	38.4	1.0	9.4	1.2	0.2	0.0	0.1
11250	Vege, Lettuce, Butterhead (Boston/Bibb) leaves, raw	3.5 grams	100	101.0	8.8	21.3	0.0	0.5	0.1	0.2
11251	Vege, Lettuce, Cos/Romaine, raw	1 small leaf	5	0.7	0.1	0.1	0.1	0.0	0.0	0.0
11252	Vege, Lettuce, Iceberg, head, raw	1 inner leaf	10	1.4	0.2	0.2	0.2	0.0	0.0	0.0
11253	Vege, Lettuce, Looseleaf, raw	1 small head	324	38.9	3.3	6.8	4.5	0.6	0.0	0.3
11796	Vege, Lotus Root, boiled w/salt, drained	1 cup, shredded	56	10.1	0.7	2.0	1.1	0.2	0.0	0.1
11974	Vege, Mushrooms, sauteed	1 tbsp, cubes	9.1	7.5	0.2	1.8	0.0	0.0	0.0	0.0
11805	Vege, Onions, boiled w/salt, chopped, drained	1 ring	10	40.7	0.5	3.8	0.1	2.7	1.1	0.5
11282	Vege, Onions, chopped, raw	1 tbsp, chopped	15	4.2	0.1	1.0	0.3	0.0	0.0	0.0
11291	Vege, Onions, Spring (tops & bulb) chopped, raw	1 tbsp	5	17.5	0.4	4.2	0.5	0.0	0.0	0.0
11298	Vege, Parsnip, peeled, raw	1 cup, slices	76	61.6	1.0	14.8	3.0	0.2	0.1	0.0
11318	Vege, Peas & Carrots, canned, regular pack, solids & liquid	½ cup	174	92.2	5.6	17.0	5.6	0.5	0.0	0.2
11323	Vege, Peas & Carrots, frozen, boiled, drained, no salt	½ cup	80	38.4	2.5	8.1	2.5	0.3	0.0	0.2
11301	Vege, Peas w/edible pod-Snow/Sugar, boiled, drained, no salt	½ cup	80	33.6	2.6	5.6	2.2	0.2	0.0	0.1
11305	Vege, Peas, Green, boiled, drained, no salt	½ cup	80	67.2	4.3	12.5	4.4	0.2	0.0	0.1
11308	Vege, Peas, Green, canned, regular pack, drained	½ cup	85	58.7	3.8	10.7	3.5	0.3	0.0	0.1
11980	Vege, Pepper, Chili, Green, canned	½ cup	62	16.7	1.0	3.3	2.1	0.3	0.0	0.2
11670	Vege, Pepper, Hot Chili, raw	½ cup	70	14.7	0.5	3.2	1.2	0.2	0.0	0.1
11632	Vege, Pepper, Jalapeno, canned, solids & liquid	1 pepper	27	7.8	0.2	1.8	0.0	0.1	0.0	0.1
11979	Vege, Pepper, Jalapeno, raw	½ cup chopped	85	23.0	0.8	4.0	2.2	0.8	0.0	0.4
11333	Vege, Pepper, Sweet, Green, chopped/sliced, raw	3.5 oz	100	18.0	1.0	3.9	0.9	0.2	0.0	0.1
11821	Vege, Pepper, Sweet, Red, raw	3.5 oz	100	18.0	1.0	3.9	0.0	0.2	0.0	0.1
11951	Vege, Pepper, Sweet, Yellow, raw	1 tbsp	9.3	2.5	0.1	0.6	0.2	0.0	0.0	0.0
11973	Vege, Pickles, Bread & Butter	10 strips	52	14.0	0.5	3.3	0.5	0.1	0.0	0.0
11937	Vege, Pickles, Cucumber, Dill	2 slices	15	13.2	1.2	2.6	0.0	0.1	0.0	0.1
11941	Vege, Pickles, Cucumber, Sour, slices/spears	1 large (4" long)	135	14.9	0.4	3.0	1.6	0.3	0.0	0.1 .
11940	Vege, Pickles, Cucumber, Sweet, Gherkins	1 large Gherkin (3" long)	35	3.9	0.1	0.8	0.4	0.1	0.0	0.0
11970	Vege, Pickles, Fresh Pack	1 medium	35	41.0	0.1	11.1	0.4	0.1	0.0	0.0
11975	Vege, Pickles, Kosher	2 slices	15	1.8	0.2	0.3	0.0	0.0	0.0	0.0
11976	Vege, Pickles, Sweet & Sour	1.0 oz	28	6.7	0.6	1.2	0.8	0.1	0.1	0.0

Sat (g)	Chol (mg)	Cal (mg)	Iron (mg)	Magn (mg)	Phos (mg)	Pota (mg)	Sodi (mg)	Zinc (mg)	Vit A (RE)	Vit C (mg)	Vit E (mg)	Thia (mg)	Ribo (mg)	Niac (mg)	Vit B-6 (mg)	Fol (µg)	Vit B-12 (µg)	Wat (g)
0.1	0.0	28.1	0.9	15.6	43.7	247.3	200.5	0.3	56.2	48.4	0.0	0.1	0.1	0.5	0.1	46.8	0.0	68.1
0.0	0.0	18.6	0.1	4.8	9.0	58.2	153.0	0.1	7.8	12.1	0.0	0.0	0.0	0.2	0.1	12.0	0.0	56.2
0.0	0.0	21.7	0.1	5.6	10.5	67.9	5.6	0.1	9.1	14.1	0.1	0.0	0.0	0.2	0.1	14.0	0.0	65.5
0.0	0.0	16.5	0.2	5.3	8.1	86.1	6.3	0.1	4.6	14.7	0.0	0.0	0.0	0.1	0.0	19.8	0.0	32.4
0.0	0.0	98.0	1.0	58.8	32.2	560.0	238.0	0.2	16.8	2.8	0.0	0.0	0.0	0.4	0.1	39.6	0.0	131.6
0.0	0.0	22.6	0.5	9.5	21.9	165.7	48.2	0.2	1792.2	1.7	0.3	0.0	0.0	0.4	0.2	10.1	0.0	63.8
0.0	0.0	20.4	0.3	7.3	19.0	115.3	215.4	0.2	1292.1	2.0	0.0	0.0	0.0	0.3	0.1	7.9	0.0	65.6
0.0	0.0	9.9	0.2	5.6	19.8	88.0	150.0	0.1	1.2	27.5	0.0	0.0	0.0	0.3	0.1	27.3	0.0	57.7
0.0	0.0	10.5	0.3	5.6	14.9	86.2	157.5	0.1	1.2	19.4	0.0	0.0	0.0	0.2	0.1	25.4	0.0	58.3
0.0	0.0	28.8	0.6	17.1	51.3	250.2	233.1	0.6	12.6	65.3	0.0	0.1	0.1	0.6	0.2	36.9	0.0	80.5
0.0	0.0	32.0	0.7	19.0	57.0	278.0	23.0	0.6	14.0	72.6	0.0	0.1	0.1	0.7	0.2	41.0	0.0	89.5
0.0	0.0	26.0	0.4	12.0	66.0	173.0	297.0	0.2	0.0	3.6	0.0	0.0	0.0	0.4	0.1	3.4	0.0	92.3
0.0	0.0	33.6	0.3	9.6	20.0	227.2	72.8	0.1	10.4	4.9	0.3	0.0	0.0	0.3	0.1	17.6	0.0	75.3
0.0	0.0	51.0	2.0	75.7	29.0	483.1	365.2	0.3	276.3	15.8	0.0	0.1	0.1	0.3	0.1	7.6	0.0	81.5
0.0	0.0	88.1	0.3	12.6	19.2	192.4	186.5	0.3	231.6	13.5	0.7	0.0	0.1	0.4	0.1	68.8	0.0	68.0
0.3	0.0	7.5	1.5	72.5	187.5	627.5	10.0	1.6	52.5	12.0	0.0	0.4	0.2	3.8	0.6	76.3	0.0	183.0
4.2	167.0	66.8	0.9	25.1	95.2	268.9	91.9	0.8	60.1	4.7	0.0	0.7	0.2	1.6	0.2	42.3	0.2	127.5
0.1	0.0	3.3	0.3	13.1	41.8	134.5	174.7	0.3	0.0	4.5	0.0	0.0	0.1	0.8	0.0	31.2	0.0	66.7
0.1	0.0	3.7	0.5	20.9	62.7	164.8	3.7	0.7	12.3	5.7	0.1	0.0	0.1	1.2	0.1	55.1	0.0	96.8
0.1	0.0	5.3	0.4	24.2	67.2	195.3	285.6	0.5	25.2	8.5	0.1	0.0	0.1	1.2	0.1	51.8	0.0	80.4
0.1	0.0	3.4	0.4	15.1	58.0	176.4	2.5	0.3	10.9	5.4	0.0	0.1	0.1	1.4	0.1	30.0	0.0	62.9
0.1	0.0	3.4	0.3	16.0	47.9	123.5	4.2	0.3	18.5	2.6	0.1	0.1	0.1	1.1	0.1	26.0	0.0	64.5
0.1	0.0	107.5	0.9	43.7	42.8	351.1	201.6	0.9	66.4	1.8	0.0	0.1	0.1	1.2	0.1	106.7	0.0	63.4
0.0	0.0	5.6	0.1	4.8	8.4	59.2	0.8	0.1	2.8	1.1	0.0	0.0	0.0	0.0	0.0	5.6	0.0	38.6
0.0	0.0	5.9	0.3	12.9	21.8	245.5	236.6	0.1	5.9	1.3	0.0	0.1	0.0	0.6	0.1	14.3	0.0	90.9
0.0	0.0	0.4	0.0	0.7	1.1	11.1	0.2	0.0	0.4	0.1	0.0	0.0	0.0	0.0	0.0	1.0	0.0	4.7
0.0	0.0	110.0	1.2	32.0	165.0	340.0	12.0	1.2	0.0	13.0	0.0	0.1	0.1	0.3	0.2	24.3	0.0	60.0
0.0	0.0	44.5	1.6	23.2	51.5	211.1	9.8	0.4	0.0	0.0	0.0	0.0	0.2	1.8	0.0	10.6	0.0	4.1
0.0	0.0	0.0	0.0	0.5	3.4	11.4	0.1	0.0	0.0	0.4	0.0	0.0	0.0	0.1	0.0	0.9	0.0	2.7
0.0	0.0	2.2	0.3	10.1	20.9	84.2	172.8	1.0	0.0	0.2	0.0	0.0	0.1	1.1	0.1	15.0	0.0	60.1
0.0	0.0	0.7	0.2	1.4	10.4	42.7	28.6	0.1	0.0	0.5	0.0	0.0	0.0	0.5	0.0	2.2	0.0	10.9
0.0	0.0	4.4	0.3	6.0	26.4	51.6	170.0	0.3	0.0	0.0	0.0	0.0	0.0	0.6	0.0	4.9	0.0	36.4
0.6	0.0	671.6	4.9	175.8	168.4	503.2	16.7	1.2	4993.2	20.5	3.7	0.1	0.7	4.4	0.7	153.6	0.0	135.6
1.9	0.0	30.4	1.5	0.0	87.2	185.6	226.1	0.0	40.5	28.8	0.0	0.1	0.3	1.8	0.0	0.0	0.0	45.4
0.0	0.0	4.7	0.3	3.1	5.3	14.3	34.5	0.1	0.0	0.6	0.0	0.0	0.0	0.0	0.0	3.2	0.0	7.3
0.0	0.0	46.8	0.6	11.7	18.2	148.2	168.4	0.2	481.0	26.7	0.0	0.0	0.0	0.3	0.1	8.6	0.0	59.3
0.0	0.0	21.3	0.3	16.2	38.3	289.0	218.5	0.3	3.4	45.9	0.0	0.0	0.0	0.3	0.1	10.3	0.0	76.8
0.0	0.0	29.2	0.1	2.6	5.1	32.5	29.9	0.0	109.6	4.2	0.0	0.0	0.0	0.1	0.0	1.5	0.0	10.0
0.0	0.0	37.2	1.4	17.4	21.1	107.9	12.4	0.1	6.2	5.2	0.0	0.0	0.0	0.2	0.1	30.1	0.0	112.6
0.0	0.0	37.2	1.4	17.4	21.1	107.9	305.0	0.1	6.2	5.2	0.0	0.0	0.0	0.2	0.1	30.1	0.0	112.6
0.1	0.0	14.0	3.1	35.0	153.0	284.0	10.0	1.6	4.0	12.6	0.0	0.2	0.1	1.2	0.2	67.0	0.0	68.7
0.0	0.0	1.6	0.0	0.7	1.2	12.9	0.3	0.0	4.9	0.4	0.0	0.0	0.0	0.0	0.0	3.7	0.0	4.8
0.0	0.0	3.6	0.1	0.6	4.5	29.0	0.8	0.0	26.0	2.4	0.0	0.0	0.0	0.1	0.0	13.6	0.0	9.5
0.1	0.0	61.6	1.6	29.2	64.8	511.9	29.2	0.7	106.9	12.6	0.9	0.1	0.1	0.6	0.1	181.4	0.0	310.7
0.0	0.0	38.1	0.8	6.2	14.0	147.8	5.0	0.2	106.4	10.1	0.2	0.0	0.0	0.2	0.0	27.9	0.0	52.6
0.0	0.0	0.7	0.0	0.9	3.6	45.0	1.1	0.0	0.0	0.0	0.0	0.0	0.0	0.0	0.0	1.1	0.0	7.0
0.9	0.0	3.1	0.2	1.9	8.1	12.9	37.5	0.0	2.3	0.1	0.0	0.0	0.0	0.4	0.0	6.6	0.0	2.9
0.0	0.0	2.4	0.0	0.9	2.9	16.2	1.8	0.0	0.5	0.4	0.0	0.0	0.0	0.0	0.0	2.0	0.0	13.8
0.0	0.0	12.9	0.1	4.6	15.2	81.1	1.1	0.1	0.0	3.8	0.1	0.0	0.0	0.0	0.1	8.3	0.0	0.2
0.0	0.0	28.1	0.4	22.0	52.4	278.9	7.6	0.2	0.0	9.9	0.8	0.1	0.0	0.6	0.1	44.2	0.0	59.1
0.1	0.0	31.3	1.8	29.6	92.2	174.0	15.7	1.2	66.1	17.1	0.7	0.2	0.1	1.5	0.1	49.6	0.0	149.5
0.1	0.0	18.4	0.8	12.8	39.2	126.4	243.2	0.4	620.8	6.5	0.0	0.2	0.1	0.9	0.1	20.8	0.0	68.6
0.0	0.0	33.6	1.6	20.8	44.0	192.0	192.0	0.3	10.4	38.3	0.0	0.1	0.1	0.4	0.1	23.3	0.0	71.1
0.0	0.0	21.6	1.2	31.2	93.6	216.8	191.2	1.0	48.0	11.4	0.0	0.2	0.1	1.6	0.2	50.6	0.0	62.3
0.1	0.0	17.0	0.8	14.5	57.0	147.1	1.7	0.6	65.5	8.2	0.3	0.1	0.1	0.6	0.1	37.7	0.0	69.4
0.0	0.0	8.7	0.3	10.5	19.8	158.7	8.1	0.2	21.1	51.3	0.4	0.1	0.0	0.8	0.2	18.0	0.0	56.9
0.0	0.0	25.2	0.9	2.8	7.7	79.1	277.9	0.1	9.1	23.9	0.0	0.0	0.0	0.4	0.1	37.8	0.0	65.3
0.0	0.0	3.2	0.1	4.3	7.8	54.5	0.3	0.1	3.8	25.1	0.0	0.0	0.0	0.3	0.1	14.3	0.0	24.7
0.1	0.0	19.6	1.6	12.8	15.3	164.1	1420.4	0.3	144.5	8.5	0.6	0.0	0.0	0.3	0.2	11.9	0.0	75.6
0.0	0.0	8.0	0.5	7.0	13.0	72.0	4.0	0.1	29.0	41.2	0.0	0.1	0.1	1.1	0.1	9.9	0.0	94.7
0.0	0.0	8.0	0.5	7.0	13.0	72.0	4.0	0.1	334.0	41.2	0.0	0.1	0.0	1.1	0.1	9.9	0.0	94.7
0.0	0.0	0.8	0.0	0.9	1.8	16.5	0.2	0.0	53.0	17.7	0.1	0.0	0.0	0.0	0.0	2.0	0.0	8.6
0.0	0.0	5.7	0.2	6.2	12.5	110.2	1.0	0.1	12.5	95.4	0.0	0.0	0.0	0.5	0.1	13.5	0.0	47.9
0.0	0.0	5.6	0.2	5.0	19.4	49.8	3.8	0.2	5.0	0.6	0.0	0.0	0.0	0.3	0.0	22.2	0.0	10.9
0.1	0.0	0.0	0.5	5.4	18.9	31.1	24.3	0.0	20.3	1.4	0.1	0.0	0.0	0.0	0.0	1.0	0.0	127.0
0.0	0.0	0.0	0.1	1.4	4.9	8.1	422.8	0.0	5.3	0.4	0.1	0.0	0.0	0.0	0.0	0.2	0.0	32.9
0.0	0.0	1.4	0.2	1.4	4.2	11.2	6.3	0.0	4.6	0.4	0.1	0.0	0.1	0.0	0.0	0.4	0.0	22.8
0.0	0.0	4.4	0.1	1.2	2.9	13.1	1.7	0.6	1.4	0.5	0.0	0.0	0.0	0.1	0.0	6.5	0.0	14.4
0.0	0.0	18.8	0.5	7.3	15.1	142.8	15.1	0.0	171.6	9.9	0.6	0.0	0.1	0.4	0.0	17.4	0.0	25.7

Code	Food Name	Unit/Amt	Wt (g)	Energy (Kcal)	Prot (g)	Carb (g)	Fiber (g)	Fat (g)	Mono (g)	Poly (g)
11383	Vege, Potato Mashed, granules w/milk, prep w/water & margarine	½ cup	100	358.0	10.9	77.7	0.0	1.1	0.2	0.3
11672	Vege, Potato Pancakes, homemade	½ cup	105	83.0	2.1	13.8	1.9	2.3	0.7	0.7
11414	Vege, Potato Salad, homemade	1 cup	128	284.2	4.3	39.0	4.1	13.7	5.6	1.0
11410	Vege, Potato Wedges, frozen, USDA Commodity	1 cup	250	357.5	6.7	27.9	3.3	20.5	6.2	9.3
11385	Vege, Potato, Au Gratin, mix, prep w/H$_2$O, whole milk & butter	⅙ of 5.5 oz package	26	81.6	2.3	19.3	1.1	1.0	0.3	0.0
11376	Vege, Potato, canned, drained	1 potato (2.5"diam)	135	116.1	2.3	27.0	2.7	0.1	0.0	0.1
11675	Vege, Potato, Flesh & Skin cooked in microwave, no salt	½ cup of whole potatoes	150	66.0	1.8	14.8	2.1	0.2	0.0	0.1
11674	Vege, Potato, Flesh & Skin, baked, no salt	1 potato: 2.33 x 4.75"	202	220.2	4.6	51.0	4.8	0.2	0.0	0.1
11363	Vege, Potato, Flesh only, baked, no salt	1 potato: 2.33 x 4.75"	156	145.1	3.1	33.6	2.3	0.2	0.0	0.1
11365	Vege, Potato, Flesh only, boiled in skin, no salt	1 potato (2.5"diam)	136	118.3	2.5	27.4	2.7	0.1	0.0	0.1
11367	Vege, Potato, Flesh only, boiled w/o skin, no salt	1 potato (2.5"diam)	136	118.3	2.5	27.4	2.4	0.1	0.0	0.1
911405	Vege, Potato, French Fries, frozen, fried in oil & lard	10 strips	65	101.4	1.6	15.8	2.0	3.8	2.4	0.4
11403	Vege, Potato, French Fries, frozen, oven heated, no salt	10 strips	50	157.5	2.0	19.8	1.6	8.3	4.0	0.5
11391	Vege, Potato, Hashed Brown, plain, frozen, cooked	4.0 oz	115	94.3	2.4	20.4	1.6	0.7	0.0	0.3
11930	Vege, Potato, Mashed, dried flakes w/o milk, prep w/whole milk & margarine	½ cup	105	118.7	2.0	15.8	2.4	5.9	1.7	0.3
11371	Vege, Potato, Mashed, homemade w/milk & margarine	½ cup	105	113.4	2.2	15.1	2.3	5.2	2.1	1.4
11396	Vege, Potato, O'Brien, frozen	½ cup	105	111.3	2.0	17.5	2.1	4.4	1.2	0.2
11387	Vege, Potato, Scalloped, mix, prep w/H$_2$O, whole milk & butter	⅙ of 5.5 oz package	26	93.1	2.0	19.2	2.2	1.2	0.0	0.5
11364	Vege, Potato, Skin only, baked, no salt	skin from 1 potato: 2.33 x 4.75"	58	114.8	2.5	26.7	4.6	0.1	0.0	0.0
11401	Vege, Potato, whole, frozen, boiled, drained, no salt	3.5 oz	100	65.0	2.0	14.5	1.4	0.1	0.0	0.1
11426	Vege, Pumpkin Pie Mix, canned	½ cup	39	7.4	1.2	0.9	0.0	0.2	0.0	0.0
11424	Vege, Pumpkin, canned, no salt	½ cup	122	41.5	1.3	9.9	3.5	0.3	0.0	0.0
11952	Vege, Radicchio, raw	1 cup	43	6.9	0.6	1.5	0.0	0.0	0.0	0.0
11676	Vege, Radish Sprouts, raw	1 cup, shredded	40	9.2	0.6	1.8	0.4	0.1	0.0	0.0
11430	Vege, Radish, Oriental (Daikon) raw	1 cup	116	314.4	9.2	73.5	0.0	0.8	0.1	0.4
11439	Vege, Sauerkraut, canned, solids & liquid	1 cup, slices	133	109.1	4.4	24.7	4.4	0.3	0.0	0.0
11677	Vege, Shallots, peeled, raw	¼ cup	3.6	12.5	0.4	2.9	0.0	0.0	0.0	0.0
11452	Vege, Soybean Sprouts, mature seeds, sprouted, raw	3.5 oz	100	72.0	2.5	16.8	0.0	0.1	0.0	0.0
11853	Vege, Soybeans, Green, boiled w/salt, drained	½ cup	47	38.1	4.0	3.1	0.4	2.1	0.5	1.2
11461	Vege, Spinach, canned, drained	½ cup	60	13.8	1.8	2.3	1.4	0.2	0.0	0.1
11463	Vege, Spinach, chopped or leaf, frozen	½ cup	117	22.2	2.5	3.4	2.6	0.4	0.0	0.2
11457	Vege, Spinach, raw	10 oz package	220	61.6	6.9	11.7	6.6	0.5	0.0	0.2
11484	Vege, Squash, Acorn, boiled, drained, no salt	1 cup	30	6.6	0.9	1.1	0.8	0.1	0.0	0.0
11486	Vege, Squash, Butternut, baked, no salt	1 cup	30	12.0	0.3	3.1	0.0	0.0	0.0	0.0
11493	Vege, Squash, Spaghetti, boiled or baked, drained, no salt	1 cup, cubes	205	55.4	1.4	13.2	2.9	0.5	0.0	0.3
11642	Vege, Squash, Summer, All Varieties, boiled, drained, no salt	½ cup	77	15.4	0.7	3.3	1.1	0.2	0.0	0.1
11641	Vege, Squash, Summer, All Varieties, slices, raw	½ cup	90	18.0	0.8	3.9	1.3	0.3	0.0	0.1
11644	Vege, Squash, Winter, All Varieties, baked, no salt	½ cup	190	74.1	1.7	16.6	5.3	1.2	0.1	0.5
11872	Vege, Succotash (corn & lima beans) frozen, boiled w/salt, drained	1 large: 3.12 x 0.6"	16	18.4	0.8	3.9	0.0	0.1	0.0	0.1
11508	Vege, Sweet Potato, baked in skin, no salt	½ cup	96	98.9	1.7	23.3	2.9	0.1	0.0	0.0
11659	Vege, Sweet Potato, Candied, homemade	½ cup	164	172.2	2.7	39.8	3.0	0.5	0.0	0.2
11647	Vege, Sweet Potato, canned w/syrup, drained	½ cup	164	224.7	1.4	45.7	3.9	5.3	1.0	0.2
11954	Vege, Tomatillos, raw	1 can (No. 3 vacuum/404 x 307)	638	280.7	26.5	43.7	0.0	4.3	0.4	1.8
11540	Vege, Tomato Juice, canned, w/salt	½ cup, sliced	68	21.8	0.7	2.4	1.3	0.7	0.1	0.3
11887	Vege, Tomato Paste, canned w/salt	½ cup, chopped	67	11.4	0.5	2.8	0.3	0.0	0.0	0.0
11888	Vege, Tomato Puree, canned w/salt	½ cup	131	395.6	16.9	97.8	21.6	0.6	0.1	0.2
11549	Vege, Tomato Sauce, canned	½ cup	123	39.4	1.6	8.7	1.7	0.5	0.1	0.2
11533	Vege, Tomato, Red, canned, stewed	1 slice or wedge	20	3.2	0.2	0.6	0.2	0.0	0.0	0.0
11531	Vege, Tomato, Red, canned, whole	1 tomato	111	31.1	1.1	7.5	1.1	0.1	0.0	0.1
11883	Vege, Tomato, Red, Cherry, ripe, raw, Jun-Oct	½ cup	123	23.4	1.1	5.4	1.2	0.2	0.0	0.1
11660	Vege, Tomato, Red, ripe, stewed	1 tbsp	15	4.1	0.2	0.9	0.2	0.1	0.0	0.0
11885	Vege, Tomato, Red, ripe, whole, canned, no added salt	1 medium	123	97.2	2.4	16.1	2.1	3.3	1.3	1.1
11529	Vege, Tomato, Red, ripe, whole, raw	yield from recipe	604	114.8	5.6	26.4	6.0	0.8	0.1	0.3
11537	Vege, Tomato, Red, w/green chilies, canned	½ cup	123	25.8	1.0	5.7	1.4	0.4	0.1	0.2
11955	Vege, Tomato, Sun-dried	½ cup	123	32.0	1.0	7.8	0.0	0.2	0.0	0.1
11956	Vege, Tomato, Sun-dried, oil packed, drained	1 cup	261	673.4	36.8	145.5	32.1	7.8	1.3	2.9
11565	Vege, Turnip, boiled, drained, no salt	1 piece	3	0.6	0.0	0.1	0.1	0.0	0.0	0.0
11590	Vege, Waterchestnut, Chinese, canned, solids & liquid	10 oz package, mashed	284	309.6	13.6	66.9	21.9	1.8	0.0	0.0
11578	Vegetable Juice Cocktail, canned	3.5 oz	100	48.0	0.6	11.0	0.2	0.2	0.0	0.0
11159	Vegetable Salad, Coleslaw, homemade	1 cup	241	48.2	1.7	10.2	1.7	0.1	0.0	0.1
11581	Vegetables, Mixed, canned, drained solids	½ cup	60	41.4	0.8	7.4	0.9	1.6	0.4	0.8
924281	Vegetarian Manicotti	10 oz package	275	162.3	7.9	36.0	12.1	0.4	0.0	0.0
22246	Vegetarian, Beef Stew, canned entree/Nestle Chef-Mate	1 serving	71	190.3	14.0	21.0	0.0	5.3	1.7	1.3
22121	Vegetarian, Better'n Burgers/Vegan Burgers, frozen/Worthington, Morningstar	1 patty	38	28.9	2.3	2.9	0.5	0.9	0.4	0.0
22126	Vegetarian, Big Franks, meatless, frozen/Worthingfoods, Loma Linda	1 patty	85	91.0	13.9	7.5	4.3	0.5	0.3	0.2
22122	Vegetarian, Breakfast Patties/Worthington, Morningstar	1 patty	38	88.2	9.0	1.1	1.1	5.3	1.1	2.7
22363	Vegetarian, Breakfast Stuff-Its, egg & cheese pockets, frozen/SunnyFresh	1 patty	38	79.4	9.9	3.7	2.0	2.8	0.7	1.3
22120	Vegetarian, Burger Crumbles/Worthington, Morningstar	1 serving	64	147.2	6.8	14.7	1.0	7.6	0.9	0.6
924269	Vegetarian, Chili Mac/Worthington	1 cup	110	231.0	22.2	6.6	5.1	12.9	4.6	4.9

Sat (g)	Chol (mg)	Cal (mg)	Iron (mg)	Magn (mg)	Phos (mg)	Pota (mg)	Sodi (mg)	Zinc (mg)	Vit A (RE)	Vit C (mg)	Vit E (mg)	Thia (mg)	Ribo (mg)	Niac (mg)	Vit B-6 (mg)	Fol (μg)	Vit B-12 (μg)	Wat (g)
0.5	2.0	142.0	3.5	74.0	237.0	1848.0	82.0	1.2	9.0	16.0	0.0	0.2	0.3	4.2	0.9	29.9	0.0	6.3
0.7	2.1	32.6	0.6	16.8	46.2	351.8	245.7	0.3	13.7	3.2	0.0	0.0	0.1	0.8	0.2	7.5	0.0	85.5
6.5	0.0	38.4	2.0	24.3	61.4	486.4	954.9	0.4	2.6	8.8	0.1	0.3	0.1	2.8	0.3	21.1	0.0	67.7
3.6	170.0	47.5	1.6	37.5	130.0	635.0	1322.5	0.8	82.5	25.0	0.0	0.2	0.2	2.2	0.4	16.8	0.0	190.0
0.6	0.0	80.9	0.4	16.6	105.0	257.4	544.7	0.2	18.7	4.0	0.0	0.0	0.1	1.1	0.0	10.5	0.0	1.3
0.0	0.0	10.8	0.4	27.0	54.0	442.8	325.4	0.4	10.0	0.1	0.1	0.1	0.0	1.8	0.4	12.0	0.0	104.6
0.0	0.0	58.5	1.1	21.0	33.0	307.5	325.5	0.6	0.0	11.4	0.1	0.1	0.0	1.3	0.2	6.8	0.0	131.7
0.1	0.0	20.2	2.7	54.5	115.1	844.4	492.9	0.6	0.0	26.1	0.0	0.2	0.1	3.3	0.7	22.2	0.0	143.8
0.0	0.0	7.8	0.5	39.0	78.0	610.0	376.0	0.5	0.0	20.0	0.0	0.2	0.0	2.2	0.5	14.2	0.0	117.7
0.0	0.0	6.8	0.4	29.9	59.8	515.4	326.4	0.4	0.0	17.7	0.1	0.1	0.0	2.0	0.4	13.6	0.0	104.7
0.0	0.0	6.8	0.4	29.9	59.8	515.4	5.4	0.4	0.0	17.7	0.1	0.1	0.0	2.0	0.4	13.6	0.0	104.7
0.6	0.0	3.9	0.6	11.1	41.6	211.9	15.0	0.2	0.0	6.4	0.1	0.1	0.0	1.1	0.2	7.8	0.0	43.3
3.4	6.5	9.5	0.4	17.0	46.5	366.0	108.0	0.2	0.0	5.2	0.0	0.1	0.0	1.6	0.1	14.5	0.0	19.0
0.2	0.0	11.5	1.1	12.7	54.1	327.8	25.3	0.2	0.0	9.4	0.0	0.1	0.0	1.9	0.1	4.8	0.0	90.7
3.6	14.7	51.5	0.2	18.9	58.8	244.7	348.6	0.2	22.1	10.2	0.7	0.1	0.1	0.7	0.0	7.8	0.1	80.1
1.3	3.2	36.8	0.2	20.0	63.0	152.3	276.2	0.3	21.0	6.3	0.0	0.1	0.1	0.8	0.0	7.4	0.0	81.4
2.9	12.6	27.3	0.3	18.9	48.3	303.5	309.8	0.3	21.0	6.4	0.0	0.1	0.0	1.1	0.2	8.3	0.0	80.1
0.3	1.3	16.1	0.5	15.3	51.2	235.3	410.3	0.2	0.0	4.3	0.1	0.0	0.0	1.2	0.0	8.2	0.0	1.6
0.0	0.0	19.7	4.1	24.9	58.6	332.3	149.1	0.3	0.0	7.8	0.0	0.1	0.1	1.8	0.4	12.5	0.0	27.4
0.0	0.0	7.0	0.8	11.0	26.0	287.0	256.0	0.3	0.0	9.4	0.0	0.1	0.0	1.3	0.0	8.4	0.0	82.8
0.1	0.0	15.2	0.9	14.8	40.6	170.0	4.3	0.1	75.7	4.3	0.0	0.0	0.0	0.4	0.1	14.1	0.0	36.2
0.2	0.0	31.7	1.7	28.1	42.7	251.3	294.0	0.2	2691.3	5.1	0.0	0.0	0.1	0.4	0.1	15.0	0.0	109.8
0.0	0.0	28.0	0.9	29.2	18.9	212.4	19.4	0.1	56.8	9.0	0.0	0.0	0.0	0.2	0.0	4.9	0.0	40.4
0.0	0.0	7.6	0.2	5.2	16.0	120.8	8.8	0.2	1.2	3.2	0.9	0.0	0.0	0.1	0.0	24.0	0.0	37.3
0.3	0.0	729.6	7.8	197.2	236.6	4053.0	322.5	2.5	0.0	0.0	0.0	0.3	0.8	3.9	0.7	341.9	0.0	22.8
0.0	0.0	79.8	0.9	30.6	99.8	505.4	26.6	0.5	0.0	10.6	0.0	0.1	0.3	0.7	0.4	35.0	0.0	102.4
0.0	0.0	6.6	0.2	3.7	10.7	59.4	2.1	0.1	202.0	1.4	0.0	0.0	0.1	0.0	0.1	4.2	0.0	0.1
0.0	0.0	37.0	1.2	21.0	60.0	334.0	12.0	0.4	119.0	8.0	0.0	0.1	0.0	0.2	0.3	34.2	0.0	79.8
0.3	0.0	27.7	0.6	28.2	63.5	166.9	4.7	0.5	0.5	3.9	0.0	0.1	0.0	0.5	0.0	37.6	0.0	37.3
0.0	0.0	81.6	2.1	52.2	33.6	279.6	42.0	0.5	491.4	5.9	0.6	0.1	0.1	0.3	0.1	87.5	0.0	54.7
0.1	0.0	97.1	1.8	65.5	37.4	269.1	87.8	0.5	752.3	15.8	1.1	0.0	0.1	0.3	0.1	67.9	0.0	109.1
0.1	0.0	321.2	3.3	151.8	105.6	655.6	708.4	1.5	1711.6	27.1	0.0	0.1	0.4	0.9	0.3	236.5	0.0	198.0
0.0	0.0	29.7	0.8	23.7	14.7	167.4	23.7	0.2	201.6	8.4	0.6	0.0	0.1	0.2	0.1	58.3	0.0	27.5
0.0	0.0	12.3	0.2	8.7	8.1	85.2	72.0	0.0	210.0	4.5	0.0	0.0	0.0	0.3	0.0	5.8	0.0	26.3
0.1	0.0	43.1	0.7	22.6	0.0	239.9	520.7	0.4	22.6	7.2	0.0	0.1	0.0	1.7	0.2	16.4	0.0	189.2
0.0	0.0	20.8	0.3	18.5	30.0	147.8	182.5	0.3	22.3	4.2	0.0	0.0	0.0	0.4	0.1	15.5	0.0	72.1
0.1	0.0	24.3	0.3	21.6	35.1	172.8	0.9	0.4	26.1	5.0	0.1	0.0	0.0	0.5	0.1	18.1	0.0	84.3
0.2	0.0	26.6	0.6	15.2	38.0	830.3	450.3	0.5	676.4	18.2	0.0	0.2	0.0	1.3	0.1	53.2	0.0	169.1
0.0	0.0	2.7	0.2	8.5	18.7	65.6	40.5	0.1	4.6	1.3	0.0	0.0	0.0	0.2	0.0	5.2	0.0	10.9
0.0	0.0	26.9	0.4	19.2	52.8	334.1	236.2	0.3	2094.7	23.6	0.3	0.1	0.1	0.6	0.2	21.7	0.0	69.9
0.1	0.0	34.4	0.9	16.4	44.3	301.8	21.3	0.4	2796.2	28.0	0.5	0.1	0.2	1.0	0.4	18.2	0.0	119.5
2.2	13.1	42.6	1.9	18.0	42.6	310.0	114.8	0.2	687.2	11.0	0.0	0.0	0.1	0.6	0.1	18.7	0.0	109.8
0.9	0.0	950.6	10.0	325.4	427.5	3974.7	1850.2	0.6	1122.9	242.4	0.0	0.3	1.3	3.1	0.7	45.9	0.0	551.6
0.1	0.0	4.8	0.4	13.6	26.5	182.2	0.7	0.1	7.5	8.0	0.3	0.0	0.0	1.3	0.0	62.3	0.0	62.3
0.0	0.0	6.0	0.4	7.4	12.7	147.4	241.9	0.1	37.5	12.3	0.6	0.0	0.0	0.5	0.1	13.3	0.0	62.9
0.1	0.0	217.5	6.0	233.2	386.5	2524.4	175.5	2.2	2259.8	152.9	0.7	1.2	1.0	12.0	0.6	157.1	0.0	4.0
0.1	0.0	12.3	0.8	24.6	51.7	458.8	18.5	0.2	98.4	26.4	0.0	0.1	0.1	1.5	0.2	11.6	0.0	109.4
0.0	0.0	1.0	0.1	1.6	5.8	42.4	8.4	0.0	30.0	3.2	0.0	0.0	0.0	0.1	0.0	5.8	0.0	19.0
0.0	0.0	36.6	0.8	13.3	22.2	264.2	245.3	0.2	59.9	12.7	0.4	0.1	0.0	0.8	0.0	6.0	0.0	101.0
0.0	0.0	36.9	0.7	14.8	23.4	271.8	182.0	0.2	73.8	17.5	0.4	0.1	0.0	0.9	0.1	9.6	0.0	115.2
0.0	0.0	0.9	0.1	2.1	4.7	41.9	1.7	0.0	11.1	3.4	0.1	0.0	0.0	0.1	0.0	2.0	0.0	13.8
0.6	0.0	32.0	1.3	18.5	46.7	303.8	559.7	0.2	82.4	22.4	1.6	0.1	0.1	1.4	0.1	13.5	0.0	99.2
0.1	0.0	181.2	3.3	72.5	114.8	1371.1	60.4	1.0	362.4	85.8	2.3	0.3	0.2	4.4	0.5	47.1	0.0	565.6
0.1	0.0	6.2	0.8	13.5	29.5	273.1	11.1	0.1	76.3	23.5	0.5	0.1	0.1	0.8	0.1	18.5	0.0	115.3
0.0	0.0	32.0	0.6	13.5	28.3	308.7	266.9	0.2	71.3	18.2	0.0	0.1	0.0	0.8	0.1	12.4	0.0	112.9
1.1	0.0	287.1	23.7	506.3	929.2	8944.5	5468.0	5.2	227.1	102.3	0.0	1.4	1.3	23.6	0.9	177.5	0.0	38.0
0.0	0.0	0.7	0.0	0.2	0.6	4.1	8.6	0.0	0.0	0.3	0.0	0.0	0.0	0.0	0.0	0.3	0.0	2.8
0.0	0.0	363.5	2.9	196.0	227.2	1613.1	48.3	4.6	14.2	119.0	0.0	0.4	0.3	2.1	0.8	51.1	0.0	196.3
0.0	0.0	12.0	0.6	22.0	78.0	90.0	362.0	1.1	22.0	4.1	0.0	0.0	0.0	0.2	0.1	15.9	30.6	87.4
0.0	0.0	31.8	1.5	0.0	67.5	508.5	732.3	0.5	611.2	49.0	0.0	0.1	0.1	1.6	0.0	0.0	0.0	0.0
0.2	4.8	27.0	0.4	6.0	19.2	108.6	13.8	0.1	49.2	19.6	0.0	0.0	0.0	0.2	0.1	15.9	0.0	48.9
0.1	0.0	68.8	2.3	60.5	140.3	464.8	96.3	1.3	1177.0	8.8	1.0	0.2	0.3	2.3	0.2	52.3	0.0	228.9
1.3	128.5	39.8	0.7	3.6	88.8	68.2	283.3	0.3	0.0	0.0	0.2	0.0	0.2	0.1	0.0	0.0	0.4	29.2
0.3	4.9	9.5	0.2	5.3	23.9	58.5	179.0	0.4	46.7	0.4	0.1	0.0	0.0	0.5	0.0	0.0	0.1	31.4
0.1	0.0	86.7	2.9	16.2	181.1	433.5	382.5	0.7	0.0	0.0	0.0	0.3	0.6	4.1	0.2	245.7	0.0	60.6
0.6	0.0	7.6	0.7	0.0	63.1	45.2	166.8	0.9	0.0	0.0	0.0	0.2	0.5	4.3	0.5	0.0	2.2	21.9
0.5	0.8	18.2	1.9	1.1	106.4	101.8	259.2	0.4	0.0	0.0	0.3	5.4	0.1	1.8	0.2	0.0	1.5	20.4
3.1	93.4	62.7	0.9	2.6	38.4	30.7	233.0	0.2	65.3	0.0	0.1	0.1	0.2	1.5	0.0	0.0	0.2	34.4
3.3	0.0	79.2	6.4	2.2	173.8	178.2	476.3	1.6	0.0	0.0	0.7	9.9	0.4	3.0	0.5	0.0	4.4	66.3

Code	Food Name	Unit/Amt	Wt (g)	Energy (Kcal)	Prot (g)	Carb (g)	Fiber (g)	Fat (g)	Mono (g)	Poly (g)
22215	Vegetarian, Chili w/beans, canned entree/Nestle Chef-Mate	1 cup	220	316.8	11.5	22.9	0.0	19.9	0.0	0.0
924060	Vegetarian, Chili w/beans/Worthington	1 cup	253	412.4	17.7	29.0	11.1	25.0	10.7	1.4
22216	Vegetarian, Chili w/o beans, canned entree/Nestle Chef-Mate	1 cup	220	323.4	14.1	20.6	6.0	20.6	0.0	0.0
22217	Vegetarian, Corned Beef Hash, canned entree/Nestle Chef-Mate	1 cup	250	430.0	18.6	17.6	3.0	31.6	13.6	1.8
22119	Vegetarian, Deli Franks/Worthington, Morningstar	1 cup	253	485.8	24.2	29.1	6.1	30.3	14.7	1.1
22118	Vegetarian, Garden Patties, frozen/Worthington, Morningstar	1 patty	67	166.2	15.5	5.5	4.1	9.2	2.9	4.9
22125	Vegetarian, Harvest Burger, Original Flavor, vege protein patty, original flavor	1 patty	90	160.2	15.1	13.7	5.4	5.1	1.4	2.9
22223	Vegetarian, Macaroni And Cheese, canned entree/Nestle Chef-Mate	1 patty	90	137.3	18.0	7.0	5.7	4.1	0.0	0.0
22127	Vegetarian, Natural Touch Garden Vege Patty, frozen/Worthington	1 cup	253	283.4	10.8	35.4	3.3	11.0	3.0	0.5
22128	Vegetarian, Natural Touch Vegan Burgers, frozen/Worthington	1 cup	252	448.6	42.2	38.4	15.1	14.2	4.0	8.1
22360	Vegetarian, Sandwich, Egg & Cheese Biscuit, pre-ckd, frozen/SunnyFresh	1 patty	85	91.0	13.9	7.5	4.3	0.5	0.3	0.2
22361	Vegetarian, Sandwich, Egg, Ham & Cheese Biscuit, pre-ckd, frozen/SunnyFresh	1 serving	99	223.7	9.9	24.6	0.0	8.9	1.1	3.7
22224	Vegetarian, Sausage N' Shells, canned entree/Nestle Chef-Mate	½ cup	121	244.4	12.3	25.3	0.1	9.8	1.2	3.8
22123	Vegetarian, Spicy Black Bean Burger/Worthington, Morningstar	1 patty	78	117.8	4.6	5.8	0.3	8.5	3.8	1.1
22218	Vegetarian, Spicy Chili With Beans, canned entree/Nestle Chef-Mate	1 cup	253	371.9	38.2	49.3	15.4	2.5	0.8	1.1
924030	Vegetarian, Stew, Beef Vegetable/Worthington	1 cup	253	422.5	16.9	32.8	4.3	24.7	10.7	1.1
18367	Waffle, Plain, homemade	1 lg	75	217.5	4.6	26.4	1.1	10.3	0.0	0.0
18365	Waffle, Plain/Buttermilk, frozen, ready-to-heat	1 sm	34	98.9	2.7	11.2	0.0	4.8	1.2	2.3
1072	Whipped Dessert Topping, Nondairy, pressurized can	2 tsbp	7	13.2	0.3	1.2	0.0	0.9	0.1	0.0
1073	Whipped Dessert Topping, Nondairy, semi solid, frozen	1 tsbp	4	10.5	0.0	0.6	0.0	0.9	0.1	0.0
901913	Whipped Topping, Nondairy/Cool Whip	2 tbsp	9	28.6	0.1	2.1	0.0	2.3	0.1	0.0
19393	Yogurt, Frozen, Chocolate, soft serve	½ cup	72	129.6	2.9	14.4	0.0	5.8	1.4	0.0
19293	Yogurt, Frozen, Vanilla, soft serve	½ cup	72	115.2	2.9	17.9	1.6	4.3	1.3	0.2
1121	Yogurt, Lowfat w/fruit, 10g protein/8 oz	8.0 oz	227	360.9	9.1	54.9	0.0	12.7	3.6	0.5
1117	Yogurt, Lowfat, Plain, 12g protein/8 oz	8.0 oz	227	225.3	9.0	42.3	0.0	2.6	0.7	0.1
1119	Yogurt, Lowfat, Vanilla, 11g protein/8 oz	8.0 oz	227	143.7	11.9	16.0	0.0	3.5	1.0	0.1
901906	Yogurt, Lowfat, Yoplait	6 oz.	170	145.3	8.4	23.5	0.0	2.1	0.6	0.1
1118	Yogurt, Nonfat, Skim, 13g protein/8 oz	8.0 oz	227	276.9	10.4	52.6	2.7	4.3	1.3	0.8
901909	Yogurt, Whole Milk w/fruit	8.0 oz	227	120.3	13.0	18.0	0.0	0.0	0.0	0.0
1116	Yogurt, Whole Milk, Plain, 8g protein/8 oz	8.0 oz	227	256.5	9.6	42.6	0.0	7.9	2.6	0.2
			0.0	0.0	0.0	0.0	0.0	0.0	0.0	0.0

Sat (g)	Chol (mg)	Cal (mg)	Iron (mg)	Magn (mg)	Phos (mg)	Pota (mg)	Sodi (mg)	Zinc (mg)	Vit A (RE)	Vit C (mg)	Vit E (mg)	Thia (mg)	Ribo (mg)	Niac (mg)	Vit B-6 (mg)	Fol (μg)	Vit B-12 (μg)	Wat (g)
0.0	0.0	28.0	1.9	28.0	136.0	337.0	854.0	2.0	490.0	4.0	0.0	0.1	0.5	3.5	0.1	40.0	2.0	154.2
10.9	55.7	88.6	4.8	45.5	167.0	511.1	1171.4	3.9	301.1	0.8	1.2	0.1	0.2	3.5	0.2	0.0	1.4	175.8
0.0	0.0	55.0	2.4	53.0	236.0	593.0	926.0	2.0	738.0	4.0	0.0	0.1	0.8	2.5	0.2	30.0	0.0	151.5
14.4	85.0	67.5	4.5	45.0	162.5	530.0	1587.5	4.5	302.5	1.8	1.6	0.1	0.3	4.8	0.3	0.0	1.8	176.4
13.4	88.6	45.5	3.0	38.0	240.4	536.4	1593.9	7.5	0.0	1.5	0.3	0.2	0.3	6.3	0.6	0.0	2.5	163.9
1.3	0.7	25.5	0.9	5.4	63.0	74.4	641.2	0.6	0.0	0.0	1.9	0.2	0.0	0.0	0.0	0.0	0.0	34.6
0.7	0.9	64.8	1.6	39.6	166.5	241.2	513.0	0.8	102.6	0.0	1.3	8.7	0.1	0.0	0.0	38.7	0.0	53.9
1.0	0.0	101.7	3.9	0.0	0.0	0.0	411.3	0.0	0.0	0.0	0.0	0.0	0.0	0.0	0.0	0.0	0.0	58.5
6.2	27.8	202.4	1.9	32.9	250.5	151.8	1343.4	1.6	55.7	0.0	0.2	0.3	0.3	2.5	0.1	0.0	0.2	191.3
2.0	2.5	181.4	4.6	110.9	466.2	675.4	1436.4	2.2	287.3	0.0	3.7	24.3	0.4	0.0	0.0	0.0	0.0	150.9
0.1	0.0	86.7	2.9	16.2	181.1	433.5	382.5	0.7	0.0	0.0	0.0	0.3	0.6	4.1	0.2	245.7	0.0	60.6
2.4	110.9	101.0	2.2	3.0	49.5	39.6	563.3	0.3	57.4	0.0	2.0	0.2	0.3	2.0	0.0	0.0	0.3	53.0
2.6	115.0	106.5	2.5	3.6	54.5	47.2	728.4	0.3	59.3	0.1	2.4	0.2	0.3	2.0	0.0	0.0	0.3	70.2
2.7	16.4	12.5	1.0	16.4	64.7	293.3	304.2	0.7	42.1	0.0	1.4	0.2	0.1	2.0	0.2	0.0	0.4	57.9
0.6	2.5	182.2	6.0	141.7	485.8	872.9	1619.2	3.0	45.5	0.0	1.2	26.1	0.5	0.0	0.7	0.0	0.2	152.9
10.7	55.7	83.5	5.4	53.1	177.1	647.7	1485.1	2.8	210.0	1.3	2.1	0.1	0.1	3.0	0.3	0.0	0.9	172.9
5.2	2.7	93.0	1.2	15.0	252.0	134.3	458.3	0.4	19.5	0.2	0.0	0.2	0.2	1.2	0.1	9.0	0.2	31.9
1.0	23.5	86.7	0.8	6.5	64.6	54.1	173.7	0.2	22.1	0.1	0.0	0.1	0.1	0.7	0.0	15.6	0.1	14.3
0.7	0.7	6.3	0.0	0.7	6.0	10.5	4.6	0.0	3.4	0.0	0.0	0.0	0.0	0.0	0.0	0.3	0.0	4.7
0.8	0.0	0.2	0.0	0.0	0.7	0.8	2.5	0.0	1.9	0.0	0.0	0.0	0.0	0.0	0.0	0.0	0.0	2.4
2.0	0.0	0.6	0.0	0.2	0.7	1.6	2.3	0.0	7.7	0.0	0.0	0.0	0.0	0.0	0.0	0.0	0.0	4.5
4.3	14.4	72.0	0.0	14.4	57.6	100.8	57.6	0.3	28.8	0.0	0.0	0.0	0.1	0.0	0.0	0.0	0.1	47.5
2.6	3.6	105.8	0.9	19.4	100.1	187.9	70.6	0.4	31.0	0.2	0.1	0.0	0.2	0.2	0.1	7.9	0.2	45.9
7.8	4.5	324.6	0.7	31.8	292.8	479.0	197.5	1.0	129.4	1.8	0.1	0.1	0.5	0.7	0.2	13.6	0.7	148.2
1.7	10.2	313.9	0.1	30.1	246.7	402.0	120.8	1.5	27.2	1.4	0.1	0.1	0.4	0.2	0.1	19.3	1.0	170.9
2.3	13.8	414.5	0.2	39.6	325.7	530.7	159.4	2.0	36.3	1.8	0.1	0.1	0.5	0.3	0.1	25.4	1.3	193.1
1.4	8.3	291.2	0.1	27.9	228.8	372.8	111.9	1.4	22.1	1.3	0.1	0.1	0.3	0.2	0.1	17.9	0.9	134.3
2.1	13.4	0.0	0.0	0.0	0.0	475.4	121.5	0.0	0.0	0.0	0.0	0.0	0.0	0.0	0.0	0.0	0.0	0.0
0.0	5.0	0.0	0.0	0.0	0.0	590.0	160.0	0.0	0.0	0.0	0.0	0.0	0.0	0.0	0.0	0.0	0.0	0.0
5.1	30.9	292.0	0.1	0.0	229.1	374.1	111.9	1.4	59.5	1.1	0.0	0.1	0.3	0.2	0.1	18.1	0.9	0.0
0.0	0.0	0.0	0.0	0.0	0.0	0.0	0.0	0.0	0.0	0.0	0.0	0.0	0.0	0.0	0.0	0.0	0.0	

CHEMISTRY: A TOOL FOR UNDERSTANDING NUTRITION

You have already completed at least one basic high school and/or college course in chemistry; consequently, this appendix serves only to review key chemistry principles that arise in the study of nutrition. The study of human nutrition requires a basic awareness of and familiarity with general chemistry, organic chemistry, and biochemistry. This appendix provides fundamental concepts regarding atoms, molecules, chemical bonds, pH, organic compounds, and biochemical structures. An understanding of basic chemistry may make the study of nutrition easier and more interesting. It helps connect nutrient characteristics with the structural and chemical attributes of the individual components of food.

One concept to keep in mind is that the physical and chemical properties of almost anything are intimately related to its structure, whether atoms, molecules, or organisms (Table B-1). A basic knowledge of chemical structures can help you visualize important fundamental concepts in nutrition.

■ Properties of Matter and Mass

All living and nonliving things are composed of matter. Two characteristics of matter are (1) it has mass and (2) it occupies space (volume). Mass is related to the amount of force it takes to move an object—it takes less force to move a paper clip than a pencil; therefore, the clip has less mass. Volume is related to the amount of space an object occupies—a pint of water occupies less space than a gallon; therefore, a pint has a smaller volume. Both of these properties depend on how much of the substance there is.

Another property of matter is density. Density is defined as the mass of an object divided by its volume:

$$\text{Density} = \frac{\text{Mass}}{\text{Volume}}$$

Density is independent of how much matter is available. The density of water in a lake is the same as in a cup.

Matter exists in three states, which are solid, liquid, or gas. An example of a solid is ice; a liquid is water, and a gas is steam. Density is commonly expressed in units as g per cubic centimeter (g/cm^3). Table B-2 lists the densities of several common substances.

You can use density to compare objects. Using the density of pure water as a comparison, lean body tissue has a density of about 1.1 g/cm^3. The density of body fat in comparison is about 0.9 g/cm^3. Substances that are less dense than water are buoyant (they tend to float), whereas substances that are more dense than water sink. The next time you are at the swimming pool, note the density of men and women. Women tend to have more body fat, so they float; men are generally more muscular (have more lean tissue), so they tend to sink deeper in the water. This physical property is used to determine the amount of body fat stored in a person (see Chapter 13).

Extensive and Intensive Properties

Properties of matter are divided into two categories: extensive and intensive. Extensive properties of matter depend on the amount of matter. Intensive properties are independent of the size of the sample. The boiling point and freezing point of a substance are intensive properties. No matter how much or how little water you have, it

TABLE B-1 Periodic Table of the Elements

Main-Group Elements

Key

1
H
1.00794

Atomic Number
Symbol
Atomic Weight

Period	1 IA	2 IIA		3 IIIB	4 IVB	5 VB	6 VIB	7 VIIB	8	9 VIIB	10	11 IB	12 IIB	13 IIIA	14 IVA	15 VA	16 VIA	17 VIIA	18 VIIIA
1	1 H 1.00794																		2 He 4.002602
2	3 Li 6.941	4 Be 9.012182												5 B 10.811	6 C 12.011	7 N 14.00674	8 O 15.9994	9 F 18.998403	10 Ne 20.1797
3	11 Na 22.989768	12 Mg 24.3050												13 Al 26.981539	14 Si 28.0855	15 P 30.973762	16 S 32.066	17 Cl 35.4527	18 Ar 39.948
4	19 K 39.0983	20 Ca 40.078	21 Sc 44.955910	22 Ti 47.88	23 V 50.9415	24 Cr 51.9961	25 Mn 54.93805	26 Fe 55.847	27 Co 58.93320	28 Ni 58.69	29 Cu 63.546	30 Zn 65.39	31 Ga 69.723	32 Ge 72.61	33 As 74.92159	34 Se 78.96	35 Br 79.904	36 Kr 83.80
5	37 Rb 85.4678	38 Sr 87.62	39 Y 88.90585	40 Zr 91.224	41 Nb 92.90638	42 Mo 95.94	43 Tc (98)	44 Ru 101.07	45 Rh 102.90550	46 Pd 106.42	47 Ag 107.8682	48 Cd 112.411	49 In 114.82	50 Sn 118.710	51 Sb 121.75	52 Te 127.60	53 I 126.90447	54 Xe 131.29
6	55 Cs 132.90543	56 Ba 137.327	57 La* 138.9055	72 Hf 178.49	73 Ta 180.9479	74 W 183.85	75 Re 186.207	76 Os 190.2	77 Ir 192.22	78 Pt 195.08	79 Au 196.96654	80 Hg 200.59	81 Tl 204.3833	82 Pb 207.2	83 Bi 208.98037	84 Po (209)	85 At (210)	86 Rn (222)
7	87 Fr (223)	88 Ra (226)	89 Ac** (227)	104 Unq (261)	105 Unp (262)	106 Unh (263)	107 Uns (262)	108 Uno (265)	109 Une (267)									

Transitional Metals (groups 3–12)

Inner-transitional Metals

*Lanthanides

58 Ce 140.115	59 Pr 140.90765	60 Nd 144.24	61 Pm (145)	62 Sm 150.36	63 Eu 151.965	64 Gd 157.25	65 Tb 158.92534	66 Dy 162.50	67 Ho 164.93032	68 Er 167.266	69 Tm 168.93421	70 Yb 173.04	71 Lu 174.967

**Actinides

90 Th 232.0381	91 Pa (231)	92 U 238.0289	93 Np (237)	94 Pu (244)	95 Am (243)	96 Cm (247)	97 Bk (247)	98 Cf (251)	99 Es (252)	100 Fm (257)	101 Md (258)	102 No (259)	103 Lr (262)

Key to Abbreviations

Name	Symbol	Name	Symbol	Name	Symbol	Name	Symbol
Actinium	Ac	Europium	Eu	Molybdenum	Mo	Samarium	Sm
Aluminum	Al	Fermium	Fm	Neodymium	Nd	Scandium	Sc
Americium	Am	Fluorine	F	Neon	Ne	Selenium	Se
Antimony	Sb	Francium	Fr	Neptunium	Np	Silicon	Si
Argon	Ar	Gadolinium	Gd	Nickel	Ni	Silver	Ag
Arsenic	As	Gallium	Ga	Niobium	Nb	Sodium	Na
Astatine	At	Germanium	Ge	Nitrogen	N	Strontium	Sr
Barium	Ba	Gold	Au	Nobelium	No	Sulfur	S
Berkelium	Bk	Hafnium	Hf	Osmium	Os	Tantalum	Ta
Beryllium	Be	Hahnium	Ha	Oxygen	O	Technetium	Tc
Bismuth	Bi	Helium	He	Palladium	Pd	Tellurium	Te
Boron	B	Holmium	Ho	Phosphorus	P	Terbium	Tb
Bromine	Br	Hydrogen	H	Platinum	Pt	Thallium	Tl
Cadmium	Cd	Indium	In	Plutonium	Pu	Thorium	Th
Calcium	Ca	Iodine	I	Polonium	Po	Thulium	Tm
Californium	Cf	Iridium	Ir	Potassium	K	Tin	Sn
Carbon	C	Iron	Fe	Praseodymium	Pr	Titanium	Ti
Cerium	Ce	Krypton	Kr	Promethium	Pm	Tungsten	W
Cesium	Cs	Lanthanum	La	Protactinium	Pa	Uranium	U
Chlorine	Cl	Lawrencium	Lw	Radium	Ra	Vanadium	V
Chromium	Cr	Lead	Pb	Radon	Rn	Xenon	Xe
Cobalt	Co	Lithium	Li	Rhenium	Re	Ytterbium	Yb
Copper	Cu	Lutetium	Lu	Rhodium	Rh	Yttrium	Y
Curium	Cm	Magnesium	Mg	Rubidium	Rb	Zinc	Zn
Dysprosium	Dy	Manganese	Mn	Ruthenium	Ru	Zirconium	Zr
Einsteinium	Es	Mendelevium	Md	Rutherfordium	Rf		
Erbium	Er	Mercury	Hg				

TABLE B-2   Densities of Some Selected Substances (g/cm³)*

State	Density	Example
Gas g/L	1.31	Oxygen
Liquids g/mL	0.92	Olive oil
	1.00	Water
Solids g/cm³	1.59	Sucrose
	2.16	Salt

*1 ml = 1cm³ = cc

still boils at 100°C (**celcius**) at one atmosphere of pressure. Intensive properties are much more useful than extensive properties, since they represent qualities associated with a particular substance.

Mass and volume of a sample are extensive properties. Energy is also an extensive property. Energy is defined as the ability to do work or to transfer heat. There are many forms of energy that can be converted into other forms of energy. For example, a potato obtains its energy from the sun in the form of solar energy, and it converts this energy into chemical energy stored in the chemical bonds of starch. Electrical energy can be converted into heat energy in order to bake a potato. Once eaten, the chemical energy in the baked potato can be converted to ATP energy to power muscle tissue. This muscle energy can be used to prepare the soil and plant more potatoes. This sequence of events is an example of the law of conservation of energy, "that energy can be converted from one form to another but it can't be created or destroyed."

Temperature is a measure of the degree of "hotness" of a material, whereas heat is a form of energy that can be transferred between two objects of different temperature.

When heat energy is added to something, its temperature rises. It takes significantly more energy to boil water than to heat an empty teakettle. Therefore, different forms of matter respond differently to heat. The specific heat of a substance is the quantity of heat energy required to change the temperature of 1 g of that substance by 1°C. Extrapolating from the definition of a calorie, the specific heat of water is 1 cal $g^{-1}°C^{-1}$. (The specific heat of water is 1.000) The specific heat of alcohol is 0.587 cal $g^{-1}°C^{-1}$; it takes only a little over half a calorie to increase the temperature of 1 gram of alcohol by 1°C.

Every substance has a characteristic set of intensive properties divided into two classes: physical and chemical properties. Physical properties can be determined without altering the chemical composition of the substance. Ice melts at 1°C. Sugar melts at 186°C. Melting and boiling points are common examples of physical properties.

Chemical properties determine the changes that a substance undergoes in **chemical reactions.** Other substances affect the chemical properties of a substance. A chemical change or reaction is a process whereby the composition of one or more substances is changed. What actually takes place is affected by the chemical properties of the participants.

$$C_6H_{12}O_6 \;+\; 6O_2 \;\rightarrow\; 6CO_2 \;+\; 6H_2O$$

Glucose   Oxygen   Carbon dioxide   Water

Units

The SI units *(Systeme International d'Units)* used for scientific measurements designate a specific metric unit. The units used most frequently in nutrition are mass (kilogram), length (meter), temperature, and amount of substance. Prefixes indicate decimal fractions or multiples of the various units. For example, *kilo* means 1×10^3 meter, or 1 kilometer, and 1 millimeter is 1×10^{-3} meter.

The temperature scale commonly used in scientific studies is the Celsius scale. On this scale, water freezes at 0°Celsius, and 32°Fahrenheit. Water boils at 100°C and 212°F. Normal body temperature is 37.0°C, and 98.6°F. For English-metric conversions for length, weight, temperature, and volume (amount) see Appendix J.

Calories and Joules

Energy is measured in calories or joules. A calorie is the amount of energy required to raise the temperature of 1 gram of water 1 degree C. The SI unit of energy is the joule (J). A mass of 1 g moving at a velocity of 1 m/s possesses the energy equivalent of 1 J. A joule is not a large amount of energy, so kilojoules (kJ) are widely used in nutrition chemistry, biology, and biochemistry. In terms of the joule, 1 calorie = 4.184J. Note that the energy content of foods is expressed as kilocalories (kcal), the amount of energy needed to raise the temperature of 1 kilogram of water 1°C.

Scientific Notation

In science, very large and very small numbers frequently must be used, but they are awkward because large numbers have a long string of trailing zeros and small numbers have a long string of leading zeros. The convenient way to express these numbers is to use the power of 10, or scientific notation.

In scientific notation, a number is expressed as a product of a coefficient multiplied by a power of 10. The coefficient is a number equal to or greater than 1 but less than 10. The power of 10 is the exponent.

$$a \times 10^b$$

where *a* is the coefficient and *b* is the exponent.

$$6.02217 \times 10^{23} = 602,217,000,000,000,000,000,000$$
$$2.99161 \times 10^{-23} = 0.0000000000000000000000299161$$

In the previous examples, the positive exponent for the number indicates that the number is very large. The negative exponent indicates a very small number.

To change a number greater than 1 into scientific notation, move the decimal point to the left until the number is greater than 1 but less than 10. This is the coefficient. The number of places that the decimal is moved becomes the exponent of 10. To change a number less than 1 into scientific notation, move the decimal point to the right until the number is greater than 1 but less than 10. This is the coefficient. The number of places that the decimal is moved is given with a negative sign and is the exponent of 10.

▪ Atoms

The smallest unit of matter that can undergo a chemical change is called an **atom**. An element is composed of atoms of only one kind. For example, the element carbon is composed of just carbon atoms. There are more than 100 different elements.

Atomic Structure

The center of the atom is a nucleus containing two (subatomic) particles: **protons,** which carry a positive charge, and **neutrons,** with no charge. The mass of the proton equals the mass of the neutron. Adding the protons and neutrons together equals the atomic mass of the atom. An atom of carbon containing 6 protons and 6 neutrons has an atomic mass of 12. The atomic mass of nitrogen is 14 and the atomic mass of oxygen is 16. What is the atomic mass of hydrogen (review Table B-1)?

The atomic number is equal to the number of protons in the nucleus. What are the atomic numbers of hydrogen, carbon, nitrogen, and oxygen?

Surrounding the nucleus of the atom are negatively charged subatomic particles called **electrons.** The nucleus is actually surrounded by an electron cloud. Electrons have about 2000 times less mass than the mass of protons or neutrons. Thus, all the mass of an atom essentially is located within the nucleus. The structure of an atom can therefore be pictured as a very tiny, highly dense nuclear core surrounded by a cloud of electrons. The number of electrons in an atom equals the number of protons, so the net charge is zero.

Electrons surrounding the nucleus have a somewhat peculiar, nonintuitive (contrary to what would be expected) behavior. For instance, it's impossible to know precisely where any given electron is located at any given moment. It is possible to define only a volume of space where the electron is most likely to be found. This volume has a specific distribution of electron density in space and is called an orbital. An orbital is a volume of space. Each orbital has its own characteristic energy and shape. Different orbitals have different energies.

Orbitals of similar energy are grouped together into electron shells. A shell can contain 1, 4, 9, or 16 different orbitals. Shells can hold a maximum of 2, 8, 18, or 32 electrons, depending on the number of orbitals in the shell, and any shell can hold less than the maximum number of electrons.

Electrons don't move from one orbital to another but reside in their orbital or energy level. The first orbital outside the nucleus has room for just two electrons. When the orbital is full, the next orbital away from the nucleus is available for electrons, and in that orbital there is room for 8 electrons. Thus, hydrogen has one electron in orbital 1. Carbon has 2 electrons in orbital 1 and 4 in orbital 2. In orbital 3, there is room for 8 electrons. Sulfur, with an atomic number of 16 has 2 electrons in the first orbital, 8 in the second, and 6 in the third (Table B-3).

Only the electron in the outermost orbital (if the orbital is incomplete) can participate in chemical reactions to form chemical bonds. The outermost electrons of an atom are known as the valence electrons.

An atom tends to bond with other atoms that will fill its outer shell and produce a stable number of valence electrons. For instance, a hydrogen atom, with only a single electron shell and one electron, will react with other atoms that provide another electron and fill the shell with a stable number of two electrons.

Isotopes and Atomic Weight

All the atoms of an element have the same number of protons in the nucleus, but the number of neutrons in the nuclei of elements such as carbon, nitrogen, oxygen may vary. All elements have varieties, called **isotopes,** that differ from each other only in number of neutrons and therefore in atomic mass. Hydrogen atoms have only one proton, but an isotope can have one or two neutrons. Tritium, a radioactive isotope, has one proton and two neutrons. Carbon nuclei, for example, can contain five, six, seven, or eight neutrons. Isotopes are distinguished by adding the number of protons and neutrons together and writing the resultant sum as a superscript to the left of the elemental symbol. For example, carbon nuclei have six protons and six neutrons, so it is written as ^{12}C. The isotope containing seven neutrons is labeled ^{13}C, and the isotope containing eight neutrons is labeled ^{14}C. Note that, because all these

TABLE B-3	Atoms Commonly Present in Organic Molecules						
Atom	Symbol	Atomic Number	Atomic Mass	Orbital 1	Orbital 2	Orbital 3	Number of Chemical Bonds
Hydrogen	H	1	1	1	0	0	1
Carbon	C	6	12	2	4	0	4
Nitrogen	N	7	14	2	5	0	3
Oxygen	O	8	16	2	6	0	2
Sulfur	S	16	32	2	8	6	2

atoms have six protons, they are all carbon atoms, but, because they possess different numbers of neutrons, they represent isotopes of carbon. All isotopes of an element behave the same way chemically.

Atomic weight considers the fact that an element is a mixture of isotopes. If all carbon were ^{12}C, the atomic weight would be the same as its atomic mass, 12. But, since carbon contains ^{13}C and ^{14}C, the atomic weight is slightly higher, 12.011. The atomic weight is based on the relative abundance of each isotope.

Although the ordinary chemical behavior of different isotopes of the same element is virtually identical, the radiochemical behavior is sometimes different. Isotopes exhibit differences in physical behavior—because they decay (break down) to more stable isotopes by giving off nuclear particles of ionizing radiation. Certain unstable isotopes (radioisotopes) are in an obvious process of decay. Every element has at least one such radioisotope. These radioisotopes have a physical half-life, which is the time required for 50% of its atoms to decay to a more stable state. Isotopes such as ^{32}P (phosphorus), emit radiation that can be measured by instruments such as Geiger counters and scintillation counters. The isotope ^{14}C decays more rapidly than other isotopes of carbon. Other isotopes are not radioactive but still can be traced in bodily fluids or tissues using other types of instruments. Examples include ^{13}C and ^{15}N; these are called stable isotopes, since they decay very slowly and do not emit radiation.

Isotope "markers," such as ^{32}P and ^{13}C, have a practical use, as they can be used to trace nutrients as they participate in the chemical pathways in the body. For example, researchers can "mark" a glucose molecule with a radioactive carbon atom (^{14}C). This allows them to see where the carbons of glucose are distributed in the body, and it helps indicate what chemical transformations glucose undergoes when metabolized. Such studies have demonstrated that glucose can become part of the lipid stored in adipose cells or form the CO_2 (detected as $^{14}CO_2$) that is exhaled. Isotope techniques are widely used in nutrition research.

Carbon Dating Using the Properties of Isotopes

Have you ever wondered how the age of plants, animals, and humans that have been dead for a long time are determined? Carbon-14 dating has been an important tool for archaeologists and other scientists in deciding when a carbon-containing species lived and died. The knowledge of the ongoing radioactive decay of ^{14}C can determine the age of ancient materials because the half-life of any radioactive substance is constant.

This method depends on the fact that carbon dioxide in the air consists of ^{12}C, with trace amounts of ^{14}C, the isotope that is radioactive and decays. The amount of ^{14}C in the air does not decrease over time because it is constantly being formed from ^{14}N by the action of cosmic rays, which captures neutrons in the upper atmosphere. ^{14}C is radioactive and undergoes decay with a half-life of 5730 years.

As long as a plant is living, it absorbs carbon dioxide from the air, and a constant fraction of the ^{14}C is incorporated into carbon-containing molecules. When animals eat plants, the ^{14}C is incorporated into them. In other words, a defined amount of ^{14}C will be present along with ^{12}C.

When the plant or animal (human) dies, there is no longer an exchange of carbon dioxide with the atmosphere. Therefore, the amount of ^{14}C in the organism decreases with time as it decays. (This method of dating cannot be used for organic material older than 50,000 years.) It is possible to estimate the age of an object by determining the ratio of ^{14}C to ^{12}C because the ratio is constantly diminishing. Using these dating techniques, it has been possible to determine the kinds and amounts of foods humans consumed thousands of years ago.

For instance, the quick-frozen "Ice Man," who was discovered in the Italian Alps in 1991, had died about 5300 years earlier, based on carbon dating analysis. When he was discovered, he was in an extraordinary state of preservation. In fact, the hikers who discovered his body assumed he had just died. The "Ice Man" was 5 feet 4

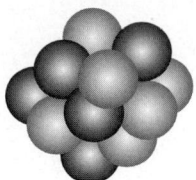

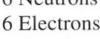

^{12}Carbon
6 Protons
6 Neutrons
6 Electrons

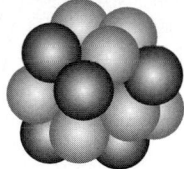

^{13}Carbon
6 Protons
7 Neutrons
6 Electrons

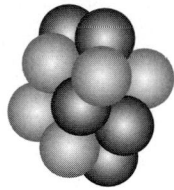

^{14}Carbon
6 Protons
8 Neutrons
6 Electrons

inches tall, weighed about 110 pounds, and was 40 to 45 years old when he died. What was remarkable about the man was that his joints were badly worn, and he had virtually no body fat, indicating a life of very hard labor. His diet certainly consisted of some cereals, since he carried evidence that he had been involved in threshing grain. Based on the contents of his stomach, it was possible to construct his last meal. Carbon dating gives scientists an opportunity to look at the health of ancient ancestors and relate these data to their diet.

Atomic and Molar Mass

Atoms are very small. One ^{12}C atom has a mass of 1.993×10^{-23} g. The units used to quantify atomic mass are called atomic mass units (amu). An amu is calculated for each element by dividing the mass of that atom by 1.6605×10^{-24}, which is essentially the mass of one proton or neutron. Performing this division on ^{12}C, the mass of such an atom is 12 amu. The amu for each element is listed in the bottom portion of each entry in the periodic table.

You are familiar with counting units, such as the number of sticks in a package of chewing gum. In chemistry, the unit of dealing with atoms, ions (an electrically charged atom), and molecules (a combination of atoms) is the mole. A mole is defined as the amount of matter that contains as many objects (things) as the number of atoms in 12 g of ^{12}C. The number of atoms in 12g of ^{12}C is

$$12 \text{ g } ^{12}C \times \frac{1 \text{ atom}}{1.993 \times 10^{-23} \text{g } ^{12}C} = 6.023 \times 10^{23} \text{ atoms}$$

It is not their weight but the *number* of molecules that determines the physiological effect of a substance. Therefore, the number of "objects" in a mole is 6.02×10^{23}, which is called Avogadro's number. This concept of g per mole can be extended directly. A mole (mol) of anything contains Avogadro's number of these objects:

$$1 \text{ mol } ^{12}C \text{ atoms} = 6.02 \times 10^{23} \, ^{12}C \text{ atoms}$$
$$1 \text{ mol of water molecules} = 6.02 \times 10^{23} \, H_2O \text{ molecules}$$
$$1 \text{ mol } NO_3^- \text{ ions} = 6.02 \times 10^{23} \, NO_3^- \text{ ions}$$

In order to relate the number of units of matter to mass, as measured by instruments, the individual mass of each unit of matter is needed. The mass of the atom is expressed as atomic weight. The molecular weight of an individual molecule is the sum of the atomic weights of its constituent atoms. The molar mass of a substance is the mass, in g, of a mole of the substance.

A single ^{12}C atom has a mass of 12 amu, but a single ^{24}Mg is twice as massive, 24 amu. Because a mole always has the same number of particles, a mole of Mg is twice as massive as a mole of ^{12}C atoms. A mole of carbon weighs 12 g; a mole of Mg weighs 24 g. The same number that refers to the mass of a single atom of an element (in amu) also represents the mass (in g) of 1 mol of atoms of that element. For example, one ^{12}C atom weighs 12 amu. One mol ^{12}C weighs 12 g. One ^{24}Mg atom weighs 24 amu, and 1 mol ^{24}Mg weighs 24 g.

The mass in g of 1 mole of a substance is called its molar mass. The molar mass (in g) of any substance is always numerically equal to its formula weight (in amu). For example, one H_2O molecule weighs 18.0 amu, and 1 mol of H_2O weighs 18.0 g. One NaCl molecule weighs 58.5 amu, and 1 mol of NaCl weighs 58.5 g.

■ Molecules, Covalent Bonds, Hydrogen Bonds, Ions and Ionic Compounds

Molecules

Molecules are formed through the interaction of the electrons, between two or more atoms in the outermost orbitals (valence electrons). When electrons are

Dalton is another term used to indicate atomic mass, such as for proteins, DNA, and RNA. This is equivalent to an amu.

shared, chemical **bonds** are formed. The term **compound** refers to molecules composed of more than one element. Water is a compound. Each molecule (or compound) possesses its own properties, such as color, taste, and density.

The number of chemical bonds that an atom can form depends on the number of electrons needed to complete the outermost orbital. Hydrogen can form just one chemical bond because it has room for just one electron in its orbital of two electrons. Carbon can form four chemical bonds, nitrogen three, oxygen two, and sulfur two (review Table B-3).

A molecular formula gives the elemental composition of a molecule or compound. This consists of the symbols of the atoms in the molecule, plus a subscript denoting the number of each type of atom.

A structural formula shows how the atoms are arranged with respect to each other. As an extension, molecular and ball-and-stick models approximate the shape of the molecule (Fig. B-1).

When molecules combine with each other, atoms do not increase or decrease in number. Atoms present in starting materials must be present in the products. For example, count the carbons hydrogen and oxygen atoms in glucose and oxygen before and after the chemical change below. This example also illustrates the process of conservation of mass.

$$C_6H_{12}O_6 + 6\,O_2 \rightarrow 6\,CO_2 + 6\,H_2O$$

Covalent Bonds

When atoms share their valence electrons, a **covalent bond** is formed. The electrons shared between atoms are bonding electrons; these represent the adhesive that holds atoms together in molecular form.

When two identical atoms share electrons, such as in the formation of hydrogen gas (H_2) or oxygen gas (O_2), the covalent bond is very strong because the electrons are shared equally. This equal distribution between the atoms makes the molecule nonpolar. Consider the simple component methane (CH_4). Hydrogen has one electron in its valence shell, and that valence shell can hold a maximum of two electrons. Carbon has four electrons in its valence shell, and that shell can hold a maximum of eight electrons. Both carbon and hydrogen fill their valence shells to the maximum by sharing electrons with each other. Notice that each hydrogen in methane contains

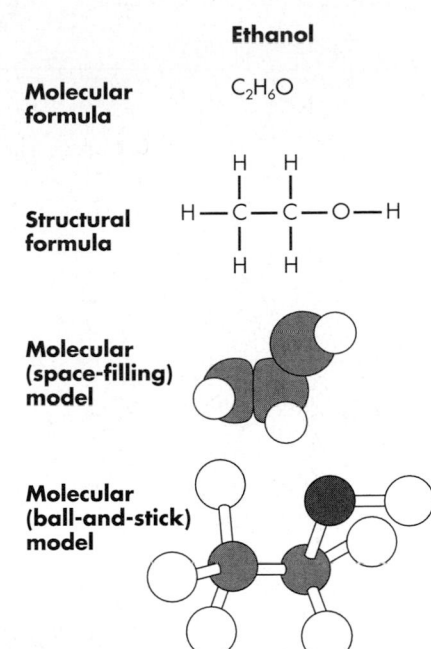

	Ethanol
Molecular formula	C_2H_6O
Structural formula	
Molecular (space-filling) model	
Molecular (ball-and-stick) model	

▌ FIGURE B-1 Examples of the molecular and structural formulas and the molecular models of ethanol. The space-filling type of model gives a more realistic feeling of the space occupied by the atoms. On the other hand, the ball-and-stick type shows the bonds and bond angles more clearly.

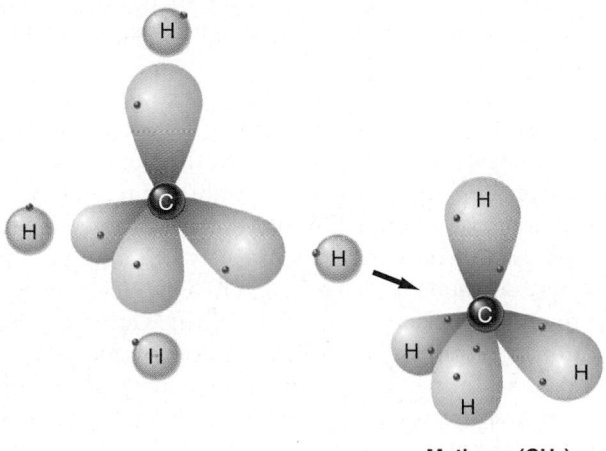

Methane (CH₄)

In each of the four bonds, one electron of the carbon is shared with the electron of a hydrogen atom in a single, sausage-shaped molecular orbital encompassing the two nuclei. Methane is the simplest organic molecule. Even the largest organic molecules are held together by strong covalent bonds like these.

two electrons and that the carbon atom has eight electrons in its valence. A good way to look at this is that the hydrogen atoms share one pair of electrons, whereas the carbon atoms share four pairs of electrons.

Guidelines that govern the formation of covalent bonds are as follows:

1. The valence shell of each element must have room to accommodate additional electrons.

2. Second-row nonmetallic elements of the periodic table (e.g., carbon, nitrogen, and oxygen) and hydrogen typically fill their valence shells by sharing the necessary number of electrons with another element.

3. Third-row nonmetals and those beyond this point in the periodic table (e.g., phosphorus, sulfur, and chloride) frequently make fewer covalent bonds than are necessary to fill the valence shell. Sulfur, for example, typically makes two bonds instead of the six that are possible. Phosphorus often forms five bonds.

A single covalent bond forms when two atoms share one electron pair. A double covalent bond forms when two atoms share two electron pairs.

When electrons spend approximately equal time around each atom nucleus, the bond is called a nonpolar covalent bond. These are the strongest chemical bonds. If the two nuclei are not equally attractive to electrons, their atoms can form a polar covalent bond in which the electrons spend more time orbiting the more attractive nucleus. For example, when hydrogen bonds with oxygen, the electrons are more attracted to the oxygen nucleus and orbit that nucleus than they do the hydrogen nucleus. Electrons carry a negative charge. This makes the oxygen region of the molecule slightly negative and the hydrogen region slightly positive. The Greek letter delta (δ) is used to symbolize a charge less than that of one electron or proton. A slightly negative region of a molecule is shown as δ^- and a slightly positive region is shown as δ^+. A molecule such as this is called a dipole because it has two charged poles. Water is a good example.

Water, the most abundant molecule in the body, serves as a good solvent because it is polar. For example, the oxygen atom pulls electrons from the two hydrogen atoms toward its side of the water molecule, so that the oxygen side is more negatively charged than the hydrogen side of the molecule.

When two different atoms form a covalent bond, the bonding electrons are never shared equally. Consider the H–O bond in water. It is unreasonable to expect that the hydrogen nucleus (containing one proton) and the oxygen nucleus (containing eight protons) have identical forces of attraction for the shared electron pair. In addition, other factors come into play, such as how many shells each atom has, how many electrons are in the shells, and the distance the shared electrons are from each nucleus. All of these factors lead to an unequal sharing of electrons in a covalent bond between different atoms.

The ability of an atom in a molecule to attract electrons in the direction of itself is called electronegativity. Elements toward the top right corner of the periodic table have the highest electronegativity, and those toward the bottom left have the lowest (electronegativity generally increases from left to right in a row of the periodic table, and decreases going down a column; the difference in the electronegativities of bonded atoms can be used to determine the polarity of a bond). Metals have low electronegativity, whereas nonmetals have relatively high electronegativity. Oxygen and nitrogen have the highest electronegativities of the elements typically found in compounds important to nutrition. The electronegativity values of atoms determine the type of chemical bond formed. If the electronegativity of two bonding atoms differs greatly, electron transfer occurs to yield an ionic bond, as in Na^+Cl^-. If the electronegativity values are not very different, a covalent bond is formed.

Polar molecules are weakly attracted both to ions and to other polar molecules. The positive end of the molecule can align itself with an anion or with the negative end of another molecule. These attractive forces, called, respectively, ion-dipole and dipole-dipole forces, are much weaker than covalent bonds individually, but, when there are many of them, they make a significant contribution to the total energy of

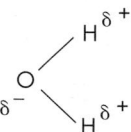

δ denotes partial charge

a collection of molecules. Water, for instance, has a much higher boiling point than expected because the molecules are glued together by such forces.

Hydrogen Bonds

Water, and most other molecules containing an O—H or N—H bond, exhibit a particularly strong interaction called hydrogen bonding (Fig. B-2). In this case, the hydrogen atom of one molecule is attracted to a nonbonded electron pair of a highly electronegative atom of a neighboring molecule, such as oxygen. Water molecules are weakly attracted to each other by hydrogen bonds. This attraction is responsible for many of the biologically important properties of water. Hydrogen bonds, such as those found in large proteins and DNA, hold the molecule together. These molecules fold or twist into three-dimensional shapes, due in part to the action of hydrogen bonds. Hydrogen bonds are usually symbolized by a dotted line between the atoms: —C—O ··· H—N—. Hydrogen bonds are the weakest of all chemical bonds. There will be much more about chemical bonds in the chapters on carbohydrate (Chapter 5), lipids (Chapter 6), and proteins (Chapter 7).

Ions and Ionic Compounds

Atoms that have an equal number of positively charged protons and negatively charged electrons are electrically neutral. Atoms or molecules that have positive or negative charges are called ions. **Ionic bonds** result when one or more valence electrons from one atom are completely transferred to another atom or molecule. Elements that have one to three valance electrons have a tendency to give up electrons, and those with four to seven electrons have a tendency to accept electrons. The electrons are not shared. Take the case of sodium chloride. One atom loses electrons, so that its number of electrons becomes smaller than its number of protons; thus, it becomes positively charged as Na^+ in sodium chloride. The other atom gains electrons, so its number of electrons is greater than its number of protons, so it becomes negatively charged as Cl^- in sodium chloride.

Positively charged ions are called cations, as they move toward negative pole in an electric field. The second atom with more electrons than protons becomes negatively charged or is an anion because it moves to the positive pole. NaCl is an example of an ionic compound.

The single electron in the outer orbital of sodium is attracted to chlorine's outer orbital with its 7 electrons. Sodium has 3 electron shells, with a total of 11 electrons. There is room for 1 more electron in the chlorine outer orbital to make up the shell of 8 electrons. Chlorine has 17 electrons, 2 in the first shell, 8 in the second shell, and 7 in the third—this creates a chloride ion. Note the name change that occurs

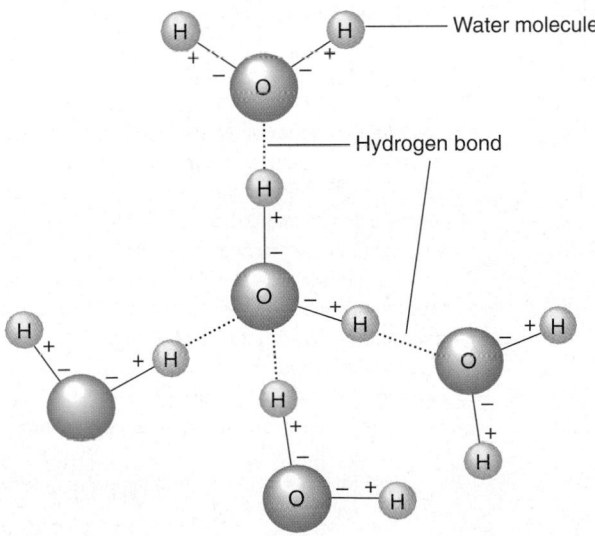

■ FIGURE **B-2** Hydrogen bonds between water molecules. The oxygen atoms of water molecules are weakly joined together by the attraction of the electronegative oxygen for the positively charged hydrogen. These weak bonds are called hydrogen bonds.

when an element gains an electron to become a negative ion; the suffix becomes *–ide*.

The electrons in metal atoms (these elements that have luster and conduct electricity) are not tightly bound to the nucleus, so, when metals undergo chemical transformations, they frequently lose one or more electrons. This results in a metallic species containing more protons than electrons, thus possessing a net positive charge. Sodium is an example.

In nonmetallic elements, the electrons are very tightly held by the nucleus and cations are rarely formed, and then only under forcing conditions. Instead, nonmetallic elements generally accept additional electrons. This results in a species with a net negative charge. Chlorine is an example.

These charged atoms, where electron(s) have been added or removed, are collectively known as ions. Sodium (Na^+), potassium (K^+), and calcium (Ca^{2+}) are found in the body as cations. Chloride (Cl^-) is a common anion in the body. See Table B-4 for a more complete list of common ions found in the body.

Ionic bonds are weaker than polar covalent bonds. Ionic compounds easily separate when dissolved in water. Table salt (NaCl) is obvious when poured out of the salt shaker, but when the salt is stirred into a cup of water it disappears. It *dissociates*. The polar water's negative side (oxygen) is attracted to the Na^+, and the positive side (hydrogen) is attracted to Cl^-. Water molecules that surround the ions, in turn, attract other water molecules to form hydration spheres around each ion. This mechanism makes ions or molecules soluble in water. Many organic molecules dissolve in water. These molecules are called hydrophilic. Molecules that are composed of nonpolar covalent bonds, such as fats, are called hydrophobic. They don't carry a charge, so they are insoluble in water.

Salts

Salts are substances composed of cations and anions. Table salt is NaCl. The Na^+ and Cl^- are attracted to each other by electrostatic force, and the resulting ionic compound is known chemically as sodium chloride. Salts are formed by the interaction of acids and bases in a neutralization reaction. Water is also formed in such a reaction. In this type of reaction, hydrogen ions of an acid are replaced by the positive ions of a base, and a salt forms. For example, when hydrochloric acid reacts with sodium hydroxide, table salt is produced:

TABLE B-4	Important Ions in the Human Body	
Common Ions	**Symbol**	**Some Functions**
Calcium	Ca^{2+}	Component of bones and teeth, necessary for blood clotting, muscle contraction, and nerve transmission
Sodium	Na^+	Helps maintain membrane potentials (electrical charge differences across a membrane) and water balance
Potassium	K^+	Helps maintain membrane potentials
Hydrogen	H^+	Helps maintain acid-base balance
Hydroxide	OH^-	Helps maintain acid-base balance
Chloride	Cl^-	Helps maintain acid-base balance
Bicarbonate	HCO_3^-	Helps maintain acid-base balance
Ammonium	NH_4^+	Helps maintain acid-base balance
Phosphate	PO_4^{3-}	Component of bone and teeth, involved in energy exchange and acid-base balance
Iron	Fe^{2+}	Necessary for red blood cell formation and function
Magnesium	Mg^{2+}	Necessary for enzyme function

$$\text{HCl} \quad + \quad \text{NaOH} \quad \rightarrow \quad \text{NaCl} \quad + \quad \text{H}_2\text{O}$$

Hydrochloric acid   Sodium hydroxide   Salt   Water

(Neutralization reaction)

The formula for salts can be misleading. For example, NaCl suggests that table salt exists as a discrete entity containing one sodium ion and one chloride ion. An inspection of the chemical structure of table salt shows that it is actually a three-dimensional stack of layers—much like having a ream of paper with all the pages glued together (Fig. B-3).

Salts separate to form positively and negatively charged ions when dissolved in water. Substances that dissolve in water and conduct electricity are called electrolytes. A solute that produces ions in solution forms an electrolytic solution that conducts an electrical current. A salt solution is a good conductor of electricity. (A sugar solution does not conduct electricity because it doesn't form ions.) Sodium (Na^+), potassium (K^+), calcium (Ca^{2+}), and chloride (Cl^-), magnesium (Mg^{2+}), phosphate (PO_4^{3-}), and bicarbonate (HCO_3^-) form various electrolytes in the body.

■ Acids, Bases, and pH Scales

We all have a pretty good idea of what acids and bases are. We know that lemon juice is acid and drain cleaners are strong bases.

Water molecules of two hydrogens and one oxygen are held together by polar covalent bonds. Although these are strong bonds, a *small* proportion of them break, releasing a hydrogen ion and a hydroxyl ion. The hydrogen ion (a proton) is transferred to another oxygen in a water molecule, forming a *hydronium ion*. This means that a pair of water molecules can act as an acid and a base, since water self-ionizes, forming hydronium ions and hydroxide ions.

$$2\text{H}_2\text{O} \quad \leftrightarrow \quad \text{H}_3\text{O}^+ \quad + \quad \text{OH}^-$$

Water   Hydronium ion   Hydroxide ion

For simplicity, ionized water will be represented by H^+ and OH^-.

The ionization of water molecules produces equal amounts of hydronium and hydroxide ions, which are both equal to a 10^{-7} molar concentration. At this concentration of ionization, water is considered neutral.

A solution that has a higher concentration of H^+ is said to be acidic, and one that is lower is basic or alkaline. An acid is defined as a substance that can ionize and release protons (H^+) into solution. It is a proton donor.

Because a hydrogen atom without its electron is a proton (H^+), any substance that releases hydrogen ions when in water is an acid. For example, hydrogen chloride

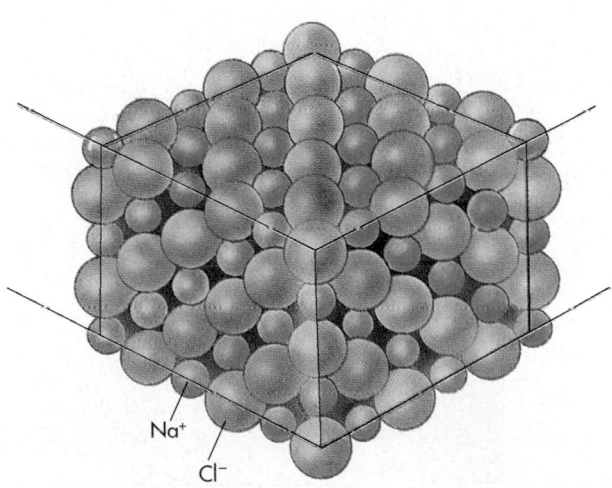

Na$^+$

Cl$^-$

■ **FIGURE B-3** Molecules of sodium chloride (table salt) in typical cube-shape formation.

(HCl) forms hydrogen and chloride ions (H⁺ and Cl⁻) in solution and therefore is an acid.

$$HCl \rightarrow H^+ + Cl^-$$

Figure B-4 lists several common acids and bases. A base is a negatively charged ion or a molecule that ionizes to produce an anion, which can combine with a proton (H⁺), removing it from solution. A base is a proton acceptor. Any substance that can accept hydrogen ions while in water is a base. Many bases can function as proton acceptors by releasing hydroxide ions (OH⁻) when dissolved in water. Most strong bases release OH⁻ into solution. The OH⁻ combines with H⁺ to form water.

$$\underset{\text{Sodium hydroxide}}{NaOH} \quad \rightarrow \quad \underset{\text{Sodium ion}}{Na^+} \quad + \quad \underset{\text{Hydroxide ion}}{OH^-}$$

The hydroxide ions are proton acceptors as they go on to combine with hydrogen ions to form water:

$$\underset{\text{Hydroxide ion}}{OH^-} \quad + \quad \underset{\text{Hydrogen ion}}{H^+} \quad \rightarrow \quad \underset{\text{Water}}{H_2O}$$

pH

Acidity is expressed in terms of pH, a measure of the molarity (the ratio of solute per liter of solution) of H⁺. Molarity is expressed by square brackets, so the molarity of H⁺ is symbolized as [H⁺]. pH is defined as the negative logarithm of the hydrogen

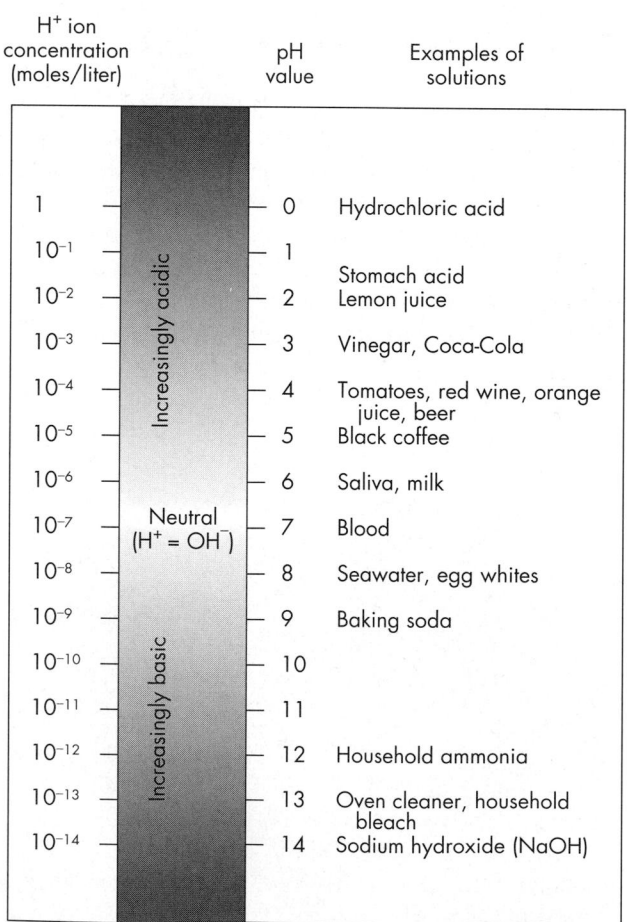

■ FIGURE B-4 The pH values of common substances. Note that tomatoes aren't really that acidic.

ion molarity, or pH $= -\log[H^+]$. The pH unit is the H^+ concentration of a solution. Pure water has a neutral pH because it contains equal amounts of hydrogen (hydronium) and hydroxyl ions. The pH scale runs from 0 to 14 (Fig. B-4).

Since pH is a logarithmic scale, a solution with 10 times the hydrogen ion concentration of 10^{-6} molar has a pH of 6. A solution with 1/10 the hydrogen ion concentration of 10^{-8} molar has a pH of 8. A solution with a pH of 4 is 10 times as **acidic** as one with a pH of 5 and 100 times as acidic as one with a pH of 6. This may be confusing because it is inversely related to the hydrogen ion concentration: A solution with a high hydrogen ion concentration has a low pH number. A solution with a low hydrogen concentration has a high pH number. Acid solutions have a pH of less than 7. Basic, or **alkaline,** solutions have a pH greater than 7.

A slight disruption of pH can seriously disturb normal physiological functions, so it is important the body be able to control pH. Blood normally has a pH range from 7.35 to 7.45. Any deviations from this range can cause dizziness, fainting, coma, paralysis, or death.

Acids and bases are classified as strong or weak. Strong acids and strong bases dissociate completely when dissolved in water. Consequently, they release all of their hydrogen ions or hydroxide ions when dissolved. In general, the more completely an acid or a base dissociates, the stronger it is. Hydrochloric acid, for example, is a strong acid because it completely dissociates in water.

Weak acids only partially dissociate in water. Consequently, they release only some of their acidic hydrogens. For example, when acetic acid ($CH_3\overset{\overset{O}{\|}}{C}-OH$, the principal component of vinegar) dissolves in water, the acetic acid only partially dissociates.

$$CH_3\overset{\overset{O}{\|}}{C}-OH \quad \leftrightarrow \quad CH_3\overset{\overset{O}{\|}}{C}-O^- \quad + \quad H^+$$

Acetic acid   Acetate ion   Proton

The equilibrium lies far to the left, so that only a small fraction of the acetic acid in the vinegar is dissociated into acetate ions and protons.

Most weak bases release hydroxide into solution by reacting with the water itself. For example, ammonia (NH_3) reacts with water to form NH_4^+ and OH^-.

$$NH_3 \quad + \quad H_2O \quad \leftrightarrow \quad NH_4^+ \quad + \quad OH^-$$

Ammonia   Water   Ammonium ion   Hydroxide ion

Buffers

Many of the biochemical reactions that occur in living tissues require tight control of pH. To prevent changes in the H^+ concentration in the body, and to control the pH, a system of buffers is maintained. The pH of the blood is between 7.35 and 7.45. Buffers are ions and molecules that stabilize the pH of a solution. In the blood (plasma), the pH is maintained by the carbonic acid–bicarbonate buffer system. The acid is formed by the combination of water and carbon dioxide. Carbonic acid separates into bicarbonate ion (HCO_3^-) and the hydrogen ion (H^+).

$$HCO_3^- \quad + \quad H^+ \quad \leftrightarrow \quad H_2CO_3 \quad \leftrightarrow \quad H_2O \quad + \quad CO_2$$

Bicarbonate   Hydrogen ion   Carbonic acid   Water   Carbon dioxide

The reaction can go either way. The direction depends on the concentration of ions on either side of the arrows. Carbon dioxide is a gas that is constantly removed from the body by exhalation. For example, if an acid were released into the blood plasma (more H^+ in solution), the reaction would be driven to the right. Acids that are present in the plasma come from cellular activities, but, despite the increase in H^+ by these acids, the blood plasma hardly changes; it is essentially constant. The buffer, bicarbonate, accomplishes this. It is constantly formed to maintain normal pH. Bicarbonate ions and carbonic acid prevent decreases or increases of pH. The kidneys also play a role by absorbing or releasing H^+ or HCO_3^-, depending on the acid-balance balance in the person. Thus, much of the excess acid leaves the body via the urine (urine has an acid pH), so lungs and kidneys keep this buffering system functioning and, in turn, are key to acid-base balance in the body.

■ Free Radicals

You are aware that atoms tend to share electron pairs when forming chemical bonds, and there is a tendency to share enough electrons to completely fill the valence shell. A consequence is that atoms or elements are rarely found with an odd number of electrons. But, when a molecule with an odd number of electrons does arise, it is called a free radical. An example is the superoxide anion. Oxygen is composed of two oxygen atoms (O_2); if an electron is added, it becomes superoxide, or $O_2^{-\bullet}$. The dot signifies an unpaired electron.

Superoxide and other free radicals are reactive, primarily because they contain an unpaired electron. Free radicals seek an electron by attacking and removing electrons from other compounds, such as at the location where hydrogens are attached to carbon. This not only damages the molecule but transforms it into a free radical.

$$R^\bullet + -CH_2 \rightarrow RH^+ -CH^{-\bullet}$$

Free radicals are also formed when a covalent bond breaks and each atom or molecule fragment recovers the electron originally used to make the bond. In this case, energy—usually in the form of sunlight, ultraviolet radiation, or heat—is used to break the bond.

$$A-B + energy \rightarrow A^\bullet + B^\bullet$$

Because free radicals are reactive, they can generate thousands of other free radicals within minutes in a chain-reaction process. The reactivity of free radicals sometimes produces detrimental effects in living systems. For instance, the development of heart disease and some types of cancer, such as skin and lung cancer, are probably promoted by free radicals. However, some normal physiological functions in the body involve free radical formation; they are used by various white blood cells to kill invading bacteria.

The body has a number of mechanisms, such as antioxidants, for neutralizing free radicals. These are substances that react with and neutralize free radicals of oxygen and nitrogen. The enzyme superoxide dismutase (SOD) converts superoxide into oxygen and hydrogen peroxide. One form of SOD contains the minerals copper and zinc, whereas another form contains manganese. Other antioxidants obtained from the diet are vitamin E and vitamin C.

Some substances are used extensively in the food industry to trap free radicals or prevent their formation. This allows for increased storage time of food by decreasing chemical breakdown. These substances are part of a class of food additives called preservatives (see Chapter 19). Vitamin E added to cooking oils protects $C=C$ bonds by trapping free radicals.

■ Organic Chemistry

Organic compounds contain carbon in combination with other elements, such as hydrogen, oxygen, and nitrogen. Carbon compounds are associated with living things, but why carbon? It is because carbon forms very stable bonds, such as single, double, and even triple bonds. Carbon forms strong covalent bonds with many other atoms. Carbon atoms can form rings and chains by bonding to other carbons. Variation in the length of the chains, and their atomic combinations, allows the formation of a wide variety of molecules. Organic molecules generally contain hydrogen to form the hydrocarbon chains and rings.

Cyclic and Chain Compounds

Cyclic organic compounds are common forms of hydrocarbons. Note the diagram of butyric acid (a chain) in the margin and compare that to the structure of glucose, which is a ring. Even though the two compounds are only carbon, oxygen, and hydrogen, each conveys a very different property. Some ring structures are referred to as aromatic compounds.

Hydrocarbons as chains or rings provide the backbone of many groups of compounds that make up important organic nutrients. Other groups are attached to these backbones. They usually contain atoms of oxygen, nitrogen, phosphorus, and sulfur. The functional or reactive groups provide the unique chemical properties of organic molecules. Classes of organic molecules are known by their functional groups (Table B-5).

Several important organic compounds contain a functional group called a carbonyl group (C=O). The carbonyl group is the parent compound for ketones, aldehydes, and many related groups. Table B-5, has a list of all these compounds that are important to nutrition.

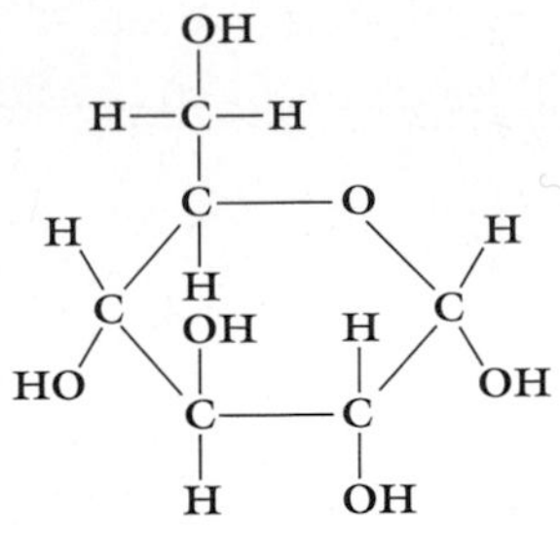

Glucose

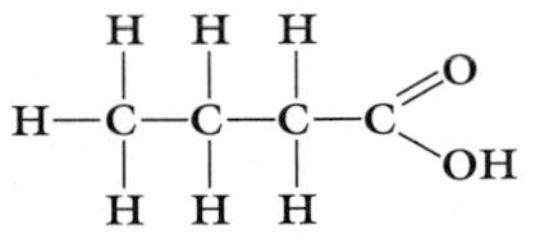

Butyric acid

TABLE B-5   Typical Chemical Groups Found in Nutrients

Functional Group	Name	Typically Found In	Example
$-OH$	Hydroxide	Alcohols	CH_3-OH
$-C=O$ (with H)	Aldehyde	Sugars	$CH_3C=O$ (with H)
$C-C=O$ (with C)	Ketone	Ketones	$CH_3C=O$ (with CH_3)
$-C=O$ (with OH)	Carboxyl	Acids	$CH_3C=O$ (with OH)
$-S-S-$	Disulfide	Proteins	$CH_3-S-S-CH_3$
$-C=O$	Carbonyl	Aldehydes, ketones, caboxylic acids, amides	$(CH_3)_2C=O$
$-C-NH_2$	Amine	Proteins	CH_3-NH_2
$-C=O$ (with NH_2)	Amide	Vitamins	$CH_3C=O$ (with NH_2)
$HO-P=O$ (with OH, OH)	Phosphate	High-energy compounds	$CH_2-O-P=O$ (with OH, $O-CH_2-$)
$-C=O$ (with $O-C$)	Ester	Triglycerides	$CH_3-C=O$ (with $O-CH_2CH_3$)
$-O-\overset{O}{\overset{\|}{C}}-CH_2-$	Acyl	Triglycerides	$-CH_2-\overset{O}{\overset{\|}{C}}-O-\overset{}{C} \begin{smallmatrix} C-O-\overset{O}{\overset{\|}{C}}-CH_2- \\ C-O-\overset{O}{\overset{\|}{C}}-CH_2- \end{smallmatrix}$

Ketones are organic compounds in which the carbonyl group occurs at the interior of a carbon chain and therefore flanked by carbon atoms. Body fat that is breaking down at a rapid rate produces ketones $\left(\begin{smallmatrix} C-C=O \\ | \\ C \end{smallmatrix}\right)$, some of which are removed from the body by way of the urine (see Chapter 4).

Aldehydes $\left(\begin{smallmatrix} -C=O \\ | \\ H \end{smallmatrix}\right)$ are organic compounds that contain a carbonyl group to which at least one hydrogen atom is attached. This active group is found in one important form of vitamin A. As an aldehyde, it plays a central role in vision.

Many of our most common substances, both in foods and in the body, contain carboxylic acids. A carboxylic acid $\left(\begin{smallmatrix} O \\ \| \\ -C-OH \end{smallmatrix}\right)$ contains the carbonyl group with an OH group attached. These acids are widely distributed in tissues and natural products. Vinegar contains acetic acid. Citrus fruits contain citric acid, and vitamin C is ascorbic acid.

The carboxyl group is an acid because it can donate a H^+ (proton) to a solution. A very common acid formed in muscle cells is known as lactic acid. When lactic acid ionizes, it releases the H^+ and becomes lactate. Since both forms of the acid (ionized and nonionized) are in solution, the proportion depends on the pH of the solution. The terms *lactic acid* and *lactate* are both correct.

An alcohol has the carbonyl group, C=O, but the O is bonded to a single hydrogen, so the double bond of the carbonyl group changes to a single bond, forming an OH or hydroxide group (ROH).

An ester $\left(\begin{smallmatrix} O \\ \| \\ R-C-O-C \end{smallmatrix}\right)$ is an organic compound that has an O-C group attached to a carbonyl group. An ester is the product of a reaction between a carboxylic acid and an alcohol. The formation of lipids called triglycerides involves the formation of ester bonds.

The carbonyl portion of a compound such as an ester is called an acyl group. Thus, removal of the hydroxyl group (OH) from an organic acid forms an acyl group.

Two sulfur atoms (S—S), each attached to a carbon, produce a disulfide group. This group is important to the structural characteristics of certain proteins.

A single carbon with an amine group attached ($-NH_2$) is a component of all amino acids (Fig. B-5).

■ Isomerism

Molecules that have identical chemical formulas but different structures are called **isomers.** A simple example of this is two compounds with the formula C_2H_6O.

$$CH_3CH_2OH \qquad CH_3OCH_3$$
Ethanol   Methyl ether

Ethanol, or alcohol, is consumed by millions of people every day. Methyl ether is a poisonous substance. This illustrates an important point about isomers: Since they have different structures, they must have different *chemical* properties.

The difference in properties between two isomers can be great (as in the preceding example) or very subtle, but the differences are there and are detectable. There are different types of isomerism but only two of the common types will be briefly reviewed in this section: structural isomers and stereoisomers.

Structural Isomers

Isomers in which the number and kinds of bonds differ are called structural isomers. Molecules containing chains of carbon atoms typically have many structural isomers. Any variation in the way the chain is branched gives rise to a new isomer. For example, pentane (C_5H_{12}) has three isomers, as shown in the margin.

Pentane $CH_3-CH_2-CH_2-CH_2-CH_3$

Neopentane $CH_3-CH_2-\underset{\underset{CH_3}{|}}{CH}-CH_3$

Isopentane $CH_3-\underset{\underset{CH_3}{|}}{\overset{\overset{CH_3}{|}}{C}}-CH_3$

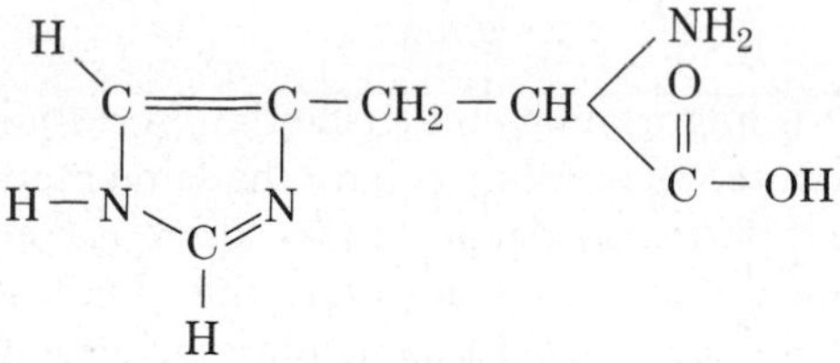

Histidine (His)
(essential)

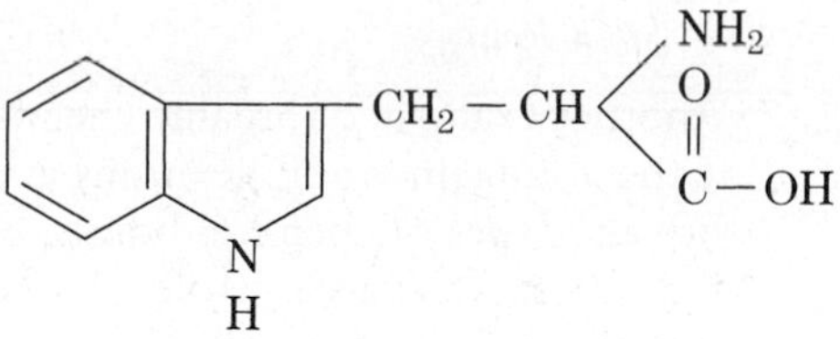

Tryptophan (Trp)
(essential)

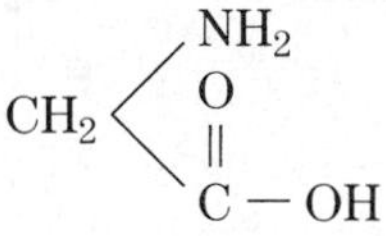

Glycine (Gly)

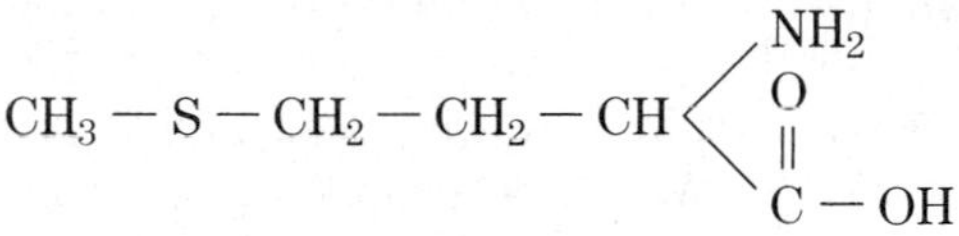

Methionine (Met)
(essential)

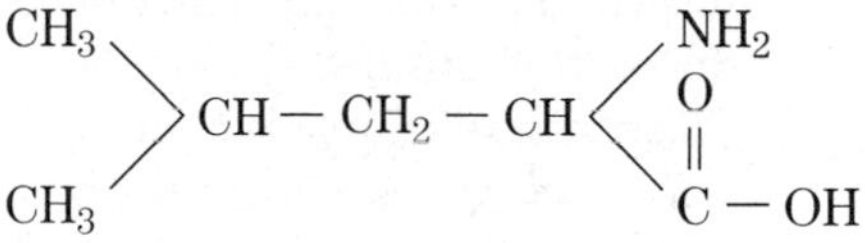

Leucine (Leu)
(essential)

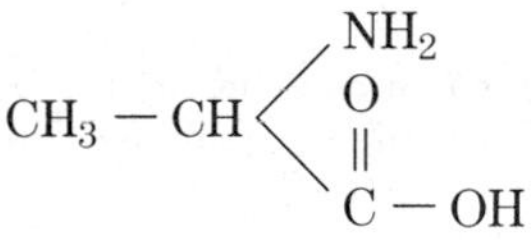

Alanine (Ala)

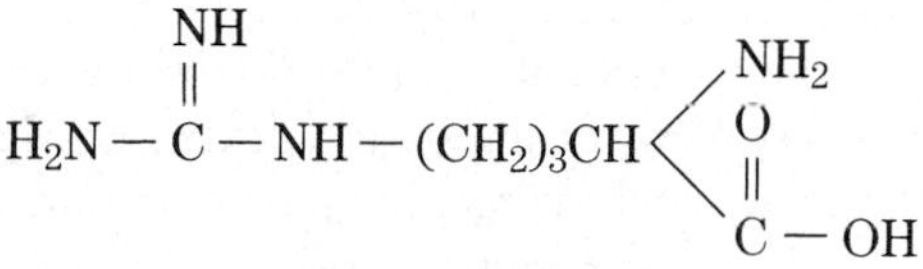

Arginine (Arg)
(essential)

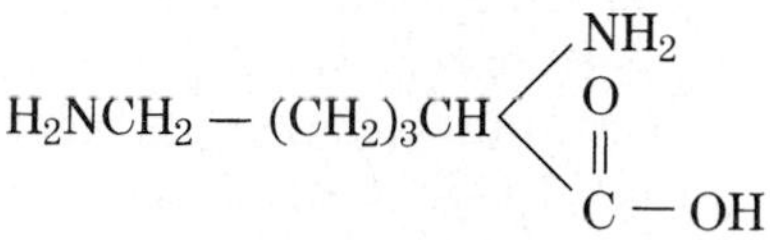

Lysine (Lys)
(essential)

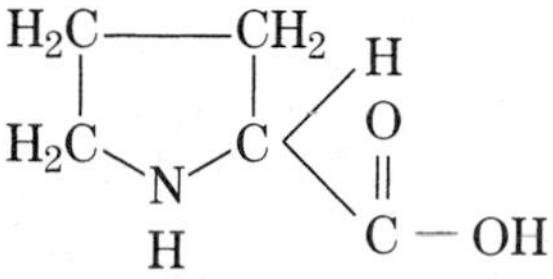

Proline (Pro)

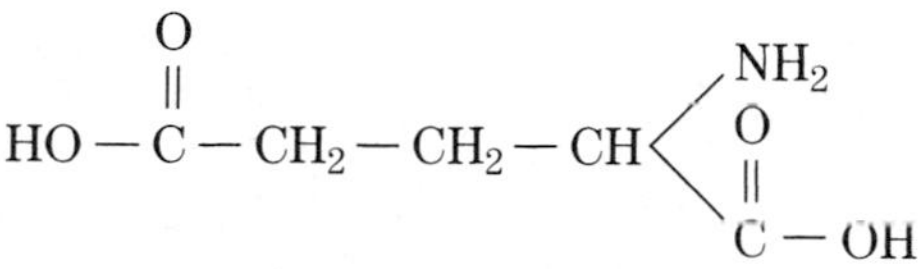

Glutamic Acid (Glu)

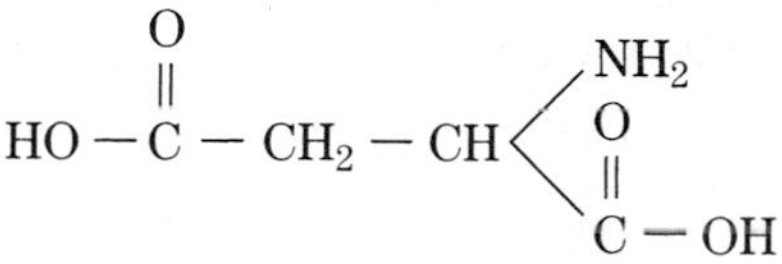

Aspartic Acid (Asp)

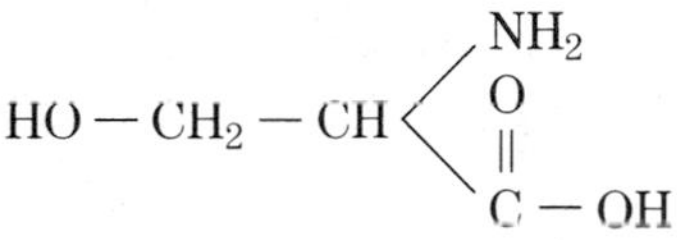

Serine (Ser)

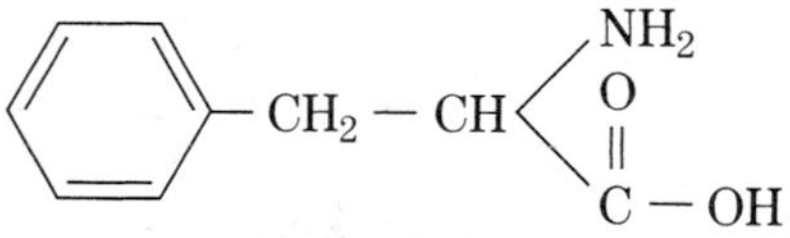

Phenylalanine (Phe)
(essential)

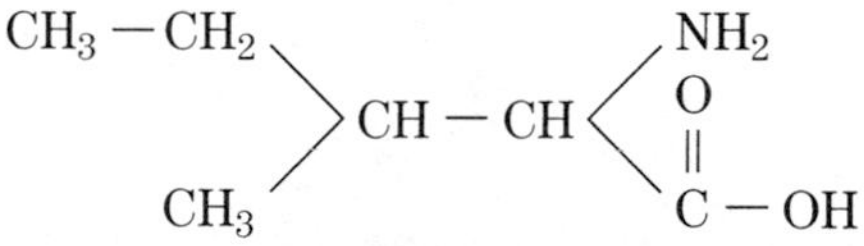

Isoleucine (Ile)
(essential)

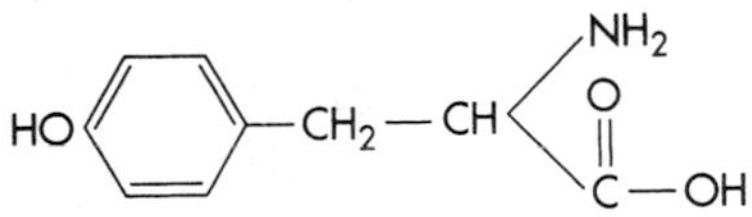

Tyrosine (Tyr)

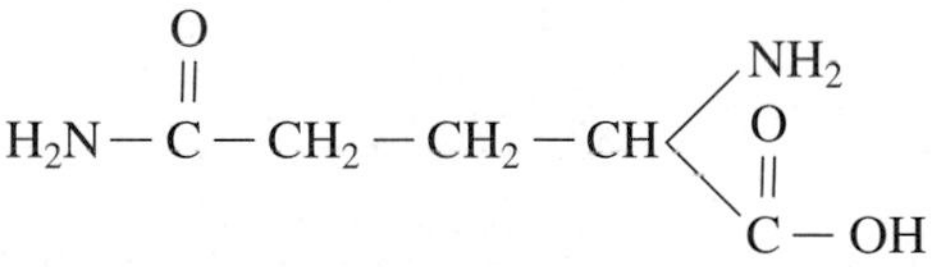

Glutamine (Gln)

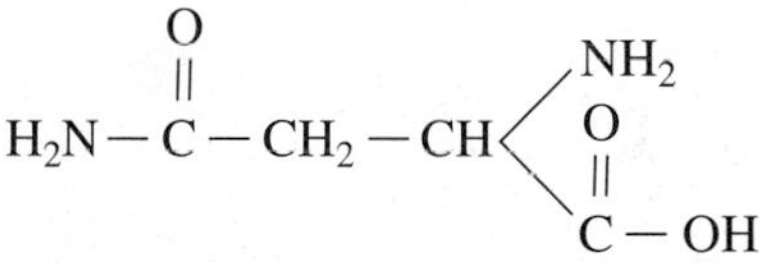

Asparagine (Asn)

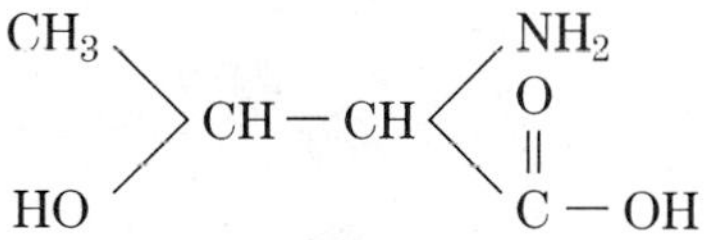

Threonine (Thr)
(essential)

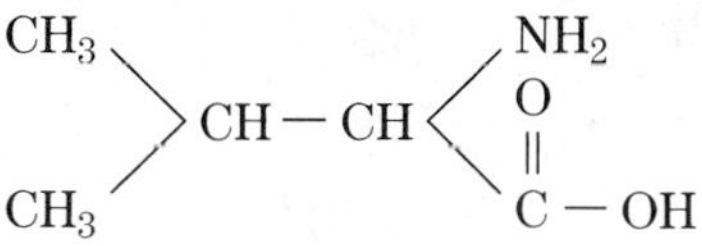

Valine (Val)
(essential)

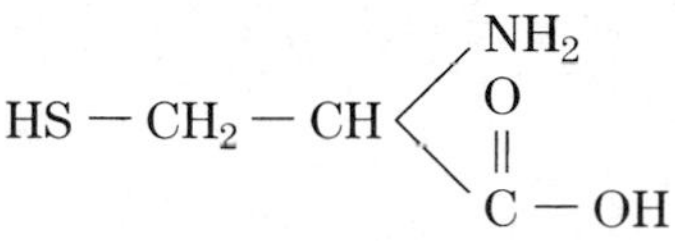

Cysteine (Cys)

■ FIGURE B-5 The 20 common amino acids in foods.

H₃C   CH₃
$C=C$
H   H

cis-2-butene; the methyl groups are
on the same side of the double bond

H   CH₃
$C=C$
H₃C   H

trans-2-butene; the methyl groups are
on opposite sides of the double bond

Stereoisomers

Another example of organic chemistry that is important to understanding nutrition is the arrangement of the atoms in the structure. Stereoisomers have the same number and types of chemical bonds, but with different spatial arranges (different configurations in space). Molecules containing double bonds illustrate this. Because there is no freedom to rotate around a C=C bond, molecules containing such bonds frequently exhibit stereoisomerism. For example, in the molecule 2-butene (CH₃CH = CHCH₃), the methyl groups (—CH₃) can be located on the same side of the bond (*cis* **isomer**) or on opposite sides of the double bond (*trans* **isomer**), as shown in the margin. The only difference between the two isomers is the location of the methyl groups.

Another example is oleic acid and its isomer elaidic acid (Fig. B-6*a*). Oleic acid is a *cis* isomer, or the form found naturally in food. With food-processing technology, such as hydrogenation, cis bonds of fatty acids are converted to trans bonds. When vegetable oils are converted to vegetable fats, such as in margarine or shortening, some of the trans isomer are formed. Elaidic acid is not the natural form. Isomers of these types are called geometric isomers. Generous intakes of trans isomers of fatty acids are associated with an increased risk of cardiovascular disease (see Chapter 6).

Stereoisomerism depends on which way the functional group is pointed with respect to other molecules. If there are two isomers, *D* stands for dextro or right-handed, and *L* stands for levo or left-handed, such as alanine in D-alanine and L-alanine (Fig. B-6*b*). Stereoisomers that can't be superimposed on their mirror images are called optical isomers. Optical isomers can be identified from each other by their reaction to plane-polarized light. One solution of an isomer that rotates the

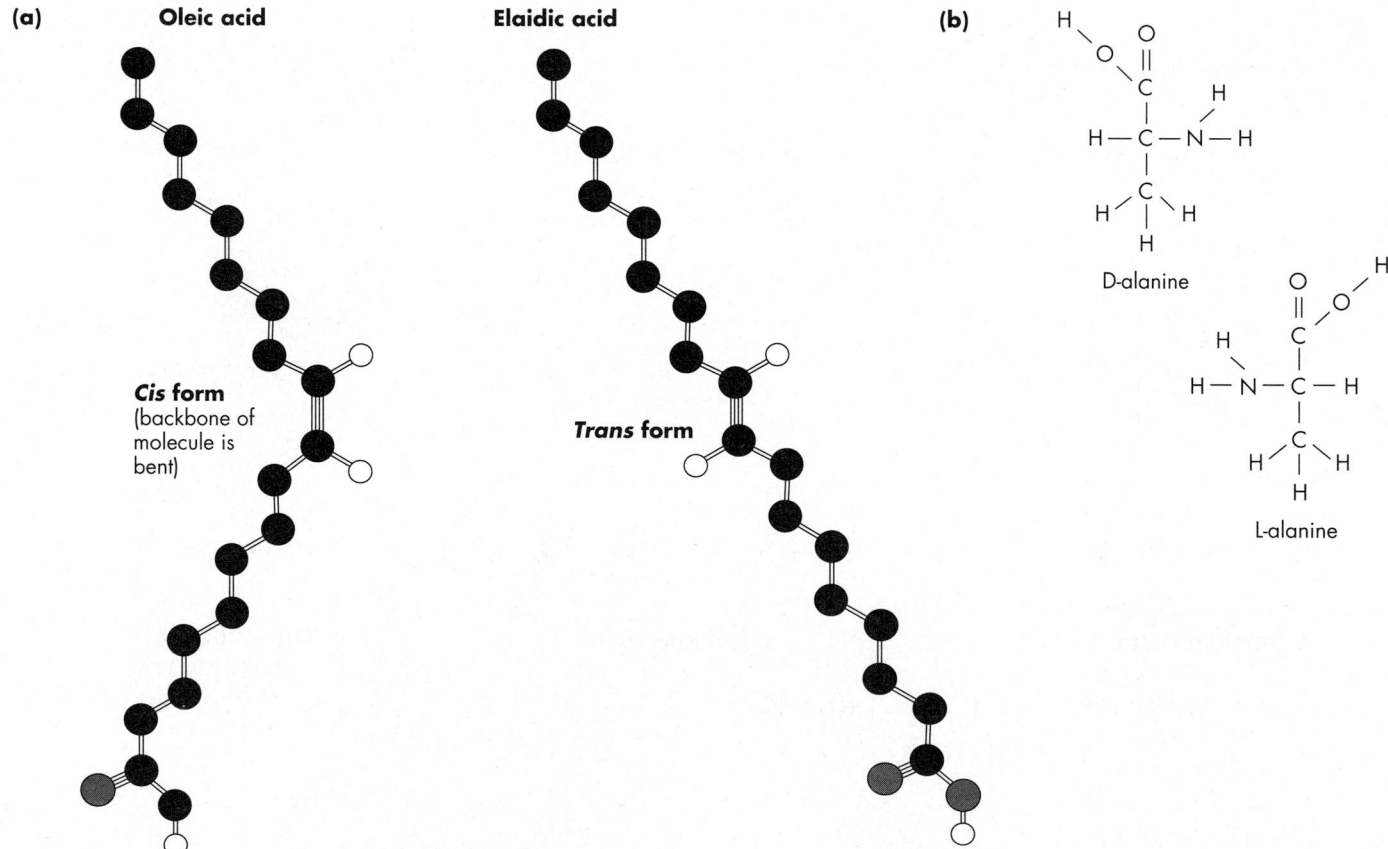

FIGURE B-6 *(a) Cis* and *trans* isomers of fatty acids. *Cis* forms are the most common forms in unprocessed foods. *(b)* Optical isomers of alanine—an amino acid. The L isomer is the most commonly found amino acid in nature.

plane of polarized light to the right is dextrorotary. And the solution of its mirror image rotates the plane of light to the left and, so, is levorotary.

The difference between these two stereoisomers of organic chemicals is "fit." This is important, since the molecule has to fit an enzyme in order to make the chemical reaction work. For example, human enzymes in all cells combine only with L-amino acids (building blocks of protein) and D-sugars. D-amino acids and L-sugars just won't function in the body. It is rather like trying to wear the left-hand glove on the right hand and do anything that requires manual skill.

A carbon atom with four different atoms or groups of atoms attached is asymmetric. Asymmetric carbons are also called chiral centers. A molecule with one chiral carbon can have two stereoisomers, such as alanine, just described. When two or more (n) chiral carbons are present, there can be 2^n stereoisomers. Some stereoisomers are mirror images of each other and are called enantiomers. When chiral molecules are rotated but cannot be superimposed on their mirror image, they are called diastereomers.

In all living organisms, many molecules are chiral.

When compounds have more than one chiral center, the "RS" system of naming is used, rather than the D and L system. The RS system allows each group attached to a chiral center be assigned a priority. Here is a list of some priorities.

$$-OCH_2 > OH > -NH_2 > -COOH > -CHO > -CH_2OH > -CH_3 > -H$$

The chiral atom has four different attachments; 1, 2, 3, and 4. Number 4 has the lowest priority (pointing away from you). If the other 3 attachments (1, 2, and 3) decrease in clockwise order, the structure is of the R configuration. If they decrease counterclockwise, they are of the S configuration. Using this configuration, every chiral carbon is either R or S.

This RS terminology is important to understanding vitamin E chemistry. It is now known that vitamin E as alpha-tocopherol has three chiral centers, and so has eight different stereoisomers (2^3). They are all found in synthetic preparations. The three chiral centers are identified as 2, 4, and 8 as related to the position on the phytal side chain (see Chapter 9). The RRR isomer (i.e., R form at each of the 3 chiral centers on the phytal tail) is the natural form. A transfer protein in the liver only recognizes the R form of the chiral center at the 2 position. Of all the eight combinations of R and S in the phytal tail of synthetic vitamin E, the only biologically active ones are RRR, RSR, RSS, RRS, as they all have the R form in the 2 position.

Biochemistry

The study of the chemistry or molecular basis of life and the reactions, structures, and composition of living materials is known as biochemistry. Biochemical reactions are possible because of enzymes. Living organisms convert the energy they extract from food and into energy for growth, maintenance, and reproduction. Energy can be stored for future use. The energy in the food is converted and used in the form of chemical energy contained in adenosine triphosphate (ATP). That fact that living organisms can self-replicate depends on deoxyribonucleic acid (DNA) and the genetic code. All forms of life store and transmit genetic information in the form of DNA.

RRR and SRR isomers of vitamin E. Of the two, only the RRR isomer contributes to vitamin E needs.

Composition of Living Organisms

Approximately 98.5% of the body's weight are composed of the elements oxygen, carbon, hydrogen, nitrogen, calcium, and phosphorus. Elements such as iron, zinc, and copper are present in trace amounts in the body, but that doesn't mean they are unimportant. For instance, iron combines with a blood protein to form hemoglobin, an oxygen carrier. Hemoglobin transports oxygen from the lungs to the tissues and assists in returning carbon dioxide from the tissues to the lungs for removal.

Water is the most abundant chemical in the body, making up to about 70% of human tissue. Other important classes of compounds in the body are the proteins, carbohydrate, lipids, and nucleic acids.

■ Biochemical Reactions

All the biochemical reactions that occur in the body are described as metabolism. The intermediate compounds in metabolism are termed *metabolites*. Metabolic reactions that build (synthesize) complex molecules are described as anabolic. An example is the synthesis of protein from amino acids. The reactions that break down (degrade) larger molecules into smaller ones are described as catabolic. An example is starch breaking down to glucose molecules.

Carbohydrates

Carbohydrates are aldehydes with hydroxyl groups and ketones, containing carbon, hydrogen, and oxygen with the general formula CH_2O. (There are twice as many hydrogen atoms as carbon and oxygen atoms.) The suffix *-ose* indicates a sugar. *Hexose* refers to a 6-carbon monosaccharide. There are three structural isomers of hexose: galactose, glucose, and fructose. All have the same formula, $C_6H_{12}O_6$, but the arrangement of their individual atoms differs in small ways.

The simplest carbohydrates are monosaccharides. When two monosaccharides are chemically bonded, they form a disaccharide, or double sugar. The table sugar sucrose is an example of a disaccharide, formed from glucose and fructose.

Polysaccharides are many monosaccharides joined by covalent bonds. Plant starch and cellulose are examples of polysaccharides. Some starches have thousands of glucose subunits. In animals, carbohydrate is stored as an animal starch called glycogen, found in liver and muscle tissue.

Di- and *poly*saccharides are assembled by a condensation reaction. Water is removed. Hydrolysis, or the splitting by the addition of water, digests di- and polysaccharides to smaller sugar units.

Lipids

Lipids are a class of nonpolar materials that are grouped according to solubility in organic solvents. They don't dissolve in water because they are nonpolar or hydrophobic.

Simple lipids include fatty acids and steroids. The lipid, cholesterol, serves as the precursor (parent) for the steroid hormones, such as testosterone, estrogen, and progesterone. Complex lipids include triglycerides (often referred to as *triacylglycerols*), which are esters of glycerol and fatty acids; phospholipids are composed of glycerol, phosphoric acid, and long-chain fatty acids; sphingolipids are composed of sphingosine, phosphorhic acid, long-chain fatty acids and choline; and glycosphingolipids are composed of sphingosine, fatty acids, and carbohydrates. Triglycerides represent fuel found in food and stored in adipose tissues. Phospholipids are part polar and part nonpolar, which allows them to interact with water and function as surfactants. They prevent the lungs from collapsing. Sphingophospholipids make up the material surrounding nerves. Glycosphingolipids are structural material for brain and nerve tissue. These complex lipids can be hydrolyzed to yield fatty acids.

Prostaglandins are a special type of fatty acid produced by almost all organs in the body and have specific regulatory functions. They are all derived from certain (dietary essential) fatty acids.

Proteins

Proteins are polymers of amino acids. Twenty of the amino acids are incorporated into the great variety of body proteins. Although the amino acids contain an amino group (NH_2) and a carboxylic acid group $\left(\begin{smallmatrix} O \\ \parallel \\ -C-OH \end{smallmatrix}\right)$; each has a distinctive structure (review Fig. B-5). Proteins typically contain many atoms, such as carbon, nitrogen, sulfur, hydrogen, and oxygen.

The genetic information found in DNA in the nucleus of the cell is the code book for constructing a protein. The sequence of amino acids in a protein follows the DNA (code) for synthesizing the protein. This protein can be made over and over again because of the code carried in the person's genes.

Nucleic Acids (DNA and RNA)

Nucleic acids include DNA, RNA, and the subunits from which they are formed, called nucleotides. The nucleotide is made of three components; a 5-carbon pentose sugar, a phosphate group, and a nitrogenous base (Fig. B-7). There are two kinds of nitrogenous base: purines and pyrimidines.

The sugar in RNA (ribonucelic acid) contains the beta-D ribose, which is a sugar. The pyrimidine bases in ribonucleic acids are uracil and cytosine, and the purine bases are cytosine and adenine. RNA is a single polynucleotide strand, not a double strand, like DNA (deoxyribonucleic acid).

DNA found in the nucleus of the cell is the basis of the genetic code. The sugar deoxyribose can be covalently bonded to the purine bases adenine and guanine and two pyrimidines, cytosine and thymine (Fig. B-8). There are four types of nucleotides that can produce the long chain that makes up a single strand of DNA. The DNA is a sugar phosphate chain made up of two strands that twist around each other to form a helix. The bases project into the center of the structure, forming a staircase structure. They are held together by hydrogen bonds (Fig. B-9).

(a)

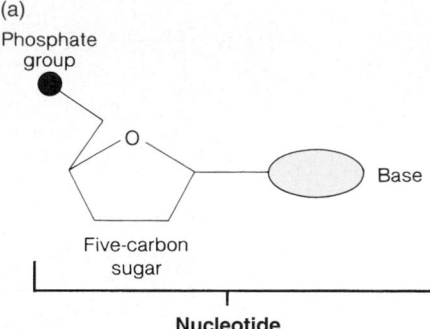

Nucleotide

(b)

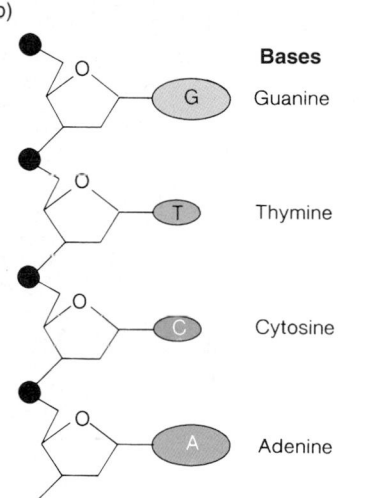

Bases

■ FIGURE **B-7** (a) The general structure of a nucleotide. (b) A polymer of nucleotides, or polynucleotide is formed by sugar-phosphate bonds between nucleotides.

Purines   **Pyrimidines**

Guanine   Cytosine

Thymine   Adenine

■ FIGURE **B-8** The four nitrogenous bases in deoxyribonucleic acid (DNA). Notice that hydrogen bonds can form between guanine and cytosine and between thymine and adenine.

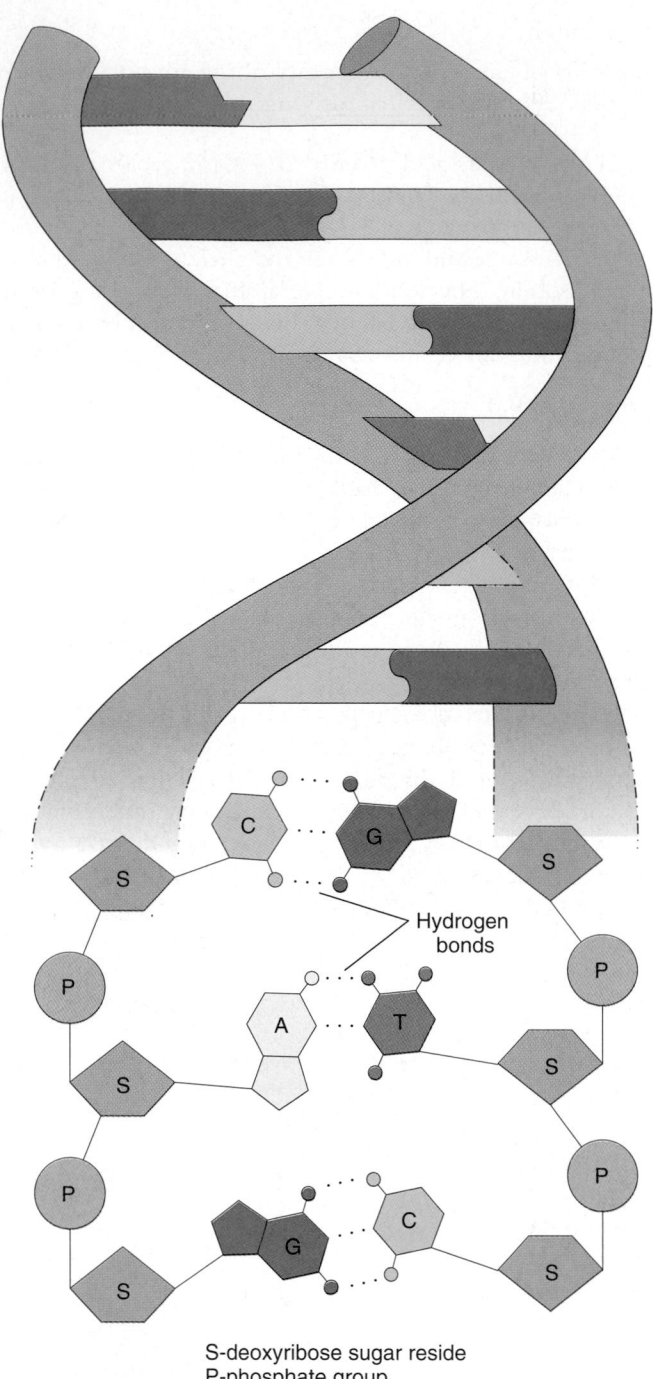

Hydrogen bonds

S-deoxyribose sugar reside
P-phosphate group

■ FIGURE B-9 The double-helix structure of DNA. The two strands are held together by hydrogen bonds between complementary bases in each strand.

DNA consists of two strands of a polynucleotide chain coiled around an axis to form a right-handed double helix. There are always an equal number of purine and pyrimidine bases. And there is something called complementary base pairing; adenine pairs only with thymine, and guanine pairs only with cytosine.

Although there are only four bases, the number of sequences of bases is endless. The total human genome consists of billions of base pairs making up about 30,000 genes. The applications of this knowledge can lead to genetic screening for breast cancer and, in the future, drugs to treat obesity and inborn errors of metabolism.

During replication, the helix uncoils and separates, so that each chain or strand serves as a template for the synthesis of its complementary chain. This is known as cell division. Each daughter chain has one strand of the original strand and one new strand.

RNA, another nucleic acid, takes its instructions from DNA. There are three types of RNA: ribosomal RNA, transfer RNA, and messenger RNA. Ribosomal RNA forms part of the structure of ribosomes where proteins are synthesized. Messenger RNA contains the code for the synthesis of a specific protein. Transfer RNA decodes the genetic message in RNA and assembles the amino acids for the protein assembly line (see Chapter 7 for details).

■ Important Chemical Reactions Related to the Study of Nutrition

One of the most important properties of chemical compounds is the type of reactions they undergo. Chemical reactions are responsible for vision, thinking, movement, and everything else that occurs in the human body.

In a chemical reaction, a compound or set of compounds (the reactants) is converted into another compound or set of compounds (the products), accompanied by the absorption or release of energy, which is typically heat in biological processes. In effect, the reactants reshuffle their atoms to form products. Clearly, then, no atoms lose their identity during a chemical reaction, and no atoms are gained, lost, or converted to another kind of atom during the course of chemical activity.

Chemists have grouped reactions according to their similarities in chemical behavior. Some of these are performed over and over within each cell. Following is a brief overview of some important reaction types.

Condensation Reactions

A condensation reaction occurs when two molecules join together to form a larger molecule and a small molecule (usually water). The two-reactant molecules typically contain hydroxyl groups, meaning that there are two OH groups. A simple example is the condensation of ethanol to make ethyl ether and water.

$$CH_3CH_2OH + CH_3CH_2OH \rightarrow CH_3CH_2-O-CH_2CH_3 + H_2O$$

Ethanol   Ethanol   Ethyl ether   Water

Although this reaction does not occur in the body, it illustrates the essential features of condensation reactions. One OH group gains a proton and forms a water molecule. The other OH group loses a proton and forms a bond with the other molecule—in exactly the same place that the water molecule leaves. Note that this is an overall description of what happens, not how it happens. Although it is typical for both molecules to contain an OH group in a condensation reaction, it is not a requirement for the reaction. A condensation reaction can occur where only one of the reactants contains an OH group.

Hydrolysis Reactions

Hydrolysis reactions are reactions that occur when water is added to a compound. In biological systems, hydrolysis reactions are very frequently the reverse of condensation reactions. That is, water is added to a large molecule, which results in the formation of two smaller molecules. This can be illustrated by the hydrolysis of lactose.

$$C_{12}H_{22}O_{11} + H_2O \rightarrow C_6H_{12}O_6 + C_6H_{12}O_6$$

Lactose   Water   Glucose   Galactose

Many important compounds in cells are formed using condensation reactions, and the breakdown of many compounds into smaller fragments occurs via hydrolysis reactions. For instance, hydrolysis of foodstuffs in the intestine yields smaller compounds, which the body can absorb, such as the breakdown of the sugar lactose in milk, by the action of the enzyme lactase, to glucose and galactose. The reverse occurs when the human mammary gland makes lactose. Also, when the carbohydrate glucose is converted to glycogen for storage, or to fat for muscle fuel, the synthetic processes use condensation reactions.

Oxidation and Reduction Reactions

Oxidation-reduction or redox reactions are important in nutrition science because they release energy from food during oxidation and synthesize carbohydrates, fatty acids, and other organic compounds during reduction. Oxidation and reactions take place with a simultaneous reduction reaction. Redox reactions follow three rules:

1. No oxidation reaction takes place without something being reduced, and no reduction takes place without something being oxidized.
2. In inorganic chemistry oxidation is the loss of electrons, and in organic chemistry oxidation is the loss of hydrogen.
3. In inorganic chemistry reduction is the gain in electrons, and in organic chemistry reduction is the gain of hydrogen.

A simple redox reaction involving iron is as follows:

$$Fe^{2+} - e^- \leftrightarrow Fe^{3+}$$

A biochemical redox reaction involving the coenzyme form of riboflavin occurs as follows:

$$\begin{array}{c} +2H \\ FAD \leftrightarrow FADH_2 \\ -2H \end{array}$$

Chapters 4, 10, and 12 provide more information about coenzymes, cofactors, and oxidation-reduction reactions.

Energy and Enzymatic Reactions

Enzymes are large proteins with varying amino acid composition that behave as organic **catalysts.** They are highly specific. Enzymes help a reaction to proceed by lowering the "energy of activation," so that the reaction can go faster (Fig. B-10). Enzymes lower this energy barrier between the reactants and the products by changing their shape. Some of the enzyme reactions that occur in the cell require coenzymes (vitamins) at the active site to make the reaction go, whereas many others don't. Fortunately, an enzyme isn't consumed by the reaction, so it can be used over and over.

Enzymatic reactions either require energy or liberate energy. The difference in energy contained in the substrate and the energy contained in the products is called the "free energy" of the enzymatic reaction. Free energy is the amount of energy available to do work and is designated G—or, more properly, ΔG—the change in free energy. ΔG is a thermodynamic property of a reaction. With a change in free energy, there is also a change in the overall order of the reaction. This change in order is the entropy, or ΔS, of the reaction. S stands for the randomness or disorder in a system. For example, ΔS can increase as disorder gets worse, or ΔS can decrease as order gets better. Think of your home; without doing any housekeeping, it becomes disordered. It has a $+\Delta S$.

In the first reaction of glycolysis, glucose and inorganic phosphate (Pi) produce glucose 6-phosphate, a product with more energy (review Fig 4-5 on page 135). The ΔG is positive. This is an endergonic reaction, as it requires an input of energy to get it going. The products contain more energy than the reactants.

An enzymatic reaction that proceeds spontaneously releases energy, $-\Delta G$. This reaction is exergonic. When ATP breaks down to ADP and Pi, the reaction is exergonic and has a negative free energy change. The net result is an increase in disorder of the system, a $+\Delta S$, and the products contain less energy than the reactants.

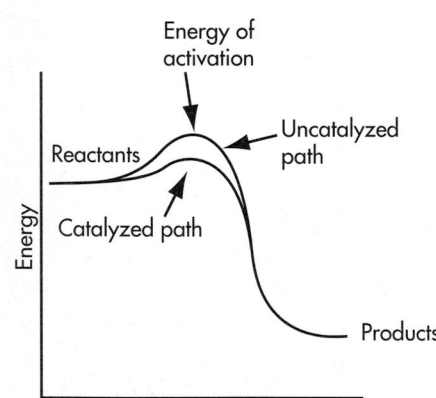

FIGURE B-10 Enzymes and other catalysts accelerate chemical reactions by reducing the energy barrier to the reaction. Reactants molecules free in solution can react only if they meet in just the right orientation and with enough energy. An enzyme holds its substrate molecules in the right orientation to react and exerts forces on them that cause chemical bonds to break and form. In this way, an enzyme lowers the energy barrier that substrates must pass and, so, increases their reaction rates.

When these two reactions are coupled, the exergonic reaction drives the endergonic reaction. The glucose +ATP produces glucose 6-phosphate + ADP. The exergonic reaction has a large $-\Delta G$. The endergonic reaction has a smaller $+\Delta S$. Because the overall reaction is a negative ΔG, the reaction proceeds spontaneously.

These coupled exergonic and endergonic reactions are a fundamental aspect of energy metabolism in living cells.

To clean your house, you must put some energy into the operation, $+\Delta G$. This reaction, when completed, will yield a product. Energy, as ATP, will be consumed by your muscles as you move furniture, vacuum, sort and discard junk, pick up trash, and wash the windows, and entropy in the reaction will decline, $-\Delta S$; there is an increase in order. You have cleaned your house. The important thing in this reaction is that the total energy within the product increases. These types of enzymatic reactions are related to nutrition and the total energy for growth, maintenance, and repair.

Common Chemical Structures

Most compounds in the body are composed of carbon, hydrogen, and oxygen, with carbon often being the predominant atom. Some commonly encountered combinations of atoms, called functional groups, have been given specific names because they appear in many molecules. You need to be familiar with them, for they are the most important features in many of our nutrients. The important ones were listed in Table B-5. You will be using these names and studying these structures throughout this course.

The Drawing of Chemical Structures

Chemists have developed a short-hand notation for writing chemical formulas, called stick structures. In stick structures, neither carbon atoms nor the hydrogens bonded to the carbon atoms are expressly shown. What are shown are the bonds between the carbon atoms and the position of all atoms other than carbon and hydrogen. Keep in mind that there are carbon atoms at the apices of every angle in the structure (with the appropriate number of hydrogens attached to the carbon) and at the terminal end of the sticks. By way of illustration, look at a stick structure of propane ($CH_3CH_2CH_3$).

The advantage of using stick structures is that it allows for a clear representation of complex molecules without cluttering up the picture. This notation will be used throughout the text. It is handy when large structures, such as fatty acids, have to be represented.

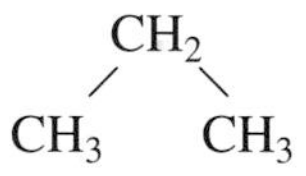

CH_2
CH_3 CH_3

Propane

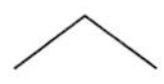

**Stick structure
of propane**

Appendix C

DIETARY ADVICE FOR CANADIANS

The following chart includes information on macronutrients from the Recommended Nutrient Intakes (RNIs) listed in *The Report of the Scientific Review Committee,* last published in 1990. Previous RNIs for micronutrients have been replaced by the Dietary Reference Intakes (DRIs) that apply to Canadian and U.S. citizens. These are listed on the inside cover. Both Canadian and American scientists worked on the various DRI committees, coming up with a set of harmonized Dietary Reference Intakes for both countries. The remaining DRIs for macronutrients are still under development, so these older RNIs for energy, protein, and omega-3 and omega-6 fatty acids, listed below, remain as the current standard for Canadians.

TABLE C-1 Summary of Examples of Recommended Macronutrient Intakes Based on Energy Expressed as Daily Rates

Age	Gender	Energy (kcal)	Protein (g)	ω-3 PUFA* (g)	ω-6 PUFA (g)
Months					
0–4	Both	600	12[†]	0.50	3.0
5–12	Both	900	12	0.50	3.0
Years					
1	Both	1100	13	0.60	4.0
2–3	Both	1300	16	0.70	4.0
4–6	Both	1800	19	1.00	6.0
7–9	M	2200	26	1.20	7.0
	F	1900	26	1.00	6.0
10–12	M	2500	34	1.40	8.0
	F	2200	36	1.20	7.0
13–15	M	2800	49	1.50	9.0
	F	2200	46	1.20	7.0
16–18	M	3200	58	1.80	11.0
	F	2100	47	1.20	7.0
19–24	M	3000	61	1.60	10.0
	F	2100	50	1.20	7.0
25–49	M	2700	64	1.50	9.0
	F	1900	51	1.10	7.0
50–74	M	2300	63	1.30	8.0
	F	1800	54	1.10[‡]	7.0[‡]
75+	M	2000	59	1.10	7.0
	F[SS]	1700	55	1.10[‡]	7.0[‡]
Pregnancy (additional)					
1st trimester		100	5	.05	0.3
2nd trimester		300	20	0.16	0.9
3rd trimester		300	24	0.16	0.9
Lactation		450	20	0.25	1.5

From Scientific Review Committee: *Nutrition recommendations.* Ottawa, Canada, 1990. Health and Welfare.

* PUFA, polyunsaturated fatty acids

[†]Protein is assumed to be from breast milk and must be adjusted for infant formula.

[‡]Level below which intake should not fall

[SS]Assumes moderate physical activity

Excellent World Wide Web resources for Canadians are Health Canada (http://www.hc-sc.gc.ca), Dietitians of Canada (http://www.dietitians.ca), and the National Institute of Nutrition (http://www.nin.ca).

■ Summary of the Nutrition Recommendations for Canadians

1. *The Canadian diet should provide energy consistent with the maintenance of body weight within the recommended range.* Physical activity should be appropriate to circumstances and capabilities. Although the importance of maintaining some activity throughout life can be stressed, it is not possible to specify a level of physical activity for the whole population. As a general guideline, it is desirable that adults, for as long as possible, maintain an activity level that permits an energy intake of at least 1800 kcal while keeping weight within the recommended range.

2. *The Canadian diet should include essential nutrients in amounts recommended in this report.* Although it is important that the diet provide the recommended amounts of nutrients, it should be understood that no evidence was found that intakes in excess of the RNI confer any health benefit. There is no general need for supplements, except for vitamin D for infants and folate during pregnancy. Vitamin D supplementation might be required for elderly persons not exposed to the sun and iron for pregnant women with low iron stores.

3. *The Canadian diet should include no more than 30% of energy as fat (33g per 1000 kcal) and no more than 10% as saturated fat (11g per 1000 kcal).* Dietary cholesterol, though not as influential in affecting blood cholesterol, is not without importance. A reduction in cholesterol intake normally will accompany a reduction in total fat and saturated fat. The recommendation to reduce total fat intake does not apply to children under the age of 2 years.

4. *The Canadian diet should provide 55% of energy as carbohydrate (138g per 1000 kcal) from a variety of sources.* Sources should be selected that provide complex carbohydrates, a variety of dietary fiber, and beta-carotene.

5. *The sodium content of the Canadian diet should be reduced.* The present food supply provides sodium in an amount greatly exceeding requirements. Although insufficient evidence exists to support a precise recommendation, potential benefit would be expected from a reduction in current sodium intake.

6. *The Canadian diet should include no more than 5% of total energy as alcohol, or two drinks daily, whichever is less.* The harmful influence of alcohol on blood pressure provides a more urgent reason for moderation. During pregnancy, it is prudent to abstain from alcoholic beverages because a safe intake is not known with certainty.

7. *The Canadian diet should contain no more caffeine than the equivalent of four regular cups of coffee per day.* This is a prudent measure in view of the increased risk for cardiovascular disease associated with high intakes of caffeine.

8. *Community water supplies containing less fluoride than 1 mg per liter should be fluoridated to that level.* Fluoridation of community water supplies has proven to be a safe, effective, and economical method of improving dental health.

In essence, suggested actions toward healthful eating as listed in Canada's Guidelines for Healthy Eating include the following:

- Enjoy a variety of foods.
- Emphasize cereals, breads, other grain products, vegetables, and fruits.
- Choose low-fat dairy products, lean meats, and foods prepared with little or no fat.
- Achieve and maintain a healthful body weight by enjoying regular physical activity and healthful eating.
- Limit salt, alcohol, and caffeine.

The *Canadian Food Guide* is a guide to help Canadians make wise food choices (Fig. C-1). The rainbow side of the Food Guide places foods into four groups: grain products; vegetables and fruit; milk products; and meat and meat alternatives. The rainbow includes information about the types of foods to choose from each food group for healthy eating.

The bar side of the Food Guide helps Canadians decide how much they need from each group every day. The guide gives a range for the number of servings for

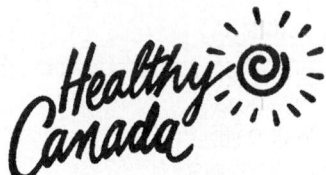

CANADA'S

Food Guide

TO HEALTHY EATING

Health and Welfare Canada

Santé et Bien-être social Canada

Enjoy a variety of foods from each group every day.

Choose lower-fat foods more often.

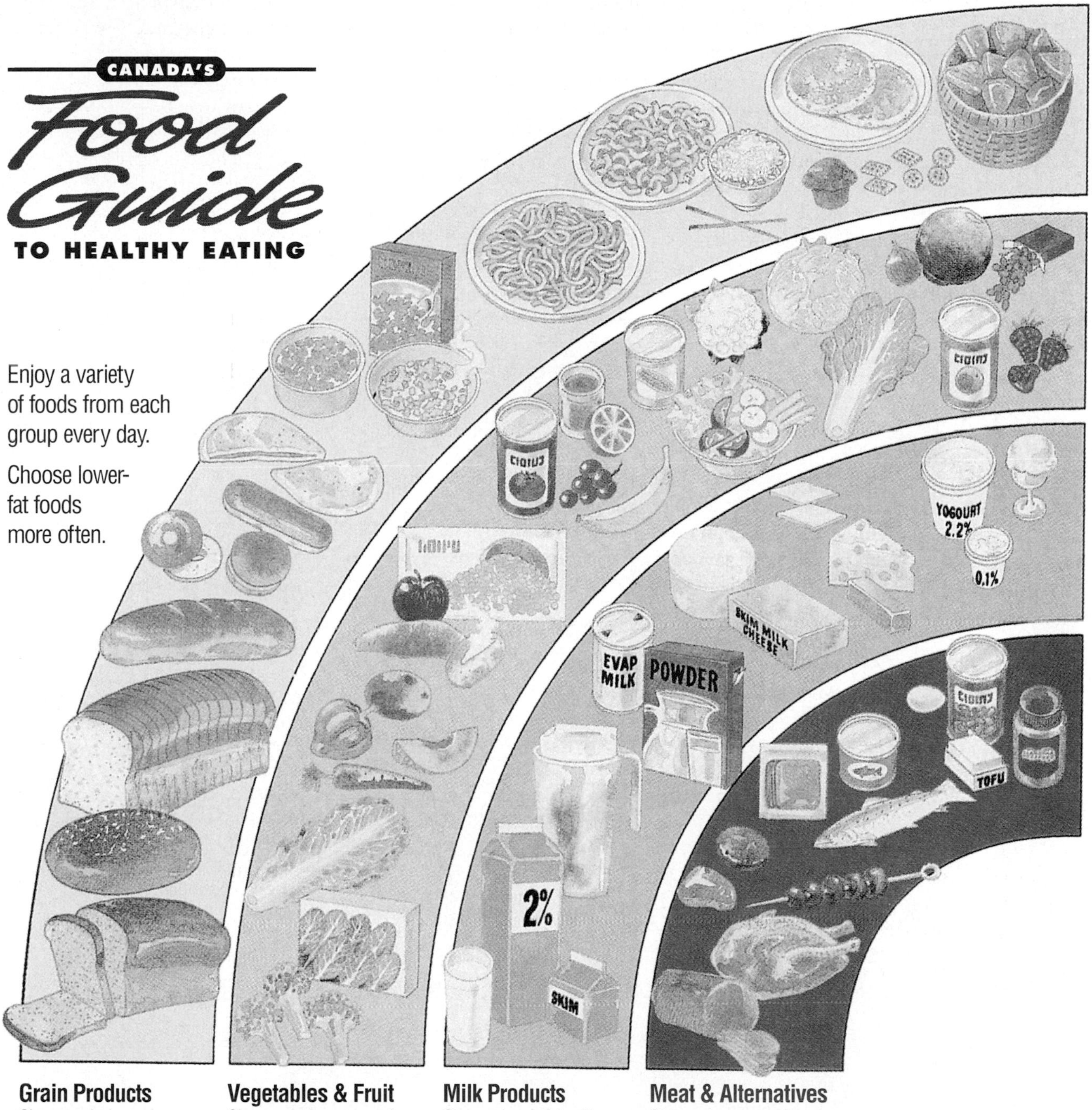

Grain Products
Choose whole-grain and enriched products more often.

Vegetables & Fruit
Choose dark green and orange vegetables and orange fruit more often.

Milk Products
Choose lower-fat milk products more often.

Meat & Alternatives
Choose leaner meats, poultry and fish, as well as dried peas, beans, and lentils more often.

Canada

FIGURE C-1 Canadian Food Guide to Healthy Eating.

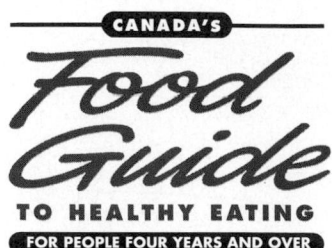

Different People Need Different Amounts of Food

The amount of food you need every day from the four food groups and other foods depends on your age, body size, activity level, whether you are male or female and if you are pregnant or breastfeeding. That's why the Food Guide gives a lower and higher number of servings for each food group. For example, young children can choose the lower number of servings, while male teenagers can go to the higher number. Most other people can choose servings somewhere in between.

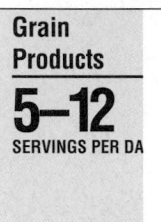

Grain Products
5–12
SERVINGS PER DA

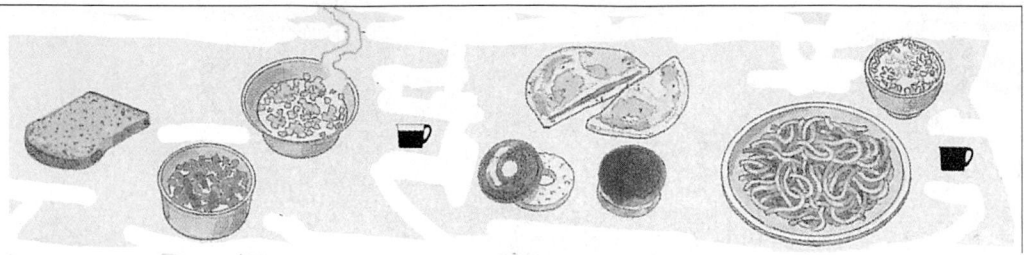

Vegetables & Fruit
5–10
SERVINGS PER DAY

1 Serving

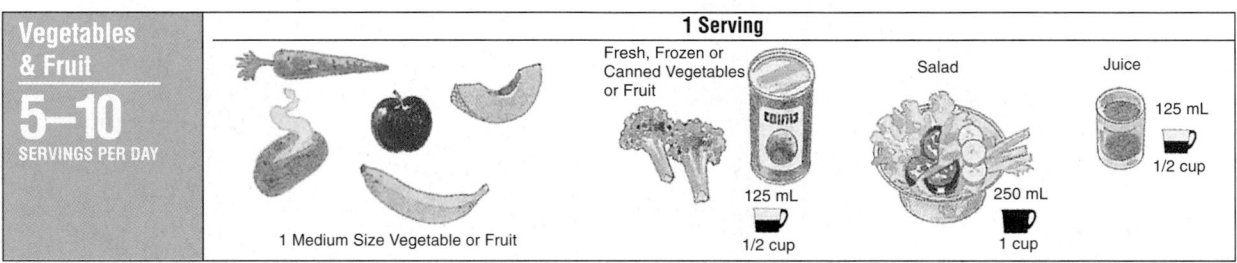

1 Medium Size Vegetable or Fruit

Fresh, Frozen or Canned Vegetables or Fruit
125 mL
1/2 cup

Salad
250 mL
1 cup

Juice
125 mL
1/2 cup

Milk Products
SERVINGS PER DAY
Children 4–9 years: 2-3
Youth 10–16 years: 3–4
Adults: 2-4
Pregnant & Breast-feeding Women: 3-4

1 Serving

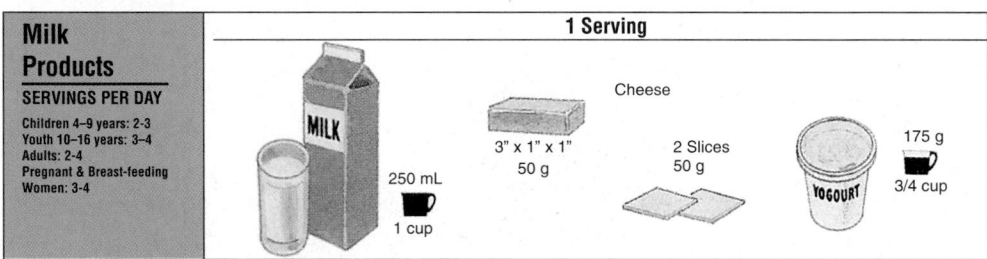

MILK
250 mL
1 cup

Cheese
3" x 1" x 1"
50 g

2 Slices
50 g

YOGOURT
175 g
3/4 cup

Other Foods

Taste and enjoyment can also come from other foods and beverages that are not part of the four food groups. Some of these foods are higher in fat or Calories, so use these foods in moderation.

Meat & Alternatives
2–3
SERVINGS PER DAY

1 Serving

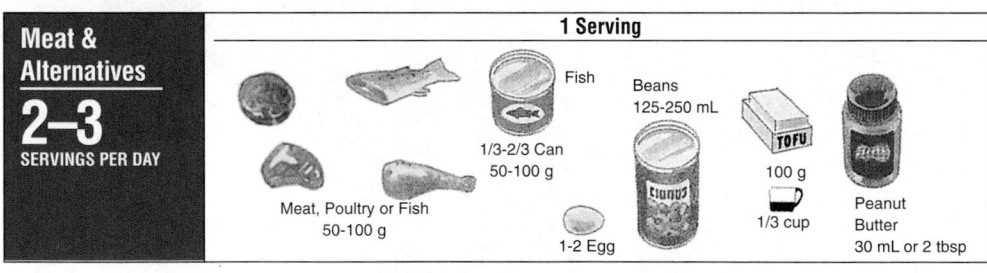

Meat, Poultry or Fish
50-100 g

Fish
1/3-2/3 Can
50-100 g

1-2 Egg

Beans
125-250 mL

TOFU
100 g
1/3 cup

Peanut Butter
30 mL or 2 tbsp

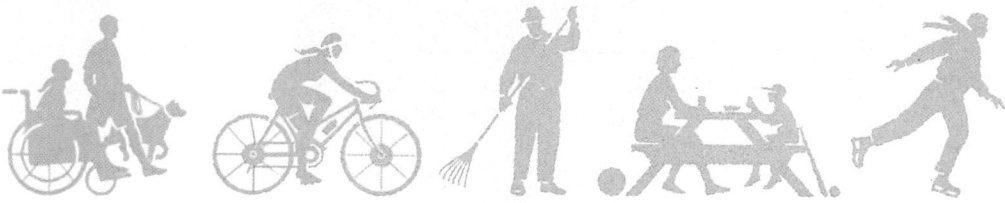

Enjoy eating well, being active, and feeling good about yourself. That's VITALIT 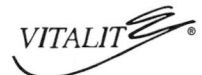 ®

© Minister of Supply and Services Canada 1992   Cat. No. H39-252 / 1992E   No changes permitted. Reprint permission not required.
ISBN 0-662-19648-1

FIGURE C-1 concluded

each food group, since different people need different amounts of food. The Food Guide also shows serving sizes for different foods.

The bar side of the Food Guide also tells how other foods that are not part of the four food groups can have a role in healthy eating. Since some of these "other foods" are higher in fat or calories, the Food Guide recommends using these foods in moderation.

■ Canada's Basic Labeling Requirements: Under the Food and Drugs Act and the Consumer Packaging and Labeling Act

In general, prepackaged products must show the following basic label information:

1. THE COMMON NAME. This is either the name by which the food is generally known (e.g., orange drink, vanilla cookies, chocolate candies) or the name prescribed by a regulation (e.g., orange juice from concentrate, 60% whole-wheat bread, milk chocolate, mayonnaise). When a prescribed common name is used, the product must conform to the compositional standard set forth in the regulations. The common name is to be shown on the principal display panel (i.e., main panel) in English and French in a minimum type height of 1.6 mm, based on the lower case letter *o*.

2. A Metric Net Quality declaration by volume (e.g., milliliters, liters), weight (e.g., grams, kilograms) or by count, as applicable. The net quantity declaration is to be shown on the principal display panel in English and French. The following symbols are considered to be bilingual:

   grams—g
   kilograms—k
   milliliters—ml or mL
   liters—l or L

   A minimum type height of 1.6 mm, based on the lowercase letter *o*, is required for all information in the net declaration, except for the numbers, which are to be shown in boldface type of not less than the following height:

   a. ¹⁄₁₆ inch (1.6 millimeters), where the principal display surface of the container is not more than 5 square inches (32 square centimeters)
   b. 1.8 inch (3.2 millimeters), where the principal display surface of the container is more than 5 square inches (32 centimeters) but not more than 40 square inches (258 square centimeters)
   c. ¼ inch (6.4 millimeters), where the principal display surface of the container is more than 40 square inches (258 square centimeters) but not more than 100 square inches (645 square centimeters)
   d. ⅜ inch (9.5 millimeters), where the principal display surface of the container is more than 100 square inches (645 square centimeters) but not more than 400 square inches (25.8 square decimeters) and
   e. ½ inch (12.7 millimeters), where the principal display surface of the container is more than 400 square inches (25.8 square decimeters)

   Additional nonmetric declarations (e.g., fluid ounces, pounds) are not required but may be shown grouped with the metric statement provided they are not false or misleading.

3. A LIST OF INGREDIENTS and their components (i.e., ingredients of ingredients) in descending order of proportion by weight. Spices, seasonings and herbs except salt, natural and artificial flavors, flavor enhancers, food additives, and vitamin and mineral nutrients may be shown at the end of the list in any order. Some components are completely exempt from a component declaration, whereas others are exempt depending on the amount used. Components of natural or artificial flavoring preparations, seasonings and spice or herb mixtures are:
   a. flavor enhancers
   b. salt
   c. Food additives that affect the finished product and

   d. Food additives listed in Table X of Division 16 of the Food and Drug Regulations must be shown in the ingredient list as if they were an ingredient of the finished food.

An ingredient or component must be shown in the list of ingredients by its common name. The list of ingredients is to be shown in English and French on any label panel except the bottom. It is required to be displayed clearly and prominently and be readily discernible. A minimum type height of 1.6 mm based on the lowercase letter *o* will usually satisfy this requirement.

4. THE NAME AND ADDRESS declaration of the responsible company. The company name must be the legal registered company name. The address should be complete enough for postal purposes and include the name of the country, if other than Canada or USA. This information is to be shown in either English or French on any label panel except the bottom, in a minimum type height of 1.6 mm based on the lowercase letter *o*. If only a Canadian company name and address are shown on an imported product that has been wholly manufactured outside of Canada, the Canadian declaration must be preceded by the appropriate terms "imported by/importÈ par" or "imported from/importÈ pour." Alternatively, the country of origin may be declared adjacent to the Canadian company name and address.

5. When a food has a DURABLE LIFE of 90 days or less, a "best before" date and storage instructions if they differ from normal room storage conditions must be declared. Additional information is available upon request.

6. When artificial flavors are used whether alone or with natural flavoring agents and a vignette on the label indicates a natural flavor source (e.g., picture of an apple), information that the added flavoring ingredient is imitation, artificial, or simulated must appear on or adjacent to the vignette in French and English in at least the same type height as required for the numbers in the net quantity.

7. Standard container sizes are specified for wine, glucose and refined sugar syrups, peanut butter, cookies, and biscuits. Specific information is available upon request.

Health Canada, a Canadian government agency, is proposing a new policy on nutrition labeling that would result in important changes to food labels. The proposal is that nutrition labeling will be mandatory on most foods (with some exceptions) and will be consistent in look, easy to find, legible, and readable. Nutrition labels will provide core information on calories, fat, saturated fat, trans fat, cholesterol, sodium, carbohydrate, fiber, sugar, protein, vitamin A, vitamins C, calcium, and iron. These changes will make nutrition information easier to find, more complete, and available on more foods and will allow Canadians to use this basic knowledge to make healthy food choices.

HOW TO READ A CANADIAN NUTRITION INFORMATION LABEL

Nutrition information is expressed per **suggested serving**. The serving size will vary according to food type and brand. Consider this fact when comparing foods.

Gives the calorie content (Cal)

Indicates the quantity of naturally occurring and added sugars as well as dietary fibre

Indicates the level of sodium from salt and all other sources

Vitamins and minerals are expressed as a percentage of the highest recommended amount

millilitres:
5 mL = 1 teaspoon

kilojoules:
metric unit of energy
1 Cal = 4.18kJ

grams: 28 g = 1 ounce

LASAGNA
Nutrition Information
per 275 g serving
(1 cup/250 mL)

Energy	275	Cal
	1140	kJ
Protein	19	g
Fat	7	g
Polyunsaturates	0.8	g
Monounsaturates	1.9	g
Saturates	2.5	g
Cholesterol	46	mg
Carbohydrate	34	g
Starch	29	g
Sugars	5	g
Dietary Fibre	0.2	g
Sodium	850	mg
Potassium	675	mg

Percentage of Recommended Daily Intake

Thiamine	20%
Riboflavin	19%
Niacin	18%
Calcium	12%
Iron	28%

EXCHANGE SYSTEM LISTS

■ Milk Exchange List

Skim and Very Low-Fat Milk

(12 grams carbohydrate, 8 grams protein, 0–3 grams fat, 90 kcal)

1 cup	skim or nonfat milk (½% and 1%)
⅓ cup	powdered (nonfat dry, before adding liquid)
½ cup	canned, evaporated skim milk
1 cup	buttermilk made from nonfat or low-fat milk
¾ cup	yogurt made from nonfat milk (plain, unflavored)
1 cup	nonfat or low-fat fruit-flavored yogurt sweetened with aspartame or nonnutritive sweetener

Low-Fat Milk

(12 grams carbohydrate, 8 grams protein, 5 grams fat, 120 kcal)

1 cup	2% milk
¾ cup	plain low-fat yogurt (added milk solids)
1 cup	sweet acidophilus milk

Whole Milk

(12 grams carbohydrate, 8 grams protein, 8 grams fat, 150 kcal)

1 cup	whole milk
½ cup	evaporated whole milk
1 cup	goat's milk
1 cup	kefir

■ Vegetable Exchange List

(5 grams carbohydrate, 2 grams protein, 0 grams fat, 25 kcal)
1 vegetable exchange equals:

½ cup cooked vegetables or vegetable juice
1 cup raw vegetables

artichoke	eggplant	radishes
artichoke hearts	green onions or scallions	salad greens
asparagus	green pepper	sauerkraut
beans (green, wax, Italian)	greens (e.g., collard)	spinach
bean sprouts	kohlrabi	squash (summer)
beets	leeks	tomato (fresh, canned, sauce)
broccoli	mixed vegetables (without corn, peas, or pasta)	tomato/vegetable juice
brussels sprouts		
cabbage	mushrooms	turnips
carrots	okra	water chestnuts
cauliflower	onions	watercress
celery	pea pods	zucchini
cucumber	peppers	

▪ Fruit Exchange List

Fruit

(15 grams carbohydrate, 0 grams protein, 0 grams fat, 60 kcal)
1 fruit exchange equals:

1	apple (small)
4 rings	apple, dried
½ cup	applesauce (unsweetened)
4	apricots, fresh
8 halves	apricots, dried
1	banana (small)
¾ cup	blackberries
¾ cup	blueberries
⅓ melon	cantaloupe (small)
1 cup cubes	cantaloupe
12	cherries (3 oz)
½ cup	cherries, canned
3	dates
2	figs, fresh (3½ oz)
1½	figs, dried
½ cup	fruit cocktail
½	grapefruit
¾ cup	grapefruit sections
17	grapes (small)
1 slice	honeydew melon (or 1 cup cubes)
1	kiwi
¾ cup	mandarin orange sections
½	mango (or ½ cup cubes)
1	nectarine (small)
1	orange (small)
½	papaya (or 1 cup cubes)
1	peach, fresh (medium)
½ cup	peaches, canned
½	pear, fresh
½ cup	pear, canned
¾ cup	pineapple, fresh
½ cup	pineapple, canned
2	plums (small)
½ cup	plums, canned
3	prunes, dried
2 tbsp	raisins
1 cup	raspberries
1¼ cup	strawberries (raw, whole)
2	tangerines
1 slice	watermelon (or 1¼ cups cubes)

Fruit Juice

½ cup	apple juice/cider
⅓ cup	cranberry juice cocktail
1 cup	cranberry juice cocktail, reduced-calorie
⅓ cup	fruit juice blends, 100% juice
⅓ cup	grape juice
½ cup	grapefruit juice
½ cup	orange juice
½ cup	pineapple juice
⅓ cup	prune juice

■ Starch Exchange List

(15 grams carbohydrate, 3 grams protein, 0–1 gram fat, 80 kcal)
1 starch exchange equals:

Bread

½ (1 oz)	bagel
2 slices (1½ oz)	bread, reduced-calorie
1 slice (1 oz)	bread, white, whole-wheat, pumpernickel, or rye
2 (⅔ oz)	bread sticks, crisp, 4 in long × 3½ in
½	English muffin
½ (1 oz)	hot dog or hamburger bun
½	pita, 6 in across
1 slice (1 oz)	raisin bread, unfrosted
1 (1 oz)	roll, plain (small)
1	tortilla, corn, 6 in across
1	tortilla, flour, 7–8 in across
1	waffle, 4½ in square, reduced-fat

Cereals and Grains

½ cup	bran cereal
½ cup	bulgur
½ cup	cereal
¾ cup	cereal, unsweetened, ready-to-eat
3 tbsp	cornmeal (dry)
⅓ cup	couscous
3 tbsp	flour (dry)
¼ cup	granola, low-fat
¼ cup	Grape-Nuts
½ cup	grits
½ cup	kasha
¼ cup	millet
¼ cup	muesli
½ cup	oats
½ cup	pasta
1½ cups	puffed cereal
½ cup	rice milk
⅓ cup	rice, white or brown
½ cup	Shredded Wheat
½ cup	sugar-frosted cereal
3 tbsp	wheat germ

Starchy Vegetables

⅓ cup	baked beans
½ cup	corn
1 (5 oz)	corn on the cob (medium)
1 cup	mixed vegetables with corn, peas, or pasta
½ cup	peas, green
½ cup	plantain
1 (3 oz)	potato, baked or boiled (small)
½ cup	potato, mashed
1 cup	squash, winter (acorn, butternut)
½ cup	yam, sweet potato, plain

Crackers and Snacks

8	animal crackers
3	graham crackers, 2½ in square
¾ oz	matzoh
4 slices	melba toast
24	oyster crackers
3 cups	popcorn (popped, no fat added or low-fat microwave)
¾ oz	pretzels
2	rice cakes, 4 in across
6	saltine-type crackers
15–20 (¾ oz)	snack chips, fat-free (tortilla, potato)
2–5 (¾ oz)	whole-wheat crackers, no fat added

Dried Beans, Peas, and Lentils

(counts as 1 starch exchange plus 1 very lean meat exchange)

½ cup	beans and peas (garbanzo, pinto, kidney, white, split, black-eyed)
⅔ cup	lima beans
½ cup	lentils
3 tbsp	miso

Starchy Foods Prepared with Fat

(counts as 1 starch exchange plus 1 fat exchange)

1	biscuit, 2½ in across
½ cup	chow mein noodles
1 (2 oz)	corn bread, 2 in cube
6	crackers, round butter type
1 cup	croutons
16–25 (3 oz)	French-fried potatoes
¼ cup	granola
1 (1½ oz)	muffin (small)
2	pancakes, 4 in across
3 cups	popcorn, microwave
3	sandwich crackers, cheese or peanut butter filling
⅓ cup	stuffing, bread (prepared)
2	taco shells, 6 in across
1	waffle, 4½ in square
4–6 (1 oz)	whole-wheat crackers, fat added

■ Other Carbohydrates Exchange List

One exchange equals 15 grams carbohydrate, or 1 starch, or 1 fruit, or 1 milk.

Exchanges per Serving

1/12th cake	angel food cake, unfrosted	2 carbohydrates
2 in square	brownie, unfrosted (small)	1 carbohydrate, 1 fat
2 in square	cake, unfrosted	1 carbohydrate, 1 fat
2 in square	cake, frosted	2 carbohydrates, 1 fat
2	cookies, fat-free (small)	1 carbohydrate
2	cookies or sandwich cookies with creme filling (small)	1 carbohydrate, 1 fat
¼ cup	cranberry sauce, jellied	1½ carbohydrates
1	cupcake, frosted (small)	2 carbohydrates, 1 fat
1 (1½ oz)	doughnut, plain cake (medium)	1½ carbohydrates, 2 fats
3¾ in across (2 oz)	doughnuts, glazed	2 carbohydrates, 2 fats
1 bar (3 oz)	fruit juice bars, frozen, 100% juice	1 carbohydrate
1 roll (¾ oz)	fruit snacks, chewy (puréed fruit concentrate)	1 carbohydrate
1 tbsp	honey	1 carbohydrate
1 tbsp	sugar	1 carbohydrate

1 tbsp	fruit spread, 100% fruit	1 carbohydrate
½ cup	gelatin, regular	1 carbohydrate
3	gingersnaps	1 carbohydrate
1 bar	granola bar	1 carbohydrate, 1 fat
1 bar	granola bar, fat-free	2 carbohydrates
⅓ cup	hummus	1 carbohydrate, 1 fat
½ cup	ice cream	1 carbohydrate, 2 fats
½ cup	ice cream, light	1 carbohydrate, 1 fat
½ cup	ice cream, fat-free, no sugar added	1 carbohydrate
1 tbsp	jam or jelly, regular	1 carbohydrate
1 cup	milk, chocolate, whole	2 carbohydrates, 1 fat
⅙ pie	pie, fruit, 2 crusts	3 carbohydrates, 2 fats
⅛ pie	pie, pumpkin or custard	1 carbohydrate, 2 fats
12–18 (1 oz)	potato chips	1 carbohydrate, 2 fats
½ cup	pudding, regular (made with low-fat milk)	2 carbohydrates
½ cup	pudding, sugar-free (made with low fat milk)	1 carbohydrate
¼ cup	salad dressing, fat-free	1 carbohydrate
½ cup	sherbet, sorbet	2 carbohydrates
½ cup	spaghetti or pasta sauce, canned	1 carbohydrate, 1 fat
1 (2½ oz)	sweet roll or Danish	2½ carbohydrates, 2 fats
2 tbsp	syrup, light	1 carbohydrate
1 tbsp	syrup, regular	1 carbohydrate
6–12 (1 oz)	tortilla chips	1 carbohydrate, 2 fats
5	vanilla wafers	1 carbohydrate, 1 fat
⅓ cup	yogurt, frozen, low-fat or fat-free	1 carbohydrate, 0–1 fat
½ cup	yogurt, frozen, fat-free, no sugar added	1 carbohydrate
1 cup	yogurt, low-fat, with fruit	3 carbohydrates, 0–1 fat

■ Meat and Meat Substitutes Exchange List

Very Lean Meat and Substitutes List

(0 grams carbohydrate, 7 grams protein, 0–1 grams fat, and 35 kcal)
One very lean meat exchange equals:

Poultry
1 oz   chicken or turkey (white meat, no skin), Cornish hen (no skin)

Fish
1 oz   fresh or frozen cod, flounder, haddock, halibut, trout; tuna, fresh or canned in water

Shellfish
1 oz   clams, crab, lobster, scallops, shrimp, imitation shellfish

Game
1 oz   duck or pheasant (no skin), venison, buffalo, ostrich

Cheese with 1 gram or less fat per ounce
¼ cup   nonfat or low-fat cottage cheese
1 oz   fat-free cheese

Other
1 oz   processed sandwich meats with 1 grams or less fat per ounce, such as deli thin, shaved meats, chipped beef, turkey ham
2   egg whites
¼ cup   egg substitute, plain
1 oz   hot dogs with 1 gram or less fat per ounce
1 oz   kidney (high in cholesterol)
1 oz   sausage with 1 gram or less fat per ounce

Counts as one very lean meat and one starch exchange:

1/2 cup	dried beans, peas, lentils (cooked)

Lean Meat and Substitutes List

(0 grams carbohydrate, 7 grams protein, 3 grams fat, and 55 kcal)
One lean meat exchange equals:

Beef

1 oz	USDA Select or Choice grades of lean beef trimmed of fat, such as round, sirloin, and flank steak; tenderloin; roast (rib, chuck, rump); steak (T-bone, porterhouse, cubed), ground round

Pork

1 oz	lean pork, such as fresh ham; canned, cured, or boiled ham; Canadian bacon; tenderloin, center loin chop

Lamb

1 oz	roast, chop, leg

Veal

1 oz	lean chop, roast

Poultry

1 oz	chicken, turkey (dark meat, no skin), chicken white meat (with skin), domestic duck or goose (well drained of fat, no skin)

Fish

1 oz	herring (uncreamed or smoked)
6	oysters (medium)
1 oz	salmon (fresh or canned), catfish
2	sardines (canned, medium)
1 oz	tuna (canned in oil, drained)

Game

1 oz	goose (no skin), rabbit

Cheese

¼ cup	4.5%–fat cottage cheese
2 tbsp	grated Parmesan
1 oz	cheeses with 3 grams or less fat per ounce

Other

1½ oz	hot dogs with 3 grams or less fat per ounce
1 oz	processed sandwich meat with 3 grams or less fat per ounce, such as turkey pastrami or kielbasa
1 oz	liver, heart (high in cholesterol)

Medium-Fat Meat and Substitutes List

(0 grams carbohydrate, 7 grams protein, 5 grams fat, and 75 kcal)
One medium-fat meat exchange equals:

Beef

1 oz	most beef products (ground beef, meatloaf, corned beef, short ribs, prime grades of meat trimmed of fat, such as prime rib)

Pork

1 oz	top loin, chop, Boston butt, cutlet

Lamb

1 oz	rib roast, ground

Veal

1 oz	cutlet (ground or cubed, unbreaded)

	Poultry
1 oz	chicken dark meat (with skin), ground turkey or ground chicken, fried chicken (with skin)

	Fish
1 oz	any fried fish product

	Cheese (with 5 grams or less fat per ounce)
1 oz	feta
1 oz	mozzarella
¼ cup (2 oz)	ricotta

	Other
1	egg (high in cholesterol, limit to 3 per week)
1 oz	sausage with 5 grams or less fat per ounce
1 cup	soy milk
¼ cup	tempeh
4 oz or ½ cup	tofu

High-Fat Meat and Substitutes List

(0 grams carbohydrate, 7 grams protein, 8 grams fat, and 100 kcal)
One high-fat meat exchange equals:

	Pork
1 oz	spareribs, ground pork, pork sausage

	Cheese
1 oz	all regular cheeses, such as American, cheddar, Monterey Jack, Swiss

	Other
1 oz	processed sandwich meats with 8 grams or less fat per ounce, such as bologna, pimento loaf, salami
1 oz	sausage, such as bratwurst, Italian, knockwurst, Polish, smoked
1 (10/lb)	hot dog (turkey or chicken)
3 slices (20 slices/lb)	bacon

Counts as one high-fat meat plus one fat exchange:

1 (10/lb)	hot dog (beef, pork, or combination)
2 tbsp	peanut butter (contains unsaturated fat)

■ Fat Exchange List

Monosaturated Fats List

(5 grams fat and 45 kcal)
One exchange equals:

⅛ (1 oz)	avocado (medium)
1 tsp	oil (canola, olive, peanut)
	olives:
8	ripe, black (large)
10	green, stuffed (large)
6 nuts	almonds, cashews
6 nuts	mixed (50% peanuts)
10 nuts	peanuts
4 halves	pecans
2 tsp	peanut butter, smooth or crunchy
1 tbsp	sesame seeds
2 tsp	tahini paste

Polyunsaturated Fats List

(5 grams fat and 45 kcal)
One exchange equals:

	margarine:
1 tsp	stick, tub, or squeeze
1 tbsp	lower-fat (30 to 50% vegetable oil)
	mayonnaise:
1 tsp	regular
1 tbsp	reduced-fat
4 halves	nuts, walnuts, English
1 tsp	oil (corn, safflower, soybean)
	salad dressing:
1 tbsp	regular
2 tbsp	reduced-fat
	Miracle Whip Salad Dressing®:
2 tsp	regular
1 tbsp	reduced-fat
1 tbsp	seeds: pumpkin, sunflower

Saturated Fats List

(5 grams fat and 45 kcal)
One exchange equals:

1 slice (20 slices/lb)	bacon, cooked
1 tsp	bacon, grease
	butter:
1 tsp	stick
2 tsp	whipped
1 tbsp	reduced-fat
2 tbsp (½ oz)	chitterlings, boiled
2 tbsp	coconut, sweetened, shredded
2 tbsp	cream, half and half
	cream cheese:
1 tbsp (½ oz)	regular
2 tbsp (1 oz)	reduced-fat
	fatback or salt pork*
1 tsp	shortening or lard
	sour cream:
2 tbsp	regular
3 tbsp	reduced-fat

■ Free Foods List

A *free food* is any food or drink that contains less than 20 kcal or less than 5 grams of carbohydrate per serving. Foods with a serving size listed should be limited to three servings per day. Foods listed without a serving size can be eaten as often as you like.

Fat-Free or Reduced-Fat Foods

1 tbsp	cream cheese, fat-free
1 tbsp	creamers, nondairy, liquid
2 tsp	creamers, nondairy, powdered
1 tbsp	mayonnaise, fat-free
1 tsp	mayonnaise, reduced-fat
4 tbsp	margarine, fat-free
1 tsp	margarine, reduced-fat

---

*Use a piece 1 in × 1 in × ¼ in if you plan to eat the fatback cooked with vegetables. Use a piece 2 in × 1 in × ½ in when eating only the vegetables with the fatback removed.

1 tbsp	Miracle Whip®, nonfat
1 tsp	Miracle Whip®, reduced-fat nonstick cooking spray
1 tbsp	salad dressing, fat-free
2 tbsp	salad dressing, fat-free, Italian
¼ cup	salsa
1 tbsp	sour cream, fat-free, reduced-fat
2 tbsp	whipped topping, regular or light

Sugar-Free or Low-Sugar Foods

1 candy —	candy, hard, sugar-free
	gelatin dessert, sugar-free
	gelatin, unflavored
	gum, sugar-free
2 tsp	jam or jelly, low-sugar, or light sugar substitutes†
2 tbsp	syrup, sugar-free

Drinks

	bouillon, broth, consommé
	bouillon or broth, low-sodium
	carbonated or mineral water
	club soda
1 tbsp	cocoa powder, unsweetened
	coffee
	diet soft drinks, sugar-free
	drink mixes, sugar-free
	tea
	tonic water, sugar-free

Condiments

1 tbsp	catsup
	horseradish
	lemon juice
	lime juice
	mustard
1½	pickles, dill (large)
	soy sauce, regular or light
1 tbsp	taco sauce
	vinegar

Seasonings

flavoring extracts
garlic
herbs, fresh or dried
pimento
spices
Tabasco® or hot pepper sauce
wine, used in cooking
worcestershire sauce

---

†Sugar substitutes, alternatives, or replacements that are approved by the Food and Drug Administration (FDA) are safe to use. Common brand names include
    Equal® (aspartame)
    Sprinkle Sweet® (saccharin)
    Sweet One® (acesulfame-K)
    Sweet-10® (saccharin)
    Sugar Twin® (saccharin)
    Sweet 'n Low® (saccharin)

■ Combination Foods List

	Entrées	Exchanges per Serving
1 cup (8 oz)	tuna noodle casserole, lasagna, spaghetti with meatballs, chili with beans, macaroni and cheese	2 carbohydrates, 2 medium-fat meats
2 cups (16 oz)	chow mein (without noodles or rice)	1 carbohydrate, 2 lean meats
¼ of 10 in (5 oz)	pizza, cheese, thin crust	2 carbohydrates, 2 medium-fat meats, 1 fat
¼ of 10 in (5 oz)	pizza, meat topping, thin crust	2 carbohydrates, 2 medium-fat meats, 2 fats
1 (7 oz)	pot pie	2 carbohydrates, 1 medium-fat meat, 4 fats
	Frozen Entrées	
1 (11 oz)	salisbury steak with gravy, mashed potato	2 carbohydrates, 3 medium-fat meats, 3-4 fats
1 (11 oz)	turkey with gravy, mashed potato, dressing	2 carbohydrates, 2 medium-fat meats, 2 fats
1 (8 oz)	entrée with less than 300 kcal	2 carbohydrates, 3 lean meats
	Soups	
1 cup	bean	1 carbohydrate, 1 very lean meat
1 cup (8 oz)	cream (made with water)	1 carbohydrate, 1 fat
½ cup (4 oz)	split pea (made with water)	1 carbohydrate
1 cup (8 oz)	tomato (made with water)	1 carbohydrate
1 cup (8 oz)	vegetable beef, chicken noodle, or other broth-type	1 carbohydrate

Fast (Quick-Service) Foods

		Exchanges per Serving
2	burritos with beef	4 carbohydrates, 2 medium-fat meats, 2 fats
6	chicken nuggets	1 carbohydrate, 2 medium-fat meats, 1 fat
1 each	chicken breast and wing, breaded and fried	1 carbohydrate, 4 medium-fat meats, 2 fats
1	fish sandwich/tartar sauce	3 carbohydrates, 1 medium-fat meat, 3 fats
20–25	French fries, thin	2 carbohydrates, 2 fats
1	hamburger (regular)	2 carbohydrates, 2 medium-fat meats
1	hamburger (large)	2 carbohydrates, 3 medium-fat meats, 1 fat
1	hot dog with bun	1 carbohydrate, 1 high-fat meat, 1 fat
1	individual pan pizza	5 carbohydrates, 3 medium-fat meats, 3 fats
1	soft-serve cone (medium)	2 carbohydrates, 1 fat
1 sub (6 in)	submarine sandwich	3 carbohydrates, 1 vegetable, 2 medium-fat meats, 1 fat
1 (6 oz)	taco, hard shell	2 carbohydrates, 2 medium-fat meats, 2 fats
1 (3 oz)	taco, soft shell	1 carbohydrate, 1 medium-fat meat, 1 fat

DIETARY INTAKE AND ENERGY EXPENDITURE ASSESSMENT

Although it may seem overwhelming at first, it is actually very easy to track the foods you eat. One tip is to record foods and beverages consumed as soon as possible after the actual time of consumption.

I. Fill in the food record form that follows. This appendix contains a blank copy (see the completed example in Table E-1). Then, to estimate the nutrient values of the foods you are eating, consult food labels and the food composition table in this book (Appendix A), or use the nutrition software package available with this book. If these resources do not have the serving size you need, adjust the value. If you drink ½ cup of orange juice, for example, but a table has values only for 1 cup, halve all values before you record them. Then, consider pooling all the same food to save time; if you drink a cup of 1% milk three times throughout the day, enter your milk consumption only once as 3 cups. As you record your intake for use on the nutrient analysis form that follows, consider the following tips:

- Measure and record the amounts of foods eaten in portion sizes of cups, teaspoons, tablespoons, ounces, slices, or inches (or convert metric units to these units).
- Record brand names of all food products, such as "Quick Quaker Oats."
- Measure and record all those little extras, such as gravies, salad dressings, taco sauces, pickles, jelly, sugar, catsup, and margarine.
- For beverages
  —List the type of milk, such as whole, skim, 1%, evaporated, chocolate, or reconstituted dry.
  —Indicate whether fruit juice is fresh, frozen, or canned.
  —Indicate type for other beverages, such as fruit drink, fruit-flavored drink, Kool-Aid, and hot chocolate made with water or milk.
- For fruits
  —Indicate whether fresh, frozen, dried, or canned.
  —If whole, record number eaten and size with approximate measurements (such as 1 apple—3 in in diameter).
  —Indicate whether processed in water, light syrup, or heavy syrup.
- For vegetables
  —Indicate whether fresh, frozen, dried, or canned.
  —Record as portion of cup, teaspoon, or tablespoon, or as pieces (such as carrot sticks — 4 in long, ½ in thick).
  —Record preparation method.
- For cereals
  —Record cooked cereals in portions of tablespoon or cup (a level measurement after cooking).
  —Record dry cereal in level portions of tablespoon or cup.
  —If margarine, milk, sugar, fruit, or something else is added, measure and record amount and type.
- For breads
  —Indicate whether whole wheat, rye, white, and so on.
  —Measure and record number and size of portion (biscuit—2 in across, 1 in thick; slice of homemade rye bread—3 in by 4 in, ¼ in thick).
  —Sandwiches: list *all* ingredients (lettuce, mayonnaise, tomato, and so on).

- For meat, fish, poultry, and cheese
  —Give size (length, width, thickness) in inches or weight in ounces after cooking for meat, fish, and poultry (such as cooked hamburger patty—3 in across, ½ in thick).
  —Give size (length, width, thickness) in inches or weight in ounces for cheese.
  —Record measurements only for the cooked, edible part—without bone or fat that is left on the plate.
  —Describe how meat, poultry, or fish was prepared.
- For eggs
  —Record as soft or hard cooked, fried, scrambled, poached, or omelet.
  —If milk, butter, or drippings are used, specify kinds and amount.
- For desserts
  —List commercial brand or "homemade" or "bakery" under brand.
  —Purchased candies, cookies, and cakes: specify kind and size.
  —Measure and record portion size of cakes, pies, and cookies by specifying thickness, diameter, and width or length, depending on the item.

Time	Minutes Spent Eating	M or S*	H† (0–3)	Activity While Eating	Place of Eating	Food and Quantity	Others Present	Reason for Choice

*M or S: Meal or snack
†H: Degree of hunger (0 = none; 3 = maximum)

TABLE E-1   One Day's Food Record—This Activity Can Help You Understand More About Your Food Habits

Time	Minutes Spent Eating	M or S*	H† (0–3)	Activity While Eating	Place of Eating	Food and Quantity	Others Present	Reason for Choice
7:10 A.M.	15	M	2	Standing, fixing lunch	Kitchen	orange juice, 1 cup Crispix, 1 cup 2% milk, ½ cup Sugar, 2 tsp Black coffee	——	Health Habit Health Taste Habit
10:00 A.M.	4	S	1	Sitting, taking notes	Classroom	Diet cola, 12 oz	Class	Weight control
12:15 P.M.	40	M	2	Sitting, talking	Student union	Chicken sandwich with lettuce and mayonnaise Pear, 1 2% milk, 1 cup	Friends	Taste Health Health
2:30 P.M.	10	S	1	Sitting, studying	Library	Regular cola, 12 oz	Friend	Hunger
6:30 P.M.	35	M	3	Sitting, talking	Kitchen	Pork chop, 1 Baked potato, 1 Margarine, 2 tbsp Lettuce and tomato salad Ranch dressing, 2 tbsp Peas, ½ cup Whole milk, 1 cup Cherry pie, 1 piece	Boyfriend	Convenience Health Taste Health Taste Health Habit Taste
9:10 P.M.	10	S	2	Sitting, studying	Living room	Apple, 1 Glass mineral water, 1	——	Weight control Weight control

*M or S: Meal or snack
†H: Degree of hunger (0 = none; 3 = maximum)

II. Now complete the nutrient analysis form as shown, using your food record. A blank copy of this form is printed on three pages ahead for your use. Note that the NutriQuest software available with this book will create such a table for you if you simply enter all food eaten.

Nutrient Analysis Form (Sample)

Name	Quantity	Kcal	Protein (g)	Carbohydrates (g)	Dietary fiber (g)	Total fat (g)	Monounsaturated fat (g)	Polyunsaturated fat (g)	Saturated fat (g)	Cholesterol (mg)	Calcium (mg)	Iron (mg)
Egg bagel, 3.5-in. diameter	1 ea.	180	7.45	34.7	0.748	1.00	0.286	0.400	0.171	44.0	20.0	2.10
Jelly	1 tbsp	49.0	0.018	12.7	——	0.018	0.005	0.005	0.005	——	2.00	0.120
Orange juice, prepared fresh or frozen	1½ cup	165	2.52	40.2	1.49	0.210	0.037	0.045	0.025	——	33.0	0.411
Cheeseburger, McDonald's	2 ea.	636	30.2	57.0	0.460	32.0	12.2	2.18	13.3	80.0	338	5.68
French fries, McDonald's	1 order	220	3.00	26.1	4.19	11.5	4.37	0.570	4.61	8.57	9.10	0.605
Cola beverage, regular	1½ cup	151	——	38.5							9.00	0.120
Pork loin chop, broiled, lean	4 oz.	261	36.2	——	——	11.9	5.35	1.43	4.09	112	5.67	1.04
Baked potato with skin	1 ea.	220	4.65	51.0	3.90	0.200	0.004	0.087	0.052		20.0	2.75
Peas, frozen, cooked	½ cup	63.0	4.12	11.4	3.61	0.220	0.019	0.103	0.039		19.0	1.25
Margarine, regular or soft, 80% fat	20 g	143	0.160	0.100	——	16.1	5.70	6.92	2.76		5.29	——
Iceberg lettuce, chopped	2 cup	14.6	1.13	2.34	1.68	0.212	0.008	0.112	0.028	——	21.2	0.560
French dressing	2 oz	300	0.318	3.63	0.431	32.0	14.2	12.4	4.94		7.10	0.227
2% low-fat milk	1 cup	121	8.12	11.7	——	4.78	1.35	0.170	2.92	22.0	297	0.120
Graham crackers	2 ea.	60.0	1.04	10.8	1.40	1.46	0.600	0.400	0.400	——	6.00	0.367
Totals		2584	99.0	300	17.9	112	44.1	24.8	33.4	266	792	15.4
RDA or related nutrient standard*		2900	58		——						1000	8
% of nutrient needs		89	170		——						79	193

Abbreviations: g = grams, mg = milligrams, μg = micrograms

*Values from inside cover. The values listed are for a male age 19 years. Note that number of kcal is just a rough estimate. It is better to base energy needs on actual energy output.

†In RAE units. Table values are in RE units since the food values have not been updated to reflect the latest vitamin A standards. RAE equal RE for foods with preformed vitamin A, such as for the pork chop, but RAE are only about half the RE listed for foods with provitamin A carotenoids, such as for the peas (see Chapter 9 for details).

‡In DFE units. Note that the table values are in micrograms for all folate forms. The specific DFE for each food has yet to be incorporated into food tables (see chapter 10 for more details on DFE units).

Nutrient Analysis Form (Sample) cont'd

Magnesium (mg)	Phosphorus (mg)	Potassium (mg)	Sodium (mg)	Zinc (mg)	Vitamin A (RE)	Vitamin C (mg)	Vitamin E (mg)	Thiamin (mg)	Riboflavin (mg)	Niacin (mg)	Vitamin B-6 (mg)	Folate (µg)	Vitamin B-12 (µg)
18.0	61.0	65.0	300	0.612	7.00	——	1.80	2.58	0.197	2.40	0.030	16.3	0.065
0.720	1.00	16.0	4.00	——	0.200	0.710	0.016	0.002	0.005	0.036	0.005	2.00	——
36.0	60.0	711	3.00	0.192	28.5	145	0.714	0.300	0.060	0.750	0.165	163	——
45.8	410	314	1460	5.20	134	4.10	0.560	0.600	0.480	8.66	0.230	42.0	1.82
26.7	101	564	109	0.320	5.00	12.5	0.203	0.122	0.020	2.26	0.218	19.0	0.027
3.00	46.0	4.00	15.0	0.049	——								
34.0	277	476	88.2	2.54	3.15	0.454	0.405	1.30	0.350	6.28	0.535	6.77	0.839
55.0	115	844	16.0	0.650	——	26.1	0.100	0.216	0.067	3.32	0.701	22.2	——
23.0	72.0	134	70.0	0.750	53.4	7.90	0.400	0.226	0.140	1.18	0.090	46.9	——
0.467	4.06	7.54	216	0.041	199	0.028	2.19	0.002	0.006	0.004	0.002	0.211	0.017
10.1	22.4	177	10.1	0.246	37.0	4.36	0.120	0.052	0.034	0.210	0.044	62.8	——
5.81	3.63	7.03	666	0.045	0.023	——	15.9	——	——	——	0.006	——	——
33.0	232	377	122	0.963	140	2.32	0.080	0.095	0.403	0.210	0.105	12.0	0.888
6.00	20.0	36.0	86.0	0.113	——	——	——	0.020	0.030	0.600	0.011	1.80	——
298	1425	3732	3165	11.7	607	204	22.5	5.52	1.79	25.9	2.14	395	3.65
400	700	2000	500	11	900†	90	15	1.2	1.3	16	1.3	400†	2.4
75	204	187	633	106	67	226	150	450	138	162	160	99	152

Nutrient Analysis Form (Sample)

Name	Quantity	Kcal	Protein (g)	Carbohydrates (g)	Dietary fiber (g)	Total fat (g)	Monounsaturated fat (g)	Polyunsaturated fat (g)	Saturated fat (g)	Cholesterol (mg)	Calcium (mg)	Iron (mg)
Totals												
RDA or related nutrient standard*												†
% of nutrient needs												

*Values from inside cover. Note that number of kcals is just a rough estimate. It is better to base energy needs on actual energy output.
†Use RAE values, even though food table is based on RE units.

Nutrient Analysis Form (Sample) cont'd

Magnesium (mg)	Phosphorus (mg)	Potassium (mg)	Sodium (mg)	Zinc (mg)	Vitamin A (RE)	Vitamin C (mg)	Vitamin E (mg)	Thiamin (mg)	Riboflavin (mg)	Niacin (mg)	Vitamin B-6 (mg)	Folate (μg)	Vitamin B-12 (μg)
					†								

III. Complete the following table as you summarize your dietary intake.

Percentage of kcal from Protein, Fat, Carbohydrate, and Alcohol

Intake

Protein (P):   ____g/day $\times$ 4 kcal/g = (P)____ kcal/day

Fat (F):   ____g/day $\times$ 9 kcal/g = (F)____ kcal/day

Carbohydrate (C):   ____g/day $\times$ 4 kcal/g = (C)____ kcal/day

Alcohol (A):   (A)____ kcal/day*

                        Total kcal (T)/day = (T)____ kcal/day

Percentage of kcal from protein:

$\dfrac{(P)}{(T)}$ _____ $\times$ 100 = ____% of total kcal

Percentage of kcal from fat:

$\dfrac{(F)}{(T)}$ _____ $\times$ 100 = ____% of total kcal

Percentage of kcal from carbohydrate:

$\dfrac{(C)}{(T)}$ _____ $\times$ 100 = ____ % of total kcal

Percentage of kcal from alcohol:

$\dfrac{(A)}{(T)}$ _____ $\times$ 100 = ____% of total kcal

NOTE: The four percentages can total 99, 100, or 101, depending on the way in which figures were rounded off earlier.

*To calculate how many kcal in a beverage are from alcohol, look up the beverage in Appendix A. Determine how many kcal are from carbohydrate (multiply carbohydrate grams times 4), fat (fat grams times 9), and protein (protein grams times 4). The remaining kcal are from alcohol.

IV. Use the following table to again record your food intake for one day, placing each food item in the correct category of the Food Guide Pyramid, with the correct number of servings (see Table 2-5 in Chapter 2). Note that a food such as toast with margarine contributes to two categories—namely, to the bread, cereal, rice, and pasta group and to the fats, oils, and sweets group. You can expect that many food choices will contribute to more than one group. Indicate the number of servings from the Food Guide Pyramid that each food yields.

Indicate the Number of Servings from the Food Guide Pyramid That Each Food Yields

Food or Beverage	Amount Eaten	Milk, Yogurt, and Cheese	Meat, Poultry, Fish, Dry Beans, Eggs, and Nuts	Fruits	Vegetables	Bread, Cereal, Rice, and Pasta	Fats, Oils, and Sweets
Group totals							
Recommended servings							In moderation
Shortages in numbers of servings							

V. Evaluation. Are there weaknesses suggested in your nutrient intake that correspond to missing servings in the Food Guide Pyramid? Consider replacing the missing servings to improve your nutrient intake.

VI. For the same day you keep your food record, also keep a 24-hour record of your activities. Include sleeping, sitting, and walking, as well as the obvious forms of exercise. Calculate your energy expenditure for these activities using Table 13-7 in Chapter 13 or the software available with this book. Try to substitute a similar activity if your particular activity is not listed. Calculate the total kcal you used for the day (total for column 3). Following is an example of an activity record. A blank form follows for your use. Ask your professor whether you are to turn in the form or the activity printout from the software.

Weight (kg)*: 70 kg

| Activity | Time (Minutes): Convert to Hours | Energy Cost | | |
		Column I kcal/kg/hr (from Table 13-7)	Column 2 (Column 1 × Time)	Column 3 (Column 2 × Weight in kg)
Brisk walking	(60 min) 1 hr	4.4	(×1) = 4.4	(× 70) = 308

*lb/2.2

Weight (kg)*:

| Activity | Time (Minutes): Convert to Hours | Energy Cost | | |
		Column I kcal/kg/hr (from Table 13-7)	Column 2 (Column 1 × Time)	Column 3 (Column 2 × Weight in kg)

Total kcal used (from adding all of column 3)

*lb/2.2

FATTY ACIDS, INCLUDING OMEGA-3 FATTY ACIDS IN FOODS

Chain Length, Number, and Site of Double Bonds for Common Fatty Acids

Common name of fatty acid	Number of carbon atoms and number and site of double bond(s), counting from methyl end ($-CH_3$) if appropriate
Saturated Fatty Acids (No Double Bonds)	
Formic	1
Acetic	2
Propionic	3
Butyric	4
Valeric	5
Caproic	6
Caprylic	8
Capric	10
Lauric	12
Myristic	14
Palmitic	16
Stearic	18
Unsaturated Fatty Acids	
Oleic	18:1 (9-10) ω-9
Linoleic	18:2 (6-7, 9-10) ω-6
Alpha-linolenic	18:3 (3-4, 6-7, 9-10) ω-3
Arachidonic	20:4 (6-7, 9-10, 12-13, 15-16) ω-6
Eicosapentaenoic	20:5 (3-4, 6-7, 9-10, 12-13, 15-16) ω-3
Docosahexaenoic	22:6 (3-4, 6-7, 9-10, 12-13, 15-16, 18-19) ω-3

Fatty Acid Composition of Selected Foods*

						Fatty Acid†				
		Saturated								
Food Item	<C12:0	C12:0	14:0	C16:0	C18:0	C18:1 ω-9	C18:2 ω-6	C18:3 ω-3	C20:5 ω-3	C22:6 ω-3
Fats and Oils		Lauric Acid	Myristic Acid	Palmitic Acid	Stearic Acid	Oleic Acid	Linoleic Acid	Alpha-Linolenic Acid	EPA‡	DHA‡
Beef tallow	——	0.90	3.70	24.9	18.9	36.0	3.1	0.60	——	——
Butter	7.0	2.20	8.10	21.3	9.8	20.4	1.8	1.20	——	——
Cocoa butter	——		0.10	25.4	33.2	32.6	2.8	0.10	——	——
Corn oil	——	——	——	11.0	2.0	25.0	58.0	0.70	——	——
Cottonseed oil	——	——	0.80	22.7	2.3	17.0	51.5	0.20	——	——
Lard	0.1	0.20	1.30	23	15.2	40.9	9.7	1.10	——	——
Olive oil	——		——	11.0	2.5	72.5	7.5	0.60	——	——
Palm kernel oil	7	47.00	16.40	8.1	2.8	11.4	1.6	——	——	——
Palm oil	——	0.10	1.00	43.5	4.3	36.6	9.1	0.20	——	——
Safflower oil	——	——	——	4.2	1.9	14.4	74.6	——	——	——
Shortenings	0.2	0.10	1.60	23.0	15.2	41.0	9.7	1.10	——	——
Margarine, stick	——	——	0.20	9.7	6.0	36.0	24.3	1.10	——	——
Margarine, tub	——	——	0.100	8.7	5.0	37.3	24.6	1.10	——	——
Canola oil	——	——	——	4.0	1.8	56.0	20.3	9.30	——	——
Soybean oil	——	——	——	14.0	4.0	29.0	45.0	3.00	——	——
Coconut oil	14.0	45.00	17.00	8.2	3.0	6.0	1.8	——	——	——
Peanut oil	——	——	0.100	9.5	2.2	44.8	32.0	——	——	——
Cod liver oil	——	——	3.6	10.6	2.8	20.6	0.9	0.9	6.9	11.0
Menhaden oil	——	——	8.0	15.1	3.8	14.6	2.2	1.5	13.2	4.9
Meat, Fish, and Poultry										
Beef, lean only, uncooked	——	0.04	0.50	4.0	2.1	6.5	0.4	0.16	——	——
Chicken, white meat, cooked	——	0.03	0.01	2.1	0.7	3.5	2.1	0.10	0.01	0.05
Salmon, coho, cooked	——	——	0.18	0.8	0.3	1.7	0.2	0.40	0.40	1.40
Tuna, light, canned in water	——	——	0.02	0.2	0.1	0.1	——	0.02	0.05	0.20
Nuts and Seeds										
Walnuts	——	——	——	4.4	1.6	8.8	38	9	——	——
Flaxseeds	——	——	——	1.8	1.4	6.9	4.3	18.1	——	——

From USDA Nutrient Database for Standard Reference, Release 13.

*Only major fatty acids are presented.

†All values represent grams per 100 g edible portion.

‡EPA eicosapentaenoic acid
 DHA docosahexaenoic acid } fish oil fatty acids

THE 1983 METROPOLITAN LIFE INSURANCE COMPANY HEIGHT-WEIGHT TABLE AND DETERMINATION OF FRAME SIZE

1983 Metropolitan Life Insurance Company Height-Weight Table*†

Women						Men					
Height		Frame				Height		Frame			
Ft.	In.	Small	Medium	Large		Ft.	In.	Small	Medium	Large	
4	10	102–111	109–121	118–131		5	2	128–134	131–141	138–150	
4	11	103–113	111–123	120–134		5	3	130–136	133–143	140–153	
5	0	104–115	113–126	122–137		5	4	132–138	135–145	142–156	
5	1	106–118	115–129	125–140		5	5	134–140	137–148	144–160	
5	2	108–121	118–132	128–143		5	6	136–142	139–151	146–164	
5	3	111–124	121–135	131–147		5	7	138–145	142–154	149–168	
5	4	114–127	124–138	134–151		5	8	140–148	145–157	152–172	
5	5	117–130	127–141	137–155		5	9	142–151	148–160	155–176	
5	6	120–133	130–144	140–159		5	10	144–154	151–163	158–180	
5	7	123–136	133–147	143–163		5	11	146–157	154–166	161–184	
5	8	126–139	136–150	146–167		6	0	149–160	157–170	164–188	
5	9	129–142	139–153	149–170		6	1	152–164	160–174	168–192	
5	10	132–145	142–156	152–173		6	2	155 168	164–178	172–197	
5	11	135–148	145–159	155–176		6	3	158–172	167–182	176–202	
6	0	138–151	148–162	158–179		6	4	162–176	171–187	181–207	

Reprinted courtesy of Metropolitan Life Insurance Company, *Statistical Bulletin.*

Permission granted courtesy of Metropolitan Life Insurance Company, *Statistical Bulletin.*

*Based on a weight-height mortality study conducted by the Society of Actuaries and the Association of Life Insurance Medical Directors of America, Metropolitan Life Insurance Medical Directors of America, Metropolitan Life Insurance Company, revised 1983.

†Weights at ages 25 to 59 based on lowest mortality. Height includes 1-in heel. Weight for women includes 3 lb for indoor clothing. Weight for men includes 5 lb for indoor clothing.

■ Using the Metropolitan Life Insurance Table to Estimate Healthy Weight

The Metropolitan Life Insurance Table is a common method for estimating healthy weight. The table lists for any height the weight that is associated with a maximum life span. The table does not tell the healthiest weight for a living person; it simply lists the weight associated with longevity.

There are many criticisms of this table. These stem from the inclusion of some people and the exclusion of others. For example, only policyholders of life insurance are included. In addition, smokers are included, but anyone over the age of 60 is excluded. Weight is only measured at the time of purchase of insurance, and there is no follow-up. All of these factors contribute to the fact that this table is to be used only as a rough screening tool; not meeting the exact recommendations should not be cause for alarm.

To diagnose overweight or obesity using the table, calculate the percentage of the Metropolitan Life Insurance Table weight. Use the midpoint of a weight range for a specific height.

$$\frac{(\text{Current wt.} - \text{wt. from table})}{\text{Weight from table}} \times 100$$

Example:

$$\frac{140 - 120}{120} \times 100 = 17\% \text{ over standard}$$

Overweight can be defined as weighing at least 10% more than the weight listed on the table. Obesity weighs in at 20% more than that listed on the table. Moreover, this measure of obesity comes in degrees. Whereas mild obesity carries little health risk, severe obesity raises overall health risk twelvefold.

Degrees of Obesity

% Over Healthy Body Weight	Form of Obesity
20–40%	Mild
41–99%	Moderate
100%+	Severe

■ Determining Frame Size

Method 1

Height is recorded without shoes.

Wrist circumference is measured just beyond the bony (styloid) process at the wrist joint on the right arm, using a tape measure.

The following formula is used:

$$r = \frac{\text{Height (cm)}}{\text{Wrist circumference (cm)}}$$

Frame size can be determined as follows:[†]

Males	Females
$r > 10.4$ small	$r > 11$ small
$r = 9.6–10.4$ medium	$r = 10.1–11$ medium
$r < 9.6$ large	$r < 10.1$ large

Method 2

The patient's right arm is extended forward, perpendicular to the body, with the arm bent so the angle at the elbow forms 90 degrees, with the fingers pointing up and the palm turned away from the body. The greatest breadth across the elbow joint is measured with a sliding caliper along the axis of the upper arm, on the two prominent bones on either side of the elbow. This is recorded as the elbow breadth. The following tables give elbow breadth measurements for medium-framed men and women of various heights. Measurements lower than those listed indicate a small frame size; higher measurements indicate a large frame size.[‡]

Men		Women	
Height in 1″ Heels	Elbow Breadth	Height in 1″ Heels	Elbow Breadth
5′2″–5′3″	2½–2⅞″	4′10″–4′11″	2¼–2½″
5′4″–5′7″	2⅝–2⅞″	5′0″–5′3″	2¼–2½″
5′8″–5′11″	2¾–3″	5′4″–5′7″	2⅜–2⅝″
6′0″–6′3″	2¾–3¼″	5′8″–5′11″	2⅜–2⅝″
6′4″ and over	2⅞–3¼″	6′0″ and over	2½–2¾″

[†]From Grant JP: *Handbook of total parenteral nutrition.* Philadelphia: WB Saunders, 1980.
[‡]From Metropolitan Life Insurance Co., 1983.

CAFFEINE CONTENT OF FOODS

Beverages	mg
Carbonated Beverages*	
Cherry Coke, Coca-Cola—12 fl oz (370 g)	46
Cherry cola, Slice—12 fl oz (360 g)	48
Cherry RC—12 fl oz (360 g)	12
Coca-Cola—12 fl oz (370 g)	46
Coca-Cola Classic—12 fl oz (369 g)	46
Cola, RC—12 fl oz (360 g)	18
Mello Yello—12 fl oz (372 g)	52
Mr. Pibb—12 fl oz (369 g)	40
Mountain Dew—12 fl oz (360 g)	54
Dr. Pepper-type soda—12 fl oz (368 g)	41
Pepsi Cola—12 fl oz (360 g)	38
Carbonated Beverages, Low-Calorie*	
Diet Cherry Coke, Coca-Cola—12 fl oz (354 g)	46
Diet cherry cola, Slice—12 fl oz (360 g)	41
Diet Coke, Coca-Cola—12 fl oz (354 g)	46
Diet cola, aspartame-sweetened—12 fl oz (355 g)	50
Diet Pepsi—12 fl oz (360 g)	36
Diet RC—12 fl oz (360 g)	48
Coffee	
Brewed—6 fl oz (177 g)	103
Instant powder—1 tsp (1.8 g)	57
Decaffeinated—1 rounded tsp (1.8 g)	2
With chicory—1 tsp (1.8 g)	37
Prepared from instant powder—6 fl oz & 1 tsp powder (179 g)	57
Amaretto, General Foods—6 fl oz & 11.5 g powder (189 g)	60
Amaretto, sugar-free, General Foods—6 fl oz water & 7.7 g powder (185 g)	60
Decaffeinated—6 fl oz water & 1 tsp powder (179 g)	2
Francais, General Foods—6 fl oz water & 11.5 g powder (189 g)	53
Francais, sugar-free, General Foods—6 fl oz water & 7.7 g powder (185 g)	59
Irish creme, General Foods—6 fl oz water & 12.8 g powder (190 g)	53
Irish creme, sugar free, General Foods—6 fl oz water & 7.1 g powder (185 g)	48
Irish mocha mint, General Foods—6 fl oz water & 11.5 g powder (189 g)	27
Irish mocha mint, sugar-free, General Foods—6 fl oz water & 6.4 g powder (189 g)	25
Orange cappuccino, General Foods—6 fl oz water & 14 g powder (191 g)	73
Orange cappuccino, sugar-free, General Foods—6 fl oz water & 6.7 g powder (184 g)	71
Suisse mocha, General Foods—6 fl oz water & 11.5 g powder (189 g)	41

Data from Pennington JAT, *Bowes and Church's Food Values of Portions Commonly Consumed*, ed. 17, 1998, JB Lippincott. Reprinted with permission.

Abbreviations: g = grams, mg = milligrams

*Caffeine-free carbonated beverages and most noncarbonated beverages contain no caffeine.

Coffee cont'd

Suisse mocha, sugar-free, General Foods—6 fl oz water & 6.4 g powder (184 g)	40
Vienna, General Foods—6 fl oz water & 14 g powder (191 g)	56
Vienna, sugar-free, General Foods—6 fl oz water & 6.7 g powder (184 g)	55
with chicory—6 fl oz water & 1 tsp powder (179 g)	38

Tea, Hot/Iced

Brewed 3 min—6 fl oz water (178 g)	36
Instant powder—1 tsp (0.7 g)	31
With lemon flavor—1 rounded tsp (1.4 g)	25
With sugar & lemon flavor—3 tsp (23 g)	29
With sodium saccharin & lemon flavor—2 tsp (1.6 g)	36
Prepared from instant powder	
1 tsp powder in 8 fl oz water (237 g)	31
Crystal Light—8 fl oz (238 g)	11
With lemon flavor—1 tsp powder in 8 fl oz water (238 g)	26
With sugar & lemon flavor—3 tsp powder in 8 fl oz water (259 g)	29
With sodium, saccharin & lemon flavor—2 tsp powder in 8 fl oz water (238 g)	36

Candy

Chocolate	
German sweet, Bakers—1 oz square (28 g)	8
Semi-sweet, Bakers—1 oz square (28 g)	13
Chocolate chips	
Bakers—¼ cup (43 g)	12
German sweet, Bakers—¼ cup (43 g)	15
Semi-sweet, Bakers—¼ cup (43 g)	14

Desserts

Frozen Desserts

Pudding pops, Jell-O	
Chocolate—1 pop (47 g)	2
Chocolate caramel swirl—1 pop (47 g)	1
Chocolate fudge—1 pop (47 g)	3
Chocolate vanilla swirl—1 pop (47 g)	2
Chocolate with chocolate coating—1 pop (49 g)	3
Double chocolate swirl pop (47 g)	2
Milk chocolate—1 pop (47 g)	2

Pies

Chocolate mousse, from mix, Jell-O—⅛ pie (95 g)	6

Puddings, from Instant Mix

Chocolate	
Jell-O—½ cup (150 g)	5
Sugar-free, D-Zerta—½ cup (130 g)	4
Sugar-free, Jell-O—½ cup (133 g)	4
Chocolate fudge	
Jell-O—½ cup (150 g)	8
Chocolate fudge mousse, Jell-O—½ cup (86 g)	12
Chocolate mousse, Jell-O—½ cup (86 g)	9
Chocolate tapioca, Jell-O—½ cup (147 g)	8
Milk chocolate, Jell-O—½ cup (150 g)	5

Milk Beverages

Chocolate flavor mix in whole milk—2–3 tsp powder in 8 fl oz milk (266 g)	8
Chocolate malted milk flavor powder	
In whole milk—3 tsp powder in 8 fl oz milk (265 g)	8
With added nutrients in whole milk—4–5 tsp powder in 8 fl oz milk (265 g)	5
Chocolate syrup in whole milk—2 tbsp syrup in 8 fl oz milk (282 g)	6
Cocoa/hot chocolate, prepared with water from mix—3–4 tsp powder in 6 fl oz water (206 g)	4

Milk Beverage Mixes

Chocolate flavor mix, powder—2–3 tsp (22 g)	8
Chocolate malted milk flavor mix, powder—¾ oz (3 tsp) (21 g)	8
Chocolate malted milk flavor mix with added nutrients, powder—¾ oz (4–5 tsp) (21 g)	6
Chocolate syrup—2 tbsp (1 fl oz) (38 g)	5
Cocoa mix powder—1 oz pkt (3–4 tsp) (28 g)	5

Miscellaneous

Baking chocolate, unsweetened, Bakers—1 oz (28 g)	25

SOURCES OF NUTRITION INFORMATION

Consider the following reliable sources of food and nutrition information:

Journals That Regularly Cover Nutrition Topics

*American Family Physician**
American Journal of Clinical Nutrition
American Journal of Epidemiology
American Journal of Medicine
American Journal of Nursing
American Journal of Obstetrics and Gynecology
American Journal of Physiology
American Journal of Public Health
American Scientist
Annals of Internal Medicine
Annual Reviews of Medicine
Annual Reviews of Nutrition
Archives of Disease in Childhood
Archives of Internal Medicine
British Journal of Nutrition
BMJ (British Medical Journal)
Cancer
Cancer Research
Circulation
Diabetes
Diabetes Care
Disease-a-Month
FASEB Journal
*FDA Consumer**
Food Chemical Toxicology
Food Engineering
Gastroenterology
Geriatrics
Gut
Human Nutrition: Applied Nutrition
Human Nutrition: Clinical Nutrition
*Journal of the American College of Nutrition**

*Journal of The American Dietetic Association**
Journal of the American Geriatric Society
JAMA (Journal of the American Medical Association)
Journal of Applied Physiology
*Journal of Canadian Dietetic Association**
Journal of Clinical Investigation
Journal of Food Service
Journal of Food Technology
JNCI (Journal of the National Cancer Institute)
Journal of Nutrition
*Journal of Nutritional Education**
Journal of Nutrition for the Elderly
Journal of Nutrition Research
Journal of Pediatrics
Lancet
Mayo Clinic Proceedings
Medicine and Science in Sports and Exercise
Nature
The New England Journal of Medicine
Nutrition
Nutrition Reviews
*Nutrition Today**
Pediatrics
The Physician and Sports Medicine
*Postgraduate Medicine**
Proceedings of the Nutrition Society
Science
*Science News**
*Scientific American**

The majority of these journals are available in college and university libraries or in a specialty library on campus, such as one designated for health services or home economics. As indicated, a few journals will be filed under their abbreviations, rather than the first word in their full name. A reference librarian can help you locate any of these sources. The asterisked (*) journals are ones you may find especially interesting and useful because of the number of nutrition articles presented each month or the less technical nature of the presentation.

Magazines for the Consumer That Cover Nutrition Topics

American Health for Women
Better Homes and Gardens
Good Housekeeping

Health
Parents
Self

Textbooks and Other Sources for Advanced Study of Nutrition Topics

Brody T: *Nutritional biochemistry.*2nd ed. San Diego: Academic Press, 1999.

Groff JL, Gropper SS: *Advanced human nutrition and metabolism*. St Paul, MN: West, 2000.

International Life Sciences Institute: *Present knowledge in nutrition*. 7th ed. Washington DC The Nutrition Foundation, 1996.

Mahan LK, Escott-Stump: *Krause's food, nutrition, and diet therapy*. 10th ed. Philadelphia: WB Saunders, 2000.

Murray RK and others: *Harper's biochemistry*. 25th ed. Norwalk, CT: Appleton & Lange, 2000.

Schils ME, Olson JA, Shike M, Ross AC: *Modern nutrition in health and disease*. 9th ed. Philadelphia: Lea & Febiger, 1999.

Stipanuk MH: *Biochemical and physiological aspects of human nutrition*. Philadephia: WB Saunders, 2000.

Newsletters That Cover Nutrition Issues on a Regular Basis

American Institute for Cancer Research (AICR) Washington, DC 20069
http://www.icr.ac.uk/

CNI Nutrition Week
Community Nutrition Institute
910 17th St. N.W., Suite 413
Washington, DC 20006
http://www.unidial.com

Dairy Council Digest
National Dairy Council
10255 West Higgins Road, Suite 900
Rosemont, IL 60018
(inexpensive)
http://www.national/dairycouncil.com

Dietetic Currents
Ross Laboratories
Director of Professional Services
625 Cleveland Ave.
Columbus, OH 43216
(free)
http://www.ross.com

Egg Nutrition Center
1819 H St. N.W., No. 510
Washington, DC 20009
(free)
http://www.enc-online.org/

Environmental Nutrition
52 Riverside Dr.
New York, NY 10024
http://www.eatright.org

Food and Nutrition News
National Cattlemen's Beef Association
444 Michigan Ave.
Chicago, IL 60611
(free)
http://www.beef.org

Harvard Medical School Health Letter
Department of Continuing Education
25 Shattuck St.
Boston, MA 02115
http://www.hms.harvard.edu/news/index.html

Mayo Clinic Health Letter
P.O. Box 53889
Boulder, CO 80322-3889
http://mayohealth.org

National Council Against Health Fraud
Newsletter (NCAHF)
P.O. Box 1276
Loma Linda, CA 92354
http://www.ncahf.org/

Nutrition Action Healthletter
1875 Connecticut Ave.
Washington, DC 20009-5728
http://www.cspinet.org

Nutrition Forum
George Stickley Co.
210 Washington Square
Philadelphia, PA 19106
http://www.quackwatch.com

Nutrition & the M.D.
Raven Press
1185 Avenue of the Americas
New York, NY 10036
http://www.lww.com

Nutrition Research Newsletter
P.O. Box 700
Pallisades, NY 10964
http://www.biz-lib.com/ZTINR.html

Soy Connection
United Soybean Board
16305 Swingley Ridge Drive
Suite 110
Chesterfield, MO 63017
(free)
http://smartsoy.ag.uiuc.edu/~usb/speced.html/

Tufts University Diet & Nutrition Letter
P.O. Box 10948
Des Moines, IA 50940
http://www.healthletter.tufts.edu/

University of California at Berkeley
Wellness Letter
P.O. Box 420148
Palm Coast, FL 32142
http://magazines.enews.com/magazines/vcbw

Professional Organizations with a Commitment to Nutrition Issues

American Academy of Pediatrics
P.O. Box 1034
Evanston, IL 60204
http://www.aap.org

American Cancer Society
90 Park Ave.
New York, NY 10016
http://www.cancer.org

American College of Sports Medicine
P.O. Box 1440
Indianapolis, IN 46204
http://www.acsm.org/

American Dental Association
211 E. Chicago Ave.
Chicago, IL 60611
http://www.ada.org

American Diabetes Association
2 Park Ave.
New York, NY 10016
http://www.diabetes.org

American Dietetic Association
216 W. Jackson Blvd.
Suite 800
Chicago, IL 60606
http://www.eatright.org

American Geriatrics Society
770 Lexington Ave.
Suite 400
New York, NY 10021
http://www.americangeriatrics.org

American Heart Association
7272 Greenville Ave.
Dallas, TX 75231
http://www.americanheart.org

American Home Economics Association
2010 Massachusetts Ave. N.W.
Washington, DC 20036
http://www.orst.edu

American Society for Nutritional Sciences
9650 Rockville Pike
Bethesda, MD 20014
http://www.faseb.org/asns

American Medical Association
Nutrition Information Section
535 N. Dearborn St.
Chicago, IL 60610
http://www.ama-assn org/

American Public Health Association
1015 Fifteenth St. N.W.
Washington, DC 20005
http://www.apha.org

American Society for Clinical Nutrition
9650 Rockville Pike
Bethesda, MD 20014
http://www.faseb.org/ajcn

The Canadian Diabetes Association
15 Toronto St.
Suite 1001
Toronto, Ontario M5C 2E3 Canada
http://www.diabetes.ca

The Canadian Dietetic Association
480 University Ave.
Suite 601
Toronto, Ontario M5G 1V2 Canada
http://www.dietitians.ca

The Canadian Society for Nutritional Sciences
Department of Foods and Nutrition
University of Manitoba
Winnipeg, Manitoba, R3T 2N2 Canada
http://www.hc-sc.gc.ca

Food and Nutrition Board
National Research Council
National Academy of Sciences
2101 Constitution Ave. N.W.
Washington, DC 20418
http://www.nas.edu/fnb/

Institute of Food Technologies
221 N. LaSalle St.
Chicago, IL 60601
http://www.ift.org

National Council on the Aging
1828 L St. N.W.
Washington, DC 20036
http://www.ncoa.org

National Institute of Nutrition
1335 Carling Ave.
Suite 210
Ottawa, Ontario K1Z OL2 Canada
http://www.nines.com

National Osteoporosis Foundation
1150 Seventeenth St. N.W., Suite 500
Washington, DC 20036
http://www.nof.org

Society for Nutrition Education
2001 Killebrew Dr., Suite 340
Minneapolis, MN 55425
http://www.sne.org

Professional or Lay Organizations Concerned with Nutrition Issues

Bread for the World Institute
1100 Wayne Ave.
Silver Springs, MD 20910
http://www.bread.org

California Council Against Health Fraud,
Inc.
P.O. Box 1276
Loma Linda, CA 92354
http://www.ncahf.org

Children's Foundation
1420 New York Ave. N.W.
Suite 800
Washington, DC 20005
http://www.childrenfoundation.com

Food Research and Action Center (FRAC)
1875 Connecticut Ave. N.W. #540
Washington, DC 20009
http://www.iglou.com/why/
resource/1100.htm

Institute for Food and Development Policy
1885 Mission St.
San Francisco, CA 94103
http://www.foodfirst.org

La Leche League International, Inc.
9616 Minneapolis Ave.
Franklin Park, IL 60131
http://www.lalecheleague.org

March of Dimes Birth Defects Foundation
(National Headquarters)
1275 Mamaroneck Ave.
White Plains, NY 10605
http://www.modimes.org

Overeaters Anonymous (OA)
2190 190th St.
Torrance, CA 90504
http://www.overeatersanonymous.org

Oxfam America
115 Broadway
Boston, MA 02116
http://www.oxfamamerica.org

Local Resources for Advice on Nutrition Issues

Cooperative extension agents in county extension offices
Dietitians (contact the state or local Dietetics Association)
Nutrition faculty affiliated with departments of food and nutrition, home economics, and dietetics
Registered dietitians (RDs) in city, county, or state agencies

Government Agencies Concerned with Nutrition Issues or That Distribute Nutrition Information

United States
The Consumer Information Center
Department 609K
Pueblo, CO 81009
http://www.pueblo.gsa.gov

Food and Drug Administration (FDA)
5600 Fishers Lane
Rockville, MD 20852
http://www.fda.gov

*Food and Nutrition Information and Education
Resources Center*
National Library of Congress
Beltsville, MD 20705
http://www.nal.usda.gov

Human Nutrition Research Division
Agricultural Research Center
Beltsville, MD 20705
http://www.usda.gov

National Center for Health Statistics
3700 East-West
Hyattsville, MD 20782
http://www.cdc.gov/nchswww

National Heart, Lung, and Blood Institute
9000 Rockville Pike, Building 31, Room
4A21
Bethesda, MD 20892
http://www.nhlbi.gov

National Institute on Aging
Information Office
Building 31, Room 5C35
Bethesda, MD 20205
http://www.nih.gov/nia/

Office of Cancer Communications
National Cancer Institute
Building 31, Room 10A18
90 Rockville Pike
Bethesda, MD 20205
http://www.nci.nih.gov

USDA, Agricultural Research Service
6505 Belcrest Rd., Room 344
Hyattsville, MD 20782
http://www.usda.gov

USDA, Food Safety & Inspection Service
Room 1180 South, 14th and
Independence Ave. S.W.
Washington, DC 20250
http://www.usda.gov

U.S. Government Printing Office
The Superintendent of Documents
Washington, DC 20402
http://www.printgovt.org

Canada
Canadian Food Inspection Agency
59 Camelot Dr.
Nepean, Ontario K1A OY9
http://www.cfia-acia.agr.ca

Health and Welfare Canada
Canadian Government Publishing Center
Minister of Supply and Services
Ottawa, Ontario K1A 0S9
http://www.hc-sc-gc.ca

Home Economics Directorate
880 Portage Ave.
Second Floor
Winnipeg, Manitoba R3G 0P1
http://www.mbnet.mb.ca

Nutrition Programs
446 Jeanne Mance Building
Tunney's Pasture
Ottawa, Ontario K1A 1B4
http://www.hc-sc.gc.ca

Nutrition Services
P.O. Box 488
Halifax, Nova Scotia B3J 3R8
http://www.fns.usda.gov

United Nations
Food and Agriculture Organization (FAO)
North American Regional Office
1001 22nd St. N.W.
Washington, DC 20437
or
Via della Terma di Caracella
0100 Rome, Italy
http://www.fao.org

World Health Organization (WHO)
1211 Geneva 27
Switzerland
http://www.who.org

Trade Organizations and Companies That Distribute Nutrition Information

American Institute of Baking
P.O. Box 1148
Manhattan, KS 66502
http://www.aibonline.org

American Meat Institute
P.O. Box 3556
Washington, DC 20007
http://www.meatami.org

Beech-Nut Nutrition Corporation
Booth 1414
Checkerboard Square
St. Louis, MO 63164
http://www.beech-nut.com/index.htm

Best Foods
Consumer Service Department
Division of CPC International
International Plaza
Englewood Cliffs, NJ 07632
http://www.bestfoods.com

Campbell Soup Co.
Food Service Products Division
Campbell Plaza
Camden, NJ 08103
http://www.campbellsoups.com

Continental Baking Company
Checkerboard Square
St. Louis, MO 63164
http://www.scisoc.org

The Dannon Company, Inc.
120 White Plains Rd.
Tarrytown, NY 10591-5536
http://www.dannon.com

Del Monte Foods
One Market Plaza
San Francisco, CA 94105
http://www.delmonte-international.com

General Mills
P.O. Box 1113
Minneapolis, MN 55440
http://www.generalmills.com

Gerber Products Co.
445 State St.
Fremont, MI 49413
http://www.gerber.com/home1.html

H.J. Heinz
Consumer Relations
P.O. Box 57
Pittsburgh, PA 15230
http://www.heinzbaby.com

Idaho Potato Commission
P.O. Box 1968
Boise, ID 83701
http://www.idahopotatoes.com

Kellogg Company
Department of Home Economics Services
Battle Creek, MI 49016
http://www.kellog.com

Kraft General Foods
Three Lakes Dr.
Northfield, IL 60093
http://www.kraftfoods.com

Mead Johnson Nutritionals
2404 Pennsylvania Ave.
Evansville, IN 47721
http://www.meadjohnson.com

National Dairy Council
10255 W. Higgins Rd.
Rosemont, IL 60018-4233
http://www.natdairycoun.org

The NutraSweet Kelco Company
1751 Lake Cook Rd.
Deerfield, IL 60015
http://www.nutrasweetkelco.com/default.htm

Pillsbury Company
1177 Pillsbury Building
608 Second Ave. S.
Minneapolis, MN 55402
http://www.pillsbury.com

Ross Laboratories
Director of Professional Services
625 Cleveland Ave.
Columbus, OH 43216
http://www.ross.com

Sunkist Growers, Inc.
14130 Riverside Dr.
Sherman Oaks, CA 91423
http://www.sunkist.com/index.html

Vitamin Nutrition Information Service
(VNIS)
Hoffmann-LaRoche
340 Kingsland Ave.
Nutley, NJ 07110
http://www.rocheusa.com

ENGLISH-METRIC CONVERSIONS AND METRIC UNITS

Metric-English Conversions

Length

English (USA)	= Metric
inch (in)	= 2.54 cm, 25.4 mm
foot (ft)	= 0.30 m, 30.48 cm
yard (yd)	= 0.91 m, 91.4 cm
mile (statute) (5280 ft)	= 1.61 km, 1609 m
mile (nautical) (6077 ft, 1.15 statute mi)	= 1.85 km, 1850 m

Metric	= English (USA)
millimeter (mm)	= 0.039 in (thickness of a dime)
centimeter (cm)	= 0.39 in
meter (m)	= 3.28 ft, 39.37 in
kilometer (km)	= 0.62 mi, 1091 yd, 3273 ft

Weight

English (USA)	= Metric
grain	= 64.80 mg
ounce (oz)	= 28.35 g
pound (lb)	= 453.60 g, 0.45 kg
ton (short—2000 lb)	= 0.91 metric ton (907 kg)

Metric	= English (USA)
milligram (mg)	= 0.002 grain (0.000035 oz)
gram (g)	= 0.04 oz (1/28 of an oz)
kilogram (kg)	= 35.27 oz, 2.20 lb
metric ton (1000 kg)	= 1.10 tons

Volume

English (USA)	= Metric
cubic inch	= 16.39 cc
cubic foot	= 0.03 m³
cubic yard	= 0.765 m³
ounce	= 0.03 liter (30 ml)*
pint (pt)	= 0.47 liter
quart (qt)	= 0.95 liter
gallon (gal)	= 3.79 liters

Metric	= English (USA)
milliliter (ml)	= 0.03 oz
liter (L)	= 2.12 pt
liter	= 1.06 qt
liter	= 0.27 gal

1 liter ÷ 1000 = 1 milliliter or 1 cubic centimeter (10^{-3} liter)

1 liter ÷ 1,000,000 = 1 microliter (10^{-6} liter)

*Note: 1 ml = 1 cc

Farenheit-Celsius Temperature Conversion Scale

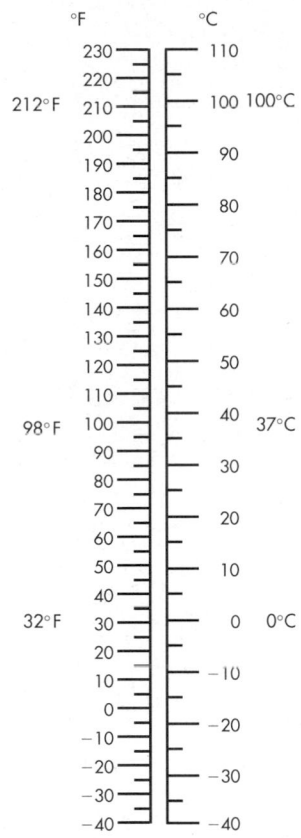

To convert temperature scales:

Fahrenheit to Celsius °C = (°F − 32) × 5/9

Celsius to Fahrenheit °F = 9/5 (°C) + 32

Additional Metric and Other Units Commonly Used in Nutrition

Unit/Abbreviation	Other Equivalent Measure
milligram/mg	1/1000 of a gram
microgram/μg	1/1,000,000 of a gram
deciliter/dl	1/10 of a liter (about 1/2 cup)
milliliter/ml	1/1000 of a liter (5 ml is about 1 tsp)
International Unit/IU	Crude measure of vitamin activity generally based on growth rate seen in animals

Overall, it is important to know what meter, gram, and liter represent, as well as the prefixes micro (1/1,000,000), milli (1/1000), centi (1/100), and kilo (1000).

Answers to Critical Thinking Questions

Chapter 1

1. Supplements purchased in a store can provide vitamins and minerals. However, that is all they provide. Foods, on the other hand, supply not only vitamins and minerals but also carbohydrates, proteins, fats, and dietary fiber. These provide energy and bulk for a healthy digestive system. The phytochemicals present are another bonus (see Chapter 2 for details). In addition, it is easy to overdose on certain vitamins and minerals when supplements are used.

2. A diet consisting primarily of foods derived from animal sources contains mostly proteins and fats, with a high percentage of fats as saturated fats. Saturated fats lead to a rise in blood cholesterol in many people. High blood cholesterol is linked to increased risk of cardiovascular disease. A diet high in fat is also related to increased risk of colon and prostate cancer in men.

   Fruits and vegetables are rich in dietary fiber, which helps decrease blood cholesterol and increases the rate of peristalsis in the gastrointestinal tract. Fruits and vegetables, for the most part, contain low amounts of fat, if any, and are low in calories, thus helping maintain healthy body weight.

   Early humans lived only 30 years or so. Today our life expectancy is more than double that. History can give us clues to improve our diets, but only actual studies—such as double-blind research—can establish the actual advantages of any diet. Subjects could be placed on one of the two diets and followed for a number of years. Tests such as blood pressure, blood cholesterol, and body weight would show how the diets affect overall health.

3. Unfortunately for Wesley, he is at high risk for developing alcoholism. He should carefully consider the consequences of alcohol use. Wesley may choose to avoid alcohol completely or consume it in moderation only. It may be helpful for him to recognize the signs of alcohol abuse to prevent any problems before they begin.

Chapter 2

1. Increasing one's fruit and vegetable intake can be easy; it just takes planning.
   - Search for fast-food restaurants with a salad bar.
   - Buy a variety of fruits and vegetables at the grocery store.
   - Include a fruit and/or vegetable at every meal.
   - Carry snacks, such as an apple, a banana, or carrots, with you so that, when you get hungry, you can avoid grabbing a candy bar.
   - Buy canned fruits and vegetables. These are convenient, and, because they are canned immediately after harvest, they retain their vitamins and minerals.
   - In the refrigerator, keep a bowl of fresh vegetables handy for snacks.
   - Drink 100% fruit and vegetable juices.

2. Since the typical American diet consists of many foods high in fat and low in dietary fiber, Athe should assess her diet with respect to these components. She should list all of the foods she eats, preferably for a whole week, and estimate how much fat and dietary fiber she consumes. She could use Appendix A in this textbook or the accompanying software. She then should change her eating habits to obtain recommended amounts of fat and dietary fiber. Most likely, Athe will need to decrease fat intake as well as increase dietary fiber.

3. A 1600-kcal diet could consist of 2 low-fat milk exchanges, 3 vegetables, 4 fruits, 8 starches, 4 lean meats, and 4 fats. Following is one sample day. There are many variations.

   Breakfast: ¾ cup shredded wheat
   1 cup 1% reduced-fat milk
   1 slice toast
   1 tsp margarine
   ½ cup orange juice

   Lunch: 2 oz turkey breast
   1 tbsp low-fat mayonnaise
   2 slices whole-wheat bread
   5 celery sticks
   5 baby carrots
   1 small banana

   Dinner: 2 oz ham
   1 cup rice
   ½ cup pineapple
   ½ cup green beans
   1 small dinner roll
   1 tsp tub margarine
   1 cup 1% reduced-fat milk

   Snack: ½ cup applesauce
   ½ bagel
   1 tbsp reduced-fat cream cheese

Chapter 3

1. Hair analysis has been used as a research tool for testing people for certain trace mineral toxicities, such as arsenic and lead. All other applications are considered unreliable at this time, primarily because people use shampoo and other related products that contaminate hair with a variety of added components, some of which are vitamins and minerals. Any coloring agents

would also effect hair composition. Overall, analyzing hair for trace mineral status would require that the hair sample be free of any hair product for several months and that the sample be collected using a specific protocol. Certainly these test results do not provide a reliable guide to her nutrient needs. She should instead speak to a registered dietitian.

2. Growth hormone and testosterone are of no value in increasing linear height after closure of the growth plates at the ends of the bones (epiphyses). This takes place generally by age 18 to 21 years. Thus, David will not benefit from this product. In addition, for testosterone treatments to function in the body, they must be administered via injection or as a patch applied to the skin. David certainly would not want to inject anything that he purchased over the Web. David should just resign himself to being 5'7".

3. The small intestine is the most important absorption site in the digestive system because of its large surface area. Since much of the young girl's small intestine was removed, many of the nutrients she consumes are escaping absorption. It is likely that only a highly refined diet or intravenous total parenteral nutrition therapy will succeed in keeping her adequately nourished.

Chapter 4

1. Mitochondria are the sites for cellular ATP synthesis—the powerhouses of the cell. Aerobic metabolism also takes place in the mitochondria. Wherever there is a need for the production of large amounts of ATP, such as in muscle cells, mitochondria will be found in greater numbers. The greater the need for energy, the greater the number of mitochondria.

2. Body fat is gained when energy consumption exceeds energy expenditure. This is true whether the energy (calories) comes from carbohydrate, protein, or fat. A great excess of carbohydrate intake can promote fat synthesis. If eaten in excess, the same is true of protein. Unless Stephanie learns to control the amount of calories she consumes, she will continue to gain fat even though she is on a "fat-free diet." Furthermore, this lack of fat can be harmful, because fat provides essential fatty acids to the body and performs a variety of other needed functions.

3. Many serious health problems do not surface until years after the harmful behavior continues. Tom's diet is lacking many essential vitamins and minerals. For example, his eyes may worsen over the years with lack of vitamin A. His colon health may suffer due to low dietary fiber intake. With so many calorically dense foods, Tom is risking obesity, cardiovascular disease, type 2 diabetes, and hypertension.

Chapter 5

1. Diet pills, even over-the-counter ones, are expensive. The psyllium in Celia's diet pills is a fiber that produces bulk, which helps make the dieter feel satiated. However, instead of buying expensive pills that make her feel full so that she will not each as much, Celia should simply change her eating habits to include more fruits and vegetables. Not only do they contain dietary fiber, but they also supply vitamins and minerals. Beans, whole grains, oats, fruits, and vegetables all contain ample dietary fiber and are great low-energy sources of nutrients.

2. Diverticulosis is a condition in which tiny pouches form in the wall of the colon. When foods are eaten that are not fully digested, such as hulls and seeds, undigested pieces may become trapped in the pouches. Bacteria then metabolize these particles into acids and gases, which irritate the diverticula, causing them to swell; this condition is called *diverticulitis*. The acids and gases in the swollen pouches cause cramping and abdominal pain.

3. Foods that remain in the mouth, usually caught between the teeth, are a source of food that bacteria can metabolize. As a by-product of this metabolism, bacteria produce acids, which can decay tooth enamel, causing caries. Chewing sugar-free gum after meals decreases the risk of caries because chewing stimulates the secretion of saliva, which helps dislodge foods that remain in the mouth. Sugar-free gums also contain sugar substitutes, which bacteria can't metabolize. In addition, saliva has a higher pH than the acids produced by bacterial metabolism. This helps neutralize the acids.

Chapter 6

1. The general term *fats* refers to lipids in foods without reference to their structure. Only dietary fats with a high proportion of saturated fatty acids (or trans fatty acids) have been associated with an increased risk of cardiovascular disease. In the body, fat (primarily in the form of triglycerides) has many beneficial functions. Triglycerides form the main energy stores in the body and can release fatty acids, which serve as fuel for many cells, such as those in muscles at rest and during light activity. Stored fat insulates the body and protects vital organs. Absorption of fat-soluble vitamins from the intestine is aided by their association with dietary fats. In addition, the two essential fatty acids, linoleic acid and alpha-linolenic acid, are not synthesized by the body and must be in the diet to maintain health. Thus, some fat is needed in the diet; moderation of intake, not elimination, is the goal.

2. Triglycerides in foods promote satiety (i.e., a feeling of fullness). Triglycerides produce this effect by influencing certain hormonal responses, which in turn affect the rate of stomach emptying. After a nonfat meal, the stomach empties rapidly, so one feels hungry in a short time. In contrast, after a meal containing some fat, the rate of stomach emptying slows, so one

feels satiated for a longer period. If dieters with limited caloric intakes would include a small amount of fat in their meals, they would not feel hungry all the time. Increasing dietary fiber intake provides the same benefit. As a result, dieters would be less likely to give up their diets quickly and would have a better chance of long-term success.

3. The amount of cholesterol carried in HDL (high-density lipoprotein) also indicates the risk of cardiovascular disease. If the one's HDL is greater than 60 mg/dl, the risk of cardiovascular disease is low. If it's less than 35 mg/dl, the risk is high. The ratio of total serum cholesterol to HDL-cholesterol is also a good indicator of one's risk. If the ratio exceeds 4 to 1, the risk is high. Since Juan's total cholesterol was 210 mg/dl and HDL cholesterol was 65 mg/dl, the ratio was 3.2 to 1 (210 mg/dl ÷ 65 mg/dl), which means he has a low risk for developing cardiovascular disease. LDL-cholesterol, which is 125 mg/dl, is also not elevated (LDL = total cholesterol − HDL − (triglycerides ÷ 5); 210 mg/dl − 65 mg/dl − [100 mg/dl ÷ 5] =125 mg/dl).

Chapter 7

1. PKU is the abbreviation for the disease *phenylketonuria*. The liver of a person with phenylketonuria cannot readily convert phenylalanine, an essential amino acid, to tyrosine, a nonessential amino acid. Insufficient enzyme action causes this defect.

   The inability to metabolize excess phenylalanine to tyrosine leads to the formation of abnormal products that arise from alternative metabolic pathways; these products can cause mental retardation. Thus, it is vital to determine which infants have PKU, since the amount of phenylalanine in their diets must be monitored. However, because it is an essential amino acid, some phenylalanine must be consumed. Since phenylalanine cannot be sufficiently metabolized to tyrosine, the

latter must be considered an essential amino acid for people with PKU.

2. Protein synthesis is a complex process by which a specific sequence and number of amino acids determine the primary structure of a protein. If a given amino acid is not present during protein synthesis, production will stop. In other words, protein is an all-or-none process: All of the amino acids necessary to make the protein must be available, or the protein will not be made at all. A mixed diet of plant products will likely contain enough of all nine essential amino acids, so the all-or-none principle won't typically be an issue in diet planning, even in vegetarianism.

3. Much of the nitrogen that is part of amino acids is converted into urea in the liver as part of amino acid metabolism. This urea is excreted by the kidneys. Samantha's mother shows evidence of kidney problems. Overall, Samantha's mother is consuming more protein than her kidney function can tolerate. Lowering protein in her diet would help.

Chapter 8

1. Many risks and diseases correlate with behaviors often combined with alcohol abuse. Unplanned sexual activity can lead to the contraction of STDs and other diseases, feelings of guilt, unplanned pregnancy, and toxicity to a fetus. If property is damaged, others can be harmed, and the persons responsible must deal with the legal and financial consequences. Both cigarettes and excessive alcohol use are carcinogenic. When alcohol is used, the liver and other gastrointestinal tract organs can be harmed. The addition of smoking can compound poor health by increasing the risk of oral cancer.

2. Typical signs of alcohol abuse in teenagers are withdrawal from family activities, poor (failing) school performance, and increased colds and other general ills. He may also be making references to suicide.

3. There is no one simple answer to the problems of campus binge drinking, but there are a number of actions you plan to take to combat the epidemic. As president of your university, you may publicize that 41% of all academic problems stem from alcohol abuse, and 28% of the students who are dropping out of the school are doing so in part because of alcohol-related course failures. You may want the students to know binge drinking has caused many injuries and even deaths on campus, and you may publicize the names of the victims and the circumstances under which they were hospitalized or died: circumstances such as car accidents, murder, suicide, rape, alcohol poisoning, and personal injures. Faculty and student leaders may be asked to schedule regular campuswide seminars for students to help them take charge of staying sober. Alcohol-free dorms may be the rule, and alcohol-free social events on campus may be considered a high priority. Alcohol counseling may be made available on a confidential basis through the student health center and local social service organizations. AA may be invited to campus to speak about its programs and institute a campus chapter.

Chapter 9

1. Some cereal manufacturers add beta-carotene to their products to reduce the risk of vitamin A toxicity. This is because the body converts beta-carotene to vitamin A only if it is needed. Once the body has enough vitamin A, the remainder stays in the beta-carotene form, which is nontoxic. Some supplement manufacturers are also using this principle by supplying some vitamin A content as beta-carotene.

2. A possible explanation for the lack of clot dissolution in Tim's leg is that he has been consuming many foods rich in vitamin K, such as dark green leafy vegetables, soybean oil, and members of the cabbage family. Vitamin K is also produced

by the intestinal bacteria. This vitamin assists in clot formation and is antagonistic to oral anticoagulant medications. If the vitamin K is not reduced in Tim's diet, the therapy won't be very effective.

3. Many vitamins, such as the water-soluble ones, can often be excreted when taken in excess; however, the fat-soluble vitamins are not as readily excreted. Vitamins A and D, in particular, can accumulate in large amounts, causing toxic effects. These effects can occur at just three times or more than the Daily Values with regular usage of such excess quantities. This is especially true in children. Excessive intakes of some water-soluble vitamins can also be toxic, but much higher doses are needed.

Chapter 10

1. People with alcoholism usually have unbalanced diets, which can impair absorption of vitamins and minerals from the GI tract. An associated problem is poor metabolism. The B-vitamins are essential for metabolism: gluconeogenesis, lipogenesis, lipolysis, and overall carbohydrate metabolism. Alcohol consumption decreases the absorption of many B-vitamins, such as thiamin, riboflavin, niacin, and folate. All of these vitamins are important in maintaining proper metabolic and nervous system function.

2. Humans must obtain vitamin C from foods, because the body cannot synthesize it. A major function of this vitamin is to promote the formation of collagen, an important protein found in connective tissue. Collagen is an integral component of bone, skin, and blood vessels. Thus, a low intake of vitamin C will impair wound healing. Deficiency can also lead to scurvy, whose symptoms include bleeding gums and pinpoint hemorrhages on the skin.

Vitamin C is an antioxidant. It works with vitamin E against free radicals and helps "reactivate" vitamin E so that it can continue to function. Vitamin C also deters certain forms of cancer, enhances iron absorption, assists in carnitine production, and synthesizes norepinephrine, a neurotransmitter.

Finally, vitamin C is essential for lymphocytic activity within the immune system. Since it assists in the production of lymphocytes, maintaining appropriate vitamin C intake gives the body the building blocks it needs to fight off infections. However, vitamin C does not *cure* the common cold or heart disease.

3. Cooking increases the concentration of vitamin C in spinach because large amounts of water are lost during the cooking process. During heating, spinach shrinks and loses much more water than other vegetables, such as brussels sprouts.

Chapter 11

1. When doing physical work, such as mowing the lawn, one perspires. The degree of perspiration varies among people and depends on the time of day. Muscle strength and endurance decline significantly when there is a 3% loss of body weight. Symptoms such as thirst may indicate a 2% loss of body weight caused by dehydration. With greater water loss, a headache and dizziness may develop. Even further water loss may induce a coma.

Any person who anticipates significant loss of body water through perspiration would benefit from hydrating before the activity, just as in preparation for an athletic event. Doing so will minimize dehydration. Drinking fluids during such exertion is also helpful.

2. Almost all foods contain sodium. Most of the sodium in our diets is added during food processing, during cooking, and at mealtimes. The American Heart Association recommends that all people limit their sodium intake to no more than 2.4 g/day. Still, sodium is essential to maintenance of normal fluid balance throughout the body and to normal nerve impulse conduction. If sodium intake is inadequate, neuromuscular symptoms will appear, including muscle weakness, headache, irritability, and confusion.

3. Calcium is needed for normal bone growth and development. Bones serve as reservoirs of calcium for blood homeostasis. Regulation of blood calcium may necessitate the resorption of bone mineral deposits for the release of calcium from bone. Thus, bone mineralization is vital before and during adolescence, when the greatest amount of bone development occurs. Manuela is already an adult, but she can still consume calcium in amounts sufficient to decrease the incidence of bone demineralization.

Some of the richest sources of calcium are milk and sardines, which Manuela, a vegan, will not eat. As an alternative, she should become aware of which vegetables contain calcium, but most are poor sources. She should also choose calcium-fortified foods, such as some brands of orange juice. However, if she cannot meet her calcium needs by modifying her diet, based on a nutrient analysis of her current intake, calcium supplements are advised.

Chapter 12

1. Vitamin C is important not only for collagen synthesis but also for treating iron deficiency anemia, since it modestly enhances iron absorption in the GI tract. Vitamin C increases absorption of nonheme iron by donating an electron to the ferric form of iron to create the ferrous form of iron, which is absorbed better, and then chelating it as well.

2. For zinc to be considered a reasonable treatment for the common cold, we need more definitive studies. Research results are quite mixed at this time. Further studies should include a greater number of participants, and determination of the presence of a cold should be standardized. Finally, researchers

should ensure that the placebo lozenge has the same flavor as the zinc lozenge. In this way, positive or negative results will not be attributed to the good or poor flavor of the lozenges. Overall, more convincing evidence is necessary for zinc lozenges to be considered a scientifically proven cold treatment.

3. The mineral selenium is a cofactor for the activity of the enzyme glutathione peroxidase. This enzyme participates in a system that metabolizes peroxides into less toxic alcohol derivatives and water. Peroxides tend to become free radicals, which in turn can attack and break down cell membranes, causing cell damage. Selenium is considered to be important in protecting heart cells and other cells against oxidative damage. In addition, because it reduces the amount of free radical damage to cells, selenium may be important in protecting against cancer.

Chapter 13

1. Energy intake must equal energy output for body weight to remain the same. Weight increases when energy intake is more than output. Since basal metabolism decreases by 2% for every decade over 30 years of age, either energy intake or energy output must be modified to maintain the same weight.

   Energy balance can be attained in this case by increasing physical activity, a facet of life that tends to decrease with aging. Taking up a sport, jogging, or even parking the car farther away from a building to increase walking distance are all good strategies. People tend to become less active and therefore expend less energy without reducing food intake as they age. By increasing physical activity, energy balance and desirable weight can be maintained.

2. Although Hal has seen a steady decrease in his weight for the duration of his diet thus far, his body has built-in mechanisms that tend to fight weight loss. One of those factors is his basal metabolism. This tends to decrease to conserve energy as the number of calories in the diet decreases. Also, lipoprotein lipase activity increases in the body, which increases lipid uptake into adipose (fat) cells. The increased activity of this enzyme allows the body to take up fats more efficiently from the blood after the dieting has stopped.

   Thus, the body resists weight loss by physiological means; however, it may finally surrender to persistent dieting, and Hal will continue to lose weight as long as he continues to diet.

3. For a weight-loss plan to be successful, the person must be mentally prepared for the time and commitment involved. Weight loss requires a certain amount of time for planning meals, purchasing more healthy foods, and devising a plan for when temptations arise. This woman obviously has her hands full with other obligations at this time. Because of her busy schedule, it would be difficult to stick to an eating plan. Weight-loss failure can be discouraging. It would be wise for this woman to wait until her schedule lightens up a bit and, instead, focus on weight maintenance.

Chapter 14

1. Marty has enhanced his cardiovascular fitness, a laudable goal. In addition, after a period of training, muscle cells worked on a regular basis will make more mitochondria. Since mitochondria are the sites of aerobic metabolism, this means that more ATP can be generated. ATP is a necessary component for muscle action.

2. Many wrestlers and other athletes lose weight quickly by losing large amounts of water, usually by sweating. By doing so, an athlete can compete in a lower weight class and thus gain an advantage over an opponent. However, losing weight this way can significantly impede performance. Over time, repeated dehydration episodes can lead to serious complications, such as kidney failure. Athletes also risk developing heat stress during the event.

   The loss of water before a competition is the quick method of losing weight. But, if an athlete is serious about his or her sport, a gradual change in diet to create the best possible weight/muscle composition should be the goal.

3. A person's appropriate dietary intake of protein should be determined using the RDA for protein: 0.8 g/kg body weight. Athletes could increase their protein intake to 1.2 to 1.8 g/kg body weight to supply the amount of protein needed for muscle growth and development. Overall, about 15% of energy intake as protein is required to meet this recommendation. About 60% of energy intake should be supplied by carbohydrates, leaving about 20 to 25% of energy intake to be supplied by fat. The high carbohydrate intake is necessary to supply glucose for glycogen synthesis; glycogen is the storage form of glucose in muscles.

Chapter 15

1. Signs that indicate an eating disorder include the following:
   a. Refusal to eat much food
   b. Obsession with being and looking thin
   c. Obsession with counting calories
   d. Not wanting to eat with others (e.g., refusing to go to a restaurant)
   e. Continually criticizing one's looks and comparing oneself to others, especially slender people
   f. Being convinced that one is fat

2. In addition to the detrimental social aspects of anorexia nervosa, such as alienation from others, there are serious physical consequences. Nutritional deficiencies may develop that can cause an imbalance of the sex hormones. Jennifer has already stopped menstruating, compromising her fertility. The disease may also prevent her from gaining enough weight to support the

developing fetus if she were to become pregnant later. Starvation leads to a loss of lean body tissue, such as muscle. The heart rate decreases as metabolism slows, which causes the person to become easily tired, increasing the need for sleep. Since tissue is lost from the heart muscle as well as from the rest of the body, heart function may also be impaired. Another potential problem is anemia caused by inadequate nutrient intake.

3. One of the most important topics Tom should discuss is proper nutrition. Using the concepts of adequacy, balance, and moderation, he can teach students about their diets. He could also present case studies of real people who have anorexia nervosa and bulimia nervosa, so that his students can see firsthand the outcome of these diseases. Tom should also focus on increasing awareness of the challenges facing these young adults. The prepuberty and teenage years are a time of self-evaluation and criticism. It is important for Tom to help his students feel good from within by emphasizing the importance of self-worth, regardless of one's physical appearance. Finally, Tom can teach his students how to cope with difficult situations by showing them how to alleviate stress in positive and constructive ways.

Chapter 16

1. Many changes occur in a woman during pregnancy. Her uterus and breasts grow, and her total blood volume increases. The placenta develops, the heart and kidneys work harder, stores of body fat increase, and, toward the latter part of the pregnancy, mammary glands prepare to produce milk. The nutrients needed to support these changes are listed below:
   a. Increased energy, about 300 more kcal/day is necessary, especially during the second and third trimesters. This amount should allow adequate weight gain (25 to 35 lb for a woman

who begins pregnancy at a healthy weight).
   b. Protein needs are also increased, by about 10 g/day for women over 24 years of age and about 15 g/day for women under 24. She likely eats this much protein already. This amount should support adequate growth.
   c. Carbohydrate intake should be at least 100 g/day to prevent ketosis.
   d. Vitamin D should be 5 μg/day either through sunlight exposure or through vitamin D–fortified milk consumption. This amount will support fetal bone growth.
   e. Folate intake should increase to 600 μg/day to support red blood cell formation and DNA synthesis.
   f. Iron intake should increase to about 27 mg/day. This will support hemoglobin synthesis.
   g. Calcium is needed to promote mineralization of fetal bones and teeth. Calcium intake should meet 1000 mg/day.
   h. Zinc is important for growth and development. Intake should increase to 11 mg/day to support this.

These nutrients should be obtained mostly from foods. However, prenatal supplements can aid in supplying these nutrients to the pregnant woman, especially in circumstances that may prevent her from adequately consuming sufficient nutrients from foods.

2. Since Hannah is below her ideal body weight, she needs to consume additional calories to feed her fetus as well as to nourish her own growing body. Her food selections should emphasize fortified whole grains, fruits, vegetables, and calcium sources. She also needs a good source of protein at each meal to build body tissues. It would be beneficial for her to visit her physician regularly throughout the pregnancy.

3. As the pregnancy advances, the uterus continues to grow to accommodate the growing fetus. As it

does, it presses against the stomach as well as the intestines. Also, hormones produced in increased amounts during pregnancy relax muscles. This explains why heartburn may occur; the lower esophageal (cardiac) sphincter relaxes somewhat, allowing some foods and acid to regurgitate back into the esophagus—hence the heartburn. It is recommended that smaller quantities of foods be ingested and that the woman not recline after eating. High amounts of fats also decrease the rate of stomach emptying; therefore, decreasing the amounts of fats in the diet should also help. Since hormones relax muscles, the rate of peristalsis may also decrease and constipation may develop. It would be wise to gradually increase the amount of dietary fiber in Sandy's diet to improve her digestive system's peristaltic activity.

Chapter 17

1. Human milk is low in iron. Although it provides many essential nutrients to the baby, it doesn't meet all of a baby's needs after about 6 months, since iron stores are depleted by this time. This iron deficiency leads to a form of *anemia*. To prevent iron deficiency anemia in infants, it is wise to begin feeding them iron-fortified cereal between 4 and 6 months of age. In addition, to prevent anemia, some pediatricians recommend giving iron supplements to breastfed infants beginning shortly after birth.

2. Typical breakfast foods include cereal, eggs, toast, and pancakes, but any food can be a breakfast, lunch, or dinner food as long as it is nutrient dense. If Tim doesn't like the traditional breakfast foods but enjoys a sandwich, macaroni and cheese, or yogurt, his parents can offer them. These nutritious foods are no more beneficial at lunchtime than they are at 7 A.M.

The depletion of carbohydrate stores that occurs during the night can cause children to be lethargic and inattentive in the morning. Eating early in the morning replenishes carbohydrate stores. Many experts believe that the nutrients consumed stimulate attention in children, allowing them to perform better in school.

3. It usually takes a few days for signs of a food allergy to develop. Common allergic symptoms are diarrhea, vomiting, runny nose, wheezing, and swelling. An infection could produce the same symptoms but is usually accompanied by a fever. If Irene and Chris's baby is indeed having an allergic reaction, ceasing to feed the food to the baby should cause the symptoms to disappear. If they do disappear, it is likely that the food caused the allergy. The food can probably be reintroduced later, since babies outgrow most food allergies. Fortunately, the baby did not have the most generalized and severe kind of allergic reaction, an often fatal condition called *anaphylactic shock*.

Chapter 18

1. Science has established a considerable link between nutrition (diet) and health. For example, very-low-fat diets have been shown to reverse atherosclerosis, and weight loss can improve type 2 diabetes in some people by reducing body fat. Although body cells will age no matter what health practices are followed, morbidity can be decreased through diet and lifestyle. A consistently healthful diet and a regimen of regular physical activity have proven effective in maintaining a healthful body: Muscles are firmer, bone fractures are less likely, and the person looks and feels better. The secret to enjoying "youth" throughout life is to establish a healthful physical, mental, and social framework.

2. Though it is true that a 30% calorie restriction in laboratory animals appears to increase life expectancy, it is too soon to know the full implications of such a restriction. As well, appetite does not appear to decrease even in animals who have been restricted for most of their lives, and maintenance of reproductive function is still in question. Most humans would be unwilling to restrict themselves to this degree, and such restriction may not be appropriate in humans. Certainly, childhood is a highly inappropriate time to restrict calories, since this is the major time for growth and development. Alexis would do more harm than good by implementing such a plan with her family.

3. The 1994 DSHEA Law allows companies to market herbal products without prior approval by FDA as long as they make vague structure/function claims. Jamila has to rely on the truthfulness of the manufacturer of the herbal product concerning any possible health benefits from use. Ideally, Jamila should make sure that any use of herbal products follow three specific guidelines:
   a. Follow label directions carefully and start with a low dose.
   b. Increase the dose gradually as needed, watching for potential side effects. These potential side effects should be listed on the label.
   c. Do not use products that contain mixtures of herbal substances. Many of these products have been especially linked to health problems with use.

Chapter 19

1. USDA recommends cutting boards with unmarred surfaces made from nonporous materials. These include plexiglass, plastic, and marble, which are easy to clean. Grooves or cuts on surfaces provide a "home" where bacteria can thrive. If Jon wants to buy a wooden cutting board, he should plan to clean it using hot, soapy water every time he cuts something. He should also try not to use the same board for both meats and vegetables or fruits. If he must use it for everything, he should cut the vegetables first, wash the board in hot, soapy water, and then cut the meats. Jon should also sanitize any board once a week in a solution of 2 teaspoons chlorine bleach per quart of water, to minimize any bacterial growth.

2. Bacteria thrive at room temperature, especially between 40° and 140°F. Some bacteria cause foodborne illness by releasing endotoxins and some by producing exotoxins. Cooling by refrigeration slows down bacterial growth, but it does not stop it or destroy toxins already produced. Foods left at room temperature for 2 hours, or even 1 hour in hot weather, provide microorganisms with the opportunity to grow. Refrigeration after that time is too late. Diana is correct in wanting to discard the food.

3. Bacteria and other microbes in foods cause more than 96% of all food-related illness. Only a small minority of people are susceptible to the health effects of food additives, such as sulfites. USDA states that most food-borne illnesses arise from poor food-handling practices by consumers. Thus, Joseph is at more risk from how he stores and prepares food rather than the food additives in the snack cakes he eats on occasion.

Chapter 20

1. Undernourished children (and adults) often show apathy, muscular weakness, and decreased physical activity and work capability. Since undernutrition decreases resistance to disease, undernourished children are likely to have more frequent infections and to recover more slowly from illness than are well-fed children.

2. Where extreme food shortages exist, there is no choice but to supply hungry people with food—they are starving and dying. However, reliance on outside help is not a long-range solution. Rather, developing countries need to develop their economies and infrastructures, so that people are able to produce or buy sufficient amounts of nutritious

food to meet their needs. Appropriate development includes many aspects: education, control of population growth (if indicated), availability of machinery and other agricultural tools, and nonfarm employment opportunities. Small farms and businesses should be encouraged. As the overall economy expands, more people will be able to afford nutritious food. Agricultural production should focus on basic food crops to be consumed by a country's own citizens, rather than primarily on cash crops for export.

3. For every supporter of biotechnology, there is an equally convinced opponent. The first list here is in support of biotechnology, and the second is in opposition of it.

Probiotechnology
- Improved quality of product
- Increased resistance to certain pests, such as the European corn borer
- Improved crop yield
- Faster, more accurate production of improved crop varieties
- Elimination of certain pests
- Increased tolerance to droughts
- Decreased incidence of food-borne illness
- Decreased need for pesticides and preservatives
- Improved nutrient content of foods

Antibiotechnology
- Rapid insect resistance to insecticides that have been genetically engineered into plants
- Possible addition of allergens to these "new" foods
- Unnecessary because we have an adequate food supply
- Unnatural and may harm the environment

There are other arguments on both sides of this issue, and it will likely be quite some time before all the questions about biotechnology are answered.

Medical Terminology to Aid in the Study of Nutrition

Term Meaning

a- Without, from

aden-, adeno- Gland

-algia Pain

aliment Food

-amine Containing nitrogen

andr-, andro- Man or male

apo-, ap- Detached

arteri-, arterio- Artery

arthr-, arthro- Joint

-ase Enzyme

-blast Immature form, embryonic

brady- Slow

buli- Ox

canc-, carcino- Malignancy

cardi-, cardio- Heart

centi- Divided into 100 parts

chol-, chole-, cholo- Bile, gall

cholecyst- Gallbladder

chondr-, chondri-, chondro- Cartilage

chrom-, chromo- Color, colored

-clast Something that breaks

col-, coli-, colo- Colon

cyano-, cyan- Blue

cyt-, cyto- Cell

derm-, dermato- Skin

dextr-, dextro- Right, on or toward the right

duoden-, duodeno- Duodenum

dys- Difficult, painful

ect-, ecto- Without, outside, external

-ectomy Excision of

-ein A protein

em- Blood

-emia In blood

encephal-, encephalo- Brain

endo-, ento-, end-, ent- Within

enter-, entero- Intestine

erythr-, erythro- Red

esophag-, esophago- Esophagus

eu- Well, easy, good

gastr-, gastro, gastri- Stomach

gen- To become or produce

gloss-, glosso- Tongue

glyco-, glyc- Sugar

gynec-, gyn-, gyne- Women or female (especially female reproductive organs)

hem-, hemat- Blood

hepat-, hepato- Liver

hexa-, hex- Six

histo-, hist- Tissue

homeo-, homoeo-, homoio- Sameness, similarity

hydr-, hydro- Water

hyper- Excessive, above, beyond

hypo-, hyp- Under, beneath, deficient

hyster-, hystero- Uterus

idio- One's own, peculiar to, separate, distinct

ile-, ileo- Ileum

inter- Between, among

intra- Within, during, between layers of

-itis Inflammation of

jenun-, jejuno- Jejunum

kilo- One thousand

lact-, lacti-, lacto- Milk

leuc-, leuk- White, colorless

lev-, levo- Left, toward the left

lip-, lipo- Fat, lipid

litho-, lith- Stone

lymph-, lympho- Waterlike

lysis Destruction

mal- Bad, badly

malac-, malaco- Soft, a condition of abnormal softness

mega-, meg- Large, great

meta- After, later; change, exchange

metallo- Containing metal

micro- Divided into 1 million parts

milli- Divided into 1000 parts

mono- One

morph-, morpho- Form, shape

my-, myo- Muscle

myel-, myelo- Marrow, spinal cord

nas-, naso- Nose, nasal

necr-, necro- Dead

nephr-, nephro- Kidney

neur-, neuro- Nerve

-oid Formed like, resembling

-ol Alcohol

olig-, oligo- Few, scant

-oma Tumor

ophthalmo-, ophthalm- Eye, eyeball

-orex Mouth

-orexis Desire, appetite

-ose Sugar, carbohydrate

-osis Action, process, result, usually abnormal or diseased

ost-, osteo-, oste- Bone

ot- Ear

ovari-, ovario- Ovary

ovo-, ovi Eggs

pan- All

pancreat-, pancreato- Pancreas

para- Beside

parieto- Wall of a cavity, parietal bone

patho-, path- Disease

ped- Child, foot

-penia Without, lack of

-phobia Fear of

-plasm, -plasma Formative, formed, cell or tissue substance

pneum-, pneumo-, pneumono- Lung

-poiesis Production, format

poly- Many, much

post- After

pre- Before

prot-, proto- First

pseud-, pseudo- False

pulmo-, pulmon-, pulmono- Lung

pyel-, pyelo- Pelvis

pyr- Fever, fire

rect-, recto- Rectum

reni-, reno- Kidney

rhin-, rhino- Nose

-rrhagia Rupture, excessive fluid discharge

-rrhea Flow, discharge

sate To fill

scler-, sclero- Hard, hardness

-scopy Viewing

seb-, sebi-, sebo- Hard fat sebum, sebaceous glands

semi- Half

-soma, somat-, somato- Body

-stasia, -stasis Slowing or stopping of

stenosis Narrowing of

stomat-, stomato- Mouth, stoma

-stomy Surgical opening

sub- Under, below

super- Over, above

tachy- Swift, fast

thi-, thio- Containing sulfur

thromb-, thrombo- Blood clot

tox-, toxi-, toxo- Poison

trache-, tracheo- Trachea

-trophy Growth or mutation

ure-, urea-, ureo- Urine

uter-, utero- Uterus

vas-, vaso- Blood vessel

ven-, veni-, veno- Vein

vita- Life

xer-, xero- Dry

GLOSSARY TERMS

absorption The process by which substances are taken up from the GI tract and enter the bloodstream or the lymph.

absorptive cells A class of cells, also called *enterocytes,* that line the villi; fingerlike projections in the small intestine that participate in nutrient absorption.

acesulfame (ay-SUL-fame) An alternative sweetener that yields no energy to the body; it is 200 times sweeter than sucrose.

acetic acid (a-See-tic) A two-compound fatty acid that is used in the synthesis of lipids.

$$CH_3 - \overset{\overset{O}{\|}}{C} - OH$$

acetylcholine (a-See-toe-coal-ene) A neurotransmitter from nerve endings.

achlorhydria (ay-clor-HIGH-dre-ah) A decrease in stomach acid primarily due to age associated loss of acid-producing gastric cells.

acidic pH A pH less than 7. Lemon juice has an acid pH.

acquired immunodeficiency syndrome (AIDS) A disorder in which a virus (human immunodeficiency virus [HIV]) infects specific types of immune system cells. This leaves the person with reduced immune function and in turn defenseless against numerous infectious agents; typically contributes to the person's death.

actin (AK-tin) A protein in muscle fiber that, together with myosin, is responsible for contraction.

active absorption transport Absorption using a carrier and expending energy. In this way, the absorptive cell absorbs nutrients, such as glucose, when a high concentration of the nutrient is already present in the absorptive cells.

acute alcohol intoxication A temporary deterioration in mental function, accompanied by muscular incoordination, and partial paralysis as a result of drinking alcoholic beverages too rapidly.

adenosine diphosphate (ADP) A breakdown product of ATP. ADP is synthesized into ATP using energy from foodstuffs and a phosphate group (abbreviated Pi).

adenosine triphosphate (ATP) (ah-DEN-o-sin try-FOS-fate) The main energy currency for cells. ATP energy is used to promote ion pumping, enzyme activity, and muscular contraction.

adequate intake (AI) Recommendations for nutrient intake when not enough information is available to establish an RDA. AIs are based on observed or experimentally determined estimates of the average nutrient intake that appears to maintain a defined nutritional state (e.g., bone health) in a specific population. Used when no RDA can be set.

adipose cells (ADD-ih-pos) Fat-storing cells.

adipose tissue A group of fat-storing cells.

ad libitum (ad-LIB-itum) At one's desire or pleasure.

adrenergic (ADD-ren-er-gic) Actions of epinephrine and norepinephrine.

aerobic (air-ROW-bic) Requiring oxygen.

alcohol Generally refers to ethyl alcohol or ethanol, CH_3CH_2OH.

alcohol dehydrogenase (dee-high-DRO-jen-ase) The enzyme used in alcohol (ethanol) metabolism; the major enzyme used in the liver when alcohol is in low concentration.

aldosterone (al-DOS-ter-own) A hormone produced by the adrenal glands that acts on the kidneys to cause sodium reabsorption and, in turn, water conservation.

alkaline pH A pH greater than 7. Baking soda in water yields an alkaline pH.

allergen A foreign protein, or antigen, that induces excess production of certain immune system antibodies; subsequent exposure to the same protein leads to allergic symptoms. Whereas all allergens are antigens, not all antigens are allergens.

allergy A hypersensitive immune response that occurs when antibodies produced by the body react with a protein foreign to the body (antigen).

alpha (α) bond A type of chemical bond that can be broken by human intestinal enzymes in digestion; drawn as C $\backsim$ C.

alpha keto acids The breakdown product of several amino acids.

alpha-linolenic acid (AL-fah-lin-oh-LE-nik) An essential omega-3 fatty acid with 18 carbons and 3 double bonds (C18:3, ω-3).

alveoli (al-VE-o-lye) Basic functional units of the lungs.

amenorrhea (A-men-or-ee-a) The absence of three or more consecutive menstrual cycles; the absence of menses in a female.

amino acid (ah-MEE-noh) The building block for proteins containing a central carbon atom with a nitrogen atom and other atoms attached.

amniotic fluid (am-nee-OTT-ik) Fluid contained in a sac within the uterus. This fluid surrounds and protects the fetus during development.

amphetamine (am-FET-ah-mean) A group of medications that stimulate the central nervous system, among other effects. Abuse is linked to physical and psychological dependence.

amylase (AM-uh-lace) Starch-digesting enzyme from the salivary glands or pancreas.

amylopectin (AM-uh-low-pek-tin) A branched-chain type of starch composed of glucose units.

amylose (AM-uh-los) A digestible straight-chain polysaccharide made of glucose units; component of starch in foods.

anabolic/anabolism (an-AH-bol-iz-um) Building compounds.

anaerobic (AN-ah-ROW-bic) Not requiring oxygen.

analog (AN-a-log) A chemical compound that differs slightly from another, usually natural, compound. Analogs generally contain extra or altered chemical groups and may have similar or opposite metabolic effects compared with the native compound.

anaphylactic shock (an-ah-fih-LAK-tic) A severe allergic response that results in lowered blood pressure and respiratory and gastrointestinal distress. This can be fatal.

androgenic (AN-dro-jenic) A general term for hormones that stimulate development in male sex organs—for example, testosterone.

android obesity (AN-droyd) Obesity in which fat storage is located primarily in the abdominal area; defined as a waist circumference of 40 in (100 cm) in men and 35 in (88 cm) in women. Android obesity is closely associated with a high risk of cardiovascular disease, hypertension, and diabetes.

anemia (ah-NEM-ee-a) Generally refers to a decreased oxygen-carrying capacity of the blood. This can be caused by many factors, such as iron deficiency or blood loss.

anergy (AN-er-jee) Lack of an immune response to foreign compounds entering the body.

angiotensin I (an-jee-oh-TEN-sin) An intermediary compound produced during the body's attempt to conserve water and sodium; it is converted in the lungs to angiotensin II.

angiotensin II A compound produced from angiotensin I, which increases blood vessel constriction and triggers production of the hormone aldosterone.

animal model Study of disease in animals that duplicates human disease. This can be used to understand more about human disease.

anorexia nervosa (an-oh-REX-ee-uh ner-VOH-sah) An eating disorder involving a psychological loss or denial of appetite and self-starvation, related in part to a distorted body image and to various social pressures commonly associated with puberty.

anthropometry (an-throw-PO-meh-tree) The measurement of body weight and the lengths, circumferences, and thicknesses of parts of the body.

antibody (AN-tih-bod-ee) Blood proteins that inactivate foreign proteins found in the body. This helps prevent and control infections.

antibody-mediated immunity Immunity provided by B lymphocytes. Also known as humoral immunity.

antidiuretic hormone (ADH) (an-tie-dye-u-RET-ik) A hormone secreted by the pituitary gland that acts on the kidney to cause a decrease in water excretion. It is also called arginine vasopressin (AVP).

antigen (AN-ti-jen) Any substance that induces a state of sensitivity and/or resistance to microbes or toxic substances after a lag period; substance that stimulates a specific aspect of the immune system.

antioxidant (an-tie-OX-ih-dant) Generally a compound that stops the damaging effects of reactive oxygen species and reactive nitrogen species. This prevents the oxidation of substances in food or the body, particularly lipids. Antioxidants are especially important in preventing the oxidation of polyunsaturated lipids in the membranes of cells. An antioxidant is able to donate electrons to electron-seeking compounds. This in turn reduces electron capture and thus breakdown of unsaturated fatty acids and other cell components by oxidizing agents. Vitamin E is one antioxidant that cells use for protection. Some compounds have antioxidant capabilities (i.e., stop oxidation) but are not electron donors per se.

aorta (a-ORT-ah) The major arterial vessel of the body leaving from the left ventricle.

apoferritin (ape-oh-FERR-ih-tin) A protein in the intestinal cell that binds with the ferric form of iron (Fe^{3+}) to form ferritin.

apolipoprotein (ape-oh-LIP-oh-pro-teen) A protein attached to the surface of a lipoprotein or embedded in its outer shell. Apolipoproteins can help enzymes function, act as a lipid-transfer protein, or assist in the binding of a lipoprotein to a cell-surface receptor.

apoptosis (ah-pop-TOE-sis) A process that occurs over time in which enzymes in a cell set off a series of events that disable numerous cell functions, eventually leading to cell death.

appetite The primarily psychological (external) influences that encourage us to find and eat food, often in the absence of obvious hunger.

arachidonic acid (ar-a-kih-DON-ik) An omega-6 fatty acid with 20 carbon atoms and four carbon-carbon double bonds (C20:4, ω-6); precursor to some eicosanoids.

areola (ah-REE-oh-lah) The circular dark area of skin at the center of the breast.

ariboflavinosis (ah-rih-bo-flay-vih-NOH-sis) A condition resulting from a lack of riboflavin. The *a* means "without," and the *osis* stands for "a condition of."

aromatherapy The use of the vapors of essential oils extracted from flowers, leaves, stalks, fruits, and roots for therapeutic purposes.

arrhythmias (ah-RITH-me-ahs) Abnormal heart rhythms which may be too slow, too early, too rapid, or irregular.

arteriole (ar-TEAR-e-ol) A tiny artery branch.

artery A blood vessel that carries blood away from the heart.

arthritis Inflammation at a point where bones join together. The disease has many possible causes.

aseptic processing (ah-SEP-tik) A method by which food and containers are simultaneously sterilized; it allows manufacturers to produce boxes of milk that can be stored at room temperature. Variations of this process are also known as *ultrahigh temperature (UHT)* packaging.

aspartame (AH-spar-tame) An alternative sweetener made of two amino acids and methanol; it is about 180 times sweeter than sucrose.

ataxia (a-TAX-ee-ah) Inability to coordinate muscle activity during voluntary movement; incoordination.

atherosclerosis (ath-e-roh-scle-ROH-sis) A buildup of fatty material (plaque) in the arteries, including those surrounding the heart.

atom Smallest combining unit of an element.

atria/atrium (A-tree-um) Either of the two upper chambers of the heart that receive venous blood.

atrophy (AT-row-fee) A wasting away of tissue or organs.

autodigestion Literally, "self-digestion." The stomach limits autodigestion by covering itself with a thick layer of mucus and producing enzymes and acid only when needed for digestion of foodstuff.

autoimmune Immune reactions against normal body cells; self against self.

avidin (AV-ih-din) A protein found in raw egg whites that can bind biotin and inhibit its absorption; cooking destroys avidin.

axon The part of a nerve cell that conducts impulses away from the main body of the cell.

bacteria Single-cell microorganisms, some of which produce poisonous substances that cause illness in humans. They contain only one chromosome and lack many of the organelles found in human cells. Bacteria produce enzymes that can digest substances around them. Some can live without oxygen and survive harsh conditions by means of spore formation.

baryophobia (bear-ee-oh-FO-bee-ah) A disorder of young children and young adults characterized by stunted growth. It results from parental underfeeding in an attempt to prevent development of obesity and cardiovascular disease.

basal metabolism The minimal energy the body requires to support itself in a fasting state when resting and awake in a warm, quiet environment. It amounts to roughly 1 kcal/kg/hr for men and 0.9 kcal/kg/hr for women; these values are often referred to as basal metabolic rate (BMR).

benign Noncancerous; tumors that do not spread.

beriberi (BEAR-ee-BEAR-ee) The thiamin deficiency disorder characterized by muscle weakness, loss of appetite, nerve degeneration, and sometimes edema.

beta (β) bond A type of bond that cannot be broken by human intestinal enzymes during digestion when it is part of a long chain of glucose molecules; drawn as C–O–C.

betaine (bee-TAINE) An oxidation product of choline metabolism and a methyl (-CH₃) donor in methionine metabolism.

beta oxidation The breakdown of a fatty acid into numerous acetyl-CoA molecules.

BHA Butylated hydroxyanisol, a synthetic antioxidant added to food.

BHT Butylated hydroxytoluene, a synthetic antioxidant added to food.

bile A liver secretion that is stored in the gallbladder and released through the common bile duct into the duodenum. It is essential for the absorption of fat.

bile acids Emulsifiers synthesized by the liver and released by the gallbladder during digestion.

binge-eating disorder An eating disorder characterized by recurrent binge eating and feelings of loss of control over eating. Binge episodes can be triggered by frustration, anger, depression, anxiety, permission to eat forbidden foods, and excessive hunger.

bioavailability The degree to which the amount of an ingested nutrient is absorbed and is available to the body.

biochemical lesion An indication of reduced biochemical function (e.g., low concentrations of nutrient by-products or enzyme activities in the blood or urine) resulting from a nutritional deficiency.

bioelectrical impedance A method to estimate total body fat that uses a low-energy electrical current. The more fat storage a person has, the more impedance (resistance) to electrical flow will be exhibited.

biological value (BV) A measure of how efficiently food protein, once absorbed from the gastrointestinal tract, can be turned into body tissues.

biotechnology A collection of processes that involve the use of advanced scientific techniques to alter and, ideally, improve characteristics of animals, plants, and other forms of life.

bisphosphonates (bis-FOS-foh-nates) Compounds primarily composed of carbon and phosphorus that bind to bone mineral and in turn reduce bone breakdown.

bleaching process The process by which light depletes the rhodopsin concentration in the eye. This fall in rhodopsin concentration allows the eye to become adapted to bright light.

B lymphocyte (LIM-fo-site) White blood cells processed by liver and spleen tissues that are responsible for antibody production. They are responsible for recognition of foreign substances (such as bacteria) in extracellular sites in the body.

blood doping A technique by which an athlete's red blood cell count is increased. Blood is taken from the athlete, and the red blood cells are concentrated and then later reinjected into the athlete.

body mass index Weight (in kilograms) divided by height squared (in meters). A normal value is 18.5 to 24.9. A value of 25 or greater indicates a risk for body weight-related health disorders. 1 BMI unit equals 6–7 pounds.

bolus (BOWL-us) A mass of food that is swallowed.

bomb calorimeter (kal-oh-RIM-eh-ter) An instrument used to determine the energy content of a food.

bond A sharing of electrons, charges, or attractions linking two atoms.

bone mass Total mineral substance (such as calcium or phosphorus) in a cross section of bone, generally expressed as grams per centimeter of length. In contrast *bone mineral density* is the total mineral content of bone at a specific bone site divided by the width of the bone at that site, generally expressed as grams per cubic centimeter.

bone remodeling A process by which bone is first resorbed by osteoclast cells and then reformed by osteoblast cells. This process allows the body to form bone where needed, such as in areas of high mechanical stress.

bronchial tree (BRON-key-al) The bronchi and the branches on the tree.

bronchioles Smallest division of lungs.

brown adipose tissue (ADD-ih-pose) A specialized form of adipose tissue that produces large amounts of heat by metabolizing energy-yielding nutrients without synthesizing much ATP. The energy is released as heat.

buffer Compound that causes a solution to resist changes in acid-base balance.

bulimia nervosa (boo-LEEM-ee-uh) An eating disorder in which large quantities of food are eaten at one time (binge eating) and then purged from the body by vomiting, or misuse of laxatives, diuretics, or enemas. Alternate means to counteract the caloric excess are fasting and excessive exercise.

calcitonin (kal-sih-TONE-in) A thyroid gland hormone that inhibits bone resorption.

calcitriol (kal-sih-TRIH-ol) The name sometimes given to the active hormone form of vitamin D [1,25(OH)$_2$D] that contains a derivative of cholesterol as part of its structure.

calmodulin (kal-MOD-ju-lyn) A cell protein that binds calcium ions. The resulting calmodulin-Ca^{2+} complex influences the activity of some enzymes in the cell.

cancer A condition characterized by uncontrolled growth of abnormal body cells.

cancer initiation The step in the process of cancer development that begins with alterations in DNA, the genetic material in a cell. This may cause the cell to no longer respond to normal physiological controls.

cancer progression The final stage in the cancer process, during which the cancer cells proliferate, forming a mass large enough to significantly affect body functions.

cancer promotion The stage in the cancer process when cell division increases, in turn decreasing the time available for repair enzymes to act on altered DNA, and encouraging cells with altered DNA to develop and grow. Anything that increases the rate of cell division decreases the chance that the repair enzymes will find the altered part of the DNA in time to do their work.

capillary (KAP-ill-air-ee) A microscopic blood vessel that connects an arteriole and a venule; the functional unit of the circulatory system.

capillary bed Minute vessels one cell thick that create a junction between arterial and venous circulation. Gas and nutrient exchange occurs here between body cells and the bloodstream.

carbohydrate (kar-bow-HIGH-drate) A compound containing carbon, hydrogen, and oxygen atoms; most are known as *sugars, starches,* and *dietary fibers.*

carbohydrate counting Diet method that assigns a certain number of food exchanges or carbohydrate grams to each meal and snack. Insulin is matched to carbohydrate intake, and carbohydrate grams can come from several combinations of exchanges.

carbohydrate loading A process in which a very high carbohydrate intake is consumed for 6 days before an athletic event while tapering exercise duration in an attempt to increase muscle glycogen stores.

carbon skeleton Amino acid after the amino group has been removed.

carcinogenic Describes a compound with the potential to cause cancer.

carcinoma Invasive malignant tumor derived from epithelial tissues that cover the body.

cardiac muscle Muscle that makes up the walls of the heart. Produces rhythmical involuntary contractions.

cardiac output (CARD-ee-ack) The amount of blood pumped by the heart.

cardiomyopathy Primary heart-muscle disease of unknown origin.

cardiovascular disease Disease of the heart and blood vessels.

cariogenic (CARE-ee-oh-jen-ik) Literally "caries producing"; a substance often carbohydrate-rich (such as caramel), that promotes dental caries.

carnitine (CAR-nih-teen) A compound used to shuttle fatty acids from the cytosol of the cell into mitochondria.

carotenoids (kah-ROT-en-oyds) Pigment materials in fruits and vegetables that range in color from yellow to orange to red; 3 yield vitamin A activity in humans and thus are called provitamin A. Many have antioxidant properties as well. One example is beta-carotene.

carpal tunnel syndrome (CAR-pull) (SIN-drom) A disease in which nerves that travel to the wrist are pinched as they pass through a narrow opening in a bone in the wrist.

case-control study Individuals who have the condition in question, such as lung cancer, are compared with individuals who do not have the condition.

casein (KAY-seen) Protein found in milk that forms curds when exposed to acid and is difficult for infants to digest.

cash crop A crop grown specifically for export, so that goods from other countries can be purchased. Cultivation of cash crops diverts agricultural resources necessary to feed a country's own citizens. Examples are coffee, tea, cocoa, and bananas.

catabolic/catabolism (cat-ah-BOL-ik) Breaking down compounds.

catalyst (CAT-ul-ist) A compound that speeds reaction rates but is not altered by the reaction.

cecum (See-come) The first portion of the large intestine, which connects to the ileum.

celiac disease (SEA-lee-ak) An immunological or allergic reaction to the protein gluten in certain cereals, such as wheat and rye. The effect is to destroy the intestinal enterocytes, resulting in a much reduced surface area due to flattening of the villi. Elimination of wheat, rye, and certain other grains from the diet typically restores the intestinal surface.

cell A minute structure; the living basis of plant and animal organization. In animals it is bounded by a cell membrane. Cells contain both genetic material and systems for synthesizing energy-yielding compounds. Cells have the ability to take up compounds from and excrete compounds into their surroundings.

cell body The part of a nerve cell that contains the nucleus; the cell body lies between the dendrites and axon.

cell differentiation The process of transforming an unspecialized cell into a specialized cell.

cell-mediated immunity T lymphocytes that do not secrete antibodies but come in actual contact with the invading cells in order to destroy it.

cell nucleus Organelle bound by its own double membrane and containing chromosomes, the genetic information for cell protein synthesis and cell replication.

cell proliferation The continuous development of cells in tissue formation.

cellulose (SELL-you-los) A straight-chain polysaccharide of glucose molecules that is undigestible because of the presence of beta bonds; part of insoluble fiber.

Celsius A centigrade measure of temperature. For conversion: (degrees in Fahrenheit − 32) × 5/9 = C°; (degrees in Celsius × 9/5) + 32 = F°.

central nervous system (CNS) The brain and spinal cord portions of the nervous system.

cerebrovascular accident (CVA) (se-REE-bro-VAS-cue-lar) Death of part of the brain tissue due typically to a blood clot.

ceruloplasmin (se-RUE-low-PLAS-min) A blue, copper-containing protein component in the blood that can remove an electron from Fe^{2+} (the ferrous form) to yield Fe^{3+} (the ferric form). The Fe^{3+} form of iron can then bind with transport and storage proteins, such as transferrin.

chain-breaking Breaking the link between two or more actions that encourage a "problem" behavior, such as overeating linked to snacking while watching television.

chelates (KEY-lates) Complexes formed between metal ions and substances with charged groups, such as proteins. The charged groups on the substance form two or more attachments with the metal ions, forming a ring structure. The metal ion is then firmly attached.

chelation The use of medicinal compounds, such as ethylenediaminetetraacetic acid (EDTA), to bind metals and other constituents in the blood.

chemical reaction An interaction between two chemicals that changes both participants.

chemical score A ratio comparing the essential amino acid content of the protein in a food with the essential amino acid content in a reference protein. The lowest amino acid ratio calculated for any essential amino acid is the chemical score.

cholecystokinin (CCK) (ko-la-sis-toe-KY-nin) A hormone that stimulates enzyme release from the pancreas and bile release from the gallbladder.

cholinergic (coal-in-NER-jic) Actions of acetylcholine.

cholesterol (ko-LES-te-rol) A waxy lipid found in all body cells; it has a structure containing multiple chemical rings (steroid structure). Cholesterol is found only in foods that contain animal products.

chromosome A single large DNA molecule and its associated proteins containing many genes; it stores and transmits genetic information.

chronic (KRON-ik) Long-standing, developing over time; slow to develop or resolve. When referring to disease, this term indicates that the disease progress, once developed, is slow and tends to remain; a good example is heart disease.

chylomicrons (kye-lo-MY-krons) Lipoprotein made of dietary fats that are surrounded by a shell of cholesterol, phospholipids, and protein. Chylomicrons are formed in the absorptive cells in the small intestine after fat absorption and travel through the lymphatic system to the bloodstream.

chyme (KIME) A mixture of stomach secretions and partially digested food.

cirrhosis (see-ROH-sis) A loss of functioning liver cells, which are replaced by nonfunctioning connective tissue. Any substance that poisons liver cells can lead to cirrhosis. The most common cause is a chronic, excessive alcohol intake.

cis isomer (sis EYE-so-mer) An isomer form seen in compounds with double bonds, such as fatty acids, in which the hydrogens on both ends of the double bond lie on the same side of the plane of that bond.

citric acid cycle A pathway that breaks down acetyl-CoA, yielding carbon dioxide, FADH$_2$, NADH + H$^+$, and GTP. The pathway can also be used to synthesize compounds.

clinical lesion A sign seen on physical examination or a symptom perceived by the patient resulting from a nutritional deficiency.

clinical symptoms Generally, a change in health status noted by the individual (such as stomach pain) or noticed by a clinician during physical examination (the latter is technically called a clinical sign).

clinician A person who works in the healthcare field.

***Clostridium botulinum* (klo-STRID-ee-um BOT-you-LY-num)** A bacterium that can cause a fatal type of food-borne illness.

coenzyme A compound that combines with an inactive protein called an apoenzyme to form a catalytically active protein called a holoenzyme. In this manner, coenzymes aid in enzyme function.

cofactor An organic or inorganic substance that binds to a specific region on an enzyme and is necessary for the enzyme's activity.

cognitive behavior therapy Psychological therapy in which the person's assumptions about dieting, body weight, and related issues are challenged. New ways of thinking are explored and then practiced by the person. In this way, the person can learn new ways to control disordered eating behaviors and related life stress.

cognitive restructuring Changing one's frame of mind regarding a behavior—for example, instead of using a difficult day as an excuse to overeat, substituting other pleasures for rewards, such as a relaxing walk with a friend.

colic (KOL-ik) Periodic, inconsolable crying in a healthy young infant associated with sharp abdominal pain.

colipase (co-LIE-pace) A protein the pancreas secretes that changes the shape of pancreatic lipase, facilitating its action.

collagen (KOL-ah-jen) The major protein of the material that holds together the various structures of the body.

colostrum (ko-LAHS-trum) The first fluid secreted by the breast during late pregnancy and the first few days after birth. This thick fluid is rich in immune factors and protein.

comorbid A disease process that accompanies another disease. For example, if hypertension develops as obesity is established, hypertension is said to be a comorbid condition accompanying the obesity.

complement A series of blood proteins that participate in a complex reaction cascade following stimulation by an antigen-antibody complex or the surface of a bacterial cell. Various activated complement proteins can enhance phagocytosis, contribute to inflammation, and destroy bacteria.

complementary proteins Two food protein sources that make up for each other's inadequate supply of specific essential amino acids; together they yield a sufficient amount of all nine and so provide high-quality (complete) protein for the diet.

complete proteins Proteins that contain ample amounts of all nine essential amino acids.

compound A group of different types of atoms bonded together in definite proportion (see also molecule). Not all chemical compounds exist as molecules. Some compounds are made up of ions attracted to each other, such as Na$^+$Cl$^-$ (table salt).

compression of morbidity The goal of delaying the onset of disabilities caused by chronic disease.

concentration gradient Gradation in concentration that occurs between two regions having different concentrations.

conceptus (kon-SEP-tus) A generic term for any developmental stage derived from the fertilized ovum (zygote) until birth. The conceptus includes the extraembryonic membranes, as well as the embryo or fetus.

congenital (con-JEN-i-tal) A term that means "present at birth." Thus, a congenital abnormality is a defect that has been present since birth. These defects may be inherited from the parents, may occur as a result of damage or infection while in the uterus, or may occur at the time of birth.

conjugase (KON-ju-gase) Enzyme systems in the intestine that enhance folate absorption; they remove glutamate molecules from polyglutamate forms of folate.

conjunctiva (kon-junk-TEA-vah) Mucous membrane covering the anterior surface of the eyeball and the posterior surface of the eyelids.

connective tissue The material that holds together the various structures of the body. Tendons and cartilages are composed largely of connective tissue. Connective tissue also forms part of bone and the nonmuscular structures of arteries and veins.

constipation A condition in which bowel movements are infrequent.

contingency management Forming a plan of action to respond to a situation in which a problem behavior is likely, such as when snacks are within arm's reach at a party.

control group Participants in an experiment who are not given the treatment being tested.

cortical bone (KORT-ih-kal) Dense, compact bone that comprises the outer surface and shafts of bone; also called compact bone.

corticosteroid (kor-ti-ko-STARE-oyd) A steroid produced by the adrenal gland, an example of which is cortisol.

cortisol (KORT-ih-sol) A hormone made by the adrenal glands that stimulates the production of glucose from amino acids, among other functions.

covalent bond (ko-VAY-lent) A union of two atoms formed by the sharing of electrons.

creatine (cree-A-tin) A compound in muscles that can exist in a high energy state, phosphocreatine. This indirectly provides energy for muscle contraction by forming ATP from ADP.

cretinism (KREET-in-ism) The stunting of body growth and poor mental development in the offspring that results from inadequate maternal intake of iodide during pregnancy.

Crohn's disease An inflammatory disease of the gastrointestinal tract, but generally more pronounced in the terminal ileum. A family history is a major risk factor. The disease limits the absorptive capacity of the small intestine.

crude fiber What remains of dietary fiber after extended acid and alkaline treatment. This consists primarily of cellulose and lignins.

cryptosporidiosis (krip-toe-spore-id-ee-O-sis) An intestinal disease, characterized by diarrhea, that originates from a protozoan parasite of the genus *Cryptosporidium*.

cyclooxygenase (sigh-cl-OXY-jen-ase) An oxygenase enzyme used to synthesize prostaglandins, thromboxanes, and other eicosanoids.

cystic fibrosis (SIS-tik figh-BRO-sis) A disease that often leads to overproduction of mucus. Mucus can invade the pancreas, decreasing enzyme output. The lack of lipase enzyme output then contributes to severe fat malabsorption.

cytochrome (SITE-o-krome) Electron-transfer compound that participates in the electron transport chain.

cytokine (SITE-o-kine) A protein secreted by a cell that regulates the activity of neighboring cells.

cytoplasm (SITE-o-plazem) The fluid and organelles (except the nucleus) in a cell.

cytotoxic T cell (site-o-TOX-ik) Type of T-cell that interacts with the infected host cell through special receptor sites on the T-cell surface.

cytotoxic test (SITE-o-TOX-ik) An unreliable test to define food allergies that involves mixing white blood cells with food proteins.

Daily Reference Intakes (DRIs) The term used to encompass the latest nutrient recommendations made by the Food and Nutrition Board of the National Academy of Sciences. These include RDAs.

Daily Reference Values (DRVs) Nutrient-intake standards established for protein and some other dietary components lacking an RDA or a related nutrient standard, including fat, saturated fat, cholesterol, carbohydrate, dietary fiber, sodium, and potassium. The DRVs for cholesterol, sodium, and potassium are constant; those for other nutrients increase as energy intake increases. The DRVs constitute part of the Daily Values used in food labeling.

Daily Values A set of standard nutrient-intake values developed by FDA and used as a reference for expressing nutrient content on nutrition labels. The Daily Values include two types of standards—Reference Daily Intakes and Daily Reference Values.

dark adaptation The process by which the rhodopsin concentration in the eye increases in dark conditions, allowing improved vision in the dark.

deamination (dee-am-ih-NA-shun) The removal of an amino group from an amino acid.

decarboxylation (dee-car-box-ih-LAY-shun) The action of removing one molecule of carbon dioxide from a carboxylic acid.

decubitus ulcers (dee-CUBE-ih-tus) Chronic ulcers that appear in pressure areas of the skin over a body prominence in patients confined to bed or immobilized (i.e., bedsores).

Delaney Clause A clause to the 1958 Food Additives Amendment of the Pure Food and Drug Act in the United States that prevents the intentional (direct) addition to foods of a compound that has been shown to cause cancer in laboratory animals or humans.

dementia (de-MEN-sha) General persistent loss or decrease in mental function.

denature (dee-NAY-ture) Alteration of a protein's three-dimensional structure, usually because of treatment by heat, enzymes, acid or alkaline solutions, or agitation.

dendrite (DEN-dright) A relatively short, highly branched nerve cell process that carries electrical activity to the main body of the nerve cell.

dental caries (KARE-ees) Erosions in the surface of a tooth caused by acids made by bacteria as they metabolize sugars.

deoxyribonucleic acid (DNA) The site of hereditary information in cells; DNA directs the synthesis of cell proteins.

depolarization Reversal of membrane potential, which triggers generation of the nerve impulse in nerve cells.

dermatitis (dur-ma-TIE-tis) Inflammation of the skin.

dermis (DUR-miss) The second, or deep, layer of the skin under the epidermis.

dextrin (DECK-strin) Partial breakdown product of starch that contains few to many glucose molecules. These appear when starch is being digested into many units of maltose by salivary and pancreatic amylase.

diabetes (DYE-uh-BEET-eez) A disease characterized by high blood glucose (hyperglycemia), resulting from insufficient insulin action in the body (see also type I diabetes and type 2 diabetes). Although this disease is commonly referred to as "diabetes," its technical name is diabetes mellitus.

diastolic blood pressure (dye-ah-STOL-ik) The pressure in the arterial blood vessels when the heart is between beats.

dietary fiber Substances in plant foods that are not digested by the processes that take place in the stomach or small intestine. These add bulk to feces.

Dietary Guidelines General goals for nutrient intake and diet composition set by government agencies—USDA and the Department of Health and Human Services (DHHS).

dietitian See registered dietitian.

diffusion The net movement of molecules or ions from regions of higher to regions of lower concentration.

digestibility (dye-JES-tih-bil-it-ee) The proportion of food substances eaten that can be broken down in the intestinal tract for absorption into the body.

digestion The process by which large ingested molecules are mechanically and chemically broken down to produce smaller forms that can be absorbed across the wall of the GI tract.

dihomo-gama-linolenic acid (die-homo-gama-lin-oh-len-ik) An omega-6 fatty acid with 20 carbons and 4 double bonds; the precursor to some eicosanoids.

direct calorimetry (kal-oh-RIM-eh-tree) A method of determining a body's energy use by measuring heat that emanates from the body, usually using an insulated chamber.

disaccharides (dye-SACK-uh-rides) Class of sugars formed by the chemical bonding of two monosaccharides.

distillation (dis-te-LAY-shun) A physical method used to separate liquids based on their boiling points.

diuretic (dye-u-RET-ik) A substance that, when ingested, increases the flow of urine.

diverticula (DYE-ver-TIK-you-luh) Pouches that protrude through the exterior wall of the large intestine.

diverticulitis (DYE-ver-tik-you-LITE-us) An inflammation of the diverticula caused by acids produced by bacterial metabolism inside the diverticula.

diverticulosis (DYE-ver-tik-you-LOW-sus) The condition of having many diverticula in the large intestine.

docosahexaenoic acid (DHA) (DOE-co-sa-hex-ee-no-ik) An omega-3 fatty acid with 22 carbons and 6 carbon-carbon double bonds ($C22:6$, ω-3). It is present in large amounts in fish oils and is synthesized in the body from alpha-linolenic acid. DHA is especially present in the retina of the eye.

dopamine (DOE-pah-mean) A type of neurotransmitter in the central nervous system that leads to feelings of euphoria, among other functions; it is also the precursor of norepinephrine, another neurotransmitter molecule.

double-blind study An experiment in which the participants and researchers are unaware of the participant's assignment (test or placebo) or the outcome of the study until it is completed. An independent third party holds the code and the data until the study is completed.

duodenum (doo-oh-DEE-num, or doo-ODD-num) First portion of the small intestine. Leads from pyloric sphincter to the jejunum.

ecchymoses (ec-ee-MOS-ease) Discoloration of an area of the skin or mucous membrane caused by blood's seeping into the tissue due to fragility of the vessel walls.

ecosystem A "community" in nature that includes plants, animals, and the environment.

ectomorph (EK-tuh-morf) A body type associated with very long, thin bones and very long, thin fingers.

edema (uh-DEE-muh) The buildup of excess fluid in extracellular spaces.

eicosanoids (eye-KOH-san-oyds) Hormonelike compounds synthesized from polyunsaturated fatty acids, such as arachidonic acid. Within this class of compounds are prostaglandins, thromboxanes, and leukotrienes.

eicosapentaenoic acid (EPA) (eye-KOH-sah-pen-tah-ee-NO-ik) An omega-3 fatty acid with 20 carbons and 5 carbon-carbon double bonds ($C20:5$, ω-3). It is present in large amounts in fish oils and is synthesized from alpha-linolenic acid. EPA is metabolized to eicosanoids.

elastin (ee-LAS-tin) Rubberband-like connective tissue protein found in lungs and large arteries where elastic properties are essential.

electrolytes (ih-LEK-tro-lites) Substances that break down into ions in water and, in turn, are able to conduct an electrical current. These include sodium, chloride, and potassium.

electron A part of an atom that is negatively charged. Electrons orbit the nucleus.

electron transport chain A series of reactions using oxygen to convert $NADH+H^+$ and $FADH_2$ molecules to free NAD and FAD molecules by the donation of electrons and hydrogen ions, yielding water and ATP.

elements Substances that cannot be broken down further by using ordinary chemical procedures.

elimination diet A restrictive diet that systematically tests foods that may cause an allergic response by first eliminating them for 1 to 2 weeks and then adding them back, one at a time.

embryo (EM-bree-oh) In humans, the developing in utero offspring from about the beginning of the third to the end of the eighth week after conception.

emulsifier (ee-MULL-sih-fire) A compound that can suspend fat in water by isolating individual fat droplets using a shell of water molecules or other substances to prevent the fat from coalescing.

endocrine gland (EN-doh-krin) A hormone-producing gland.

endocytosis (phagocytosis/pinocytosis) Forms of active absorption in which the absorptive cell forms an indentation in its membrane and particles (phagocytosis) or fluids (pinocytosis) entering the indentation are then engulfed by the cell.

endometrium (en-doh-ME-tree-um) The membrane that lines the inside of the uterus. It increases in thickness during the menstrual cycle until ovulation occurs. The surface layers are shed during menstruation if conception does not take place.

endomorph (EN-doh-morf) A body type characterized by short, stubby bones, a short trunk, and short fingers.

endoplasmic reticulum (ER) (en-doh-PLAZ-mik re-TIK-u-lum) An organelle in the cytoplasm composed of a network of canals running through the cytoplasm. **Rough ER** contains ribosomes. **Smooth ER** contains no ribosomes.

endorphins (en-DOR-fins) Natural body tranquilizers that may be involved in the feeding response and function in pain reduction.

endothelial cells (en-doh-THEE-lee-al) A layer of flat cells lining the blood and lymphatic vessels and the chambers of the heart.

energy balance A state in which energy intake, in the form of food and/or alcohol, matches the energy expended, primarily through basal metabolism and physical activity.

energy density Determined by comparing the energy (kcal) content of a food to its weight.

enriched A term generally meaning that the vitamins thiamin, niacin, riboflavin, and folate and the mineral iron have been added to a grain product to improve nutritional quality.

enterocytes (en-TER-oh-sites) Villi are lined with these epithelial cells, which are highly specialized for digestion and absorption.

enterohepatic circulation (EN-ter-oh-heh-PAT-ik) Recycling of compounds between the small intestine and the liver over and over again, as happens with bile acids.

enzyme (EN-zime) A compound that speeds the rate of a chemical process but is not altered by the chemical process. Almost all enzymes are proteins.

epidemiology (ep-uh-dee-me-OLL-uh-gee) The study of how disease patterns vary between different population groups, such as the cases of stomach cancer in Japan compared with that in Germany.

epidermis (ep-ih-DUR-miss) The outermost layer of the skin, composed of epithelial layers.

epigenetic carcinogens (promoters) (ep-ih-je-NET-ik car-SIN-oh-jens) Compounds that increase cell division and thereby increase the chance that a cell with altered DNA will develop into cancer.

epiglottis (ep-ih-GLOT-iss) Flap that folds down over the trachea during swallowing.

epinephrine (ep-ih-NEF-rin) A hormone (also known as adrenaline) that is released by the adrenal gland. The related hormone, norepinephrine, is released from various nerve endings in the body. Both hormones increase glycogen breakdown in the liver, among other functions.

epiphyseal line (ep-ih-FEES-ee-al) When bone growth is complete, a line replaces the plate.

epiphyseal plate A cartilage-like layer in the long bone. It functions in longitudinal growth.

epiphyses (e-PIF-ih-seas) Ends of long bones. The epiphyseal plate—sometimes referred to as the growth plate—is made of cartilage and allows growth of the bone to occur. During childhood, the cartilage cells multiply and absorb calcium, to develop into bone.

epithelial cells (ep-ih-THEE-lee-ul) Cells that cover the surface of the body and line body cavities.

epithelial tissue The covering in internal and external surfaces of the body, including the lining of vessels and other small cavities. It consists of epithelial cells joined by a small amount of cementing material.

equilibrium (ee-kwih-LIB-ree-um) In nutrition, a state in which nutrient intake equals nutrient losses. Thus, the body maintains a stable condition.

ergogenic (ur-go-JEN-ic) Work-producing. An ergogenic acid is a physical, mechanical, nutritional, psychological, or pharmacological substance or treatment that is intended to directly improve exercise performance.

erythrocyte (eh-RITH-row-site) Mature red blood cell. This has no nucleus and a life span of about 120 days; it contains hemoglobin, which transports oxygen and carbon dioxide.

erythropoietin (eh-REE-throw-POY-eh-tin) A hormone secreted mostly by the kidneys that enhances red blood cell synthesis and stimulates red blood cell release from bone marrow.

esophagus (eh-SOF-ah-gus) A tube in the GI tract that connects the pharynx with the stomach.

essential fatty acids Fatty acids that must be present in the diet to maintain health. Currently only linoleic acid and alpha-linolenic acid are classified as essential fatty acids.

essential (indispensable) amino acids Amino acids that cannot be synthesized by humans in sufficient amounts and therefore must be included in the diet; there are nine essential amino acids. These are also called indispensable amino acids.

essential nutrient In nutritional terms, a substance that, when left out of a diet, leads to signs of poor health. The body either can't produce this nutrient or can't produce them fast enough to meet its needs. Then, if added back to a diet before permanent damage occurs, the affected aspects of health are restored.

esterification (e-ster-ih-fih-KAY-shun) With regard to fats, the process of attaching fatty acids to a glycerol molecule, creating an ester bond and releasing water. Removing a fatty acid is called deesterification; reattaching a fatty acid is called reesterification.

estimated average requirement (EAR) An amount of nutrient intake that is estimated to meet the needs of 50% of the individuals in a specific age and gender group.

eustachian tubes (you-STAY-shun) Thin tubes connected to the middle ear that open into the throat.

exchange The serving size of a food on a specific exchange list.

exchange system A system for classifying foods into numerous lists based on their macronutrient composition and establishing serving sizes, so that one serving of each food on a list contains the same amount of carbohydrate, protein, fat, and energy content.

exocrine gland (EK-so-krin) A cluster of epithelial cells specialized for secretion. They have ducts that lead to an epithelial surface.

exocytosis (ek-so-sigh-TOE-sis) The process of cellular secretion in which the secretory products are contained within a membrane-enclosed vesicle. The vesicle fuses with the cell membrane and is open to the extracellular environment.

experiment A test made to examine the validity of a hypothesis.

extracellular Not contained in the cells.

extracellular fluid Fluid present outside the cells; this includes intravascular and interstitial fluids; it represents one-third of all body fluid.

extracellular space The space outside cells.

facies (FAY-sheez) The appearance of the face of a person with alcoholism when blood vessels break near the surface, causing a blushed look.

facilitated diffusion The carrier-mediated transport of molecules through the cell membrane along the direction of their concentration gradients. It does not require the expenditure of energy.

failure to thrive Inadequate gains in height and weight in infancy, often due to an inadequate food intake.

famine An extreme shortage of food that leads to massive starvation in a population; often associated with crop failures, war, and political strife.

fasting hypoglycemia (HIGH-po-gligh-SEE-me-ah) Low blood glucose that follows about a day of fasting.

fat-soluble vitamins Vitamins that dissolve in such substances as ether and benzene, but not readily in water. These vitamins are A, D, E, and K.

fatty acid A chain of carbons linked together and surrounded by hydrogen atoms. These hydrocarbons are found in lipids and contain a carboxyl (acid group) ($-\overset{\overset{\displaystyle O}{\|}}{C}-OH$) at one end and a methyl group ($-CH_3$) at the other.

feces (FEE-seas) Substances discharged from the bowel during defecation, consisting of the undigested residue of food, dead GI tract cells, mucus, bacteria, and other waste material. Another term for feces is *stool*.

feeding center A group of cells in the hypothalamus that, when stimulated, causes hunger.

female athlete triad A condition characterized by disordered eating, lack of menstrual periods, and osteoporosis.

fermentation The metabolism, without the use of oxygen, of carbohydrates to alcohols, acids, and carbon dioxide.

ferritin (FERR-ih-tin) A protein compound that serves as the storage form of iron in the blood and tissues.

fetal alcohol effect (FAE) Hyperactivity, attention deficit disorder, poor judgment, sleep disorders, and delayed learning as a result of being prenatally exposed to alcohol.

fetal alcohol syndrome (FAS) (FEET-al) A group of irreversible physical and mental abnormalities in the infant that result from the mother's consuming alcohol during pregnancy.

fetus (FEET-us) The developing life form from about the beginning of the ninth week after conception until birth.

filaments (FILL-ah-ments) Parts of a muscle fiber.

fluoroapatite (fleur-oh-APP-uh-tite) A tooth crystal containing fluoride ions. Presence of this crystal makes the tooth relatively acid resistant.

fluorosis (flo-ROW-sis) A condition caused by excessive fluoride intake, characterized by poor tooth structure and discoloration.

folk medicine A medical treatment based on the beliefs, traditions, or customs of a particular society or ethnic/cultural group.

follicular hyperkeratosis (fo-LICK-you-lar high-per-ker-ah-TOE-sis) A condition in which keratin, a protein, accumulates around hair follicles. This skin change occurs in a vitamin A deficiency.

food-borne illness Sickness caused by the ingestion of food containing toxic substances produced by microorganisms.

food diary A written record of sequential food intake for a period of time. Details associated with the food intake are often recorded as well.

food intolerance An adverse reaction to food that does not involve an allergic reaction.

food sensitivity A mild reaction to a substance in a food that might be expressed as slight itching or redness of the skin.

fore milk The first breast milk delivered in the nursing session.

fortified A term generally meaning that vitamins, minerals, or both have been added to a food product in excess of what was originally found in the product.

fraternal twins Offspring that develop from two separate ova and sperm and therefore have separate genetic identities, although they develop simultaneously in the mother.

free erythrocyte protoporphyrins (FEP) (eh-RITH-row-site pro-toe-POR-fir-ins) Immature red blood cells released from the bone marrow. An elevated blood FEP reflects a decreased ability to make red blood cells and suggests iron deficiency anemia. Lead poisoning also raises blood FEP.

free radical Short-lived form of compounds that exist with an unpaired electron in the outer electron shell. This causes an electron-seeking nature, which can be very destructive to electron-dense areas of a cell, such as DNA and cell membranes.

free water The water not bound to the compounds in a food. This is available for microbial use.

fructose (FROOK-tose) A monosaccharide with six carbons that form a five-membered or six-membered ring with oxygen in the ring; found in fruits and honey.

fruitarian (froot-AIR-ee-un) A person who eats primarily fruits, nuts, honey, and vegetable oils.

functional foods Foods that provide health benefits beyond those supplied by the traditional nutrients they contain. For example, a tomato contains the phytochemical lycopene, so it can be called a functional food.

fungi Simple parasitic life forms, including molds, mildews, yeasts, and mushrooms. They live on dead or decaying organic matter. Fungi can grow as single cells, like yeast, or as multicellular colonies, as seen with molds.

galactose (gah-LAK-tos) A six-carbon monosaccharide; an isomer of glucose.

galactosemia (gah-LAK-toh-SEE-mee-ah) A rare genetic disease characterized by the buildup of the single sugar galactose in the bloodstream, resulting from the inability of the liver to metabolize it. If present at birth and left untreated, this disease causes severe mental and growth retardation in the infant.

gallbladder The organ attached to the underside of the liver and in which bile is stored and secreted.

gastric inhibitory peptide (GIP) (GAS-trik in-HIB-ih-tor-ee PEP-tide) A hormone that slows gastric motility and stimulates insulin release from the pancreas.

gastrin (GAS-trin) A hormone that stimulates enzyme and acid secretion in the stomach.

gastroesophageal reflux disease (GERD) (gas-troh-eh-SOF-ah-jee-al) Disease that results from stomach acid backing up into the esophagus. The acid irritates the lining of the esophagus, causing pain.

gastrointestinal distention (gas-troh-in-TEST-in-al) Expansion of the wall of the stomach or intestines due to pressure caused by the presence of gases, food, drink, or other factors. This contributes to a feeling of satiety brought on by food intake.

gastrointestinal (GI) tract The main sites in the body used for digestion and absorption of nutrients. It consists of the mouth, esophagus, stomach, small intestine, large intestine, rectum, and anus.

gastroplasty (GAS-troh-plas-tee) Surgery performed on the stomach to limit its volume to approximately 30 milliliters, about the size of a shot glass.

genes (JEANs) The hereditary material on chromosomes that makes up DNA. Genes provide the blueprint for the production of cell proteins.

gene expression Use of information on a gene via transcription and translation leading to production of a protein. Thought to be a major determinant of cellular differentiation.

generally recognized as safe (GRAS) A list of food additives that in 1958 were considered safe for consumption. Manufacturers were allowed to continue to use these additives, without special clearance, when needed for food products. FDA bears responsibility for proving they are not safe but can remove unsafe products from the list.

genetic engineering Alteration of genetic material in plants or animals with the intent of improving growth, disease resistance, or other characteristics.

genotoxic carcinogen (initiator) (JEH-no-TOK-sik car-SIN-oh-jen) A compound that directly alters DNA or is converted in cells to metabolites that alter DNA, thereby providing the potential for cancer to develop.

gestation (jes-TAY-shun) The period of intrauterine development of offspring, from conception to birth; in humans, gestation lasts for about 40 weeks after the woman's last menstrual period.

gestational diabetes (jes-TAY-shun-al) Elevated blood glucose that develops during pregnancy and returns to normal after birth; one cause is placental production of hormones that antagonize regulation of blood glucose by insulin.

glomerulus (glo-MER-you-lus) The capillaries in the kidney that filter urine from the blood.

glucagon (GLOO-kuh-gon) A hormone made by the pancreas that stimulates the breakdown of glycogen in the liver into glucose; this raises blood glucose. Glucagon also performs other functions.

gluconeogenesis (gloo-ko-nee-oh-JEN-uh-sis) The production of new glucose molecules by metabolic pathways in the cell. Amino acids derived from protein usually provide the carbons for this glucose.

glucose (GLOO-kos) A six-carbon carbohydrate found in blood, and in table sugar bound to fructose; also known as *dextrose*, it is one of the simple sugars.

glucose polymer A carbohydrate source used in some sports drinks that consists of a few glucose molecules bonded together.

glutathione (gloo-tah-THIGH-on) A reducing agent. It can remove toxic peroxides that form in the cell during aerobic metabolism.

glutathione peroxidase (gloo-tah-THIGH-on per-OX-ih-dase) A selenium-containing enzyme that can destroy peroxides. It acts in conjunction with vitamin E to reduce free-radical damage to cells.

glycemic index (gli-SEA-mik) A ratio used to measure the relative ability of a carbohydrate to raise blood glucose compared with the ability of white bread (or glucose) to raise blood glucose.

glycerol (GLIS-er-ol) A three-carbon alcohol used to form triglycerides.

glycocalyx (gli-ko-KAL-iks) Hairlike projections on the extracellular surface of the plasma membrane of cells; consists of short, branched carbohydrate chains.

glycogen (GLI-ko-jen) A carbohydrate made of multiple units of glucose with a highly branched structure; sometimes known as *animal starch*. It is the storage form of glucose in humans and is synthesized (and stored) in the liver and muscles.

glycolipid (gli-ko-LIP-id) A lipid (fat) containing a carbohydrate group.

glycolysis (gli-KOL-ih-sis) The metabolic pathway that converts glucose into two molecules of pyruvic acid, with the net gain of two ATP and two $NADH+H^+$.

glycoprotein (gli-ko-PRO-teen) A protein containing a carbohydrate group.

glycosylation (gli-COS-ih-lay-shun) The process by which glucose attaches to (glycates) other compounds, such as proteins.

goiter (GOY-ter) An enlargement of the thyroid gland, which can be caused by a lack of iodide in the diet.

goitrogens (GOY-troh-jens) Substances in food and water that interfere with thyroid gland metabolism and thus may cause goiter if consumed in large amounts.

Golgi complex (GOAL-jee) The cell organelle near the nucleus that processes newly synthesized protein for secretion or distribution to other organelles.

green revolution Increases in crop yields accompanying the introduction of new agricultural technologies in less developed countries, beginning in the 1960s. The key technologies were high-yielding, disease-resistant strains of rice, wheat, and corn; greater use of fertilizer and water; and improved cultivation practices.

growth hormone A pituitary hormone that stimulates body growth and release of fat from storage; it also has other effects.

gums Dietary fiber containing chains of galactose, glucuronic acid, and other monosaccharides; characteristically found in exudates from plant stems.

gynecoid obesity (GI-nih-coyd) Obesity in which fat storage is located primarily in the buttocks and thigh area.

H₂ blockers Medications, such as cimetidine (Tagamet), that block the stimulation of stomach acid production cause by histamine.

Harris-Benedict equation An equation that predicts resting metabolic rate based on a person's weight, height, and age.

heart attack Rapid fall in heart function caused by reduced blood flow through the heart's blood vessels. Often part of the heart dies in the process. It is technically called a myocardial infarction.

heartburn A pain emanating from the esophagus, caused by stomach acid backing up into the esophagus and irritating the esophageal tissue.

heart disease A disease usually caused by the deposition of fatty material in the blood vessels that serve the heart, often called hardening of the arteries. These deposits restrict blood flow through the heart, which in turn can lead to heart damage and death. Also termed *coronary heart disease* (CHD), as the vessels of the heart are the primary site of disease; part of *cardiovascular disease.*

heat cramps Heat cramps are a frequent complication of heat exhaustion. They usually occur in individuals exercising for several hours in a hot climate who have experienced large sweat losses and have consumed a large volume of unsalted water. The cramps occur in skeletal muscles and consist of contractions for 1 to 3 minutes at a time.

heat exhaustion The first stage of heat-related illness that occurs because of depletion of blood volume from fluid loss by the body. This increases body temperature and can lead to headache, dizziness, muscle weakness, and visual disturbances, among other effects.

heat-labile (LAY-bile) A structure or activity that is changed by heating.

heatstroke Heatstroke can occur when internal body temperature reaches 105°F. Sweating generally ceases if left untreated, and blood circulation is greatly reduced. Nervous system damage may ensue and death is likely. Often in individuals who suffer heatstroke the skin is hot and dry.

helper T-cell Type of T-cell that interacts with macrophages and secretes substances to signal an invading pathogen. Stimulates B lymphocytes to proliferate.

hematocrit (hee-MAT-oh-krit) The percentage of total blood volume made up of red blood cells.

heme iron (HEEM) Iron provided from animal tissues as hemoglobin and myoglobin. Approximately 40% of the iron in meat is heme iron; it is readily absorbed.

hemicellulose (hem-ih-SELL-you-los) A dietary fiber containing xylose, galactose, glucose, and other monosaccharides bonded together.

hemochromatosis (heem-oh-krom-ah-TOE-sis) A disorder of iron metabolism characterized by increased iron absorption and deposition in the liver and heart tissue. This eventually poisons the cells in those organs.

hemoglobin (HEEM-oh-glow-bin) The iron-containing part of the red blood cell that carries oxygen to the cells and some carbon dioxide away from the cells. It is also responsible for the red color of blood.

hemolysis (hee-MOL-ih-sis) Destruction of red blood cells caused by the breakdown of the red blood cell membranes. This causes the cell contents to leak into the fluid portion (plasma) of the blood.

hemopoiesis (heem-oh-po-EE-sis) Production of red blood cells. Also called hematopoiesis

hemorrhagic stroke (hem-oh-RAJ-ik) Damage to part of the brain resulting from rupture of a blood vessel and subsequent bleeding within or over the internal surface of the brain.

hemorrhoid (HEM-or-oyd) A pronounced swelling in a large vein, particularly veins found in the anal region.

hemosiderin (heem-oh-SID-er-in) An insoluble iron-protein compound found in the liver. Hemosiderin stores iron when the amount of iron in the body exceeds the storage capacity of ferritin.

hepatic portal system (vein) (he-PAT-ik) The vein that conveys blood from capillaries in the intestines and portions of the stomach to capillaries in the liver.

hepatic vein (he-PAT-ik) The vein that drains the liver.

herbicide (ERB-ih-side) A compound that reduces the growth and reproduction of plants.

hexose (HEK-sos) A general term describing a carbohydrate containing six carbon atoms.

high-density lipoprotein (HDL) Lipoprotein, synthesized in part by the liver and intestine, that picks up cholesterol from dying cells and other sources and transfers it to the other lipoproteins in the bloodstream, as well as directly to the liver. A low blood HDL value increases the risk for cardiovascular disease.

high-fructose corn syrup A corn syrup that has been manufactured to contain between 40% and 90% fructose.

high-quality (complete) proteins Dietary proteins that contain ample amounts of all nine essential amino acids.

hind milk (HYND) The milk secreted at the end of a nursing session; it is higher in fat than fore milk.

histamine (HISS-tuh-meen) A breakdown product of the amino acid histidine that stimulates acid secretion by the stomach and has other effects on the body, such as contraction of smooth muscles, increased nasal secretions, relaxation of blood vessels, and changes in relaxation of airways. It appears to decrease hunger and food intake.

homeostasis (home-ee-oh-STAY-sis) A series of adjustments that act to prevent change in the internal environment in the body.

hormone A compound secreted into the bloodstream that acts to control the function of distant target organ cells. Hormones can be either amino acid-like (epinephrine), proteinlike (insulin), or fatlike (estrogen).

hospice units (HAHS-pis) A facility offering care that emphasizes comfort and dignity in death.

human immunodeficiency virus (HIV) The virus that leads to acquired immune deficiency syndrome. There are 10 forms of HIV worldwide, called clades.

hunger The primarily physiological (internal) drive to find and eat food, mostly regulated by innate cues to eating.

hydrogenation (high-dro-jen-AY-shun) Addition of hydrogen to a carbon-carbon double bond, producing a single bond. Because hydrogenation of unsaturated fatty acids in a vegetable oil increases its hardness, this process is used to convert liquid oils into more solid fats, which are used in making margarine and shortening. Trans fatty acids are a by-product of hydrogenation of vegetable oils.

hydrolysis (high-DROL-ih-sis) A chemical reaction in which a compound is broken down by the addition of water. One product receives a hydrogen ion (H^+), while the other product receives a hydroxyl ion (OH^-). Hydrolytic enzymes break down compounds using water in the manner just described.

hydrophilic (high-dro-FILL-ik) Attracts water; literally means "water loving."

hydrophobic (high-dro-FO-bik) Repels water; literally means "water fearing."

hydroxyapatite (high-drox-ee-APP-uh-tite) A compound, composed primarily of calcium and phosphate, that is deposited into the bone protein matrix to give bone strength and rigidity ($Ca_{10}[PO_4]_6OH_2$).

hyperactivity A poorly defined term generally used to label inattention, irritability, and excessively active behavior in children. Technically referred to as Attention Deficit Hyperactive Disorder.

hypercalcemia (high-per-kal-SEE-mee-ah) A high concentration of calcium in the bloodstream. This can lead to loss of appetite, calcium deposits in organs, and other health problems.

hypercarotenemia (high-per-car-oh-teh-NEEM-ee-ah) High amounts of carotenoids in the bloodstream, usually caused by consuming a diet high in carrots or squash or by taking beta-carotene supplements.

hyperglycemia (HIGH-per-gligh-SEE-me-uh) High blood glucose, above 125 mg per 100 ml (dl) of blood.

hypergymnasia (high-per-jim-NAY-zee-ah) Exercising more than is required for physical fitness or maximum performance in a sport; excessive exercise.

hyperlipidemia (high-per-lip-ih-DEE-me-ah) The presence of an abnormally large amount of lipids in the circulating blood.

hyperplasia (high-per-PLAY-zee-uh) An increase in cell number.

hypertension (high-per-TEN-shun) A condition in which blood pressure remains persistently elevated. Obesity, inactivity, excess alcohol intake, and excess salt (sodium) intake all can contribute to the problem; also called high blood pressure.

hypertrophy (high-PURR-tro-fee) An increase in tissue or organ size.

hypervitaminosis (HIGH-per-vi-tah-mi-NO-sis) Condition resulting from intake of excessive amounts of one or more vitamins.

hypocalcemia (HIGH-po-kal-SEE-me-ah) Low blood calcium, typically arising from inadequate parathyroid hormone release or action.

hypochromic (high-po-KROM-ik) Describing pale red blood cells lacking sufficient hemoglobin as a result of iron deficiency. Hypochromic cells have a reduced oxygen-carrying ability.

hypoglycemia (HIGH-po-gligh-SEE-me-uh) Low blood glucose, below 40 to 50 mg per 100 ml (dl) of blood.

hypothalamus (high-po-THALL-uh-mus) A region at the base of the brain that contains cells that play a role in the regulation of hunger, respiration, body temperature, and other body functions.

hypothesis (high-POTH-eh-sis) An "educated guess" by a scientist to explain a phenomenon.

hysterectomy (hiss-te-RECK-toe-mee) Surgical removal of the uterus.

identical twins Two offspring that develop from a single ovum and sperm and, consequently, have the same genetic makeup.

ileocecal sphincter (ill-ee-oh-SEE-kal SFINK-ter) Ring of smooth muscle between the ileum of small intestine and the colon.

ileum (ILL-ee-um) Terminal portion of the small intestine.

immunoglobulins (em-you-no-GLOB-you-lins) Proteins found in the blood that are responsible for anti-body-mediated immunity, and bind specifically to antigen. Also called *antibodies*. Immunoglobulins are produced by B-lymphocytes in response to a foreign substance (antigen) in the bloodstream.

incidence The number of new cases of a disease in a defined population over a specific period of time, such as 1 year.

incidental food additives Additives that appear in food products indirectly, from environmental contamination of food ingredients or during the manufacturing process.

incomplete (lower-quality) protein Food protein that lacks ample amount of one or more of the essential amino acids needed to support human protein needs.

indirect calorimetry (kal-oh-RIM-eh-tree) A method to measure the energy use by the body by measuring oxygen uptake. Formulas are then used to convert this gas exchange value into energy use.

infectious disease (in-FEK-shus) Any disease caused by an invasion of the body by microorganisms, such as bacteria, fungi, or viruses.

infrastructure (IN-fra-struck-sure) The basic framework of a system or organization. For society, this includes roads, bridges, telephones, and other basic technologies.

innervate (INN-ur-vate) To supply with nerve fiber.

inorganic (in-or-GAN-ik) Anything lacking carbon atoms bonded to hydrogen atoms in the chemical structure.

insensible In this case, not perceived by the person, such as water lost with each breath.

insoluble fibers Fibers that mostly do not dissolve in water and are not metabolized by bacteria in the large intestine. These include cellulose, some hemicelluloses, and lignins.

insulin (IN-su-lynn) A hormone produced by the beta cells of the pancreas. Insulin increases the synthesis of glycogen in the liver and the movement of glucose from the bloodstream into muscle and adipose cells, among other processes.

integumentary (in-teg-you-MEN-tah-ree) The organ system having to do with the skin, nails, and sweat glands; the largest organ in the body.

intentional food additive Additives knowingly (directly) incorporated into food products by manufacturers.

interferons (in-ter-FEAR-ons) A group of proteins released by virus-infected cells that bind to other cells, stimulating synthesis of antiviral proteins, which in turn inhibit viral multiplication.

intermediate A chemical compound formed in one of many steps in a metabolic pathway. For example, pyruvate is an intermediate in the glycolysis pathway.

international unit (IU) A crude measure of vitamin activity, often based on the growth rate of animals. Today these units have generally been replaced by precise measurement of actual quantities in milligrams or micrograms.

interstitial fluid (in-ter-STISH-al) Fluid between cells.

intracellular (in-tra-SELL-you-lar) Within a cell.

intracellular fluid Fluid contained within a cell; represents about two-thirds of all body fluid.

intravascular fluid (in-tra-VAS-kyu-lar) Fluid within the bloodstream (i.e., in the arteries, veins, capillaries, and lymph vessels).

intrinsic factor (in-TRIN-zik) A substance present in gastric juice that enhances vitamin B-12 absorption.

in utero (in-YOU-ter-oh) "In the uterus," or during pregnancy.

in vitro (in-VEE-troh) Refers to experiments performed outside the body, such as in a test tube—literally, *in glass*.

in vivo (in-VEE-vo) Within the living body.

ion (EYE-on) An atom with an unequal number of electrons and protons. Negative ions have more electrons than protons; positive ions have more protons than electrons.

ionic bond (eye-ON-ik) A union between two atoms formed by an attraction of a positive ion to a negative ion, as seen in table salt (NA^+Cl^-).

irradiation (ir-RAY-dee-AY-shun) A process in which radiation energy is applied to foods, creating compounds (free radicals) within the food that destroy cell membranes, break down DNA, link proteins together, limit enzyme activity, and alter a variety of other proteins and cell functions that would otherwise lead to food spoilage. This process does not make the food radioactive.

ischemia (ih-SKI-mee-ah) Lack of blood flow due to mechanical obstruction of the blood supply, mainly from arterial narrowing.

ischemic stroke (ih-SKI-mik) A stroke caused by the absence of blood flow to a part of the brain.

isomers (EYE-so-mers) Different chemical structures for compounds that share the same chemical formula.

isotope (EYE-so-towp) An alternate form of a chemical element. It differs from other atoms of the same element in the number of neutrons in its nucleus.

jaundice (JOHN-diss) A yellow staining of the skin and sclera (white of the eye) resulting from a buildup of bile pigments in the bloodstream. Liver or gallbladder disease is often the cause.

jejunum (je-JOO-um) The first half of the small intestine (minus the first 12 in., which is the duodenum).

ketogenic (kee-toe-JEN-ik) A name often given to diets that lead to the abundant production of ketone bodies by the liver. This can be caused by a low carbohydrate intake.

ketone bodies (KEE-tone) Incomplete breakdown products of fat, containing three or four carbons. Most contain a chemical group called a ketone, hence the name. An example is acetoacetic acid.

ketosis (kee-TOE-sis) The condition of having a high concentration of ketone bodies and related breakdown products in the bloodstream and tissues.

kidney nephrons (NEF-rons) Units of kidney cells that filter wastes from the bloodstream and deposit them in the urine.

kilocalorie (kill-oh-KAL-oh-ree) (kcal) The heat needed to raise the temperature of 1000 g (1 L) of water 1 degree Celsius; also written as Calories, with a capital *C*.

kilojoule (KIL-oh-jool) (kJ) A measure of work. A mass of one kilogram moving at a velocity of 1 meter/sec possesses the energy of 1 kJ. One kcal equals 4.18 kJ.

kwashiorkor (kwash-ee-OR-core) A disease occurring primarily in young children who have an existing disease and who consume a marginal amount of energy and considerably insufficient protein in relation to needs. The child suffers from infections and exhibits edema, poor growth, weakness, and an increased susceptibility to further illness.

lacteal (LACK-tee-al) A small lymphatic duct associated with a villus of the small intestine.

lactic acid (LAK-tik) A three-carbon acid; also called *lactate*, formed during anaerobic cell metabolism; a partial breakdown product of glucose.

lactobacillus bifidus factor (lak-toe-bah-SIL-us BIFF-id-us) A protective factor secreted in the colostrum that encourages growth of beneficial bacteria in the newborn's intestines.

lacto-ovo-pesco vegetarian (lak-toe-o-vo-pes-co-vej-eh-TEAR-ree-an) A person who consumes only plant products, dairy products, eggs, and fish.

lacto-ovo-vegetarian (lak-toe-o-vo-vej-eh-TEAR-ree-an) A person who consumes only plant products, dairy products, and eggs.

lactose (LAK-tose) A sugar composed of glucose linked to another sugar called galactose.

lactose intolerance (primary and secondary) Primary lactose intolerance occurs when lactase production declines for no apparent reason. Secondary lactose intolerance occurs when a specific cause, such as long-standing diarrhea, results in a decline in lactase production.

lacto-vegetarian (lak-toe-vej-eh-TEAR-ree-an) A person who consumes only plant products and dairy products.

lanugo (lah-NEW-go) Downlike hair that appears after a person has lost much body fat through semi-starvation. The hair stands erect and traps air, acting as insulation for the body to compensate for the relative lack of body fat, which usually functions as insulation. Fetuses also have lanugo.

larva (LAR-va) An early developmental stage in the life history of some microorganisms, such as parasites.

larynx (LAYR-ingks) Structure located between the pharynx and trachea that contains the vocal cords; also called *voice box*.

laxative A medication or other substance that stimulates evacuation of the intestinal tract.

lean body mass The part of the human body that is free of all but essential body fat; calculated as body weight minus fat storage weight. This includes organs such as the brain, muscles, and liver, as well as blood and other body fluids.

lecithin (LESS-uh-thin) A group of phospholipids containing two fatty acids, a phosphate group, and a choline molecule. Lecithins are a group of compounds, since they can differ based on the types of fatty acids found on each lecithin molecule.

leptin (LEP-tin) A hormone made by adipose tissue that influences long-term regulation of fat mass. Leptin also influences reproductive functions, as well as other physiological processes, such as insulin release.

"let-down reflex" A reflex stimulated by infant suckling that causes the release (ejection) of milk from milk ducts in the mother's breasts.

leukemia (loo-KEY-mee-ah) A malignant neoplasm of blood-forming tissues, the bone marrow.

leukocyte (LOO-ko-site) A white blood cell.

leukotriene (LT) (loo-ko-TRY-een) An important mediator of many diseases involving inflammatory or hypersensitivity reactions, such as asthma; it is derived from fatty acids.

life expectancy The average length of life for a given group of people born in a certain year, such as this year.

life span The potential oldest age to which a person can reach.

lignins (LIG-nins) Insoluble fiber made up of a multiringed alcohol (noncarbohydrate) structure.

limiting amino acid The essential amino acid in the lowest concentration in a food or diet relative to body needs.

linoleic acid (lin-oh-LEE-ik) An essential omega-6 fatty acid with 18 carbon atoms and two double bonds (C18:2, ω-6).

lipase (LYE-pase) Fat-digesting enzyme; gastric lipase is produced by the stomach and pancreatic lipase by the pancreas.

lipid (LIP-id) A compound composed of much carbon and hydrogen, little oxygen, and sometimes other elements. Lipids dissolve in ether or benzene and include triglycerides, cholesterol, and phospholipids.

lipid peroxidation (per-OX-ih-day-shun) A process initiated by an environmental component that induces the formation of an organic free radical, R•. In the formation of a fatty acid of this type, first a carbon-carbon double bond is broken. The resulting breakdown products react with oxygen to form peroxides (a) or free radicals (b):

a.

```
    H H
    | |
—C—C—O—O—H
    | |
    H H
```

b.

```
    H H
    | |         •
—C—C—O—O
    | |
    H H
```

lipofuscin (lip-oh-FEW-shun) A brown pigment characteristically found in aging cells. It is present in lysosomes and is the product of the breakdown of unsaturated fatty acids and perhaps membrane damage.

lipogenesis (lye-poh-JEN-eh-sis) The building of fatty acids using derivatives of acetyl-CoA.

lipogenic (lye-poh-JEN-ik) Creating lipid. The liver is the major organ with lipogenic potential in the human body.

lipolysis (lye-POL-ih-sis) The breakdown of triglycerides to glycerol and fatty acids.

lipoprotein (ly-poh-PRO-teen) A compound found in the bloodstream containing a core of lipids with a shell of protein, phospholipid, and cholesterol.

lipoprotein lipase (lye-poh-PRO-teen LYE-pase) An enzyme attached to the outside of endothelial cells that line the capillaries in the blood vessels; it breaks down triglycerides into free fatty acids and glycerol.

lipoxin (LX) (lih-POX-in) Eicosanoids made by white blood cells that are involved in the immune system and allergic responses.

lipoxygenase (lih-POX-ih-jen-ace) An oxygenase enzyme used to synthesize leukotrienes and lipoxins, two types of eicosanoids.

liter (LEE-ter) (L) A measure of volume in the metric system. One liter equals 0.96 quarts.

lobules (LOB-you-els) Saclike structures in the breast that store milk.

long-chain fatty acids Fatty acids that contain 12 or more carbons.

low birth weight (LBW) Referring to any infant weighing less than 2.5 kg (5.5 lb) at birth; most commonly results from preterm birth; these infants are at higher risk for health problems.

low-density lipoprotein (LDL) The lipoprotein in the blood containing primarily cholesterol; elevated LDL-cholesterol is strongly linked to cardiovascular disease risk.

lower-body obesity The type of obesity, also called gynoid, in which fat storage is primarily located in the buttocks and thigh area.

lower esophageal sphincter (en-sof-ah-GEE-al-SFINK-ter) A circular muscle that constricts the opening of the esophagus to the stomach.

lower-quality (incomplete) proteins Dietary proteins that are low in or lack an ample amount of one or more of the amino acids essential for human protein needs.

lumen (LOO-men) The inside cavity of a tube, such as the GI tract or a blood vessel.

lymph (limf) A clear, plasmalike fluid that flows through lymph vessels.

lymph duct A large lymphatic vessel that empties lymph into the circulatory system.

lymph node A small tissue located along the course of the lymph vessels.

lymphatic system (lim-FAT-ick) System of vessels that can accept fluid surrounding cells and large particles, such as products of fat absorption. This lymph fluid eventually passes into the bloodstream via the lymphatic system.

lymphatic vessel (lim-FAT-ick) Vessel that carries lymph.

lymphocyte (LIM-fo-site) A class of white blood cells involved in the immune system, generally composing about 25% of all white blood cells. There are several types of lymphocytes with diverse functions, including antibody production, allergic reactions, graft rejections, tumor control, and regulation of the immune system.

lymphoma (lim-FO-ma) A malignant tumor arising from lymph nodes or other lymph tissues.

lysosome (LYE-so-som) A cellular organelle that contains digestive enzymes for use inside the cell for turnover of cell parts.

lysozyme (LYE-so-zime) A set of enzyme substances produced by a variety of cells; it can destroy bacteria by rupturing cell membranes.

macrocytic anemia (mack-ro-SIT-ik ah-NEM-ee-a) Anemia characterized by the presence of abnormally large red blood cells. A typical cause is folate or vitamin B-12 deficiency.

macrophage (MACK-ro-faj) Any large mononuclear phagocytic cell that is found in the tissues and is derived from a monocyte in the blood. Besides functioning as important phagocytes, macrophages secrete numerous cytokines and act as antigen-presenting cells.

major mineral A mineral vital to health that is required in the diet in amounts greater than 100 mg/day.

malignant (ma-LIG-nant) Essentially, to do anything malicious. In reference to a tumor, the property of spreading locally and to distant sites.

malnutrition Failing health that results from long-standing dietary practices that do not coincide with nutritional needs.

malonyl-CoA (MAL-o-kneel) A chemical intermediate in fatty-acid synthesis. The vitamin biotin participates in its synthesis.

maltose (MALL-tos) Glucose bonded to glucose.

mannitol (MAN-ih-tol) An alcohol derivative of fructose.

marasmus (ma-RAZ-mus) A disease that results from consuming a grossly insufficient amount of protein and energy; one of the diseases classed as protein-energy malnutrition. Victims have little or no fat stores, little muscle mass, and poor strength. Death from infection is common.

mass movement A peristaltic wave that simultaneously coordinates contraction over a large area of the large intestine. Mass movements propel material from one portion of the large intestine to another and from the large intestine into the rectum.

meconium (me-KO-nee-um) The first thick, mucuslike stool passed by the infant after birth.

medium-chain fatty acid A fatty acid that contains 6 to 10 carbons.

megadose Intake of a nutrient in excess of 10 times human need.

megaloblast (MEG-ah-low-blast) A large, nucleated, immature red blood cell that results from the inability of a precursor cell to divide when it normally should.

memory cells B lymphocytes that remain after an infection to convey permanent immunity.

menarche (men-AR-kee) The onset of menstruation. Menarche usually occurs around age 13, 2 or 3 years after the first signs of puberty start to appear.

menopause (MEN-oh-paws) The cessation of menses in women, usually beginning at about 50 years of age.

mesomorph (MEZ-oh-morf) A body type associated with average bone size, trunk size, and finger length.

metabolism (meh-TAB-oh-lizm) Chemical processes that occur in the body, enabling cells to release energy from foods, convert one substance into another, and prepare end products for excretion; in sum, the processes that allow for life.

metallothionein (meh-TAL-oh-THIGH-oh-neen) A protein that binds and regulates the release of zinc and copper in intestinal and liver cells.

metastasize (ma-TAS-tah-size) The spreading of disease from one part of the body to another, even to parts of the body that are remote from the site of original tumor. Cancer cells can spread via blood vessels, the lymphatic system, or direct growth of the tumor.

meter A measure of length in the metric system. One meter equals 39.4 in.

micelles (my-SELLS) Water-soluble spherical structures formed by lecithin and bile acids, in which the hydrophobic parts of the molecules face inward and the hydrophilic parts face outward. Lipids enclosed within micelles do not separate out into an oily layer, as they normally do when mixed with water.

microcytic (my-kro-SIT-ik) Literally means "small cell." Microcytic red blood cells are smaller than normal.

microcytic hypochromic anemia An anemia exhibiting small, pale red blood cells lacking sufficient hemoglobin and thus having reduced oxygen-carrying ability. It is often caused by an iron deficiency.

microfractures Small fractures, undetectable by X rays or other bone scans, that may develop constantly in bones.

microsomal ethanol oxidizing system (my-kro-SO-mol) An alternative pathway for alcohol metabolism when alcohol is in high concentration in the liver; uses rather than yields energy for the body, in contrast to alcohol dehydrogenase activity.

microvilli (my-kro-VIL-eye) Microscopic, hairlike projections of cell membranes of certain epithelial cells.

minerals The basic chemical elements used in the body to help form body structures and regulate body processes. Examples are calcium and iron.

miscarriage Termination of pregnancy that occurs before the fetus can survive; also called *spontaneous abortion.*

mitochondria (my-toe-KON-dree-ah) The main sites of energy production in a cell. They also contain the pathway for oxidizing fat for fuel, among other metabolic pathways.

modified food starch A product consisting of chemically linked starch molecules that are more stable than normal, unmodified starches.

molecule A group of atoms chemically linked together—that is, tightly connected by attractive forces (see also compound).

monoamine (MON-oh-ah-MEAN) A molecule containing one amide group.

monoglyceride (mon-oh-GLIS-er-ide) A breakdown product of a triglyceride consisting of one fatty acid bonded to a glycerol backbone.

monosaccharide (mon-oh-SACK-uh-ride) A class of simple sugars, such as glucose, that can be absorbed into the body without further chemical alteration.

monounsaturated fatty acid (mon-oh-un-SAT-ur-ated) A fatty acid containing one carbon-carbon double bond.

morbidity A disease condition or state; illness.

mortality This represents a population's death rate. The term *morbidity* refers to the amount of sickness present.

mottling (MOT-ling) The discoloration or marking of the surface of teeth from fluorosis.

mucilages (MYOU-sih-laj) Dietary fiber consisting of chains of galactose, mannose, and other monosaccharides; characteristically found in seaweed.

mucopolysaccharide (MYOO-ko-POL-ee-SAK-ah-ride) Substance containing protein and carbohydrate parts; found in bone and other organs.

mucosa (MYOO-co-saw) Mucous membrane consisting of cells and supporting connective tissue. In the digestive tract, there is also a layer of smooth muscle supporting the mucosa. Mucosa lines cavities that open to the outside of the body, such as the stomach and intestine, and generally contains glands that secrete mucus.

mucous membranes (MYOO-cuss) Also called mucosae, these line passageways open to the exterior environment.

mucus (MYOO-cuss) A thick fluid secreted by glands throughout the body. It contains a compound that has both carbohydrate and protein parts. It acts as a lubricant and means of protection for cells.

muscle fiber Component of a muscle cell.

muscle tissue A type of tissue adapted to contract.

mutagen (MYOO-tah-jen) Any agent that promotes a mutation (e.g., radioactive substances, X rays, or certain chemicals).

mutagenitity An agent that can induce or increase the frequency of mutation in an organism.

mutase (MYOO-tace) An enzyme that rearranges the functional groups on a molecule.

mutation (myoo-TAY-shun) A change in the chemistry of a gene that is perpetuated in subsequent divisions of the cell in which it occurred; a change in the sequence of the DNA base pairs.

mycotoxin (MY-ko-tok-sin) A group of toxic compounds produced by molds, such as aflatoxin B-1 found on moldy grains.

myelin (MY-eh-lyn) A combined lipid and protein (lipoprotein) that covers nerve fibers.

myocardial depression Decreased activity of the heart muscle.

myocardial infarction (MY-oh-CARD-ee-ahl in-FARK-shun) Death of part of the heart muscle.

myofibrils (my-oh-FIB-rils) A bundle of contractile fibers within a muscle cell.

myoglobin (my-oh-GLOW-bin) The iron-containing protein that controls the rate of diffusion of oxygen (O_2) from red blood cells into the muscle cells.

myosin (MY-oh-sin) A thick filament protein that connects with actin to cause a muscle contraction.

negative balance The state in which nutrient losses from the body exceed intake, as in cases of starvation.

negative energy balance The state in which energy intake is less than energy expended, resulting in weight loss.

neoplasm (KNEE-oh-plaz-em) New and abnormal growth of tissues, which may be benign or cancerous.

nephron (NEF-ron) The functional unit of the kidney.

nerve A bundle of nerve axons outside the central nervous system.

nervous tissue Tissues composed of highly branched, elongated cells that transport nerve impulses from one part of the body to another.

neural tube defect A defect in the formation of the neural tube occurring during early fetal development. These are seen in about 2500 infants per year in the United States. This type of defect results in various nervous system disorders, such as spina bifida. Folate deficiency in the pregnant woman increases the risk of the fetus's developing this disorder.

neuroendocrine (nyoo-row-EN-do-krin) Substances or functions linked to combined action of both endocrine glands and the nervous system. Examples include substances released from glands in response to nerve stimulation.

neuroglia (nyoo-row-GLEE-ah) Specialized support cells of the central nervous system.

neuromuscular junction (nyoo-row-MUS-kyo-lar) A chemical synapse between a motor neuron and a muscle fiber.

neuron (NYOUR-on) The structural and functional unit of the nervous system. Consists of cell body, dendrites and axon.

neuropeptide Y (nyoo-row-PEP-tide) A small protein (36 amino acids) that increases food intake and reduces energy expenditure when injected into the brain of experimental animals.

neurotransmitter (nyoo-row-TRANS-mit-er) A compound made by a nerve cell that allows for communication between it and other cells.

neutron (NEW-tron) The part of an atom that has no charge.

neutrophil (NEW-tro-fil) A type of phagocytic white blood cell, normally constituting about 60% to 70% of the white blood cell count. Forms highly toxic compounds, which destroy bacteria.

nicotinamide adenine dinucleotide (NAD) A compound that readily accepts and donates electrons and hydrogen ions; made from the vitamin niacin.

night blindness A vitamin A deficiency condition in which the retina in the eye cannot adjust to low amounts of light.

nitrate (NI-trait) A nitrogen-containing compound used to cure meats. Its use contributes a pink color to meats and confers some resistance to bacterial growth.

nitrosamine (ni-TROH-sa-mean) A carcinogen formed from nitrates and breakdown products of amino acids; can lead to stomach cancer.

nonessential (dispensable) amino acids Amino acids that can be synthesized by a healthy body in sufficient amounts; there are 11 nonessential amino acids. These are also termed dispensable amino acids.

nonexercise activity thermogenesis (NEAT) Adaptive energy expended via increased heat production, such as when one is subjected to overfeeding.

nonheme iron (non-HEEM) Iron provided from plant sources and animal tissues other than hemoglobin and myoglobin. Nonheme iron is less efficiently absorbed than heme iron, as absorption is also more closely dependent on body needs.

nonpolar A neutral compound; no positive or negative poles present.

nonspecific immunity Defenses that stop the invasion of pathogens. Requires no previous encounter with a pathogen.

no-observable-effect level (NOEL) The highest dose of an additive that produces no deleterious health effects in animals.

norepinephrine (nor-ep-ih-NEF-rin) A neurotransmitter from nerve endings and a hormone from the adrenal gland. It is involved in hunger regulation, blood glucose regulation, and other body processes.

nuclear receptor A site on the DNA in a cell where compounds (such as hormones) bind. Cells that contain DNA receptors for a specific compound are affected by that compound.

nucleoli, nucleolus (NEW-klee-o-lie) Center for production of ribosomes within the cell nucleus.

nucleus (NEW-klee-us) In chemistry, the core of an atom; it contains protons and neutrons.

nutrient density The ratio calculated by dividing a food's contribution to the needs for a nutrient by its contribution to energy needs. When the contribution to nutrient needs exceeds its energy contribution, the food is considered to have a favorable nutrient density.

nutrient receptors Proposed sites in the small intestine that contribute signals to the brain that in turn elicit a feeling of satiety. These receptors are stimulated by nutrient exposure in the lumen of the small intestine

nutrients Chemical substances in food that nourish the body by providing energy, building materials, and factors to regulate needed chemical reactions in the body. The body either can't make these nutrients or can't make them fast enough for its needs.

nutrition The Council on Food and Nutrition of the American Medical Association defines nutrition as "the science of food; the nutrients and the substances therein; their action, interaction, and balance in relation to health and disease; and the process by which the organism (i.e., body) ingests, digests, absorbs, transports, utilizes, and excretes food substances."

nutritionist A person who advises about nutrition and/or works in the field of food and nutrition. In many states in the United States, a person does not need formal training to use this title. Some states reserve this title for registered dietitians.

nutrition label A label containing "Nutrition Facts" that must be included on most foods. It depicts nutrient content in comparison to the Daily Values set by FDA.

nutrition status The nutritional health of a person as determined by **a**nthropometric measures (height, weight, circumferences, and so on), **b**iochemical measures of nutrients or their by-products in blood and urine, a **c**linical (physical) examination, and a **d**ietary analysis (ABCD).

nystagmus (ni-STAG-mus) Involuntary, rapid, rhythmic movement of the eyeball.

obesity (oh-BEES-ih-tee) A condition characterized by excess body fat, typically defined in clinical settings as body mass index (BMI) $\geq$ to 30.

oleic acid (oh-LAY-ik) An omega-9 fatty acid with 18 carbons and one double bond (C18:1, ω-9).

olfactory (ol-FAK-toe-ree) Sense of smell.

olfactory cells Cells in the nasal region that discriminate numerous chemical molecules and transmit that information to the brain. This information represents one of the components of flavor.

oligosaccharides (ol-ih-go-SAK-ah-rides) Carbohydrates containing 2 to 10 monosaccharide units.

omega-3 (ω-3) fatty acid Unsaturated fatty acid with the first double bond on the third carbon atom from the methyl end ($-CH_3$).

omega-6 (ω-6) fatty acid Unsaturated fatty acid with the first double bond on the sixth carbon atom from the methyl end ($-CH_3$).

omnivore (AHM-nih-voor) A person who consumes foods from both plant and animal sources.

oncogene (AHN-ko-jeen) Gene that codes for a protein that in turn leads to cellular growth and development.

oncotic force (ahn-KAH-tik) The osmotic potential exerted by blood proteins in the bloodstream.

opportunistic infection An infection that arises primarily in people who are already ill because of another disease.

organ A group of tissues designed to perform a specific function—for example, the heart. It contains muscle tissue, nerve tissue, and so on.

organelles (OAR-gan-ells) A compartment, particle, or filament that performs specialized functions within a cell.

organic Anything that contains carbon atoms chemically bonded to hydrogen atoms in the structure.

organism A living thing. The human body is an organism consisting of many organs, which act in a coordinated manner to support life.

osmolality (oz-mo-LAL-ih-tee) A measure of the total concentration of a solution; the number of particles of solute per kilogram of solvent.

osmosis (oz-MO-sis) The passage of a solvent (water) through a semipermeable membrane from a less concentrated solution to a more concentrated compartment.

osmotic pressure The exerted pressure needed to keep particles in a solution from drawing liquid toward them across a semipermeable membrane.

osteoblast (OS-tee-oh-blast) Cells in bone that secrete mineral and bone matrix.

osteocalcin (OS-tee-oh-KAL-sin) A protein produced in bone that is thought to bind calcium; synthesis of osteocalcin is aided by vitamin K.

osteoclasts (OS-tee-oh-klasts) Bone cells that arise originally from a type of white blood cell. Osteoclasts secrete substances that lead to bone erosion. This erosion can set the stage for subsequent bone mineralization.

osteomalacia (OS-tee-oh-mal-AY-shuh) Softening of the bones that occurs in adults as the result of bone decalcification linked to inadequate vitamin D status.

osteopenia (os-tee-oh-PEE-nee-ah) Decreased bone mass caused by cancer, hyperthyroidism, or other reasons.

osteoporosis (os-tee-oh-po-ROH-sis) Decreased bone density where no outward causes can be found. This bone loss is related to the effects of aging, poor diet, and hormonal effects of menopause in women.

ostomy (OS-toe-me) A surgically created short-circuit in intestinal flow where the end point usually opens from the abdominal cavity rather than the anus—for example, a colostomy.

overnutrition A state in which nutritional intake exceeds the body's needs.

ovum (OH-vum) The egg cell from which a fetus eventually develops if the egg is fertilized by a sperm cell.

oxalic acid (oxalate) An organic acid found in spinach, rhubarb, and other leafy green vegetables that can depress the absorption of certain minerals present in the food, such as calcium.

oxidation (ox-ih-DAY-shun) Loss of an electron by an atom or a molecule; in metabolism, often associated with a gain of oxygen or loss of hydrogen. Oxidation (loss of an electron) and reduction (gain of an electron) take place simultaneously in metabolism, because an electron that is lost by one atom is accepted by another.

oxidize (OX-ih-dize) Specifically, to lose an electron or gain an oxygen atom.

oxidizing agent In one sense, a substance capable of capturing an electron from another compound. A compound is "oxidized" when it loses an electron.

oxygenase (OK-si-jen-ace) Enzyme that incorporates oxygen directly into a molecule.

oxytocin (ok-si-TO-sin) A hormone secreted by the posterior part of the pituitary gland. It causes contraction of the musclelike cells surrounding the ducts of the breasts and the smooth muscle of the uterus.

p53 gene A tumor suppressant gene that can prevent inappropriate cell division.

pacemaker A group of cells in the heart that regulates contractions.

palatable (PAL-it-ah-bull) Pleasing to taste.

parasthesia (para-STEE-zya) An abnormal spontaneous sensation, such as of burning, prickling, and numbness.

parathyroid hormone (PTH) A hormone made by the parathyroid glands that increases synthesis of the vitamin D hormone and aids calcium release from bone and calcium uptake by the kidneys, among other functions.

passive absorption (transport) Absorption that uses no energy. It requires permeability for the substance through the wall of the small intestine and a concentration gradient higher in the lumen of the intestine than in the absorptive cell. The higher concentration of the substance in the lumen of the intestine in comparison with that in the absorptive cells promotes the absorption of the nutrient.

pasteurizing (PAS-tur-i-zing) Heating food products rapidly to kill pathogenic microorganisms.

pathway A metabolic progression of individual steps from starting materials to ending products, such as $C_6H_{12}O_6$ (glucose) + O_2 yielding CO_2 + H_2O.

pectin (PEK-tin) Dietary fiber containing chains of galacturonic acid and other monosaccharides; characteristically found between plant cell walls.

peer-reviewed journal A journal that publishes research only after two or three scientists who were not part of the study agree it was well conducted and the results are fairly represented. Thus, the research has been approved by peers of the research team.

pellagra (peh-LAHG-rah) A disease characterized by inflammation of the skin, diarrhea, and eventual mental incapacity; results from an insufficient amount of the vitamin niacin in the diet.

pepsin (PEP-sin) A protein-digesting enzyme produced by the stomach.

peptide A few amino acids chemically bonded together; often two to four.

peptide bond A chemical bond formed to link amino acids in a protein.

percentile Classification of a measurement of a unit into divisions of 100 units.

peripheral nervous system (PNS) (peh-RIF-er-al) The nerves of the central nervous system that lie outside the brain and spinal cord.

peripheral neuropathy (peh-RIF-er-al nyoo-ROP-ah-thee) Impaired sensory, motor, and reflex actions affecting arms and legs, and causing calf muscle tenderness and difficulty in rising from a squatting position.

peristalsis (per-ih-STALL-sis) A coordinated muscular contraction that is used to propel food down the gastrointestinal tract.

pernicious anemia The anemia that results from the inability to absorb sufficient vitamin B-12; it is associated with nerve degeneration, which can result in eventual paralysis and death.

peroxisome (per-OK-si-som) Cell organelle that destroys toxic products within the cell.

peroxyl radical (per-OK-syl) Compounds containing O-O are peroxides. The radical has one unpaired electron designated ROO•.

pesticide A general term for an agent that can destroy bacteria, fungi, insects, rodents, or other pests.

pH A measure of relative acidity or alkalinity of a solution. The pH scale is 0–14. A ph below 7 is acidic; a pH above 7 is alkaline.

phagocytic cells (fag-oh-SIT-ick) Cells that engulf substances; these cells include neutrophils and macrophages.

phagocytosis (FAG-oh-sigh-TOW-sis) A form of active absorption in which the absorptive cell forms an indentation, and particles or fluids entering the indentation are then engulfed by the cell.

pharynx (FAIR-ingks) The organ of the digestive tract and respiratory tract located at the back of the oral and nasal cavities.

phenylalanine (fen-ihl-AL-ah-neen) An essential (indispensable) amino acid.

phenylketonuria (PKU) (fen-ihl-kee-toh-NEW-ree-ah) A disease caused by a defect in the ability of the liver to metabolize the amino acid phenylalanine into the amino acid tyrosine. Toxic by-products of phenylalanine can then build up in the body and lead to mental retardation.

phosphocreatine (PCr) (fos-fo-CREE-a-tin) A high-energy compound that can be used to re-form adenosine triphosphate (ATP) from adenosine diphosphate (ADP).

phospholipid Any of a class of fat-related substances that contain phosphorus, fatty acids, and a nitrogen-containing base. The phospholipids are an essential part of every cell.

photoisomerization (foto-eye-SOM-er-eye-zay-shun) Molecular isomerization of a compound by the energy of light.

photon (FO-ton) A unit of light intensity at the retina, having the brightness of one candle.

photosynthesis (foto-SIN-tha-sis) The process by which plants use solar energy from the sun to produce energy-yielding compounds, such as glucose.

phylloquinone (fil-oh-KWIN-own) A form of vitamin K that comes from plants; also called vitamin K_1.

physiological anemia The normal increase in blood volume in pregnancy that dilutes the concentration of red blood cells, resulting in anemia; also called *hemodilution*.

phytic acid (phytate) (FY-tick, FY-tate) A constituent of plant fibers that binds positive ions to its multiple phosphate groups.

phytobezoar (fy-tow-BEE-zor) A pellet of fiber characteristically found in the stomach.

phytochemical A chemical found in plants. Some phytochemicals may contribute to a reduced risk of cancer or cardiovascular disease in people who consume them regularly.

pica (PIE-kah) The practice of eating nonfood items, such as dirt, laundry starch, or clay.

placebo (plah-SEE-bo) A fake medicine used to disguise the roles of participants in an experiment; if fake surgery is performed, that is called a *sham operation*.

placenta (plah-SEN-tah) An organ that forms in pregnant women. Through this organ, oxygen and nutrients from the mother's blood are transferred to the fetus and fetal wastes are removed. The placenta also releases hormones that maintain the pregnant state.

plaque (PLACK) In terms of cardiovascular disease, a cholesterol-rich substance deposited in the blood vessels; it contains various white blood cells, smooth muscle cells, connective tissue, cholesterol and other lipids, and eventually calcium; sometimes called *atherosclerotic plaque* to distinguish it from bacterial plaque, which forms on teeth.

plasma The fluid, extracellular portion of the circulating blood. This includes the blood serum plus all blood-clotting factors. In contrast, serum is the fluid that results after the blood is first allowed to clot before being centrifuged; this will not contain the blood-clotting factors.

plasma cells Mature B lymphocytes; these can produce 2,000 antibodies proteins per second.

polar A compound with distinct positive and negative charges (poles) on it. These charges act like poles on a magnet.

polyglutamate form of folate (POL-ee-GLOO-tah-mate) Folate with more than one glutamate molecule attached.

polyneuropathy (POL-ee-nyoo-ROP-ah-thee) A disease process involving a number of peripheral nerves.

polypeptide (POL-ee-PEP-tide) Fifty to 100 amino acids bonded together.

polysaccharide (POL-ee-SACK-uh-ride) Carbohydrate containing many glucose units, up to 3000 or more; also known as complex carbohydrates.

polyunsaturated fatty acid A fatty acid containing two or more carbon-carbon double bonds.

pool The amount of a nutrient found within the body that can be easily mobilized when needed.

portal vein A large vein that distributes blood from the intestine to the liver through capillaries.

post-translational Occurring or formed after protein synthesis is completed by the ribosomes.

positive balance A state in which nutrient intake exceeds losses. This causes a net gain of the nutrient in the body, such as when tissue protein is gained during growth.

positive energy balance State in which energy intake is greater than energy expended, generally resulting in weight gain.

power stroke The process by which the thick filament pulls alongside the thin filament in a muscle cell, causing muscle contraction.

precursor A compound that comes before; to precede.

preeclampsia (pre-ee-KLAMP-see-ah) Part of the disease pregnancy-induced hypertension. This serious disorder can include high blood pressure, kidney failure, convulsions, and even death of the mother and fetus. Mild cases are known as preeclampsia: more severe cases are called eclampsia or, more correctly, toxemia.

pregnancy-induced hypertension A serious disorder that can include high blood pressure, kidney failure, convulsion, and even death of the mother and the fetus. A poor diet (especially a deficient calcium intake) increases the risk for developing this disease.

premenstrual syndrome A disorder (also referred to as *PMS*) found in some women a few days before the onset of menses and characterized by depression, anxiety, headache, bloating, and mood swings. Severe cases are currently termed premenstrual dysphoric disorder (PDD).

preservatives Compounds that extend the shelf life of foods by inhibiting microbial growth or minimizing the destructive effect of oxygen and metals.

preterm An infant born before 37 weeks of gestation; also referred to as premature.

prevalence The number of people at any one time who have a specific disease, such as obesity or cancer.

previtamin D$_3$ Precursor of vitamin D$_3$. Formed as a result of sunlight opening a ring on 7-dehyrocholestrol.

primary disease A disease process that is not simply caused by another disease process.

primary prevention The attempt to prevent a disease from developing in the first place—for example, following a diet low in saturated fat and cholesterol in an attempt to prevent cardiovascular disease.

primary structure of a protein The order of amino acids in the protein molecule.

progestins (pro-JES-tins) Hormones, including progesterone, that are necessary for maintaining pregnancy and lactation.

prognosis (prog-NO-sis) A forecast of the course and end of a disease.

prohormone Precursor of a hormone.

prolactin (pro-LACK-tin) A hormone secreted by the mother that stimulates the synthesis of milk.

prospective Research that follows individuals during a current course of treatment. This is in contrast to retrospective research, which examines the past habits of individuals.

prostacyclin (PGI) (prost-tah-SIGH-klin) Eicosanoid made by the blood vessel walls that is a potent inhibitor of blood clotting, (PGI$_2$).

prostaglandin (PG) (pros-tah-GLAN-din) One of several potent hormonelike compounds made of polyunsaturated fatty acids that produce diverse effects in the body.

prostate gland (PROS-tait) A solid, chestnut-shaped organ surrounding the first part of the urethra in the male. The prostate gland is situated immediately under the bladder and in front of the rectum. The prostate gland secretes substances into the semen as the fluid passes through ducts leading from the seminal vesicles into the urethra.

protein Food and body components made of amino acids; they contain carbon, hydrogen, oxygen, nitro-

gen, and sometimes other elements, in a specific configuration. Proteins contain the form of nitrogen most easily used by the human body.

protein-efficiency ratio (PER) A measure of protein quality in a food, determined by the ability of a protein to support the growth of a young animal.

protein-energy malnutrition (PEM) A condition resulting from regularly consuming insufficient amounts of energy and protein. The deficiency eventually results in body wasting of primarily lean tissue and an increased susceptibility to infection.

protein quality A measure of the ability of a food protein to support body growth and maintenance.

prothrombin (pro-THROM-bin) One of the numerous proteins that participate in the formation of blood clots. Conversion of its precursor protein to the active blood-clotting factor in the liver requires vitamin K.

proton (PRO-ton) The part of an atom that is positively charged.

protooncogenes (pro-toe-ON-ko-jeans) Genes that code for proteins that in turn cause a resting cell to divide.

psyllium (SIL-ee-um) A mostly soluble type of dietary fiber found in the seeds of the plantain plant.

pulmonary circulation (pulmonary circuit) The system of blood vessels from the right ventricle of the heart to the lungs and back to the left atrium of the heart.

pyloric sphincter (pi-LOR-ik SFINK-ter) Ring of smooth muscle between the stomach and the duodenum.

racemase Enzymes that catalyze reactions involving structural rearrangement of a molecule (e.g., conversion of D-alanine isomer to L-alanine isomer).

radiation Literally, energy that is emitted from a center in all directions. Various forms of radiation energy include X rays and ultraviolet rays from the sun.

raffinose (RAF-ih-nos) An indigestible oligosaccharide made of three monosaccharides (galactose-glucose-fructose).

rancid (RAN-sid) Containing products of decomposed fatty acids; they yield unpleasant flavors and odors.

reactive hypoglycemia (HIGH-po-gligh-SEE-mee-uh) Low blood glucose that may follow a meal high in simple sugars, with corresponding symptoms of irritability, headache, nervousness, sweating, and confusion; actually called *postprandial hypoglycemia*. The actual number of cases of this disease in the population is low.

reactive oxygen species Several oxygen derivatives produced during the formation of ATP. Formed constantly in the human body and shown to kill bacteria and inactivate proteins, they are also implicated in a number of diseases. They have been linked to inflammatory processes and cancer development.

receptive framework for learning The process by which a person opens up to learning more about a problem; it usually involves seeking more information about the issue from books and people. In the case of seeking behavior changes, it involves examining background experience to evaluate whether a behavior change is feasible.

receptor (ri-SEP-ter) A site in a cell at which compounds (such as hormones) bind. Cells that contain receptors for a specific compound are partially controlled by that compound.

receptor pathway for cholesterol uptake A process by which LDL particles (cholesterol-containing) are bound by cell receptors and incorporated into the cell.

recombinant DNA (re-KOM-bih-nant) A molecule composed of the DNA of two different species spliced together, such as a combination of bacterial and human DNA used to produce unique bacteria that now can synthesize human proteins.

Recommended Dietary Allowances (RDAs) Recommended intakes of nutrients that meet the needs of nearly all (97 to 98 percent) healthy individuals of similar age and gender. These are established by the Food and Nutrition Board of the National Academy of Sciences.

Recommended Nutrient Intake (RNI) The Canadian version of RDA published in 1990.

redox agents (RE-doks) Chemicals that can readily undergo both oxidation (loss of an electron) and reduction (gain of an electron).

reducing agent A compound capable of donating electrons (also hydrogens) to another compound.

reduction In chemical terms, the gain of an electron by an atom; takes place simultaneously with oxidation (loss of an electron by an atom) in metabolism because an electron that is lost by one atom is accepted by another. In metabolism, reduction is often associated with the gain of hydrogen.

Reference Daily Intake (RDI) Nutrient-intake standards set by FDA based on the 1968 RDA standards for various vitamins and minerals. RDIs have been set for four categories of people: infants, toddlers, people over 4 years of age, and pregnant or lactating women. Generally the highest RDA value in each category is used as the RDI. The RDIs constitute part of the Daily Values used in food labeling.

registered dietitian (rd) (dye-eh-TISH-shun) A person who has completed a baccalaureate degree program approved by The American Dietetic Association, performed at least 900 hours of supervised professional practice, and passed a registration examination.

reinforcement A reaction by others in response to a person's behavior. Positive reinforcement entails encouragement; negative reinforcement entails criticism or penalty.

relapse prevention A series of strategies used to help prevent and cope with weight-control lapses, such as recognizing high-risk situations and deciding beforehand on appropriate responses.

remodeling The constant building and breakdown of bone throughout life.

renin (REN-in) An enzyme formed in the kidney in response to low blood pressure; it acts on a blood protein to produce angiotensin I.

requirement The amount of a nutrient required by one person to maintain health. This varies between individuals. We do not know our individual requirements for each nutrient.

reserve capacity The extent to which an organ can preserve essentially normal function despite decreasing cell number or cell activity.

resorption The loss of a substance by physiologic or pathologic means.

respiration The utilization of oxygen; in the human organism, the inhalation of oxygen and the exhalation of carbon dioxide; in cells, the oxidation (electron removal) of food molecules, particularly in the citric acid cycle, to obtain energy.

restraint A feeling that occurs as a result of restricted food intake, often associated with the belief that there are good and bad foods.

retinoids (RET-ih-noyds) A collective term for the biologically active forms of vitamin A, including retinol, retinal, and retinoic acid.

reverse transport of cholesterol The process by which cholesterol is picked up by HDL particles and transferred to the liver or to other lipoproteins that can dispose of it in the liver.

rhodopsin (row-DOP-sin) Photoreceptor in the rod cells composed of 11-cis retinal and opsin.

riboneucleic acid (RNA) (RI-bow-new-CLAY-ik) Single-stranded nucleic acid involved in the transcription of genetic information and translation of that information into protein structure; contains the sugar ribose. Comes in three forms: messenger RNA, ribosomal RNA, and transfer RNA.

ribose (RIGH-bos) A five-carbon sugar found in genetic material— specifically, RNA.

ribosomes (RI-bow-soms) Cytoplasmic particles that mediate the linking together of amino acids to form proteins; attached to endoplasmic reticulum as bound ribosomes, or suspended in cytoplasm as free ribosomes.

rickets (RIK-its) A disease characterized by softening of the bones caused by poor calcium deposition. This deficiency disease arises in infants and children with a poor vitamin D status.

risk factor A term used frequently when discussing diseases and factors contributing to their development. A risk factor is an aspect of our lives—such as heredity, lifestyle choices (e.g., smoking), or nutritional habits—that make us more likely to develop a disease.

R-protein A protein produced by the salivary glands that enhances absorption of vitamin B-12, possibly protecting the vitamin during its passage through the stomach.

RXR, RAR Abbreviation for retinoid X receptor and retinoic acid receptor. These subfamilies of retinoid receptors interact with retinoic acid and bind to specific sites on DNA. This allows for cell differentiation.

saccharin (SACK-ah-rin) An alternate sweetener that yields no energy to the body; it is 300 times sweeter than sucrose.

saliva (sah-LIGH-vah) A watery fluid, produced by the salivary glands in the mouth, that contains lubricants, enzymes, and other substances.

salivary amylase (SAL-ih-var-ee AM-ih-lace) Starch-digesting enzyme produced by salivary glands.

salt Generally refers to a compound of sodium and chloride in a 40:60 ratio.

sarcoma (sar-KO-mah) A malignant tumor arising from connective tissues.

sarcomere (SAR-ko-meer) A portion of a muscle fiber that is considered the functional unit of a myofibril.

satiety (suh-TIE-uh-tee) State in which there is no longer a desire to eat; a feeling of satisfaction.

saturated fatty acid A fatty acid containing no carbon-carbon double bonds.

scavenger pathway for cholesterol uptake A process by which LDL particles (cholesterol-containing) are taken up by scavenger cells embedded in the blood vessels.

scurvy (SKER-vee) The deficiency disease that results after a few weeks to months of consuming a diet that lacks vitamin C; pinpoint hemorrhages on the skin are an early sign.

sebum (SEA-bum) A substance secreted by sebaceous glands consisting of keratin and cellular material.

secondary deficiency A deficiency caused not by lack of the nutrient in question but by lack of a substance or process that is needed for that nutrient to function.

secondary disease A disease process that develops as a result of another disease.

secondary prevention Interventions to prevent further development of a disease so as to reduce the risk of further damage to health; for example, smoking cessation for a person who has already suffered a heart attack.

secretin (SEE-kreh-tin) A hormone that causes bicarbonate ion release from the pancreas.

secretory vesicles (see-KRE-tor-ee VES-ih-kels) Membrane-bound vesicles produced by the Golgi apparatus; contains protein to be secreted by cell.

segmentation Contractions of the circular muscles in the intestines that lead to a dividing and mixing of the intestinal contents. This action aids digestion and absorption of nutrients.

self-monitoring A process of tracking a behavior and conditions affecting that behavior; actions are usually recorded in a diary, along with location, time, and state of mind. This can be a tool to help people understand more about their eating habits.

self-talk The internal dialogue that we carry on in our heads as we sort out beliefs, feelings, attitudes, and events happening in our lives.

semiessential amino acids Amino acids that, when consumed, spare the need to use an essential amino acid for their synthesis. Tyrosine in the diet, for example, spares the need to use phenylalanine for tyrosine synthesis.

sequesterants (see-KWES-ter-ants) Compounds that bind free metal ions. By so doing, they reduce the ability of ions to cause rancidity in foods containing fat.

serotonin (ser-oh-TONE-in) A neurotransmitter synthesized from the amino acid tryptophan that appears to both decrease the desire to eat carbohydrates and to induce sleep.

serum (SEER-um) The portion of the blood fluid remaining after (1) the blood is allowed to clot and (2) the red and white blood cells and other solid matter are removed by centrifugation.

set point Often refers to the close regulation of body weight. It is not known what cells control this set point or how it actually functions in weight regulation. There is evidence, however, that mechanisms exist that help regulate weight.

sexually transmitted disease (STD) A contagious disease usually acquired by sexual intercourse or genital contact. Common examples include gonorrhea and syphilis; also called venereal disease.

short-chain fatty acids Fatty acids that contain fewer than eight carbon atoms.

sickle cell disease (sickle cell anemia) An anemia that results from a malformation of the red blood cell because of an incorrect primary structure in part of its hemoglobin protein chains. The disease can lead to episodes of severe bone and joint pain, abdominal pain, headache, convulsions, paralysis, and even death.

sign A change in health status that is apparent on physical examination.

skeletal muscle Muscle responsible for voluntary body movements.

slough (SLUF) To shed or cast off.

small-for-gestational age (SGA) (jes-TAY-shun-al) Referring to infants who weigh less than the expected weight for their length of gestation. This corresponds to less than 2.5 kg (5.5 lb) in a full-term newborn. A preterm infant who is also SGA will most likely develop some medical complications.

smooth muscle Muscle under involuntary control; found in GI tract, artery walls, respiratory passages, urinary tract and reproductive tract.

sodium bicarbonate (SO-dee-um bi-KAR-bow-nait) An alkaline substance made basically of sodium and carbon dioxide ($NaHCO_3$).

soft palate (PAL-it) The fleshy posterior portion of the roof of the mouth.

soluble fibers (SOL-you-bull) Fibers that either dissolve or swell in water and are metabolized (fermented) by bacteria in the large intestine. These include pectins, gums, and mucilages.

solvent A substance that other substances dissolve in.

sorbitol (SOR-bih-tol) An alcohol derivative of glucose that yields about 3 kcal/g but is slowly absorbed from the small intestine. It is used in some sugarless gums and dietetic foods.

specific heat Heat required to raise the temperature of 1 g of a substance 1°C. Water has a high specific heat, meaning that a relatively large amount of heat is required to raise its temperature; therefore, it tends to resist large temperature fluctuations.

specific immunity Function of lymphocytes directed at specific antigens.

sphincter (SFINK-ter) A muscular valve that controls flow of foodstuff in the GI tract.

spontaneous abortion Any cessation of pregnancy and expulsion of the embryo or nonviable fetus as the result of natural causes, such as a genetic defect or developmental problem; also called *miscarriage*.

spores Dormant reproductive cells capable of forming into adult organisms without the help of another cell. Various fungi and bacteria form spores.

sports anemia (ah-NEE-me-ah) A decrease in the blood's ability to carry oxygen, found in athletes, which may be caused by iron loss through perspiration and feces, red blood cell destruction due to the impact of exercise as the foot strikes the ground, or increased blood volume.

stable isotope An isotope is a specific form of a chemical element. It differs from atoms of other forms (isotopes) of the same element in the number of neutrons in its nucleus. "Stable" means that the isotope is not radioactive, in contrast to some other types of isotopes.

stachyose (STACK-ee-os) An indigestible oligosaccharide made of four monosaccharides (galactose-galactose-glucose-fructose).

starch A carbohydrate made of multiple units of glucose attached together in a form the body can digest; also known as *complex carbohydrate.*

stem cell Cell that, in an adult body, divides continuously and forms a supply of cells for differentiation.

stenosis (ste-NO-sis) Narrowing or stricture of a duct or canal.

steroids (STARE-oyds) A group of hormones and related compounds that are derivatives of cholesterol.

sterol (STARE-ol) A compound containing a multiring (steroid) structure and a hydroxyl group (-OH).

stimulus control Altering the environment to minimize the stimuli for a "problem" behavior—for example, removing foods from sight and storing them in kitchen cabinets.

stress fracture A fracture that occurs from repeated jarring of a bone. Common sites include bones of the foot.

stroke The loss of body function that results from a blood clot or other change in the brain that affects blood flow. This in turn causes the death of brain tissue. Also called a cerebrovascular accident.

subclinical Not seen on a clinical (physical) examination.

subclinical disease Disease or disorder that is present but not severe enough to produce symptoms that can be detected or diagnosed.

submucosal layer (sub-myoo-KO-sal) A layer of blood and lymph vessels along with nerve fibers and connective tissue that stretch the whole length of the GI tract.

sucralose (SOO-kra-los) An alternative sweetener that has chlorines in place of some hydroxyl (-OH) groups on sucrose. It is 600 times sweeter than sucrose.

sucrose (SOO-kros) Fructose bonded to glucose; table sugar.

sugar Simple carbohydrate form with a chemical composition $(CH_2O)_n$. Most sugars form ringed structures when in solution.

superoxide dismutase (soo-per-OX-ide DISS-myoo-tase) An enzyme that can quench (deactivate) a superoxide negative free radical $(O_2^{•})$. This can contain the mineral manganese, copper, or zinc.

sympathetic nervous system Part of the nervous system that regulates involuntary vital functions, including the activity of the heart, smooth muscles, and adrenal glands. The sympathetic nervous system specifically accelerates heart rate, constricts blood vessels, and raises blood pressure. The parasympathetic nervous system slows heart rate, increases intestinal peristalsis and gland activity, and relaxes sphincters.

symptom A change in health status noted by the person with the problem, such as a stomach pain.

synapse (SIN-aps) The space between axon of one neuron and the dendrite of another neuron.

syndrome X A condition in which the person has insulin resistance, hypertension, increased blood triglycerides, and decreased HDL levels. This condition is usually accompanied by obesity, lack of physical activity, and a diet high in refined carbohydrates.

system A collection of organs that work together to perform an overall function.

systemic circulation (system circuit) The part of the circulatory system concerned with the flow of blood from the left ventricle to the body and back to the right atrium.

systolic blood pressure (sis-TOL-lik) The pressure in the arterial blood vessels associated with the pumping of blood from the heart.

telomerase (teh-LO-mer-ace) Enzyme that maintains length and completeness of chromosomes.

telomeres (TELL-oh-meers) Caps at the end of chromosomes.

tendon (TEN-don) Dense regular connective tissue that attaches a muscle to a bone.

teratogenic (ter-A-toe-jen-ic) Tending to produce physical defects in a developing fetus.

tertiary structure of a protein (TER-she-air-ee) The three-dimensional structure of a protein, formed by interactions of amino acids placed far apart in the primary structure.

tetany (TET-ah-nee) A state marked by sharp contraction of muscles with failure to relax afterward; usually caused by abnormal calcium metabolism.

theory An explanation for a phenomenon that has numerous lines of evidence to support it.

thermic effect of food (TEF) The increase in metabolism that occurs during the digestion, absorption, and metabolism of energy-yielding nutrients. This represents 5 to 10% of energy consumed.

thrifty metabolism A metabolism that characteristically conserves more energy than normal, such that it increases risk of weight gain and obesity.

thromboxane (TX) (throm-BOK-sane) A stimulant of blood clotting made in the blood from polyunsaturated fatty acids.

thyroid-stimulating hormone (TSH) The hormone that regulates the uptake of iodide by the thyroid gland and release of thyroid hormone. TSH is secreted in response to a low concentration of circulating thyroid hormone (thyroxine).

tissue (TISH-you) A group of cells designed to perform a specific function; muscle tissue is an example.

T lymphocyte (tee-LYMF-oh-site) A type of white blood cell that recognizes intracellular antigens (e.g.,

viral antigens in infected cells), fragments of which move to the cell surface. T cells originate in the bone marrow but must mature in the thymus gland.

tocopherols (tuh-KOFF-er-alls) A group of four structurally similar compounds that have vitamin E activity. The "RRR" isomer of alpha-tocopherol is the most active form.

tocotrienols (toe-co-TRY-en-ols) A group of four compounds with the same basic chemical structure as the tocopherols but containing slightly altered side chains. They exhibit much less vitamin E activity than the corresponding tocopherols.

tolerable upper intake level (UL) Maximum chronic daily intake of a nutrient that is unlikely to cause adverse health effects in almost all people in a population. This number applies to a chronic daily use.

total parenteral nutrition The intravenous provision of all necessary nutrients, including the most basic forms of protein, carbohydrates, lipids, vitamins, minerals, and electrolytes. This solution is generally infused for 12 to 24 hours/day in a volume of about 2 to 3 L.

toxic Poisonous; caused by a poison.

toxicity The capacity of a substance to produce injury or illness at some dosage.

toxin Poisonous compounds produced by an organism that can cause disease.

trabecular bone (trah-BEK-you-lar) The spongy, inner matrix of bone, found primarily in the spine, pelvis, and ends of bones; also called cancellous bone.

trace mineral A mineral vital to health that is required in the diet in amounts less than 100 mg per day.

trachea (TRAY-key-ah) The airway leading from the larynx to the bronchi.

transamination (trans-am-ih-NAY-shun) The transfer of an amino group from an amino acid to a carbon skeleton to form a new amino acid.

trans **fatty acids** A form of an unsaturated fatty acid, usually a monounsaturated one when found in food, in which the hydrogens on both carbons forming that double bond lie on opposite sides of that bond. A *cis* fatty acid has the hydrogens lying on the same side of the carbon-carbon double bond.

trans isomers Compound where the hydrogens lie opposite each other across a carbon-carbon double bond.

transferrin (trans-FER-in) A blood protein that transports iron in the blood.

transketolase (trans-KEY-toe-lace) An enzyme whose functional component is TPP (thiamin pyrophosphate); converts glucose to pentose sugars.

triglyceride (try-GLISS-uh-ride) The major form of lipid in the body and in food. It is composed of three fatty acids bonded to glycerol, an alcohol. May also be called a triacylglycerol, since the form of fatty acid attached exists as an acyl group.

trimesters Three 13- to 14-week periods into which the normal pregnancy of 38 to 40 weeks is divided somewhat arbitrarily for purposes of discussion and analysis. Development of the embryo and fetus, however, is continuous throughout pregnancy, with no specific physiological markers demarcating the transition from one trimester to the next.

trophic hormone (TROW-fic) Hormone that stimulates the secretion of another secreting gland.

trypsin (TRIP-sin) A protein-digesting enzyme secreted by the pancreas in a inactive form into the small intestine that contributes to protein digestion.

tryptophan (TRIP-toe-fan) An essential amino acid, a precursor of serotonin.

tumor Mass of cells; may be cancerous (malignant) or noncancerous (benign).

tumor suppressor genes Genes that prevent cells from dividing.

type 1 diabetes A form of diabetes in which the person with the disease is prone to ketosis and requires insulin therapy.

type 2 diabetes A form of diabetes in which ketosis is not commonly seen. Insulin therapy can be used but often is not required; often associated with obesity.

tyrosine (TIE-row-seen) A nonessential amino acid and precursor of dopamine, norepinephrine, and epinephrine.

ulcer (UL-sir) Erosion of the tissue lining, usually in the stomach (gastric ulcer) or the upper small intestine (duodenal ulcer). These are generally referred to as *peptic ulcers.*

umami (you-MA-mee) A brothy, meaty, savory flavor in some foods. Monosodium glutamate enhances this flavor when added to foods.

undernutrition Failing health that results from a longstanding dietary intake that does not meet nutritional needs.

underwater weighing A method of estimating total body fat by weighing the individual on a standard scale and then weighing him or her again submerged in water. The difference between the two weights is used to estimate total body fat.

underweight A body mass index below 18.5. The cutoff is less precise than for obesity because this condition has been studied less.

upper-body obesity The type of obesity, also called android, in which fat is stored primarily in the abdominal area; defined as a waist circumference > 40 inches in men and >35 inches in women; closely associated with a high risk of cardiovascular disease, hypertension, and type 2 diabetes.

urea (yoo-REE-ah) Nitrogenous waste product of protein metabolism; major source of nitrogen in the

urine, chemically $H_2N-\overset{\overset{\displaystyle O}{\|}}{C}-NH_2$

ureter (YOUR-ih-ter) Tube that transports urine from the kidney to the urinary bladder.

urethra (yoo-REE-thra) Tube that transports urine from the urinary bladder to the outside of the body.

uvula (YOO-vyo-la) The fleshy portion of the soft palate that prevents food from being expelled through the nose during swallowing.

vagus nerves (VAY-guss) Nerves arising from the brain that branch off to other organs and are essential for control of speech, swallowing, and gastrointestinal function.

vegan (VEE-gun) A person who eats only plant foods.

vegetarian A person who avoids eating animal products to a varying degree, ranging from consuming no animal products to simply not consuming four-footed animal products.

vein A blood vessel that conveys blood to the heart.

ventricle (VEN-tri-kel) Either of the two lower chambers of the heart that contain blood to be pumped from the heart. The term is also used to describe the four interconnecting cavities in the brain.

venule (VEN-yool) A tiny vessel that carries blood from the capillary to a vein.

very-low-calorie diet (VLCD) Known also as *protein-sparing modified fast* (PSMF), this diet allows a person 400 to 800 kcal per day, often in liquid form. Of this, 120 to 480 kcal is carbohydrate; the rest is mostly high-biological value protein.

very-low-density lipoprotein (VLDL) The lipoprotein created in the liver that carries both the cholesterol and lipids newly synthesized by the liver.

villi (VIL-eye) Fingerlike protrusions into the small intestine that participate in digestion and absorption of foodstuff.

virus (VI-rus) The smallest known type of infectious agent, many of which cause disease in humans. They do not metabolize, grow, or move by themselves. They reproduce by the aid of a living cellular host. Viruses are essentially a piece of genetic material surrounded by a coat of protein.

visual cycle A chemical process in the eye that participates in vision. Forms of vitamin A participate in the process.

vitamin D Fat-soluble vitamin responsible for maintenance of bone, in part by increasing calcium absorption in the GI tract.

vitamins Compounds needed in very small amounts in the diet to help regulate and support chemical reactions in the body. Absence from the diet must result in a disease that timely replacement of the vitamin will cure.

VO₂max Maximum volume of oxygen that can be consumed per unit of time.

water The universal solvent of life; chemically, H_2O. The body is composed of about 60% water. Water (fluid) needs are about 8 cups per day.

water-soluble vitamins Vitamins that dissolve in water. These vitamins are the B-vitamins and vitamin C.

Wernicke-Korsakoff syndrome Thiamin-deficiency disease caused by excessive alcohol consumption. Symptoms include eye problems, difficulty walking, and deranged mental functions.

whey (WAY) Proteins, such as lactalbumin, that are found in great amounts in human milk and are easy to digest.

white blood cells One of the formed elements of the circulating blood system; also called *leukocytes.* Five types of leukocytes are lymphocytes, monocytes, neutrophils, basophils, and eosinophils. White blood cells are able to squeeze through intracellular spaces and migrate. Leukocytes phagocytize bacteria, fungi, and viruses, as well as detoxify proteins that may result from allergic reactions, cellular injury, and other immune system cells.

white matter Brain tissue composed of myelin-coated nerve cell fibers, which carries information between nerve cells in the brain and spinal cord.

whole grains Grains containing the entire seed of the plant, including the bran, germ, and endosperm (starchy interior). Examples are whole wheat and brown rice.

withdrawal With regard to alcohol, ranges from anxiety, decreased cognition, tremulousness, increased irritability, and hyperreactivity to full-blown delirium tremens. Symptoms can begin about 8 hours after the last drink and usually pass by the third day.

xanthine dehydrogenase (ZAN-thin de-HY-droj-eh-nase) An enzyme containing molybdenum and iron, which functions in the formation of uric acid and the mobilization of iron from liver ferritin stores.

xenobiotic (ZEE-no-bye-OT-ic) Compound that is foreign to the body. The principal classes are drugs, chemical carcinogens, and environmental substances such as pesticides.

xerophthalmia (zer-op-THAL-mee-uh) A condition marked by dryness of the cornea and eye membranes that results from vitamin A deficiency and can lead to blindness. The specific cause is a lack of mucus production by the eye, which then leaves it more vulnerable to surface dirt and bacterial infections.

xylitol (ZIGH-lih-tol) An alcohol derivative of the five-carbon monosaccharide, xylose.

zygote (ZIGH-goat) The fertilized ovum; the cell resulting from union of an egg cell (ovum) and sperm until it divides.

zymogen (zigh-MO-gin) An inactive form of an enzyme that requires the removal of a minor part of the chemical structure for it to work. The zymogen is converted into an active enzyme at the appropriate time, such as when released into the stomach or small intestine.

Credits

Chemistry—*Cont.*
 of ions and ionic compounds, A-81–A-82
 isomerism and, A-88–A-92
 matter and mass properties and,
   A-71–A-75
 molecules and, A-78–A-79
 organic, A-86–A-88
 reactions related to study of nutrition and,
   A-95–A-97
 of salts, A-82–A-83
Chicken fat, 205
Child Care Food Program, 799
Childhood. *See also* Adolescence; Infancy
 baryophobia during, 616, 620
 breakfast, fat intake, and snacks during,
   692–93
 calcium needs during, 694–95
 children of alcoholics and, 309, 310
 diabetes during, 693
 fat intake during, 232
 homelessness during, 801
 hyperactivity during, sugar and, 182, 690
 iron deficiency anemia during, 475
 kwashiorkor during, 281–84
 lead toxicity during, 777
 obesity during, 525–26, 529, 693–96
 orphaning by AIDS and, 820
 pesticide risks during, 787
 preschool children and. *See* Preschool
   children
 protein needs during, 261–62
 rickets during, 338, 342
 school-age children and. *See* School-age
   children
 scurvy during, 400
 shift to urban life and, 808
 single parents and, 801
 undernutrition during, 796
 veganism during, 293
 vitamin A deficiency during, 331, 333
 vitamin E needs during, 352
 zinc deficiency during, 482
China, famine in, 795
Chinese cuisine, 75
Chinese medicine, 742, 746
Chloride, 436–37, 453
 absorption, transport, and excretion
   of, 436
 deficiency of, 437
 in foods, 436
 functions of, 436
 needs for, 45, 436
 toxicity of, 437
Chloride ions, A-82
Chlorothiazide (Diuril), for
   hypertension, 462
Cholecystokinin (CCK), 115, 223, 268
 fat digestion and, 216
 hunger and satiety and, 518
Cholesterol, 214–15, A-92
 absorption of, 177
 blood. *See* Blood cholesterol
 in cell membrane, 81
 definition of, 5

Cholesterol—*Cont.*
 dietary. *See* Dietary cholesterol
 formation of, 215
 HDL. *See* High-density lipoproteins
   (HDL)
 LDL. *See* Low-density lipoproteins (LDL)
 receptor pathways for uptake of, 220–21
 vitamin D production from, 86
Cholestin, for cardiovascular disease, 252
Cholestyramine (Questran)
 to lower LDL-cholesterol, 251
 nutritional problems related to, 727
Choline, 13, 325, 394–95, 403
 absorption, metabolism, and excretion
   of, 394
 deficiency of, 394
 in foods, 394
 functions of, 394
 needs for, 395, 396–97
Cholinergic effect, 100
Chondroitin, 745
Chromium, 494–95, 497, 504–5
 absorption, transport, storage, and
   excretion of, 494
 deficiency of, 494
 for diabetes, 505
 DRI for, 45
 as ergogenic aid, 595
 essentiality of, 504
 in foods, 494
 functions of, 494
 misleading claims for supplements
   and, 505
 needs for, 495, 505
 toxicity of, 495
Chromium picolinate, 559, 560
Chromosomes, 84, 117
Chronic diseases
 as cause of death, 4, 5
 definition of, 5
Chylomicrons, 218
Chyme, 107, 268
Chymotrypsin, 268
Cigarette smoking. *See* Smoking
Ciguatera fish poisoning, 768
Cimetidine (Tagamet)
 for heartburn, 123
 nutritional problems related to, 727
 for ulcers, 122
Circulatory system, 86, 89–94
Cirrhosis, 5
 alcohol and, 299, 306–7
 definition of, 5
cis isomers, A-90–A-91
Citric acid (citrate)
 as food additive, 775
 formation of, 137
Citric acid cycle, 136–39, 147, 369, 378
Civil unrest, undernutrition and, 806
Clinical lesions, undernutrition and, 156
Clinicians, 671
Clostridium, 112, 755
Clostridium botulinum, 753, 756, 757,
   764–65, 773

Clostridium botulinum—Cont.
 in honey, 188, 681
Clostridium perfringens, 753, 759, 763
CNS (central nervous system), 99
CoA (coenzyme A), 376, 377
Cocaine, pregnancy outcome and, 644
Coconut oil, 206, 232
Codons, 263
Coenzyme(s), 132
 B-vitamins as, 366
 vitamin B-6 as, 379
Coenzyme A (CoA), 376, 377
Coenzyme Q, 139
Coenzyme Q-10, 139, 719, 745
 as ergogenic aid, 595
Cofactors, 353
 zinc as, 480
Coffee. *See also* Caffeine
 cardiovascular disease and, 249
Cognitive behavior therapy, for eating
   disorders, 609, 612
Cognitive function, vitamin B-6 and, 380
Cognitive restructuring, 539, 540
Cohort studies, 24
Colestipol (Colestid), to lower LDL-
   cholesterol, 251
Colic, 683–84
Colipase, 216–17
Collagen, 483
 in bones, 88
 synthesis of, 396–97, 399
Colon, 111–14
Colon cancer, diet and, 414, 415
 dietary fiber and, 176
 high-protein diets and, 276
Colors, as food additives, 773
Color vision, 331
Colostrum, 651
Combination foods, exchange list for, A-116
Commodity Supplemental Food Program,
   799
Common cold, zinc as remedy for, 480
Community nutrition services, 734–35
Companies, as information sources,
   A-139–A-140
Complement, 97
Complementary alternative medicine
   (CAM), 741–47. *See also* Herbal
   products; Vitamin supplements
Complementary proteins, 261
Complete proteins, 261
Compression of morbidity, 710–11
Compulsive overeating, 616, 617–20
Concentration gradient, 81
Conceptus, 632
Condensation reactions, A-95
Conditionally dispensable amino acids, 259
Cones, vitamin A and, 330, 331
Congo, undernutrition in, 806
Congregate meal programs, for older adults,
   735, 799, 800
Congregate Meals for the Elderly, 799
Conjugates, 383
Conjunctiva, 333

Formula feeding—*Cont.*
  excessive, avoiding, 681
  recommendations for, 681
Fortified, meaning of term on food
    labels, 60
FOS (fructooligosaccharides), 37, 113
Four Day Wonder Diet, 558
4-9-4 estimates, 10–11
Fractures, stress, 581
Frame size, determining, A-130
Fraternal twins, 527
Free erythrocyte protoporphyrins
    (FEP), 472
Free foods
  exchange list for, A-114–A-115
  in Exchange System, 64
Free radicals, 307, 345, A-86
  aging and, 718
  neutralization of. *See* Antioxidants
Free to Be Me Girl Scout badge
    program, 697
Freshness date, 770
Fructooligosaccharides (FOS), 37, 113
Fructose, 162–63
  absorption of, 170
  sweetness of, 174, 175
Fruit(s)
  during adulthood, 712
  exchange list for, A-108
Fruitarians, 291
FSH (follicle-stimulating hormone),
    101, 102
Functional foods, 37
Functional groups, A-87–A-88
Fungi, 750
  causing food-borne illness, 754, 768–69
Furosemide (Lasix), nutritional problems
    related to, 727

■ **G**

GABA (gamma-aminobutyric acid),
    synthesis of, 380
Galactose, 162, 163
  absorption of, 170
Galactosemia, 272
  breastfeeding and, 656
Gallbladder
  age-related changes in function of, 723
  role in digestion, 114
Gametes, 117
Gamma-aminobutyric acid (GABA),
    synthesis of, 380
Gamma hydroxybutyric acid (GHB), as
    ergogenic aid, 595
Garcinia cambogia, as ergogenic aid, 596
Garlic, 744
Gas, intestinal, with beans, 165, 277
Gastric inhibitory peptide (GIP), 115, 223
Gastric juice, 107
Gastrin, 115, 223
Gastroesophageal reflux disease
    (GERD), 123

Gastrointestinal distention, hunger and
    satiety and, 518
Gastrointestinal (GI) tract, 105. *See also*
    Digestive system
Gastroplasty, 543–44
Gelatins, 261
  as food additives, 775
Gemfibrozil (Lopid)
  to lower LDL-cholesterol, 252
  to raise HDL-cholesterol, 251
Gender. *See also* Female athletes; Girls; Men;
    Women
  alcohol metabolism and dependency
    and, 311
Gene(s), 84
  cancer and, 411–12
Gene chips, 29
Gene expression, 329
Generally recognized as safe (GRAS)
    list, 770
Gene therapy, 31–32
Genetically-altered foods, 779, 812–13
  safety of, 812–13
Genetic counseling, 32–33
Genetic diseases, sickle cell disease, 266, 267
Genetic engineering, 812–14
Genetics
  of alcohol dependency, 310
  of cancer, 413
  cardiovascular disease risk related to, 247
  of eating disorders, 601, 603
  family trees and, 31
  of longevity, 710–11
  malnutrition and, 794
  nutritional diseases and, 29–30
  of obesity, 527, 529
Genetic testing, 32–33
Genistein, anticancer effects of, 279
Genograms, 31
Genotoxic carcinogens, 412
GERD (gastroesophageal reflux
    disease), 123
Gestation, 635. *See also* Pregnancy
Gestational diabetes, 648
GHB (gamma hydroxybutyric acid), as
    ergogenic aid, 595
GI (glycemic index), 184–85
  cardiovascular disease and, 249
Giardia, 756
Ginger, 744
Ginkgo biloba, 744
Ginseng, 744
GIP (gastric inhibitory peptide), 115, 223
Girls
  adolescent, diets of, 697–98
  calcium needs of, 695
  iron deficiency anemia in, 475
GI (gastrointestinal) tract, 105. *See also*
    Digestive system
Glial cells, 99–100
Glipizide (Glucotrol), for diabetes
    mellitus, 200
Glomerulus, 117

Glossitis, vitamin deficiencies causing,
    372, 374
Glucagon, 103
  blood glucose regulation by, 196, 197
  gluconeogenesis and, 196
Gluconeogenesis, 144–45, 146, 148,
    173–74, 196
Glucosamine, 745
Glucose, 7, 162. *See also* Blood glucose
  absorption of, 170, 176
  chromium and, 494–95
  as energy source, 146, 147, 172–73
  formation of, 272
  glycolysis and, 132–33, 134, 135, 147,
    569–70
  as muscle fuel, 569–72, 571
  production of, 144–45
  protein sparing and, 173–74
  sugars in RNA and DNA synthesized
    from, 174
  sweetness of, 174, 175
Glutamic acid, 260, A-89
  in gluconeogenesis, 144
Glutamine, A-89
  as ergogenic aid, 594
Glutathione, 398
Glutathione peroxidase, 346, 486
Glycated hemoglobin, blood glucose
    measurement using, 199
Glycemic index (GI), 184–85
  cardiovascular disease and, 249
Glycerol, 132
  as ergogenic aid, 596
  as food additive, 774
  in gluconeogenesis, 145
  in lipolysis, 143
Glycine, A-89
Glycocalyx, in cell membrane, 82
Glycogen, 132, 163
  metabolism of, 141
  as muscle fuel, 570–71
  production by muscles, 88
  structure and function of, 166–67
Glycolipids, in cell membrane, 82
Glycolysis, 132–36, 147, 296–97,
    569–70, A-96
  ATP in, 133–34, 147, 569
  glucose to pyruvate in, 132–33, 134, 135,
    147, 569–70
  lactate production in, 134, 136
Glycoprotein(s), in cell membrane, 82
Glycoprotein hormones, 101, 102
Glycosphingolipids, A-92
Glycosylation, of proteins, aging and, 719
Glycyrrhizin, 37
Goat's milk, 675
Goblet cells
  of small intestine, 111
  of stomach, 268
Goiter, 490, 491, 794
Goitrogens, 491
Golgi complex, 84
Good source, meaning of term on food
    labels, 60

Lactose, 163, 165, 181
  digestion of, 169
  sweetness of, 174, 175
Lactose intolerance, 112, 170, 185–86
  in older adulthood, 722
Lactovegetarians, 291
  pregnancy and, 640
Laetrile, 406
La Leche League, 656
Lanugo, 213, 606
Lard, 206
Large intestine, 111–14
  absorption in, 213
  cancer of, 176, 276, 414, 415
Larvae, of *Trichinella spiralis,* 766–67
Larynx, 98, 99, 106
Latin America. *See also specific countries*
  external debt of, 810
Latin American Diet Pyramid, 74, 75
Lauric acid, A-127, A-128
Laxatives, 124
  in bulimia nervosa, 611
  nutritional problems related to, 727
  in older adulthood, 722
Lay organizations, as information sources,
  A-138
LBW (low-birth-weight) infants, 635, 636,
  643, 644
LDL. *See* Low-density lipoproteins (LDL)
L-DOPA, vitamin-6 requirement and, 382
Lead, bone concentrations of, hypertension
  and, 460
Lead toxicity, 777–78
  calcium supplements and, 444
Lean, meaning of term on food labels, 60
Lean body mass, 511
  age-related decrease in, 724–25
Leavening agents, 774
Lecithins, 213, 214
  polyunsaturated, for alcohol abuse, 315
Legumes, as protein source, 277, 280
Leptin, 103, 518, 528
Let-down reflex, 650–51
Leucine, A-89
Leukemias, 334, 410–11
Leukocytes, 91, 95–96
Leukotrienes (LT), 208, 210–11
Levulose. *See* Fructose
LH (luteinizing hormone), 101, 102
Life expectancy, 710, 715–16
  diet and, 54–55
Life span, 715
Lifestyle
  cardiovascular disease and, 244
  healthy, 710–11
  pregnancy outcome related to, 644
Light, meaning of term on food labels, 60
Lignans, 37, 443, 745
Lignins, 167
Limiting amino acids, 261, 262
Lind, James, 398
Linoleic acid, A-127, A-128
Linolenic acid, 207, 233

Lipase, 216
  hormone-sensitive, 141
Lipectomy, suction, 537
Lipid(s), 7–8, 202–38. *See also* Adipose
    tissue; Body fat; Dietary fat; Oils
  absorption of, 218
  biochemical reactions of, A-92
  common properties of, 204
  definition of, 6
  digestion of, 216–17, 351
  fatty acids. *See* Essential fatty acids; Fatty
    acids
  in foods, 223–28, 232–37
  metabolism of, 141–44, 149, 380
  phospholipids, 204, 213–14
  recommendations for intake of, 229–32
  sterols, 204, 214–15. *See also* Blood
    cholesterol; Cholesterol
  transport in bloodstream, 218–23
  triglycerides. *See* Triglycerides
Lipid peroxidation, 346
Lipogenesis, 143–44
Lipoic acid, 405
Lipolysis, 141–43
  carbohydrates and, 142
  ketogenesis and, 142–43
Lipoprotein(s), 218. *See also*
    Apolipoproteins; High-density
    lipoproteins (HDL); Low-density
    lipoproteins (LDL)
  cardiovascular disease and, 249
Lipoprotein(a), cardiovascular disease
  and, 249
Lipoprotein lipase, 218
Lipoxins (LX), 208, 210
Lipoxygenase, 208
Listeria, 755
Listeria monocytogenes, 753, 756, 763–64
  pregnancy outcome and, 645
Lite, meaning of term on food labels, 60
Lithium carbonate (Lithane), for bulimia
    nervosa, 615
Liver
  age-related changes in function of, 723
  alcohol effects on, 298, 304, 723
  alcohol metabolism in, 299
  blood glucose regulation by, 196
  cancer of, diet and, 414
  choline deficiency and, 394
  cirrhosis of, 5, 299, 306–7
  disease of, as cause of death, 4, 5
  lipid production by, 218–19
  role in digestion, 114
  vitamin A storage in, 329
Lobules, in breast, 650
Local governments, pesticide regulation
    by, 786
Local information sources, A-138
Loneliness, cardiovascular disease
    and, 249
Long bones, 87
Long-chain fatty acids, 206
Lönnerdal, Bo, 652–53

Lovastatin (Mevacor)
  for cardiovascular disease, 252
  to lower LDL-cholesterol, 251
Low-birth-weight (LBW) infants, 635, 636,
    643, 644
Low-carbohydrate diets, 127, 143, 144, 558
Low-density lipoproteins (LDL), 184,
    218–22, 232
  atherosclerosis and, 245–46
  calculation of, 247
  cardiovascular disease and, 249
  diet changes to reduce, 248, 250
  lowering, 250
  in older adulthood, 725
Lower-body obesity, 525, 526
Lower esophageal sphincter, 106
  heartburn and, 123
Lower-quality proteins, 261
"Low-fat," on food labels, 235
Low-fat diets, 558
LT (leukotrienes), 208, 210–11
Lumen, of gastrointestinal tract, 105, 106
Lungs
  age-related changes in function of, 724
  diseases of, as cause of death, 5
Lutein, 332, 335
Luteinizing hormone (LH), 101, 102
LX (lipoxins), 208, 210
Lycopene, 332, 335
Lymph, 95
Lymphatic system, 86, 94–95
Lymphatic vessels, 91, 92, 93
Lymph ducts, 95
Lymph nodes, 94
Lymphocytes, 94, 95, 96
Lymphomas, 411
Lysine, 262, A-89
Lysosomes, 84
Lysozyme, in human milk, 653

■ M

Maalox
  for heartburn, 123
  nutritional problems related to, 727
Machado, Alice, 611
Macrocytic anemia, 385–86
Macrophages, 95–96
Macular degeneration
  estrogen in prevention of, 447
  in older adulthood, 724
  vitamin A and, 334
Mad cow disease, 766–67
Magazines, as information sources, A-135
Magnesium, 450–52, 453
  absorption, transport, storage, and
    excretion of, 450
  alcohol and, 306
  blood pressure and, 461
  deficiency of, 306, 452
  DRI for, 45
  in foods, 451, A-1–A-70
  functions of, 450
  needs for, 451
  toxicity of, 123, 452

Estimated minimum sodium, chloride, and potassium
requirements for healthy persons

Age	Weight (kg)	Sodium (mg)*†	Chloride (mg)*†	Potassium (mg)‡
Months				
0–5	4.5	120	180	500
6–11	8.9	200	300	700
Years				
1	11	225	350	1000
2–5	16	300	500	1400
6–9	25	400	600	1600
10–18	50	500	750	2000
>18§	70	500	750	2000

*No allowance has been included for large, prolonged losses from the skin
through sweat.

†There is no evidence that higher intakes confer any additional health benefit.

‡Desirable intakes of potassium may considerably exceed these values
(~3500 mg for adults).

§No allowance has been included for growth. Values given for people under
18 years of age assume a growth rate corresponding to the
50th percentile reported by the National Center for Health Statistics
and averaged for males and females.

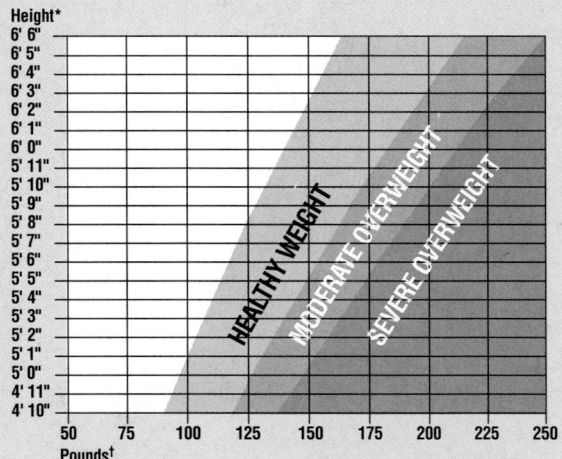

* Without shoes.
† Without clothes. The higher weights apply
   to people with more muscle and bone,
   such as many men.

Dietary Reference Intakes (DRIs): Tolerable Upper Intake Levels (UL[a]), Vitamins
Food and Nutrition Board, Institute of Medicine, National Academies

Life Stage Group	Vitamin A (µg/d)[b]	Vitamin C (mg/d)	Vitamin D (µg/d)	Vitamin E (mg/d)[c,d]	Vitamin K	Thiamin	Riboflavin	Niacin (mg/d)[d]	Vitamin B-6 (mg/d)	Folate (µg/d)[d]	Vitamin B-12	Pantothenic Acid	Biotin	Choline (g/d)	Carotenoids[e]
Infants															
0–6 mo	600	ND[f]	25	ND	ND	ND	ND	ND	ND	ND	ND	ND	ND	ND	ND
7–12 mo	600	ND	25	ND	ND	ND	ND	ND	ND	ND	ND	ND	ND	ND	ND
Children															
1–3 y	600	400	50	200	ND	ND	ND	10	30	300	ND	ND	ND	1.0	ND
4–8 y	900	650	50	300	ND	ND	ND	15	40	400	ND	ND	ND	1.0	ND
Males, Females															
9–13 y	1,700	1,200	50	600	ND	ND	ND	20	60	600	ND	ND	ND	2.0	ND
14–18 y	2,800	1,800	50	800	ND	ND	ND	30	80	800	ND	ND	ND	3.0	ND
19–70 y	3,000	2,000	50	1,000	ND	ND	ND	35	100	1,000	ND	ND	ND	3.5	ND
>70 y	3,000	2,000	50	1,000	ND	ND	ND	35	100	1,000	ND	ND	ND	3.5	ND
Pregnancy															
≤18 y	2,800	1,800	50	800	ND	ND	ND	30	80	800	ND	ND	ND	3.0	ND
19–50 y	3,000	2,000	50	1,000	ND	ND	ND	35	100	1,000	ND	ND	ND	3.5	ND
Lactation															
≤18 y	2,800	1,800	50	800	ND	ND	ND	30	80	800	ND	ND	ND	3.0	ND
19–50 y	3,000	2,000	50	1,000	ND	ND	ND	35	100	1,000	ND	ND	ND	3.5	ND

[a] UL = The maximum level of daily nutrient intake that is likely to pose no risk of adverse effects. Unless otherwise specified, the UL represents total intake from food, water, and supplements. Due to lack of suitable data, ULs could not be established for vitamin K, thiamin, riboflavin, vitamin B-12, pantothenic acid, biotin, or carotenoids. In the absence of ULs, extra caution may be warranted in consuming levels above recommended intakes.

[b] As preformed vitamin A only.

[c] As α-tocopherol; applies to any form of supplemental α-tocopherol.

[d] The ULs for vitamin E, niacin, and folate apply to synthetic forms obtained from supplements, fortified foods, or a combination of the two.

[e] β-Carotene supplements are advised only to serve as a provitamin A source for individuals at risk of vitamin A deficiency.

[f] ND = Not determinable due to lack of data of adverse effects in this age group and concern with regard to lack of ability to handle excess amounts. Source of intake should be from food only to prevent high levels of intake.

SOURCES: *Dietary Reference Intakes for Calcium, Phosphorous, Magnesium, Vitamin D, and Fluoride* (1997); *Dietary Reference Intakes for Thiamin, Riboflavin, Niacin, Vitamin B₆, Folate, Vitamin B₁₂, Pantothenic Acid, Biotin, and Choline* (1998); *Dietary Reference Intakes for Vitamin C, Vitamine E, Selenium, and Carotenoids* (2000); and *Dietary Reference Intakes for Vitamin A, Vitamin K, Arsenic, Boron, Chromium, Copper, Iodine, Iron, Manganese, Molybdenum, Nickel, Silicon, Vanadium, and Zinc* (2001). These reports may be accessed via www.nap.edu.